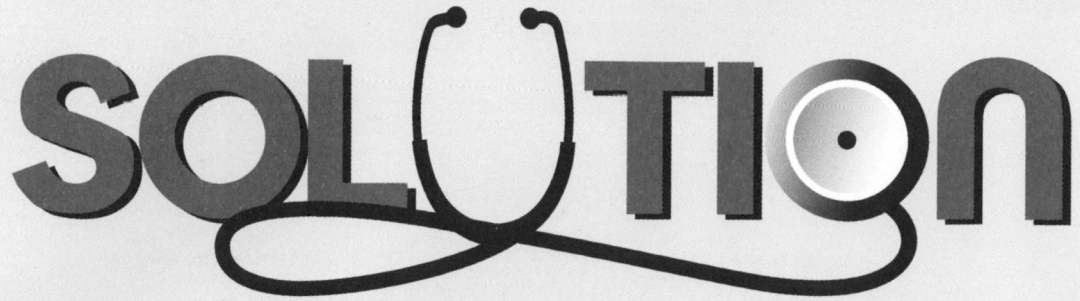

SOLUTION

Activate your online access today!

This text comes with access to the complete contents online, fully searchable, plus other valuable features.

Three simple steps to gain instant access...

1) Visit **www.manualofsurgicalprocedures.com**
2) Click on Register Now
3) Follow the instructions and then enter your access code found below when prompted

This website is for individual use only. If you are interested in multi-user access, please contact customer service. For technical assistance, email customerservice@lww.com or call 1-800-468-1128 (inside the US) or 1-410-528-4000 (outside the US).

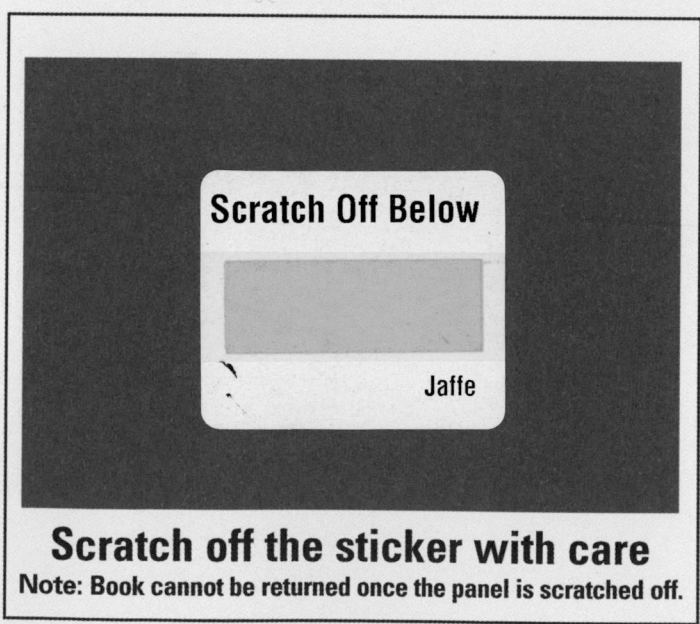

Scratch Off Below

Jaffe

Scratch off the sticker with care

Note: Book cannot be returned once the panel is scratched off.

Wolters Kluwer Health | Lippincott Williams & Wilkins

ANESTHESIOLOGIST'S MANUAL OF SURGICAL PROCEDURES

Fourth Edition

EDITORS

Richard A. Jaffe, MD, PhD
Professor of Anesthesia and Neurosurgery

Stanley I. Samuels, MD
Clinical Professor of Anesthesia, Emeritus

ASSOCIATE EDITORS

Clifford A. Schmiesing, MD
Clinical Associate Professor of Anesthesia

Brenda Golianu, MD
Assistant Professor of Anesthesia

Stanford University School of Medicine
Stanford, California

Wolters Kluwer | Lippincott Williams & Wilkins
Health
Philadelphia • Baltimore • New York • London
Buenos Aires • Hong Kong • Sydney • Tokyo

This book is respectfully dedicated to
our friend, mentor, teacher, and colleague,
C. Philip Larson, Jr., MD, MS

Acquisitions Editor: Brian Brown
Managing Editor: Nicole Dernoski
Project Manager: Jennifer Harper
Senior Manufacturing Manager: Benjamin Rivera
Senior Marketing Manager: Angela Panetta
Creative Director: Doug Smock
Production Services: Aptara, Inc.

530 Walnut Street
Philadelphia, PA 19106 USA
LWW.com

Printed in China

Library of Congress Cataloging-in-Publication Data

Anesthesiologist's manual of surgical procedures / editors, Richard A. Jaffe, Cliff Schmiesing, Brenda Golianu. — 4th ed.
p. ; cm.
Includes bibliographical references and index.
ISBN-13: 978-0-7817-6670-8
ISBN-10: 0-7817-6670-2
1. Anesthesiology—Handbooks, manuals, etc. 2. Surgery, Operative—Handbooks, manuals, etc. 3. Operations, Surgical—Handbooks, manuals, etc. I. Jaffe, Richard A. II. Schmiesing, Cliff. III. Golianu, Brenda.
[DNLM: 1. Anesthesia—methods. 2. Surgical Procedures, Operative. WO 235 A5795 2009]
RD82.2.A54 2009
617.9′6—dc22

2008043783

10 9 8 7 6

CONTENTS

CONTRIBUTING AUTHORS

Vernon J. Adams, Jr., DMD
Assistant Clinical Professor of Pediatrics
Plastic and Dental Surgery
Palo Alto, California
Office-Based Dental Procedures

John R. Adler, MD
Professor of Neurosurgery
Stanford University Medical Center
Department of Neurosurgery
Stanford, California
Stereotactic Neurosurgery

Craig Albanese, MD
Professor of Surgery and, by courtesy, of Obstetrics & Gynecology and Pediatrics
Stanford University Medical Center
Stanford, California

D.M. Alcorn, MD
Associate Professor of Ophthalmology and Pediatrics
Department of Ophthalmology
Pediatric Ophthalmic Surgery

Sophoclis P. Alexopoulos, MD
Clinical Instructor of Surgery–Multi-Organ Transplantation
Stanford University Medical Center
Stanford, California

Timothy Angelotti, MD, PhD
Associate Professor
Department of Anesthesia/CCM
Stanford University
Stanford, California
Kidney, Pancreas Transplantation; Multiorgan Procurement

Martin S. Angst, MD
Associate Professor of Anesthesia
Department of Anesthesia
Stanford University School of Medicine
Stanford, California
Pancreatic, Peritoneal Surgery

Sandra Leigh Bardas, BSP, RPH, FCSHP
Clinical Pharmacist
Stanford Hospitals and Clinics
Stanford, California
Drug Interactions

Michael J. Bellino, MD
Assistant Professor of Orthopaedic Surgery
Stanford University Medical Center
Department of Orthopaedic Surgery
Stanford, California
Orthopedic Surgery - Hip, Pelvis, Upper Leg

Melissa T. Berhow, MD, PhD
Clinical Assistant Professor
Stanford University Medical Center
Department of Anesthesia
Stanford, California
Burn Surgery

David A. Berman, MD
Medical Director
Dermatologic Surgeon
Berman Skin Institute
Palo Alto, California
Active Staff
Sequoia Hospital
Redwood City, California
Office-Based Dermatologic/Laser Surgery

Scott Berta, MD
Clinical Instructor of Neurosurgery
Stanford University Medical Center
Stanford, California

Nikolas H. Blevins, MD
Associate Professor
Chief, Division of Otology/Neurotology
Medical Director, LPCH
Stanford Cochlear Implant Center Department
Stanford University
Stanford, California
Otology; Neurotology

M. Gail Boltz, MD
Clinical Professor of Anesthesia
Stanford University Medical Center
Department of Anesthesia
Stanford, California
Pediatric Cardiovascular Surgery; Pediatric Cardiac Catheterization

C. Andrew Bonham, MD
Associate Professor of Surgery
Stanford University Medical Center
Stanford, California
Biliary Surgery

John Brock-Utne, MD, MSc, PhD
Professor (Clinical) of Anesthesia, Emeritus
Stanford University Medical Center
Stanford, California

Jay B. Brodsky, MD
Professor, Department of Anesthesia
Stanford University School of Medicine
Medical Director - Perioperative Services
Stanford University Medical Center
Stanford, California
Thoracic, Stomach, Laparoscopic Surgery; Adult Out-of-OR Procedures

Stephan Busque, MD, MSc, FRCSC
Associate Professor of Surgery
Stanford University
Director, Adult Kidney and Pancreas Transplant Program
Stanford Hospital and Clinics
Stanford, California
Kidney, Pancreatic Transplantation

Walter B. Cannon, MD
Clinical Professor of Cardiothoracic and Thoracic Surgery
Medical Director - Perioperative Services
Stanford University Medical Center
Department of Cardiothoracic Surgery
Stanford, California
Thoracic Surgery

Eugene J. Carragee, MD, FACS
Professor and Vice-Chairman
Chief, Spinal Surgery Section
Department of Orthopaedic Surgery
Stanford University School of Medicine
Director, Orthopaedic Spine Clinic
Stanford University Hospital and Clinic
Stanford, California
Orthopedic Spine Surgery

Ian Carroll, MD, MS
Clinical Instructor
Anesthesia and Pain Management
Stanford University
Stanford, California
Pain Management

Brendan Carvalho, MBBCh, FRCA, MDCH
Assistant Professor
Department of Anesthesia
Stanford University
Stanford University Medical Center
Stanford, California
Laparoscopic, Gynecologic, Obstetric Surgery

Michael W. Champeau, MD
Adjunct Clinical Professor of Anesthesia
Associated Anesthesiologists
Palo Alto, California
Surgery for Sleep Disorders

James Chang, MD
Professor of Surgery (Plastic Surgery) and Orthopedic Surgery
Stanford University Medical Center
Chief of Plastic Surgery
Stanford Hospital and Clinics
Stanford, California
Functional Restoration; Pediatric Hand Surgery

Kay W. Chang, MD
Professor, Otolaryngology
Stanford University
Associate Professor, Division of Pediatric Otolaryngology
Lucile Packard Children's Hospital at Stanford
Palo Alto, California
Pediatric Otolaryngology

Steven D. Chang, MD
Professor of Neurosurgery
Stanford University Medical Center
Department of Neurosurgery
Stanford, California
Intracranial, Stereotactic Neurosurgery

Bertha Chen, MD
Associate Professor of Obstetrics and Gynecology
Stanford University Medical Center
Department of Obstetrics and Gynecology
Stanford, California
Gynecologic Surgery

Michael Chen, MD
Clinical Assistant Professor of Anesthesia
Stanford University Medical Center
Stanford, California

Emilie V. Cheung, MD
Assistant Professor of Orthopaedic Surgery
Stanford University Medical Center
Stanford, California

Benjamin Chung, MD
Assistant Professor of Urology
Palo Alto Veteran's Administration Health Care System
Palo Alto, California

Rebecca E. Claure, MD
Clinical Assistant Professor
Department of Anesthesia
Stanford University Medical Center
Lucile Salter Packard Children's Hospital
Stanford, California

Lee Coleman, MD
Staff Anesthesiologist
Cedars Sinai Medical Center
Los Angeles, California

George W. Commons, MD
Clinical Assistant Professor of Functional Restoration
Stanford University School of Medicine
Plastic Surgery Center
Palo Alto, California
Liposuction

Waldo Concepcion, MD
Associate Professor of Surgery
Multi-Organ Transplantation
Stanford University Medical Center
Stanford, California

Tara Cornaby, MD
Clinical Assistant Professor of Anesthesia
Stanford University Medical Center
Department of Anesthesia
Stanford, California
Cosmetic Facial Surgery, Craniofacial Surgery, Functional Restoration

John J. Csongradi, MD
Orthopedic Surgery
Santa Clara Valley Medical Center
San Jose, California
Orthopaedic Surgery-Knee, Lower Leg, Hand and Foot

Myriam J. Curet, MD, FACS
Professor, Department of Surgery
Stanford University
Chief, Section of Minimally Invasive Surgery
Stanford Hospitals and Clinics
Stanford, California
Bariatric Surgery, Laparoscopic General Surgery

Michael P. Dake, MD
Professor, Cardiothoracic Surgery
Stanford University Medical Center
Stanford, California
Endovascular Surgery

Edward J. Damrose, MD
Assistant Professor
Chief, Division of Laryngology
Stanford University School of Medicine
Stanford, California
Laryngology

Charles DeBattista, MD
Associate Professor of Psychiatry and Behavioral Sciences
Stanford University Medical Center
Department of Psychiatry and Behavioral Sciences
Stanford, California
Electroconvulsive Therapy

Steven A. Deem, MD
Associate Professor of Anesthesia
University of Washington
Department of Anesthesia
Harborview Medical Center
Seattle, Washington
Urology

Jennifer L. De la Pena, MD
Assistant Professor
Surgical Oncology Division
University of Nevada
Las Vegas, Nevada
Breast Surgery

Dev M. Desai, MD, PhD, FACS
Associate Professor
Department of Surgery
University of Texas Southwestern Medical School
Chief, Division of Pediatric Transplantation
Children's Medical Center
Dallas, Texas
Liver Transplantation; Multiorgan Procurement

Robert L. Dodd, MD, PhD
Assistant Professor of Neurosurgery and of Radiology
Stanford University Medical Center
Department of Neurosurgery/Neuroradiology
Stanford, California
Intracranial, Extracranial Neurosurgery

Sarah S. Donaldson, MD, FACR
Catharine and Howard Avery Professor
Stanford School of Medicine
Radiation Oncology-Radiation Therapy
Stanford, California
Pediatric Radiation Therapy

Anne M. Dubin, MD
Associate Professor of Pediatrics (Pediatric Cardiology)
Lillian Packard Childrens Hospital
Department of Pediatrics - Cardiology
Stanford, California
Pediatric Cardiac Surgery

Sanjeev Dutta, MD, MA
Assistant Professor of Surgery and Pediatrics
Department of Surgery
Lucile Salter Packard Children's Hospital
Stanford, California

Alice A. Edler, MD
Assistant Professor of Anesthesia
Stanford University Medical Center
Department of Anesthesia
Stanford, California
Pediatric Ophthalmic, Orthopedic Surgery

Michael Edwards, MD
Lucile Packard Children's Hospital Professor in Pediatric Neurosurgery and, Professor, by courtesy, of Pediatrics
Department of Neurosurgery
Stanford University Medical Center
Stanford, California

Peter R. Egbert, MD
Professor of Ophthalmology
Department of Ophthalmology
Stanford University
Stanford, California
Ophthalmic Surgery

Christoph Egger-Halbeis, MD, MBA
Director of Medical Affairs
Bern, Switzerland

Yasser Y. El-Sayed, MD
Associate Professor and Associate Chief
Division of Maternal-Fetal Medicine and Obstetrics
Department of Obstetrics and Gynecology
Stanford University
Stanford, California
Obstetric Surgery

Carlos O. Esquivel, MD, PhD
Professor of Surgery
Department of Surgery
Chief, Division of Transplantation
Stanford University
Stanford, California
Liver Transplantation; Multi-organ procurement

James I. Fann, MD
Associate Professor
Department of Cardiothoracic Surgery
Stanford University
Stanford, California
Minimally Invasive Cardiac Surgery, Vascular Surgery

Ruth M. Fanning, MB, BCh, MRCPI, FFARCSI
Clinical Assistant Professor
Department of Anesthesia
Stanford University Medical Center
Stanford, California
Laparoscopic General Surgery

William W. Feaster, MD
Clinical Professor of Anesthesia and Pediatrics
Department of Anesthesia
Stanford University Medical Center
Stanford, California
Pediatric Neurosurgery

William E. Fee, Jr., MD
Edward C. and Amy H. Sewall Professor II
Stanford School of Medicine
Department of Otolaryngology/Head and Neck Surgery
Stanford, California
Otolaryngology

Jeffrey A. Feinstein, MD, MPH
Associate Professor of Pediatrics
Lucile Packard Childrens Hospital
Department of Pediatrics – Cardiology
Stanford, California
Pediatric Cardiac Catheterization

Gordon Finlayson, MD, FRCPC
CCM Fellow
University of British Columbia
Vancouver, British Columbia, Canada

Stephen P. Fischer, MD
Associate Professor of Anesthesia
Stanford University Medical Center
Stanford, California
Preoperative Testing/Diagnostics

Linda E. Foppiano, MD
Clinical Associate Professor of Anesthesia
Stanford University Medical Center
Stanford, California
Cardiac Surgery, Heart-Lung Transplantation

Joan K. Frisoli, MD, PhD
Assistant Professor of Radiology
Department of Radiology-Diagnostic Radiology
Stanford University Medical Center
Stanford, California
TIPS

Louise Furukawa, MD
Clinical Assistant Professor in Anesthesia
Stanford University Medical Center
Stanford, California
Repair of Craniofacial Malformations

Raymond R. Gaeta, MD
Associate Professor of Anesthesia
Medical Director, Division of Pain Management
Stanford University Medical Center
Stanford, California
Pain Management

James G. Gamble, MD, PhD
Professor of Orthopaedic Surgery
Department of Orthopaedic Surgery
Stanford University Medical Center
Stanford, California

Harcharan S. Gill, MD
Associate Professor of Urology
Department of Urology
Stanford University Medical Center
Stanford, California
Urology

Brenda Golianu, MD
Assistant Professor of Anesthesia (Pediatric Anesthesia)
Stanford University Medical Center
Stanford, California
Pediatric General Surgery; Standard Pediatric Pain Management

Julie Good, MD
Clinical Assistant Professor in Anesthesia
Pediatric Pain and Symptom Management/Palliative Care
Department of Anesthesia
Stanford University
Stanford, California
Pediatric Pain Management

Stuart B. Goodman, MD, PhD, FRCSC, FACS
Professor of Orthopaedic Surgery
Stanford University Medical Center
Department of Orthopaedic Surgery
Stanford, California
Orthopedic Surgery: Hip, Pelvis, Upper Leg, Knee

Ralph S. Greco, MD
Johnson and Johnson Professor of Surgery and Professor, by courtesy, of Mechanical Engineering
Department of Surgery
Stanford University Medical Center
Stanford, California
Endocrine Surgery

Cosmin Guta, MD
Clinical Assistant Professor
Department of Anesthesia
Stanford University Medical Center
Stanford, California
ENT Surgery

Alvin Hackel, MD
Professor (Clinical) of Anesthesia and Pediatrics, Emeritus
Stanford University
Stanford, California
Latex Allergy Considerations

Bruce D. Halperin, MD
Adjunct Clinical Associate Professor
Department of Anesthesia
Stanford University Medical Center
Stanford, California
Liposuction

Gregory B. Hammer, MD
Professor of Anesthesia and, by courtesy, of Pediatrics
Stanford University Medical Center
Stanford, California
Pediatric Otolaryngology; General; Urology; Surgery for Craniofacial Malformations; Pediatric Out-of-OR Procedures; Pediatric Anesthetjc Protocols and Postoperative Pain Management

Frank L. Hanley, MD
Lawrence Crowley, MD, Endowed Professor in Child Health
Department of Cardiothoracic Surgery, Pediatric Cardiac Surgery
Stanford University Medical Center
Stanford, California
Pediatric Cardiovascular Surgery

Leland H. Hanowell, MD
Associate Professor
Department of Anesthesia
Stanford University Hospital
Stanford, California
Adult Out-of-OR Procedures

Gary E. Hartman, MD
Clinical Professor of Pediatric Surgery and Surgical Education
Lucile Packard Childrens Hospital
Stanford, California
ECMO

Gary Heit, MD, PhD
Staff Neurosurgeon
Kaiser Permanente
Redwood City, California

Jamie M. Henderson, MD
Associate Professor of Neurosurgery
Department of Neurosurgery
Stanford University Medical Center
Stanford, California
Functional Neurosurgery

Vincent R. Hentz, MD
Professor of Plastic and Reconstructive Surgery
Chief, Hand and Upper Limb Service
Stanford University Medical Center
Stanford, California
Hand Surgery

Jerome E. Hester, MD
Attending Surgeon, Department of Surgery
Stanford University Medical Center
Facial Reconstructive Surgical and Medical Center
Palo Alto, California
Surgery for Sleep Disorders

Charles C. Hill, MD
Clinical Assistant Professor in Anesthesia
Department of Anesthesia
Stanford University Medical Center
Stanford, California
Trauma Surgery

Terri D. Homer, MD
Associated Anesthesiologist
Palo Alto, California
Office-Based Anesthesia

Anita Honkanen, MD
Clinical Associate Professor in Anesthesia
Chief, Pediatric Anesthesia Service
Stanford University Medical Center
Stanford, California

Vincent Hsieh, MD
Resident in Anesthesia
Stanford University School of Medicine
Stanford, California
Colorectal Surgery

James I. Huddleston, MD
Assistant Professor
Department of Orthopaedic Surgery
Stanford University, School of Medicine
Stanford, California

Stephen L. Huhn, MD
Associate Professor of Neurosurgery
Department of Neurosurgery
Stanford University Medical Center
Stanford, California
Pediatric Neurosurgery

Amreen Husain, MD
Assistant Professor of Obstetrics and Gynecology
Stanford University Medical Center
Stanford, California
Gynecologic Oncology

Peter H. Hwang, MD
Associate Professor
Chief, Rhinology, Otolaryngology Head & Neck Surgery
Stanford University School of Medicine
Stanford, California
Endoscopic Sinus Surgery

Robert K. Jackler, MD
Professor
Sewall Professor and Chair, OHNS, Associate Dean CME
Stanford University School of Medicine
Stanford, California
Otology; Neurotology

Richard A. Jaffe, MD, PhD
Professor of Anesthesia and
Professor by courtesy, of Neurosurgery
Chief, Neurosurgical Anesthesia Service
Stanford University Medical Center
Stanford, California
Neurosurgery: Intracranial, functional, and carotid; Ophthalmic Surgery; Dental Surgery; Craniofacial Surgery; Adult Out-of-OR Procedures; Adult Anesthetic Protocols

Stefanie S. Jeffrey, MD, FACS
Associate Professor
Department of Surgery, Division of Surgical Oncology
Stanford University School of Medicine
Stanford, California
Breast Surgery

David M. Kahn, MD
Clinical Associate Professor
Department of Surgery - Plastic and Reconstructive Surgery
Stanford University Medical Center
Stanford, California
Facial Cosmetic Surgery; Nonfacial Aesthetic Surgery; Functional Restoration

Komal Kamra, MD
Clinical Assistant Professor
Department of Anesthesia
Stanford University Medical Center
Stanford, California
Cardiac Catheterization, Pediatric Orthopedic Surgery

Michael J. Kaplan, MD
Professor
Chief, Head and Neck Surgery
Department of Otolaryngology-Head and Neck Surgery
Stanford University School of Medicine
Stanford, California
Head and Neck Surgery

Daniel S. Kapp, MD
Professor of Radiation Oncology
Stanford University Medical Center
Stanford, California
Gynecologic Oncology

Andrew C. Karich, MD
Orthopedic Surgeon
Saint Jude Heritage Healthcare
Fullerton, California

Stephen T. Kee, MD
Chief Interventional Radiology
UCLA Medical Center
Department of Interventional Radiology
Los Angeles, California
Endovascular and Tracheobronchial Stent-Graphing; RF Ablation

Mark Koransky, MD
Surgeon
Palo Alto Medical Foundation
Fremont Center
Fremont, California
Endocrine Surgery

Vivekanand Kulkarni, MD
Clinical Assistant Professor
Department of Anesthesia
Stanford University Medical Center
Stanford, California

Trang H. La, MD
Resident, Department of Radiation Oncology
Stanford University School of Medicine
Stanford, California

Eleonora G. Lad, MD, PhD
Research Fellow, Department of Ophthalmology
Stanford University Medical Center
Stanford, California

Amy L. Ladd, MD
Professor, Department of Orthopaedic Surgery
Chief, Robert A. Chase Hand & Upper Limb Center
Chief, Pediatric Hand Clinic
Stanford University Medical Center
Lucile Packard Children's Hospital
Stanford, California
Shoulder/Arm Surgery; Pediatric Hand Surgery

Azeem K. Lakha, DMD
Private Practice, Dentist
Palo Alto, California
Office-based Dental Procedures

Cathy R. Lammers, MD, FAAP
Associate Professor of Pediatric Anesthesiology
UC Davis Children's Hospital
Sacramento, California
Pediatric Otolaryngology, Urology; Pediatric Out-of-OR Procedures, Latex Allergy Considerations

Kathleen L. Larkin MD
Clinical Assistant Professor in Anesthesia
Stanford University Medical Center
Stanford, California

C. Philip Larson, Jr., MD, CM
Professor of Anesthesia and Neurosurgery, Emeritus
Stanford University Medical Center
Professor of Clinical Anesthesiology
University of California, Los Angeles
Los Angeles, California
Adult Anesthetic Protocols, Spine Surgery

Edward R. Laws, MD, FACS
Professor, Department of Neurosurgery
Stanford University Hospital
Stanford, California
Pituitary Surgery

Hendrikus J. M. Lemmens, MD, PhD
Professor of Anesthesia
Department of Anesthesia
Stanford University School of Medicine
Stanford, California
Hepatic, Biliary Surgery; Liver Transplantation

L. Bing Liem, DO
Cardiology
Albuquerque, New Mexico
DC Cardioversion; ICD Placement

Angeline F. Lim, MD
Duet Plastic Surgery, A Medical Corporation
Mt. View, California

Eva D. Littman, MD
OBGYN/Infertility Specialist
Nevada Fertility CARES Center
Summerlin Medical Center
Las Vegas, Nevada
Infertility Surgery

Jens Lohser, MD, MSc, FRCPC
Clinical Assistant Professor, University of British Columbia
Department of Anesthesia
Vancouver, British Columbia
Canada
Thoracic Surgery

Eliza Long, MD
Staff Physician
Department of Surgery
Stanford University Medical Center
Stanford, California
Endocrine Surgery

Joseph F. Looby, DO
Craniofacial Surgery Fellow
Plastic and Reconstructive Surgery
Stanford University Medical Center
Stanford, California

Sean C. Mackey, MD, PhD
Associate Professor
Chief, Division of Pain Management
Stanford School of Medicine
Stanford, California
Pain Management

Hari Mallidi, MD
Instructor, Cardiothoracic Surgery
Stanford University
Stanford, California
Director, Cardiothoracic Surgery
Regional Medical Center of San Jose
San Jose, California

Kevin A. Malott, MD
Clinical Assistant Professor
Department of Anesthesia
Stanford University Hospital
Stanford, California
Stomach, Intestinal Surgery

Neyssa Marina, MD
Professor of Pediatrics Hematology/Oncology
Lucile Packard Children's Hospital
Stanford University Medical Center
Stanford, California

Michael P. Marks, MD
Chief, Interventional Neuroradiology
Professor of Radiology and, by courtesy, of Neurosurgery
Stanford University Medical Center
Stanford, California
Interventional Neuroradiology

Jeffrey Marotte, MD
Urologist
Conway Urology
Little Rock, Arkansas

Marc L. Melcher, MD, PhD
Assistant Professor, Department of Surgery
Stanford University Medical Center
Stanford, California
Liver, Kidney Transplantation

Anna H. Messner, MD
Associate Professor of Otolaryngology and Pediatrics
Stanford University Medical Center
Lucile Packard Childrens Hospital
Stanford, California
Pediatric Otolaryngology

Frederick G. Mihm, MD
Professor of Anesthesia
Stanford University Medical Center
Stanford, California
Endocrine Surgery; Orthopedic Surgery of Lower Extremities; Emergency Procedures for Anesthesiologists

Amin A. Milki, MD
Professor of Obstetrics and Gynecology (Reproductive Endocrinology and Infertility)
Stanford University Medical Center
Stanford, California
Infertility Surgery

R. Scott Mitchell, MD
Professor of Cardiothoracic Surgery
Stanford University Medical Center
Stanford, California
Cardiac, Vascular Surgery

Darius M. Moshfeghi, MD
Assistant Professor
Department of Ophthalmology
Stanford University Medical Center
Stanford, California

Sam P. Most, MD
Associate Professor
Chief, Facial Plastic Surgery Division
Stanford University School of Medicine
Stanford, California
Facial Surgery

Vladimir Nekhendzy, MD
Clinical Associate Professor of Anesthesia and Otolaryngology
Chief, ENT Anesthesia Division
Director, Difficult Airway Management Program
Department of Anesthesia
Stanford University Medical Center
Stanford, California
Otolaryngology Surgery

Camran Nezhat, MD, FACOG, FACS
Fellowship Director
Center for Special Minimally Invasive and Robotic Surgery
Clinical Professor of OB/GYN
University of California at San Francisco
Clinical Professor of OB/GYN and Surgery
Stanford University Medical Center
Stanford, California
Laparoscopic Procedures for Gynecologic Surgery

Jeffrey A. Norton, MD
Professor of Surgery
Chief, Surgical Oncology and General Surgery
Stanford University Medical Center
Stanford, California
Laparoscopic Procedures for Gynecologic Surgery

Harry A. Oberhelman, MD, FACS
Professor of Surgery, Emeritus
Stanford University Medical Center
Stanford, California
Intestinal, Hepatic, Peritoneal Surgery

Ronald G. Pearl, MD, PhD
Chairman, Professor of Anesthesia
Stanford University Medical Center
Stanford, California
Urology

Stanton B. Perry, MD
Clinical Associate Professor of Cardiology
Lucile Salter Packard Children's Hospital
Stanford, California
Pediatric Cardiac Catheterization

Carlos E. Pineda, MD
Fellow in Surgery
Department of Surgery
Stanford University School of Medicine
Stanford, California
Colorectal Surgery

Nelson B. Powell, MD
Adjunct Clinical Professor
Department of Otolaryngology/Head & Neck Surgery
Stanford University
Stanford, California
Surgery for Sleep Disorders

Chandra Ramamoorthy, MD
Professor of Anesthesia
Stanford University Medical Center
Stanford, California
Pediatric Cardiovascular Surgery; Pediatric Cardiac Catheterization

Radhamangalam J. Ramamurthi, MD, FRCA
Clinical Assistant Professor
Department of Anesthesiology
Stanford University Medical Center
Stanford, California

Emily Ratner, MD
Clinical Professor in Anesthesia
Stanford University Medical Center
Stanford, California

V. Mohan Reddy, MD
Associate Professor of Cardiothoracic Surgery (Pediatric Cardiac Surgery) and Pediatrics
Lucile Packard Childrens Hospital
Stanford, California
Pediatric Cardiovascular Surgery

Bruce A. Reitz, MD
Norman E. Shumway Professor
Department of Cardiothoracic Surgery
Stanford University Medical Center
Stanford, California
Heart/Lung Transplantation

Robert W. Riley, DDS, MD
Adjunct Clinical Professor
Department of Otolaryngology/Head & Neck Surgery
Stanford University Medical Center
Stanford, California
Surgery for Sleep Disorders

Lawrence A. Rinsky, MD
Professor (Clinical) of Orthopaedic Surgery
Department of Orthopaedic Surgery
Stanford University Medical Center
Stanford, California
Pediatric Orthopedic Surgery

Daniel J. Riskin, MD
Consulting Assistant Professor of Surgery
Department of Surgery
Stanford University Hospital
Trauma Surgery

Myer H. Rosenthal, MD, FACCP
Professor (Clinical) of Anesthesia, Medicine, and Surgery, Emeritus
Stanford University Medical Center
Stanford, California
Gynecologic Oncology, Emergency Procedures for Anesthesiologists

Lonny L. Ross, MD, FRCSC
Assistant Professor of Plastic Surgery
Children's Hospital at University of Manitoba
Winnipeg, Manitoba, Canada
Malformations

Stephen I. Ryu, MD
Clinical Assistant Professor
Department of Neurosurgery
Stanford University Medical Center
Stanford, California

Gordon T. Sakamoto, MD
Resident in Neurosurgery
Departmet of Neurosurgery
Stanford School of Medicine
Stanford, California
Intracranial Neurosurgery

Steven A. Schendel, MD, DDS, FACS
Professor Emeritus
Department of Surgery
Stanford University
Stanford, California
Dental Surgery; Craniofacial Surgery; Surgery for Craniofacial Malformation

Clifford A. Schmiesing, MD
Clinical Associate Professor of Anesthesia
Stanford University Medical Center
Stanford, California
Preoperative Anesthesia Considerations

Don M. Sesso, DO
Center for Facial and Airway Reconstructive Surgery
Palo Alto, California
Sleep Disordered Breathing

Jeannie Seybold, MD
Clinical Instructor of Anesthesia
Department of Anesthesia
Stanford University Medical Center
Stanford, California

Steven Shafer, MD
Professor of Anesthesia
Stanford University Medical Center
Stanford, California
TIVA

Andrew A. Shelton, MD
Assistant Professor of Surgery (General Surgery)
Stanford University Medical Center
Stanford, California
Colorectal Surgery

Linda M. Dairiki Shortliffe, MD
Professor and Chair of Urology
Stanford School of Medicine
Stanford, California
Pediatric Urology

Lawrence M. Shuer, MD
Professor, Department of Neurosurgery
Stanford University
Chief of Staff
Stanford Hospital and Clinics
Stanford, California
Intracranial, Functional, Spinal, Extracranial neurosurgery; Surgery for Craniofacial Malformations

Lawrence C. Siegel, MD
Professor of Anesthesia
Stanford University Medical Center
Veterans Administration Hospital
Palo Alto Health Care System
Palo Alto, California
Heart-Lung Transplantation, Cardiac Surgery, Minimally Invasive Cardiac Surgery

Eric J. Sirulnick, MD
Cardiologist
Cardiovascular Consultants of Nevada
Henderson, Nevada
DC Cardioversion, ICD Placement

Baird M. Smith, MD
Assistant Professor of Surgery and Pediatrics
Santa Clara Valley Medical Center
San Jose, California
Pediatric General Surgery

Samuel K. S. So, MD, FACS
Lui Hac Minh Professor
Department of Surgery - General Surgery
Stanford School of Medicine
Stanford, California
Hepatic Surgery

David A. Spain, MD
Professor of Surgery
Stanford University Medical Center
Stanford, California
Trauma Surgery

Gary K. Steinberg, MD, PhD
Bernard and Ronni Lacroute-William Randolph Hearst Professor of Neurosurgery and the Neurosciences
Chairman, Department of Neurosurgery
Stanford University School of Medicine
Stanford, California
Intracranial, Extracranial Neurosurgery

Brian P. Struyk, MD
Fellow in Anesthesia
Department of Anesthesia
Stanford University School of Medicine
Stanford, California
Pediatric Neurosurgery

Naiyi Sun, MD
Fellow in Anesthesia
Department of Anesthesia
Stanford University School of Medicine
Stanford, California
Special Considerations for Latex Allergy

Sarmela T. Sunder, MD
Stanford University School of Medicine
Stanford, California
Endoscopic Sinus Surgery

Daniel Y. Sze, MD, PhD
Associate Professor
Interventional Radiology
Stanford University Medical Center
Stanford, California
Imaging, Image-Guided Procedures

M. Mark Taslimi, MD
Clinical Professor of Obstetrics & Gynecology
Lucile Packard Children's Hospital
Stanford University Medical Center
Stanford, California
Medical Director, Santa Cruz PDC
Santa Cruz, California
Obstetric Surgery

Nelson N. Teng, MD, PhD
Associate Professor in Obstetrics and Gynecology
Stanford University Medical Center
Stanford, California
Gynecologic Oncology

Kalyani R. Trivedi, MD
Pediatrics, Pediatric Cardiology
California Pacific Medical Center
San Francisco, California
Pediatric Cardiac Catheterization

Pieter Van der Starre, MD, PhD
Associate Professor of Anesthesia
Stanford University Medical Center
Stanford, California
Vascular Surgery

Lindsey Vokach-Brodsky, MB, ChB, FFARCSI
Clinical Associate Professor of Anesthesia
Stanford University Medical Center
Stanford, California
Breast Surgery; Laparoscopic Procedures for Gynecologic Surgery; Nonfacial Aesthetic Surgery

Geoffrey Brant Walton, MD
Clinical Instructor in Anesthesia
Stanford University Medical Center
Stanford, California
Trauma Surgery

Irene L. Wapnir, MD, FACS
Associate Professor
Chief of Breast Surgery
Department of Surgery
Stanford University Medical Center
Stanford, California
Breast Surgery

Mark Lane Welton, MD
Associate Professor of Surgery
Stanford University Medical Center
Stanford, California
Colorectal Surgery

Lynn M. Westphal, MD
Associate Professor
Department of Obstetrics and Gynecology
Stanford University Medical Center
Stanford, California
Infertility Surgery

Richard I. Whyte, MD
Professor of Cardiothoracic Surgery
Stanford University Medical Center
Stanford, California
Thoracic Esophageal Surgery

Kimberley Wirsing, MD
Hand Fellow
Department of Orthopaedics
Stanford University School of Medicine
Stanford, California

Ilene Y. Wong, MD
Resident in Urology
Stanford University School of Medicine
Stanford, California
Pediatric Urology

Sherry M. Wren, MD
Professor of Surgery
Stanford University Medical Center
Palo Alto Veterans Hospital
Palo Alto, California
Stomach Surgery

Imad M. Yamout, MD
Clinical Assistant Professor
Department of Anesthesia
Stanford University Medical Center
Stanford, California
Pediatric Urology

O. W. Stephanie Yap, MD
Southeastern Gynecologic Oncology
Atlanta, Georgia
Gynecologic Oncology

Kenneth K. Yim, MD, FACS
Plastic Surgeon
Santa Clara Valley Medical Center
San Jose, California
Burn Surgery

FOREWORD

The first edition of *The Anesthesiologist's Manual of Surgical Procedures* was published in 1994 and became an instant classic, fulfilling a major need among anesthesiologists for a textbook which allowed them to provide optimal care for the extensive range of procedures which are performed daily in the operating room. Although an individual anesthesiologist may have expertise in one or more subspecialty areas, it is common for that same individual to provide anesthesia for general surgery, thoracic surgery, neurosurgery, orthopedic surgery, plastic surgery, pediatric surgery, obstetric and gynecologic surgery, vascular surgery, and even cardiac surgery in his or her normal practice. Since each of these subspecialty surgery areas has an array of different procedures with unique anesthetic challenges, the individual anesthesiologist needed an easy method for preparing for this wide range of cases. The first edition of *The Anesthesiologist's Manual of Surgical Procedures* fulfilled that need, providing expert advice on the anesthesia issues relevant to each case that an anesthesiologist might encounter throughout the year.

Fifteen years after publication of the first edition of *The Anesthesiologist's Manual of Surgical Procedures,* the need for such a textbook has only increased. Although there has been a trend towards increased subspecialization within anesthesia, the majority of anesthesiologists continue to provide anesthesia for multiple subspecialty areas. The field of surgery has also advanced, with many procedures having new anesthetic implications and new procedures being developed. The anesthetic challenges have only increased during the past 15 years, both with the development of more complex surgical procedures and with development of "less invasive" surgical procedures (such as robotic surgery, video-assisted thoracic surgery, and off-pump coronary artery bypass procedures) which pose unique anesthetic challenges.

In the current age of information technology, it is reasonable to ask whether a textbook such as this one is needed since primary and review articles are readily accessible from any computer. I believe that *The Anesthesiologist's Manual of Surgical Procedures* fulfills a need which is not normally met by these other sources. The book is unique since each chapter is written jointly by a surgeon and an anesthesiologist who both have knowledge and experience in that surgical area. In contrast to many published articles, this book focuses on the information which the anesthesiologist needs to know. For each procedure, the surgical considerations, the procedural issues, and the preoperative, intraoperative, and postoperative anesthetic considerations are reviewed in a concise, easy-to-follow manner. This consistent format throughout the entire book allows the reader to develop a rapid approach to finding the information that is most relevant to a specific procedure. In my experience, such critical information takes much longer to identify or is often not included in published articles.

The Fourth Edition of this now classic textbook is again extensively revised and updated, while still continuing the format which has been invaluable for anesthesiologists during the past 15 years. This edition includes almost 40 new surgical procedures and demonstrates the advances in laparoscopic surgery and the increased use of regional anesthesia. Anesthesia has advanced since the prior edition was published, and these changes can be seen in the descriptions of anesthetic management for many specific procedures.

For the past 15 years, *The Anesthesiologist's Manual of Surgical Procedures* has been the textbook which I have used most extensively in my practice. Similar to the way propofol has replaced pentothal, each edition has replaced the prior one, documenting the advances which have been made in anesthetic management throughout this time. The new Fourth Edition now replaces the dog-eared Third Edition on my bookshelf, providing me with invaluable assistance as I contemplate the challenges on the daily anesthesia schedule.

Ronald G. Pearl, MD, PhD
Professor and Chair
Department of Anesthesia
Stanford University School of Medicine

ACKNOWLEDGMENTS

We would like to thank our many surgical and anesthesia colleagues for their generous contribution of time and expertise, our families for their patience and support, Donna J. Allison, Ph.D. for a remarkable job of proofreading under adverse circumstances, and the editorial staff at Lippincott Williams and Wilkins—most particularly our Executive Editor Brian Brown, and our Managing Editor Nicole Dernoski, for their patient and enthusiastic support of this project.

This edition is built upon the foundation of its predecessors and, thus, includes material from prior editions. We remain grateful to our former contributors, some of whose words continue to live on in the present edition.

PREFACE

The goals of the fourth edition remain unchanged from those of the first—that is, to provide an easily accessible source of clinically relevant information about a wide variety of both common and not so common surgical procedures. As with the first edition, this edition does not pretend to be either a textbook of anesthesia or a textbook of surgery. Indeed, in the formulation of an anesthetic plan, there is no substitute for experience and sound clinical judgment.

Those familiar with the preceding editions will notice that the format and organization of this edition remain largely unchanged. Color has been added to improve readability of the tables and clarity of the figures. Along with new chapters and new procedures, every existing procedure was reviewed and revised as necessary to reflect current practices.

Once again we have made extensive use of abbreviations, medical symbols, and telegraphic sentence structure to present a large quantity of information in a condensed format. While we realize that it may be aesthetically more pleasing to read: "hypoxia or hypercapnia can lead to the development of tachycardia and hypertension", it takes up a lot less space to write: $\downarrow P_aO_2$ or $\uparrow P_aCO_2 \rightarrow \uparrow$HR + $\uparrow$BP.

This will be the last edition to benefit from the unique talents of my long-time colleague Stanley Samuels. His retirement, however, does give me the opportunity to review his important contributions to this textbook. First a bit of history; I was a resident in Anesthesiology when I developed the concept for this book, and it did not take long to realize that I had no idea how to go about getting a textbook published. The most successful medical textbook author I knew was my former chairman, William F. Ganong. So, shortly after I joined the faculty at Stanford, I approached him for advice. He liked the concept and agreed to put me in contact with one of his publishers. About this same time I had another realization—that it might be difficult to convince a large number of my new surgical and anesthesia colleagues to contribute their valuable time and talent to what they might view as a not particularly rewarding endeavor. Fortunately as a resident I had many occasions to work with Stanley, and had quickly come to realize that he possessed a certain Irish charm and almost magical ability to elicit the cooperation of others. Recognizing how important these special talents would be for the successful completion of the book, I approached him regarding collaboration. He agreed, and some 2 1/2 years later the first edition was published, an accomplishment that was in no small part a result of his persuasive powers.

This edition also marks another transition at the editorial level with the addition of two associate editors. Cliff Schmiesing and Brenda Golianu, both faculty members in the Department of Anesthesia at Stanford, bring special expertise in areas of adult and pediatric anesthesia respectively. I am thankful that they kindly agreed to assist with the time-consuming and complex editorial process involved in the production of this new edition.

Unlike previous editions, this edition was edited almost entirely online. While advantageous in theory, the translation to practice was much more difficult than anyone anticipated. Computer software no matter how well-intentioned is no substitute for a dedicated, thoughtful, and talented editorial assistant. Dee Mosteller, our editorial assistant for the previous editions, was sorely missed.

As always, the editorial team welcomes the comments and suggestions of our readers (email: TheAnesthesiologistsManual.Jaffe@Stanford.edu), and we hope that this 4th edition will become a useful resource in their clinical practice.

Richard A. Jaffe
Stanford University
School of Medicine
August 2008

SECTION

1.0 NEUROSURGERY

CHAPTER

1.1 Intracranial Neurosurgery

SURGEONS

Gary K. Steinberg, MD, PhD (*Neurovascular surgery*)
Robert L. Dodd, MD, PhD (*Neurovascular surgery*)
Gordon T. Sakamoto, MD (*General neurosurgery*)
Lawrence M. Shuer, MD (*General neurosurgery*)
Steven D. Chang, MD (*General neurosurgery, Stereotactic neurosurgery*)
Edward R. Laws, MD (Pituitary surgery)

ANESTHESIOLOGIST

Richard A. Jaffe, MD, PhD

CRANIOTOMY FOR INTRACRANIAL ANEURYSMS

SURGICAL CONSIDERATIONS

Gary K. Steinberg and Robert L. Dodd

Description: Intracranial aneurysms are focal protrusions arising from vessel wall weaknesses at major bifurcations of the arteries at the base of the brain (some frequent sites of aneurysms are shown in Fig. 1.1-1), and are most commonly treated by microsurgical clip ligation. The high rate of mortality and morbidity from aneurysmal rupture necessitates treatment for symptomatic lesions. Treatment for asymptomatic lesions generally is recommended when the lifetime risk of rupture exceeds the risk of treatment. The most important surgical considerations include: clinical presentation, aneurysm size and location, patient age and neurologic status, and medical comorbidities. Aneurysm rupture into the subarachnoid spaces is the most common clinical presentation; however, symptoms from the mass effect of enlarging aneurysms or ischemic symptoms from emboli also may occur. Aneurysm morphology, size, and location are important in determining the surgical approach, and these aneurysm characteristics, as well as patient age, condition, and comorbidities, affect the overall outcome. The **Hess and Hunt clinical grading system** (Table 1.1-1) has been proven useful in describing patients with ruptured intracranial aneurysms because it has been shown to have prognostic value in terms of ultimate clinical outcome. Grading is based on the neurologic examination and ranges from grade I (minimal headache, no neurologic deficit) to grade V (moribund).

Through a **craniotomy** or **craniectomy,** using microscopic techniques, the parent vessel giving rise to the aneurysm is identified. The aneurysm neck is isolated, and a small, nonferromagnetic alloy spring clip is placed across the aneurysm neck, excluding it from the circulation. A **frontotemporal (pterional) craniotomy** normally is used to approach anterior circulation aneurysms. This requires extensive drilling of the medial sphenoid wing (pterion) and

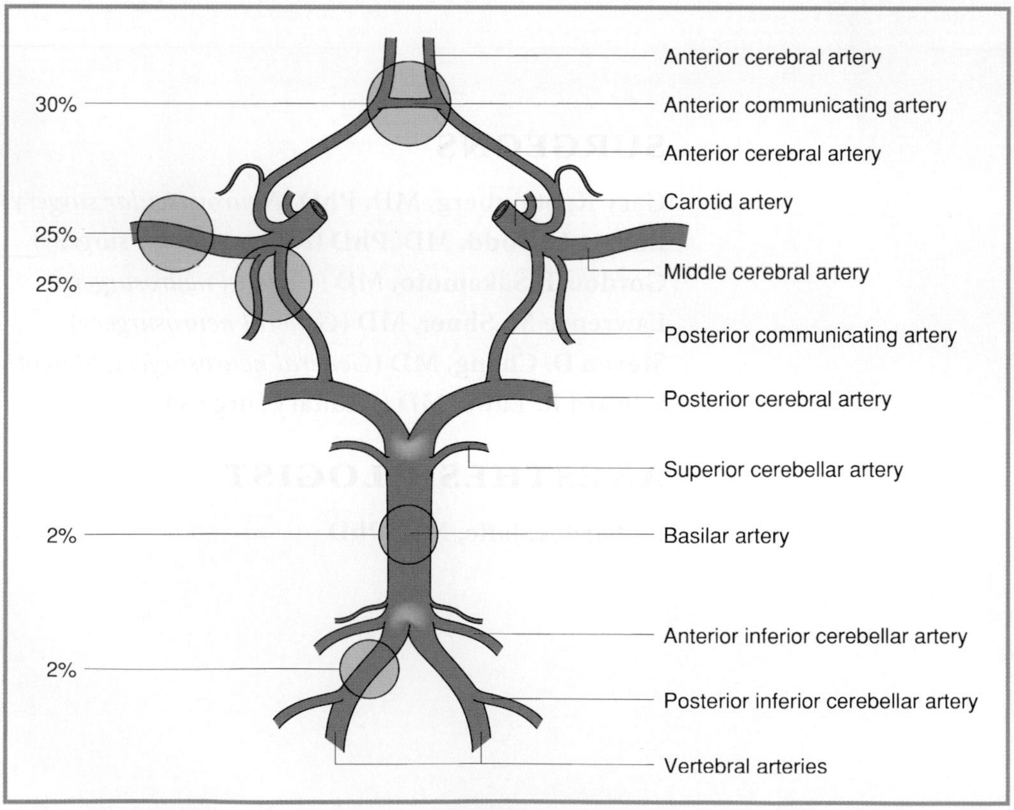

Figure 1.1-1. Locations of aneurysms of the circle of Willis and their relative occurrence. (Reproduced with permission from Greenfield LJ, Mulholland MW, Lillemore KD, et al: *Surgery: Scientific Principles and Practice,* 3rd edition. Lippincott Williams & Wilkins, Philadelphia: 2001.)

Table 1.1-1. Hunt-Hess Grading System for Aneurysmal SAH*

Grade	Description
I	Asymptomatic or minimal headache and slight neck stiffness (mortality ~2%)
II	Moderate-to-severe headache, neck stiffness, no neurological deficit (except cranial nerve palsy)—(mortality ~5%)
III	Drowsiness, confusion, or mild focal deficit (mortality 15–20%)
IV	Stupor, moderate-to-severe hemiparesis, possible early decerebrate rigidity, and vegetative disturbances (mortality 30–40%)
V	Deep coma, decerebrate rigidity, moribund (mortality 50–80%)

* The presence of serious systemic disease—such as hypertension, diabetes, severe arteriosclerosis, chronic pulmonary disease, and angiographic vasospasm—results in placement in the next less-favorable category.

allows access to most aneurysms on the anterior and lateral Circle of Willis vessels: internal carotid-paraclinoid/superior hypophyseal artery; internal carotid-ophthalmic artery; posterior communicating artery; anterior choroidal artery; internal carotid artery bifurcation; middle cerebral artery; and anterior communicating artery. Posterior circulation aneurysms are approached via a pterional or subtemporal exposure (upper basilar artery, posterior cerebral artery, superior cerebellar artery), a suboccipital exposure (vertebral artery, posterior inferior cerebellar artery), or a combined subtemporal and suboccipital exposure (basilar trunk, vertebrobasilar junction). Circulatory arrest under CPB with deep hypothermia (16–20°C) is used for repairing some giant (> 2.5 cm) aneurysms.

Usual preop diagnosis: Cerebral aneurysm; subarachnoid hemorrhage (SAH); intracerebral hemorrhage; progressive neurological deficits (mass effect on cranial nerves or CNS structures); TIAs; cerebral infarct

SUMMARY OF PROCEDURES

	Anterior Circulation Aneurysms	Posterior Circulation Aneurysms	Circulatory Arrest (CPB) W/Deep Hypothermia
Position	Supine, head in Mayfield headrest, turned 30–45° to side away from aneurysm, vertex dropped (Fig. 1.1-5)	⇐ Or lateral decubitus, head lateral in Mayfield headrest	⇐ + Both groins must be accessible for arterial + venous cannulation; access to chest for defibrillation
Incision	Frontotemporal	⇐ Or temporal, temporosuboccipital, or suboccipital	⇐
Special instrumentation	Operating microscope; aneurysm clips; radiolucent table, and headrest for intraop angiography	⇐ + Aperture clips to accommodate cranial nerves and critical vessels	⇐ + CPB pump; femoral cannulae; defibrillator; CUSA for partially thrombosed aneurysms
Unique considerations	Temporary arterial clipping; mild hypothermia (33°C); intraop angiography with access to femoral artery; electrophysiological monitoring (SEPs, BAERs); brain relaxation; ± lumbar subarachnoid CSF drainage; dexamethasone 8–12 mg iv	⇐	⇐ + No manipulation of brain retractors after systemic heparinization; meticulous attention to hemostasis
Antibiotics	Ceftriaxone 1–2 g iv q d (avoid Ca^{++} containing solutions)	⇐	⇐
Surgical time	3–5 h	3–6 h	6–8 h
Closing considerations	Rewarming	⇐	⇐
EBL	250–1000 mL	⇐	2000–4000 mL

SUMMARY OF PROCEDURES (cont'd)

	Anterior Circulation Aneurysms	Posterior Circulation Aneurysms	Circulatory Arrest (CPB) W/Deep Hypothermia
Postop care	ICU 1–7 d; postop CBF monitoring. Transcranial Doppler (TDC) monitor	⇐	⇐ + ICP monitoring
Mortality	Unruptured: 0.5%	1.5%	5–10% (giant aneurysms)
	Ruptured:		
	Hunt and Hess grades I–III: < 10% (See Table 1.1-1.)	15%	5–15%
	Hunt and Hess grades IV–V: 20–40% (See Table 1.1-1.)	20–50%	15–50%
Morbidity	Neurological: 5–20%	10–30%	10–50%
	Cranial nerve injury	⇐	⇐
	Stroke	⇐	⇐
	Hydrocephalus: 15–25%	⇐	⇐
	Hyponatremia	⇐	⇐
	Respiratory failure: Rare	⇐	⇐
	Seizures: 2–20%	⇐	⇐
	Thromboembolism: Rare	⇐	⇐
	CSF leak: Rare	⇐	⇐
	Infection: Rare	⇐	⇐
	Massive blood loss: Rare	⇐	⇐
Pain score	3–4	3–4	4–5

PATIENT POPULATION CHARACTERISTICS

Age range	30–70 yr (Peak incidence in 5th and 6th decades)
Male:Female	44:56
Incidence	8–16/100,000/yr for ruptured aneurysms with SAH (highest in Japan and Finland) Overall incidence of rebleeding is ~11% (4% in the first 24 h).
Etiology	Idiopathic (probably acquired and related to hemodynamic stress at arterial branch points, although may have congenital predisposition to loss of internal elastic lamina); traumatic; infectious; familial
Associated conditions	Polycystic kidney disease; coarctation of the aorta; Marfan syndrome; Ehlers-Danlos syndrome; intracranial AVMs; aortic aneurysm; fibromuscular dysplasia; pseudoxanthoma elastica; Rendu-Osler-Weber syndrome; cocaine/amphetamine use

ANESTHETIC CONSIDERATIONS

(Procedures covered: craniotomy for intracranial aneurysms; craniotomy for cerebral embolectomy)

PREOPERATIVE

Aneurysms may occur in any age group, although they generally become symptomatic and are diagnosed in young or middle-aged adults who are usually in otherwise good health. Most patients have warning Sx before the first major bleed, but these tend to be mild and nonspecific (e.g., headache, dizziness, orbital pain, slight motor or sensory disturbances). The symptoms are generally disregarded by both patients and physicians. Most patients with SAH will be receiving nimodipine; SBP should be maintained between 100 and 160 mmHg using pressors if necessary. Patients with symptomatic vasospasm may benefit from triple-H therapy (see below).

Respiratory	Respiratory complications (e.g., neurogenic pulmonary edema (up to 23%), pneumonia, ARDS, PE) are the most common non-neurologic causes of death following SAH. Pulmonary aspiration may have occurred as the result of a neurological deficit from an intracranial hemorrhage. **Tests:** As indicated from H&P. Elevated cTnI may predict pulmonary complications.

Cardiovascular	Generally, these patients do not have other cardiovascular diseases, although intracerebral aneurysms occur more commonly in patients with certain congenital disorders, such as polycystic disease of the kidneys, coarctation of the aorta, fibromuscular hyperplasia, and Marfan and Ehlers-Danlos syndromes. Patients who have had a recent intracranial hemorrhage from leaking or rupture of a cerebral aneurysm are prone to develop systemic HTN, hypovolemia, and ECG abnormalities. The HTN is thought to be due to autonomic hyperactivity, and is generally treated with antihypertensive medication, which should be continued up to the time of anesthesia and surgery. Why hypovolemia occurs following SAH is not clear, but may be due in part to cerebral vasospasm and to sustained bed rest. ECG abnormalities occur in most patients following an intracranial hemorrhage and may represent subendocardial injury 2° catecholamine release. Dysrhythmias (most commonly PVCs) occur in 30–80% of patients, and ischemic changes (typically T-wave inversion and S–T-segment depression) are seen in > 50%. Appropriate preop preparation includes ECG characterization of the abnormality. If patient has Hx of ischemic heart disease, ECHO and cardiac enzyme studies may be helpful in determining whether the myocardial injury and consequent ECG changes are likely to be of clinical significance. **Tests:** ECG; others (e.g., cardiac enzymes) as indicated from H&P.
Neurological	Seldom do aneurysms produce neurological Sx by enlarging to the point that they compress adjacent neural tissue or cause ↑ ICP. If an intracranial hemorrhage occurs, the neurological dysfunction will vary, depending on the site and extent of the hemorrhage. Typically, SAH → ↑↑ ICP → Sudden severe HA ± confusion and disorientation, ± motor deficit, ± coma. Admission GCS < 12 predicts ↑ mortality. Subsequent cerebral vasospasm (~70% incidence) may cause worsening of the neurological deficits. Clinically detectable vasospasm commonly begins on day 1 reaching a maximum at 6–8 d, and usually is resolved within 2–3 wk. The precipitating agent is believed to be free Hb → release of vasospastic substances from brain tissue. Treatment of vasospasm usually involves support of BP (occasionally, induced HTN), hydration to normovolemia, and systemic Ca^{++} antagonists (e.g., nimodipine (60 mg PO q 4 h) or iv (3–15 mg/h iv)). Triple H therapy (↑ volume, ↑ BP, ↓ Hct) does not appear to confer any additional advantage in most patients. Control of BP is important: any substantial ↑ BP may → serious rebleed, permanent neurological deficits or death; any substantial ↓ BP may → cerebral ischemia and infarction. Arterial catheterization and continuous beat-to-beat monitoring of BP prior to induction of anesthesia is essential in these patients. **Tests:** CT; MRI; CTA, which the anesthesiologist should examine preop to identify the nature and site of the aneurysm.
Hydrocephalus	Acute hydrocephalus occurs in 15–20% of patients within 24 h of SAH. External ventricular drainage may be necessary.
Hematologic	Thrombocytopenia may develop following SAH. **Tests:** Hct; PT; PTT
Radiographic findings	CT: Blood in basal cisterns (~95% of patients) or ventricles; CTA (replacing conventional angiography): anatomical characteristics of the aneurysm.
Laboratory	Cardiac enzymes if ECG changes observed (↑ cTnI predicts ↓ neurologic outcome and ↑ mortality); others as indicated from H&P.
Hepatic	Hepatic dysfunction following SAH is not uncommon (24% in one series). **Tests:** LFTs, as indicated from H&P.
Premedication	Small doses of midazolam 1–3 mg iv are preferable to opiates. Detailed discussion with the patient about the anesthetic plan, with appropriate reassurance, is essential. Should an intracranial aneurysm leak or rupture in the immediate preop period, its signs may be difficult to distinguish from those associated with excessive response to premedication.

INTRAOPERATIVE

Anesthetic technique: GETA. The goals of anesthesia for this operation are to: (a) maintain optimum CPP (cerebral MAP minus cerebral venous pressure or ICP, whichever is greater), although it may be necessary to ↓ CPP rapidly if intracranial hemorrhage occurs during surgery; (b) decrease intracranial volume (blood and tissue) to optimize working space for surgeons within the cranial compartment, thereby minimizing the need for surgical retraction of brain tissue; and (c) decrease metabolic rate and $CMRO_2$ with the expectation that the brain will tolerate hypotension and ischemia if sudden decreases in MAP and, hence, CPP become necessary.

Induction	Smooth induction is essential. STP 2–5 mg/kg (or propofol 1–2 mg/kg iv) to provide amnesia and ↓ cerebral blood volume by inducing cerebral vasoconstriction. Fentanyl 7–10 mcg/kg iv to blunt response to intubation and provide analgesia for the first hours of surgery. Pancuronium 0.1 mg/kg, vecuronium 0.15 mg/kg, or rocuronium 0.7–1 mg/kg to provide muscle relaxation for tracheal intubation and positioning patient. Patients on nimodipine may require pressors (e.g., phenylephrine) during and after induction. Poor H-H grade patients (IV–V) may not tolerate ↓ MAP during induction. These patients may benefit from moderate hyperventilation during induction.	
Maintenance	Isoflurane or sevoflurane (1/2 MAC if EP monitoring is used), inspired with O_2. Avoid N_2O > 50% and entirely in patients with ↑↑ ICP. Propofol (75–100 mcg/kg/min) may be used to further ↓ cerebral blood volume, ↓ cerebral metabolism, and ↓ $CMRO_2$. Generally, if pancuronium is used, no additional NMBs are needed; however, if movement is of concern, rocuronium 10 mcg/kg/min will provide adequate neuromuscular blockade. A remifentanil infusion (0.05–0.1 mcg/kg/min) can be used to supplement the anesthetic without interfering with EP monitoring. TIVA is not necessary for monitoring SSEPs or MEPs.	
Emergence	H-H grade IV–V patients are not extubated and should be kept sedated on ventilator support postop. For grade I–III patients, with the start of dural closure, consider using low-dose sevoflurane (e.g., 0.5%) in 50% N_2O, supplemented with a low-dose remifentanil infusion (e.g., 0.05 mcg/kg/min). As recovery from anesthesia occurs, the patient's BP generally will increase in response to the emergence stimuli. Titration of β-adrenergic blocking drugs (e.g., labetalol or esmolol) with vasodilators (e.g., SNP) may be needed; if so, the dose should be stabilized before transport to ICU. (See Control of BP, below.) The inhalation agent can be D/C'd at the time of dressing application. Most patients will breathe spontaneously and can be extubated uneventfully while on the remifentanil infusion. If the brain has not been injured by the surgical procedure, the patient should awaken within 10 min after cessation of remifentanil administration. As the patient is awakening, it is important to assure full reversal from neuromuscular blockade and close regulation of BP. If the patient begins to cough on ETT, either it should be removed or cough reflex suppressed with iv lidocaine (0.5–1 mg/kg). Patient is placed in bed in a 30° head-up position and transported to ICU for monitoring overnight. Supplemental O_2 should be administered and close regulation of BP maintained. Prophylactic antiemetics (e.g., metoclopramide 10–20 mg and ondansetron 4 mg or dolasetron 12.5 mg) should be given 30 min before extubation.	
Blood and fluid requirements	IV: 14–18 ga × 2 NS @ <10 mL/kg + UO	Maintain euvolemia. If blood volume is normal, crystalloid fluid should not exceed 10 mL/kg beyond that required to replace UO. Rapid, massive blood loss is possible.
	Expand blood volume with albumin 5% if Hct >30%. Albumin + PRBC if Hct <30% Maintain colloid oncotic pressure	If blood volume is low because of vasospasm or prolonged bed rest, albumin 5% is given if Hct > 30%; combinations of albumin and blood, if Hct is < 30%.
	Hetastarch may → coagulopathy.	Hetastarch 6% may be used in place of albumin, but limit use because of potential for coagulopathy.
Brain relaxation	Hyperventilate to $PaCO_2$ = 30 mmHg ($PetCO_2$ = 25 mmHg). PaO_2 > 100 mmHg	↓ $PaCO_2$ → ↓cerebral vascular volume (better surgical access) + ↑ CBF to ischemic areas ("Robin Hood" effect) + ↓ anesthetic requirements + ↑ lactic acid buffering.

Brain relaxation (cont'd)	↓ fluids < 10 mL/kg + UO Consider propofol infusion to replace N_2O ↓ isoflurane/sevoflurane to < 1/2 MAC Mannitol 0.5–1 g/kg	Remifentanil infusion (0.05–0.2 mcg/kg/min) may be required to provide adequate analgesia Mannitol/furosemide → ↓K^+; monitor level and replace as necessary. If mannitol is administered too rapidly, ↓ BP may occur, probably from peripheral vasodilation.
	± Furosemide 0.3 mg/kg ± Steroids (e.g., 8 mg dexamethasone)	
	± Lumbar CSF drain Head up to provide venous drainage Minimize neck flexion/rotation	CSF drain may be placed after induction of anesthesia, avoid rapid drainage → rupture
Monitoring	Standard monitors (see p. B-1). Arterial line Bladder temperature Blood glucose (100–180 mg/dl)	Direct monitoring of arterial BP is essential because marked fluctuations may occur, necessitating drug therapy, as well as need for ABGs. Transducers should always be at the level of the head rather than the heart.
	CVP line UO (Foley catheter) ± Evoked potentials	Monitoring CVP is desirable in virtually all patients to assess adequacy of fluid therapy, for infusion of vasoactive drugs both intraop and postop, and for aspiration of VAE. Localization of the catheter can be determined by CXR, ECG tracing (noting P-wave changes), or pressure-wave contour and value as the catheter is withdrawn from the right atrium.
Hypothermia	Water-circulating pads Cold OR Bladder irrigation	Mild hypothermia (33–34°C) is used in some centers to ↓$CMRO_2$ and to ↓ susceptibility to ischemic injury during temporary clip application. $CMRO_2$ decreases ~30%@ 33°C. This level of hypothermia has minimal effect on coagulation or the incidence of cardiac dysrhythmias. Rewarming using surface means can be quite slow. The use of bladder irrigation (40°C saline) or an InnerCool-type device is useful.
	InnerCool or equivalent	A heat-exchange catheter may be placed in the vena cava (via femoral vein) to facilitate patient cooling and rewarming.
	IHAST Study	Although it implied that mild hypothermia was not useful in aneurysm surgery, the IHAST study was not designed to assess the effectiveness of mild hypothermia in the patient group most likely to benefit: patients requiring temporary clip times > 3 min. Generalizing the IHAST findings to all aneurysm patients is an unfortunate disservice to many of them.
	↓ superficial blood flow	Administer drugs through CVP line in hypothermic patients to ensure prompt effect.
Triple H therapy (if requested)	Hypervolemia Hypertension	Goal: CVP = 10–12; PCWP = 12–16 Goal: SBP 120–150 mmHg (preclipping); 160–200 mmHg (postclipping)
	Hemodilution	Goal: HCT = 30–35%

Control of BP	During application of head fixation device (Mayfield): remifentanil: 100–200 mcg iv bolus 1–2 min in advance. During exposure: ↓ MAP to ~80% of baseline. Temporary clipping: ↑ MAP to ~120% of baseline.	Control of BP is critical to the successful outcome of the case. ↑↑ BP → ↑↑ transmural pressure across the aneurysmal wall → rupture of the aneurysm. Many neurosurgeons apply a temporary clip on the major feeding vessel(s) in advance of clipping the aneurysm. This technique collapses the aneurysm and makes the clipping easier and less likely to cause inadvertent rupture. If this technique is used, it is essential for the anesthesiologist to ↑ BP ~20% above baseline pressure to maximize collateral flow while the feeding vessel(s) is occluded. Phenylephrine is preferred because it has minimal dysrhythmogenic potential.
	Postclipping: MAP typically 70–90 mmHg	If it becomes necessary to ↓ BP, use esmolol 50–200 mcg/kg/min to ↓ HR to ~60 supplemented as necessary with SNP 0.1–4 mcg/kg/min to desired effect. Responses to vasoactive drugs are much easier to regulate if a normal blood volume has been established and maintained throughout the anesthetic period. Labetalol (5–100 mg total dose) is a useful adjunct for postop pressure control.
Aneurysmal rupture	↓ MAP to 40–50 mmHg, if necessary. Consider carotid compression	Bolus SNP: ~20 mmHg ↓ MAP/15 mcg SNP. Ipsilateral or bilateral carotid occlusion is often effective in controlling hemorrhage while a temporary clip is applied.
	Adenosine 12 mg iv (CVP line)	Adenosine will produce asystole, allowing time for the application for a temporary clip. An external pacemaker should be available.
Positioning	For most aneurysms: Supine, head turned Three-point fixation (beware of marked ↑ BP with use of pins). Use shoulder roll. ✓ and pad pressure points. ✓ eyes.	Anesthetic gas hoses and all monitoring and vascular catheter lines are directed to patient's side or feet, where the anesthesiologist is positioned during surgery. SCDs used to minimize DVT. Shoulder roll to ↓ brachial plexus stretch. Remifentanil (100–200 mcg bolus) to minimize ↑ BP during skull pinning.
Complications	Aneurysm rupture (intraop)	6–18% incidence; up to 2% rupture during induction.
	Hypothermia (mild)	Many patients can be extubated safely at core T ≥ 35°C with active rewarming in progress.

POSTOPERATIVE

Complications	Intracranial hemorrhage Stroke Cerebral vasospasm	New deficits or delayed emergence may necessitate urgent transport to CT scanner and/or return to the OR Prophylactic triple H therapy (↑ volume, ↑ BP, ↓Hct) may have no advantage over simple euvolemia.
Pain management	Meperidine (10–20 mg iv prn) Codeine (30–60 mg im q 4 h prn)	Meperidine will ↓ postop shivering. Avoid oversedation → interferes with neuro exam.
Tests	CT scan, if any change in neurological status	Be prepared to re-secure airway.

Suggested Readings

1. Chang SD, Steinberg GK: Management of intracranial aneurysm. *Vascular Medicine* 1998; 3:315–26.
2. Cully MD, Larson CP Jr, Silverberg GD: Hetastarch coagulopathy in a neurosurgical patient. *Anesthesiology* 1987; 66(5):706–7.
3. Dashti R, Hernesniemi J, Niemela M, et al: Microneurosurgical management of middle cerebral artery bifurcation aneurysms. *Surg Neurol* 2007; 67(5):441–56.
4. Dodd RL, Steinberg GK: Aneurysms. In: Aminoff MJ, Daroff RB (eds) *Encyclopedia of the Neurological Sciences*. Academic Press, San Diego: 2003, 161–172.
5. Lopez JR, Chang SD, Steinberg GK: The use of electrophysiological monitoring in the intraoperative management of intracranial aneurysms. *J Neurol Neurosurg Psychiatry* 1999; 66:189–96.
6. Mayer SA, LiMandri G, Sherman D, et al: Electrocardiographic markers of abnormal left ventricular wall motion in acute subarachnoid hemorrhage. *J Neurosurg* 1995; 83:889–96.
7. Mayer SA, Lin J, Homma S, et al: Myocardial injury and left ventricular performance after subarachnoid hemorrhage. *Stroke* 1999; 30:780–6.
8. Mocco J, Rose JC, Komotar RJ, et al: Blood pressure management in patients with intracerebral and subarachnoid hemorrhage. *Neurosurg Clin N Am* 2006; 17(suppl 1):25–40.
9. Molyneux A, Kerr R, Stratton I, et al: International Subarachnoid Aneurysm Trial (ISAT) of neurosurgical clipping versus endovascular coiling in 2143 patients with ruptured intracranial aneurysms: a randomized trial. *Lancet* 2002; 360(9342):1267–74.
10. Priebe HJ: Aneurysmal subarachnoid haemorrhage and the anaesthetist. *Br J Anaesth* 2007; 99(1):102–18.
11. Qureshi AI, Janardhan V, Hanel RA, et al: Comparison of endovascular and surgical treatments for intracranial aneurysms: an evidence-based review. *Lancet Neurol* 2007; 6(9):816–25.
12. Randell T, Niemela M, Kytta J, et al: Principles of neuroanesthesia in aneurysmal subarachnoid hemorrhage: the Helsinki experience. *Surg Neurol* 2006; 66(4):1271–6.
13. Steinberg GK, Drake CG, Peerless SJ: Deliberate basilar or vertebral artery occlusion in the treatment of intracranial aneurysms. Immediate results and long-term outcome in 201 patients. *J Neurosurg* 1993; 79:161–73.
14. Sundt TM Jr: *Surgical Techniques for Saccular and Giant Intracranial Aneurysms.* Williams & Wilkins, Baltimore: 1990.
15. Todd MM, Hindman BJ, Clarke WR, et al: Mild intraoperative hypothermia during surgery for intracranial aneurysm. *N Engl J Med* 2005; 352(2):121–4.
16. Weir B: *Aneurysms Affecting the Nervous System.* Williams & Wilkins, Baltimore: 1987.

ANESTHETIC CONSIDERATIONS FOR CRANIOTOMY FOR GIANT INTRACRANIAL ANEURYSMS

(Requiring deep hypothermic circulatory arrest)

PREOPERATIVE

Aneurysms are classified as "giant" when they are > 2.5 cm in diameter. These represent ~5% of all aneurysms. They occur twice as often in women, usually become symptomatic in the 4th or 5th decade of life, and present particularly difficult surgical challenges: (a) their large size makes direct visualization of the vascular anatomy difficult; (b) vascular branches essential to maintaining flow to normal brain may be an integral part of the giant aneurysm and cannot be included in the clipping without causing permanent neurological injury; (c) standard aneurysm clips may not occlude a large, turgid aneurysm, or may slip or move, once applied; and (d) giant aneurysms may rupture during dissection or clip application, resulting in severe neurological morbidity or mortality. Many of these aneurysms are amenable to coiling or other interventional radiologic techniques. For those requiring craniotomy, a special anesthetic and surgical management, using deep hypothermia to 18°C, achieved with fem-fem CPB and temporary circulatory arrest, is employed. These techniques decompress the aneurysm, making it easier to clip, and protect the brain during circulatory arrest. The duration of cardiac arrest may be as long as 45 minutes.

Respiratory	None unless patient has Hx of smoking or has sustained pulmonary aspiration as a result of a neurological deficit from an intracranial hemorrhage. **Tests:** As indicated from H&P; elevated cTnI may predict pulmonary complications.
Cardiovascular	Generally, these patients do not have other cardiovascular diseases. (See Anesthetic Considerations for Intracranial Aneurysms, p. 6.) **Tests:** ECG; others as indicated from H&P.
Neurological	These patients usually present with complaints of intermittent or persistent headaches or visual disturbances that are probably due to aneurysmal compression of adjacent neural

Neurological (cont'd)	tissue or ↑ ICP. If an intracranial hemorrhage occurs, neurological dysfunction varies, depending on site and extent of the hemorrhage. Cerebral vasospasm is a major complication of intracranial hemorrhage (see discussion in Anesthetic Considerations for Intracranial Aneurysms, p. 6). **Tests:** CT; MRI; angiogram. The anesthesiologist should examine the cerebral angiogram preop to visualize the size and site of aneurysm.
Hematologic	T&C for 6 U PRBCs. **Tests:** Hct; PT; PTT; hemogram; others as indicated from H&P.
Laboratory	Other tests as indicated from H&P.
Premedication	If premedication is desirable, small doses of midazolam (e.g., 1–2 mg) are preferable to opiates. Detailed discussion with patient about the anesthetic plan, with appropriate reassurance, is effective in reducing premedication requirements. Should an intracranial aneurysm leak or rupture in the immediate preop period, it may be difficult to distinguish this event from changes associated with excessive responses to premedication.

INTRAOPERATIVE

Anesthetic technique: GETA. The goals of anesthesia for this procedure are to: (a) provide adequate surgical anesthesia; (b) ↓ intracranial volume (blood and tissue) and optimize working space within the cranial compartment, thereby minimizing the need for surgical retraction of brain tissue; and (c) ↑ tolerance of the brain to ischemia by decreasing $CMRO_2$, which occurs with the use of deep hypothermia, barbiturate therapy, and isovolemic hemodilution.

Induction	STP 2–5 mg/kg or propofol 2–3 mg/kg iv to provide amnesia and ↓ CBV by inducing cerebral vasoconstriction. Fentanyl 7–10 mcg/kg iv to provide analgesia for the first hours. Vecuronium 0.15 mg/kg or rocuronium 0.7–1 mg/kg to provide relaxation for intubation and positioning.	
Maintenance	Propofol 100–200 mcg/kg/min administered by constant-infusion pump. These doses provide additional amnesia and ↓ CBV and $CMRO_2$. Isoflurane ≤ 1%. N_2O not used. An additional dose of NMB is administered just prior to the start of CPB.	
Emergence	Because of the length and nature of the operation, and the potential for temporary neurological injury, it is advisable to leave the ETT in place immediately postop, and send patient to the ICU on controlled ventilation. If patient begins to cough, the reflex should be suppressed with opiates, NMBs, and/or LTA sprayed down the ETT. The patient is placed in bed in a 30° head-up position and transported to ICU for overnight monitoring. Supplemental O_2 should be administered and close regulation of BP maintained. Prophylactic antiemetic (e.g., droperidol 0.625 mg or metoclopramide 10–20 mg, and ondansetron 4 mg) should be given 30 min before extubation.	
Blood and fluid requirements	IV: 14–16 ga × 2 NS @ 1–2 mL/kg/h PRBC 4–6 U	Maintain euvolemia Cold NS up to 10 mL/kg, + a volume equal to UO, is administered during surgery.
Isovolemic hemodilution	5% albumin 8 × 250 mL NS 4 × 1000 mL	Albumin and NS are placed in a refrigerator at 4°C the night before surgery to be used as necessary for cooling during isovolemic hemodilution.
	CPD bags	After induction of anesthesia, a 2nd arterial or large-vein cannula is placed for removal of blood into CPD bags. Generally, about 1000 mL of blood are removed and replaced with 1 L of cold albumin 5%. This usually → ↓Hct to 22–26%. Frequent intraop Hct checks are appropriate. The withdrawn blood is held at room temperature for reinfusion at the conclusion of operation. In addition, the perfusate from the CPB unit is spun down and packed cells are returned to patient.

Control of ICP (brain relaxation)	Hyperventilate to $PaCO_2$ = 25–30 mmHg Limit crystalloid < 10 mL/kg + UO Limit isoflurane ≤ 1%. Mannitol 0.5–1 g/kg ± Furosemide 0.3 mg/kg Dexamethasone 8–12 mg	Ventilation is controlled and TV and RR adjusted such that $PaCO_2$ ranges from 25–30 mmHg. There are several advantages to hypocarbia, including: ↓ CBV to provide more surgical working space, thereby lessening the need for vigorous retraction of brain tissue; improving regional distribution of CBF by preferentially diverting blood to potentially ischemic areas of the brain; better buffering of brain lactic acid that may form as a result of focal ischemia; and decreasing anesthetic requirement.
	± Lumbar CSF drainage Position head to promote venous drainage	Elevate head of bed and minimize neck flexion/rotation if possible.
Monitoring	Standard monitors (see p. B-1). Temperature = esophageal, bladder and brain surface Arterial line	Frequent checks are made of Hct, electrolytes, ACT values, before, during, and after CPB.
	CVP (triple-lumen) line	CVP line is used for infusions of esmolol, SNP, and phenylephrine.
	Blood glucose	Keep glucose between 80 and 180 mg/dl.
	UO	Keep UO > 0.5 mL/kg/h.
Control of BP	Maintain BP normal-to-20% below normal.	BP control is critical to successful surgery. ↑ BP during induction or prior to CPB will ↑ transmural pressure across the aneurysmal wall and ↑ likelihood of rupture. Prior to CPB, BP is generally kept to normal-to-20% below normal for patient, using anesthetic agents alone or with an esmolol infusion to ↓ HR to a range of 50–60 bpm. If desired level of BP is not achieved with this combination, SNP or propofol infusion may be added. SNP also facilitates both cooling and rewarming because of its vasodilatory effect.
	Phenylephrine	If a vasoconstrictor is needed, particularly during CPB while patient is still cold, phenylephrine is preferred because of its minimal dysrhythmogenic potential.
Positioning	Shoulder roll 180° table rotation ✓ and pad pressure points. ✓ eyes. Circuit extension tubes	Anesthetic gas hoses and all monitoring and vascular catheter lines are directed to patient's feet. Make sure that all will reach the foot of operating table.
	SCD	SCDs used to minimize DVT.
Deep hypothermia and CPB	Initial cooling: Circulating water Thermal blankets Ice packs SNP infusion	Surface cooling, and/or central cooling is begun as soon as induction is complete, using either a central venous heat exchange device (e.g., INNERCOOL) or thermal blankets above and below patient, ice packs and infusion of cold fluids during establishment of isovolemic hemodilution.
	Innercool-type device	A SNP infusion (if tolerated) will promote surface cooling.
	ACT monitoring Heparinization	Once the aneurysm is exposed and the decision is made that CPB is required, systemic **heparinization** (load: 300 U/kg; maintenance: 100 U/kg/h) is established, and patient is put on CPB using fem-fem bypass and cooled to ~18°C. During CPB

Deep hypothermia and CPB (cont'd)		cooling, the heart will usually fibrillate between 22–26°C. After 18°C is reached, the CPB unit is shut off to deflate the aneurysm; it may be activated and shut off several times during clipping to evaluate adequacy of the surgical occlusion of the aneurysm and to apply additional clips. **Total circulatory arrest time should not exceed 45 min.**
	Rewarming	When clipping is complete, CPB is resumed and warming instituted. Partial CPB is continued until normal cardiac rhythm is established, and body temperature reaches ~36°C. Once partial CPB is D/C, patient will tend to cool unless vigorous efforts at warming are continued. Warming the OR and iv fluids, and use of warming lights, Bair-Hugger, and an Innercool-type device will facilitate the warming process. ACT analysis is performed to establish that heparin reversal is complete 5–10 min after protamine (1 mg/100 U heparin activity). Blood is sent for clotting studies, and Plts, FFP, and calcium gluconate are administered as needed. Hetastarch 6% is not used in these patients because of its potential for inducing a coagulopathy.
Complications	↓↓ BP 2° failure to maintain circulating volume Dysrhythmias 2° ↓ K^+ from diuresis and cold	

POSTOPERATIVE

Complications	HTN Vasospasm Intracranial hemorrhage, stroke Hypothermia Hypervolemia Coagulopathy DVT Seizures PE	HTN Rx: esmolol + SNP titrated to effect. Vasospasm Rx: fluid-loading Patient should be rewarmed to 36–37°C before terminating CPB. ✓ coag status. Sz Rx: Phenytoin (1 g iv slowly to avoid ↓BP). WB: Phenytoin is incompatible with dextrose containing solutions.
Pain management	Meperidine (10–20 mg iv prn) Codeine (30–60 mg im q 4 h prn)	Meperidine minimizes postop shivering.
Tests	CT scan Coag panel	If any question about neurological status arises, a CT scan is performed postop. Coagulation studies are needed early postop to assure normal coagulation.

Suggested Readings

1. Cully MD, Larson CP Jr, Silverberg GD: Hetastarch coagulopathy in a neurosurgical patient. *Anesthesiology* 1987; 66(5):706–7.
2. Larson CP Jr. Anesthetic management for surgical ablation of giant cerebral aneurysms. *Int Anesthesiol Clin* 1996; 34(4):151–160.
3. Lawton MT, Raudzens PA, Zabramski JM, et al: Hypothermic circulation arrest in neurovascular surgery: evolving indications and predictors of patient outcome. *Neurosurgery* 1998; 43:10–20.
4. Parkinson RJ, Eddleman CS, Batjer JJ, et al: Giant intracranial aneurysms: endovascular challenges. *Neurosurgery* 2006; 59(5 suppl 3):S103–12; discussion S3–13.

5. Steinberg GK, Chung M: Giant cerebral aneurysms: morphology and structural pathology. In *Giant Cerebral Aneurysms.* Olwad IA, Barrow DL, eds. American Association of Neurological Surgeons, Park Ridge: 1995, 1–11.
6. Whittle IR, Dorsch NW, Besser M: Giant intracranial aneurysms: diagnosis, management, and outcome. *Surg Neurol* 1984; 21(3):218–0.
7. Young WL, Lawton MT, Gupta DK, et al: Anesthetic management of deep hypothermic circulatory arrest for cerebral aneurysm clipping. *Anesthesiology* 2002; 96:497–503.

CRANIOTOMY FOR CEREBRAL EMBOLECTOMY

SURGICAL CONSIDERATIONS

Gary K. Steinberg and Robert L. Dodd

Description: While intravenous or endovascular intra-arterial thrombolysis is the current standard therapy for intracranial intravascular clots, embolic occlusion of a major intracranial vessel occasionally requires microsurgical embolectomy. In particular, when the embolus is a large atherosclerotic plaque or foreign body (such as a balloon or microcoil from endovascular treatment), surgery may be the treatment of choice. Because cerebral ischemia often proceeds to irreversible infarction before the surgeon can restore blood flow, early diagnosis is of the utmost importance, and several studies have demonstrated that the best results from embolectomy occur when the procedure is performed within 6 h following the onset of a neurologic deficit.

A standard craniotomy is fashioned as previously described for other lesions involving the vasculature at the skull base (see p. 4), and the occluded intracranial artery is exposed using microsurgical techniques. The involved arterial segment is isolated, temporarily occluded with miniature clips, and an arteriotomy is performed to remove the thrombus or embolus (Fig. 1.1-2). The arteriotomy is then closed and blood flow reestablished.

Usual preop diagnosis: Stroke; TIA; intracranial arterial occlusion; catheter embolization to intracranial artery

SUMMARY OF PROCEDURE	
Position	Supine or lateral decubitus
Incision	Frontal, temporal, or occipital
Special instrumentation	Microscopic instruments (fine forceps, miniature vascular clips, operating microscope)
Unique considerations	Neuroprotective agents during arterial segment occlusion (barbiturates, mannitol), mild hypothermia (33°C)
Antibiotics	Ceftriaxone 1–2 gm iv (avoid Ca^{++} containing solutions)
Surgical time	3–4 h
Closing considerations	Avoid ↓BP (MAP 80–100 mmHg). Induced mild HTN (MAP 90–110) during temporary arterial occlusion.
EBL	100–250 mL
Postop care	Control BP (MAP 80–100 mmHg); start aspirin postop d 1; ICU: 1–2 d.
Mortality	5–10%
Morbidity	Intracerebral hemorrhage Stroke MI: Rare Thromboembolism: Rare Respiratory failure: Rare Infection: Rare
Pain score	3–4

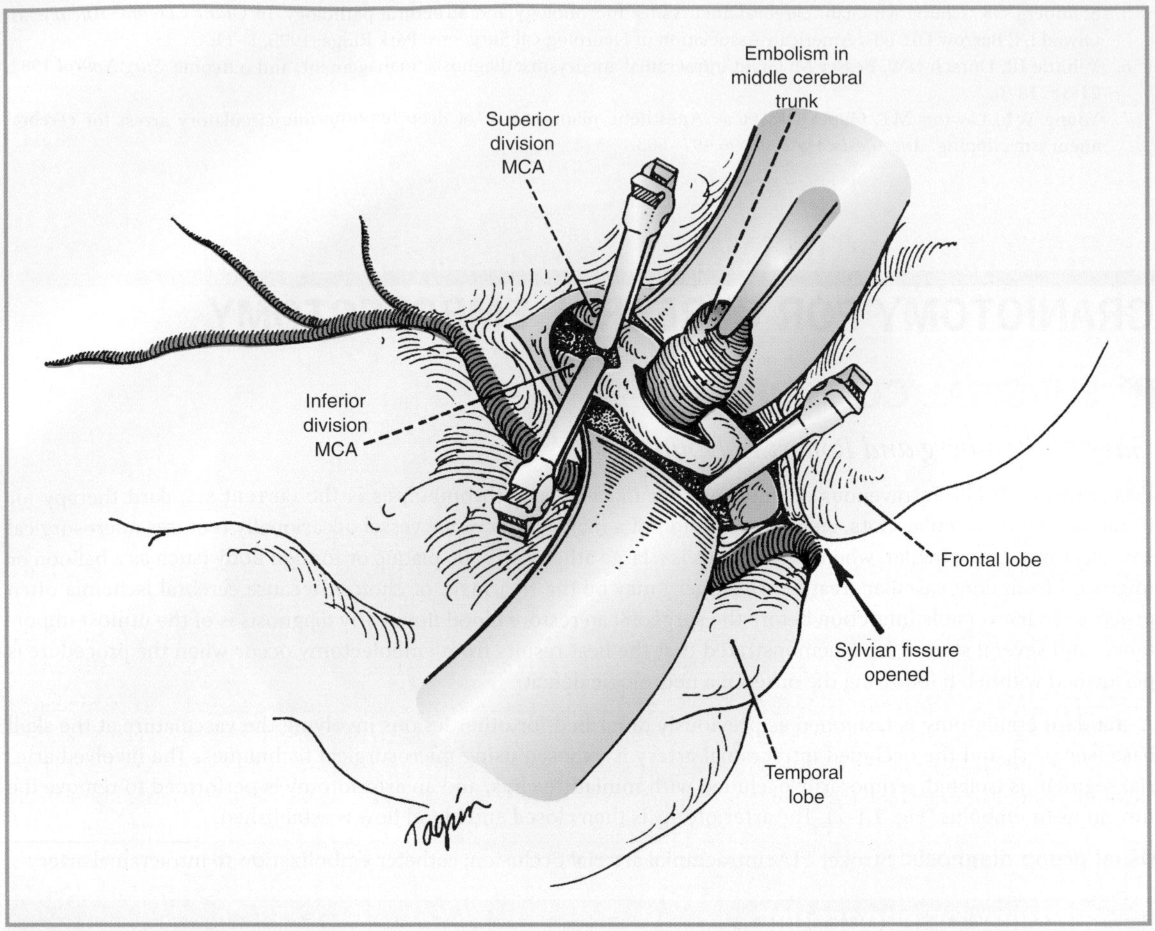

Figure 1.1-2. Middle cerebral artery (MCA) embolectomy. Exposure of right MCA in the sylvian fissure and removal of an embolus from the MI segment. (Reproduced with permission from Ojemann RG, Ogilvy CS, Crowell RM, et al: *Surgical Management of Neurovascular Disease,* 3rd edition. Williams & Wilkins, Philadelphia: 1995.)

PATIENT POPULATION CHARACTERISTICS	
Age range	50–80 yr
Male:Female	1:1
Incidence	Rare
Etiology	Atherosclerosis; carotid artery disease; atrial fibrillation; iatrogenic endovascular catheter complication
Associated conditions	HTN; CAD; PVD; carotid artery disease; hyperlipidemia; smoking; alcohol abuse; obesity; atrial fibrillation

ANESTHETIC CONSIDERATIONS

See Anesthetic Considerations for Craniotomy for Intracranial Aneurysms, p. 6.

Suggested Readings

1. Gomez CR, Orr SC, Soto RD: Neuroendovascular rescue: interventional treatment of acute ischemic stroke. *Curr Treat Options Cardiovasc Med* 2002; 4:405–19.
2. Kakinuma K, Ezuka I, Takai N, et al: The simple indicator for revascularization of acute middle cerebral artery occlusion using angiogram and ultra-early embolectomy. *Surg Neurol* 1999; 51:332–41.
3. Pikus HJ, Heros RC: Stroke: indications for emergent surgical intervention. *Clin Neurosurg* 1999; 45:113–27.

4. Schmidek HH, Sweet WH, eds: *Operative Neurosurgical Techniques: Indications, Methods, and Results,* Vols I-II. WB Saunders, Philadelphia: 2000.
5. Sundt TM Jr: *Surgical Techniques for Saccular and Giant Intracranial Aneurysms.* Williams & Wilkins, Baltimore: 1990, 467–76.
6. Touho H, Morisako T, Hashimoto Y, et al: Embolectomy for acute embolic occlusion of the internal carotid artery bifurcation. *Surg Neurol* 1999; 51:313–20.

CRANIOTOMY FOR INTRACRANIAL VASCULAR MALFORMATIONS

SURGICAL CONSIDERATIONS

Gary K. Steinberg

Description: Intracranial vascular malformations are congenital abnormalities that cause intracranial hemorrhage, seizures, headaches, progressive neurological deficits, or audible bruits. Intracranial vascular malformations comprise high-flow, arteriovenous malformations (AVMs); low-flow, angiographically occult vascular malformations (AOVMs), including cavernous malformations (a collection of enlarged capillaries with thin inelastic walls prone to leaking), "cryptic" AVMs, capillary telangiectasias and transitional malformations; and low-flow, venous angiomas (developmental venous anomalies). **Microsurgical resection** is the optimal treatment for these lesions, although preop endovascular embolization and preop or postop focused **stereotactic radiosurgery** (heavy particle or photon) may be useful adjuncts.

Most moderate-sized and large **AVMs** (> 3 cm diameter) are resected using a standard **scalp flap** and with **craniotomy** centered over the area of the AVM using image-guidance techniques. The patient is positioned appropriately to place the craniotomy site uppermost in the field and parallel to the floor. For example, a patient with a left frontal AVM would be positioned supine, head turned to the right, a left frontal or bicranial scalp flap raised and a left frontal craniotomy bone flap removed. A patient with a right medial occipital AVM would be positioned in the left lateral decubitus position with head turned semiprone and a right occipital scalp flap and craniotomy performed. Smaller AVMs (< 3 cm diameter), many low-flow AOVMs, and many deep-seated vascular malformations (AVMs and AOVMs) require a small, **stereotactic craniotomy.** This is performed by attaching fiducial markers or (less frequently) a stereotactic base frame to the patient's skull (using local anesthetic and sedation). Next, a CT or MRI scan is obtained. The location of the AVM in relation to the markers (or frame) is calculated, using a computer and stereotactic geometric principles. The patient is taken to the OR, intubated (fiber optically if a frame is used), and positioned for surgery. The surgical navigation system reference is attached to the headrest and microscope and calibrated. A small scalp flap and a small craniotomy (a few cm in diameter) can be fashioned precisely for microscopic exposure of the malformation. Microsurgical resection of brain stem and thalamic vascular malformations often necessitate special positioning. In frame-based surgery, a three-dimensional arc frame is fixed to the base frame, and coordinates are set to localize the vascular malformation within the brain.

Usual preop diagnosis: Cerebral AVM; dural AVM; cavernous malformation; angiographically occult vascular malformation; intracerebral hemorrhage; subarachnoid hemorrhage; seizures; epilepsy; progressive neurological deficit; migraine or vascular headaches

SUMMARY OF PROCEDURES

	Standard Craniotomy (High-Flow AVM)	Stereotactic Craniotomy (Low-Flow AOVM)	Brain Stem/Thalamic Vascular Malformations
Position	Supine, lateral, Concorde (modified prone) (Fig. 1.1-3)	⇐	Lateral, Concorde, or semi-sitting (Fig. 1.1-4)
Incision	Frontal, temporal, parietal, occipital, suboccipital, or combination	⇐	Suboccipital (midline), paramedian or occipital
Special instrumentation	Operating microscope; irrigating bipolar coagulation; radiolucent table and headrest. Sundt mini aneurysm and micro AVM clips. Access to femoral artery for intraop angiography.	⇐ + Surgical navigation system	⇐

SUMMARY OF PROCEDURES (cont'd)

	Standard Craniotomy (High-Flow AVM)	Stereotactic Craniotomy (Low-Flow AOVM)	Brain Stem/Thalamic Vascular Malformations
Unique considerations	Induced hypotension (MAP 60–65 mmHg) during resection, use of neuroprotective agents (see Craniotomy for Aneurysms, pp. 6–7). Relaxed brain. Mild hypothermia (33°C); ± lumbar CSF drain.	Use of neuroprotective agents and relaxed brain (see Craniotomy for Aneurysms, pp. 8–9).	⇐
Antibiotics	Ceftriaxone 1 gm iv (avoid Ca^{++}-containing solutions)	⇐	⇐
Surgical time	4–10 h	2–5 h	3–6 h
Closing considerations	Maintain MAP 65–75 mmHg. Avoid ↑ venous pressure. For supratentorial vascular malformations, administer additional anticonvulsants; give loading dose of phenytoin (1 g iv for adults) if not previously on anticonvulsants.	Keep MAP 70–90 mmHg. ⇐ ⇐	⇐ ⇐ No anticonvulsants necessary
EBL	500–3000 mL	< 250 mL	⇐
Postop care	ICU × 1–2 d. Maintain MAP 65–75 mmHg for 1 d. ICP monitoring, ventricular drain; normovolemic in ICU.	ICU × 1 d; normovolemic in ICU	⇐
Mortality	1–10%, depending on AVM size, location, and venous drainage pattern	< 0.5%	< 2%
Morbidity	Overall: 5–30% Breakthrough bleeding: < 5% Intracranial hemorrhage Cerebral edema Stroke < 15% Hydrocephalus Massive blood loss: Occasional Thromboembolism: Rare Infection: Rare	< 5% ⇐ ⇐ ⇐ ⇐ ⇐ ⇐ ⇐	10–50% (transient) < 5% ⇐ ⇐ ⇐ ⇐ ⇐ ⇐ ⇐
Pain score	3–4	3–4	3–4

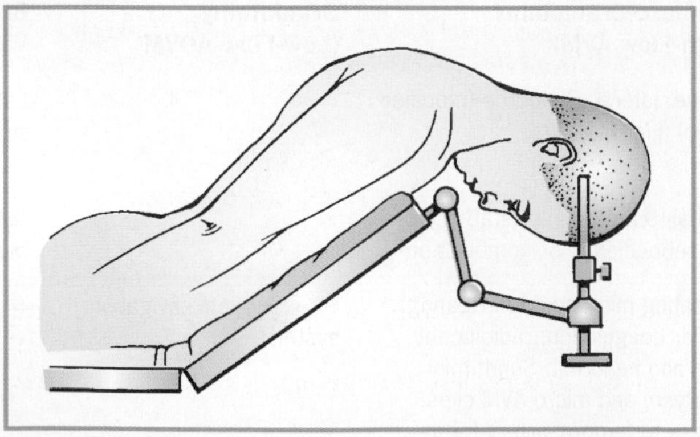

Figure 1.1-3. Concorde (modified prone) position for resection of posterior fossa vascular malformations.

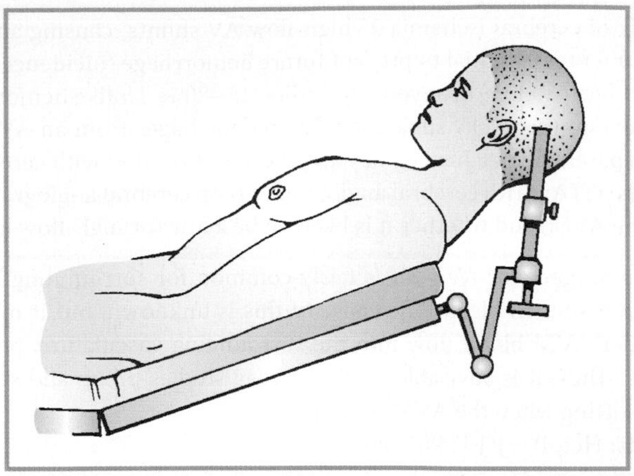

Figure 1.1-4. Semisitting position for resection of deep posterior corpus callosum or thalamic vascular malformations.

PATIENT POPULATION CHARACTERISTICS

Age range	15–40 yr (most common), 41–60 yr (less frequent)
Male:Female	1:1
Incidence	0.5–1% of the U.S. population
Etiology	Congenital; traumatic for dural AVM
Associated conditions	Intracranial aneurysm (~10% of AVM patients [up to 58% in some studies]); Von Hippel-Lindau disease; Rendu-Osler-Weber syndrome; familial cavernous malformation syndrome

ANESTHETIC CONSIDERATIONS

PREOPERATIVE

AVMs are direct arterial-to-venous communications without intervening normal capillary circulation. On histological exam, the vessel walls are thin and lack a muscular layer; consequently, the vessels exhibit loss of normal vasomotor control or responsiveness to changes in $PaCO_2$. **Stereotactic localization** is essential for safe excision of deep-seated AVMs (e.g., those located in the corona radiata, basal ganglia, visual center, cerebellar white matter, or corpus callosum). Untreated, the overall risk of rupture is ~2–4% per year. AVMs > 6 cm in maximum diameter and located near eloquent areas of cortex or with deep venous drainage (grade IV and V) have a high complication rate and may not be suitable for surgical resection.

Respiratory	Not usually significant unless patient has Hx of smoking, or has pulmonary aspiration as a result of a neurological deficit from an intracranial hemorrhage. **Tests:** As indicated from H&P.
Cardiovascular	Generally, these patients do not have other cardiovascular diseases. Occasionally, ECG changes are noted following intracranial hemorrhage and may represent subendocardial injury 2° catecholamine release. **Tests:** ECG; others as indicated from H&P.
Neurological	Presenting Sx depend on location and size of AVM, and whether it is a low- or high-flow lesion. Hemorrhage with resultant headache and/or neurological deficit is the most common Sx, although patients also may present with intractable seizure disorder, recurrent HAs,

Neurological (cont'd)	or Sx of cerebral ischemia 2° high-flow AV shunts, causing an intracerebral steal. Surgical treatment is essential to prevent future hemorrhage (incidence of 2–4%/yr) with substantial mortality (6–30%) or severe morbidity (15–80%). Unlike hemorrhages from an intracerebral aneurysm (generally subarachnoid), hemorrhages from an AVM are usually ventricular or intraparenchymal; hence, they are seldom associated with cerebral vasospasm. **Tests:** CTA; MRI; cerebral angiogram. Preop cerebral angiogram indicates size and location of the AVM, and whether it is likely to be a low- or high-flow lesion.
Hematologic	After surgery for AVM, it is fairly common for surrounding brain tissue to swell and resection sites to bleed. The cause of this is unknown, but it may be related to diversion of former AVM blood flow into the surrounding vasculature, producing a fragile hyperemic state. Thus, it is advisable to obtain coag studies preop and stage excision over more than one sitting when the AVM is large. **Tests:** Hct; PT; PTT; Plt count
Laboratory	CBC; other tests as indicated from H&P.
Premedication	If medication is desirable, small doses of midazolam (e.g., 1–3 mg iv) are useful. Detailed discussion with patient about the anesthetic plan, with appropriate reassurance, is essential.

INTRAOPERATIVE

Anesthetic technique: GETA. The goals of anesthesia for this operation are to: (a) ↓ $CMRO_2$ to lessen the dependence of normal brain on vessels feeding the AVM; (b) decrease intracranial volume (blood and tissue) to optimize surgical working space within the cranial compartment and minimize the need for surgical retraction of brain tissue; and (c) maintain a somewhat decreased (10–20% below normal) CPP to lessen blood loss during excision of the AVM (CPP = cerebral arterial pressure minus cerebral venous pressure or ICP, whichever is greater). For stereotactic surgery, scalp localizing markers are attached. The patient is then sent to MR or CT, where the exact coordinates defining the AVM and critical adjacent structures are established. The patient is brought to OR and anesthesia is induced.

Induction	STP 2–5 mg/kg or propofol 2–3 mg/kg iv provides amnesia and ↓ CBV by inducing cerebral vasoconstriction. Fentanyl 7–10 mcg/kg iv blunts the response to laryngoscopy and provides analgesia for the first hours. High-dose opiates used as a primary anesthetic technique do not alter CBF or $CMRO_2$ enough to provide any special benefits. Vecuronium (0.15 mg/kg), rocuronium (0.6–1 mg/kg), or pancuronium (0.1 mg/kg), provide muscle relaxation for intubation and patient positioning. Occasionally the patient may be in a stereotactic frame and ET intubation must be accomplished before anesthesia is induced, because the frame partially occludes the mouth, making conventional laryngoscopy impossible. Awake oral fiber optic intubation of the trachea is the easiest method for accomplishing this (see p. B-5).
Maintenance	Isoflurane ≤ 1% or sevoflurane ≤ 2% (limit to 1/2 MAC maximum if EP monitoring is used) with 1:1 O_2/N_2O. With EP monitoring, a remifentanil infusion (0.05–0.15 mcg/kg/min) may be necessary to supplement the anesthetic. Propofol (75–150 mcg/kg/min) by continuous infusion may be administered to provide ↓ CBV and ↓ $CMRO_2$, and allow for reduction in inhalation agent concentration or elimination of N_2O. Mild hypothermia (33°C) provides additional cerebral protection (see below). Additional neuromuscular blocking drugs are usually not necessary, but can be administered if patient movement is of concern. Induced hypotension is often useful during AVM resection. Following resection, induced hypertension (e.g., 90 mmHg) may be requested to inspect hemostasis.
Emergence	With the start of dural closure, consider changing the anesthetic to low-dose sevoflurane (e.g., 0.5%) in 50% N_2O, supplemented with a low-dose remifentanil infusion (e.g., 0.05 mcg/kg/min). A propofol infusion (if used) should be discontinued at the start of the scalp closure. The patient's BP generally will increase and titration of β-adrenergic blocking drugs (e.g., labetalol or esmolol) and/or vasodilators (e.g., SNP) may be needed. (See Control of BP, below.) The inhalation agents can be D/C'd at the time of dressing application.

Emergence (cont'd)	Most patients will breathe spontaneously and can be extubated uneventfully while on the remifentanil infusion. If the brain has not been injured by the surgical procedure, the patient should awaken within 10 min after cessation of remifentanil administration. Close regulation of BP is essential. If the patient begins to cough on ETT, either it should be removed or cough reflex suppressed with iv lidocaine (0.5–1 mg/kg). Patient is placed in bed in a 30° head-up position and transported to ICU for monitoring overnight. Supplemental O_2 should be administered and close regulation of BP maintained (typically at ~10% below baseline values). Prophylactic antiemetics (e.g., metoclopramide 10–20 mg and ondansetron 4 mg) should be given 30 min before extubation.	
Blood and fluid requirements	IV: 14–16 ga × 2 NS @ < 10 mL/kg + UO Massive blood loss possible Maintain euvolemia Maintain colloid oncotic pressure	If blood volume is normal, NS—not to exceed 10 mL/kg beyond that required to replace UO—is given. If hypovolemic, albumin 5% is given if Hct > 30%; combinations of albumin and blood, if Hct < 30%.
Hypothermia	Thermal blankets Cool air blower Cold OR InnerCool-type device Bladder irrigation	Mild hypothermia (33°–34°C) is used in some centers for cerebral protection and to ↓ brain size. This level of hypothermia does not interfere appreciably with coagulation, nor is it generally associated with cardiac dysrhythmias. Warming is begun as soon as possible after lesion resection and is greatly facilitated by the use of a central warming device (e.g., InnerCool).
Brain Relaxation (control of ICP)	Hyperventilate to $PaCO_2$ = ~30 mmHg or $PetCO_2$ = 25 mmHg. Limit isoflurane ≤ 1%. Maintain euvolemia Consider propofol infusion to replace N_2O Mannitol 0.5–1 g/kg Furosemide 0.3 mg/kg Lumbar CSF drainage	↓ $PaCO_2$ →↓ cerebral vascular volume →↑ working space and lessens need for vigorous retraction of brain tissue. ↓ $PaCO_2$ also improves the regional distribution of CBF by preferentially diverting blood to potentially ischemic areas of the brain. If AVM is superficial, decreasing brain volume is less important, and the first four techniques listed (at left) are usually sufficient. If AVM is deep, the additional listed therapies may be needed.
Monitoring	Standard monitors (see p. B-1). Core temp: deep esophageal best Arterial line CVP line, triple lumen UO Blood glucose (100–180 mg%)	Direct monitoring is essential for rapid control of BP. Transducer should always be placed at the level of the head rather than the heart, since CPP is arterial pressure at the brain level minus CVP or ICP, whichever is higher. Monitoring CVP via a near right atrial catheter is desirable in virtually all patients to assess adequacy of fluid therapy, for infusion of vasoactive drugs and aspiration of VAE. Localization of the catheter can be determined by CXR, ECG tracing, noting P-wave changes, or pressure-wave contour and value as the catheter is withdrawn from the right atrium. **NB**: If patient has a high-flow AVM causing a large AV shunt, venous blood may appear arterialized (bright red) during central venous catheterization.
Control of BP	Isoflurane/sevoflurane Esmolol infusion SNP infusion Maintain normovolemia. Labetolol (emergence)	Close regulation of BP during induction and prior to excision of AVMs is important, both to prevent bleeding (↑ BP) and to avoid ischemia 2° steal (↓ BP). After surgical excision is under way, however, modest decreases in MAP (≤ 20% below normal) using isoflurane, alone or in combination

Control of BP (cont'd)		with esmolol and/or SNP, should be used to prevent excessive bleeding. Responses to vasoactive drugs are much easier to regulate if the patient is euvolemic.
Positioning	Shoulder roll Three-point fixation ✓ and pad pressure points. ✓ eyes. 180° rotation SCDs	For most AVMs, patient is supine, head turned laterally in three-point fixation, a roll under shoulder on the side of operation (Fig. 1.1-5). Anesthetic hoses and all monitoring/vascular catheter lines are directed toward patient's feet or side. Make sure that all will reach the foot of operating table. SCDs are used to minimize DVT. Remifentanil (2–4 mcg/kg iv bolus) should be used to minimize ↑ BP during skull pinning.

POSTOPERATIVE

Complications	Neurological deficits	If these complications occur, the patient likely will have to be reintubated and transported to the CT scanner for further neurological evaluation or possible reoperation.
	Cerebral edema and ↑ ICP Intracerebral hemorrhage Seizures	Careful regulation of BP is essential to avoid postop hemorrhage. *Sz Rx: Phenytoin (1 g loading dose). **NB**: Incompatible with dextrose-containing solutions.
Pain management	Meperidine 10–20 mg iv/70 kg Codeine (30–60 mg im q 4 h prn)	At this dose, meperidine minimizes postop shivering without producing excessive sedation.
Tests	CT scan	If neurological status changes.

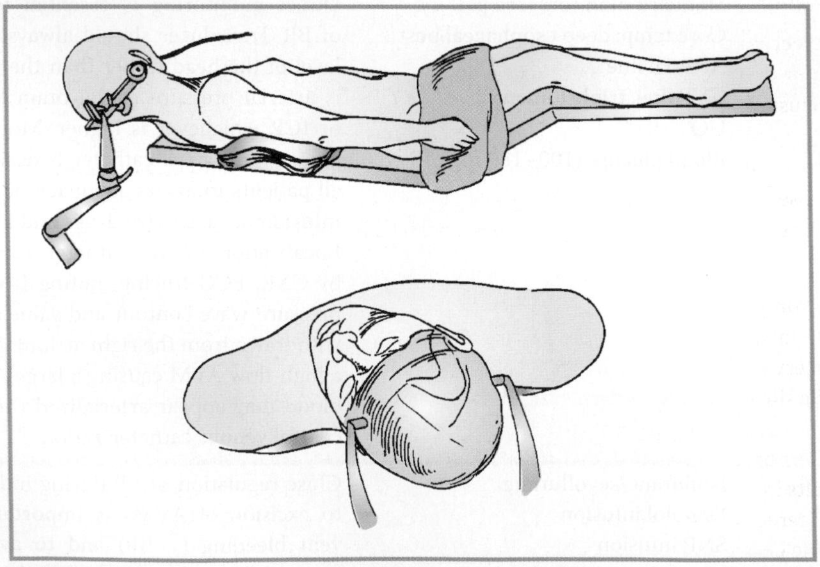

Figure 1.1-5. Supine position, head elevated above heart, turned 30–45° to side, vertex dropped for approach to anterior circulation aneurysms and frontal vascular malformations. (Reproduced with permission from Long DM: *Atlas of Operative Neurosurgical Technique*, Vol 1. Williams & Wilkins, Philadelphia: 1989.)

Suggested Readings

1. Al-Rodhan NR, Sundt TJ, Piepgras DG, et al: Occlusive hyperemia: a theory for the hemodynamic complications following resection of intracerebral arteriovenous malformations. *J Neurosurg* 1993; 78:167.
2. Chang SD, Lopez JR, Steinberg GK: The usefulness of electrophysiologic monitoring during resection of central nervous system vascular malformations. *J Stroke Cerebrovasc Dis* 1999; 8:412–22.
3. Cully MD, Larson CP Jr, Silverberg GD: Hetastarch coagulopathy in a neurosurgical patient [Letter]. *Anesthesiology* 1987; 66(5):706–7.
4. Fleetwood IG, Steinberg GK: Arteriovenous malformations. *Lancet* 2002; 359:863–73.
5. Friedlander RM. Arteriovenous malformations of the brain. *N Engl J Med* 2007; 356(26):2704–2712.
6. Hashimoto T, Young WL. Anesthesia-related considerations for cerebral arteriovenous malformations. *Neurosurg Focus* 2001;11(5):e5.
7. Sano T, Drummond JC, Patel PM, et al: A comparison of the cerebral protective effects of isoflurane and mild hypothermia in a model of incomplete forebrain ischemia in the rat. *Anesthesiology* 1992; 76(2):221–8.
8. Schmidek HH, Sweet WH, eds: *Operative Neurosurgical Techniques: Indications, Methods, and Results,* Vols I–II. WB Saunders, Philadelphia: 2000.
9. Steinberg GK, Chang SD, Gerwitz RJ, et al: Microsurgical resection of brain stem, thalmic and basal ganglia angiographically occult vascular malformation. *Neurosurgery* 2000; 46:260–71.
10. Steinberg GK, Stoodley MA: Surgical management of intracranial arteriovenous malformations. In *Operative Neurosurgical Techniques,* 4th edition. Schmidek HH, ed. WB Saunders, Philadelphia: 2000, 1363–91.
11. Szabo MD, Crosby G, Sundaram P, et al: Hypertension does not cause spontaneous hemorrhage of intracranial arteriovenous malformations. *Anesthesiology* 1989; 70(5):761–3.
12. Wilkins RH: Natural history of intracranial vascular malformations: a review. *Neurosurgery* 1985; 16(3):421–30.
13. Young WL, Kader A, Ornstein E, et al: Cerebral hyperemia after arteriovenous malformation resection is related to "breakthrough" complications but not to feeding artery pressure. The Columbia University Arteriovenous Malformation Study Project. *Neurosurgery* 1996; 38:1085–95.

CRANIOTOMY FOR EXTRACRANIAL-INTRACRANIAL REVASCULARIZATION (EC-IC BYPASS)

SURGICAL CONSIDERATIONS

Gary K. Steinberg and Robert L. Dodd

Description: **Extracranial-intracranial (EC-IC) revascularization** procedures are performed when: (a) deliberate occlusion of a major cervical artery (carotid or vertebral) is necessary and inadequate collateral CBF is available or (b) stenosis or occlusion of major cervical or intracranial arteries causes TIA or stroke, despite the use of maximum medical therapy (e.g., antiplatelet drugs, heparin, or Coumadin). The chief causes of stenosis or occlusion are atherosclerotic disease, radiation injury, and moyamoya disease. The subset of patients who benefit from revascularization are those whose radiographic and metabolism studies demonstrate that they have ↓ CBF and poor or absent vascular reserve. The most important surgical considerations include site of stenosis, adequacy of donor graft, and patient age.

A standard craniotomy is fashioned as previously described for other lesions involving the vasculature around the skull base, and the intracranial site of anastomosis is exposed using microscopic techniques. Typically, a donor extracranial scalp artery (e.g., superficial temporal artery) is anastomosed to an intracranial artery (e.g., middle cerebral artery) distal to the site of stenosis. When scalp vessels are inadequate, an interposition vein segment can be sutured to a cervical artery and then anastomosed to the designated intracranial artery. The most common EC-IC procedure is a **superficial temporal artery (STA)-to-middle cerebral artery (MCA) branch anastomosis** (See Figs 1.1-6 to 1.1-10). Other grafts include STA-to-posterior cerebral artery, STA-to-superior cerebellar artery, occipital artery-to-posterior inferior cerebral artery or interposition saphenous vein segment graft from the cervical external carotid artery to the middle cerebral artery, posterior cerebral artery, or superior cerebellar artery.

Variant procedure or approaches: **Indirect revascularization** is commonly employed in patients in whom the graft vessels are too small for direct anastomosis. Vascular source tissues include a temporalis muscle flap and a flap of dura folded under so that its outer vascular surface is apposed to the cortical surface. **Encephalo-duro-arterio-synangiosis (EDAS)** is an indirect variant procedure wherein the STA is dissected circumferentially with its

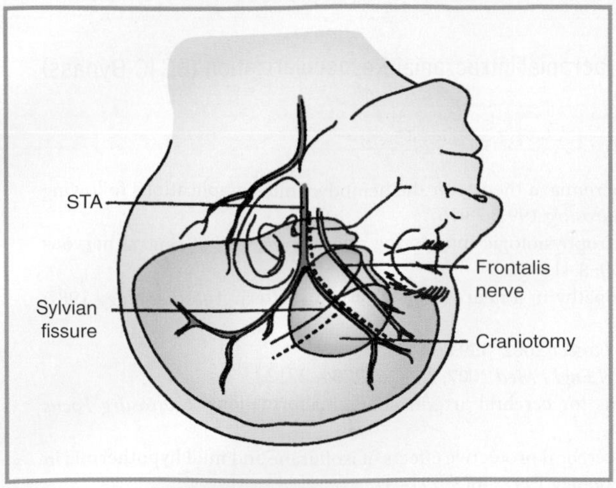

Figure 1.1-6. Typical skin incision for EC-IC bypass. The main incision is planned over the superficial temporal artery (STA) with a T extension to allow exposure of the bone. (Reproduced from Chang SD, Steinberg GK: Superficial temporal artery to middle cerebral artery anastomosis. *Tech Neurosurg* 2000; 6(2):86–100.)

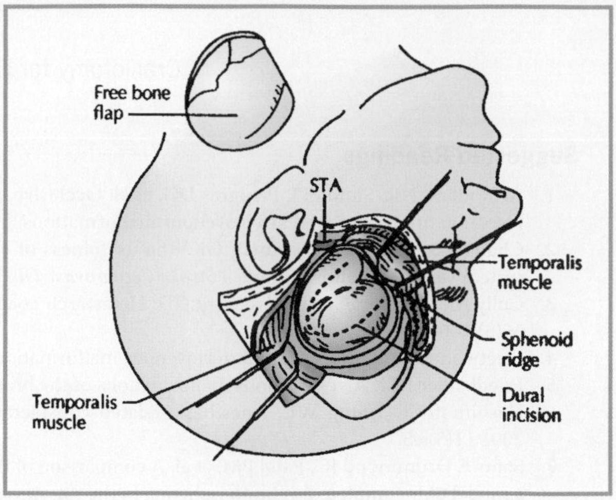

Figure 1.1-7. After the STA is dissected out, the temporalis muscle is divided and the bone flap is made to allow exposure of the brain over the anterior sylvian fissure. (Reproduced from Chang SD, Steinberg GK: Superficial temporal artery to middle cerebral artery anastomosis. *Tech Neurosurg* 2000; 6(2):86–100.)

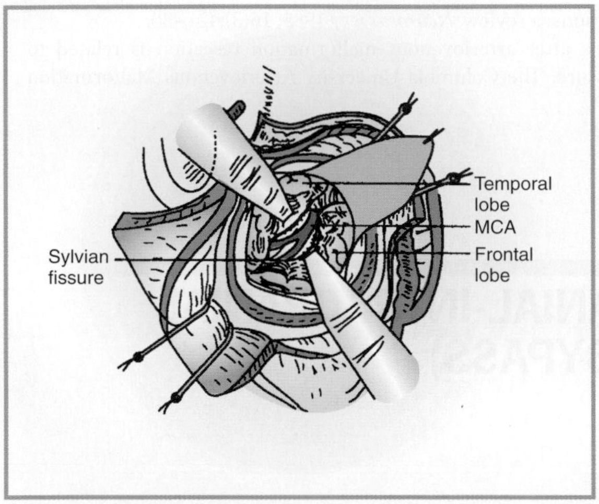

Figure 1.1-8. A middle cerebral artery (MCA) recipient vessel is identified. The sylvian fissure can be split to allow identification of a larger, more proximal branch of the MCA, preferably an M3 branch. (Reproduced from Chang SD, Steinberg GK: Superficial temporal artery to middle cerebral artery anastomosis. *Tech Neurosurg* 2000; 6(2):86–100.)

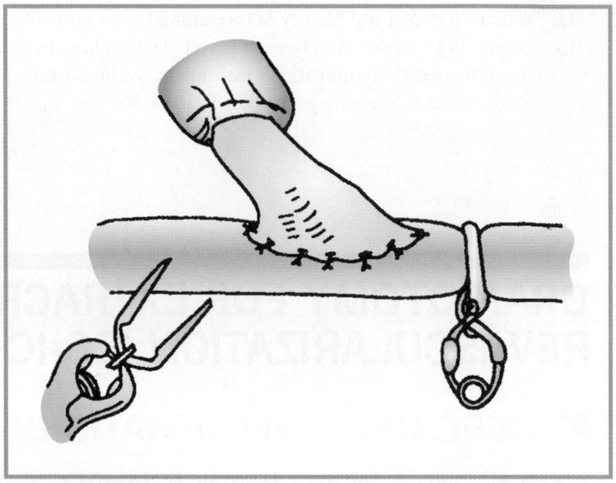

Figure 1.1-9. When the anastomosis is complete, the vascular clips are removed. (Reproduced from Chang SD, Steinberg GK: Superficial temporal artery to middle cerebral artery anastomosis. *Tech Neurosurg* 2000; 6(2):86–100.)

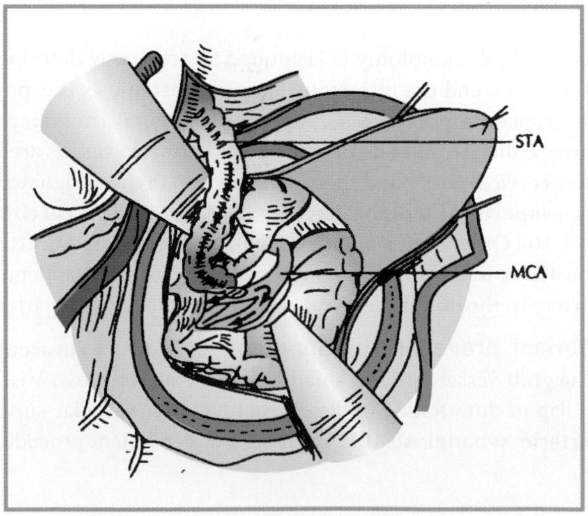

Figure 1.1-10. The completed anastomosis shows the STA positioned such that flow is directed toward the proximal portions of the MCA. (Reproduced from Chang SD, Steinberg GK: Superficial temporal artery to middle cerebral artery anastomosis. *Tech Neurosurg* 2000; 6(2):86–100.)

adventitia in the scalp, left in continuity and laid on the surface of the brain after opening the dura. **Omentum-to-brain transposition** is a rarely used variant, wherein the omentum, with its luxuriant blood supply, is lengthened, left attached to the right gastroepiploic artery, tunneled subcutaneously in the chest and neck, and laid over a large area of poorly vascularized cerebral cortex after opening the dura. Sometimes a free omental graft is transposed to the brain by anastomosing the omental gastroepiploic artery and vein to the superficial temporal artery and vein. Revascularization is induced by angiogenesis factors and growth substances secreted by the brain and omentum.

Usual preop diagnosis: Moyamoya disease (cerebral ischemia due to occlusion of vessels at base of the brain); stroke; TIA; carotid artery stenosis (inaccessible to carotid endarterectomy); carotid artery occlusion; middle cerebral artery stenosis or occlusion; vertebral artery stenosis or occlusion; basilar artery stenosis or occlusion.

SUMMARY OF PROCEDURES

	EC-IC Bypass	EC-IC Bypass with Vein Graft	Indirect Procedures
Position	Supine or lateral decubitus	⇐	⇐
Incision	Frontal, parietal, temporal, occipital, or a combination of these, depending on area to be vascularized.	⇐ + Medial aspect of leg and thigh for harvesting greater saphenous vein	⇐ + possible abdominal incision for harvesting omentum and chest/ neck incision for tunneling
Special instrumentation	Microscopic instruments; microvascular Doppler to identify scalp donor artery course and confirm graft patency.	⇐ + Tunneling instruments	⇐
Unique considerations	Neuroprotective agents (barbiturates, mannitol) and induced mild HTN (MAP 90–110 mmHg) during cross-clamp of recipient intracranial artery. Avoid excessive brain relaxation. Mild hypothermia (33°C). Dexamethasone 8–12 mg iv.	⇐ + Attention to proper alignment of vein when tunneled, to avoid kinking; heparinization if major cervical artery (carotid, vertebral) is temporarily occluded.	⇐ + Avoid devascularizing source tissue during dissection or compromise to blood supply during closure.
Antibiotics	Ceftriaxone 1–2 gm iv q d (avoid Ca^{++} containing solution)	←	⇐
Surgical time	3–5 h	⇐	⇐
Closing considerations	Careful attention to hemostasis. Avoid compromise of graft with dural closure, bone replacement or scalp closure.	⇐	⇐
EBL	< 100 mL	⇐	100–500 mL
Postop care	Start aspirin on POD 1; monitor for subdural hygroma (CSF fluid collection in subdural space); ICU × 1 d.	⇐	⇐
Mortality	< 0.5%	⇐	⇐
Morbidity	Transient neurologic deficit: ~20–40% Subdural hygroma: Rare Wound infection: Rare Stroke: Rare	⇐ ⇐ ⇐	 ⇐ ⇐ Abdominal hernia: Rare
Pain score	3	3	3

PATIENT POPULATION CHARACTERISTICS	
Age range	40–80 yr; 2–20 yr for moyamoya disease
Male:Female	1:1 for atherosclerotic disease; 1:1.4 for moyamoya disease
Incidence	Thromboembolic stroke common, but indications for EC-IC bypass rare; 1/million/yr for moyamoya disease
Etiology	Atherosclerosis; embolism from heart or carotid artery
Associated conditions	HTN; CAD; PVD; hyperlipidemia; smoking; alcohol abuse; obesity; moyamoya disease

ANESTHETIC CONSIDERATIONS

PREOPERATIVE

Patients range in age from pediatric (classic moyamoya disease) to adult. These patients may have significant pre-existing neurologic deficits. HTN in these patients is often an adaptation to cerebral vascular insufficiency → hypoperfusion. Inappropriate treatment of this compensatory HTN → cerebral ischemia and stroke. Patients with symptomatic moyamoya disease or bilateral carotid stenosis or occlusion may be good candidates for EC-IC bypass, especially since there are no alternative forms of therapy that have proven to be effective. Most patients present with h/o TIAs or stroke and most are receiving antiplatelet medication.

Respiratory	None unless patient has Hx of smoking or has sustained pulmonary aspiration 2° neurological deficit. **Tests:** As indicated from H&P.
Cardiovascular	HTN is a common adaptive mechanism to maintain cerebral perfusion; therefore "normalization" of BP preop may be undesirable. Adult patients may have generalized vascular disease, including CAD, so a careful cardiac Hx, physical exam, and ECG analysis should be done. If findings are positive, consider a more complete evaluation, including ECHO and coronary angiography. Be aware that cardiac insufficiency is the cause of about half of the deaths in patients with cerebrovascular disease. **Tests:** Consider ECG, others as indicated from H&P.
Neurological	Patients present with Sx of focal ischemic lesions. Cerebral angiography is necessary to r/o other causes of TIAs and characterize collateral circulation. Regional CBF studies are generally not helpful, because measurement does not distinguish between low flow due to cerebrovascular obstruction from that due to low metabolic demands 2° prolonged cerebral ischemia. Pre-existing deficits should be well-characterized. **Tests:** CTA; MRI; angiogram
Hematologic	For most patients: a platelet-suppressive dose of aspirin should be continued through the day of surgery; drugs affecting PT/PTT should be D/C'd at least 1 wk before surgery to avoid excessive bleeding; Clopidogrel (Plavix) should be D/C'd 5 d before surgery. **Tests:** Hct; PT; PTT; hemogram
Laboratory	Tests as indicated from H&P.
Premedication	If medication is desirable, small doses of midazolam (e.g., 1–3 mg iv) are useful. Detailed discussion with the patient about the anesthetic plan with appropriate reassurance is essential.

INTRAOPERATIVE

Anesthetic technique: GETA. The goals of anesthesia for this procedure are to: (a) maximize flow to the ischemic area through collateral channels by maintaining BP at normal or somewhat elevated values; (b) ↑ tolerance of the brain to ischemia by decreasing $CMRO_2$ with the use of mild hypothermia (33–34°C) and barbiturate therapy; (c) ↓ intracranial volume (blood and tissue) to optimize working space within the cranial compartment, thereby minimizing the need for surgical retraction of brain tissue; and (d) provide adequate surgical anesthesia.

Induction	STP 2–5 mg/kg (or propofol 1–2 mg/kg iv) to provide amnesia and ↓ cerebral blood volume by inducing cerebral vasoconstriction. Fentanyl 7–10 mcg/kg iv to blunt response to intubation and provide analgesia for the first hours of surgery. Pancuronium (0.1 mg/kg; helps offset ↓ HR/BP 2° induction drugs), vecuronium 0.15 mg/kg, or rocuronium 0.7–1.0 mg/kg to provide muscle relaxation for tracheal intubation. Bolus ephedrine and/or phenylephrine are often necessary to maintain CPP during induction.	
Maintenance	Isoflurane ≤ 1% or sevoflurane ≤ 2% (1/2 MAC maximum if EP monitoring is used) with 1:1 O_2/N_2O. A phenylephrine infusion is usually necessary to maintain CPP during the procedure. STP (2–5 mg/kg) is given just before surgical occlusion of the cerebral vessel in preparation for anastomosis. A bolus dose of phenylephrine and/or ephedrine is often given concomitantly to offset the hypotensive effects of STP. If mild hypothermia was employed, rewarming should start as soon as revascularization is complete.	
Emergence	With the start of dural closure, consider changing the anesthetic to low-dose sevoflurane (e.g., 0.5%) in 50% N_2O, supplemented with a low-dose remifentanil infusion (e.g., 0.05 mcg/kg/min). A propofol infusion (if used) should be discontinued at the start of the scalp closure. The patient's BP generally will increase and titration of β-adrenergic blocking drugs (e.g., labetalol or esmolol) and/or vasodilators (e.g., SNP) may be needed. (See Control of BP, below.) The inhalation agents can be D/C'd at the time of dressing application. Most patients will breathe spontaneously and can be extubated uneventfully while on the remifentanil infusion. If the brain has not been injured by the surgical procedure, the patient should awaken within 10 min after cessation of remifentanil administration. Close regulation of BP is essential. If the patient begins to cough on ETT, either it should be removed or cough reflex suppressed with iv lidocaine (0.5–1.0 mg/kg). Patient is placed in bed in a 30° head-up position and transported to ICU for monitoring overnight. Supplemental O_2 should be administered and close regulation of BP maintained (typically at ~10% below baseline values). Prophylactic antiemetics (e.g., metoclopramide 10–20 mg, ondansetron 4 mg) should be given 30 min before extubation.	
Blood and fluid requirements	IV: 18 ga × 2 NS @ < 10 mL/kg + UO	In hypothermic patients, IV drugs should be administered through the central line to ensure timely entry into the central circulation.
	CVP (triple-lumen)	CVP use low volume (1 mL) extension for drug infusions. Reserve distal lumen for pressure monitoring and air aspiration.
Control of brain volume (ICP)	Avoid hypovolemia ↓ isoflurane ≤ 0.5%, or sevoflurane < 1% N_2O ≤ 50% ± Furosemide 10–20 mg iv ± Mannitol 0.5–1.0 g/kg	Maintain normovolemia. Generally, vigorous control of brain volume is not necessary since surgeon is working with cerebral vessels on the surface of the brain. Keep $PaCO_2$ = ~30 mmHg. Excessive hypocarbia may cause unwanted cerebral vasoconstriction in these patients.
Monitoring	Standard monitors (see p. B-1). Core temperature Arterial line CVP (triple-lumen catheter) UO	Core temperature is best approximated by a deep esophageal temperature probe. Bladder temp tends to lag behind core temp. The distal CVP lumen is used for pressure monitoring.
Control of BP	Maintain normal BP (MAP). Phenylephrine infusion	Maintenance of normal MAP is important because cerebral autoregulation is often impaired in these patients, particularly during temporary occlusion of the surgical vessel being anastomosed. If a vasoconstrictor is needed, a pure α-adrenergic agonist, such as phenylephrine, is preferred because it has minimal dysrhythmogenic potential.

Control of BP (cont'd)	Normovolemia	Responses to vasoactive drugs are much easier to regulate if a normal blood volume has been maintained throughout the anesthetic period.
Positioning	✓ and pad pressure points. ✓ eyes. Shoulder roll SCDs	Anesthetic hoses and monitoring and vascular lines directed to patient's feet where anesthesiologist is positioned during surgery. Used to minimize DVT.
Hypothermia	Cold-water circulating blankets. Core temp goal: 33–34°C. InnerCool-type device Bladder irrigation	Surface cooling is quite effective in patients with high surface-to-volume ratios, and should be started as soon as induction of anesthesia is complete, using a cold-water circulating blanket underneath and above the patient. When anastomosis is nearly complete, vigorous efforts at warming, including bladder irrigation, are initiated. Cooling, and especially rewarming are greatly facilitated by the use of a central heat-exchange device (e.g., InnerCool) placed in the inferior vena cava through a femoral vein introducer.
Complications	Seizures Stroke Hemorrhage at anastomosis Brain swelling	*Sz Rx: Phenytoin (1 g loading dose). **NB**: Incompatible with dextrose-containing solutions. May be 2° hyperemia in revascularized territory.

POSTOPERATIVE

Complications	Localized scalp necrosis Brain swelling	Major complications uncommon; localized scalp necrosis unique to this procedure. May be 2° to delayed hyperemia. Careful control of BP is important.
Pain management	Meperidine (10–20 mg iv prn) Codeine (30–60 mg im q 4 h prn)	Useful to suppress shivering Postop pain is usually not severe.
Tests	Cerebral angiogram Regional blood flow studies CT scan	Cerebral angiography documents patency of graft and collateral flow. Some centers have the capability of performing regional blood flow studies. If any question about neurological status, a CT scan is performed.

Suggested Readings

1. Adams HP, Powers WJ, Grubb RL, et al: Preview of a new trial of extracranial-to-intracranial arterial anastomosis. *Neurosurg Clin North Am* 2000;36:613–24.
2. Baykan N, Ozgen S, Ustalar ZS, et al: Moyamoya disease and anesthesia. *Paediatr Anaesth* 2005; 15(12):1111–5.
3. Chang SD, Steinberg GK: Superficial temporal artery to middle cerebral artery anastomosis. *Techniques in Neurosurgery* 2000; 6:86–100.
4. Crowley RW, Mendel R, Dumont AS: Evolution of cerebral revascularization techniques. *Neurosurg Focus* 2008; 24(2):E3.
5. Firlick AD, Newell DW, Steinberg GK, eds: Cerebral revascularization. *Neurosurg Clin North Am* 2001; 12(3).
6. Fujimura M, Kaneta T, Mugikura S, et al: Temporary neurologic deterioration due to cerebral hyperperfusion after superficial temporal artery-middle cerebral artery anastomosis in patients with adult-onset moyamoya disease. *Surg Neurol* 2007; 67(3):273–82.
7. Kato R, Terui K, Yokota K, et al: Anesthetic management for cesarean section in moyamoya disease: a report of five consecutive cases and a mini-review. *Int J Obstet Anesth* 2006; 15(2):152–158.
8. Kikuta K, Takagi Y, Nozaki K, et al: Effects of intravenous anesthesia with propofol on regional cortical blood flow and intracranial pressure in surgery for moyamoya disease. *Surg Neurol* 2007; 68(4):421–4.

9. Ohue S, Kumon Y, Kohno K, et al: Postoperative temporary neurological deficits in adults with moyamoya disease. *Surg Neurol* 2007; Epub ahead of print.
10. Schmidek HH, Sweet WH, eds: *Operative Neurosurgical Techniques: Indications, Methods, and Results,* Vols I-II. WB Saunders, Philadelphia: 2000.
11. Schmiedek P, Piepgras A, Leinsinger G, et al: Improvement of cerebrovascular reserve capacity by EC-IC arterial bypass surgery in patients with ICA occlusion and hemodynamic cerebral ischemic. *J Neurosurg* 1994; 81:236–44.
12. Steinberg GK, ed: Cerebral revascularization techniques. *Techniques in Neurosurgery* 2000; 6(2).

CRANIOTOMY FOR TUMOR

SURGICAL CONSIDERATIONS

Gordon T. Sakamoto, Lawrence M. Shuer, and Steven D. Chang

Description: Many classification systems exist for brain tumors. Generally, brain tumors can be classified by their location and a differential diagnosis can be generated based on tumor location and patient age. Brain tumors are either supratentorial or infratentorial (Table 1.1-2), or intraaxial or extraaxial (Table 1.1-3). The surgical approach depends on the location of the lesion, the need for brain relaxation, and whether exposure will require brain resection. Patient positioning generally depends on the location and surgical approach to the tumor (Table 1.1-4). Once positioned, the patient's head typically is placed in a Mayfield pin fixation system to prevent head movement during surgery and to allow for intraoperative image-guided stereotactic navigation.

Several types of incisions are used for these procedures. **Linear incisions** can be used to resect small tumors over the convexity or when using a midline approach to the posterior fossa, and often have the advantage of a more rapid wound closure. **Curvilinear** or **horseshoe-shaped incisions** are commonly used for larger tumors. After the skull is exposed, burr holes are made with a drill and the bone flap is cut with the craniotome. Some surgeons routinely use a **free-bone flap**, in which the bone is completely removed and stored for the duration of the case. Other surgeons turn an **osteoplastic flap**, where the bone is left attached to muscle and/or pericranium to keep it partially vascularized.

Table 1.1-2. Common Tumor Location (Supratentorial vs Infratentorial)

Supratentorial	Infratentorial
Metastatic tumors	Metastatic tumors
Astrocytoma/glioblastoma	Acoustic neuromas
Oligodendroglioma	Meningiomas
Ependymoma	Hemangioblastoma
Meningioma	Medulloblastoma
Choroid plexus papilloma	
Craniopharyngioma	
Primitive neuroectodermal tumor (PNET)	

Table 1.1-3. Intraaxial (Within-the-Brain Parenchyma) vs Extraaxial (Outside-the-Brain Parenchyma)

Intraaxial Tumors	Extra-axial Tumors
Astrocytoma/glioblastoma	Meningioma
Metastatic tumors	Acoustic neuroma
Oligodendroglioma	Choroid plexus papilloma
Ependymoma	Craniopharyngioma
Hemangioblastoma	Hemangiopericytoma
Medulloblastoma	
PNET	

Table 1.1-4. Common Patient Positions Based on Tumor Location

Supine:	Most supratentorial tumors in the frontal, temporal, or anterior parietal lobe. Tumors of the lateral ventricles and 3rd ventricle. Tumors of the anterior 2/3 of the interhemispheric fissure.
Lateral:	Tumors of the posterior or lateral parietal lobe, posterior temporal lobe, cerebellopontine angle, or lateral cerebellum. Tumors of the posterior ventricular horn.
Prone:	Tumors of the occipital lobe, most midline cerebellar tumors, and tumors of the 4th ventricle. Tumors of the posterior 1/3 interhemispheric fissure and the tentorium.
Sitting:	Tumors of the pineal region. Tumors of the 4th ventricle or midline cerebellum.

When performing certain posterior fossa resections (e.g., a retromastoid craniotomy or low suboccipital craniotomy), the surgeon may choose to remove the bone without replacement, performing a **craniectomy** instead of a craniotomy. After the bone is removed, a few small holes are drilled near the edge of the craniotomy. These holes are used to suspend the dura using sutures. This helps prevent blood from accumulating in the epidural space during the rest of the case. The dura is then opened either in a stellate or curvilinear fashion. The method of dural opening generally is based on the size of the bone opening and its proximity to venous sinuses. The surgeon then proceeds with tumor removal if it is on the surface or with brain retraction/resection if the tumor is deep to the surface. At this point, the surgeon may request anesthetic interventions for brain relaxation (osmotic diuresis, hyperventilation) and specific BP control. After the tumor is removed, hemostasis is achieved and the dura is closed. The bone flap is replaced and fixated, the galea is closed with sutures, and the skin incision is closed with staples. During closure, the surgeon may ask for specific BP parameters to ensure that there is hemostasis in the resection bed and surgical field. Patients typically are extubated after cranial surgery, because it is paramount to obtain a neurologic exam as soon after surgery as possible. Patients undergoing a craniotomy almost always require a postoperative ICU course.

Electrophysiologic monitoring detects changes in SSEP, brain stem auditory evoked potentials (BAEP), and motor cranial nerve EMGs. Such monitoring is commonly used for tumors of the brain stem and skull base, or when resecting tumors in critical locations. Early changes in electrophysiologic monitoring potentials may alert the anesthesiologist to manipulate BP and may help the surgeon to further define the extent of safe retraction and tumor resection to minimize the likelihood of a postoperative deficit.

Image-guided navigation involves the use of a computerized workstation that can track the position of specific instruments before and during the operation. This allows the surgeon to: (a) plan appropriate skin and bone openings, (b) choose an optimal trajectory to the tumor, and (c) achieve a volumetric resection of the tumor. Image-guided navigation involves obtaining a CT or MRI scan prior to the start of the surgical procedure; the time required to obtain this study is usually offset by a shorter operative time. Data from the operative microscope can also be incorporated into the navigation system to aid in tumor dissection.

Mild hypothermia is often utilized when resecting tumors in eloquent areas of the brain, because hypothermia has been shown to provide neuroprotection.

CSF drainage usually is accomplished by use of a lumbar drain. Lumbar drainage typically is used for tumors in the cerebellopontine angle, in the pineal region, or tumors associated with significant edema. CSF drainage can also be accomplished by placing a ventriculostomy or by draining various cisterns during the operation.

Awake craniotomies typically are reserved for tumors adjacent to or within the speech areas of the dominant cortex. Patients are sedated during cranial opening, and are awakened once the dura is open. Direct cortical stimulation is performed to determine the relationship between the tumor and the speech centers. The surgeon then maps out eloquent and non-eloquent areas of the brain prior to beginning the tumor resection. The patient continues to converse during the tumor resection to ensure that language function is not altered.

Interstitial chemotherapy or brachytherapy can be performed after the tumor resection by implanting chemotherapy impregnated wafers or radioactive seeds in the resection cavity. Additionally, a balloon tip catheter can be placed in the resection bed and injected with radioactive material at a later date.

Variant procedure or approaches: Patient position varies depending on tumor location and surgeon preference (Table 1.1-4). Tumors on the convexity, or surface, of the brain may require minimal brain relaxation or exposure. Deep tumors, or tumors around the brain stem or skull base, may require substantial brain relaxation and retraction for optimal exposure. For deep tumors or tumors within or adjacent to critical structures, the operating microscope is commonly used. Large vascular tumors may undergo preoperative embolization of the tumor blood supply in order to minimize intraoperative blood loss.

Usual preoperative diagnosis: Glioma; glioblastoma multiforme; astrocytoma; oligodendroglioma; ependymoma; PNET; meningioma; craniopharyngioma; choroid plexus papilloma; hemangioblastomas; medulloblastoma; acoustic neuroma; brain metastasis; hemangiopericytoma

SUMMARY OF PROCEDURE

Position	Supine, lateral, prone, or sitting, based on location of tumor
Incision	Linear or curvilinear, based on location of tumor
Special instrumentation	Operating microscope, laser, CUSA, electrophysiologic monitoring, image-guided navigation, lumbar drain, ventriculostomy
Unique considerations	ETT must be taped securely in a location satisfactory to the surgeon; anode or RAE tube is helpful in certain situations. Decadron is usually given preoperatively and dosed every 6 h to minimize brain edema. Brain relaxation techniques may be required. The patient with ↑ ICP may require special consideration for induction of anesthesia. Awake craniotomy (see p. 34) may be required for tumors involving eloquent brain areas.
Antibiotics	Ceftriaxone 1–2 g iv (avoid Ca^{++} containing solutions)
Surgical time	3–5 h typically
Closing considerations	Possible requirement for dural graft. Drain often left in the epidural or subgaleal space. Good BP control during closing and extubation to prevent hemorrhage into tumor resection bed.
EBL	50–500 mL (Meningiomas and renal cell mets are highly vascular tumors and blood loss may be substantial.)
Postoperative care	ICU or close observation unit X 1–3 d. Fluid and electrolytes require frequent monitoring. BP may need to be controlled with antihypertensives.
Mortality	0–5% (mortality higher for tumors in critical locations)
Morbidity	Infection: 1% Neurological: neurologic disability, nerve injury: 0–10% CSF leak: 1–3% Venous sinus injury, air embolus Endocrine disorder Massive blood loss
Pain score	2–7

PATIENT POPULATION CHARACTERISTICS

Age range	Infant to 85 yr (usually 20–60 yr)
Male:Female	~1:1
Incidence	Common neurosurgical procedure (~40,000 dx/yr in the United States)
Etiology	Neoplastic

ANESTHETIC CONSIDERATIONS

(Procedures covered: craniotomy for tumor; craniotomy for skull tumor)

PREOPERATIVE

Typically this is a healthy patient population, apart from Sx attributable to intracranial pathology (↑ ICP, Sz, HA, N/V, visual disturbances). Discuss surgical approach, positioning, tumor type and potential for blood loss with surgeon. These patients are often receiving steroids to ↓ ICP.

Respiratory	Occasionally neurogenic pulmonary edema may occur. H/o chemotherapy or radiation therapy may affect pulmonary function and airway management. Otherwise no special considerations, unless indicated from H&P.
Cardiovascular	Benign or malignant brain tumors cause edema formation in adjacent normal brain tissue, which may →↑ ICP. If ICP increases sufficiently to cause herniation of the brain stem, patients develop the "Cushing triad" of HTN, bradycardia, and respiratory irregularity. These changes will resolve when ICP is reduced, so vigorous attempts to regulate BP and HR prior to craniotomy are not warranted. After the diagnosis of brain tumor is made, most patients are placed on high-dose steroid therapy to lessen edema in surrounding normal brain. Steroids are extremely effective in this setting, and Sx of ↑ ICP will often abate. **Tests:** Consider ECG; others as indicated from H&P.
Neurological	Patients may present with complaints related to ↑ ICP (e.g., HA, N/V, visual changes, recent onset of Sz), neurological deficits from compression of motor area, or as a result of hemorrhage from the tumor or edema in surrounding normal brain. Document preop physical findings. **Tests:** A CT scan or MRI will delineate the site and size of the tumor, especially if iv contrast material, such as gadolinium, is administered to enhance the margins of the tumor. for intracranial mass effects: midline shift, ↓ ventricular volume, ↓ peri-brainstem (basal cisterns) CSF space, obstructive hydrocephalus.
Laboratory	Coags should be normal. Hct, electrolytes, and other tests as indicated from H&P.
Premedication	Standard premedication (except for patients with the possibility of ↑ ICP: no sedation).

INTRAOPERATIVE

Anesthetic technique: Small tumors, particularly those located in deeper brain structures, may be localized and resected using stereotactic or image-guidance techniques. Generally, scalp markers (fiducials) or a stereotactic frame are placed on the patient's head; then the patient is taken to CT/MR for determination of the exact tumor site. GETA is almost invariably used for tumor removal, although MAC (see Awake Craniotomy, p. 34) is used on rare occasions when the surgeon needs to assess motor or sensory function during the resection of the tumor adjacent to critical motor or speech areas.

Induction	If the patient is in a stereotactic frame, or a difficult intubation is anticipated, orotracheal intubation will need to be accomplished before induction of GA. Awake fiber optic intubation (see p. B-5) is the best choice, because fitting a mask on the face with the stereotactic frame in place is impossible. After the airway is secured, anesthesia usually is induced with STP (2–5 mg/kg) or propofol (1–3 mg/kg) and fentanyl (3–5 mcg/kg) in combination with a NMR (e.g., vecuronium 0.1 mg/kg or rocuronium 0.6 mg/kg). To minimize ↑↑ BP and ↑ ICP with ET intubation, it is important that the patient be well anesthetized (and paralyzed) before undertaking laryngoscopy. Induction doses of STP, propofol, or midazolam may not be sufficient to abolish increases in MAP, CPP, and, hence, ↑ ICP is associated with laryngoscopy and tracheal intubation. Consider hyperventilating the patient and using remifentanil (2–3 mcg/kg) as part of the induction technique to further blunt the response to laryngoscopy in patients with ↑ ICP.
Maintenance	Isoflurane or sevoflurane ≤1 MAC (≤1/2 MAC if EP monitoring is used), inspired with 50:50 O_2/N_2O. Propofol (50–100 mcg/kg/min) can replace N_2O and may be used to further ↓cerebral blood volume, ↓ cerebral metabolism, and ↓ $CMRO_2$. Generally, if pancuronium is used, no additional NMBs are needed; however, if movement is of concern, rocuronium 10 mcg/kg/min will provide adequate neuromuscular blockade. A remifentanil infusion (0.05–0.2 mcg/kg/min) can be used to supplement the anesthetic without interfering with EP monitoring.
Emergence	Surgeons should request transient ↑ MAP to 90–100 mmHg to test hemostasis after the tumor has been resected. With the start of dural closure, consider changing the anesthetic

Emergence (cont'd)	to low-dose sevoflurane (e.g., 0.5%) with 50% N_2O (or propofol replacement), supplemented with a low-dose remifentanil infusion (e.g., 0.05 mcg/kg/min). The patient's BP generally will increase and titration of β-adrenergic blocking drugs (e.g., labetalol or esmolol) and/or vasodilators (e.g., SNP) may be needed. (See Control of BP, below.) Reverse NMB as necessary. The anesthetic agent can be D/C'd at the time of dressing application while continuing the remifentanil infusion. Most patients will breathe spontaneously and can be extubated uneventfully while on 0.05 mcg/kg/min remifentanil. If the brain has not been injured by the surgical procedure, the patient should awaken within 10 min after cessation of remifentanil administration. Keep close regulation of BP. Patient is placed in bed in a 20–30° head-up position and transported to ICU for monitoring overnight. Supplemental O_2 should be administered and BP control maintained. Prophylactic antiemetics (e.g., metoclopramide 10–20 mg and ondansetron 4 mg) should be given iv ~30 min before extubation.	
Blood and fluid requirements	IV: 16–18 ga × 2 NS @ 2–3 mL/kg/h	Brain tumors (e.g., meningioma) can be highly vascular. To minimize postop cerebral edema, limit NS to ≤ 10 mL/kg + replacement of UO. If volume is needed, administer albumin 5% as required.
Monitoring	Standard monitors (see p. B-1). Arterial line CVP line ± Precordial Doppler ± BAER, SSEP, MEP UO	If the head of the OR table is significantly elevated (≥ 30°) or if the patient is in the seated position, a precordial Doppler monitor is necessary to monitor for VAE. Evoked potentials can be monitored in the presence of inhaled anesthetics (e.g. ≤ 0.6% isoflurane with 50% N_2O).
Positioning	Supratentorial: supine/lateral Posterior fossa: prone/sitting ✓ and pad pressure points. ✓ eyes.	For brain tumors in the frontal, parietal, or temporal lobes, patient will be supine with head in Mayfield-Kees skeletal fixation, turned to the side and a roll under the shoulder on the operative side (Fig. 1.1-5). For occipital or posterior fossa tumors, patient may be prone or, occasionally, sitting (see Anesthetic Considerations for Cervical Neurosurgical Procedures, Positioning, p. 109). Acoustic neuromas are generally most easily removed with patient in the lateral ("park-bench") position with a roll under the axilla. The patient generally lies on a "bean bag" which holds her/him firmly in the lateral position.
Control of ICP	Maintain normovolemia Control BP in normal range for patient PaO_2 > 100 mmHg Limit isoflurane or sevoflurane to 1/2 MAC Steroids: 8–12 mg decadron iv	Patients with intracranial tumors may be on the steep portion of the intracranial compliance curve such that any increase in intracranial volume may →↑↑ ICP. Transient increases in ICP—even up to 50–60 mmHg—are tolerated, provided they are promptly terminated. Sustained increases in ICP > 25–30 mmHg are associated with severe neurologic injury and poor outcome.
	$PaCO_2$ = 25–30 mmHg	↓ $PaCO_2$ →↓ CBV (providing better surgical access) + ↑ CBF to ischemic areas ("Robin Hood" effect) + ↓ anesthetic requirements.
	Replace N_2O with propofol infusion	If further reduction in ICP is needed consider replacing N_2O with a propofol infusion.
	Mannitol 0.5–1.0 g/kg ± Furosemide 10–20 mg	Mannitol/furosemide → ↓ K^+; monitor level and replace as necessary. If mannitol is administered too rapidly, profound ↓ BP will occur, probably from peripheral vasodilation.

Control of ICP (cont'd)	± Lumbar CSF drain Head up 20–30°	CSF drain often placed after induction of anesthesia, and may be opened as required to ↓ CSF volume and pressure.

POSTOPERATIVE

Complications	Seizures Neurologic deficits Tension pneumocephalus Hemorrhage requiring reexploration Edema and ↑ ICP	* Sz Rx: Phenytoin (1 g loading dose). **NB**: Incompatible with dextrose-containing solutions. In seated position, additional rare, but possible complications include quadriplegia from excessive flexion of head or tension pneumocephalus from air in cerebral cavities. Severe tension pneumocephalus may delay emergence from anesthesia or cause postop neurologic deficits. CT scan may be necessary for Dx.
Pain management	Meperidine (10–20 mg iv prn) Codeine (30–60 mg im q 4 h)	Meperidine minimizes postop shivering. Avoid excessive sedation.
Tests	CT scan	If patient exhibits any delay in emergence from anesthesia and surgery, or any new neurologic deficits emerge postop, a CT scan is invariably obtained.

Suggested Readings

1. Apuzzo MLJ: *Brain Surgery: Complication, Avoidance and Management.* Churchill Livingstone, New York: 1993, 175–688.
2. Buckner JC, Brown PD, O'Neill BP, et al: Central nervous system tumors. *Mayo Clin Proc* 2007, 82(10): 1271–86.
3. Domaingue CM, Nye DH: Hypotensive effect of mannitol administered rapidly. *Anaesth Intensive Care* 1985; 13(2):134–6.
4. Domino KB, Hemstad JR, Lam AM, et al: Effect of nitrous oxide on intracranial pressure after cranial-dural closure in patients undergoing craniotomy. *Anesthesiology* 1992; 77(3):421–5.
5. Eng C, Lam AM, Mayberg TS, et al: The influence of propofol with and without nitrous oxide on cerebral blood flow velocity and CO_2 reactivity in humans. *Anesthesiology* 1992; 77(5):872–9.
6. Grady RE, Horlocker TT, Brown RD, et al: Neurologic complications after placement of cerebrospinal fluid drainage catheters and needles in anesthetized patients: implications for regional anesthesia. Mayo Perioperative Outcomes Group. *Anesth Analg* 1999; 88:388–92.
7. Manninen PH, Raman SK, Boyle K, et al: Early postoperative complications following neurosurgical procedures. *Can J Anaesth* 1999; 46:7–14.
8. Minton MD, Grosslight KR, Stirt JA, et al: Increases in intracranial pressure from succinylcholine: prevention by prior nondepolarizing blockade. *Anesthesiology* 1986; 65(2):165–9.

ANESTHETIC CONSIDERATIONS FOR AWAKE CRANIOTOMY

PREOPERATIVE

These patients typically are otherwise healthy except for a tumor (or AVM) involving eloquent (speech) areas of the brain. In some centers, awake craniotomies are still used for epilepsy surgery. Awake craniotomies for functional procedures (e.g., deep brain electrode placement) usually involve 1 or 2 burr holes with small dural punctures, and are discussed on page 71.

In addition to the preoperative anesthetic considerations for brain tumors (see p. 31) or vascular malformations (see p. 19), it is essential that these patients (and family) meet with their anesthesiologist and monitoring neurologist to discuss in detail both the anesthetic and surgical aspects of the procedures, as well as the specific speech mapping techniques that will be used. The patient should be warned that a Foley catheter will be placed while they are sedated;

however after the sedation is stopped, the catheter will become annoying, and the patient will be convinced that he/she has a full bladder. Intraoperative cooperation is critical, and there is no pharmacologic substitute for a well-informed patient.

Premed	Midazolam 1–3 mg iv is usually tolerated. Beware of respiratory depression →↑ ICP. Antiemetic: e.g., ondansetron 4 mg iv slowly and q 2–3 h during the procedure

INTRAOPERATIVE

Anesthetic technique: Although some centers use an asleep-awake-asleep technique with airway control (ETT or LMA) during the sleep phases, we prefer the following technique that minimizes airway manipulation and its inherent risk of coughing and bucking.

Premapping	Most patients with space-occupying lesions will benefit from the early administration of mannitol 0.5 gm/kg by slow iv infusion (check with surgeon for possible contraindications). With the patient in a beach-chair position and following the application of standard monitors and nasal prong O_2, initial sedation is provided by incremental midazolam titrated by effect (1–10 mg iv). A loading dose of dexmedetomidine (1 mcg/kg iv over 10–15 min as tolerated) is given while the sites for arterial line and central line (subclavian or antecubital long-line) placement are infiltrated with local anesthetic. Following the loading dose, a maintenance infusion of dexmedetomidine (0.2–0.7 mcg/kg/h) typically 0.4 mcg/kg/h is started. The dexmedetomidine produces cooperative sedation and analgesia without respiratory depression. A ↓ BP and ↓ HR are common and occasionally will require treatment with vagolytics and/or pressors. If necessary the sedation can be deepened with a propofol infusion (25–75 mcg/kg/min) to cover the more painful aspects of the procedure. A nasal airway may be useful in some patients. Scalp blocks (supraorbital, temporal, and occipital nerves) are placed using 0.5% bupivacaine with epinephrine. Arterial line, cerebral line, and Foley catheter are placed. Pin sites for the Mayfield skull clamp are infiltrated with local anesthetic and the clamp is applied. The incision is infiltrated with local anesthetic and, after patient comfort has been assured, the craniotomy is allowed to proceed. Drapes should be arranged so that the anesthesiologist and neuromonitoring team have an unobstructed view of, and access to, the patient's face and airway.
Mapping	The dexmedetomidine (and propofol) infusions are stopped at the end of the craniotomy. Initial mapping (e.g., phase-reversal localization) can be accomplished while the patient is recovering from the sedation. Some direct cortical stimulation can produce seizures; it is important that sterile, iced saline be immediately available for cortical irrigation to suppress the seizure activity. If seizure activity spreads, it will be necessary to administer a bolus dose of STP (25–75 mg iv) through the central line. Airway support (e.g., LMA) may be necessary in the post-ictal phase. The patient should be awake and cooperative ~20 min after the dexmedetomidine and propofol infusions have stopped. Occasionally, flumazenil may be necessary to remove residual midazolam effects. Detailed speech-mapping can then be readily accomplished. We use a miniature wireless microphone taped below the patient's mouth to amplify the patient's voice during testing and tumor resection.
Resection	If the lesion is located safely away from the mapped speech areas, the resection can be accomplished after reinstituting the dexmedetomidine and propofol infusions. Otherwise, the patient must be kept awake and talking throughout the resection. Often the patient will benefit from a low-dose remifentanil infusion (e.g., < 0.05 mcg/kg/min) to improve ability to tolerate positional discomfort.
Closing	Closing is best accomplished by resuming the previously effective infusions of dexmedetomidine and propofol. The infusions should be stopped during the final phase of wound closure. Careful control of BP may require the use of labetalol, esmolol, and SNP, which should be titrated during emergence. Typically, the patient will be awake and alert for transport to the ICU.

CRANIOTOMY FOR SKULL TUMOR

SURGICAL CONSIDERATIONS

Gordon T. Sakamoto, Lawrence M. Shuer, and Steven D. Chang

Description: Tumors of the skull fall into the classification of other bony tumors. Examples of types of skull tumors often requiring surgery include eosinophilic granuloma, histiocytosis, hemangioma, osteoma, epidermoid, dermoid, metastases, osteosarcoma, fibrous dysplasia, chordoma, chondrosarcoma, and meningioma. These tumors may occur anywhere on the skull, except chordoma and chondrosarcoma, which usually arise from the skull base. The exact positioning of the patient depends on the location of tumor. For example, the sitting or prone position often is used for tumors in the occipital or suboccipital regions and the supine position is used for frontal, temporal, or parietal tumors. Some surgeons prefer the lateral position for temporal or parietal bone lesions and the prone position for occipital and some suboccipital bone lesions. Complete immobilization of the head is often not necessary, so the patient's head can be placed in a horseshoe or a Shea headrest. If complete immobilization is required, Mayfield pin fixation is used. The tumor is removed by placing burr holes near or around the tumor. Then the affected skull is removed by cutting a bone flap around the tumor with the craniotome. In a suboccipital or posterior fossa craniectomy, the bone often is removed piecemeal with either a drill or a series of rongeurs. The dura usually is not opened unless it is involved with the tumor. The surgeon may elect to perform a **cranioplasty** to cover the defect, depending upon the size and location. The defect can be repaired using a variety of methods, which include the use of a polymer, such as methylmethacrylate, or a bone cement, such as hydroxyapatite. Additionally, autologous bone may be harvested from another location on the skull or another site (hip or rib) for reconstruction. Lastly, the surgeon may elect to repair the cranial defect at a later date, using a custom implant made from titanium, methylmethacrylate, or polyethylethylketone (PEEK). After the tumor is removed and the reconstruction is completed, the skin incision is closed. Occasionally, the skull tumor will be approached intracranially, if its location favors that approach. Examples include tumors of the petrous portion of the temporal bone, fibrous dysplasia involving the optic canal, or skull base tumors, such as chordomas and chondrosarcomas.

Usual preop diagnosis: Eosinophilic granuloma; histiocytosis; hemangioma; osteoma; epidermoid; dermoid tumor; metastatic tumors; osteosarcoma; fibrous dysplasia; chordoma; chondrosarcoma; meningioma

SUMMARY OF PROCEDURE

Position	Supine, lateral, prone, or sitting, based on the location of the tumor
Incision	Dependent on location of tumor
Special instrumentation	Neuro drill, craniotome, image-guided navigation (if intracranial)
Unique considerations	ETT must be taped securely in a location satisfactory to the surgeon. Anode or RAE tube may be helpful in certain situations.
Antibiotics	Cefazolin 1 g iv (if dura not opened)
Surgical time	1–4 h
Closing considerations	Drain often left in epidural space. Surgeon often requests control of BP to avoid hemorrhage into the bed of tumor.
EBL	25–500 mL
Postop care	ICU or close observation unit
Mortality	0–2% (higher for tumors in critical locations)
Morbidity	Usually < 5% Infection Neurological disability CSF leak Massive blood loss 2° venous sinus injury
Pain score	2–5

PATIENT POPULATION CHARACTERISTICS	
Age range	Infant–85 yr (usually 20–60 yr)
Male:Female	~1:1
Incidence	Unknown
Etiology	Neoplastic

ANESTHETIC CONSIDERATIONS

See Anesthetic Considerations following Craniotomy for Tumor, p. 31. Note, however, that patients with skull tumors rarely have problems with ICP.

Suggested Readings

1. Sawaya RE, Kroll S, Wecht DA, et al: Tumors of the scalp and skull. In *The Practice of Neurosurgery.* Tindall GT, Cooper PR, Barrow DL, eds. Williams & Wilkins, Baltimore: 1996, 1371–84.
2. Scolozzi P, Martinez A, Jaques B: Complex orbito-fronto-temporal reconstruction using computer-designed PEEK implant. *J Craniofac Surg* 2007; 18(1):224–8.
3. Verret DJ, Ducic Y, Oxford L, et al: Hydroxyapatite Cement in Craniofacial Reconstruction. *Otolaryngol Head Neck Surg* 2005; 133(6):897–9.

CRANIOTOMY FOR TRAUMA

SURGICAL CONSIDERATIONS

Gordon T. Sakamoto, Lawrence M. Shuer, and Steven D. Chang

Description: Head injuries occasionally require emergent surgical procedures to evacuate mass lesions or débride contused or contaminated brain. The majority of these injuries are supratentorial. The surgical procedure depends on the exact type and location of the injury (e.g., epidural, subdural, intraparenchymal hematomas, or depressed skull fracture); however, most traumatic injuries can be addressed through a wide frontotempoparietal craniotomy. Often the entire head is shaved and placed in a headrest (pins, suction cups, or horseshoe). If the C-spine has not been cleared, the patient may be placed in a lateral position to minimize neck involvement. Timing is often important for these procedures, because the patient usually has a component of ↑ ICP, either from a hematoma or from cerebral edema due to the trauma. Hyperventilation, mannitol, hypertonic saline, and diuresis may be necessary to control the patient's ICP until the patient can be taken into the operating room and undergo a wide decompressive hemicraniectomy (frontotempoparietal craniectomy). For a standard trauma craniotomy, the scalp incision starts anterior to the tragus and continues superiorly in a question-mark type path, ending in the frontal area (Fig. 1.1-11). This incision can be modified according to the location and extent of the injury. The skin is reflected and the skull is perforated with a cranial drill. The temporal burr hole should be placed first, because if the patient's condition deteriorates rapidly, the temporal burr hole can be enlarged quickly to a craniectomy for decompression before continuing with the craniotomy. A chronic subdural hematoma may be drained through burr holes. However, if there is an acute subdural hematoma, epidural hematoma, intraparenchymal hemorrhage, depressed fracture, or penetrating wound, a formal bone flap is elevated. Wide exposure is used to visualize and control sources of bleeding. Gentle warm irrigation may be used to aid in removal of an acute subdural hematoma. Mass lesions and associated contused brain parenchyma are identified and removed (Fig. 1.1-12). For penetrating head injuries or depressed skull fractures, the wound is débrided, foreign bodies are removed, bleeding is controlled, and the dura is repaired if lacerated. It is important to débride the wound as much as possible, but it is often not possible to safely remove all fragments from the wound. Depending on the injury and the presence of brain swelling, it may be necessary to close the dura with autologous pericranium, or fascia lata. If these are not available, a synthetic dural substitute or bovine pericardium can be used. Alternatively, the dura may be left open, or multiple relaxing incisions may be made in the dura to allow for brain swelling. The surgeon can often repair and reconstruct a depressed skull fracture after removing a bone flap that surrounds the fracture. Additionally, the bone flap may be left out to compensate for brain swelling and replaced later. A subgaleal drain may be inserted and brought out through a separate incision. An ICP monitor or a ventriculostomy may be placed at the end of the procedure.

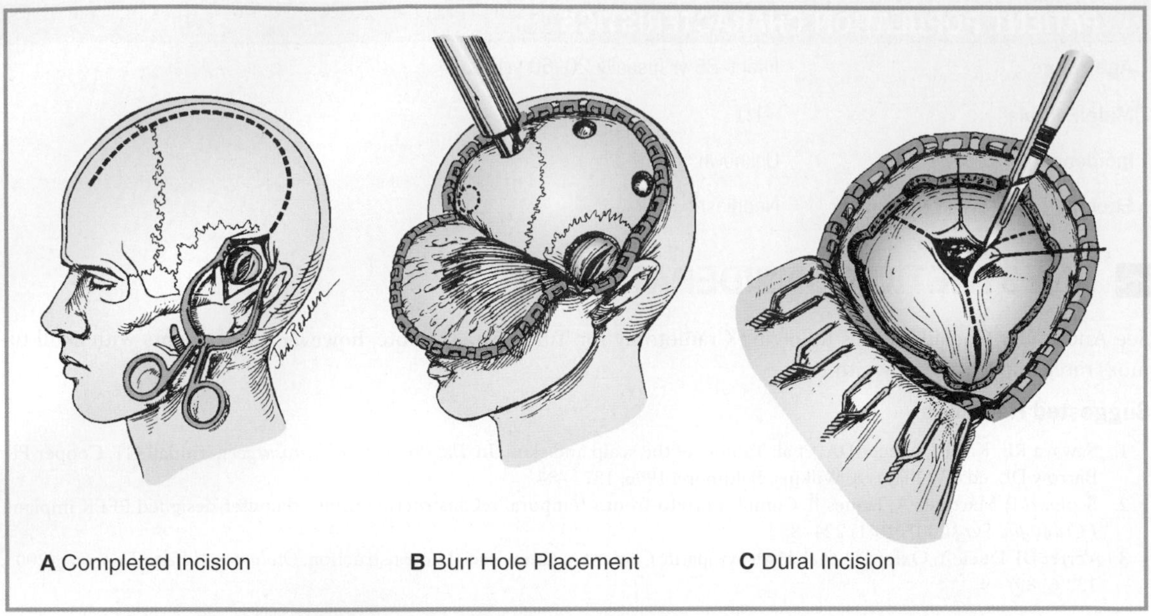

Figure 1.1-11. In an acute subdural hematoma: **A:** burr hole is made, followed by craniectomy, and the incision is extended upward to form a large question mark, the medial extent of which follows the midline. **B:** Additional burr holes are made, with the medial ones 1.5 cm off the midline to avoid injury to the major venous structures and granulations. The anterior burr hole is placed above the frontal sinus (the size of which can be estimated from preop radiographs). **C:** The dura can be opened with a Y- or X-shaped incision, with a flap being based on the superior sagittal sinus. (Reproduced with permission from Grossman RG, Loftus CM: *Principles of Neurosurgery,* 2nd edition. Lippincott-Raven, Philadelphia: 1999.)

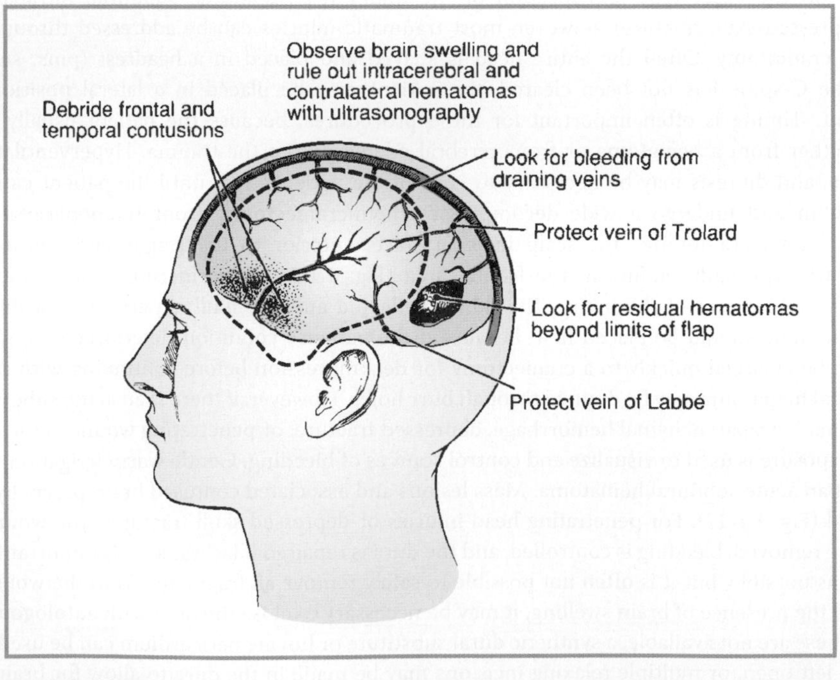

Figure 1.1-12. Precautions to be taken during a craniotomy for subdural hematoma. (Reproduced with permission from Grossman RG, Loftus CM: *Principles of Neurosurgery,* 2nd edition. Lippincott-Raven, 1999.)

Frontal sinus fracture: If a skull fracture involves the frontal sinus and/or there is a CSF leak, the sinus may need to be obliterated or cranialized. Obliteration involves removal of the mucosa of the sinus and filling the sinus with antibiotic soaked Gelfoam sponges. Cranialization of the frontal sinus involves removing the posterior bony wall of the sinus and removing the mucosa. If there is a CSF leak, the dura will need to be repaired.

Variant indication: Some patients, after having a large ischemic stroke, will develop malignant cerebral edema, which may necessitate a decompressive hemicraniectomy (frontotempoparietal craniectomy) in order to control rising ICPs and prevent herniation.

Usual preop diagnosis: Epidural hematoma; acute subdural hematoma; intracerebral hematoma; depressed skull fracture; cerebral contusion; gunshot wound of the brain; malignant cerebral edema

SUMMARY OF PROCEDURE

Position	Supine, lateral, prone, or sitting, depending on site of injury
Incision	Varies with location of injury (typical incision shown in Fig. 1.1-11)
Unique considerations	The patient may have ↑↑ ICP. Because incipient herniation and/or associated injuries may be a concern, timing is critical. C-spine precautions may be necessary. Patients may also be on anti-coagulation medications, necessitating transfusions of blood products or recombinant activated factor VII.
Antibiotics	Ceftriaxone 1 g iv (avoid Ca^{++} containing solutions)
Surgical time	1.5–6 h
Closing considerations	Application of head dressing may jostle ETT at end of case →↑ BP. Patient may stay intubated postop. ICP monitor or external ventricular drain may be placed. Antiepileptic medications may be given for prophylaxis, if the patient had a seizure.
EBL	25–500 mL
Postop care	ICU or close observation unit until stable. Fluid and electrolytes require frequent monitoring, as the patient may develop SIADH. BP may need to be controlled with vasodilator and β-blocker infusions.
Mortality	10–50%, depending on lesion; higher for acute subdural hematomas, lower for epidural hematomas.
Morbidity	Morbidity depends on lesion; morbidity from craniotomy itself is low. Infection Neurologic disability Nerve injury CSF leak Endocrine disorders: SIADH Panhypopituitarism Diabetes insipidus (DI) Massive blood loss: venous sinus injury
Pain score	2–4

PATIENT POPULATION CHARACTERISTICS

Age range	Infant–85 yr (usually 15–40 yr)
Male:Female	2:1
Incidence	Relatively common
Etiology	Trauma
Associated conditions	Abdominal injuries; C-spine fractures

ANESTHETIC CONSIDERATIONS

PREOPERATIVE

Traumatic brain injury (TBI) is the leading cause of death of persons < 24 years old. A penetrating injury of the skull usually will cause major damage to the brain as a result of both focal and diffuse neuronal injury with hemorrhage into brain tissue. Surgery is necessary to evacuate hematomas, control intracranial bleeding, to débride the wound, and to remove bone fragments, foreign material, and damaged brain so that the cranial vault can better accommodate the brain swelling that inevitably occurs. Epidural hematomas form between the skull and dura, and are usually due to bleeding from an artery (e.g., anterior cerebral or middle meningeal). Hence, time is of the essence and rapid evacuation and control of the bleeding is essential if permanent neurological injury is to be avoided. Subdural bleeding occurs between the dura and the leptomeninges lining the brain surface. This bleeding is usually venous in origin, and usually occurs more gradually. Focal intracranial hemorrhages may be either arterial or venous, and, as with subdural hematomas, must be evacuated if they are enlarging.

Respiratory	Ensure a secure airway and adequate ventilation. Localized injuries to the frontal or parietal lobes may not cause any respiratory changes. If ↑ ICP, respirations may become slow (< 10 min) and deep, and result in substantial hypocapnia. Many patients with head injuries demonstrate partial airway obstruction from the tongue falling back into the posterior pharyngeal space. If this occurs, or if the patient is comatose and unable to protect the airway and prevent aspiration of gastric contents, immediate tracheal intubation should be performed. Head injuries in the region of the occipital lobes may → hypoventilation or apnea. Neurogenic pulmonary edema may occur in up to 20% of TBI patients. **Tests:** As indicated from H&P and as time allows.
Cardiovascular	Most patients with head injuries evidence ↑ BP and ↑ HR. Relative hypotension (SBP < 90 mmHg) →↑ morbidity and mortality. If ICP increases sufficiently to cause herniation of brain stem, patients develop the "Cushing triad" of ↑ BP, ↓ HR and irregular respiration. These changes resolve when ↑ ICP is relieved, so vigorous attempts to regulate BP prior to craniotomy are not warranted. However, the patient should be taken to OR as quickly as possible. **Tests:** As indicated from H&P, and as time allows.
Neurological	Neurological evaluation of the head-injured patient is based on the Glasgow Coma Scale (Table 1.1-5). The scale involves evaluation of three functions: eye opening, verbal response, and motor response. Using this scoring system, the severity of brain injury may be classified as mild (13–15 points), moderate (9–12 points), or severe (8 points or less). By definition, any patient having 8 points or less is in coma. Additional useful neurological examinations include assessment of pupillary size and reactivity to the light, reflex responses, and evidence of asymmetry or flaccidity of the extremities or decerebrate (e.g., rigid arm extension) or decorticate (e.g., rigid arm flexion) posturing. Head-injured patients whose neurological function is deteriorating rapidly, and in whom an epidural or subdural hemorrhage is suspected, should be taken to OR immediately. Hyperventilation is appropriate if herniation is eminent. **Tests:** CT scan
Hematologic	Severe head injury may be associated with a progressively worsening coagulopathy, resulting in a clinical picture similar to that of DIC. The reason for this is not known, but the brain is rich in thromboplastin and other coagulation factors. **Tests:** Hct; PT; PTT; others as indicated from H&P.
Associated Injuries	Multiple organ system injury must be considered. Evidence of intrathoracic or intraperitoneal hemorrhage should be sought and repaired first if the patient is hemodynamically unstable. **Tests:** may include MRI, CT, ultrasound and others as indicated.
Laboratory	Other tests as indicated from H&P, and as time permits.
Premedication	Usually none

Table 1.1-5. Glasgow Coma Scale (GCS)

Category	Score
I. Eyes open:	
Never	1
To pain	2
To verbal stimuli	3
Spontaneously	4
II. Best verbal response:	
None	1
Incomprehensible sounds	2
Inappropriate words	3
Patient disoriented and converses	4
Patient oriented and converses	5
III. Best motor response:	
None	1
Extension (decerebrate rigidity)	2
Flexion abnormal (decorticate rigidity)	3
Flexion withdrawal	4
Patient localizes pain	5
Patient Obeys	6
	I+II+III Total = 3–15

INTRAOPERATIVE

Anesthetic technique: GETA

Induction

↑ ICP is likely in most patients with head injury requiring operation, and induction of anesthesia is best accomplished with drugs that ↓ ICP. A mannitol infusion (0.25–1 mg/kg iv over 20 min) may be necessary to control ICP. If the patient is hemodynamically stable and not hypovolemic, titrated induction with STP (2–5 mg/kg) or propofol (1.5–3 mg/kg) + fentanyl (2–5 mcg/kg) is satisfactory. If hemodynamically unstable, etomidate (0.1–0.4 mg/kg) is suitable for induction. Ketamine is not used because of its ability to ↑ ICP. If the patient is comatose, anesthetic requirement is less, needing only O_2 and muscle relaxant, or low-dose isoflurane (0.5%) or sevoflurane (< 1%). A nondepolarizing muscle relaxant (vecuronium [0.1 mg/kg] or rocuronium [1 mg/kg]) is administered for ET intubation. Succinylcholine may ↑ ICP transiently, but is still appropriate for emergency airway management. A defasciculating dose of a non-depolarizing NMB may attenuate the ICP ↑. Nasotracheal intubation is not recommended for patients with the possibility of maxillary and/or basilar skull fractures because of the potential for inserting the tube through the fracture site into the brain. To minimize ↑↑ BP and ↑↑ ICP with ET intubation, consider bolus remifentanil (2–5 mcg/kg iv) 1–2 min before laryngoscopy. In hypovolemic patients, hydration with a mixture of crystalloid (e.g., NS) and colloid (e.g., 5% albumin) should be initiated prior to induction.

Maintenance

The ideal drug for maintenance of anesthesia decreases ICP and $CMRO_2$, maintains cerebral autoregulation, redistributes flow to potentially ischemic areas, and provides protection for the brain from focal ischemia. Unfortunately, there is no ideal anesthetic.

Both isoflurane and sevoflurane are good choices for patients undergoing neurosurgical procedures. Although these agents cause dose-dependent increases in CBF and volume, and hence ↑ ICP, these effects tend to be mitigated by the prior administration of STP (or propofol), hyperventilation, and by limiting the inspired concentrations to < 1 MAC. At these concentrations, CBF responses to changes in $PaCO_2$ are maintained, and cerebral autoregulation remains intact.

N_2O is best avoided in patients with significantly elevated ICP. A propofol infusion is a reasonable alternative although its use has been associated with a ↓ CBF >↓ $CMRO_2$ →↑ potential for ischemia. Jugular bulb O_2 saturation may be reduced during propofol anesthesia, consistent with an unfavorable supply-demand balance.

Maintenance (cont'd)	BP Goals: Keep SBP ~90 mmHg and CPP 60–70 mmHg. Avoid prophylactic hyperventilation. Mild hypothermia may be beneficial if maintained > 48 h. DVT prophylaxis is recommended. High-dose steroid administration is associated with worsened outcomes. Muscle relaxation can be maintained as necessary.	
Emergence	Because recovery from head injury is so unpredictable, it is generally advisable to leave the ETT in place and maintain controlled ventilation until there is sufficient clinical evidence that normal neurological recovery is occurring. Postop sedation can be accomplished using propofol (20–75 mcg/kg/min) not to exceed 5 mg/kg/h to minimize the occurrence of propofol-related infusion syndrome (including: metabolic acidosis, ↑ K^+, rhabdomyolysis).	
Blood and fluid requirements	Possible marked blood loss IV: 14–16 ga × 1 NS @ 2–4 mL/kg/h ± Albumin 5%	Blood transfusion to keep Hct > 30. Minimize postop cerebral edema by limiting crystalloid volume to < 10 mL/kg + replacement of UO. Glucose-containing solutions should be avoided; blood glucose levels should be maintained between 80–180 mg%. If volume is needed, albumin 5% should be administered.
Control of blood loss	Keep CPP 60–70 mmHg Keep SBP > 90 mmHg Maintain normovolemia	Controlled hypotension generally is not used unless bleeding becomes profuse and difficult to control. ↓ BP is better treated initially with volume replacement than vasopressors.
Monitoring	Standard monitors (see p. B-1). ± Arterial line ± CVP line ± UO	If the injury is extensive or unknown, or if the patient is unstable, invasive monitoring is mandatory. Monitor for VAE if head is elevated above heart. Level the arterial line at the head. EEG, EP, and SjO_2 monitoring may be desirable.
Positioning	✓ and pad pressure points. ✓ eyes.	For occipital or posterior fossa lesions, patient may be prone or sitting (see Anesthetic Considerations for Cervical Neurosurgical Procedures, Positioning, p. 107). Otherwise, patient will be supine with head in Mayfield-Kees skeletal fixation and turned to the side, and a roll placed under the shoulder on the operative side.
Control of ICP	Adequate anesthesia Head up 20–30° Keep SBP ≥ 90 mmHg STP or propofol infusion	Transient increases in ICP—even up to 50–60 mmHg—are generally tolerated, provided they are promptly terminated. Sustained increases in ICP > 25–30 mmHg are associated with severe neurologic injury and poor outcome. Patients with skull fractures or intracranial bleeding may be on the steep portion of intracranial compliance curve such that any increase in intracranial volume may cause ↑↑ ICP.
	Hyperventilation to $PaCO_2$ = 25–30 mmHg PaO_2 > 100 mmHg	↓ CO_2 → cerebral vasoconstriction →↓ CBV, ↓ CBF, and ↓ ICP. Patients with diffuse brain injury may have lost cerebrovascular sensitivity to $PaCO_2$. Despite maintaining adequate ventilation, oxygenation and BP, patients with diffuse head injury often exhibit arterial and CSF lactic acidosis, a further indication of the metabolic derangement that exists in the brain from the injury.
	Keep CPP 60–70 mmHg	Control MAP and cerebral venous pressure so that CPP = 60–70 mmHg. In severe, diffuse head injury with loss of autoregulation, some parts of the brain may exhibit 'luxury perfusion', while other areas exhibit severe ischemia.

Control of ICP (cont'd)	Mannitol 0.25–1.0 g/kg	Vigorous diuresis will commence in about 30 min (if blood volume is adequate) and brain shrinkage will follow. It is often necessary to provide supplemental potassium (20–30 mEq iv slowly).
	Furosemide 10–20 mg	Simultaneous administration of furosemide (10–20 mg) is recommended to avoid the transient ↑ CBV and ↑ ICP following mannitol. If mannitol is administered too rapidly, profound hypotension will occur, probably from peripheral vasodilatation.

POSTOPERATIVE

Complications	Seizures	* Sz Rx: phenytoin (1 g loading dose). **NB:** Incompatible with dextrose-containing solutions.
	Neurologic deficits Hemorrhage SIADH/DI	Some patients with severe head injury remain unconscious for weeks or months, without evidencing any substantial neurological recovery. A late complication of head injury is hydrocephalus requiring a shunt procedure.
	NPE ↑ICP DIC	Neurogenic pulmonary edema may result from massive sympathetic discharge 2° ↑↑ ICP. Rx: ↓ ICP, alpha-blockers to control BP, respiratory support. TBI is a risk factor for DIC.
Pain management	Fentanyl/propofol infusion	Most patients will remain intubated and sedated postop.
Tests	CT scan ICP monitor	Unless neurological recovery is rapid, periodic CT scans are obtained postop to follow the intracranial changes. In addition, in many institutions, a device for monitoring ICP postop is placed at the time of operation.

Suggested Readings

1. Adembri C, Venturi L, Pellegrini-Giampietro DE: Neuroprotective effects of propofol in acute cerebral injury. *CNS Drug Rev* 2007; 13(3):333–351.
2. Baumann A, Audibert G, McDonnell J, et al: Neurogenic pulmonary edema. *Acta Anesthesiol Scand* 2007; 51(4):447–55.
3. Brain Trauma Foundation; American Association of Neurological Surgeons; Congress of Neurological Surgeons; Joint Section on Neurotrauma and Critical Care, AANS/CNS: Guidelines for the management of severe traumatic brain injury. XI. Anesthetics, analgesics, and sedatives. *J Neurotrauma* 2007; 24(Suppl 1):S71–6.
4. Corbett SM, Montoya ID, Moore FA: Propofol-related infusion syndrome in intensive care patients. *Pharmacotherapy* 2008; 28(2):250–8.
5. Domaingue CM, Nye DH: Hypotensive effect of mannitol administered rapidly. *Anaesth Intensive Care* 1985; 13(2):134–6.
6. Hutchinson P, Timofeev I, Kirkpatrick P: Surgery for brain edema. *Neurosurg Focus* 2007; 22(5):E14.
7. Kawana Y, Kawaguchi M, Inoue S, et al: Jugular bulb oxygen saturation under propofol or sevoflurane/nitrous oxide anesthesia during deliberate mild hypothermia in neurosurgical patients. *J Neurosurg Anesthesiol* 2004; 16(1):6–10.
8. Kelly DF, McBride DQ, Becker DP: Surgical management of severe closed head injury in adults. In *Operative Neurosurgical Techniques: Indications, Methods, and Results.* Schmidek HA, Sweet WH, eds. WB Saunders, Philadelphia: 2000, 61–90.
9. King LR, McLaurin RL, Knowles HC Jr: Acid-base balance and arterial and CSF lactate levels following human head injury. *J Neurosurg* 1974; 40(5):617–25.
10. Marion DW, Penrod LE, Kelsey SE, et al: Treatment of traumatic brain injury with moderate hypothermia. *N Engl J Med* 1997; 336:540–6.
11. Minassian AT, Dube L, Guilleux AN, et al: Changes in intracranial pressure and cerebral autoregulation in patients with severe traumatic brain injury. *Crit Care Med* 2002; 30:1616–22.
12. Pasternak JJ, Hertzfeldt DN, Stanger SR, et al: Disseminated intravascular coagulation after craniotomy. *J Neurosurg Anesthesiol* 2008; 20(1):15–20.
13. Piek J: Medical complications in severe head injury. *New Horiz* 1995; 3:534–9.
14. Powner DJ, Hartwell EA, Hoots WK: Counteracting the effects of anticoagulants and antiplatelet agents during neurosurgical emergencies. *Neurosurgery* 2005; 57(5):823–31.

MICROVASCULAR DECOMPRESSION OF CRANIAL NERVE

SURGICAL CONSIDERATIONS

Gordon T. Sakamoto, Lawrence M. Shuer, and Steven D. Chang

Description: Microvascular decompression is used to treat various disorders of the cranial nerves, including trigeminal neuralgia, hemifacial spasm and, more rarely, glossopharyngeal neuralgia. Trigeminal neuralgia is characterized by brief episodes of intense, stabbing facial pain along the distribution of the trigeminal nerve. This pain usually can be elicited by gentle stimulation of the affected area. Hemifacial spasm is characterized by paroxysmal repetitive twitching of the facial muscles. The twitching usually starts with the muscles around the eye and can progress to involve the rest of the facial muscles. Glossopharyngeal neuralgia is characterized by paroxysmal pain that involves the ear and throat. Typically, the pain is described as 'stabbing' and radiates from one site to the other. Swallowing, drinking cold beverages, talking, or coughing can elicit the pain.

All of these conditions are usually unilateral and are often caused by compression of a cranial nerve by a vascular structure. In trigeminal neuralgia, the superior cerebellar artery is the usual culprit. In hemifacial spasm, usually the anterior inferior cerebellar or vertebral artery is compressing the facial nerve. In glossopharyngeal neuralgia, the posterior inferior cerebellar or vertebral artery is usually the offending artery. Large veins can also compress the cranial nerves. The goal of a microvascular decompression is to remove the pressure on the cranial nerve. To perform a microvascular decompression, a linear incision is made behind the ear on the affected side (Fig. 1.1-13A). Dissection is taken down to the skull, and several burr holes are made. The burr holes can be enlarged into a **craniectomy** (Fig. 1.1-13B) or used for elevation of a bone flap. The craniectomy is placed below the transverse sinus and medial to the sigmoid sinus to allow access to the cerebellopontine angle. Any venous sinus bleeding is controlled and the dura is opened (Fig. 1.1-13C). With brain relaxation, the cerebellum is retracted. The operating microscope allows the surgeon to explore the involved cranial nerve. If an offending vessel is identified, it is carefully dissected away from the nerve and shredded Teflon felt or a small, plastic sponge is placed to keep the vessel away from the cranial nerve. In the case of trigeminal or glossopharyngeal neuralgia, if no offending vessel is identified, a **partial section of the nerve** may be performed. Partial section of the 9th or 10th cranial nerve may cause some vasomotor instability. BAERs, facial nerve monitoring, and EMGs can be measured intraop to protect the cranial nerves. Once the cranial nerve has been decompressed, the dura is closed, and the wound is closed in layers. The main variations in this procedure are in patient positioning and surgeon's preference of monitoring modalities. Patient positioning may be lateral, prone, supine, or sitting. Intraop, mannitol (0.5–1 g/kg) and a lumbar drain (for CSF removal) may be needed for brain relaxation. Success rate is typically 75–95%, with a recurrence rate as high as 3.5% per year.

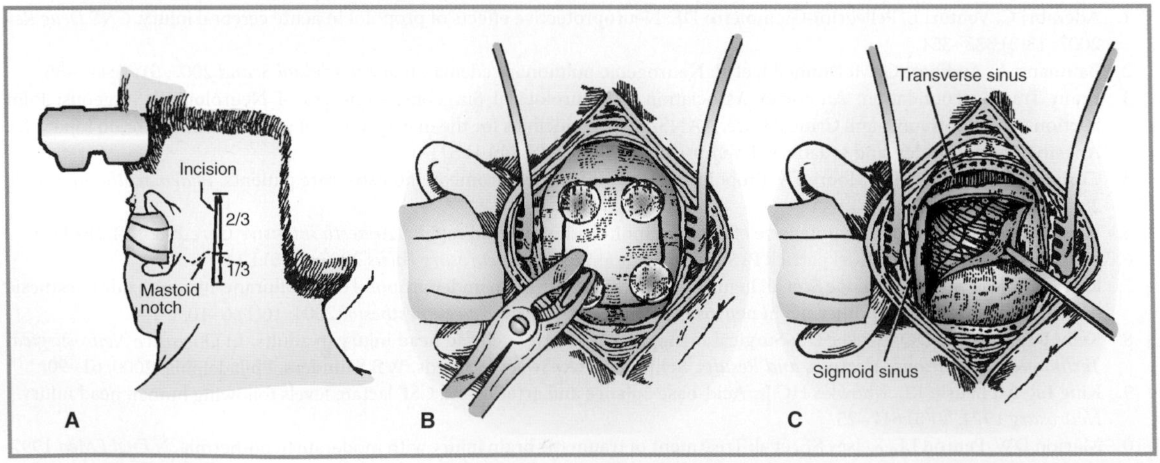

Figure 1.1-13. Microvascular decompression: **A.** Location of incision. **B.** Enlargement of burr holes into craniectomy with a rongeur. **C.** Dural opening on the left side. Note position of venous sinuses. (Reproduced with permission from Wilson CB: *Neurosurgical Procedures: Personal Approaches to Classic Operations.* Williams & Wilkins, Philadelphia: 1992.)

Alternative Procedure: Gamma Knife surgery is less effective than microvascular decompression, but may be appropriate for patients unwilling or unable to undergo surgery. Other options include radiofrequency rhizotomy (see p. 86), glycerol injection, and balloon compression.

Usual preop diagnosis: Trigeminal neuralgia; tic douloureux; hemifacial spasm; tinnitus; glossopharyngeal neuralgia

SUMMARY OF PROCEDURE

Position	Normally, lateral ("park-bench"), head elevated 30°; upper shoulder retracted caudally
Incision	Retroauricular (mastoid) (See Fig. 1.1-13A.)
Special instrumentation	Operating microscope; cranial perforator; ± facial nerve monitoring; ± EMG; ± BAER
Unique considerations	Risk of air embolus in head-elevated positions
Antibiotics	Ceftriaxone 1–2 gm iv q d (avoid Ca^{++}-containing solutions)
Surgical time	2–3 h
EBL	25–250 mL
Postop care	ICU or close observation unit. Observe for change in neurologic status (e.g., level of alertness, response to commands), usually for 12–24 h.
Mortality	0.2–2%
Morbidity	Facial sensory deficit: 25% (often transient) Aseptic meningitis: ≤ 20%, usually occurring 3–7 d postop Hearing loss: 3% Diplopia (usually transient) Facial weakness: 2% Deafness: 1% Infection CSF leak Massive blood loss due to vertebral artery injury or sinus laceration
Pain score	4–6

PATIENT POPULATION CHARACTERISTICS

Age range	40–85 yr (usually 60–70 yr)
Male:Female	~2:3
Incidence	4/1,000,000 (trigeminal neuralgia); 0.06/100,000 (glossopharyngeal neuralgia)
Etiology	Vascular compression of cranial nerve; multiple sclerosis plaque
Associated conditions	HTN; multiple sclerosis

ANESTHETIC CONSIDERATIONS

PREOPERATIVE

Microvascular decompression involves a full craniotomy for decompression of a cranial nerve that is causing facial pain and/or spasm of facial muscles. Generally, these patients have trigeminal neuralgia or tic douloureux that has not been responsive to medical management (e.g., carbamazepine [Tegretol] therapy) and percutaneous rhizotomy or glycerol injection has failed.

Respiratory	None unless the patient has a long-standing Hx of smoking and has COPD.
Cardiovascular	Many patients will have Hx of idiopathic HTN requiring antihypertensive medications. Good preop control of BP is important because it will make intraop and postop management of BP easier. Anticipate exaggerated hemodynamic response to anesthetic medications.
Neurological	The presenting symptom is pain ± muscle spasm in the maxillary and/or mandibular division of the trigeminal nerve, unaccompanied by any motor or sensory deficits. Identify trigger points so that they may be avoided during mask placement and induction.
Laboratory	None, except for routine preop studies.
Premedication	Generally, patients for these procedures are elderly and do not require any special premedication. Midazolam 1–3 mg iv will provide amnesia for the preop events, if that is desired by patient or surgeons.

INTRAOPERATIVE

Anesthetic technique: GA is necessary because a full craniotomy is performed. ICP is not increased in these patients. Brain volume reduction, however, is important to provide the surgeon with sufficient space to identify and relieve the pressure on the offending nerve without requiring excessive brain retraction in the process.

Induction	Induction is best accomplished with drugs that cause brain volume reduction, including STP (2–5 mg/kg) or propofol (1–2 mg/kg), followed by neuromuscular blockade and ET intubation.	
Maintenance	Standard maintenance (p. B-2) is usually satisfactory. Desflurane has been associated with ↑ PONV. BP is maintained in the normal range during the operation. Hyperventilation to achieve a $PaCO_2$ of 25–30 mmHg is helpful to ↓ brain volume and ↑ workspace. Once the nerve has been isolated, stop hyperventilation. A spinal drain may be used to remove CSF during the operation and improve exposure. The drain usually is opened at the time of dural opening and closed as soon as surgery on the nerve is complete.	
Emergence	The ETT is removed at the conclusion of operation. Postop HTN may need to be controlled with esmolol and/or SNP by continuous pump infusion. Prophylactic antiemetic (e.g., metoclopramide 10 mg and ondansetron 4 mg) should be given 30 min before extubation. The incidence of PONV is high following this procedure.	
Blood and fluid requirements	Large blood loss is rare IV: 18 ga × 1 NS @ 2–4 mL/kg/h	Mannitol 0.5–1 mg/kg is sometimes necessary to provide sufficient brain volume reduction to permit adequate surgical exposure.
Monitoring	Standard monitors (see p. B-1). Arterial line CVP line ± EMG and/or SSEP	Invasive monitoring will facilitate intraop and postop BP management. Sometimes EMG and/or SSEP monitoring of the facial nerve is performed.
Positioning	Lateral, "park bench" Pillow between legs ✓ and pad pressure points. ✓ eyes.	Patients usually will be positioned laterally in the "park-bench" position. Padding of the axillae and elbows and placing a pillow between the legs are necessary. A bean bag is often used to hold patient stable in the lateral position.

POSTOPERATIVE

Complications	PONV Bleeding Brain edema	PONV is common and usually requires multimodal treatment (see p. C-1). Major complications from this operation are uncommon, and postop recovery is usually uneventful. On rare occasion, significant brain edema or bleeding may be experienced.
Pain management	Codeine (30–60 mg im q 4 h)	
Tests	CT scan, if neurological recovery is delayed.	

Suggested Readings

1. Ashkan K, Marsh H: Microvascular decompression for trigeminal neuralgia in the elderly: a review of the safety and efficacy. *Neurosurgery* 2004; 55(4):840–8; discussion 848–50.
2. Cheshire WP: Trigeminal neuralgia: for one nerve a multitude of treatments. *Expert Rev Neurother* 2007; 7(11):1565–79.
3. Elias WJ, Burchiel KJ: Microvascular decompression. *Clin J Pain* 2002; 18(1):35–41.
4. Jannetta PJ: Supralateral exposure of the trigeminal nerve in the cerebellopontine angle for microvascular decompression. In *Brain Surgery: Complication, Avoidance and Management.* Apuzzo MLJ, ed. Churchill Livingstone, New York: 1993, 2085–96.
5. Lonser RR, Arthur AS, Apfelbaum RI: Neurovascular decompression in surgical disorders of cranial nerves V, VII, IX. In *Operative Neurosurgical Techniques: Indications, Methods, and Results.* Schmidek HA, Sweet WH, eds. WB Saunders, Philadelphia: 2000, 1576–88.
6. Meng L, Quinlan JJ: Assessing risk factors for postoperative nausea and vomiting: a retrospective study in patients undergoing retromastoid craniectomy with microvascular decompression of cranial nerves. *J Neurosurg Anesthesiol* 2006; 18(4):235–9.
7. Sheehan J, Pan HC, Stroila M, et al: Gamma Knife surgery for trigeminal neuralgia: outcomes and prognostic factors. *J Neurosurg* 2005; 102(3):434–41.

BIFRONTAL CRANIOTOMY FOR CSF LEAK

SURGICAL CONSIDERATIONS

Gordon T. Sakamoto, Lawrence M. Shuer, and Steven D. Chang

Description: Trauma (44% accidental; 29% surgical) is the leading cause of CSF leaks. CSF leaks can also be caused by tumors (22%), congenital malformations, or as a result of transsphenoidal surgery. Most CSF leaks involve the floor of the anterior cranial fossa (e.g., cribriform plate: 35%), with drainage through the auditory canal (otorrhea), nasopharynx (rhinorrhea), sinus air cells, or other less common routes. CSF leaks can occasionally stop on their own or by management with a lumbar drain. However, to lessen the risk of meningitis, surgical repair is the usual treatment.

The surgical repair of CSF leaks has changed with the advent of the endoscope. The success rates of endoscopic closure are similar to open surgical approaches while avoiding the morbidity associated with craniotomies. Although it is common to attempt closure of a CSF leak endoscopically before proceeding on to an open repair, selected patients may benefit by proceeding directly to an open surgical approach.

An open surgical repair is typically done through a bifrontal craniotomy. The patient is placed in a supine position, and the head is stabilized with a Mayfield clamp. A bicoronal skin incision (Fig. 1.1-14) is made, and the pericranium is often turned as a separate flap and kept moist during the case. Next, burr holes are drilled and a bifrontal free-bone flap is elevated. Care is taken to avoid injury to the underlying superior sagittal sinus. If the frontal sinuses are entered, the mucosa is stripped and the sinus is packed with antibiotic-soaked

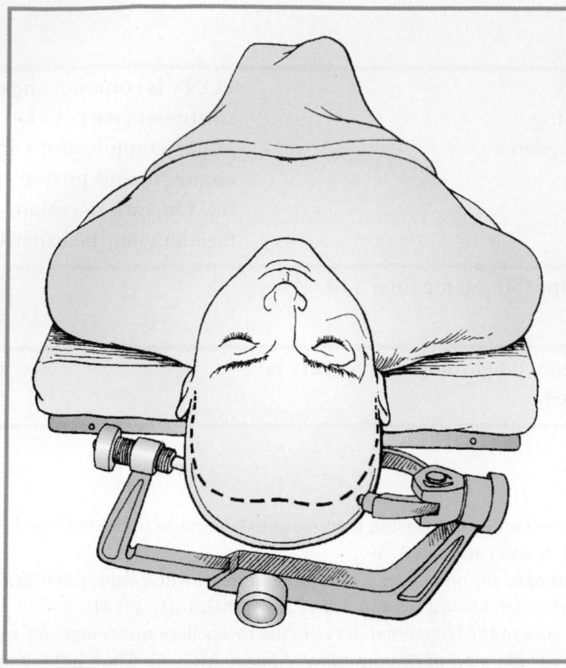

Figure 1.1-14. Patient positioning for bifrontal craniotomy with bicoronal skin incision outlined. This position allows the frontal lobes to separate from the anterior cranial fossa with minimal retraction on the frontal lobes. (Reproduced with permission from Tindall GT, Cooper PR, Barrow DL: *The Practice of Neurosurgery.* Williams & Wilkins, Philadelphia: 1996.)

Gelfoam. The dura is opened over the inferiomedial frontal lobes and the sagittal sinus is ligated. An intradural exploration is undertaken to determine the site of the leak. Identification of the leak site is essential for successful outcome. Brain relaxation is usually necessary to reduce the need for mechanical retraction, and may require mannitol, hyperventilation, and/or the placement of a lumbar drain. The frontal lobes are elevated, and the olfactory tracts may be sacrificed. If the site of the leak can be determined, the dural repair can be performed using fascia lata, pericranium, bovine pericardium, or a synthetic dural substitute. It usually is necessary to strip the dura off the anterior cranial fossa to complete the repair. Defects in the bone can be plugged with a variety of materials (e.g., pericranial flap, fat, muscle, bone, or wax). After the repair is complete, the dura can be closed and the bone flap replaced, often with a drain left in the epidural space. Additionally, tissue sealants such as fibrin glue can be sprayed over the dural suture line to help create a watertight seal. At this point, brain relaxation is no longer required. The wound is closed with stitches and skin is closed with staples.

A combined approach may be used for CSF leaks 2° to a tumor that invades the dura and the cribriform plate. In these cases, the procedure often is performed with an otorhinolaryngologist. The intracranial part of this procedure is identical to the bifrontal craniotomy, except that bone and tumor are removed at the floor of the anterior cranial fossa. The extracranial part of this procedure is performed by the otorhinolaryngologist, who approaches the sinonasal region endoscopically or through a lateral rhinotomy or degloving gingival incision. The extracranial approach is chosen to complement the cranial exposure and a common space is created between the two operative fields. Closure involves isolating the two operative fields once again. The dural repair is as above. The mucosa of the nasal cavity is replaced with the use of a skin graft.

Alternate Procedure: Transnasal endoscopic repair of selected CSF leaks has been shown to be effective with significantly ↓ morbidity compared with craniotomy.

Usual preop diagnosis: CSF leak or rhinorrhea; fracture of the anterior cranial fossa; intracranial encephalocele; cribriform plate tumor; olfactory neuroblastoma (tumor of the olfactory epithelium). β-2 transferrin is a relatively sensitive and specific marker for CSF and can be used to establish the diagnosis.

SUMMARY OF PROCEDURE	
Position	Supine
Incision	Bicoronal (Fig. 1.1-14); Transnasal for endoscopic
Special instrumentation	Operating microscope; endoscope; image-guidance system
Unique considerations	Brain relaxation desired; lumbar subarachnoid catheter; fascia lata graft
Antibiotics	Ceftriaxone 1–2 g iv q d (avoid Ca^{++} containing solutions)
Surgical time	2–3.5 h, depending on extent of leak or lesion
Closing considerations	Drain often left in epidural space. Anticipate that the application of a full head dressing will jostle patient and ETT →↑ BP + coughing/bucking.
EBL	75–500 mL
Postop care	ICU or close observation unit; Valsalva maneuver, coughing and vomiting can cause ↑↑↑ ICP → recurring CSF leak
Mortality	≤ 5%
Morbidity	Usually < 5% for all complications Infection (ascending meningitis) Recurrent CSF leak Neurologic disability Nerve injury Massive blood loss: venous sinus injury
Pain score	3–5

PATIENT POPULATION CHARACTERISTICS	
Age range	15–65 yr
Male:Female	~3:2
Incidence	Relatively uncommon neurosurgical procedure
Etiology	Traumatic (73%); congenital; neoplastic

ANESTHETIC CONSIDERATIONS

See Anesthetic Considerations following Transsphenoidal Resection of Pituitary Tumor, p. 54.

NB: Positive pressure mask ventilation in patient with an anterior CSF leak may produce severe pneumocephalus.

Suggested Readings

1. Abuabara A: Cerebrospinal fluid rhinorrhea: diagnosis and management. *Med Oral Patol Oral Cir Bucal* 2007; 12(5):E397–400.
2. Couldwell WT, Weiss MH: Cerebrospinal fluid fistulas. In *Brain Surgery: Complication, Avoidance and Management.* Apuzzo MLJ, ed. Churchill Livingstone, New York: 1993, 2329–42.
3. Kerr JT, Chu FWK, Bayles SW: Cerebrospinal Fluid Rhinorrhea: Diagnosis and Management. *Otolaryngol Clin North Am* 2005; 38(4):597–611.
4. Martin TJ, Loehrl TA: Endoscopic CSF leak repair. *Curr Opin Otolaryngol Head Neck Surg* 2007; 15(1):35–39.
5. Martin TJ, Loehrl TA: Endoscopic CSF leak repair. *Curr Opin Otolaryngol Head Neck Surg* 2007;15(1):35–9.
6. Osguthorpe J, Patel S: Craniofacial approaches to tumors of the anterior skull base. *Otolaryngol Clin North Am* 2001; 34(6):1123–42.

TRANSORAL APPROACH TO THE CERVICOMEDULLARY JUNCTION AND ODONTOID

SURGICAL CONSIDERATIONS

Gordon T. Sakamoto, Lawrence M. Shuer, and Steven D. Chang

Description: The transoral approach provides excellent access to the odontoid process of the C2 vertebral body, as well as the skull base just anterior to the brain stem (Fig. 1.1-15). This is important for conditions where there is pressure on the ventral brain stem or spinal cord → Sx: HA, impaired ambulation, hyperreflexia, paresthesias, neurogenic bladder, etc. Common indications for this approach include basilar impression (upward translocation of the odontoid process) (Fig. 1.1-16A); degeneration of the odontoid due to rheumatoid disease (Fig. 1.1-17A); fracture of

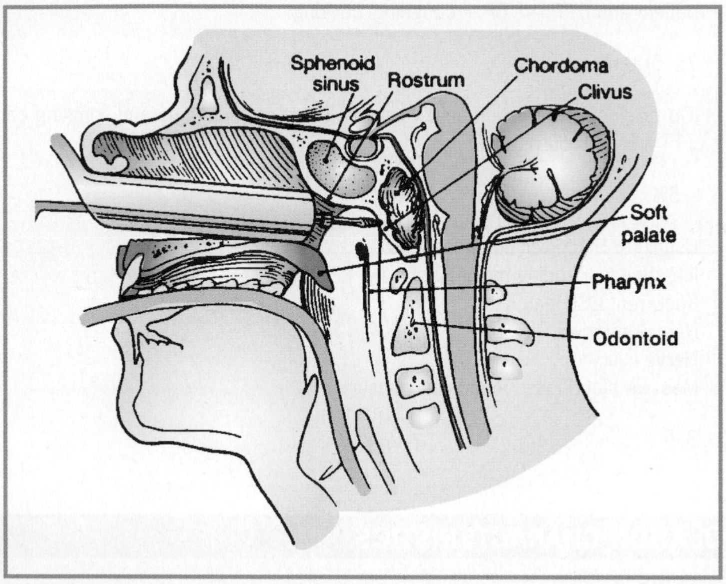

Figure 1.1-15. Inferior exposure of the clivus and chordoma. (Reproduced with permission from Grossman RG, Loftus CM: *Principles of Neurosurgery,* 2nd edition. Lippincott-Raven, Philadelphia: 1999.)

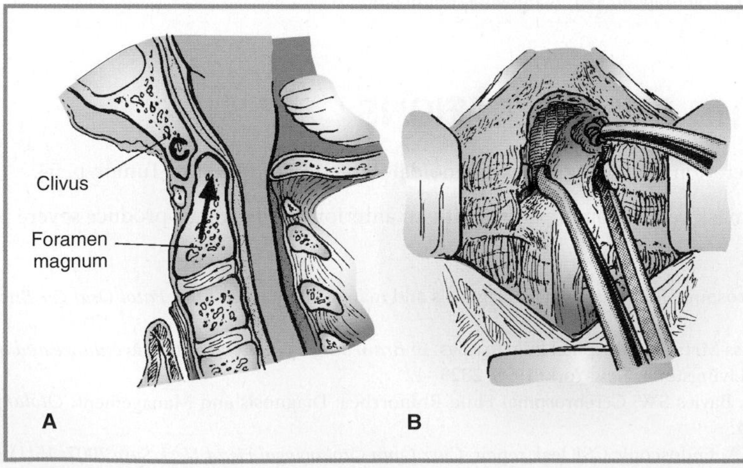

Figure 1.1-16. **A.** Basilar impression. The dens has moved superiorly into the foramen magnum (*arrow*). **B.** Removal of the dens with a drill. The arch of C1 and a portion of the clivus have been removed. (Reproduced with permission from Donald PJ: *Surgery of the Skull Base.* Lippincott-Raven, Philadelphia: 1998.)

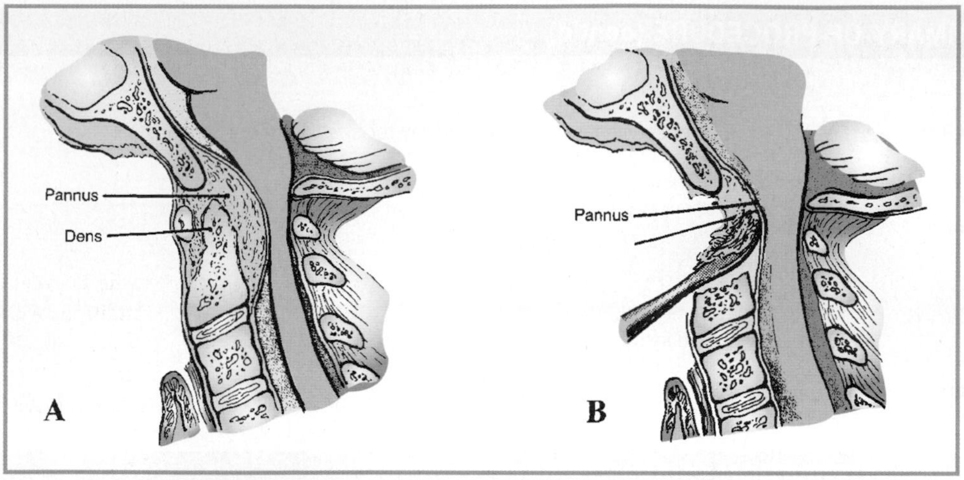

Figure 1.1-17. **A.** Pannus formation in a patient with rheumatoid arthritis. **B.** Removal of pannus. (Reproduced with permission from Donald PJ: *Surgery of the Skull Base.* Lippincott-Raven, Philadelphia: 1998.)

the odontoid, and resection of extradural tumors, such as chordomas and metastases. In these cases, the operation is performed through the oral cavity with an incision in the posterior wall of the pharynx. Special retractors hold the mouth open and keep the tongue out of the way. Fluoroscopic or image guidance helps the surgeon maintain proper trajectory. Intraop monitoring of evoked potentials (i.e., SSEP or BAER) and use of the operative microscope help avoid injury to the brain stem and spinal cord. The dissection is carried down to expose the anterior arch of C1 and body of C2. To decompress the region, the anterior arch of C1 and the odontoid process are removed. For basilar impression, a portion of the clivus may need to be removed to gain access to the dens (Fig. 1.1-16B). For rheumatoid arthritis, the pannus (thickened fibrous tissue) surrounding the dens is also removed (Fig. 1.1-17B). If an extradural tumor is found, it is resected in a piecemeal fashion. If a CSF leak occurs, the dura can be closed with fascia, muscle, fibrin glue, or thrombin-soaked Gelfoam. Upon completion of the decompression, the mucosa is closed. It may be necessary to fuse the occiput to the upper C-spine to correct any cervical instability. This may take place at the same time, or at a later date. C-spine precautions normally are used during and after the case. The patient may be in traction with tongs or a halter.

Variations in procedure: A fiber optic nasal intubation or tracheostomy may be necessary to gain adequate exposure and maintain ventilation. It also may be necessary to split the soft palate, hard palate, tongue, and/or mandible to obtain adequate exposure.

Usual preop diagnosis: Basilar impression (platybasia); odontoid fracture; rheumatoid arthritis with atlantoaxial instability and anterior impingement of the cord; chordoma; metastatic tumor

SUMMARY OF PROCEDURE

Position	Supine; head in traction or pins
Incision	Back of oropharynx
Special instrumentation	Operating microscope; I.I.; intraop monitoring = SSEP or BAER; micro drill; intraoral retractors for exposure; image-guided navigation system (optional)
Unique considerations	FOL may be necessary. ETT must be taped securely in a location satisfactory to surgeon. Anode or RAE tube may be helpful. Occasionally, a **tracheostomy** is performed in advance.
Antibiotics	Ceftriaxone 1g iv (avoid Ca^{++} containing solutions)
Surgical time	2.5–3 h
Closing considerations	Patient may remain intubated postop. C-spine precautions may be necessary.

SUMMARY OF PROCEDURE (cont'd)	
EBL	25–250 mL
Postop care	ICU or close observation unit; monitor airway for swelling (✓ for stridor).
Mortality	0–3%
Morbidity	All < 5%: Infection CSF leak Neurological Massive blood loss
Pain score	2–4

PATIENT POPULATION CHARACTERISTICS	
Age range	18–85 yr (usually 20–60 yr)
Male:Female	~1:2
Incidence	Rare
Etiology	Neoplastic; traumatic; congenital; degenerative
Associated conditions	Rheumatoid arthritis (atlantoaxial subluxation in 25%; basilar compression in 8%); traumatic injury

ANESTHETIC CONSIDERATIONS

See Anesthetic Considerations following Transsphenoidal Resection of Pituitary Tumor, p. 54.

Suggested Readings

1. Hadley MN, Spetzler RF, Sonntag VKH: The transoral approach to the superior cervical spine. *J Neurosurg* 1989; 71(1):16–23.
2. Vangilder JC, Menezes AH: Craniovertebral abnormalities and their neurosurgical management. In *Operative Neurosurgical Techniques: Indications, Methods, and Results.* Schmidek HA, Sweet WH, eds. WB Saunders, Philadelphia: 2000, 1934–45.

TRANSSPHENOIDAL RESECTION OF PITUITARY TUMOR

SURGICAL CONSIDERATIONS

Edward R. Laws, Gordon T. Sakamoto, Lawrence M. Shuer, and Steven D. Chang

Description: The transsphenoidal approach to the sella turcica is a direct procedure used to gain access to the pituitary gland and sella region and is associated with relatively fewer complications than a craniotomy. The procedure usually is performed transnasally; although a sublabial transeptal approach is out of favor it may be used in patients with large tumors. An otorhinolaryngologist may participate in obtaining the exposure, which typically involves creating a tunnel to the sphenoid sinus. Once the sphenoid sinus is reached, it is entered by removing the face and rostrum. The thin bone of the lateral wall of the sphenoid sinus protects portions of the optic nerve and carotid artery. The sella is entered by removing a portion of the sellar floor (Fig. 1.1-18A). Under image guidance and with the aid of the operating microscope and/or endoscope, the surgeon can operate safely upon the pituitary gland, respecting the midline and avoiding injury to the carotid arteries in the cavernous sinus on either side of the exposure. After the sellar floor is removed, the dura is opened and the tumor is removed with a series of microdissectors and curettes. Following tumor removal, if there is a CSF leak, the surgeon may harvest fat, muscle, or fascia from the thigh or abdomen to pack into the sella to reduce free intrasellar space and serve as a graft to prevent a leak (Fig. 1.1-18B). Resorbable materials, such as Gelfoam and fibrin glue, also may be used to obliterate dead space within the sella. The

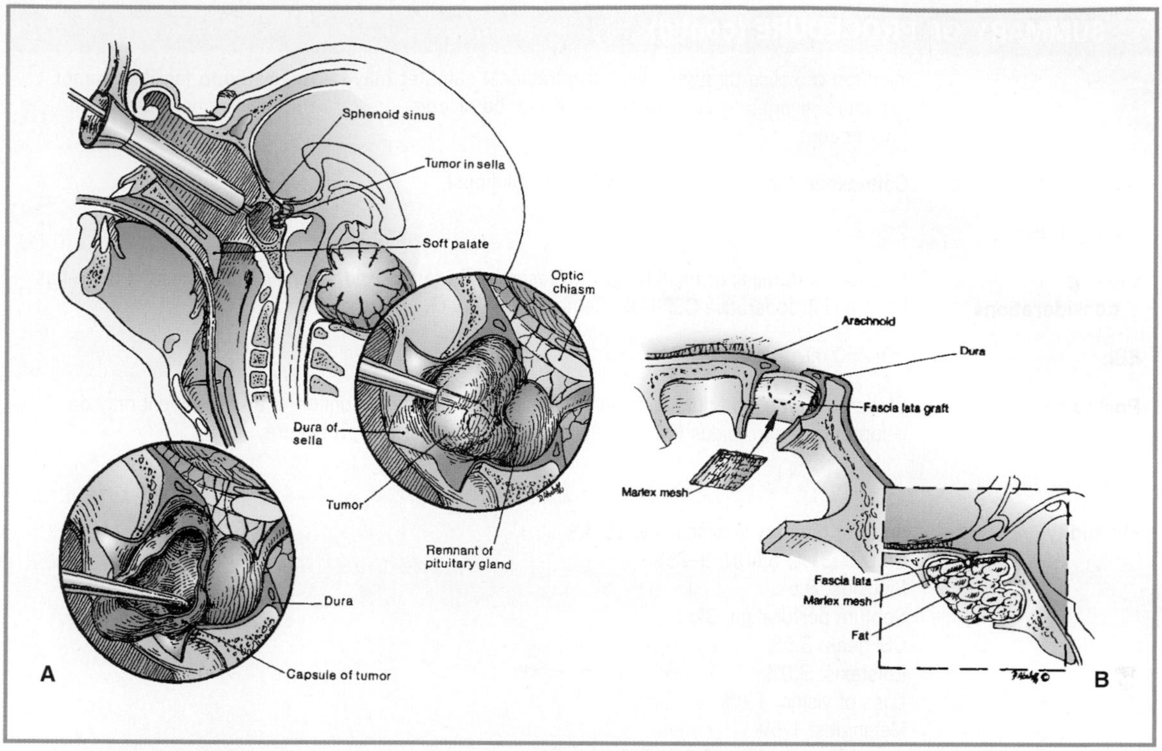

Figure 1.1-18. The transnasal/transsphenoidal removal of a pituitary tumor. **A.** The rostrum of the sphenoid is removed (*upper*). The floor of the sella is removed, the dura opened, and the tumor removed using microcurettes (*middle and lower*). **B.** Fat taken from the subcutaneous tissue at the time of the fascial resection is utilized to fill the sphenoid and hold the graft material in position. (Reproduced with permission from Grossman RG, Loftus CM: *Principles of Neurosurgery,* 2nd edition. Lippincott-Raven, Philadelphia: 1999.)

floor of the sella can be reconstructed with bone salvaged from the exposure or artificial material. During the closure, the sphenoid sinus also may be packed and sealed with the same materials used to close the sella. The nostrils may or may not be packed, depending on the details of the technique used.

Alternative Procedure: Endoscopic transsphenoidal approach has several advantages (improved surgical view and access, fewer complications and more rapid recovery).

Usual preop diagnoses: Pituitary tumor; prolactin-secreting tumor; growth hormone-secreting tumor (acromegaly); ACTH-secreting tumor (Cushing's disease); visual compromise, intrasellar tumor; craniopharyngioma; meningioma; Forbes-Albright syndrome (galactorrhea-amenorrhea syndrome)

SUMMARY OF PROCEDURE

Position	Supine, head elevated 20–30°
Incision	Endonasal; + abdomen (or thigh) for fat graft; occasionally sublabial, maxillary gingiva;
Special instrumentation	Operating microscope; operating endscope; micro drill; neuronavigation (image guidance) Throat packs may be used but are usually unnecessary.
Unique considerations	ETT must be taped securely in a location away from the surgeon (usually left side of mouth). Anode or RAE tube may be helpful but is not essential. The generous use of topical vasoconstrictors and the injection of epinephrine-containing solutions may →↑ BP and dysrhythmias. Dissection in the nasal cavity can be painful →↑ BP and ↑ ICP. There is a risk of VAE following inadvertent entry into the cavernous sinus. Valsalva maneuver, jugular compression, or

SUMMARY OF PROCEDURE (cont'd)

	injection of saline through a lumbar intrathecal catheter may be requested to facilitate tumor exposure. Injuries to sphenopalatine or carotid arteries are rare but may be dramatic when they occur.
Antibiotics	Ceftriaxone 1 g iv (avoid Ca^{++} containing solutions)
Surgical time	2.5–3 h
Closing considerations	Possible abdominal or thigh-fat graft. Closure quite fast. Avoid straining and bucking if there has been an intraoperative CSF leak. Remove throat pack before operation.
EBL	25–250 mL
Postop care	Close observation of fluid and electrolytes require frequent monitoring as the patient may develop diabetes insipidus (DI), usually transient, following this procedure.
Mortality	1%
Morbidity	Anterior pituitary insufficiency: 19.4% DI: 0.5–31%; SIADH: 9–25% Sinusitis: 8.5% Septum perforation: 3% CSF leak: 3.5% Epistaxis: 3.0% Loss of vision: 1.8% Meningitis: 1.5% Carotid artery injury: 1.1% stroke (rare) **Prolactin Secreting:** Few anesthetic implications beyond possible mass effect and ↑ ICP **ACTH Secreting:** HTN is very common and is often associated with diastolic dysfunction. OSA is common and may have implications for postop airway management. Hyperglycemia is common and should be treated if blood glucose > 180 mg/dL. ↑ cortisol → fragile skin and veins → difficult iv access. **Growth Hormone Secreting:** Hypertrophy of the mandible, tongue and other facial tissues is common and complicates airway management. Hoarseness suggests laryngeal stenosis or recurrent laryngeal nerve dysfunction. OSA is very common with its attendant risk of postop airway compromise. HTN and diastolic dysfunction (with a need for ↑ filling pressure) are very common. The incidence of intraop ventricular ectopy and SVT is higher in these patients. ECG changes (e.g., ST/T wave changes, conduction abnormality) are common. **Pituitary Apoplexy:** Acute hemorrhagic infarction of the pituitary → severe HA, shock, coma, death. Urgent surgical decompression required.
Pain score	2–4

PATIENT POPULATION CHARACTERISTICS

Age range	18–85 yr (usually 30–50 yr)
Male:Female	2:3 (microadenomas)
Incidence	16.7% (autopsy studies); 1.5/100,000/yr diagnosed
Etiology	Neoplastic; traumatic
Associated conditions	Cushing's disease (ACTH); acromegaly (GH); amenorrhea/galactorrhea (prolactin); hyperthyroidism (TSH); hypergonadotropism (FSH; LH); multiple endocrine neoplasia I

ANESTHETIC CONSIDERATIONS

(Procedures covered: bifrontal craniotomy for CSF leak; transoral approach to cervicomedullary junction, odontoid; transsphenoidal resection of pituitary tumor)

PREOPERATIVE

Endocrine	Tumors of the pituitary gland are either nonfunctional or secretory. If nonfunctional, they will produce Sx either by their mass effect on adjacent pituitary tissue, or because of extension outside of the sella turcica. Rarely, the mass effect may cause the clinical picture of panhypopituitarism requiring preop treatment with thyroxine, glucocorticoid, and vasopressin. Functional tumors commonly secrete prolactin (→ lactation), ACTH (→ adrenal hyperplasia), or growth hormone (→ acromegaly). Hyperprolactinemia may occur with any tumor 2° loss of inhibition of prolactin secretion. **Tests:** Preop endocrine studies, including serum and urinary levels of pituitary, thyroid, and adrenal hormones; appropriate replacement therapy established before proceeding with surgery. "Stress-dose" hydrocortisone (e.g., 100 mg iv q.8.h) is often unnecessary; treatment should be guided by symptoms and periop cortisol levels. Dexamethasone will not interfere with cortisol assays.
Respiratory	No special requirements, unless patient has acromegaly, in which case large facial features, long neck, large tongue, and redundant soft tissue in the oropharynx may make mask fit and ET intubation difficult. If these patients evidence hoarseness or inspiratory stridor, they should have a full clinical and radiological evaluation of the upper airway. **Tests:** As indicated from H&P.
Cardiovascular	No special requirements unless patient has acromegaly, in which case they may have HTN, ischemic heart disease, and diabetes. **Tests:** As indicated from H&P.
Neurological	Secretory tumors of the pituitary are usually small, confined to the sella, rarely cause ↑ ICP (2° direct tumor effects or by obstruction of 3rd ventricle), and commonly produce Sx of endocrine dysfunction early in their growth. In contrast, nonfunctional pituitary tumors may not produce Sx until they extend beyond the boundaries of the sella, causing HA's (the most common presenting symptom) or compression of the optic chiasm, producing visual field defects (temporal or bitemporal hemianopsia). **Tests:** A CT or MRI will delineate the site and size of the tumor, especially if iv contrast material, such as gadolinium, is administered to enhance the margins of the tumor.
Musculoskeletal	If growth hormone is the primary secretant, patient will exhibit Sx of acromegaly, including large hands, feet, head, and tongue. Cushing's myopathy (UE proximal muscle weakness) may affect apparent recovery from muscle relaxant. **Tests:** As indicated from H&P.
Laboratory	Metabolic panel, HCT, and others as indicated from H&P. ↓ Na^+ may indicate DI; ↑↑ Ca^{++} may indicate MEN I.
Premedication	If ↑ ICP is not a concern, patients may benefit from midazolam 1–2 mg iv. In patients with ↑ ICP consider pretreatment with mannitol (e.g., 0.25 gm/kg 20 min before induction). Acromegalic patients may develop airway obstruction following even small doses of sedatives or narcotics.

INTRAOPERATIVE

Anesthetic technique: GETA is required for this operation, since the surgical approach is through either the nose or the mouth above the maxillary gum line and behind the nose. A lumbar drain may be placed to permit intraop management of ICP and access to the tumor.

Induction	If a difficult intubation is anticipated (e.g., severe acromegalic patients), orotracheal intubation will need to be accomplished before induction of GA. LMA placement may be difficult and awake FOL is often the best choice (see p. B-5). Because pituitary tumors generally

Induction (cont'd)	are confined to the sella turcica and, hence, ICP usually is not increased, a standard induction technique with standard ETT is appropriate (see p. B-2). An oral RAE tube may be preferred by oral surgeons. If increased ICP is of concern, induction should be similar to that used for patients with other kinds of brain tumors (see Anesthetic Considerations for Craniotomy for Tumor, p. 31). Because the surgeon will be working from the patient's right side, the ETT must be positioned at the far left side of the mouth. The surgeon may infiltrate the nasal mucosa with lidocaine and epinephrine →↑ BP + dysrhythmias → possible myocardial ischemia.	
Maintenance	Standard maintenance with sevoflurane (or propofol infusion) supplemented with remifentanil (see p. 1539). Generally, no further NMBs are administered beyond ET intubation. With adequate anesthesia, and the head in Mayfield clamp, patient movement of any consequence is highly unlikely. Ventilation is controlled with $PaCO_2$ maintained in the normal range. Hyperventilation is not desirable, because it makes it more difficult to access the tumor in the sella and establish that it has been removed in its entirety. Following the resection, the surgeon may request a Valsalva maneuver to check for CSF leak.	
Emergence	If the patient evidences normal emergence from anesthesia, the ETT should be removed before vigorous coughing ensues. Before removing the ETT, however, make certain that all blood accumulated in the back of the throat is suctioned out, and that oropharyngeal packs which may have been placed in the back of the throat have been removed. An OG tube should be used to suction out the stomach. The surgeon may have packed the nose at the end of operation, forcing the patient to be an obligatory mouth breather. If there is any question about airway patency because of a large tongue, small mouth, or soft-tissue redundancy in the oropharynx, the ETT should be left in place until patient is fully awake from anesthesia. Prophylactic antiemetics (e.g., metoclopramide 20 mg and ondansetron 4 mg) should be given 30 min before extubation.	
Blood and fluid requirements	Minimal blood loss usual Potential large blood loss IV: 16–18 ga × 1 NS @ 4–8 mL/kg/h	Blood loss is minimal, unless the surgeon inadvertently enters the internal carotid artery or cavernous sinus. Additional iv access may be necessary.
Monitoring	Standard monitors (see p. B-1). ± Arterial line ± UO ± CVP line ± precordial Doppler	Monitor for VAE in semisitting position if > 30°. Ulnar artery flow may be compromised in acromegaly—document Alan test before placing radial artery catheter. CVP line should be placed in patients at significant risk for VAE or as medically indicated.
Positioning	✓ and pad pressure points. ✓ eyes. Shoulder roll Table turned 90–180°	The surgeon will use an operating microscope or endoscope, which means that the anesthesiologist will be positioned at the side or foot. Anesthetic hoses and intravascular lines must be long enough to be accessible.
Complications	Carotid injury VAE	Potential for large volume hemorrhage and intraop stroke. Deliberate hypotension may facilitate repair. Carotid compression may →↓ CBF → ischemia.

POSTOPERATIVE

Complications	Hypopituitarism Diabetes insipidus (24–48h postop) CSF leak SIADH Cranial nerve injury	Replacement therapy with steroids is necessary in hypopituitary patients until normal pituitary function returns. Occasionally, patients will develop DI postop → polyuria and ↓ urine specific gravity < 1.005. Rarely, this may occur in the PACU necessitating fluid replacement and/or DDAVP.

Pain management	Codeine (30–60 mg im q 4 h)	HA is the most common complaint.
Tests	CT scan Serum cortisol Visual acuity/fields	If a patient exhibits any delay in emergence from anesthesia and surgery, or any new neurologic deficits emerge postop, a CT scan is ordinarily obtained.

Suggested Readings

1. Burton CM, Nemergut EC: Anesthetic and critical care management of patients undergoing pituitary surgery. *Front Horm Res* 2006; 34:236–55.
2. Chan VWS, Tindal S: Anesthesia for transsphenoidal surgery in a patient with extreme giantism. *Br J Anaesth* 1998; 60:464–8.
3. Ciric I, Ragin B, Baumgartner C, et al: Complications of transsphenoidal surgery: Results of a national survey, review of the literature, and personal experience. *Neurosurgery* 1997; 40(2):225–36.
4. Elias JW, Laws ER Jr: Transsphenoidal approaches to lesions of the sella. In *Operative Neurosurgical Techniques: Indications, Methods, and Results.* Schmidek HA, Sweet WH, eds. WB Saunders, Philadelphia: 2000, 373–84.
5. Fahlbusch R, Honegger KR, Paulus W, et al: Surgical treatment of craniopharyngiomas: experience with 168 patients. *J Neurosurg* 1999; 90:237–50.
6. Lim M, Williams D, Maartens N: Anaesthesia for pituitary surgery. J Clin Neurosci 2006;13(4):413–8.
7. Nemergut EC, Dumont AS, Barry UT, et al: Perioperative management of patients undergoing transsphenoidal pituitary surgery. *Anesth Analg* 2005; 101(4):1170–81.
8. Semple PL, Laws ER: Complications in a contemporary series of patients who underwent transsphenoidal surgery for Cushing's Disease. *J Neurosurg* 1999; 91:175–9.
9. Sethi DS, Leong JL: Endoscopic pituitary surgery. *Otolaryngol Clin North Am* 2006;39(3):563–83.

VENTRICULAR SHUNT PROCEDURES

SURGICAL CONSIDERATIONS

Gordon T. Sakamoto, Lawrence M. Shuer, and Steven D. Chang

Description: Many conditions exist where it is necessary to shunt CSF from the ventricles to another body cavity where it can be absorbed readily. The most common condition is hydrocephalus, where there is dilation of the ventricular system due to an obstruction in the flow of CSF or decreased absorption of CSF by the arachnoid villi. Hydrocephalus is commonly treated by diverting CSF to the peritoneal cavity via a ventriculoperitoneal shunt (**VP shunt**). Most shunt systems have a one-way, pressure-dependent valve to regulate the flow of CSF. These valves usually have a preset pressure setting (e.g., low, medium, high) at which they open and allow CSF to flow. Newer valves have externally adjustable opening pressures, flow-regulating devices, and/or antisiphon systems to prevent overshunting. Additionally, antibiotic impregnated catheters can be used to reduce the risk of infection.

To insert a VP shunt, the patient is positioned so that the cranial incision and abdominal incision are aligned in the same plane. The scalp is shaved (usually over the frontal or parietal region), and a continuous surgical field is created from head to abdomen. The cranial incision is made over the intended region of cannulation of the ventricle, and a burr hole is made in the cranium. A subgaleal pocket is created for the valve, usually behind the ear. A separate incision is made in the abdomen, and the dissection is carried down to the level of the peritoneum. A catheter is then passed subcutaneously from the abdominal incision to the cranial incision with a special tunneling instrument (Fig. 1.1-20A). Alternatively, the catheter can be threaded from the cranial incision to the abdominal incision. It may be necessary to use one or more incisions between the head and the abdomen to thread the catheter. The valve is connected to the peritoneal catheter and placed in the subgaleal pocket. A ventricular catheter is then inserted into the ventricle (Fig. 1.1-20B) and a small amount of CSF is drained to check placement and patency of the catheter. The ventricular catheter is then connected to the valve, and CSF flow through the entire shunt system is checked by draining some CSF from the distal end of the peritoneal catheter. The distal end is then placed into the peritoneal cavity and all wounds are closed.

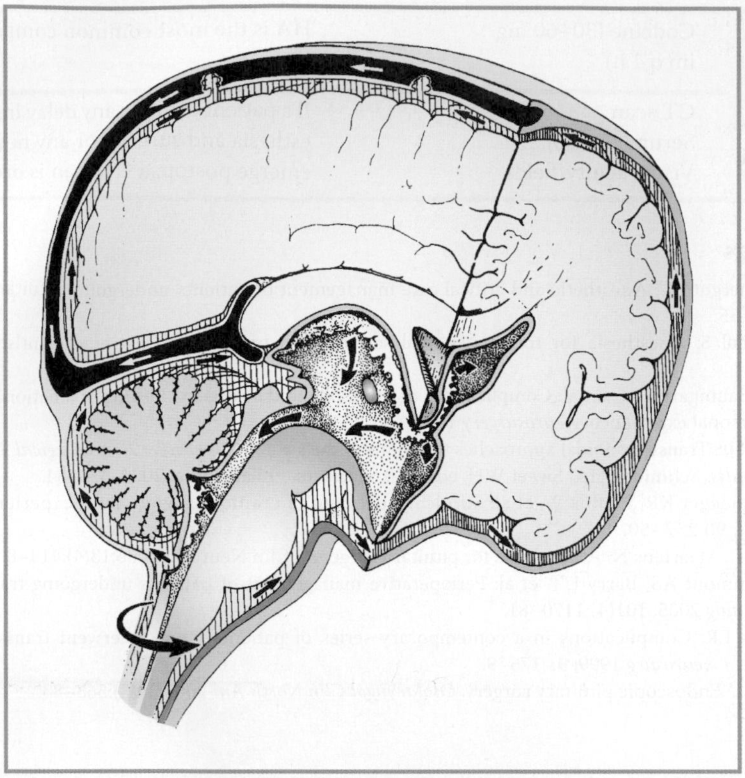

Figure 1.1-19. Pathways of CSF flow and potential sites of obstruction. (Reproduced with permission from Tindall GT, Cooper PR, Barrow DL: *The Practice of Neurosurgery,* Vol III. Williams & Wilkins, 1996. Orig. from Scott RM: *Hydrocephalus. Concepts in Neurosurgery,* Vol III. Williams & Wilkins, Philadelphia: 1990.)

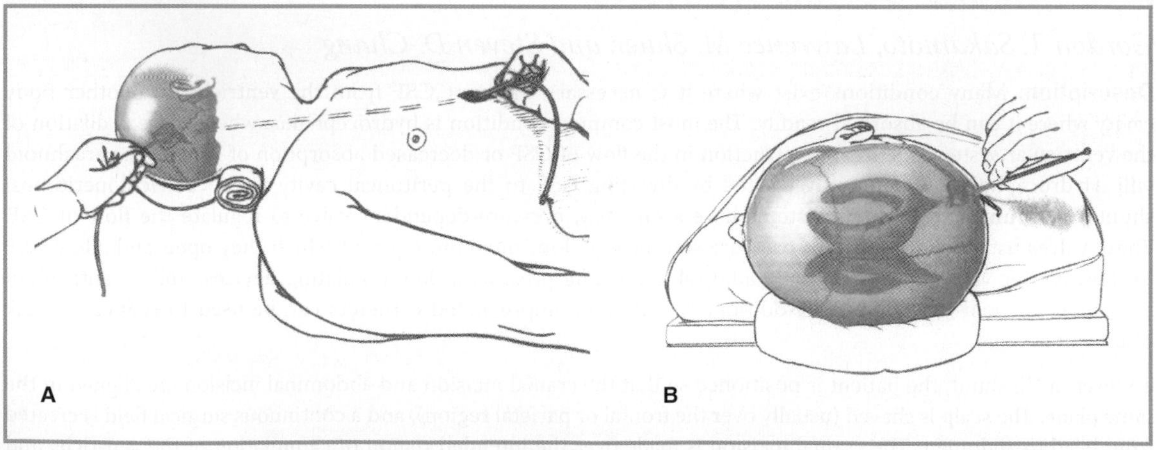

Figure 1.1-20. **A.** The catheter is threaded from the abdominal incision to the cranial incision. **B.** Insertion of the ventricular catheter. (Reproduced with permission from Meyer FB: *Atlas of Neurosurgery: Basic Approaches to Cranial and Vascular Procedures.* Churchill Livingstone, 1999).

Any component of the shunt may malfunction; thus, it may be necessary to test each component at the time of revision to identify the problem. To test the patency of the ventricular catheter, it is disconnected from the valve and CSF should flow freely through it. A saline-filled manometer can be attached to the valve to measure the opening pressure of the valve. The manometer should drain spontaneously until the opening pressure of the valve is reached. An elevated opening pressure may indicate a valve malfunction or a distal occlusion. If a distal occlusion is suspected, gentle irrigation may clear it, but externalization may be necessary.

Variant procedure or approaches: Endoscopy, fluoroscopy, ultrasound, image-guided navigation, or intraoperative MRI may be used to help place the catheter into the ventricle. The ventricular catheter can be placed in either lateral ventricle; occasionally, both lateral ventricles are cannulated. This procedure also is used to shunt the 4th ventricle and sometimes, subarachnoid cysts and subdural hygromas. The distal end alternatively may be placed in the pleural cavity or the right atrium (ventriculoatrial or **VA shunt**). If the distal end of the catheter is placed into the pleural cavity, a Valsalva maneuver is performed upon closure to reinflate the lung. To place the distal end into the atrium, a vein is cannulated in the neck (usually IJ, EJ, or facial vein), and the catheter is fed into the atrium under fluoroscopic guidance. It may be necessary to inject radiopaque contrast to verify proper placement. Rarely, the distal end of the catheter can be placed in an intracranial venous sinus, the gallbladder, or the ureter.

Endoscopic Third Ventriculostomy (ETV): Endoscopic third ventriculostomy is being used with increasing frequency to treat both obstructive and communicating forms of hydrocephalus. Head fixation is generally not needed and the procedure involves a small skin incision over the frontoparietal lobe to gain access to the skull. A small burr hole is then made. The dura is opened over the burr hole, permitting the insertion of the endoscope into the lateral ventricle. Under endoscopic guidance, the tuber cinereum is then fenestrated with a balloon tip catheter. CSF is diverted through the membranous floor of 3rd ventricle into the basal cisterns. The endoscope is then removed and the wound is closed.

Usual preop diagnosis: Hydrocephalus; obstructive or communicating hydrocephalus; aqueductal stenosis; Dandy-Walker malformation (cystic dilation of the 4th ventricle and incomplete formation of the cerebellar vermis); occult hydrocephalus; normal-pressure hydrocephalus; subarachnoid cyst; subdural hygroma; pseudotumor cerebri.

SUMMARY OF PROCEDURES

	VP Shunt	VA Shunt	ETV
Position	Supine, with head turned to contralateral side	⇐	
Incision	Scalp, either coronal and retroauricular, or parietal; + neck and abdomen	Scalp, either coronal and retroauricular or parietal; + neck	
Special instrumentation	Ventricular endoscope (optional)	⇐ + I.I.	
Unique considerations	Patient to be treated as if there is ↑ ICP.	⇐	
Antibiotics	Ceftriaxone 1–2 g iv q d (avoid Ca^{++} containing solutions)	⇐	
Surgical time	1 h	⇐	
EBL	5–25 mL	⇐	
Postop care	PACU → room; usually kept flat for 24 h.	⇐	
Mortality	< 1%	⇐	
Morbidity	Infection: < 15% Neurological: Intracranial bleed: < 1% Subdural hematoma: < 1% Hardware failure: < 1%	⇐	Basilar artery injury ↑↑ ICP →↓↓ HR or asystole
Pain score	4–6	2–4	

PATIENT POPULATION CHARACTERISTICS

Age range	Newborn-elderly
Male:Female	1:1
Incidence	Common
Etiology	Congenital (3–4/1000 live births); acquired; neoplastic; infectious; posthemorrhagic
Associated conditions	Subarachnoid hemorrhage; myelodysplasia; spina bifida (95% incidence); intraventricular hemorrhage; intraventricular tumor

ANESTHETIC CONSIDERATIONS

PREOPERATIVE

Ventricular shunts are inserted to ameliorate hydrocephalus or cyst formation, which may be either congenital or acquired.

Cardiovascular	↑ ICP →↑ BP + ↓↓ HR (Cushing's response) **Tests:** As indicated from H&P.
Neurological	The most common presenting Sx is HA. If hydrocephalus is severe, Sx of ↑ ICP (> 15 mmHg) (e.g., N/V, drowsiness, papilledema, Sz, and focal neurological defects) develop.
Laboratory	Tests as indicated by H&P.
Premedication	Usually not required; should be avoided in patients with ↑ ICP.

INTRAOPERATIVE

Anesthetic technique: GETA

Induction	If ↑ ICP, iv induction with STP (2–5 mg/kg) or propofol (1–2 mg/kg) is preferred, because of their ability to decrease cerebral blood volume and, hence, to decrease ICP. ET intubation is accomplished with the use of a NMB (e.g., vecuronium [0.1 mg/kg]; or rocuronium [0.6–1 mg/kg]).	
Maintenance	Isoflurane ≤ 1% or sevoflurane < 2%, inspired with 50:50 N_2O/O_2 mixture. Depending on duration of operation, additional doses of vecuronium (0.1 mg/kg) or rocuronium (0.2 mg/kg) may be needed. Maintain normal temperature in children by keeping OR warm (78F) and using a forced-air warming blanket. Ventilation should be controlled. TV and frequency should be adjusted such that the $PetCO_2$ = 35–40 mmHg. Hyperventilation and hypocarbia are undesirable because they make cannulation of the ventricle(s) more difficult. Maintain normotension. During endoscopic 3rd ventriculostomy (ETV), puncture of the floor of the 3rd ventricle may be associated with significant ↓↓ HR or asystole. The surgeon should be immediately informed if bradycardia occurs.	
Emergence	ETT is removed at the conclusion of the anesthetic. Prophylactic antiemetic (e.g., metoclopramide 10–20 mg and ondansetron 4 mg) should be given 30 min before extubation.	
Blood and fluid requirements	IV: 18–20 ga × 1 NS @ 4–6 mL/kg/h	Administer crystalloid, usually NS. Blood is rarely, if ever, necessary.
Monitoring	Standard monitors (see p. B-1).	Invasive monitors as indicated
Positioning	Table turned 180° ✓ and pad pressure points. ✓ eyes.	Supine with a bolster under the shoulder on the operative side. The head, chest, and abdomen are prepped, so all anesthesia equipment and lines must be at the sides of the patient.

Complications	Valve malfunction	Major intraop complications from this operation are rare.
	↓↓ HR or asystole Basilar artery injury	ETV may be associated with severe bradycardia and injury to the basilar artery or its branches.

POSTOPERATIVE

Pain management	Children < 2 yr: Tylenol suppositories (10–15 mg/kg q 4 h) Adults: meperidine 10–20 mg iv prn

Suggested Readings

1. Aryan HE, Meltzer HS, Park MS, et al: Initial experience with antibiotic impregnated silicone catheters for shunting of cerebrospinal fluid in children. *Child's Nerv Syst* 2005; 21(1):56–61.
2. Drake JM, Iantosca MR: Current systems for cerebrospinal fluid shunting and management of pediatric hydrocephalus: Endoscopic and image-guided surgery in hydrocephalus. In *Operative Neurosurgical Techniques: Indications, Methods, and Results.* Schmidek HA, Sweet WH, eds. WB Saunders, Philadelphia: 2000, 573–94.
3. Drake JM, Kestle JRW, Tuli S: CSF shunts 50 years on past, present and future. *Childs Nerv Syst* 2000;16:800–4.
4. Drake JM, Sainte-Rose C: *The Shunt Book.* Blackwell Scientific, New York: 1995.
5. Woodworth GF, McGirt MJ, Elfert P, et al: Frameless stereotactic ventricular shunt placement for idiopathic intracranial hypertension. *Stereotact Funct Neurosurg* 2005; 83(1):12–6.
6. Wu Y, Green NL, Wrensch MR, et al: Ventriculoperitoneal shunt complications in California: 1990–2000. *Neurosurgery* 2007; 61(3):557–562.

CRANIOCERVICAL DECOMPRESSION (CHIARI MALFORMATION)

SURGICAL CONSIDERATIONS

Gordon T. Sakamoto, Lawrence M. Shuer, and Steven D. Chang

Description: Historically, congenital hindbrain abnormalities characterized by cerebellar descent were known collectively as **Arnold-Chiari malformations**; now they are known as **Chiari malformations**. In these abnormalities, portions of the cerebellum protrude through the foramen magnum and may compress the brain stem and upper cervical spinal cord. Frequently, the malformation is accompanied by **syringomyelia**, a condition in which CSF is located abnormally within the spinal cord. In **Type I Chiari** malformation, the cerebellar tonsils are herniated through the foramen magnum. In **Type II Chiari** malformation, the tonsils, vermis, 4th ventricle, pons, and medulla are displaced caudally through the foramen magnum. Type II Chiari malformations are usually found in infants and are associated with myelomeningoceles. In **Type III Chiari** malformations there is a defect in the back of the head or neck through which the cerebellum and/or brainstem is herniated. Patients with **Type IV Chiari** malformations usually do not survive past infancy.

In order to make room for the brainstem and caudally displaced cerebellum, decompression of the craniocervical junction is necessary. This procedure may be performed in either the prone, 3/4 prone, or seated position. The head is placed in Mayfield pin fixation. A midline incision is made, and the dissection is carried down to the skull and the posterior arch of C1. Paramedian burr holes are placed to aid in the suboccipital craniectomy. The craniotome is then used to remove an approximately 4 cm by 3 cm bone flap that includes the foramen magnum. Care is taken to avoid injury to the underlying venous sinuses when performing the craniectomy.

The posterior arch of C1 is removed and as many upper cervical lamina as are needed to fully decompress the Chiari malformation are removed. Next, any constricting fibrous bands are cut and the dura is opened. Any subarachnoid adhesions should be lysed to allow the free flow of CSF. The tonsils are dissected apart under microscopic guidance

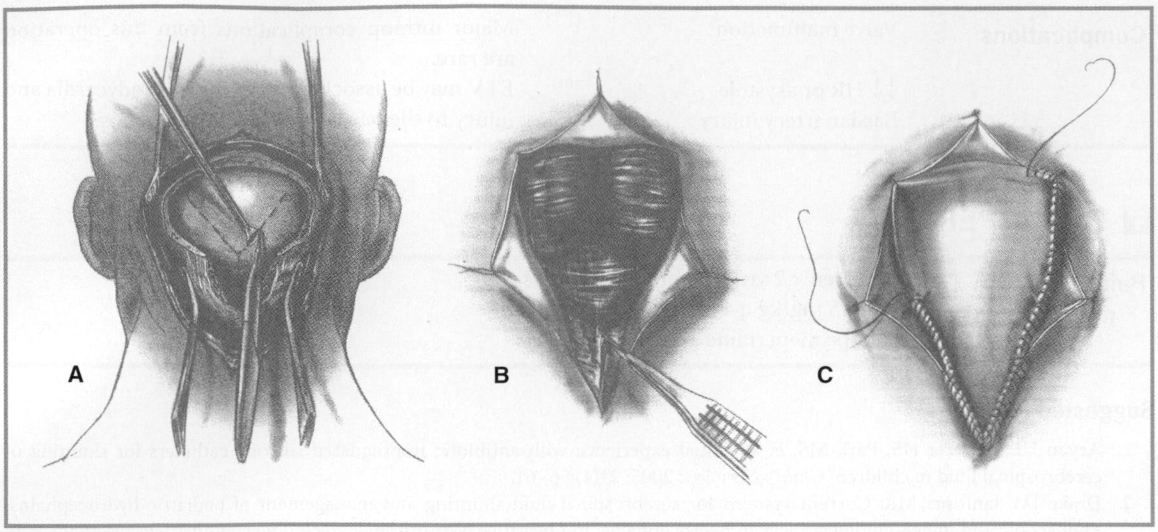

Figure 1.1-21. **A.** A Y-shaped dural incision is made through the occipital craniectomy and laminectomy. **B.** Opening the arachnoid mater to gain access to the cerebellar tonsils and fourth ventricle. **C.** Loose closure of dura with graft. (Reproduced with permission from Meyer F: *Atlas of Neurosurgery: Basic Approaches to Cranial and Vascular Procedures.* Churchill Livingstone, 1999.)

to gain an opening to the 4th ventricle (Figure 1.1-21A,B). The cerebellar tonsils can be reduced with electrocautery or by resection in order to facilitate the outflow of CSF from the 4th ventricle. A stent or a shunt may be placed in the 4th ventricle and brought out to the subarachnoid space to ensure adequate drainage of the 4th ventricle. The dura is closed loosely with autologous pericranium, fascia lata, or bovine pericardium (Fig. 1.1-21C). This creates a widely patent cisterna magna and prevents constriction at the cervicomedullary junction.

Usual preop diagnosis: Chiari Malformation I or II, Arnold-Chiari malformation; syringomyelia

SUMMARY OF PROCEDURE

Position	Prone or sitting
Incision	Midline posterior, posterolateral thigh for fascia lata graft (optional)
Special instrumentation	Operating microscope
Unique considerations	Risk of air embolus; brain stem manipulation can cause BP and pulse instability; dural patch used to expand dura at foramen magnum
Antibiotics	Ceftriaxone 1–2 g iv q d (avoid Ca^{++} containing solutions)
Surgical time	2.5–3.5 h
Closing considerations	BP control to ensure adequate hemostasis
EBL	25–250 mL
Postop care	ICU or constant observation unit; neurological function monitored.
Mortality	0–3% (usually respiratory arrest)
Morbidity	Respiratory depression: 14% up to 5 d postop All others < 5%: Infection Neurological: dysphagia and ↓ gag reflex

SUMMARY OF PROCEDURE (cont'd)	
	Aseptic meningitis CSF leak Massive blood loss; vertebral artery or transverse sinus injury
Pain score	5–7

PATIENT POPULATION CHARACTERISTICS	
Age range	Infant–70 yr; Chiari I: average age = 41 yr
Male:Female	~1:1
Incidence	Relatively rare neurosurgical procedure
Etiology	Congenital; acquired, S/P lumboperitoneal shunting
Associated conditions	Hydrocephalus; syringomyelia; scoliosis; myelodysplasia

ANESTHETIC CONSIDERATIONS

See Anesthetic Considerations for Cervical Neurosurgical Procedures, p. 106.

Suggested Readings

1. Hankinson TC, Klimo P Jr, Feldstein NA, et al. Chiari malformations, syringohydromyelia and scoliosis. *Neurosurg Clin N Am* 2007; 18(3):549–68.
2. Klekamp J, Batzdorf U, Samii M, et al: The surgical treatment of Chiari I malformation. *Acta Neurochir* 1996; 138:788–801.
3. Rhoton AL: Microsurgery of syringomyelia and the syringomyelia-Chiari complex. In *Operative Neurosurgical Techniques: Indications, Methods, and Results.* Schmidek HA, Sweet WH, eds. WB Saunders, Philadelphia: 2000, 1955–69.

STEREOTACTIC NEUROSURGERY

SURGICAL CONSIDERATIONS

Steven D. Chang and John R. Adler

Description: Stereotaxis applies simple rules of geometry to radiographic images to allow precise localization within the brain. Such techniques can be applied to a variety of neurosurgical procedures, providing up to 1-mm accuracy. This precision makes it possible to perform certain intracranial procedures less invasively. Methods include both frame-based and frameless navigation systems, as well as specific stereotactic applications for functional neurosurgery and radiosurgery.

Frame-based stereotaxy: Stereotactic localization was developed using frames; however, with the widespread use of image-guided, 'frameless' stereotactic systems, frame-based stereotaxy is rarely used. These procedures begin with the attachment of a frame to the patient's head using four screws that anchor it to the skull. This is typically done outside the OR, using local anesthetic and, sometimes, light sedation. In the cooperative adult, frame application takes only 5–10 min; however, GA typically is used for children. Once the frame is in place, access to the patient's airway is restricted. A key for emergency removal of the frame must be kept with the patient at all times. With the stereotactic frame in place, CT, MRI, and/or cerebral angiography are used for target identification and localization. During imaging, a set of fiducials (radiographically visible markers) is attached to the frame. These fiducials provide the geometric reference points needed for localization. Data from imaging studies are used to calculate the spatial coordinates of the target(s). In nearly all cooperative patients, there is no need for sedation or analgesia during this stage of the procedure.

Frame-based stereotaxy is used most frequently for brain biopsies; however, drainage of cystic lesions or placement of a catheter or depth electrodes also can be performed. These common procedures involve relatively minor surgery, usually requiring only light sedation and local anesthesia. After prepping and draping, specialized operating tools are attached to the stereotactic frame. These instruments provide spatial guidance throughout the surgical procedure. A burr or twist drill hole is the usual form of intracranial access. Maximal sedation is needed during drilling and dural opening. Anesthetic considerations include ensuring adequate oxygenation and ventilation, which may be compromised by the sterile drapes. Additionally, sedation should be light enough at times to allow the neurosurgeon to test gross neurologic function, such as extremity movement, both during and immediately after biopsy. At the completion of the case, the frame is removed and the patient is brought to the recovery room.

Image-guided "frameless" stereotaxy: Over the last several years, techniques have been developed to provide neurosurgeons with a real-time computer display of position and trajectory. Spatial information is displayed on high-speed computer work stations as two-dimensional images and three-dimensional renderings obtained from CT and/or MRI. These devices have the added advantage of being frameless; instead of a frame providing a system of reference, small markers (fiducials) are affixed to the scalp and forehead with adhesive. Advances in image-guided navigation also allow the incorporation of ultrasound and endoscopy to provide intraoperative updating of the preoperative radiographic images.

Image-guided surgery begins with an imaging study performed with fiducials in place. The remainder of the case is performed in the OR, usually under GA. After the patient's head is appropriately fixed and positioned, the locations of the fiducials are entered into a computer, using any one of several different commercially available digitizing techniques. The most common system uses triangulation of infrared light from LEDs to determine the position of a pointer in space. The computer calculates the position of the pointer with respect to the patient and displays on the monitor the images from the scan with a representation of the pointer superimposed. Because the process of localization assumes a constant frame of reference, it is important that fiducials do not move between the time of imaging and registration in the OR. A further refinement, the dynamic reference frame, may be affixed to the craniotomy headrest to allow intraoperative repositioning of the patient. The OR must be set up to accommodate the computer and monitor as well as to allow a direct line-of-sight between the operative site and an array of infrared sensors. (See Fig. 1.1-22.) Care must be taken to avoid patient movement during the initial registration of the fiducials, because this induces a component of error with respect to the accuracy of the navigation system. The camera system can be repositioned during the case and still maintain accuracy.

The spatial information provided to neurosurgeons by image guidance can be used to access deep or critically located lesions through the most direct trajectory and a smaller craniotomy. These techniques have been used primarily during craniotomy for tumor or vascular malformation; however, image guidance also can be used for brain biopsy,

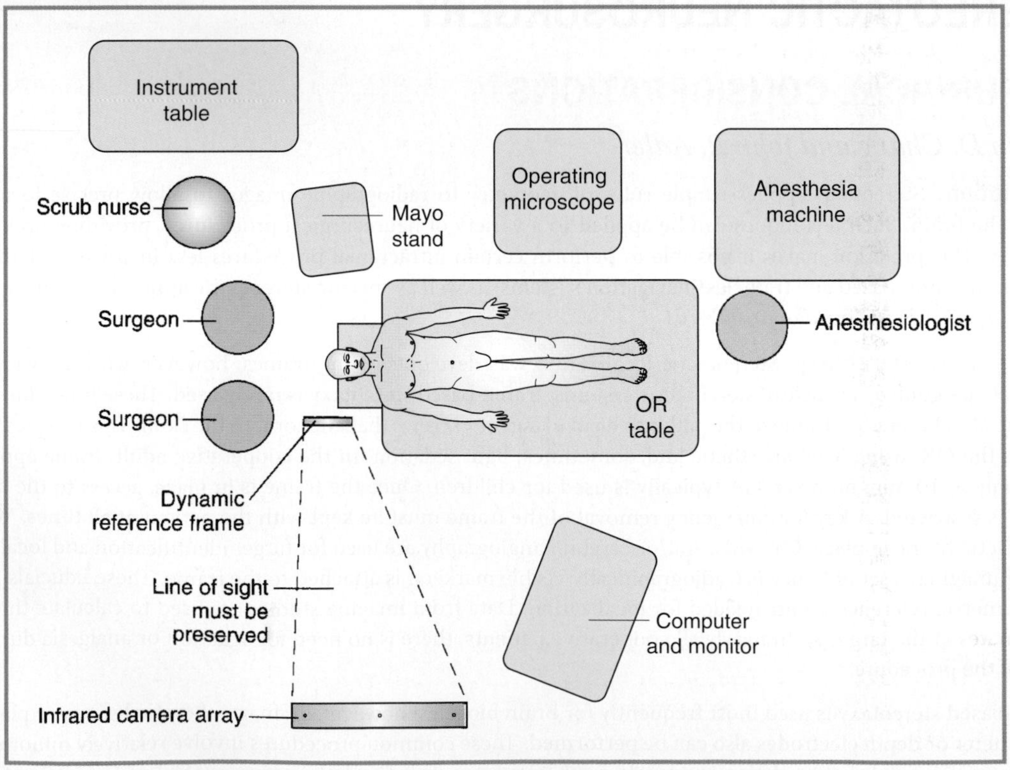

Figure 1.1-22. OR layout for frameless stereotactic surgery.

shunt placement, cyst drainage or other smaller procedures. As with most craniotomies, GA is used. Maneuvers that alter the spatial relationship of the intracranial contents, such as hyperventilation, diuresis or CSF drainage, will result in brain shift relative to the presurgical images and should be avoided if possible, particularly during the early stages of surgery.

Radiosurgery: This technique uses focused radiation to ablate small or residual tumors and vascular malformations. It can also be used to treat some pain, psychiatric and movement disorders. In contrast to other stereotactic operations, radiosurgery is performed outside the OR, using a linear accelerator or other specialized irradiation device. Cooperative adults need little or no sedation during the procedure. Children, however, almost always require GA from the beginning of frame placement through the actual treatment, which may last from 5–8 h. Consequently, anesthesia must be administered at several locations in the hospital, as well as during transport between these sites. Ideally, GA is initiated in the imaging suite just prior to frame placement. After transport to the recovery unit, the child is maintained under anesthesia while radiosurgical treatment is being planned, which takes from 1–3 h. The patient is then transported to the radiosurgery suite, still anesthetized, and treatment is performed. Depending on complexity, radiosurgery itself may last from 1–2 h. At the completion of treatment, the stereotaxic frame is removed and the child is awakened.

Newer, frameless radiosurgical systems can obviate the need for GA and most children can be set up and treated with iv sedation alone. However, the set-up and treatment are usually performed on different days and the child can go home while the treatment plan is created. These systems also allow for fractionation of the total dose, which may spare damage to surrounding critical structures.

Functional Neurosurgery: (See p. 70 for additional discussion of these procedures) Surgery using precisely placed lesions (e.g., **pallidotomy**, **thalamotomy**) or deep-brain stimulators for the treatment of movement disorders, pain, and certain psychiatric syndromes are encompassed by the term "**functional stereotaxy**." These techniques depend on absolutely precise localization of specialized instruments. These surgeries traditionally have required the use of a stereotactic frame. However, advances in imaging and image-guided navigation have obviated the need for a stereotactic frame. Concurrent neuroanatomic localization using electrophysiologic techniques is routinely used, regardless of the stereotactic system employed. In order to preserve neural potentials and allow the patient to cooperate with neurologic testing, GA is not used. Frameless procedures begin with placement of the fiducials (small screws) and imaging. Typically the fiducials are implanted in the patient's skull using local anesthetic and a special screwdriver. Then the patient undergoes a CT scan, which is uploaded into the image-guided navigation system. The surgeon can then plan the trajectory in the computer. In the OR, the patient's head is placed in Mayfield pins, and the imaged-guided navigation system is set up and the fiducials are registered. A small skin incision is made, and a burr hole is placed with the patient under iv sedation. The patient is then awakened and must remain awake and cooperative throughout a several-hour procedure, which may require patient participation in various neurologic tests. The recording electrodes are positioned using the image-guided navigation system and the electrophysiologic monitoring. After the proper electrophysiologic position is obtained, the recording electrode is removed and the deep brain stimulator is placed in the exact same position and depth. After the deep-brain stimulator is placed, a subgaleal pocket may be created to house the leads until they can be connected to the pulse generator. Frame based procedures begin with the attachment of a rigid frame to the patient's skull with local anesthesia. The stereotactic frame provides an immobile reference which aids in targeting. The remainder of the procedure is similar to the frameless procedure previously described.

Usual preop diagnosis: Brain disease requiring biopsy; brain tumor; vascular malformation; Parkinson's disease; hydrocephalus; pseudotumor cerebri; pain syndromes; psychiatric syndromes; cyst drainage

SUMMARY OF PROCEDURES

	Frame-Based Stereotaxy	Frameless Stereotaxy	Radiosurgery	Functional Neurosurgery
Position	Supine or prone	Sitting, supine, prone, or lateral	Supine or prone	Supine, head fixed to floor stand
Incision	0.5–2 cm, scalp	1–12 cm, scalp	None	1–3 cm, scalp
Special instrumentation	Stereotactic treatment arc	Sensor array, pointer, computer, monitor, dynamic reference frame	Linear accelerator (LINAC) Cyberknife	Electrophysiologic monitoring equipment, image-guided navigation, C-arm

SUMMARY OF PROCEDURES (cont'd)

	Frame-Based Biopsy	Frameless Craniotomy	Pediatric Radiosurgery	Functional Neurosurgery
Unique considerations	Key for emergency: removal of frame	1. Minimize brain shift. 2. No patient movement during registration. 3. Clear line-of-sight between camera and dynamic reference frame.	Extended anesthesia in several different locations	Patient must be awake, able to cooperate with testing.
Antibiotics	Ceftriaxone 1g iv (avoid Ca++ containing solutions)	Ceftriaxone 1g iv (avoid Ca^{++} containing solutions)	None	Ceftriaxone 1g iv (avoid Ca++ containing solutions)
Surgical time	0.5–1.5 h	2–6 h	5–8 h	2–6 h
EBL	< 10 mL	20–1000 mL	None	< 100 mL
Postop care	PACU	ICU	PACU	Neuroobservation unit
Mortality	< 0.5%	1%	None	< 1%
Morbidity	Overall: < 1% Symptomatic intracerebral hemorrhage	Infection Air emboli Hemorrhage Stroke Sz Worsening edema	N/V: 2–3%	N/V: 1–10% Intracerebral hemorrhage New neurologic deficits
Pain score	2	4	2	2

PATIENT POPULATION CHARACTERISTICS

Age range	All ages	⇐	0–12 yr	18–90 yr
Male:Female	1:1	⇐	⇐	⇐
Incidence	Uncommon	Unusual	⇐	Rare
Etiology	Tumor; infection; AIDS; demyelinating syndromes	Tumor; vascular malformations; epilepsy	⇐	Parkinson's disease; pain syndromes; psychiatric syndromes

ANESTHETIC CONSIDERATIONS

PREOPERATIVE

Neurosurgical procedures are performed using stereotactic control when the lesion is small and/or is located deep within brain tissue, or as a means of obtaining a biopsy of a lesion for diagnosis. For example, focal, deep-seated AVMs may be resected under stereotactic, or image-guided, control. These patients are often otherwise healthy.

Neurological	Neurological Sx vary (depending on site and size of the lesion) and they should be carefully documented. In addition to the usual tests, a CT or MRI scan is obtained preop with the frame in place to determine stereotactic coordinates. Once the coordinates are established, the frame or fiducial markers must not be moved until the operation is complete.
Laboratory	Tests as indicated from H&P.

INTRAOPERATIVE

Anesthetic technique: GETA or MAC. In adults, fiducial markers or a stereotactic frame are placed before surgery and the patient is taken to the radiologic suite for CT/MRI scan to determine stereotactic coordinates. The patient is then brought to OR with the frame or fiducial markers in place. The key for removing the stereotactic frame must be readily available in the event of an airway emergency. Biopsies generally are done under local anesthesia with MAC. If a complete resection is planned (e.g., AVM resection), GETA is used. In children, it is usually necessary to induce GA before placing the frame, thus necessitating the maintenance of GA during the CT/MRI scan. The child is then moved to the OR, still anesthetized, and the operation is completed.

Induction	If MAC is planned, O_2 by nasal prongs is administered, and the patient is lightly sedated with combinations of propofol 25–50 mcg/kg/min ± midazolam 1–4 mg/kg in divided doses to provide amnesia ± remifentanil 0.02–0.05 mcg/kg/min to provide analgesia. It is important that the patient be able to communicate with the surgeon as needed throughout the operation. For functional neurosurgery (e.g., pallidotomy), sedation should be minimized to preserve normal electrophysiological activity essential for mapping. If GETA is needed in a framed stereotactic procedure, FOL is necessary before inducing anesthesia because the frame precludes intubation by direct laryngoscopy (see p. B-5). After ET intubation is established, anesthesia may be induced with STP 2–5 mg/kg or propofol 1–2 mg/kg, followed by a nondepolarizing NMB to facilitate positioning of patient.	
Maintenance	If GA is used, maintenance is the same as for a tumor (see Anesthetic Considerations for Craniotomy for Tumor, p. 31) or AVM (see Anesthetic Considerations for Craniotomy for Intracranial Vascular Malformations, p. 19). If children are to be transported from the site of placement of the stereotactic frame to the radiologic suite and then to the OR, it is best to use a propofol infusion (e.g., 75–150 mcg/kg/min) with spontaneous or controlled ventilation to assure adequate ventilation and oxygenation during transport and study. Opiates and nondepolarizing NMBs should not be administered until the child is in the operating suite.	
Emergence	ETT generally is removed at the conclusion of the operation. Prophylactic antiemetic (e.g., metoclopramide 10–20 mg and ondansetron 4 mg) in adults should be given 30 min before extubation.	
Blood and fluid requirements	IV: 16–18 ga × 2 (adults); 20–22 ga (children) NS @ 4–6 mL/kg/h	Blood loss is minimal because the volume of tissue removed is small.
Monitoring	If local anesthesia: standard monitors (see p. B-1). If GA: Arterial line CVP line UO	
Positioning	✓ and pad pressure points. ✓ eyes.	

POSTOPERATIVE

Complications	Bleeding	Focal bleeding may occur postop, causing onset of a neurological deficit.
Pain management	Vicodin (1–2 mg po q 4 h prn)	
Tests	CT or MRI scan, if a new neurological deficit occurs.	

Suggested Readings

1. Baker KC, Isert PR: Anaesthetic considerations for children undergoing stereotactic radiosurgery. *Anaesth Intensive Care* 1997; 25(6):691–5.
2. Burchiel KJ: Image-based functional neurosurgery. *Clin Neurosurg* 1992; 39:314–30.
3. Chang SD, Adler JR, Hancock SL: Clinical uses of radiosurgery. *Oncology* 1998; 12(8):1181–91.
4. Glidenberg PL, Tasker RR, eds: *Textbook of Sterotactic and Functional Neurosurgery.* McGraw-Hill, New York: 1997.
5. Glidenberg PL, Woo SY: Multimodality program involving stereotactic surgery in brain tumor management. *Stereotact Funct Neurosurg* 2000; 75(2–3):147–52.
6. Glidenberg PL: Stereotactic surgery: the past and the future. *Stereotact Funct Neurosurg* 1998; 70(2–4):57–70.
7. Heilbrun MP, ed: *Stereotactic Neurosurgery.* Williams & Wilkins, Baltimore: 1988.
8. Holloway KL, Gaede SE, Starr PA, et al: Frameless stereotaxy using bone fiducial markers for deep brain stimulation. *J Neurosurg* 2005; 103(3):404–13.
9. Kondziolka D: Functional neurosurgery. *Neurosurgery* 1999; 44(l):12–20.
10. Maciunas, RJ: Stereotactic radiosurgery. *Nat Med* 1996; 2(6):712–13.
11. Ohye C: The idea of stereotaxy toward minimally invasive neurosurgery. *Stereotact Funct Neuorsurg* 2000; 74(3–4):185–93.
12. Ross DA: Minimalism through stereotactic technique. *Clin Neurosurg* 1996; 43:317–23.
13. Vannier MW, Marsh JL: Three-dimensional imaging, surgical planning, and image-guided therapy. *Radiol Clin North Am* 1996; 34(3):545–63.
14. Venkatraghavan L, Manninen P, Mak P, et al: Anesthesia for functional neurosurgery: review of complications. *J Neurosurg Anesthesiol* 2006; 18(1):64–67.
15. Woodworth GF, McGirt MJ, Samdani A, et al: Frameless image guided stereotactic brain biopsy procedure: diagnostic yield, surgical morbidity, and comparison with the frame based technique. *J Neurosurg* 2006; 104(2):233–7.

CHAPTER

1.2 Functional Neurosurgery

SURGEONS

Jamie M. Henderson, MD
Gary Heit, MD, PhD
Lawrence M. Shuer, MD

ANESTHESIOLOGIST

Richard A. Jaffe, MD, PhD

FUNCTIONAL NEUROSURGERY—INTRODUCTION: THE SURGICAL TREATMENT OF PAIN, MOVEMENT DISORDERS, AND EPILEPSY

INTRODUCTION

Gary Heit, PhD, MD, Jamie M. Henderson, MD

Functional neurosurgery differs from most surgical subspecialties in that it aims to alter the function of the nervous system, rather than addressing anatomical abnormalities. In 2008, the three most common treatment areas are chronic pain, epilepsy, and movement disorders. Each of these disease states has a distinctive anesthetic requirement dictated by the specific pathophysiology and subsequent intraop objectives. Procedures may be performed under local anesthesia, conscious sedation, or GA, and can be divided into ablative (destructive) or augmentative (nondestructive) techniques. With the exception of the treatment of epilepsy and some specific chronic pain disorders, ablative techniques are now seldom performed because of their unpredictable duration of effect and irreversible nature of the lesion. Neuroaugmentation (electrical stimulation or continuous local drug administration) tends to produce more lasting benefits and, more importantly, can be changed to meet fluctuations in the patient's symptoms.

The key to successful functional neurosurgical therapies is target identification. Many targets can be identified anatomically on appropriate radiographic studies, whereas others may be difficult to visualize even with special techniques. However, even areas that can be targeted anatomically may vary in terms of their physiological function. Thus, it is important to incorporate physiological testing in many functional neurosurgical procedures. For pain management, this involves the identification of a target nucleus, as well as the appropriate somatotopic location

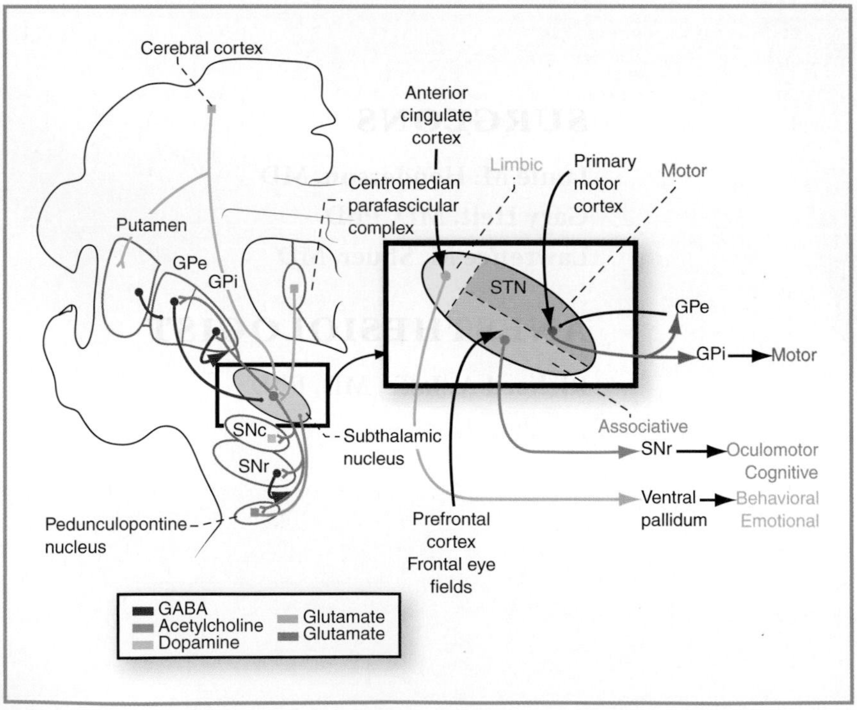

Figure 1.2-1. Topographical anatomy of the ventrolateral thalamus. CM = centrum medianum; GPe = external segment of globus pallidus; GPi = internal segment of globus pallidus; Put = putamen; LPO = lateropolaris; VOA = ventrooralis anterior; VOP = ventrooralis posterior; VIM = ventrali intermedius; Vce and Vci = ventralis caudalis externus and internus. (Reproduced with permission from Grossman RG, Loftus CM: *Principles of Neurosurgery,* 2nd edition. Lippincott-Raven, 1999.)

matching the patient's complaints. In the case of movement disorders, target location is often the region that is involved in the generation of tremor or abnormal movements. These regions may also be closely associated with areas involved in higher cognitive behavior. Thus, the need for physiological identification often dictates a specific anesthetic technique.

STEREOTACTIC PROCEDURES: DEEP BRAIN STIMULATION, PALLIDOTOMY, AND THALAMOTOMY

SURGICAL CONSIDERATIONS

Description: Many procedures are currently performed with **frame-based stereotactic techniques,** with intracranial access achieved via a burr hole or twist drill. There is a growing trend to use 'frameless' stereotactic approaches, with two major systems currently in use. Real-time frameless localization can be achieved by replacing the stereotactic frame with rigidly attached skull markers ("fiducials") that provide a fixed reference. Another innovative alternative is to produce a fixed trajectory guide using rapid prototyping techniques. Both of these approaches have been used successfully and appear to be equivalent in accuracy to a stereotactic frame.

Two approaches to identification of the functional target are used following initial stereotactic CT or MRI radiographic localization; both require patient cooperation. In one approach, the target is confirmed by assessing symptomatic resolution during high-frequency macrostimulation and by identifying surrounding structures using their characteristic stimulation-evoked responses. In the other approach, before stimulation testing, single-neuron recordings are performed to localize the appropriate target through somatotopic kinesthetic and/or somatosensory responses. In an awake patient, appropriate stimulation is delivered to the skin, or by passive and active movement of the joints. This technique utilizes specialized high-impedance microelectrodes and amplifiers susceptible to interference from monitoring equipment, which may necessitate manual measurements of BP and clinical assessment of oxygenation. Anesthesia or sedation can modify neuronal activity significantly and, thus, interfere with functional mapping. For example, propofol has been shown to inhibit globus pallidus neurons for several minutes beyond its behavioral effects. Additionally, many of these agents have been shown to change evoked potential (EP) responses, raising the possibility that they could alter stimulation thresholds for either the internal capsule or optic tract.

Thermal ablation for pallidotomy or thalamotomy typically is performed with a radiofrequency (RF) lesion generator operating at 500 kHz, which may interfere with some types of monitoring equipment; however, the ablation process only lasts approximately 12–30 sec.

A variety of movement disorders are amenable to surgical treatment. They can be divided into akinetic (e.g., Parkinson's) and hyperkinetic (e.g., dystonias, tremor, spasticity) syndromes. Idiopathic **Parkinson's disease** is best treated with **deep brain stimulation (DBS)** targeted to a functional subcomponent of either the subthalamic nucleus or globus pallidus interna (posteroventral **pallidotomy,** or PVP, Fig 1.2-2). Tremor syndromes are treated by DBS, targeting the ventral intermedius thalamic nucleus (**thalamotomy** or stimulation), whereas dystonias are treated by stimulation of the globus pallidus interna. **Spasticity** is not treated stereotactically, but through the administration of intrathecal baclofen (GABA-like synaptic inhibition) in the lumbar cistern via an internalized pump system. Abrupt loss of intrathecal infusion of baclofen, however, can quickly lead to a serious withdrawal syndrome with dysautonomia, circulatory collapse, and death within hours. Spasticity refractory to intrathecal baclofen may be amenable to selective dorsal root rhizotomy performed through an open laminectomy.

For **DBS,** mapping and implantation of the intracranial stimulating electrode is performed under local anesthesia to permit monitoring of behavioral and physiologic responses. A 2–3 cm linear incision (burr-hole access) or stab wound (twist-drill access), generally is placed near the coronal suture and 10–50 mm from the midline in the frontal bone. This can be accomplished under propofol sedation for patient comfort. Subsequently, minimal or no sedation is used, as patient cooperation is necessary during the functional mapping component of the case. If single-neuron recordings are used, propofol should be discontinued at least 20 min in advance of mapping, because it can produce prolonged suppression of target neuronal activity. If sedation is needed, use a low-dose (0.01–0.05 mcg/kg/min) remifentanil infusion. Local anesthetics should not contain epinephrine. Avoid central-acting β-blockers (e.g., propranolol), which suppress tremor activity in target neurons. Sedation with meperidine in patients taking

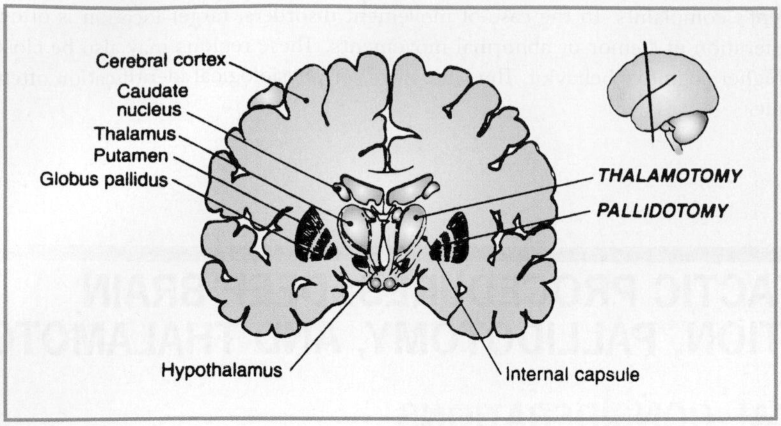

Figure 1.2-2. Anatomical locations for therapeutic lesions (thalamotomy and pallidotomy) for the surgical treatment of Parkinson's disease. Inset shows the plane of the coronal section through the diencephalon, identifying the lesions. (Reproduced with permission from Mason LJ, Cojocaru TT, Cole DJ: Surgical intervention and anesthetic management of the patient with Parkinson's disease. In *International Anesthesiology Clinics: Topics in Neuroanesthesia.* Jaffe RA, Giffard RG, eds. Little, Brown, Boston: 1996; 4(34):141.)

selegiline is contraindicated. No dopaminergic antagonist (e.g., metoclopramide, droperidol) should be given to Parkinsonian patients or patients with dopamine-responsive dystonia. To enhance single-cell responses, withhold medications prescribed for target symptoms for 8–24 h. In some cases (e.g., Parkinson's disease), this may result in a rebound HTN requiring active treatment; however, patients will resume their medications postop (often in the post-anesthesia recovery area) and the HTN will resolve. The **implantable pulse generator (IPG)** may be placed in an infraclavicular subcutaneous pocket at the time of the intracranial electrode implantation. Implantation of the IPG and subcutaneous tunneling of the electrode lead can be done under MAC, but is best tolerated under GETA. To facilitate intubation, the calvarial wound is closed temporally and the stereotactic localizing apparatus is removed. Closure consists of a single, interrupted suture for stab wounds or two-layer suture/staple closure for a burr hole. IPG pockets are closed in two layers. The subcutaneous layer is closed with absorbable sutures, and the skin is closed with staples or sutures.

Usual preop diagnosis: Medically intractable idiopathic Parkinson's disease with disabling L-Dopa-induced dyskinesia, bradykinesia, or rigidity; severe fluctuations in medication responses; dystonia musculorum deformans; post-CVA dystonia; occasionally, torticollis; tremor; movement disorders

SUMMARY OF PROCEDURE	
Position	Supine
Incision	Linear (burr holes); stab-wound (twist drill)
Unique considerations	Minimal/no sedation. BP ↑ in patients who have their antihypertensive medications withheld. Manual vital sign monitoring as electronic monitors may interfere with single-cell recordings.
Antibiotics + other meds	Cefazolin 1 g; dexamethasone 6–8 mg
Surgical time	3–6 h
EBL	25–150 mL
Postop care	Continue antibiotics, Parkinson's medications. BP may ↓. Maintain MAP <90 mmHg to prevent postop bleeding. ICU vs. step-down.
Mortality	<0.5%

SUMMARY OF PROCEDURE (cont'd)	
Morbidity	Overall: 8–27% Infection Hardware failure: Rare Intracranial hemorrhage Cognitive disturbances
Pain score	2–3

PATIENT POPULATION CHARACTERISTICS	
Age range	12–80 yr
Male:Female	1:1
Incidence	Becoming common
Etiology	Idiopathic; genetic
Associated conditions	Dystonia

ANESTHETIC CONSIDERATIONS

Parkinson's disease is the most common movement disorder, affecting ~1% of the population > 60 yr. It is caused by the loss of dopaminergic neurons in the substantia nigra → ↓ dopamine (dopamine/acetylcholine imbalance) in basal ganglia → movement disorder. Medical treatment is directed primarily to restoring dopamine levels by increasing the availability of the dopamine precursor (L-dopa), inhibiting liver dopa decarboxylase (carbidopa, usually given in combination with L-dopa as Sinemet), by releasing endogenous dopamine (amantadine [Symmetrel]) and by blocking MAO-B (selegiline [Eldepryl]). Medical treatment also may include dopamine agonists (pergolide [Permax]; bromocriptine [Parlodel]), and acetylcholine antagonists (amantadine [Symmetrel], benztropine [Cogentin]) to correct the dopamine/acetylcholine imbalance. Patients presenting for surgery have failed medical therapy and will have been taken off their antiparkinsonian medications 8–24 h before surgery. This will maximize their symptoms to help assess treatment effects intraop; thus, preop assessment on the day of surgery will be difficult.

PREOPERATIVE

Respiratory	Autonomic dysfunction → esophageal dysfunction →↑ risk of aspiration. Patients typically have ↓ vital capacity 2° rigidity, dyskinesia →↓ respiratory function and ↓ cough. Laryngospasm and respiratory failure may occur following withdrawal of antiparkinsonian medications. **Tests:** CXR; consider ABG; PFTs may be difficult to obtain.
Cardiovascular	Autonomic dysfunction → orthostatic hypotension. Dopamine replacement therapy → cardiac dysrhythmias, ↓ BP, and hypovolemia. In patients taking selegiline (MAOI): avoid meperidine →↑↑ BP, rigidity, agitation; sympathomimetics → exaggerated ↑ BP.
Neurological	The primary Sx of Parkinson's disease include rigidity, tremor, bradykinesia, muscle weakness. Secondary symptoms include dementia, depression, and speech difficulty. Patients may alternate between a state of immobility and one of exaggerated tremor (which may interfere with intraop monitoring).
Renal	Urinary retention is common.
Gastrointestinal	Autonomic dysfunction → gastroparesis, ↑ incidence of reflux. Poor nutrition. Pharyngeal muscle dysfunction → dysphagia.
Laboratory	As indicated from H&P.
Premedication	None. These patients may have received small doses of fentanyl and/or midazolam to facilitate placement of the stereotactic frame. For frameless procedures, fiducial markers or mounting screws will have been placed before surgery.

INTRAOPERATIVE

Anesthetic technique: MAC, with minimal or no sedation, as patient cooperation and typical neuronal activity are essential for the success of the procedure.

Induction	Low-dose remifentanil (0.01–0.05 mcg/kg/min) or propofol (25–75 mcg/kg/min) may be used for sedation during burr-hole placement only. If propofol is used, it should be discontinued 20–30 min before electrophysiologic recording or mapping. In the event of an airway emergency in framed procedures, a means of releasing the patient from the stereotactic frame must be readily available.	
Maintenance	BP control is important to decrease the risk of intracranial hemorrhage during passage of the recording and stimulating electrodes. If not otherwise contraindicated, MAP should be kept 10–20% below normal for that patient. This usually can be accomplished without an arterial line by using an infusion of NTG titrated to effect or by using small doses of atenolol (0.5–1 mg increments iv). Atenolol is preferred over other parenteral β-blockers, because its CNS penetration is limited → minimal effect on central tremor.	
Emergence	Postop BP control can be continued by using atenolol or labetalol titrated to effect at the end of the procedure. The patient is usually transported to the PACU, then to the neurology ward for postop monitoring. Antiparkinsonian medication should be given in the PACU.	
Blood and fluid requirements	Minimal blood loss IV: 18–20 ga ×1 NS/LR @ 1–2 mL/kg/h	For unilateral procedures, IV should be placed in the ipsilateral arm (relative to side of surgery).
Monitoring	Standard monitors (see p. B-1)	Exaggerated tremors and/or neurologic testing in these patients may interfere with monitoring. It may be helpful to place the BP cuff on a leg (less tremor). For unilateral procedures, monitors should not be placed on the contralateral arm, which must be kept free for testing.
Positioning	✓ and pad pressure points. ✓ stereotactic frame clearance.	Patient comfort may be improved by placing pillows under the knees to relieve lower back strain. A massage therapist can greatly improve patient comfort during the procedure.
Complications	Intracerebral hemorrhage Loss of airway in stereotactic frame	Dx: ↓ mental status and hemiparesis. CT scan usually required to confirm Dx. Emergency craniotomy may be necessary. Rx: remove stereotactic frame and secure airway.

POSTOPERATIVE

Complications	Intracranial hemorrhage Motor deficit Visual field deficit Aphasia	Intracranial hemorrhage may require emergency craniotomy. The surgeon should be notified immediately if any new deficits are noted.
Tests	None	Unless otherwise indicated.
Pain management	Usually not necessary	

References:

1. Benabid A, Pollak P, Gao D, Hoffman D, Limousin P, Gay E, Payen I, Benazzouz A: Chronic electrical stimulation of the ventralis intermedius nucleus of the thalamus as a treatment of movement disorders. *J Neurosurg* 1996; 84:203–14.
2. Guridi J, Lozana A: A brief history of pallidotomy. Neurosurgery 1997; 41(5):1169–83.

3. Heit G. Murphy G, Jaffe R, Golby A, Silverberg GS: The effects of propofol on human globus pallidus neurons. *Stereotact Funct Neurosurg* 1997; 67(1–2):74.
4. Joint C, Nandi D, Parkin S, Gregory R, Aziz T: Hardware-related problems of deep brain stimulation. *Move Disord* 2002; 17(Suppl 3):S175–80.
5. Pereira EA, Green AL, Nandi D, Aziz TZ. Deep brain stimulation: indications and evidence. *Expert Rev Med Devices* 2007; 4(5):591–603.
6. Deuschl G, Schade-Brittinger C, Krack P, et al. A randomized trial of deep-brain stimulation for Parkinson's disease. *N Engl J Med* 2006; 355(9):896–908.
7. Krack P, Fraiz V, Mendes A, et al. Postoperative management of subthalamic nucleus stimulation for Parkinson's disease. *Mov Disord* 2002; 17(Suppl 3):S188–97.
8. Volkmann J. Deep brain stimulation for the treatment of Parkinson's disease. *J Clin Neurophysiol* 2004; 21(1):6–17.
9. Moro E, Lang AE. Criteria for deep-brain stimulation in Parkinson's disease: review and analysis. *Expert Rev Neurother* 2006; 6(11):1695–705.

SURGICAL ANALGESICS: SPINAL CORD STIMULATION, INTRATHECAL PUMPS, AND CORTICAL STIMULATION

SURGICAL CONSIDERATIONS

Description: Chronic pain arises from a variety of etiologies. It can involve both neuropathic and nociceptive processes and occur in a variety of anatomical distributions (e.g., radicular versus a hemibody pattern). Therapeutic interventions are dictated by the pathophysiology of the pain, its qualitative nature, etiology, and the patients' prognosis. Common procedures for chronic pain are directed at the spinal cord, and may consist of epidural or intrathecal medications or electrical stimulation.

For **chronic spinal cord stimulation** (e.g., postlaminectomy syndrome) an epidural electrode is implanted either percutaneously or via an open laminectomy. **Percutaneous electrodes** are easier to implant and have less associated surgical pain. The surgical electrode (implanted via laminectomy) confers greater mechanical stability in the epidural space. Additionally, given its larger contact size, it can generate higher current densities with less drain on the implanted system. For percutaneous electrodes, a small skin incision is made two to three vertebral levels caudal to the target region of the spinal cord. For **'surgical paddle' electrodes,** the skin incision is made one to two levels caudal to the target zone of the spinal cord, and a laminectomy is performed to provide access to the epidural space. Incisions are closed in the standard fashion.

In either technique, patient cooperation is required during intraop test stimulation. The procedures are done in the prone or lateral position with consequent implications for airway management in the sedated patient. Localization of the electrodes is accomplished initially based on radiographic criteria; however, these localizations are only approximate, and it is recommended that the electrode placement be confirmed by intraop stimulation. The patient needs to be sufficiently alert to communicate the quality, distribution, and intensity of the stimulation-induced paresthesias. To assess efficacy, the electrode may be externalized and percutaneous stimulation used for assessment. If there is ≥50% reduction in pain, the patient may return to the OR for internalization of the implantable pulse generator (IPG). Postop, these patients can have an exacerbation of pain, particularly if neuropathic in nature. They may require iv lidocaine or ketamine infusions to return them to their preop baseline, even with a functioning and appropriately located stimulating electrode.

For **pain of central origin** (e.g., poststroke, multiple sclerosis, and trigeminal nerve pathology), surgical procedures are directed at the thalamus and cortex. Thalamic interventions include stereotactic insertion of stimulating electrodes into sensory thalamus. **Thalamic DBS** requires awake mapping of the somatotopic representation of the affected body part through either microelectrode mapping or stimulation-induced paresthesias. For medically intractable neuropathic pain syndromes, **epidural motor cortex stimulation** has shown great promise. Functional mapping of the motor cortex for epidural stimulation can be done with anatomical and physiological mapping under GA via a craniotomy, with the anesthetic tailored to minimize interference with EP recording. The incision consists of a 5–10-cm linear or 5 × 10 cm trapezoidal incision placed over and paralleling the motor cortex.

Identification of the appropriate location on the motor strip can be done initially with epidural mapping using SSEPs elicited from the part of the body where the pain originates. In cases of denervation syndromes, SSEP may not be present and the minimum intensity point for epidural stimulation-induced movements is used. In rare cases, the surgeon may elect to perform the surgery awake to facilitate mapping. To assess efficacy, the electrode may be externalized and percutaneous stimulation assessed for overall therapeutic efficacy. If there is ≥ 50% reduction in pain, the patient will return to the OR for internalization of the IPG. Closure consists of calvarial reconstruction with externalization of leads. The craniotomy incision is closed in the standard fashion. If a percutaneous trial is done, the IPG implant requires a second GETA with reopening of wounds.

The surgical treatment of trigeminal neuralgia is **microvascular decompression of the trigeminal nerve** in the prepontine cistern (see p. 44). In patients who are poor surgical candidates, treatment is accomplished with ablative procedures aimed at the gasserian ganglia, using hemolytic, mechanical, or RF techniques. Patients who fail gasserian ganglion interventions or have atypical facial pain are candidates for **thalamic DBS** or **motor cortex stimulation.** Surgical treatments for trigeminal neuralgia, however, may become obsolete, given the advent of **stereotactic radiosurgical ablative techniques.** These systems utilize multiple beams of radiation focused on the nerve to achieve pain relief equivalent to microvascular decompression without the attendant complications of an invasive neurosurgical procedure.

For pain unresponsive to spinal cord stimulation or because of unacceptable side effects of parental medications, continuous intrathecal administration of analgesics can be accomplished with an **implantable medication delivery system.** An incision is made over the L3–L4, L4–L5, or L5–S1 spinous process and a second incision is placed in the RLQ of the abdomen. A tunnel tool is used to bring the catheter from the lumbar spinal region to the abdomen. This tunnel is rarely tolerated without GETA or deep sedation. A reservoir or continuous-delivery pump is then placed in the abdomen and attached to the catheter. Both incisions are closed in two layers.

Intrathecal narcotics (typically morphine), can produce satisfactory results, since therapeutic drug concentrations can be achieved at the level of spinal opiate receptors without influencing higher CNS opiate systems. This therapeutic intervention can be assessed through a percutaneous catheter trial. Patients who experience ≥ 50% reduction in pain are candidates for a **totally implanted pump system.** These are low-morbidity procedures (5–10%) with infections and hardware failures constituting the greatest problems. Abrupt cessation of medications—through either patient noncompliance with refill schedules (10–12 wk) or hardware failure—however, can lead to a serious withdrawal syndrome.

Usual preop diagnosis: Chronic pain

SUMMARY OF PROCEDURE

Position	Prone/lateral
Incision	2–3 levels above target area (spinal cord stimulation) + laminectomy; L3, 4, 5 (intrathecal pump) + 2nd incision RLQ of abdomen.
Unique considerations	Patient communication important; therefore, avoid oversedation. Copious use of local anesthetics (avoid overdosing).
Antibiotics	Cefazolin 1 g
Surgical time	1.5–3 h
EBL	25 mL
Postop care	May have ↑ pain
Mortality	0.5%
Morbidity	Overall: 5–10% Infection Hardware failure Withdrawal Sx
Pain score	3–8

PATIENT POPULATION CHARACTERISTICS

Age range	20–75 yr
Male:Female	1:1
Incidence	Common
Etiology	Iatrogenic; neuropathic; traumatic
Associated conditions	Opiate dependency

ANESTHETIC CONSIDERATIONS

PREOPERATIVE

Patients with chronic pain often present unique challenges to the anesthesiologist and surgeon. They may be intolerant of any additional pain (e.g., iv placement, positioning on the OR table, postop pain) and seemingly immune to typical doses of systemic analgesics while remaining vulnerable to opioid overdose. In most cases, patients should continue their usual pain medications and co-analgesics until ~2 h before surgery. Typically any transdermal fentanyl patch should be left in place unless its location will be subject to intraoperative heating, compression, or other manipulation. A detailed H/o of patient pain, effective (and ineffective) pain management techniques and drugs, and the current medication regime (including the use of both over and under the counter drugs and herbals) is essential.

Respiratory	Chronic pain →↓ physical activity →↓ respiratory reserve.
Cardiovascular	Ventricular dysrhythmias have been associated with methadone at doses > 200 mg/day. Chronic pain →↓ physical activity →↓ cardiovascular reserve.
Neurological	A careful neurologic assessment is essential to detect pre-existing deficits.
Psychological	These patients often benefit from a detailed explanation of the surgical and anesthetic procedures including expectations and contingency plans for intraop pain management if an awake procedure is planned. These patients may have a higher incidence of co-existing psychiatric disease and often have high scores on standardized measures of hysteria and hypochondria. Patients on antipsychotic medication may develop neuroleptic malignant syndrome.
Gastrointestinal	Chronic opioid use may →↓ gastric emptying and ↓ GI motility with chronic constipation. Inactivity 2° chronic pain → obesity.
Laboratory	As indicated from H&P. For patients on anticonvulsants, drug levels are useful to exclude toxic effects.
Premedication	Chronic opioid use may make the patients at risk for gastric aspiration 2° ↓ bowel motility. Consider metoclopramide 10–20 mg iv 30 min preinduction with Na citrate 30 mL po on transport to the OR. Midazolam iv titrated to effect can be beneficial.

INTRAOPERATIVE

Anesthetic technique: The placement of intrathecal pumps and cortical stimulators is often best accomplished under GA using anesthetic techniques appropriate for spinal or intracranial procedures. Accurate electrode placement may require an awake patient during at least a portion of the procedure. For intracranial electrode placement, see the anesthetic technique for awake craniotomy (p. 34). These same general principles can also be used for spinal cord electrode placement, although regional techniques are usually simpler and just as effective.

Thoracic epidural	Following the application of standard monitors and with an iv catheter in place, the patient should be seated carefully on the edge of the operating table. Provide support for feet and arms as necessary. The epidural injection should be at the level of the surgery (usually 2–3 levels below the electrode target site). A single bolus injection of 10 mL of 0.75% bupivacaine usually provides excellent surgical anesthesia without compromising the ability to map the more rostral portion of the spinal cord. It is important to avoid oversedation and to minimize the use of systemic analgesics in order to ensure accurate spinal cord mapping.	
Blood and fluid requirements	IV: 18 ga ×1 NS/LR @ 2–4 mL/kg/h	After replacement of preop deficit
Monitoring	Standard monitors (see p. B-1).	
Positioning	Prone ✓and pad pressure points. ✓eyes	The patient should self-position on bolsters (hips and upper chest) or Wilson frame.
Complications	Spinal cord injury	

POSTOPERATIVE

Complications	Spinal cord injury Epidural hematoma Respiratory distress Drug withdrawal symptoms	Prompt postop neurologic assessment is essential. May occur in response to the patient's usual opiate dose if the spinal stimulation has produced significant pain relief.
Tests	None unless otherwise indicated	Surgeons may request specific tests.
Pain management	Typically complex and multimodal	Patient often intolerant of postop pain while remaining susceptible to narcotic overdose. Acute pain service consult recommended.

References:

1. North RB: Spinal cord stimulation patient selection. In *Surgical Management of Pain.* Burchiel KJ, ed. Thieme Medical Pub, NY: 2002, 527–34.
2. Pagura JR, Rabello JR, Cerueira de Lima W: Microvascular decompression for trigeminal neuralgia. In *Textbook of Stereotactic and Functional Neurosurgery.* Gildenberg PL, Tasker RK, eds. McGraw Hill, NY: 1998, 1715–21.
3. Tsubokawa T: Motor cortex stimulation for the relief of central deafferented pain. In *Surgical Management of Pain.* Burchiel KJ, ed. Thieme Medical Pub, NY; 2002, 555–64.
4. Kopf A, Banzhaf A, Stein C. Perioperative management of the chronic pain patient. *Baillieres Best Pract Clin Anesthesiol* 2005; 19:59–77.
5. Brill S, Ginosar Y, Davidson EM. Perioperative management of chronic pain patients with opioid dependency. *Curr Opin Anaesth* 2006; 19:325–31.

VAGAL NERVE STIMULATION

SURGICAL CONSIDERATIONS

Description: The surgical treatment of medically intractable epilepsy consists of either **surgical resection** of the epileptic site (see p. 81) or **vagal nerve stimulation (VNS).** For patients who are not candidates for resective surgery, VNS can be a viable surgical strategy. Although it is a low-morbidity procedure, its efficacy also is low. VNS tends to produce a 50% or greater reduction of Sz in ~48% of patients after 18 mo of stimulation.

By contrast, **temporal lobectomy** for patients with medial temporal lobe epilepsy has an 80–85% chance of making the patient seizure-free, while using only one anticonvulsant medication, or none at all. Surgery for **extratemporal epilepsy** originating in neocortex has a 50% chance of making the patient seizure-free, in the absence of a structural lesion. (If an anatomical abnormality is present, then that figure increases to ~75%.) In general, the complication rate is ~7%, dependent on the exact location of the Sz focus and its relationship to eloquent cortex.

Left vagal nerve stimulation is also used to treat some types of medically refractory **depression**. As with its use in epilepsy, the exact mechanism of action remains unclear.

Two incisions are used for VNS: one left anterior cervical, placed approximately at the C6–C7 level, with a second incision in the left infraclavicular region for placement of the implantable pulse generator (IPG). Most surgeons perform the procedure through a carotid-type incision and place the IPG caudally through blunt dissection. The left vagus nerve is isolated, and the electrode assembly is wrapped around the nerve below the origin of the superior and inferior cervical cardiac branches. During surgery, the interface between the vagal nerve and the electrode is tested with electrical stimulation. Fortunately, this is associated with a very low incidence of bradycardia and extremely rare reports of asystole. All resolve with cessation of stimulation and administration of atropine. The surgeon should inform the anesthesiologist when vagal stimulation is about to begin. The incisions are closed using the standard technique; however, because many patients are developmentally delayed, the final skin layer is often closed with a subcutaneous technique that does not require subsequent suture removal.

Usual preop diagnosis: Partial onset seizures refractory to medication; chronic or recurrent depression refractory to other medical treatment

SUMMARY OF PROCEDURES

Position	Supine
Incision	Anterior cervical (C6–7) + infraclavicular pocket (for IPG)
Unique considerations	Bradycardia → asystole during stimulation phase
Antibiotics	Cefazolin 1 g
Surgical time	1.5 h
EBL	<50 mL
Postop care	Observe for ↑ Sz activity postop × 8 h
Mortality	<0.5%
Morbidity	Hoarseness: ~50%, may be 2° nerve injury or fatigue, device malfunction Cough: ~40% in first 3 mo after surgery Infection: 2% Dysphagia during stimulation →↑ aspiration risk Dyspnea during stimulation; patients with OSA may have ↑ apneic events Nerve/vascular injury (similar to carotid surgery)
Pain score	1–2

PATIENT POPULATION CHARACTERISTICS

Age range	12–80 yr (≥18 yr for treatment of depression)
Male:Female	1:1
Incidence	>30,000 patients treated worldwide thru 2007
Etiology	Idiopathic, typically
Associated conditions	Developmental delay; severe depression

ANESTHETIC CONSIDERATIONS

PREOPERATIVE

Antiepileptic medication, such as phenytoin, will abolish seizure disorders in most patients, but some develop intolerable side effects; others are refractory to medical therapy. Surgical ablation of the Sz focus may be the only effective therapy for some patients. For patients who are not candidates for ablative procedures, the placement of a vagal nerve stimulator may be a viable alternative. These patients typically take multiple antiepileptic medications that should be continued throughout the morning of surgery. These same general considerations are also applicable to patients with refractory depression.

Neurologic	The only common neurological finding in epilepsy patients is a Hx of uncontrollable Sz, either focal or generalized. Obtain a description of Sz and prodromal Sx.
Psychiatric	Medications used to treat depression (e.g., MAOI, SSRI) may have significant interactions with other drugs (e.g., meperidine → serotonin syndrome)
Gastrointestinal	Abnormal liver function may be associated with use of valproate and carbamazepine. **Tests:** LFT and others as indicated from H&P.
Hematologic	Phenytoin/phenobarbital →↓ Hct; carbamazepine/valproate/ethosuximide/primidone →↓ Plt; carbamazepine/primidone →↓ WBC. **Tests:** CBC and others as indicated from H&P.
Laboratory	Tests as indicated from H&P.
Premedication	Standard premedication (see p. B-1) is usually appropriate.

INTRAOPERATIVE

Anesthetic technique: GETA. Chronic use of antiepileptic medications may cause hepatic enzyme induction → accelerated drug metabolism; resistance to muscle relaxants including succinylcholine.

Induction	Standard induction (see p. B-2). Once anesthesia is induced, a nondepolarizing NMR is administered.	
Maintenance	Standard maintenance (see p. B-2). Generally, no further NMBs are administered beyond those used for tracheal intubation. Hyperventilation may promote Sz activity. Sevoflurane and enflurane can induce epileptiform EEG activity.	
Emergence	No special considerations. Prophylactic antiemetic (e.g., ondansetron 4 mg) should be given 30–60 min before extubation.	
Blood and fluid requirements	Minimal blood loss IV: 18 ga NS/LR @ 4–6 mL/kg/h	Possibility of injury to carotid artery or jugular vein may result in significant blood loss.
Monitoring	Standard monitors (see p. B-1). EEG monitoring not necessary	O_2 sat and $ETCO_2$ monitoring will indicate the adequacy of ventilation and oxygenation.
Positioning	✓and pad pressure points. ✓eyes.	Head turned to the right with neck extension
Complications	Asystole	Rarely (<1%), the SA node is innervated by the left vagus nerve. In those patients, vagal stimulation may result in severe bradycardia or asystole. Rx: stop stimulation; atropine 0.5 mg iv ± CPR.
	Bronchospasm	Bronchospasm may occur as a result at vagal nerve stimulation.
	Sz	
	Vascular injury	

POSTOPERATIVE

Complications	Seizure Vocal cord paralysis Hoarseness Peritracheal hematoma	Sz precautions may be necessary. Monitor carefully for altered mental status. Airway obstruction may occur.
Pain management	Usually mild discomfort	Rx: See p. C-2.
Tests	No routine tests	

References:

1. Augustinsson LE, Ben-Menachem E: Vagal nerve stimulation for the treatment of refractory seizures. In *Textbook of Stereotactic and Functional Neurosurgery.* Gildenberg PL, Tasker RK, eds. McGraw Hill, NY: 1998, 1715–21.
2. Mason LJ, Cojocaru TT, Cole DJ: Surgical intervention and anesthetic management of the patient with Parkinson's disease. In *Topics in Neuroanesthesia.* Jaffe RA, Giffard RG, eds. Little, Brown, Boston: 1996; 34(4):133–50.
3. Hatton KW, McLarney JT, Pittman T, Fahy BG. Vagal nerve stimulation: overview and implications for anesthesiologists. *Anesth Analg* 2006; 103(5):1241–9.
4. Multon S, Schoenen J. Pain control by vagus nerve stimulation: from animal to man...and back. Acta Neurol Belg 2005; 105(2):62–7.
5. Shafique S, Dalsing MC. Vagus nerve stimulation therapy for treatment of drug-resistant epilepsy and depression. *Perspect Vasc Endovasc Ther* 2006; 18(4):323–7.

EPILEPSY SURGERY

SURGICAL CONSIDERATIONS

Lawrence M. Shuer and Gary Heit

Description: In the United States, the prevalence of epilepsy is ~5–20/1,000 (0.5–2%), meaning that at least 1.5 million people have epilepsy. In childhood, the incidence and prevalence is higher, with 90% of all new cases occurring before the age of 20. Intractable epilepsy is defined as persistent seizure activity of such frequency or severity that prevents normal function and/or development. This diagnosis is made only after an adequate trial of anticonvulsant medication(s), with therapeutic levels, has been documented. Of all those with epilepsy, 10–20% prove to be intractable; it is estimated that ~20–30% of patients with intractable epilepsy may benefit from a surgical procedure.

The causes of epilepsy are varied, ranging from idiopathic to neoplastic. Epilepsy surgery is most beneficial in patients with partial epilepsy 2° a structural lesion. Most commonly, this lesion is located in the temporal lobe, and the most common operation is a **temporal lobectomy,** in both children and adults. Cerebral dominance and, hence, the location of speech, must be determined using a preop Wada test (intracarotid amobarbital injection to localize language function), although functional MRI mapping of speech centers may eventually replace this invasive test. Studies to define the epileptogenic focus include simultaneous recordings of video/EEG and high-resolution MRI and PET scans. Temporal lobe surgery may involve removal of only the structural lesion and associated epileptogenic cortex, cortical resection alone, excision of the amygdala and hippocampus, or removal of the entire anterior temporal lobe, with the extent of posterior resection dependent on dominance. Depending on the involved center, intraop electrocorticography may be used, requiring neurolept anesthesia (tranquilizer, opiate and N_2O). In addition, the speech center may need to be identified intraop, necessitating an awake procedure. These differing options will significantly alter the choice of anesthesia and must be established before surgery.

For a standard **temporal lobectomy,** the patient is placed supine on the operating table with the head turned 90° and held with pin fixation. A 'question mark' temporal incision is often used, and hemostasis is achieved with skin clips.

A flap—either a free temporal bone flap or an osteoplastic flap, based on the temporalis muscle—is elevated with a high-speed craniotome. A **subtemporal craniectomy** allows visualization of the entire anterior temporal lobe. The dura is opened, widely exposing the anterior 6–6.5 cm of the temporal lobe. Labbe's vein must be preserved. At this point, surface and/or depth electrocorticography may be employed and **inhalation anesthetics must not be used.** After mapping the lesion, amygdala and hippocampus or anterior temporal lobe is removed. Temporal lobectomy involves resection of both the lateral and medial temporal structures, and is commonly performed in two steps. Often an operating microscope will be used to completely resect medial structures, including the uncus and hippocampal formation. Injury to the brain stem, 3rd and 4th cranial nerves, and either the middle cerebral or posterior cerebral arteries can occur; these are known complications of this surgery. Closure of the dura, bone flap, and scalp concludes the surgery.

Variant procedure or approaches: There are four common variant procedures. The first is sectioning of the corpus callosum, known as a **corpus callosotomy.** This is commonly used for patients with atonic seizures or partial seizures with secondary generalization. Either the anterior two-thirds or the entire corpus callosum is divided in the midline. The approach is the same as any transcallosal, intraventricular procedure, and uses a bifrontal, paramedian scalp incision and elevation of free-bone flap adjacent to the midline in the region of the coronal suture. Injury to the sagittal sinus is possible and may result in massive VAE or hemorrhage. In addition, numerous bridging veins across the interhemispheric fissure must be preserved to avoid venous congestion and possible infarction. The right cerebral hemisphere is gently retracted from the falx, exposing the paired anterior cerebral arteries and underlying corpus callosum. If an anterior two-thirds transection is performed, an intraop x-ray is required to determine the posterior border.

The second variant involves either a **frontal, temporal,** or **occipital craniotomy** for resection of a structural, epileptogenic focus, such as a tumor or AVM. This procedure may use **stereotaxic localization** and the resultant craniotomy may be performed with image guidance, or in a stereotaxic head frame, which affects the method of intubation. The subsequent craniotomy is similar to the excision of any structural lesion, with the exception of intraop electrocorticography of surrounding cortex, which if used will affect the choice of anesthetic.

The third variant is most common and consists of a diagnostic procedure involving placement of **surface and/or depth electrodes.** This may be performed with or without stereotaxic localization. Often only burr holes, outlining the future craniotomy flap, are used. After placement, the electrodes are externalized, and postop the patient's naturally occurring Sz are recorded, in conjunction with video monitoring, to register the clinical presentation with the onset of ictal activity. This recording/observation period may last for several days. The patient is then returned to the OR and the epileptogenic focus resected as described earlier.

The fourth alternative is **selective amygdalohippocampectomy,** a variation of the standard anterior temporal lobectomy. In this procedure, the surgeon makes a cortical incision in the anterior temporal lobe and exposes and resects the amygdala and hippocampus, sparing the remaining portions of the temporal lobe. This procedure is sometimes used on the dominant side of the brain in an effort to lower the risk of postop speech and language dysfunction.

Usual preop diagnosis: Temporal lobe epilepsy; partial epilepsy; intractable epilepsy

SUMMARY OF PROCEDURES	
Position	Supine, rarely prone for occipital lesions; table turned 180°
Incision	Temporal question mark, reverse question mark, paramedian, frontal, or occipital
Special instrumentation	Operating microscope; Cavitron; bipolar cautery; surface electrode grids and strips; depth electrode
Unique considerations	Electrocorticography requiring neuroleptic anesthesia; awake procedures for mapping of temporal and/or frontal speech areas; stereotaxic craniotomy and lesionectomy
Antibiotics	Ceftriaxone 1 g iv (avoid administration with calcium-containing solutions)
Surgical time	3 h
EBL	Minimal for diagnostic procedures; 250–500 mL with craniotomy (adults)
Postop care	After craniotomy, ICU for 12–24 h

SUMMARY OF PROCEDURES (cont'd)	
Mortality	<1%
Morbidity	Hemiplegia Dysphasia Ophthalmoplegia Brain stem injury
Pain score	2–4

PATIENT POPULATION CHARACTERISTICS	
Age range	New onset Sz: pediatric and geriatric populations
Male:Female	1:1
Incidence	180,000/yr (new cases of epilepsy): ~10% eventually present for surgery/yr
Etiology	Idiopathic (mesial temporal sclerosis); infectious (brain abscess, encephalitis); traumatic (glial scar); vascular (AVM, infarct); neoplastic (glioma, hamartoma, ganglioglioma); congenital (cortical dysplasia)
Associated conditions	Tuberous sclerosis; Sturge-Weber syndrome; infantile hemiplegia; encephalitis; hemimegalencephaly

ANESTHETIC CONSIDERATIONS

PREOPERATIVE

Epilepsy is a common neurologic disorder among young adults. Antiepileptic medication, such as phenytoin, will abolish seizure disorders in most patients, but some develop intolerable side effects to such medications; others are refractory to medical therapy. Surgical ablation of the seizure focus may be the only effective therapy for these patients if they are to become self-sufficient. Several operations may be done, the most common being placement of surface or depth electrodes to determine the focus of the Sz, with subsequent temporal lobectomy for removal of the focus. In some cases, the lesion may be very focal and amenable to stereotactic localization and removal. At some centers both seizure mapping and subsequent resection are carried out during the course of an awake craniotomy (see p. 34). If wake-up testing is planned, the procedure should be explained to the patient in detail including what the patient should expect to hear and feel during the test.

Neurological	Usually the only neurological finding is a Hx of uncontrollable seizures, either focal or generalized. Obtain a description of Sz and prodromal Sx. Sz medications should be continued through the morning of surgery. **Tests:** A preop Wada test (intracarotid injection of sodium amytal) and/or fMRI mapping is performed to determine whether the area of proposed surgery has any cerebral dominance or speech function.
Gastrointestinal	Abnormal liver function may be associated with valproate and carbamazepine use. **Tests:** LFT and others as indicated from H&P.
Hematologic	Phenytoin/phenobarbital →↓ Hct; Carbamazepine/valproate/ethosuximide/primidone →↓ Plt; Carbamazepine/primidone →↓ WBC **Tests:** CBC and others as indicated from H&P.
Laboratory	Tests as indicated from H&P.
Premedication	Standard premedication (see p. B-1) is usually appropriate.

INTRAOPERATIVE

Anesthetic technique: GETA (± wake-up testing) or local anesthesia (awake craniotomy). The placement of surface or depth electrodes is done under GETA, as is a temporal lobectomy in the nondominant hemisphere. If the seizure focus is in the dominant hemisphere and/or if there is any question about possible injury to speech or motor areas, the procedure may be performed under local anesthesia (awake craniotomy, see p. 34), with intraop localization of the seizure focus.

Induction	Standard induction (see p. B-2). If a difficult intubation is anticipated (e.g., stereotactic frame), orotracheal intubation is best accomplished before induction of GA. An awake fiber optic intubation is the best technique (see p. B-5). After anesthesia is induced, a nondepolarizing neuromuscular relaxant is administered.
Maintenance	Standard maintenance (see p. B-2). Generally, no further NMBs are administered beyond that used for tracheal intubation. With adequate anesthesia, and the head fixed in the Mayfield-Kees skeletal fixation, patient movement of any consequence is highly unlikely. Furthermore, it is useful to see movement of an extremity as an indicator of inadequate depth of anesthesia.
Emergence	No special considerations. Prophylactic antiemetic (e.g., ondansetron 4 mg iv, ±metoclopramide 10–20 mg iv) should be given 30 min before extubation. Surgeon should infiltrate wound with 0.5% bupivacaine (max = ~30 mL) or 0.75% ropivacaine (max = ~40 mL) with epinephrine to improve post-op analgesia.

Wake-up testing: At some institutions, an asleep-awake-asleep technique is used in which the patient is placed under GETA for positioning and craniotomy. After surgical exposure of the seizure area, the patient is allowed to awaken to assess neurologic function while areas of the brain are stimulated. When the seizure focus has been adequately delineated, GA is reinstituted for the remainder of the operation. An excellent anesthetic technique under these circumstances includes the use of sevoflurane (± 50% N_2O) for amnesia, and remifentanil (0.05–2 mcg/kg/min) by continuous infusion for analgesia. The advantage of these drugs is that they are quickly eliminated, allowing for rapid emergence for the awake component of the procedure, followed by rapid reinduction of anesthesia when the testing period is over. To allow the patient to talk during the awake portion of the procedure, the ETT must be removed. This is best accomplished by inserting a small or medium-sized tube changer through the ETT before it is removed. The tube changer can then be used as a guide for reinsertion of the ETT, and it will not prevent normal vocalization by the patient during the awake phase. Alternatively, an LMA can be used to secure the airway initially, removed for the awake testing and reinserted for closure.

Blood and fluid requirements	Moderate blood loss IV: 18 ga ×2 NS @ 4–6 mL/kg/h	Two iv cannulae are useful: one for fluid administration, another for infusion of anesthetic and other drugs. Alternatively, one peripheral iv and a CVP cannula are inserted. Blood transfusions are seldom needed.
Monitoring	Standard monitors (see p. B-1). Arterial line ± CVP line UO	O_2 sat and $ETCO_2$ monitoring will indicate the adequacy of ventilation and oxygenation in awake patients.
Positioning	Table rotated 180° ✓and pad pressure points ✓eyes	Semisitting position with head held in Mayfield-Kees 3-pin clamp and rotated laterally with a roll under the shoulder on the operative side. Anesthetic hoses and intravascular lines must be long enough to be accessible.
Complications	Anxiety Agitation Sz	Local anesthetic toxicity may produce agitation and seizures. Iced NS should be immediately available to flood cortical surface for Sz control.

POSTOPERATIVE

Complications	Seizure Bleeding Cerebral edema	Monitor carefully for altered mental status. May require urgent reexploration and removal of electrode grid if present.
Pain management	Codeine 30–60 mg im q 4 h PCA (selected patients)	Avoid oversedation. LA infiltration of the incision effectively reduces postop pain. Morphine PCA (e.g., 1.5 mg, 8 min lockout, 40 mg/4 h max) combined with ondansetron 4 mg iv q 4 h
Tests	CT scan	If a patient exhibits any delay in emergence from anesthesia and surgery, or any new neurologic deficits appear, a CT scan is invariably obtained.

References:

1. Blume WT, Grabow JD, Darley FL, Aronson AE: Intracarotid amobarbital test of language and memory before temporal lobectomy for seizure control. *Neurology* 1973; 23(8):812–19.
2. Kofke WA, Tempelhoff R, Dasheiff RM: Anesthetic implications of epilepsy, status epilepticus, and epilepsy surgery. *J Neurosurg Anesthesiol* 1997; 9:349–72.
3. NIH Consensus Development Conference. *Consensus Statement: Surgery for Epilepsy.* 1990; 8(2):2; *JAMA* 1990; 264: 729–33.
4. Zimmerman RS, Sirven JI: An overview of surgery for chronic seizures. *Mayo Clinic Proc* 2003; 78(1):109–17.
5. Tanriverdi T, Poulin N, Olivier A. Life 12 years after temporal lobe epilepsy surgery: A long-term prospective clinical study. *Seizure* 2008; 17(4):339–49.
6. Duncan JS. Epilepsy surgery. Clin Med 2007;7(2):137–42.
7. Soriano SG, Bozza P. Anesthesia for epilepsy surgery in children. *Childs Nerv Syst* 2006; 22(8):834–43.
8. Frost EA, Booij L. Ansethesia in the patient for awake craniotomy. *Curr Opin Anaesthesiol* 2007; 20:331–5.

SURGERY FOR SPASTICITY

SURGICAL CONSIDERATIONS

Description: Neurologic conditions associated with spasticity of the extremities include spinal cord injury, multiple sclerosis, stroke, etc. The spasticity is often managed with oral medications. An alternative approach is to infuse baclofen (GABA-agonist that decreases frequency and amplitude of tonic impulses to the muscle spindles) into the subarachnoid space via an implanted pump. When these therapeutic modalities fail, it may be necessary to perform surgery. Some of the procedures are destructive in that a lesion is placed in certain nerves or the spinal cord to destroy the reflex arc that is contributing to the spasticity. There are both percutaneous and open techniques for placing the lesion. In the **open procedures,** a **laminectomy** is performed (see Posterior Lumbar Spine Surgery, p. 119). In a case where a **myelotomy** is to be performed, the lower spinal cord is exposed and incised at the appropriate location to interrupt the reflex arc. In certain cases, selective electrical stimulation can be performed on isolated dorsal rootlets from the involved extremity. Abnormal responses in the extremities are monitored via EMG and direct observation. When abnormal responses are detected, that particular rootlet is divided (**dorsal rhizotomy**). This procedure is somewhat tedious and requires that stable anesthetic conditions be maintained so that appropriate monitoring can be carried out during the procedure. The surgeon usually must sacrifice 40–60% of the dorsal rootlets in cases of spastic diplegia found in cerebral palsy.

Variant procedure or approaches: Percutaneous **RF rhizotomy** is another procedure used for spasticity. A thermal lesion is placed in the appropriate dorsal roots with a RF generator. Needles are passed into the neural foramen via a posterolateral trajectory for levels L1–L5, and then from a midline approach to the S1 root. The needle position is determined by A-P and lateral fluoroscopy and by stimulus mapping. Stimulating current is delivered via an electrode passed through the needle. A low-level stimulating current causes muscle twitching in the appropriate leg if the needle is in the proper location. Once placed and verified, the RF generator is used to produce the lesion. At the termination of this procedure, the patient's legs should be flaccid. Patients with spinal cord injury producing anesthesia below T10 may not require additional anesthetic for the procedure.

Usual preop diagnosis: Spasticity; multiple sclerosis; spinal cord injury

SUMMARY OF PROCEDURES

	Open Rhizotomy or Myelotomy	RF Rhizotomy
Position	Prone	⇐
Incision	Midline	Needles placed in lumbar region
Special instrumentation	EMG monitor; nerve stimulator	RF generator; fluoroscope
Unique considerations	Anesthetic that allows EMG recordings	May not require anesthesia if anesthetic below waist (2° spinal cord surgery).
Antibiotics	Ceftriaxone 1 g iv (avoid administration with calcium-containing solutions)	None
Surgical time	4 h	2 h
Closing considerations	Surgeon may wish to test dural closure with Valsalva maneuver.	
EBL	50–250 mL	Negligible
Postop care	Head flat; PACU room	⇐
Mortality	<1%	⇐
Morbidity	All <5%: CSF leak Infection Hemorrhage Neurological impairment	⇐
Pain score	4	2

PATIENT POPULATION CHARACTERISTICS

Age range	3–55 yr
Male:Female	~3:2
Incidence	Relatively uncommon neurosurgical procedure
Etiology	Hyperactivity of gamma stretch reflex
Associated conditions	Multiple sclerosis; cerebral palsy; spinal cord injury

ANESTHETIC CONSIDERATIONS

See Anesthetic Considerations for Surgical Correction of Spinal Dysraphism, Pediatric Neurosurgery, p. 1162.

References:

1. Kennemore DE: Percutaneous electrocoagulation of spinal nerves for the relief of pain and spasticity. In *Radionics Procedure Technique Series.* Radionics, Burlington MA: 1978.
2. Peacock WJ, Staudt LA, Nuwer MR: A neurosurgical approach to spasticity: selective posterior rhizotomy. In *Neurosurgery Update,* Vol II. Wilkins RH, Rengachary SS, eds. McGraw-Hill, New York: 1991, 403–7.
3. Steinbok P. Selective dorsal rhizotomy for spastic cerebral palsy: a review. *Childs Nerv Syst* 2007; 23(9):981–90.

PERCUTANEOUS PROCEDURES FOR TRIGEMINAL NEURALGIA

SURGICAL CONSIDERATIONS

Lawrence M. Shuer

Description: Three percutaneous procedures are commonly used to treat trigeminal neuralgia (a well-defined pain disorder of the face). Each involves placing a needle percutaneously from the cheek into the foramen ovale at the base of the skull under a light iv anesthetic. For **glycerol injection,** it is necessary for the surgeon to verify that the needle is placed in the cistern of the trigeminal (AKA Gasserian) ganglion. This usually is done via I.I. or x-ray films with contrast instilled into the cistern by the surgeon. There should be free flow of CSF through the needle. The patient is then placed in the seated position with head flexed and sterile glycerol is injected into the cistern (a potentially painful event). The patient is taken to the recovery room with the head still flexed for 1 h. The glycerol damages neurons in the ganglion, which usually causes mild sensory loss and relieves the tic pain in most cases. **Percutaneous balloon compression** of the ganglion is a procedure done in some centers for this condition. The needle is placed similarly to the previously mentioned procedure, but, in this case, a balloon catheter is placed through the needle, and the balloon is inflated after it is successfully located in the Gasserian ganglion cistern. The patient may be kept sedated throughout this procedure. Compression of the ganglion will relieve the pain in many patients.

Radiofrequency (RF) rhizotomy is the most common percutaneous procedure used for trigeminal neuralgia. This procedure differs from glycerol injection in that a RF generator is used to place a thermal lesion in the appropriate portion of the Gasserian ganglion. The needle is actually an insulated electrode with a portion of the tip exposed. The proper needle position is determined by applying stimulating current, with the patient awake, while assessing patient's responses. Multiple brief periods of anesthesia will be required to adjust the needle position or to lesion the nerve. It is important for the patient to awaken quickly and be able to cooperate with the stimulus localization throughout this procedure. This same approach may be used to place a stimulating electrode in the ganglion with the leads subsequently tunnelled to an implantable pulse generator. Direct stimulation has been shown to provide pain relief in many patients.

Usual preop diagnosis: Trigeminal neuralgia; tic douloureux

SUMMARY OF PROCEDURES

	Glycerol Injection	Balloon Compression	RF Rhizotomy
Position	Supine	⇐	⇐
Incision	Needle placed lateral to mouth on cheek	⇐	⇐
Special instrumentation	I.I.	⇐	⇐ + RF generator

SUMMARY OF PROCEDURES (cont'd)

	Glycerol Injection	Balloon Compression	RF Rhizotomy
Unique considerations	Hypertensive response to needle placement	⇐	⇐ + Requirement for periodic deep sedation with rapid awakening for RF lesioning.
Antibiotics	Usually none	⇐	⇐
Surgical time	0.5 h	1 h	1–1.5 h
EBL	None	⇐	⇐
Postop care	Seated position with head flexed for 1 h	PACU	PACU
Mortality	~1%	⇐	⇐
Morbidity	Usually < 5%: Infection Complete facial numbness (anesthesia dolorosa) Extraocular muscle paresis (diplopia) CSF leak Carotid puncture Facial hematoma	⇐	⇐
Pain score	3–7	2–4	2–4

PATIENT POPULATION CHARACTERISTICS

Age range	40–85 yr (usually 60–70 yr)
Male:Female	1:2
Incidence	Trigeminal neuralgia: 4.3/100,000/yr [~25/100,000/yr > 70 yrs]
Etiology	Vascular compression of trigeminal nerve; multiple sclerosis plaque; cerebellopontine angle tumor; AVMs
Associated conditions	HTN; multiple sclerosis; rheumatoid arthritis; Charcot-Marie-Tooth disease; Sjogren syndrome

ANESTHETIC CONSIDERATIONS

PREOPERATIVE

Trigeminal neuralgia, or tic douloureux, is a condition that develops in adults usually > 60 yr old. It is more common in women in whom an intermittent, severe, lancinating pain arises over the maxillary and/or mandibular divisions of the trigeminal nerve. The ophthalmic division of the trigeminal nerve is rarely involved. The pain is unilateral and often can be precipitated by stimulating a trigger point, such as by rubbing the cheek, mastication, or brushing the teeth. The cause of this condition is not known. Medical management consists of therapy with carbamazepine (Tegretol) or oxcarbazepine (Trileptal), anticonvulsants, and analgesics specific for this condition. The failure rate for medical treatment is 50–60%. Stereotactic radiosurgery (dose = ~60 Gy) has been shown to have long-term effectiveness in ~50% of patients who failed drug therapy. Surgery is considered when medical or radiotherapy management fails to control pain or complications of drug therapy develop (anemia, bleeding disorders, dizziness, etc.). One of three types of percutaneous procedures is performed: either **glycerol injection, RF rhizotomy** of the symptomatic branches of the trigeminal ganglion or direct ganglionic stimulation. If these treatments fail, microvascular decompression of the trigeminal nerve is considered.

Respiratory	No common associations or special considerations, unless patient has a longstanding Hx of smoking and has COPD. **Tests:** As indicated from H&P.
Cardiovascular	Most patients have Hx of idiopathic HTN and take antihypertensive medications. Good control of BP preop is important because most patients become hypertensive during the operative procedure. Intraop HTN is often unavoidable because of the surgical need to have the patient awake during much of the procedure. **Tests:** As indicated by H&P.
Neurological	The presenting symptom is pain in the maxillary and/or mandibular division of the trigeminal nerve, unaccompanied by motor or sensory deficits. (Dx should be questioned in the presence of sensory deficits).
Laboratory	As indicated from H&P. CBC/platelets if Rx carbamazepine. Anticonvulsant drug levels.
Premedication	Midazolam (1–2 mg iv) ± glycopyrrolate 0.2 mg iv shortly before induction of anesthesia to minimize oral secretions while the surgeon is working in the mouth, positioning the needle.

INTRAOPERATIVE

Anesthetic technique: GA, regardless of which percutaneous technique is to be used. O_2 by nasal cannula should be administered before induction of anesthesia. To keep the cannula out of the surgeon's field, it must be taped above the eye on the side of operation.

Induction	Because the surgeon will want the patient awake to check for pain distribution as soon as the needle or electrode is in place, the induction drug must be potent, but short-acting. Methohexital (0.5–1 mg/kg) is preferred for this purpose, but propofol (1–2 mg/kg) alone or at a reduced dose in combination with remifentanil (0.5 mcg/kg) has been used successfully. The drug should be injected by bolus into a rapidly flowing iv to achieve a high concentration in the brain quickly. Continuous infusion of the drugs is not satisfactory, because it fails to achieve a high brain concentration quickly, and its continuous administration prolongs the time before the patient is sufficiently able to communicate with the surgeon. In experienced hands, the needle is placed within a matter of 2–3 min. If difficulty is encountered in placing the needle, additional bolus doses of induction drug may be needed. Patients often develop apnea for 1–2 min, followed by partial or total airway obstruction, while the surgeon has his hand in the mouth positioning the needle. Prior to induction of anesthesia, therefore, it is essential that the anesthesiologist optimize ventilation and oxygenation by asking the patient to take a series of deep breaths through the nose with the mouth closed. This will ↑ the O_2 level and ↓ the CO_2 level in the lungs before induction. To maintain adequate spontaneous ventilation and oxygenation, it is usually necessary to institute forward displacement of the mandible while the surgeon inserts the needle. Another alternative is to insert a nasal airway. If **glycerol injection** is used, needle position is verified by radiological imaging, using a radio-opaque dye. Patient is awakened and placed in a seated position with head flexed. The glycerol is injected, causing severe pain. Patient is then moved to recovery room still in seated position with the head forward to keep the glycerol localized to the region of the trigeminal ganglion. If **RF rhizotomy** stimulator electrode placement is performed, the patient is awakened and the position of the electrode is verified by stimulating the ganglion with heat or directly and determining the site of pain. The patient is then reanesthetized with a smaller bolus of the same drug to permit electrode adjustment or local heating for ~1 min. This procedure may be repeated several times. Each time, the patient needs less anesthetic, because of both the cumulative effects of the drug, and the fact that the ganglion is becoming damaged by the heat and manipulation.

Emergence	Following glycerol injection patients are maintained in a seated position with an ice pack on the cheek at the site of needle insertion to minimize postop bleeding and swelling. These patients often complain of pain in the face, requiring opiate analgesics. Following RF rhizotomy, the face is usually numb, which is the end point for concluding the operation.	
Blood and fluid requirements	IV: 18–20 ga ×1 NS/LR @ 4–6 mL/kg/h	
Monitoring	Standard monitors (see p. B-1).	HTN patients may require an arterial line.
Control of BP	Labetalol Clonidine patch SNP infusion may be necessary	Patients almost invariably become hypertensive during this therapy. Attempts to lessen these episodes with a clonidine patch preop or use of intermittent doses of labetalol prophylactically or therapeutically are only partially successful.
Positioning	Table turned 180° ✓ and pad pressure points. ✓ eyes.	Patient in reclining position with head in the midline.
Complications	Failure of needle placement Bleeding Respiratory arrest Oculocardiac reflex	Major complications from this operation are uncommon, but include: (1) Failure to identify the foramen ovale, through which the needle must be inserted to reach the trigeminal ganglion. If the needle cannot be placed within 30–40 min, the procedure usually is aborted until another day. (2) Bleeding into cheek from puncture of a branch of the facial artery. (3) Apnea from spillover of the neurolytic solution into circulating CSF, presumably affecting the respiratory center in the 4th ventricle.

POSTOPERATIVE

Pain management	Parenteral opiates (see p. C-2).

References

1. Bennetto L, Patel NK, Fuller G. Trigeminal neuralgia and its management. *BMJ* 2007; 334(7586):201–5.
2. Jorns TP, Zakrzewska JM. Evidence-based approach to the medical management of trigeminal neuralgia. *Br J Neurosurg* 2007; 21(3):253–61.
3. Monstad P. Microvascular decompression as a treatment for cranial nerve hyperactive dysfunction—a critical view. *Acta Neurol Scand Suppl* 2007; 187:30–3.
4. Young RF: Stereotactic procedures for facial pain. In: *Brain Surgery: Complication, Avoidance and Management.* Apuzzo MU, ed. Churchill Livingstone, New York: 1993, 2097–113.

CHAPTER

1.3 Spinal Neurosurgery

SURGEONS

Stephen Ryu, MD
Scott Berta, MD

ANESTHESIOLOGIST

C. Philip Larson, Jr., MD, MS

ANTERIOR FUSION/FIXATION OF THE UPPER CERVICAL (C1-C2) SPINE

SURGICAL CONSIDERATIONS

Description: **Transoral odontoid excision**: The **transoral approach** is indicated primarily to relieve ventral irreducible compression of the cervicomedullary junction due to extradural lesions involving the lower part of the clivus, C1 and C2 vertebral bodies. This approach provides direct access to the C1 anterior arch and odontoid process of C2. The anesthetized patient is positioned supine usually with cervical traction. A Dingman or similar retractor is used to facilitate surgical access. The soft palate is retracted upwards with stay sutures. Through a posterior midline incision over the pharyngeal wall, the C1 anterior arch and C2 vertebra are exposed (Fig 1.3-1). Using fluoroscopic guidance, bony decompression of the clivus, C1 anterior arch, odontoid process, and C2 vertebral body is performed. Instrumentation of C1-C2 may be performed with plate and screws. The wound is closed in two layers after securing hemostasis. As the procedure often results in significant instability at the craniovertebral junction, posterior occipitocervical fusion often is required.

Variants of the transoral procedure: **Transpalatal exposure** with removal of hard palate or a **tongue-splitting transmandibular approach** may be required for adequate exposure of the clivus or upper C-spine, respectively. A **high cervical anterior retropharyngeal approach** is rarely used to approach C1-C3 without traversing the oral cavity and with less destabilization. A transcervical approach to the C2 body can be performed using an endoscope and a highly beveled tubular retractor.

Transodontoid screw fixation: Fractures of the odontoid process of C2 account for 10–20% of all C-spine fractures and are classified (**Anderson and D'Alonzo**) into three types, based on anatomical location. **Type I fractures**, which occur at the tip of dens, are treated conservatively. **Type II fractures**, which occur through the waist of the odontoid process, are the most common and are often inherently unstable, requiring surgical treatment. **Type III fractures** occur through the body of C2 and can be treated surgically or with external immobilization. Internal instrumented fixation is the ideal treatment for Type II fractures, because it provides immediate stability while preserving C1-C2 rotation.

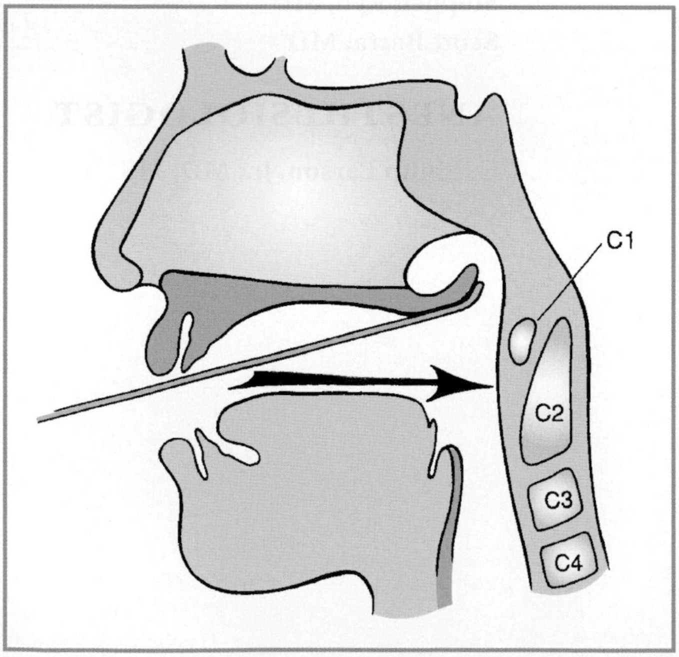

Figure 1.3-1. The transoral approach. (Reproduced with permission from An HS, Cotler JM: *Spinal Instrumentation.* Williams & Wilkins, Philadelphia: 1992.)

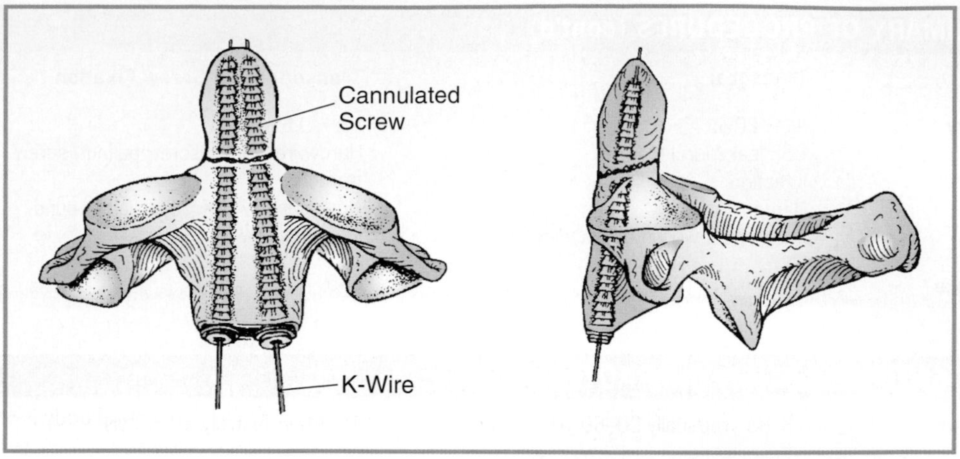

Figure 1.3-2. Screw fixation technique, using cannulated screws. K-wire provides provisional stabilization and allows guided tapping and screw placement. (Reproduced with permission from An HS, Cotler JM: *Spinal Instrumentation*. Williams & Wilkins, Philadelphia: 1992.)

The anesthetized patient is placed in a supine position with traction of 5–10 lb. The mouth may be kept open using a radiolucent jaw distractor. A horizontal skin incision is made at approximately C5 level, and the platysma is cut along the skin incision. The anterior C-spine is exposed by opening the natural plane between the trachea and esophagus medially and carotid sheath laterally. Using a guide tube, a hole is drilled under fluoroscopy through the body of C2, the odontoid process, and its apex, through the fracture. The drilled hole is tapped, and an appropriately sized screw is placed (Fig 1.3-2). At this point, fluoroscopy of the patient's neck in flexion and extension is done to exclude C1-C2 instability.

Usual Preop diagnosis: Basilar impression (telescoping of C-spine into posterior fossa); odontoid fracture; rheumatoid arthritis with atlantoaxial instability; traumatic irreducible atlantoaxial instability; Type II odontoid fractures (recent or remote)

SUMMARY OF PROCEDURES

	Transoral	Transodontoid Screw Fixation
Position	Supine, head in mild extension with traction	Supine; head in mild extension with traction
Incision	Posterior oropharynx	Transverse skin incision in the anterolateral neck at C5 level
Special instrumentation	Operating microscope, I.I., Dingman retractor	K-wire, drill, odontoid screw instrumentation
Unique considerations	Requires ≥ 3 cm mouth opening; armored ETT must be taped securely away from surgical field. Tracheostomy is needed occasionally. Fiber optic intubation may be required.	Fiber optic intubation in patients with C1-C2 instability; biplanar fluoroscopy is mandatory.
Surgical time	2–4 h	2–3 h
Closing considerations	Extubation may be delayed due to lingual swelling.	Routine wound closure
EBL	25–200 mL	25–200 mL
Postop care	ICU or close observation unit. Monitor airway for respiratory obstruction. ± Postop immobilization. Will require leaving NG tube in postop.	PACU → room; cervical collar
Mortality	0–3%	1%

SUMMARY OF PROCEDURES (cont'd)		
	Transoral	Transodontoid Screw Fixation
Morbidity	All < 20%: CSF leak/dural tear Infection Neural injury Pharyngeal wound dehiscence	All: < 15% Hardware failure (screw pullout, screw fracture): 10% Nonunion: 5–10% Superficial wound infection: 2%
Pain score	3–5	3–5

PATIENT POPULATION CHARACTERISTICS		
Age range	18–85 yr (usually 20–60 yr)	15–90 yr (usually 20–60 yr)
Male:Female	1:2	1.5:1
Incidence	Rare	Common (10–20% of C-spine fractures)
Etiology	Neoplastic; traumatic; congenital; degenerative	Traumatic
Associated conditions	Rheumatoid arthritis	-

ANESTHETIC CONSIDERATIONS

See Anesthetic Considerations for Cervical Neurosurgical Procedures, p. 106.

Suggested Readings

1. Apelbaum RI, Lonser RR, Veres R, et al: Direct anterior screw fixation for recent and remote odontoid fractures. *J Neurosurgery (Spine 2)* 2000; 93:227–36.
2. Crockard AH: Transoral approach to intra/extradural tumors. In *Surgery of Cranial Base Tumors*. Sekhar LN, Janecka ID, eds. Raven Press, New York: 1993, 225–34.
3. Fountas KN, Kapsalaki EZ Nikolakakos LG, et al: Anterior cervical discectomy and fusion associated complications. *Spine* 2007; 32(21):2310–7.
4. Menezes AH: Transoral approach to the clivus and upper cervical spine. In *Neurosurgery*. Wilkins RH, Rengachary SS, eds. McGraw-Hill, New York: 1995, 306–13.
5. Vender JR, Harrison SJ, McDonnell DE: Fusion and instrumentation at C1–3 via the high anterior cervical approach. *J Neurosurgery (Spine 1)* 2000; 92:24–9.

POSTERIOR FUSION/FIXATION OF THE UPPER CERVICAL SPINE

SURGICAL CONSIDERATIONS

Description: **Craniocervical (occipitocervical, craniovertebral) fusion/fixation** or instrumentation involves stabilization of the occiput and upper three or four cervical vertebrae, while **atlantoaxial fusion/fixation** involves stabilization of the atlas (C1) and axis (C2). Instability may be caused by congenital, traumatic, degenerative, neoplastic, or infectious conditions resulting in compression of the lower brain stem or cervical spinal cord. Symptoms may include paresthesias and/or weakness of the upper and lower extremities.

Atlantoaxial techniques: **Atlantoaxial (C1-C2) fusion** is performed in the prone position, with or without traction. Through a posterior midline incision, the occiput and upper C-spine are exposed. A posterior iliac or rib graft may be harvested and fashioned appropriately. The bone graft can be secured with wires to the decorticated segments to be fused. Traditionally, the fixation has been performed with sublaminar wires alone; however, other fixation techniques—such as **C1-C2 transarticular screw fixation** and more recently the **C1-C2 lateral mass fusion**

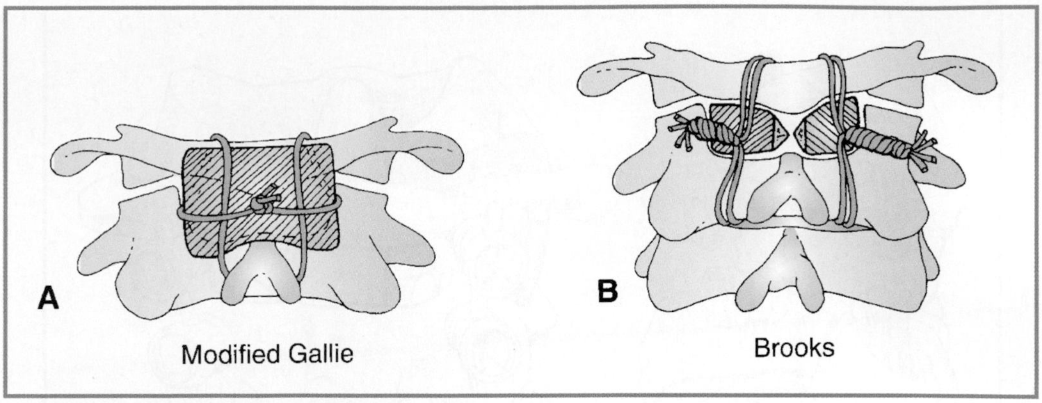

Figure 1.3-3. Posterior wiring techniques. **A.** Modified Gallie using an H-shaped bone graft from the iliac crest, contoured to fit over the posterior arches of C1 and C2. A double U-shaped 18- or 20-ga wire is passed under the arch of C1 from inferior to superior. **B.** Brooks-type fusion with doubled-twisted 24-ga wires passed under the arch of C1 and then under the lamina of C2. Rectangular iliac crest bone grafts are fitted in the intervals between the arch of C1 and each lamina of the axis. (Reproduced with permission from An HS, Cotler JM: *Spinal Instrumentation.* Williams & Wilkins, Philadelphia: 1992.)

techniques are being used more often because they are biomechanically stronger and permit early ambulation with minimal orthotic support.

In **C1-C2 posterior wiring techniques**, the posterior arches of C1 and C2 laminae are exposed through a midline incision. Of the various wiring techniques used, **Gallie's** and **Brooks'** are the most widely accepted. In **Gallie's fusion** (Fig 1.3-3A), a wire loop or cable is passed underneath the C1 arch and brought over a bone graft wedged between C1 and C2 and then tightened over the C2 spinous process. In **Brooks' technique** (Fig 1.3-3B), wires are passed beneath the C2 lamina and C1 posterior arch on each side and tightened over a bone graft placed between C1 and C2. The posterior aspects of C1 and C2 are decorticated to facilitate the bony fusion. Wiring techniques are simpler, but carry the risk of cord injury during wire placement.

C1-C2 transarticular screw fixation was initially popular because of its greater biomechanical stability, higher fusion rates (87–100%), and superior fixation of atlantoaxial rotation. The occiput and C1-C3 vertebrae are exposed

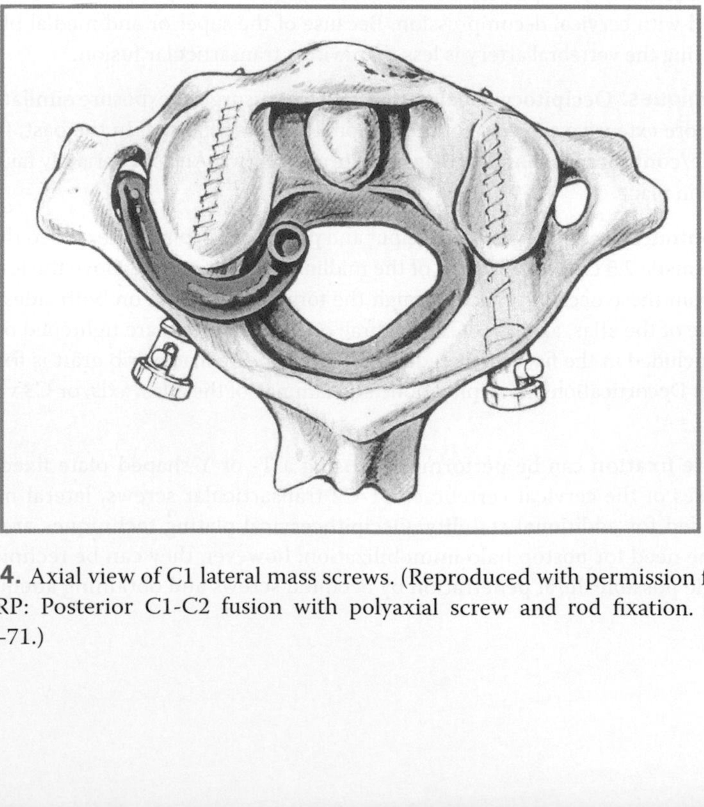

Figure 1.3-4. Axial view of C1 lateral mass screws. (Reproduced with permission from Harms J, Melcher RP: Posterior C1-C2 fusion with polyaxial screw and rod fixation. *Spine* 2001; 26(22):2467–71.)

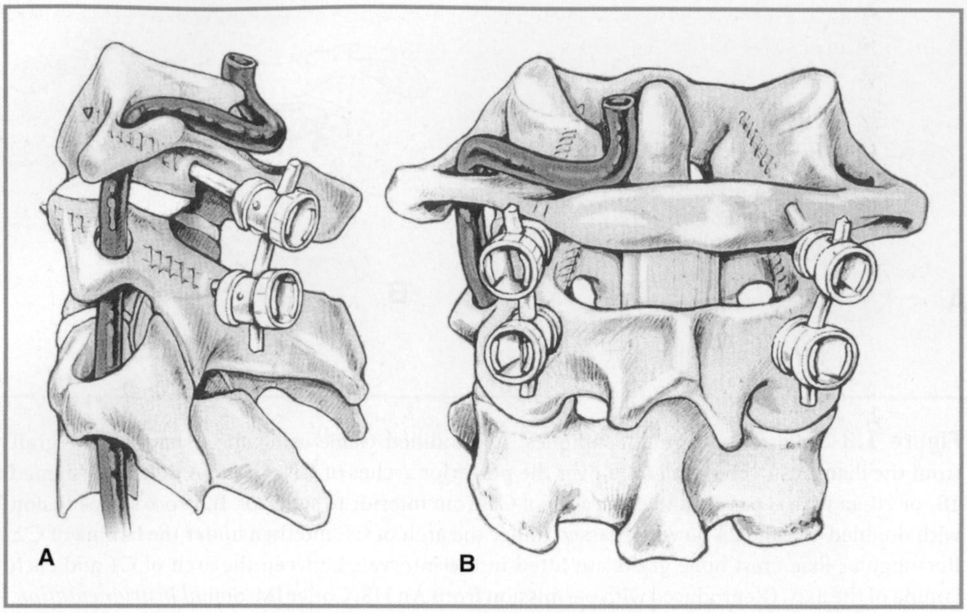

Figure 1.3-5. Lateral (**A**) and AP view (**B**) of C1-C2 fusion. (Reproduced with permission from Harms J, Melcher RP: Posterior C1-C2 fusion with polyaxial screw and rod fixation. *Spine* 2001; 26(22):2467–71.)

by a conventional posterior approach. Screws are placed from each lateral mass toward the anterior tubercle of C1 under fluoroscopic guidance. The major risks of this technique include injury to the vertebral artery (4.1%), malposition of screws, or instrumentation failure. Twenty percent of patients will have an anomalous vertebral artery, demonstrated by radiographic studies, precluding use of this technique.

In **C1-C2 lateral mass fusion**, the C-spine is exposed subperiosteally from occiput to C3-4 vertebrae by a conventional posterior approach. In this technique, polyaxial screws are passed into the lateral mass of C1 (Fig 1.3-4). Additionally, C2 pedicle screws are also placed and then attached to the C1 screws by connecting rods (Fig 1.3-5). If required, a reduction maneuver is carried out by repositioning the head or by direct manipulation of the C1 and C2 vertebrae. C1-C2 interfacetal fusion or posterior interlaminar fusion may be performed with wiring. The C1-C2 construct can be combined with cervical decompression. Because of the superior and medial placement of C2 pedicle screws, the risk of injuring the vertebral artery is less than with a transarticular fusion.

Craniocervical techniques: **Occipitocervical fusion** involves a surgical exposure similar to that of atlantoaxial fusion, except that a more extensive exposure of the occipital bone is required. In the past, fixation was performed with a **Luque rectangle/contoured rod and wiring** or plate and screws. An appropriately fashioned rib or iliac crest graft was then secured in place.

In **occipitocervical contoured rod fixation**, the occiput and posterior C-spine are exposed through a posterior incision, and trephines are made 2.5 cm to either side of the midline and about 2 cm above the foramen magnum. Wires or cables are passed from these occipital holes through the foramen magnum on both sides. Sublaminar wires are passed beneath laminae of the atlas, axis, and C3 vertebrae on each side, and are tightened over a rod. Other cervical vertebrae may be included in the fixation as required. A tricorticate iliac or rib graft is fixed with wires over the occipitocervical region. Decortication of occipital bone and laminae of the atlas, axis, or C3 vertebrae is essential for bony fusion.

Occipitocervical plate fixation can be performed by using a T- or Y-shaped plate fixed by screws to the occiput and lateral masses of the cervical vertebrae. C1-C2 transarticular screws, lateral mass screws, or wiring techniques can be added for additional stability. Occipitocervical plating techniques are biomechanically stable, often obviating the need for postop halo immobilization; however, they can be technically challenging. The major concerns include possible dural penetration by occipital screws and obtaining adequate contouring of the construct.

Usual preop diagnosis: Transoral odontoid resection; occipitoatlantal instability; atlantoaxial instability; odontoid fractures; spinal fractures; cervical instability; previous failed fusions

SUMMARY OF PROCEDURES

	Atlantoaxial (C1-C2) Fusion/Fixation	Occipitocervical Fusion/Fixation
Position	Prone, head in tong traction or pins	⇐
Incision	Posterior midline incision	⇐
Special instrumentation	Fluoroscopy; drills; wires/cables; lateral mass plate and/or screws; transarticular screws	Fluoroscopy; drills; rods, wires/cables; plates and screws
Unique considerations	Iliac/rib autograft ± posterior ilium for graft. Fiber optic intubation and SSEPs	⇐
Surgical time	2–3 h	3–4 h
Closing considerations	Routine wound closure	Halo vest may be needed in selected cases.
EBL	100–500 mL	⇐
Postop care	PACU, then → room	⇐
Mortality	< 1%	⇐
Morbidity	Vertebral artery injury: 4.1% CSF leak Instrumentation failure Nonunion	Neural injury ⇐ ⇐ ⇐
Pain score	5–9	5–10

PATIENT POPULATION CHARACTERISTICS

Age range	18–85 yr (usually 20–60 yr)
Male:Female	1:2
Incidence	Rare
Etiology	Neoplastic; traumatic; congenital; degenerative; infections; rheumatoid arthritis

ANESTHETIC CONSIDERATIONS

See Anesthetic Considerations for Cervical Neurosurgical Procedures, p. 106.

Suggested Readings

1. Harms J, Melcher R: Posterior C1-C2 fusion with polyaxial screw and rod fixation. *Spine* 2001;26:2467–71.
2. Menendez JA, Wright NM: Techniques of posterior C1-C2 stabilization. *Neurosurgery* 2007; 60(suppl 1):S103–11.
3. Vangilder JC, Menezes AH: Craniovertebral abnormalities and their neurosurgical management. In: *Operative Neurosurgical Techniques.* Schmidek HH, Sweet WH, eds. WB Saunders, Philadelphia: 2000, 1934–45.
4. Wright N, Lauryssen C: Vertebral artery injury in C1–2 transarticular screw fixation: results of a survey of the AANS/CNS section on disorders of the spine and peripheral nerves. *J Neurosurg* 1998; 88:634–40.

ANTERIOR FUSION/FIXATION OF THE MID AND LOWER CERVICAL SPINE

SURGICAL CONSIDERATIONS

Description: The first description of the anterior approach for excision of a cervical disc was made by Smith and Robinson in 1958. This approach permits easy and safe access to the entire C-spine below C2. **Anterior cervical discectomy** is commonly indicated for the removal of herniated discs or osteophytes compressing the spinal cord or nerve roots. Multisegmental cervical spondylosis (narrowing of spinal canal) may require single- or multi-level corpectomy (removal of a vertebral body). During anterior cervical discectomy, an approach from the left side of the neck is often preferred because it minimizes the chances of injury to the recurrent laryngeal nerve. The dissection is carried along the avascular plane between the trachea and esophagus medially, and the carotid sheath laterally (Figs 1.3-6 and 1.3-7). The fascia is incised to expose the longus colli muscles and anterior C-spine. The disc level is confirmed using fluoroscopy. The annulus is incised, and the disc is removed in piecemeal fashion with the use of an operating microscope. **Fusion and instrumentation** are often performed after discectomy to maintain disc space height, restore normal cervical lordosis, prevent graft extrusion, facilitate early ambulation, and possibly prevent delayed deformity and pain due to collapse of the disc space. After the discectomy, osteophytes are removed from the vertebral bodies, and an appropriately sized bone graft or prosthesis is placed in the intervertebral space. PEEK and carbon-fiber cages are radiolucent and allow good assessment of bony fusion. Fusion with instrumentation is often essential for immediate stability and early ambulation.

Anterior screw-plate fixation (with MRI-compatible titanium) is the preferred method of fixation for C2-C7. It provides stable fixation after discectomy or corpectomy, prevents bone graft migration, improves fusion rate, corrects spinal deformities, and may restore anterior and middle column function following cervical trauma. Plates and screws are placed under fluoroscopic guidance to prevent dural penetration or malposition. Hemodynamic changes should be monitored closely during the procedure, because ↓ HR or ↓ BP during the instrumentation may suggest cord compression.

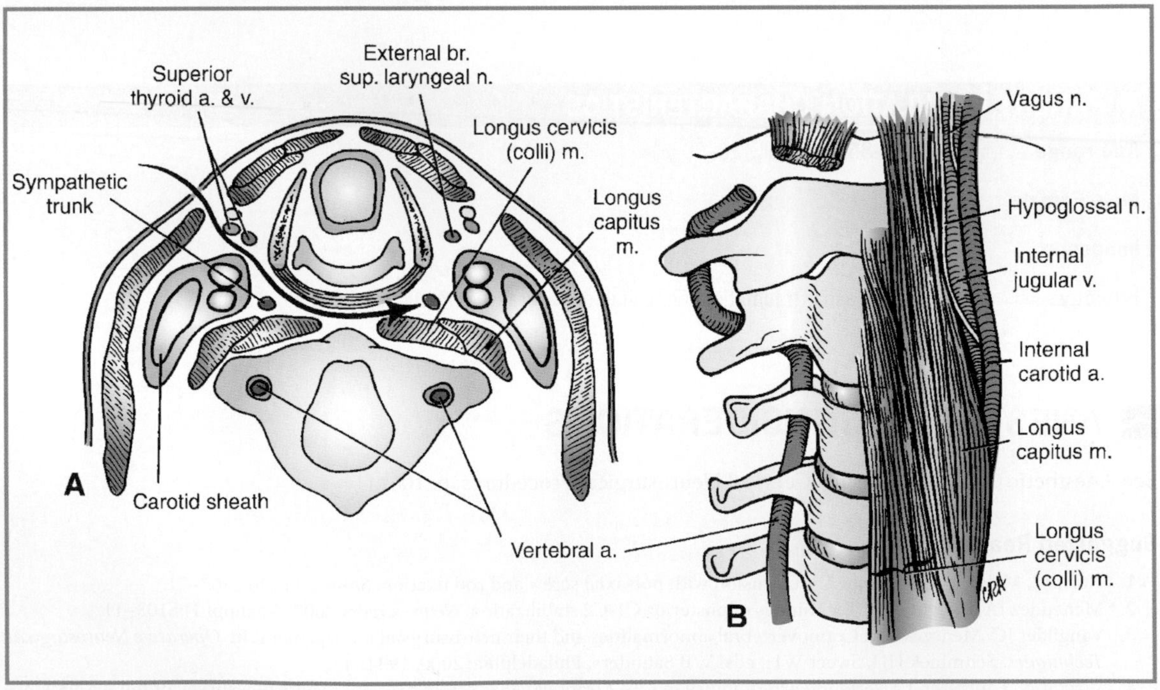

Figure 1.3-6. Upper C-spine. **A.** Cross-section showing the anteromedial approach. **B.** Anterior aspect, after stripping the longus collis muscle. (Reproduced with permission from An HS, Cotler JM: *Spinal Instrumentation.* Williams & Wilkins, Philadelphia: 1992.)

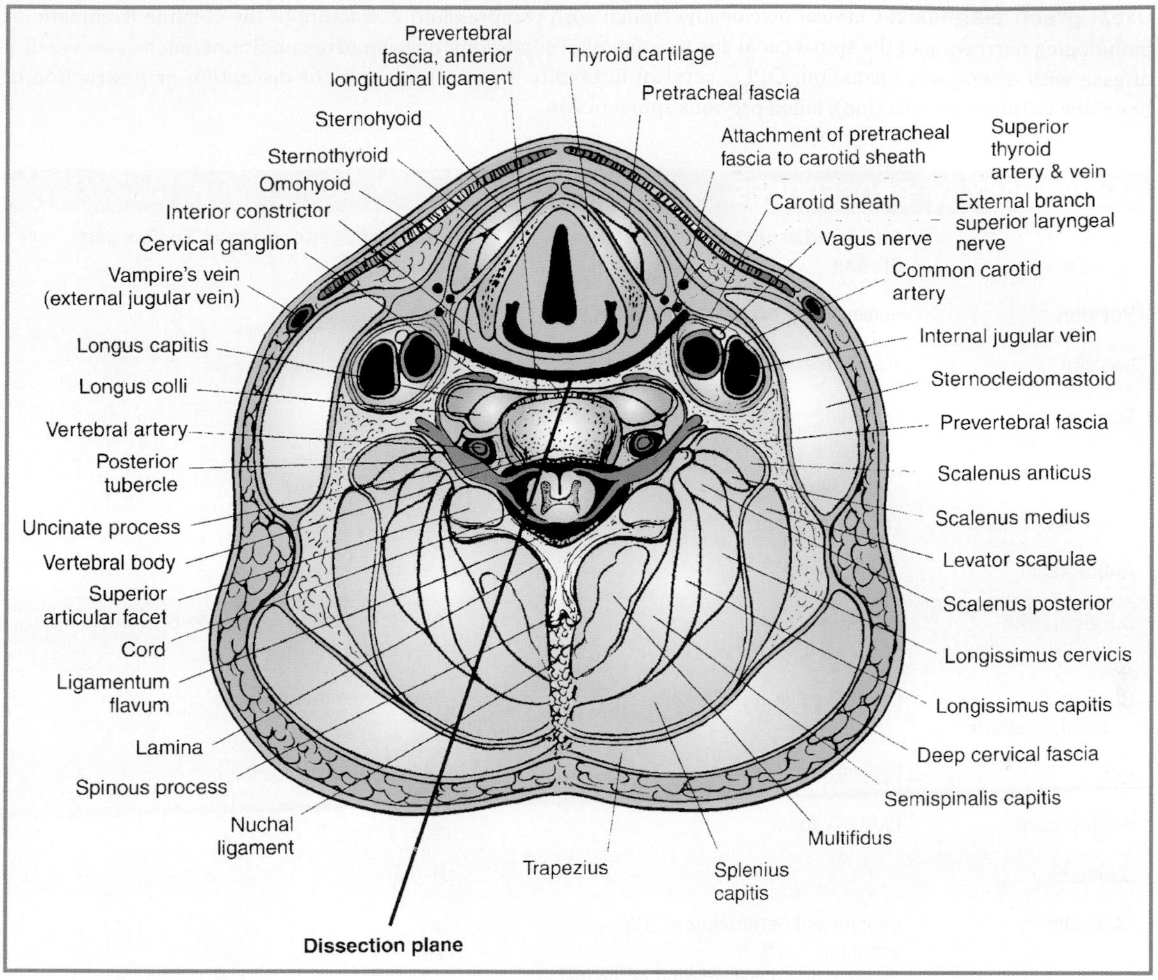

Figure 1.3-7. Cross-section of the C-spine at C5 level. Note the deep cervical fascia, the pretracheal fascia, and the prevertebral fascia. Note the relationship of the pretracheal fascia to the carotid sheath. Dissection plane is shown. (Modified with permission from Hoppenfeld S, deBoer P: *Surgical Exposures in Orthopaedics: The Anatomic Approach,* 2nd edition. Lippincott Williams & Wilkins, Philadelphia: 1994.)

Usual preop diagnosis: Cervical radiculopathy (nerve-root compression due to disc herniation or osteophytic compression); cervical myelopathy (spinal-cord compression by disc/osteophytes); cervical instability (ligamentous laxity or disruption)

Variant procedure: Cervical (vertebral) corpectomy and fusion are used to treat conditions in which there is anterior impingement of the spinal cord or narrowing of the spinal canal at the level of the vertebral body, including multisegmental cervical spondylitic compression, ossification of the posterior longitudinal ligament (OPLL), tumors, infections (e.g., TB, osteomyelitis), or C-spine injury. The surgical exposure is similar to that for anterior cervical discectomy. A transverse neck incision is preferred for corpectomy involving two or three vertebrae; however, a vertical skin incision along the anterior border of the sternomastoid may be used if more than three vertebrae are involved. Before the removal of a vertebral body, adjacent discs are resected. The posterior part of the vertebra and osteophytes at the posterior margins are excised. Reconstruction is accomplished with an autograft, allograft, or cages (metal or carbon fiber spaces filled with bone fragments). Some of the newer cages are expandable, facilitating a good fit. Supplemental fixation with plates and screws is essential to prevent graft extrusion, to facilitate fusion, and to permit early ambulation.

Usual preop diagnosis: Cervical myelopathy (spinal cord compression) 2° fracture of the C-spine (traumatic or pathologic); narrowing of the spinal canal due to congenital conditions; degenerative conditions, such as severe disc disease with osteophyte formation; OPLL; cervical instability (ligamentous laxity or disruption or destruction of bone due to tumor or infection); failed previous spinal fusion

SUMMARY OF PROCEDURES

	Cervical Discectomy ± Fusion and Plating	Cervical Corpectomy ± Fusion and Plating
Position	Supine, head extended on headrest	⇐
Incision	Transverse anterolateral	⇐ or vertical anterolateral
Special instrumentation	Operating microscope; anterior cervical plates	⇐
Unique considerations	Fiber optic intubation may be necessary; ± cervical traction	⇐
Antibiotics	Cefazolin 1 g	⇐
Surgical time	1–2 h (+ 1h for fusion/plating)	1.5–3 h for single level; add 20–30 min for each additional level.
Closing considerations	Cervical collar (soft/hard)	Cervical collar (soft/hard)
EBL	25–250 mL	50–1000 mL
Postop care	PACU → room	⇐
Mortality	< 1%	0–5%
Morbidity	Esophageal perforation: < 1% Infection: < 1% Massive blood loss–carotid or jugular injury, : < 1% Myelopathy: < 1% Nerve injury: Recurrent laryngeal nerve: 5% Root: < 1% Sympathetic chain: < 1% Postop instability: < 1% Instrument failure: < 1% Slipped graft: < 1%	⇐ ⇐ ⇐ ⇐ ⇐ ⇐ ⇐ ⇐ ⇐ 1–15% ⇐
Pain score	3–5	3–5

PATIENT POPULATION CHARACTERISTICS

Age range	18–85 yr (usually 20–60 yr)	⇐
Male:Female	1:2	⇐
Incidence	Rare	⇐
Etiology	Neoplastic; traumatic; congenital; degenerative; OPLL	⇐

ANESTHETIC CONSIDERATIONS

See Anesthetic Considerations for Cervical Neurosurgical Procedures, p. 106.

Suggested Readings

1. Brislin BT, Hilibrand AS: Avoidance of complications in anterior cervical spine revision surgery. *Curr Opin Orthop* 2001; 12(3):257–64.
2. Dickman CA, Marciano FF: Principles and techniques of screw fixation of the cervical spine. In *Principles of Spinal Surgery.* Menezes AH, Sonntag VKH, eds. McGraw-Hill, New York: 1995; 123–39.

POSTERIOR FUSION/FIXATION OF THE MID AND LOWER CERVICAL SPINE

SURGICAL CONSIDERATIONS

Description: **Posterior cervical laminectomy** (removal of lamina), **foraminotomy** (opening of the neural foramina), and **laminotomy** (removal of a portion of the lamina) are posterior procedures for decompression of the neural elements in the C-spine. These procedures are used to treat cervical radiculopathy 2° degenerative disc disease (e.g., herniated discs, osteophytes). The major advantage of **foraminotomy** over an anterior approach is that it does not require fusion and, thus, preserves the motion of the involved vertebral segments and obviates the need for immobilization for fusion. It also permits decompression of multiple levels, if required. Disadvantages of foraminotomy include an increased incidence of neck pain and the fact that it is not an effective approach to midline disc herniation. **Decompressive laminectomy** can be used to treat cervical canal stenosis (congenital or degenerative) and for removal of intraspinal masses (tumors, AVMs, infective granulomas), which may be extradural, intradural, extramedullary, or intramedullary. Depending on the location of the tumor, the surgeon may need to open the dura and/or spinal cord. Obviously, the intradural intramedullary tumors involve more risk and are more delicate to remove. Many laminae may be removed to expose and excise the tumor. Surgical adjunctive tools (e.g., CUSA, laser, surgical microscope, etc.) may be used to aid in removal of the tumor. Intraop evoked potential monitoring may be used during these procedures to test the integrity of the dorsal columns. After the tumor has been removed, the wound is closed in layers, as in a simple laminectomy.

Surgery is performed in the prone or sitting position through a posterior midline incision over the involved vertebrae. The paraspinal muscles are dissected off the spinous processes, and lamina and bone are removed piecemeal. The extent of the procedure depends on the indications for treatment. Hemostasis is achieved with bipolar cautery, and raw bone surfaces are sealed with bone wax. Topical hemostatic agents are used to aid in hemostasis in the epidural gutters. If the patient has an intradural tumor or process, such as syringomyelia, the dura is opened and the operating microscope is used for this portion of the procedure. After the intradural procedure is complete, the dura is closed, and the surgeon may wish to test the integrity of the closure with a Valsalva-like maneuver (sustained inspiration to 30–40 cmH_2O). The wound is closed in layers, and a drain may be left in the epidural space. Multilevel laminectomies with foraminotomies (involving partial removal of cervical facet joints) can result in late-onset cervical kyphosis, an extremely difficult condition to treat. These patients are usually considered for concomitant posterior fusion and instrumentation, especially in the presence of cervical segmental instability.

Newer less traumatic techniques can be used to perform foraminotomies and discectomies in the cervical spine in a **minimally invasive (MIS)** fashion. These use one of many tubular retractor systems [e.g., **METRx** (Medtronic, Memphis, TN, USA)]. These afford similar exposure but minimize blood loss, scar, and pain by spreading the muscles. The disadvantage is unfamiliar exposure, difficulty with retractor placement, and potential of neurological injury by inadvertent penetration of the interlaminar space.

Posterior cervical wiring techniques include: (a) **interspinous wiring** (Fig 1.3-8) (wires are passed through drilled holes in the base of adjacent spinous processes and then tightened); (b) **sublaminar wiring** with Luque rods or rectangles (sublaminar wires are passed at each level on both sides and are tightened over the rods or rectangles); and (c) **a triple-wire technique** with the first wire being passed through drill holes at the base of each spinous process, and the second and third wires passed through the same holes and then through drill holes in the previously placed

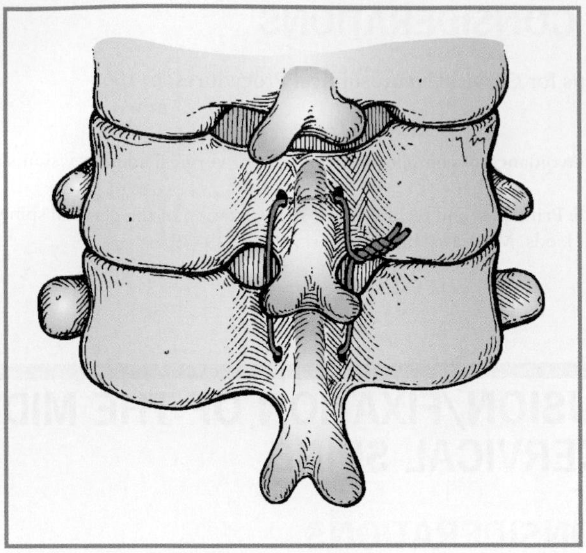

Figure 1.3-8. Intraspinous wiring. Wires passed through drilled holes in base of adjacent spinous processes and tightened. (Reproduced with permission from An HS, Cotler JM: *Spinal Instrumentation*, 2nd edition. Lippincott Williams & Wilkins, Philadelphia: 1999.)

bone grafts. This latter technique is biomechanically sound, because it places the bone grafts in compression. Wiring techniques, while stable in flexion, however, are less stable in extension and rotation, and they cannot be performed in patients with prior laminectomy or requiring laminectomy.

In the **posterior cervical lateral mass screw fixation** technique, the C-spine is exposed through a midline incision over the involved vertebral segments. The lateral mass (bony column between facet joints) is identified, drilled, and tapped. Cortical screws are passed into the lateral mass and fixed with plates or rods. The trajectory of the screws in the lateral mass is to the upper outer corner in the classic Magerl technique. The entry point should be approximately 1 mm medial to the midpoint of the lateral mass (Fig 1.3-9). The axial trajectory angulation should be 25°, and the

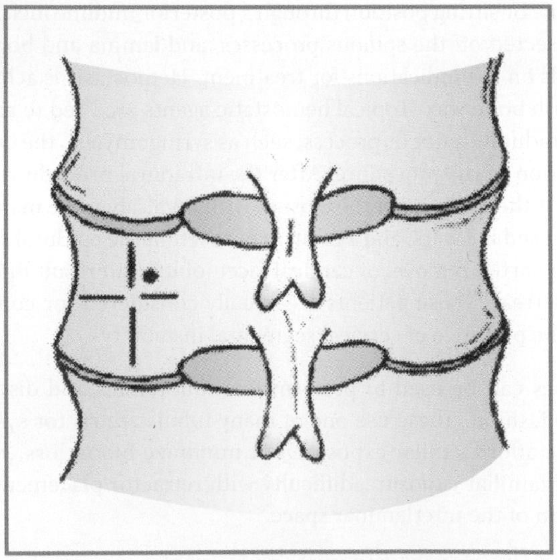

Figure 1.3-9. Magerl technique lateral mass screw entry point. (Reproduced with permission from Barrey C, Mertens P, et al: Quantitative anatomic evaluation of cervical lateral mass fixation with a comparison of the Roy-Camille and the Magerl Screw techniques. *Spine* 2005; 30(6):E140–7.)

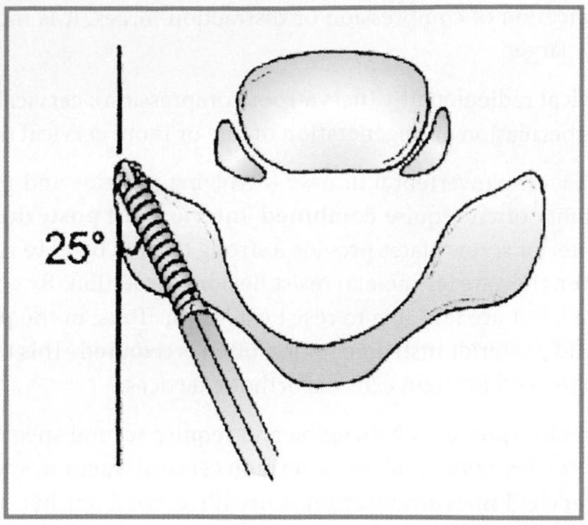

Figure 1.3-10. Magerl technique lateral mass screw axial trajectory angulation. (Reproduced with permission from Barrey C, Mertens P, et al: Quantitative anatomic evaluation of cervical lateral mass fixation with a comparison of the Roy-Camille and the Magerl Screw techniques. *Spine* 2005; 30(6):E140–7.)

sagittal angulation should be 45°, which is inline with the facet joints (Figs 1.3-10 and 1.3-11). Adjacent facet joints are decorticated and bone grafts are placed. Lateral mass plating provides a rigid multisegmental fixation and can be performed in patients with prior laminectomy. The major risks involved with this procedure are nerve-root and vertebral artery injuries.

Cervical pedicle screw plate fixation is an effective alternative to lateral mass fixation. In this technique, screws are passed under fluoroscopic guidance into the cervical pedicles and secured to plates or rods. This procedure is technically demanding, as the cervical pedicles are narrow and in close proximity to nerve roots, vertebral artery, and spinal cord and their trajectories are typically unfamiliar. This technique is biomechanically stable and permits the

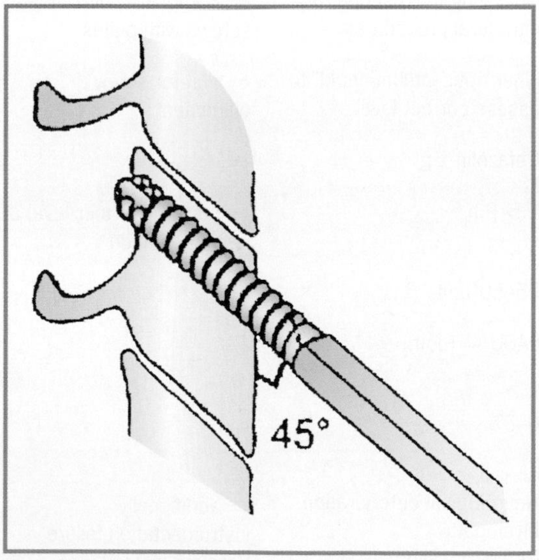

Figure 1.3-11. Magerl technique lateral mass screw sagittal trajectory angulation. (Reproduced with permission from Barrey C, Mertens P, et al: Quantitative anatomic evaluation of cervical lateral mass fixation with a comparison of the Roy-Camille and the Magerl Screw techniques. *Spine* 2005; 30(6):E140–7.)

correction of deformity by application of compression or distraction forces. It is most commonly performed at C2 where the pedicles are relatively larger.

Usual preop diagnosis: Cervical radiculopathy (nerve-root compression); cervical myelopathy (spinal-cord compression); cervical disc disease (herniation or degeneration of one or more cervical discs); C-spine injury

Variant procedures: Patients with panvertebral disease (involving anterior and posterior elements of the spine) and three-column spinal instability often require **combined anterior and posterior decompression, reconstruction, and instrumentation**. Anterior screw plates provide a strong tension band to resist vertical/horizontal translation and neck extension; however, they are less able to resist flexion or rotation. By contrast, posterior cervical plates strongly resist flexion or rotation, but are less able to resist extension. Thus, in the presence of three-column spinal instability, combined anterior and posterior instrumentation often is required. This technique provides rigid fixation of spinal segments and avoids the need for rigid external orthotic devices.

Combined instrumentation techniques are challenging and require several special considerations. Patients with any unstable C-spine may require fiber optic intubation, intraop cervical traction, and electrophysiological monitoring. **Anterior and posterior cervical instrumentation** is usually carried out in a single surgical session although may be staged. The transition between the anterior and posterior approaches requires a specialized operating table (e.g., Jackson spinal table or Stryker frame) and careful coordination among the entire OR team. The long duration of surgery may be associated with increased incidence of respiratory complications, blood loss, and prolonged ICU stays. In rare instances, an additional anterior or posterior approach may be performed ("540-degree procedure").

Usual preop diagnosis: C-spine injury causing three-column (severe, unstable) injuries; cervicothoracic junctional pathologies; correction of kyphotic deformities; panvertebral disorders involving C-spine (neoplasms, infection, spondylitic myelopathy); failed symptomatic anterior cervical fusions

SUMMARY OF PROCEDURE

	Cervical Laminotomy/ Foraminotomy	Cervical Laminectomy with Instrumentation	Combined Anterior/ Posterior Cervical Instrumentation
Position	Prone or sitting; pin fixation or horseshoe headrest	Prone; pin fixation or horseshoe headrest	⇐ + supine
Incision	Posterior midline neck	⇐	⇐ + transverse or longitudinal anterolateral
Special instrumentation	Operating microscope for intradural procedures	⇐ + implants, pedicle screws with plates	Implants; anterior and posterior plates with screws
Unique considerations	Fiber optic intubation; I.I. to assess correct level	⇐ ; I.I. for screw placement	Implants; anterior and posterior plates with screws
Antibiotics	Cefazolin 1 g	⇐	⇐
Surgical time	1.5–2 h	⇐ Add 30–45 min/level of instrumentation	4–5 h
EBL	25–500 mL	⇐	250–600 mL
Postop care	PACU → room	⇐	⇐; sometimes needs short ICU stay
Mortality	0–3%	⇐	⇐
Morbidity	All < 5%: Neurological deterioration Myelopathy Nerve-root injury CSF leak Postop instability Infection	⇐ ⇐ additionally: Instrumentation failure Vascular injury Nerve-root injury 2° screws	5–10% ⇐ additionally: Bone graft dislodgement Respiratory problems
Pain score	2–6	5–10	7–10

PATIENT POPULATION CHARACTERISTICS	
Age range	18–85 yr (usually 20–60 yr)
Male: Female	1:2
Incidence	Rare
Etiology	Neoplastic; traumatic; congenital; degenerative; infections; rheumatoid arthritis

ANESTHETIC CONSIDERATIONS

See Anesthetic Considerations for Cervical Neurosurgical Procedures, p. 106.

Suggested Reading

1. Collias JC, Roberts MP: Posterior surgical approaches for cervical disk herniation and spondylitic myelopathy. In *Operative Neurosurgical Techniques.* Schmidek HH, ed. WB Saunders, Philadelphia: 2000, 2016–28.

ANTERIOR CERVICOTHORACIC SPINE SURGERY

SURGICAL CONSIDERATIONS

Description: The **anterior approach** to the **cervicothoracic junction** (CTJ-C7-T3) is performed for discectomy, stabilization of spinal fractures, tumor resection, spinal reconstruction, and instrumentation. Anterior approaches to the CTJ often are challenging, as this area represents a rapid transition from cervical lordosis to thoracic kyphosis, resulting in abrupt increase in the depth of the wound. The confluence of great vessels, and visceral (trachea, esophagus) and neural structures at the thoracic inlet makes them susceptible to injury. The modified anterior approach utilizes a "hockey stick" incision to allow greater access to the lower cervical and upper thoracic spine. This technique does not require any additional bone resection during the approach. The **transsternal** approach involves a longitudinal incision along the anterior border of the sternomastoid, extended over the midline of the sternum to the xiphisternum. The sternum is divided using an oscillating saw and retracted to expose the anterior aspect of the CTJ. The wide exposure available with this approach permits vertebral resection, reconstruction, and instrumentation. The **transclavicular** approach involves a T-shaped incision over the clavicles, with a vertical limb extending down the midline of the sternum. Subplatysmal flaps are elevated; and the sternal and clavicular heads of the sternomastoid are detached from their origin and retracted superolaterally. The medial third of the clavicle and manubrium are resected to provide an excellent direct anterior approach to the CTJ for vertebral decompression, reconstruction, and stabilization.

Variant procedure and approaches: **Axillary thoracotomy and high transthoracic thoracotomy** approaches permit an anterolateral exposure to CTJ. As these procedures involve entering the thoracic cavity, they typically require OLV during the procedure.

Usual preop diagnosis: C7-T3 disc disease, fracture, tumor, and deformity

SUMMARY OF PROCEDURES

	Transsternal Approach	Transclavicular Approach	Axillary/High Thoracotomy
Position	Supine	⇐	Lateral
Incision	Longitudinal incision along anterior border of sternomastoid	T-shaped incision over clavicles with a vertical limb down the midline of sternum	Lateral chest wall

SUMMARY OF PROCEDURES (cont'd)			
	Transsternal Approach	**Transclavicular Approach**	**Axillary/High Thoracotomy**
Special instrumentation	Anterior cervical plates Special oscillating saw for sternal opening	⇐ Special blades for clavicular resection	⇐
Unique considerations	OLV not necessary	⇐	OLV necessary
Antibiotics	Cefazolin 1 g iv	⇐	⇐
Surgical time	3–4 h	⇐	⇐
Closing considerations	Soft cervical collar	⇐	⇐
EBL	200–500 mL	⇐	⇐
Postop care	PACU → room	⇐	⇐
Mortality	1–2%	⇐	⇐
Morbidity	Wound infection/breakdown Injury to great vessels at thoracic inlet	⇐ ⇐ Cosmetic deformity	⇐ ⇐ Respiratory problems
Pain score	7–10	7–10	7–10

PATIENT POPULATION CHARACTERISTICS	
Age range	30–50 yr
Male:Female	1:1
Incidence	Uncommon
Etiology	Disc herniations; trauma; tumor; infections

Suggested Reading

1. Kim DH, Beck CE, Dietz DD, et al: Surgical approaches to the cervicothoracic junction. In: *Operative Neurosurgical Techniques.* Schmidek HH, ed. WB Saunders, Philadelphia: 2000, 2107–21.

ANESTHETIC CONSIDERATIONS FOR CERVICAL NEUROSURGICAL PROCEDURES

(Procedures covered: anterior/posterior fusion/fixation of upper and mid/lower C-spine; anterior cervicothoracic spine surgery)

PREOPERATIVE

Surgery of the C-spine is common, primarily because of the frequency of herniation of a cervical intervertebral disc causing compression of the adjacent spinal nerve roots. Other, less frequent indications for cervical surgery include: acute or chronic instability of the neck requiring fusion; removal of a tumor of the spinal cord; or craniocervical decompression for Arnold-Chiari malformation.

Respiratory	Acute fractures of the C-spine may be associated with sufficient trauma to the spinal cord to cause acute respiratory insufficiency and inability to handle oropharyngeal secretions. If this occurs, immediate tracheal intubation is necessary. Before initiating intubation, the neck must be stabilized, preferably in Gardner-Wells tongs or a body jacket; lacking those, a tight neck collar with sandbags on each side of the head will suffice. The objective is to **not flex or extend the head or move it laterally** during the course of tracheal intubation. Fiberoptic intubation techniques that secure the airway with minimal or no manipulation of the cervical spine should be used. **Tests**: Consider ABG to substantiate degree of respiratory impairment, if present.
Cardiovascular	Acute fractures of the C-spine and associated spinal cord trauma may → loss of sympathetic tone, which, in turn, may cause peripheral vasodilation and bradycardia. Generally, this condition can be treated effectively with crystalloid and/or colloid infusion, and atropine to ↑ HR. Rarely is it necessary to use vasopressors to maintain BP or HR. If spinal cord injury is suspected an A-line must be placed and MAP should be maintained above 80 at all times to avoid vascular insufficiency of the spinal cord. **Tests:** As indicated from H&P.
Neurological	Patients with herniation of a cervical disc generally complain first of pain in the neck, particularly with lateral rotation of the head. The pain may radiate down one or, rarely, both arms. As nerve compression continues, patients begin to develop weakness and atrophy of specific muscle groups in the arm. These Sx, however, are not specific to herniation of a disc and may be caused by a spinal cord tumor or cyst. Patients with acute fractures of the neck and attendant spinal cord trauma at the T1 level may be paraplegic to some degree, whereas fractures above C5 may result in quadriplegia and loss of phrenic nerve function. Injuries between these two levels result in variable loss of motor and sensory functions in the upper extremities. A careful documentation of preop sensory and motor deficits is important. **Tests:** MRI has replaced myelography as the primary diagnostic test because it distinguishes disc from tumor from cyst. Emergency CT is invaluable in the assessment of patients with acute neck injuries and suspected cervical fracture; if not available, A-P and lateral x-rays of the neck generally will reveal the site and extent of bony injury.
Hematologic	Antiplatelet agents should be stopped 10 d before elective surgery. At least 2 units of PRBCs should be ready along with a type and screen if large amounts of blood loss are anticipated, as can occur in some posterior cervical surgeries. **Tests**: Hct; T&C, others as indicated from H&P.
Laboratory	Other tests as indicated from H&P.
Premedication	Premedication is very useful in this patient population. Midazolam 2–4 mg iv and meperidine 20–40 mg iv in divided doses prior to entering the OR makes patients amnestic and tractable. Also, antibiotics (usually 1 g of cefazolin if not PCN allergic) should be given at least **30 min** prior to skin incision for them to be effective against infection.

INTRAOPERATIVE

Anesthetic technique:	GETA
Induction	For patients with a stable neck, orotracheal intubation using standard laryngoscopy is acceptable. If the operation is to be performed transorally or at C1–2; if the patient's neck is unstable; if the head is in tongs, a halo device, or a body jacket; or if the findings on the H&P suggest that tracheal intubation may be difficult, the ETT should be placed using FOL. FOL can be performed under local anesthesia before induction of GA, but this requires topicalization of the airway, which will cause coughing and potential injury to the spinal cord. A much better method is to perform a Plan C under general anesthesia. (For details of fiberoptic intubation and Plan C, see p. B-5.) Consider using

Induction (cont'd)	a wire-reinforced tube as it allows for maximal bending of the tube to remove it from the surgical field, and it will not be compressed by the Dingman retractor. A wire-reinforced tube is also desirable when the surgical procedure is to be done in the prone position. Most importantly, it is vital to discuss the severity of the surgical lesion and the planned intubation with the surgeon before proceeding. Nasotracheal intubation is rarely needed for this type of surgery. After the ETT is in place, anesthesia is induced with propofol 0.5–2.5 mg/kg or STP 3–5 mg/kg. FOI should be performed when there is any question that the neck is unstable or if positioning could potentially cause injury to the spine. The patient remains awake during positioning and FOI, then a post-intubation neuro exam is performed, and only then is the patient anesthetized. This applies even for cases where the patient is in a Mayfield head-holder.
Maintenance	Standard maintenance (see p. B-2). Neuromuscular blockade with rocuronium 0.6 mg/kg or vecuronium 0.1 mg/kg is helpful for positioning the patient and insertion of the Dingman retractor. After the retractor is in place and the operation is under way, further use of relaxants is usually not necessary.
Emergence	If a cervical fusion has been performed and the patient has been returned to a halo device or body jacket, it is desirable to leave ETT in place until the patient is fully awake, responding to commands, and able to manage his/her own airway. **NB:** Immediate airway obstruction 2° soft-tissue occlusion or superior laryngeal nerve damage may occur on extubation. A useful way to test for airway patency is to deflate the cuff of the tracheal tube and determine that the patient is able to breathe around the tube as well as through it. If there is any question about adequacy of the airway, it is prudent to leave the ETT in place and spray lidocaine 4% 4 mL down the trachea using a laryngotracheal anesthesia device (LTA) before emergence. This technique will usually prevent or minimize coughing or bucking on the ETT for about 15–30 min. One also should consider inserting an airway exchange catheter (AEC) through the ETT tube before its removal. AECs are well tolerated, and can be left in place until one is confident that no further airway compromise will occur. So long as the AEC is not touching the carina, it will not induce coughing or bucking, and the patient can talk without difficulty. This catheter will provide a conduit for immediate reinsertion of an ETT if airway obstruction from early or delayed swelling, bleeding, or hematoma formation should occur.
Blood and fluid requirements	iv: 16–18 ga × 1 NS/LR @ 4–6 mL/kg/h Blood transfusion is rarely needed for operations on the C-spine.
Monitoring	Standard monitors (see p. B-1). ± Arterial line ± CVP line ± Doppler ± Urinary catheter If a standard BP cuff is to be used, consider placing it on a leg at the ankle. If placed on an arm without rigid protection (e.g., sleds), the surgeons tend to lean on the cuff, making it difficult to take consistent, reliable measurements. If the patient has a CV, respiratory, or metabolic disorder (e.g., insulin-dependent diabetes) consider inserting an arterial catheter. During cases of spinal cord injury or severe stenosis, it is important to keep in mind that an arterial line should be placed prior to induction when hypotension is most likely. If a posterior surgical approach with patient in seated position is planned, an arterial catheter is useful for monitoring BP, and a CVP catheter is necessary for monitoring CVP and aspiration of air, if VAE occurs. If patient is seated, an ultrasonic Doppler flow probe also should be placed on the anterior chest wall, with confirmation of its performance by injecting

Monitoring (cont'd)		1 mL of agitated NS into CVP line and listening for the characteristic change in Doppler sound.
	SSEP	If SSEP monitoring is planned, the combination of sevoflurane (1 MAC or less), O_2, opiates (fentanyl or meperidine), and neuromuscular blockade (rocuronium) is an appropriate anesthetic regimen for optimizing the potentials. More than 50% N_2O and 0.5 MAC isoflurane make SSEP monitoring less satisfactory.
Positioning	Supine: ✓and pad pressure points. ✓ eyes. Shoulder roll Cervical traction	For **anterior cervical discectomy** and/or fusion, patient is positioned supine with a roll under the shoulders or neck, and the head is moderately extended. A cervical strap may be placed below the chin and behind the occiput, and attached to a weight of 5–10 lb hung over the head of the bed. If patient is in a halo or tongs, 5–10 lb of weight are attached to the device. Alternatively, the surgeon may request traction intermittently during insertion of bone plugs for fusion. The surgical incision can be made on either side of the neck at the discretion of the surgeon.
	Prone: ✓and pad pressure points. ✓ eyes. ✓ genitalia.	A **posterior approach** is used if the operation is for spinal stenosis or craniocervical decompression. With this approach, patient is usually positioned prone (on a Wilson frame or on bolsters), or more rarely sitting, with the head in 3-point fixation.
	Sitting: ✓ and pad pressure points. ✓ eyes. VAE monitoring: ✓ ETT position.	Although seldom used today, there are advantages to the neurosurgeon, the anesthesiologist, and, thus, the patient as well, in using a seated position. Advantages for the neurosurgeon: (a) easier access to the lesion; (b) less blood loss, since both arterial and venous pressures are lower than if patient were prone; (c) less interference from CSF, since it readily drains away from the operative site; and (d) lower incidence of postop neurological injury. Advantages to the anesthesiologist are: (a) less chance that ETT and other arterial and venous catheters will become dislodged than with patient prone; (b) less chance for inadvertent pressure injury; (c) easier assessment and management of ventilation; and (d) easier access to patient for insertion of additional catheters, if necessary.
Complications	VAE	The major disadvantage of the sitting position is the risk of VAE, particularly paradoxical air embolism to the left side of the heart through a PFO (or, rarely, through the pulmonary circulation) → CNS or coronary emboli. Incidence of VAE is 25–45% in patients operated on in the seated position. VAE is easily detected using a combination of Doppler, $ETCO_2$, and ETN_2 analysis; and complications are rare. If VAE is suspected (Sx =↓$ETCO_2$, ↑ETN_2, ↓BP, dysrhythmias), notify the surgeon and aspirate the right atrial

Complications (cont'd)	VAE (cont'd)	catheter using a 10-mL syringe. This generally will confirm the Dx as well as provide treatment. If VAE continues, and the surgeon has difficulty identifying the site of air entrainment, consider using PEEP ≤ 10 cm H_2O or bilateral jugular compression to increase CVP and cerebral venous pressure. Low levels of PEEP applied and released gradually will not promote paradoxical air embolism.
	Esophagus perforation	A possible complication of anterior cervical surgery is esophageal perforation. One way to assess for this type of injury is to flood the operative field with water and then force air though the oropharynx and look for any signs of bubbling. These can be occult and manifest post-op as fistulas as well.
	Retraction nerve injury	Another potential complication of anterior surgery is retraction injury to various nerves including the recurrent laryngeal. Pressure can be taken off of the nerve by reducing the cuff pressure once the retractors are in place to mitigate any compression due to the nerve being trapped between the retractor and the ET cuff.
	Hypotension	↓ BP caused by venous pooling, inadequate venous return to the heart, and ↓ CO can be treated by wrapping lower extremities while patient is supine, infusing adequate fluid volume to maintain right heart filling pressure, and avoiding excessive depth of anesthesia. Any **acute** drop in MAP may be due to a vascular injury, either obvious (vertebral artery injury) or occult (deep great vessel injury) until proven otherwise. The source of bleeding should be identified.

POSTOPERATIVE

Complications	Airway obstruction, edema Hematoma Neurologic deficit	The cause of airway obstruction is usually from soft tissue falling back against the posterior pharyngeal wall, which cannot be corrected by forward displacement of the mandible because of the neck fusion or postop traction/stabilization device. May require oral or nasal airway. Consider inserting an airway exchange catheter (AEC) before removing the ET tube.
	Tension pneumothorax	Delayed respiratory insufficiency usually is caused by either development of a tension pneumothorax from entrainment of air via the surgical wound or an unsuspected oropharyngeal laceration during tracheal intubation, or from bleeding into the neck at the surgical site, with progressive compression and occlusion of the airway. If a tension pneumothorax is suspected and circulatory signs are stable, immediate CXR should confirm the Dx. If circulation is failing,

Complications (cont'd)	Tension pneumothorax (cont'd)	an 18- or 20-ga needle catheter should be inserted immediately anteriorly at the 2nd intercostal space on the suspected side to relieve the pneumothorax. If the Dx is airway obstruction from bleeding into the neck, the wound should be opened immediately and clots and blood removed. This should be done before any attempts at intubation, because direct laryngoscopy may not be possible if tracheal deviation distorts the view. Emergent tracheostomy or cricothyrotomy can be lifesaving in patients with significant soft tissue swelling. If the Dx is soft tissue swelling, then exploration usually results in very little blood being found. These patients are given high-dose short-course steroid and have a good prognosis. It is sometimes difficult to distinguish airway obstruction from tension pneumothorax by physical signs. One useful way is to check for the "puff sign." With airway obstruction from any cause, what gas moves in and out of the airway does so very slowly because of an obstruction. In contrast, with tension pneumothorax, gas moves out of airway with great speed because of high intrapleural pressure. By applying positive pressure to the airway and listening at the patient's mouth for the sound of gas escaping as airway pressure is released, one hears either a puff or jet of air escaping (tension pneumothorax) or slow, gradual exit of air (airway obstruction).
Pain management	PCA	(see p. C-3).
Tests	CXR Hct	Repeat neurological exam prior to discharge from PACU.

Suggested Readings

1. Black S, Cucchiara RF, Nishimura RA, et al: Parameters affecting occurrence of paradoxical air embolism. *Anesthesiology* 1989; 71(2):235–41.
2. Black S, Ockert DB, Oliver WC Jr, et al: Outcome following posterior fossa craniectomy in patients in the sitting or horizontal positions. *Anesthesiology* 1988; 69(1):49–56.
3. Cucchiara RF, Nugent M, Seward JB, et al: Air embolism in upright neurosurgical patients: detection and localization by two-dimensional transesophageal echocardiography. *Anesthesiology* 1984; 60(4):353–5.
4. Larson CP: A safe, effective, reliable modification of the ASA difficult airway algorithm for adult patients. *Curr Rev Clin Anesth* 2002, 23:1–12.
5. Pearl RG, Larson CP Jr: Hemodynamic effects of positive end-expiratory pressure during continuous venous air embolism in the dog. *Anesthesiology* 1986; 64(6):724–9.
6. Sonntag VKH, Hadley MN: Management of upper cervical spinal instability. In *Neurosurgery Update*, Vol II. Wilkins RH, Rengachary SS, eds. McGraw-Hill, New York: 1991, 222–33.
7. Zasslow MA, Pearl RG, Larson CP Jr, et al: PEEP does not affect left atrial-right atrial pressure difference in neurosurgical patients. *Anesthesiology* 1988; 68(5):760–3.

ANTERIOR THORACIC SPINE SURGERY

SURGICAL CONSIDERATIONS

Description: The **anterior approach** to the mid and lower thoracic spine (T4-T12/L1) is performed for spinal fracture, scoliosis/kyphosis, tumor, and infection. The **anterior transthoracic approach** provides a wide and easy exposure of the thoracic spine from T4-T10. The patient is placed in a lateral decubitus position (right or left, based on spinal pathology). An incision is made over the involved vertebrae and extended rostrally one or two intercostal spaces. The muscles and ribs are retracted, the pleura are opened, and lungs retracted to expose the vertebral bodies. Discectomy, corpectomy, bony reconstruction, and stabilization can be performed as required under radiographic guidance. The risk of spinal cord injury depends on the extent of surgery and reconstruction. The complex vasculature can be challenging. Hemostasis is vital to prevent hemothorax. Chylothorax and lymphatic injury are rare.

The **transition zone** at the thoracolumbar (TL) spine (T11-L1) is somewhat difficult to expose and requires a combined transthoracic and retroperitoneal approach through the diaphragm **(thoracolumbar transdiaphragmatic approach)**. A left-sided approach is preferred, since it is easier to retract the spleen and stomach than the liver. The skin incision is made over the 10th rib, down to thoracic muscles, and the rib is resected subperiosteally to provide wide exposure. Blunt dissection separates the peritoneum from the undersurface of the diaphragm and lateral and posterior abdominal walls. With gentle retraction of the lung and abdominal contents, the diaphragm is well visualized and is sectioned circumferentially from the chest wall. This provides an excellent exposure of the anterior aspect of the TL junction. Most procedures can be performed with minimal retraction of lung tissue at this level; thus, OLV is not typically required. Vertebral resection, reconstruction, and stabilization are performed with radiographic guidance. Reconstruction of the diaphragm is important to prevent hernation. This is rare with pure retroperitoneal approaches.

Variant procedure or approach: **An 11th rib extrapleural-retroperitoneal approach** offers an alternative approach to the TL junction. It provides excellent exposure without the need to incise the diaphragm, resulting in less morbidity and reduced risk of pulmonary complications. Since the pleural cavity is not entered, chest drains and OLV are not needed.

Thoracoscopic spine surgery: This technically challenging procedure is performed in the lateral position with GA, using OLV. Four or more 10–15 mm portals are made, with the working portal centered over the target vertebra. The optical (scope) portal is placed two or three intercostal spaces cranial to the target vertebra. Separate portals anterior to the working channel allow suction/irrigation and retraction. When using **thoracoscopic instrumentation**, hardware is placed through the portals in the chest wall under fluoroscopic guidance. Blood loss must be minimized as hemostasis is difficult with this approach. Since instrumentation requires a wide exposure of the spine, OLV is essential. The major advantages of thoracoscopic surgery include minimal rib retraction; minimal blood loss, with consequent early removal of chest drain; reduced wound pain; early ambulation; and low morbidity. These factors combine to reduce hospital stay.

Usual preop diagnosis: Fractures (usually at the TL junction); scoliosis; primary and metastatic tumors of the spine; pyogenic and tuberculous osteomyelitis; Scheuermann's kyphosis

SUMMARY OF PROCEDURES

	Transthoracic (T4-T10)	Transdiaphragmatic (T11-L1),10th Rib	Thoracoscopic
Position	Lateral decubitus + axillary roll	⇐	⇐
Incision	Over involved vertebrae	Along 10th rib	3–4 portals (10–15 mm)
Special instrumentation	Anterior thoracic instrumentation/cages	⇐	Thoracoscopic spinal instrumentation
Unique considerations	DLT ± OLV	⇐	DLT; OLV mandatory
Antibiotics	Cefazolin 1 g iv	⇐	⇐
Surgical time	2–6 h	⇐	⇐

SUMMARY OF PROCEDURES (cont'd)

	Transthoracic (T4-T10)	Transdiaphragmatic (T11-L1),10th Rib	Thoracoscopic
Closing considerations	Transfer to bed before emergence. **NB:** sudden movement may dislodge grafts or implants.	⇐	⇐ + May need closure of diaphragm.
EBL	200–5,000 mL; nontumor cases: 200–400 mL	⇐	50–200 mL
Postop care	Chest tube to water seal	⇐	⇐
	Chest physiotherapy/incentive spirometer Short ICU stay is usual. Bleeding > 200 mL/h → re-exploration		Shorter period of chest drain/ ICU stay
Mortality	3–5%	⇐	⇐
Morbidity	Overall: 5–15%	⇐	⇐ + Problems with OLV
	DVT	⇐	
			Conversion to open surgery: 4%
	Neurological: 1–2%	⇐	
	Infection	⇐	–
	Vascular injury	⇐	–
	Sepsis	⇐	–
	Atelectasis	⇐	⇐
	Pneumonia	⇐	⇐
Pain score	7–10	7–10	5–8

PATIENT POPULATION CHARACTERISTICS

Age range	12–30 yr (scoliosis surgery); > 40 yr (tumor and infection surgery)
Male:Female	1:1; except for > scoliosis surgery in females
Incidence	20,000/yr
Etiology	Scoliosis, idiopathic (50%); trauma (20%); scoliosis, neuromuscular (15%); infections, tumors (10%); scoliosis, congenital (5%)
Associated conditions	See Etiology

ANESTHETIC CONSIDERATIONS

See Anesthetic Considerations for Thoracolumbar Neurosurgical Procedures, p. 124.

Suggested Readings

1. Francaviglia N, Maiello M: Anterolateral techniques for stabilization in the thoracic spine. In: *Operative Neurosurgical Techniques.* Schmidek HH, Sweet WH, eds. WB Saunders, Philadelphia: 2000, 2141–5.
2. Johnson MR, Murphy JM, Southwick OW: Surgical approaches to the spine. In: *The Spine.* Herkowitz NH, Garfin RS, eds. WB Saunders, Philadelphia: 1999, 1463–1571.
3. Kim M, Nolan P, Finkelstein JA: Evaluation of 11th rib extrapleural-retroperitoneal approach to the thoracolumbar junction. *J Neurosurgery (Spine)* 2000; 93:168–74.
4. Kumar R, Dunsker SB: Surgical management of thoracic disc herniation. In *Operative Neurosurgical Techniques.* Schmidek HH, Sweet WH, eds. WB Saunders, Philadelphia: 2000, 2122–40.
5. Kurz LT, Pursel SE, Herkowitz HN: Modified anterior approach to the cervicothoracic junction. *Spine* 1991; 16(10 Suppl): S542–47.
6. Sundaresan N, Shah J, Feghali JG: A transsternal approach to the upper thoracic vertebrae. *Am J Surg* 1984; 148:473–7.
7. Sunderesan N, Shah J, Foley KM, et al: An anterior approach to upper thoracic vertebrae. *J Neurosurg* 1984; 61: 686–90.

POSTERIOR THORACIC SPINE SURGERY

SURGICAL CONSIDERATIONS

Description: Thoracic laminectomy (midline removal of the lamina) and **costotransversectomy** (off midline removal of the rib head and transverse process) are procedures for decompressing the neural elements of the thoracic spine via a posterior approach. (Commonly used approaches are shown in Fig 1.3-12.)

Thoracic laminectomy is used to treat spinal cord compression due to disc herniation, neoplasm, or trauma. It also is used to gain access to the spinal canal or spinal cord for various intradural mass lesions, including syringomyelia. Thoracic laminectomy is done through a posterior midline incision centered over the involved vertebrae. The paraspinal muscles are retracted subperiosteally from the spinous processes and laminae on both sides. Laminae are removed piecemeal with rongeurs or drills. Extensive laminectomy involving several segments or requiring removal of facet joints may require stabilization with transpedicular screws or hooks. Intradural procedures are performed with an operating microscope and microneurosurgical instruments. After completion of the intradural procedure, watertight closure of the dura is obtained and tested with Valsalva maneuver (sustained inspiration at 30–40 cmH_2O).

A **transpedicular approach** may be indicated for removal of herniated discs, excision or decompression of tumors, and the treatment of infection involving vertebral bodies. This procedure is performed in the prone position through a posterior midline incision centered over the affected vertebrae. The paraspinal muscles are retracted subperiosteally on both sides to expose laminae and facet joints. Facet joints and the superior half of the involved pedicle are drilled out to expose the lateral limits of the thecal sac and the nerve roots. A laterally herniated disc can be removed in a piecemeal fashion. If required, total removal of the pedicle is done to facilitate adequate bony decompression. Posterior instrumentation by pedicle screws, sublaminar wiring with rods, or a hook-rod construct may be performed.

The **lateral extracavitary approach** is a modification of a **costotransversectomy** and provides access to the anterior and posterior elements of the spine, thereby avoiding the need for a thoracotomy. This approach is performed with the patient in the prone position. A midline skin incision is made three levels above and below the involved vertebrae. The lower part of the incision may be curved over the involved side, if needed. A myocutaneous flap is developed by dissecting the scapular muscles (trapezius, rhomboids, etc.) laterally. Paraspinal muscles are freed from

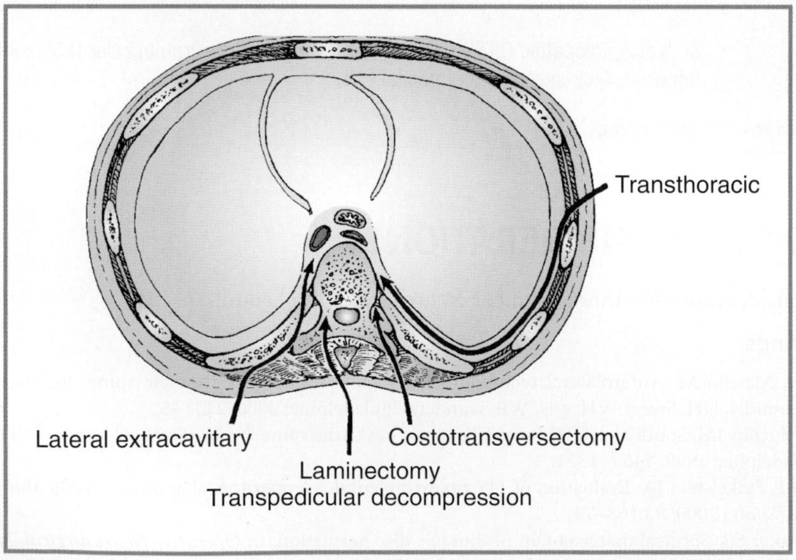

Figure 1.3-12. Surgical approaches to the thoracic spine. (Reproduced with permission from Tindall GT, Cooper PR, Barrow DL: *The Practice of Neurosurgery*, Vol. II. Williams & Wilkins, Philadelphia: 1996.)

the spinous processes and dorsal spinal elements to enable retraction, which exposes the entire rib cage and dorsal vertebral elements. Subperiosteal resection, from its costovertebral tip to the posterior bend of the appropriate rib is done. The parietal pleura are gently separated from the ribs and the vertebrae to expose the posterolateral aspect of the vertebral bodies. The transverse process, pedicle, and laminae are removed, as required, to permit direct visualization of the cord during decompression of the vertebral body. Discectomy/corpectomy, vertebral reconstruction, and instrumentation are performed as required. Complete spondylectomy and anterior reconstruction is possible with this approach with minimal retraction to the cord. Combined anterior-posterior instrumentation can be used to leverage off each other for deformity correction. At the end of the procedure, the operative field is filled with saline to check for any evidence of air leak. A small chest tube can be placed if an air leak is present. A layered wound closure with drain is performed.

Thoracic pedicle screws have largely replaced the older hook-rod construct and **Harrington** rods as the fixation of choice. These can be technically challenging because the thoracic pedicles tend to be rather narrow and variable. Potential complications include injury to surrounding nerves, spinal cord, blood vessels (both local and great vessel), and lung parenchyma.

Usual preop diagnosis: Thoracic radiculopathy (nerve-root compression); thoracic disc disease (herniation or degeneration of thoracic disc); thoracic myelopathy (spinal cord compression); thoracic canal stenosis (degenerative); infections (TB, pyogenic osteomyelitis) and tumors to spine (primary bone tumors or metastatic); intraspinal tumors; syringomyelia

SUMMARY OF PROCEDURES

	Thoracic Laminectomy	Transpedicular Approach	Lateral Extracavitary Approach
Position	Prone	⇐	⇐
Incision	Posterior midline	⇐	⇐; with/without hockey-stick extension
Special instrumentation	Operating microscope ± EP monitoring ± Pedicle screws/hooks	⇐	⇐ ± anterior and posterior spinal instrumentation
Unique considerations	I.I. localization	⇐	⇐
Surgical time	2–3 h	⇐ Add 30–45 min for bony/tumor decompression	3–7 h, based on need for anterior bony resection/reconstruction
Closing considerations	Often no cast	TL support/orthosis	⇐
EBL	100–1000 mL	200–1000 mL	300–3000 mL
Postop care	PACU → room	⇐	⇐ ± ICU
Mortality	0–5%	⇐	⇐
Morbidity	All $<$ 5% Neurological: Myelopathy Nerve-root injury Massive blood loss CSF leak	⇐ ⇐	⇐ ⇐
Pain score	6–10	6–10	8–10

PATIENT POPULATION CHARACTERISTICS	
Age range	18–85 yr (usually 20–60 yr)
Male:Female	1:2
Incidence	Rare
Etiology	Neoplastic; traumatic; congenital; degenerative

ANESTHETIC CONSIDERATIONS

See Anesthetic Considerations for Thoracolumbar Neurosurgical Procedures, p. 124.

Suggested Readings

1. Fessler RG: Lateral extracavitary and extrapleural approaches to the thoracic and lumbar spine. In: *The Principles of Spine Surgery.* Menezes AH, Sonntag VKH, eds. McGraw-Hill, New York: 1995, 1279–91.
2. Kim DH, Beck CE, Dietz DD, et al: Surgical approaches to the cervicothoracic junction. In: *Operative Neurosurgical Techniques.* Schmidek HH, Sweet WH, eds. WB Saunders, Philadelphia: 2000, 2107–21.
3. Kumar R, Dunsler SB: Surgical management of thoracic disc herniation. In: *Operative Neurosurgical Techniques.* Schmidek HH, Sweet WH, eds. WB Saunders, Philadelphia: 2000, 2122–31.

ANTERIOR LUMBAR/LUMBOSACRAL SPINE SURGERY

SURGICAL CONSIDERATIONS

Description: The use of anterior procedures is steadily increasing among spine surgeons. Most procedures permit short-segment instrumentation of the spine, which often obviates the need for subsequent posterior fixation. The most significant disadvantage of these procedures involves the risk of injury to the great vessels; thus, these procedures are commonly done in association with a vascular or general surgeon. There is also risk of injury to the peritoneal contents and the neural plexus around the lumbosacral spine. Anterior instrumentation systems generally fall

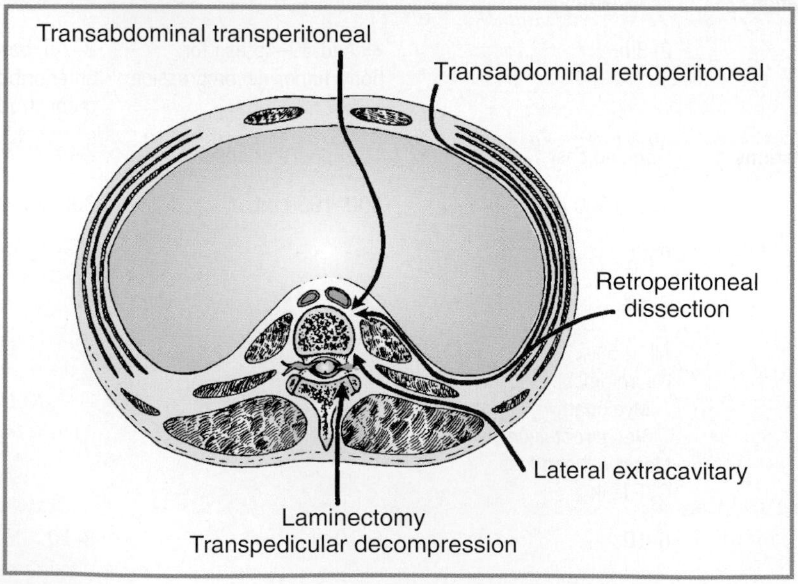

Figure 1.3-13. Surgical approaches to the lumbar spine. (Reproduced with permission from Tindall GT, Cooper PR, Barrow DL: *The Practice of Neurosurgery,* Vol. II. Williams & Wilkins, Philadelphia: 1996.)

into three categories: (a) **plating systems** (e.g., Z plating, anterior locking plates, and MACS-TL); (b) **rod systems** (e.g., Kostuik-Harrington, Kaneda, and Moss-Miami); and (c) **interbody devices** (e.g., cages and allografts).

An **anterior lumbar interbody fusion** (ALIF) can be done with artificial cages or bone. After exposure of the disc space, the exact midline of the space is marked and verified with fluoroscopy. A spacing guide determines the exact position for pilot holes; and a partial discectomy is performed through these pilot holes, which are distracted and later reamed. Bone or cage is then attached to a specialized implant driver for insertion under fluoroscopic guidance. Harvested bone chips and other fusion enhancers are placed into the cages or around the bone dowel. Anterior lumbar interbody fusion provides immediate mechanical stability and long-term load support, with the ability to heal through the disc space. Its primary disadvantages include bleeding and possible major vessel injury.

A **lumbar artificial disc** can be placed via this approach. The approach is similar to that of the ALIF but instead of placing a bone graft or cage, a mobile prosthetic disc is placed according to manufacturer's instruction. No additional stabilization or bone grafting is required. Accurate placement of this disc is absolutely critical to the success of this procedure. Fluoroscopy is used extensively to ensure this. There is immediate stability and because motion is preserved, early mobilization is recommended.

Anterior instrumentation after ALIF can be done with a variety of screws and/or plates. These include a screw and screw/plate combination to buttress the graft from falling out. Other devices provide plate stabilization across interspaces. These can be used alone or with a posterior stabilization surgery. These add time to the anterior case and run the risk of hardware failure, but have the advantage of potentially improving the overall fusion rate and decreasing the graft related complications.

A **transperitoneal approach** involves laparotomy through a Pfannenstiel's or subumbilical vertical midline incision. After opening the peritoneum, intestines are retracted to expose the anterior aspect of lower lumbar and lumbosacral spine, an exposure that is often difficult to achieve with the retroperitoneal approach. Exposure of L4-L5 disc spaces requires mobilization of the aorta and inferior vena cava, along with its bifurcations.

Variants of the transperitoneal approach: **A laparoscopic transperitoneal approach** often is used at the L5-S1 level. With the patient supine, Trendelenburg position is used to move the small intestine away from the operative field. The procedure is performed through one 10 mm portal for a 30° endoscope, two 5 mm portals for retraction, and one 20 mm working portal for instruments. For access to the L5-S1 level, the posterior peritoneum is incised at the base of the sigmoid mesocolon with endoscopic scissors. Laparoscopic interbody fusion and instrumentation is performed as required, using specially designed long-alignment tubes, distraction plugs, and a reamer, as in the open procedure. The peritoneum is closed with endoscopic sutures or clips. The major advantages of this technique are related to the minimal manipulation of abdominal viscera required and minimal trauma to the abdominal wall. Additionally, postop pain, recovery time, and length of hospitalization are often less, permitting an early return to the patient's normal activities.

Variants of the retroperitoneal approach: A lateral retroperitoneal approach provides an excellent exposure of the lumbar spine from L1-S1 through a flank incision. The procedure is performed in the lateral decubitus position. The skin incision is made from the lateral border of the paravertebral muscles at the midlumbar level to the lateral border of the rectus abdominis. The incision is angulated below the umbilicus for exposure of the lower lumbar and lumbosacral junction, and is carried down to the peritoneum.

The **supine retroperitoneal approach** is accomplished through a left paramedian incision, and the peritoneum and abdominal contents are retracted. This is one of the most common approaches. Ligation of lumbar intersegmental arteries and tributaries of the iliac vein may be required to allow a direct anterior exposure from L3-S1. An approach surgeon trained in vascular or general surgery can often expose even more. With blunt dissection, the peritoneum is peeled off the lateral and posterior abdominal walls, diaphragm, and iliopsoas, exposing the anterior aspect of the lumbar spine. Vertebral resection and reconstruction are carried out in the routine manner. During this procedure, the great vessels, ureter, and sympathetic trunk need to be protected. Monopolar cautery is avoided, because it can cause injury to the presacral plexus, which can result in retrograde ejaculation.

A **laparoscopic retroperitoneal approach** can be used for performing an anterior lumbar interbody fusion following discectomy in patients with lumbar segmental instability. This procedure is performed in the right lateral decubitus position. A 10–12 mm port is made in the posterior axillary line midway between the 12th rib and iliac crest, and a trochar is advanced into the peritoneum. Retroperitoneal dissection is accomplished by balloon inflation, with 1,000 mL of air or saline, through a trochar. This procedure is carried out under direct vision through the laparoscope. Discectomy, fusion, or instrumentation requires two additional working portals. Retroperitoneal insufflation with CO_2 may be required during the procedure.

Usual preop diagnosis: Degenerative disc disease; segmental instability; vertebral fractures; benign and neoplastic diseases of lumbar spine; vertebral osteomyelitis; TB

SUMMARY OF PROCEDURES

	Transperitoneal Instrumentation	Retroperitoneal Instrumentation	Endoscopic Approach
Position	Supine	Supine/lateral decubitus	Right lateral decubitus
Incision	Pfannenstiel's/vertical subumbilical	Flank incision	3–4 ports
Special instrumentation	Z plates, Kaneda instrumentation, MACS-TL, femoral rings, cages; intervertebral disc replacements	⇐	Endoscopic instrumentation; balloon dissector
Unique considerations	NG tube, preop bowel prep	⇐	⇐
Antibiotics	Cefazolin 1 g iv	⇐	⇐
Surgical time	3–4 hrs	⇐	⇐
Closing considerations	Transfer to bed while anesthetized. Smooth emergence necessary to avoid graft/implant disruption.	⇐	Rapid closure of ports
EBL	200–600 mL	200–5000 mL; nontumor cases: 200–400 mL	100–500 mL
Postop care	PACU → ward; patients with infections/tumors → ICU. Postop ileus common.	⇐	⇐
Mortality	Malignancy and sepsis: 1–2% Elective: < 1%	⇐ ⇐	–
Morbidity	Neurological injury: 2–6% Vascular injury: 2–15% Retrograde ejaculation: 5–35%	⇐ ⇐ < 5%	– – –
Pain score	6–7	6–7	4–6

PATIENT POPULATION CHARACTERISTICS

Age range	Variable, infant-adult (usually 20–60 yr)
Male:Female	1:1 (usually)
Incidence	Uncommon
Etiology	Degenerative; lumbar segmental instability; neoplastic; traumatic; infectious

ANESTHETIC CONSIDERATIONS

See Anesthetic Considerations for Thoracolumbar Neurosurgical Procedures, p. 124.

Suggested Readings

1. Harrington FJ, Friehs G, Epstein MH: Surgical management of segmental spinal instability. In: *Operative Neurosurgical Techniques.* Schmidek HH, Sweet WH, eds. WB Saunders, Philadelphia: 2000, 2280–2302.
2. Kostuik JP, Carl A, Ferron S: Anterior Zielke instrumentation for spinal deformity in adults. *J Bone Joint Surg* 1989; 71(6):898–906.
3. Kozak JA, O'Brien JP: Simultaneous combined anterior and posterior fusion. An independent analysis of a treatment for the disabled low-back pain patient. *Spine* 1990; 15(4):322–8.
4. Leong JCY: Anterior interbody fusion. In: *Lumbar Interbody Fusion.* Lin PM, Gill K, eds. Raven Press, New York: 1989, 133–47.

POSTERIOR LUMBAR SPINE SURGERY

SURGICAL CONSIDERATIONS

Description: **Lumbar laminotomy** (partial removal of lamina) and **laminectomy** (complete removal of lamina) are procedures for decompressing the neural elements of the lumbar spine via a posterior approach. They can be used to treat lumbar radiculopathy 2° degenerative disc disease (e.g., herniated discs or osteophytes). **Decompressive laminectomy** can be used to treat compression of the cauda equina, usually 2° degenerative disease, congenital stenosis, neoplasm, and, occasionally, trauma. Lumbar laminectomy is also used to gain access to the spinal canal for dealing with intradural tumors, arteriovenous malformations (AVMs), and other spinal cord lesions.

Through a vertical midline incision, the lumbodorsal fascia is exposed, and then the paraspinal muscles are dissected off the spinous process and lamina of the segments intended for decompression. The level may need to be checked by intraop x-ray or fluoroscopy if the surgeon is not able to identify location based on visual confirmation of anatomic level. The bone landmarks are identified and ligamentous attachments are cut. The bone is removed piecemeal with rongeurs, gouges, or power drills. Care is taken not to injure the underlying dura. If a dural tear is found, it usually must be repaired. The surgeon may want a **Valsalva-like maneuver** (sustained inspiration at 30–40 cmH_2O) performed to test the integrity of the repair. If disc is to be removed, the dura is retracted and the annulus incised. The disc is removed piecemeal with a series of curettes and disc-biting rongeurs. There is a risk of damage to retroperitoneal structures (e.g., great vessels or intestines) during this portion of the procedure. More commonly, there may be troublesome epidural bleeding, which may be difficult to control and will necessitate transfusion. Hemostasis is obtained prior to closure. The wound is closed in layers and a drain may be left in the epidural space. The patient is rolled supine onto a bed at the completion of the procedure.

Minimally invasive surgery (MIS) lumbar surgery is performed through a short paramedian incision at the level of the affected disc. Under radiographic guidance, a series of soft tissue dilators are inserted over a previously placed guide wire to create an operative corridor through the paraspinous musculature. A tubular retractor is inserted over the dilators and connected to a flexible support arm assembly. Endoscope or microscope is used to perform laminotomy and discectomy and/or decompressive laminectomy. As the retractor is withdrawn at the end of the procedure, the paraspinal muscles resume their normal anatomic position, obliterating the dead space. Skin margins are closed with subcuticular sutures. Although all the major risks of surgery are still present, the blood loss, postoperative pain, and hospital stay are reduced. In theory, less trauma to the paraspinous muscles compromises less the post-operative function of the spine.

Usual preop diagnosis: Lumbar radiculopathy (nerve-root compression); lumbar disc disease (herniation or degeneration of lumbar discs); lumbar canal stenosis; lateral recess stenosis; neurogenic claudication; herniated disc; metastatic tumor to spine; lumbar spine tumor; lumbar spondylosis (degeneration of lumbar spine); spondylolysis (structural defect in the pars interarticularis of the vertebra); spondylolisthesis (slipping of one vertebra over another)

SUMMARY OF PROCEDURES

	Lumber Laminectomy	Lumbar Laminotomy	MIS
Position	Prone	⇐	⇐
Incision	Posterior midline	⇐	Paramedian port over disc
Special instrumentation	± Operative microscope	⇐	Endoscopic instrumentation (optional)
Unique considerations	I.I. localization to assess the correct level	⇐	⇐
Antibiotics	Cefazolin 1 g iv	⇐	⇐
Surgical time	1–2 h for single level; add 0.5–1 h/additional level	2 h for single level; add 0.5 h/additional level	⇐
EBL	25–500 mL	50–1000 mL	10–50 mL
Postop care	PACU →room	⇐	⇐
Mortality	0.5%	⇐	⇐
Morbidity	All < 5%: CSF leak Nerve root injury Infection Postop instability Massive blood loss Injury to retroperitoneal structures	⇐ ⇐ ⇐ ⇐ – – ⇐	⇐ ⇐ ⇐ – – – ⇐
Pain score	4–7	4–9	3–6

PATIENT POPULATION CHARACTERISTICS

Age range	15–85 yr (usually 30–60 yr)
Male:Female	3:2
Incidence	Common
Etiology	Degenerative; traumatic; neoplastic; infectious

ANESTHETIC CONSIDERATIONS

See Anesthetic Considerations for Thoracolumbar Neurosurgical Procedures, p. 124.

Suggested Readings

1. Finneson BE, Schmidek HH: Lumbar disc excision. In: *Operative Neurosurgical Techniques.* Schmidek HH, Sweet WH, eds. WB Saunders, Philadelphia: 2000, 2219–31.
2. Foley KT, Smith MM, Raja Rampersaud Y: Microendoscopic discectomy. In *Operative Neurosurgical Techniques.* Schmidek HH, Sweet WH, eds. WB Saunders, Philadelphia: 2000, 2246–56.

POSTERIOR LUMBAR FUSION AND INSTRUMENTATION

SURGICAL CONSIDERATIONS

Description: **Posterior lumbar spinal fusion** may relieve low-back pain resulting from intervertebral movement. This surgery is often indicated for segmental lumbar instability, spondylolisthesis, or iatrogenic instability due to extensive laminectomy or facetectomy.

The **pedicle screw stabilization** technique provides rigid three-column spinal fixation and is the preferred mode of instrumentation in lumbar spinal surgery (Fig. 1.3-14). Pedicle screws are passed after tapping the entry site, and are fixed with rods or plates on each side of each vertebral segment. The major risks with pedicle screw fixation include screw malposition and nerve-root injury. Pedicle screws may be combined with hooks to provide fixation of the lumbar/thoracolumbar spine, an approach that improves the stability of the construct and minimizes the risk of instrumentation failure. Facet screw stabilization can also be performed to fix levels together. This is usually not used in a stand alone fashion but in combination with anterior fixation. Instrumentation can be placed via percutaneous techniques that decrease blood loss and patient pain; however, complications often go undetected and unseen.

Posterolateral fusion (PLF) is performed through a posterior midline incision, with the paraspinal muscles retracted subperiosteally from the affected lumbar vertebrae. Decompressive laminectomy and discectomy are performed as needed. Posterolateral fusion is performed by decorticating the facet joints and transverse processes. Bone graft is then placed over the decorticated bone. Instrumentation with pedicle screws and plate/rod constructs often is done for stability and to facilitate fusion.

Posterior lumbar interbody fusion (PLIF) consists of a bilateral laminectomy and removal of the inferior facet and the medial portion of the superior facet. The dural sac is retracted, and a total discectomy, together with the removal of cartilaginous end plates, is performed. The anterior disc space is packed with bone graft. Appropriately sized rectangular bone grafts or cages are inserted into the posterior half of the disc space on both sides to provide structural support close to the center of rotation. The nerve roots above and below the disc space should be visualized during the procedure to avoid excessive retraction. Instrumentation with pedicle screws, and a rod/plate construct is often added to facilitate early fusion and ambulation, while preventing the extrusion of the graft. The major advantage of this procedure is that it provides the ability to achieve combined anterior and posterior spinal fusion, while avoiding

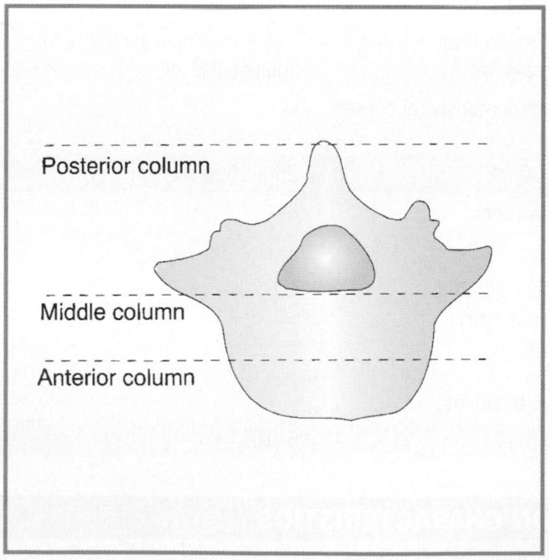

Figure 1.3-14. Spinal three-column model developed by F. Denis. Disruption of elements of two or more columns renders the spine unstable. (Reproduced with permission from Tindall GT, Cooper PR, Barrow DL: *The Practice of Neurosurgery*, Vol. II. Williams & Wilkins, Philadelphia: 1996.)

the significant morbidity often associated with anterior lumbar surgery. Its major disadvantages include the potential risk of nerve-root injury and compromise of the structural integrity of both facet joints.

Tansforaminal lumbar interbody fusion (TLIF) is a modification of the PLIF, using a unilateral posterolateral approach. A **hemilaminectomy and total facetectomy** is performed on one side. A near total discectomy is performed and the first bone graft or cage is inserted across the disc space to the contralateral side. A second bone graft may be inserted into the ipsilateral posterior disc space, and satisfactory placement of the bone grafts is confirmed by fluoroscopy. Supplemental pedicle screw stabilization is indicated as in PLIF. This approach has been adopted to be performed with MIS techniques to afford circumferential lumbar decompression and stabilization via an all posterior approach.

Direct/Extreme Lateral Interbody Fusion (DLIF/XLIF) is an MIS (minimally invasive surgery) procedure performed by having the patient positioned on his/her side where the surgeons approach to the spine will be directly laterally through the retroperitoneal cavity. A specialized retractor is used with multiple long blades that allow for visualization of the spine through the deep layers of tissue. **Neuromonitoring** (EMG nerve root mapping) is essential in the procedure to help avoid nerve injury. Therefore, when this neuromonitoring is being performed, minimal or no paralytic should be used as they may confound monitoring.

Transaxial Lumbo-sacral fusion (Trans1) is an **MIS** procedure performed by having the patient positioned prone. A complete L5-S1 discectomy and fusion with screw instrumentation is performed. This is done via a 1-cm incision at the base of the sacrum. Specialized tubular dilators and shims protect the visceral contents while a reamer and disc remover tools are used to remove disc. There is minimal blood loss, but occult injury to peritoneal contents including the viscera and blood vessels can occur acutely or present in a delayed fashion.

Usual Preop diagnosis: Lumbar segmental instability; spondylolisthesis; iatrogenic lumbar instability; lumbar disc disease, spondylolysis; mechanical back pain syndrome

SUMMARY OF PROCEDURES

	Posterolateral Fusion	PLIF	TLIF (DLIF/XLIF)
Position	Prone	⇐	⇐ (DLIF/XLIF: Lateral)
Incision	Posterior midline	⇐	⇐ (DLIF/XLIF: Lateral)
Special instrumentation	Drills, pedicle screws, or hooks	⇐ ;osteotomes, curettes, bone plugs, or cages	⇐ ; angled curettes, angled impactors
Unique considerations	I.I. localization and guidance	⇐	⇐ (DLIF/XLIF: EMG)
Antibiotics	Cefazolin 1 g iv	⇐	⇐
Surgical time	2 h for single level + 0.5 h/ additional level	3–4 h for single level + 1 h/ additional level	2–3 h for single level + 1 h/ additional level
Closing considerations	No brace/lumbosacral corset	⇐	⇐
EBL	250–500 mL	250–1000 mL	250–750 mL (less with MIS)
Postop care	PACU → room	⇐	⇐
Mortality	0–5%	⇐	⇐
Morbidity	Nonunion: 20–30% Nerve-root injury CSF leak Infection Massive blood loss	10–20% ⇐ ⇐ ⇐	⇐ ⇐ ⇐ ⇐
Pain score	6–10	6–10	6–10 (4–7 with MIS)

PATIENT POPULATION CHARACTERISTICS

Age range	15–85 yr (usually 30–60 yr)
Male:Female	3:2
Incidence	Common
Etiology	Degenerative; traumatic; neoplastic; infectious

ANESTHETIC CONSIDERATIONS

See Anesthetic Considerations for Thoracolumbar Neurosurgical Procedures, p. 124.

COMBINED ANTERIOR AND POSTERIOR INSTRUMENTATION OF THE THORACIC AND LUMBAR SPINE

SURGICAL CONSIDERATIONS

Description: Patients with multilevel vertebral collapse, unstable three-column injuries, severe kyphosis or scoliosis, and/or neoplastic or infective conditions involving multiple spinal levels often require **combined anterior and posterior instrumentation**. This approach provides: (a) complete circumferential neural decompression, which facilitates maximal neuronal recovery; (b) rigid short-segment spinal fixation, which facilitates early ambulation with minimal orthotic support; and (c) maximal correction of deformities with low instrumentation failure and high fusion rates. The combined approach maximizes the possibility of complete resection of the neoplastic or infective process. Patients with major systemic disease or poor marrow reserve may require staged procedures. Combined instrumentation procedures are often lengthy, requiring 5–10 h of surgery. Major related morbidities include infection, wound breakdown, respiratory complications, and significant blood loss. The transition between anterior and posterior procedures should be performed carefully to minimize disruption of the instrumentation.

Usual preop diagnosis: Lumbar segmental instability; spondylolisthesis; iatrogenic lumbar instability; spondylolysis; mechanical back pain syndrome

SUMMARY OF PROCEDURE	
Position	Prone + supine/lateral
Incision	Posterior midline skin incision + transverse
Special instrumentation	Anterior and posterior spinal implants and instrumentation sets
Unique considerations	OLV for anterior thoracic approaches; radiological localization; intraop EP monitoring (optional)
Antibiotics	Cefazolin 1 g
Surgical time	4–10 h
EBL	500–5000 mL
Postop care	PACU → room; sometimes needs short ICU stay.
Mortality	0–3%
Morbidity	Respiratory problems: atelectasis, pneumonia Infection Bone graft dislodgement
Pain score	7–10

PATIENT POPULATION CHARACTERISTICS	
Age range	15–85 yr (usually 30–60 yr)
Male:Female	3:2
Incidence	Common
Etiology	Congenital, degenerative; traumatic; neoplastic; infectious >; infectious

Suggested Readings

1. Denis FF: The three column spine and its significance in the classification of acute thoracolumbar spinal injuries. *Spine* 1983;8:817–31 .
2. Harrington FJ, Friehs G, Epstein MH: Surgical management of segmental spinal instability In *Operative Neurosurgical Techniques.* Schmidek HH, Sweet WH, eds. WB Saunders, Philadelphia: 2000, 2280–2302.
3. Leong JCY: Anterior interbody fusion. In: *Lumbar Interbody Fusion.* Lin PM, Gill K, eds. Raven Press, New York: 1989, 133–47.
4. Lowe TG, Tahernia D: Unilateral transforaminal posterior lumbar interbody fusion. *Clin Ortho* 2002; 394:227–36.
5. Sundaresan N, Steinberger AA, Moore F, et al: Surgical management of primary and metastatic tumors of the spine. In: *Operative Neurosurgical Techniques.* Schmidek HH, Sweet WH, eds. WB Saunders, Philadelphia: 2000, 2146–70.

ANESTHETIC CONSIDERATIONS FOR THORACOLUMBAR NEUROSURGICAL PROCEDURES

(Procedures covered: anterior/posterior thoracic spine surgery; anterior lumbar/lumbosacral spine surgery; posterior lumbar spine surgery; posterior lumbar fusion and instrumentation; combined anterior/posterior instrumentation of the thoracic and lumbar spine)

PREOPERATIVE

Surgery of the lumbar or thoracic spine is common as a result of a variety of spinal disorders, including herniation of lumbar or thoracic intervertebral disks causing compression of the adjacent spinal cord or nerve roots; spinal stenosis from bony overgrowth causing compression of the nerve roots or spinal cord; spondylolisthesis; traumatic injury to the spine; and removal of a spinal tumor or placement of a shunt from a spinal cord cyst into the subarachnoid or peritoneal spaces. Because these diseases span a wide age range, the patients may be healthy, or they may have severe cardiovascular and/or respiratory disorders. Generally, the surgical incision is made in the thoracic or lumbar region, but the surgeon may elect to approach a lumbar disk retroperitoneally using an abdominal or flank incision. Sometimes both anterior and posterior approaches are used sequentially. Finally, some anterior abdominal or thoracic procedures are performed thoracoscopically.

Neurologic	Patients with a herniated disk or spinal stenosis generally complain of pain, often in the pelvis or radiating down one or both legs. As nerve or spinal cord compression continues, patients develop motor weakness and atrophy of muscle groups in the legs as well as sensory deficits and/or bowel/bladder dysfunction. These changes also may result from a spinal cord tumor or cyst, so an MRI must be obtained to establish the cause. The MRI may be enhanced by the use of gadolinium or other contrast material. **Tests:** MRI
Hematologic	Blood loss may be substantial if the surgeon plans both an anterior and posterior approach in the same patient, or if the operation includes both spinal cord decompression and posterior spinal instrumentation. For these operations, at least 2 U autologous, directed-donor, or bank blood should be available at all times. Consideration should also be given to utilizing a cell saving device. Many of these patient will have been taking aspirin or NSAIDs, which may have been stopped ≥ 1 wk before surgery, and bleeding can be excessive even if coagulation studies are normal.
Laboratory	Preop Hct if autologous donations made and to assess baseline. Other tests as indicated from H&P.
Premedication	Adequate premedication is important. Many of these patients will have had prior back operations and dread having another one. Also, they often come to the preop suite complaining of pain because they were instructed not to take their daily analgesic medication. Midazolam 2–4 mg and sometimes meperidine 20–30 mg will increase their preop comfort level.

INTRAOPERATIVE

Anesthetic technique: GA is almost invariably used for these operations because it maximizes patient comfort, provides airway control, and permits use of controlled hypotension. Spinal and epidural anesthesia are, in principle, excellent techniques for lumbar surgery, particularly for removal of a lumbar intervertebral disc, but they are seldom used because of the medicolegal concern that the regional anesthetic may be blamed for a new neurological deficit, if one should occur as a result of the surgery. Regional anesthesia is generally not suitable for lumbar fusion or removal of a spinal cord tumor or cyst because the duration of operation is usually unpredictable, and may be prolonged.

Induction	Standard induction (p. B-2). Use of a wire-reinforced tube should be considered if the patient is to be turned prone to avoid tube kinking and occlusion. If the surgeon elects to approach isolated disease of the thoracic spine through the chest, a DLT will be necessary to deflate the lung on the operative side Avoid use of N_2O for thorascopic or anterior intra- or retroperitoneal approaches to prevent hypoxemia and bowel enlargement with impingement on the operative site.	
Maintenance	Standard maintenance (see p. B-2). A combination of N_2O, opiate, sevoflurane or isoflurane, and NMB will provide adequate anesthesia. Once exposure is completed with the posterior approach, muscle relaxation is no longer needed. If an anterior and then a posterior approach are to be used in the same patient, one can either move the patient to a gurney after the anterior portion is completed, and then roll the patient onto the same operating table, or transfer the patient from one OR table to another. Another alternative is to perform the operation on a Jackson table, which allows the patient to be turned from supine to prone without having to move them. If this table is used, it is advisable for the anesthesiologist to disconnect all iv lines and electrical wires so they are not inadvertently pulled out during the 180° rotation. For thorascopic or anterior abdominal approaches, neuromuscular blockade should be maintained until the spine surgery is complete and closure is under way. If both SSEP and motor evoked potentials are to be monitored, which is standard in scoliosis surgery, the anesthetic management must be tailored to avoid the use of nitrous oxide or volatile agents. The usual technique is total intravenous anesthesia (TIVA), generally using continuous infusions of propofol (75–200 mcg/kg/min) and remifentanil (0.1–0.5 mcg/kg/min). The higher doses of both are used at the start of the anesthetic, and gradually tapered over time to the lower doses. Depending upon the duration of the operation, it is advisable to terminate the propofol 30–60 min before its conclusion. The remifentanil will need to be continued in low dose until the closure is complete. Be prepared to administer fentanyl to provide prompt analgesia until a blood level of longer acting opiates (morphine, dihydromorphone) can be established. During induction in these patients, it is prudent to administer midazolam 5 mg or more to prevent recall until the propofol and remifentanil blood levels can be established. Also, it is useful to administer a small dose of rocuronium (20–30 mg) or succinylcholine to facilitate endotracheal intubation. After the baseline SSEP and motor evoked potentials have been established, some surgeons will request NMB during dissection of the muscles from the bones. This can be accomplished safely with rocuronium (20–40 mg).	
Emergence	Standard emergence (p. B-3), after the patient has been returned to the supine position on a bed or gurney. If the intubation was difficult, or the operation was prolonged and airway edema or respiratory depression is possible, it may be advisable to leave the patient's trachea intubated overnight.	
Blood and fluid requirements	iv: 16–18 ga × 1 NS/LR @ 5 mL/kg/h up to a maximum of 40 mL/kg.	To perhaps lessen the chance of postop blindness from ischemic optic neuropathy, do not administer more than 40 mL/kg of crystalloid regardless of the duration of surgery if the operation is performed with the patient in the prone position. If additional fluid is needed, administer hetastarch 6% up to a

Blood and fluid requirements (cont'd)		maximum of 20 mL/kg, albumin 5% or blood. Blood transfusion is usually necessary when there has been extensive bony decompression and fusion. Cell Saver®; is used by some if large blood loss is anticipated.
Control of blood loss	Controlled hypotension	In the absence of severe cord compression, modest decreases in BP are helpful to ↓blood loss when extensive surgery is anticipated. This may be accomplished with combinations of sevoflurane or isoflurane and opiates, or by the use of α- and β-blockers (e.g., labetalol, esmolol) and SNP. BP values ~20% < the patient's lowest recorded pressure when awake are usually satisfactory, but should not be < 60 mmHg MAP in young adults or 80 mmHg in elderly patients. After the bony dissection is complete, the benefit of controlled ↓ BP wanes, and a more normal BP is advisable.
Monitoring	Standard monitors (see p. B-1). ± Arterial line ± CVP line ± Urinary catheter	For simple back surgery, standard monitors are sufficient. If controlled ↓ BP or if an extensive posterior or anterior and posterior approach are planned, an arterial catheter is essential to monitor BP, and a CVP catheter is recommended for infusion of vasoactive drugs and monitoring of CVP. A urinary drainage catheter is also desirable if surgery is expected to last several h or substantial fluid shifts are anticipated. Do not administer excessive crystalloid volumes to promote urine output. For reasons not yet determined, urine output is often less than expected when patients are positioned prone. These patients will not develop severe renal insufficiency because of decreased urine output during surgery.
Positioning	✓ and pad pressure points. ✓ eyes and ears frequently. ✓ breasts and genitals. ✓ free abdominal movement. Neutral C-spine	Except for syringoperitoneal shunts, which are performed with the patient in the lateral position, patients are positioned prone on a Wilson frame or on bolsters, or in the knee-chest position on an Andrews table. The head is placed in a neutral position using a foam pillow with cutouts for the eyes, nose, and chin (e.g., Andrews Gentle-Rest pillow). Whenever possible maintain the patient's head at or above the level of the heart to lessen the development of facial and intracranial edema. If the patient also has cervical disk disease, it is advisable to place a cervical collar before turning the patient prone. Other options are to use a horseshoe headrest or place the head in Gardner-Wells tongs or in a Mayfield head clamp. When placed in a headrest, the ET should be strain-relieved near the mouth with a penrose drain tied around the head clamp to prevent gradual extubation due to gravity. Elbows, knees, feet, and any pressure points need padding.
Complications	↓ BP Bowel or ureteral injury Hemorrhage	↓ BP may be 2° abdominal compression and ↓venous return. ↑ blood loss may occur 2° epidural vein engorgement, abdominal compression or vascular injury.

POSTOPERATIVE

Complications	↓ BP Hemorrhage Nerve-root injury Blindness	Any acute drop in BP may be due to a vascular injury, either obvious (segmental artery) or occult (deep great vessel injury) until proven otherwise. The source of bleeding should be identified. If ↓BP persists despite vigorous blood and fluid administration, suspect bleeding into the retroperitoneal space or abdomen. Alert the surgeon of this possibility and prepare for immediate exploration.
Pain management	PCA (p. C-3) Epidural opiate (p. C-2)	Some surgeons may place a mixture consisting of Duramorph ± fentanyl, ± steroid, in Avitene® hemostat into the epidural space before closing. This provides excellent postop analgesia.
Tests	Hct; document neurological status.	If postop bleeding is suspected, serial Hct determinations are useful.

Suggested Reading

1. Sonntag VRH, Hadley MN: Surgical approaches to the thoracolumbar spine. In *Clinical Neurosurgery*, Vol 36. Williams & Wilkins, Baltimore: 1990, 168–85.

CHAPTER

1.4 Carotid Endarterectomy

SURGEONS

Gary K. Steinberg, MD, PhD
Robert L. Dodd, MD, PhD

ANESTHESIOLOGIST

Richard A. Jaffe, MD, PhD

CAROTID ENDARTERECTOMY

SURGICAL CONSIDERATIONS

Gary K. Steinberg and Robert L. Dodd

Description: **Carotid endarterectomy** (CEA) is frequently used to treat severe atherosclerotic occlusive disease involving internal carotid arteries at the common carotid artery bifurcation. Atherosclerotic carotid artery disease commonly causes thromboembolic or hemodynamic stroke and transient ischemic attacks (TIAs). Recent studies proved the efficacy of this operation, compared with medical treatment for symptomatic high-grade stenosis (70–99%), symptomatic moderate stenosis (50–69%), and asymptomatic high-grade stenosis (≥ 60%).

The operation involves opening the common carotid artery and the proximal internal carotid artery in the neck (Fig 1.4-1), removing atherosclerotic plaque from the inside of the artery, and repairing the wall of the arteries (media and adventitia). Opening the carotid artery (**arteriotomy**) requires temporary occlusion of the proximal common carotid artery, distal internal carotid artery, external carotid artery and, usually, its first branch, the superior thyroid artery. The entire procedure can be achieved under continued occlusion of these vessels if the collateral blood flow to the territory supplied by the occluded internal carotid is deemed adequate (on the basis of intraop EEG monitoring, internal carotid artery back-bleeding, stump pressures, CBF studies, or angiography). Alternatively, an internal shunt between the proximal common carotid artery and distal internal carotid artery can be placed after the arteriotomy for use during the endarterectomy. Often a synthetic graft (e.g., Dacron) or, occasionally, a vein graft, is used to reconstruct ("patch") the arteriotomy site and increase the luminal diameter.

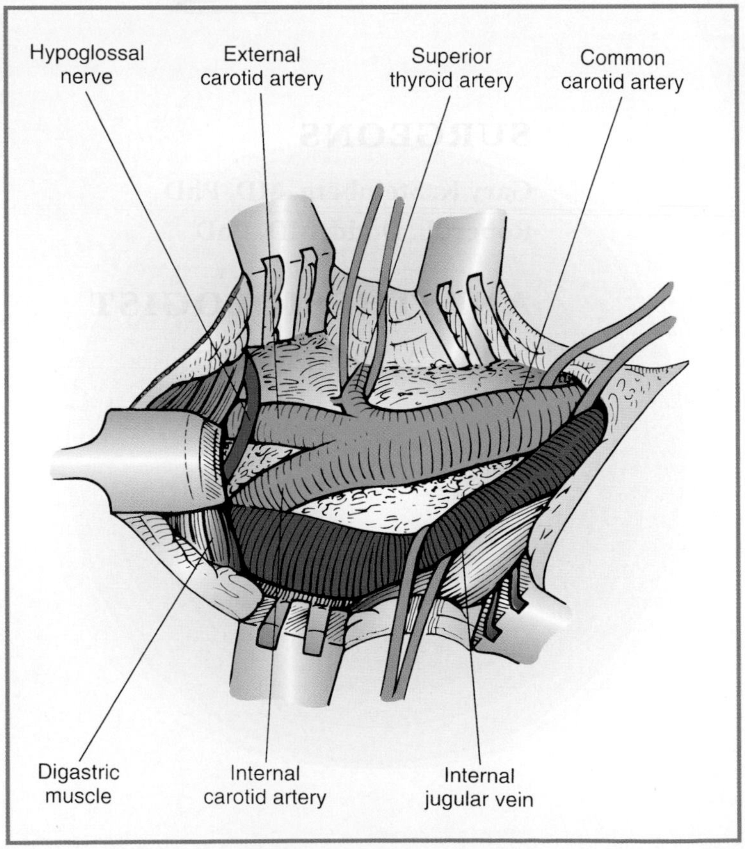

Figure 1.4-1. Exposure and control of carotid artery. (Reproduced with permission from Calne R, Pollard SG: *Operative Surgery*. Gower Medical Pub: 1992.)

Variant Procedure or Approaches: The vascular surgeon's approach to CEA is described in chapter 6.3. Carotid stenting is described in the Intracranial Neurology section (13.1). EC-IC Bypass for treatment of carotid occlusion is described in Section 1.1.

Usual preop diagnosis: Stroke; TIAs; carotid artery stenosis; carotid artery dissection

SUMMARY OF PROCEDURE

Position	Supine
Incision	Anterolateral neck; occasionally, if "patching" arteriotomy, may have to harvest portion of greater saphenous vein from leg.
Special instrumentation	Magnification loupes; vascular instruments ± shunt (Bard, Javid, Pruitt-Inahara)
Unique considerations	Techniques for monitoring cerebral blood flow: EEG-spectral analysis or raw EEG, somatosensory evoked potentials (SEPs), back-bleeding or internal carotid artery stump pressure (> 50 mmHg), CBF measurements using Xenon, transcranial Doppler. Full anticoagulation with heparin (typically 7500–10,000 U iv) during arterial occlusion ± reversal with protamine (typically 35–50 mg iv) 10 min after repair and reopening of carotid arteries. Maintaining mild HTN during internal carotid artery occlusion (MAP 90–110). Use of intraop neuroprotective agents during internal carotid artery occlusion (e.g., iv STP 2–5 mg/kg to produce EEG burst-suppression).
Antibiotics	Cefazolin (1 g iv q 6 h)
Surgical time	~3 h
Closing considerations	Avoid ↑BP or ↓BP (typical MAP 80–100); meticulous hemostasis.
EBL	50–150 mL
Postop care	Control of BP (MAP 80–100 mmHg); start aspirin on postop d 1; ICU or other monitored bed × 6–24 h.
Mortality	0.3–1.1% (combined CABG/CEA: up to 17.7%)
Morbidity	0.5–4% with postop MI Cranial nerve injury: Up to 39% (Typically 8%) Stroke: 1–3% (~2/3 postop) MI: 1–2% Postop bleeding: 1.7–2.7% Wound infection: Rare
Pain score	3

PATIENT POPULATION CHARACTERISTICS

Age range	50–90 yr
Male:Female	1:1
Incidence	150,000 CEAs/yr in the United States
Etiology	Atherosclerosis; occasionally, traumatic (dissection)
Associated conditions	HTN; CAD; PVD; smoking; obesity; alcohol abuse; hyperlipidemia

ANESTHETIC CONSIDERATIONS

(Procedure covered: carotid endarterectomy)

PREOPERATIVE

The incidence of occlusive or ulcerative lesions of the extracranial or intracranial vasculature increases with advancing years. Generally, these lesions are asymptomatic until the cross-sectional area of the vessel is decreased by at least 50%. This is because in most patients the cerebral vasculature has excellent collateral circulation, most importantly the Circle of Willis (normal in only 50% of patients), but also the carotid-basilar anastomosis via the trigeminal artery and the extra- to intracranial collateral flow via the ophthalmic artery or branches of the vertebral artery. Patients presenting for CEA generally fall into one of three categories: (1) Those with TIAs, presenting with symptoms that may be focal or generalized. (2) Patients with completed stroke. If the stroke is recent (< 2–4 wk), some surgeons will not operate on the patient for fear of converting an ischemic infarct into a hemorrhagic infarct; however, if the infarct is small and clinical deficit minor, early surgery may be indicated. Angiographic evaluation usually demonstrates a stenotic and/or ulcerative lesion at the carotid bifurcation. (3) Patients with asymptomatic bruit, which usually is found during a routine physical examination of the neck. These are of concern because they may signal the development of carotid stenosis and may benefit from surgical intervention.

Respiratory	Patients should be asked to stop smoking prior to anesthesia, even if only the night before. Although cessation of smoking for such a short time will not lessen the volume of secretions appreciably or make the airways less irritable to a foreign body, such as an ETT, it will provide sufficient time for the carbon monoxide levels in the blood to decrease, thereby enhancing O_2-carrying capacity. Any Hx of pulmonary disease should be evaluated with spirometry, ABGs, and CXR. If there is evidence of pulmonary infection, appropriate antibiotic therapy should be instituted. If secretions are excessive, preop pulmonary physiotherapy, including bronchodilator therapy, may be indicated. **Tests:** ABGs; spirometry; CXR, if indicated from H&P.
Cardiovascular	Careful evaluation of cardiovascular status is essential and should include a detailed Hx of cardiovascular function and serial determinations of BP in both arms to establish the range of pressures that normally occur, and whether there are regional differences. If BP is different in the two arms, it should be measured intraop and postop in the arm with the higher values. Also, a preop ECG is mandatory. The reason for concern about cardiovascular function is twofold: (1) It is often necessary to administer vasoactive drugs to regulate BP during CEA, either to maintain it at a normal value, or sometimes to increase it as much as 20% above the highest resting pressure to maintain optimal collateral circulation during surgical carotid occlusion. (2) The incidence of perioperative MI in this surgical population is > 1%, and represents the most common major postop complication in this operation. Except in the case of emergencies, anesthesia and operation should not proceed in the face of severe, uncontrolled HTN, diabetes, or recent MI. Antihypertensive medications should be continued up to the time of anesthesia. **Tests:** ECG; others as indicated from H&P.
Neurological	The Sx of cerebrovascular insufficiency are due to either critical stenosis or occlusion of cerebral vessels, combined with inadequate collateral circulation. The degenerative plaques or mural thrombi readily break off from the vessel wall and cause focal ischemic lesions. Manual occlusion of the carotid arteries is not an appropriate test of tolerance to temporary circulatory occlusion, as it may endanger the patient by precipitating embolization from an ulcerative lesion or by inducing bradycardia and ↓BP from activation of the carotid sinus reflex. It is desirable, however, to position the patient's head in the operative position as a test of the effect of that position on CBF. It is well-documented that hyperextension and lateral rotation of the head may occlude vertebral-basilar flow and, if sustained, contribute to postop cerebral ischemia. Sx of dizziness or diplopia will emerge with this maneuver if CBF is compromised. **Tests:** Carotid and cerebral angiography will identify type of lesion (ulcerative or stenotic), its location, and extent of collateral circulation. Other commonly used techniques include MR angiography, CT angiography, and duplex ultrasonography. As part of the preop evaluation, the anesthesiologist should examine the angiograms of the patient or discuss the case with the surgeon in order to understand with type, location, and extent of the lesion.

Hematologic	Aspirin or other anti-Plt therapy usually is begun preop to ↓ the risk of periop thromboembolic complications. **Tests:** PT; PTT
Laboratory	Tests as indicated from H&P.
Premedication	Use of premedication in patients undergoing CEA is controversial. Should a new TIA or stroke occur in the immediate preop period, its Sx may be difficult to distinguish from those associated with excessive responses to premedication. In this population, detailed discussion about the anesthetic and surgical plan, with appropriate reassurance, is usually sufficient. If medication is desired, midazolam 1–3 mg is preferable to opiates.

INTRAOPERATIVE

Anesthetic technique (regional): Historically, regional anesthesia—in the form of superficial and deep cervical plexus blocks, supplemented as needed by a local field block—was used for most CEAs. It provided the opportunity to evaluate cerebral function during a trial occlusion of 2–3 min. If the patient showed no adverse effects, the operation was completed under regional anesthesia. If the patient developed neurological changes, a shunt was inserted or GA was induced and ET intubation performed, following which the operation was completed. Regional anesthesia, however, has several disadvantages: absence of cerebral protection, patients may tolerate carotid occlusion for 10 min or more before suddenly losing consciousness or developing a Sz; and conversion to GETA may be technically difficult. Nevertheless, the technique still has some advocates among anesthesiologists and surgeons. It is claimed that: (1) it decreases the need for a surgical shunt and, thereby, avoids the complications of shunt insertion; (2) it decreases the length of stay in the ICU; and, (3) as an anesthetic technique, it is well-accepted by some patients.

Anesthetic technique (GETA): GETA offers both direct and indirect advantages for patients undergoing CEA: cerebral protection by decreasing $CMRO_2$ and redistributing flow toward the potentially ischemic area; greater patient comfort; and the ability to regulate PO_2, PCO_2, and MAP. Despite these arguments favoring GA, recent studies comparing regional and GA suggest that there is no clear outcome advantage of one technique over the other.

Induction	Both STP (3–5 mg/kg) and propofol (1–2 mg/kg), when carefully titrated, are suitable for induction agents, as arterial BP will generally remain at acceptable levels (± 20% of baseline) in normovolemic patients. These agents will ↓ $CMRO_2$, constrict normally reactive cerebral vessels, and → a redistribution of CBF toward potentially ischemic areas. Etomidate (0.1–0.4 mg/kg) may be useful for induction of anesthesia in hemodynamically unstable patients. A muscle relaxant, such as vecuronium (0.15 mg/kg), cisatracurium (0.1–0.2 mg/kg), or rocuronium (0.5–0.6 mg/kg) is administered for tracheal intubation. An analgesic, such as fentanyl (2–5 mcg/kg), or remifentanil (1–3 mcg/kg), may be given to minimize the cardiovascular responses to ET intubation. These opiates have minimal effects on CBF or $CMRO_2$.
Maintenance	Isoflurane (up to 0.6%) or sevoflurane (up to 1%) inspired, in combination with N_2O 50% and remifentanil (0.05–0.2 mcg/kg/min), is satisfactory and will not interfere with EEG or EP monitoring. Just before cross-clamping of the carotid artery, an additional dose of STP sufficient to produce burst suppression on the EEG (usually 1–3 mg/kg) may be administered for its cerebral protective effects. Frawley et al. have suggested that STP adequately protects the brain during CEA, and that a surgical shunt is obsolete and not needed.
Emergence	Upon removal of the carotid cross-clamps, total carotid occlusion time should be noted on the anesthetic record. After 10 min and once bleeding from the arteriotomy site has been controlled, protamine (typically 0.5 mg/100 U heparin) is administered iv slowly over at least 10 min. If ↓BP occurs, rate of protamine administration should be slowed. If vasopressors were used during surgery, patient should be weaned from them during emergence, because HTN is likely as patient awakens from anesthesia. The need to control BP with a combination of esmolol and SNP/NTG is likely in the emergence phase. Antiemetic prophylaxis (e.g., ondansetron 4 mg iv 30 min before end of case) is usually appropriate. Prophylactic β-blockers may be quite useful in this patient population.

Blood and fluid requirements	IV: 18 ga × 2 NS/LR @ 5–10 mL/kg/h	Blood replacement is seldom an issue. Studies indicate that elevated blood glucose may ↓ tolerance of brain to ischemia; thus, it is prudent to avoid glucose-containing solutions and treat levels > 180 mg/dL. One iv is dedicated to drug infusions.
	Hetastarch 6% < 20 mL/kg	If volume expansion is needed, hetastarch stays in the intravascular compartment longer (2–3 d) than crystalloid solutions (1–3 h).
Monitoring	Standard monitors (see p. B-1). Arterial line (often pre-induction) UO CVP (if otherwise indicated)	Marked fluctuations in BP may occur, necessitating vasoactive drug therapy. The arterial pressure transducer should be placed at the level of the head to accurately assess CPP. A CVP catheter is seldom necessary. Vasoactive drugs usually can be given safely through a second iv placed in the proximal arm. A second pressure transducer set-up may be needed for stump pressure measurements. Monitors incorporating EASI ECG analysis technology can provide 12-lead ECGs using only five actual leads.
Cerebral perfusion monitoring	rCBF	Regional CBF (rCBF) ≥ 25 mL/min/100 g brain is satisfactory, and < 20 mL/min/100 g indicates potential for cerebral ischemia; however, capability for making rCBF measurements is not generally available in OR.
	EEG	A variety of spectral compression techniques permit computerized EEG analysis in OR. The major disadvantages are: the EEG may not identify small focal areas of ischemia; the depth of anesthesia and arterial CO_2 must be stable or the EEG will not be interpretable; and there is a high incidence of false positives and negatives.
	Stump pressure	Stump pressure (pressure distal to the carotid clamp—also called "back pressure"— is used to evaluate the adequacy of cerebral perfusion. Cerebral ischemia rarely occurs at stump pressures > 60 mmHg. The major criticism of stump pressure is the large number of false positives. This occurs in ~1/3 of patients and results in a shunt being placed when none is needed. The simplicity of the measurement and its relative validity when pressure is > 60 mmHg still make it a useful clinical method for ensuring adequate perfusion.
	Cerebral oximetry	Cerebral oximetry (e.g., Somanetics Invos) is being used with increasing frequency to evaluate cerebral perfusion during CEA. Cerebral oximeter sensors are placed on the forehead, where it is presumed they measure O_2 sat in the superficial frontal cortex. With carotid occlusion, ipsilateral oximetric values may decrease suggesting inadequate cerebral perfusion. The method is nonquantitative and a portion of the signal may originate from structures superficial to the cortex

Cerebral perfusion monitoring (cont'd)		perfused by branches of the external carotid artery. False positive and false negative results can occur.
	SSEP	SSEPs are being used with increasing frequency as a means of determining the adequacy of cerebral perfusion during temporary occlusion of the carotid artery. This technique requires continuous monitoring by personnel with special training. Areas of focal ischemia may not be detected. False positive and false negative results can occur.
	Transcranial Doppler (TCD)	TCD scanning alone or combined with EEG monitoring is a useful method for detecting microemboli (air or particulate matter) during CEA. It also has been suggested that TCD can be used as a guide for regulating BP postop to minimize the occurrence of post-CEA cerebral hyperperfusion states. This technique requires continuous monitoring by personnel with special training, and may be technically difficult to implement intraop.
Control of BP	Keep MAP ≥ awake levels. Autoregulation Vasopressors: Phenylephrine infusion	It is highly desirable to maintain MAP at or slightly above the patient's highest recorded resting pressure while awake. Volatile anesthetics impair autoregulation; therefore, the higher the pressure, the more likely it is that cerebral perfusion will be adequate during surgical occlusion. A pure a-adrenergic agonist (e.g., phenylephrine) is ideal to support BP, because it has minimal dysrhythmogenic potential. A V-4 or V-5 lead usually will indicate if ↓ BP is causing myocardial ischemia.
	Coronary vasodilation NTG infusion	A simultaneous infusion of NTG (0.2–0.4 mcg/kg/min) may improve coronary flow during periods of induced ↑ BP. If hypertensive episodes occur during surgery, infusions of esmolol ± NTG/SNP work well to control BP.
	Labetalol (pre-emergence)	Long duration effect makes intraop titration difficult
Positioning	✓ and pad pressure points. ✓ eyes.	

POSTOPERATIVE

Complications	Circulatory instability: ↓ BP	Circulatory instability is common. ↓ BP may be due to hypovolemia, depression of circulation by anesthetic or other drugs, dysrhythmias, or exposure of the baroreceptor mechanism to a new higher pressure, causing an exaggerated reflex response. Rx by volume expansion and pressors.
	HTN MI Stroke	HTN may be due to loss of the normal carotid baroreceptor mechanism. It may → excessive bleeding, increased myocardial O_2 consumption, dysrhythmias, MI, intracerebral hemorrhage and ↑ICP from cerebral edema.

Complications (cont'd)	Loss of carotid body function	Ipsilateral chemoreceptor function is lost in most patients after CEA, → ↓ventilatory and circulatory responses to hypoxia and a modest increase in resting arterial $PaCO_2$. These patients should be given supplemental O_2 postop. Special attention must be directed toward preventing atelectasis or other pulmonary or circulatory abnormalities that might cause hypoxemia.
	Respiratory insufficiency	Acute respiratory insufficiency may occur 2° hematoma formation with tracheal deviation, vocal cord paralysis from surgical traction on laryngeal nerves, or tension pneumothorax from dissection of air through the wound into the mediastinum and pleural space. Unexpected respiratory distress should immediately bring these three possibilities to mind, with appropriate Dx and therapy. A hematoma that causes respiratory distress always should be evacuated before reintubation is attempted.
	Tension pneumothorax	If there is evidence of circulatory insufficiency, a tension pneumothorax should be relieved immediately by needle evacuation.
	Intimal flap → stroke	Should a patient emerge from anesthesia with a new neurological deficit, immediate surgical exploration of the operative site or immediate cerebral angiography should be performed to determine if an intimal flap has formed at the site of operation. This is a surgically correctable lesion and, if corrected immediately, may lessen the severity of the subsequent neurological deficit.
Pain management	Meperidine (10 mg iv prn) Codeine (30–60 mg im q 4 h)	
Tests	Cerebral angiography Carotid ultrasound	

Suggested Readings

1. Allen BT, Anderson CB, Rubin BG, Thompson RW, Flye MW, Young-Beyer P: The influence of anesthetic technique on perioperative complications after carotid endarterectomy. *J Vasc Surg* 1994; 19:834–42.
2. Archer DP, Tang TKK: The choice of anaesthetic for carotid endarterectomy: does it matter? *Can J Anaesth* 1995; 42:566–70.
3. Fiori L, Parenti G, Marconi F: Combined transcranial Doppler and electrophysiologic monitoring for carotid endarterectomy. *J Neurosurg Anesthesiol* 1997; 9:11–6.
4. Frawley JE, Hicks RG, Gray LJ, Niesche JW: Carotid endarterectomy without a shunt for symptomatic lesions associated with contralateral severe stenosis or occlusion. *J Vasc Surg* 1996; 23:421–7.
5. Guay J. Regional or general anesthesia for carotid endarterectomy? Evidence from published prospective and retrospective studies. *J Cardiothorac Vasc Anesth* 2007; 21(1):127–32.
6. Kearse LA Jr, Lopez-Bresnahan M, McPeck K, Zaslavsky A: Preoperative cerebrovascular symptoms and electroencephalographic abnormalities do not predict cerebral ischemia during carotid endarterectomy. *Stroke* 1995; 26:1210–4.
7. Luebke T, Aleksic M, Brunkwall J. Meta-analysis of randomized trials comparing carotid entarterectomy and endovascular treatment. *Eur J Vasc Endovasc Surg* 2007; 34(4):470–9.
8. Mutch WAC, White IWC, Donin N, Thomson IR, Rosenbloom M, Cheang M, West M: Haemodynamic instability and myocardial ischaemia during carotid endarterectomy: a comparison of propofol and isoflurane. *Can J Anaesth* 1995; 42:577–87.

9. Sajid MS, Vijaynager B, Singh P et al.: Leterature review of cranial nerve injuries during carotid endarterectomy. *Acta Surg Belg,* 2007; 107(1): 25–8.
10. Sejersten M, Wagner GS, Pahlm O et al.: Detection of acute ischemia from the EASI-derived 12-lead electrocardiogram acquired in clinical practice. *J Electrocardiol* 2007; 40:120–6.
11. Wade, JG, Larson CP Jr, Hickey RF, Ehrenfeld WK, Severinghaus JW: Effect of carotid endarterectomy on carotid chemoreceptor and baroreceptor function in man. *N Engl J Med* 1970; 282(15):823–9.
12. Warner DS, Hindman BJ, Todd MM, Sawin PD, Kirchner J, Roland CL, Jamerson BD: Intracranial pressure and hemodynamic effects of remifentanil versus alfentanil in patients undergoing supratentorial craniotomy. *Anesth Analg* 1996; 83:348–53.

SECTION

2.0 OPHTHALMIC SURGERY

SURGEONS

Eleonora M. Lad, MD, PhD
Peter R. Egbert, MD
Darius M. Moshfeghi, MD

ANESTHESIOLOGIST

Richard A. Jaffe, MD, PhD

CATARACT EXTRACTION WITH INTRAOCULAR LENS INSERTION

SURGICAL CONSIDERATIONS

Description: Cataract–the leading cause of treatable blindness in the world–is defined as opacification of the crystalline lens. **Cataract surgery** is among the most common surgical procedures, with more than 1.3 million performed in the United States each year. Several approaches to cataract removal have evolved as a result of advances in both instrumentation and artificial intraocular lenses (IOL). Most modern cataract surgery is performed using the **extracapsular technique,** which involves removal of the crystalline lens through an opening made in the anterior lens capsule (known as a **capsulectomy**). Removal of the lens nucleus can then be accomplished intact, which requires an 8-10 mm corneal incision, or by **phacoemulsification** wherein ultrasound energy is used to fragment the lens, allowing aspiration of the lens material. The advantage to phacoemulsification is that the entire procedure can be performed through a much smaller, clear corneal incision (usually ~3 mm in length). With both approaches, the softer, more peripheral cortical lens material is then removed by aspiration, leaving the posterior capsular bag intact to support an IOL implant (Fig. 2-1). If the lens capsule is torn or is for any reason unable to support an IOL, the lens can be fixated with sutures in the posterior chamber (behind the iris), or an anterior chamber IOL can be placed in front of the iris. Presently, the most popular materials for IOL implants are polymethylmethacrylate, silicon, and acrylic. Only silicon and acrylic are foldable, which allows their insertion through a small corneal incision and, therefore, are the most commonly used. The wound is closed with nylon or Vicryl suture (9-0 or 10-0) to achieve a watertight seal, although when small incisions are used, the wounds are often self-sealing and do not require sutures.

Variant procedure or approaches: **Intracapsular cataract extraction** involves removal of the crystalline lens with its surrounding capsular bag intact. To accomplish this, the zonules that normally stabilize and center the lens must be broken, and a cryoprobe often is used to remove the lens from the eye through a large incision. This procedure is performed infrequently, given the superior visual outcomes of extracapsular techniques. It may be indicated in situations where capsular bag support has been compromised by either trauma or inherited disorders.

Usual preop diagnosis: Cataract

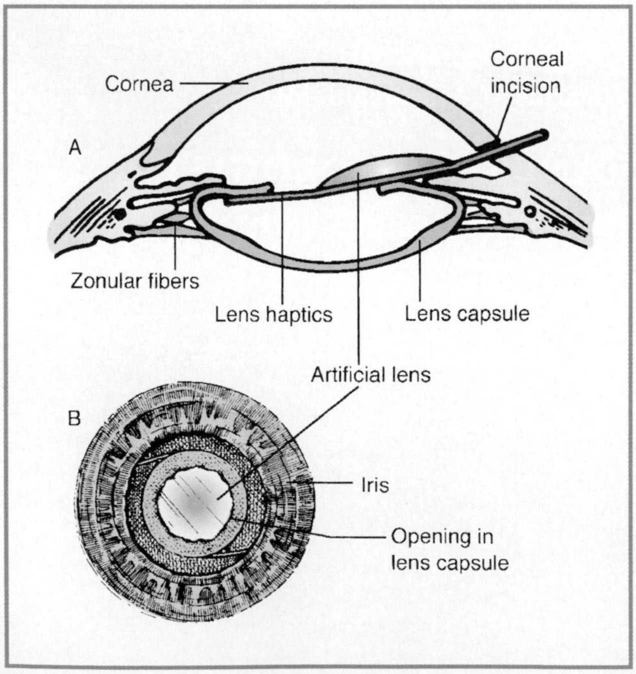

Figure 2-1. (**A**) Placement of intraocular lens into remaining capsular bag. (**B**) "In-the-bag" insertion.

SUMMARY OF PROCEDURE	
Position	Supine, table rotated 90–180°
Incision	2.8 mm peripheral cornea (phacoemulsification) or 8–10 mm (corneoscleral junction)
Special instrumentation	Surgical microscope; phacoemulsification machine
Antibiotics	Subconjunctival cefazolin (50–100 mg) or gentamicin (20–40 mg) or a topical fluoroquinolone
Surgical time	15–60 min
EBL	None
Postop Care	Possible eye patch/shield for 24 h, topical medications
Mortality	Rare
Morbidity	Posterior capsule rupture: 3.1% Corneal edema: < 2% Macular edema: 1–2% Retinal detachment: < 1% Choroidal hemorrhage: 0.3% Endophthalmitis: < 0.2 %
Pain score	1–2

PATIENT POPULATION CHARACTERISTICS	
Age range	3 mo–75 yr
Male:Female	1:1
Incidence	> 1,000,000/yr in the United States
Etiology	Congenital; metabolic; traumatic; senile; medication-induced (steroids)
Associated conditions	Systemic diseases of elderly patients–common; cardiovascular disease; diabetes; HTN Patients may be on antiplatelet or anticoagulant therapy. It is generally accepted that these drugs do not need to be discontinued before cataract surgery (especially if INR ≤ 1.5)

ANESTHETIC CONSIDERATIONS

Cataract surgery is performed worldwide using various regional, local, or topical anesthetic techniques and agents and general anesthesia. At the 2002 Congress of the International Council of Ophthalmology in Sydney, Australia, it was reported that almost all cataract surgeries worldwide were performed using regional anesthesia. Surgeons performed just over half of the anesthetic procedures, whereas anesthetists performed the rest of the procedures. The most frequently employed techniques were the peribulbar block followed by topical anesthesia.

At the present time in the United States, cataract surgery is most commonly performed using only topical anesthetic agents (e.g., preservative-free 2–4% lidocaine, levobupivacaine 0.75%, ropivacaine 1%, oxybuprocaine 1%, or tetracaine 0.5%) to block trigeminal nerve endings in the cornea and conjunctiva. Iris and ciliary body anesthesia depend on local anesthetic penetration into the anterior chamber. Thus, in a few patients, there may be a need for supplemental anesthetic administration (e.g., intracameral, 1% lidocaine) as well as systemic analgesic and sedative drugs. Inadvertent eye and lid movement should be expected. Adverse reactions to topical anesthetics are extremely rare and typically allergic in nature. A recent prospective randomized double-blind series demonstrated that combining topical anesthesia with intracameral lidocaine anesthesia was safe and effective in phacoemulsification with intraocular lens implantation. This technique avoided potential sequelae of retrobulbar or peribulbar anesthesia for cataract surgery. However, patients undergoing cataract surgery using topical anesthesia reported greater intraoperative and postoperative discomfort than those given a sub-Tenon block. Use of intravenous sedation increased the incidence of adverse events as compared with topical anesthesia without sedation.

Anesthesia-trained personnel monitored most patients during cataract surgery, and the most commonly used local anesthetic was lidocaine. The anesthetic method associated with the lowest degree of pain, dissatisfaction, drowsiness, or nausea and vomiting was a regional block technique with administration of sedatives and diphenhydramine.

See Anesthetic Considerations for Ophthalmic Surgical Procedures under MAC (adult), p. 154, or for Pediatric Ophthalmic Surgery, p. 1175.

Suggested Readings

1. Borazan M, Karalezli A, Akova YA, Algan C, Oto S: Comparative clinical trial of topical anaesthetic agents for cataract surgery with phacoemulsification: lidocaine 2% drops, levobupivacaine 0.75% drops, and ropivacaine 1% drops. *Eye* 2008; 22(3):425–9.
2. Chuang LH, Yeung L, Ku WC, et al: Safety and efficacy of topical anesthesia combined with a lower concentration of intracameral lidocaine in phacoemulsification: paired human eye study. *J Cataract Refract Surg* 2007; 33(2):293–6.
3. Coelho RP, Weissheimer J, Romão E, et al: Pain induced by phacoemulsification without sedation using topical or peribulbar anesthesia. *J Cataract Refract Surg* 2005; 31(2):385–8.
4. Eichel R, Goldberg I: Anaesthesia techniques for cataract surgery: a survey of delegates to the Congress of the International Council of Ophthalmology, 2002. *Clin Experiment Ophthalmol* 2005; 33(5):469–72.
5. Eke T, Thompson JR: Serious complications of local anaesthesia for cataract surgery: a 1 year national survey in the United Kingdom. *Br J Ophthalmol* 2007; 91(4):470–5.
6. Ezra DG, Allan BD: Topical anaesthesia alone versus topical anaesthesia with intracameral lidocaine for phacoemulsification. *Cochrane Database Syst Rev* 2007; 3:CD005276.
7. Kallio H, Rosenberg PH: Advances in ophthalmic regional anaesthesia. *Best Pract Res Clin Anaesthesiol* 2005; 19(2):215–27.
8. Katz J, Feldman MA, Bass EB, et al: Injectable versus topical anesthesia for cataract surgery: Patient perceptions of pain and side effects. *Ophthalmology* 2000; 107:2054–60.
9. Navaleza JS, Pendse SJ, Blecher MH: Choosing anesthesia for cataract surgery. *Ophthalmol Clin North Am* 2006; 19(2): 233–7.
10. See Suggested Reading following Ophthalmic Surgery section, p. 171
11. Srinivasan S, Fern AI, Selvaraj S, et al: Randomized double blind clinical trial comparing topical and sub-Tenon's anaesthesia in routine cataract surgery. *Br J Anaesth* 2004; 93:683–6.
12. Tan CS, Au Eong KG, Kumar CM: Visual experiences during cataract surgery: what anaesthesia providers should know. *Eur J Anaesthesiol* 2005; 22(6):413–19.
13. Vann MA, Ogunnaike BO, Joshi GP: Sedation and anesthesia care for ophthalmologic surgery during local/regional anesthesia. *Anesthesiology* 2007; 107(3):502–8.

CORNEAL TRANSPLANT

SURGICAL CONSIDERATIONS

Description: **Corneal transplantation (penetrating keratoplasty [PKP])** involves replacing a portion of the host cornea with tissue from a donor eye (allograft). The primary goals of this procedure are to restore both the integrity of the cornea and to establish a clear visual axis. The ideal death-to-preservation time of the donor cornea is < 18 h, and the donor cornea can be stored for up to 2 wks before transplantation. The procedure often begins with the placement of a scleral fixation ring (Flieringa ring), just beyond the corneoscleral junction, which is secured with 7-0 Vicryl sutures. This provides additional scleral support that is especially helpful in children or patients who have undergone previous cataract surgery. The donor corneal button is removed from the surrounding corneoscleral rim with a trephine and kept in storage medium until the recipient bed is prepared. The host cornea is then trephined in a previously marked central location, using either manual or vacuum-assist techniques. After the eye is opened, it is critical to avoid patient movement, coughing, bucking, or any Valsalva maneuvers to prevent expulsion of the intraocular contents through the wound. The size of the donor button is generally cut ~0.25 mm larger than the host bed. The donor cornea is then sutured into place with 10-0 nylon sutures, which can be accomplished using 16 interrupted sutures, running sutures, or a combination, depending on a number of factors unique to each patient. Great care is taken during manipulation of the allograft to avoid trauma to the inner surface of the graft, as damage to the endothelial cells in this location can result in primary graft failure.

Variant procedure or approaches: PKP may be combined with **cataract extraction** or exchange of a previously placed intraocular lens (IOL). Additionally, PKP may be combined with **limbal stem-cell transplantation** (autograft from less injured eye) in cases where the most superficial corneal epithelial layer is unable to regenerate following damage (e.g., chemical burn injuries) to the limbal stem cells. **Partial-thickness transplants,** called **lamellar keratoplasty,** also can be performed in certain clinical situations.

Usual preop diagnosis: Persistent corneal edema; inherited corneal dystrophy; keratoconus; corneal scar

SUMMARY OF PROCEDURE

Position	Supine, table rotated 90–180°
Incision	Corneal
Special instrumentation	Surgical microscope
Unique considerations	Open-globe precautions: Avoid coughing, bucking, or Valsalva maneuvers to prevent expulsion of intraocular contents.
Antibiotics	Subconjunctival cefazolin (50–100 mg) or gentamicin (20–40 mg)
Surgical time	60–90 min
EBL	Minimal
Postop care	Patch/shield for 24 h, long-term topical immunosuppression to prevent graft rejection
Mortality	Rare
Morbidity	Graft rejection: ~5% Suprachoroidal hemorrhage: < 1% (higher for MAC: ~4%) Infection: < 1%
Pain score	2

PATIENT POPULATION CHARACTERISTICS

Age range	Any age
Male:Female	1:1
Incidence	> 40,000 cases/yr in the United States and Canada
Etiology	Corneal opacity or decompensation resulting from endothelial failure; inherited dystrophy; keratoconus; scarring related to trauma/chemical burn/infection
Associated conditions	Congenital malformations; sleep apnea; atopic disease/asthma; Down syndrome

ANESTHETIC CONSIDERATIONS

Corneal transplants commonly require GA or a retrobulbar/peribulbar block to prevent movement of the eyelids or extraocular muscles that could lead to distortion of the globe during the procedure. However, in patients with significant coagulopathy, a history of perforated corneal ulcers, severe systemic disease, or other conditions that make the use of these forms of anesthesia less preferable, PKP can be performed with topical anesthesia in cooperative patients.

See Anesthetic Considerations for Ophthalmic Surgical Procedures under MAC (adult), p. 154, or for Pediatric Ophthalmic Surgery, p. 1175.

Suggested Readings

1. Kallio H, Rosenberg PH: Advances in ophthalmic regional anaesthesia. *Best Pract Res Clin Anaesthesiol* 2005; 19(2):215–27.
2. Riddle HK Jr, Price MO, Price FW Jr: Topical anesthesia for penetrating keratoplasty. *Cornea* 2004; 23(7):712–4.
3. See Suggested Readings following Ophthalmic Surgery section, p. 171.
4. Thompson RW Jr, Price MO, Bowers PJ, et al: Long-term graft survival after penetrating keratoplasty. *Ophthalmology* 2003; 110:1396–1402.

TRABECULECTOMY

SURGICAL CONSIDERATIONS

Description: **Glaucoma** is a disorder characterized by progressive optic neuropathy in which elevated intraocular pressure (IOP) is the most modifiable risk factor. It is the second most common cause of blindness in the United States and accounts for more than 5.1 million cases of blindness throughout the world. **Trabeculectomy** (glaucoma filtration procedure) is the most common surgical procedure used to reduce IOP and is often undertaken only after medical therapy has failed. In trabeculectomy, a drainage fistula is created from the anterior chamber to the subconjunctival space, allowing aqueous humor to drain from the eye. (Normal anatomy relevant for aqueous fluid production is shown in Fig. 2-2). First, an incision is created in the conjunctiva and Tenon's layer, exposing the underlying bare sclera. A partial-thickness (4–5 mm) scleral flap, hinged at the limbus, is then created. Because scarring is the most common cause of surgical failure, antimetabolites, such as mitomycin-C or 5-fluorouracil, are often applied to the surgical site to slow or prevent fibroblast proliferation. Next, an incision into the anterior chamber is created at the base of the scleral flap and converted to a sclerotomy by removing an approximate 1 × 4 mm piece of corneoscleral tissue. To prevent the iris from entering the fistula as well as to protect against future angle closure, an **iridectomy** is performed, followed by closure of the overlying scleral flap with 10-0 nylon sutures. Before closure, it is important to avoid coughing, bucking, or Valsalva maneuvers, which might cause suprachoroidal hemorrhage or expulsion of intraocular content. The conjunctiva is then reapposed, using running 8-0 or 9-0 Vicryl suture.

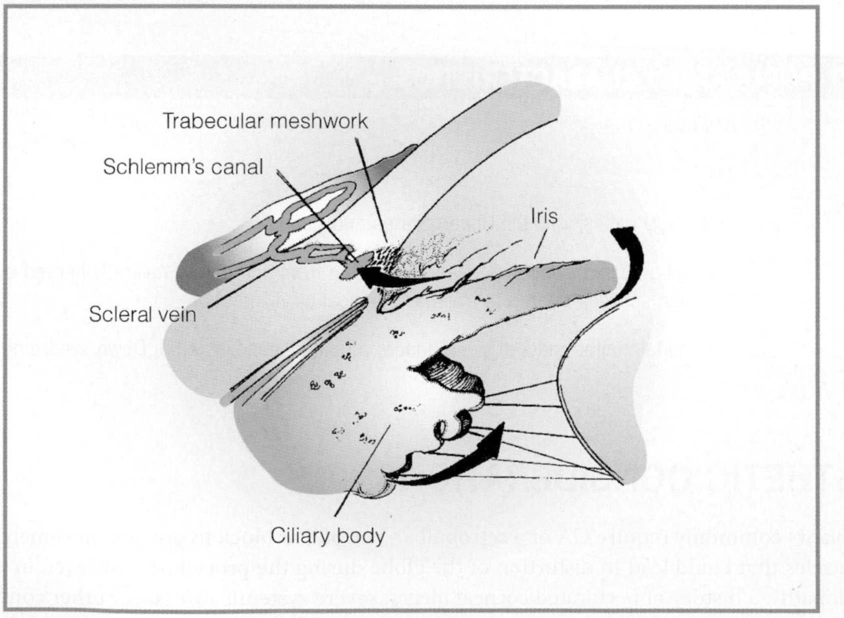

Figure 2-2. Ocular anatomy concerned with control of IOP. (Reproduced with permission from Barash PG, Cullen BF, Stoelting RK, eds: *Clinical Anesthesiology,* 4th edition. Lippincott Williams & Wilkins, 2001.)

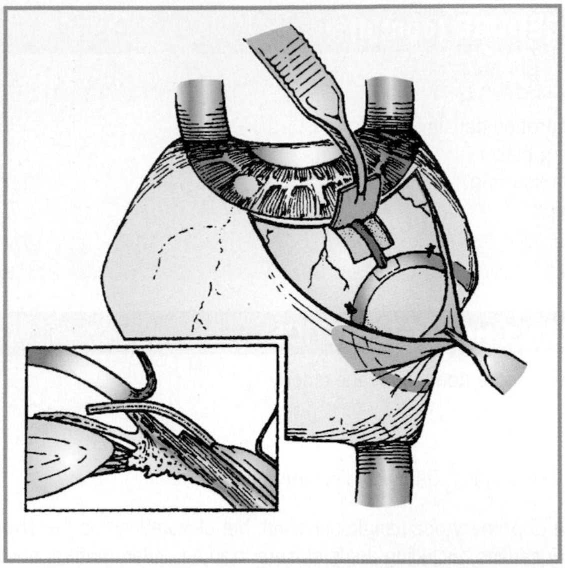

Figure 2-3. Basic technique of inserting Molteno implant. Silicone tube is inserted into anterior chamber via needle track and is connected to a subconjunctival acrylic plate that is attached to the sclera near the equator. (Reproduced with permission from Shields MB: *Textbook of Glaucoma,* 4th edition. Williams & Wilkins, Philadelphia, 1998.)

Variant procedure or approaches: In patients for whom trabeculectomy has failed, a variety of drainage implants have been created to maintain the patency of the drainage fistula. These devices (e.g., **Ahmed, Molteno, Krupin, Baerveldt**) consist of plastic reservoirs that are placed in the sub-Tenon's space and are connected to a tube that enters the anterior chamber (Fig. 2-3). These devices differ in implant size and whether or not there is an internal valve to prevent excessive drainage. Long-term IOP reduction with drainage implants is not as successful as trabeculectomy.

In infants and children with congenital glaucoma (see Pediatric Ophthalmic Surgery, p. 1174), the anterior chamber angle, which normally allows outflow of aqueous, develops abnormally and often requires surgical intervention. Goniotomy (opening Schlemm's canal) is usually the initial procedure of choice. An alternative procedure is a trabeculotomy performed by exposing Schlemm's canal (the drainage system) in a corneoscleral cutdown. A trabeculotome is then threaded into this canal and is rotated, creating a tear in the trabecular meshwork and allowing direct communication between the anterior chamber and Schlemm's canal.

Usual preop diagnosis: Glaucoma

SUMMARY OF PROCEDURE

Position	Supine, table rotated 90–180°
Incision	Superior portion of eye
Special instrumentation	Surgical microscope
Unique considerations	Prevent coughing, bucking, Valsalva maneuvers while globe is open, to prevent expulsion of intraocular contents.
Antibiotics	Subconjunctival cefazolin (50–100 mg) or gentamicin (20–40 mg)
Surgical time	30–60 min
EBL	Minimal
Postop care	Patch/shield × 24 h; long-term topical immunosuppression to reduce scarring. Scleral flap sutures can be cut with a laser postop to increase flow.

SUMMARY OF PROCEDURE (cont'd)	
Mortality	Rare
Morbidity	Overfiltration causing hypotony Leaking bleb Fistula scarring Infection
Pain score	1–2

PATIENT POPULATION CHARACTERISTICS	
Age range	Any age; more common in the elderly
Male:Female	1:1
Incidence	1.7% Caucasians; 5.6% African-Americans
Etiology	Cause of primary open angle unknown, but elevated IOP is the strongest risk factor. Many secondary causes, including angle closure, trauma, inflammation, neovascularization, and congenital abnormalities
Associated conditions	Diseases of the elderly, including cardiovascular disease, HTN, and diabetes. Children may have multiple congenital anomalies.

ANESTHETIC CONSIDERATIONS

Trabeculectomy is typically accomplished using sub-Tenon anesthesia, which allows monitoring of conjunctival mobility when selecting the surgical site. Alternatively, it can be done using topical anesthetics. GA is usually reserved for pediatric patients, patients unlikely or unable to cooperate during the procedure, or if low intraocular pressure from anesthesia is desirable.

Subconjunctival anesthesia at the bleb site may be associated with a poorer outcome, because it may stimulate fibroblasts to cause scarring due to hemorrhage and tissue damage. Peribulbar and retrobulbar injections in patients with advanced glaucoma may be associated with increased intraocular pressure, which can be prevented by decreasing anesthetic volumes and avoiding the use of orbital Honan balloons.

Topical and intracameral anesthesia are being increasingly employed for trabeculectomy to avoid injection pain and potential complications, such as conjunctival button holes and hemorrhage. However, topical agents have the following limitations: inferior duration and intensity of anesthetic effect and lack of ocular akinesia, which is necessary to prevent globe compression in patients with prominent eyelid squeezing. Topical gels are not ideal in trabeculectomy because they can interfere with the surgical site. Intracameral lidocaine as a supplement to topical anesthesia has the theoretical advantage of increasing depth of anterior chamber, but it poses the risk of damaging the phakic lens and excessive iridectomy enlargement. To avoid these possible complications, intracameral acetylcholine or topical pilocarpine can be used in conjunction with intracameral lidocaine.

See Anesthetic Considerations for Ophthalmic Surgical Procedures under MAC (adult), p. 154, or for Pediatric Ophthalmic Surgery, p. 1175.

Suggested Readings

1. Carrillo MM, Buys YM, Faingold D, et al: Prospective study comparing lidocaine 2% jelly versus sub-Tenon's anaesthesia for trabeculectomy surgery. *Br J Ophthalmol* 2004; 88(8):1004–7.
2. Edmunds B, Bunce CV, Thompson JR, et al: Factors associated with success in first-time trabeculectomy for patients at low risk of failure with chronic open-angle glaucoma. *Ophthalmology* 2004; 111:97–103.
3. Jones E, Clarke J, Khaw PT: Recent advances in trabeculectomy technique. *Curr Opin Ophthalmol* 2005; 16(2):107–13.
4. Sauder G, Jonas JB: Topical anesthesia for penetrating trabeculectomy. *Graefes Arch Clin Exp Ophthalmol* 2002; 240: 739–42.
5. See Suggested Readings following Ophthalmic Surgery section, p. 171.
6. Zabriskie NA, Ahmed IIK, Crandall AS, et al: A comparison of topical and retrobulbar anesthesia for trabeculectomy. *J Glaucoma* 2002; 11:306–14.

ECTROPION REPAIR

SURGICAL CONSIDERATIONS

Description: Ectropion is a malposition of the eyelid, in which the lid margin is everted away from the globe. The surgical approach depends on the underlying anatomic abnormality, which can be congenital, involutional, cicatricial (scarring), or due to mechanical traction from masses or facial nerve palsy. A lateral **tarsal strip procedure** is often used, with the lateral canthal tendon first released by performing a **lateral canthotomy and cantholysis** of the crus (Fig. 2-4). A lateral portion of tarsus is then dissected free of overlying skin, muscle, and conjunctiva. This strip of tarsus is trimmed to the appropriate length and is secured to the periosteum of the lateral orbital rim with suture. Excess skin is removed and the defect is closed.

Variant procedure or approaches: Cicatricial ectropion from a contracting scar can sometimes be released with a Z-plasty incision that releases vertical skin tension. Alternatively, a full-thickness skin graft may be required and can be harvested from the upper lid or the postauricular or supraclavicular regions.

Usual preop diagnosis: Ectropion of the eyelid

SUMMARY OF PROCEDURE	
Position	Supine, table rotated 90–180°
Incision	Lateral canthal region or area of scarring
Special instrumentation	Surgical loupes
Antibiotics	None intraop
Surgical time	0.5–1 h
EBL	Minimal
Postop care	Topical antibiotic ointment
Mortality	Rare
Morbidity	Lid malposition Infection: Very rare
Pain score	1–2

PATIENT POPULATION CHARACTERISTICS	
Age range	Any age
Male:Female	1:1
Incidence	Common
Etiology	Congenital; aging; malignancy; facial nerve palsy
Associated conditions	Systemic diseases of elderly patients common; cardiovascular disease; diabetes; HTN

ANESTHETIC CONSIDERATIONS

See Anesthetic Considerations for Ophthalmic Surgical Procedures under MAC (adult), p. 154, or for Pediatric Ophthalmic Surgery, p. 1175.

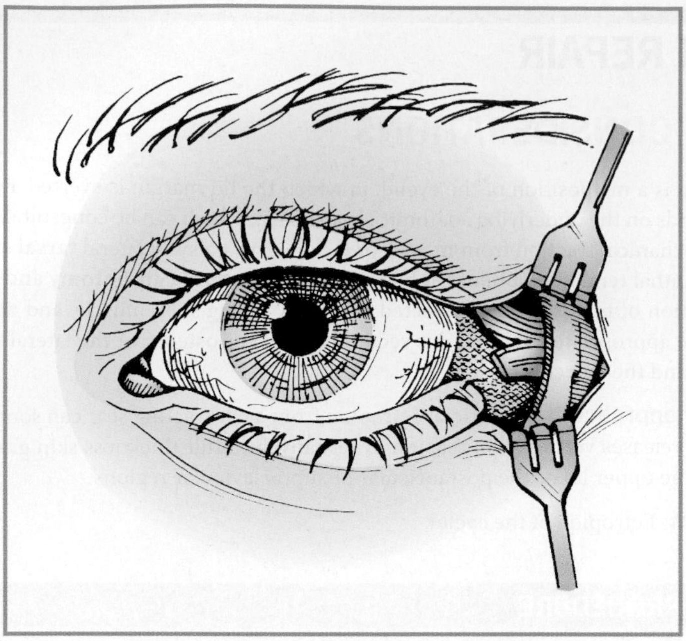

Figure 2-4. In the tarsal strip procedure, the lower eyelid is incised laterally. The entire lower crus of the canthal tendon must be severed. (Redrawn with permission from *Duane's Clinical Ophthalmology,* Vol. 5. Williams & Wilkins, Philadelphia, 2000.)

Suggested Reading

1. See Suggested Reading following Ophthalmic Surgery section, p. 171.

ENTROPION REPAIR

SURGICAL CONSIDERATIONS

Description: Entropion is a condition characterized by an inward rotation of the eyelid margin. The surgical approach depends on the underlying anatomic abnormality, which can be congenital, spastic, involutional, or cicatricial (scarring). For the more common involutional or age-related cases, the primary defect involves horizontal lid laxity, disinsertion of the lower lid retractors and/or an overriding orbicularis muscle. Correction often involves use of the **lateral tarsal strip procedure** (see description under Ectropion Repair) to achieve tightening of the lower lid. Reattachment of the eyelid retractor muscles/aponeurosis may also be used in certain cases, either alone or in addition to a tarsal strip procedure.

Variant procedure or approaches: **Cicatricial entropion** results from a contracting scar of the tarsus and/or conjunctiva pulling the lid margin inward. Correction requires release of this tension and either a **lid-splitting procedure** with tarsal advancement, rotational grafts, or free mucosal grafts harvested from hard palate. In the latter case, nasal intubation will be required to allow access to the graft site. **Quickert procedure** involves the placement of 2–3 sutures under local anesthesia to evert the eyelid. Entropion frequently recurs after this procedure.

Usual preop diagnosis: Entropion of eyelid

SUMMARY OF PROCEDURE	
Position	Supine, table rotated 90–180°
Incision	Lateral canthal region or area of conjunctival scarring. Mucosal graft may be harvested from hard palate.

SUMMARY OF PROCEDURE (cont'd)	
Special instrumentation	Surgical loupes
Antibiotics	Non intraop
Surgical time	0.5–1 h
EBL	Minimal
Postop Care	Topical antibiotic ointment
Mortality	Rare Lid malposition
Morbidity	Infection: Very rare
Pain score	1–2

PATIENT POPULATION CHARACTERISTICS	
Age range	Any age
Male:Female	1:1
Incidence	Common
Etiology	Congenital; aging; inflammation
Associated conditions	Cicatricial entropion can be associated with pemphigoid; Stevens-Johnson syndrome (a sometimes fatal form of erythema multiforme); chemical burns; trachoma.

ANESTHETIC CONSIDERATIONS

Entropion repair can usually be accomplished as an outpatient procedure using local anesthesia and MAC.

See Anesthetic Considerations for Ophthalmic Surgical Procedures under MAC (adult), p. 154, or for Pediatric Ophthalmic Surgery, p. 1175.

Suggested Reading

1. See Suggested Reading following Ophthalmic Surgery section, p. 171.

PTOSIS REPAIR

SURGICAL CONSIDERATIONS

Description: **Ptosis** (drooping of the upper eyelid margin) can be severe enough to obstruct the visual axis. Causes include congenital maldevelopment, mechanical traction, myogenic conditions (e.g., dystrophies, myasthenia gravis), neurogenic conditions (e.g., Horner's syndrome, cranial nerve III palsy), and aponeurotic dehiscence. The surgical approach depends primarily on the presence or absence of adequate levator muscle function that is responsible for elevating the upper eyelid. The most common etiology is age-related dehiscence or disinsertion of the levator aponeurosis from its normal attachment to the tarsus. Because levator muscle function is usually satisfactory in these patients, surgical correction involves reinserting the aponeurosis to the anterior tarsus alone or in combination with shortening of the aponeurosis by advancement or resection. Access is obtained by an incision in the upper eyelid crease. Removal of excess skin and orbicularis muscle (**blepharoplasty**) may be performed simultaneously. Although several formulas have been devised to determine the amount of aponeurotic shortening, intraop measurement usually is performed to ensure that the appropriate lid position and contour are achieved. This requires that the procedure be performed under local anesthesia and that the patient be positioned and draped in a way that allows him/her to sit upright during surgery.

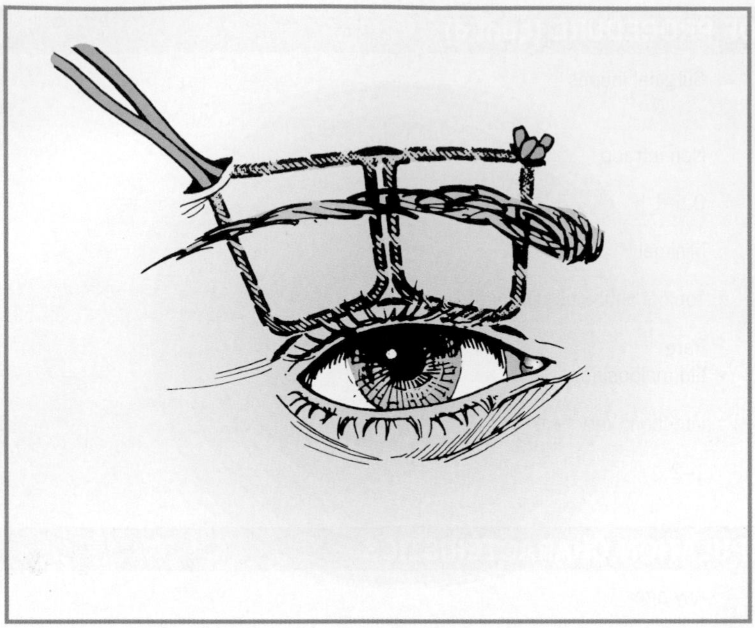

Figure 2-5. Frontalis sling (modified Crawford technique). Note location of brow and lid incisions and double rhomboid fascial slings. (Redrawn with permission from *Duane's Clinical Ophthalmology,* Vol. 5. Williams & Wilkins, Philadelphia, 2000.)

Variant procedure or approaches: In patients with levator muscle function that is not adequate to achieve eyelid elevation, a **frontalis sling procedure** is performed to elevate the upper eyelid (Fig. 2-5). More commonly required in children with congenital ptosis, this allows the patient to open the eye by elevating the brow. A variety of materials can be used to accomplish this suspension, including silicon rods or fascia. In children < 3 yr, autologous fascia lata can be harvested from the outer thigh from hip to knee. The material is tunneled beneath the skin and muscle from the brow incisions to the anterior tarsal region of the eyelid using Wright needles. After appropriate contour and height are achieved, the sling is secured and incisions are closed. Frontalis suspension usually is performed under GA in both adults and children.

Usual preop diagnosis: Ptosis

SUMMARY OF PROCEDURE	
Position	Supine, table rotated 90–180°
Incision	Upper eyelid crease; brow; and lateral thigh (frontalis sling)
Special instrumentation	Surgical loupes
Antibiotics	Cefazolin 1 g iv
Surgical time	0.5–1 h
EBL	Minimal
Postop care	Topical antibiotic ointment; cool compresses
Mortality	Rare
Morbidity	Lid malposition (overcorrection, undercorrection, asymmetry) Corneal exposure Infection: More common with silicone rods
Pain score	1–2

PATIENT POPULATION CHARACTERISTICS	
Age range	Any Age
Male:Female	1:1
Incidence	Common
Etiology	Congenital; aponeurotic; neurogenic; myogenic; mechanical
Associated conditions	Neurogenic causes associated with myasthenia gravis; myogenic causes include chronic external ophthalmoplegia (can have dysrhythmias and SZ disorders); oculopharyngeal dystrophy

ANESTHETIC CONSIDERATIONS

Ptosis repair typically requires GA for infants and children and can be accomplished with local anesthesia and MAC as an outpatient procedure in adults. The need for patient cooperation during the surgery should be discussed with the surgeon and patient in advance. See Anesthetic Considerations for Ophthalmic Surgical Procedures under MAC, p. 154.

Suggested Reading

1. See Suggested Reading following Ophthalmic Surgery section, p. 171.

EYELID RECONSTRUCTION

SURGICAL CONSIDERATIONS

Description: Given the relatively small tissue area of the eyelids and their importance in both ocular health and cosmesis, excision of lid tumors often requires some form of reconstructive surgery. For lesions suspected of being malignant, **frozen-sections** are often performed prior to closing the defect. Additionally, **Mohs technique** (microscopically controlled serial excision) may be performed (usually by a dermatologist) to achieve clear margins, with reconstruction undertaken during a separate operation. During closure of full-thickness defects that involve the eyelid margin, attention is focused on aligning the lid in all dimensions (Fig. 2-6), while avoiding exposed sutures on the conjunctival surface that might damage the cornea. For small lid defects involving < ¼ of the lid length, direct closure often can be accomplished with release of the lateral canthal tendon (**canthotomy and cantholysis**) to reduce wound tension, if necessary.

Variant procedure or approaches: Larger excisions often require grafting techniques that are designed to replace both the anterior (skin/orbicularis) and posterior (tarsus/conjunctiva) lamellae of the eyelid. This can be accomplished with rotational grafts, a tarsoconjunctival advancement flap or free grafts of cartilage, hard palate, cadaver sclera, or composite grafts as posterior lamellar replacement materials.

Usual preop diagnosis: Basal-cell carcinoma; squamous-cell carcinoma; melanoma; sebaceous carcinoma; or trauma

SUMMARY OF PROCEDURE	
Position	Supine, table rotated 90–180°
Incision	Upper and/or lower eyelid. Postauricular, supraclavicular, or hard palate if graft harvesting required
Special instrumentation	Surgical loupes
Antibiotics	Cefazolin 1 g iv
Surgical time	0.5–2 h
EBL	Minimal

SUMMARY OF PROCEDURE (cont'd)	
Postop care	Topical antibiotic ointment; cool compresses; pressure dressing
Mortality	Rare
Morbidity	Graft failure Lid deformity Corneal exposure Infection: < 1%
Pain score	2–3

PATIENT POPULATION CHARACTERISTICS	
Age range	Usually elderly
Male:Female	1:1
Incidence	Common
Etiology	Sun exposure-related malignancy
Associated conditions	Diseases of the elderly, including cardiovascular disease, HTN, and diabetes

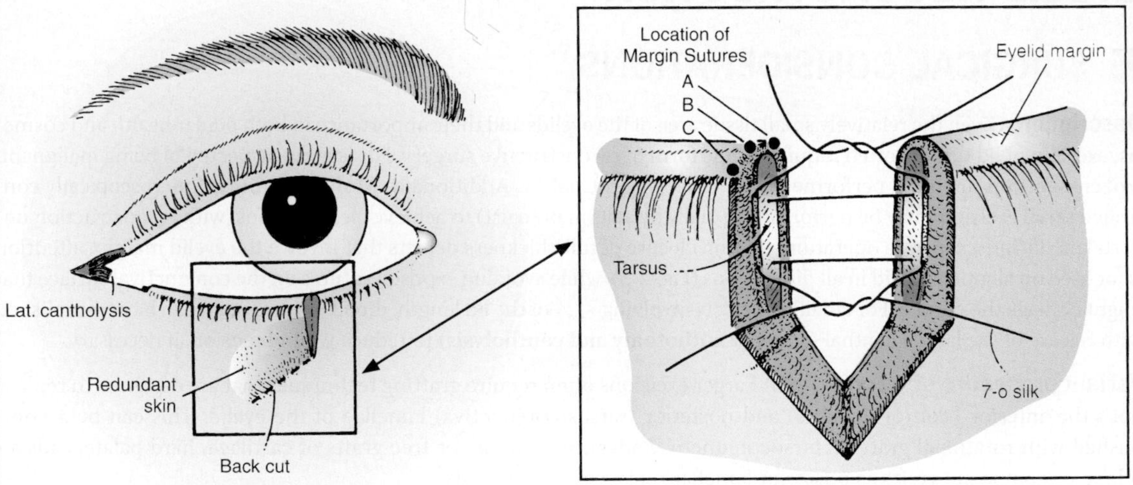

Figure 2-6. Closure of full-thickness defect in the lower lid. The tarsal sutures and half-thickness tarsus are placed first, with the secondary closures at points A, B, C, and the eyelid margin. (Reproduced with permission from McCord CD, Tanenbaum M, eds: *Oculoplastic Surgery,* 2nd edition. Raven Press, New York, 1987.)

ANESTHETIC CONSIDERATIONS

Eyelid reconstruction can often be accomplished with local anesthesia and MAC. See Anesthetic Considerations for Ophthalmic Surgical Procedures under MAC, p. 154.

Suggested Readings

1. Codner MA, WEinfeld AB: Comprehensive eyelid reconstruction. *ANZ J Surg* 2007; 77(Suppl 1):A71.
2. See Suggested Readings following Ophthalmic Surgery section, p. 171.

PTERYGIUM EXCISION

SURGICAL CONSIDERATIONS

Description: Pterygia are fibrovascular growths that originate in the interpalpebral conjunctiva and grow into the superficial layer of the cornea. They often produce refractive changes and/or obstruct the central visual axis and, thus, require removal. Although this procedure is often performed in the clinic or minor-procedure room, larger lesions may require an OR. In both settings, local anesthesia is applied both topically (tetracaine 0.5%) and subconjunctivally (lidocaine 2%). The lesion is dissected from the cornea and from the surrounding healthy conjunctiva, leaving a bed of bare sclera that may or may not be closed primarily (Fig. 2-7).

Variant procedure or approaches: For larger excisions and to decrease the rate of recurrence, **conjunctival transposition** or **free-graft techniques** can be used to cover the area of bare sclera. Topical antimetabolites, such as mitomycin-C, also may be applied to prevent recurrence.

Preop diagnosis or indications: Pterygium

SUMMARY OF PROCEDURE	
Position	Supine, table rotated 90–180°
Incision	Interpalpebral area adjacent to involved limbus
Special instrumentation	Operating microscope
Antibiotics	Topical postop
Surgical time	15–45 min
EBL	Minimal
Postop care	Topical antibiotic ointment
Mortality	Rare
Morbidity	Recurrence: 37%, without adjunctive therapy or grafting Extraocular muscle injury (higher risk in re-op eyes)
Pain score	1–2

PATIENT POPULATION CHARACTERISTICS	
Age range	Usually young-to-middle age
Male:Female	1:1
Incidence	Common
Etiology	Related to sun exposure

References

1. Ang LP, Chua JL, Tan DT: Current concepts and techniques in pterygium treatment. *Curr Opin Ophthalmol* 2007; 18(4):308–13.

ANESTHETIC CONSIDERATIONS FOR OPHTHALMIC SURGICAL PROCEDURES UNDER MAC

(Procedures covered: cataract extraction and other procedures; corneal transplant; trabeculectomy; ectropion-entropion repair; ptosis surgery; eyelid reconstruction; pterygium excision)

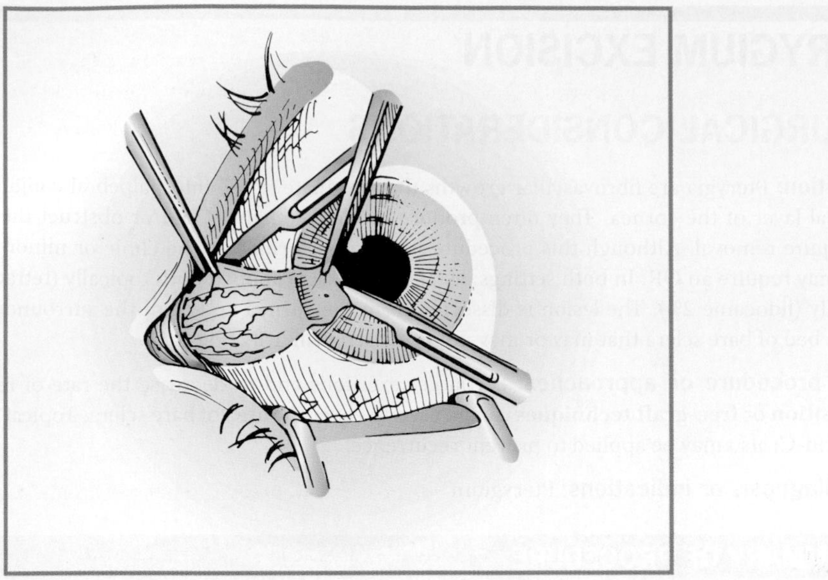

Figure 2-7. Bare sclera excision can be started from the corneal apex or by incising around the conjunctival body of the pterygium. (Redrawn with permission from *Duane's Clinical Ophthalmology*, Vol 6. Williams & Wilkins, Philadelphia, 2000.)

PREOPERATIVE

Ophthalmic procedures that are of relatively short duration and those that result in minimal blood loss are being performed increasingly more often on an outpatient basis, usually with topical or regional anesthesia (e.g., retrobulbar or peribulbar blocks) under MAC (see p. B-3). **Retrobulbar and peribulbar injections** achieve excellent anesthesia and provide equal degrees of akinesia. Given the associated risk of inadvertent intrathecal injection of anesthetic, orbital hemorrhage, need for heavy sedation during injection, and delayed return of visual function postop, many cataract surgeries are performed using **topical anesthesia**. An additional benefit is that the bleeding risk is lower and the procedure can be performed safely in patients taking anticoagulants or with bleeding disorders. Although satisfactory pain relief usually is achieved with this method, the lack of akinesia requires a highly cooperative patient to prevent sudden eye movements during surgery. Some surgeons will supplement topical anesthesia with **intracameral lidocaine** (injections into the anterior chamber) although this has not been proven better than topical anesthetics alone in terms of patient comfort and satisfaction. **Sub-Tenon's injection** is another anesthetic technique used by many surgeons as a compromise between topical application and orbital injections. After preop application of topical anesthetics, a small incision is made in the bulbar conjunctiva, exposing the sub-Tenon's space. A blunt cannula is inserted under direct visualization and local anesthetic injected into the retrobulbar space. The main benefit is that no sharp needle is used, thereby reducing the risk of intrathecal injection and orbital hemorrhage from vessel injury. The onset of akinesia, however, is often delayed, and this technique still has the disadvantage of delayed return of postop visual function.

The pain on injection is slightly less with peribulbar blocks or sub-Tenon blocks as compared with retrobulbar techniques. The placement of the intravenous cannula was reported to represent the worst discomfort during cataract surgery, thus indicating that the eye blocks were not uncomfortable. Intraoperative pain is significantly less during retrobulbar blocks and peribulbar blocks than during topical anesthesia. Rates of ocular perforation following injection blocks are low (1 in 1000–10,000). A great majority (70%) of patients preferred peribulbar/retrobulbar anesthesia, 10% preferred topical, and 18% indicated no preference.

Because the majority of ocular procedures are performed on elderly patients, multiple coexisting medical illnesses are often present. A thorough preop H&P, along with appropriate ancillary studies are mandatory even though local anesthesia/MAC is planned. Contraindications to regional anesthesia/MAC for ocular surgery may include bleeding diathesis, open-eye injuries, claustrophobia, chronic cough, inability to lie flat, or patient refusal.

Respiratory	Elderly patients have increased incidence of hiatal hernia and, therefore, are at increased risk for pulmonary aspiration. Assess the patient's ability to lie flat for the duration of the procedure. Patients with chronic cough may require GA. **Tests:** As indicated from H&P

Cardiovascular	Hx of HTN, CAD, CHF, or poor exercise tolerance should prompt a thorough investigation into the patient's cardiac status, including efficacy of current medications and recent ECG (compared with previous ECGs). Consultation with a cardiologist may be appropriate to optimize the patient's condition before surgery. **Tests:** ECG; others (e.g., ECHO) as indicated from H&P
Diabetes	Diabetic patients are at increased risk for silent myocardial ischemia. Pulmonary aspiration 2° diabetic gastroparesis is also a risk in this population. Patients usually take 1/2 of their normal NPH (or other intermediate or long acting) insulin dose (on the morning of surgery); fasting blood sugar is checked; and an iv infusion of D5 LR is started if glucose $<$ 90 mg/dl, or treated with regular insulin if glucose $>$ 200 mg/dl. Blood sugar is checked intraop and postop. Patients on insulin pumps should maintain their basal infusion rate, and eliminate preprandial boluses. The anesthesiologist should ask the patient about their insulin sensitivity (the amount of insulin necessary to ↓ blood glucose by 50 mg/dl). Blood glucose should be monitored hourly.
Musculoskeletal	Arthritic changes make lying flat difficult for some patients. Careful positions and padding are essential. A low-level remifentanil infusion (~0.05 mcg/kg/min) may be helpful in some cases
Hematologic	✓ for antiplatelet or anticoagulant drug use, particularly in patients undergoing lid or orbital procedures. **Tests:** As indicated from H&P. (e.g., PT if patient is on anticoagulant)
Laboratory	Cr usual in patients $>$ 64 yr; in other patients, as indicated from H&P
Premedication	Patients will benefit from a detailed explanation of events prior to surgery (including iv placement, application of monitors, performance of local block, ocular pressure, prepping eye, draping of the whole face, and provision of supplemental O_2) and the assurance that the anesthesiologist will always be nearby, monitoring them. Midazolam (0.5–1 mg iv) is often beneficial. For patients with increased risk of aspiration (e.g., with hiatal hernia or diabetic gastroparesis) and for obese and/or very anxious patients, metoclopramide 10 mg iv may enhance gastric emptying.

INTRAOPERATIVE

Anesthetic technique: MAC (see p. B-3). Topical anesthesia typically is accomplished by the ophthalmologist, often using tetracaine or other long lasting LA, supplemented with 2% lidocaine, injected subconjunctivally. Placement of retrobulbar or peribulbar blocks may be painful and very short-acting agents (e.g., remifentanil 0.5–1 mcg/kg, alfentanil 5–7 mcg/kg, or propofol 30–50 mg) should be administered to minimize patient discomfort. Dose requirements vary significantly among patients, and the anesthesiologist should be prepared to treat ↓BP and apnea. Usually, further sedation is unnecessary and may interfere with patient cooperation during the surgery. Coughing should be avoided during the procedure, and the anesthesiologist must always be prepared to administer GA if necessary.

Retrobulbar block: Using a 25- or 27-ga needle (1.5"), the retrobulbar space is approached from the infratemporal quadrant of the orbit. The eye should be in a neutral or downward and medial position. Once the needle is positioned and there is no return of blood or CSF on aspiration, 3–5 mL of anesthetic solution is injected slowly. A facial nerve block is necessary to prevent eyelid movement. This can be accomplished by injecting 4-8 mL of anesthetic solution above and below the lateral aspect of the orbit. Typically, the anesthetic solution consists of a 50:50 mixture of 0.5% bupivacaine and 2% lidocaine with hyaluronidase.

Peribulbar block: Using a 25- or 27-ga needle (5/8"–1"), 5–6 mL of anesthetic solution is injected into the peribulbar space, entering just superior to the inferior rim of the orbit at the junction of the lateral and middle thirds of the lower lid. Although perforation of the globe and hemorrhage are still possible, direct injury to the optic nerve and subdural injection are not likely due to the length and position of the needle. Peribulbar blocks generally have a slower onset than retrobulbar blocks and are more likely to cause conjunctival swelling, which may interfere with surgery.

Sub-Tenon's Anesthesia: Injection of LA (often lidocaine ± epi) through a 22-ga cannula into the space below Tenon's capsule (episcleral membrane) produces ocular anesthesia in many ways similar to retrobulbar block. However, the onset is slower and akinesia is less reliable. The usual injection volume is 3–5 mL with more necessary if akinesia is required. Unlike retrobulbar block, significant complications with the technique are extremely rare.

Blood and fluid requirements	IV: 18–20 ga × 1 NS/LR @ 1.5–3 mL/kg/h	Excessive fluids → bladder distention → ↑BP, agitation
Monitoring	Standard monitors (see p. B-1). Verbal response	It is important to remain in communication with the patient throughout the procedure. (Take care to avoid evoking head movement).
Positioning	✓ and pad pressure points. ✓ nonoperated eye.	Place pillows under knees to relieve back strain
Complications	Dysrhythmias, especially ↓HR	Usually 2° traction on ocular/periocular tissues (see OCR, p. 1111)
	↑BP	2° anxiety, pain, etc. Rx: reassurance, local anesthetics, labetalol 5 mg or hydralazine 4-mg increments, as appropriate
	Retrobulbar hemorrhage (1–3%)	Rx: pressure bandage; usually cancel surgery
	Globe perforation	If a needle perforation, usually no repair is necessary
	Convulsions 2° iv local anesthetic	Supportive treatment with IPPV; cancel surgery
	Respiratory arrest	2° subarachnoid injection. Rx: CPR
	Oculocardiacreflex(OCR)→↓↓HR, ↓↓BP	Rx: Stop stimulation; use atropine (see OCR, p. 1111)

POSTOPERATIVE

Complications	Myocardial ischemia	Rx: Provide O_2; ✓ BP; sublingual NTG; ✓ ECG; cardiology consultation
	Corneal abrasion	
	Photophobia	
	N/V	Rx: Ondansetron 4 mg iv, ± metoclopramide, 10 mg iv
	Diplopia	
Pain management	Acetaminophen 325–1000 mg po	

Table 2-1. Commonly Used Ophthalmic Drugs and Their Systemic Effects

Phenylephrine	An α-adrenergic agonist that causes mydriasis (pupillary dilation) and vasoconstriction to aid ocular surgery; however, it also can precipitate significant HTN and dysrhythmias.
Echothiophate	An irreversible cholinesterase inhibitor used in glaucoma treatment to cause miosis and ↓IOP. Its systemic absorption can reduce plasma cholinesterase activity and thereby prolong paralysis 2° to succinylcholine (usually not more than 20–30 min).
Timolol	A nonselective β-blocker that decreases production of aqueous humor →↓IOP. Rarely, it may be associated with atropine-resistant bradycardia, asthma, CHF, and ↓BP.
Acetazolamide	A carbonic anhydrase inhibitor used to ↓IOP. It also can cause diuresis and a hypokalemic metabolic acidosis.
Betaxolol	A relatively oculospecific β-blocker used to ↓IOP. Effects may be additive to systemic β-blockers.
Cyclopentolate	A commonly used mydriatic with the potential for CNS toxicity, including Sz, psychotic reactions, and dysarthria.
Atropine	An anticholinergic that produces mydriasis to aid with ocular examination and surgery. It also can precipitate central anticholinergic syndrome. (Sx range from dry mouth, tachycardia, agitation, delirium, and hallucinations to unconsciousness.) Physostigmine 0.01–0.03 mg/kg will increase central acetylcholine and reverse the symptoms. (It may be repeated after 15–30 min).

Suggested Readings

1. Ahmad S, Ahmad A: Complications of ophthalmologic nerve blocks: a review. *J Clin Anesth* 2003; 15(7):564–9.
2. Friedman DS, Bass EB, Lubomski LH, et al: Synthesis of the literature on the effectiveness of regional anesthesia for cataract surgery. *Ophthalmology* 2001; 108:519–29.
3. McGoldrick KE, Gayer S: Anesthesia and the eye. In *Clinical Anesthesia*, 5th edition. Barash PG, Cullen BF, Stoelting RK, eds. Lippincott Williams & Wilkins, Philadelphia: 2006, 974–96.
4. Vann MA, Ogunnaike BO, Joshi GP: Sedation and anesthesia care for ophthalmologic surgery during local/regional anesthesia. *Anesthesiology* 2007; 107(3):502–8.

REPAIR OF RUPTURED OR LACERATED GLOBE

SURGICAL CONSIDERATIONS

Description: A ruptured globe involves a tear of either the corneal or scleral layers of the eye and can occur in the setting of blunt, penetrating, or perforating trauma. The primary goal of surgical repair is to replace extruded intraocular contents, close defects, and remove any foreign body. Orbital CT scans are performed preop to aid in the identification of the latter. To reduce the risk of causing further damage, complete examination of the eye is often delayed until the patient is in the controlled setting of the OR under GA. Although anterior injuries are readily identifiable, posterior injuries may require extensive exploration that can require a 360° opening of the conjunctiva and isolation of each extraocular muscle to allow adequate inspection of the entire scleral surface. Corneal lacerations usually are closed with 10-0 nylon sutures while 8-0 nylon or Vicryl may be used for scleral tissue. Until these wounds are closed, it is crucial that Valsalva maneuvers (which raise IOP), be avoided to prevent further extrusion of intraocular contents.

Variant procedures or approaches: After globe integrity has been established, other associated injuries may be addressed, including repair of conjunctival lacerations, extraocular muscle injuries/detachments, retinal detachments, or removal of a traumatic cataract.

Usual preop diagnosis: Ruptured globe

SUMMARY OF PROCEDURE	
Position	Supine, table rotated 90–180°
Incision	Conjunctival peritomy (360° conjunctival incision) to allow exposure of posterior sclera
Special instrumentation	Operating microscope
Antibiotics	IV gentamicin (80 mg) and cefazolin (1 g); subconjunctival and topical antibiotics
Closing considerations	Avoid Valsalva-like maneuvers (coughing, bucking, etc.)
Surgical time	1–2 h
EBL	Minimal
Postop care	Hospital admission for iv antibiotics
Mortality	Rare
Morbidity	Wound leak Infection: Rate depends on injury Sympathetic ophthalmia: Rare
Pain score	4

PATIENT POPULATION CHARACTERISTICS	
Age range	Usually < 40 yr
Male:Female	9:1
Incidence	Common
Etiology	Work- or sports-related injury; motor vehicle accidents
Associated conditions	Intoxication; orbital/facial trauma; head injury

ANESTHETIC CONSIDERATIONS

PREOPERATIVE

This is a generally healthy patient population; however, patients with penetrating eye injuries present the anesthesiologist with two special challenges: (1) They invariably have full stomachs, resulting in risk of aspiration. (2) They are at risk of blindness 2° ↑IOP and loss of ocular contents, which may be a result of coughing, crying, and/or struggling during induction. Normal IOP ranges from 10–22 mmHg, depending on the rate of formation and drainage of aqueous humor, choroidal blood volume, scleral rigidity, extraocular muscle tone, as well as extrinsic pressure on the eye (e.g., a poorly fitting mask or retrobulbar hematoma). Patient movement, coughing, straining, vomiting, hypercarbia, HTN, and ET intubation also may ↑IOP to 40 mmHg or more.

Full-stomach precautions	Consider patient to have a full stomach if the injury occurred within 8 h of the last meal. Pain and anxiety due to trauma will delay gastric emptying. Goal is to minimize risk of aspiration pneumonitis by decreasing gastric volume and acidity. Consider premedication with metoclopramide (10–20 mg iv), antacids such as Na citrate (15–30 mL po, immediately prior to induction), and H_2-histamine receptor antagonists (ranitidine [50 mg iv]). H_2-histamine receptor antagonists, however, have no effect on the pH of gastric secretions present in the stomach prior to administration and are, therefore, of limited value in patients presenting for emergency surgery. If patient has Hx of smoking or is an asthmatic, consider preop use of inhalers such as albuterol (2–4 puffs).
Associated Injuries	A ruptured globe may be only one of multiple injuries to the head and neck or other structures. Other injuries should be excluded preoperatively.
Laboratory	Tests as indicated from H&P
Premedication	Patients often are very anxious and may benefit from benzodiazepines (e.g., for pediatric population, midazolam 0.5–0.75 mg/kg po in cola or apple juice, 15–30 mL). Avoid narcotic premedication, which may ↑ nausea and possibility of emesis.

INTRAOPERATIVE

Anesthetic technique: GETA. Regional anesthesia (e.g., retrobulbar block) is contraindicated in patients with open-eye injury because of ↑IOP, which may accompany injection of local anesthetic behind the globe. Thus, in spite of the increased risk of aspiration from a full stomach, GETA is recommended. In patients where the risk of GA is unacceptably high (e.g., extensive pulmonary or unstable cardiac disease) surgical repair can be accomplished using topical anesthesia (see Auffarth GU et al.).

Induction	To protect the airway and prevent ↑IOP, a rapid-sequence induction with cricoid pressure and a smooth intubation are required. Although the choice of induction agent is relatively straightforward—propofol 1–2 mg/kg or STP 3–5 mg/kg—the choice of neuromuscular blocking agents for facilitating intubation is controversial.

Induction (cont'd)	Succinylcholine provides a rapid onset, short duration of action, and excellent intubating conditions, but it also transiently increases IOP. This ↑IOP is not always attenuated by pretreatment with a nondepolarizing agent (e.g., d-tubocurarine). Rocuronium (1 mg/kg) produces muscle relaxation in 1–2 min and may be a satisfactory alternative to succinylcholine; however, a premature attempt at intubation may significantly ↑IOP as a result of coughing and straining. Of interest, there are no reports in the literature documenting exacerbation of eye injuries with the use of succinylcholine following pretreatment with a NMR. Given that the anesthesiologist's main concern is safe airway management, the following is a suggested induction plan: (1) Preoxygenation, avoiding external pressure on the eye from face mask (2) Pretreatment with a nondepolarizing relaxant (e.g., d-tubocurarine 0.06 mg/kg or equivalent), followed by iv lidocaine (1 mg/kg) and fentanyl (2–3 mcg/kg) to blunt the cardiovascular response to laryngoscopy and intubation (3) 4 min later, with cricoid pressure, induce with STP (3–5 mg/kg) or propofol (1–2 mg/kg) and succinylcholine (1.5 mg/kg). Intubate with oral RAE tube. Note: for pediatric patients, it might be appropriate to induce with sevoflurane while maintaining cricoid pressure and intubating when the patient is deeply anesthetized. Trying to start an iv prior to induction may precipitate struggling and crying, leading to further eye injury.	
Maintenance	Standard maintenance or TIVA (see p. B-2). Avoid hypercapnia, which →↑IOP. Muscle relaxation is mandatory until the eye is surgically closed. Humidify gases for pediatric patients.	
Emergence	Decompress the stomach with OG tube. Goal is smooth emergence and extubation with patient awake with intact airway reflexes. IV lidocaine (1.5 mg/kg) 5 min before extubation; posterior pharyngeal suctioning with patient deeply anesthetized, combined with a small amount of narcotic (remifentanil ~1 mcg/kg), may blunt cough reflex prior to extubation. The common occurrence of PONV requires administration of intraop antiemetics (e.g., metoclopramide 10 mg iv, and ondansetron 4 mg iv 30 min before end of surgery).	
Blood and fluid requirements	IV: 18–20 ga ×1 (adult) 20 ga ×1 (child) NS/LR @ 5–10 mL/kg/h Warm fluids	
Monitoring	Standard monitors (see p. B-1)	Neuromuscular blockade must be monitored closely and additional relaxant given as necessary to prevent patient movement during surgery.
Positioning	✓ and pad pressure points ✓ nonoperated eye	
Complications	↑ IOP with extrusion of intraocular contents Aspiration of gastric contents	IOP (normal = ~10–22 mmHg) increased by: blink = 10–15 mmHg; forced closure = > 70 mmHg.

POSTOPERATIVE

Complications	N/V	Rx: Metoclopramide 10 mg iv, droperidol 0.625 mg iv (with due respect to the black-box warning), ondansetron 4 mg iv
	Aspiration pneumonitis	Provide O_2 by face mask, if not intubated. Follow O_2 sat. ✓ CXR
	Photophobia Diplopia Hemorrhagic retinopathy Corneal abrasion	
Pain management	Acetaminophen	Occasionally, parenteral opiates (see p. C-2)

Suggested Readings

1. Auffarth GU, Vargas LG, Klett J, et al: Repair of a ruptured globe using topical anesthesia. *J Cataract Refract Surg* 2004; 30(3):726–9.
2. Boscia F, La Tegola MG, Columbo G, et al: Combined topical anesthesia and sedation for open-globe injuries in selected patients. *Ophthalmology* 2003; 110(8):1555–9.
3. Chidiac EJ, Raiskin AO: Succinylcholine and the open eye. *Ophthalmol Clin North Am* 2006; 19(2):279–85.
4. Kumar C, Doods C, Fanning G, eds: *Ophthalmic Anaesthesia*. Lisse: Swets and Zeitlinger BV, 2002.
5. McGoldrick KE, Gayer S: Anesthesia and the eye. In *Clinical Anesthesia*, 5th edition. Barash PG, Cullen BF, Stoelting RK, eds. Lippincott Williams & Wilkins, Philadelphia, 2006.
6. Vachon CA, Warner DO, Bacon DR: Succinylcholine and the open globe. Tracing the teaching. *Anesthesiology* 2003; 99:220–3.

DACRYOCYSTORHINOSTOMY (DCR)

SURGICAL CONSIDERATIONS

Description: **Dacryocystorhinostomy (DCR)** is performed for patients with symptomatic obstruction of the nasolacrimal duct (NLD) and is commonly associated with chronic dacryocystitis. The procedure is designed to create a fistula from the common canaliculus to the nasopharynx, which bypasses the site of obstruction. DCR can be performed under GA or local anesthesia (subcutaneous and nasal cavity cocaine 4%). Intranasal phenylephrine and/or cocaine pledgets are often placed to decrease mucosal bleeding. A skin incision is made below the medial canthal tendon that is extended to the lacrimal fossa with blunt dissection. Bleeding can be excessive if the angular vessels are injured. The now exposed periosteum is incised and a 1.5 cm × 1.5 cm osteotomy is created with a burr and/or Kerrison punch, exiting at the level of the middle meatus. A Crawford lacrimal probe attached to silicone tubing is inserted into the superior punctum and advanced into the lacrimal sac, which is then opened along its medial wall. Following incision of the nasal mucosa through the osteotomy, the posterior flap of the lacrimal sac is sutured to the posterior nasal mucosa flap. The probe is advanced through the osteotomy and into the middle meatus, where it is retrieved through the nare. The second end of the probe is advanced along the same path but beginning through the inferior punctum. The ends of the silicone tubing are tied together in the nare and the anterior flaps of lacrimal sac and nasal mucosa are sutured together. Thrombin and gel foam can be used to control mucosal bleeding and the skin is reapproximated after ensuring hemostasis.

Variant procedures or approaches: If the lacrimal obstruction is more proximal to the lacrimal sac, a **Jones tube** can be placed (Fig. 2-8), creating an artificial lumen from the conjunctiva to the nasopharynx to bypass the entire nasolacrimal drainage system. An endonasal approach using a rigid endoscopic ± laser offers the advantage of no skin incision, good visualization of intranasal pathology and less post-op discomfort.

Usual preop diagnosis: NLD obstruction

SUMMARY OF PROCEDURE	
Position	Supine, table rotated 90–180°
Incision	15 mm, just below medial canthus (Fig. 2-9)
Special instrumentation	Headlight; surgical loupes
Unique considerations	Nasal packing with phenylephrine/cocaine. Blood may drain into upper airway during surgery
Antibiotics	Cefazolin 1 g iv
Surgical time	1–1.5 h

SUMMARY OF PROCEDURE (cont'd)	
EBL	100–200 mL
Postop care	Outpatient
Mortality	Rare
Morbidity	Failure to drain Bleeding: 5% Infection: < 1%
Pain score	3–4

PATIENT POPULATION CHARACTERISTICS	
Age range	30–70 yr
Male:Female	1:1
Incidence	Common
Etiology	Usually scarring from prior infection or trauma
Associated conditions	Deviated septum; nasal polyps; nasopharyngeal masses

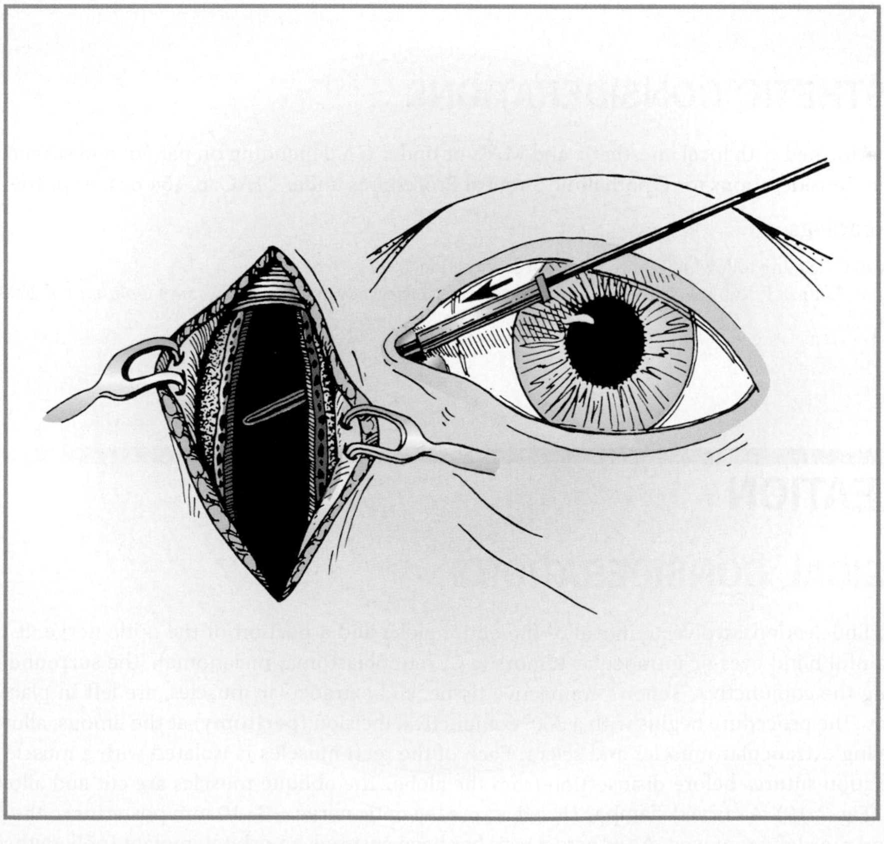

Figure 2-8. Insertion of a Pyrex Jone's tube. (Reproduced with permission from McCord CD, Tanenbaum M, Nunery WR: *Oculoplastic Surgery.* Raven Press, 1995.)

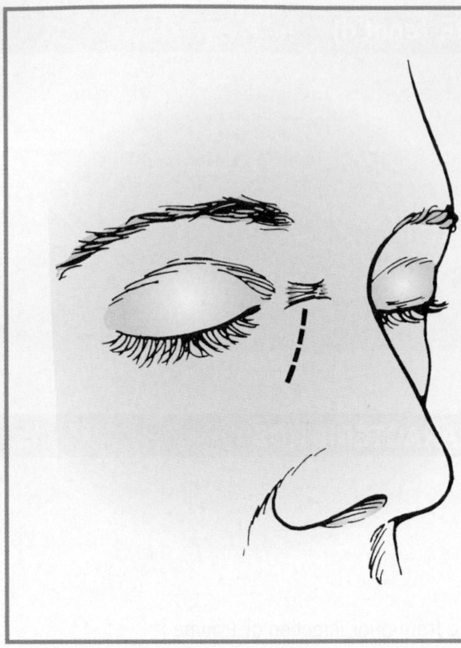

Figure 2-9. Linear skin incision for a standard DCR. (Reproduced with permission from Wright KW: *Textbook of Ophthalmology.* Williams & Wilkins, Philadelphia, 1997.)

ANESTHETIC CONSIDERATIONS

DCR can be performed with local anesthetic and MAC or under GA depending on patient and surgeon preferences. See Anesthetic Considerations for Ophthalmic Surgical Procedures under MAC: p. 154 or GA: p. 165.

Suggested Readings

1. See Suggested Reading following Ophthalmic Surgery section, p. 171.
2. Watkins LM, Janfaza P, Rubin PA: The evolution of endonasal dacryocystorhinostomy. *Surg Ophthalmol* 2003; 48(1):73–84.

ENUCLEATION

SURGICAL CONSIDERATIONS

Description: Enucleation involves removal of the entire globe and a portion of the optic nerve. It usually is performed for painful blind eyes or intraocular tumors (e.g., retinoblastoma, melanoma). The surrounding ocular adnexa, including the conjunctiva, Tenon's connective tissue, and extraocular muscles, are left in place to secure an orbital implant. The procedure begins with a 360° conjunctival incision (**peritomy**) at the limbus, allowing exposure of the underlying extraocular muscles and sclera. Each of the recti muscles is isolated with a muscle hook and secured with fixation sutures before disinsertion from the globe. The oblique muscles are cut and allowed to retract into the orbit (Fig. 2-10). A curved clamp is closed across the optic nerve ~3–10 mm posterior to the globe, and the nerve is cut and the globe removed. After hemostasis has been ensured, an orbital implant (polymethylmethacrylate

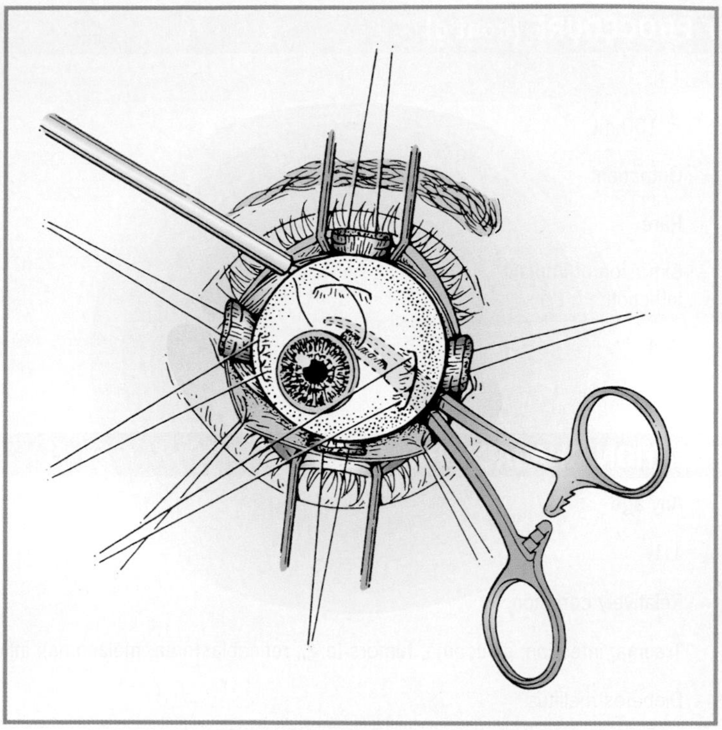

Figure 2-10. Each of the four recti is isolated with 6-0 Dexon suture. The superior oblique tendon is detached. The inferior oblique is sutured to the inferior border of the lateral rectus. 4-0 silk traction sutures are in place over the medial and lateral rectus stump. The globe is rotated laterally, while a curved clamp is introduced from the medial direction. Either a curved scissors or an enucleation snare may be used to transect the optic nerve. (Reproduced with permission form McCord, CD Jr, Tanenbaum M, Nunery WR: *Oculoplastic Surgery.* Raven Press, Philadelphia, 1995.)

or hydroxyapatite) is placed into the socket. The overlying muscles, connective tissue, and conjunctiva are closed to improve motility and prevent extrusion.

Variant procedure or approaches: **Evisceration** involves removing all intraocular contents through a corneoscleral incision, leaving the scleral shell with the attached adnexa in place. This usually is performed in cases of endophthalmitis, but never if malignancy is suspected. **Exenteration** is a more extensive procedure for the management of aggressive malignant tumors or infections where all orbital tissue, often including surrounding orbital bone and adjacent sinuses, is removed.

Usual preop diagnosis: Painful blind eye; intraocular tumors; sympathetic ophthalmia

SUMMARY OF PROCEDURE	
Position	Supine, table rotated 90–180°
Incision	360° conjunctival (peritomy)
Special instrumentation	Surgical loupes
Antibiotics	Irrigate socket with gentamicin postop

SUMMARY OF PROCEDURE (cont'd)	
Surgical time	1 h
EBL	< 100 mL
Postop care	Outpatient
Mortality	Rare
Morbidity	Extrusion of implant Infection: < 1%
Pain score	3–4

PATIENT POPULATION CHARACTERISTICS	
Age range	Any age
Male:Female	1:1
Incidence	Relatively common
Etiology	Trauma; infection; glaucoma; tumors (e.g., retinoblastoma, melanoma); inflammation
Associated conditions	Diabetes mellitus

ANESTHETIC CONSIDERATIONS

See Anesthetic Considerations for Ophthalmic Surgical Procedures under GA, p. 165.

Suggested Reading

1. See Suggested Reading following Ophthalmic Surgery section, p. 171.

ORBITOTOMY—ANTERIOR AND LATERAL

SURGICAL CONSIDERATIONS

Description: Surgical access to the orbit is required for biopsy/excision of masses, drainage of orbital abscesses, removal of a foreign body, or repair of orbital fractures, among other procedures. The orbit may be divided into several compartments and the surgical approach will vary by the location and size of the lesion. In general, an **anterior orbitotomy** is used for small tumors in the anterior orbit and can be approached from a transconjunctival, transseptal, or transperiosteal incision. By contrast, a **lateral orbitotomy** allows for removal of larger masses located further posteriorly in the orbit, as well as those lesions involving the lacrimal gland. In this procedure, the skin incision can be placed just under the brow (**Stallard-Wright**), in the lid crease with lateral extension, or higher in the eyebrow (**coronal**). The dissection is carried down to the periosteum, which is then incised and reflected. The lateral orbital wall is exposed and an osteotomy is performed using an oscillating saw, after preplacing suture holes with a power drill. The section of bone is removed with a clamp and the periorbita is opened, allowing intraorbital dissection. After biopsy or removal of the mass, the periorbita is closed and the bone fragment replaced.

Variant procedures or approaches: A **medial orbitotomy** is often required to access lesions that are located medial to the optic nerve.

Usual preop diagnosis: Orbital mass; fractures; foreign body; abscess

SUMMARY OF PROCEDURE	
Position	Supine, table rotated 90–180°
Incision	Variable (see above)
Special instrumentation	Surgical loupes
Antibiotics	Cefazolin 1 g iv
Surgical time	1–3 h
EBL	Usually minimal, unless vascular tumor
Mortality	Rare
Morbidity	Orbital hemorrhage Impaired ocular motility Secondary infection Loss of vision Infection: $< 1\%$
Pain score	3–6

PATIENT POPULATION CHARACTERISTICS	
Age range	Any age
Male:Female	1:1
Incidence	Fairly common
Etiology	Tumor, such as hemangioma, lymphangioma, lymphoma; lacrimal gland tumors; infection; fracture; foreign body

ANESTHETIC CONSIDERATIONS

[Procedures covered: dacryocystorhinostomy (DCR); enucleation; anterior and lateral orbitotomy.]

PREOPERATIVE

Patients presenting for DCR, enucleation, and orbitotomy represent a diverse population. These patients are generally healthy, aside from the infection, tumor, or trauma underlying their ocular or periocular pathology. Preop evaluation should focus on possible coexisting disease and the systemic manifestations of previous therapeutic interventions (e.g., chemotherapy and drugs used to treat glaucoma).

Laboratory	Tests as indicated from H&P
Premedication	Standard premedication (see p. B-1)

INTRAOPERATIVE

Anesthetic technique	GETA
Induction	Standard induction (see p. B-2). An oral RAE ETT may be preferred.
Maintenance	Standard maintenance (see, p. B-2). Muscle relaxation is not required.
Emergence	No special considerations. The common occurrence of PONV requires the administration of intraop antiemetics (e.g., metoclopramide 10 mg iv, and ondansetron 4 mg iv).

Blood and fluid requirements	Blood loss variable IV: 18-20 ga ×1 NS/LR @ 4–6 mL/kg/h	
Monitoring	Standard monitors (see p. B-1)	
Positioning	Table rotated 90° ✓ and pad pressure points ✓ nonoperated eye	
Complications	Oculocardiac reflex (OCR) → ↓↓HR	See discussion in Anesthetic Considerations for Strabismus Surgery, p. 1175

POSTOPERATIVE

Complications	PONV	Rx: Metoclopramide 10 mg iv, and/or ondansetron 4 mg iv
Pain management	Acetaminophen	Occasionally parenteral opiates (see p. C-2)

RETINAL SURGERY

SURGICAL CONSIDERATIONS

Description: Retinal surgery is performed for a wide variety of conditions (see Usual preop diagnoses, below). Most **retinal detachments** are due to one or more small tears in the retina. Retinal detachments are classified as traction, exudative (not usually treated with surgery), or rhegmatogenous (rupture, tear). Children, especially those with ROP or trauma, may develop retinal detachments. In adults, retinal detachments are most frequently associated with diabetes, myopia, trauma, and previous cataract surgery. Rhegmatogenous retinal detachments (more common in adults) start off with a small retinal tear, which allows the vitreous to seep in between the retina and pigment epithelium, forcing retinal separation. Sx range from floaters and flashes to showers of black specks and, ultimately, to a dark shadow that impinges on the field of vision. Retinal detachments may be complicated by proliferative vitreoretinopathy (PVR), in which scar tissue grows along the surface of the retina, rendering it stiff and difficult to reattach. Less commonly, retinal detachments are induced by other forms of vitreoretinal traction, or by trauma involving an open globe. Care must be taken to avoid any increase in intraocular pressure (IOP) in an eye that may be ruptured. On rare occasion, retinal detachments are due to the formation of a giant retinal tear. Just as rarely, retinal surgery may be done on premature infants in an effort to prevent or repair retinal detachments. The ultimate aim of retinal surgery is the preservation or recovery of vision through the restoration of normal posterior segment anatomy. (Anatomy of the eye is shown in Fig. 2-11.)

Retinal surgery may involve various procedures alone or in combination, including scleral buckling, vitrectomy, gas-fluid exchange, and injection of vitreous substitutes. **Scleral buckles** are silicone rubber appliances sutured to the sclera to indent the eye wall, thereby relieving vitreous traction and functionally closing retinal tears. This is an external procedure in which the eye may either not be entered at all or entered with a small needle puncture through the sclera for drainage of subretinal fluid.

Cryotherapy or lasers are used frequently to establish chorioretinal adhesions around retinal tears. Cryotherapy is applied to the sclera; a laser is applied with a fiber optic cable introduced into the vitreous cavity during vitrectomy surgery, often in combination with a wide-field viewing system. It also can be administered with an indirect ophthalmoscope delivery system for those eyes not undergoing vitrectomy.

Simple detachments frequently can be repaired by a pneumatic retinopexy, in which retinal tears are treated with cryotherapy and/or laser, and an expanding gas is injected into the vitreous cavity. This technique usually is done in

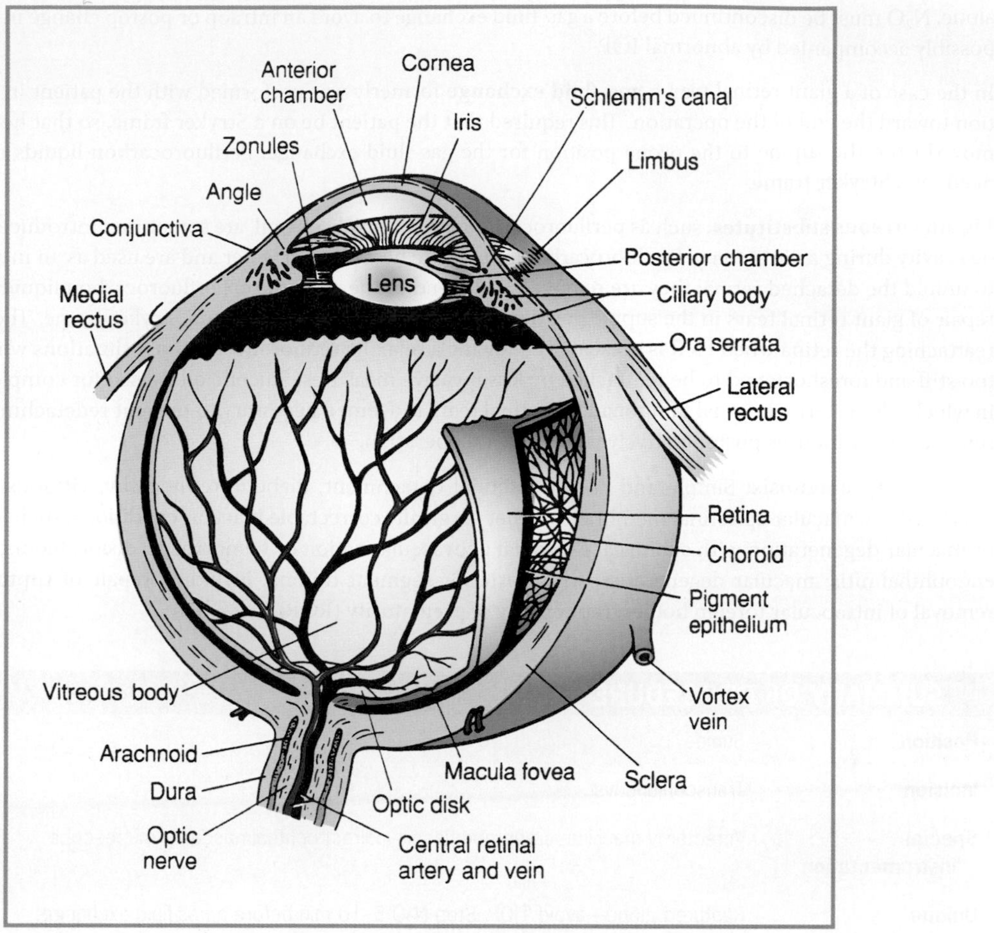

Figure 2-11. Eye anatomy. (Reproduced with permission from Langston D, ed: *Manual of Ocular Diagnosis and Therapy,* 2nd edition. Little, Brown, Boston: 1985.)

phakic eyes (eyes with intact lens) with tears between the 9 o'clock and 4 o'clock positions. Pneumatic retinopexy usually is done as an outpatient office procedure, with local anesthesia, or, less commonly, MAC. The other procedures discussed usually are done with MAC, although GA may be used, according to surgeon's preference and the patient's systemic condition. Some surgeons inject retrobulbar or subconjunctival bupivacaine at the end of a procedure done under GA to decrease postop pain.

Vitrectomy (removal of vitreous) is commonly performed to reduce traction on the retina (↓retinal detachment), clear blood and debris and remove scar tissue. It is an intraocular procedure in which three 20–25-ga openings are made into the vitreous cavity with a myringotomy blade 3–4 mm posterior to the limbus (junction of the cornea and sclera.) One of these openings in the inferotemporal quadrant is used for infusion of balanced salt solution via a sutured or transconjunctival trochar-based cannula. The remaining openings are at the 9:30 and 2:30 o'clock positions. One is used for a hand-held fiber optic light; the other, for insertion of a variety of manual and automated instruments, including suction cutters, scissors, and forceps, used to remove and section abnormal tissue within the vitreous cavity.

Visualization of the retina during vitrectomy is made possible by a contact lens, which is either sutured to the eye or held in position by an assistant. Some of these lenses provide a wide-field, inverted view of the retina, necessitating an image inverter on the microscope. Alternatively, a noncontact, wide-field lens may be positioned just above the cornea, suspended from the microscope. Balanced salt solution replaces the vitreous and other tissues removed during the operation. A bubble of gas is sometimes introduced into the vitreous cavity during a scleral buckle or a vitrectomy when the surgeon wants an internal tamponade of retinal tears that cannot be closed adequately by a scleral buckle alone. N_2O must be discontinued before a gas-fluid exchange to avoid an intraop or postop change in gas bubble size, possibly accompanied by abnormal IOP.

In the case of a giant retinal tear, a **gas-fluid exchange** formerly was performed with the patient in the prone position toward the end of the operation. This required that the patient be on a Stryker frame, so that he or she could be moved from the supine to the prone position for the gas-fluid exchange. Perfluorocarbon liquids now obviate the need for a Stryker frame.

Liquid vitreous substitutes, such as perfluorocarbon liquids or silicone oil, are sometimes introduced into the vitreous cavity during a vitrectomy. Perfluorocarbon liquids are heavier than water and are used as an intraoperative tool to unfold the detached retina; they are removed at the end of the procedure. Perfluorocarbon liquids make possible repair of giant retinal tears in the supine position, thus eliminating the need for a Stryker frame. They also facilitate reattaching the retina when PVR is present, by allowing a relaxing retinotomy for those situations where the retina is too stiff and foreshortened to be reattached by less invasive measures. Silicone oil is used for complex detachments in which a long-term, internal tamponade of retinal tears is deemed necessary to prevent redetachment. It usually is removed a few months postoperatively with a second operation.

Usual preop diagnosis: Simple and complex retinal detachment; diabetic retinopathy; vitreous hemorrhage or opacification; macular epiretinal membranes; other surgically correctable macular conditions, such as macular holes or macular degeneration with subfoveal choroidal neovascularization or hemorrhage; dislocated intraocular lenses; endophthalmitis; macular degeneration with posterior segment trauma, including repair of ruptured globes and removal of intraocular foreign bodies; retinopathy of prematurity (ROP).

SUMMARY OF PROCEDURE

Position	Supine
Incision	Transconjunctival
Special instrumentation	Vitrectomy machine; cryoprobe; laser; indirect ophthalmoscope; microscope
Unique considerations	Ruptured globe—avoid ↑IOP. Stop N_2O 5–10 min before a gas-fluid exchange.
Antibiotics	May use iv antibiotics at the start of surgery, in addition to subconjunctival antibiotics at conclusion of surgery.
Surgical time	Pneumatic retinopexy: 20 min Scleral buckle: 30 min to 2 h Vitrectomy: 1–4+ h
Closing considerations	Try to avoid postop bucking or vomiting
EBL	None
Postop care	Prone positioning, if gas was injected
Mortality	Extremely rare
Morbidity	Hemorrhage: $< 5\%$ Retinal detachment: $< 5\%$ Infection: $< 1\%$
Pain score	6

PATIENT POPULATION CHARACTERISTICS

Age range	Usually adults; occasionally premature infants (ROP) and children (retinal detachment or trauma)
Male:Female	1:1

PATIENT POPULATION CHARACTERISTICS (cont'd)	
Incidence	1/20,000 phakic; 1/250 pseudophakic (postcataract extraction with placement of intraocular lens)
Etiology	Majority idiopathic; some related to systemic disease or induced by trauma
Associated conditions	Idiopathic: retinal detachment, epiretinal membrane, macular hole Diabetic retinopathy: vitreous hemorrhage or traction retinal detachment Macular degeneration: subfoveal choroidal neovascularization or hemorrhage Trauma: vitreous hemorrhage, retinal detachment, ruptured globe Intraocular foreign body (IOFB) HTN: vitreous hemorrhage Extreme prematurity: ROP, retinal detachment

ANESTHETIC CONSIDERATIONS

PREOPERATIVE

In MAC cases, the need for anxiolytics can often be reduced or eliminated by discussing in detail what will happen to the patient during the procedure and by addressing patient concerns (e.g., claustrophobia, positional pain, supine dyspnea, etc.). Most vitreous and retinal procedures can be accomplished using regional anesthetic techniques (retrobulbar, peribulbar, or sub-Tenon's block with MAC. Procedures requiring more than 2 hrs and patients (or surgeons) with special needs (e.g., claustrophobia, uncooperative, immature) may benefit from GA. With MAC, the anesthesiologist's goal should be a comfortable, cooperative patient who can lie completely still without falling asleep (uncontrolled movement when suddenly awakened) for 1–2 hours.

Cardiovascular	Mannitol decreases IOP by increasing plasma oncotic pressure relative to aqueous humor pressure. It usually is given just before or during surgery. Total dosage should not exceed 1.5–2 g/kg iv over a 30–60 min period. Rapid infusion of large doses of mannitol may precipitate CHF, pulmonary edema, electrolyte abnormalities, HTN, and, possibly, myocardial ischemia; hence, the importance of a thorough evaluation of the patient's renal and cardiovascular status prior to administering mannitol. **Tests:** As indicated from H&P
Diabetes	Diabetic patients are at increased risk for silent myocardial ischemia. Pulmonary aspiration 2° diabetic gastroparesis is also a risk in this population. Patients usually take 1/2 or 1/3 of their normal NPH insulin dose (on the morning of surgery); fasting blood sugar is checked; and an iv infusion of D5 LR is started if glucose < 90 mg/dl, or treated with regular insulin if glucose > 200 mg/dl. Blood sugar is checked intraop and postop.
Renal	Acetazolamide, a carbonic anhydrase inhibitor, decreases secretion of aqueous humor. It also inhibits renal carbonic anhydrase, thereby facilitating the loss of HCO_3, Na^+, K^+, and water. Thus, patients on chronic therapy may be acidotic, hypokalemic, and hyponatremic. **Tests:** Electrolytes; others as indicated from H&P
Hematologic	✓ for sickle-cell disease. Sickle-cell trait is not commonly associated with periop complications. Patients with sickle-cell anemia should be well hydrated and transfused preop, as necessary to increase HbA concentration $> 40\%$.
Laboratory	Tests as indicated from H&P
Premedication	Midazolam 0.5 mg/kg po for pediatric patients (~30 min to peak effect; ~30 min duration of effect) and midazolam 1–2 mg iv incrementally for adults, will help alleviate anxiety. Avoid excessive sedation (respiratory depression) in sickle-cell patients. Surgeons prefer a normal IOP during retinal reattachment surgery and, therefore, patients may be given acetazolamide or mannitol to decrease IOP.

INTRAOPERATIVE

Anesthetic technique: Retinal detachment surgery may be performed under regional anesthesia (e.g., retrobulbar or peribulbar block); however, if the surgery is expected to be > 2 h, GETA may be preferable.

Induction	Standard induction (see p. B-2) is appropriate for these patients with care being taken not to put pressure on the affected eye with the face mask.	
Maintenance	Standard maintenance (see p. B-2). Ophthalmologists, however, may use expanding gases, such as sulfur hexafluoride (SF_6) or perfluoropropane (C_3F_8), for internal tamponade of the retinal tears and, if N_2O is used, the injected bubble may expand rapidly, causing a dramatic rise in IOP. This can impair retinal blood flow. N_2O, if used at all, should be D/C'd at least 15 min before gas injection. If the patient needs a second surgery and GA after the first gas injection, N_2O should be avoided for at least 5 d after the air injection, 10 d after the SF_6 injection, and 15–30 d after the C_3F_8. Given the importance of patient immobility, nondepolarizing muscle relaxants may be advantageous, especially if N_2O is D/C'd.	
Emergence	Use narcotics for pain control and iv lidocaine 1.0–1.5 mg/kg 5 min prior to extubation to provide smooth emergence. The common occurrence of PONV requires the administration of intraop antiemetics (e.g., metoclopramide 10 mg iv and ondansetron 4 mg iv 30 min before the end of surgery).	
Blood and fluid requirements	IV: 18–20 ga ×1 (adult) 20 ga ×1 (child) NS/LR @ 4-6 mL/kg/h	
Monitoring	Standard monitors (see p. B-1)	Processed EEG may be useful in monitoring level of sedation Care should be taken to avoid CO_2 accumulation under the drapes in MAC cases. A suction line can be used to improve air circulation under the drape
Positioning	✓ and pad pressure points ✓ and pad nonsurgical eye	For long MAC cases, short "time-outs" should be taken to allow patients to reposition themselves
Complications	Oculocardiac reflex (OCR)	See Intraoperative Complications under Anesthetic Considerations for Strabismus Surgery, p. 1175

POSTOPERATIVE

Complications	PONV Corneal abrasion Vitreous hemorrhage Glaucoma Ptosis Diplopia Loss of vision Infection	Rx: Ondansetron 4 mg iv ± Metoclopramide 10 mg iv; however, eye pain (e.g., 2° to corneal abrasion) may also cause N/V. If this is the case, treat pain (ophthalmology consult). Persistently low BP → retinal ischemia and central retinal artery occlusion
Pain management	Retrobulbar anesthesia	Meperidine 0.5–1 mg/kg/h iv
Tests	None routinely required	

Suggested Readings

1. Charles S, Fanning GL: Anesthesia considerations for vitreoretinal surgery. *Ophthalmol Clin North Am* 2006; 19(2):239–43.
2. Hamilton RC: Techniques of orbital regional anaesthesia. *Brit J Anaesth* 1995; 75:88–92.
3. McGoldrick KE, Gayer SI: *Anesthesia and the Eye.* In Clinical Anesthesia, 5th edition. Barash PG, Cullen BF, Stoelting RK, eds. Lippincott Williams & Wilkins, Philadelphia: 2006, 969–88.
4. Ryan SJ, Hinton DR, et al., ed: *Retina,* 4th edition. CV Mosby Co, St. Louis: 2005.

General Ophthalmic Surgery Suggested Readings

1. Ahmad S, Ahmad A: Complications of ophthalmologic nerve blocks: a review. *J Clin Anesth* 2003; 15(7):564–9.
2. Albert DM, Jakobiec FA, eds: *Principles and Practice of Ophthalmology.* WB Saunders, Philadelphia: 2000;1463–76.
3. External Disease and Cornea: *Basic and Clinical Science Course.* The Foundation of the American Academy of Ophthalmology 1998; 8:411–36.
4. Greenbaum G, ed: *Ocular Anesthesia.* WB Saunders, Philadelphia: 1997.
5. Krachmer JH, Mannis MJ, Holland EJ: *Cornea.* Mosby-Year Book, St. Louis: 1997.
6. Lens and Cataract. *Basic and Clinical Science Course.* The Foundation of the American Academy of Ophthalmology 2001;11:66–186.
7. Levine MR, ed: *Manual of Oculoplastic Surgery,* 2nd edition. Butterworth-Heinmann, New York: 1996.
8. Moster MR, Azura-Blanco A, eds: Ocular anesthesia. *Ophthalmol Clin North Am* 2006;19:151–322.
9. Nesi FA, Smith BC, eds: *Ophthalmic Plastic and Reconstructive Surgery,* 2nd edition. Mosby-Year Book, St. Louis: 1997.
10. Phelps CD, Hansjoerg EJ, eds: *Manual of Common Ophthalmic Surgical Procedures.* Churchill Livingstone, New York: 1986.
11. Pokhrel PK, Loftus SA: Ocular emergencies. *Am Fam Physician* 2007; 76(6):829–36.
12. Shields MB: *Textbook of Glaucoma,* 4th edition. Williams & Wilkins, Baltimore: 1998.
13. Waltman SR, Keates RH, Hoyt CS, et al, eds: *Surgery of the Eye.* Churchill Livingstone, New York: 1988.

SECTION

3.0 OTOLARYNGOLOGY—HEAD AND NECK SURGERY

SURGEONS

Michael J. Kaplan, MD (*Head & Neck Surgery*)
Edward Damrose, MD (*Laryngology*)
Nikolas H. Blevins, MD (*Otology & Neurotology*)
Robert K. Jackler, MD (*Otology & Neurotology*)
Peter Hwang, MD (*Endoscopic Sinus Surgery*)
Sarmela T. Sunder (*Endoscopic Sinus Surgery*)
Sam P. Most, MD (*Nasal Surgery*)
Willard E. Fee, Jr. MD (*Head & Neck Surgery*)
Jerome E. Hester, MD (*Surgery for Sleep Disorders*)
Robert W. Riley, DDS, MD (*Sleep-disordered breathing*)
Nelson B. Powell, MD (*Sleep-disordered breathing*)
Donald M. Sesso, DO (*Sleep-disordered breathing*)

ANESTHESIOLOGISTS

Vladimir Nekhendzy, MD
Cosmin Guta, MD (*Neurotology*)
Michael W. Champeau, MD (*Sleep-disordered breathing*)

INTRODUCTION—SURGEON'S PERSPECTIVE

Interdisciplinary cooperation is nowhere more critical than where the priority of airway maintenance is confronted both with abnormalities in the airway and with adjacent surgical goals. An anesthesiologist versed both in the management of the difficult airway and an ability to accurately anticipate the issues confronting the surgeon is critical. Similarly, a communicative surgeon fully aware of the problems the anesthesiologist is likely to encounter is critical to minimizing complications. Important issues that require mutual understanding include:

(a) Airway management: anesthesia induction, endotracheal tube size, head range of motion with shared airway space, a well-secured ETT, postop airway edema, and smooth emergence from anesthesia
(b) Muscle relaxation, patient immobility, patient positioning
(c) Deliberate relative hypotensive anesthesia and management of bradycardia
(d) Antiemetics and pain management postop
(e) Patient population considerations: frequent cardiac and pulmonary issues associated with older patients, especially with alcohol and tobacco use; degenerative c-spine issues and prior irradiation affecting neck mobility.

Airway management: An initially compromised airway is not uncommon in many otolaryngology head and neck procedures. Many others may develop airway loss at induction or if premature extubation occurs. Communication between the surgeon and anesthesiologist is essential, as is a discussion of a plan and backup plan should an emergency arise. Availability of a sliding Jackson scope and tracheotomy equipment, as well as plans for fiberoptic intubation, awake intubation, or retrograde intubation should be discussed as indicated.

For procedures within the airway, an endotracheal tube no larger than 6 mm should be adequate, and will reduce postop airway edema. An armored tube is helpful when the surgical procedure is intraoral and the tube may be compressed. A nasotracheal intubation should be discussed as an alternative in this situation. If laser surgery is planned, maintaining the FiO_2 at < 0.3 is indicated. If fiberoptic bronchoscopy is planned, then a 7.0- or 7.5-mm ETT will facilitate passage of the bronchoscope through the ETT, after which for a longer case, changing to a smaller tube may be warranted.

As the patient is generally turned 90° or 180° away from the anesthesiologist, a very secure airway is important. If the surgeon needs access in the mouth, securing the tube via a wire to several teeth may work better than tape.

Muscle relaxation and patient positioning: Avoidance of muscle relaxation is important if a motor nerve, such as the facial nerve, is to be dissected. Muscle relaxation is important, on the other hand, in esophagoscopy and tongue surgery. Communicate and coordinate timing of drug administration. Frequently the surgeon will need to turn the patient's head during surgery. Anticipating this movement when initially securing the endotracheal tube and its connections will prevent disconnection. In neck surgery, the neck is often rotated away from the surgeon; over-rotation presents the risk of brachial plexus stretch injuries. If a radial free flap is anticipated, then positioning of the arm as well as rotation of the head should be carefully coordinated to avoid injury while still providing needed access and a secure airway.

Deliberate relative hypotensive anesthesia, to a SBP of <100 mmHg, depending on individual patient's needs, is often a boon to the surgeon operating in the highly vascular fields of the head and neck, or operating with a microscope. For selected cases the patient also will have had preop embolization of a tumor and its blood supply (e.g., angiofibromas and skull base paragangliomas). **Bradycardia** may occur if the surgeon operates near the vagus nerve or carotid bifurcation. If this occurs, it is usually sufficient for the anesthesiologist to communicate this and the surgeon can desist for a period of time. Occasionally topical or locally injected anesthetics will be necessary.

INTRODUCTION—ANESTHESIOLOGIST'S PERSPECTIVE

Vladimir Nekhendzy

Patients with head and neck cancer are often older smokers with an ↑ incidence of CAD, HTN, chronic renal insufficiency, and COPD. Careful H&P must be performed to ensure that the patient's functional status is optimized before surgery.

Otolaryngology patients commonly present difficult airway problems. Some of the common features of the H&P, which may be associated with difficult airway include: (a) specific anatomic characteristics (e.g., ↓ C-spine ROM, large tongue, receding jaw, etc.); (b) Hx of stridor and hoarseness (airway narrowing and possible vocal cord dysfunction); (c) previous Hx of neck surgery, trauma, or XRT (↓ compliance of the tissues, ↓ neck ROM, ↓ mouth opening); (d) previous Hx of difficult intubation; (e) oropharyngeal infections (e.g., epiglottitis, retropharyngeal abscess, Ludwig's angina) or tumors. Meticulous examination of the airway must be performed, and an abnormal airway assessment should heighten the anesthesiologist's level of concern.

There should be a low threshold for an awake intubation if the airway is questionable. If a conventional DL after induction of GA is chosen and there is any question about airway management, at least two clearly defined alternative airway management backup plans should be in place with all the corresponding airway equipment prepared prior to induction. The patient's head position should be optimized and simple intubating aids (e.g., stylets, gum elastic bougie, Trachlight), as well as ETTs of different sizes should be available. Video laryngoscopy (e.g., Glidescope) plays an increasingly important role in difficult airway management, and the use of LMA Fastrach reliably provides rescue ventilation with 95–100% success rate in many difficult airway management situations.

For the majority of otolaryngological surgical procedures, the patient's airway must be shared with the surgeon, while immediate access to the airway is difficult because the patient is turned 90° or 180° away from the anesthesiologist. The ETT must be well secured to prevent an accidental extubation, or withdrawal of the ETT to the subglottic area which may result in direct pressure on the recurrent laryngeal nerves by the ETT cuff. For certain procedures (e.g., excision of tumors of the base of the tongue, tongue suspension for obstructive sleep apnea [OSA]), and other intraoral procedures, nasal intubation may be required for surgical access, and the surgeon should be consulted before induction.

The essential anesthesia management requirements for the majority of the otolaryngological procedures include:

(a) Assurance of good intraop and postop analgesia (most of the procedures are performed on highly reflexogenic areas).

(b) Clear surgical field (the operated areas are highly vascular). Moderate controlled hypotension is widely employed: ↓ SBP < 100 mmHg, MAP = 60–70 mmHg, unless contraindicated 2° concurrent medical conditions.

(c) Patient immobility (for certain procedures profound muscle relaxation may be required, while for others (e.g., nerve monitoring) administration of non-depolarizing muscle relaxants must be avoided).

(d) Smooth emergence. One of the most challenging tasks, as every attempt should be made to avoid or minimize patient reaction to the ETT during tracheal extubation. Straining, bucking, or coughing may provoke bleeding (↑ venous and arterial pressure), disrupt delicate suture lines (e.g., facial nerve repair), dislodge surgical grafts (e.g., tympanoplasty), or cause additional trauma to the vocal cords (VC) after VC surgery. Many ENT surgeons have their own "list" of procedures where the patient's reaction to the ETT should be completely avoided during extubation, and an anesthesiologist should be familiar with the surgeon's preferences.

With the possible exception of patients presenting for OSA surgery (see Anesthetic Considerations for Reconstructive Surgery for Sleep-Disordered Breathing, p. 255), the **opioid-based anesthetic techniques** are especially advantageous for achieving or facilitating the previously stated anesthetic objectives. The opioid-based techniques also result in significant ↓ MAC and facilitate early elimination of volatile agents, while blunting the tracheal response to the ETT. The choice of an opioid analgesic depends on several factors: the anticipated degree of intraop surgical stimulation, immediate postop pain, duration of surgery, patient's concomitant medical conditions, underlying physical status, and prior opioid use. Highly potent opioids (e.g., fentanyl: loading dose 3–10 mcg/kg; sufentanil: loading dose 0.5–1.5 mcg/kg iv); followed by either intermittent boluses or continuous infusion are the author's preferred choice for major ENT surgery. Continuous iv infusions of opioids offer advantages over intermittent boluses, resulting in ↓ total dose, greater hemodynamic stability, more rapid emergence, less pain in the immediate postop period, and ↓ times to discharge from the recovery room. For highly stimulating procedures followed by minimal or absent postop discomfort (e.g., laser surgery of the airway), shorter-acting opioids are preferred: remifentanil (loading dose 0.5–1.0 mcg/kg iv, infusion 0.1–0.25 mcg/kg/min iv) or alfentanil (loading dose 20–40 mcg/kg iv, infusion 0.25–1.0 mcg/kg/min iv). Total intravenous anesthesia (TIVA) is commonly employed, especially for endoscopic procedures.

Maintenance of **controlled hypotension** can be easily facilitated by administration a potent inhalational anesthetic and/or intermittent iv boluses of the vasoactive drugs (e.g., esmolol 0.3–1.0 mg/kg, labetalol 0.1–0.3 mg/kg,

Table 3-1. Advantages of the LMA Compared with the ETT

Adverse Event	ETT %	LMA %	Ratio
Clinically significant problems	3.4	0.9	3.8
Laryngeal spasm	0.38	0.12	3.2
Aspiration	0.017	0.02	0.85
Sore throat	50	10	5
Laryngeal trauma	6.2	? (< 1)	> 6
Coughing on emergence	60	2	30

*Modified from Brimacombe JR, Brain AJ: *The Laryngeal Mask Airway. A Review and Practical Guide.* WB Saunders, Philadelphia: 1997.

hydralazine 0.07–0.15 mg/kg). IV infusion of NTG or SNP (0.25–1 mcg/kg/min) is rarely necessary. Additional doses of iv labetalol are almost always beneficial at the end of surgery to prevent rebound hypertension in the early postop period.

Antiemetic prophylaxis should be routine, and most commonly is achieved by iv administration of a 5-HT_3 blocker. Multimodal antiemetic prophylaxis should be employed for patients at high risk for PONV. The addition of metoclopramide (10–20 mg iv) may be beneficial for patients who have undergone procedures resulting in accumulation of blood in the stomach (e.g., nasal or intraoral surgery).

GETA is most widely employed. Use of an LMA type device for the ENT surgery, when feasible, is often beneficial. An LMA is associated with less stimulating emergence from anesthesia, and a reduction in the number of episodes of coughing, laryngospasm, and laryngeal trauma (Table 3-1).

LMA use is associated with decreased patient morbidity, which otherwise commonly manifests as feelings of "fullness" (25%), transient dysphagia (4–24%), bacteremia (4%), and minor pharyngeal abrasions (2%). The single most limiting feature of the LMA is the potential for aspiration of stomach contents.

A flexible laryngeal mask airway (FLMA) is most frequently used in ENT anesthesia, because its shaft can be bent away from the surgical field and moved freely inside the patient's mouth to find an optimal angle for connection to the anesthesia circuit. Movement of the FLMA shaft is not transmitted to the cuff, and the FLMA provides a stable airway during maintenance of anesthesia. The FLMA has been used successfully in different ENT procedures, including adenotonsillectomy, ear and nasal surgery, facial plastic surgery and head and neck surgery. Close communication between the surgeon and anesthesiologist is essential, because even a properly placed FLMA can become dislodged during surgical manipulations.

Use of the standard LMA insertion technique is crucial for adequately protecting the larynx from possible aspiration and minimizing the risk of gastric insufflation if positive pressure ventilation (PPV) is planned. Although it may be difficult to predict the optimal FLMA size for the patient, the largest size (FLMA #5) should be used for PPV whenever possible, to minimize the incidence of oropharyngeal leak and gastric insufflation. Gastric insufflation is further avoided by ↓ Vt to 6–10 mL/kg and by keeping PIP < 20 cm H_2O. The absence of gastric insufflation should be documented in the anesthesia record after auscultating the epigastric area. Maintaining neuromuscular blockade during PPV through the FLMA is not essential, but may offer the advantages of ↑ chest wall compliance and ↓ incidence of reflux and regurgitation 2° patient movement or reaction to the FLMA. Suggested use of the FLMA for selected ENT procedures is discussed below.

Suggested Readings

1. Asai T, Murao K, Yukawa H, et al: Re-evaluation of appropriate size of the laryngeal mask airway. *Br J Anaesth* 1999; 83:478–9.
2. Benumof J: Laryngeal mask airway and the ASA difficult airway algorithm. *Anesthesiology* 1996; 84:686–96.
3. Brimacombe J, Berry A: Insertion of the laryngeal mask airway–a prospective study of four techniques. *Anaesth Intensive Care* 1993; 21:89–92.
4. Brimacombe JR, Berry A: The incidence of aspiration associated with the laryngeal mask airway: a meta-analysis of published literature. *J Clin Anesth* 1995; 7:297–305.
5. Brimacombe JR, Brain AJ: The Laryngeal Mask Airway: A Review and Practical Guide. WB Saunders, London: 1997.
6. Brimacombe JR: Positive pressure ventilation with the size 5 laryngeal mask. *J Clin Anesth* 1997; 9:113–7.
7. Brown BR: Anaesthesia for ear, nose, throat and maxillofacial procedures. In *International Practice of Anaesthesia*. Prys-Roberts C, Brown BR, eds. Oxford, Butterworth-Heinemann: 1996, 2–9.
8. Cook TM: A new practical classification of laryngeal view. *Anaesthesia* 2000; 55:274–9.

9. Cooper RM, Pacey JA, Bishop MJ, et al: Early clinical experience with a new videolaryngoscope (GlideScope) in 728 patients. *Can J Anaesth* 2005; 52:191–8.
10. Dimitriou V, Voyagis GS, Brimacombe JR: Flexible lightwand-guided tracheal intubation with the intubating laryngeal mask Fastrach™ in adults after unpredicted failed laryngoscope-guided tracheal intubation. *Anesthesiology* 2002; 96:296–9.
11. Dougherty TB: The difficult airway in conventional head and neck surgery. In *Airway Management: Principles and Practice.* Benumof JL, ed. Mosby, St. Louis: 1996, 686–97.
12. Ferson DZ, Rosenblatt WH, Johansen MJ, et al: Use of the intubating LMA-Fastrach in 254 patients with difficult-to-manage airways. *Anesthesiology* 2001; 95:1175–81.
13. Gataure PS, Vaughan RS, Latto IP: Simulated difficult intubation: comparison of the gum elastic bougie and the stylet. *Anaesthesia* 1996; 51:935–8.
14. Hung OR, Pytka S, Morris I, et al: Lightwand intubation: II–clinical trial of a new lightwand for tracheal intubation in patients with difficult airways. *Can J Anaesth* 1995; 42:826–30.
15. Joo HS, Kapoor S, Rose FK, et al: The intubating laryngeal mask airway after induction of general anesthesia versus awake fiberoptic intubation in patients with difficult airways. *Anesth Analg* 2001; 92:1342–6.
16. Lim Y, Yeo SW: A comparison of the GlideScope with the Macintosh laryngoscope for tracheal intubation in patients with simulated difficult airway. *Anaesth Intensive Care* 2005; 33:243–7.
17. Montes FR, Trillos JE, Rinc—n IE, et al: Comparison of total intravenous anesthesia and sevoflurane-fentanyl anesthesia for outpatient otorhinolaryngeal surgery. *J Clin Anesth* 2002; 14:324–8.
18. Nair MB, Bailey PM: Review of uses of the laryngeal mask in ENT anesthesia. *Anaesthesia* 1995; 50:898–900.
19. Silk JM, Hill HM, Calder I: Difficult intubation and the laryngeal mask. *Eur J Anaesthesiol Suppl* 1991; 4:47–51.
20. Wuesten R, Van Aken H, Glass PS, et al: Assessment of depth of anesthesia and postoperative respiratory recovery after remifentanil- versus alfentanil-based total intravenous anesthesia in patients undergoing ear-nose-throat surgery. *Anesthesiology* 2001; 94:211–7.

LARYNGOSCOPY/BRONCHOSCOPY/ESOPHAGOSCOPY

SURGICAL CONSIDERATIONS

Description: **Laryngoscopy** is used for inspection of the pharynx, hypopharynx, or larynx for diagnostic and/or therapeutic benefit. The patient is supine with cervical spine flexed and atlantoaxial joint extended (this position is best achieved with a headrest); and the teeth are protected with a mouth guard. The laryngoscope is introduced (Fig. 3-1); then, with a lifting motion, a thorough examination of the oropharynx, hypopharynx, laryngopharynx, and larynx is carried out and biopsies can be taken. Any bleeding normally can be controlled easily with pressure. Laryngoscopy often is combined with esophagoscopy, bronchoscopy, or direct nasopharyngoscopy to survey the aerodigestive tract for malignancy. If the procedure is diagnostic, the surgeon may need to visualize the airway before intubation and/or muscle relaxation. If a laser is to be utilized, a special laser ETT, < 30% FiO_2, and avoidance of N_2O are required.

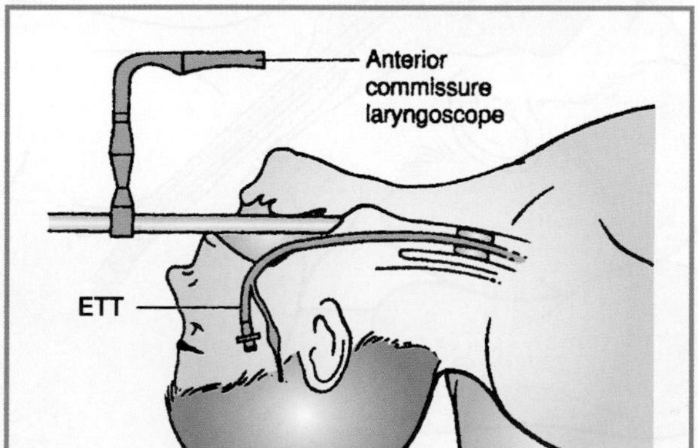

Figure 3-1. Placement of anterior commissure laryngoscope for laryngoscopy.

Usual preop diagnosis: Oropharyngeal, hypopharyngeal, or laryngeal tumors

Description: **Operative micolaryngoscopy.** A variety of laryngeal lesions, including papilloma, cysts, and polyps, can be removed endoscopically. Because of their close apposition to the delicate tissues of the vocal fold, a high degree of precision may be needed to remove the growth without damaging the underlying membrane. To this end, specialized endoscopes, such as the Dedo operating laryngoscope, are deployed transorally to allow the surgeon a binocular view of the vocal fold and the target lesion. They can be suspended from a Mayo stand in order to free both of the surgeon's hands for operating. Using the microscope, a variety of specialized endoscopic instruments and the CO_2 laser, the surgeon may be afforded excellent visualization of and unobstructed access to the vocal folds for diagnostic and therapeutic purposes. Operative microlaryngoscopy may necessitate several hours of work. Because of the precision involved in such procedures and the high degree of stimulation to the patient, general anesthesia (± jet ventilation) with muscle relaxation is required. Intubation with a small-caliber microlaryngeal or laser-safe tube (5 or 6 mm) may be required for these procedures. In cases where jet ventilation is to be performed, an endoscope suitable for this technique should be available. Intermittent apnic ventilation is also a possibility, although this involves periodic interruption of surgery, which can be cumbersome and distracting.

Usual preop diagnosis: Vocal fold neoplasm; vocal fold paralysis

Description: **Bronchoscopy** is used for visualization of the tracheobronchial tree for both diagnostic and therapeutic purposes. The patient is supine with head elevated and neck extended at the upper cervical level. The bronchoscope is directed along the right side of the tongue forward toward the midline to visualize the epiglottis. Next, the bronchoscope tip is used to lift the epiglottis and advance the bronchoscope through the vocal cords, into the trachea and bronchus (Fig. 3-2). The scope can be directed for inspection of the carina, main bronchi, and, with the aid of telescopes, the segmental bronchi.

Flexible fiberoptic bronchoscopy is more commonly performed than rigid bronchoscopy. The endoscope is usually connected to a monitor, and suction, irrigation, and biopsy channels are self-integrated. Spontaneous ventilation

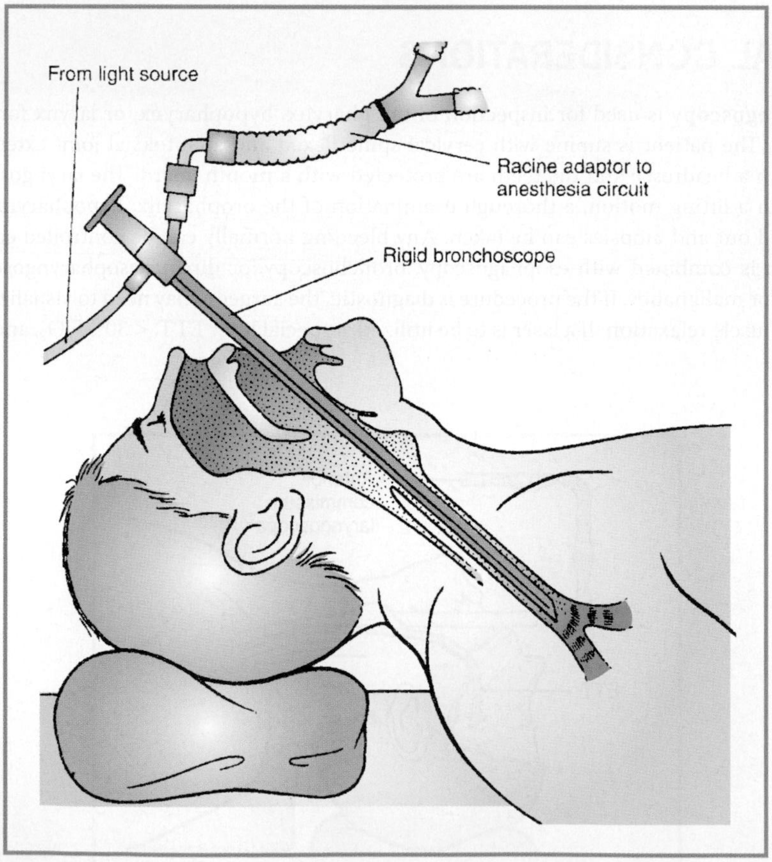

Figure 3-2. Rigid bronchoscopy showing adaptor (Racine) for anesthesia machine. Note neck flexion and head extension to align oropharyngeal and tracheal axes.

can be maintained which can allow the procedure to be performed without an ETT in place, affording unobstructed visualization of the entire upper airway. A bite block is usually placed to protect the endoscope from dental trauma and to allow easier advancement through the oropharynx into the larynx.

Usual preop diagnosis: Head and neck squamous-cell carcinoma; foreign body (FB) in bronchus

Description: **Esophagoscopy** is used for visualization of the esophagus for either diagnostic or therapeutic benefit. The patient is supine with head elevated and neck extended at the upper cervical level. The esophagoscope (held in the right hand) is advanced through the mouth behind the arytenoids, gently using the left thumb. The bevel of the scope is then used to advance through the cricopharyngeal muscle (upper esophageal sphincter) with an upward lifting movement, entering the cervical esophagus. As the scope advances, the head may have to be lowered or the neck extended and the scope directed slightly toward the left. It should be advanced only when a visible lumen is seen all the way down to the cardia. **Flexible fiberoptic esophagoscopy** is performed in an essentially identical manner. Superior visualization has made this the technique of choice for many surgeons. Biopsies may be taken and percutaneous gastrostomy tubes may be placed using the fiberoptic esophagoscope.

Usual preop diagnosis: Head and neck squamous-cell carcinoma; FB ingestion

Description: **Panendoscopy**, or triple endoscopy, is the combination of laryngoscopy, bronchoscopy, and esophagoscopy. It is usually performed as part of the evaluation of patients with newly diagnosed cancer of the head and neck for several reasons: (a) to gauge the extent of the primary tumor and to evaluate resectability; (b) to evaluate for the presence of synchronous tumors in other locations within the upper aerodigestive tract; (c) to identify the source of the primary lesion in patients who present with secondary cervical metastases. In the 3rd case, after PET-CT, endoscopy is supplemented with directed biopsies from those locations most likely to contain the occult primary lesion, including the nasopharynx, tonsillar fossae, and tongue base, with tonsillectomy commonly done as well. Identification of the source of the primary lesion allows for more directed therapy, tailoring irradiation fields with improved local control and overall.

Usual preop diagnosis: Head and neck squamous-cell carcinoma.

SUMMARY OF PROCEDURES

	Laryngoscopy	Bronchoscopy	Esophagoscopy	If Therapeutic Procedure Added
Position	Supine	⇐	⇐	⇐
Special instrumentation	Endoscopes, video monitors, suction	⇐	⇐	Laser, laser-safe ETT, gastroscope and G-tube (abdominal prep)
Unique considerations	Dexamethasone 4–8 mg if airway edema	⇐	⇐	⇐ If laser ablation, keep O_2 < 30%
Antibiotics	None	None	None	cefazolin 1gm and metronidazole 500 mg or clindamycin 600 mg
Surgical time	10–30 min	⇐	⇐	30–120+ min
EBL	Minimal	⇐	⇐	typically minimal
Postop care	PACU; rarely 23 h stay 2° airway issues	⇐	⇐	⇐; depends on specific intervention, if G-tube: monitor for abdominal signs
Mortality	< 1%	⇐	⇐	⇐
Morbidity	With MDL, Incisor trauma < 1%	⇐	⇐	⇐ ; if G-tube placement, <2% abdominal bleed or free air; if MDL with laser of laser bronchoscopy < 1% pneumothorax, < 5% airway compromise

SUMMARY OF PROCEDURES (cont'd)

	Laryngoscopy	Bronchoscopy	Esophagoscopy	If Therapeutic Procedure Added
Morbidity (cont'd)	Airway obstruction or postprocedure edema requiring reintubation: < 1%	⇐	⇐	
	Esophageal perforation < 1%	⇐	⇐	
	Laryngospasm: < 5%	⇐	⇐	
Pain score	1–2	1–2	1–2	1–2

PATIENT POPULATION CHARACTERISTICS

Age range	Newborn–90+	⇐	⇐	⇐
Male:Female	1:1	⇐	⇐	⇐
Incidence	Common	⇐	⇐	⇐
Etiology	Tumors, foreign bodies, congenital webs	⇐	⇐	⇐ ; nutritional need (G-tube)
Association Conditions	Other congenital issues; if malignancy, prior RT or chemotherapy and the conditions associated with that malignancy	⇐	⇐	⇐

ANESTHETIC CONSIDERATIONS

(Procedures covered: bronchoscopy, esophagoscopy, panendoscopy, operative microlaryngoscopy, Zenker's diverticulectomy, laser surgery of the airway)

PREOPERATIVE

Many of these patients are elderly and have a Hx of smoking and ETOH abuse with corresponding implications for intraop management. Patient fluid and nutritional status may be further compromised by pre-existing malignancy. Meticulous attention to airway management is paramount in these procedures, and close communication with the surgeon is essential. Some patients presenting for esophagoscopy may have obstructing lesions of the esophagus or **Zenker's diverticulum**, active GI bleeding, or require the removal of a FB, putting them at ↑ risk of aspiration.

Airway	Although rare, the airway may be compromised in these patients at both the upper and lower airway levels; thus a thorough preop airway assessment is essential. A clear backup plan for securing the airway should be devised and discussed with the surgeon before induction of GA. Stridor at rest suggests an airway narrowing ≤4.5 mm, although the airway diameter can be seriously reduced even without stridor being present. Inspiratory stridor usually is associated with supraglottic lesions, while expiratory stridor suggests airway narrowing below the glottis. Glottic lesions are characterized by both inspiratory and expiratory stridor. Patients with lesions in the mediastinum may have involvement of the recurrent laryngeal nerve, presenting with hoarseness and potential airway management problems (e.g., difficult mask ventilation, difficult intubation, ↑aspiration risk, aspiration risk). (See also Anesthetic Considerations for Laryngectomy, p. 202)

Respiratory	These patients may have a high incidence of COPD and ↓respiratory reserve. The nature and characteristics of a productive cough must be noted. Wheezing on exam must be treated with bronchodilators before induction. Patients presenting with vocal cord (VC) paralysis or achalasia may have had the repeated episodes of pulmonary aspiration. **Tests:** CXR; other tests as indicated from H&P.
Dental	Physical exam should include a careful dental assessment and documentation of any missing, loose or damaged teeth. Patients (or parents, as appropriate) should be informed that dental trauma may occur as a result of surgical instrumentation of the patient's mouth during the procedure.
Cardiovascular	Adrenergic responses during endoscopy may be associated with up to a 4% incidence of myocardial ischemia. Careful preop Hx and thorough physical exam should be undertaken in patients with Hx of CAD and CHF, or those with cardiac risk factors (including age > 40 yrs, male, HTN, hypercholesteremia, long Hx of smoking, obesity, and family Hx). The volume status of debilitated patients who are unable to eat because of obstructing lesions of the esophagus should be assessed by measuring orthostatic BP changes. **Tests:** ECG; Other tests as indicated from H&P.
Neurologic	Some patients may have Hx of ETOH abuse, which may result in ↑ anesthetic requirements 2° hepatic enzyme induction. Symptoms of alcohol withdrawal (e.g., tremulousness, ↑ sympathetic activity, and altered mental status), if present, should be controlled before surgery.
Hematologic	Patients with malignancy or chronic disease may have evidence of anemia or coagulopathy. **Tests:** CBC; coagulation studies as indicated from H&P
Gastrointestinal	In some patients (e.g., with malignant tumors), significant electrolyte abnormalities may be present 2° malnutrition. Hypokalemia and hypomagnesemia should be corrected preop. In patients with Hx of ETOH abuse, liver disease and cirrhosis may be present. **Tests:** Electrolytes; BUN; Cr; LFT; coag studies, as indicated from H&P.
Premedication	An antisialogogue (e.g., glycopyrrolate 0.2 mg iv) may be desired by the surgeon to faciliate panendoscopy, especially in patients with copious secretions. Sedative premedication is routine, but should be minimized in the elderly and avoided in patients with symptoms of upper airway obstruction.

INTRAOPERATIVE

Anesthetic technique: GETA. Airway management requires careful planning and continuous communication with the surgeon. Surgical requirements include adequate muscle relaxation (movement, coughing, or bucking during endoscopy may have disastrous consequences) and immobile vocal cords for vocal cord surgery. Cardiovascular stability is important: laryngeal, tracheal, and carinal reflexes may provoke severe ↑ BP and ↑ HR, which can be detrimental in some patients. Adequate depth of anesthesia is essential, but the requirements for rapid awakening and return of laryngeal reflexes present additional challenges in anesthetic management. Short-acting β-blockers (e.g., esmolol) may be indicated to treat break-through sympathetic responses, especially in patients with cardiac disease. Use of short-acting opioids (see Introduction, p. 174) is useful for these procedures which, although highly stimulating, are characterized by minimal or absent postop pain, and the majority of patients are discharged home from the recovery room.

Special considerations: If **flexible bronchoscopy** is planned, the patient's trachea is intubated in routine fashion by the anesthesiologist with a large diameter ETT (7.5–8.0 mm ID) to acommodate a flexible video bronchoscope. The ETT is usually taped midline. As an alternative, in selected patients, flexible bronchoscopy can be performed without tracheal intubation through the **Patil-Syracuse mask** during manual bag-mask ventilation. Placement and manipulation of the flexible bronchoscope by the surgeon will be facilitated by the concomitant use of one of the hollow oral airways used for the fiberoptic intubation (e.g., **Williams airway**). This approach is useful when intraoral surgical manipulation is planned, as the patient can then be tracheally intubated with a smaller diameter ETT (e.g., 6.0 mm ID), to facilitate surgical access.

Flexible esophagoscopy is rarely performed as an isolated procedure, but if done, would also be facilitated by tracheal placement of a small diameter (e.g., 6.0 mm ID) ETT; the ETT is usually moved over to the left corner of the mouth and taped to the lower jaw, to provide more room for the esophagoscope advancement and manipulation.

If **rigid bronchoscopy** is planned first, GA is induced, and the patient is hyperventilated through the face mask with FiO_2=1.0. Following muscle relaxation, the surgeon may proceed, without securing an airway. Quick and gentle DL for application of topical lidocaine to the larynx and upper trachea (LTA, 4% lidocaine 3–4 cc) before rigid bronchoscopy may help blunt hemodynamic responses to the subsequent surgical manipulation. DL with LTA should be avoided in patients with tumors at the base of the tongue (↑ risk of bleeding) (see Anesthetic Considerations for Glossectomy, p. 209) or when pre-existing copious secretions or bleeding are present in the upper airway 2° ↑ risk of pulmonary aspiration on emergence from anesthesia. It is advisable to demonstrate to the surgical team and document in the chart absence of dental damage after DL has been performed.

After the rigid bronchoscope is introduced into the patient's trachea, it is connected to an anesthesia circuit through a flexible side port adapter (Racine, Fig. 3-1), and the patient is ventilated manually. High flows are usually required because of the leak around the bronchoscope. Close communication with the surgeon is essential for adjusting ventilation when the bronchoscope is introduced into the mainstem bronchus to avoid high inflating pressures and to assure complete exhalation (↓ risk of barotrauma). After rigid bronchoscopy is completed, mask ventilation with FiO_2=1.0 before intubation is advisable to assure adequate oxygenation and normocapnia. A reinforced ETT is useful for **rigid esophagoscopy** to avoid possible compression of the ETT. The ETT should be moved to the left side of the patient's mouth to facilitate introduction of the surgical instruments, and taped to the lower jaw because full opening of the patient's mouth is required.

For **operative microlaryngoscopy,** a small-diameter (usually 5.0 mm ID), cuffed long microlaryngeal tube (MLT) is used to facilitate visualization of the larynx. The CO_2 laser, which can precisely vaporize superficial tissue, is widely used for vocal cord **laser surgery**, while the Nd:YAG (neodymium-yttrium-aluminum-garnet) laser is usually employed for airway tumor debulking because of its ability to coagulate deeper lesions. The Nd:YAG can be used through the suction channel of the fiber optic or video bronchoscope, whereas the CO_2 laser must be aimed directly at the targeted tissue. Both the CO_2 and Nd:YAG wavelengths lie outside the visible spectrum, and a separate, lower energy visible beam is used for aiming. The patient must be motionless, the patient's eyes must be protected with tape and moistened gauze, and OR personnel must wear protective goggles.

An **intermittent apnea technique** involves hyperventilation, followed by intermittent tracheal extubation for 1–5 min, during which the laser is used. This approach is time-consuming and may be associated with a higher incidence of airway trauma and edema 2° repeated intubations. Careful pulse oximeter monitoring is essential for this technique.

Jet ventilation (Fig. 3-3) may be necessary when an ETT cannot be used (e.g., some supraglottic and subglottic lesions). For supraglottic jet ventilation, the ventilating laryngoscope is most commonly employed. The axis of the jet should be in line with the trachea, and full egress of air (complete chest deflation) should be assured between the jet ventilator "puffs." Close communication with the surgeon is essential. The jet should be triggered during pauses between laser firings to keep the vocal cords immobile. If jet ventilation is used for laser resection of papillomas, there is a risk of spreading the virus to OR personnel, and special face masks should be worn in the OR. Jet ventilation generally provides adequate ventilation without introducing flammable material or obstructing the surgical field. Its use, however, may be associated with potentially severe complications, including barotrauma, pneumothorax and gastric distension (risk of regurgitation), and is hindered by ↓ chest-wall or lung compliance. Full muscle relaxation is absolutely essential with this technique, to facilitate precise laser firing. High-frequency jet ventilation can also be used through a catheter passed below the vocal cords into the patient's trachea, but this requires special equipment that is not widely available. Its advantages include excellent operating conditions and improved cardiovascular stability, but it may be associated with a higher incidence of barotrauma, laryngospasm and hypoventilation.

For laser cases, precautions must be taken to prevent **airway fire**, including:

- Use special laser ETT (e.g., Mallinkrodt Laser-Flex, Xomed Laser Shield), although none of them provides 100% protection from all types of lasers. Small (5.0 mm ID and smaller) diameter laser ETTs are preferred to facilitate surgical access.
- Use the lowest possible FiO_2 (≤ 0.3–0.4 strongly preferred), that will assure adequate oxygenation (dilute O_2 with air, N_2, or helium) and avoid N_2O (both O_2 and N_2O promote combustion).
- Use colored (methylene blue-tinged) NS in the ETT cuff (will immediately alert the surgeon in case of a laser hit).
- Place the ETT sufficiently deep into the trachea for the cuff to be out of surgical sight.

Similar considerations apply in patients undergoing endoscopic **Zenker's diverticulectomy**, when the CO_2 laser is used.

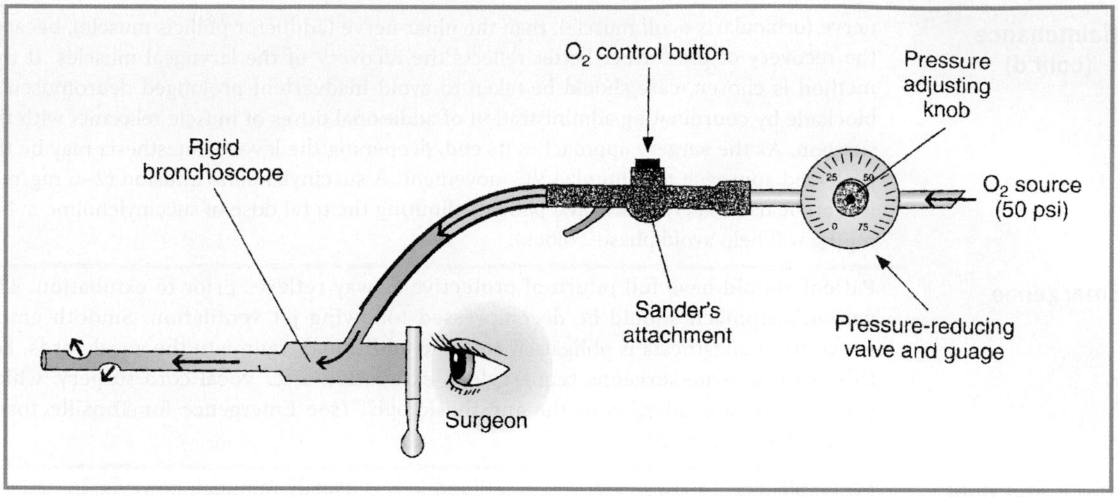

Figure 3-3. Rigid bronchoscope with modified Sanders jet ventilation technique. The wall oxygen supply at 50 psi is connected to a reducing valve that allows the pressure to be adjusted from 0 to 50 psi. The side port of the bronchoscope is used as the Venturi injector site, and the open end can be used for continuous viewing by the endoscopist.

Induction	Patients at risk for aspiration (e.g., **Zenker's diverticulum**) may require RSI with cricoid pressure (CP) if symptoms of active gastroesophageal reflux disease are present. Otherwise, anatomical location of the diverticulum (above the cricoid cartilage) makes application of CP largely ineffective. With the possible exception of endoscopic Zenker's diverticulectomy, fentanyl use should be minimized (1–2 mcg/kg) or even completely avoided in favor of the short-acting opioids (remifentanil or alfentanil IV (see Introduction, p. 174), 2° minimal postop pain. Propofol (1–2 mg/kg) is the ideal induction agent. Patients with mobile, floppy, supraglottic tumors (e.g., papillomatosis, epiglottic cancer, large vocal cord polyps) are at ↑ risk for complete airway obstruction after induction of GA with or without neuromuscular blockade. Anesthetic management of these patients requires careful planning and meticulous preparation (see Anesthetic Considerations for Laryngectomy, p. 202.) The surgeon should be consulted about the extent of the disease and the potential need for a tracheostomy. If the disease is severe, the surgeon should be present during induction for the possible need to perform urgent or emergent rigid bronchoscopy or cricothyrotomy/tracheostomy.
Maintenance	TIVA (e.g., propofol: 80–180 mcg/kg/min; remifentanil 0.1–0.25 mcg/kg/min) is widely used, especially when rigid bronchoscopy or jet ventilation/intermittent apnea techniques are planned. Compared to alfentanyl, the use of remifentanil during TIVA is associated with the increased hemodynamic stability, reduction in propofol dose and faster respiratory recovery. When the ETT is used throughout the case, delivery of anesthetic gases may be used instead of a propofol infusion, especially if a bronchodilating effect is desirable. Desflurane and sevoflurane are the preferred agents because of their low blood:gas solubility; sevoflurane may be favored in patients with pre-existing cardiac disease to minimize the risk of a dose-dependent tachycardia. Break-through sympathetic responses can be managed safely by administration of β-blockers IV or small boluses of a short-acting opioid (see Introduction, p. 174). With intermittent apnea or jet ventilation techniques, it may be difficult to avoid hypercapnia and hypoxemia, which may provoke intraop dysrhythmias. Full muscle relaxation is routine: vocal cord immobility is essential for microlaryngeal and laser surgery. Monitoring the neuromuscular blockade may be more accurate at the facial

Maintenance (cont'd)	nerve (orbicularis oculi muscle), than the ulnar nerve (adductor pollicis muscle), because the recovery of the former better reflects the recovery of the laryngeal muscles. If this method is chosen, care should be taken to avoid inadvertent prolonged neuromuscular blockade by coordinating administration of additional doses of muscle relaxants with the surgeon. As the surgery approaches its end, deepening the level of anesthesia may be the preferred approach to minimize VC movement. A succinylcholine infusion (2–6 mg/min iv) can be used safely in selected patients (limiting the total dose of succinylcholine ≤ 4–6 mg/kg will help avoid phase 2 block).	
Emergence	Patient should have full return of protective airway reflexes prior to extubation. The patient's stomach should be decompressed following jet ventilation. Smooth emergence from anesthesia is obligatory to avoid additional trauma to the vocal cords. For this reason, some surgeons request deep extubation after vocal cord surgery, which presents extra challenges to the anesthesiologist (see Emergence for Tonsillectomy, Adenoidectomy, p. 205).	
Blood and fluid requirements	IV: GI bleeder: 14–16 ga × 2 Others: 20 ga × 1 NS/LR @ 2–3 mL/kg/h For esophagoscopy: NS/LR @ 4–6 mL/kg/h	Blood loss is usually minimal; however, in patients with ↑ risk of GI bleed, blood loss may be massive. T&C these patients for 2 U PRBC with blood immediately available in OR.
Monitoring	Standard monitors (p. B-1). ± arterial line	In patients with ↑ risk of GI bleed, an arterial line is desirable
Positioning	OR table rotated 90° or 180° away from the anesthesiologist ✓ and pad pressure points. ✓ eyes.	A shoulder roll is placed and the patient's neck is extended to facilitate endoscopy. Special attention should be paid to prevent compression of the patient's shoulder by the vertical bar of the Mayo stand which is frequently employed for suspending the operating laryngoscope or endoscope.
Complications	Inadequate ventilation Loss of airway	Hypoxia and hypercarbia may be difficult to avoid with jet ventilation
	Perforation of airway Dysrhythmias Pneumothorax	Mechanical or laser perforation of the airway may → bronchospasm or uncontrollable hemorrhage. Dx: ↑RR, ↓BP, ↑CVP, wheezing, ↓O_2 saturation, ↑PIP, SOB, chest pain, ↓breath sounds, ↓ECG amplitude, dullness on percussion. Rx: chest tube or needle aspiration, FiO_2=1.0, ventilation and volume expansion.
	Eye trauma Bleeding post-biopsy	Eye trauma from surgical instruments used during endoscopy may require ophthalmology consult.
Airway fire (steps taken **simultaneously** by the anesthesiologist and surgeon)	Disconnect the inspiratory limb of the anesthesia circuit. Extinguish fire with NS. Remove ETT after deflating cuff. Extinguish and remove all burning material.	This is an acute, life-threatening emergency. NB: turning ventilator off only may not be sufficient due to continued delivery of fresh gas to the patient's lungs. Rigid or flexible bronchoscopy is required to ✓ extent of damage, presence of ETT fragments, and airway edema. All inhaled gases should be humidified. Patients are usually reintubated and monitored in the ICU.
	Resume ventilation by face mask with FiO_2 = 1.0. Flexible fiberoptic bronchoscopy. Save ETT for later examination.	

POSTOPERATIVE

Complications	Dental trauma Bleeding Eye trauma	Dental trauma may result from surgical manipulation of the airway, and the anesthesiologist must check the teeth immediately after airway access is gained. If dental trauma is detected, notify the surgeon to discuss management options, both immediate and subsequent.
	Postop airway compromise	Has a higher incidence than in general surgery patient population. Patients with T3 lesions and those with associated laryngeal biopsy (↑ airway swelling) after panendoscopy may be at high risk for reintubation in PACU. Delayed upper airway edema after laser surgery has been described, when the coagulation (Nd:YAG) laser is used.
	Esophageal perforation	Complaints of painful swallowing as well as fever, tachycardia, neck/chest/back pains postop may suggest an esophageal perforation.
	Pneumothorax Pneumomediastinum Hemothorax Aspiration	Pneumothorax (see above), mediastinal air or hemothorax from esophageal perforation may present as ↓ BP and cardiovascular collapse.
Pain management	Short acting opiod	Fentanyl 25–50 mcg iv prn is usually sufficient.
Tests	✓ CXR	For evidence of pneumothorax, hemothorax, mediastinal air.

Suggested Readings

1. Abdelmalak B, Ryckman JV, AlHaddad S, et al: Respiratory arrest after successful neodymium:yttrium-aluminum-garnet laser treatment of subglottic tracheal stenosis. *Anesth Analg* 2002; 95:485–6.
2. Ayuso A, Luis M, Sala X, et al: Effects of anesthetic technique on the hemodynamic response to microlaryngeal surgery. *Ann Otol Rhinol Laryngol* 1997; 106(10Pt1):863–8.
3. Bacher A, Lang T, Weber J, et al: Respiratory efficacy of subglottic low-frequency, subglottic combined-frequency, and supraglottic combined-frequency jet ventilation during microlaryngeal surgery. *Anesth Analg* 2000; 91:1506–12.
4. Braverman I, Sichel JY, Halimi P, et al: Complication of jet ventilation during microlaryngeal surgery. *Ann Otol Rhinol Laryngol* 1994; 103:624–7.
5. Donati F, Meistelman C, Benoit P: Vecuronium neuromuscular blockade at the adductor muscles of the larynx and adductor pollicis. *Anesthesiology* 1991; 74:833–7.
6. Donlon JV: Anesthetic and airway management of laryngoscopy and bronchoscopy. In *Airway Management: Principles and Practice.* Benumof JL, ed. Mosby, St. Louis: 1996, 666–85.
7. Dougherty TB: The difficult airway in conventional head and neck surgery. In *Airway Management: Principles and Practice.* Benumof JL, ed. Mosby, St. Louis: 1996, 686–97.
8. Gaumann DM, Tassonyi E, Fathi F, et al: Effects of topical laryngeal lidocaine on the sympathetic response to rigid panendoscopy under general anesthesia. *J Otorhinolaryngol Relat Spec* 1992; 54:49–53.
9. Hill RS, Koltai PJ, Parnes SM: Airway complications from laryngoscopy and panendoscopy. *Ann Otol Rhinol Laryngol* 1987; 96:691–4.
10. Jaquet Y, Monnier P, Van Melle G, et al: Complications of different ventilation strategies in endoscopic laryngeal surgery: a 10-year review. *Anesthesiology* 2006; 104:52–9.
11. McRae K: Anesthesia for airway surgery. *Anesthesiol Clin North Am* 2001; 19:497–541.
12. Ozkose Z, Yalcin Cok O, Tuncer B, et al: Comparison of hemodynamics, recovery profile, and early postoperative pain control and costs of remifentanil versus alfentanil-based total intravenous anesthesia (TIVA). *J Clin Anesth* 2002; 14:161–8.
13. Sosis MB: Anesthesia for laser airway surgery. In *Airway Management: Principles and Practice.* Benumof JL, ed. Mosby, St. Louis: 1996, 698–735.

TRACHEOTOMY/TRACHEOSTOMY AND CRICOTHYROIDOTOMY

SURGICAL CONSIDERATIONS

Description: When an airway needs to be obtained right away and intubation is not an option, a cricothrotomy is indicated. A vertical incision is made in the midline through the cricothyroid membrane, an initial influx of air is facilitated if the patient is spontaneously breathing, and a small ETT placed. It is wise to convert this to a tracheostomy as soon as it is convenient to do so as this reduces the subsequent incidence of subglottic stenosis and cricoid chondritis.

A tracheotomy is generally done in a controlled setting, either under general anesthesia in an intubated patient or under local anesthesia. Either a short transverse incision 1–2 cm inferior to the cricoid or a midline vertical incision beginning at the same location may be used. Strap muscles are retracted laterally, the thyroid isthmus is divided if necessary, and in adults an inferiorly based tracheal flap consisting of the 2nd or 3rd tracheal ring is made and secured to the skin inferiorly. In small children, it is better to make only a vertical midline incision to minimize the incidence of stenosis; left and right stay sutures are then placed to assist in reintubation in the event of accidental dislodgment of the tracheotomy tube. The tracheotomy tube in all patients is secured to the skin with sutures. Trach ties supplement this securing of the tube unless these circumferential ties would interfere with venous drainage of a flap used in the head and neck reconstruction.

When prolonged use of a tracheotomy is anticipated and it is unlikely that mechanical ventilation will be needed, there are specialized silicon tracheotomy tubes with minimal intraluminal plastic and may be associated with fewer intaluminal potential complications.

Usual preoperative diagnosis: Indications for tracheostomy are numerous, but share the common theme of securing a safe airway either in anticipation of postop airway edema, inability to protect the airway from aspiration, or as an urgent need to obtain an upper airway in pending obstruction. The fastest way to obtain an airway in an outright emergency when intubation is not an option is a cricothrostomy. Another 3rd general inidication is to protect the larynx from injury if prolonged intubation is anticipated, such as in a prolonged ICU setting or in paralysis associated with cervical spinal cord trauma. Rarer indications are bilateral vocal cord paralysis or a history of recurrent allergy associated with larynogspasm.

SUMMARY OF PROCEDURES

	Tracheostomy	Cricothyrotomy
Position	Supine, head extended	⇐
Incision	Transverse or vertical	Stab incision through cricothyroid membrane
Special instrumentation	None (most institutions have a "trach set")	Scalpel is all that is initially needed in this emergency setting
Unique considerations	Local or general, intubated or not. Specialized equipment and silicon trach cannulas selectively arranged for.	⇐
Antibiotics	None	⇐
Surgical Time	3–20 min	30 sec–2 min
EBL	Minimal	⇐
Postop Care	Warm humidification; suctioning; changing inner cannula; skin care; monitor for bleeding and dislodgement; in emergency remove entire tracheotomy tube	⇐; convert to tracheotomy as soon as convenient
Mortality	<1%	⇐

■ SUMMARY OF PROCEDURES (cont'd)		
Morbidity	Bleeding <5% cellulitis/tracheitis <5% tracheal stenosis <1%	Subglottic stenosis risk if not converted
Pain score	1–2	2–4

■ PATIENT POPULATION CHARACTERISTICS		
Age range	All	⇐
Male:Female	Dependent on underlying condition	⇐
Incidence	Common	⇐
Etiology	Anticipated airway obstruction, airway obstruction, prolonged intubation	Trauma
Associated conditions	Dependent on underlying c ondition, but typically cardiopulmonary or neurological conditions	Trauma

ANESTHETIC CONSIDERATIONS

PREOPERATIVE

Typically, there are three patient populations presenting for tracheostomy: (a) critically ill intubated patients in chronic respiratory failure or following major trauma; (b) patients for whom tracheostomy is part of a scheduled procedure (e.g., laryngectomy); (c) patients with impending or total upper airway obstruction (e.g., Ludwig's angina, retropharyngeal abscess). If the latter constitutes life-threatening emergency, tracheotomy/cricothyroidotomy may be the preferred approach. Aside from an occasional otherwise healthy patient in the 3rd category, all patients presenting for tracheostomy are usually debilitated, have associated cardiac or pulmonary disease, with neurological and metabolic abnormalities.

Respiratory	Patients in group 1 usually require mechanical ventilation with PEEP to maintain adequate oxygenation. The continued application of PEEP may be an important consideration during their transport from ICU to OR. Patients in group 2 require a careful airway evaluation (see Anesthetic Considerations for Neck Dissection, p. 216, and Laryngectomy, p. 202). Based on the assessment, the anesthesiologist must decide whether to choose a DL, an awake FOI, or a tracheostomy under local anesthesia to secure the airway. Patients in group 3 will usually require semi-emergent or emergent tracheostomy. Patients in all three groups should be evaluated for the presence of possible recurrent aspiration. **Tests:** CXR; ABG, as indicated from H&P
Cardiovascular	All patients may have significant cardiac risk factors, including smoking, ETOH abuse, male gender, ↑ cholesterol, family Hx, and HTN. Some patients may have recently undergone major cardiac surgery, and may be on pharmacological inotropic support, with full invasive monitoring, including PA line. **Tests:** ECG, and other tests as indicated, in patients of the 2nd group.
Neurological	Preop neurological deficits should be fully documented
Hematologic	In cases of malignancy or chronic disease, coagulopathies or anemia may be present **Tests:** CBC; Coagulation studies
Laboratory:	Other tests as indicated from H&P
Premedication	Standard premedication (p. B-1) in elective cases. Premedication is best avoided in critically ill patients and patients with symptoms of upper airway obstruction

INTRAOPERATIVE

Anesthetic technique: GETA in intubated patients, or in patients who pose no problems for conventional DL and tracheal intubation. In the presence of significant airway compromise or anticipated very difficult intubation local anesthesia may be required. Most tracheostomies are elective or semiurgent, and are performed under GA. Patients with ↑ mucosal swelling (e.g. generalized edema, prolonged intubation) and ↑ tissue fragility (e.g. chronic steroid therapy) are at risk for tracheal mucosal separation → creation of a false passage during tracheostomy. This will constitute a true emergency (see Postoperative Complications, below).

Induction	If already intubated (group 1, above), convert pre-existing ICU sedation to GA, using carefully titrated induction (e.g., etomidate 0.2–0.3 mg/kg iv) or an inhalational agent. If not intubated, and no airway problems are anticipated, a standard induction (p. B-2) may be appropriate. If airway problems are anticipated, an awake FOI or tracheostomy performed under local anesthesia may be the techniques of choice (see Anesthetic Considerations for Neck Dissection, p. 216, and Laryngectomy, p. 202). In any event, the anesthesiologist should be prepared to deal with a failed intubation, and have a surgeon immediately available to perform cricothyrotomy/tracheostomy if ventilation proves impossible.	
Maintenance	Standard maintenance (see p. B-2). Full muscle relaxation is required. FiO_2=1.0 usually is required before insertion of the tracheostomy tube. This high O_2 concentration, combined with electrocautery, may precipitate airway fire (see Postoperative Complications, below). A cuffed ETT should be used to prevent O_2 from leaking into the surgical site. In order to avoid inadvertent ETT cuff puncture, consider advancing the ETT closer toward the carina, before the trachea is opened. The trachea is usually opened above the cuff, and the ETT is slowly retracted cephalad, under direct vision by the surgeon (NOTE: Do not remove the ETT completely!). Sterile gas sampling tubing, extra ETTs and anesthesia circuit should be readily available (see Maintenance for Laryngectomy, p. 203). After the tracheostomy tube is secured, it should be suctioned and connected to the anesthesia circuit. Verify the $ETCO_2$ tracing, ✓ the inflation pressures, and remove the ETT.	
Emergence	Considerations for group 2 and 3 patients are described above. Patients in the first group will continue on ventilatory support in the ICU. The tracheostomy tube must be carefully suctioned and the delivered O_2 should be humidified. Opioid sedation will minimize reaction to suctioning in the early postop period. Tracheostomy tubes should not be removed for at least the first 5–7 days until a track is formed.	
Blood and Fluid Requirements	IV: 18ga × 1 NS/LR @ 2–3 mL/kg/h	EBL is typically minimal, when the tracheostomy is performed as an isolated procedure
Monitoring	Standard monitors (p. B-1)	Avoid ECG pad placement in the prepped area. Invasive monitoring may be appropriate depending on the patient's condition.
Positioning	Shoulder roll ✓ and pad pressure points. ✓ eyes.	A shoulder roll is usually placed, and patient's neck extended, which may result in ETT cuff migrating cephalad, closer to the incision site (danger of inadvertent perforation by the surgeon on entering the trachea!). Make sure the ETT is positioned at the sufficient depth and taped securely.
Complications	Pneumothorax Pneumomediastinum Hemorrhage Aspiration of blood	Pneumothorax may occur with a low neck dissection, or if a false passage (see Postop Complications, below) has been created during the tracheostomy tube insertion. Dx and Rx – see Anesthetic Considerations for Laryngoscopy/Bronchoscopy/Esophagoscopy, p. 180.
	False tracheal passage/tracheal disruption Difficult ETT insertion/reinsertion	This is an airway emergency, and must be quickly recognized (absent CO_2, ↑ PIP, absent or very distant breath sounds). Reintroduction of the existing ETT from the proximal trachea should be attempted.

Complications (cont'd)	Difficult ETT insertion/reinsertion (cont'd)	Rigid bronchoscope should be available to reestablish the airway, in case of a failed reintubation. An alternative approach is to insert a large bore iv catheter into the tracheal lumen distal to the tracheostomy site and jet-ventilate the patient. Insertion of an airway exchange catheter through the bronchoscopy elbow adapter attached to the existing ETT has been advocated prior to tracheostomy tube insertion in patients at high risk for this complication.
	Airway Fire	Tracheostomy fires are usually not as catastrophic as other airway fires, possibly because the tracheostomy acts as a vent. Rx: immediately disconnect the patient from the anesthesia machine, extinguish the fire with NS and ventilate the lungs with room air using a self-inflating bag. Removing or changing the existing ETT at this point may be more risky than leaving it in, especially if the patient was previously difficult to intubate or the airway has become edematous.

POSTOPERATIVE

Complications	Pneumothorax Pneumomediastinum Hemorrhage	See Postoperative complications after Laryngoscopy/Bronchoscopy/Esophagoscopy, p. 185.
	Occlusion of the tracheostomy tube	This could be due to secretions, mucus plug, blood or positioning of the tube in the mainstem bronchus or against the tracheal wall.
	Tracheostomy tube displacement	Reintubate orally or through the tracheostomy site
Pain management	PCA (p. C-3) IV opioids	
Tests	CXR	✓ tracheostomy tube position and ✓ for evidence of either pneumothorax or pneumomedias-tinum

Suggested Readings

1. Brown BR: Anaesthesia for ear, nose, throat and maxillofacial procedures. In International Practice of Anaesthesia. Prys-Roberts C, Brown BR, eds. Butterworth-Heinemann, Oxford: 1996, 2–9.
2. Chee WK, Benumof JL: Airway fire during tracheostomy: extubation may be contraindicated. *Anesthesiology* 1998; 89:1576–8.
3. Donlon JV, Feldman MA: Anesthesia for eye, ear, nose, and throat surgery. In *Miller's Anesthesia,* 6th edition. Miller RD, ed. Elsevier, Philadelphia: 2005, 2527–49.
4. Mcguire G, El-beheiry H, Brown D: Loss of the airway during tracheostomy: rescue oxygenation and re-establishment of the airway. Can *J Anesth* 2001; 48:697–700.
5. Rogers ML, Nickalls RWD, Brackenbury ET, et al: Airway fire during tracheostomy: prevention strategies for surgeons and anaesthetists. Ann *R Coll Surg Engl* 2001; 83:376–80.

INTUBATION FOR EPIGLOTTITIS

ANESTHETIC CONSIDERATIONS

PREOPERATIVE

Epiglottitis is an acute inflammation and swelling of the epiglottis, associated with a generalized systemic toxicity, usually due to *Haemophilus influenza* Type B. It also can be caused by β-hemolytic streptococci, staphylococci, pneumococci, or unusual pathogens among immunocompromised individuals and drug/alcohol abusers. It occasionally results in total laryngeal obstruction and death 2° asphyxia. At one time, the typical patient was a previously healthy child 3–5 yr old; however, since the advent of the H-flu vaccine, epiglottitis is more common in adults (predominantly males). The most common presenting symptoms are sore throat, dysphagia/odynophagia, fever, respiratory difficulty, and drooling. Pediatric patients may appear toxic on presentation.

Airway	Enlarged epiglottis seen frequently on neck x-ray. Neck tenderness or swelling also observed in some patients. Patients with stridor are at high risk for upper airway obstruction.
Respiratory	The patient, typically sitting upright, may display hoarseness, muffled voice, dyspnea, and chest-wall retractions. **NB:** Rapid treatment should be instituted instead of performing time-consuming investigations. The sudden development of respiratory obstruction in the x-ray suite could have a disastrous outcome.
Hematologic	A high leukocyte count usually is found in these patients. **Tests:** Blood drawing before the airway is secured may be inadvisable.
Premedication	None

INTRAOPERATIVE

Anesthetic technique: GETA. Patients presenting with imminent or actual airway obstruction should be intubated immediately. Airway management for **adult** patients presenting with **mild-to-moderate** symptoms is controversial. Although routine prophylactic intubation of these patients may not be necessary, 18% subsequently develop complete airway obstruction; thus, close monitoring is mandatory if intubation is deferred. It is imperative to realize that total airway obstruction can occur suddenly and without warning.

An experienced anesthesiologist should be present for this procedure. In the pediatric patient, it is critical that neither visualization of the epiglottis nor other maneuvers be attempted to confirm the Dx before anesthesia. In adults, it has been suggested that indirect laryngoscopy or FOB may be performed without the risk of precipitating complete airway obstruction, although this approach is controversial.

Induction	If an iv is in place, atropine 0.02 mg/kg may be given to the pediatric patient to prevent vagal reflexes resulting from manipulation of the inflamed epiglottis. If no iv access is available, inhalation induction (sevoflurane in FiO_2=1.0) with the patient in the sitting position should be used. Intramuscular injection should be avoided to prevent agitation, crying, and subsequent total airway obstruction (iv line is placed after induction of anesthesia). An experienced ENT surgeon, ready to perform an emergency tracheostomy, must be present at induction. Early application of CPAP is essential to maintain the upper airway patency. Inhalation induction may be prolonged and intubation extremely difficult. Different sizes of ETTs must be available.
Maintenance	Standard maintenance (see p. B-2).
Emergence	The patient will remain intubated for 24–48 h and should be kept sedated and restrained to prevent accidental extubation.

Blood and fluid requirements	IV: 18–20 ga (adult) 22–26 ga (child) NS/LR @ 3–5 mL/kg/h (adult); @ 1.5 mL/kg/h (child)	Minimal blood loss Fluid requirements may be ↑ 2° fever and dehydration.
Monitoring	Standard monitors (p. B-1)	
Positioning	✓ and pad pressure points. ✓ eyes.	
Complications	POPE (postobstructive pulmonary edema)	A short-lived POPE occasionally occurs after relief of the obstruction and must be treated with IPPV.

POSTOPERATIVE

Complications	Accidental extubation ETT blockage	These complications can prove fatal. The blockages are sometimes due to crusting of the ETT 2° insufficient humidification.
Pain management	PCA (p. C-3) IV opioids	Postop sedation and manual restraints are often required

Suggested Readings

1. Brown BR: Anaesthesia for ear, nose, throat and maxillofacial procedures. In *International Practice of Anaesthesia*. Prys-Roberts C, Brown BR, eds. Butterworth-Heinemann, Oxford: 1996, 2–9.
2. Crockett DM, Healy GB, McGill TJ, et al: Airway management of acute supraglottitis at the Children's Hospital, Boston: 1980–1985. *Ann Otol Rhinol Laryngol* 1988; 97(2Pt1):114–19.
3. Donlon JV, Feldman MA: Anesthesia for eye, ear, nose, and throat surgery. In *Miller's Anesthesia*, 6th edition. Miller RD, ed. Elsevier, Philadelphia: 2005, 2527–49.
4. Dort JC, Frohlich AM, Tate RB: Acute epiglottis in adults: diagnosis and treatment in 43 patients. *J Otolaryngol* 1994; 23:281–5.
5. Park KW, Darvish A, Lowenstein E: Airway management for adult patients with acute epiglottitis. *Anesthesiology* 1998; 88:254–61
6. Senior BA, Radkowski D, MacArthur C, et al: Changing patterns in pediatric supraglottitis: a multi-institutional review, 1980 to 1992. *OHNS* 1994; 110:203–10.

ZENKER'S DIVERTICULECTOMY

SURGICAL CONSIDERATIONS

Description: Zenker's diverticulum is a herniation of mucosa through the posterior hypopharyngeal wall immediately above the cricopharyngeus muscle and below the inferior constrictor in an area called Killian's dehiscience. This is an acquired disorder, usually seen in the 6th to 9th decades of life and felt secondary to tonic spasm or achalasia of the cricopharyngeus muscle. Clinically, patients may experience dysphagia, globus, coughing, and regurgitation of undigested food. Weight loss and aspiration pneumonia can be seen in severe cases. Barium swallow is usually diagnostic. Endoscopy will reveal the presence of a pouch of variable size posterior to the cricopharyngeus muscle often filled with undigested debris. Cricopharyngeal achalasia may present in the absence of a well-formed diverticulum with much the same symptom complex. Treatment is usually aimed at division of the cricopharyngeus muscle and eradication of the pouch.

Variant approaches. Open: Under GA with muscle relaxation, an incision is made in the left side of the neck to expose the diverticulum and cricopharyngeus muscle. The muscle is cut, the diverticulum resected, and the hypopharyngeal defect closed. In patients with pure cricopharyngeal spasm, the muscle alone is cut. A drain is placed and the wound is closed. A nasogastric tube may be placed for postop feeding. Aspiration precautions should be observed at both induction and reversal of anesthesia, as this is a common comorbidity in patients with Zenker's diverticulum. **Endoscopic:** Selected patients may be candidates for endoscopic treatment of a Zenker's diverticulum. This is better described as diverticulotomy rather than diverticulectomy, because the redundant hypopharyngeal mucosa is not removed, and the cricopharyngeus muscle is not divided in its entirety. Rather, the common wall separating the diverticulum from the esophagus is reduced so as to prevent food and debris from collecting within the confines of the diverticulum. With the patient under general anesthesia and muscle relaxation, an esophagodiverticuloscope is placed transorally and advanced into the hypopharynx. The endoscope is deployed so as to visualize clearly the opening into the diverticulum. The common wall separating the diverticulum from the true esophageal inlet is then cut, either with a stapler or with a CO_2 laser.

Usual preop diagnosis: Dysphagia; Zenker's diverticulum; cricopharyngeal spasm

SUMMARY OF PROCEDURES

	Open	Endoscopic
Position	Supine; table 90°; head extended	Supine
Special instrumentation	Anode or laser ETT; microscope	⇐ ; endoscopic stapler or CO_2 laser
Unique considerations		Keep O_2 < 30 % and avoid N_2O if lasering.
Antibiotics	Cefazolin 1gm and metronidazole 500 mg; clindamycin 600 mg	
Surgical time	1–2 h	30 min to 1 h
EBL	< 25 mL	0–25 mL
Postop care	Reflux precautions should be observed; patients may require nasogastric tube feeding for several days	Reflux precautions should be observed
Mortality	< 1%	< 1%
Morbidity	Fistula formation < 5% Vocal cord paralysis Hematoma 1–5% Infection 1–5% Aspiration	Perforation < 5% Aspiration
Pain score	3–5	3–5

PATIENT POPULATION CHARACTERISTICS

Age range	60–90
Male:Female	1.5:1
Incidence	1 in 50,000; Caucasians
Etiology	GERD; neurogenerative disorders
Associated conditions	GERD

ANESTHETIC CONSIDERATIONS

(See page 180)

Suggested Readings

1. Aly A, Devitt PG, Jamieson GG: Evolution of surgical treatment for pharyngeal pouch. *Br J Surg* 2004; 9(6):657–64.
2. Dohlman G, Mattsson L: The endoscopic operation for hypopharyngeal diverticula: a roentgencinematographic study. *Arch Otolaryngol* 1960; 71:744–52.
3. Feeley MA, Righi PD, Weisberger EC, et al: Zenker's diverticulum: analysis of surgical complications from diverticulectomy and cricopharyngeal mytomoy. *Laryngoscope* 1999; 109(6):858–61.
4. Huang B, Payne WS, Cameron AJ: Surgical management for recurrent pharygoesophageal (Zenker's) diverticulum. *Ann Thoracic Surg* 1984; 37(3):189–91.
5. van Overbeek JJ: Pathogenesis and methods of treatment of Zenker's diverticulum. *Ann Otol Rhinol Laryngol* 2003; 112(7):583–93.
6. Witterick IJ, Gullane PJ, Yeung E: Outcome analysis of Zenker's diverticulectomy and criopharyngeal mytomy. *Head Neck* 1995; 17(5):382 –8.

LARYNGEAL FRAMEWORK SURGERY (THYROPLASTY, ARYTHENOID ADDUCTION, INJECTION LARYNGOPLASTY)

SURGICAL CONSIDERATIONS

Description: **Thyroplasty** is a surgical technique of medializing a paralyzed vocal fold via placement of an implant inserted through the cartilage of the thyroid ala. Under local anesthesia with intravenous sedation, a skin incision is made at the level of the larynx and the thyroid cartilage exposed. Using a small saw, drill bit, or knife, a window is cut in the cartilage to the level of the inner perichondrium. Lateral pressure is then applied to the paralyzed side to gauge the amount of medialization necessary to improve phonation. Because the shape and size of the implant is created based on the location and degree of medialization needed to improve the voice, it is important for the patient to be awake and able to phonate during the procedure. Often the patient is kept in a state of deeper sedation in the beginning of the case and then is lightened as the case proceeds to allow the patient to be responsive and interactive with the surgeon. This can be a challenge for the anesthesiologist to strike a happy medium between patient comfort and coherence. After the desired degree of medialization is obtained, the implant is secured in place and the wound closed over a drain.

Description: **Arytenoid adduction** is often performed in conjunction with thyroplasty. This involves placement of a suture around the muscular process of the arytenoid cartilage which, when tightened, causes posteromedial rotation of the vocal process and adduction of the vocal fold. Usually the technique is employed when there is a persistent gap between the vocal folds posteriorly.

Description: **Injection laryngoplasty** refers to medialization of a paralyzed vocal fold by means of injection, whether percutaneous or endoscopic. Its minimally invasive nature is its chief advantage over thyroplasty or arytenoid adduction. However, the longevity of the injected material as well as its side effect profile are major determinants as to whether or not this procedure should be considered. Traditionally, Teflon has been the injectable material of choice. However, because of the potential for a foreign body reaction, Teflon has been largely replaced by more biocompatible materials, such as collagen, acellular human dermis, fat, gelfoam, and calcium hydroxylapatite to name a few. Because of the low viscosity of material such as collagen, many patients are candidates for percutaneous injection, which can be performed in the office or procedure room under simple topical anesthetic. The patient is seated upright and the nasal cavity topically anesthetized with lidocaine 2% and neosynephrine. A fiberoptic rhinolaryngoscope attached to a camera and television monitor is then passed transnasally to the level of the glottis. Through a 25- or 27-gauge needle, the desired material is injected either transcartilagenously, through the cricothyroid membrane, or under the thyroid ala into the paraglottic space. Observing on the monitor, the material is injected until the desired degree of medialization is obtained. This is well tolerated by patients with minimal pain. Airway obstruction or bleeding are exceedingly rare.

For those who request or require injection under GETA a 5.0 microlaryngeal tube is desirable. Jet ventilation and apneic techniques can also be used. An operating laryngoscope is advanced to the level of the glottis and suspended from a Mayo stand. The paryalyzed vocal fold is then injected, usually at the mid and posterior aspects, until adequate medialization is seen. Usually this entails slight overcorrection such that the medialized fold will now be slightly across midline. Hemostasis if needed is usually obtained with epinephrine-soaked pledgets placed directly on the vocal fold. The scope is then withdrawn and the procedure terminated.

It is important for the anesthesiologist to be aware if a patient has undergone a prior medialization procedure. This is not a contraindication to orotracheal intubation for subsequent procedures requiring GETA. However, traumatic intubation or the use of a tube larger than 6 mm may cause trauma to the adducted fold. A laceration of the vocal fold can potentially expose or dislodge a thyroplasty implant, making it more likely to become infected and potentially extrude.

Usual preop diagnosis: Vocal fold paralysis.

SUMMARY OF PROCEDURES

	Thyroplasty	Arytenoid Adduction	Injection Laryngoplasty
Position	Supine	⇐	⇐
Special instrumentation	Head and neck set; headlights	–	Dedo operating laryngoscope; laryngeal injection needles; Jet ventilation setup.
Unique considerations	Overmedialization of the vocal fold can potentially cause stridor and dyspnea; Coordination between the surgeon and anesthesiologists is essential to time lightening of anesthesia; ETT stimulation can cause coughing.	If GETA is requested, intubate with 5.0 microlaryngeal tube.	Overmedialization of the vocal fold can potentially cause stridor and dyspnea.
Antibiotics	Cefazolin 1gm	⇐	⇐
Surgical Time	1–2 h	⇐	30 min
EBL	< 10 mL	10–20 mL	Minimal
Postop care	Decadron intravenously for 24 h; racemic epinephrine; cool mist.	⇐	racemic epinephrine; cool mist as needed
Mortality	Rare	⇐	⇐
Morbidity	Need for revision: 10–20% Transient dyspnea or laryngospasm Infection: < 5% Airway obstruction requiring tracheostomy: 1% Extrusion: rare	⇐ ⇐ ⇐ ⇐	Need for repeat injection common 5–10% rare ⇐
Pain score	3–4	4–5	1–2

PATIENT POPULATION CHARACTERISTICS

Age range	18 and over
Male:Female	1:1
Incidence	Common
Etiology	Surgical trauma to recurrent laryngeal nerve; cancer; trauma; idiopathic
Associated conditions	Cancer; coronary artery disease; lung disease; tumors of skull base

Suggested Readings

1. Cotter CS, Avidano MA, Crary MA, et al: Laryngeal complications after type 1 thyroplasty. *Otolaryngol Head Neck Surg* 1995; 113(6): 671–3.
2. Damrose EJ, Berke GS: Advances in the management of glottic insufficiency. *Curr Opin Otolaryngol Head Neck Surg* 2003; 11(6):480–4.
3. Flint PW, Purcell LL, Cummings CW: Pathophysiology and indications for medialization thyroplasty in patients with dysphagia and aspiration. *Otolaryngol Head Neck Surg* 1997; 116(3):349–54.
4. Herman C: Medialization thyroplasty for unilateral vocal cord paralysis. *AORN J* 2002; 75(3):512–22.
5. Isshiki N, Morita H, Okamura H, et al: Thyroplasty as a new phonosurgical technique. *Acta Otolaryngol* 1974; 78(5–6): 451–7.
6. Isshiki N, Taira T, Tanabe M: Surgical alteration of the vocal pitch. *J Otolarygnol* 1983; 12(5):335–40.
7. Isshiki N, Tsuji DH, Yamamoto Y, et al: Midline lateralization thyroplasty for adductor spasmodic dysphonia. *Ann Otol Rhinol Laryngol* 2000; 109(2):187–93.
8. Pou AM, Carrau RL, Eibling DE et al: Laryngeal framework surgery for the management f aspiration in high vagal lesions. *Am J Otolaryngol* 1998; 19(1):1–7.
9. Weinman EC, Maragos NE: Airway compromise in thyroplasty surgery. *Laryngoscope* 2000; 110(7):1082–5.

ANESTHETIC CONSIDERATIONS

PREOPERATIVE

The laryngeal framework surgery (LFS) is the surgery of choice for dysphonias resulting from incomplete glottic closure or inadequate vocal fold tension. With thyroplasty, direct surgery on the vocal folds is avoided, eliminating the possibility of scarring and voice aggravation. Type I (medialization) thyroplasty is most commonly performed for the unilateral VC paralysis or bowing (in elderly patients), and involves placement of a small silicon implant within the larynx on the affected side.

Airway	No airway problems are usually encountered in these patients
Cardiovascular	Elderly patients may present with advanced cerebrovascular, cardiovascular, or pulmonary disease. Preop pulmonary aspiration due to glottic incompetence is uncommon, but may be seen when the VC paralysis is of central origin, affecting both motor and sensory components of the VC innervation.
Tests	EKG; other tests as indicated from H&P
Laboratory	Tests, as indicated from H&P
Premedication	Standard premedication with iv midazolam can frequently be reduced or avoided, especially in the elderly.

INTRAOPERATIVE

Anesthetic technique: Most commonly, thyroplasty is performed under MAC, which allows the surgeon to achieve optimal improvement in the patient's voice quality (sometimes facilitated by visualization of the VC movement through a nasally introduced flexible fiberoptic endoscope) before locking the laryngeal implant in place. It can also be performed under GA, when the concomitant use of the LMA and flexible fiberoptic bronchoscope allows a real-time assessment of VC positioning. **Arythenoid adduction** and **injection laryngoplasty** are usually performed under GETA with the use of a small (5.0 mm ID) MLT ETT.

The essential surgical requirements for **thyroplasty** performed under MAC include: patient immobility for an effective injection of a local anesthetic; alternating levels of MAC sedation, depending on the part of the surgery (deep level of sedation during the surgical approach to the cartilage, light for the implant placement, and deep again during the surgical closure); absence of straining/bucking/coughing during the implant placement and manipulation on the thyroid cartilage necessitates the use of iv opioids.

GETA for **arythenoid adduction** and **injection laryngoplasty** requires full muscle relaxation with quick return of protective airway reflexes and smooth emergence from anesthesia.

When providing MAC for thyroplasty, a quick patient transition to the "light" state for the implant placement is required. A combination of a small dose (1–2 mcg/kg) of iv fentanyl with the iv propofol infusion, or iv midazolam with iv remifentanil infusion (typically, 0.05–0.1 mcg/kg/min to avoid severe respiratory depression), will achieve the stated objective. For a thyroplasty performed under GA, as well as for the GETA employed for a **arythenoid adduction** and **injection laryngoplasty** surgery, the use of TIVA (see Introduction, Anesthesiologist's Perspectives, p. 174) has been shown to be highly beneficial. The **injection laryngoplasty** procedures can be very short, and, if properly coordinated with the surgeon, can occasionally be performed without tracheal intubation, using an apnea technique following IV induction, administration of a relatively large dose of succinylcholine (1.5–2 mg/kg) and brief mask hyperventilation with $FiO_2 = 1.0$.

Blood and fluid Requirements	IV: 20 ga × 1 LR @ 2 cc/kg/h	EBL is minimal during all the LFS procedures
Monitoring	Standard monitors (p. B-1) ± arterial line	Even in patients with pre-existing significant CV disease, A-line monitoring is usually not necessary
Positioning	Table may be turned 90–180° ✓ and pad pressure points ✓ eyes	To prevent claustrophobia, inform the patient presenting for the thyroplasty under MAC, that his/her face will be partially covered with surgical towels.
Complications	Overmedialization stridor and dysphonia	Can be quickly corrected by the surgeon

POSTOPERATIVE

Complications	Wound hematoma. Airway obstruction Stridor Extrusion of the prosthesis
Pain management	Short-acting parenteral opioids (p. C-1) are usually sufficient

Suggested Readings

1. Grundler S, Stacey MR: Thyroplasty under general anesthesia using a laryngeal mask airway and fibreoptic bronchoscope. *Can J Anaesth* 1999; 46(5Pt1):460–3.
2. Hoffman H, McCabe D, McCulloch T, et al: Laryngeal collagen injection as an adjunct to medialization laryngoplasty. *Laryngoscope* 2002; 112(8 Pt1):1407–13.
3. LinksOdland RM, Wigley T, Rice R: Management of unilateral vocal fold paralysis. *Am Surg* 1995; 61:438–43.
4. Lundy DS, Casiano RR, Xue JW: Can maximum phonation time predict voice outcome after thyroplasty type I? *Laryngoscope* 2004; 114:1447–54.
5. Razzaq I, Wooldridge W: A series of thyroplasty cases under general anaesthesia. Br J Anaesth 2000;85:547–9.
6. Remacle M, Lawson G, Jamart J, et al: Treatment of vocal fold immobility by injectable homologous collagen: short-term results. *Eur Arch Otorhinolaryngol* 2006; 263:205–9.
7. Remacle M, Lawson G, Mayné A: Use of a laryngeal mask during medialization laryngoplasty. *Rev Laryngol Otol Rhinol (Bord)* 2003; 124:335–8.

TRACHEAL AND CRICOTRACHEAL RESECTION

SURGICAL CONSIDERATIONS

Description: Prolonged endotracheal intubation and complications from tracheotomy account for most cases of subglottic or tracheal stenosis. Wegener's disease commonly affects the subglottic airway and secondary dyspnea may be the first presenting sign of the disease. In females in the 4th to 6th decades of life, subglottic stenosis can be idiopathic. Whatever the etiology, subglottic and tracheal stenosis can be a major source of morbidity for afflicted patients, resulting in dyspnea, dysphonia, and tracheostomy dependence. In selected individuals, resection of the stenotic region with primary repair can often produced marked and sustained relief of symptoms in a single stage procedure, often without need for a temporary tracheostomy.

Tracheal resection is the treatment of choice in patients with isolated tracheal stenosis. Up to four to five rings of cartilage can be resected, more if releasing maneuvers to mobilize the larynx and intrathoracic trachea are performed. Induction of anesthesia is simplest in patients with pre-existing tracheostomies. For those patients who present without a tracheostomy, a tracheostomy under local anesthesia can be performed at or immediately below the stenotic segment. If possible, it is preferable to dilate the stenosis and proceed to endotracheal intubation so as to avoid further injury to the trachea with a fresh tracheotomy. With the patient in the supine position, a transverse cervical incision is made. The thyroid isthmus is divided and separated from the cervical trachea. Careful blunt dissection on the lateral aspects of the diseased segment is performed to avoid injury to the recurrent laryngeal nerves. A vertical incision is made along the face of the stenotic segment until a healthy complete ring of cartilage is identified above and below the stenotic segment. The anesthesiologist withdraws the ETT up into the subglottis and the diseased segment of trachea is resected. At this time, the surgeon may intubate the distal segment of trachea in order to afford better access to the superior aspect of the diseased segment. In this case, the breathing circuit will need to be switched from the orotracheal tube to the distal tube. The distal trachea can be more easily mobilized superiorly following blunt finger dissection along the anterior tracheal wall into the mediastinum. The orotracheal tube is then advanced inferiorly into the distal healthy segment. The healthy distal and proximal segments of trachea are then reanastomosed over the ETT using interrupted sutures. The wound is closed and a drain placed. If the patient is to remain intubated overnight, it is important to ensure that the cuff of the endotracheal tube remains inferior to the suture line so as not to put tension on the repair. If the patient is to be extubated in the OR, care should be taken to minimize coughing or bucking so as not to rupture the repair site. Endoscopy can be performed prior to transport from the operating room to ensure that at least one vocal fold is mobile. If neither vocal fold is mobile, a bilateral recurrent laryngeal nerve injury should be suspected and a tracheostomy performed. Regardless of whether or not the patient is extubated immediately or later, fiberoptic laryngoscopy to assess vocal fold motion postop is standard of care. Voice quality is not an adequate assesment of vocal fold function. A paralyzed vocal fold can be midline with complete compensation by the mobile fold and no overt dysphonia. In bilateral vocal fold paralysis, the voice is often normal, and the patient's only symptoms will be dyspnea and stridor.

Cricotracheal resection allows single-stage repair of subglottic or a combined subglottic/tracheal stenosis. The procedure is similar to that of tracheal resection with several caveats. It is important to carefully gauge the relationship of the stenosis to the vocal folds. Stenosis that involves the vocal folds is a contraindication to cricotracheal resection. The anterior arch of the cricoid cartilage is usually resected, along with the subglottic soft tissue component of the stenosis, preserving the cricoid plate. This creates a cradle into which the trachea will slide superiorly. No more than one-third of the inferior aspect of the cricoid plate can be resected. More than this will disrupt the posterior cricoarytenoid muscles and prevent vocal fold abduction during inspiration. As resection proceeds, the ETT will be withdrawn above the glottis. It is helpful at this point to attach an umbilical tape to the distal tip of the ETT to allow the surgeon to assist the anesthesiologist in advancing the tube back through the glottis and into the trachea when the resection is complete. The trachea is sutured to the thyroid cartilage anteriorly and the cricoid ring laterally; the wound is closed; and a drain may be placed. The patient is extubated in the OR and vocal fold mobility checked. Tracheostomy is only required in the setting of bilateral vocal fold paralysis and should otherwise be avoided. As with tracheal resection, a preop assesment of vocal fold motion is critical in planning surgery. If unilateral paralysis is present preop, great care is needed to minimize potential injury to the contralateral recurrent laryngeal nerve.

Usual preop diagnosis: Subglottic stenosis; tracheal stenosis

SUMMARY OF PROCEDURES

	Tracheal Resection	Cricotracheal Resection
Position	Supine	Supine
Incision	Transverse cervical	Transverse cervical
Special instrumentation	Major head and neck tray; headlights	⇐

SUMMARY OF PROCEDURES (cont'd)

	Tracheal Resection	Cricotracheal Resection
Unique considerations	Intubation may be difficult owing to degree of stenosis; dilation may be required prior to intubation; awake tracheostomy under local anesthesia may be necessary in select cases.	⇐
Antibiotics	Cefazolin 1gm and metronidazole 500 mg; clindamycin 600 mg; vancomycin 1gm; piperacillin/tazobactam 3.375 gm	⇐
Surgical time	3 h	⇐
EBL	50–100 mL	⇐
Postop care	Most patients can be extubated at the conclusion of surgery; coughing and stimulation should be minimized; if significant edema is expected, patients may remain intubated for 24 to 48 h then extubated; patients may require temporary NG tube feedings if laryngeal releasing maneuvers performed; monitoring in ICU setting for airway compromise or subcutaneous emphysema required postop	⇐
Mortality	1–2%	⇐
Morbidity	Restenosis: 10% Vocal cord paralysis: 2–3% Dehiscience: 5% Subcutaneous emphysema: 1–2% Airway edema requiring tracheotomy: 2%	10–15% 3–5% < 5% 1–2% 5%
Pain score	5–6	5–6

PATIENT POPULATION CHARACTERISTICS

Age range	All ages
Male:Female	2:1
Incidence	1% of all patients requiring intubation
Etiology	Prolonged intubation; prior tracheostomy; Wegener's disease; external trauma; neoplasm; radiation; gastroesophageal reflux; idiopathic.
Associated conditions	Atherosclerosis; asthma; gastroesophageal reflux.

Suggested Readings

1. Brown BR: Anaesthesia for ear, nose, throat and maxillofacial procedures. In *International Practice of Anaesthesia*. Prys-Roberts C, Brown BR, eds. Butterworth-Heinemann, Oxford: 1996, 2–9.
2. Chee WK, Benumof JL: Airway fire during tracheostomy: extubation may be contraindicated. *Anesthesiology* 1998; 89:1576–8.
3. Donlon JV, Feldman MA: Anesthesia for eye, ear, nose, and throat surgery. In *Miller's Anesthesia*, 6th edition. Miller RD, ed. Elsevier/Churchhill Livingstone, Philadelphia: 2005, 2527–49.
4. McGuire G, El-Beheiry H, Brown D: Loss of the airway during tracheostomy: rescue oxygenation and re-establishment of the airway. *Can J Anesth* 2001; 48:697–700.
5. Rogers ML, Nickalls RWD, Brackenbury ET, et al: Airway fire during tracheostomy: prevention strategies for surgeons and anaesthetists. *Ann R Coll Surg Engl* 2001; 83:376–80.

LARYNGECTOMY: PARTIAL AND TOTAL

SURGICAL CONSIDERATIONS

Description: Either radiation, chemoradiation or surgery is commonly employed as primary treatment of laryngeal squamous cell carcinoma. Selected tumors can be removed endoscopically, as reviewed above. Open procedures, which may be primary or following recurrence after irradiation, are designed to fit tumor extent. If at least one cricoarytenoid unit (innervated posterior cricoarytenoid muscle and working cricoarytenoid joint) is uninvolved by tumor, the patient may be a candidate for less than a total laryngectomy.

A **vertical partial laryngectomy** (VPL) involves removal of the true and false vocal cord, and up to one-third of the contralateral same structures including the anterior commissure. The contralateral cricoarytenoid unit is preserved, and reconstruction often includes a pedicled sternohyoid muscle as well as thyroid cartilage perichondrium. Exposure and anesthetic considerations are similar to that of a total laryngectomy (discussed below) other than the fact that a temporary tracheotomy is used in the partial laryngectomy.

A **supraglottic laryngectomy** (Fig. 3-4 and Fig. 3-5) or **anterior horizontal partial laryngectomy** (AHPL) (Fig. 3-6) involves removal of laryngeal structures superior to the true vocal cords. The amount of retained false vocal cord tissue is variable. One or both cricoarytenoid units remain. The resection may include some of the base of tongue. Exposure and anesthetic considerations are the same as for for a VPL, including the need for a temporary tracheotomy.

A **supracricoid laryngectomy** involves removal of the larynx from the cricoid ring to the hyoid bone with preservation of at least one arytenoid. A temporary tracheostomy is required. Cuts are made above the thyroid ala, through the cricothyroid membrane, and anterior to the arytenoid cartilages. The epiglottis may be included in the resection if necessary, depending upon the extent of the tumor. Blunt finger dissection anterior to the trachea into the mediastinum is performed to allow for superior mobilization of the trachea. A cricohyoidopexy, involving the suturing of the cricoid ring to the hyoid bone, is then performed with three heavy sutures. If the epiglottis has been preserved, a cricohyoidoepiglottopexy is performed. The strap muscles are then used to reinforce the closure, and drains are placed.

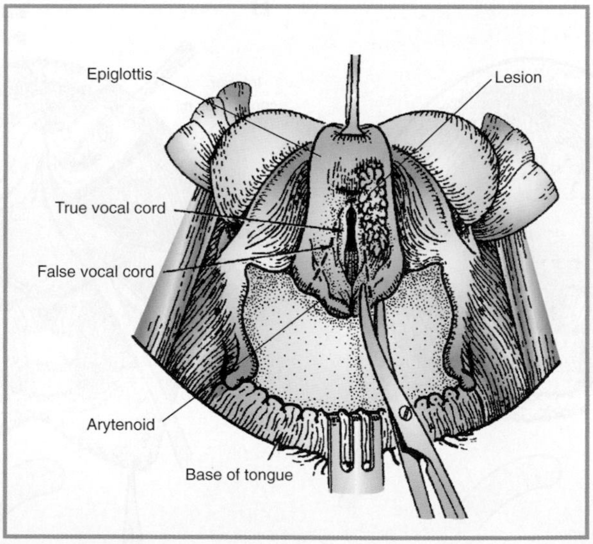

Figure 3-4. The larynx is viewed from the midline, as seen by the surgeon standing at the head of the operating table. Unless the lesion extends posteriorly to the arytenoid, the aryepiglottic fold is transected on each side by placing one blade of the dissecting scissors into the laryngeal ventricle or above the false vocal cord and the other blade in the pyriform sinus. The arytenoid on one side can be resected if the tumor extends posteriorly to involve this structure. (Reproduced with permission from Montgomery WW: *Surgery of the Upper Respiratory System,* 3rd edition. Williams & Wilkins, Baltimore: 1996.)

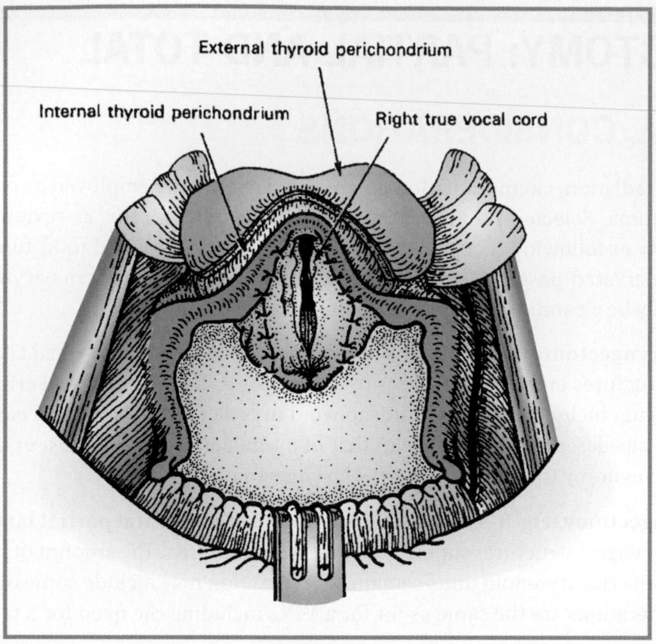

Figure 3-5. The repair following supraglottic partial laryngectomy begins by carefully approximating the margin of the mucous membrane of the pyriform sinus to the lateral margin of the laryngeal ventricle, or to the margin of resection above the false vocal cord. There is usually some distortion of the true vocal cord when the repair is accomplished, as is shown on the patient's right side. The repair is continued anteriorly by placing multiple interrupted 3-0 chromic catgut sutures. (Reproduced with permission from Montgomery WW: *Surgery of the Upper Respiratory System,* 3rd edition. Williams & Wilkins, Baltimore: 1996.)

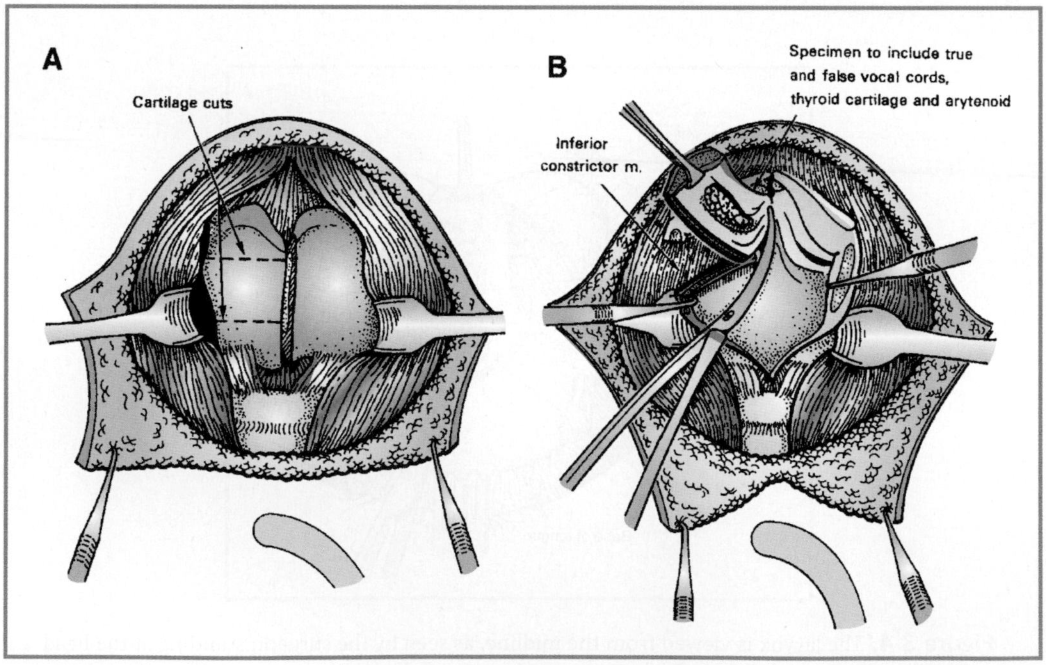

Figure 3-6. **(A)** Horizontal incisions, corresponding to the mucosal incision, are made through the thyroid lamina. **(B)** The specimen—including true and false vocal cords, the arytenoid, and a portion of the thyroid lamina—is resected en bloc. (Reproduced with permission from Montgomery WW: *Surgery of the Upper Respiratory System,* 3rd edition. Williams & Wilkins, Baltimore: 1996.)

A **total laryngectomy (TL)** involves the resection of the entire larynx, and can be done via an incision about 8 cm long, low in the midline neck. An apron incision is often used instead, or the low incision is extended toward a mastoid tip in order to provide exposure for a neck dissection if indicated. The thyroid gland is often preserved, pedicled on its superior and inferior vasculature after dividing the isthmus; but if indicated a partial thyroidectomy may be included. The thyoid is resected with the specimen and the pharynx closed primarily. A nasogastric tube is used for nutrition for all open laryngeal tumor surgery, unless the surgeon opts to provide nutrition via a tracheoesphageal puncture, discussed below. As the remaining trachea is sutured to the anterior skin in a true tracheostoma, no tracheotomy tube or ETT is required postop unless there is marked stomal edema or mechanical ventilaton is required, which is not common.

If a TL is performed, a **tracheoesphageal puncture** (TEP) may be performed simultaneously. This involves the creation of a tract or fistula between the trachea and the esophagus for placement of a voicing prosthesis (a one-way valve that allows airflow from the trachea into the pharynx for alaryngeal speech). The voicing prosthesis may be placed at the time of the laryngectomy or as a secondary procedure at a later date. If performed secondarily, it is placed using the technique of rigid esophagoscopy (see previous section). If TEP is performed at the time of laryngectomy, the valve can be placed simultaneously. Some surgeons prefer to place a red rubber catheter instead, which can allow the patient to be fed via this route in lieu of a nasogastric or gastrostomy tube. After the patient is deemed fit to start oral intake, the catheter can be exchanged secondarily for the voice prosthesis. If a rubber catheter is used, the tube will protrude from the stoma, and care must be taken not to dislodge it during suctioning or while removing or replacing the laryngectomy tube if one is temporarily used during the period of postop edema.

A TL can be extended to include part of the hypopharynx or oropharynx as dictated by tumor extent. If flap reconstruction is necessary because of the extent of the tumor, options include use of a pectoralis major myocutaneous flap or a free flap, such as a radial free flap, to reconstruct less than a circumferential defect. If a circumferential defect following resection exists (e.g. after resection of the superior cervical esophagus and the larynx), options for reconstruction include use of a laparascopically harvested jejunal free flap, gastric pullup, or a tubed radial free flap reinforced with a pectoralis major myogenous flap.

Postop care: Inpatient admission for 5–10 d; monitored bed or ICU for tracheostomy care or following more extensive pharyngeal reconstruction; a cuffed trachestomy tube (and a temporary tracheotomy) will usually be required for partial laryngectomy patients or if the patient will require postop mechanical ventilation. A shorter tracheostomy tube following a TL will be needed if there is significant peristomal edema or if mechanical ventilation is required. General and drain management is similar to a neck dissection.

Usual preop diagnosis: Cancer of larynx; intractable aspiration with resultant pneumonia unresponsive to other techniques.

SUMMARY OF PROCEDURES

	Total or Partial	Pharyngolaryngectomy
Position	Supine, head extended	⇐
Special instrumentation	Major head/neck set; headlights	⇐
Unique considerations	Laryngeal tumors may distort airway. Fiberoptic intubation or other management of the difficult airway should be considered. May be combined with neck dissection.	⇐
Antibiotics	Cefazolin 1 gm and metronidazole 500 mg; clindamycin 600 mg	⇐
Surgical time	2–4 h; 4–8 if neck dissection added	4–8 + h
EBL	50–300 mL With neck dissection: up to 500 mL. Transfusions rarely indicated.	⇐ ⇐ ⇐
Postop care	Tracheotomy care, drain management; tube feedings	⇐
Mortality	< 1%	⇐

SUMMARY OF PROCEDURES (cont'd)

Morbidity	Fistula formation: 5%: 15–20% if prior irradiation Hematoma: < 4% Infection: < 5% DVT/PE: < 1%	1% ⇐ ⇐ ⇐
Pain score	4–6	4–7

PATIENT POPULATION CHARACTERISTICS

Age range	40–80, occasionally older and younger
Male:Female	3:1
Incidence	Common
Etiology	Smoking; alcohol
Associated conditions	COPD; atherosclerosis; diabetes

ANESTHETIC CONSIDERATIONS

PREOPERATIVE

See preop considerations for Neck Dissection, p. 216.

Airway	If a stridor at rest is pressent, its severity must be carefully evaluated. Patients with symptoms and signs of severe obstruction (complaints of difficulty breathing, nocturnal symptoms, sleeping upright, use of accessory muscles on inspiration at rest) will likely be difficult to ventilate and intubate.
Respiratory	Patients with severe stridor may manifest baseline hypoxemia (with or without hypercarbia) 2° ↓ airway diameter and atelectases caused by ↓ ability to effectively handle secretions.

INTRAOPERATIVE

Anesthetic technique: GETA. Although tracheostomy is universally performed in these patients, smooth emergence is still important 2° delicate suture lines. Full muscle relaxation is essential. Moderate ↓ BP (see Introduction, p. 174) is desirable, but may be limited by concomitant cardiovascular disease.

Induction	There is no universal recipe for management of the partially obstructed airway. One approach is outlined below. If stridor is **absent** and airway assessment is normal, standard induction followed by DL is appropriate. In patients with pre-existing stridor, attempts to secure an airway while awake (including awake FOI) may precipitate complete upper airway obstruction. In patients with **moderate stridor,** in whom intubation is considered possible (larynx visible on preop nasal endoscopy, tumor not too large, absence of gross anatomical distortion, absence of fixed hemilarynx), inhalational induction, followed by gentle DL or asleep FOI, is the technique of choice. The ENT surgeon should be present in the OR, ready to perform rigid bronchoscopy or emergent tracheostomy. If the airway cannot be secured after 2–3 attempts, tracheostomy must be performed under controlled conditions with the patient breathing spontaneously. In patients with **severe stridor** and low probability of successful intubation, a preliminary tracheostomy must be performed under local anesthesia without any sedation.

Induction (cont'd)	Although in the majority of patients presenting for laryngectomy the location of tumor is submucosal, exophytic tumor growth may be present (e.g., VC). In this circumstance, direct visualization of the passage of the ETT through the VC (DL or video laryngoscopy) is essential to eliminate or greatly diminish the risk of tumor fragmentation and bleeding. Other anesthetic considerations are similar to those in Neck Dissection, p. 216.
Maintenance	See Anesthetic Considerations for Neck Dissection, p. 216. After tracheostomy, a sterile reinforced ETT (6.0–7.0 mm ID) is inserted by the surgeon and connected to a sterile anesthesia breathing circuit. Proper ETT placement should be confirmed by presence of $ETCO_2$ equal bilateral breath sounds and normal airway compliance. Following tracheostomy, ↑ FiO_2 to at least 50%, because the surgeon will continue working around the ETT, occasionally removing it from the patient's trachea for suture application. The position of the ETT in the tracheostoma should be monitored closely to prevent the ETT from slipping into the right mainstem bronchus.
Emergence	See Anesthetic Considerations for Neck Dissection, p. 216.

For further discussion, see Intraoperative Considerations for Neck Dissections, p. 216.

POSTOPERATIVE

See Postop Considerations for Neck Dissections, p. 218.

Suggested Readings

1. Bonner S, Taylor M: Airway obstruction in head and neck surgery. *Anaesthesia* 2000; 55:290–1.
2. Donlon JV, Feldman MA: Anesthesia for eye, ear, nose, and throat surgery. In *Miller's Anesthesia*, 6th edition. Miller RD, ed. Elsevier/Churchhill Livingstone, Philadelphia: 2005, 2527–49.
3. Dougherty TB, Nguyen DT: Anesthetic management of the patient scheduled for head and neck cancer surgery. *J Clin Anesth* 1994; 6:74–82.
4. Mason RA, Fielder CP: The obstructed airway in head and neck surgery. *Anaesthesia* 1999; 54:625–8.
5. See Suggested Readings for Neck Dissection, p. 218.

TONSILLECTOMY AND/OR ADENOIDECTOMY

SURGICAL CONSIDERATIONS

Description: The dissection for **tonsillectomy** is carried out with the patient supine, shoulders elevated on a small pillow (Fig. 3-7). A mouth gag is inserted; and, if an **adenoidectomy** is being done concurrently, adenoids are removed first with a curette, and the nasopharynx packed. The tonsillectomy is accomplished by firmly grasping the upper pole of the tonsil and drawing it medially, allowing a mucosal incision to be made over the anterior faucial pillar. The tonsil is dissected from its bed and removed. A snare may be used to snip the dissected tonsil off at the lower pole. Hemostasis is secured with gauze packs and the use of electrocautery. Packs are removed from the nasopharynx and tonsillar beds before extubation. Tonsillectomy may be combined with **palatopharyngoplasty** in cases of obstructive sleep apnea (OSA) or stertorous breathing (see p. 249).

Variant procedure or approaches: **Guillotine technique** (rarely used)

Usual preop diagnosis: Chronic tonsillitis and/or adenoiditis (most common); OSA; asymmetric enlargement of tonsils (to r/o cancer); nasal airway obstruction; snoring; peritonsillar abscess.

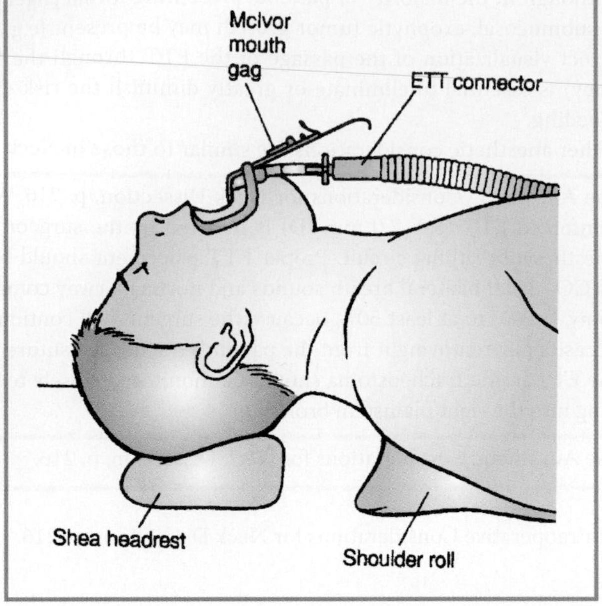

Figure 3-7. The "Rose" position for tonsillectomy.

SUMMARY OF PROCEDURE

Position	"Rose" (supine, shoulder roll, head extended); surgeon at head of table (turned 90–180°)
Incision	Intraoral mucosal
Special instrumentation	Mouth gag (McIvor)
Unique considerations	Use of armored ETT prevents compression of tube by mouth gag. Tube should be secured to lower lip in midline.
Antibiotics	Amoxicillin po
Surgical time	30–60 min
Closing considerations	If patient has OSA, a heightened sensitivity to narcotics and sedatives may make emergence more difficult. Avoid hypercapnia on emergence to prevent vasodilation and resultant bleeding. Awake extubation will provide maximum airway protection.
EBL	25–200 mL. Monitor suction bottle contents and irrigation as an indication of blood loss.
Postop care	Lateral position; head down; gentle suctioning
Mortality	Rare
Morbidity	Bleeding: 4% Infection: 4% Delayed bleeding: 3.2% Aspiration: Rare Tooth damage: Rare
Pain score	4–6

PATIENT POPULATION CHARACTERISTICS

Age range	2+ yr
Male:Female	1:1

■ PATIENT POPULATION CHARACTERISTICS (cont'd)	
Incidence	50 per 10,000 children in the United States
Etiology	Chronic infection; OSA (most common indication); peritonsillar abscess; snoring; cancer
Associated conditions	Nonspecific

ANESTHETIC CONSIDERATIONS

PREOPERATIVE

Most patients are young and otherwise healthy; however, a subset of both pediatric and adult patients may present with Sx of OSA or URI. For many children, this is their first anesthetic; therefore, it is imperative to ✓ family Hx for anesthetic problems. Most adult and pediatric patients are discharged from the hospital on the day of surgery.

Airway	In patients with a Hx of snoring or OSA, the probability of difficult mask ventilation and/or intubation may be high, 2° airway characteristics peculiar to these patients (see Anesthesia for Reconstructive Surgery for Sleep-Disordered Breathing, p. 255). In children with short-stature syndrome, including achondroplastic dwarfism and selected cases of Down syndrome, atlantoaxial subluxation and stenosis of the spinal canal may be present, and neck extension in these patients should be avoided.
Respiratory	In patients presenting with Sx of acute URI (purulent sputum or nasal secretions, fever, etc.), the general recommendation is to postpone any elective procedure until symptoms have abated, usually within 7–14 d. **Tests:** As indicated from H&P.
Dental	The presence of chipped, loose, or broken teeth should be documented preop and the patient (or parents, if appropriate) should be informed that there is a possibility of further tooth damage/dislodgement by the mouth gag applied by the surgeon.
Cardiovascular	Rarely, chronic airway obstruction (e.g., OSA) with hypoxemia may → pulmonary HTN and right heart failure. Patients with Down syndrome may have concomitant CHD. **Tests:** As indicated from H&P.
Hematologic	✓ for recent aspirin use and Hx of excessive bleeding following minor trauma or tooth extraction.
Laboratory	CBC; other tests as indicated from H&P.
Premedication	Sedative premedication is routine (see p. B-1), but should be avoided in OSA patients and patients with Sx of upper airway obstruction. Some surgeons request preop administration of an antisialagogue to achieve a dry surgical field.

INTRAOPERATIVE

Anesthetic technique: Balanced GETA is most commonly used in adults. (For pediatric anesthetic considerations, see p. 943.) Adequate muscle relaxation is an essential surgical requirement: it facilitates surgical exposure and prevents patient from swallowing. Continuous control and protection of the airway is another major objective, along with smooth emergence from anesthesia and prevention of early postop laryngospasm. Specific airway considerations include the possibility of difficult mask ventilation and/or difficult intubation 2° large tonsils and ↓ pharyngeal space, as well as the possibility of intraop obstruction of the ETT with the mouth gag placed by the surgeon.

Induction	An **intravenous induction** with propofol (2 mg/kg) and fentanyl (2–3 mcg/kg) is suitable for the majority of patients. If difficulty with mask ventilation is encountered, an oral airway is preferred to a nasal airway, 2° the possibility of trauma to the hypertrophied adenoid tissue and the resultant brisk bleeding. Patients with peritonsillar abscess may

Induction (cont'd)	have trismus, which usually resolves after induction of anesthesia and administration of a muscle relaxant. Great care should be exercised with introduction and manipulation of laryngoscope blade to avoid bleeding 2° inadvertent trauma to the enlarged tonsils, and to prevent soiling of the airway in patients with a peritonsillar abscess. The lightwand technique of tracheal intubation should be used with caution or avoided in these patients. The use of a small (6.0 mm ID) reinforced ETT is preferred over an oral RAE ETT, because of better resistance to kinking/obstruction by the mouth gag. The use of a FLMA can safely protect the airway during adenotonsillectomy and reduce the incidence of postextubation complications in adults and children. Its use for this procedure, however, has not become popular in the United States.
Maintenance	Opening of a mouth gag and the tonsillectomy itself constitute powerful noxious stimuli; therefore, an adequate depth of anesthesia must be maintained. It is essential to verify the ETT position before and after Boyle-Davis or McIvor mouth gag application (e.g., chest movement, bilateral and equal breath sounds, and nomal PIP): the ETT may be obstructed, dislodged, kinked, or inadvertently advanced into a mainstem bronchus, or the patient's trachea can be prematurely extubated when the mouth gag is repositioned/removed. Moderate ↓ BP is desirable but not obligatory; and judicious use of vasoactive drugs (see Introduction, p. 174) is preferred to deep levels of anesthesia 2° short duration of the procedure. Low-dose remifentanil infusion (see Introduction, p. 174) as part of either balanced or TIVA technique will provide superior hemodynamic stability and facilitate smooth emergence from anesthesia. For a balanced inhalational technique, desflurane and sevoflurane are the preferred agents for these short surgical procedures. Isoflurane may be favored in pediatric patients 2° ↓ agitation on emergence. The mouth gag may be repositioned several times during the procedure and is removed only at the end of the case. Vigorous patient movement while the mouth gag is hooked on the Mayo stand may cause C-spine injury; thus, neuromuscular blockade should usually be maintained until the end of the surgery. Prevention of PONV is of major importance. If a throat pack is not used by the surgeon, the patient's stomach should be suctioned at the end of the case, and further gastric emptying may be facilitated by administration of metoclopromide (1–2 mg/kg up to 20 mg iv). Administration of 5-HT_3 blockers (e.g., ondansetron 0.1 mg/kg up to 4 mg iv), with or without steroids (e.g., dexamethasone 4–10 mg iv), will usually provide adequate antiemetic prophylaxis.
Emergence	Removal of a throat pack (if used by the surgeon) should be verified before extubation. Care must be exercised while suctioning the oropharynx to avoid bleeding. The use of the rubber-tipped vs. Yankauer tip suction catheter may be preferred. Extubation should be smooth and performed after the patient is able to follow commands, because this usually signifies return of protective airway reflexes. If extubation is to be performed at deeper levels of anesthesia (e.g., in small children), the patient should be placed in the lateral decubitus, head-down position ("tonsillar position") to protect the airway from soiling 2° postop bleeding or aspiration of gastric contents. The patient should remain in this position until fully awake. This method of extubation is time- and labor-consuming, requires adequate depth of anesthesia to prevent postextubation laryngospasm, and does not prevent postextubation upper airway obstruction. Careful attention is required to protect patient's pressure points and to prevent the patient from rolling supine. Furthermore, with the head-down position, venous pressure in the surgical wound is increased with the possibility of provoking postop bleeding. This method of extubation cannot be advocated for routine use in adults.
Blood and fluid requirements	IV: 18 ga × 1 (adult) 20 ga × 1 (child) NS/LR @ 4–6 mL/kg/h (adult) Blood loss is typically minimal. Adequate hydration should continue in the immediate postop period.
Monitoring	Standard monitors (p. B-1)

Positioning	✓ and pad pressure points. ✓ eyes.	See Anesthetic Considerations for Panendoscopy, p. 180.
Complications	ETT obstruction dislodgement Bleeding	ETTs of different sizes should be readily available. Blood loss sometimes may be difficult to assess 2° drainage into stomach, especially if a throat pack is not used. Careful observation of suction canisters and close communication with the surgeon are essential.

POSTOPERATIVE

Complications	Retention of throat pack	Manifested by immediate symptoms of upper airway obstruction. Under direct laryngoscopy, remove pack with Magill forceps.
	Laryngospasm	A relatively common complication, particularly in the pediatric population. Rx: 100% O_2 via mask ventilation with jaw thrust and CPAP. Rapid-sequence induction (RSI) and direct laryngoscopy/intubation for persistent laryngospasm.
	Bleeding tonsil	Bleeding usually occurs at a slow pace; large volumes of blood may be swallowed and hypovolemia may occur before any bleeding is detected. Frequent swallowing should alert to the possibility of ongoing hemorrhage. ET intubation (RSI) may prove difficult due to poor visualization secondary to bleeding (effective suction must always be available) and upper airway edema. (See Pediatric section on Anesthesia for Tonsillectomy, p. 943.)
	Postobstructive (negative pressure) pulmonary edema (POPE)	POPE is a rare complication; however, it may occur in patients with pre-existing symptoms of severe upper airway obstruction. Although most cases resolve spontaneously, some patients may require reintubation and postop ventilatory support.
Pain management	See p. C-1	Adult tonsillectomy is a painful procedure, however, most patients are discharged home unless unable to sustain PO intake. Fentanyl is the preferred PACU drug, but the addition of morphine or Dilaudid may be necessary in some patients.
Tests	Hct	If blood loss is suspected

Suggested Readings

1. Brimacombe JR, Keller C, Gunkel AR, et al: The influence of the tonsilar gag on efficacy of seal, anatomic position, airway patency, and airway protection with the flexible laryngeal mask airway: a randomized, cross-over study on fresh adult cadavers. *Anesth Analg* 1999; 89:181–6.
2. Brown BR: Anaesthesia for ear, nose, throat and maxillofacial procedures. In *International Practice of Anaesthesia*. Prys-Roberts C, Brown BR, eds. Butterworth-Heinemann, Oxford: 1996, 2–9.
3. Davis L, Cook-Sather SD, Schreiner MS: Lighted stylet tracheal intubation: a review. *Anesth Analg* 2000; 90:745–56.
4. Dougherty TB: The difficult airway in conventional head and neck surgery. In Airway Management: Principles and Practice. Benumof JL, ed. Mosby, St. Louis: 1996, 686–97.
5. Ebert TJ, Robinson BJ, Uhrich TD, et al: Recovery from sevoflurane anesthesia. A comparison to isoflurane and propofol anesthesia. *Anesthesiology* 1998; 89:1524–31.
6. Sunkhani R, Pappas AL, Lurie J, et al: Ondansetron and dolasetron provide equivalent postoperative vomiting control after ambulatory tonsillectomy in dexamethasone-pretreated children. *Anesth Analg* 2002; 95:1230–5.
7. Webster AC, Morley-Forster PK, Dain S, et al: Anaesthesia for adenotonsillectomy: a comparison between tracheal intubation and the armored laryngeal mask airway. *Can J Anesth* 1993; 40:1171–7.

GLOSSECTOMY

SURGICAL CONSIDERATIONS

Description: **Glossectomy,** either **partial** or **total,** is performed for neoplastic lesions of the tongue. During this procedure, nasal intubation is helpful, but not mandatory. Complete muscle relaxation is necessary. Additionally, a drying agent, such as scopolamine or glycopyrrolate, helps reduce oral secretions and facilitates surgery. A side-biting or Dingman mouth gag is used to gain adequate surgical exposure. The lesion is resected with electrocautery and usually can be closed primarily. Depending on the extent of resection, and location on the tongue, a **tracheostomy** may be indicated; or oral intubation alone may suffice for a period of 24–48 h. If neither is done, a short course of steroids helps reduce the lingual edema. A NG tube is placed for postop feeding. A **total glossectomy** is performed in similar fashion, but frequently is combined with a **laryngectomy** because of ensuing aspiration.

Variant procedure or approaches: Glossectomy can be done with a **neck dissection** or **mandibulectomy** and (on occasion) also can be combined with a **total laryngectomy.**

Usual preop diagnosis: Neoplastic disease of the tongue or adjacent structures (e.g., alveolus, floor of mouth) with involvement of the tongue.

SUMMARY OF PROCEDURES

	Partial	Total
Position	Supine	⇐
Incision	Intraoral	⇐ + suprahyoid approach/neck approach
Special instrumentation	Dingman mouth gag	⇐
Unique considerations	Hypotensive anesthesia Nasal intubation Postop tracheostomy Steroids, if tracheostomy not performed.	⇐ ⇐ ⇐ (required)
Antibiotics	Cefazolin 1 g, metronidazole 500 mg	⇐
Surgical time	30 min–1 h	2–4 h
Closing considerations	Usually primary closure. May keep patient intubated 24–48 h if minimal tongue edema expected.	Flap repair required; laryngeal suspension usually required. Tracheostomy mandatory postop.
EBL	50–100 mL	200–400 mL
Postop care	Intubated 24–48 h	Tracheostomy care
Mortality	< 1%	⇐
Morbidity	Bleeding Infection Aspiration	Aspiration Bleeding Infection
Pain score	1–2	2–4

PATIENT POPULATION CHARACTERISTICS

Age range	Adults
Male:Female	3:1

■ PATIENT POPULATION CHARACTERISTICS (cont'd)	
Incidence	Uncommon
Etiology	Neoplasia
Associated conditions	Nonspecific

ANESTHETIC CONSIDERATIONS

PREOPERATIVE

For preop considerations, see Preoperative considerations for Neck Dissection, p. 255.

Airway	Thorough airway assessment is mandatory. Nasal intubation may or may not be required, depending on location of tumor (side vs base of tongue) and surgeon's preference (inquire preop).
Premedication	Standard. (see p. B-1) Preop administration of antisialagogue (e.g., glycopyrrolate 0.2 mg iv) may improve operating conditions—check with the surgeon.

INTRAOPERATIVE

Anesthetic technique: GETA. Complete muscle relaxation is an essential surgical requirement. For partial glossectomy, smooth extubation is desirable but not mandatory unless skin graft was used for closure (graft hematomas are the primary cause of skin graft failure). Intraop infiltration with a local anesthetic effectively supplements intraop and postop analgesia.

Induction	With a normal airway and submucosal location of tumor on the side of the tongue, standard induction (p. B-2) is appropriate. With mobile, fungating tumors located at the base of the tongue, inhalational induction with subsequent DL or video laryngoscopy may be a safer approach to avoid the risk of the upper airway obstruction. Similar to the considerations for laryngectomy (see Anesthetic Considerations for Laryngectomy, p. 202), direct visualization of the passage of the ETT through the VC (DL or video laryngoscopy) is essential, to eliminate or greatly diminish the risk of tumor fragmentation or bleeding. Large immobile tumors may make ET intubation by conventional means extremely difficult or impossible. Awake nasal FOI may be the technique of choice in these cases.	
Maintenance	During a partial glossectomy, surgical closure is quick, and short-acting inhalational agents (desflurane, sevoflurane) may be favored; TIVA may also be employed. ↓ BP (see Introduction, p. 174), although desirable, is not mandatory for partial glossectomy. If tracheostomy is performed as part of the planned procedure, the usual considerations apply (see Anesthetic Considerations for Laryngectomy, p. 202, and Tracheostomy, p. 187).	
Emergence	With prolonged procedures, especially involving tumors located at the base of the tongue, it is prudent to assess the degree of upper airway edema prior to extubation (it may be impossible to reintubate the patient if postextubation upper airway obstruction occurs). Rapid recovery with full return of protective airway reflexes is essential in patients after partial glossectomy.	
Complications	Vagal reflexes: ↓ HR, ↓ BP, mediated by surgical manipulation at the base of the tongue	Rare. Rx: notify surgeon; deepen anesthetic; iv atropine (0.4 mg).

For further discussion, see Intraoperative Considerations for Neck Dissection, p. 216.

POSTOPERATIVE

Complications	Postop airway obstruction	May occur 2° ↑ airway edema; emergent tracheostomy may be required. Prophylactic intraop steroids are beneficial.
Pain management	PCA (p. C-3) Parenteral opiates (p. C-2)	

For further discussion, see Neck Dissection, p. 216.

Suggested Readings

1. Donlon JV, Feldman MA: Anesthesia for eye, ear, nose, and throat surgery. In *Miller's Anesthesia*, 6th edition. Miller RD, ed. Elsevier/Churchhill Livingstone, Philadelphia: 2005, 2527–49.
2. Doughrty TB, Nguyen DT: Anesthetic management of the patient scheduled for head and neck cancer surgery. *J Clin Anesth* 1994; 6:74–82.

MAXILLECTOMY AND ORBIT EXENTERATION

SURGICAL CONSIDERATIONS

Description: Transfacial approaches to the paranasal sinuses may also include a maxillectomy or orbital exenteration or both. In an **orbital exenteration** the contents of the orbit are removed, including the eyeball and its attached extraocular muscles posterior toward the conus. This can be done via an incision that is made around the upper and lower eyelashes, occasionally with an extension that includes a limited incision for an external ethmoidectomy; no lateral rhinotomy incision is needed. If the eyelid skin is not involved by tumor it is preserved other than the eyelashes and lid margins. Bradycardia may occur with dissection near the optic nerve.

A **maxillectomy** may be done with the orbit exenteration. If the palate is to be preserved, the incision is the same, because access to the superior maxilla is provided by the exenteration. If the orbit is to be preserved, but the hemipalate is to be resected, then the resection can often be done fully through intraoral incisions. For example, if the anterior palate is to be resected, the approach is essentially the same as the Caldwell-Luc. If the anterior maxilla is to be preserved, but the posterior maxillary alveolar ridge is to be resected (as for a tumor involving the alveolar ridge and extending into the maxillary sinus), then the resection of the alveolar ridge usually provides adequate access for the complete resection. If necessary, either a transfacial incision, or endoscopic equipment may be used to supplement the access. Rarely is a full Weber-Ferguson incision (that involves an ethmoidectomy incision, lateral rhinotomy incison, and lip splitting incision) necessary. Osteotomies are generally made with power equipment, though osteotomes and rongeurs may at times be adequate.

Reconstruction of palate defects are generally done with an obdurator with a split thickness skin graft placed intraop on exposed soft tissue. There are a number of options to reconstruct orbit defects depending on whether skin was also resected. These options include the pericranial-galeal flap discussed for anterior cranial base surgery, a free myogenous flap such as the rectus abdominus, covered with a skin graft (as the subcutaneous fat associated with using abdominal skin generally is too bulky fot this site), or if there is extensive skin loss, then a radial free flap or lateral thigh free flap.

SUMMARY OF PROCEDURES

	Maxillectomy	Orbital Resection
Position	Head raised 30°, back raised (reduces bleeding)	⇐
Incision	Same as external sinus approach; combinable with intraoral incisions.	Eyelash incision; if necessary add external ethmoidectomy
Special instrumentation	Paranasal sinus set; headlight	⇐

SUMMARY OF PROCEDURES (cont'd)

	Maxillectomy	Orbital Resection
Unique considerations	Nasal packing	⇐; see reconstruction
Antibiotics	Cefazolin 1 gm + metronidazole 500 mg; or clindamycin 600 mg	Cefazolin 1 gm
Surgical time	2–4 h	1.5–3 h
EBL	100–300 mL	25–100 mL
Postop care	Same as endoscopic surgery	Reconstruction-dependent
Mortality	Rare	Very rare
Morbidity	Bleeding: 5% Transient Diplopia: 5% Infection: 5%	⇐ ⇐
Pain score	2–3 if no oral entry; 4–6 if palate	2–4

PATIENT POPULATION CHARACTERISTICS

Age range	50–70	40–80
Male:Female	3:1	2:1
Incidence	Common	⇐
Etiology	malignant tumors, selected benign tumors	Malignancies, rare benign proceses
Associated Conditions	Tobacco, alcohol, rare others	⇐

ANESTHETIC CONSIDERATIONS

PREOPERATIVE

Typically, these patients are older males who may have concomitant cardiopulmonary disease. Their nutritinal status is not usually affected.

Airway	For patients presenting for maxilloectomy, careful inspection is warranted, although it is unlikely that the disease process will → airway compromise. With large tumors, space available for laryngoscope blade manipulation may be somewhat decreased. XRT typically is done postop.
Cardiovascular	Preop evaluation should focus on the patient's suitability for controlled ↓ BP: may be contraindicated in patients with advanced cerebrovascular or cardiovascular disease. **Tests:** ECG; other tests as indicated from H&P.
Laboratory	Tests as indicated from H&P.
Premedication	Standard premedication (p. B-1).

INTRAOPERATIVE

Anesthetic technique: GETA. Frequently, the typical anterior cranial base surgery begins with bifrontal craniotomy (usual craniotomy considerations apply), followed by the surgical work on the paranasal sinuses, occasionally supplemented with a transethmoid incision. With that approach, the intraop surgical navigation set is frequently used, and a lumbar drain is placed after induction of anesthesia. Four percent cocaine is usually applied to the nasal passages by the surgeon →↑ BP & dysrhythmias. These procedures can be lengthy and very stimulating; the use of potent opioids (see Introduction, p. 174) is beneficial. The essential surgical requirement is ↓ bleeding into the field. Intraop hemorrhage may occasionally be brisk and substantial (in excess of 500 cc) during maxillectomy. Maintaining adequate circulating volume is crucial. Promotion of rapid awakening with full return of protective airway reflexes presents additional challenges to the anesthesiologist.

Induction	An opioid-based technique, as outlined previously (see Introduction, p. 174). Any iv induction agent can be safely used; ↓ dose in elderly and patients with significant cardiac disease. Oral tracheal intubation is performed with a small (6.0 mm ID) reinforced ETT to facilitate surgical manipulation inside patient's mouth. With large tumors, especially on the right side, care is necessary when performing DL to avoid bleeding. ETT can be secured with a short piece of tape over the chin. Placement of a small diameter esophageal temperature probe will not interfere with the surgical field.	
Maintenance	Moderate ↓ BP (unless contraindicated) usually is accomplished by titration with an inhalational agent and/or β-blockers. It is the author's preference to use desflurane for these procedures to rapidly adjust the depth of anesthesia. The use of IV remifentanil for the purpose of facilitating hemodynamic stability and controlled hypotension is highly beneficial. After the specimen has been removed, surgical stimulation decreases and the inhalational anesthetic should be significantly reduced to promote rapid awakening.	
Emergence	The stomach should be routinely suctioned at the end of the case (throat pack is removed only by the surgeon to facilitate placement of a dental prosthesis). Stomach emptying should be facilitated by administration of IV metoclopromide (10–20 mg). Nasal passages may be packed → obligate mouth breathing; oropharynx must be suctioned thoroughly and carefully. No dressing is applied postop. Washing blood off patient's face at the end of surgery is frequently accompanied by vigorous movement/shaking of the patient's head and the in-situ ETT. If sufficient doses of opioids have been used, patient will tolerate this well, without coughing/gagging/straining, while breathing spontaneously. Extubation must be smooth, with full return of protective airway reflexes. Hemoptysis may occur after extubation and the patient's mouth should be promptly covered with an O_2 mask, to avoid contamination.	
Blood and fluid requirements	IV: 16 ga × 1	Blood loss minimal-to-severe. It can be sudden and substantial.
Monitoring	LR @ 5–7 cc/kg/h Standard monitors (p. B-1) ± Arterial line	A-line monitoring is warranted for anterior cranial base surgery or in patients with significant cardiovascular disease.
Positioning	Head elevated 20–30° Table may be turned 90–180°. ✓ and pad pressure points. ✓ eyes.	
Complications	VAE	A risk of air embolism, with surgery on the paranasal sinuses should be kept in mind.
	Dysrhythmias	Dysrhythmias may occur 2° significant surgical stimulation and break-through adrenergic responses.
	Hypotension	↓ BP may be sudden 2° brisk blood loss.
	↓↓ HR	Trigeminocardiac reflex may occur during intraoperative manipulation of the trigeminal nerve.
	Brain edema	Careful fluid management, not to promote/exacerbate brain edema associated with the bifrontal craniotomy.

POSTOPERATIVE

Complications	Occult postop bleeding	Postop bleeding may cause the patient to swallow large quantities of blood, which represent an aspiration risk and may manifest as ↓ BP.
	Pneumocephalus	Persistent pneumocephalus (if the paranasal sinuses were opened) with symptoms of increased ICP.
Pain management	PCA (p. C-3) Parenteral opioids (p. C-2)	Pain is moderate

Suggested Readings

1. Donlon JV, Feldman MA: Anesthesia for eye, ear, nose, and throat surgery. In *Miller's Anesthesia,* 6th edition. Miller RD, ed. Philadelphia: Elsevier/Churchhill Livingstone, Philadelphia: 2005, 2527–49.
2. Dougherty TB, Nguyen DT: Anesthetic management of the patient scheduled for head and neck cancer surgery. *J Clin Anesth* 1994; 6:74–82.

COMPOSITE RESECTION WITH MARGINAL OR SEGMENTAL MANDIBULECTOMY (AND NECK DISSECTION)

SURGICAL CONSIDERATIONS

Description: A composite resection means that part of the mandibular alveolar ridge is resected, often along with the floor of mouth and a part of the tongue, generally for advanced squamous cell carcinoma, though occasionally for osteoradionecrosis following complications of prior irradiation or for other malignancies such as osteosarcoma. In a **marginal mandibulectomy** bone inferior to the plane of the inferior alveolar nerve (which runs just below the teeth and provides dental innervation and cutaneous sensation to the lower lip and chin) is preserved. In a **segmental mandibulectomy** a through-and-through segment of bone is removed such that there is a bone gap. A marginal mandibulectomy may at times be reconstructed with intraoral advancement flaps in an edentulous patient, or a pectoralis major myocutaneous flap or radial free flap may be indicated. A segmental resection requires either bone replacement, such as fibula free flap, or a titanium bridging bar beneath a pectoralis major myocutaneous flap. A composite resection generally requires a tracheostomy although an intraoral marginal mandibulectomy repaired locally may allow a 2–3 d intubation, thereby avoiding tracheostomy.

SUMMARY OF PROCEDURE

	Composite Resection (often with MRND)	. . . and Free Flap
Position	Supine, head extended and turned to opposite side.	⇐ + Preparation of 2nd sterile site, such as arm or leg; two surgical teams
Incision	Intraoral and neck	⇐ and donor site
Special Instrumentation	Depends on technique used; headlights, suction or suction cautery, mouth gag.	Surgeon-specific, but point cautery, mouth gag, and plastic bilateral cheek retractor common.
Unique Considerations	Armored ETT converted to, or initial, tracheostomy.	Dependent on 2nd site
Antibiotics	Common is ampicillin or cefazolin 1gm [± metronidazole 500 mg]; or clindamycin 600 mg	⇐

SUMMARY OF PROCEDURE (cont'd)

	Composite Resection (often with MRND)	. . . and Free Flap
Surgical time	6–8 h	⇐ Add 3–6 h
EBL	200–400 mL; transfusions uncommon	⇐ ; little additional loss
Postop care	Drain management, monitor for wound breakdown	⇐ + ICU for flap surveillance
Mortality	<1%	⇐
Morbidity	Bleeding: < 4% Infection ± fisuta: < 10% DVT/PE: < 1% medical: MI < 1% pneumonia: < 3%	⇐ flap failure requiring return to OR < 5% donor site morbidity
Pain Score	4–8	⇐

PATIENT POPULATION CHARACTERISTICS

Age range	40–70, occasionally older and younger	⇐
Male:Female	3:1	⇐
Incidence	Common	⇐
Etiology	SCC and other malignancy	⇐
Associated conditions	Smoking and alcohol; COPD, atherosclerostic heart disease	⇐

NECK DISSECTION

Description: The goal of a neck dissection is a lymphadenectomy either to remove known cervical metastases (an N_+ neck) or as a staging procedure in a patient apparently without clinically or radiologically involved nodes (an N_0 neck) but at significant risk nevertheless. The most common indication by far is in the management of squamous cell carcinoma (SCC) of the head and neck. For the purpose of discussing a neck dissection, the neck can be divided into five levels. Level 1 is the tissue that is inferior to the mandible, anterior to the posterior belly of the digastric muscle, and superior to the hyoid bone, including the submental triangle between the left and right anterior belly of the digastric muscles. The most prominent structure in level 1 is the submandibular gland. Level 2 through 4 includes the tissue beneath and anterior to the sterncleidomastoid muscle (SCM): level 2 is superior to the hyoid bone, level 3 between the hyoid and cricoid bone, and level 4 is inferior to the cricoid. Level 5 contains the tissue between the posterior edge of the SCM and the anterior edge of the trapezius muscle.

There are several different kinds of neck dissection, depending on which levels are removed:

(a) **Radical neck dissection (RND)** or **modified radical neck dissection** (**MRND**): this involves the removal of levels 1–5. Except in markedly advanced disease, seldom is a RND (which removes the internal jugular vein, SCM, and accessory (XI) nerve) necessary. A MRND preserves one or more of those three structures, generally at least the XI nerve. The term *functional* neck dissection is sometimes used to indicate preservation of all three of these three structures. A MRND (or RND) is generally done when there is N_+ disease. Similar surgery may also be necessary to remove extensive tumors other than SCC, such as a sarcoma or paraganglioma. An extended neck dissection involves removal of additional tissue, such as muscles deep to the superficial layer of the deep cervical fascia. MRND is a common additional procedure done for an N_+ neck at the time of removal of a primary SCC of the head and neck.

(b) **Selective neck dissection** (SND) removes less than all five levels, generally for N_0 disease when adjacent surgery is planned or in an effort to ascertain there is no histologically demonstrable disease, thereby avoiding postop irradiation to the primary site and neck. The two most common types of SND are:

i. **Supraomohyoid neck dissection (SOHND)**: this removes levels 1–3, generally in a patient with an oral cavity SCC with a depth of greater than 3.5- to 5-mm at risk for nodal involvement despite a clinically N_0 neck.

ii. **Lateral neck dissection:** removes levels 2–4, generally in N_0 patient with glottic or supraglottic carcinoma in whom, again, it is hoped that postop RT may be avoided.

SUMMARY OF PROCEDURES

	MRND (or RND)	SOHND
Position	Supine, head extended and turned to opposite side; table 90° or 180°.	⇐
Incision	Common incisions include a reverse hockey (submandibular RSTL to mastoid tip then extended inferiorly); utility/hockey; superior and inferior neck RSTL (McFee).	~7 cm RSTL (resting skin tension line) incision 3 cm inferior to the mandible, beginning anterior to SCM extending toward the mentum.
Special Instrumentation	Major head & neck set; headlights	⇐
Unique Considerations	Avoid paralysis until after marginal mandibular nerve and XI identified. If bilateral, laryngeal edema may occur; dissection near carotid body and vagus may produce transient bradycardia.	⇐
Antibiotics	Cefazolin 1gm [and metronidazole 500 mg if UADT entry planned]; or clindamycin 600 mg	⇐
Surgical time	2–4 h	1.5 h
EBL	50–250 mL; transfusions rarely indicated	⇐
Postop care	Drain management	⇐
Mortality	< 1%	⇐
Morbidity	Unanticipated neuropathy (e.g., XII, X, VII marginal branch, recurrent laryngeal nerve and phrenic nerve) < 1%; chyle leak < 2% Hematoma < 4% Infection < 5% DVT/PE ~1% XI weakness expected Shoulder pain ~20%	⇐
Pain Score	4–8	2–4

PATIENT POPULATION CHARACTERISTICS

Age range	40–80, occasionally older and younger	⇐
Male:Female	3:1	⇐
Incidence	Common	⇐
Etiology	1° site SCC; Smoking and alcohol	⇐
Associated conditions	COPD, atherosclerostic heart disease	⇐

ANESTHETIC CONSIDERATIONS

PREOPERATIVE

Many of these patients are older males with a long Hx of heavy smoking and ETOH use, and have a high incidence of associated cardiopulmonary diseases. Nutritional status of the patients may be poor and should be optimized before surgery. Neck dissections are lengthy, but are rarely associated with significant blood loss, except in patients who have undergone radiation therapy.

Airway	Airway management may be difficult 2° limited head and neck mobility, ↓ mouth opening, distorted airway, ↓ pharyngeal space and fixation of tissues 2° tumor expansion, radiation fibrosis or previous surgeries. Backup plans for airway management are essential, and a review of preop findings on indirect laryngoscopy and/or CT scan with the surgeon may be helpful in planning a strategy for intubation. If a difficult intubation is foreseen, awake FOI may be the technique of choice (see Anesthetic Considerations for Laryngectomy, p. 202). Emergent tracheostomy may technically be very difficult 2° advanced disease, neck edema, previous surgeries and distorted anatomy.
Respiratory	High incidence of chronic bronchitis and COPD. **Tests:** CXR; preop ABG in patients with advanced COPD, CO_2 retention and O_2-dependence. Flow-volume loops may be helpful in patients with symptoms of partial airway obstruction.
Cardiovascular	Careful assessment of cardiac risk factors and functional status. Documenting asymptomatic neck bruits or existing carotid artery stenosis, as well as any Sx of compromised cerebral circulation is important (see Emergence, below). HTN must be controlled preop especially in patients presenting for radical neck dissection and flap reconstruction. Uncontrolled HTN in these patients carries additional risk of exaggerated hemodynamic responses postop 2° surgical denervation of the carotid sinus (discussed below). **Tests:** ECG. Consider carotid ultrasound, cardiac stress testing and imaging studies if indicated from H&P.
Neurologic	See Preoperative Considerations for Laryngoscopy/Bronchoscopy/Esophagoscopy, p. 180). **Tests:** As indicated from H&P.
Hematologic	In cases of malignancy or chronic disease, anemia or coagulopathies may be present. **Tests:** CBC, coagulation studies.
Laboratory	LFTs, electrolytes, albumin, BUN and creatinine. Other tests as indicated from H&P.
Premedication	Standard premedication (p. B-1). Avoid premedication in patients with symptoms of partial airway obstruction.

INTRAOPERATIVE

Anesthetic technique: The anesthetic considerations for **composite resection and neck dissection** are similar. The use of deep and superficial cervical plexus blocks, as well as cervical epidural anesthesia, either alone or in combination with light GETA, has been described in the literature, but used rarely. GETA is virtually universally employed. The specific surgical requirements for the anesthetic technique are outlined above (see Introduction, p. 174). Straining or coughing/gagging on the ETT during emergence from anesthesia is particularly undesirable in neck surgery 2° easily provoked bleeding and swelling at the surgical site. Smooth emergence from anesthesia is essential. Use of a FLMA in major cancer neck surgery is dubious.

Induction	Choice of induction will depend on the degree of the airway compromise and anatomical location of any obstructing lesion. The airway may need to be secured asleep, with the patient breathing spontaneously, awake (FOI), or a tracheostomy may need to be

Induction (cont'd)	performed pre-induction. In patients with uncompromised airways, potent opioids (see Introduction, p. 174) can be safely used for induction. The induction dose of a hypnotic agent frequently must be reduced because of the patients' age, pre-existing medical conditions, and hypoalbuminemia.	
Maintenance	Maintaining moderate ↓ BP (see Introduction, p. 174) and aggressive treatment of ↑ BP are necessary. In patients with flap reconstruction, ↑ BP may overcome vasospasm, dislodging a hemostatic blood clot or poorly tied ligature → formation of a flap hematoma. Muscle relaxation is usually avoided to facilitate identification of nerves. All inspired gases should be humidified to minimize ↓ T° and propensity for mucous plugging in this patient population. However, the use of low gas flows is preferred to use of an in-circuit humidifier. Venous air embolism (VAE) during radical neck surgery occurs very rarely; maintaining adequate intravascular volume and PPV will further ↓ the incidence of this complication. If a large collection of air bubbles is observed by the surgeon in the internal jugular vein, the anesthesiologist should be notified immediately; these bubbles can be safely aspirated with a fine needle by the surgeon. Vagal reflexes from the carotid sinus may cause ↓ HR and ↓ BP. Transient prolongation of the QT interval during right radical neck dissection has been described, and may potentially progress to ventricular arrhythmias and even cardiac arrest. Tracheostomy can be performed as part of the radical neck dissection with implications for anesthesia management (see Anesthetic Considerations for Tracheostomy, p. 187).	
Emergence	If airway compromise is present preop, but tracheostomy was **not** performed, consider extubating the patient over an airway exchange catheter to facilitate for possible re-intubation. The majority of patients with microvascular flap reconstruction will have a tracheostomy placed and continued on overnight ventilatory support in the ICU. Other patients with a tracheostomy should be awakened in the OR, to exclude possible intraop embolic stroke (carotid atherosclerosis) before their transfer to the PACU or ICU. Administration of iv labetalol before awakening may prevent rebound hypertension. Up to 10% of patients may develop a sustained hypertensive response postop, probably 2° denervation of the carotid sinus; Rx aggressively 2° ↑ risk of stroke.	
Blood and fluid requirements	IV: 16(18) ga x 1 NS/LR @ 5–7mL/kg/h Fluid warmer ± humidifier	Blood loss is typically gradual. Sudden blood loss resulting from injury to the internal jugular vein or carotid artery can be surgically controlled.
Control of blood loss	Surgical hemostasis Deliberate ↓ BP	Continue aggressive Rx of ↑ BP in the PACU.
Monitoring	Standard monitors (p. B-1) ± Arterial line ± CVP line Foley catheter	A-line may be indicated for patients with pre-existing severe cardiac and pulmonary disease, chronic renal insufficiency (CRI), symptoms of cerebrovascular insufficiency, location of tumor near the carotid artery, or in patients presenting for lengthy procedures, including microvascular flap reconstruction. CVP monitoring may be warranted in severely malnourished patients, patients with severe COPD, patients with CRI and patients presenting for microvascular flap reconstruction.
Positioning	Usually supine, head elevated 30° Table turned 180° ✓ and pad pressure points. ✓ eyes.	
Complications	Vagal reflexes: ↓ HR and ↓ BP	2° carotid sinus stimulation; Rx: stop surgery; lidocaine infiltration of the carotid sinus by the surgeon; iv atropine.

Complications (cont'd)	↑ QT interval (with right radical neck dissection) Dysrhythmias	Probably caused by interruption of cervical sympathetic outflow to heart. Due to either the carotid sinus stimulation or the ↑ QT interval.
VAE	↓ $ETCO_2$ ↑ ETN_2 ↓ BP ↑ ST segment "Mill wheel" murmur Dysrhythmias	With large veins open in the neck, VAE is possible, and may account for unexplained ↓ BP and/or dysrhythmia. Rx: notify surgeon (compress open neck veins); flood field with NS; left lateral decubitus/head-down position; aspirate CVP; FiO_2=1.0; circulatory support (fluid, pressors, as required).

POSTOPERATIVE

Complications	↑ BP and ↑ HR	2° carotid sinus denervation; Rx: aggressive pharmacological intervention.
	Nerve injury Diaphragmatic paralysis	Facial nerve injury → facial droop. Recurrent laryngeal nerve injury can result in VC dysfunction. Phrenic nerve injury → respiratory problems 2° diaphragmatic paralysis.
	Pneumothorax	Pneumothorax may occur with low neck dissection. Dx and Rx: see Postop Complications after Laryngoscopy/Bronchoscopy/Esophagoscopy, p. 187
	Agitation	Agitation → ↑$PaCO_2$, ↓PaO_2, ↑HR. Rx: ✓ restrictive neck dressings; evacuate any hematoma; reestablish airway with ETT; FiO_2=1.0; ventilatory support, if required.
Pain management	PCA (p. C-3) Parenteral opiates (p. C-1)	
Tests	CXR	For position of tracheostomy tube, evidence of pneumothorax and CVP line placement.
	ECG	For diagnosis of rhythm disturbances.

Suggested Readings

1. Bonner S, Taylor M:Airway obstruction in head and neck surgery. *Anaesthesia* 2000; 55:290–1.
2. Brown BR: Anaesthesia for ear, nose, throat and maxillofacial procedures. In *International Practice of Anaesthesia*. Prys-Roberts C, Brown BR, eds. Butterworth-Heinemann, Oxford: 1996, 2–9.
3. Dougherty TB, Nguyen DT: Anesthetic management of the patient scheduled for head and neck cancer surgery. *J Clin Anesth* 1994; 6:74–82.
4. Mason RA, Fielder CP: The obstructed airway in head and neck surgery. *Anaesthesia* 1999; 54:625–8.
5. McGuirt WF, May JS: Postoperative hypertension associated with radical neck dissection. *Arch Otolaryngol Head Neck Surg* 1987; 113:1098–110.
6. Prasad KC, Shanmugam VU: Major neck surgeries under regional anesthesia. *Am J Otol* 1998; 19:163–9.
7. Rice JH, Gonzalez RM: Large visible gas bubbles in the internal jugular vein: a common occurrence during supine radical neck surgery? *J Clin Anesth* 1992; 4:21–4.
8. Rice M, Turner M, Carapiet D: The use of the laryngeal mask airway in maxillofacial surgery. *Anaesthesia* 2002; 57:826.
9. Wittich DJ, Berny JJ, Davis RK: Cervical epidural anesthesia for head and neck surgery. *Laryngoscope* 1984; 94:615–9.

LYMPH NODE BIOPSY

SURGICAL CONSIDERATIONS

Description: An open cervical node biopsy is indicated when a fine needle aspiration biopsy (FNA) has proven inadequate or is felt likely to be inadequate (as in determining a type of lymphoma). This can be done under local anesthesia, with or without monitoring, or under general anesthesia. A node is chosen based on its likelihood to answer the clinical question and minimization of operative risk to adjacent structures, especially, for example, the accesory nerve that runs in level 5 (posterior triangle) from about the midportion of the posterior border of the SCM toward the posterior clavicle and may be quite superficial.

Operative and anesthesia considerations are similar to that of a SOHND, except that the incision should be only a few cm and its location is variable though still in a RSTL (resting skin tension line), pain should be low, a small drain or no drain is used, and the patient should be able to go home the day of surgery. Often the surgeon will request a frozen section to be sure there is diagnostic tissue available.

SUMMARY OF PROCEDURE	
Position	Supine, head extended and turned to opposite side
Incision	small (often requiring only local anesthesia)
Antibiotics	Cefazolin 1gm
Surgical Time	10 min
EBL	minimal
Postop Care	Drain management
Mortality	Very rare
Morbidity	rare injury to adjacent structures (e.g., accessory nerve)
Pain Score	1–3

PATIENT POPULATION CHARACTERISTICS	
Age range	wide range
Male:Female	1:1
Incidence	Common
Etiology	In adults: 80% benign: pleomorphic adenoma (benign mixed tumor) 75% of these. 20% malignant: low grade mucoepidermoid carcinoma, adenoid cystic carcinoma, other. Chronic sialadenitis/stone rare In children: a greater % malignancy; 60% benign, 35% malignant. Chronic sialadenitis/stone <5%
Associated conditions	none

Suggested Reading

1. Nair MB, Bailey PM: Review of uses of the laryngeal mask in ENT anesthesia. *Anaesthesia* 1995; 50:898–900.

PAROTIDECTOMY: SUPERFICIAL, TOTAL, OR RADICAL

SURGICAL CONSIDERATIONS

Description: A **superficial parotidectomy** (more accurately a lateral or a **supraneural parotidectomy**) removes tissue of the parotid lateral to the facial nerve, dissecting and protecting the facial nerve (Fig. 3-8). It usually is performed for a tumor, but occasionally is performed for infectious disorders or to enable the surgeon to approach tumors of the deep lobe. A **total parotidectomy** is performed for either infectious disorders or for parotid tumors that arise in or extend medial to the facial nerve. The integrity of the facial nerve is preserved during total parotidectomy, as long as it is not involved with malignancy. It may be combined with a neck dissection or with a modified temporal bone resection when the tumor extends into the ear canal or middle ear or invades the facial nerve at the base of the skull.

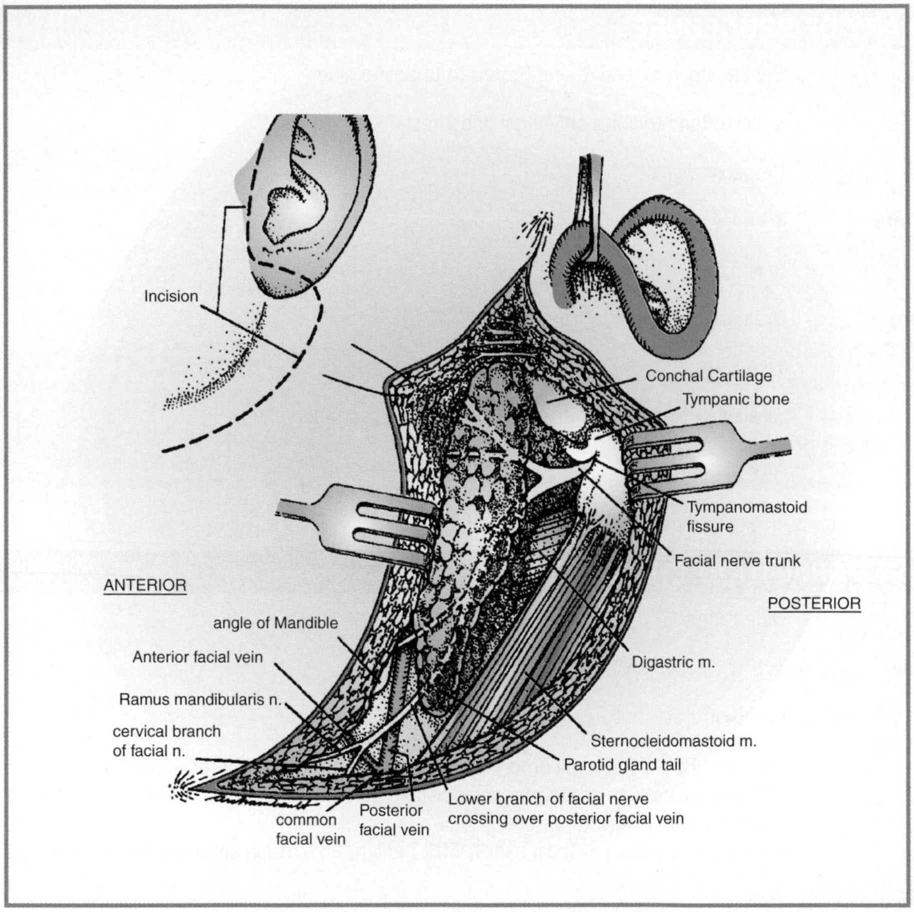

Figure 3-8. Inferior approach to facial nerve. The lower branch of the facial nerve is found immediately external to the posterior facial vein as it exits the lower pole of the parotid gland. The lower branch may divide into the ramus mandibularis and cervical branches before or after crossing the posterior facial vein. The lower branch of the facial nerve is dissected proximally to the facial-nerve trunk. The posterior facial vein should not be confused with the external jugular vein, as the facial vein runs deep to the sternocleidomastoid muscle, whereas the external jugular vein lies superficial to this muscle. Elevation of the tail of the parotid gland greatly facilitates this dissection, which must be accomplished in a plane between the posterior facial vein and the parotid gland. (Reproduced with permission from Montgomery WW: *Surgery of the Upper Respiratory System,* 3rd edition. Williams & Wilkins, Baltimore: 1996.)

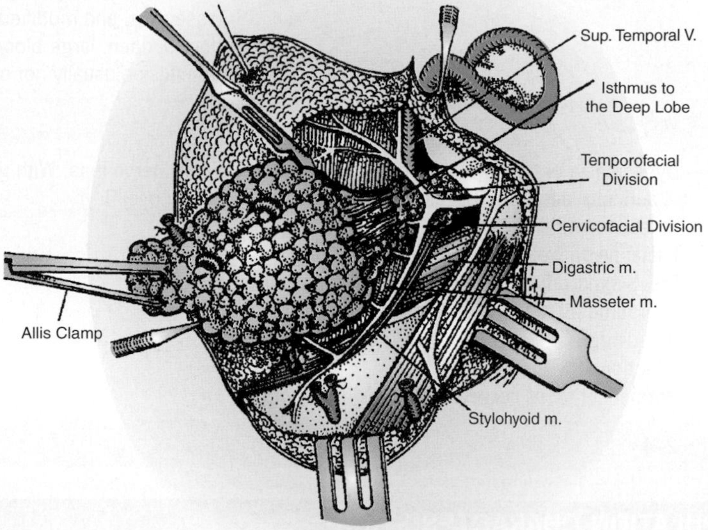

Figure 3-9. The parotid gland has been dissected from the trunk, divisions, and branches of the facial nerve. The anterior projection of the gland has been dissected free, and the parotid duct is being ligated. This dissection is conducted, for the most part, with a hemostat clamp. First, tunnels are created lateral to the branches; and the fascia between tunnels is incised as the gland is dissected forward. The facial-nerve stimulator is a useful adjunct to this dissection. (Reproduced with permission from Montgomery WW: *Surgery of the Upper Respiratory System,* 3rd edition. Williams & Wilkins, Baltimore: 1996.)

A **radical parotidectomy** removes the total parotid gland, together with the facial nerve, (which usually is reconstructed with a facial-nerve graft). The mastoid may have to be drilled to get a healthy proximal end of the facial nerve. **Microsurgical techniques** are then used to graft the resected nerve. The donar nerve may be the greater auricular nerve or the sural nerve.

Usual preop diagnosis: Benign or malignant tumor; occasionally infectious.

SUMMARY OF PROCEDURES

	Superficial/Total	Radical
Position	Supine; head turned slightly to opposite side	⇐
Incision	Preauricular, extending into neck; has many variations, including modified face-lift incision.	May require postaural extension for mastoid access.
Special instrumentation	Facial nerve stimulator, facial nerve monitor.	⇐+ drill for mastoidectomy; microscope/microsurgical instruments and 9-0 nylon for nerve reanastomosis.
Unique considerations	Initial muscle relaxation is not indicated 2° facial nerve identification. Tape oral ETT to the opposite side of the mandible.	⇐
Antibiotics	Cefazolin 1 g	⇐
Surgical time	1.5–4 h	4–8 h

SUMMARY OF PROCEDURES (cont'd)

	Superficial/Total	Radical
EBL	25–200 mL	500–700 mL for total parotidectomy, neck dissection, and modified temporal bone resection. Sudden, large blood losses do not occur; transfusion usually not necessary.
Mortality	Very rare	⇐
Morbidity	Dysesthesia or anesthesia of the greater auricular nerve: 100% (almost all will recover within 1 yr). Facial nerve weakness (temporary): 20–50% Frey's syndrome: < 5% will have clinically both ersome gustatory sweating. Bleeding: 4% Infection: 4% Permanent facial nerve paralysis: < 1%	Facial nerve loss: With graft, function returns slowly over 1 yr. ⇐ ⇐ ⇐ ⇐ ⇐
Pain score	2–4	4–6

PATIENT POPULATION CHARACTERISTICS

Age range	Infants–old age
Male:Female	1:1
Incidence	Common
Etiology	Benign mixed tumor (pleomorphic adenoma) (75%); variety of low- to high-grade malignant cancers (25%); chronic sialoadenitis (results from ductal strictures and/or stones) (rare)
Associated conditions	Nonspecific

SUBMANDIBULAR GLAND EXCISION

SURGICAL CONSIDERATIONS

Description: Removal of the submandibular gland is performed for either chronic sialoadenitis due to ductal strictures and/or stones or benign or malignant tumors of the submandibular gland. (General anatomy of the area is shown in Fig. 3-10.) The patient lies supine with a pillow under the shoulder, and head turned slightly to the opposite side. A skin crease incision is made below the mandible and skin flaps elevated. The marginal mandibular nerve is identified or may be avoided by identifying the facial vein and dissecting deep to its plane, employing the **Hayes-Martin maneuver.** Dissection is carried out within the capsule of the submandibular gland, which is then excised and removed. Frozen section usually is performed; and, if necessary, further excision, including a neck dissection for high-grade malignancies, is done.

Variant procedure or approaches: Occasionally, it may be necessary to perform a **neck dissection** (radical or functional) in the case of high-grade malignancy.

Usual preop diagnosis: Chronic sialoadenitis; stones; benign or malignant tumors

SUMMARY OF PROCEDURE

Position	Supine
Incision	Upper neck skin crease

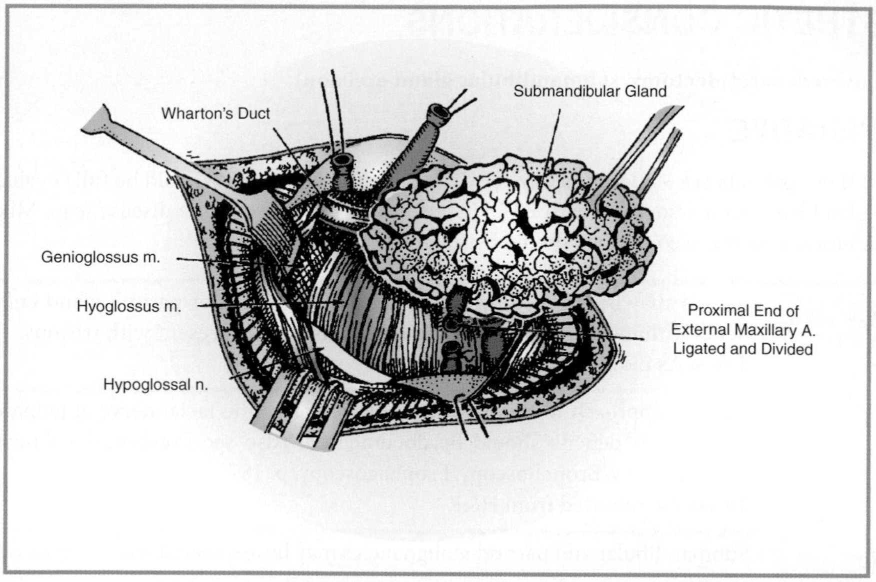

Figure 3-10. Exposure of the submandibular gland. (Reproduced with permission from Montgomery WW: *Surgery of the Upper Respiratory System,* 3rd edition. Williams & Wilkins, Baltimore: 1996.)

SUMMARY OF PROCEDURE (cont'd)

Special instrumentation	Occasionally, facial nerve stimulator
Unique considerations	If surgeon plans to use facial nerve stimulator, muscle relaxation is contraindicated.
Antibiotics	Usually not indicated
Surgical time	0.5–1 h
EBL	25 mL (400 mL if neck dissection is done)
Postop care	PACU → room or home
Mortality	Minimal
Morbidity	Marginal mandibular nerve paresis or paralysis: 20% Bleeding: 4% Infection: 4% Lingual dysesthesia: 1% XIIth nerve paresis or paralysis: ≤1%
Pain score	2–4

PATIENT POPULATION CHARACTERISTICS

Age range	Unlimited
Male:Female	1:1
Incidence	Rare
Etiology	Chronic infection Neoplasia: ~60% of tumors are benign with the remaining being low- and high-grade malignancies.
Associated conditions	Nonspecific

Otolaryngology—Head and Neck Surgery

ANESTHETIC CONSIDERATIONS

(Procedures covered: parotidectomy, submandibular gland excision)

PREOPERATIVE

The majority of these patients are > 40 yr, and any coexisting medical conditions should be fully evaluated. Diseases of the parotid gland have been associated with ETOH abuse and with autoimmune disease (e.g., Mikulicz-Sjögren syndrome); therefore, Sx of these conditions should be sought.

Respiratory	Airway may be affected by impaired mouth opening or parotid gland enlargement. Patients with involvement of the masseter muscle may present with trismus. **Tests:** As indicated from H&P.
Neurological	Surgical approach to the parotid gland will place the facial nerve at jeopardy; any preop facial nerve deficits should be documented. Also see Preoperative Considerations for Laryngoscopy/Bronchoscopy/Esophagoscopy, p. 187. **Tests:** As indicated from H&P.
Hematologic	Submandibular and parotid malignancies may be associated with chronic debilitation and anemia. **Tests:** CBC
Laboratory	Other tests as indicated from H&P. Liver panel and coags in patients with Hx of ETOH abuse.
Premedication	Standard premedication (p. B-1)

INTRAOPERATIVE

Anesthetic technique: GETA is most commonly used. Use of a FLMA also has been advocated, but does not represent the author's preference due to the possibility of distorted surgical anatomy by the inflated FLMA cuff. The FLMA also may be displaced 2° surgical intrusion into the submandibular space and occasional intraoral surgical manipulation. These procedures involve meticulous surgical dissection and are characterized by alternating levels of stimulation: relatively long, stable levels of stimulation, with sudden adrenergic responses when surgery progresses into deeper fascial planes. (For essential surgical requirements, see Introduction, p. 174.) Emergence should be rapid enough to allow immediate patient cooperation for assessment of facial nerve function by the surgeon. Muscle relaxation with nondepolarizing NMB may or may not be contraindicated, depending on the surgeon's preference and type of surgery performed (inquire preop). Patients after **submandibular gland resection** may be discharged home the same day, while parotidectomy patients are admitted to the ward.

Induction	Opioid-based techniques (see Introduction, p. 174) are beneficial. Standard IV induction with propofol (1–2 mg/kg) is typically employed. ETT should be carefully secured on the nonoperative side. Nasal intubation may be requested by the surgeon (inquire preop) for selected cases, to allow full manipulation of the patient's jaw.	
Maintenance	Moderate ↓ BP (see Introduction, p. 174) will greatly improve operating conditions and speed up the surgery. Anticipate ↑ anesthetic requirements in patients with Hx of ETOH abuse. If nondepolarizing NMBs are used, maintain one twitch to permit quick reversal of the block if requested.	
Emergence	Smooth emergence is extremely desirable and absence of reaction to the ETT is obligatory if facial nerve repair has been performed.	
Blood and fluid requirements	EBL typically ~200 mL IV: 18 ga × 1 NS/LR @ 3–5 mL/kg/h	3rd spacing is usually minimal.
Monitoring	Standard monitors (p. B-1)	

Positioning	Table usually is rotated 90–180° away from the anesthesiologist. ✓ pad pressure points. ✓ eyes.

POSTOPERATIVE

Complications	Facial paralysis 2° surgical trauma	Notify surgeons.
Pain management	Parenteral opiates (p. C-2) PCA (p. C-3)	

Suggested Readings

1. Donlon JV, Feldman MA: Anesthesia for eye, ear, nose, and throat surgery. In *Miller's Anesthesia*, 6th edition. Miller RD, ed. Elsevier, Philadelphia: 2005, pp…
2. Nair MB, Bailey PM. Review of uses of the laryngeal mask in ENT anesthesia. Anaesthesia 1995;50:898–900.

ENDOSCOPIC SINUS SURGERY

Peter H. Hwang and Sarmela T. Sunder

SURGICAL CONSIDERATIONS

Description: Sinus surgery is performed most often for the management of chronic sinus disease, nasal polyps, recurrent sinus infections, or for neoplastic conditions that may cause obstruction of the sinus cavities. This surgery includes either external procedures, through the skin or oral cavity, or endoscopic approaches, through the nostrils. The endoscopic approach—the preferred technique for most surgeons—is called **endoscopic sinus surgery (ESS)** or **functional ESS (FESS).** Other surgical procedures—including septoplasty, turbinate reduction, and, occasionally, sleep apnea surgery involving the tonsils, palate, and oropharynx—may be combined with FESS.

Endoscopic Sinus Surgery: ESS or FESS is a minimally invasive technique that utilizes telescopes intranasally to visualize and access the paranasal sinuses and anterior skull base. The primary indication for ESS is chronic sinusitis that has failed to clear with aggressive medical therapy. The goal of ESS is to open the sinuses through a transnasal minimally invasive approach. Inflamed bone and tissue are cleared from the outflow tracts of the sinuses under direct endoscopic illumination and magnification. By surgically enhancing the drainage and ventilation of the sinuses, normal mucociliary clearance can be restored. Depending on the extent of disease, surgery may involve the maxillary, ethmoid, sphenoid and/or frontal sinuses. If all four sinuses are being treated, a maxillary antrostomy is typically performed first, followed by an ethmoidectomy. A sphenoidotomy and frontal sinusotomy usually follow thereafter.

Providing openings (drainage, aeration) to the sinus cavities and obtaining tissue for pathological evaluation are the main aims of ESS. Patients are orally intubated and a throat pack can be placed in the pharynx to decrease the amount of blood swallowed. Oral gastric tubes are recommended if more than minimal bleeding is expected. Following induction of anesthesia, local medications are applied to the nasal cavity, including injection of 1% lidocaine with 1:100,000 epinephrine and/or topical application of 4% cocaine. It is important that these local medications be noted in the anesthesia record, as complications (HTN, dysrhythmias, seizures) from local application have been reported. Patients with a history of illicit cocaine use should be warned of potential drug interactions, and the intraop use of vasoactive drugs should be limited to avoid unexpected cardiovascular events.

At the end of the procedure, packing may be placed. It is imperative that any pharyngeal or throat pack be removed before the end of the procedure to avoid airway destruction.

Sinus surgical procedures may use **image guidance or surgical navigation tools.** These computer-assisted techniques involve a preop CT or MRI scan to create a navigational map for the surgeon to localize disease, normal tissues, and the boundaries of the surgical dissection. Surrounding the sinuses are several vital structures, including the periorbital tissues (e.g., orbital muscles, lacrimal apparatus, and the optic nerve), the sphenopalatine artery, ethmoid arteries, the carotid artery, as well as the skull base.

Variant procedure or approaches: For **external approaches** to sinus surgery, see External Sinus Surgery, p. 231.

Usual preop diagnosis: Nasal polyps; chronic sinusitis; recurrent acute sinus infections, benign and malignant tumors, inverted papilloma, and management of previous surgical complications (e.g., repair of CSF leak, lacrimal duct injury, and persistent or remnant ethmoid cells, scar tissue formation)

Preoperative Management: Patients should receive a decongestant nasal spray, such as oxymetazoline, preop to reduce nasal edema. This is generally given 30 min. before the start of the case, with repeat administration every 10–15 min. Preop antibiotics or steroids will vary depending on surgeon preference. Typically, an antibiotic with gram-positive and some gram-negative coverage (such as cephalexin) and an intravenous steroid such as dexamethasone are administered.

Intraoperative Management: ESS is usually performed under GA, using either endotracheal intubation or an LMA. The LMA offers the potential advantages of reducing the entry of blood into the stomach and causing less bucking or coughing during emergence, (which may provoke unnecessary bleeding from the surgical site). The tube should be taped securely to the left side or midline of the patient's mouth. The OR table is routinely turned 90° or 180°, and the patient is positioned with the head slightly elevated. The surgeon sits or stands at the patient's right and operates from a video monitor positioned at the patient's head.

The eyes are taped but should remain visible in the surgical field throughout the procedure so that the status of the orbits may be noted by the surgeon. The presence of ecchymosis or proptosis suggests a transgression of the thin bony orbital wall and requires immediate attention. Throughout the procedure, the surgeon may palpate the orbit externally while endoscopically evaluating for dehiscences of the orbital wall, which if present will reveal transmitted movement of orbital fat or periorbita.

In more complex FESS or endoscopic skull base surgery, the surgeon may use a stereotactic navigation system to map out the surgical field according to a preoperatively acquired CT or MRI scan. During preparation of the patient, a localizing headset is placed over the patient's forehead, and a computer workstation tower is positioned adjacent to the head of the patient. After a registration process, a navigating probe communicates with the workstation via electromagnetic or infrared technology to provide triplanar localization of the probe tip relative to critical anatomic structures in and adjacent to the sinuses.

Hemostasis is critical in endoscopic sinus surgery, where the small lens of the endoscope (4 mm) can be easily obscured by blood. When possible, a hypotensive anesthesia regimen can reduce bleeding and thereby optimize the surgeon's view of the operative field. It may be reasonable to maintain blood pressure at approximately 80% of the preop level.

To improve hemostasis, the surgeon may place pledgets soaked in a vasoconstrictive agent such as cocaine, oxymetazoline, or epinephrine in the nasal cavity before starting the case. A transoral or transnasal sphenopalatine ganglion block may be performed using 1% lidocaine with 1:100,000 epinephrine, which will provide vasoconstriction of the sphenopalatine artery. The lateral nasal wall and middle turbinate are also infiltrated with lidocaine/epinephrine. Additional vasoconstrictor-soaked pledgets may be placed in the operative field during the procedure to control oozing.

Complications of Endoscopic Sinus Surgery: Along the boundaries of the paranasal sinuses lie important structures that may be injured in the course of the procedure.

Maxillary Sinus: Just anterior to the maxillary sinus ostium lies the **nasolacrimal duct**. Injury to this structure, manifesting as excessive tearing, will not usually be evident until postop.

Ethmoid Sinus: Two critical boundaries of the ethmoid sinus are the medial orbital wall laterally and the skull base superiorly. **Transgression of the orbit** may result in medial rectus injury, prolapse of orbital fat, or orbital hemorrhage. If orbital hemorrhage progresses to the point of marked proptosis, vision may be threatened and an emergent decompression of the orbit may be required via lateral canthotomy and cantholysis.

The superior extent of the ethmoid dissection is the cribriform plate and the anterior skull base. A breach through the ethmoid roof may result in a **cerebrospinal fluid leak**. Cerebrospinal fluid leaks require immediate repair using autogenous tissue grafts and require an inpatient recovery period. Vigorus bag mask ventilation should be avoided in patients with known skull base defects because of the risk of creating a pneumocephalus.

Sphenoid Sinus: The sphenoid sinus, the posterior most of the paranasal sinuses, lies adjacent to critical structures of the parasellar region. The **carotid artery** and **optic nerve** run along the superolateral wall of the sphenoid sinus. Any significant bleeding on entry into or while working in the sphenoid sinus is concerning for potential carotid injury. Carotid artery injury requires emergent tamponade possible, fluid resuscitation, and angiography with embolization.

Frontal Sinus: Endoscopic approaches to the frontal sinus are especially challenging because of the narrowness of the region. Violation of the cribiform plate medially or the orbital wall laterally may lead to complications of **CSF leak** or **eye injury**, respectively.

Postop Management: In the PACU, patients s/p ESS require continued monitoring for possible delayed manifestation of complications. Maintaining normotensive hemodynamics is extremely helpful in controlling postop bleeding. Changing nasal dressings for oozing every 20–30 min is expected, but brisker bleeding should be evaluated by the surgeon for possible arterial sources requiring intervention.

Orbital injury can also present in the postop period with significant pain, diminished visual acuity, diplopia, proptosis, or ecchymosis. Any complaints of eye pain or visual changes need to be addressed urgently. The surgeon must be alerted immediately and an ophthalmology consult should be considered.

Altered mental status, focal neurologic exam, or severe headache may indicate a possible intracranial complication. Clear rhinorrhea, especially unilateral, should be closely evaluated for the possibility of cerebrospinal fluid leak.

SUMMARY OF PROCEDURE

Position	Supine; table 90° or 180°
Incision	Mucosal, intranasal
Special instrumentation	4 mm nasal endoscopes, camera monitor, computer-guided navigation system
Premedication	Cefazolin 1gm, dexamethasone 8–12 mg
Surgical time	1–3 h
EBL	50–300 mL; transfusions rare
Postop care	PACU monitoring for surgical complications; discharge home from PACU
Mortality	Rare
Morbidity	1% major complication rate (see complications of ESS above)
Pain Score	2–3

PATIENT POPULATION CHARACTERISTICS

Age range	15–80
Male:Female	1:1.5
Incidence	Common
Etiology	Medically refractory chronic sinusitis
Associated conditions	Asthma, allergic rhinitis, migraine

Other Applications of Endoscopes in Sinonasal Surgery: Although the most common indication for endoscopic sinus surgery is medically refractory chronic sinusitis, endoscopic techniques can be applied to wide range of sinonasal and skull base pathology. OR setup and patient positioning is identical to that for ESS (except as noted).

Turbinate Reduction: The inferior turbinate is the largest of the nasal turbinates (inferior, middle, superior) and when hypertrophied can cause nasal obstruction. Various methods exist for inferior turbinate reduction and include radiofrequency ablation, cauterization, submucosal resection, partial resection and out-fracture. Both turbinate cauterization and RF ablation involve inserting a probe into the soft tissue of the turbinate and producing a coagulative lesion, which ultimately contracts to reduce the turbinate soft tissue. Similarly, submucosal reduction involves making an incision through the mucosa and mechanically reducing the underlying soft tissue. Partial resection of the turbinate involves cutting through the bone, soft tissue and mucosa of the anterior one-third of the turbinate. At the conclusion, the cut edges are cauterized. The main adverse event from the majority of procedures on the turbinate is bleeding, which is usually controlled with cautery or nasal packing.

Septoplasty: Septal deviation may arise congenitally or during periods of rapid craniofacial growth, or as well from nasal trauma. Septoplasty is indicated when the septal deviation causes obstructed nasal breathing. Through an incision in the nasal vestibule, a mucoperichondrial septal flap is elevated to reveal deflections in the underlying septal cartilage and bone. Selective excision of bone and cartilage allows the septum to return to a midline position. Although the procedure may be performed using direct visualization with a headlight, nasal endoscopy provides superb visualization and allows for precise surgical maneuvering.

Control of Epistaxis: Control of epistaxis can usually be performed in the clinic; however, the OR provides a controlled environment suitable for high risk patients and patients with profuse bleeding. Under endoscopic visualization, bleeding sites can be readily identified and controlled with cautery or laser. A more definitive procedure to control posterior epistaxis is sphenopalatine artery ligation. The artery is identified at the posterior-most aspect of the middle turbinate through a mucoperiosteal incision. The artery is then cauterized or ligated with surgical clips.

Orbital Decompression: Endoscopic orbital decompression is performed for Grave's ophthalmopathy to preserve diminishing vision and to improve cosmesis associated with exophthalmos. An ethmoidectomy is performed first, followed by removal of the medial orbital wall. After adequate exposure is achieved, the orbital periosteum is incised, causing the orbital fat to prolapse into the ethmoid cavity, thereby decompressing the orbit contents. Decompression may be extended to the floor of the orbit if medial decompression alone is insufficient.

Repair of CSF leak: Discontinuity of the anterior skull base, occurring traumatically or spontaneously, may result in CSF rhinorrhea. The defect may be a small crack in the skull base or a larger defect with prolapse of meninges or brain tissue through the defect. The majority of anterior skull base CSF leaks can be closed effectively with endoscopic approaches. Meningoencephaloceles that protrude through a bony skull base defect are reduced with bipolar cautery. After endoscopic visualization of the bony defect, a layered repair is performed using bone or cartilage, followed by a free mucosal graft.

A lumbar subarachnoid drain may be placed prior to starting the case. Fluorescein can be placed through the drain to aid in identifying the leak site during surgery. If fluorescein is used, it must be carefully measured and administered to avoid the neurotoxic effects overdose (accepted dose is 0.1 cc of 10% fluorescein mixed in 10cc of nonbacteriostatic saline, administered slowly over 5 min). Postop, patients remain at bedrest for 1–3 d, typically as an inpatient.

Pituitary Surgery: The application of endoscopic technique to transnasal transphenoidal approaches to the sella provides an excellent panoramic view unavailable with microscopic approaches. Pituitary adenomas, craniopharyngiomas, and other sellar masses are suitable for endoscopic resection. The operating team consists of a neurosurgeon and an otolaryngologist working in concert. The approach is performed by the otolaryngologist, while the tumor resection is performed by the neurosurgeon under endoscopic guidance by the otolaryngologist ("four hands technique"). After performing intraoral greater palatine blocks and topically decongesting the nasal mucosa, the surgeon performing the approach creates bilateral sphenoidotomies. The posterior portion of the septum is then resected, allowing for the subsequent removal of the remainder of the sphenoid rostrum. This provides wide exposure of the sella and parasellar anatomy. The sella is then entered and tumor resection is performed endoscopically.

The dissection of the sella risks injury to the adjacent optic nerve, cavernous sinus, and carotid artery. The anesthesiologist should be prepared to hemodynamically resuscitate the patient in the rare event of a carotid injury. Additional monitoring such as an arterial line may be indicated at the discretion of the anesthesiologist.

A CSF leak may occur if the arachnoid is breached during the tumor resection. This is repaired easily with abdominal fat, fibrin glue, and an absorbable reconstruction plate. In the event of a CSF leak, a lumbar subarachnoid drain may be placed.

ANESTHETIC CONSIDERATIONS

PREOPERATIVE

The majority of these procedures are performed on an outpatient basis. Patients with extensive polypoid disease may be at risk for substantial (> 400 mL) blood loss. Many of these patients will have received a short preop course of steroid therapy to decrease tissue swelling and reduce bleeding intraop. Routine intraop administration of decadron (8–12 mg iv) to minimize postop edema, makes additional stress-dose of glucocorticoids unnecessary.

Respiratory	Many patients with nasal polyposis have a high incidence of reactive airway disease (up to 26%) as well as a hypersensitivity to aspirin, which can precipitate bronchospasm (triad patients). In these patients, NSAIDs, including ketorolac, should be avoided. In general, ketorolac administration for postop pain relief is not recommended in these patients because it may promote microvascular bleeding. **Tests:** CXR, as indicated by H&P.
Cardiovascular	See Anesthetic Considerations for Nasal Surgery, p. 234.
Premedication	See Anesthetic Considerations for Nasal Surgery, p. 234.

INTRAOPERATIVE

Anesthetic technique: **FESS** can be performed under local anesthesia with sedation (MAC) or GA. The essential surgical requirements are similar to those for other types of nasal surgery (see Anesthetic Considerations for Nasal Surgery, p. 234), although more meticulous control of intraop BP is crucial. Local anesthesia offers the advantage of reduced blood loss, but GA is performed more frequently and may be associated with less incidence of surgical complications. Patients with extensive sinus disease, history of multiple previous nasal and sinus surgeries, patients feeling uneasy about being awake, and those with reactive airway disease, or labile HTN may not be candidates for MAC. Use of a FLMA instead of an ETT offers significant advantages (see Introduction, p. 174), including decreasing airway reactivity and improving mucociliary clearance.

Maintaining intraop controlled hypotension (see Introduction, p. 174) is essential for improving surgical visibility and operating conditions. While MAP may largely affect the arterial inflow, other factors including the condition of the vascular network, local mechanisms regulating functional nasal capillary density, and local venous pressure also play a significant role in regulating overall nasal capillary perfusion. As with other types of nasal surgery, these procedures are typically characterized by minimal immediate postop pain 2° submucosal infiltrative local anesthesia used by the surgeon.

Induction	(See Anesthetic Considerations for Nasal Surgery, p. 234). The patient's eyes should be protected in a manner that allows the surgeon to quickly diagnose proptosis in case of inadvertent orbital wall penetration and intraorbital hemorrhage.	
Maintenance	(See Anesthetic Considerations for Nasal Surgery, p. 234). TIVA, with or without nitrous oxide, promotes superior hemodynamic stability and minimizes direct peripheral vasodilation. When additional ↓ BP is required esmolol is preferred over SNP. Break-through adrenergic responses occur more frequently with FESS compared to other types of nasal surgery, because many reflexogenic areas (e.g., skull base) cannot be blocked by infiltrative local anesthesia. These responses can be effectively controlled by vasoactive agents or additional boluses of remifentanil (0.5–1.0 mcg/kg iv). The anesthesiologist should frequently observe the video monitor for signs of possible complications - prolapse of periorbital fat (orbital injury), "wash-out" of blood in the surgical field (CSF leak).	
Emergence	(See Anesthetic Considerations for Nasal Surgery, p. 234). If a dural injury has occurred, a smooth extubation is mandatory.	
Blood and fluid requirements	IV: 20 ga × 1 (unilateral FESS)	Blood loss can be substantial in high- risk patients (as described above).

Blood and fluid requirements (cont'd)	18 ga × 1 (bilateral FESS) NS/LR @ 3–4 cc/kg/h Blood loss generally 100–150 mL	Meticulous surgical technique and the use of injectable vasoconstrictors are essential in reducing intraop bleeding. An IV is usually placed at the side where the surgeon is positioned (patient's right upper extremity).
Monitoring	Standard monitors (p. B-1) BP cuff left arm	Prevent BP cuff from inflating against the surgeon's hands during delicate endoscopic manipulation.
Positioning	Table turned 90–180° Head elevated 15–30° ✓ and pad pressure points ✓ eyes	Patient's arms usually tucked and carefully padded.
Complications	Dysrhythmias Tachycardia	Usually related to use of vasoconstrictor agents; and may present a problem in patients with CAD. Short-acting β-blocker (esmolol 0.5–1.0 mg/kg iv boluses) should be available to blunt these hemodynamic effects.

POSTOPERATIVE

Complications	Occult bleeding	Occult postop bleeding may cause the patient to swallow large quantities of blood (↑ aspiration risk), and repacking the nostrils may be required.
Pain management	Fentanyl 25–50 mcg iv prn is usually sufficient.	Occasionally, pain after FESS may be significant. If external approaches to the sinuses were utilized, higher doses of opioids may be necessary.

Suggested Readings

1. Bhatti MT, Stankiewicz JA: Ophthalmic complications of endoscopic sinus surgery. *Surv Ophthalmol* 2003; 48:389–402.
2. Blackwell KE, Ross DA, Kapur P, et al: Propofol for maintenance of general anesthesia: a technique to limit blood loss during endoscopic sinus surgery. *Am J Otolaryngol* 1993; 14:262–6.
3. Boezaart AP, Van der Merwe J, Coetzee A: Comparison of sodium nitroprusside- and esmolol-induced hypotension for functional endoscopic sinus surgery. *Can J Anesth* 1995; 42:373–6.
4. Bolger WE, Kennedy DW: Surgical complications and postoperative care. In: *Diseases of the Sinuses: Diagnosis and Management.* DW Kennedy, WE Bolger, SJ Zinreich, eds. B.C. Decker, Hamilton: 2001, 303–16.
5. Eberhart LH, Folz BJ, Wulf H, et al: Intravenous anesthesia provides optimal surgical conditions during microscopic and endoscopic sinus surgery. *Laryngoscope* 2003; 113:1369–73.
6. Endrich B, Franke N, Peter K, et al: Induced hypotension: action of sodium nitroprusside and nitroglycerin on the microcirculation. A micropuncture investigation. *Anesthesiology* 1987; 66:605–13.
7. Enoki T, Tsuchiya N, Shinomura T, et al: Effect of hypercapnia on arterial hypotension after induction of anaesthesia. *Acta Anaesthesiol Scand* 2005; 49:687–91.
8. Gittelman PD, Jacobs JB, Skorina J: Comparison of functional endoscopic sinus surgery under local and general anesthesia. *Ann Otol Rhinol Laryngol* 1993; 102:289–93.
9. Harkin CP, Schmeling WT, Kampine JP, et al: The effects of hyperand hypocarbia on intraparenchymal arterioles in rat brain slices. *Neuroreport* 1997; 8:1841–4.
10. Howarth PH: Leukotrienes in rhinitis. *Am J Respir Crit Care Med* 2000; 161:S133–6.
11. Jacobi KE, Bohm BE, Rickauer AJ, et al: Moderate controlled hypotension with sodium nitroprusside does not improve surgical conditions or decrease blood loss in endoscopic sinus surgery. *J Clin Anesth* 2000; 12:202–7.
12. Kinsella JB, Calhoun KH, Bradfield JJ, et al: Complications of endoscopic sinus surgery in a residency training program. *Laryngoscope* 1995; 105:1029–32.
13. Lung MA, Wang JC: Effects of hypercapnia and hypoxia on nasal vasculature and airflow resistance in the anaesthetized dog. *J Physiol* 1986; 373:261–75.
14. May M, Levine HL, Mester SJ, et al: Complications of endoscopic sinus surgery: analysis of 2108 patients – incidence and prevention. *Laryngoscope* 1994; 104:1080–3.
15. Nair S, Collins M, Hung P, et al: The effect of beta-blocker premedication on the surgical field during endoscopic sinus surgery. *Laryngoscope* 2004; 114:1042–6.
16. Nekhendzy V, Lemmens HJ, Vaughan WC, et al: The effect of deliberate hypercapnia and hypocapnia on intraoperative blood loss and quality of surgical field during functional endoscopic sinus surgery. *Anesth Analg* 2007; 105:1404–9.

17. Pavlin JD, Colley PS, Weymuller EA Jr, et al: Propofol versus isoflurane for endoscopic sinus surgery. *Am J Otolaryngol* 1999; 20:96–101.
18. Tominaga M, Stekiel TA, Bosnjak ZJ, et al: Contribution of carotid chemoreceptors to mesenteric venoconstriction during acute hypercapnia in rabbits. *Am J Physiol* 1999; 277:H2305–10.
19. Webster AC, Morley-Foster PK, Janzen V, et al: Anesthesia for intranasal surgery: a comparison between tracheal intubation and the flexible reinforced laryngeal mask airway. *Anesth Analg* 1999; 88:421–5.
20. Wormald PJ, Van Renen G, Perks J, et al: The effect of the total intravenous anesthesia compared with inhalational anesthesia on the surgical field during endoscopic sinus surgery. *Am J Rhinol* 2005; 19:514–20.

EXTERNAL SINUS SURGERY

SURGICAL CONSIDERATIONS

Description: Transfacial approaches to the paranasal sinuses include a transoral sublabial approach to the maxillary sinus and pterygomaxillary space (**Caldwell-Luc**), external ethmoidectomy (often with medial orbitotomy, and/or medial maxillectomy), and osteoplastic approaches to the frontal sinus via a bicoronal incision just behind the hairline. The usual indication for such approaches are resection of malignant and occasionally benign locally extensive tumors such as angiofibroma, especially when for technical reasons (e.g., angle of access or extension into the orbit) it is felt that an endoscopic approach is not indicated. The continued improvement in endoscopic equipment along with increasing surgical experience makes endoscopic resection increasingly more common, safe, and appropriate.

Anterior cranial base surgery: When tumors transgress the anterior cranial base at the cribriform plate and ethmoid roof, an anterior cranial base resection is often done. If the extent of the anticipated dural resection is limited, then the resection can be accomplished endoscopically. In more extensive rsections most surgeons opt for an open approach. Rarely is a central facial incision required as adequate exposure may be obtained via a bicoronal incision

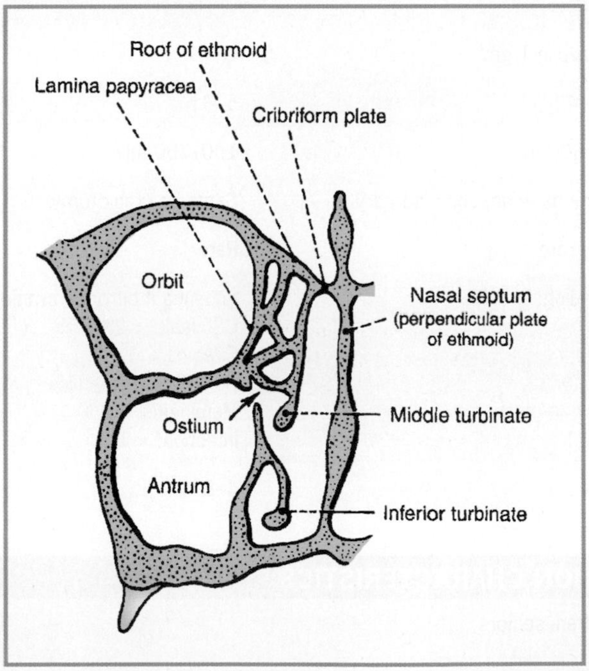

Figure 3-11. Diagrammatic representation of the relationships of the orbit, maxillary antrum, ethmoid labyrinth, and nasal cavity. Note that the medial wall of the ethmoid labyrinth is an upper extension of the attachment of the middle turbinate. The attachment of the upper extension separates the roof of the ethmoid and the cribriform plate. (Reproduced with permission from Montgomery WW: *Surgery of the Upper Respiratory System,* 3rd edition. Williams & Wilkins, 1996.)

and bifrontal craniotomy. The CSF leak is addressed by a combination of dural substitution (autologous tissue, such as temporalis fascia, bovine pericardium, or manufactured substitutes) and a pericranial-galeal flap. A lumbar subarachnoid drain is sometimes used in this setting.

Variant approaches: Approaches to the middle cranial base include an orbitozygomatic approach to the infratemporal fossa. The zygomatic arch and part of the zygomatic body is temporarily removed, the temporalis major muscle is transposed inferiorly. The lateral orbital bone with or without the orbital rim may be temporarily removed. A middle fossa craniotomy or craniectomy is usually done. This provides access to the foramen ovale, foramen rotundum, and carotid artery at the skull base, as well as the lateral orbit and superior infratemporal fossa and pterygomaxillary fossa to the pterygoid plates, and, as needed, lateral sphenoid sinus and maxillary sinus. Following tumor resection, part of the temporalis muscle may be used to assist in CSF leak managmement.

Usual preoperative diagnosis: Malignant and some benign tumors

SUMMARY OF PROCEDURES

	External Sinus Surgery	Anterior Cranial Base Surgery
Position	Head up 30°, back raised (reduces bleeding).	⇐ Also reduces intracranial pressure
Incision	Access to the ethmoid and maxilla is via a 3–4 cm incision midway between the medial canthal ligament and the midline, in the shadow of the nasal bone; a lateral rhinotomy incision is not needed.	A bicoronal incision posterior to the hairline masks the scar. A supplemental facial incision is rarely needed.
Special Instrumentation	Paranasal sinus set; headlight	⇐ + craniotomy set
Unique considerations	Nasal packing	⇐ see frontal craniotomy
Antibiotics	Cefazolin 1 gm	⇐
Surgical time	1.5–4 h	5–8 h
EBL	25–300 mL	150–750 mL
Postop care	Same as endoscopic surgery	Same as craniotomy
Mortality	Very rare	Rare
Morbidity	Bleeding: < 5%	Anosmia if bifrontal craniotomy CSF leak: < 2% CVA: <1% Bone flap loss: < 1% Memingitis: < 1% Infection: < 1%
Pain score	4–6	4–6

PATIENT POPULATION CHARACTERISTICS

Age range	Children–seniors
Male:Female	1:1
Incidence	Common
Etiology	Malignant tumors, selected benign tumors, occasionally infectious
Associated conditions	Dependent on specific tumor; also see Endoscopic Sinus Surgery

ANESTHETIC CONSIDERATIONS

See Anesthetic Considerations following Endoscopic Sinus Surgery, p. 229.

NASAL SURGERY (RHINOPLASTY, SEPTOPLASTY, SEPTORHINOPLASTY)

Sam P. Mosr

SURGICAL CONSIDERATIONS

Description: Nasal surgery is performed for cosmetic and functional restoration of the airway. Functional restoration is usually performed for either congenital or posttraumatic deviations of the septum. The nasal cavity is first cocainized with 4% cocaine-soaked pledgets placed in each nostril for 5–10 min. **Septoplasty** (reconstruction of the nasal septum) usually can be carried out under sedation with local anesthesia, using 1% lidocaine with 1:100,000 epinephrine. **Rhinoplasty-septorhinoplasty** usually is carried out under local anesthesia, but if GA is used, a mouth pack is inserted. Local infiltration with 1% lidocaine with 1:100,000 epinephrine is used to ensure vasoconstriction and to minimize bleeding. Intranasal incisions are made and septal problems corrected. Generally, an anterior hemitransfixion incision is made down to the cartilage, and a submucoperichondrial flap is elevated the length of the septum. A similar flap may be elevated on the contralateral side. Bony deformities are resected with an osteotome, while cartilaginous deformities are either resected or weakened by morselizing, either in situ or after removal, and then replaced. The incision is closed with interrupted absorbable sutures. In **rhinoplasty,** tip remodelling, hump reduction, and bony osteotomies are performed to remodel the nasal contour. Surgery on the inferior turbinates in the form of intramural cautery, resection of turbinate bone, resection of turbinate mucosa or, in some cases, complete turbinectomy may be required to produce a satisfactory airway. After the surgery is complete, both nasal cavities are packed and external splints may be used for rhinoplasty and septorhinoplasty cases. For the plastic surgeon's perspective see Chapter 11.1.

Usual preop diagnosis: Nasal deformity or deviation; deviated septum

SUMMARY OF PROCEDURE	
Position	Head up 30° to bleeding. Table may be turned 90–180°.
Incision	Intranasal, usually; extended only in open septorhinoplasty
Unique considerations	Nose initially cocainized; use of 1% lidocaine with 1:100,000 epinephrine to ↓ bleeding.
Antibiotics	Cefazolin 1 g iv; routinely used as long as nasal packs are in place.
Surgical time	1–2.5 h
Closing considerations	Nose often packed postop, necessitating oral airway after extubation.
EBL	50–100 mL (excessive blood loss rare)
Postop care	PACU
Mortality	Minimal
Morbidity	Septal perforation: 5% Bleeding: 4% Infection: 4%
Pain score	4–6

PATIENT POPULATION CHARACTERISTICS	
Age range	Young teens–young adults
Male:Female	1:1
Incidence	Common
Etiology	Congenital/traumatic septal and/or nasal deviation

ANESTHETIC CONSIDERATIONS FOR NASAL SURGERY

PREOPERATIVE

These cases typically are performed on an outpatient basis. Most of the patients are young and otherwise healthy, but some patients presenting for rhino/septoplasty and turbinate reduction surgery may have OSA with the corresponding implications for intraop management (see p. 256). Older patients may present for major reconstructive nasal surgery following resections of a basal cell carcinoma of the nose. Patients presenting for closed reduction of nasal fractures may have suffered concomitant closed head trauma. If the nose injury is recent, blood may have been swallowed, and the patient should be considered "full stomach."

Respiratory	Some patients may present with a Hx of reactive airway disease; their functional status should be checked and optimized preop. **Tests:** As indicated from H&P.
Cardiovascular	In patients with pre-existing cardiac disease, cocaine use by the surgeon for topical anesthesia or control of bleeding may be contraindicated. **Tests:** ECG in older population; others as indicated from H&P.
Neuro	Psychological disturbances are common in patients presenting for rhinologic surgery.
Premedication	Standard premedication (p. B-1). Sedation should be avoided or used with caution in patients with OSA.

INTRAOPERATIVE

Anesthetic technique: Septorhinoplasty may be performed under local anesthesia with MAC, although GA is used more commonly. The essential surgical requirements are: patient immobility; clear surgical field (nasal mucosa is extremely vascular); and smooth emergence from anesthesia to avoid postop hemorrhage.

Spontaneous or controlled ventilation can be used intraoperatively, and FLMA is strongly preferred over tracheal intubation (see above).

Induction	Standard induction with propofol (1–2 mg/kg) is an ideal induction agent because of its short duration and intrinsic antiemetic effect. For GETA, the use of an oral RAE or reinforced ETT will facilitate surgical access. Both ETT and FLMA are usually taped midline.
Maintenance	All GA techniques (balanced, inhalational, or TIVA) can be used safely, although TIVA is preferred. Propofol infusion (80–150 mcg/kg/min) may offer the advantage of ↓BP without compensatory ↑HR, and ↓ PONV. Remifentanil infusion (0.1–0.25 mcg/kg/min) will improve hemodynamic stability and facilitate rapid and smooth emergence. Maintaining moderate degree of ↓BP is essential.
Emergence	Antiemetic prophylaxis is obligatory. Emergence from anesthesia after nasal surgery presents significant challenges to the anesthesiologist. Nasal passages may be packed at the end of surgery, making the patients obligate mouth-breathers; the oropharynx should be suctioned carefully. No pressure on the patient's nose with the face mask should be allowed after tracheal extubation or FLMA removal. Full return of airway reflexes should occur before extubation, which must be accomplished smoothly without excessive bucking and coughing. The FLMA is superior to the ETT in this regard.

Blood and fluid requirements	Blood loss usually minimal IV: 20 ga × 1 NS/LR @ 2–3 cmL/kg/h	Blood loss controlled with surgical hemostasis and topical applications of vasoconstrictor (epinephrine), but also may also include cocaine.
Monitoring	Standard monitors (p. B-1)	
Positioning	Head elevated 15–30° Table turned 90–180° ✓ and pad pressure points. ✓ eyes	Patient's arms usually tucked in and should be carefully padded. For rhinoplasty, patient's eyes should be protected in a way that would allow for early recognition of an orbital injury (e.g., scleral shields, eye ointment).
Complications	Tachycardia, dysrhythmias	These are usually related to use of vasoconstrictor agents and may present a problem in patients with CAD. Short-acting β-blocker (esmolol, 0.5–1 mcg/kg in boluses) should be available to blunt these hemodynamic effects.

POSTOPERATIVE

Complications	Occult bleeding	Occult postop bleeding may caue the patient may swallow large quantities of blood (↑ aspiration risk); and repacking the nostrils may be required.
Pain management	Fentanyl 25–50 mcg iv prn is usually sufficient.	

Suggested Readings

1. Abdulatif M: Sodium nitroprusside induced hypotension: haemodynamic response and dose requirements during propofol or halothane anaesthesia. *Anaesth Intens Care* 1994; 22:155–60.
2. Brown BR: Anaesthesia for ear, nose, throat and maxillofacial procedures. In International Practice of Anaesthesia. Prys-Roberts C, Brown BR, eds. Butterworth-Heinemann, Oxford: 1996, 2–9.
3. Donlon JV, Feldman MA: Anesthesia for eye, ear, nose, and throat surgery. In *Miller's Anesthesia*, 6th edition. Miller RD, ed. Elsevier, Philadelphia: 2005, 2527–49.
4. Hinni ML, Kern EB: Psychological complications of septo-rhinoplasty. *Facial Plast Surg* 1997; 13:71–5.
5. Van Den Berg AA, Savva D, Honjol NM, et al: Comparison of total intravenous, balanced inhalational and combined intravenous-inhalational anaesthesia for tympanoplasty, septorhinoplasty and adenotonsillectomy. *Anaesth Intens Care* 1995; 23:574–82.
6. Webster AC, Morley-Foster PK, Janzen V, et al: Anesthesia for intranasal surgery: a comparison between tracheal intubation and the flexible reinforced laryngeal mask airway. *Anesth Analg* 1999; 88:421–5.
7. Williams PJ, Thompsett C, Bailey PM: Comparison of the reinforced laryngeal mask airway and tracheal intubation for nasal surgery. *Anaesthesia* 1995; 50:987–9.

FACIAL PLASTIC SURGERY

Overview: Facial plastic surgery encompasses both reconstructive and aesthetic surgery of the face and neck. Typically, surgeons are trained in either otolaryngology-head & neck surgery/facial plastic surgery or general plastic surgery (see Chapter 11.1) or both. The procedures to be covered in this section are rhinoplasty, rhytidectomy (facelift) and blepharoplasty (eyelid rejuvenation).

SURGICAL CONSIDERATIONS

RHINOPLASTY

Description: Rhinoplasty has traditionally been considered an aesthetic procedure. However, when combined with a septoplasty (rhinoseptoplasty, septorhinoplasty) it is both a functional and aesthetic operation. In some cases, a purely functional operation (functional rhinoplasty) is performed in order to improve the ability to breathe through the nose. The approach and anesthetic requirements for these can be considered together.

Technique: A septoplasty involves a unilateral intranasal incision along the anterior septum with minor variations in the placement of the incision in the antero-posterior plane. The approaches to rhinoplasty can be intranasal, extranasal or both. Frequently, the external (or "open") approach to rhinoplasty is employed. The intranasal approach involve incisions along the septum anteriorly and some combination of incisions in the nasal vestibule. The external approach combines these approaches with a midcolumellar incision. In both functional and aesthetic rhinoplasty, the maneuvers include cartilage remodeling or resection, and possibly osteotomies to manipulate the bony pyramid of the nose.

Usual preop diagnosis: For aesthetic patients, the typical preop diagnosis is nasal deformity. However, many patients also complain of nasal obstruction, and some rhinoplasty patients have purely functional concerns. Patients with significant nasal obstruction may have some component of sleep disordered breathing or even OSA. Because of this, patients with nasal obstruction are routinely asked about snoring and daytime somnolence (if they have not already had a diagnostic sleep study).

Preop and intraop preparation: Preoperatively patients receive a nasal decongestant spray (0.05% oxymetazoline spray, 3 doses 10 min. apart) to reduce intraop bleeding. Preop corticosteroid (4–8 mg Decadron iv) and antibiotics (cefazolin, 1 gm iv) are administered. Intraop, we prefer LMA for protection of the airway and esophageal inlet, as some bleeding in the nasopharynx is expected. If an endotracheal tube is used, a throat pack can be placed to reduce blood entrance into the esophagus/stomach. The tube should be secured to the *midline of the lower lip* to avoid distortion of the nose/nasal base.

Postop care: At the end of the procedure, prior to extubation, the surgeon will place an external splint of some type on the nose. Any mask placed on the patient should be done in such a fashion as to not place pressure on the nose. We prefer the transport oxygen mask be cut off such that no contact occurs. Any Valsalva can result in epistaxis and/or bleeding under the septal or nasal skin flaps. Thus, any manuevers to reduce bucking or coughing during extubation are in order.

SUMMARY OF PROCEDURE	
Position	Supine
Incision	Intranasal + columella (external rhinoplasty)
Special instrumentation	Headlight
Unique considerations	Nasal obstruction postop
Antibiotics	Often administered preop: cefazolin 1 gm iv
Other Preoperative Meds	Nasal decongestant spray, dexamethasone 4–8 mg iv
Surgical Time	1–3 h
EBL	25–50 cc
Mortality	Minimal
Morbidity	Epistaxis, septal perforation, unsatisfactory aesthetic result
Pain Score	1–4, typically mild

PATIENT POPULATION CHARACTERISTICS	
Age Range	15+ yr
Male:Female	1:1
Incidence	Common
Etiology	Nasal obstruction, desire for change in nasal form.

RHYTIDECTOMY (FACELIFT)

Description: Rhytidectomy (facelift) is almost always an aesthetic procedure. In the common vernacular, "facelift" is often used to describe total surgical facial rejuvenation (including eyelids and forehead). Strictly speaking, rhytidectomy involves aesthetic miprovement of the lower half of the face and upper neck. For this reason, some have called it a "necklift" or "lower facelift" to avoid confusion. Perhaps the latter term is more appropriate, as a separate 'necklift' procedure does exist. In any event, the anesthetic requirements for these are similar.

Technique: Rhytidectomy incisions are bilateral, extending pre and postauricularly with minor variations. In addition, the surgeon may place a small (0.5–2 cm) incision submentally for access to submental fat and/or platysma muscle. As dissection may be near branches of the facial nerve, ***avoidance of muscle relaxants*** is required.

Usual preop diagnosis: For aesthetic patients, the typical preop diagnosis is simply desire for reduction in nasolabial and labiomandibular lines, jowling, and neck skin laxity. Patients are typically over the age of 40, and usually in good health. Smoking is a contraindication due to the risk of poor wound healing and/or skin flap necrosis.

Preop and intraop preparation: Preop patients receive corticosteroid (4–8 mg Decadron iv) and antibiotics (cefazolin, 1 gm iv). Intraop, we prefer LMA for protection of the airway and esophageal inlet, though an ETT can be used. The tube should be secured to the ***midline of the lower lip*** to avoid distortion of the lower face/neck. The tube is prepped in to the field and may be manipulated side-to-side during the procedure as the submental incision is accessed. In addition, the head may be turned about 30–45° to the side opposite the surgeon. Typically, dissection near the branches of the facial nerve is undertaken, and visual monitoring for any twitches is performed by the assistant, thus ***avoidance of muscle relaxants is imperative.***

Postop care: At the end of the procedure, prior to patient extubation, the surgeon will place a circumferential external pressure dressing of some kind on the face. Typically, cotton balls soaked in antibiotic ointment are placed in the ears. The patient may have difficulty hearing due to this dressing. Drains may have been placed on each side of the neck. Any Valsalva can result in bleeding under the skin flaps. Hematoma is one of the most common periop complications and requires evacuation. Thus, any maneuvers to reduce bucking or coughing during extubation are in order.

SUMMARY OF PROCEDURE

Position	Supine
Incision	Pre/postauricular and submental
Special instrumentation	Headlight
Unique considerations	Facial nerve is monitored (visually); avoid paralytics
Antibiotics	Often administered preop: cefazolin 1 gm iv
Other preoperative meds	Dexamethasone: 4–8 mg iv
Surgical Time	3 h
EBL	25–50 cc
Mortality	Minimal
Morbidity	Hematoma, facial paralysis, unsatisfactory aesthetic result
Pain Score	1–4, typically mild

PATIENT POPULATION CHARACTERISTICS

Age range	40+
Male:Female	1:8
Incidence	Common

PATIENT POPULATION CHARACTERISTICS (cont'd)	
Etiology	Desire for change in facial aesthetics
Associated conditions	Other facial aesthetic considerations

BLEPHAROPLASTY

(For the plastic surgeon's perspective see Chapter 11.1)

Description: Blepharoplasty (eyelid rejuvenation surgery) is, in the overwhelming marjority of cases, an anesthetic procedure. In some cases, *functional upper lid blepharoplasty* may be performed to reduce visual field obstruction, and is typically covered by insurance. These procedures are often performed under local anesthesia with sedation. However, as they are often combined with other procedures (browlift, facelift), the patients are often under general anesthesia.

Technique: Upper blepharoplasty incisions are placed on curvilinear fashion along the upper eyelid creases with minor variations. The amount of skin to be excised is marked by the surgeon, and local anesthetic with epinephrine is administered. The evolution of upper eyelid blepharoplasty has led to a more conservative approach with less muscle and fat excision being performed. As the procedure becomes more skin-only, many are being performed under local anesthesia as an isolated procedure.

Lower blepharoplasty is generally performed transcutaneously with a subciliary incision or transconjunctivally via the inner portion of the lower eyelid. In the former approach, a small amount of lower lid skin and muscle is typically excised. With both approaches, the surgeon removes or repositions a small amount of the intraorbital fat pockets for the desired aesthetic result.

Usual preop diagnosis: For aesthetic patients, the typical preop diagnosis is simply desire for reduction upper lid skin excess, which may obstruct their vision (see above). In the lower lid, the most common complaint is "puffiness" of the lower eyelid, which is often due to pseudoherniation of orbital fat and descent of the midface fat with age. Patients are typically over the age of 30 and usually in good health.

Preop and intraop preparation: Preop patients receive corticosteroid (4–8 mg Decadron i.v.) and antibiotics (cefazolin, 1 gm iv). Intraop, we prefer LMA for protection of the airway and esophageal inlet. The tube should be secured to the midline of the lower lip to avoid distortion of the lower face/neck.

Postop care: At the end of the procedure, prior to patient extubation, the surgeon will confirm satisfaction with symmetry and aesthetic result. No dressings are used. Any Valsalva can result in bleeding under the skin flaps. More importantly, intraorbital pressure must be avoided as it may result in a serious complication, placing the patient's vision at risk. Thus, any maneuvers to reduce bucking or coughing during extubation are in order.

SUMMARY OF PROCEDURE	
Position	Supine
Incision	Upper lid crease, lower lid via transconjunctival or transcutaneous approaches
Special instrumentation	None
Unique considerations	None
Antibiotics	Often administered preop: cefazolin 1 gm iv
Other preoperative meds	Dexamethasone: 4–8 mg iv
Surgical Time	1.25 h (upper or lower only); 2 h (both upper and lower)
EBL	< 5 cc
Mortality	Minimal
Morbidity	Asymmetry, dry eye, ectropion, corneal abrasion, blindness (rare)
Pain Score	1–4, typically mild

PATIENT POPULATION CHARACTERISTICS	
Age range	30+
Male:Female	1:8
Incidence	Common
Etiology	Desire for change in facial aesthetics; in some cases upper blepharoplasty is performed for functional reasons
Associated conditions	Other facial aesthetic considerations

ANESTHETIC CONSIDERATIONS

(see Anesthetic Considerations for Office based procedures and Anesthetic Considerations for Facial Cosmetic Surgery p. 858)

OTOLOGY AND NEUROTOLOGY

SURGICAL CONSIDERATIONS

Otologic Surgery: Otologic surgery is indicated for a spectrum of disorders, including traumatic, developmental, infectious, and neoplastic disease. Procedures involving the external auditory canal, middle ear, and inner ear will be considered in this section. Surgery confined to the pinna or that requiring craniotomy is considered elsewhere.

The temporal bone is as complex as any region of human anatomy (Fig. 3-12 and Fig. 3-13). Multiple vital neurovascular structures interrelate in a small confined space. These include the organs of hearing and balance, the facial nerve, the carotid artery, jugular vein, and the delicate mechanisms of the middle ear. The density and complexity of the anatomy dictate the delicate nature of otologic procedures and hence many of its anesthetic requirements. Most procedures are either performed via a transcanal approach (through the natural meatus of the external ear), a retroauricular incision, or a combination of the two.

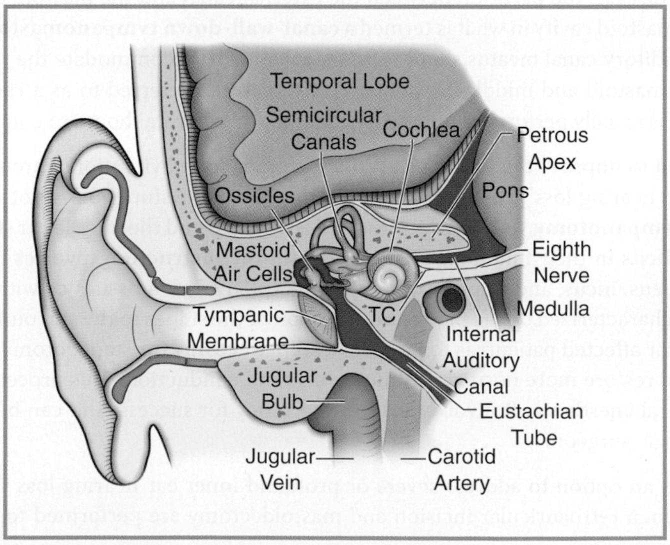

Figure 3-12. Coronal diagram of right ear

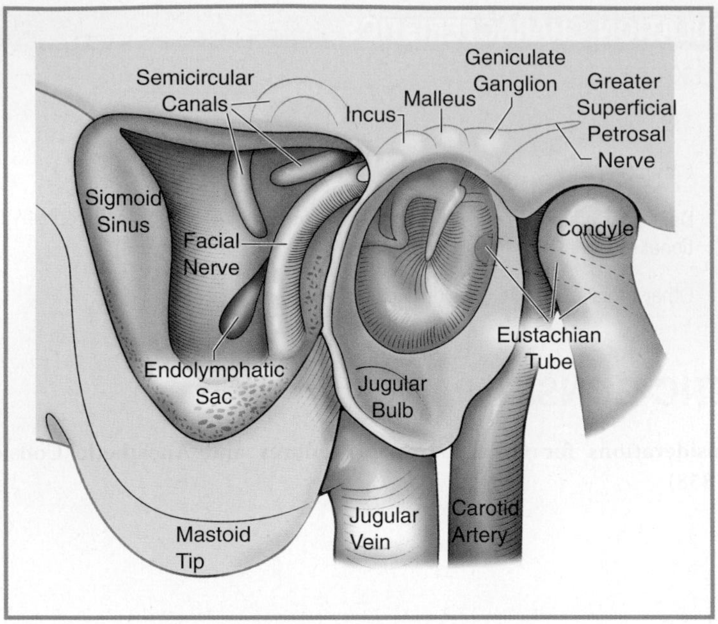

Figure 3-13. Lateral diagram of right ear

Many otologic procedures are undertaken to control recurrent or chronic ear infections (otomastoiditis). The simplest of these is the **myringotomy**, in which the tympanic membrane (TM) is incised through the ear canal, and the middle ear contents are aspirated. In most cases, a myringotomy tube is also placed to maintain middle ear aeration and drainage. This procedure usually takes just a few minutes, and is performed under mask GA. A myringoplasty involves the repair of a persistent TM perforation, and usually involves placement of autologous tissues as a patch to enable healing. When combined with repair of chronic middle ear changes, the procedure is termed a tympanoplasty.

The mastoid is an area of bone and air spaces situated behind the middle ear and external auditory canal. The removal of this bone, through a **simple mastoidectomy**, enables the removal of loculated infection, diseased tissue, and provides access to additional anatomy. This is often combined with tympanoplasty **(tympanomastoidectomy)** to address the changes from chronic infection. This is the standard surgical approach to resect a **cholesteatoma**, which is a keratin-containing epithelial cyst originating from the TM that has grown into the middle ear and mastoid cavity. When the posterior bony wall of the external auditory canal is left in place to keep the mastoid cavity anatomically distinct from the external auditory canal, the procedure is called a **canal-wall-up tympanomastoidectomy**. In contrast, for more aggressive disease, the partition between the external canal and the mastoid cavity can be removed, thereby exteriorizing the mastoid cavity in what is termed a **canal-wall-down tympanomastoidectomy**. During this procedure, the external auditory canal meatus should also be enlarged to accommodate the resulting mastoid bowl. The complete removal of mastoid and middle ear contents is sometimes referred to as a **radical mastoidectomy**. Tympanomastoid surgery is usually performed under GA, and may take several hours to complete.

Surgery is often performed to improve the mechanical conduction of sound vibrations through the middle ear into the inner ear ("conductive hearing loss"). If the cause of the mechanical dysfunction is not clear, the surgeon may perform an **exploratory tympanotomy**, during which the TM is elevated and the middle ear structures are inspected and palpated to reveal deficits in their function. **Ossicular chain reconstruction** involves rebuilding or replacing the bones of hearing (malleus, incus, and stapes) with either the patient's own tissues or with aloplastic prostheses. Otosclerosis is a disorder characterized by the progressive fixation of the stapes to the surrounding bone, resulting in hearing loss. One option for affected patients is to perform a **stapedectomy** (or stapedotomy) in which the stapes is replaced by a prosthesis to restore more normal continuity of sound conduction. This procedure can be performed either under local or general anesthesia. It involves extreme accuracy for success, and can be one of the most challenging cases for the otologic surgeon.

Cochlear implantation is an option to address severe or profound inner ear hearing loss ("sensorineural hearing loss"). During implantation, a retroauricular incision and mastoidectomy are performed to provide a pathway for device placement into the inner ear. A receiver-stimulator is placed under the skin behind the ear, and a flexible electrode array is threaded into the turns of the cochlea to later be used to stimulate the cochlear nerve directly, and thereby bypass the dysfunctional inner ear. The devices are activated usually several weeks following placement, at which time hearing function is expected to increase.

A number of procedures address disorders specifically confined to the external auditory canal. Patients may develop extra bone growths (exostoses) in the ear canal that obstruct the canal. **Exostoses resection** can be performed through a retroauricular incision or via a transcanal approach if the disease is limited. Patients may lack an ear canal (canal atresia) as the result of a congenital disorder, from chronic inflammation, or post-traumatic scarring. In such patients, a **canalplasty**, involving obstructing skin, bone, and scar can be performed. Similarly, patients may require the resection of a number of neoplastic lesions of the ear canal, most commonly of cutaneous origin. Such resections may require additional resection of adjacent tissues affected by the neoplastic process. A skin graft may be used to reconstruct the external auditory canal. This may be harvested from the retroauricular region, the inner aspect of the arm, or from the hip or thigh.

The majority of otologic surgery requires the use of a surgical microscope. The presence of the microscope has a number of implications for anesthesia. Often, the OR table is turned 180°. Of critical importance is that the patient remain entirely motionless. Any adjustment of equipment or position can have profound consequences during microdissection. Therefore, the surgeon must be made aware of any plans that may result in patient motion–even those that would otherwise seem insignificant. During microsurgery, even small amounts of bleeding can have dramatic implications, thus maintenance of a stable low blood pressure is useful.

One common theme to otologic procedures is the need to identify and preserve the **facial nerve.** The 7th cranial nerve winds its way through the temporal bone from its origin in the brainstem to the stylomastoid foramen. It passes through the middle ear, and is at risk during almost all otologic procedures. The use of an EMG-based neural monitor is now commonplace to assess neural function. The monitor will not function if paralytic agents are in use, and their untimely use can prevent the surgeon from receiving critical warnings regarding nerve activity. As a standard rule, always check with the surgeon prior to the administration of any paralytic agents during otologic procedures.

Although the internal carotid artery and jugular bulb pass through the middle ear, significant vascular injury is quite rare. Most if not all bleeding can be readily controlled with packing in the surgical field. The use of absorbable gelatin sponges (e.g., Gelfoam) is routine to hold reconstructive materials in place, and also can help with hemostasis. Venous injury, such as laceration of the sigmoid sinus during mastoidectomy, can usually be controlled using bone wax or with other hemostatic materials (e.g., Surgicel) held with pressure against the site of bleeding. In the case of a large venous injury, a **venous air embolism** can potentially result, and timely communication between the surgical and anesthesia teams can facilitate its identification and treatment. More severe arterial injury, may require additional neuroradiologic or neurosurgical intervention. Even in these rare instances, hemodynamically significant blood loss can usually be avoided with prompt and secure packing.

The temporal bone abuts the dura of the middle fossa above and the posterior fossa behind. Rarely, transgression of the dura can result either as the result of pathology or from dissection of adjacent tissues. When this occurs, the surgeon can usually close the leak using autologous tissues. The surgeon may request administration of a Valsalva maneuver to check the integrity of the repair.

Usual preop diagnoses: Acute or chronic otitis media, cholesteatoma, hearing loss (conductive or sensorineural), otosclerosis, aural atresia (acquired or congenital), tympanic membrane perforation, temporal bone fracture, temporal bone neoplasm.

SUMMARY OF PROCEDURE	
Position	Supine
Incision	Postauricular or transcanal
Special instrumentation	Binocular surgical microscope, otologic micro-instruments, otologic drill, laser
Unique considerations	Complex microanatomy, no paralytics given need for facial nerve monitoring, Possible avoidance of nitrous oxide
Antibiotics	Often administered preoperatively

SUMMARY OF PROCEDURE (cont'd)	
Surgical Time	< 1 h to > 4 h
EBL	Usually minimal
Mortality	Minimal
Morbidity	Infection, hearing loss, vertigo, facial nerve dysfunction, spinal fluid leak
Pain Score	1–6, typically mild

PATIENT POPULATION CHARACTERISTICS	
Age range	all ages
Male:Female	1:1
Incidence	Common
Etiology	Infectious, traumatic, congenital, neoplastic
Associated conditions	Heavy loss, head trauma

ANESTHETIC CONSIDERATIONS

(See Anesthetic Considerations following Maxillectomy, p. 211.)

Suggested Readings

1. Dal D, Celiker V, Ozer E, et al: Induced hypotension for tympanoplasty: a comparison of desflurane, isoflurane and sevoflurane. *Eur J Anaesthesiol* 2004; 21:902–6.
2. Donlon JV, Feldman MA: Anesthesia for eye, ear, nose, and throat surgery. In *Miller's Anesthesia,* 6th edition. Miller RD, ed. Elsevier, Philadelphia: 2005, 2527–49.
3. Fujii Y, Toyooka H, Tanaka H: Prophylactic antiemetic therapy with a combination of granisetron and dexamethasone in patients undergoing middle ear surgery. *Br J Anaesth* 1998; 81:754–6.
4. Jellish WS, Leonetti JP, Avramov A, et al: Remifentanil-based anesthesia versus a propofol technique for otologic surgical procedures. *Otolaryngol Head Neck Surg* 2000; 122:222–7.
5. Jellish WS, Leonetti JP, Fahey K, et al: Comparison of 3 different anesthetic techniques on 24-hour recovery after otologic surgical procedures. *Otolaryngol Head Neck Surg* 1999; 120:406–11.
6. Jellish WS, Leonetti JP, Murdoch JR, et al: Propofol-based anesthesia as compared with standard anesthetic techniques for middle ear surgery. *Otolaryngol Head Neck Surg* 1995; 12:262–7.
7. Jellish WS, Owen K, Edelstein S, et al: Standard anesthetic technique for middle ear surgical procedures: a comparison of desflurane and sevoflurane. *Otolaryngol Head Neck Surg* 2005; 133:269–74.
8. Liu YH, Li MJ, Wang PC, et al: Use of dexamethasone on the prophylaxis of nausea and vomiting after tympanomastoid surgery. *Laryngoscope* 2001; 111:1271–4.
9. Munson SE: Transfer of nitrous oxide into body air cavities. *Br J Anaesth* 1974; 46:202–9.
10. Ruby RF, Webster AC, Morley-Forster PK, et al: Laryngeal mask airway in paediatric otolaryngologic surgery. *J Otolaryng* 1995; 24:288–91.
11. Wang JJ, Wang PC, Liu YH, et al: Low-dose dexamethasone reduces nausea and vomiting after tympanomastoid surgery: a comparison of tropisetron with saline. *Am J Otol* 2002; 23:267–71.
12. Watcha MF, Garner FT, White PF, et al: Laryngeal mask airway vs face mask and Guedel airway during pediatric myringotomy. *Arch Otolaryngol Head Neck Surg* 1994; 120:877–80.

NEUROTOLOGICAL SKULL BASE SURGERY

SURGICAL CONSIDERATIONS

The skull base refers to the floor of the cranial cavity and can be divided into anterior, middle, and posterior fossae. It is formed by the frontal, ethmoid, sphenoid, temporal, and occipital bones. Neurotologists primarily deal with lesions in the posterior fossa which is bordered by the clivus (anterior), temporal bone (lateral), and occipital bone (posterior). An axial view of the skull identifying these structures is shown in Fig. 3-14.

The term **skull base surgery** is a misnomer as the majority of lesions treated are located adjacent to the brainstem and not intrinsic to the skull base itself. Removal of the skull base bone allows exposure to these lesions while minimizing cerebral and cerebellar retraction.

The cerebellopontine angle (CPA) is a fluid-filled space containing the facial nerve (VII) and vestibulocochlear nerve (VIII) coursing laterally towards the internal auditory canal. A depiction of the CPA and associated cranial nerves is shown in Fig. 3-15. This is one of the most commonly approached areas in skull base surgery and lesions include

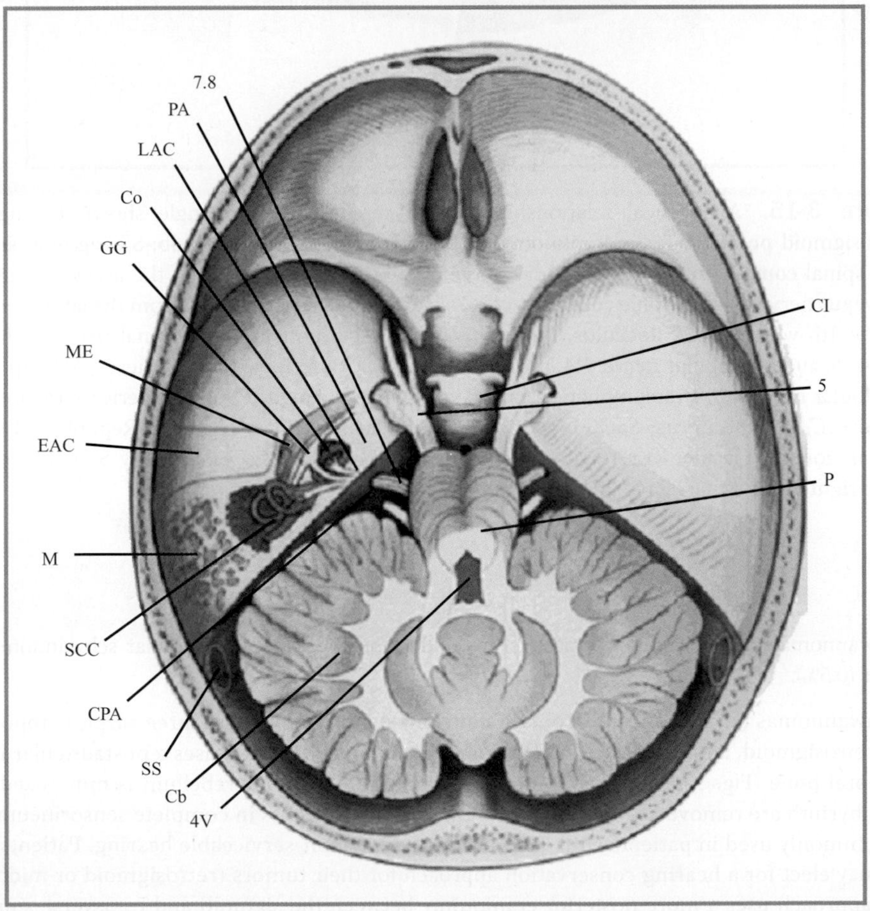

Figure 3-14. An axial view of the skull through the level of the internal auditory canal and cerebellopontine angle. *5*, Trigeminal nerve; *7*, facial nerve; *8*, audiovestibular nerve; *PA*, petrous apex; *IAC*, internal auditory canal; *Co*, cochlea; *GG*, geniculate ganglion of the facial nerve; *ME*, middle ear; *EAC*, external auditory canal; *M*, mastoid air cell system; *SCC*, semicircular canals; *CPA*, cerebellopontine angle; *SS*, sigmoid sinus; *4V*, 4th ventricle; *Cl*, clivus; *P*, pons; *Cb*, cerebellum. Republished with permission from Jackler RK: *Atlas of Neurotology and Skull Base Surgery*. Mosby, St. Louis: 1996. Copyright Dr. R. K. Jackler © 2007.

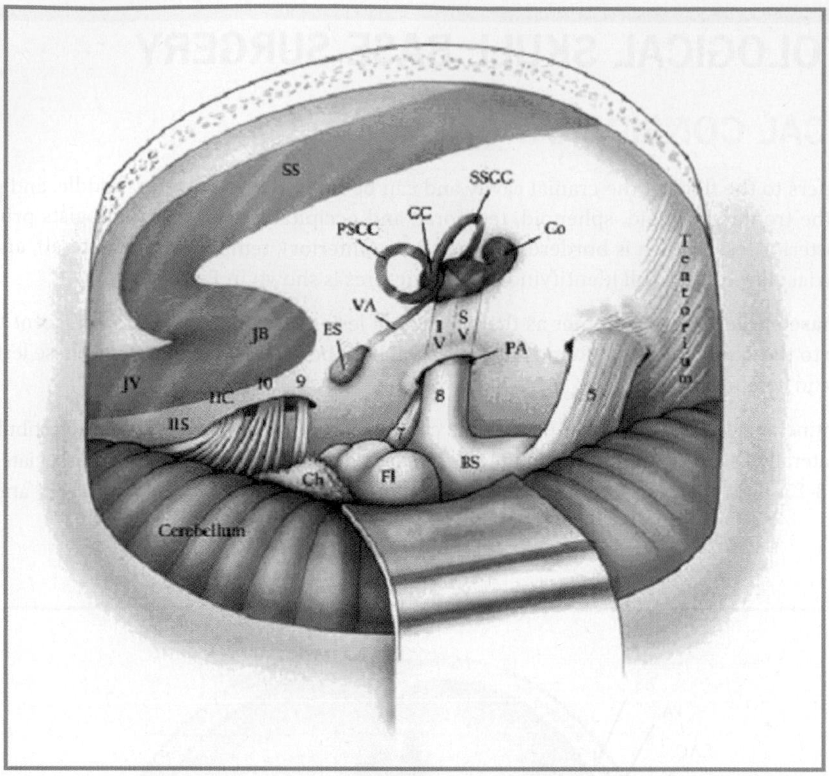

Figure 3-15. Anatomical relationships of the cerebellopontine angle shown through a retrosigmoid posterior fossa craniotomy. *JV*, jugular vein; *JB*, jugular bulb; SS, sigmoid sinus; *11s*, spinal component of the accessory nerve; *11c*, cranial component of the accessory nerve; *10*, vagus nerve; *9*, glossopharyngeal nerve; *Ch*, choroid plexus emanating from the lateral recess of the 4th ventricle; *Fl*, flocculus; *BS*, brainstem surface (pons); *5*, trigeminal nerve; *7*, facial nerve; *8*, audiovestibular nerve; *PA*, porus acousticus; *IV*, inferior vestibular nerve; *SV*, superior vestibular nerve; *ES*, endolymphatic sac; *VA*, vestibular aqueduct; *PSCC*, posterior semicircular canal; *CC*, common crus; *SSCC*, superior semicircular canal; *Co*, cochlea. (Republished with permission from Jackler RK: *Atlas of Neurotology and Skull Base Surgery*. Mosby, St. Louis: 1996. Copyright Dr. R. K. Jackler © 2007.)

vestibular schwannomas (91.3%), meningiomas (3.1%), epidermoids (2.4%), nonvestibular schwannomas (1.4%), and arachnoid cysts (0.5%).

Vestibular schwannomas (also known as **acoustic neuromas**) are removed via three surgical approaches: translabyrinthine, retrosigmoid, and middle fossa. The translabyrinthine approach uses a postauricular incision to access the temporal bone (Fig. 3-16). Retraction of the temporal lobe and cerebellum is minimized as the entire mastoid and labyrinth are removed to create access. This approach results in complete sensorineural hearing loss and is most commonly used in patients with large tumors and/or non-serviceable hearing. Patients with serviceable hearing may elect for a hearing conservation approach for their tumors (retrosigmoid or middle fossa). The retrosigmoid approach uses a more posterior craniotomy between the sigmoid and transverse sinuses. The cerebellum is retracted posterior away from the petrous face of the temporal bone (Fig. 3-15). Disadvantages include the increased incidence of postop headache and the need for rigid skull fixation (e.g., Mayfield). The middle fossa approach places the craniotomy above the ear and requires retraction of the temporal lobe (Fig. 3-17). This approach has the highest rate of hearing conservation, but can only be used in smaller tumors without increasing the risk of postop facial palsy.

Another commonly approached area is the jugular foramen which lies at the junction of the petrous apex and occipital bone. This foramen connects the intracranial compartment to the neck and contains the glossopharyngeal nerve

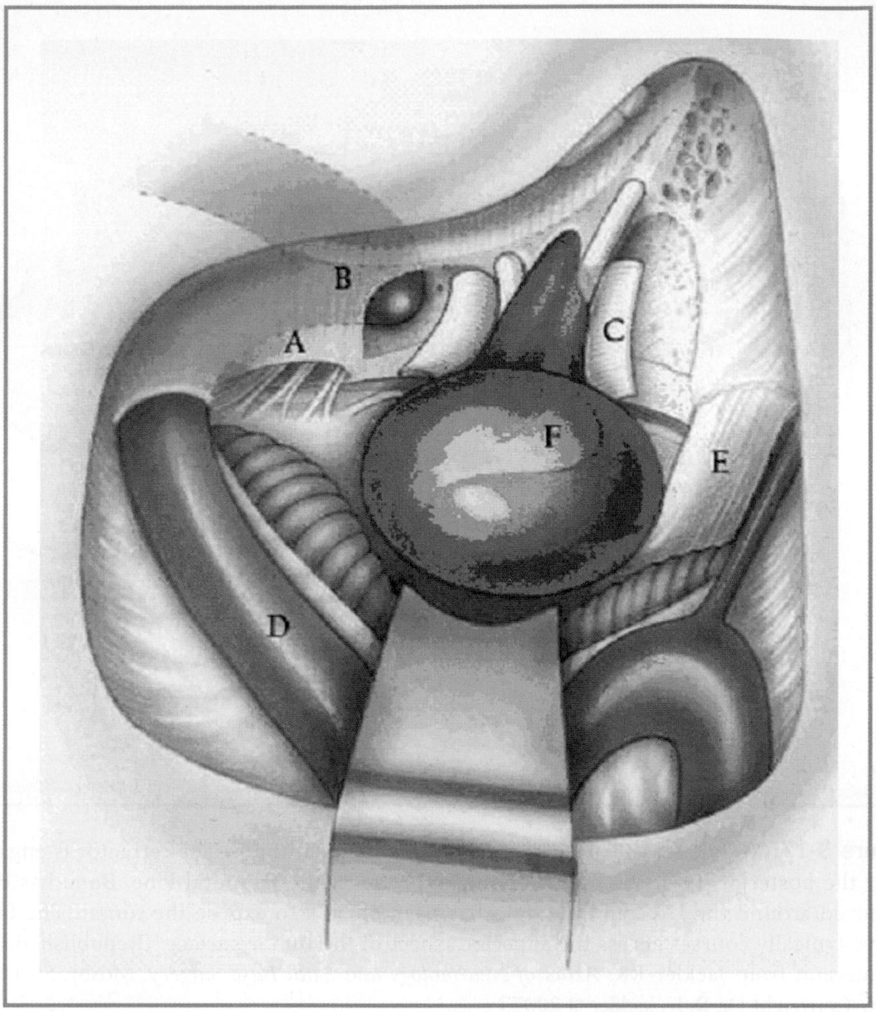

Figure 3-16. Typical left translabyrinthine posterior fossa craniotomy exposure of a medium-sized tumor. Inferiorly, the lower cranial nerves **(A)** are visible and the jugular bulb **(B)** has been identified. Troughs have been drilled above and below the IAC, and the dura **(C)** has been reflected off the tumor surface. The sigmoid sinus **(D)** and cerebellum are gently retracted posteriorly. The trigeminal nerve **(E)** is located superiorly. The facial nerve **(F)** takes a variable and often serpentine course across the medial side of the tumor. (Republished with permission from Jackler RK: Atlas of Neurotology and Skull Base Surgery. Mosby, St. Louis: 1996. Copyright Dr. R. K. Jackler © 2007.)

(IX), vagus nerve (X), accessory nerve (XI), jugular bulb, and inferior petrosal sinus. The most common tumors in this area are paragangliomas. Paragangliomas are divided into two groups: (a) adrenal paragangliomas (also known as pheochromocytomas) and (b) extraadrenal paragangliomas located in the abdomen, chest, and head and neck regions. In the jugular foramen, these tumors are often referred to as **glomus jugulare**. Less common pathologies in this area include meningiomas and lower cranial nerve schwannomas.

Glomus jugulare tumors are highly vascular and patients undergo preop embolization before surgery. Two to 4 U of autologous or crossmatched blood are kept available depending on the size and extent of the tumor. Large-bore ivs should be placed in case rapid transfusion is needed. In addition to a lateral craniotomy similar to the translabyrinthine approach, a limited neck dissection is performed in order to gain vascular control of the jugular vein and carotid artery. This transjugular craniotomy exposes the entire jugular fossa and involves resection of the involved sigmoid sinus and jugular vein (Fig. 3-18). New lower cranial nerve deficits occur

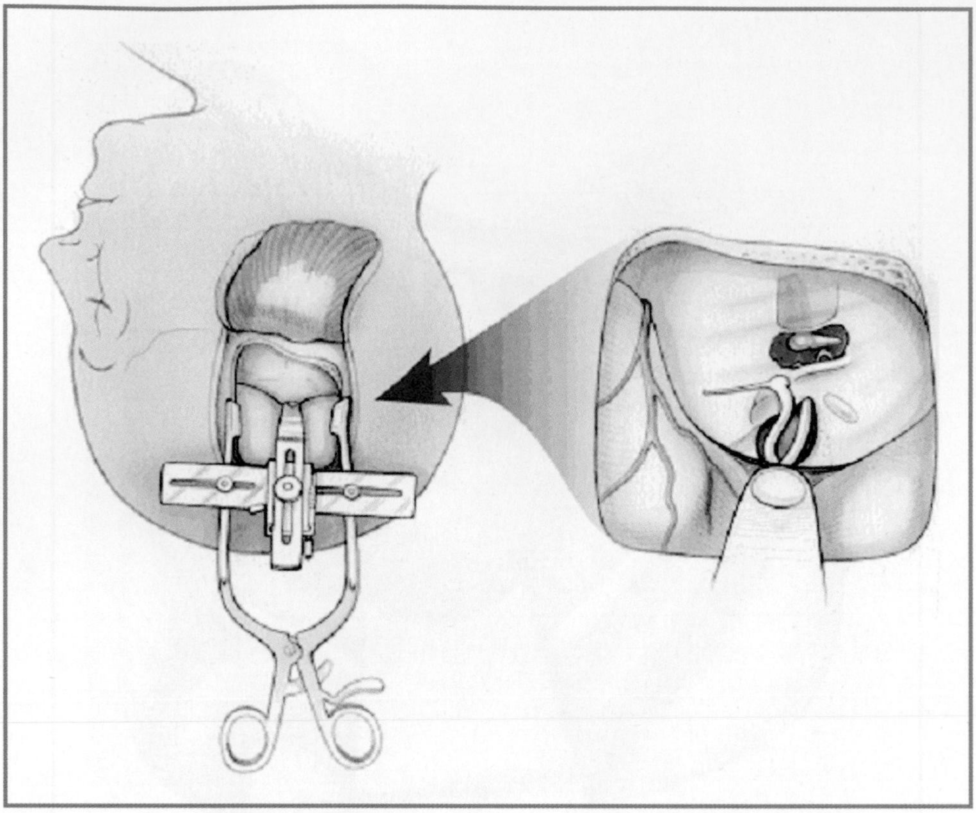

Figure 3-17. Middle fossa exposure of a small right-sided tumor. The retractor is engaged over the posterior lip of the petrous bone and retracts the temporal lobe. Bone has been removed around the IAC, and the dura has been opened to expose the tumor. The facial nerve typically courses across the superior aspect of the tumor surface. (Republished with permission from Jackler RK: *Atlas of Neurotology and Skull Base Surgery*. Mosby, St. Louis: 1996. Copyright Dr. R. K. Jackler © 2007.)

in 25–50% of patients, therefore appropriate airway and aspiration precautions must be taken. Rehabilitation often involves speech therapy and vocal cord medialization. Tracheotomy and PEG tube placement are rarely necessary.

In all of the preceding craniotomies, the patient is turned 180° away from the anesthesiologist. This allows room for the operating microscope, scrub assistant, and surgeon to all be placed around the head of the patient (Figs. 3-19 and 3-20). The patient's head is turned to one side to allow exposure of the lateral cranium and neck. In the retrosigmoid craniotomy, a Mayfield is used for rigid skull fixation. As lateral table rotation is often used during these cases, three straps should be used to secure the patient and the contralateral arm should be well padded in order to avoid ulnar neuropathy. Neurophysiologic monitoring (EMG, auditory brainstem reponses, and SSEPs) is used throughout the case; therefore, muscle relaxants should be avoided.

Stimulation of the trigeminal or vagus nerves can cause bradycardia; therefore, the surgeon should be informed of any unexpected physiologic changes occurring with the patient. Stable low blood pressure is useful in controlling slow bleeding in the surgical field. Significant hemodynamic blood loss is rare and can usually be controlled with secure packing. Large venous injuries may result in air embolism and arterial injuries may require the assistance of interventional neuroradiology. Having 1 U of cross-matched blood available is prudent in most craniotomies, whereas 2–4 U may be required in glomus jugulare cases. Cerebrospinal fluid (CSF) leaks are controlled using an abdominal fat graft.

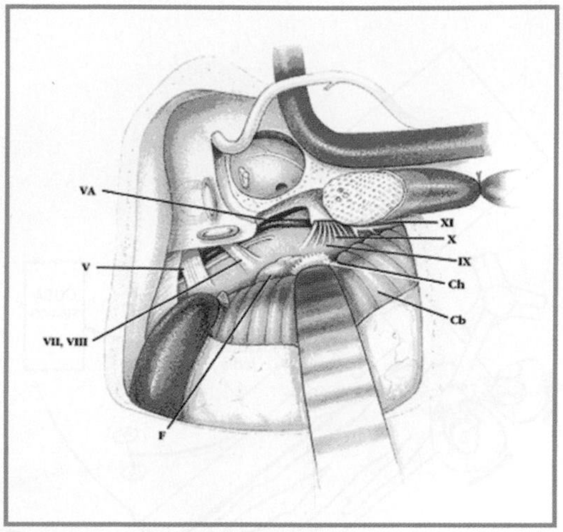

Figure 3-18. Transjugular craniotomy illustrating the degree of intracranial exposure obtained following resection of the sigmoid-jugular system and wide opening of the posterior fossa dura. Note the multiple small rootlets of the lowers cranial nerves emanating from the lateral surface of the medulla. In contrast to extracranial procedures, the sigmoid sinus is ligated proximally rather than packed extralumenally. While this illustration depicts anterior rerouting of the facial nerve, this is not necessary in most intracranial jugular foramen tumors. The sigmoid sinus has been controlled with a suture ligature just distal to the transverse-sigmoid junction. (VA–vertebral artery, F–flocculus, Ch–choroid, Cb–cerebellum, V–trigeminal nerve, VII–facial nerve, VIII–audiovestibular nerve, IX–glossopharyngeal nerve, X–vagus nerve, XI–accessory nerve). (Republished with permission from Jackler RK: *Atlas of Neurotology and Skull Base Surgery.* Mosby, St. Louis: 1996. Copyright Dr. R. K. Jackler © 2007.)

Usual Preop Diagnoses: Vestibular schwannoma (acoustic neuroma); meningioma; paraganglioma (glomus jugulare); lower cranial nerve schwannoma; epidermoid cyst; arachnoid cyst; cholesterol granuloma; chondrosarcoma; chordoma

SUMMARY OF PROCEDURE	
Position	Supine, turned 180° from anesthesia (Figs 3-19 and 3-20). Three straps to secure patient and arms well padded. Mayfield rigid fixation in retrosigmoid craniotomies
Incision	Postauricular or temporal with possible extension into neck depending on approach.
Special instrumentation	Microscope, neurophysiologic monitoring team, ultrasonic aspirator, neck dissection and vascular instruments (transjugular), middle fossa retractor (middle fossa), otologic drill
Antibiotics	Ceftriaxone 2 g iv or vancomycin 1 g iv for CSF penetration
Procedure Time	4–12 h
Closing Considerations	Minimize coughing and ↑ICP. Abdominal fat often harvested for CSF leak closure. Head dressing may be placed.
EBL	100–1000 mL depending on approach and tumor. One unit of cross-matched or autologous blood for craniotomies (2–4 U for glomus jugulare tumors) should be available.
Postop Care	Extubation in majority of cases. Monitoring in ICU for the first night. Minimal sedatives to allow neurological monitoring. Airway and aspiration precautions in patients with possible lower cranial nerve palsies.
Mortality	Rare

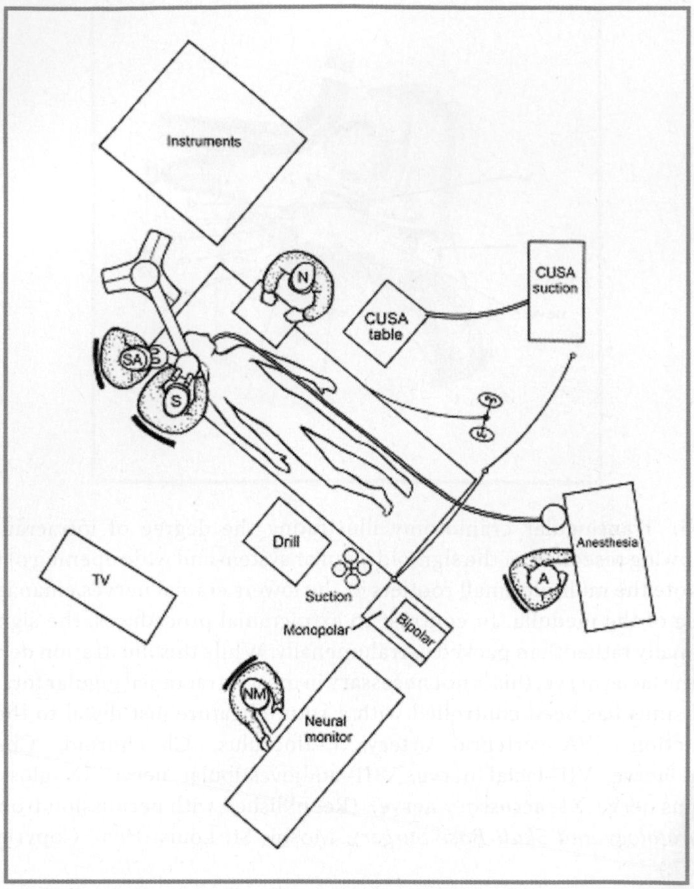

Figure 3-19. Operating room setup for posterior fossa craniotomy (translabyrinthine, retrosigmoid, and transjugular). (Republished with permission from Jackler RK: *Atlas of Neurotology and Skull Base Surgery*. Mosby, St. Louis: 1996. Copyright Dr. R. K. Jackler © 2007.)

SUMMARY OF PROCEDURE (cont'd)

Morbidity	Hearing loss (approach dependent) Vertigo Facial nerve dysfunction Hoarseness Aspiration CSF leak Meningitis Stroke (rare)
Pain Score	4–6

PATIENT POPULATION CHARACTERISTICS

Age range	5th to 6th decades for most pathology Younger patients in tumors associated with neurofibromatosis (NF-2)
Male:Female	1:1 for vestibular schwannoma
Incidence	1/100,000
Etiology	Neoplastic
Associated conditions	Hearing loss (use assistive devices when possible), vertigo, lower cranial nerve dysfunction (aspiration precautions), neurofibromatosis

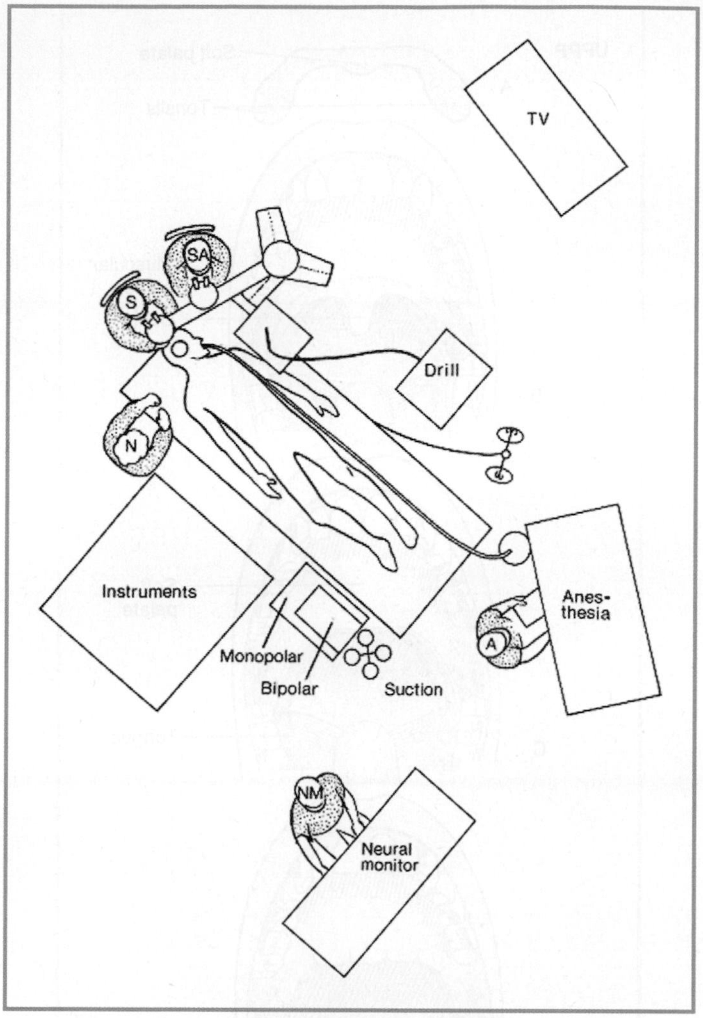

Figure 3-20. Operating room setup for middle fossa craniotomy. (Republished with permission from Jackler RK: *Atlas of Neurotology and Skull Base Surgery*. Mosby, St. Louis: 1996. Copyright Dr. R. K. Jackler © 2007.)

ANESTHETIC CONSIDERATIONS

(See Anesthetic Considerations for Maxillectomy, p. 211)

Suggested Readings

1. Brackmann DE, Bartels LJ: Rare tumors of the cerebellopontine angle. *Otolaryngol Head Neck Surg* 1980; 88:555–9.
2. Lustig LR, Jackler RK: The variable relationship between the lower cranial nerves and jugular foramen tumors: implications for neural preservation. *Am J Otol* 1996; 17:658–68.

RECONSTRUCTIVE SURGERY FOR SLEEP-DISORDERED BREATHING

SURGICAL CONSIDERATIONS

Jerome E. Hester, Robert W. Riley, Nelson B. Powell, and Donald Sesso

Description: The surgical approaches to the upper airway attempt to relieve obstruction occurring most commonly at the level of the palate, base of tongue, or pharynx. These fall into three categories: (a) classic procedures

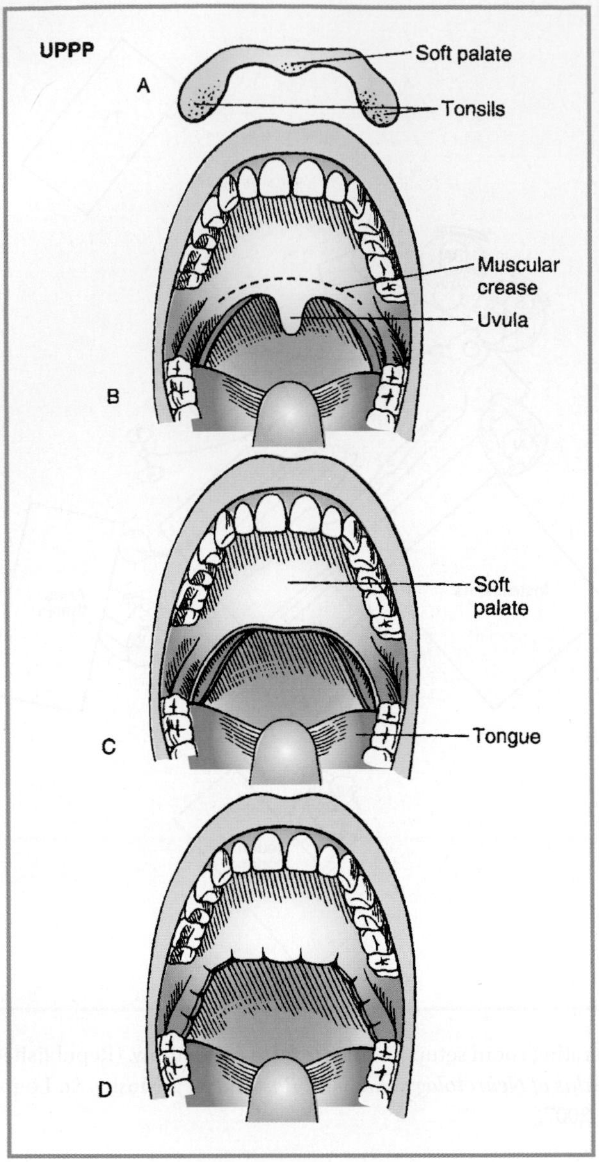

Figure 3-21. Uvulopalatopharyngoplasty (UPPP): **(A&B)** tonsils and redundant soft palate are excised; **(C)** mucosal flaps are prepared for closure; **(D)** the soft palate is closed to itself, and the anterior and posterior tonsillar pillars are sutured to each other.

that directly enlarge the upper airway; (b) specialized procedures that directly enlarge the upper airway; and (c) tracheotomy to bypass the pharyngeal portion of the upper airway. The surgeon performs a preop evaluation, including complete head and neck exam, fiber optic examination of the upper airway, and cephalometric radiographs. This, together with the results of the polysomnogram, will enable the surgeon to determine what levels of the airway need to be surgically modified. Individuals with severe obstruction may require a multistage approach to treatment.

Uvulopalatopharyngoplasty (UPPP) (Fig. 3-21) is a procedure that removes a rim of the soft palate, including the uvula. This shortens and tightens this tissue, thus preventing collapse during sleep. The tonsils, if present, are removed. The muscular crease of the palate is used as a landmark to prevent overly aggressive resection, which could → velopharyngeal insufficiency (VPI), an uncommon but serious complication. The wound is then closed, using interrupted absorbable sutures.

Uvulopalatal flap (UPF) (Fig. 3-22) is a variation of UPPP, used for treating palatal obstruction. Rather than excising a rim of the soft palate, the mucosa of the anterior aspect of the uvula is removed, along with a corresponding area of

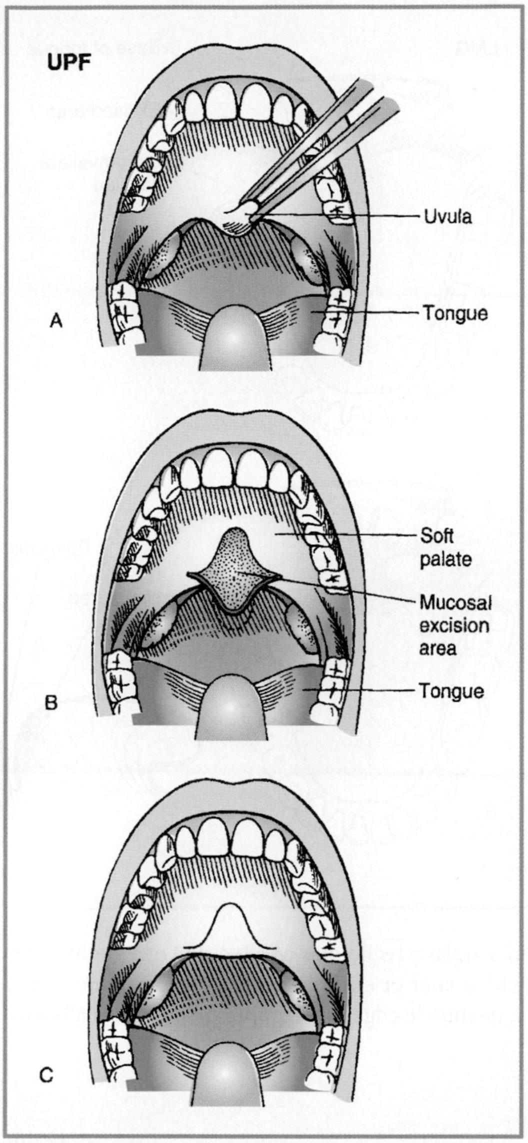

Figure 3-22. Uvulopalatal flap (UPF): **(A)** uvula is reflected back to the hard palate to identify the muscular crease; **(B)** mucosa on the oral side of the uvula and soft palate are removed, and part of the uvula is amputated; **(C)** mucosal incisions are closed with absorbable suture.

the soft palate. The uvula is then reflected superiorly and sutured into place with absorbable suture. This procedure may be done in combination with a tonsillectomy. UPF is theoretically reversible if signs of VPI become evident. UPF also may be somewhat less painful than UPPP.

Uvulopalatopharyngoglossoplasty (UPPGP) is a rarely performed, intraoral procedure incorporating a modified UPPP with limited resection of the base of tongue for both retropalatal and retrolingual collapse.

Laser midline glossectomy (LMG) is used to enlarge the retrolingual airway by excision of ~2.5 cm × 5 cm of midline tongue tissue through an intraoral approach. This also may require lingual tonsillectomy, reduction of the aryepiglottic folds, and partial epiglottectomy (Fig. 3-23). LMG usually is combined with a tracheotomy for airway protection.

Lingualplasty (LP) is the same procedure as LMG, except that additional tongue tissue is extirpated posteriorly and laterally to that portion removed by LMG (Fig. 3-23). It is usually combined with a tracheotomy (see below) for airway protection.

Inferior sagittal mandibular osteotomy and genioglossal advancement (MOGA) (Fig. 3-24) is an intraoral approach designed to enlarge the retrolingual area. This procedure relies on the firm attachment of the

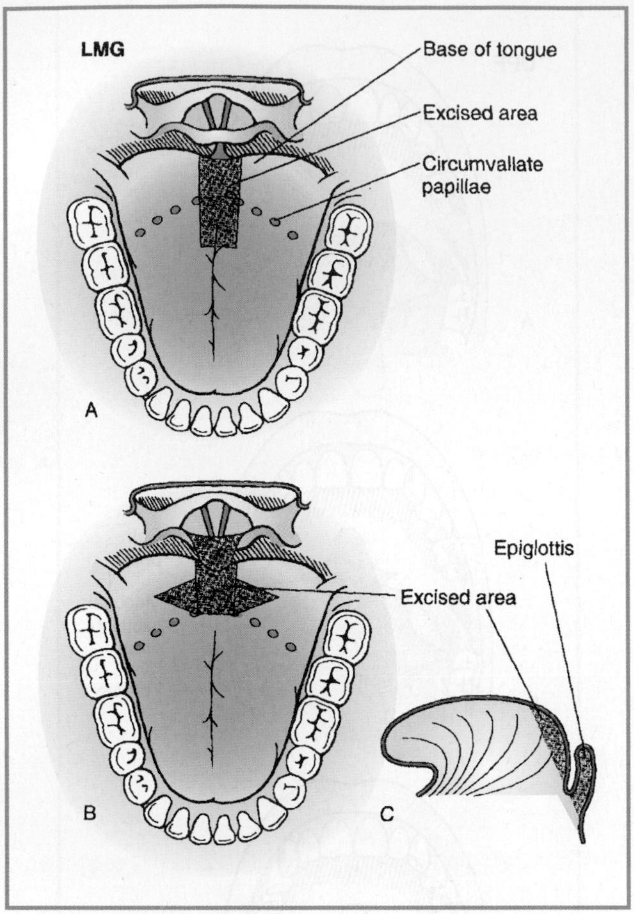

Figure 3-23. LMG/lingualplasty technique: **(A)** Excision of a midline segment of the base of the tongue is performed with a laser or electrocautery; this excision occasionally is carried lateral. **(B)** The remaining tongue muscle edges are reapproximated with absorbable suture. **(C)** Lateral view of tongue.

genioglossus muscle to the geniotubercle, a bony protuberance on the medial (lingual) aspect of the mandible. A mucosal incision is made intraorally and soft tissue, including the mentalis muscle, is elevated off the mandible. Osteotomies, which include the geniotubercle on the inner cortex, are then performed. The segment is advanced and rotated to lock it in place. The outer cortex is removed and the fragment is fixated to the inferior mandible with a titanium screw. The advancement is limited by the width of the mandible and laxity in the genioglossus muscle.

Hyoid myotomy and suspension (HM) is a retrolingual procedure that alleviates obstruction by redundant lateral pharyngeal tissue or a retrodisplaced epiglottis. A horizontal cervical incision above the hyoid bone is performed, and the dissection is carried down to the suprahyoid musculature. The midline hyoid bone is isolated and then advanced over the thyroid ala. It is then immobilized with two medial and two lateral permanent sutures (Fig. 3-25). The wound is closed, a drain placed, and a pressure dressing applied.

Maxillomandibular osteotomy and advancement (MMO) prevents retropalatal collapse through stenting of the superior pharyngeal muscles and widening of the nasopharyngeal inlet. It also minimizes retrolingual obstruction by placing the genioglossus muscle under tension, providing more room in the oral cavity for soft tissues, and stenting the lateral pharyngeal wall. An outer-table cranial bone graft usually is performed, along with arch-bar placement (or orthodontic banding in an outpatient setting) prior to the osteotomies. A LeFort I maxillary osteotomy and bilateral sagittal-split mandibular osteotomy are performed. The skeletal arches are advanced forward ~10 mm and secured with the aid of a methylmethacrylate dental splint (Fig. 3-26). Immobilization with wires, plates and screws follows, then wound closure, intermaxillary fixation, and pressure dressing application.

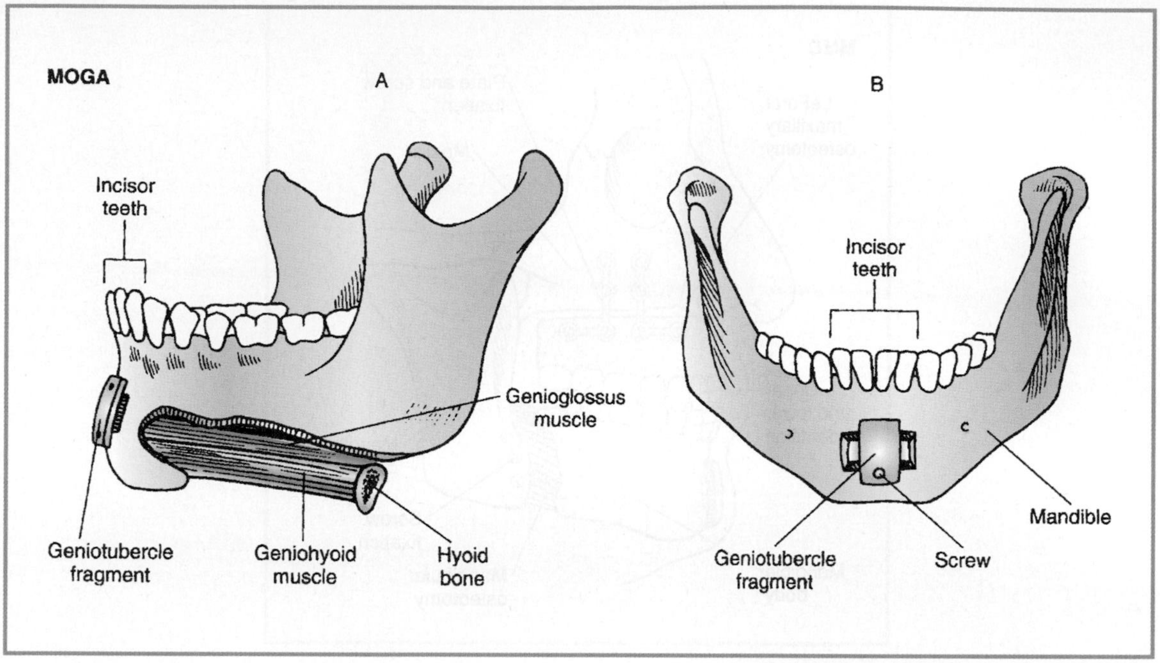

Figure 3-24. The mandibular osteotomy and genioglossus advancement (MOGA) technique: **(A)** Lateral view. **(B)** Anterior view. A rectangular anterior mandibular osteotomy below the incisor teeth is advanced, rotated, and immobilized.

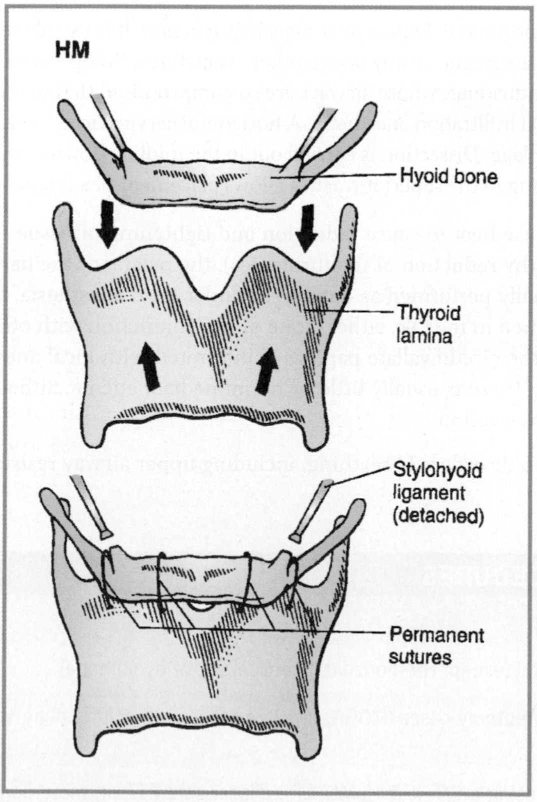

Figure 3-25. The hyoid myotomy (HM) and suspension technique: the hyoid is advanced over the thyroid lamina and immobilized.

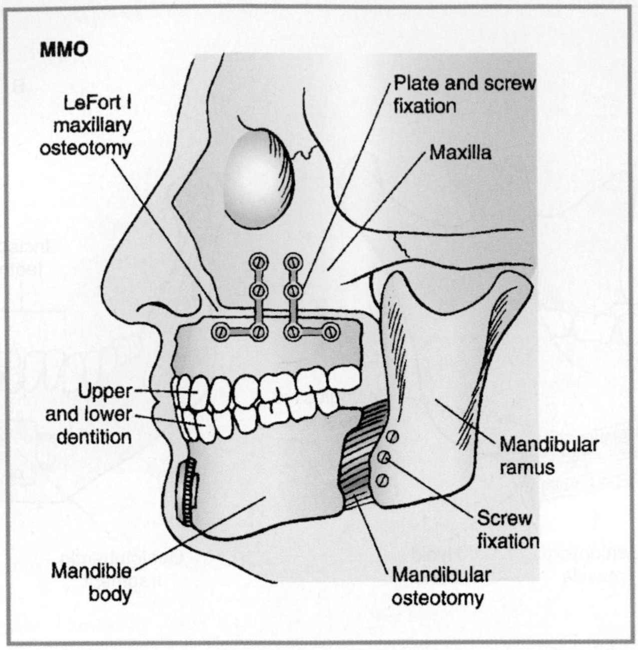

Figure 3-26. Maxillomandibular osteotomy (MMO) and advancement surgery technique.

This procedure usually is performed if previous upper airway procedures have not completely relieved the sleep-related obstruction.

Tracheotomy is a procedure performed to bypass pharyngeal obstruction. It is usually reserved for those individuals with severe OSA and may be used to secure the airway before other procedures. Preop evaluation, including fiber optic examination, will help identify those individuals whose airways are so compromised that the tracheotomy should be done with the patient awake and under local infiltration anesthetic. A horizontal cervical incision is performed midway between the manubrium and the cricoid cartilage. Dissection is carried out in the midline down to the trachea, frequently transecting the thyroid gland; then, an opening in the superior trachea allows placement of a tracheotomy tube (see p. 186).

Radiofrequency (RF) probes use heat to cause reduction and tightening of tissue. This may be used to enable the airway at the level of the nose (by reduction of the turbinates), the palate, or the base of tongue. Whereas the nasal and palatal procedures are usually performed as outpatient under local anesthesia, the initial treatment of the base of tongue commonly is performed in the OR, either alone or in conjunction with other airway procedures. The area of the tongue just anterior to the circumvallate papillae is infiltrated with local anesthetic. A needle-like RF probe is then used to heat the tissue. There is usually little or no immediate edema, although the surgeon may admit the patient overnight for airway observation.

Usual preop diagnosis: Sleep disordered breathing, including upper airway resistance syndrome and obstructive sleep apnea (OSA) syndrome

SUMMARY OF PROCEDURES

Position	Supine
Incision	Intraoral (except HM–horizontal cervical above hyoid bone)
Special instrumentation	For osteotomy cases (MOGA, MMO), sagittal and reciprocating saws, drills
Unique considerations	When using a CO_2 laser (LMG, LP), a laser-safe ETT or, more commonly, a tracheotomy tube is required. MMO requires a nasal intubation. Tracheotomy may be performed with patient sitting with iv sedation and/or local infiltration. Dexamethasone 8 mg iv.
Antibiotics	Cefazolin 1 g iv

SUMMARY OF PROCEDURES (cont'd)	
Surgical time	UPPP, UPF: 20–60 min UPPGP, LMG, LP: 1–3 h MOGA, HM: 30–60 min MMO: 3–5 h
EBL	UPPP, UPF, MOGA, HM: 0–100 mL UPPGP, LMG, LP: 50–250 mL MMO: 100–500 mL
Postop care	UPPP, UPF: PACU → ward Multiple procedures, MMO, labile HTN: ICU → ward
Mortality	Rare
Morbidity	Paresthesias: 10% HTN: 5% Wound dehiscence: 5% Bleeding: 1–2% Infection: 1–2% Hematoma/seroma: 1–2% Upper airway obstruction: 1%
Pain score	UPPP, UPPGP, LMG, LP: 8–10 UPF, MOGA, HM, MMO: 6–8

PATIENT POPULATION CHARACTERISTICS	
Age range	Children, adolescents, adults
Male:Female	3–10:1
Incidence	4–10% of adult males; 2–4% of adult females
Etiology	Upper airway collapse by frank obstruction or muscular relaxation
Associated conditions	Systemic and pulmonary HTN; CAD; cardiac arrhythmias; GERD; depression; obesity; polycythemia

ANESTHETIC CONSIDERATIONS

Michael W. Champeau

PREOPERATIVE

Patients with OSA often present with a variety of related medical conditions. These may range from chronic fatigue to conditions that place the patient at an increased risk of sudden death. Some patients have OSA associated with morbid obesity (see p. 502). Typically, patients with OSA are exquisitely sensitive to sedative drugs. Preop evaluation should include their ability to tolerate the supine position without obstructing.

Respiratory	Chronic OSA → hypoxia/hypercarbia → pulmonary HTN → right heart failure. Careful assessment of the airway is essential (suitability for mask ventilation vs. need for awake FOL or tracheostomy). Typically, 25% of patients will present with airway management problems that may require awake FOL (4%) or tracheostomy (3%). Preop evaluation should include a discussion with the surgeon of the results of preop fiber optic nasopharyngoscopy. **Tests:** PFT; ABG and CXR, if indicated from H&P.
Cardiovascular	Patients are at ↑ risk for systemic and pulmonary HTN (Sx: loud P_2, clubbing, ↑ JVD, cyanosis, RVH, right-axis deviation), cardiac arrhythmias, cerebrovascular disease, and CAD. Patients may have dyspnea on exertion and at rest, making routine assessment of cardiovascular function and reserve difficult. **Tests:** ECG; stress ECHO if abnormal ECG; others as indicated from H&P.

Neurologic	These patients may be chronically fatigued and irritable due to disrupted sleep patterns. Daytime sleepiness also may be associated with hypothyroidism or anemia, which should be ruled out. **Tests:** As indicated by H&P.
Hematologic	Chronic hypoxia → polycythemia (Sx: clubbing, cyanosis) →↑ risk of CVA. **Test:** Hct
Gastrointestinal	This patient population has a higher incidence of GERD and hiatal hernia; thus, full-stomach precautions (see p. B-4) may be required.
Laboratory	**Tests:** As indicated from H&P.
Premedication	Typically, sedative medications should be kept to a minimum in this patient population. If sedative premedication is given, the anesthesiologist **must** remain with the patient and be prepared to manage the airway.

INTRAOPERATIVE

Anesthetic technique: Typically GETA; however, patients undergoing UPF, MOGA, and HM may only require MAC.

Induction	Consideration must be given to securing the airway before induction of anesthesia if a difficult intubation is anticipated. Fiber optic intubation with meticulous topical anesthesia and minimal sedation is recommended for these patients (see Awake FOI, p. B-5); otherwise, standard induction with no muscle relaxant until ability to mask ventilate is assured. An intermediate-acting (e.g., vecuronium 0.1 mg/kg) muscle relaxant may be administered after mask ventilation is established. MMO requires nasal intubation.	
Maintenance	Maintenance with N_2O, propofol, and narcotics, in conjunction with low-dose inhalational agents (e.g., sevoflurane 0.4%), will facilitate a rapid and smooth emergence compared to maintenance with higher doses of other inhalational agents. The use of propofol (75–125 mcg/kg/min) and remifentanil (0.05–0.125 mcg/kg/min) infusions in conjunction with N_2O and low-dose sevoflurane has been particularly successful in providing the smooth, rapid emergence required for safe extubation of these patients. Anticipate ↑ BP in response to the surgical procedure, especially in patients with pre-existing HTN, during UPPP, and with down-fracture of pterygoid plate in MMO. Resist temptation to treat ↑ BP with ↑ inhalational anesthetics alone, as the quality of emergence will be compromised. Labetalol (5 mg increments) and hydralazine (5 mg increments) usually are required, whereas esmolol and SNP infusions are needed occasionally. Dexamethasone 0.1–0.15 mg/kg is recommended to ↓ postop airway edema.	
Emergence	The patient must remain intubated until sufficiently awake to respond to a series of verbal commands. Premature extubation can cause complete loss of airway (2° glossopalatal obstruction) or laryngospasm. Airway is likely to be worse upon emergence than preop 2° surgically induced edema. Extubation over a tube changer may be appropriate in rare cases. Anticipate pain and ↑ BP during emergence, which will continue into first postop day. Narcotic analgesics (e.g., morphine 0.1–0.15 mg/kg) should be administered before emergence. Antihypertensive agents usually required, as postop HTN can cause bleeding, particularly from osteotomy sites.	
Blood and fluid requirements	IV: 16–18 ga × 1 NS/LR @ 1–3 mL/kg/h	Minimal-to-little blood loss with all except MMO. EBL with MMO is 100–500 mL. Attempt to minimize fluids to reduce severity of postop airway edema (< 1000 mL of NS/LR for all except MMO; < 2000 mL for MMO).

Monitoring	Standard monitors (p. B-1) Arterial line (MMO)	Arterial line also suggested for postop BP control in all patients with pre-existing HTN and in any patient who displays labile BP intraop. Control of BP in the postop period is an extremely high priority.
Positioning	✓ and pad pressure points. ✓ eyes.	Occasional requests for minimal Trendelenburg or semi-sitting positioning.
Complications	ETT damage Hemorrhage Dysrhythmias	ETT may become dislodged or kinked during surgical manipulations. Vagally-mediated severe bradycardia/asystole may occur with maxillary or mandibular advancement during MMO.

POSTOPERATIVE

Complications	Airway compromise Airway obstruction	Airway compromise 2° hematoma, edema, excessive sedation, or underlying disease. Consider observation in ICU for patients having multiple procedures, MMO, or labile HTN.
	HTN Aspiration	Postop HTN is extremely common and can contribute significantly to likelihood of postop airway obstruction 2° hematoma.
Pain management	Minimize iv narcotics.	Avoid excessive postop sedation. UPPP patients, in particular, should be warned preop of anticipated significant postop discomfort.

Suggested Readings

1. American Society of Anesthesiologists Task Force on Management of the Difficult Airway: Practice guidelines for management of the difficult airway: an updated report by the American Society of Anesthesiologists Task Force on Management of the Difficult Airway. *Anesthesiology* 2003; 98(5):1269–77.
2. Burgess L, Derderian S, Morin G, et al: Postoperative risk following uvulopalatopharyngoplasty for obstructive sleep apnea. *Otolaryngol Head Neck Surg* 1992; 106:81–6.
3. Conway W, Fujita S, Zorick F, et al: Uvulopalatopharyngoplasty. One-year followup. *Chest* 1985; 88:385–7.
4. Escalamado RM, Glenn MG, McCulloch TM, et al: Perioperative complications and risk factors in the surgical treatment of obstructive sleep apnea. *Laryngoscope* 1989; 99:1125–9.
5. Fairbanks DN: Snoring: Surgical vs nonsurgical management. *Laryngoscope* 1984; 94:1188–92.
6. Fujita S, Conway W, Zorick F, et al: Surgical correction of anatomic abnormalities in obstructive sleep apnea syndrome: Uvulopalatopharyngoplasty. *Otolaryngol Head Neck Surg* 1981; 89:923–34.
7. Gross JB, Bachenberg KL, Benumof JL, et al; American Society of Anesthesiologists Task Force on Perioperative Management. Practice guidelines for the perioperative management of patients with obstructive sleep apnea: a report by the American Society of Anesthesiologists Task Force on Perioperative Management of patients with obstructive sleep apnea. *Anesthesiology* 2006; 104(5):1081–93.
8. Johnson JT, Pollack GL, Wagner RL: Transoral radiofrequency treatment of snoring. *Otolaryngol Head Neck Surg* 2002; 127:235–7.
9. Li KK, Powell NB, Riley RW, et al: Radiofrequency volumetric tissue reduction for treatment of turbinate hypertrophy: a pilot study. *Otolaryngol Head Neck Surg* 1998; 119:569–73.
10. Li KK, Powell NB, Riley RW, et al: Temperature controlled radiofrequency tongue base reduction for sleep-disordered breathing: long term outcomes. *Otolaryngol Head Neck Surg* 2002; 127:230–3.
11. Mickleson SA, Rosenthal L: Midline glossectomy and epiglottidectomy for obstructive sleep apnea syndrome. *Laryngoscope* 1997; 107:614–9.
12. Powell N, Riley R, Guilleminault C, et al: A reversible uvulopalatal flap for snoring and sleep apnea syndrome. *Sleep* 1996; 19(7):593–9.
13. Riley R, Powell N, Guilleminault C: Obstructive sleep apnea and the hyoid: a revised surgical procedure. *Otolaryngol Head Neck Surg* 1994; 111:717–21.

14. Riley R, Powell N, Guilleminault C: Obstructive sleep apnea syndrome: a review of 306 consecutively treated surgical patients. *Otolaryngol Head Neck Surg* 1993; 108:117–25.
15. Riley RW, Powell NP, Guilleminault C, et al: Obstructive sleep apnea surgery: risk management and complications. *Otolaryngol Head Neck Surg* 1997; 117(6):648–52.
16. Sher A, Schechtman K, Piccirillo J: The efficacy of surgical modifications of the upper airway in adults with obstructive sleep apnea syndrome. *Sleep* 1996; 19(2):156–77.
17. Woodson BT, Fujita S: Clinical experience with lingualplasty as part of the treatment of severe obstructive sleep apnea. *Otolaryngol Head Neck Surg* 1992; 107:40–8.

SECTION

4.0 DENTAL SURGERY

SURGEONS

Stephen A. Schendel, MD, DDS, FACS
Joseph Looby, DO

ANESTHESIOLOGIST

Richard A. Jaffe, MD, PhD

TEMPOROMANDIBULAR JOINT ARTHROSCOPY/ ARTHROTOMY

SURGICAL CONSIDERATIONS

Description: **Temporomandibular joint (TMJ)** surgical procedures include both open and closed surgical techniques.

TMJ arthrotomy involves a preauricular, postauricular, or endaural incision to gain access to the joint compartment. It usually is performed for severe fibrous adhesion removal in the TMJ, bony or fibrous ankylosis, tumor resection, chronic dislocation, painful nonreducing disc dislocation, and severe osteoarthritis. **Open TMJ** surgery may range from discoplasty; discectomy; arthroplasty; and/or eminoplasty (reshaping of articular eminentia) to optimize the fit of the disc, condyle, and fossa; to total joint replacement utilizing costochondral grafts or vitallium metal implants. For the open treatment of condylar fractures, extraoral approaches (e.g., preauricular, retromandibular, and submandibular) are used. All extraoral approaches to the TMJ have the risks of facial nerve damage and the creation of visible scars. Due to those possible complications, endoscopically assisted transoral approaches for open reduction and miniplate fixation of condylar mandible fractures are used increasingly more often.

TMJ arthroscopy is a minimally invasive technique that has reduced the need for open surgery of the TMJ. Arthroscopic TMJ surgery is indicated for treatment of internal derangements and intracapsular disorders. The major advantage is that it results in less periarticular tissue disruption and better preservation of vascular supply and lymphatic drainage of the joint. The procedure involves insertion of a TMJ miniscope through a preauricular puncture on the canthus-tragus line and insertion of an outflow needle. The joint compartment is continually lavaged with LR. A second cannula can be inserted. Arthroscopic procedures are performed using a triangulation technique. Arthroscopic TMJ procedures include lysis of adhesions and lavage, partial synovectomy, and abrasion arthroplasty. Sometimes a holmium:YAG laser is used to make intraarticular incisions anterior to displaced discs and to treat inflamed synovial tissue. Usually, at the end of the procedure, 2 mg dexamethasone is injected into the joint space. Injection of 2 mL 0.5% bupivacaine mixed with 1 mL sterile saline solution has been shown to significantly reduce postop pain. Arrhythmia, reflex bradycardia, and pulmonary edema have been reported as general complications in TMJ arthroscopy.

Usual preop diagnosis: Internal derangement, subluxation, and ankylosis of TMJ

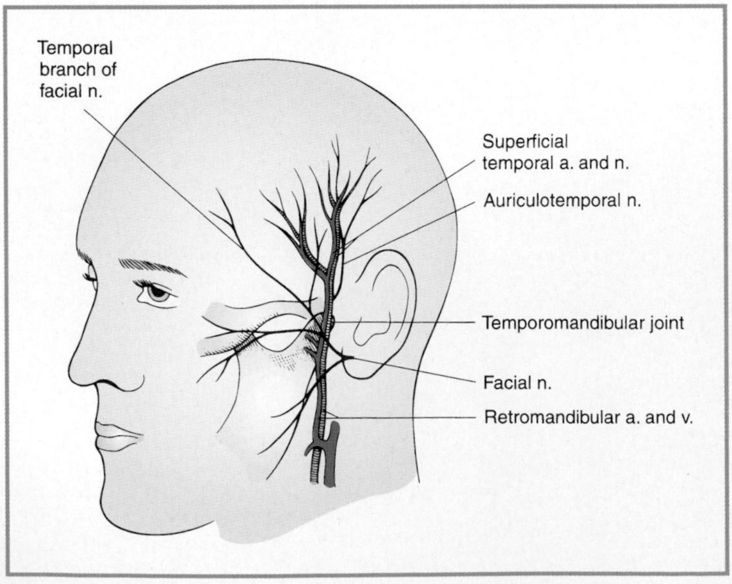

Figure 4-1. Anatomy for TMJ procedure.

SUMMARY OF PROCEDURES

	Arthroscopy	Arthrotomy
Position	Supine	⇐
Incision	Preauricular	⇐
Special instrumentation	Arthroscope; laser	Power tools, endoscope, implant plates
Antibiotics	Cefazolin 1 g	⇐
Surgical time	0.5 h	1.5–3.5 h/side
EBL	Minimal	Minimal-moderate
Postop care	Outpatient procedure	24 h stay
Mortality	Minimal	⇐
Morbidity	VII nerve damage V nerve damage Hemorrhage Partial hearing loss Ear fullness Vertigo	⇐ ⇐ ⇐
Pain score	5	5

PATIENT POPULATION CHARACTERISTICS

Age range	20–40 yr
Male:Female	1:9
Incidence	20% of adult population suffers from TMJ dysfunction (TMJD)
Etiology	TMJD possibly 2° muscle spasm, bruxism, osteoarthritis; idiopathic; trauma
Associated conditions	Psychiatric problems (typically depression); trismus; pain on opening mouth; stress

ANESTHETIC CONSIDERATIONS

See Anesthetic Considerations for Dental/Oral Surgery, p. 264.

Suggested Readings

1. Al-Ani Z, Gray R. TMD current concepts: 1. An update. *Dent Update.* 2007; 34(5):278–80, 282–4, 287–8.
2. Fricton JR, Look JO, Schiffman E, et al: Long-term study of temporomandibular joint surgery with alloplastic implants compared with nonimplant surgery and nonsurgical rehabilitation for painful temporomandibular joint disc displacement. *J Oral Maxillofac Surg* 2002; 60(12):1400–11.
3. Furst IM, Kryshtalskyj B, Weinberg S: The use of intra-articular opioids and bupivacaine for analgesia following temporomandibular joint arthroscopy: a prospective, randomized trial. *J Oral Maxillofac Surg* 2001; 59(9):979–83.
4. Indresano AT: Surgical arthroscopy as the preferred treatment for internal derangements of the temporomandibular joint. *J Oral Maxillofac Surg* 2001; 59(3):308–12.
5. Laskin DM: Temporomandibular disorders: the past, present and future. *Odontology* 2007; 95(1):10–5.
6. Mazzonetto R, Spagnoli DB: Long-term evaluation of arthroscopic discectomy of the temporomandibular joint using the Holmium YAG laser. *J Oral Maxillofac Surg* 2001; 59(9):1018–23.
7. Schon R, Schramm A, Gellrich NC, et al: Follow-up of condylar fractures of the mandible in 8 patients at 18 months after transoral endoscopic-assisted open treatment. *J Oral Maxillofac Surg* 2003; 61(1):49–54.
8. Tsuyama M, Kondoh T, Seto K, et al: Complications of temporomandibular joint arthroscopy: a retrospective analysis of 301 lysis and lavage procedures performed using the triangulation technique. *J Oral Maxillofac Surg* 2000; 58(5):500–5.

ORAL SURGERY

SURGICAL CONSIDERATIONS

Description: The most common surgeries of the oral cavity are third-molar removal, surgical extractions, apicoectomies, orthodontic exposures of teeth, osseointegrated implants, bone grafting, treatment of oral pathologic conditions, and preprosthetic surgery. **Surgical extractions** of teeth involve intraoral exposure of the roots through a mucosal incision and removal of overlying bone with a surgical drill. Risks associated with removal of teeth in the mandible are damage to the inferior alveolar nerve (anesthetic numb lip), lingual nerve (anesthetic numb tongue), and, rarely, mandibular fracture. In the posterior maxilla, oroantral fistulas can occur and are closed with a mucoperiosteal flap. **Exposure of teeth** for orthodontic therapy involves creation of a mucoperiosteal flap and attachment of a bracket with a small gold chain, on which the orthodontist can pull to integrate the tooth into the dental arch. **Bone grafting** to the maxilla and mandible is done for augmentation of the atrophied alveolar ridge and the maxillary sinus and in cases of cleft lip and palate. A second team usually harvests the bone at the same time. Possible extraoral harvesting sites include the anterior or posterior iliac crest, the tibia, and the skull. **Preprosthetic surgery** of the oral soft tissue in preparation for dentures has been replaced largely by insertion of **osseointegrated implants** for retention of individual teeth and dentures. Surgical treatment of **oral pathology** can range from removal of dentigerous cysts, with and without bone graft, to laser or surgical removal of mucosal lesions.

SUMMARY OF PROCEDURES

	Dental Surgery	Dental Implants	Oral Pathology	Bone Grafting
Position	Supine	⇐	⇐	Supine or prone
Incision	Intraoral	⇐	⇐	Intraoral and donor site
Special instrumentation	Surgical drill	Implant drill and kit	Surgical drill, laser	–
Antibiotics	None	Penicillin 1 g	Cefazolin 1 g	⇐
Unique considerations	Nasotracheal intubation Throat pack	⇐ ⇐	⇐ ⇐	⇐ ⇐
Surgical time	0.5 h/tooth	0.5 h/implant	1–3 h	2–3 h
EBL	Minimal	⇐	⇐	Moderate
Postop care	Outpatient	⇐	⇐ or 24 h stay	24 h stay
Mortality	Minimal	⇐	⇐	⇐
Morbidity	V nerve damage Aspiration of dental debris	⇐ ⇐	⇐	Hemorrhage
Pain score	3	2	3–5	5

PATIENT POPULATION CHARACTERISTICS

Age range	12–40 yr	> 16 yr	All ages	> 8 yr
Male:Female	1:1	⇐	⇐	⇐
Etiology	Idiopathic	Tooth loss	Various	⇐
Associated conditions	Craniofacial syndromes			

ANESTHETIC CONSIDERATIONS

See Anesthetic Considerations for Dental/Oral Surgery, p. 264.

Suggested Readings

1. Bataineh AB: Sensory nerve impairment following mandibular third molar surgery. *J Oral Maxillofac Surg* 2001; 59(9):1012–7.
2. Bilkay U, Tokat C, Ozek C, et al: Cancellous bone grafting in alveolar cleft repair: new experience. *J Craniofac Surg* 2002; 13(5):658–63.
3. Coulthard P, Esposito M, Worthington HV, et al: Interventions for replacing missing teeth: preprosthetic surgery versus dental implants (Cochrane Review). *Cochrane Database Syst Rev* 2002; (4):CD003604.
4. Kaufman E: Maxillary sinus elevation surgery. *Dent Today* 2002; 21(9):96–101.
5. Perry PA, Goldberg MH: Late mandibular fracture after third molar surgery: a survey of Connecticut oral and maxillofacial surgeons. *J Oral Maxillofac Surg* 2000; 58(8):858–61.

RESTORATIVE DENTISTRY

SURGICAL CONSIDERATIONS

Description: Multiple dental restorative procedures are performed under GA when there is rampant caries, and an extensive amount of dental work must be performed at one time. The second most common indication for GA is for procedures that need to be performed on mentally retarded patients who are not candidates for a local anesthetic. The actual amount of restorative dentistry is quite variable, depending on the individual case; thus, surgical time can be quite variable. Generally, blood loss is not a problem.

SUMMARY OF PROCEDURE	
Position	Supine
Incision	Intraoral
Special instrumentation	Dental armamentarium
Unique considerations	Nasal intubation; throat pack
Antibiotics	Penicillin ×5 d po
Surgical time	0.5–3 h
EBL	Minimal
Postop care	PACU →home
Mortality	Minimal
Morbidity	Pain Aspiration of dental debris Swelling
Pain score	1–3

PATIENT POPULATION CHARACTERISTICS	
Age range	2 yr–adult
Male:Female	1:1

PATIENT POPULATION CHARACTERISTICS (cont'd)	
Incidence	Unknown
Etiology	Idiopathic or congenital anomalies
Associated conditions	Mental retardation (majority); Down syndrome, seizures

ANESTHETIC CONSIDERATIONS FOR DENTAL/ORAL SURGERY

PREOPERATIVE

Most patients presenting for dental or oral surgery usually will require only local anesthesia provided by the dentist/oral surgeon. Deep sedation or GA may be required, however, for several unique patient groups: (1) young children (some with systemic diseases such as CHD, hemophilia); (2) the mentally retarded; (3) those with poorly controlled seizure disorders; (4) those presenting for TMJ procedures; and (5) those with an oral septic focus, who may be quite ill. If the patient does not fall into one of these readily identifiable categories, the reasons for GA should be ascertained. An LMA with a flexible wire-reinforced airway tube (LMA-Flexible) has been used successfully for a variety of oral surgical procedures. The use of an LMA should be discussed with the surgeon in advance since its presence may interfere with the planned procedure.

Airway	Patients presenting for TMJ procedures may have problems with mouth opening (2° pain, trismus, and arthritis), making airway examination difficult. Mouth opening may not improve with GA and muscle relaxation. Nasotracheal intubation using FOL (done awake in patients with difficult airways) should be planned. Examine nares for patency; check for loose teeth.
Respiratory	Surgery should be postponed (at least 2 wk) in patients presenting with Sx of acute RTI (fever, coughing, purulent sputum, etc.). Sx of chronic respiratory disease should be sought and treated before surgery. LMA use has been reported to decrease respiratory complications in children with upper RTIs. **Tests:** As indicated from H&P
Cardiovascular	Patients with dysrhythmias may be sensitive to the epinephrine used in local anesthetic solutions administered intraop. As with other types of elective surgery, preexisting cardiovascular problems should be treated before surgery. Prophylactic antibiotics for endocarditis are not required in most patients, exceptions include patients with prosthetic valves, congenital heart disease, h/o infective endocarditis, or heart transplant. **Tests:** As indicated from H&P
Neurological	Patients with seizure disorders should be on optimal medical therapy before surgery. Discuss precipitating factors and prodromal Sx with the patient. **Tests:** ✓ therapeutic levels of anticonvulsant (e.g., phenytoin = 10–20 mcg/mL; carbamazepine = 3–12 mcg/mL; phenobarbital = 10–40 mcg/mL)
Musculoskeletal	In addition to TMJ problems, rheumatoid arthritis is associated with cricoarytenoid joint immobility and cervical spine immobility/instability that may complicate intubation.
Laboratory	Other tests as indicated from H&P
Premedication	Standard premedication (see p. B-1) usually is appreciated, although in patients with limited airway access, sedation may be inappropriate. If FOL is planned, pretreatment with an antisialagogue (e.g., glycopyrrolate 4 mcg/kg) is useful. Metoclopramide (e.g. 10–20 mg iv adult) will reduce the incidence of PONV 2° swallowed blood.

INTRAOPERATIVE

Anesthetic technique: GETA. Typically a nasotracheal intubation is required, using an ETT 0.5–1 mm smaller than for oral intubation. In patients with difficult airways, an awake nasal FOL is indicated. (See general discussion of Awake FOL, p. B-5.)

Induction	In patients with normal airways, a standard induction (see p. B-2) with nasal intubation is appropriate. Following loss of consciousness, topical intranasal cocaine may be applied (4% on pledgets, 4 mL maximum) to shrink the nasal mucosa and for vasoconstriction. Side effects are rare, but may include ↑BP, ↑ or ↓HR, dysrhythmias, and Sz. Other topical vasoconstrictors (e.g., 0.05% oxymetazoline) may be used; however, they are also associated with cardiovascular side effects. The well-lubricated ETT is passed through the nose into the trachea, either blindly or assisted by McGill's forceps under direct laryngoscopy. The ETT is often sewn to nasal septum. The successful use of a flexible reinforced LMA in both adult and pediatric dental patients has been reported. Claimed advantages include no risk of epistaxis and no need for a throat pack, laryngoscopy or muscle relaxation. Disadvantages include interference with the procedure, throat trauma (e.g. swelling of the epiglottis) and aspiration risk.
Maintenance	Standard maintenance (see p. B-2)
Emergence	**NB: throat packs must be removed prior to extubation.** An LMA is typically removed after the patient is awake and able to follow commands.
Blood and fluid requirements	IV: 18 ga ×1 NS/LR @ 4–6 mL/kg/h
Monitoring	Standard monitors (see p. B-1)
Positioning	✓ and pad pressure points ✓ eyes

POSTOPERATIVE

These patients may swallow blood, with consequent N&V. Rx: metoclopramide 10 mg iv.

Complications	Airway obstruction 2° retained throat pack PONV	Always check for retained throat pack in patients exhibiting symptoms of airway obstruction
Pain management	Oral analgesics (see p. C-2)	

Suggested Reading for Dental/Oral Surgery

1. Atan S, Ashley P, Gilthrope MS, et al: Morbidity following dental treatment of children under intubation general aneaesthesia in a day-stay unit. *Int J Paediatr Dent* 2004; 14(1):9–16.
2. Boren E, Teuber SS, Naguwa SM, et al: A critical review of local anesthetic sensitivity. *Clin Rev Allergy Immunol* 2007; 32(1):119–28.
3. Dolwick MF, Kretzschmar DP: Morbidity associated with the preauricular and perimeatal approaches to the temporomandibular joint. *J Oral Maxillofac Surg* 1982; 40(11):699–700.
4. Finder RL, Moore PA: Adverse drug reactions to local anesthesia. *Dent Clin North Am* 2002; 46(4):747–57.
5. Gupta A, Epstein JB, Cabay RJ: Bleeding disorders or importance in dental care and related patient management. *J Can Dent Assoc* 2007; 73(1):77–83.
6. Jackson DL, Johnson BS: Conscious sedation for dentistry: risk management and patient selection. *Dent Clin North Am* 2002; 46(4):767–80.
7. Jackson DL, Johnson BS: Inhalational and enteral conscious sedation for the adult dental patient. *Dent Clin North Am* 2002; 46(4):781–802.
8. Krohner RG: Anesthetic considerations and techniques for oral and maxillofacial surgery. *Int Anesthesiol Clin* 2003; 41(3):67–89.

9. Mayhew JF: Airway management for oral and maxillofacial surgery. *Int Anesthesiol Clin.*2003; 41(3):57–65.
10. Rollert MK: The case against the laryngeal mask airway for anesthesia in oral and maxillofacial surgery. *J Oral Maxillofac Surg* 2004; 62(6):739–41.
11. Sakamoto H, Karakida K, Otsuru M, et al: Antibiotic prevention of infective endocarditis due to oral procedures: myth, magic, or science? *J Infect Chemother* 2007; 13(4):189–95.
12. Smith MH, Lung KE: Nerve injuries after dental injection: a review of the literature. *J Can Dent Assoc* 2006; 72(6):559–64.
13. Stapleton M, Sheller B, Williams BJ, et al: Combining procedures under general anesthesia. *Pediatr Dent* 2007; 29(5):397–402.
14. Todd DW: Anesthetic considerations for the obese and morbidly obese oral and maxillofacial surgery patient. *J Oral Maxillofac Surg* 2005; 63(9):1348–53.
15. Webb MD, Moore PA: Sedation for pediatric dental patients. *Dent Clin North Am* 2002; 46(4):803–14, xi.
16. Wilson W, Taubert KA, Gewitz M, et al: Prevention of infective endocarditis: guidelines from the American Heart Association: a guideline from the American Heart Association Rheumatic Fever, Endocarditis and Kawasaki Disease Committee, Council on Cardiovascular Disease in the Young, and the Council on Clinical Cardiology, Council on Cardiovascular Surgery and Anesthesia, and the Quality of Care and Outcomes Research Interdisciplinary Working Group. *J Am Dent Assoc* 2007; 138(6):739–45, 747–60.

SECTION

5.0 THORACIC SURGERY

SURGEONS

Richard I. Whyte, MD
Walter B. Cannon, MD

ANESTHESIOLOGISTS

Gordon Finlayson, MD, FRCPC
Jens Lohser, MD, MSc, FRCPC
Jay B. Brodsky, MD

INTRODUCTION—SURGEON'S PERSPECTIVE

AIRWAY AND LUNG ACCESS CONFLICTS

As in Chapter 3, induction and maintenance of anesthesia for thoracic surgery requires interdisciplinary cooperation. Perioperative communication between the surgeon and anesthesiologist is required for a satisfactory outcome. For example, during periods of OLV, significant hypoxia and hypotension may occur. Surgery may need to be stopped temporarily while the hypoxia is corrected by reinflation of the unventilated lung. Hypotension in the absence of bleeding can be corrected by less vigorous retraction of the lung and heart by the surgeon. Quick and timely communication between the anesthesiologist and the surgeon can be life-saving. Occasionally, during critical parts of the dissection, cessation of all respiration for short periods of time can make the surgeon's job much easier. Testing the changes is an option.

TUBES AND TUBE SIZES

Although the size of the ETTs may not be particularly critical for most types of surgery, thoracic surgical procedures are often different. Fiber optic bronchoscopy (FOB) through the ETT is a common event. The standard FOB just fits through an 8.0 ETT. The fiber optic laryngoscope (FOL) used for difficult intubations will fit smaller ETTs and DLTs. Proper lubrication of the bronchoscope with a polyethylene glycol-based ointment (e.g., Carbowax rather than an aqueous jelly, which will dry out quickly) makes manipulation quite easy. The FOL can be used for correct positioning of the DLT. If the bronchial portion of the DLT cannot be advanced into the left main bronchus, the bronchoscope can be advanced through the bronchial side of the DLT into the left main bronchus. Then, through use of the bronchoscope as a stent, the DLT can be advanced over the bronchoscope into the left bronchus. The depth of the tube can be determined by bronchoscopic observation of the right main bronchus through the tracheal side of the DLT. If a laser is to be involved, have a laser-compatible ETT available, keep FiO_2 to < 0.3 and do not use N_2O.

PATIENT POSITIONING AND SURGICAL INCISIONS

Patient positioning for these procedures is dictated by the type of incision used. The incisions used most often by thoracic surgeons are the **posterolateral thoracotomy** (and its variations) (Fig. 5-1A), the **median sternotomy** (Fig. 5-1B), and the anterior thoracotomy (often bilateral) (Fig. 5-1C). For procedures where excellent exposure of both lungs is mandatory (e.g., bipulmonary lung transplantation), the **"clamshell" incision** (Fig. 5-2) has become popular. Generally, patients are in the **supine position** for anterior incisions (sternotomy, cervical, and anterior thoracotomy) and in the **lateral position** for lateral and posterolateral thoracotomies. Thoracoscopic procedures (VATS) typically are performed in the lateral position. (Note: A review of a recent CXR in the OR will help ensure that the thoracotomy is performed on the correct side.)

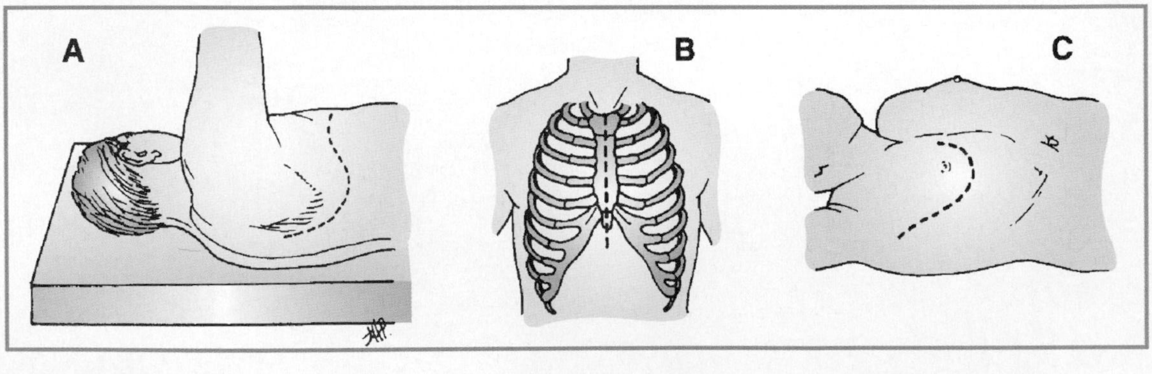

Figure 5-1. Primary incisions for thoracic surgery. **A.** Posterolateral thoracotomy, in lateral position. The incision curves in an S shape, passing under the tip of the scapula over in the fifth interspace anteriorly. **B.** Median sternotomy, in supine position, arms at side: the incision is made from the suprasternal notch to a point between the xiphoid process and umbilicus. **C.** Anterior thoracotomy in supine position. (Reproduced with permission from Fry WA: Thoracic incisions. In *General Thoracic Surgery,* 5th edition. Shields TW, LoCicero J III, Ponn RB, eds. Lippincott Williams & Wilkins, Philadelphia: 2000.)

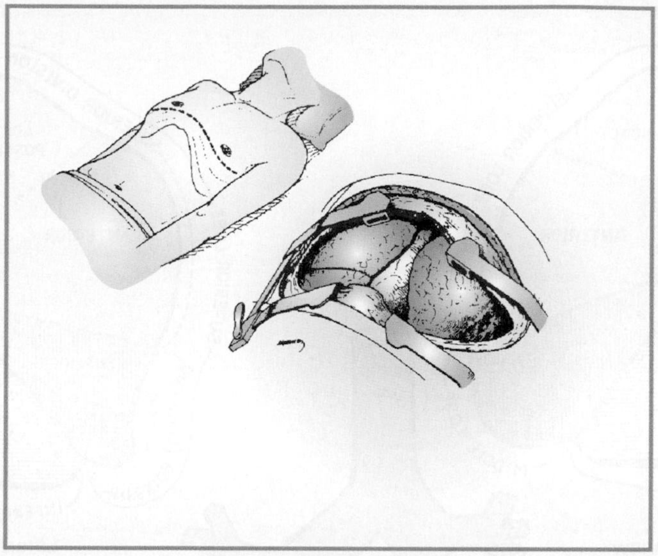

Figure 5-2. The "clamshell" incision, in classic supine position, affords excellent exposure, especially for bilateral lung procedures. (Reproduced with permission from Fry WA: Thoracic incisions. In *General Thoracic Surgery*, 5th edition. Shields TW, LoCicero J III, Ponn RB, eds. Lippincott Williams & Wilkins, Philadelphia: 2000.)

Patients undergoing surgery in the **lateral position** are initially placed on a bean bag. When GA is induced, the patient is rolled onto his/her side with the kidney rest being positioned at the level of the lower ribs. An axillary roll is placed to prevent axillary compression, and the table is flexed to assist in spreading the ribs. The head and neck must be aligned in a neutral position to avoid brachial plexus injuries. The lower arm can be either extended on an arm board or flexed and placed next to the patient's head (Fig. 5-3A). The upper arm is

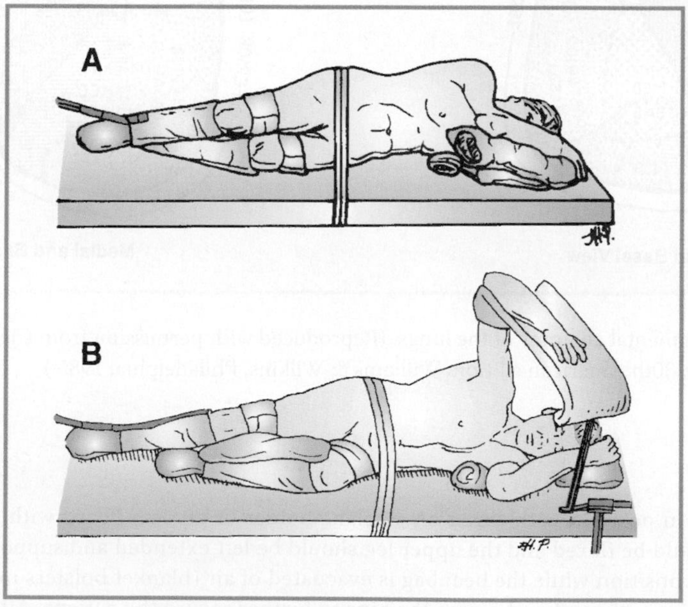

Figure 5-3. Lateral positioning for thoracic lateral and posterolateral procedures. **A.** Patient on his side, with kidney rest, axillary roll, pillows between knees, and padding under elbows. Wide adhesive tape secures the position. **B.** Upper arm abducted 90% on arm board. (Reproduced with permission from Fry WA: Thoracic incisions. In *General Thoracic Surgery*, 5th edition. Shields TW, LoCicero J III, Ponn RB, eds. Lippincott Williams & Wilkins, Philadelphia: 2000.)

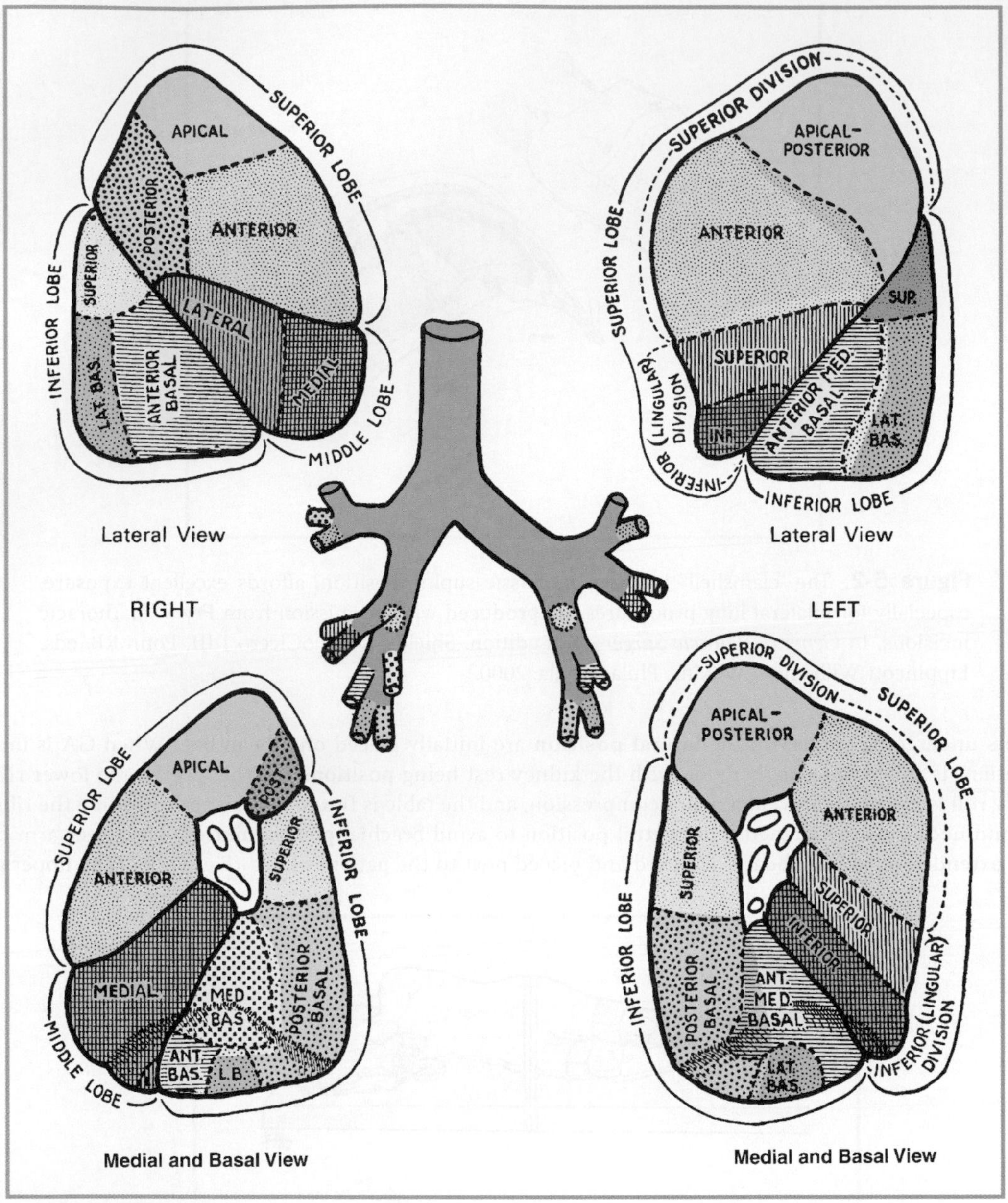

Figure 5-4. Segmental anatomy of the lungs. (Reproduced with permission from Clemente CD: *Gray's Anatomy,* 30th American edition. Williams & Wilkins, Philadelphia: 1985.)

then extended and held in position with either an airplane holder or an arm board with several pillows (Fig. 5-3B). The lower leg should be flexed and the upper leg should be left extended and supported by pillows. The back is kept in a vertical position while the beanbag is evacuated of air (blanket bolsters may be placed next to the patient). Wide adhesive tape is placed across the hips to further secure the patient. A lower-body warming blanket (e.g., Bair Hugger) should be used to avoid hypothermia. To facilitate closure, the table can be returned to the flat position. Ideally, this is accompanied by inflation, and subsequent deflation, of the beanbag. The anesthesiologist may be asked to exert downward pressure on the patient's shoulder to diminish tension on the latissimus dorsi closure.

Although the standard posterolateral thoracotomy involves division of the latissimus dorsi and serratus anterior muscles, **muscle-sparing incisions**—either transverse or vertical—are gaining in popularity because they are perceived to decrease pain and provide a more rapid recovery. Variations on the posterolateral thoracotomy all have position requirements similar to those of the standard posterolateral incision.

For an anterior incision, the patient is placed supine. A small roll placed under the shoulder blades will serve to extend the neck and facilitate access to the upper mediastinum. This is particularly important for an operation on the upper trachea, and improves visualization for cervical mediastinoscopy. In general, the arms should be tucked at the patient's sides. Having an arm extended during a sternotomy can place undue stretch on the brachial plexus → injury.

The probability of DVT in general thoracic cases is controversial, whereas the risks of prophylaxis are minimal. Given that patients undergoing thoracotomy often have protracted periods of immobility, both during and after surgery, and often have a Dx of a malignant disease (hypercoagulability), use of DVT prophylaxis is good practice. We use SCDs for all patients, except those undergoing short video-assisted procedures, and reserve subcutaneous heparin for those at higher than normal risk (e.g., with prolonged postop immobility).

POSTOPERATIVE ISSUES

The most common postop issues relevant to anesthesiologists are:

- The need for postop mechanical ventilation;
- Airway management;
- Hemodynamic instability; and
- Pain control.

The majority of patients undergoing thoracotomy can be extubated immediately postop. The most common exceptions are patients requiring preop mechanical ventilation, lung transplant patients, and those with "difficult" airways. Patients undergoing prolonged surgery may require postop mechanical ventilation. With shorter procedures, and those performed using minimally invasive techniques, even patients undergoing lung-volume-reduction surgery for severe emphysema generally can be extubated at the conclusion of the procedure.

Because DLTs are larger than standard ETTs, there is greater potential for laryngeal trauma and airway edema → loss of airway following extubation. By exchanging the DLT for a single-lumen ETT over a tube changer, this potentially catastrophic complication can be avoided.

Hemodynamic instability following surgery may be 2° several causes, the most important being ongoing blood loss (or inadequate intraop fluid replacement) and cardiac dysfunction. Use of epidural anesthesia may accentuate ↓ BP both intraop and postop.

With the use of epidural anesthesia and systemic analgesics (e.g., ketorolac) postop pain can be managed effectively. It is important for the anesthesiologist to communicate to the surgeon (and postop care team) which agents have been used, how the patient responded to them, and what types of hemodynamic, pulmonary, and neurological effects can be expected in the postop period.

LOBECTOMY, PNEUMONECTOMY

SURGICAL CONSIDERATIONS

Description: Surgery remains the most appropriate form of treatment for early-stage lung cancer. Other less common indications include infection (particularly mycobacterial disease and bronchiectasis), developmental abnormalities such as sequestrations, and trauma. Patients with Stage I or II non–small-cell lung cancer (disease confined to the lung or those with intrapulmonary node involvement only) generally are offered surgery, unless their pulmonary function is prohibitively poor or their comorbidities pose an unacceptable risk. Patients with Stage IIIA disease often receive preop chemotherapy and/or radiation; and those with Stage IIIB or IV disease are rarely offered an operation.

Table 5-1. Spirometric Criteria for Pulmonary Resection

Spirometry	Operable	Further Study Suggested
Forced vital capacity (FVC)	> 60% predicted	< 60% predicted
Forced expired volume in 1 see (FEV_1)	> 60% predicted	< 60% predicted
FEV_1 FVC ratio	> 50%	< 50%
Maximum voluntary ventilation	> 50% predicted	< 50% predicted
Gas exchange		
Diffusing capacity for carbon monoxide	> 60% predicted	< 60% predicted
Articrial carbon dioxide tension	< 45 mmHg	> 45 mmHg

Used with permission from Olson GN: Pulmonary physiologic assessment of operative risk. In: *General Thoracic Surgery*, 5th edition. Shields TW, LoCicero J III, Ponn RB, eds. Lippincott Williams & Wilkins, Philadelphia, 2003.

Regardless of the underlying disease, the preoperative evaluation should include an assessment of pulmonary function (Table 5-1). Spirometry is adequate for most patients with little or no functional impairment, but more elaborate tests—such as measurement of diffusion capacity, quantitative ventilation/perfusion scans, or formal exercise testing (Fig. 5-5)—are appropriate for others.

Following induction of general anesthesia, many surgeons perform a preoperative bronchoscopy. In patients with tumors in the trachea or mainstem bronchi, this step may be important in determining whether the patient should undergo a lobectomy, sleeve lobectomy, or pneumonectomy. Most patients undergoing **lobectomy** or **pneumonectomy** are placed in the lateral decubitus position. This approach permits a lateral or posterolateral thoracotomy (Fig. 5-1A)—the incision that provides optimal exposure of the pulmonary hilum. A more limited, **muscle-sparing incision** may be used; however, the exposure may be somewhat limited. Occasionally, a **median sternotomy approach** (Fig. 5-1 B) is used–particularly when there is significant involvement of the anterior mediastinum by the tumor.

Over the past several years, video-assisted thoracoscopic lobectomy (VATS-lobectomy) has become more widely available. Although the anesthetic and surgical details of VATS techniques are described later in the chapter, early experiences with this procedure have demonstrated similar outcomes to those associated with the more traditional open techniques. Although a limited "access" thoracotomy is necessary to remove the mobilized lobe from the chest cavity, the technique has the advantages of minimizing soft tissue trauma and the pain associated with spreading the ribs.

Following entry into the chest, the lung on the operative side is allowed to deflate. If the lung remains inflated, a flexible bronchoscope should be used to verify correct positioning of the ETT (Fig. 5-6). Alternatively, the surgeon may be able to feel the tip of the ETT and guide it into the correct position. After stable OLV has been obtained, the lung is mobilized and the bronchovascular structures are identified. Generally, the vascular structures are divided first, although when exposure is limited, it may be best to divide the bronchus first. Hypotension and arrhythmias may occur when the hilar structures or pericardium are retracted vigorously. Such aberrations generally resolve quickly on restoration of normal anatomic relationships. Inadvertent entry into a branch of the pulmonary artery during dissection can result in rapid blood loss. Because these vessels are usually under low pressure, bleeding generally can be controlled with direct pressure on the bleeding site, while the anesthesiologist resuscitates the patient and the surgeon obtains more definitive vascular control. During a lobectomy, the surgeon will ask the anesthesiologist to reinflate the lung while the bronchus leading to the lobe that will be removed is occluded. This will ensure that the remaining lobes inflate appropriately. Thorough suctioning immediately before the lobectomy eliminates secretions as a cause of continued atelectasis. Once the lung or lobe has been resected, positive pressure is applied to the bronchial stump (and lobe) to check that there is no significant postop air leak. Large air leaks are best addressed at the time of surgery, rather than waiting for them to resolve postop.

Chest drainage is standard following lobectomy and involves placement of one or two 28–36 Fr chest tubes attached to underwater seal or suction. Placing the tubes to suction typically increases observed air leak, whereas extubating the patient in the supine position typically decreases the leak. Following pneumonectomy, chest drainage is not uniformly carried out; however, if a chest tube is to be placed, a balanced drainage system must be used or the

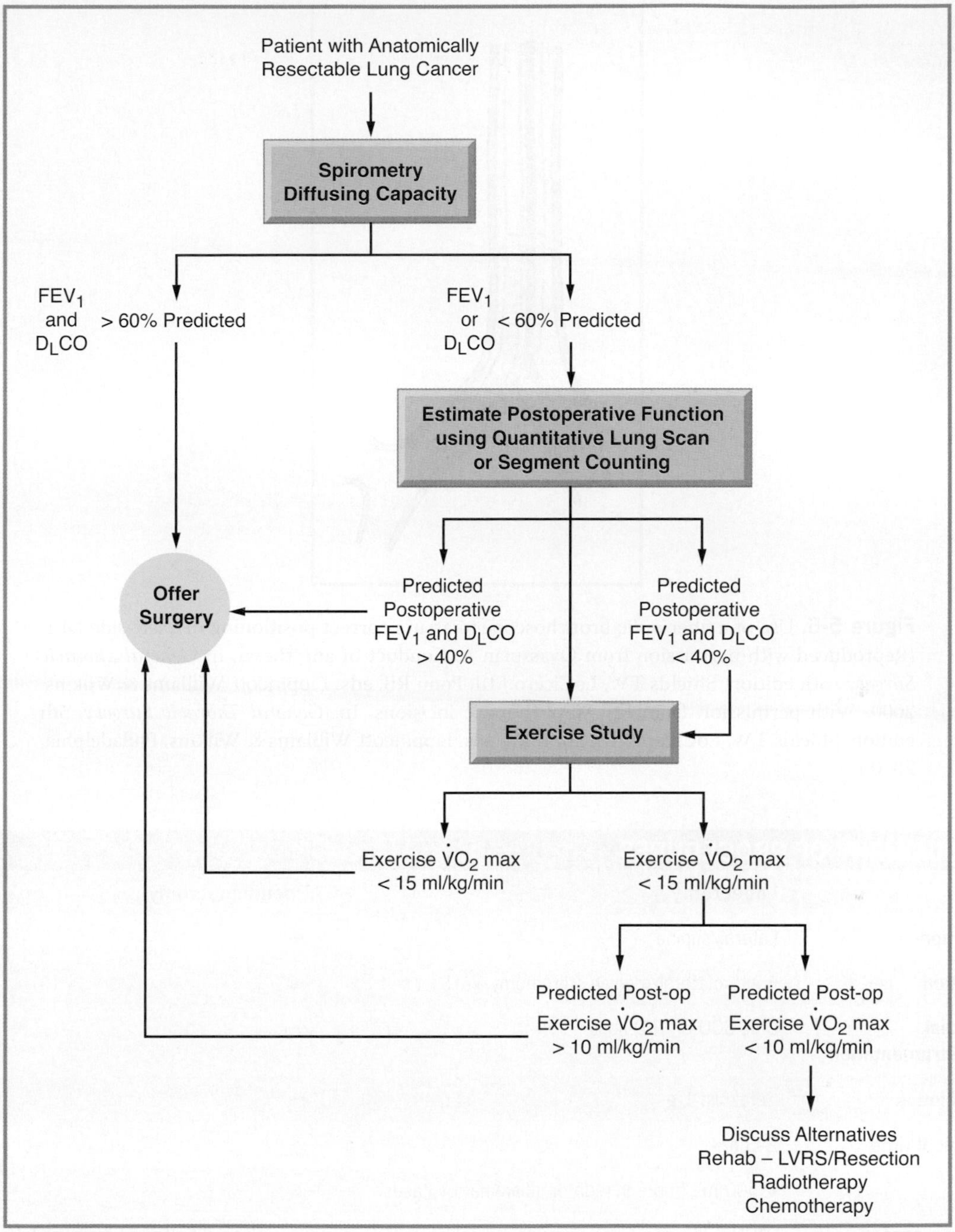

Figure 5-5. Physiologic assessment of patients with compromised lung function. (Reproduced with permission from Olson GN: Pulmonary physiologic assessment of operative risk. In *General Thoracic Surgery*, 5th edition. Shields TW, LoCicero J III, Ponn RB, eds. Lippincott Williams & Wilkins, Philadelphia, 2000.)

mediastinum will shift to the operative side, thus creating adverse hemodynamic consequences. An alternative to drainage (after the patient is placed supine) is to aspirate air from the operative pleural space until a slight negative pressure is obtained.

Usual preop diagnosis: Carcinoma of the lung; infection; developmental abnormalities; trauma

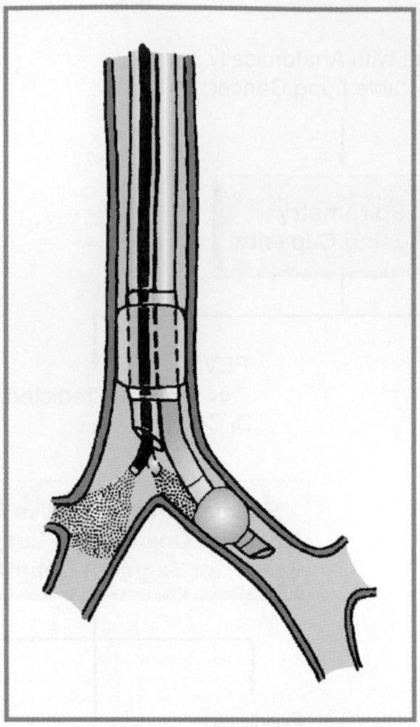

Figure 5-6. Use of a fiber optic bronchoscope to assure correct positioning of a left-side DLT. (Reproduced with permission from Ovasspian A: Conduct of anesthesia. In *General Thoracic Surgery*, 5th edition. Shields TW, LoCicero J III, Ponn RB, eds. Lippincott Williams & Wilkins, 2000. With permission from Fry WA: Thoracic incisions. In: *General Thoracic Surgery*, 5th edition. Shields TW, LoCicero J III, Ponn RB, eds. Lippincott Williams & Wilkins, Philadelphia, 2000.)

SUMMARY OF PROCEDURES

	Lobectomy	Pneumonectomy
Position	Lateral/supine	⇐
Incision	Posterolateral/median sternotomy/VATS	⇐
Special instrumentation	DLT; SCD or TED hose	⇐
Antibiotics	Cefazolin 1 g	⇐
Surgical time	2–3 h	⇐
EBL	< 500 mL (more in redo or inflammatory cases)	⇐
Postop care	PACU ± ICU; careful attention to pulmonary toilet; chest tube output	⇐ + Special balanced drainage tube
Mortality	± 1%	± 5%
Morbidity	Dysrhythmias: 10–20% DVT: 5–20% ARDS PE MI Bronchopleural fistula Chylothorax Subcutaneous emphysema Phrenic nerve injury Recurrent laryngeal nerve injury	30–40% ⇐ ⇐ ⇐ ⇐ ⇐ ⇐ ⇐ ⇐ ⇐
Pain score	7–8	7–8

Thoracic Surgery

PATIENT POPULATION CHARACTERISTICS

Age range	0–80 yr
Male:Female	15:1
Incidence	Common thoracic procedure; increasing in females
Etiology	Smoking
Associated conditions	Cardiopulmonary disease; PVD

ANESTHETIC CONSIDERATIONS

PREOPERATIVE

The main indication for lung resection is neoplasm. Other indications include infection, hemorrhage, or air-leak. The majority of patients have a Hx of cigarette smoking with associated emphysema and/or chronic bronchitis. As most patients are older, other comorbidities are common (CAD, DM). Morbidity and mortality following thoracotomy is increased with pre-existing pulmonary, cardiovascular, and neurologic disease. Lung resections are increasingly being performed via thoracoscopy, which decreases patient morbidity. Lung isolation (DLT or BB) and OLV are mandatory for surgical exposure.

Respiratory	Question patient about exercise tolerance, dyspnea, productive cough and cigarette smoking. Examine patient for cyanosis, clubbing, RR, and pattern. Listen to chest for wheezes, rhonchi, rales. Timely cessation of smoking (> 8 wk), adequate management of bronchospasm with bronchodilator treatment ± steroids, and prompt treatment of pre-existing lung infections are important to reduce postop pulmonary complications. **Tests:** PFT (see below and Table 5-2); CXR; chest CT (if available), always examine chest imaging re: ease of lung isolation; ABG (only if indicated from H&P).
Pulmonary function	Nonsmoker with normal lungs may not require any studies for simple lobectomy. Any pre-existing respiratory disease (or possibility of pneumonectomy) should trigger lung function studies. Whole-lung tests (ABG, spirometry) are sufficient in most cases. Split-function lung tests (V/Q scan) should be considered if the patient has heterogeneous disease, or a planned pneumonectomy or borderline lung resection is planned. Many variables have been shown to correlate with poor outcome. The most important are FEV_1, D_LCO, and VO_2 max, which focus on different aspects (mechanics, parenchymal function, and cardiopulmonary reserve, respectively). Postoperative predictive values of FEV_1 < 40%, D_LCO < 40%, or baseline VO_2max < 15 mL/kg/min predict ↑ risk for postop complications following pulmonary resection. Preop hypercapnia or PHTN/ RV dysfunction are relative contraindications to lung resection, except for specific circumstances (e.g., combined with LVRS in severe emphysema). Trial pneumonectomy with PA balloon occlusion is frequently discussed, but not used in clinical practice. Preop optimization of respiratory function with bronchodilator therapy should be routine.
Cardiovascular	RV dysfunction is a relative contraindication to lung resection (particularly pneumonectomy). Prophylactic digoxin or amiodarone to ↓ risk of postop atrial fibrillation have limited efficacy. **Tests:** ECG—look for evidence of RV hypertrophy, conduction problems, ischemia, and prior MI. ECHO to evaluate ventricular function; others as indicated from H&P.
Neurological	✓ Hx of previous back surgery, peripheral neuropathy. Examine thoracolumbar area for skin lesions, infection, deformities.
Musculoskeletal	Patients with lung cancer may have myasthenic (Eaton-Lambert) syndrome with resistance to depolarizing muscle relaxants and ↑ sensitivity to NDMRs. Monitor relaxation with peripheral nerve stimulator.

Table 5-2. Assessment of Risk of Postop Pulmonary Complications Following Thoracic and Abdominal Procedures

Category	Point
I. Expiratory Spirogram	
a. Normal (%FVC + %FEV_1/FVC > 150)	0
b. %FVC + %FEV_1/FVC = 100–150	1
c. %FVC + %FEV_1/FVC < 100	2
d. Preop FVC < 20 mL/kg	3
e. Post-bronchodilator FEV_1/FVC < 50%	3
II. Cardiovascular System	
a. Normal	0
b. Controlled HTN, MI sequelae for more than 2 yr	0
c. Dyspnea on exertion, orthopnea, paroxysmal nocturnal dyspnea, dependent edema. CHF, angina	1
III. ABGs	
a. Acceptable	0
b. $PaCO_2$ >50 mmHg or $PaCO_2$ < 60 mmHg on room air	1
c. Metabolic pH abnormality > 7.50 or < 7.30	1
IV. Nervous System	
a. Normal	0
b. Confusion, obtundation, agitation, spasticity, discoordination, bulbar malfunction	1
c. Significant muscular weakness	1
V. Postop Ambulation	
a. Expected ambulation (minimum, sitting at bedside) within 36 h	0
b. Expected complete bed confinement for at least 36 h	1
0 Points = Low Risk; 1–2 Points = Moderate Risk; 3 Points = High Risk	

Shapira BA, Harrison RA, Kacmarek RM, Cane RD: *Clinical Application of Respiratory Care.* 3rd edition. Year Book Medical Publishers, Chicago: 1985. (With permission.)

Hematologic	Adequate O_2-carrying capacity is important. Optimize Hb preoperatively if possible (iron, EPO), consider transfusion with Hb < 7 g/dl (<10 g/dl with CAD), depending on vital signs. Although rare, bleeding can be profuse, so blood should be immediately available. Coagulopathy may preclude neuraxial anesthesia. **Tests:** Hct; PT; PTT (if epidural anesthesia planned)
Laboratory	Other tests as indicated from H&P.
Premedication	Midazolam 0.5–2 mg iv if patient anxious (unless respiratory compromise). When epidural opioids are planned, avoid additional systemic opioid or sedative premedication that can potentiate postop respiratory effects of neuraxial opioids.

INTRAOPERATIVE

Anesthetic technique: Combined GA with continuous regional technique (epidural or paravertebral). Anesthesia for lobectomy/pneumonectomy relies on OLV techniques to improve surgical exposure and minimize damage to the operative lung in the case of lobectomy or bi-lobectomy. The challenges to the anesthesiologist include maintaining adequate oxygenation in patients with poor pulmonary reserve and ensuring that the patient is comfortable, warm, and awake at the end of surgery.

Preinduction	Placement of a regional analgesia catheter is important for postop pain control. Continuous epidural (lumbar or thoracic) and paravertebral blocks have been shown to be effective. Epidural catheters should be placed in the awake patient, whereas paravertebral catheters can be sited asleep or intraop under direct vision. The catheter tip should be as close as possible to the level of incision in order to minimize the sympathectomy. Intraop use of

Preinduction (cont'd)	regional analgesia reduces the amount of systemic anesthetics/analgesics required and, therefore, facilitates rapid emergence. An adequate block can be established with lidocaine or bupivacaine; however, higher concentrations will be required for intraop anesthesia than postop analgesia.	
Induction	Standard induction (p. B-2). If flexible bronchoscopy is planned prior to lung resection, intubate with an ETT (≥ 8 mm), which will be replaced with DLT after bronchoscopy (see below). Otherwise, proceed to intubation with an appropriate sized DLT (check imaging, rough guideline: adult male, 39–41 Fr; adult female, 35–37 Fr) after induction.	
Maintenance	Air/O_2 and isoflurane/desflurane/sevoflurane (around 0.5–0.7 MAC if neuraxial block established). Avoid N_2O. Use high FiO_2 = 0.8–1.0 at onset of OLV; titrate to lowest possible after HPV well established and operative lung collapsed. A local anesthetic (e.g., 2% lidocaine or 0.25–0.5% bupivacaine) can be infused or injected hourly into a thoracic (1–3 mL) or lumbar (5–10 mL) epidural catheter. Continuous infusion of local anesthetic generally provides better hemodynamic stability than hourly bolus injection. To enhance the effect of epidural analgesia, a loading dose of epidural opiate (e.g., hydromorphone 200–500 mcg [thoracic] or 1–1.5 mg [lumbar]) can be administered prior to incision. Epidural hydromorphone has a superior side-effect profile over morphine at equipotent doses. IV (compared to inhalational) anesthetics have a clinically insignificant benefit on OLV oxygenation (particularly if volatile agents are limited to < 1 MAC) and are, therefore, not necessary in the majority of cases.	
Emergence	Before chest closure, lungs are inflated gradually to 20–30 cmH_2O pressure to reinflate atelectatic areas and to ✓ for significant air leaks. Surgeon inserts chest tubes to drain pleural cavity and aid lung re-expansion. Patient is extubated in OR. If postop ventilation is required (rare), DLT exchanged for single-lumen ETT. Patient transferred in head-elevated position to PACU or ICU, breathing mask O_2. If hemodynamically unstable, monitor ECG, pulse oximetry, and arterial pressure during transfer.	
Blood and fluid requirements	IV: 18 ga × 1 + 14 or 16 ga × 1 Maintain stable hypovolemia, Limit fluid to 10–15 mL/kg if possible Blood: available, but rarely required; use vasopressor (ephedrine 5–10 mg iv bolus or phenylephrine 50–100 mcg iv bolus) if hypotensive.	Postop, PVR is increased in proportion to the amount of lung tissue removed. An overhydrated patient is at risk of RV failure and pulmonary edema. Replace blood loss with colloid (1:1) to minimize volume load. Third-space loss is negligible and need not be replaced. Use of epidural local anesthetics can cause ↓ BP in a volume-restricted patient; vasopressor may be needed.
Monitoring	Standard monitors (p. B-1) Arterial line Urinary catheter ± CVP line ± PA line or TEE (rare)	It is mandatory to follow oxygenation continuously during OLV. Typically, this can be done with pulse oximetry, although continuous intraarterial PO_2 monitoring is now commercially available. CVP and/or PA line optional for pneumonectomy and for patients with coexisting cardiac disease. CVP monitoring may be inaccurate intraop and is mostly placed for postop care. PA lines are rarely necessary and may interfere with PA stapling or endanger the PA stump. TEE may be of benefit in the borderline pneumonectomy to check for RV tolerance of PA cross-clamp.
Positioning	Axillary roll, "airplane" for upper arm Avoid hyperextending arms. ✓ and pad pressure points. ✓ eyes, ears, genitals.	✓ radial pulses to ensure correct placement of axillary roll (if misplaced, will compromise distal pulses). Placing the oximeter probe on the down arm may assist in monitoring arm perfusion.

Fiber optic bronchoscopy	FOB performed immediately before thoracotomy to evaluate resectability of lesion. Patient intubated with large ETT (≥ 8 mm), replaced with DLT or BB following bronchoscopy (see Bronchoscopy, p. 306).	Use the largest DLT that atraumatically passes through the glottis (typically, 39–41 Fr for men, 35–37 Fr for women). DLT can be placed accurately by careful auscultation ±confirmation by FOB. Fiberoptic confirmation is most commonly done through the tracheal lumen, but can be performed through the bronchial lumen via trans-illumination. For small children, the balloon of a Fogarty embolectomy catheter is used as a BB; for adults, either a BB or a Univent tube may be used if the proper size DLT cannot be placed. BB not ideal as FOB always needed to confirm placement, lung collapse delayed, suction and CPAP not effective and repeated inflation and collapse may be difficult.
Lung isolation	Separate lungs to prevent contralateral contamination (infection, pus, blood, tumor), allow selective ventilation and facilitate operation.	
OLV	Two lung vent: Vt = 8–10 mL/kg, normocapnia, PEEP 3–5 cm H_2O OLV: Vt = 4–8 mL/kg, permissive hypercapnia ($PaCO_2$ 50–70 mmHg), PEEP 3–8 cm H_2O (unless BPF), FiO_2: 0.6–1.0, PIP < 35 cm H_2O and plateau pressures < 25 cm H_2O, consider PCV.	Issues during OLV are: oxygenation, ventilation and lung injury. Oxygenation is rarely an issue if the DLT is adequately placed and derecruitment is avoided in the nonoperative lung. Ventilation is impaired by the smaller lumen of the DLT and the fact that only one lung is ventilated, resulting in higher ventilatory pressures. However, permissive hypoventilation allows for limiting the ventilatory stress. Acute lung injury may result in post-pneumonectomy pulmonary edema, which may occur even after lesser resections. Limiting Vt, peak and plateau pressures, FiO_2, duration of OLV and atelectasis formation help to minimize the risk.
Complications	Hypoxemia	Hypoxemia is now relatively infrequent due to better lung isolation techniques and anesthetic agents with less suppression of HPV. If hypoxemia occurs, tube position should immediately be confirmed and FiO_2 increased towards 1.0. Suctioning of secretions and lung recruitment maneuvers are often all that is required. If derecruitment has occurred, higher levels of PEEP should be employed; however, this may potentially worsen oxygenation. CPAP to the (recruited) operative lung is always helpful, as is clamping of the PA to exclude shunt flow. Return to two-lung ventilation (if possible) will always improve oxygenation (even if used intermittently only) and should be considered with refractory hypoxemia.
	Hypercarbia	Mild hypercarbia is well tolerated except in the setting of severe PHTN. CO_2 levels above 70 mmHg may be associated with tachycardia, dysrhythmias and cardiac depression. Treat with higher minute ventilation.
	Arrhythmia	✓ for mechanical compression of heart or great vessels.
	Hypotension	✓ volume status (but always hypovolemic) and cardiac function. Consider neosynephrine for BP support if ↓ BP is 2° epidural.

Thoracic Surgery

Complications (cont'd)	Airway rupture	✓ integrity of intubated bronchus after re-expanding lung.
	DVT	Preventive measures: TED hose or SCD.
	Airway trauma from intubation, tracheobronchial rupture	Force should NEVER be used during insertion of a DLT, as it may result in catastrophic airway disruptions. Do not overdistend bronchial balloon or DLT cuffs. DLT bronchial cuff usually requires < 2 mL air for airtight seal, if an appropriate (large) DLT is used.

POSTOPERATIVE

Complications	Injuries related to lateral positioning	Pressure damage to ear, eye, nose, deltoid muscle, iliac crest, brachial plexus, and radial, ulnar, common peroneal, and sciatic nerves have all been reported.
	Structural injuries related to thoracotomy	Neurologic (phrenic and recurrent laryngeal nerves), thoracic duct, spinal cord; bronchopleural fistula, tracheobronchial disruption
	Surgical complications	Cardiac herniation, tension pneumothorax, bleeding, torsion of residual lobe, acute lung injury/ARDS
	Cardiopulmonary complications	Supraventricular dysrhythmias, SVT, acute RV failure, atelectasis, BPF, pneumonia, PE. For SVT, treat underlying cause and correct electrolyte abnormalities. Most postop SVTs are 2° atrial fibrillation or 2° catecholamine surge and may resolve spontaneously. Hemodynamically unstable patients will require cardioversion. Beta blockers, amiodarone, Ca^{++} channel blockers, and overdrive cardiac pacing are effective in patients with unstable AF.
Pain management	Neuraxial opioids—epidural or intrathecal Parenteral opioids (iv, im, continuous iv, PCA [p. C-3]) Intercostal blocks. Interpleural analgesia	Effective analgesia via epidural or paravertebral route is essential in order for patient to cough, deep breathe, and ambulate early. Epidural infusions consist of a local anesthetic + opioid mixture (smaller volume and higher concentration with thoracic placement). Paravertebral infusions are local anesthetic only, thereby avoiding
	Epidural local anesthetics Cryoanalgesia	opioid side-effects. Paravertebral analgesia interferes less with postop lung function than epidural analgesia.
	NSAID (ketorolac)	Ketorolac (10–15 mg) is helpful as adjunct analgesic, particularly with referred shoulder pain.
Tests	Hct, CXR, ABG and others as indicated.	

Suggested Readings

1. Alam N, Flores RM: Video-assisted thoracic surgery (VATS) lobectomy: the evidence base. *JSLS* 2007; 11(3):368–74.
2. Amar D: Perioperative atrial tachyarrhythmias. *Anesthesiology* 2002; 97(6):1618–23.
3. Beckles MA, Sprio SG, Colice GL, et al: Initial evaluation of the patient with lung cancer: symptoms, signs, laboratory tests, and paraneoplastic syndromes. *Chest* 2003; 123:S1, 97S–104S.
4. Beckles MA, Sprio SG, Colice GL, et al: The physiologic evaluation of patients with lung cancer being considered for resectional surgery. *Chest* 2003; 123:S1, 105S–14S.

5. Brodsky JB, Macario A, Mark JBD: Tracheal diameter predicts double-lumen tube size: a method for selecting left double-lumen tubes. *Anesth Analg* 1996; 82:861–4.
6. Davies RG, Myles PS, Graham JM: A comparison of the analgesic efficacy and side-effects of paravertebral vs epidural blockade for thoracotomy–a systematic review and meta-analysis of randomized trials. *Br J Anaesth* 2006; 96(4):418–26.
7. Fortier G, Cote D, Bergeron C, et al: New landmarks improve the positioning of the left Broncho-Cath double-lumen tube-comparison with the classic technique. *Can J Anaesth* 2001; 48(8):790–4.
8. Kavanagh BP, Katz J, Sandler AN, et al: Pain control after thoracic surgery. A review of current techniques. *Anesthesiology* 1994; 81:737–59.
9. Lohser J: Evidence-based management of one-lung ventilation. *Thorac Anesth Anesthesiol Clin North America* 2008; 26(2): accepted.
10. McKenna RJ Jr, Houck W, Fuller CB: Video-assisted thoracic surgery lobectomy: experience with 1,100 cases. *Ann Thorac Surg* 2006; 81(2):421–5; discussion 425–6.
11. Slinger PD, Johnston MR: Preoperative assessment: an anesthesiologist's perspective. *Thorac Surg Clin* 2005; 15(1):11–25.
12. Slinger PD: Postpneumonectomy pulmonary edema: good news, bad news. *Anesthesiology* 2006; 105(1):2–5.

WEDGE RESECTION OF LUNG LESION

SURGICAL CONSIDERATIONS

Description: **Wedge resection** (removal of a mass in a manner that does not remove an entire anatomical pulmonary segment) may be carried out for a number of reasons. A known or suspected cancer may be removed by this limited resection. There is general agreement that this is an appropriate operation for patients with peripheral non–small-cell tumors and who have pulmonary reserve limited to the point that they are unable to tolerate lobectomy. Wedge resection also is used for resection of single- or multiple-metastatic lesions from various primary neoplasms. A single metastasis may be removed through a limited thoracotomy incision. At the other extreme, a **median sternotomy** may be used to remove bilateral lesions. Wedge resection also is indicated for diagnostic and therapeutic purposes in lesions which defy diagnosis by less invasive techniques. Incisions vary with location, number of lesions, and technique used. **Limited thoracotomy, standard thoracotomy,** or **median sternotomy** may be used under different circumstances. **Stapling** (Fig. 5-7), **clamp and suture** technique, or **excision and**

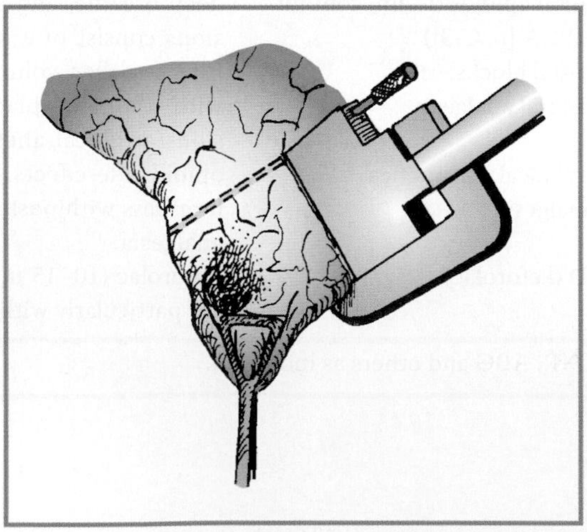

Figure 5-7. Stapler used to perform wedge incision. (Reproduced with permission from Scott-Conner CEH, Dawson DL: *Operative Anatomy.* Lippincott Williams & Wilkins, Philadelphia, 2003.)

suture technique may be used for lesions in different locations. Wedge resection is best performed in the lateral position and with OLV. Small nodules on the edge of the lung and diagnostic biopsies for interstitial lung disease often can be performed with the thoracoscope, thereby avoiding a thoracotomy. In patients who cannot tolerate OLV (e.g., with ARDS), it may be necessary to keep the patient supine and ventilate both lungs. The wedge resection itself generally is carried out with a surgical stapling device (Fig. 5-7) that simultaneously staples the lung parenchyma and cuts between staple lines. Alternatively, the lung tissue can be clamped and oversewn—a technique applicable to particularly indurated lung tissue that is too thick for a stapler. A final option is to perform a pneumonotomy, enucleate the nodule, and suture the lung closed. A single chest tube usually is placed for postop chest drainage.

Variant approach: Video-assisted thoracoscopy surgery (VATS) (see p. 313).

Usual preop diagnosis: Metastatic tumor to the lungs; primary lung cancer (typically, lobectomy); unknown pulmonary lesion

SUMMARY OF PROCEDURE

Position	Lateral or supine
Incision	Limited and related to location of solitary lesion; sternotomy for bilateral lesions
Special instrumentation	DLT
Antibiotics	Cefazolin 1 g (or other antibiotic as indicated from culture and sensitivity)
Surgical time	< 1–3 h, depending on number of lesions
EBL	< 500 mL
Postop care	PACU ± ICU; careful attention to pulmonary toilet, chest tube output
Mortality	Minimal
Morbidity	Air leaks Cardiac dysrhythmias
Pain score	2–6

PATIENT POPULATION CHARACTERISTICS

Age range	30–60 yr most common
Male:Female	1:1
Incidence	Common thoracic procedure
Etiology	Variable – neoplasm or inflammatory disease
Associated conditions	COPD; cardiovascular disease; malignancy; infection

ANESTHETIC CONSIDERATIONS

PREOPERATIVE

The anesthetic considerations for this procedure are very similar to those for lobectomy/ pneumonectomy, although most wedge resections are easily accomplished via thoracoscopy. Wedge resection of the lung may be performed for diagnosis of interstitial process/lesion or for resection of neoplasm in patients with poor pulmonary reserve, who may not tolerate an anatomic resection.

Respiratory	PFTs similar to major thoracotomy. Further evaluation directed toward an underlying disease (e.g., immuno-compromised patient for open-lung biopsy, patient with metastatic lesions, etc.). **Tests:** PFTs (see Lobectomy, Pneumonectomy, p. 275); CXR; chest CT (if available), always examine chest imaging for airway problems that might interfare with lung isolation, airway compression/obstruction; ABG (only if indicated from H&P).
Cardiovascular	**Tests:** ECG—look for evidence of RV hypertrophy, conduction problems, ischemia, and previous MI.
Neurological	Hx of previous back surgery or peripheral neuropathy. Examine thoracolumbar area for skin lesions, infection, deformities. The placement of an epidural catheter in patients with neurologic problems is controversial.
Musculoskeletal	Patients with lung cancer may have myasthenic (Eaton-Lambert) syndrome with resistance to depolarizing muscle relaxants and ↑ sensitivity to NMRs. Monitor relaxation with a peripheral nerve stimulator.
Hematologic	Patients are often anemic from primary disease. Consider preop blood transfusion or erythropoietin therapy. **Tests:** Hct
Laboratory	Other tests as indicated from H&P.
Premedication	Midazolam 0.5–2 mg iv if patient anxious. When epidural opioids are planned, avoid additional systemic opioid or sedative premedication, which can potentiate postop respiratory effects of central neuraxial opioids.

INTRAOPERATIVE

Anesthetic technique: GETA, often combined with epidural or paravertebral blocks for thoracotomy approach. Thoracoscopy approach does not usually require a regional anesthetic. DLT or BB required for lung isolation.

Induction	Standard induction. Short acting paralytic (succinylcholine 1–1.5 mg/kg or vecuronium 0.1 mg/kg or rocuronium 0.3–0.6 mg/kg for tracheal intubation)	
Maintenance	**Balanced technique:** Air-O_2, isoflurane, and iv opioids (usually fentanyl). No N_2O. Pain is highly variable after thoracoscopic procedures, dependent on degree of lung dissection. If a regional catheter is used, management should be similar to pneumonectomy/lobectomy (consider lower dose of opioid). If parenteral analgesia is insufficient, useful adjuncts include intercostal block, paravertebral block and/or intrapleural local anesthetic (given through the chest tube after the lung is inflated [maximum 0.5 mL/kg of bupivacaine 0.25% with epinephrine]).	
Emergence	Ensure complete recruitment of operative lung. Extubate in OR, transfer in head-up position to PACU or ICU, breathing O_2 by mask.	
Blood and fluid requirements	IV: 16–14 ga × 1 NS/LR @ 2 mL/kg/h (maintenance fluid)	Replace blood loss with colloid (1:1). Third-space loss is negligible and does not need to be replaced.
Monitoring	Standard monitors (p. B-1) ± Arterial line	 Depending on comorbidities.
Positioning	Lateral decubitus or supine, with wedge under back on operated side. ✓ and pad pressure points. ✓ eyes, ears, genitals.	

Ventilation	Lung isolation (DLT or BB) usually required, except for easily accessible/ peripheral lesions. DLT superior in regards to rapidity of lung collapse.	For OLV technique, see Anesthetic Considerations for Lobectomy/Pneumonectomy, p. 275.
Complications during OLV	See OLV under Intraop Anesthetic Considerations for Lobectomy/ Pneumonectomy, p. 278.	

POSTOPERATIVE

Complications	Same as for lobectomy, pneumonectomy Pain	See Postop Complications for Lobectomy, Pneumonectomy, p. 279. Pain may at times be poorly controlled with parenteral agents alone. May require neuraxial technique for rescue. More common with extensive resections than simple wedge
Complications during OLV	See OLV under Intraop Anesthetic Considerations for Lobectomy/ Pneumonectomy, p. 279.	
Pain management	Parenteral opioids (iv, im, continuous iv, PCA [p. C-3]). Epidural Intercostal blocks Interpleural analgesia NSAID (ketorolac 10–15 mg)	See Pain Management for Lobectomy, Pneumonectomy, p. 279.

Suggested Readings

1. McKenna RJ Jr, Mahtabifard A, Pickens A, et al: Fast-tracking after video-assisted thoracoscopic surgery lobectomy, segmentectomy, and pneumonectomy. *Ann Thorac Surg* 2007; 84(5):1663–7.
2. See Pneumonectomy/ Lobectomy Suggested Readings p. 279–280.
3. Shah JS, Bready LL: Anesthesia for thoracoscopy. *Anesthesiol Clin North Am* 2001; 19(1):153–71.

CHEST-WALL RESECTION

SURGICAL CONSIDERATIONS

Description: Removal of portions of the thoracic cage may be required under several circumstances with the two most common indications being (a) lung cancer that has invaded the chest wall and (b) primary chest-wall tumors (the notable exceptions being Ewing's sarcoma and rhabdomyosarcoma). Although preoperative chemotherapy is not standard treatment for chest-wall sarcomas, some patients may have received Adriamycin, which is associated with cardiotoxicity at high doses. If the tumor process involves the skin, an appropriate area of skin—typically, 4 cm around the tumor—must be resected along with the specimen. Underlying subcutaneous tissue and muscle should always be resected in continuity; however, the tumor itself must not be exposed. Wide skin flaps are frequently necessary as well. Limited resection (1–5 cm segments of one or two ribs) generally requires no specific reconstructive measures, but resection of larger areas of the chest wall may require extensive reconstruction including the use of plastic mesh replacement with or without methylmethacrylate, rib grafts and muscle, or myocutaneous flaps. Removal of anterolateral or anterior portions of the chest wall, particularly resections that include the sternum, are associated with greater postoperative instability than are resections of posterior portions of the chest wall, which are protected by the back muscles and scapula. Larger defects can be tolerated posteriorly without reconstruction, as the scapula provides chest-wall stabilization and prevents lung herniation. If a prosthesis is required, it must be covered by viable muscle so as to avoid erosion through the skin. Extensive reconstruction of the chest wall is often carried out in conjunction with plastic surgeons.

Usual preop diagnosis: Lung cancer with a chest-wall attachment; primary tumor of the chest wall (bone, cartilage, or soft tissue); radiation necrosis

SUMMARY OF PROCEDURE	
Position	Supine or lateral
Incision	Over mass to be resected
Special instrumentation	Bone instruments; Marlex (or other) mesh; methylmethacrylate
Antibiotics	Cefazolin 1 g (or as indicated by culture and sensitivity)
Surgical time	1–8 h
Closing considerations	May require help of plastic surgeon in extensive cases.
EBL	100–2000 mL
Postop care	PACU or ICU; some patients require temporary ventilatory support.
Mortality	< 5%
Morbidity	Paradoxical chest-wall motion (less in posterior resections) Pneumothorax Wound complications
Pain score	3–8

PATIENT POPULATION CHARACTERISTICS	
Age range	Adults of all ages; children, rarely
Male:Female	1:1
Incidence	Relatively rare
Etiology	Unknown
Associated conditions	Lung cancer; metastatic disease; smoking-related diseases; cardiovascular disease

ANESTHETIC CONSIDERATIONS

See Anesthetic Considerations following Repair of Pectus Excavatum or Carinatum, p. 287.

Suggested Readings

1. Baue AE, ed: *Glenn's Thoracic and Cardiovascular Surgery*, 6th edition, Volume II. Geha AS, Hammond GL, Laks H, et al., eds. Appleton & Lange, Norwalk: 1996.
2. Sellke FW, Swanson S, del Nido P: *Sabiston & Spencer: Surgery of the Chest. Section I: Chest Wall*, 7th edition. Elsevier Saunders, Philadelphia: 2004.

REPAIR OF PECTUS EXCAVATUM OR CARINATUM

SURGICAL CONSIDERATIONS

Description: Standard bony and cartilaginous repair of a pectus excavatum (funnel chest) or carinatum (pigeon breast) deformities is usually elective surgery with the aim of improving contour and body image. Evidence that these repairs have any positive effect on cardiopulmonary function is controversial, although some surgeons feel that it can be more than a cosmetic procedure–particularly in patients with prominent deformities. Recent evidence suggests that, although resting cardiopulmonary function tests do not improve after pectus repairs, maximal exercise capacity may improve.

To **repair pectus excavatum,** enough pairs of costal cartilages—usually four to six—must be removed to be able to mobilize and elevate the sternum. Depending on the severity of the defect and patient's age, fixation of the sternum in the corrected position may be necessary. **Repair of pectus carinatum** is somewhat more complicated because the defects are more varied–often with a rotational component as well as anteroposterior displacement; however, removal of cartilages and correction of the position of the sternum are still the mainstays of treatment.

A midline incision provides the most satisfactory access to the cartilages and sternum. For cosmetic reasons, however, it may be important to use a curvilinear transverse incision, particularly in females. This incision requires extensive mobilization of subcutaneous and muscle flaps. The wound complication rate is somewhat greater after transverse incisions. The costal cartilages are moved by subperichondrial dissection. This may be tedious and time-consuming, especially because four or five, or even more, pairs of cartilages need to be removed. The elevation of the sternum is usually fairly straightforward, and usually is accompanied by a transverse sternal osteotomy (Fig. 5-8). Intercostal muscle bundles may be left attached to the sternum or may be detached and reattached for

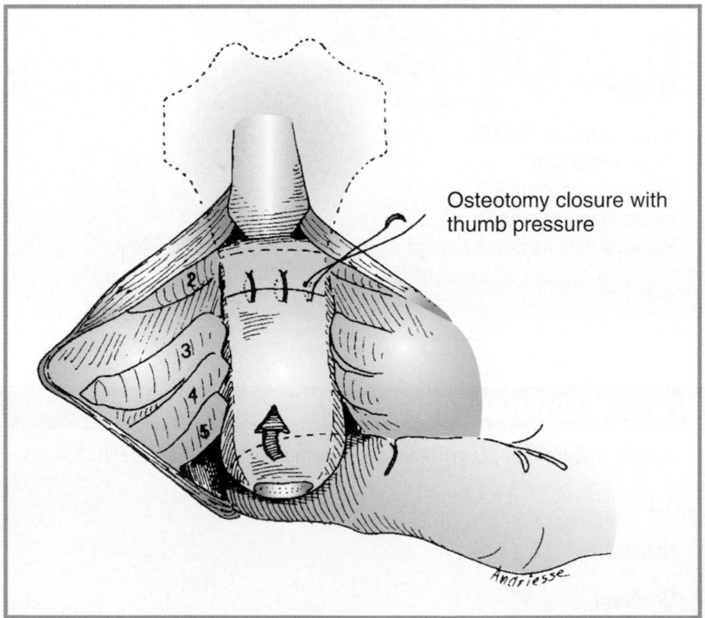

Figure 5-8. Correction of a pectus excavatum defect in a child. After subperichondrial resection of the involved costal cartilages, a wedge osteotomy permits anterior mobilization of the lower portion of the sternum. (Reproduced with permission from Shamberger RC: Chest wall deformities. In *General Thoracic Surgery*, 5th edition. Shields TW, LoCicero J III, Ponn RB, eds. Lippincott Williams & Wilkins, Philadelphia: 2000.)

better positioning of the sternum. Sternal support normally is not used in infants, but may be used in older children. One common method of support is the use of a temporary transverse metal strut resting on the ribs, but beneath the sternum. The final position of the sternum is easier to predict following repair of the pectus carinatum than following repair of pectus excavatum. Because of the negative intrathoracic pressure, it is easier to hold the sternum down than up. Ideally, patients for repair of pectus excavatum are just under school age. Satisfactory repair, however, may be carried out at almost any time during childhood. As full growth is attained, results tend to be less favorable. Pectus carinatum generally has its onset during adolescence, and it is well to let the patient complete his or her growth spurt prior to undertaking repair. (Also see Repair of Pectus Excavatum/Carinatum in Pediatric General Surgery, p. 1270.)

Variant procedure or approaches: In certain circumstances, particularly in teenage girls and patients who do not engage in strenuous sports, subcutaneous, custom-made implants may be placed to improve body contour without necessitating major bony and cartilaginous repairs. These are usually carried out by plastic surgeons.

Usual preop diagnosis: Pectus excavatum or carinatum

SUMMARY OF PROCEDURE

Position	Supine
Incision	Transverse or vertical
Special instrumentation	Bone instruments; sometimes metal struts or wires for reconstruction
Antibiotics	Cefazolin 1 g iv q 8 h × 36–48 h
Surgical time	2–3 h
Closing considerations	Pleural and wound drainage common
EBL	100–500 mL
Postop care	ICU
Mortality	Minimal
Morbidity	Pneumothorax: 5–10% Wound infection Sternum necrosis Immigration of strut Paradoxical chest-wall motion → hypoventilation/atelectasis
Pain score	4–5

PATIENT POPULATION CHARACTERISTICS

Age range	Usually children, 5–10 yr; teenagers, sometimes; adults, rarely
Male:Female	1:1
Incidence	Unusual
Etiology	Unknown
Associated conditions	Marfan syndrome; MVP

ANESTHETIC CONSIDERATIONS

(Procedures covered: chest-wall resection; repair of pectus excavatum/carinatum)

PREOPERATIVE

Patients for chest-wall resection often have extensive cancer and may be weak and debilitated. A very large resection may create a "flail chest" situation, compromising postop ventilation.

Respiratory	Mild pectus seldom interferes with ventilation; no special studies indicated. Severe pectus deformity can be associated with restrictive lung defects. **Tests:** CXR; PFT, ABG, if indicated from H&P.
Cardiovascular	With severe pectus, the heart is displaced to the left and compressed; arrhythmias and RVOTO can occur 2° impaired filling, especially during exercise or in upright position. ECG may show right axis deviation, atrial and ventricular arrhythmias. A functional murmur may be detected. ECHO may reveal ↓ SV with MVP. **Tests:** ECG; cardiac catheterization if indicated. Echocardiogram if symptoms or signs suggest MVP or RVOTO.
Hematologic	**Tests:** Hct
Musculoskeletal	Chest-wall resection performed for invasive or metastatic cancer; patient may be markedly debilitated: pectus repair of chest-wall deformity for cosmetic, orthopedic, or cardiopulmonary indications: pectus deformity usually asymptomatic.
Laboratory	Other tests as indicated from H&P.
Premedication	Consider anxiolysis with short acting benzodiazepine. When epidural opioids are planned, minimize systemic opioid or sedative premedication to avoid potentiating postoperative respiratory depression from central neuroaxial opioids.

INTRAOPERATIVE

Anesthetic technique: GETA, occasionally combined with epidural for minimal chest-wall resection; however, epidural anesthesia is an excellent adjunct for extensive chest-wall resections or repair of pectus deformities.

Induction	Standard induction (see p. B-2). In the setting of RVOTO avoid myocardial depressants, hypovolemia and a short diastolic filling time (e.g., tachycardia). Lung isolation (DLT or BB) usually required for chest wall resections.	
Maintenance	Standard maintenance (see p. B-2) or high-dose opioid technique (fentanyl 10–25 mcg/kg) for patient with severe RVOTO. Patients with MVP will require prophylactic antibiotics for bacterial endocarditis. OLV, if necessary, as outlined for lobectomy/ pneumonectomy.	
Emergence	Extubate in OR; if high-dose opioid →ICU for later extubation.	
Blood and fluid requirements	IV: 18–16 ga × 1 NS/LR @ 1–2 mL/kg/h	Usually minimal blood loss. Fluid restriction unnecessary as this is extrapulmonary operation.
Monitoring	Standard monitors (p. B-1) ± Arterial line	Close monitoring with arterial and central venous catheters may be required in patients with significant cardiopulmonary compromise.
Positioning	✓ and pad pressure points. ✓ eyes.	
Complications	Pneumothorax	Unintentional pleural tear can cause pneumothorax. Intraop deterioration characterized by ↑ ventilatory pressure, hypotension, and hypoxemia suggests pneumothorax. Increase FiO_2; D/C N_2O.

Complications (cont'd)	Pneumothorax (cont.)	Ensure pleural space is decompressed appropriately with needle or tube thoracostomy.
	Cardiac perforation	Rare, catastrophic event reported with aberrant bar placement during minimally invasive approach. Heralded by signs of hemorrhagic or obstructive shock. Supporting bar may interfere with external cardiac compressions.

POSTOPERATIVE

Complications	Hypoventilation Flail chest Atelectasis/pneumonia	Although most patients do not require postop ventilatory support, with extensive chest-wall resection, patient may hypoventilate. Respiratory stimulants, such as doxapram, should be avoided as they may → deep inspirations that can → severe sternal retractions. Paradoxical chest-wall movement may occur during spontaneous ventilation with flail chest; postop atelectasis 20 splinting. Obtain postop CXR.
	Pericarditis	Similar to post pericardotomy syndrome; usually responsive to NSAIDs though occasionally corticosteroids or percutaneous drainage required.
	Bar displacement	Following minimally invasive repair (Nuss) the bar may become displaced and require repositioning. Inadequate analgesia and absence of a stabilizing bar often cited as contributing factors.
Pain management	Depends on site and extent of chest wall resected. Parenteral or epidural opioids with local anesthetic.	Epidural opioids and local anesthetics are particularly useful if flail chest is present—reduces need for ventilatory support.

Suggested Readings

1. Baue AE, ed: *Glenn's Thoracic and Cardiovascular Surgery,* 6th edition, Volume II. Geha AS, Hammond GL, Laks H, et al., assoc. eds. Appleton & Lange, Norwalk: 1996.
2. Garcia VF, Seyfer AE, Graeber GM: Reconstruction of congenital chest-wall deformities. *Surg Clin North Am* 1989; 69(5): 1103–18.
3. Ghory MJ, James FW, Mays W: Cardiac performance in children with pectus excavatum. *J Pediatr Surg* 1989; 24(8):751–5.
4. Gips H, Konstantin Z, Hiss J: Cardiac perforation by a pectus bar after surgical correction of pectus excavatum: case report and review of the literature. *Pediatr Surg Int* 2007.
5. Jacobs JP, Quintessenza JA, Morell VO, et al: Minimally invasive endoscopic repair of pectus excavatum. *Eur J Cardiothorac Surg* 2002; 21(5): 869–73.
6. Mansour KA, Thourani VH, Odessey EA, et al: Thirty-year experience with repair of pectus deformities in adults. *Ann Thorac Surg* 2003;76(2):391–5; discussion 395.
7. McBride WJ, Dicker R, Abajian JC, et al: Continuous thoracic epidural infusions for postoperative analgesia after pectus deformity repair. *J Pediatr Surg* 1996; 31(1): 105–7.
8. Nuss D, Croitoru DP, Kelly RE, et al: Review and discussion of the complications of minimally invasive pectus excavatum repair. *Eur J Pediatr Surg* 2002; 12(4):230–4.
9. Robicsek SA, Lobato EB: Repair of pectus excavatum. Anesthesia considerations. *Chest Surg Clin North Am* 2000; 10(2): 253–9.
10. Sellke FW, Swanson S, del Nido P: *Sabiston & Spencer: Surgery of the Chest. Section I: Chest Wall,* 7th edition. Elsevier Saunders, Philadelphia: 2004.

11. Shamberger RC: Chest wall deformities. In: *General Thoracic Surgery,* 5th edition. Shields TW, LoCicero J III, Ponn RB, eds. Lippincott Williams & Wilkins, Philadelphia: 2000, 535–62.
12. Sullivan EA, Bussieres JS, Tschernko EM: In: *Thoracic Anesthesia,* 3rd edition. Kaplan JA, Slinger PD, eds. Churchill Livingstone, Philadelphia: 2003.

THORACOPLASTY

SURGICAL CONSIDERATIONS

Description: The objective of a **thoracoplasty** (removal of several ribs) is to permanently obliterate an existing pleural space or to collapse a portion of the lung. Formerly, this operation was used in the treatment of tuberculosis (TB); however, because of better drug therapy, appropriate pulmonary resection and the decrease in incidence of TB, thoracoplasty is now rare. The procedure also was used for obliterating empyema spaces and helping to close bronchopleural fistulas (BPFs). The use of **pedicled muscle flaps** (serratus anterior, pectoralis major, and latissimus dorsi are the most common) or an **omental transposition** have largely replaced thoracoplasty for filling empyema spaces and encouraging closing of BPFs. These operations are less deforming and better tolerated physiologically because they do not result in paradoxical motion of the chest wall.

For patients whose lungs will never expand to fill the space—such as those who have had a pneumonectomy or who have a permanently noncompliant lung—resection of multiple overlying ribs may be necessary (Fig. 5-9). Thoracoplasty is accomplished by removing several ribs in a subperiosteal fashion, allowing the underlying chest wall to collapse. This collapse is aided by the normally negative intrapleural pressure. Because the periosteum is left intact, the ribs will regenerate, resulting in a permanent, bony collapse of the chest wall. If the objective of the thoracoplasty is to obliterate a relatively small space (meaning that segments of only two to three ribs need be removed), the procedure may be done in a single stage, with little postop physiologic impairment of respiration. If extensive thoracoplasty is necessary, however, the procedure may be done in stages to minimize postop chest-wall instability and resultant respiratory problems.

Usual preop diagnosis: Pulmonary TB; BPF; empyema

SUMMARY OF PROCEDURE	
Position	Usually lateral
Incision	Along rib line
Special instrumentation	Bone instruments
Unique considerations	TB or fungal infection may be present
Antibiotics	As indicated by culture and sensitivity
Surgical time	2–3 h
EBL	500 mL or more
Postop care	ICU
Mortality	Minimal
Morbidity	Paradoxical chest-wall motion → atelectasis → hypoxemia: 10% Pneumothorax: Rare
Pain score	7–8

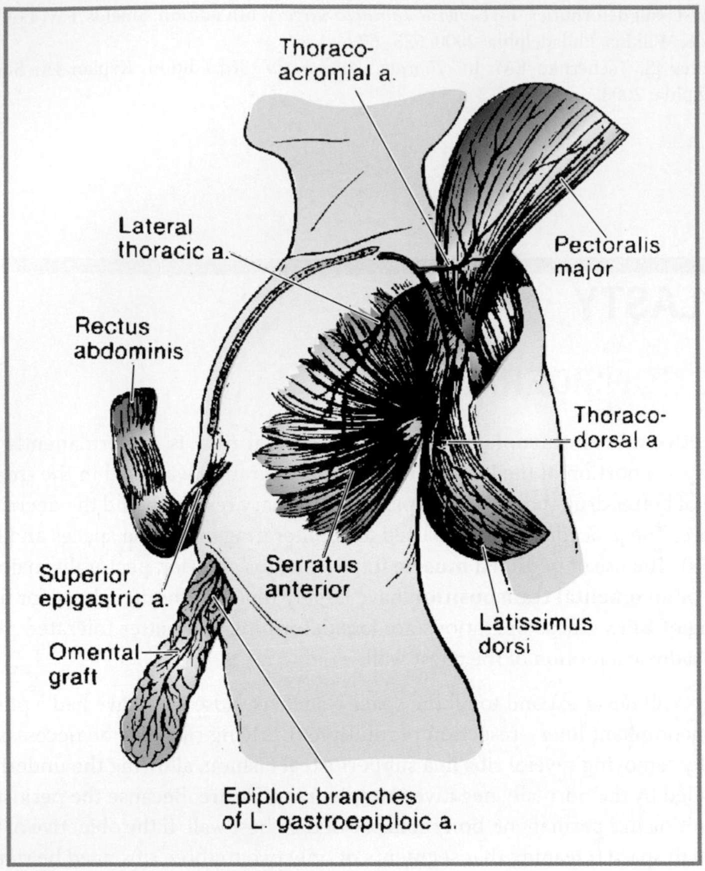

Figure 5-9. Extrathoracic muscle flaps that may be used to obliterate a postpneumo-nectomy empyema cavity. (Reproduced with permission from Miller JI Jr: Postsurgical empyema. In *General Thoracic Surgery,* 5th edition. Shields TW, LoCicero J III, Ponn RB, eds. Lippincott Williams & Wilkins, Philadelphia: 2000.)

PATIENT POPULATION CHARACTERISTICS	
Age range	Middle-aged or older adults
Male:Female	1:1
Incidence	Rare
Etiology	TB; pneumococcal infection; neoplasm; complication of pneumonectomy
Associated conditions	Immunosuppression

ANESTHETIC CONSIDERATIONS

See Anesthetic Considerations following Drainage of Empyema, p. 292.

Suggested Readings

1. Baue AE, ed: *Glenn's Thoracic and Cardiovascular Surgery,* 6th edition, Volume II. Geha AS, Hammond GL, Laks H, et al., assoc. eds. Appleton & Lange, Norwalk, CT: 1996.

2. Sellke FW, Swanso S, del Nido P: *Sabiston & Spencer: Surgery of the Chest. Section I: Chest Wall,* 7th edition. Elsevier Saunders, Philadelphia: 2004.
3. Seify H, Mansour K, Miller J, et al: Single-stage muscle flap reconstruction of the postpneumonectomy empyema space: the Emory experience. *Plast Reconstr Surg* 2007; 120(7):1886–91.

DRAINAGE OF EMPYEMA

SURGICAL CONSIDERATIONS

Description: Empyema is infection within the pleural space, and the primary treatment for it is drainage. Patients may be acutely ill or they may have a history of prolonged infirmity. The most common cause of empyema is extraparenchymal extension of a pneumonia, although other causes include trauma, iatrogenic, and esophageal perforation. The three phases of an empyema are the exudative phase, the fibrinopurulent phase, and the organized phase. The early, or exudative, phase of an empyema is usually associated with fever, dyspnea, and a pleural effusion, with the diagnosis generally being made by thoracentesis. In more established infections, patients may complain of chronic symptoms, such as pain, dyspnea, and chest heaviness, and their medical history may include several previous courses of antibiotics.

Treatment of empyemas is based on the stage and the underlying cause of the infection. Except in its earliest phase, chest tube drainage alone rarely provides adequate therapy. In the fibrinopurulent stage, thoracoscopic drainage with disruption of loculations and removal of the fine peel on the lung is enough to drain the infected fluid and allow the underlying lung to expand. This procedure typically is done with the patient in the lateral position and involves three thoracoscopy ports. Blood loss is generally small, although large volumes of irrigation fluid may be necessary to thoroughly débride the thoracic cavity.

As the empyema becomes more established, the peel becomes thicker and more difficult to remove thoracoscopically. In such cases, an **open thoracotomy** is necessary. Due to the extensive intrapleural inflammation, blood and fluid losses may be substantial. To identify the correct plane between the lung and the thickened pleura, the lung may need to be re-expanded frequently throughout the procedure. Satisfactory drainage is accomplished when the infected fluid is removed and the lung expands freely. Because the peel often intimately adheres to the underlying lung, there may be a moderate postop air leak.

In patients too ill to undergo thoracotomy, **rib resection** with subsequent open drainage tube will permit the underlying lung to expand over a period of several weeks. Although this may be done under local anesthesia, a brief general anesthetic is often easier on the patient. In this operation, the patient is placed in the lateral position and an incision is made over the rib corresponding to the most dependent portion of the empyema cavity. A 6-cm length of the rib is excised and a large-diameter (≥ 50 Fr) tube is inserted into the empyema cavity. More permanent open drainage is obtained by fashioning an **Eloesser flap.** In this procedure, a U-shaped flap of skin is rotated into the empyema cavity after rib resection. This creates a long-term, skin-lined tube that will last indefinitely. A varient of this procedure—the **Claggett procedure**—is carried out for empyema (with or without bronchopleural fistula) following pneumonectomy, since closed drainage rarely suffices in that situation. The principle is the same: drainage is accomplished through an epithelial-lined permanent opening. The opening is made anterolaterally and dependently so that drainage is effective and the patient can handle dressing changes without assistance. Segments of 2-3 ribs are removed and the skin is sutured to the parietal pleura, leaving a permanent opening for drainage and irrigation. Without an underlying lung, and with a relatively fixed mediastinum, this procedure is well tolerated physiologically.

Usual preop diagnosis: Nontuberculosis empyema (typically pneumococcal)

SUMMARY OF PROCEDURES

	Eloesser or Clagett	Tube Thoracostomy
Position	Usually lateral	Lateral
Incision	Over empyema pocket for Eloesser	Lateral
Special instrumentation	None	Large tubes

SUMMARY OF PROCEDURES (cont'd)

	Eloesser or Clagett	Tube Thoracostomy
Unique considerations	Patient may have BPF	Local or GA
Antibiotics	As indicated by culture and sensitivity	⇐
Surgical time	1 h; occasionally more	< 1 h
Closing considerations	Wound left open	None
EBL	100 mL	Minimal
Postop care	PACU → room	⇐
Mortality	Minimal	⇐
Morbidity	Fluid drainage Bleeding: Rare	Air leak
Pain score	3–4	2–3

PATIENT POPULATION CHARACTERISTICS

Age range	Usually adults
Male:Female	1:1
Incidence	Decreasing
Etiology	Pneumonia; esophageal or bronchial leak; lymphatic or hematogenous spread of infection; post-trauma or thoracic surgery
Associated conditions	Bronchopleural fistula (BPF); sepsis; malnutrition

ANESTHETIC CONSIDERATIONS

(Procedures covered: thoracoplasty; drainage of empyema)

PREOPERATIVE

The guiding principle in the anesthetic management of empyema is to protect the nonaffected lung from soiling by the affected side. These patients are often chronically ill with sepsis and cachexia; and there is usually an underlying BPF (which may require awake intubation).

Respiratory	Patients usually have pre-existing pulmonary disease. Preop pulmonary findings may include collapse of the ipsilateral lung, impaired hypoxic pulmonary vasoconstriction 2° infection, and mediastinal shift to the ipsilateral side. Procedure often is performed for empyema in the presence of BPF following lung resection (particularly pneumonectomy), penetrating injury to chest, or rupture of a cyst or bulla. When possible, surgeon should drain empyema under local anesthesia before induction, with patient sitting upright. If empyema is loculated, complete drainage may not be possible. **Tests:** Consider PFTs; ABG; obtain CXR to determine efficacy of preop chest drainage; if chest CT available, look for airway obstruction that could interfere with DLT placement.
Cardiovascular	There may be ECG changes because of mediastinal shift to the affected side. **Tests:** As indicated from H&P.

Neurological	✓ Hx of back surgery, peripheral neuropathy. Examine lumbar area for skin lesions, infection, deformities. Avoid placement of epidural catheter in patient with neurologic problems or if obviously bacteremic or septic.
Musculoskeletal	Patients with lung cancer may have myasthenic (Eaton-Lambert) syndrome with resistance to depolarizing muscle relaxant and ↑sensitivity to NDMRs. Monitor relaxation with peripheral nerve stimulator.
Hematologic	Transfuse patients with preop Hct < 25% or Hct < 30% in patients with CAD. (Hb level necessary to maintain adequate O_2 content.) Obtain autologous blood during the month before surgery or consider preop erythropoietin therapy in anemic patients.
Laboratory	Other tests as indicated from H&P.
Premedication	Midazolam 0.5–2 mg iv if patient anxious. When epidural opioids are planned, avoid systemic opioid or sedative premedication, which can potentiate postop respiratory effects of central neuraxial opioids.

INTRAOPERATIVE

Anesthetic technique: GETA; combined with epidural anesthesia/analgesia if thoracotomy is indicated and patient is not bacteremic or septic.

Induction	Consider inhalational induction (e.g., sevoflurane) if patient has significant BPF. Rapid-sequence induction with cricoid pressure is an alternative (p. B-4). Intubate with DLT; isolate lungs to protect from aspiration and tension pneumothorax. Consider using DLT with bronchial lumen to side opposite BPF. Contamination of the healthy lung from aspiration of pus is a major concern; thus, proper tube position should be verified by FOB, and adequate cuff inflation should be checked. Large DLT provides snug fit in bronchus and limits aspiration. Pus may appear in tracheal lumen (lumen to the diseased lung); suction frequently to avoid soiling good lung.
Maintenance	O_2 and isoflurane (1.0–1.5%); less required if epidural local anesthetics used. No N_2O. Use FiO_2 = 0.5–1.0. A local anesthetic (e.g., 2% lidocaine with 1:200,000 epinephrine or 0.25% bupivacaine) can be infused or injected hourly into a thoracic (3–5 mL) or lumbar (5–10 mL) epidural catheter. Continuous infusion of local anesthetic generally provides better hemodynamic stability than hourly bolus injection. To enhance the effect of epidural analgesia, a loading dose of opiate (e.g., hydromorphone 0.4–1 mg [thoracic] or 1–1.5 mg [lumbar]) can be administered early in the surgery and at least 1 h before conclusion. Following intubation, isolate lung with DLT or BB. The chest tube is then removed while the chest is prepped for the operation. Ventilate only the healthy lung. Because BPF is an abnormal communication between the bronchial tree and pleural cavity, if no chest tube is present, conventional intubation with IPPV can produce tension pneumothorax. Keep unclamped and do not remove a functioning chest tube until the lung is isolated and ventilation to the diseased lung is stopped. After the chest is opened, there is no chance of pneumothorax, but the large air leak through BPF may prevent satisfactory ventilation of that lung. High-frequency ventilation (HFV) is recommended by some, but studies show no benefit; in some patients the BPF is actually increased with HFV. See OLV Management under Anesthetic Considerations for Lobectomy, Pneumonectomy, p. 278.
Emergence	Before closing the chest, lungs are inflated gradually to 30 cmH_2O pressure to reinflate atelectatic areas and to check for significant air leaks. The surgeon will insert chest tubes to drain pleural cavity and aid lung re-expansion. Patient is extubated while still in OR. If postop ventilation is required (rare), the DLT is exchanged for an ETT. If BPF is still open, consider selective ventilation postop through DLT. It may be necessary to ventilate each lung separately; use smaller TVs to lung with BPF. Alternatively, pressure-controlled ventilation may be used to avoid major air leaks through BPF.

Blood and fluid requirements	IV: 16–18 ga × 1 Avoid hypervolemia. Use vasopressor (ephedrine 5–10 mg iv bolus or phenylephrine 50–100 mcg iv bolus) if hypotensive.	An overhydrated patient is at increased risk of right-heart failure and pulmonary edema. Replace blood loss with crystalloid (1:3) or colloid (1:1). Third-space losses are negligible and do not need to be replaced. Use of epidural local anesthetics can cause ↓ BP in a volume-restricted patient; vasopressor often needed.
Monitoring	Standard monitors (p. B-1) ± CVP and/or PA line ± Arterial line	
Positioning	Axillary roll, "airplane" for upper arm Avoid hyperextending arms. ✓ and pad pressure points. ✓ eyes, ears, genitals.	Placing the oximeter probe on the down side may help detect inadequate perfusion from compression.

POSTOPERATIVE

Complications	Tension pneumothorax Aspiration pneumonia ("down" lung)	Functioning chest tube necessary to prevent tension pneumothorax.
Pain management	Analgesic requirements minimal Parenteral opioids (iv, im, PCA [p. C-3]), epidural, NSAID	See Pain Management under Anesthetic Considerations for Lobectomy, Pneumonectomy, p. 279.

Suggested Readings

1. Baue AE, ed: *Glenn's Thoracic and Cardiovascular Surgery,* 6th edition, Volume II. Geha AS, Hammond GL, Laks H, et al., assoc. eds. Appleton & Lange, Norwalk: 1996.
2. Benjaminsson E, Klain M: Intraoperative dual-mode independent lung ventilation of a patient with bronchopleural fistula. *Anesth Analg* 1981; 60(2):118–19.
3. Bishop MJ, Benson MS, Sato P, et al: Comparison of high-frequency jet ventilation with conventional mechanical ventilation for bronchopleural fistula. *Anesth Analg* 1987; 66(9):833–8.
4. Langston HT: Thoracoplasty: the how and the why. *Ann Thorac Surg* 1991; 52(6):1351–3.
5. Miller JI Jr: Postsurgical empyema. In *General Thoracic Surgery,* 5th edition. Shields TW, LoCicero J III, Ponn RB, eds. Lippincott Williams & Wilkins, Philadelphia: 2000, 709–16.
6. Sellke FW, Swanson S, del Nido P: *Sabiston & Spencer: Surgery of the Chest,* 7th edition. Elsevier Saunders, Philadelphia: 2004.

TRACHEAL RESECTION

SURGICAL CONSIDERATIONS

Description: The primary indications for **tracheal resection** are benign stricture and primary tracheal neoplasm. Benign strictures often are related to previous intubation or tracheostomy, whereas the most common malignant tumors include squamous cell carcinoma and adenoid cystic carcinoma. Proximal tracheal resections may also be required for trauma or idiopathic laryngotracheal stenosis. The preoperative assessment of patients with tracheal disease generally involves imaging with either CT or MRI. Important considerations include the length and position of the lesion and the caliber of the airway. Although up to 50% of the trachea can be resected with a successful primary anastomosis, shorter segment resections are technically simpler and do not require special techniques to maximize tracheal mobility.

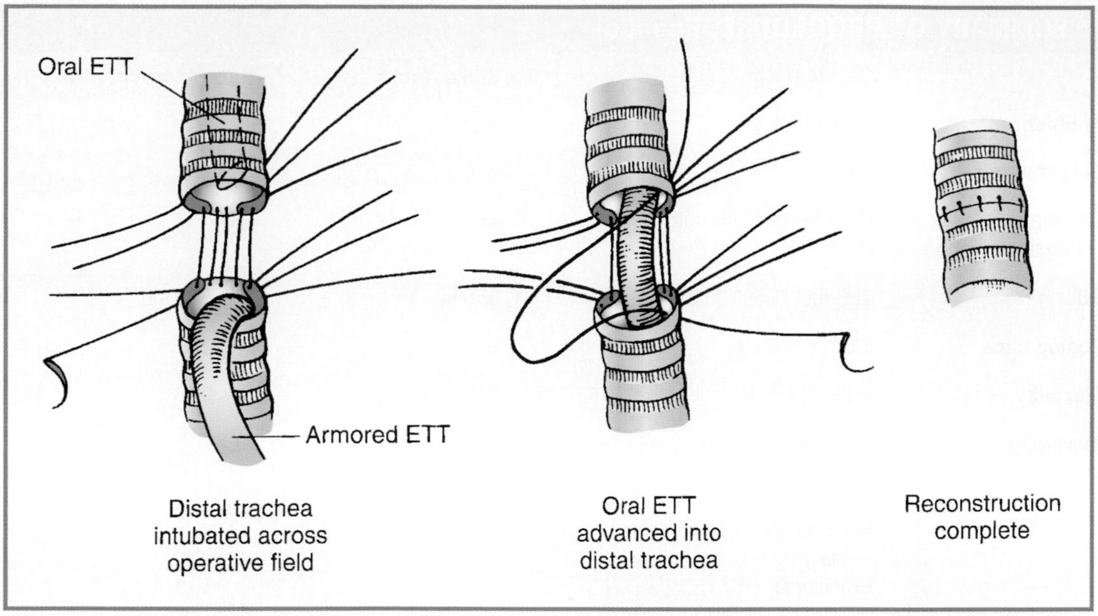

Figure 5-10. Stages of tracheal reconstruction. Note ETT in distal trachea. (Reproduced with permission from Grillo HC: *Current Problems in Surgery*. Year Book Medical Publishers, 1970.)

Lesions of the upper and midtrachea can be approached through the neck, whereas lesions of the lower trachea and carina must be approached through the right chest. When using the **cervical approach,** the patient is positioned with the neck extended. A transverse collar incision is used and subplatysmal planes are developed. The trachea is then extensively mobilized anteriorly and posteriorly. To minimize the risk of devascularizing the trachea, only the region to be removed should be circumferentially dissected. During this portion of the operation, care is taken to avoid injury of the recurrent laryngeal nerves. The trachea is then opened, the oral ETT is withdrawn into the proximal trachea, and a sterile armored ETT is passed across the operative field. Fine, interrupted, absorbable sutures are placed, but not tied. Once all sutures are in place, the armored tube is removed and the oral ETT is positioned across the anastomosis. The ends of the trachea are approximated with minimal tension and the sutures are tied (Fig. 5-10). To provide minimal tension, it may be necessary to flex the neck for this portion of the procedure. A suture may be placed from the chin to the chest wall to maintain neck flexion for several days postop. At the end of the procedure, the patient should be extubated to minimize airway irritation and disruption of the anastomosis.

Lesions of the lower trachea must be approached thought the right chest, where the same techniques as discussed above are used. To facilitate exposure of the distal trachea, OLV using either a DLT or a single-lumen tube advanced into the left main bronchus is helpful.

As is apparent from the above discussion, all tracheal procedures require cooperation and frequent communication between the surgeon and anesthesiologist. Occasionally, special techniques, such as jet ventilation or CPB, may be necessary for tracheal surgery.

Usual preop diagnosis: Tracheal stenosis or tumor (adenoid cystic carcinoma or squamous cell carcinoma most common)

SUMMARY OF PROCEDURES

	Cervical Approach	Sternotomy	Right Thoracotomy
Position	Supine	⇐	Left lateral decubitus
Incision	Transverse low cervical	Cervical + sternotomy	Right thoracotomy

SUMMARY OF PROCEDURES (cont'd)

	Cervical Approach	Sternotomy	Right Thoracotomy
Antibiotics	Cefazolin 1 g	⇐	⇐
Surgical time	3 h	3–4 h	4 h
Closing considerations	Neck flexion (chin stitch)	⇐	⇐
EBL	200 mL	350 mL	350–500 mL
Postop care	ICU	⇐	⇐
Mortality	< 5%	5%	⇐
Morbidity	Retained secretions Dehiscence Recurrent stenosis Recurrent/superior laryngeal nerve injury Granuloma	⇐	⇐
Pain score	3–4	5–6	7–9

PATIENT POPULATION CHARACTERISTICS

Age range	Wide variation
Male:Female	1:1
Incidence	Rare
Etiology	Stenosis usually 2° to intubation or injury; tumor, either primary (e.g., smoking) or secondary (e.g., esophageal, lung, thyroid cancer)
Associated conditions	Carcinoid syndrome; cardiopulmonary disease; tracheoesophageal fistula (TEF)

ANESTHETIC CONSIDERATIONS

PREOPERATIVE

Respiratory	Initial presentation may involve Sx of airway obstruction (stridor, cough, dyspnea), which may be misdiagnosed as asthma or pneumonitis. Patients presenting for tracheal resection almost exclusively have fixed obstruction, but may have an associated dynamic component. A careful preop evaluation of the airway usually includes bronchoscopic delineation of lesion site and size. This in combination with a review of CT images will help to determine a plan including type of induction, size of ETT and location of ETT tip. **Tests:** PFT with flow/volume loops; bronchoscopy; CT scan to determine extent of tracheal obstruction
Laboratory	Other tests as indicated from H&P.
Premedication	Patients with stridor or critical airway lesions should not receive preop sedation. It is probably best to avoid sedation in all patients. Patients may be unable to lie flat 2° respiratory distress. Low-density helium-oxygen mixtures (Heliox) have the clinical advantage of reducing airway resistance to flow past the obstruction, which may be beneficial in optimizing the patient prior to the procedure.

INTRAOPERATIVE

Anesthetic technique: GETA, combined with epidural or paravertebral catheter if sternotomy or thoracotomy approach is used. Surgery is divided into five phases: induction, dissection, open trachea, closure and emergence. Induction, open trachea, and emergence are the critical and potentially dangerous stages. Close communication between surgeon and anesthesiologist is required.

Induction	Be prepared for airway emergency. Surgeon must be present and prepared for emergency rigid bronchoscopy and/or to perform tracheostomy below lesion. Induction depends on the site and degree of airway narrowing. Proximal or narrow lesions usually require inhalation induction or awake FOI, whereas distal or mild lesions may be approached with a rapid sequence i.v. induction. Sevoflurane/O_2 is preferred for smooth inhalation induction with depression of cough reflex; avoid N_2O. High concentrations of sevoflurane may be necessary. Heliox (79% helium in oxygen) has been recommended to decrease resistance to flow past the obstruction; however, helium is not widely available and limits the FiO_2 that can be administered. Have a variety of laryngeal blades and uncut ETTs of various sizes, including small 5 mm tubes available. If ETT passes beyond lesion, can begin IPPV. If ETT cannot be passed, spontaneous ventilation with 100% O_2 and sevoflurane will be required if there is a dynamic obstruction, while patients with fixed lesions will tolerate PPV through a proximal tube. Careful and gradual dilation of the stenotic lesion may be required, using different sizes of ETTs or rigid bronchoscopy to facilitate placement of an adequate size ETT for ventilation. For carinal resections, use a sterile ETT, which can be placed by surgeon directly into each bronchus during resection for cross-field ventilation. An armored tube is preferable because it avoids kinking during repeated manipulations by the surgeon. Another option is to place jet ventilation catheters into the mainstem bronchi and jet-ventilate the patient during the open trachea stage.	
Maintenance	Inhalational anesthesia can be unreliable (and may pollute the OR environment) due to frequent tube changes and intermittent apnea. TIVA is preferable: use propofol (25–100 mcg/kg/min) and remifentanil (0.05–0.2 mcg/kg/min) infusions. After the airway is secured, muscle relaxation should be given to avoid movement or coughing during the procedure. Standard maintenance (p. B-2). FiO_2 = 1.0 if using apneic oxygenation; continuous monitoring with pulse oximetry mandatory. Consider HFJV through a small-diameter catheter if ETT interferes with operation. HFJV will require iv anesthesia, because inhalational agents cannot be delivered predictably; CPB can be used (rare). Analgesia requirements are highly dependent on surgical approach. Standard parenteral opioids are sufficient for the cervical approach, whereas epidural of paravertebral analgesia (similar to lobectomy) are used for open intrathoracic procedures.	
Emergence	Early extubation; presence of ETT and IPPV can disrupt fresh suture line. Remove ETT as soon as patient is awake enough to protect airway and breathing spontaneously, but before bucking and coughing occur. Presence of a "guardian suture" (chestwall to chin) will make reintubation more difficult. Assess integrity of recurrent laryngeal nerve after high tracheal resections.+	
Blood and fluid requirements	IV: 16–18 ga × 1 (left arm) NS/LR @ 3 mL/kg/h	✓ innominate artery compression, affects a right arm perfusion.
Monitoring	Standard monitors (p. B-1) ± Arterial line	Left radial artery cannulation permits uninterrupted monitoring of BP during periods of innominate artery compression. Placement of iv in left arm allows unimpeded infusion. Right-extremity pulse oximetry will help detect innominate artery occlusion (which otherwise could lead to stroke.)
Positioning	✓ and pad pressure points. ✓ eyes.	
Airway management	ETT replaced with sterile ETT and circuit intraop.	Ater the trachea is divided, the surgeon places a sterile ETT in the distal trachea. The original ETT is withdrawn above the surgical site. The surgeon attaches a sterile anesthesia circuit to distal ETT

Airway management (cont'd)		for ventilation. Then, the surgeon places a suture through the distal tip of the original ETT. Before reanastomosis of trachea, the distal trachea is suctioned to remove accumulated blood and secretions. After a posterior suture line is completed, the original ETT is pulled through the trachea and the distal tube (which is below the resection) is removed. Reattach and ventilate patient through original ETT.
Complications	Tracheal edema	Corticosteroids (dexamethasone 6–8 mg iv) to ↓ tracheal edema.
	Injury to neck	Any structure in the neck can be damaged, including superior and recurrent laryngeal nerves, trachea, and thoracic duct.

POSTOPERATIVE

Complications	Tracheal disruption	Neck swelling, subcutaneous emphysema, and inability to ventilate indicate loss of air-tight anastomosis. Immediate re-exploration of neck is essential. May be fatal.
	Recurrent laryngeal nerve injury	Bilateral (occasionally unilateral) laryngeal nerve damage may → airway obstruction, necessitating reintubation. Mask ventilation may be ineffective.
Position	Airway edema Keep head flexed to reduce tension on tracheal suture line.	Place patient in head-up, neck-flexed position. Treat with nebulized racemic epinephrine if airway compromise occurs. If reintubation is required, a small ETT should be placed under direct vision or fiberoptic guidance, to avoid disruption of the anastomosis.
Pain management	Parenteral opioids (p. C-2) ± Epidural	After patient is fully awake.

Suggested Readings

1. Ashiku SK, Mathisen DJ: Idiopathic laryngotracheal stenosis. *Chest Surg Clin North Am* 2003;13(2):257–69.
2. Gaissert HA, Grillo HC, Shadmehr MB, et al: Long-term survival after resection of primary adenoid cystic and squamous cell carcinoma of the trachea and carina. *Ann Thorac Surg* 2004;78(6):1889–96, discussion 1896–7.
3. McRae K: Anesthesia for airway surgery. *Anesthesiol Clin North Am* 2001; 19(3):497–541.
4. Perera ER, Vidic DM, Zivot J: Carinal resection with two high-frequency jet ventilation delivery systems. *Can J Anaesth* 1993; 40(1): 59–63.
5. Sandberg W: Anesthesia and airway management for tracheal resection and reconstruction. *Int Anesthesiol Clin* 2000; 38(1): 55–75.

EXCISION OF MEDIASTINAL TUMOR

SURGICAL CONSIDERATIONS

Description: Mediastinal tumors are characterized by their location (anterior, middle, and posterior) and their size. Common anterior mediastinal tumors include thymic tumors (benign or malignant thymoma and thymic carcinoma), germ-cell tumors, lymphoma, and substernal goiters. Typically, thymic and germ-cell tumors are resected, whereas lymphomas are biopsied. Substernal goiters usually can be resected through the neck. Tumors in the anterior mediastinum usually are removed through a **median sternotomy,** whereas tumors in the middle and posterior mediastinum usually are removed through a **lateral thoracotomy or thoracoscopy (VATS).** Although middle and posterior mediastinal tumors usually do not present airway management problems, the issue of functioning neuroendocrine tissue must be considered. Mediastinal pheochromocytomas are uncommon middle mediastinal tumors however, as with pheochromocytomas arising in other locations, appropriate preop adrenergic management is necessary. Some cysts or small tumors may be excised using **video thoracoscopy** (see Video-Assisted Thoracoscopy, p. 313).

Mediastinal tumors that are well encapsulated generally are removed in a straightforward fashion. If anterior mediastinal tumors are not well encapsulated and are attached to pericardium or lung on either side, appropriate portions of these attached structures may be removed in continuity with the tumor. If there is attachment to phrenic nerves on either side, one nerve may be sacrificed if necessary to remove the tumor completely. In patients with anterior mediastinal tumors, invasion of the major vascular structures, particularly the aorta and arch vessels, presents an even greater problem.

Germ-cell tumors of the anterior mediastinum–particularly nonseminomatous tumors–are often treated with chemotherapy initially. A common regimen for these patients consists of cisplatin, etoposide, and bleomycin, and because bleomycin is associated with pulmonary toxicity–particularly in conjunction with high concentrations of inhaled oxygen–care must be taken to keep the $FiO_2 < 40\%$ when conducting these operations.

Another common issue with patients with large anterior mediastinal masses is that of intrathoracic airway obstruction at the time of anesthetic induction. Although most mediastinal masses do not cause obstruction of the trachea or tracheobronchial tree, large mediastinal masses in the anterior mediastinum, in conjunction with muscle relaxation, can lead to complete obstruction of the airway with inability to ventilate the patient. Although rigid bronchoscopy may permit ventilation through the obstruction, it cannot be counted on to relieve the obstruction; therefore, only short-acting or no muscle relaxants (spontaneous ventilation) should be used in these patients.

Usual preop diagnosis: Thymoma; teratodermoid; ganglioneuroma; lymphoma; schwannoma; substernal goiter

SUMMARY OF PROCEDURE

Position	Supine or lateral
Incision	Median sternotomy or lateral thoracotomy
Special instrumentation	Sternal or rib retractors
Antibiotics	Cefazolin 1 g
Surgical time	≤ 2 h
EBL	< 500 mL
Postop care	Frequently ICU
Mortality	Minimal
Morbidity	Bleeding
Pain score	5–8

PATIENT POPULATION CHARACTERISTICS

Age range	All ages
Male:Female	1:1
Etiology	**Anterior mediastinum:** Thymoma; teratoma; pericardial cyst; lymphoma; parasternal (Morgagni) hernia; lipoma **Superior mediastinum:** Goiter; aneurysm; parathyroid tumor; esophageal tumor; angiomatous tumor **Middle mediastinum:** Lymphoma; lymph node inflammation; bronchogenic tumor; bronchogenic cyst **Posterior mediastinum:** Neurogenic tumor; aneurysm (enteric cyst); esophageal tumor; bronchogenic tumor
Associated conditions	SVC syndrome; myasthenia gravis; recurrent laryngeal nerve damage; airway obstruction; dyspnea; Horner's syndrome

ANESTHETIC CONSIDERATIONS

See Anesthetic Considerations following Mediastinoscopy, p. 302.

Suggested Readings

1. Baue AE, ed: *Glenn's Thoracic and Cardiovascular Surgery,* 6th edition, Volume II. Geha AS, Hammond GL, Laks H, et al., assoc. eds. Appleton & Lange, Norwalk, CT: 1996.
2. de Wit R: Refining the optimal chemotherapy regimen in good prognosis germ cell cancer: interpretation of the current body of knowledge. *J Clin Oncol* 2007; 25(28):4346–9.
3. Lewer BM, Torrance JM: Anaesthesia for a patient with a mediastinal mass presenting with acute stridor. *Anaesth Intensive Care* 1996; 24(5):605–8.
4. Narang S, Harte HB, Body SC: Anesthesia for patients with a mediastinal mass. *Anesthesiol Clin North Am* 2001; 19(3): 559–79.
5. Sellke FW, Swanson S, del Nido P: *Sabiston & Spencer: Surgery of the Chest,* 7th edition. Elsevier Saunders, Philadelphia: 2004.
6. Viswabathans S, Campbell CE, Cork RC: Asymptomatic undetected mediastinal mass: a death during ambulatory anesthesia. *J Clin Anesth* 1995; 7(2):151–5.

MEDIASTINOSCOPY

SURGICAL CONSIDERATIONS

Description: Mediastinoscopy is used for biopsy of mediastinal lymph nodes. The most common indication for this procedure is bronchogenic carcinoma, although lymphadenopathy associated with lymphoma, sarcoidosis, and infectious granulomatous diseases are also indications for mediastinoscopy. **Cervical mediastinoscopy** provides access to the pretracheal, paratracheal, and anterior subcarinal nodes (Fig. 5-11), whereas **transthoracic mediastinoscopy** (also known as **anterior mediastinotomy** or **Chamberlain's procedure**) provides access to the aortopulmonary lymph nodes. Previous mediastinoscopy and radiation are relative contraindications to this procedure. If

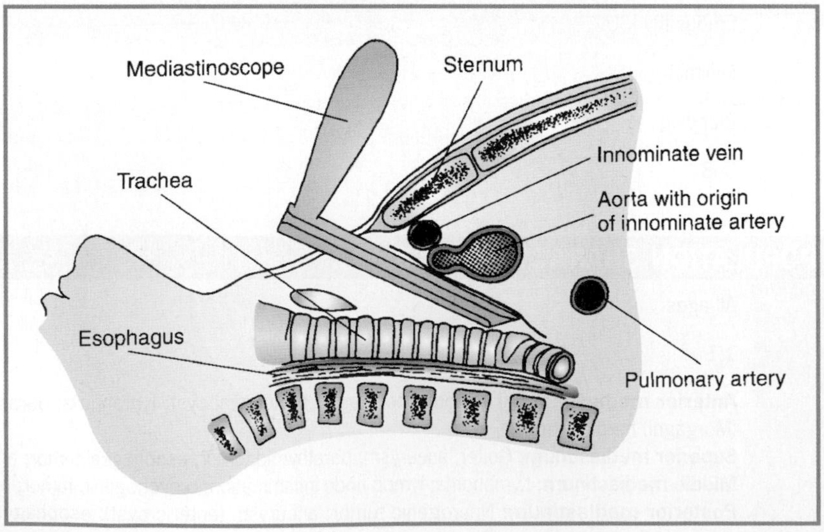

Figure 5-11. Mediastinoscope is inserted through a small cervical incision into the middle mediastinum, along the pretracheal plane. (Reproduced with permission from Baker RJ, Fischer JE: *Mastery of Surgery.* Lippincott Williams & Wilkins, Philadelphia: 2001.)

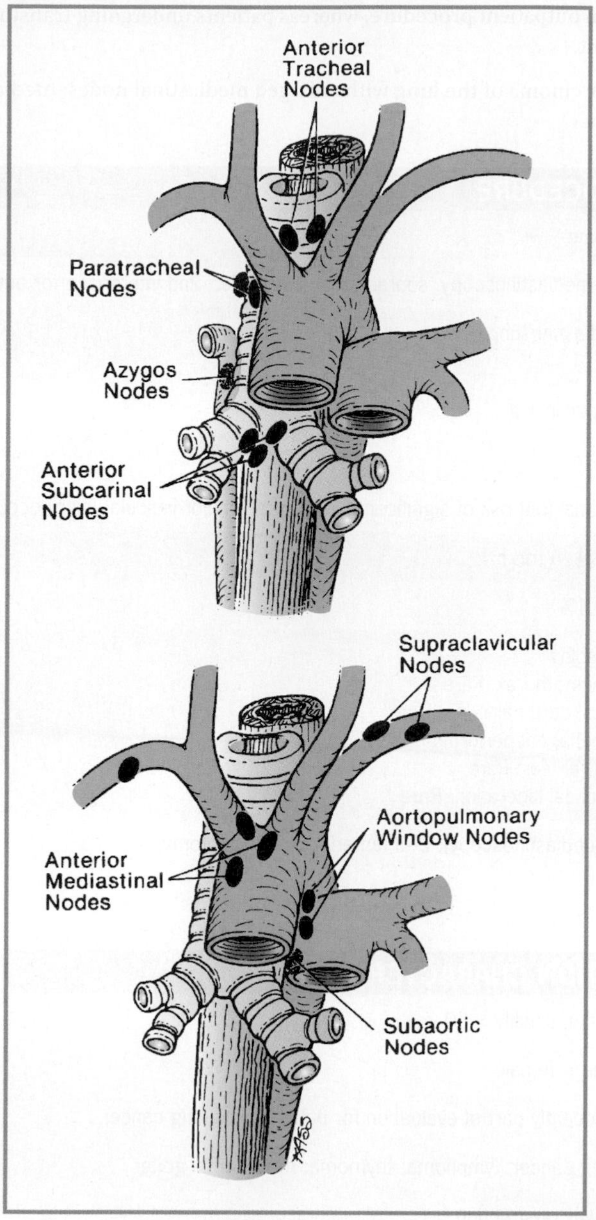

Figure 5-12. Lymph node sites accessible to mediastinoscope biopsy. Many of these can be reached by standard cervical mediastinoscopy. Anterior and aortopulmonary window nodes, however, require extended or anterior mediastinoscopy, VATS, or needle biopsy. (Reproduced with permission from Bocage J-P, Mackenzie JW, Nosher JL: Invasive diagnostic procedures. In *General Thoracic Surgery,* 5th edition. Shields TW, LoCicero J III, Ponn RB, eds. Lippincott Williams & Wilkins, Philadelphia: 2000.)

a thoracic aneurysm is present or SVC is obstructed, mediastinoscopy is contraindicated, because the anatomy is distorted and vessels can be punctured inadvertently by the mediastinoscope.

Variant procedure or approaches: For nodes on the left side of the mediastinum, **transthoracic mediastinoscopy** is performed through a limited anterior thoracotomy. In the classic **Chamberlain's procedure,** the 3rd costal cartilage is resected and the mediastinum is explored without entering the pleural space. As with cervical mediastinoscopy, visualization is often limited and lymph nodes should be aspirated before biopsy. If the pleural space is entered during the course of the procedure, either a chest tube can be placed postop or the pleural space can be aspirated immediately before wound closure. Patients should be extubated at the end of the operation. Cervical mediastinoscopy is usually an outpatient procedure, whereas patients undergoing transthoracic mediastinoscopy are usually hospitalized overnight.

Usual preop diagnosis: Carcinoma of the lung with enlarged mediastinal nodes; mediastinal node enlargement 2° lymphoma, thymoma, or other

SUMMARY OF PROCEDURE	
Position	Supine
Incision	For mediastinoscopy, suprasternal; usually left 2nd interspace for anterior mediastinotomy.
Special instrumentation	Mediastinoscope
Antibiotics	Cefazolin 1 g
Surgical time	≤ 1 h
EBL	Minimal (but risk of significant blood loss if major vascular injury occurs).
Postop care	PACU → room
Mortality	< 0.1%
Morbidity	Bleeding Pneumothorax: Rare Vocal cord paralysis: Rare Esophageal perforation: Rare Pleural tear: Rare Tracheal laceration: Rare
Pain score	2 (mediastinoscopy); 2–3 (anterior mediastinotomy)

PATIENT POPULATION CHARACTERISTICS	
Age range	Adults, usually > 50 yr
Male:Female	Male > female
Incidence	Frequently part of evaluation for patients with lung cancer.
Etiology	Lung cancer; lymphoma; thymoma; retrosternal goiter
Associated conditions	Airway obstruction

ANESTHETIC CONSIDERATIONS

PREOPERATIVE

(Procedures covered: excision of mediastinal tumor; mediastinoscopy)

Typically, these patients can be divided into two populations, depending on the presence or absence of a significant mediastinal mass (with the potential for catastrophic airway obstruction or cardiovascular collapse on induction of anesthesia). The preop assessment must focus on the differentiation of these two populations. Close consultation with the surgeon is essential in formulating the anesthetic plan. On occasion, patients with critical airway or cardiac compression may require a tissue biopsy for diagnostic purposes only. If general anesthesia poses a significant physiologic threat to the patient, search for an alternative, less invasive biopsy site.

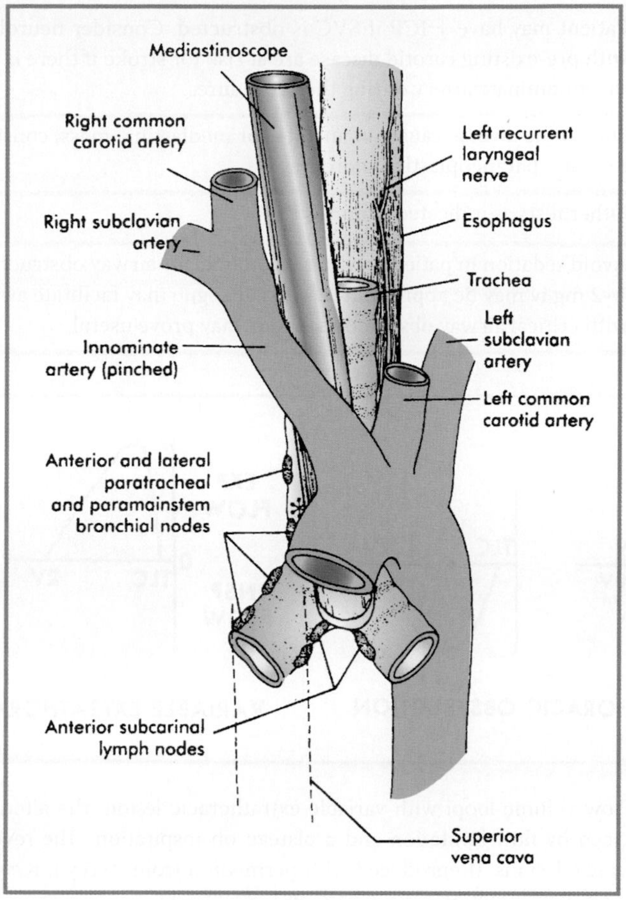

Figure 5-13. Relationship of mediastinoscope to trachea and great vessels. (Reproduced with permission from Petty C: Right radial artery pressure during mediastinoscopy. *Anesth Analg* 1979; 58:428. Modified in Rogers MC: *Principles & Practices of Anesthesiology.* Mosby-Year Book, St. Louis: 1993.)

Respiratory	Question patient with anterior mediastinal mass about ability to lie supine and the presence of cough or dyspnea. Change in position may cause superior vena caval obstruction or cardiac and airway compression by mediastinal mass (which may be apparent only following induction or on emergence from anesthesia). On PE, ✓ for the presence of cyanosis, wheezing, or stridor in the upright and supine positions. If significant airway compression or SVC obstruction is present, the surgeon may delay surgery for radiation or chemotherapy. Patients with SVC syndrome (edema; venous engorgement of head, neck, and upper body; supine dyspnea; ± headache; mental status change) may have significant airway edema. **Tests:** Classic teaching has recommended PFTs with flow volume loops in upright and supine positions (Fig. 5-14 shows flow volume loop) in patients with suspected central airway obstruction. These investigations demonstrate airflow obstruction during inspiration in patients with an extrathoracic mass and during expiration in patients with an intrathoracic mass. CT scans obtained with the patient supine delineate the location and extent of both airway and cardiac ± vascular compression. These images may predict patients at higher risk (> 50% tracheal compression).
Cardiovascular	Intrathoracic vascular structures (e.g., right heart, PA, SVC) may be compressed → ↓ BP, hypoxia, SVC syndrome. Involvement of the pericardium may → tamponade. **Tests:** ECHO, CT/MRI if indicated by H&P.
Musculoskeletal	Patients with lung cancer may have myasthenic (Eaton-Lambert) syndrome with resistance to depolarizing agents and ↑ sensitivity to NDMRs. Monitor relaxation with peripheral nerve stimulator.

Neurologic	Patient may have ↑ ICP if SVC is obstructed. Consider neurology consultation. Patients with pre-existing carotid disease are at risk for stroke if there is significant compression of the innominate artery during the procedure.
Endocrine	Due to the diverse causes of an anterior mediastinal mass, consider comorbid thyroid disease and paraneoplastic syndromes.
Laboratory	Other tests as indicated from H&P.
Premedication	Avoid sedation in patients with the potential for airway obstruction; otherwise, midazolam 1–2 mg iv may be appropriate. Antisialogogue may facilitate awake intubation. In patients with critical airway obstruction, heliox may prove useful.

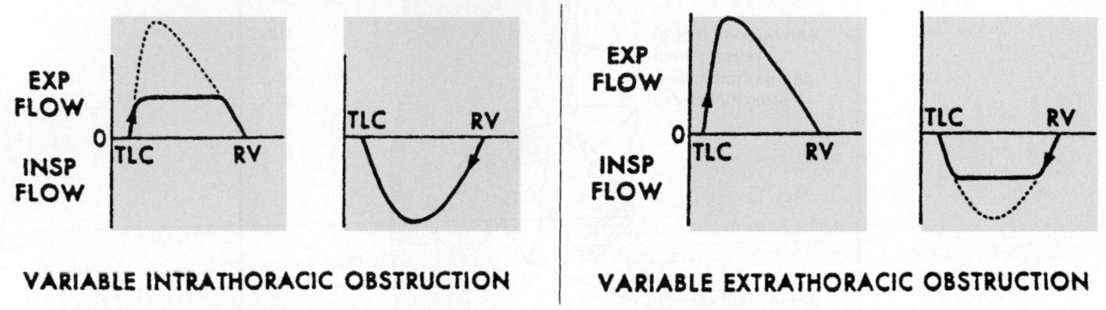

Figure 5-14. Flow volume loop: with variable extrathoracic lesion, the alteration in the flow volume loop is seen by flow limitation and a plateau on inspiration. The reverse occurs with variable intrathoracic lesions. (Reproduced with permission from Acres J, Kryger MH: Clinical significance of pulmonary function tests. *Chest* 1981; 80:207–11.)

INTRAOPERATIVE

Anesthetic technique: GETA, combined with epidural if thoracotomy is planned.

Induction	Consider awake FOI (e.g., if symptomatic in supine position). Alternatively, a mask induction with sevoflurane/O_2 in a spontaneously breathing patient may be safe. Use of neuromuscular blockers in high risk patients may precipitate airway obstruction and CV collapse. Select a reinforced endotracheal tube when intubating patients with airway compression. Complete or partial airway obstruction by anterior mediastinal mass can also be due to changes in lung and chest-wall mechanics associated with changes in the patient's position (sitting to supine during procedure) or to muscle relaxation. Consider placing the patient in the lateral or prone position in the event of central airway compression. A surgeon familiar with rigid bronchoscopy must be in the OR ready to bypass any obstruction. In rare instances, percutaneous cardiopulmonary bypass (CPB) may be necessary to complete the procedure safely. If this is indicated, it must be employed electively, not as a rescue measure. Salvage or emergent use of CPB in these patients is rarely successful.	
Maintenance	O_2 (100%) and isoflurane (1–1.5%) or sevoflurane (1.5–2.5%). Avoid N_2O, especially during OLV. Short-acting muscle relaxant and opioid as indicated.	
Emergence	Extubation in OR	
Blood and fluid requirements	IV: 14–16 ga × 1 NS/LR @ 1–2 mL/kg/h Blood in OR	Have blood for transfusion available in OR prior to surgery. Patients with SVC syndrome may have impaired venous return from upper-limb iv's. In these patients a large-bore iv cannula should be placed in lower limb for fluid and blood transfusions.

Monitoring	Standard monitors (p. B-1) ± Arterial line ± CVP/PA	Invasive monitors are appropriate in patients with large mediastinal masses. In the presence of SVC syndrome, CVP/PA catheters should be placed, using the femoral vein. BP cuff on left arm; radial artery line (if used) and pulse oximeter on right. Mass or mediastinoscope can compress innominate artery, causing reduction in right-radial pulse and right-arm BP. If only right-arm BP is measured, patients may be treated inappropriately for "hypotension" or cardiac arrest. Suspect great vessel compression if right-arm pressure is lower than left or if right-arm BP disappears in the presence of a normal ECG. Arterial compression can compromise cerebrovascular perfusion → cerebral ischemia → stroke.
Positioning	Head-up position ✓ and pad pressure points. ✓ eyes.	In patients with an anterior mediastinal mass, the head-up position reduces mass compression effect on airway and vascular structures, but may subject the patient to ↑ risk of VAE if venous bleeding occurs during the procedure. Patients with SVC obstruction, if placed in head-down position with IPPV (further impedes venous return of thoracic cavity), are at ↑ risk of airway edema and airway obstruction following extubation.
Complications	Bleeding	Surgical tamponade through mediastinoscope may be indicated. For major hemorrhage, emergency thoracotomy or median sternotomy may be required to stop bleeding. Can occur from laceration of mediastinal vein.
	Air embolism	Head elevation increases risk of embolism, particularly if patient breathes spontaneously. Monitor $ETCO_2$ and ETN_2.
	Airway rupture or obstruction	Requires immediate thoracotomy.
	Tracheal collapse	Acute obstruction may require rigid bronchoscope to reopen airway.
	Recurrent laryngeal nerve injury	If recurrent laryngeal nerve injury is suspected, the vocal cords should be examined during spontaneous breathing at the time of extubation.

POSTOPERATIVE

Complications	Pneumothorax	(see Postop Complications for Cervical Neurosurgical Procedures, p. 108).
	Phrenic/recurrent laryngeal nerve damage	Bilateral laryngeal nerve damage may result in airway obstruction, necessitating reintubation. Mask ventilation may be ineffective.
	Bleeding Tracheomalacia	May occur in patients with longstanding mediastinal mass (e.g., retrosternal goiter)
Pain management	Parenteral opioids (p. C-2) ± Epidural	
Tests	CXR on all patients to r/o pneumothorax.	See Postop Complications for VATS, p. 315.

Suggested Readings

1. Barash PG, Tsai B, Kitahata LM: Acute tracheal collapse following mediastinoscopy. *Anesthesiology* 1976; 44(1):67–8.
2. Baue AE, ed: *Glenn's Thoracic and Cardiovascular Surgery,* 6th edition, Volume II. Geha AS, Hammond GL, Laks H, et al., assoc. eds. Appleton & Lange, Norwalk: 1996.
3. Bechard P, Letourneau L, Lacasse Y, et al: Perioperative cardiorespiratory complications in adults with mediastinal mass. *Anesthesiology* 2004; 100(4):826–34.
4. Hnatiuk OW, Corcoran PC, Sierra A: Spirometry in surgery for mediastinal masses. *Chest* 2001; 120(4):1152–6.
5. Narang S, Harte BH, Body S: Anesthesia for patients with mediastinal mass. *Anesthesiol Clin North Am* 2001; 19(3):559–79.
6. Neuman GG, Weingarten AE, Abramowitz RM, et al: The anesthetic management of the patient with an anterior mediastinal mass. *Anesthesiology* 1984; 60(2):144–7.
7. Petty C: Right radial artery pressure during mediastinoscopy. *Anesth Analg* 1979; 58(5):428–30.
8. Plummer S, Hartley M, Vaughan RS: Anesthesia for telescopic procedures of the chest. *Br J Anaesth* 1998; 80(2):223–34.
9. Pullerits J, Holzman R: Anesthesia for patients with mediastinal masses. *Can J Anaesth* 1989; 36(6):681–8.
10. Sellke FW, Swanson S, del Nido Pl: *Sabiston & Spencer: Surgery of the Chest*, 7th edition. Elsevier Saunders, Philadelphia: 2004.
11. Slinger P, Karsli C: Management of the patient with a large mediastinal mass: recurring myths. *Curr Opin Anaesthesiol* 2007; 20(1):1–3.
12. Vaughan RS: Anesthesia for mediastinoscopy. *Anaesthesia* 1978; 33(2):195–8.
13. Vueghs PJ, Schurink GA, Vaes L, et al: Anesthesia in repeat mediastinoscopy: a retrospective study of 101 patients. *J Cardiothorac Vasc Anesth* 1992; 6(2):193–5.

BRONCHOSCOPY—FLEXIBLE AND RIGID

SURGICAL CONSIDERATIONS

Description: Bronchoscopy can be performed using either rigid or flexible instrumentation. **Flexible fiber optic bronchoscopy (FOB)** is used for the diagnosis and evaluation of a variety of pulmonary conditions and can be accomplished using topical anesthesia and sedation without an anesthesiologist. Transbronchial biopsies can be performed in sedated patients, although more extensive interventions—such as laser ablation of a tumor, stent placement, and balloon dilation—generally require general anesthesia. When performed under general anesthesia, the bronchoscope should be passed through a size 8 or larger ETT.

Rigid bronchoscopy is more appropriate for evaluating hemoptysis and for intrabronchial procedures such as mechanical dilation of tracheal or bronchial strictures, laser or mechanical tumor debridement, and removal of foreign bodies that cannot be extracted with basket forceps through a flexible bronchoscope. Rigid bronchoscopy is performed under general anesthesia. With the patient's head and neck extended, the eyes, teeth, and gums must be protected, and the bronchoscope is inserted into the posterior pharynx until the epiglottis is visualized. The epiglottis is lifted anteriorly, with care being taken not to use the patient's teeth as a fulcrum. The bronchoscope is then advanced into the trachea (Fig. 5-15) and the diagnostic or therapeutic procedure is carried out. Ventilation is through the sidearm of the bronchoscope and, as there is no cuff to prevent escape of anesthetic gases, high ventilatory volumes may be required. Because interventions (e.g., biopsy or tumor debridement) require removal of the bronchoscope viewing lens, the anesthesiologist must time ventilation appropriately. A Venturi ventilator may be useful when the viewing lens must be off for prolonged periods.

Laser bronchoscopy can be performed using either flexible or rigid bronchoscopes. The CO_2 laser is characterized by limited tissue penetration. As such, it is useful for superficial lesions of the upper airway. The Nd:YAG lasers use higher energies, can be directed by fiber optic light guides, and can be used for tumor ablation. As both of these types of lasers rely on thermal damage to tissues, precautions—particularly $FiO_2 \leq 40\%$—must be taken to prevent the devastating complication of airway fire. **Photodynamic therapy** uses visible light to activate a photosensitive compound into a locally toxic drug. Because no thermal energy is involved, airway fires are not an issue.

Usual preop diagnosis: Carcinoma of the lung, primary or recurrent; hemoptysis; obstruction; foreign body; benign tumor; respiratory papillomatosis

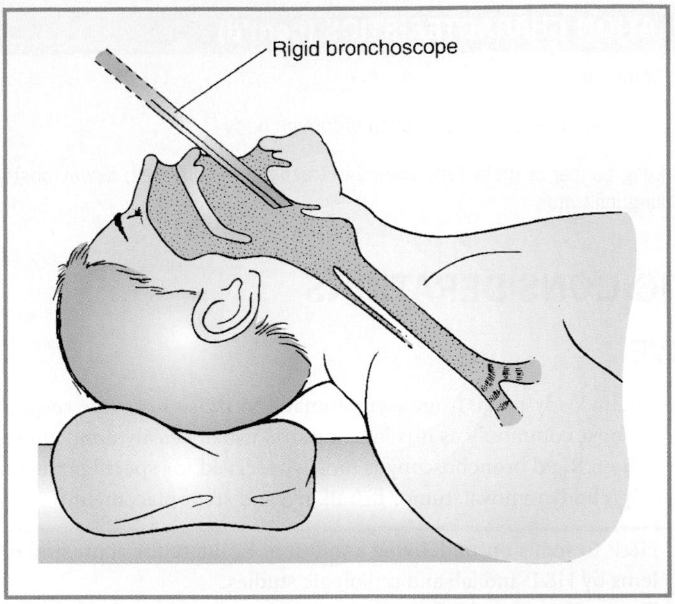

Figure 5-15. Patient positioning for rigid bronchoscopy.

SUMMARY OF PROCEDURES

	Fiber Optic Bronchoscopy	Rigid Bronchoscopy	Laser Bronchoscopy
Position	Supine	⇐ (see fig 5-15)	⇐
Special instrumentation	FOB and instruments	Rigid bronchoscope and instruments	Nd:YAG laser and bronchoscope
Unique considerations	None	Shared airway	⇐ + Keep $FiO_2 \leq 0.4$ during use of laser.
Antibiotics	Usually none	± Cefazolin 1 g	⇐
Surgical time	< 30 min	⇐	1 hr
EBL	Minimal	⇐	⇐
Postop care	PACU → room	⇐	⇐
Mortality	Minimal	⇐	5%
Morbidity	Barotrauma Airway obstruction Pneumothorax	⇐ ⇐ ⇐ Tooth damage Tracheal laceration Pneumomediastinum Esophageal perforation	⇐ Airway fire Hemorrhage Perforation
Pain score	1	1	1

PATIENT POPULATION CHARACTERISTICS

Age range	Usually adults > 50 yr
Male:Female	1:1

PATIENT POPULATION CHARACTERISTICS (cont'd)	
Incidence	Common
Etiology	Smoking; hemoptysis; aspiration of foreign body
Associated conditions	Lung cancer or metastatic spread to tracheobronchial tree; airway obstruction 2° tumor or FB; lung infiltrates

ANESTHETIC CONSIDERATIONS

PREOPERATIVE

Patients presenting for bronchoscopy range from asymptomatic to those in severe respiratory distress. Fiberoptic bronchoscopy is performed most commonly as it is less invasive, usually easily done under sedation and allows for more distal airway examination. Rigid bronchoscopy is mostly reserved for specific interventional procedures such as hemorrhage control, foreign body removal, tumor debulking, and stent placement.

Respiratory	H&P to focus on underlying condition. Evaluate for acute and chronic pulmonary problems by H&P and lab and radiologic studies. **Tests:** Consider ABG in patient with respiratory distress, SOB at rest, or poor exercise tolerance. PaO_2 < 70 mmHg and/or $PaCO_2$ > 45 mmHg indicate significant respiratory impairment and predict increased risk); PFT with flow-volume loop (for airway lesions); CXR.
Cardiovascular	Many patients have Hx of cardiac disease. Cardiology consultation should be obtained for active/unstable cardiac issues or for patient with poorly controlled chronic disease. **Tests:** Consider ECG; others as indicated from H&P.
Musculoskeletal	Patients with lung cancer may have myasthenic (Eaton-Lambert) syndrome with resistance to depolarizing muscle relaxants and ↑ sensitivity to NDMRs. Monitor relaxation with peripheral nerve stimulator.
Hematologic	Type & cross rarely required unless high risk of hemorrhage from biopsy (✓ with surgeon). Adequate O_2-carrying capacity (Hct) important. **Tests:** Hb/Hct
Laboratory	Other tests as indicated from H&P.
Premedication	Antisialagogue (glycopyrrolate 0.2 mg iv, avoids central anticholinergic effects). Light sedation with midazolam 1–2 mg iv and/or fentanyl, 50–100 mcg iv. Avoid heavy sedation that might impair postop ventilation.

INTRAOPERATIVE

Flexible bronchoscopy: Anesthetic technique for flexible FOB requires sedation or GA. Anxious patients and those with respiratory compromise may not tolerate sedation for awake FOB; and patients with Hx of gastric reflux or aspiration are not candidates for awake FOB. Local anesthetic toxicity is a distinct possibility; ensure availability of resuscitative equipment.

Sedation with topical anesthesia	Sedate patient as necessary to ensure comfort and cooperation (midazolam 1–2 mg iv and/or fentanyl 50–100 mcg iv). Bronchoscopy often better tolerated if using nasal route. Airway anesthesia can be provided with direct nerve blocks or topical anesthesia. **Nerve blocks:** Transtracheal local anesthesia; Pass needle through cricothyroid membrane, aspirate air into syringe, and then inject lidocaine (2%) 2 mL. Remove needle quickly because injection causes cough (spreads the anesthetic). Perform superior laryngeal nerve blocks: Insert needle anterior to superior cornu of thyroid cartilage. After resistance is felt, aspirate gently, then inject lidocaine (2%) 2 mL; repeat on other side.

Sedation with topical anesthesia (cont'd)	**Topical anesthesia:** Spray palate, pharynx, larynx, vocal cords, and trachea with lidocaine (4%), using nebulizer, or have patient gargle viscous lidocaine (4%). hold base of tongue forward and, using Krause's forceps, place pledgets soaked in local anesthetic in each pyriform fossa to block the internal branch of superior laryngeal nerve. Laryngeal structures are well topicalized with having the patient gargle 4% lidocaine. The trachea can be topicalized by administering 1% lidocaine through the working channel of the fiberoptic scope. Patient can hold a suction catheter in the mouth to remove oral secretions. A special face mask (Patil-Syracuse) incorporates a diaphragm through which the FOB can pass while patient breathes 100% O_2. Use a special oral airway (Ovassapian) to guide FOB over back of tongue into trachea to prevent damage to FOB by teeth. Limit amount of suctioning by surgeon, because suctioning through FOB decreases FiO_2 and FRC, $\rightarrow \downarrow PaO_2$.

General anesthesia: Almost any anesthetic technique is acceptable, including use of an LMA. A large ETT has less resistance to air flow; minimum size is 8 mm (ID) for adult FOB. If patient requires ETT < 8 mm, use a pediatric FOB. Placing an LMA allows for examination of the proximal airway and a size 2.5 or larger ProSeal LMA has an airway caliber equivalent to or larger than a size 8.0 ETT. Presence of a FOB in the ETT or LMA increases airway resistance and may result in intrinsic PEEP and dynamic hyperinflation/ pulmonary tamponade (hypotension).

Rigid bronchoscopy: Requires relatively deep GA and usually paralysis for scope insertion.

Induction	Preoxygenate well. Standard induction. Consider short-acting paralytics (e.g., succinylcholine 1 mg/kg or rocuronium 0.3–0.6 mg/kg). Use only small amount of iv opioids, because postop analgesic requirements are minimal; consider remifentanil (1 mcg/kg) to avoid postop respiratory depression.	
Maintenance	Commonly inhalation anesthesia with isoflurane, or sevoflurane and 100% O_2, however, the adequacy of inhaled agent delivery may be hampered by ongoing suctioning. TIVA is an alternative (p. B-2): propofol (50–150 mcg/kg/min) and remifentanil (0.1–0.3 mcg/kg/min). Paralysis is usually used for ETT placement and is required during rigid bronchoscopy. May be provided with short-acting, nondepolarizing agents (atracurium, vecuronium, or rocuronium) or alternatively a succinylcholine drip (1 g/250 mL NS, titrated to effect; be aware of onset of phase II block at doses > 5–6 mg/kg). Manual IPPV through side-arm of rigid bronchoscope. High flow (up to 20 L/min) to compensate for leak. Hyperventilate patient in preparation for periods of apnea. Ventilation must be interrupted whenever surgeon removes eyepiece to suction or biopsy. Manually ventilate to compensate for compliance changes that occur when bronchoscope is in trachea (ventilating both lungs) and when it is in bronchus (ventilating one lung). O_2 flush is used to compensate for leak; bypasses anesthetic vaporizer. Frequent flushing lowers anesthetic concentration. Sanders Jet Ventilator using Venturi effect—is an alternative. Allows for uninterrupted ventilation and may shorten the length of the procedure (fewer interruptions). Requires TIVA (p. B-2). Entrainment of air results in variable FiO_2. Adequacy of ventilation is hard to determine as no $EtCO_2$ monitoring is available; prolonged procedures may require intermittent blood gas analysis or transcutaneous CO_2 monitoring.	
Emergence	Place ETT or LMA at conclusion of rigid bronchoscopy. Patient must be fully awake before extubation with no residual neuromuscular blockade. Emergence can be "stormy." Patient may cough violently to clear secretions and blood. Wake-up from remifentanil infusion tends to be smoother, other considerations include early suctioning of the airway, lidocaine (1 mg/kg iv) to decrease airway reactivity. Provide postop O_2 supplementation (preferably humidified).	
Blood and fluid requirements	Blood usually not required. IV: 18 ga × 1 NS/LR @ 2 mL/kg/h	Transfusion unnecessary unless complicated by massive hemorrhage; may require emergency thoracotomy. Usually restrict iv fluids to avoid fluid overload.
Monitoring	Standard monitors (p. B-1)	***NB:** $ETCO_2$ not accurate during rigid bronchoscopy because of dilution effect at sample port.

Positioning	✓ and pad pressure points. ✓ eyes. Shoulder roll for rigid bronchoscopy	
Complications	Hypoxemia	Monitor pulse oximetry continuously. If patient hypoxemic, surgeon must withdraw bronchoscope into trachea. If problem persists, remove bronchoscope and ventilate by mask or ETT.
	Hypercapnia	Common, due to hypoventilation. Mild hypercarbia is well tolerated except for the setting of severe pulmonary HTN. CO_2 levels above 70 mmHg may be associated with tachycardia, dysrhythmias and cardiac depression. Easily treated with higher minute ventilation/hyperventilation. IV lidocaine for dysrhythmias.
	Bleeding Tracheobronchial injury Aspiration of debris	Requires frequent suctioning. For major hemorrhage, place uncut ETT down healthy bronchus and ventilate good lung. Consider DLT. May require thoracotomy using DLT or BB to isolate and/or tamponade bleeding site.

POSTOPERATIVE

Complications	Hypoxemia	Rx: Supplemental O_2. Nebulized racemic epinephrine and steroids may ↓ airway edema. Humidified O_2 may ↓ airway irritation.
	Hypoventilation Dental damage Airway trauma Pneumothorax Hemorrhage	Incomplete reversal of muscle relaxants or opioid overdosage can cause hypoventilation. Obtain ABG if patient has difficulty breathing or is oversedated. Be prepared to reintubate patient.
	Risk of aspiration Airway obstruction (bronchospasm, bleeding, dislodged tumor, FB)	If nerve blocks used to depress gag reflex, no eating or drinking for several hours postbronchoscopy.
Pain management	Minimal pain; easily treated with iv opioids.	
Tests	CXR	Obtain CXR in recovery room to ✓ for atelectasis, pneumothorax, mediastinal emphysema.

Suggested Readings

1. Bolliger CT, Sutedja TG, Strausz J, et al: Therapeutic bronchoscopy with immediate effect: laser, electrocautery, argon plasma coagulation and stents. *Eur Respir J* 2006; 27(6):1258–71.
2. Conacher ID, Curran E: Local anaesthesia and sedation for rigid bronchoscopy for emergency relief of central airway obstruction. *Anaesthesia* 2004; 59(3):290–2.
3. Conacher ID: Anaesthesia and tracheobronchial stenting for central airway obstruction in adults. *Br J Anaesth* 2003; 90(3):367–74.
4. Graham DR, Hay JG, Clague J, et al: Comparison of three different methods used to achieve local anesthesia for fiber optic bronchoscopy. *Chest* 1992; 102(3):704–7.
5. Lohser J, Brodsky JB: Bronchial stenting through a ProSeal laryngeal mask airway. *J Cardiothorac Vasc Anesth* 2006; 20(2):227–8.
6. McRae K: Anesthesia for airway surgery. *Anesthesiol Clin North Am* 2001: 19(3):497–541.
7. Moghissi K, Dixon K, Thorpe JA, et al: Photodynamic therapy (PDT) in early central lung cancer: a treatment option for patients ineligible for surgical resection. *Thorax* 2007; 62(5):374–5.
8. Wain JC: Rigid bronchoscopy: the value of a venerable procedure. *Chest Surg Clin North Am* 2001; 11(4):691–9.

AIRWAY LASER SURGERY

ANESTHETIC CONSIDERATIONS

PREOPERATIVE

Patients usually present with complications related to long-term smoking and an airway mass (endobronchial, carinal, or tracheal). Resection tends to be a misnomer, as the laser is most commonly used for debulking of an unresectable lesion. Central airway obstruction is a primary concern when providing anesthesia.

Respiratory	It is imperative to define the exact location and magnitude of any central airway obstruction. This helps to estimate an appropriate ETT size and quantify the potential for obstruction during induction. CXR and CT scan must be studied. PFTs and flow volume loops may also characterize the lesion. **Tests:** PFTs; ABGs; CXR; CT scan (to delineate airway anatomy, including site and severity of airway lesion)
Musculoskeletal	Although there may be no clinically detectable muscle weakness, some of these patients will have Eaton-Lambert syndrome → ↓ sensitivity to NDMRs and ↑ resistance to depolarizing muscle relaxants.
Hematologic	Transfuse patients with preop Hct < 25% (or < 30%, if CAD present). **Tests:** Hct
Laboratory	Other tests as indicated from H&P.
Premedication	Minimal; avoid respiratory depressants; consider antisialagogue (e.g., glycopyrrolate).

INTRAOPERATIVE

Anesthetic technique: Usually GA. Unexpected patient movement may be disastrous, which is why sedation and local anesthesia are rarely practical. Nd:YAG laser can be transmitted through a flexible quartz monofilament passed through either a rigid bronchoscope or FOB. Rigid bronchoscope provides improved visibility and better debris retrieval. It also maintains the airway with less chance of fire, although it can reflect the laser beam, causing tissue damage. Manual ventilation through the side-arm may be difficult. FOB is used with local anesthesia or through ETT under GA. Laser-safe ETTs (required for surgery in the proximal trachea) include regular ETTs wrapped in metallic tape or commercially available "laser" tubes (usually some combination of aluminum, stainless steel, Teflon, and/or silicon). Fill cuff with saline (+ methylene blue to facilitate leak detection) and avoid any petroleum-based lubricants on ETT. Steps also must be taken to protect the OR staff from laser injury. These include safety glasses to avoid ocular damage and specially designed and properly fitted filter face masks to protect from inhalation of vaporized viral particles. Photodynamic therapy is simpler in its considerations and risks: routine GETA with large ETT, immobile patient, and no risk of fire.

Induction	**Without or with distal airway obstruction** (past carina): Standard induction (see p. B-2). **With proximal airway obstruction:** Awake bronchoscopy may help to determine the feasibility of tracheal intubation. Awake fiberoptic intubation is the safest route. In patients with less severe obstruction, an inhalation induction with spontaneous ventilation may be appropriate. Avoid muscle relaxants until the airway has been secured. Several special laser ETTs are available though none guarantee against airway fire. The risk is minimized with Nd:YAG lasering of central airway lesions as the beam is directed distal to the tip of the ETT. **With rigid bronchoscopy:** GA with standard or rapid sequence induction.
Maintenance	Use isoflurane/desflurane/sevoflurane, air–O_2 mixture. Keep $FiO_2 < 0.4$. Avoid N_2O, which supports combustion. TIVA (p. B-2) with propofol (50–150 mcg/kg/min) and remifentanil (0.1–0.3 mcg/kg/min) infusion is preferable during rigid bronchoscopy as it avoids anesthetic contamination of the OR. Frequent suctioning during bronchoscopic examination may make

Maintenance (cont'd)	inhalation techniques unreliable. Short-acting, nondepolarizing relaxant or succinylcholine infusion should be used to provide an immobile patient during laser use. If the patient becomes hypoxemic, ventilate the lungs with higher FiO_2 and ask the surgeon to stop.	
Emergence	Following rigid bronchoscopy, the patient usually is intubated until awake and breathing well and protective airway reflexes have returned. Emergence can be "stormy," with bleeding and secretion clearance a problem. Patient should be recovered in the sitting position.	
Blood and fluid requirements	IV: 14–16 ga × 1–2 NS/LR @ 1–2 mL/kg/h	There is a potential for massive blood loss following inadvertent perforation of a major blood vessel.
Monitoring	Standard monitors (p. B-1).	Continuous pulse oximetry essential; monitor $ETCO_2$ to assess adequacy of ventilation ($ETCO_2$ value may be inaccurate, consider ABG during long cases). Keep alveolar $PAO_2 < 40\%$.
Positioning	✓ and pad pressure points. ✓ eyes and laser shields.	
Complications	Airway obstruction	From tumor, blood, tissue debris, etc.
	Hypoxemia/hypercarbia	From inadequate ventilation.
	Bleeding	Can be massive from perforation of blood vessel by laser. Apply topical epinephrine following laser photocoagulation to control bleeding.
	Perforation of tracheobronchial tree	May be catastrophic secondary to pneumothorax/pneumomediastinum, cardiac tamponade; lung isolation may be life saving.
	Airway fire	Rx: stop ventilation, remove O_2 source, extubate trachea to decrease inhalation of toxic products. Douse fire with saline. Suction all debris from airway. Ventilate patient by mask, then reintubate. Prior to extubation, perform bronchoscopy to reevaluate airway damage and suction debris. Consider steroids.
	Venous Air Embolism	Rx: Inform surgeon, d/c laser, prevent further entrainment. If access present, attempt to aspirate air. Immediately volume load and support circulation with vasopressors.

POSTOPERATIVE

Complications	Airway edema	Edema formation is difficult to appreciate simply based on epithelial changes during bronchoscopy. May progress dramatically after the procedure resulting in airway obstruction and need for emergency reintubation. Steroids are routinely given to minimize edema formation (dexamethasone 6–8 mg iv). Nebulized racemic epinephrine is helpful. Complications such as hemorrhage or obstruction can be delayed up to 48 h.
Pain management	Minimal pain; rarely requires analgesic.	
Tests	Continuous pulse oximetry.	

Suggested Readings

1. Conacher ID, Pae LL, McMahon CC, et al: Anesthetic management of laser surgery for central airway obstruction, a 12-year case series. *J Cardiothorac Vasc Anesth* 1998; 12(2):153–6.
2. McRae K: Anesthesia for airway surgery. *Anesthesiol Clin North Am* 2001; 19(3):497–541.
3. Ochroch EA: Laser endobronchial treatment does not need to occur in the operating room, *J Cardiothorac Vasc Anesth* 2005; 19(1):118–20.
4. Sullivan EA: Anesthetic considerations for special thoracic procedures. *Thorac Surg Clin* 2005; 15(1):131–42.
5. Vaitkeviciute I, Ehrenwerth J: Bronchial stenting and laser airway surgery should not take place outside the operating room. *J Cardiothorac Vasc Anesth* 2005; 19(1):121–2.

VIDEO-ASSISTED THORACOSCOPY SURGERY (VATS)

SURGICAL CONSIDERATIONS

Description: **Video-assisted thoracoscopy surgery** (VATS) refers to the extension of laparoscopic and other minimally invasive techniques to thoracic surgery. Although initially used for the assessment of pleural processes of unknown etiology (e.g., pleural effusion that has defied diagnosis), VATS techniques are now accepted for treatment of spontaneous pneumothorax due to apical blebs, biopsy of peripheral infiltrates or nodules, talc pleurodesis, drainage of pleural effusions and other fluid collections, decortication of early empyemas, evaluation and evacuation of traumatic hemothorax, and standard pulmonary resections, such as wedge resection and lobectomy. Although not appropriate for all non–small-cell lung cancers, small, peripheral tumors without significant hilar of mediastinal lymph node involvement are often appropriate for VATS lobectomy. VATS also has been used for lung-volume reduction surgery (see p. 323), **esophageal (Heller) myotomy**, and **upper dorsal sympathectomy**. Less well-accepted procedures include **pneumonectomy** and **esophagectomy.**

In all VATS cases, use of a DLT to provide collapse of the ipsilateral lung is mandatory, because satisfactory visualization of the pleural cavity is impossible without this collapse of the lung. The patient is usually in the lateral position. Several small incisions are used—usually three, sometimes four or more. The video thoracoscope is placed through the first incision and the pleural cavity is inspected. Other small incisions are then made for insertion of instruments. The position of the video thoracoscope and instruments may be interchanged, depending on the location of the problem.

Usual preop diagnosis: Pleural disease (e.g., effusions); recurrent empyema; recurrent pneumothorax; localized lung masses; achalasia; pulmonary infiltrates; hyperhidrosis; reflex sympathetic dystrophy (RSD)

SUMMARY OF PROCEDURE	
Position	Lateral
Incision	Usually 3 to 5 small incisions (portals) (Fig. 5-16)
Special instrumentation	Video thoracoscope with thoracoscopy instruments; DLT required.
Antibiotics	Cefazolin 1 g
Surgical time	1–3 h
Closing considerations	Chest tube placed
EBL	Minimal, although there is a risk for major bleeding.
Postop care	Chest tube
Mortality	Minimal
Morbidity	Major vascular injury: Rare Conversion to open thoracotomy: 4% Pneumothorax/persistent air leak
Pain score	2–3

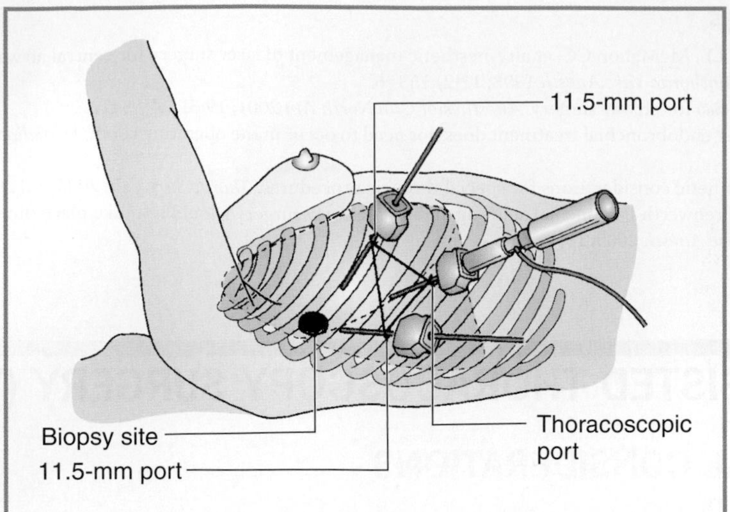

Figure 5-16. Example of thoracoscopic port placement. Positioning varies for individual need, but the principle of triangulation used for laparoscopic surgery is equally applicable in the thorax. (Reproduced with permission from Greenfield LJ, Mulholland MW, Oldham KT, et al., eds: *Surgery: Scientific Principles and Practice.* Lippincott-Raven Publishers, Philadelphia: 1997, 741.)

PATIENT POPULATION CHARACTERISTICS	
Age range	All age groups
Male:Female	1:1
Associated conditions	Pleural effusions; lung mass; pneumothorax

ANESTHETIC CONSIDERATIONS

PREOPERATIVE

As VATS is used for both diagnostic and therapeutic purposes, this patient population is quite diverse: patients may be of any age group and may present with an asymptomatic mass or be in respiratory distress due to undiagnosed interstitial disease. VATS is also used for nonthoracic procedures such as sympathectomy, pericardial window and minimally invasive cardiac surgery.

Respiratory	The preop evaluation should focus on the patient's ability to tolerate OLV, as well as the postop effects of the planned surgery. PFTs and ABG are useful prognostic tests. Question patient about dyspnea, productive cough, and cigarette smoking; examine for cyanosis, clubbing, RR, and pattern. Listen to chest for wheezes, rhonchi, and rales. Preop lung function may be improved by treating respiratory tract infections, stopping smoking for several weeks, and treatment with bronchodilators and steroids, as indicated. **Tests:** PFT; CXR; if chest CT available, look for airway anomalies that could interfere with DLT placement; ABG.
Cardiovascular	Directed at any underlying disease process.
Laboratory	As indicated from H&P.
Premedication	Standard premedication (see p. B-1). Avoid heavy sedation that might impair postop respiratory function.

INTRAOPERATIVE

Anesthetic technique: GETA, typically with OLV, using DLT or BB (see OLV, p. 278). OLV may be difficult to achieve in pediatric patients, so chest insufflation with CO_2 has been described, but is fraught with risks. Thoracoscopy has also been described in the awake, sedated patient under local or regional anesthetic technique. Although tissue trauma is significantly less than with the open thoracotomy, pain scores are not insignificant and chronic pain syndromes are common. Referred pain due to lung dissection, chest wall pain due to decortication and intercostal nerve impingements secondary to trocar insertion may cause marked postop pain. Multimodal therapy with opioid and NSAID is sufficient in many, but PCA may on occasion be required. Regional techniques (epidural or paravertebral) should be considered in compromised patients, in procedures with high conversion risk or in procedures with significant tissue trauma (e.g., decortication).

Regional anesthesia: The incision site is infiltrated with local anesthetics, and intercostal nerve blocks are performed at the level of incision and at several levels above and below incision. The same effect can be accomplished by multiple-level single-shot paravertebral nerve blocks which can be performed awake or asleep in the lateral position. Alternatively, continuous paravertebral or epidural catheters can be placed.

General anesthesia: The patient is intubated with DLT or BB to selectively collapse the operative lung. Anesthetic choice optional, but $FiO_2 = 1$ in anticipation of OLV to accelerate lung collapse. Lung collapse is slower than with thoracotomy due to lack of surgical pneumothorax. High FiO_2, early OLV, gentle suction and opening of trocar (to allow air inflow) can help to accelerate lung collapse. GA allows IPPV with complete re-expansion of lung without pain, if pleurodesis performed.

Induction	Standard induction (see p. B-2). Placement of DLT is discussed on p. 278.	
Maintenance	O_2 (60–100%) and isoflurane, desflurane or sevoflurane (0.6–1 MAC). No N_2O. Short-acting muscle relaxant and opioids as required. Consider remifentanil infusion (0.1–0.2 mcg/kg/min).	
OLV	See pneumonectomy/ lobectomy for OLV technique. p. 278	
Emergence	Extubation in OR	
Blood and fluid requirements	IV: 16–18 ga × 1 NS/LR @ 2 mL/kg/h	
Monitoring	Standard monitors (p. B-1) ± Arterial line	 Arterial catheter generally not required, unless indicated by patient's medical condition.
Positioning	✓ and pad pressure points. ✓ eyes, ears, genitals.	See p. 268 for proper positioning.
Complications	Air leak from lung Hemorrhage Injury to intrathoracic structures Air embolism	Air leak observed on re-expansion of lung. Excessive blood drainage via chest tube; falling Hct Repair may require open thoracotomy.

POSTOPERATIVE

Complications	Tension pneumothorax	In the absence of chest tube, air leak can → pneumothorax that can progress to tension pneumothorax if not treated. This may manifest as hyperresonance, ↓ chest-wall movement, dyspnea, subcutaneous emphysema, tracheal shift, dysrhythmias, cardiovascular collapse, ↓ PO_2, and ↓ SaO_2. CXR diagnostic, but need to diagnose clinically if hemodynamically unstable. Requires immediate decompression of tension pneumothorax with 14-ga iv catheter through 2nd intercostal space @ midclavicular line, followed by chest tube and continuous suction.

Pain management	IV opioids, ketorolac (30 mg)	Analgesic requirements less than for lateral thoracotomy, but moderate to severe pain may occur and chronic pain is not uncommon.
	Intrapleural anesthesia	Intrapleural local anesthetics (0.25% bupivacaine + 1:200,000 epinephrine 0.5 mL/kg) via thoracostomy drainage tube after lung is reinflated but before chest tube suction applied.
	Epidural or paravertebral	Indicated in patients with significant comorbidities and/or for procedures with significant tissue trauma (decortication, lobectomy).
Tests	CXR postop	

Suggested Readings

1. Conacher ID: Anaesthesia for thoracoscopic surgery. *Best Pract Res Clin Anaesthesiol* 2002; 16(1):53–62.
2. Harris RJ, Benveniste G, Pfitzner J: Cardiovascular collapse caused by carbon dioxide insufflation during one-lung anaesthesia for thoracoscopic dorsal sympathectomy. *Anaesth Intensive Care* 2002; 30(1):86–9.
3. Hutter J, Miller K, Moritz E: Chronic sequels after thoracoscopic procedures for benign diseases. *Eur J Cardithorac Surg* 2000; 17(6): 687–90.
4. Mineo TC: Epidural anesthesia in awake thoracic surgery. *Eur J Cardiothorac Surg* 2007; 32(1):13–9.
5. Shah JS, Bready LL: Anesthesia for thoracoscopy. *Anaesthesiol Clin North Am* 2001; 19(1):153–71.
6. Taylor R, Massey S, Stuart-Smith K: Postoperative analgesia in video-assisted thoracoscopy: the role of intercostals blockade. *J Cardiothorac Vasc Anesth* 2004; 18(3):317–21.
7. Tobias JD: Anaesthesia for minimally invasive surgery in children. *Best Pract Res Clin Anaesthesiol* 2002; 16(1):115–30.

THYMECTOMY

SURGICAL CONSIDERATIONS

Description: The two most common indications for **thymectomy are myasthenia gravis** and **thymoma.** The severity of myasthenia gravis can be classified using the Osserman scheme, which assigns Stage I to patients with ocular symptoms only, with Stages II-IV for progressive degrees of bulbar and systemic symptoms. Indications for surgery versus medical management remain controversial, with some neurologists referring nearly all patients with myasthenia gravis for surgery, whereas others referring only those with the most refractory symptoms. Patients referred for surgery often take a combination of pyridostigmine (Mestinon) and immunosuppressants (steroids and azathioprine). In cases of severe myasthenia gravis, preop plasmapheresis may be helpful in minimizing periop muscle weakness. Patients with thymoma may be asymptomatic, although ~10–20% of them have a Hx of myasthenic symptoms.

Thymectomy can be a performed through a **complete sternotomy,** an upper sternal split (manubrium only), or via a cervical approach. The value of a complete sternotomy is that it allows for removal of all anterior mediastinal tissue that may harbor small thymic rests. This is the most invasive approach, however, and the one associated with the greatest degree of intraop tissue injury. An **upper sternal split** is performed with the neck extended and a roll placed under the shoulder blades. Either a short vertical incision or a transverse incision at the level of the sternal angle may be used. Division of only the manubrium provides adequate exposure for identification, dissection, and removal of the thymus. Mobilization of the thymus can be accomplished without entering the pleural space. Care must be taken to avoid injuring the phrenic nerves. In contrast with the removal of anterior mediastinal tumors, thymectomy usually does not require OLV.

Transcervical thymectomy is performed through a collar incision similar to that used for thyroidectomy (Fig. 7.11-3). The cervical extensions of the thymus are identified and the dissection is advanced progressively into the neck. Attachments of the gland are cauterized, and a clip is placed on the thymic vein (which drains directly into the innominate vein). Exposure is aided by a special retractor that elevates the sternum anteriorly and exposes the anterior mediastinum.

At the conclusion of the operation—whether it is done through the chest or the neck—the thymic bed is drained with a small suction drain. Preop medications should be resumed as soon as possible.

Usual preop diagnosis: Myasthenia gravis; thymoma

SUMMARY OF PROCEDURES

	Sternotomy	Cervical Approach
Position	Supine	⇐
Incision	Median sternotomy	Suprasternal
Special instrumentation	None	Special sternal retractor
Antibiotics	Cefazolin 1 g	⇐
Surgical time	1–2 h	⇐
EBL	< 500 mL	⇐
Postop care	ICU — special attention to muscle strength, related to respiratory function	⇐
Mortality	< 5%	⇐
Morbidity	Infection Pneumothorax Hemothorax	⇐
Pain score	5–7	2

PATIENT POPULATION CHARACTERISTICS

Age range	Usually young adults
Male:Female	Females > males
Incidence	Infrequent
Etiology	Unknown
Associated conditions	Myasthenia gravis; benign or malignant thymoma; other autoimmune diseases (e.g., rheumatoid arthritis)

ANESTHETIC CONSIDERATIONS

PREOPERATIVE

Patients presenting for thymectomy may have myasthenia gravis, an autoimmune disease of the neuromuscular junction characterized by muscle weakness and easy fatiguability. Thymomas (benign or malignant) also may be associated with myasthenia gravis. The anesthesiologist needs to be aware of the possible compression effects of the tumor (see Excision of Mediastinal Tumor, p. 298), the potential for respiratory failure, and anticipate complications of various treatment modalities.

Respiratory	Patient may have marked reduction in VC 2° muscle weakness; establish baseline spirometry values. Classic (Leventhal) criteria predicting the need for postop ventilation include: duration of disease > 6 yr; chronic comorbid pulmonary disease; pyridostigmine dose > 750 mg/d; VC < 2.9 L. Others include preop use of steroids; and previous episode of respiratory failure. These predictors have not been widely validated. Inform the patient of the potential requirement for prolonged ventilation. **Tests:** PFTs, others as indicated from H&P.

Cardiovascular	There is a rare association between myasthenia gravis and cardiomyopathy. Consider ECG and cardiac consult if indicated from H&P.
Neurological	Review neurological assessment. Patients often exhibit diplopia, ptosis, and easy fatiguability of muscles. Difficulties with swallowing and speech are common. Review tests (EMGs, Tensilon test) done by neurologist to evaluate the adequacy of drug therapy (steroids, anticholinesterases, azathioprine, and cyclosporin A). Azathioprine (Imuran) may actually antagonize neuromuscular blockade by inhibiting phosphodiesterase. Cyclosporin A is reserved for severe disease because of the side effects of renal insufficiency and HTN. It may prolong neuromuscular blockade. 10–50% of the patients with thymomas will have myasthenia gravis and >85% of myasthenics will have thymus abnormalities.
Musculoskeletal	Determine adequacy of anticholinesterase medication. Evaluate hand strength, inspiratory efforts and PFTs. Note that an excess of anticholinesterase agents can cause weakness and respiratory failure (cholinergic crisis). A deleterious response (weakness) to Tensilon®; administration (10 mg), as well as the presence of cholinergic side effects (e.g., pupil constriction), characterize a cholinergic crises. Plasmapheresis may offer temporary (days to weeks) improvement in symptoms. Typically, patients with worsening symptoms receive 4–8 treatments prior to surgery. There should be a 24-h delay between the last plasmapheresis and surgery to restore clotting factors and immunoglobulins. Plasmapheresis also may transiently decrease plasma cholinesterase, which could prolong the effects of succinylcholine, mivacurium, and ester-type local anesthetics.
Endocrine	Other autoimmune phenomena occur in 10–15% of myasthenic patients. Elucidate symptoms of thyroid or adrenal disease. Tests: TSH; evaluate screening test if indicated from H&P.
Laboratory	Other tests as indicated from H&P.
Premedication	Avoid premedication; for the anxious patient, give a small dose of midazolam (0.5–1 mg); avoid opioids or any other sedatives that may depress ventilation. Current recommendations for anticholinesterases suggest that, in mild disease without physiological dependence, the morning dose can be held or halved. Patients with severe disease or with marked anticholinesterase dependence should receive their regular morning dose. For patients on steroids—depending on dosage and duration of steroid therapy—hydrocortisone (up to 100 mg iv bolus) before induction, then 100 mg q 8 h × 24 h, may be helpful. Note that acute steroid exposure in naïve patients may paradoxically exacerbate neuromuscular weakness. Consider aspiration prophylaxis.

INTRAOPERATIVE

Anesthetic technique: GETA, combined with thoracic or lumbar epidural if transsternal thymectomy. DLT may be requested by surgeon.

Induction	Inhalational induction with sevoflurane to avoid muscle relaxants entirely; however, patients with profound muscle weakness are at risk for aspiration 2° inadequate airway protective mechanism. Alternatively, iv propofol induction with remifentanil 1–2 mcg/kg (without muscle relaxants). If absolutely necessary, succinylcholine may be used to facilitate intubation, although myasthenic patients are considered resistant and require a dose of 1.5–2.0 mg/kg to obtain adequate conditions, which then will result in prolonged muscle weakness. Anticholinesterase therapy may prolong the duration of action of succinylcholine.
Maintenance	Standard maintenance (see p. B-2). Patients with myasthenia gravis have ↑ sensitivity to nondepolarizing NMBs, which are rarely ever needed, as maintenance with inhalational agents provides adequate neuromuscular relaxation when combined with the existing baseline weakness. If relaxants are needed, titrate small amounts (1/10 ED_{95}) of drug, using a peripheral nerve stimulator to maintain a single twitch. Cisatracurium (20–30 mcg/kg q 15–20 min or infusion 1–3 mcg/kg/min) is useful because it is rapidly eliminated. Alternatively, potent inhalation agents may provide adequate muscle relaxation, and avoid

Maintenance (cont'd)	the need for any muscle relaxant. Avoid drugs with neuromuscular blocking effects (e.g., antidysrhythmics, calcium channel blockers, diuretics, aminoglycosides, Mg^{+2}, iodinated contrast agents). Extremes of temperature, hypokalemia and hypophosphatemia may also aggravate neuromuscular weakness and should be prevented. If the patient has normal ventilatory function, then spontaneous ventilation during cervical thymectomy may be appropriate. Patients undergoing sternotomy, and any patient with ↓ pulmonary reserve, require mechanical ventilation.	
Emergence	Criteria for extubation include: head lift (5 sec); MIF > −25 cmH_2O; TV > 5 mL/kg; and full reversal evidenced by twitch monitor. Extubate when fully awake; usually immediate postop ventilation is not necessary. Because of the variable response to muscle relaxation and delayed benefits of the surgery, some patients may require postop ventilation. Whether intubated or not, monitor patient for pulmonary function by measuring MIF and spirometry (Vt). Avoid residual pharmacologic neuromuscular blockade, which will → hypoventilation and ↑ risk of gastric aspiration if protective airway reflexes are inadequate.	
Blood and fluid requirements	IV: 18 ga × 1 NS/LR @ 1–2 mL/kg/h	Consider lower extremity iv access when hemorrhage anticipated.
Monitoring	Standard monitors (p. B-1)	Avoid muscle relaxants if possible; use nerve stimulator.
Positioning	✓ and pad pressure points. ✓ eyes.	
Complications	Hemorrhage Dysrhythmia Compression of mediastinal structures Pneumothorax	

POSTOPERATIVE

Complications	Pneumothorax Respiratory failure Phrenic nerve damage Myasthenic or cholinergic crises	Pleura can be entered–usually the right side; if so, chest tube needed. (For Dx and Rx, see VATS, p. 315)
Pain management	Parenteral opioids (p. C-2) Epidural opioids (p. C-2)	Avoid respiratory depression; parenteral opioids for cervical incision; epidural opioids for median sternotomy. Of note, anticholinesterases are reported to potentiate the effect of morphine.
Drug management	Usually ↓ anticholinesterase requirement in the immediate postop period.	Reduce daily anticholinesterase by 20%. Beware of 'cholinergic' crisis. Sx include ↑ salivation, sweating, lacrimation, abdominal cramps, urinary frequency, fasciculations, and weakness 2° anticholinesterase overdose. Rx: anticholinergic agent (e.g. atropine) ± intubation and mechanical ventilation.
Tests	Tensilon (edrophonium)	Tensilon test may differentiate between myasthenic (↑ strength) and cholinergic (↓ strength) crises.
	Muscle strength	Determine muscle strength postop (grip strength and sustained head lift).
	Pupil exam	Pupil dilation (myasthenic crisis); pupil constriction (cholinergic crisis).

Suggested Readings

1. Baraka A: Anesthesia and critical care of thymectomy for myasthenia gravis. *Chest Surg Clin North Am* 2001; 11(2):337–61.
2. Baue AE, ed: *Glenn's Thoracic and Cardiovascular Surgery,* 6th edition, Volume II. Geha AS, Hammond GL, Laks H, et al., assoc. eds. Appleton & Lange, Norwalk: 1996.
3. Burgess FW, Wilcosky B Jr: Thoracic epidural anesthesia for transsternal thymectomy in myasthenia gravis. *Anesth Analg* 1989; 69(4):529–31.
4. Dillon F: Anesthesia issues in the perioperative management of myasthenia gravis. *Sem Neurol* 2004; 24(1):83–94.
5. Eisenkraft JB, Neustein SM: *Thoracic Anesthesia,* 3rd edition. Kaplan JA, Slinger PD, eds. Churchill Livingstone, Philadelphia: 2003.
6. Naquib M, el Dawlatly AA, Ashour M, et al: Multivariate determinants of the need for postoperative ventilation in myasthenia gravis. *Can J Anaesth* 1996; 43(10):1006–13.
7. OíNeill GN: Acquired disorders of the neuromuscular junction. *Int Anesthesiol Clin* 2006; 42(2):107–21.
8. Sellke FW, Swanson S, del Nido P: *Sabiston & Spencer: Surgery of the Chest,* 7th edition. Elsevier Saunders, Philadelphia: 2004.
9. Shrager JB, Nathan D, Brinster CJ, et al: Outcomes after 151 extended transcervical thymectomies for myasthenia gravis. *Ann Thorac Surg* 2006;82(5):1863–9.
10. Smith CE, Donati F, Bevan DR: Cumulative dose-response curves for atracurium in patients with myasthenia gravis. *Can J Anaesth* 1989; 36(4):402–6.

EXCISION OF BLEBS OR BULLAE

SURGICAL CONSIDERATIONS

Description: Pulmonary blebs or bullae requiring surgical treatment may vary from small, apical blebs—most usually seen in young people with spontaneous pneumothorax—to expanding, giant bullae causing respiratory distress. Specific indications for bullectomy include large size (> 30% of the lung), recurrent pneumothorax, dyspnea in conjunction with compressed adjacent parenchyma, and recurrent infection of the bullae. The small blebs can be excised through **video thoracoscopy** (see p. 313), although some surgeons still prefer an open technique for this procedure. Giant bullae are generally removed by **open thoracotomy,** although these lesions also may be excised by VATS techniques. In either case, the goal is to resect the nonfunctional bullae and allow the compressed, yet relatively preserved lung tissue to re-expand and contribute to gas exchange. The surgical technique generally involves **stapling** across the base of the bulla with reinforcing strips being applied to the staple line to minimize air leak. Alternatively, a **clamp and suture** technique may be used. However the most important point is that an airtight closure should be obtained as a prolonged air leak can be very debilitating. Patients undergoing operation for giant bullae frequently have limited pulmonary reserve and present formidable operative risks. Because the operation is planned to improve their pulmonary function, however, these patients frequently do well following operation. **Pleural abrasion** or, rarely, **pleurectomy** may accompany the excision of blebs or bullae. The blebs in young patients with recurrent spontaneous pneumothorax usually are located at the apex of the upper lobe. Bullae in patients with emphysema are usually in the upper lobe, but may be anywhere in the lung. Preop localization by CT scan is usually sufficient. If a thoracotomy is done, the approach is usually lateral.

Variant procedure or approaches: Patients with more generalized emphysema may be candidates for lung-volume reduction surgery (see p. 323).

Usual preop diagnosis: Spontaneous pneumothorax 2° ruptured blebs; giant bullae causing respiratory distress

SUMMARY OF PROCEDURE

Position	Usually lateral
Incision	Axillary
Special instrumentation	Staplers
Antibiotics	Cefazolin 1 g

SUMMARY OF PROCEDURE (cont'd)	
Surgical time	1–3 h
EBL	< 500 mL
Postop care	PACU → room; ICU or IIC for giant bullae
Mortality	Minimal
Morbidity	Air leak: 20% or more in giant bullae
Pain score	5–7

PATIENT POPULATION CHARACTERISTICS	
Age range	Young adults (blebs/small bullae); elderly (large bullae)
Male:Female	3:1
Incidence	Not uncommon
Etiology	Emphysema (usually 2° smoking); congenital; infectious
Associated conditions	Spontaneous pneumothorax; emphysema; long smoking Hx; α-antitrypsin deficiency

ANESTHETIC CONSIDERATIONS

PREOPERATIVE

Patients with apical blebs tend to be young with normal lung function and otherwise healthy. Bleb resection in these patients tends to be a routine thoracoscopic wedge-resection procedure. Patients with bullous emphysema on the other hand, may have end-stage lung disease, often with pulmonary hypertension and RV dysfunction. The risk of rupture of a bulla/bleb on the nonoperated side, with resultant tension pneumothorax, must be considered throughout the procedure. The majority of considerations and concerns therefore relate to the patient with bilateral disease. Most procedures are done thoracoscopically.

Respiratory	Cysts may be bronchogenic, postinfective, infantile, or emphysematous. With blebs, elicit Hx of repeat pneumothoraces. Bullae usually result from destruction of alveolar tissue; they represent end-stage emphysematous disease associated with severe COPD. Patients may have incapacitating dyspnea and limited pulmonary reserve. CO_2 retention ± hypoxia may be present. Obtain PFTs and ABG for baseline. **Tests:** CXR; presence of pneumothorax; if chest CT available, look for bilateral bullous disease and rule out airway anomalies that could interfere with DLT placement; ABG, as indicated from H&P.
Cardiovascular	**Tests:** ECG
Neurological	✓ Hx for previous back surgery, peripheral neuropathy. Examine thoracolumbar area for skin lesions, infection, deformities.
Hematologic	Transfuse patient with preop Hct < 25% (Hct < 30% if patient has CAD). Cross-match 2 U of blood or obtain 1–2 U of autologous blood during the month before surgery, or consider erythropoietin therapy in patients who are anemic. **Tests:** Hct
Laboratory	Other tests as indicated from H&P.
Premedication	Midazolam 1–2 mg iv if patient anxious and not in respiratory distress. Minimize sedation if planning epidural placement, as the combination of parenteral sedation and epidural opioid may result in significant respiratory depression.

INTRAOPERATIVE

Anesthetic technique: GETA—combined with regional technique if open thoracotomy.

Induction	**Minor Bleb:** standard induction (see p. B-2) **Major bullae (particularly bilateral):** main issue is risk of pulmonary tamponade/tension pneumothorax secondary to bulla expansion by PPV. Best to establish lung isolation prior to instituting PPV (DLT essential in bilateral disease, to allow for ventilation/exclusion of either side; BB sufficient for unilateral disease). Strategies include awake intubation (difficult with DLT), spontaneous ventilation induction (inhalational or iv), or, in patients with easy airway anatomy, a true rapid sequence intubation. Lung isolation should immediately be confirmed with FOB prior to providing PPV. Rapid placement of a chest tube is essential should a bulla rupture.	
Maintenance	Patients with severe COPD may have significant auto-PEEP. To avoid worsening dynamic hyperinflation of lung, treat bronchospasm aggressively and allow adequate expiratory time (↓ I:E ratio, low RR). Caution with applied PEEP: it may increase total PEEP (and therefore air trapping). Minimize risk of bulla rupture by reducing ventilatory pressures (low tidal volumes, permissive hypercapnia and pressure-control ventilation @ < 20cmH_2O). Inhalational anesthesia supplemented with epidural, local anesthetics, or iv opioids. Avoid N_2O at all times, because bullae may be filled with air.	
Emergence	Re-expand lung under direct vision to check for major air leaks. Extubate patient early. Post-bullectomy, unlike other lung resections, patients have greater functional lung tissue than preop.	
Blood and fluid requirements	IV: 16 ga × 1 NS/LR @ 1–2 mL/kg/h Use vasopressors if hypotensive.	Excess fluid predisposes to right heart failure. Epidural local anesthetics can ↓ BP in a volume-restricted patient; vasopressor often needed (e.g. ephedrine 5–10 mg iv bolus or phenylephrine 50–100 mcg iv bolus).
Monitoring	Standard monitors (p. B-1) Arterial line ± CVP, ± PA line, ± TEE	 for patients with coexisting severe cardiac disease
Positioning	✓ and pad pressure points. ✓ eyes, ears, genitals. Axillary roll; "airplane" for upper arm	See Positioning, p. 268.
Ventilation	DLT or BB needed to separate the lungs.	Allows PPV of the nonoperative lung. Use gentle PPV (pressure control) with low Vt, permissive hypercapnea ($PaCO_2$ 50–70 mmHg). Inspiratory pressure should be as low as possible (~10 cmH_2O), to reduce likelihood of rupture of bullae in nonoperative lung. Treat intraop hypoxemia with CPAP to "up" lung. In extreme cases consider CPB (rare).
Complications	Tension pneumothorax	Can occur on either side during induction, only on nonoperated side after chest is open, and again on either side postop. Presents with ↑ ventilatory pressure, progressive tracheal deviation, wheezing, cardiovascular collapse. CXR to r/o tension pneumothorax. Rx: insertion of chest tube.
	Broncho-pleural-cutaneous fistula	Placement of a chest tube can create a broncho-pleural-cutaneous fistula. Rx: low Vt, spontaneous ventilation; may require DLT for differential ventilation.
	Hypoxia Hypercardia Dysrhythmias	✓ position of DLT, suction DLT, avoid hypoventilation.

POSTOPERATIVE

Complications	Hypoventilation Dental damage Airway trauma Pneumothorax Hemorrhage Risk of aspiration Airway obstruction (bronchospasm, bleeding, dislodged tumor, FB)	Ensure complete reversal of muscle relaxants, and patient wide-awake with good respiratory effort prior to extubation. Obtain ABG if patient has difficulty breathing or is overly sedated. If nerve blocks used to depress gag reflex for awake FOI, keep patient NPO for several hours postop.
Pain management	Epidural opioids (see p. C-2). Parenteral opioids	Parenteral opioids + intrapleural local anesthetics (0.5% bupivacaine + 1:200,000 epinephrine, 0.5 mL/kg) + single-shot paravertebral blocks are adequate for thoracoscopy.
Tests	CXR	ABG if indicated.

Suggested Readings

1. Barker SJ, Clarke C, Trivedi N, et al: Anesthesia for thorascopic laser ablation of bullous emphysema. *Anesthesiology* 1993; 78(l):44–50.
2. Lohser J: Evidence-based management of one-lung ventilation. *Anesthesiol Clin North Am* 2008; 26(2): accepted.
3. Palla A, Desideri M, Rossi G, et al: Elective surgery for giant bullous emphysema: a 5-year clinical and functional follow-up. *Chest* 2005; 128(4):2043–50.
4. Pompeo E, Tacconi F, Mineo D, et al: The role of awake video-assisted thoracoscopic surgery in spontaneous pneumothorax. *J Thorac Cardiovasc Surg* 2007;133(3):786–90.
5. Tiong LU, Davies R, Gibson PG, et al. Lung volume reduction surgery for diffuse emphysema. *Cochrane Database Syst Rev* 2006;18(4): CD001001.

LUNG-VOLUME REDUCTION SURGERY

SURGICAL CONSIDERATIONS

Description: Lung-volume reduction surgery (LVRS) was initially described by Brantigan in 1958 but reintroduced by Joel Cooper in 1995 for the treatment of severe emphysema. Typically, patients referred for LVRS are chronically ill, requiring steroids, bronchodilators, and supplemental O_2. With appropriate preoperative selection and perioperative care, these patients survive surgery and demonstrate improved pulmonary function. Physiologically, reducing the volume of the lung by resecting diseased tissue improves elastic recoil and decreases airway resistance. The chest cavity also is reduced in size, thereby improving chest-wall and diaphragmatic function.

The procedure can be carried out either through a median sternotomy or endoscopically. The **open approach** begins with a median sternotomy. OLV is initiated following opening of the pleurae. Often the diseased portions of the lung remain inflated, whereas healthy areas develop absorption atelectasis. These diseased portions are resected with the aid of a linear stapler. The visceral pleura are very thin; the stapling is done with bovine pericardium to bolster the staple line; and high inspiratory pressures (> 20 cmH_2O) must be avoided. From 15–30% of the lung volume may be removed. Following careful examination for air leaks, the pleurae and chest wall are closed.

The **endoscopic approach** is carried out using standard VATS techniques and instrumentation. Diseased tissue will have been identified preop using V/Q and CT scans. Endoscopic forceps are used to guide this diseased tissue into the jaws of the stapler. Again, 15–30% of lung tissue may be removed by this means. At some centers, the anesthesiologist may be asked to measure inspiratory and expiratory volumes. Any difference between these volumes may represent an air leak requiring further exploration. Following this, access ports and the thoracotomy are closed, and chest tubes are placed. The patient is turned over to the opposite side, reprepped and redraped, and the surgery is repeated. With either approach, patients should be extubated in the OR so that no unnecessary ventilatory pressures are put on the lungs. There is usually no suction on the chest tubes and, thus, a water seal is the primary method of controlling the pleural cavity pressures. A small pneumothorax (≤ 10%) is acceptable if the patient is not in respiratory distress. A functional epidural catheter, early extubation, and the avoidance of chest tube suction are important to the success of this procedure, especially in the very ill patient. Pleural drainage consists of two chest tubes per side; in contrast with lobectomy, however, they are often left to water seal so as not to exert excessive negative pressure on the lung and disrupt the staple lines. Ideally, patients are extubated at the conclusion of the operation. Because their respiratory status is often tenuous, close monitoring, vigorous pulmonary toilet, and good pain control are essential in the postop period.

Usual preop diagnosis: COPD (emphysema)

SUMMARY OF PROCEDURES

	Open LVRS	Endoscopic LVRS
Position	Supine	Lateral decubitus
Incision	Sternotomy	Minilateral thoracotomy
Special instrumentation	Stapling devices; DLT	⇐+ Endoscopic instrumentation
Unique considerations	Bovine pericardium to bolster staple line	⇐
Antibiotics	Cefazolin 1 g	⇐
Surgical time	2 h	45–60 min/side
Closing considerations	Avoid high PIPs (> 20 cmH_2O)	⇐
EBL	Minimal	⇐
Postop care	Extubated in OR; avoid chest tube suction	⇐
Mortality	≤ 5–10%	⇐
Morbidity	Pneumothorax Infection Tearing of suture line Wound healing problems	⇐ ⇐ ⇐ ⇐
Pain score	6–8	4–6

PATIENT POPULATION CHARACTERISTICS

Age range	> 50 yr
Male:Female	Male > female
Incidence	Although the incidence of emphysema is high in the general population, only a fraction of these patients will be candidates for LVRS.
Etiology	Smoking; genetic factors
Associated conditions	CAD; pulmonary HTN; PVD; cerebrovascular disease

Table 5.3. Suggested Selection Criteria for LVRS

Medical history	Severe COPD (emphysema rather than chronic bronchitis) Age < 75 yr No cigarette smoking for 6 mo Lowest effective prednisone dose No previous chest surgery
Pulmonary function	FEV_1 >30–35% of predicted $PaCO_2$ < 50 mmHg TLC > 120% of predicted
Cardiac function	Mean PAP < 35 mmHg (if pulmonary HTN is suspected). No evidence of LV dysfunction on dobutamine stress testing (if Hx of angina or CHF is present)
Radiographic	Hyperinflation; flatted diaphragm (CXR) Decreased upper lobe perfusion (Ventilation-Perfusion scan) Emphysema, with upper lobe predominance (CT scan)
Relative exclusion criteria	Continued smoking Illness other than emphysema that may cause severe dyspnea (e.g. CAD; CHF; cancer; interstitial lung disease; bronchiectasis) Severe malnutrition Obliteration of pleural space (e.g., pleurodesis or pleurectomy) Previous thoracic surgery Morbid obesity Severe pulmonary HTN (mean PAP > 35) Chest-wall deformity with restrictive lung disease (e.g. kyphoscoliosis; severe pectus deformity; $PaCO_2$ > 55 mmHg

ANESTHETIC CONSIDERATIONS

PREOPERATIVE

LVRS involves either laser thermal contraction or surgical resection of emphysematous lung tissue. Patients have end-stage emphysema with associated pulmonary HTN and RV dysfunction. These patients are a great challenge to the anesthesiologist, because it may be difficult to maintain relatively normal physiologic parameters intraop, and to have an awake, comfortable, and spontaneously breathing patient at the completion of surgery.

Respiratory	These patients have advanced pulmonary emphysema. Examine patient for cyanosis, clubbing, RR and pattern. Listen to chest—breath sounds are often very distant or absent. Hx should include use of O_2 supplementation, recent infection, severe bronchospasm, prior surgery on the chest, and other associated diseases, such as CAD or CHF. **Tests:** PFT (± bronchodilators). Hyperinflation usually is indicated by TLC and RV value > 120%; V/Q scan; CXR; chest CT scan; noninvasive exercise test (6-min walk); preop ABG—check for hypoxemia, hypercarbia.
Cardiovascular	These patients often have coexisting cardiac disease with pulmonary HTN. **Tests:** right heart function can be determined by echocardiography or selective right heart catheterization, if indicated by H&P.
Premedication	Avoid premedication with sedative or opioids—cannot have respiratory depressants—patients have severe COPD, often are CO_2 retainers.

INTRAOPERATIVE

Anesthetic technique: GETA (with DLT or BB) ± epidural anesthesia. Place and test epidural catheter before surgery. (See Lobectomy, Pneumonectomy, pp. 276–279.)

Induction	Standard induction (see p. B-2). DLT or BB absolutely necessary during surgery to selectively ventilate each lung. DLT preferable if severe bilateral disease with increased risk of pneumothorax (See Lobectomy, Pneumonectomy, p. 277).	
Maintenance	Inhalational agent and/or propofol. IV opioids and sedative agents should not be used (exception, remifentanil infusion intraop). Anesthesia may be supplemented by continuous or bolus administration of epidural anesthetics. Mechanical ventilation with O_2 and inhalation agent only. During TLV: Vt = 6–10 mL/kg, limit PIP to < 25 cmH_2O (best to use PCV). Respiratory rate and inspiratory flow should be adjusted to minimize air trapping (low RR, long E-time). Beware of overinflation and 'breath stacking,' which can → pulmonary tamponade with severe ↓ BP and ↑ airway resistance. ABG to determine $ETCO_2$-$PaCO_2$ gradient. During OLV use PCV for Vt = 4–8 mL/kg, long E-time, RR 6–10, and permissive hypercapnia ($PaCO_2$: 50–70 mmHg); monitor lung compliance closely because the ventilated lung also has emphysema/bullous disease. Avoid overdistention with hyperinflation (→ pneumothorax) on ventilated, nonoperated lung. Patients with severe COPD may have significant auto-PEEP. To avoid dynamic hyperinflation of lung, treat bronchospasm aggressively, allow adequate expiratory time (↓ I:E ratio), limit PIP to 15–20 cmH_2O, and cautiously use applied PEEP, as it may increase total PEEP (best managed with in-line spirometry). Moderate hypercapnia is well tolerated, but higher levels may result in significant pulmonary HTN, RV dysfunction, and tachydysrhythmias. CPAP to nonventilated lung may be necessary to maintain oxygenation. Maintenance of hemodynamic stability may require pressor support (e.g., ephedrine, phenylephrine, dopamine). Dynamic hyperinflation of the lung (pulmonary tamponade) during mechanical ventilation should be suspected if ↓ BP with ↑ PIP occurs.	
Emergence	Emergence is a critical time for these patients. All physiologic parameters need to be optimized. Air leaks are common and may be worsened by prolonged mechanical ventilation, coughing or straining on the ETT. Different options are available to achieve those goals, including deep extubation or deep conversion to spontaneous pressure-support ventilation. Either way, ventilation has to be assisted until patients are wide-awake, comfortable, warm and maintaining adequate respiration with minimal support. These patients are critically dependent on good analgesia, upright/sitting position, and suctioning to ↓ mucous plugging (can be catastrophic). Recovery from GA occurs in the OR and may take 1–2 h. Ventilatory assistance via face mask with supplemental O_2 is usually necessary. ABG and CXR may be useful. When spontaneous ventilation and analgesia are satisfactory, the patient is transported to ICU. If postop mechanical ventilation is required, consider using pressure support ventilation with low levels of CPAP. The CPAP may help minimize the inspiratory work of breathing caused by lung hyperinflation. The pressure support mode of ventilation will permit control of airway pressure, while allowing patient control of $PaCO_2$. If postop intubation is anticipated, changing from DLT to ETT is required.	
Blood and fluid requirements	IV: 14–16 ga × 1 LR @ 1–2 mL/kg/h Autologous PRBC	Fluid management to restore preop deficit and provide maintenance fluid, but restrict fluids similar to lung resection surgery. Replace minor blood loss with colloid. Transfuse autologous blood for Hct < 30.
Monitoring	Standard monitors (see p. B-1). Arterial line Urinary catheter	(See Lobectomy, Pneumonectomy, p. 277). ✓ ABGs: baseline (preop) during sternotomy; 15 min after initiation of OLV; 15 min after initiation of OLV on the second lung; during closure of sternotomy; prior to extubation.
	CVP and/or PA line	Useful for postop fluid management. Depending on level of PHTN, RV dysfunction and co-morbid CAD
Positioning	✓ and pad pressure points. ✓ eyes, ears, genitals.	Axillary roll and support for upper airway is necessary for the lateral decubitus position. (See Lobectomy, Pneumonectomy, p. 277.)

POSTOPERATIVE

Complications	Hypercarbia Hypoxemia Air leak/pneumothorax Hemorrhage	
Pain management	Lumbar or thoracic epidural opioids ± local anesthetics (see p. C-2).	Essential that patient be comfortable. Begin infusion of epidural opioids and local anesthetics (see Lobectomy, Pneumonectomy, p. 279). Breakthrough pain treatment options include iv hydromorphone (cautious boluses of 0.2–0.5 mg) and/or ketorolac (10–30 mg).

Suggested Readings

1. Brantigarn OC, Mueller E, Kress MB: A surgical approach to pulmonary emphysema. *Am Rev Respir Dis* 1959; 80:194–202.
2. Brodsky JB, ed: Thoracic anesthesia. In *Problems in Anesthesia.* JB Lippincott, Philadelphia: 1990.
3. Buettner AU, McRae R, Myles PS, et al: Anaesthesia and postoperative pain management for bilateral lung volume reduction surgery. *Anaesth Inten Care* 1999; 27(5):503–8.
4. Cooper JD, Trulock EP, Triantafillou AN, et al: Bilateral pneumonectomy (volume reduction). *J Thorac Cardiovasc Surg* 1995; 109:106–19.
5. Fishman A, Martinez F, Naunheim K, et al: A randomized trial comparing lung-volume-reduction surgery with medical therapy for severe emphysema. *N Engl J Med* 2003; 348(21):2059–73.
6. Geddes D, Davies M, Koyama H, et al: Effect of lung-volume-reduction surgery in patients with severe emphysema. *N Engl J Med* 2000; 343(4):239–45.
7. Miller JI, Lee RB, Mansour KA: Lung volume reduction surgery: lessons learned. *Ann Thorac Surg* 1996; 61:1464–9.
8. National Emphysema Treatment Trial Research Group: Patients at high risk of death after lung-volume-reduction surgery. *N Engl J Med* 2001; 345(15):1075–83.
9. Pearson FG, et al: *Thoracic Surgery.* Churchill Livingstone, New York, 1995.
10. Tschernko EM: Anesthesia considerations for lung volume reduction surgery. *Anesthesiol Clin North Am* 2001; 19(3):591–609.
11. Wakabayashi A: Thoracoscopic laser pneumonectomy in the treatment of diffuse bullous emphysema. *Ann Thorac Surg* 1995; 60(4):936–42.

BRONCHOPULMONARY LAVAGE

SURGICAL CONSIDERATIONS

Description: Whole-lung bronchopulmonary lavage is occasionally required for patients with pulmonary alveolar proteinosis–a condition characterized by excessive (or abnormal) surfactant production with resultant flooding of the lungs with proteinaceous fluid. Although the underlying cause of the condition is unclear, treatment consists of periodic whole lung lavage and, more recently, GM-CSF administration. It is our practice to perform **unilateral lavage** only, although single-session, bilateral lavage has been reported. After induction of GA, a DLT is placed, and the correct position is confirmed bronchoscopically. The lung is then lavaged in aliquots of 500–1000 mL NS or 0.5–1.0 L NS to dilute and wash out excess alveolar surfactant, pus, or mucus, and to obtain material for cytological and histochemical examination. Care should be taken not to overdistend the lung, and a running tally of fluid instilled and withdrawn should be performed to avoid overhydrating the patient. Frequently, 9–12 L of fluid are used, with the initial effluent being very cloudy and the final effluent being clear. Techniques that may improve the distribution of the lavage fluid include external chest percussion and tilting the operating table (laterally as well as in the craniocaudal directions).

Usual preop diagnosis: Pulmonary alveolar proteinosis; refractory asthma; cystic fibrosis; bronchiectasis; lipoid pneumonitis; silicosis; alveolar microlithiasis; inhalation of radioactive dust

SUMMARY OF PROCEDURE	
Position	Supine or lateral decubitus
Special instrumentation	Bronchoscope; DLT; lavage fluids
Antibiotics	None
Surgical time	45 min/side
EBL	None
Postop care	PACU → home
Mortality	Rare
Morbidity	Aspiration of lavage fluid Pneumothorax/hydrothorax Atelectasis
Pain score	1–2

PATIENT POPULATION CHARACTERISTICS	
Age range	17–35 yr
Male:Female	1:1
Incidence	Uncommon
Etiology	Pulmonary alveolar proteinosis; cystic fibrosis; bronchiectasis; lipoid pneumonitis; silicosis
Associated conditions	Asthma and other abnormalities of lung function

ANESTHETIC CONSIDERATIONS

PREOPERATIVE

Although whole-lung lavage is primarily a treatment for pulmonary alveolar proteinosis, it is also used as a therapeutic modality for many other lung-related conditions (see Usual preop diagnosis, above). Respiratory dysfunction of variable symptomatology is expected in these patients. Indications for whole-lung lavage include dyspnea on exertion, resting room air PaO_2 < 60 mmHg, or shunt fraction > 10–12%. Because the procedure requires GA with OLV, it is recommended that preop V/Q scans be obtained so that unilateral lung irrigation can be performed first on the more severely affected lung. If both lungs are equally diseased, lavage should be performed on the left lung initially to allow the larger right lung to be used for ventilation to provide better gas exchange. Patients then return in subsequent days or weeks for therapeutic lavage of the contralateral lung. A nonoperative treatment option for pulmonary alveolar proteinosis using granulocyte-macrophage colony-stimulating factor (GM-CSF), has shown promise for some patients with the acquired form of pulmonary alveolar proteinosis.

Respiratory	Patients with pulmonary alveolar proteinosis generally present with cough (nonproductive > productive), dyspnea, and fatigue. Physical findings consist of diffuse rales ± clubbing or cyanosis. CXR typically reveals diffuse bilateral patchy airspace consolidation. Pulmonary compliance is reduced 2° the restrictive disease pattern. PFTs show ↓ TLC, ↓ RV, ↓ VC, and ↓ D_LCO. Though nonspecific, baseline ABGs classically demonstrate respiratory alkalosis and hypoxemia, with a calculated elevation in A-a DO_2 gradient. Some patients may be O_2-dependent or have concomitant COPD 2° Hx of smoking. Secondary infections, especially in the respiratory tract, are well recognized risks in these patients. Cessation of smoking (> 6–8 wk) and prompt treatment of any underlying infections before whole-lung lavage may be prudent. **Tests:** CXR; PFT; ABG; V/Q scans; ± CT

Cardiovascular	Directed at any underlying disease process.
Laboratory	Abnormal elevation of serum LDH has been reported in some patients and has been shown to correlate with the severity of A-a DO_2. Tests: LDH; other tests as indicated from H&P.
Premedication	Standard premedication (see p. B-1). Avoid heavy sedation that might impair adequate gas exchange before induction. O_2 supplementation may be required after premedication.

INTRAOPERATIVE

Anesthetic technique: GETA is required with OLV (see p. 278) using a DLT. In pediatric patients or small adults where appropriate sized DLT is not available, and in patients who cannot tolerate OLV, the use of partial venoarterial CPB, venovenous bypass, or even ECMO has been reported. In some cases, sequential lobar lavage with smaller volume of lavage fluid has been achieved under conscious sedation for those patients in whom OLV is not possible.

Induction	Standard induction (see p. B-2) with thorough preoxygenation. The largest DLT should be used to facilitate infusion and drainage of the lavage fluid. (Placement of DLT is discussed on p. 278.) Due to the underlying impaired respiratory function in these patients, instituting OLV will further compromise gas exchange. It is imperative to avoid spillage of lavage fluid into the ventilated lung during the procedure. This is achieved by verifying the correct position of the DLT with FOB and confirming the competency of the cuff seal by testing it against pressures as high as 50 cmH_2O. Baseline individual lung compliance, airway pressures, and ABG should be ✓'d after DLT placement.	
Maintenance	100% FiO_2 with inhalational agent (e.g., sevoflurane) or TIVA using propofol and remifentanil infusions. Muscle relaxation is necessary to avoid movement or coughing that can cause leakage of lavage fluid into the ventilated lung. Because chest physiotherapy, including vibration and percussion, is required after each cycle of lavage filling, any deleterious change from baseline lung compliance decrease or airway pressure increase of the ventilated lung should prompt the anesthesiologist to look for evidence of spillage. Filling the nonventilated lung with lavage fluid can → ↓ pulmonary shunting (→ improved O_2 sat) and ↑PVR (→↓ CO). Draining the lavage fluid can → ↑ pulmonary shunting (→↓ O_2 sat) and ↓ PVR (→ ↑ CO). Accurate inflow and outflow volume of the lavage fluid should be recorded to ensure return volumes are 90%.	
Emergence	At the conclusion of surgery, the lavaged lung should be adequately suctioned to remove any residual fluid. Bilateral lung ventilation should be reinstituted. Because the compliance of the lavaged lung is greatly reduced, higher airway pressures are required to re-expand it, but at the risk of causing barotrauma to the nonlavaged lung. A brief period of OLV to the lavaged lung, using large TVs or ↑ airway pressure, may be necessary to recruit the collapsed alveoli (higher pressure, including PEEP, is needed to counter the increase in surface tension after the removal of significant amounts of surfactant). The patient's trachea should be extubated after adequate reversal of muscle relaxation; however, if prolonged postop ventilation is anticipated (e.g., in those who aspirated lavaged fluid to the ventilated lung), changing the DLT to single lumen tube is indicated. DLT should be maintained for patients in whom differential lung ventilation is required postop.	
Blood and fluid requirements	IV: 18 ga × 1 NS/LR @ 1–2 mL/kg/h	
Monitoring	Standard monitors (p. B-1) Arterial line	Although warmed lavage fluid is used, some patients may become hypothermic after several hours of lavage under GETA.
	± CVP line ± PA line	CVP or PA line only needed as indicated by comorbid conditions. Consider fluoroscopic or TEE guided positioning of a PA catheter to the lavaged lung.

Monitoring (cont'd)		In doing so, the therapeutic potential of the catheter may be realized. Selective occlusion of pulmonary arterial blood flow can improve matching of blood flow to ventilation.
Positioning	Supine ✓ and pad pressure points. ✓ eyes.	Some prefer the lavaged lung to be dependent to minimize the risk of contaminating the contralateral lung with lavage fluid. Others prefer the lavaged lung to be nondependent because, in this position, perfusion will more closely match ventilation in the dependent lung. As a compromise, we perform lavage with the patient supine. However, intermittent manipulation of the patient position may be required to facilitate the lavage and drainage of any retained fluid. Prevention of DLT displacement during repositioning is paramount.
Complications	Hypoxemia	Hypoxemia during OLV is most commonly 2° luminal obstruction (by blood or pulmonary secretions) of the DLT, worsening of shunting, or malposition of DLT. Rx: suctioning of the DLT; PEEP to ventilated lung (may ↑ shunting); return to two-lung ventilation; and ✓ DLT position. In extreme cases, temporarily inflating the balloon of the PA catheter (if available) may be necessary to improve shunting and, thus, oxygenation. Inadequate positioning of the DLT demands stopping further installation of fluid. Most authors recommend suspending the lavage fluid 30 cm above the midaxillary line. Instilling fluid from excessive height or under pressure may precipitate pulmonary edema.
	Hypercarbia	Ensure adequate TV and RR.
	Aspiration	✓ DLT position. Turn patient to lavaged side down and head down, suction the ventilated lung, reinstitute bilateral lung ventilation with PEEP, after the lavaged lung is thoroughly drained and suctioned. Termination of procedure may be needed in severe cases. Patient may need to be kept intubated after the procedure.

POSTOPERATIVE

Complications	Pneumothorax Hydrothorax	Obtain CXR; conservative measures if small pneumothorax or hydrothorax. Otherwise, chest tube placement will be required.
	Atelectasis	Decrease in surfactant after lavage will → airspace collapse. Most patients will experience moderate coughing, which will help re-expand the atelectatic lung units.
Pain management	Parental opioids or NSAID (ketorolac 30 mg iv)	Some patients may experience chest pain due to vigorous intraop percussion.

Suggested Readings

1. Ben-Abraham R, Greenfeld A, Rozenman J, et al. Pulmonary alveolar proteinosis: step-by-step perioperative care of the whole lung lavage procedure. *Heart Lung* 2002; 31(1):43–9.
2. Bussieres JS: Whole lung lavage. *Anesthesiol Clin North Am* 2001; 19(3):543–58.
3. Cohen E, Eisenkraft JB: Bronchopulmonary lavage: effects on oxygenation and hemodynamics. *J Cardiothorac Anesth* 1990; 4(5):609–15.

4. Cohen ES, Elpern E, Silver MR: Pulmonary alveolar proteinosis causing severe hypoxemic respiratory failure treated with sequential whole-lung lavage utilizing venovenous extracorporeal membrane oxygenation. A case report and review. *Chest* 2001; 120(3):1024–6.
5. Rogers RM, Levin DC, Gray BA, et al: Physiologic effects of bronchopulmonary lavage in alveolar proteinosis. *Am Rev Respir Dis* 1978; 118(2):255–64.
6. Seymour JF, Presneill JJ: Pulmonary alveolar proteinosis: progress in the first 44 years. *Am J Respir Crit Care Med* 2002; 166(2):215–35.
7. Venkateshiah SB, Yan TD, Bonfield TL, et al: An open-label trial of granulocyte macrophage colony stimulating factor therapy for moderate symptomatic pulmonary alveolar proteinosis. *Chest* 2006; 130(1):227–37.
8. Whitsett JA, Weaver TE: Hydrophobic surfactant proteins in lung function and disease. *N Eng J Med* 2002; 347(26):2141–8.

LUNG TRANSPLANT

SURGICAL CONSIDERATIONS

Description: The most common indications for lung transplantation include emphysema, pulmonary fibrosis, cystic fibrosis, and pulmonary hypertension. Patients with the first three of these diagnoses have marked abnormalities in mechanical pulmonary function, whereas patients with pulmonary HTN often have normal lung mechanics but very abnormal cardiac function. Patients with emphysema and pulmonary fibrosis often receive single-lung transplants, and those with cystic fibrosis require double-lung transplants. The best operation for patients with pulmonary hypertension continues to be debated, with options including single-lung, double-lung, and heart-lung transplantation (see p. 456). Although candidates for lung transplantation, by definition, have end-stage lung disease, their overall state of health and functional abilities vary considerably. Furthermore, although these patients all have poor pulmonary function, many with multisystem disease are eliminated during the preop screening process. Thus, the remaining patients are generally well motivated and free of significant cardiac, renal, and vascular disease.

Single-lung transplants generally are carried out through a thoracotomy incision. Patients with emphysema as the underlying disease rarely require CPB, whereas those with pulmonary fibrosis ↓ pulmonary reserve and ↑ incidence of pulmonary HTN) more commonly require bypass. Although the need for bypass can be assessed at the outset of the operation by instituting OLV, a CPB circuit and perfusionist should always be available. The route for vascular access for bypass (transthoracic or through the groin vessels) must be considered by the surgeon at the start of the case.

Double-lung transplants generally are done through bilateral anterior thoracotomies or a single bilateral 'clamshell' incision (Fig. 5-2). Mobilization of the lung is facilitated by use of a DLT. If the patient does not tolerate OLV, CPB can be established using aortic and atrial cannulation. Some surgeons routinely use a single-lumen ETT, with a defined plan for using CPB.

The procedure for both single- and double-lung transplantation is the same for each side. The native lung is mobilized, and the bronchovascular structures are divided. Mediastinal adenopathy and extensive pleural adhesions are the rule, rather than the exception, for patients with cystic fibrosis. Such pneumonectomies take significantly longer than those for emphysema. Once the native lung is removed, the donor lung is brought into the surgical field. The bronchial anastomosis is created first, and the lung is allowed to fall into the posterior costovertebral gutter. The venous anastomosis (atrial cuff anastomosis) is fashioned next. The final sutures are placed but left untied for later deairing. The arterial anastomosis is created last. Upon removal of the arterial clamp, the lung is perfused and deaired. The venous sutures are then tied and the atrial clamp is removed. After ensuring that the vascular anastomoses are hemostatic and that there is no air leak at the bronchial site, the incision is closed or, in the case of double-lung transplant, attention is directed to the other side.

The anesthesiologist should be aware that hypotension is not uncommon on reperfusion of the donor lung, but that it usually resolves spontaneously. Specific immunosuppression protocols vary from institution to institution, but intravenous administration of steroids immediately before lung reperfusion is a common practice. Lung transplant patients typically are left intubated following surgery; however, changing from a DLT to a single-lumen tube at the conclusion of the operation facilitates postop ET suctioning.

Usual preop diagnosis: COPD; pulmonary fibrosis; cystic fibrosis; pulmonary HTN; Eisenmenger's syndrome.

For Summary of Procedure and Anesthetic Management, see Surgery for Lung and Heart/Lung Transplantation, p. 456, and Anesthetic Considerations for Lung Transplantation, p. 458.

SECTION

6.0 CARDIOVASCULAR SURGERY

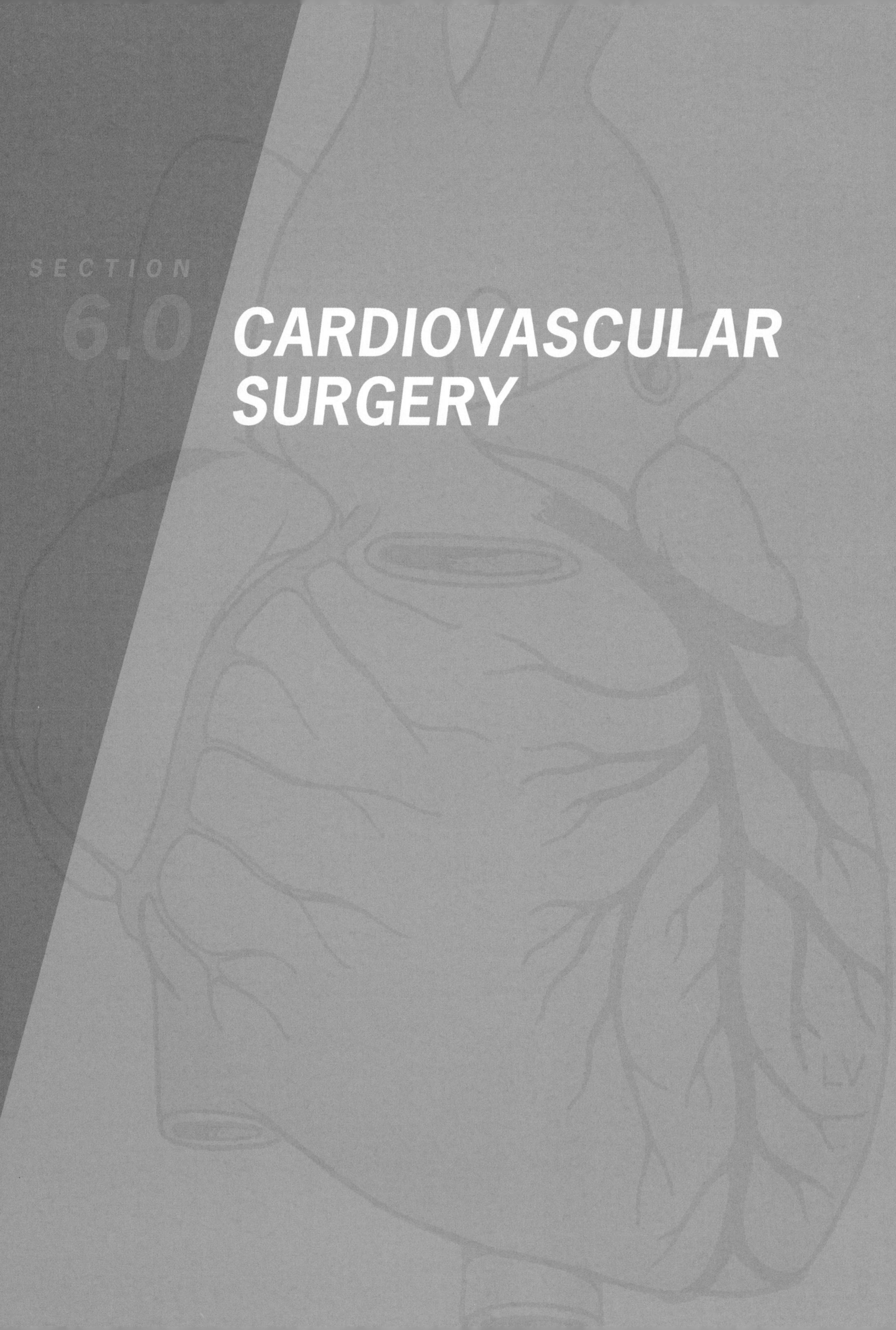

CHAPTER

6.1 Cardiac Surgery

SURGEON

R. Scott Mitchell, MD

ANESTHESIOLOGISTS

Linda E. Foppiano, MD
Lawrence C. Siegel, MD

CARDIOPULMONARY BYPASS

SURGICAL CONSIDERATIONS

The development of cardiopulmonary bypass (CPB) technology has allowed the repair of many congenital and acquired lesions of the heart and great vessels. Designed to replace cardiac and pulmonary functions, full CPB requires a blood pump and oxygenator. The pump may be of the roller-head or centrifugal variety with the latter producing less trauma to formed blood elements. The oxygenator may bubble gases (O_2 and CO_2) through a blood-filled reservoir (bubble oxygenator), or allow O_2 and CO_2 to diffuse through a thin membrane into the surrounding blood (membrane oxygenator). Utilization of any blood pump requires at least partial heparinization (ACT > 180 sec), and introduction of an oxygenator mandates full heparinization (ACT > 400 sec).

Full CPB typically drains systemic venous return via the right atrium into a venous reservoir, from which the blood is pumped through an oxygenator and then returned to the aorta or femoral artery, completely bypassing the heart and lungs (Figs 6.1-1 and 6.1-2). **Partial CPB** usually supports only a portion of the body—typically the infradiaphragmatic portion—and may use the patient's lungs as an oxygenator (left atrium → femoral artery) or a mechanical oxygenator (femoral vein → femoral artery). Full CPB is utilized during a sternotomy for work on the heart, ascending aorta, and transverse arch. Partial CPB, in which some systemic venous blood returns to the heart and is ejected into the aorta, is normally used for work on the descending or thoracoabdominal aorta. Heparin-coated components, which partially eliminate the necessity for heparin, are available.

After exposure of the relevant organs (heart or descending thoracic aorta), and after heparinization, venous and arterial cannulae must be placed intraluminally. **Cannulation of the heart** usually involves venous drainage from the right atrium, with either two cannulae inserted through the atrium into the SVC and IVC (bicaval), or via a larger, dual-stage cannula draining the right atria and IVC. Bicaval cannulation reduces venous return (and rewarming) to the heart, and allows caval snares to be placed so that the right atrium can be opened without introducing air into the venous return. Occasionally, atrial manipulation for cannulation can depress CO with resultant hypotension. This usually can be reversed with volume replacement. Aortic cannulation usually is not associated with any physiologic perturbation, although HTN must be avoided to minimize aortic complications. After the cannulae are in place and connections are made to the bypass circuit, CPB may be instituted electively. Most cardiac operations are conducted under mild hypothermia (28°C), unless profound hypothermic circulatory arrest is to be utilized. In that case, a target temperature of 16–18°C is desirable. For operations on the descending thoracic aorta, normothermia is maintained.

Cessation of CPB is accomplished by gradually decreasing pump flows, allowing for right heart filling, and gradually replenishing the circulating blood volume. Pulmonary and coronary vasodilations are mandatory during this phase, as there appears to be heightened vasoreactivity after periods of ischemia and hypothermia. For periods of cardiac arrest, during which the heart is deprived of its arterial blood supply, the metabolic demands of the myocardium must be minimized. This usually is accomplished by achieving diastolic arrest with a hyperkalemic cardioplegic solution, and also by lowering myocardial temperature to < 15°C. Frequent reinfusions of cardioplegia maintain hypothermia, prevent lactic acid accumulation, and deliver some minimally available dissolved O_2.

The **physiologic response to CPB** is complex and is associated with a massive catecholamine release which resolves after its cessation. Subsequent changes include abnormal bleeding tendencies, increased capillary permeability, leukocytosis, renal dysfunction, and impairment of the immune response. Hemodilution, nonpulsatile flow, hypothermia, exposure of formed elements to nonendothelial surfaces, complement activation, protein denaturation, cascading effects within the coagulation and fibrinolytic system, and activation of the kallikrein-bradykinin cascade, all contribute to this unphysiologic state, and account for much of the morbidity and mortality after CPB.

Many physiologic variables are now controlled by the anesthesiologist, perfusionist, and surgeon, including systemic flow and perfusion pressure, arterial O_2 and CO_2, temperature, and Hct. Other physiologic parameters follow either directly or indirectly. Thus, physiologic monitoring for the anesthesiologist and perfusionist include, at a minimum, arterial pressure, CVP, ABG determination (preferably on-line during CPB), CO, UO, and ECG. Constant communication among surgeons, perfusionist, and anesthesiologist is mandatory for a smooth operation. Transesophageal echocardiography (TEE) is rapidly becoming standard practice for cardiac surgery.

Secondary effects of CPB demand some special considerations during the final stages of the procedure and chest closure. Adverse effects on coagulation have already been mentioned, and vigorous attention to maintenance and replacement of coagulation factors is essential. The capillary leak phenomenon results in interstitial myocardial and pulmonary edema. Decreased myocardial performance and compliance mandate an increased preload, especially

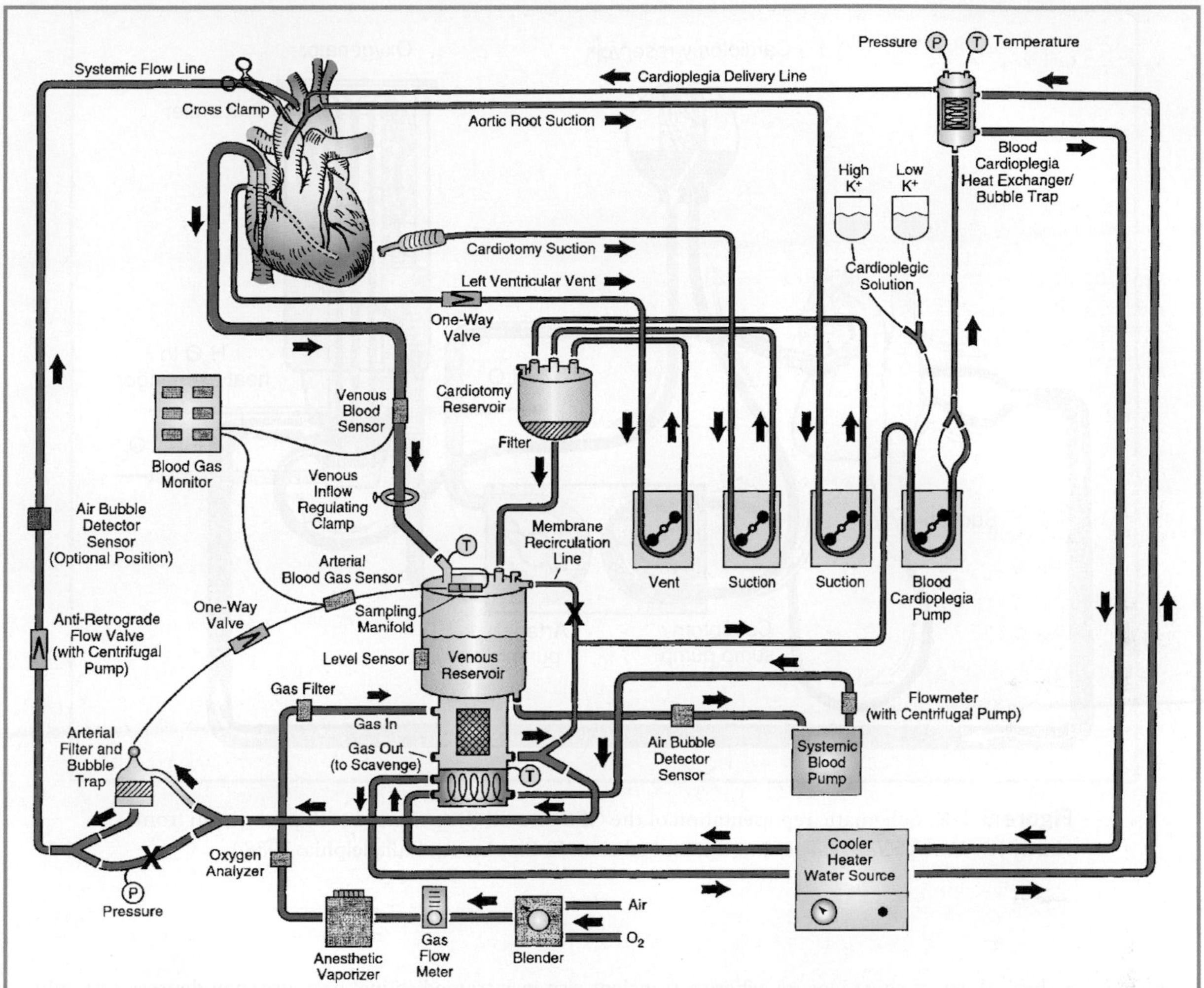

Figure 6.1-1. Detailed schematic diagram of the arrangement of a typical cardiopulmonary bypass circuit using a membrane oxygenator with integral hard-shell venous reservoir (**lower center**) and external cardiotomy reservoir. Venous cannulation is by a cavoatrial cannula and arterial cannulation is in the ascending aorta. Some circuits do not incorporate a membrane recirculation line; in these cases, the cardioplegia blood source is a separate outlet connector built into the oxygenator near the arterial outlet. The systemic blood pump may be either a roller or centrifugal type. The cardioplegia delivery system (**right**) is a one-pass combination blood/crystalloid type. The cooler-heater water source may be operated to supply water to both the oxygenator heat exchanger and cardioplegia delivery system. The air bubble detector sensor may be placed on the line between the venous reservoir and systemic pump, between the pump and membrane oxygenator inlet, or between the oxygenator outlet and arterial filter (neither shown), or on the line after the arterial filter (optional position on drawing). One-way valves prevent retrograde flow (some circuits with a centrifugal pump also incorporate a one-way valve after the pump and within the systemic flow line). Other safety devices include an oxygen analyzer placed between the anesthetic vaporizer (if used) and the oxygenator gas inlet and a reservoir level sensor attached to the housing of the hard-shell venous reservoir (on the **left center**). *Arrows*, directions of flow; *X*, placement of tubing clamps; *P* and *T* (within circles), pressure and temperature sensors. Hemoconcentrator (described in text) not shown.

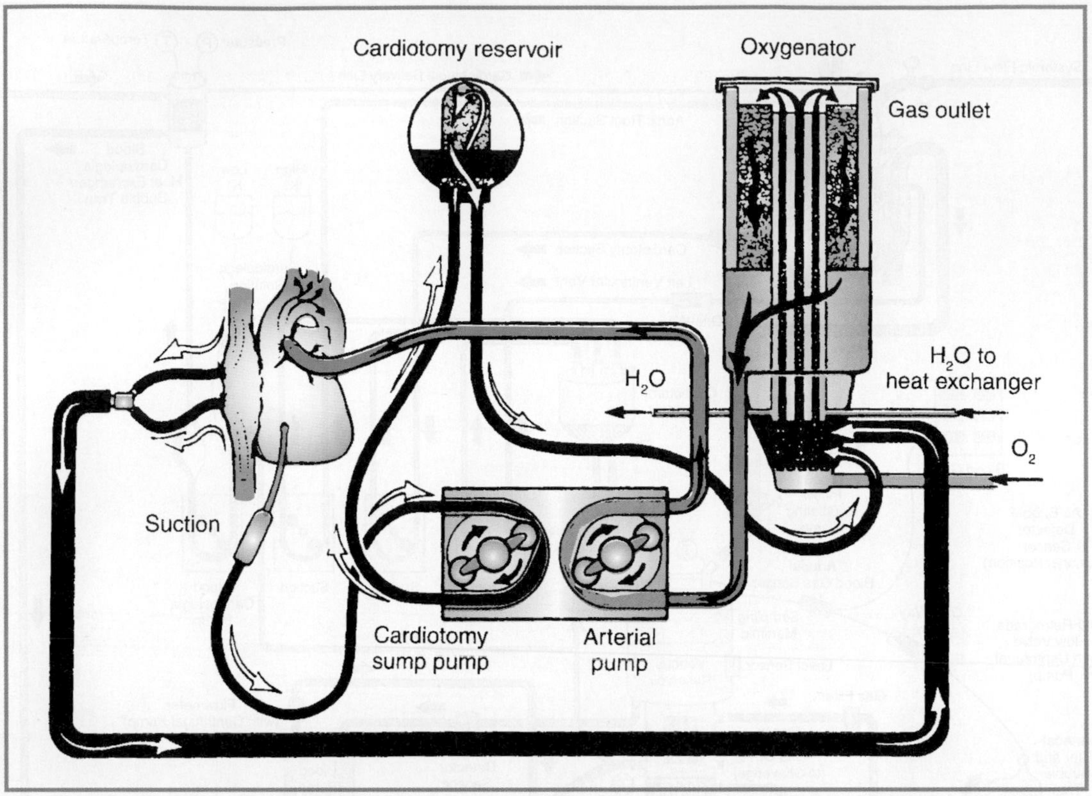

Figure 6.1-2. Schematic representation of the CPB circuit. (Reproduced with permission from Hardy JD: *Hardy's Textbook of Surgery,* 2nd edition. JB Lippincott, Philadelphia: 1988.)

during the physical act of chest closure, where a transient rise in intramediastinal pressure may depress systemic venous return. Similarly, decreased pulmonary compliance and gas exchange mandate vigilance over inspiratory pressures and lung volumes during chest closure, because mediastinal volume is physically decreased.

ANESTHETIC CONSIDERATIONS FOR CARDIOPULMONARY BYPASS (CPB)

This segment is not meant to be a definitive text on CPB, but rather a guide to the anesthetic management of bypass. Communication among surgeons, anesthesiologists, and pump technicians is of vital importance in carrying out this procedure.

PREPARATION FOR BYPASS	
Prebypass/ anticoagulation	✓ baseline ACT (normal = 90–130 sec). Heparin (3 mg [~300 U]/kg) is administered via a central vein (✓ back-bleeding to verify intravascular position) or by the surgeon directly into the atrium (preferred). ✓ ACT 3 min after heparin. It is essential to ensure adequate anticoagulation (ACT > 400 sec).
Aortic cannulation	Control MAP to ~70 mmHg for cannulation to ensure that the aortotomy does not extend. If needed, vasodilators may be used. The arterial line should be inspected for air bubbles.
Venous cannulation	Venous cannulation may be associated with atrial dysrhythmias. Blood loss can be excessive. Be prepared to infuse volume boluses, if necessary.
Pupils	Assess pupil symmetry for later comparison.

TRANSITION ONTO CPB

Stop ventilation	Commencing bypass is a dangerous period for the patient as a result of the many hemodynamic changes that occur. D/C ventilation once there is no pulmonary blood flow.
Withdraw PA catheter	Withdraw PA catheter 4–5 cm.
Stop infusions	Stop iv drugs and reduce iv fluid infusions to TKO.
Anticoagulation	ACT should be ✓'d after 5 min on CPB to ensure anticoagulation (ACT > 400 sec).
Oxygenation	Verify oxygenation by checking arterial inflow color and inline sensors and by ABG within 5 min of beginning CPB.
Flow	✓ for adequate venous drainage (CVP falls to a low level). Ensure adequate arterial inflow. Initial pressures may be very low, but usually will increase. View the descending thoracic aorta on TEE to verify flow (no aortic dissection).
Anesthesia	Anesthetics (e.g., fentanyl and midazolam) may be needed. A repeat dose (e.g., 10 mg pancuronium or 50 mg of rocuronium) should be given to prevent movement or shivering (increases O_2 requirements).
Pupils	Assess pupils. Unilateral dilation may indicate arterial inflow into the innominate artery (unilateral carotid perfusion).

BYPASS PERIOD

Anticoagulation	ACT levels should be checked regularly (q 20–30 min) and kept at > 400. Add heparin (5000–10,000 U), if needed.
Pressure/flow	There is controversy about safe flows and pressures. Generally, flows of 1.2–3 L/m^2/min are used, with pressures of 30–80 mmHg. A MAP of 50–60 mmHg is probably best for cerebral perfusion and does not result in excessive noncoronary blood flow.
Acid-base status	α-stat (ABG measured and interpreted at 37°, regardless of actual patient temperature) regulation of acid-base status is preferred because of maintenance of normal cerebral flow and autoregulation on CPB.
Hct/Electrolytes	Generally, Hct will fall to ~20, which may be acceptable (however, Hct ≥ 25 is preferable) in most patients. Hypokalemia is common and should be corrected. A K^+ > 4.5 mEq/L is desirable. Blood glucose levels should be monitored q 1 h. Treat blood glucose ↑ 125 mg/dl with iv regular insulin. (See Table 6.1-2)
UO	Keep UO >1 mL/kg/h. If needed, mannitol and/or furosemide should be given (assuming pump flow is adequate).
Temperature	During bypass, T is usually maintained at ~28°C.

Table 6.1-1. Difference Between α-Stat and pH-Stat Management During CPB

α–Stat (Temperature-uncorrected)	pH Stat (Temperature-corrected)
Plasma pH maintained at 7.4 (when measured at 37°C).	Plasma pH maintained at 7.4 at actual patient temperature.
Arterial PCO_2 maintained at 40 mmHg (when measured at 37°C).	Arterial PCO_2 maintained at 40 mmHg at actual patient temperature. Requires addition of CO_2 to inspired gases
Relative respiratory alkalosis during hypothermia	Relative normocapnia during hypothermia
Cerebral autoregulation preserved—CBF maintained.	Results in loss of cerebral autoregulation.

Table 6.1-2. Continuous Insulin Infusion in Intraoperative Adult Cardiac Surgery Patients

1. Bolus and start infusion pump as follows:

Blood Glucose	Insulin Bolus units	Insulin Drip units/h
< 125	0	0
125–175	5	1
175–225	10	2
> 225	15	3

2. Frequency of blood glucose determination: every 30 min intraoperatively!

3. Insulin titration:

Blood Glucose	Action
< 75	Stop insulin; give D50w and recheck blood glucose in 30 min. When blood glucose > 150, restart with rate 50% of previous rate.
75–100	Stop insulin; recheck blood glucose in 30 min. When blood glucose > 150, restart with rate 50% of previous rate, unless the dose is < 0.25 u/h.
101–125	If < 10% lower than last test, decrease rate by 0.5 U/h. If > 10% lower than last test, decrease rate by 50%. If neither continue current rate.
126–175	Same rate
176–225	If lower than last test—same rate. If higher than last test—increase rate by 0.5 U/h.
> 225	If > 19% lower than last test— same rate. If < 10% lower than last test OR if higher than last test increase rate by 1 U/h. If blood glucose > 225 and has not dcreased after 3 hourly increases in insulin, then double the insulin rate.

TERMINATION OF BYPASS

Rewarming	Prior to discontinuing CPB, the patient should have a core temperature of at least 36°C.
Anesthesia/ relaxation	Patient awareness may be a problem during rewarming. Volatile agents ± benzodiazepine (e.g., midazolam 3–5 mg) ± a narcotic to prevent awareness. In addition, a muscle relaxant also should be given.
Acid-base/ electrolytes/Hct	✓ electrolytes, acid-base status, and Hct. Correct acidosis. K^+: 4.5–5.5, normal ionized Ca^{++}, and Hct ≥ 20 should be assured.
Air maneuvers	Air maneuvers (to remove intracardiac and intraaortic air) are carried out when the heart is opened. Ventilation is commenced after there is pulmonary blood flow and will aid in the evacuation of air. Pleural fluid should be removed.

WEANING FROM BYPASS

Prior to weaning	Prior to weaning from CPB, the aortic cross-clamp should have been off for 30 min to allow rewarming and reperfusion of the heart. Defibrillation is often needed and pacing may be required. NSR or AV pacing is preferred. Vasoactive drugs should be available. After normal T, ventilation, cardiac rhythm, and reperfusion are established, bypass may be terminated. The heart is gradually volume-loaded (transfused from oxygenator) to adequate filling pressures and bypass flow slowly decreased over 15–45 sec until it is off. Return to bypass in the event of progressive cardiac distension or dysfunction. Assess CO and BP, and adjust vascular resistance as necessary. Inotropic agents often are required at this stage.
Reversal of anticoagulation	After the patient is off CPB, anticoagulation must be reversed with protamine (1–1.3 mg/100 U heparin), administered slowly over 10–20 min, because rapid administration can be associated with ↓ BP (treat with volume, calcium, α-agonists as necessary). Other reactions include pulmonary HTN and true allergic reactions. ✓ ACT to ensure that it has returned to control (90–130 sec).
BP management	Vasoactive support often is needed in the postbypass period; the need varies with surgical procedure, disease process, and underlying cardiac function. In general, SBP should be limited to 120 mmHg to avoid stress on the aortotomy site.

COAGULATION AND CPB

General	Bleeding is common post-CPB and may be considerable. Both preop and intraop factors contribute to this. Knowledge of these factors and the tests involved will aid with the management of these patients (Table 6.1-3).
Preop factors	Hx of previous bleeding during surgery is important. Many drugs may contribute to bleeding: aspirin/NSAIDs/clopidogrel (Plt dysfunction), anticoagulants (heparin, Coumadin) and fibrinolytic agents. These should be stopped preop, if possible, or their action reversed. Other pathological processes (e.g., liver failure/congestion, renal failure, or hemophilia) also play a role. Preop testing is important and should include PT, PTT, Plt count and bleeding time, as a minimum.
Intraop factors	CPB is associated with ↓ Plt count and function. Circulating clotting factors are decreased and fibrinolysis occurs. Many surgical teams routinely use either Amicar (5–10 g loading dose; 1 g/h, maintenance) or Aprotinin (1 mL, test dose; 1–2 million KIU, loading; 0.25–0.5 million KIU/h, maintenance) prophylactically during cardiac surgery to inhibit the fibrinolytic process. Aprotinin also has anti-inflammatory properties that may offset the inflammatory response to CPB. Recent studies have associated aprotinin (and not aminocaproic acid or tranexamic acid) with increased risk of CV events, including MI and heart failure, cerebrovascular events and renal dysfunction/failure in patients undergoing CABG surgery.
Post-CPB bleeding	The common causes of post-CPB bleeding are: surgical causes, inadequate heparin reversal, ↓ number of Plt and Plt dysfunction, ↓ clotting factors, fibrinolysis, DIC, excessive BP, and hypothermia. Surgical causes and inadequate heparin reversal (✓ ACT) should be ruled out. If no surgical cause is found and ACT is normal, Plt (1–2 plateletpheresis units) should be infused. PT, PTT, Plt count, TT, reptilase time, fibrinogen, and FSP should be checked. TEG may prove very useful. (See Fig 7.12-9 and Table 7.12-3 in Liver/Kidney Transplantation, p. 703.)

Table 6.1-3 A Treatment Plan for Excessive Bleeding After Cardiac Surgery

Action	Dosage	Indication
Rule out surgical cause	—	Absence of oozing at puncture sites and incision
More protamine	0.5–1 mg/kg	ACT > 150 sec or aPTT > 1.5 times control
Warm the patient	—	"Core" temperature < 35°C
Apply positive end-expiratory pressure (PEEP)*	5–10 cm H_2O	
Desmopressin	0.3 mcg/kg IV	Prolonged bleeding time
Aminocaproic acid	50 mg/kg, then 25 mg/kg/h	Elevated D-dimer or teardrop shaped TEG tracing
Tranexamic acid	10 mg/kg, then 1 mg/kg/h	Elevated D-dimer or teardrop shaped TEG tracing
Platelet transfusion	1 U/10 kg	Platelet count < 100,000/mm^3
Fresh frozen plasma	15 mL/kg	PT or aPTT > 1.5 times control
Cryoprecipitate	1 U/4 kg	Fibrinogen < 1 g/L or 100 mg/dL

* PEEP is contraindicated in hypovolemia.

Suggested Readings

1. Conlon N, Grocott HP, Mackensen GB: Neuroprotection during cardiac surgery. *Expert Rev Cardiovasc Ther* 2008; 6(4):503–20.
2. De Somer F: What is optimal flow and how to validate this? *J Extra Corpor Technol* 2007; 39(4):278–80.
3. Ganapathy S, Murkin JM: Pathophysiology and management of cardiopulmonary bypass. In: *Cardiac Anesthesia: Principles and Clinical Practice,* 2nd edition. Estafanous FG, Barash PG, Reves JG, eds. Lippincott Williams & Wilkins, Philadelphia: 2001, 415–46.
4. Hessel EA II: Cardiopulmonary bypass equipment. In: *Cardiac Anesthesia: Principles and Clinical Practice,* 2nd edition. Estafanous FG, Barash PG, Reves JG, eds. Lippincott Williams & Wilkins, Philadelphia: 2001, 335–86.
5. Mangano DT, Tudor IC, Dietzel C, et al: The risk associated with aprotinin in cardiac surgery. *N Engl J Med* 2006; 336(4):353–65.

6. McCloskey G: Termination of cardiopulmonary bypass and postbypass hemodynamic management. In: *Cardiac Anesthesia: Principles and Clinical Practice,* 2nd edition. Estafanous FG, Barash PG, Reves JG, eds. Lippincott Williams & Wilkins, Philadelphia: 2001, 447–64.
7. Rosenkranz ER: Myocardial preservation. In: *Cardiac Anesthesia: Principles and Clinical Practice,* 2nd edition. Estafanous FG, Barash PG, Reves JG, eds. Lippincott Williams & Wilkins, Philadelphia: 2001, 387–414.
8. Slaughter TF: The coagulation system and cardiac surgery. In: *Cardiac Anesthesia: Principles and Clinical Practice,* 2nd edition. Estafanous FG, Barash PG, Reves JG, eds. Lippincott Williams & Wilkins, Philadelphia: 2001, 319–34.

CORONARY ARTERY BYPASS GRAFT SURGERY

SURGICAL CONSIDERATIONS

Description: **Coronary artery bypass grafting (CABG)** is the most frequently performed cardiac operation. Since the discovery that coronary thrombosis is the causative event for MI, many schemes have been devised to augment the restricted coronary blood flow, including collateral pericardial blood flow to epicardial arteries and implantation of the internal mammary artery (IMA) with unligated side branches into the LV muscle. With the discovery by Favaloro that saphenous veins can be anastomosed to the epicardial coronary arteries, a new era of myocardial revascularization began. Basically, the technique involves bypass to a narrowed or occluded epicardial coronary > 1 mm in diameter with a small-diameter conduit (usually reversed saphenous vein or IMA) distal to the narrowed segment, with the proximal arterial inflow source being the ascending aorta. The IMA may be mobilized from the chest wall, leaving its proximal origin with the subclavian artery intact (pedicled graft), or the IMA may be transected and its proximal end anastomosed to the aorta or saphenous vein as a "free mammary graft." An "**all-arterial revascularization,**" using the right IMA and nondominant RA, is being utilized with increasing frequency.

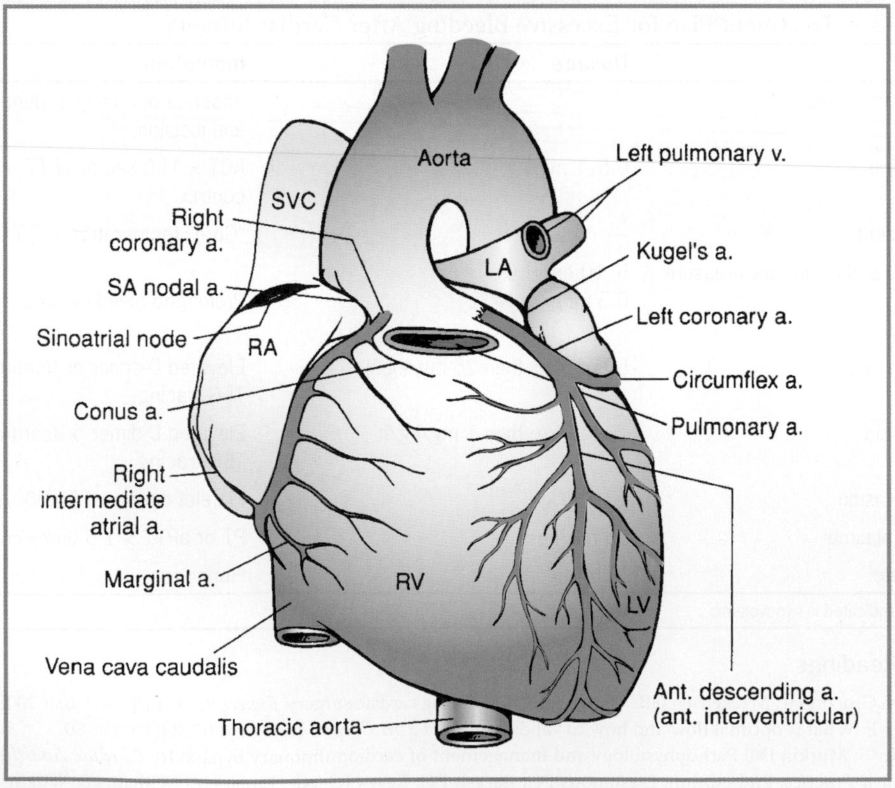

Figure 6.1-3. Coronary artery circulation—anterior view. (Reproduced with permission from Edwards EA, Malone PD, Collins JJ Jr: *Operative Anatomy of the Thorax.* Lea & Febiger, Philadelphia: 1972.)

The heart is approached through a median sternotomy, with the patient supported on full **CPB** (see separate section on CPB, p. 336). Although various operative strategies may be used, the most common regimen is for all distal (epicardial) anastomoses to be performed during a single period of aortic cross-clamping and cardiac arrest. During that period of induced asystole, myocardial protection is achieved by hypothermia and occasional reperfusion via antegrade or retrograde cardioplegia. Cardiac standstill and a bloodless field are mandatory to allow these very demanding small-diameter anastomoses to be constructed, with no obstruction to flow, in a minimal amount of time. The cross-clamp is then removed and the heart allowed to resume beating. A partially occluding aortic cross-clamp can then be applied to allow construction of the proximal aortic anastomoses. After a sufficient period of resuscitation, the patient is weaned from CPB, and decannulation, heparin reversal, and chest closure are allowed to proceed as previously noted.

The choice of conduit depends on availability and durability. Historically, the saphenous vein was the first small vessel conduit with acceptable patencies; but with prolonged experience it appears that 50% of vein grafts will be significantly diseased or occluded at 10 yr. The IMA appears to have superior long-term performance with ~90% 10-yr patency rates. Other arterial conduits, such as the left gastroepiploic artery, superficial epigastric artery, and the radial artery, are being investigated as to their long- and short-term durability. Typical target arteries include the distal right coronary and its major terminal branch, the posterior descending artery. From the left circulation, the left anterior descending (LAD), with its diagonal and septal branches, is the most important, having been estimated to supply blood to 60% of the left ventricle.

The left circumflex coronary artery courses in the posterior atrioventricular groove, and is not easily accessible for bypass, which is usually performed to its obtuse marginal or posterolateral branches.

In a randomized study on coronary artery surgery (CASS), coronary bypass was noted to be superior to medical management for relief of angina, and to prolong life in patients with left main CAD and in those with three-vessel disease and impaired LV function. Other patients may receive bypass for intractable angina refractory to medical management.

Variant procedure or approaches: **port access coronary artery revascularization** (see p. 378); **off-pump and minimally invasive coronary artery bypass** (see p. 378).

Usual preop diagnosis: CAD with Class 3 or 4 angina (angina with minimal exertion or at rest)

SUMMARY OF PROCEDURE

Position	Supine
Incision	Median sternotomy with legs prepped for saphenous vein harvest
Special instrumentation	Complete hemodynamic monitoring; TEE
Unique considerations	CPB
Antibiotics	Cefazolin 2 g iv prior to incision, then 1 g q 4 h
Surgical time	3.5–4.5 h
Closing considerations	Prevention of coagulopathy; maintenance of preload
EBL	500–600 mL
Postop care	ICU: 1–3 d, intubated 6–24 h.
Mortality	2–4%
Morbidity	Cognitive decline in patients > 60 yr: 26% MI: 3–6% Pneumonia: 5% CVA/stroke: 2–4% ↓ renal function
Pain score	7–8

PATIENT POPULATION CHARACTERISTICS	
Age range	60–80 yr (mean = 74 yr)
Male:Female	2:1
Incidence	Common
Etiology	Coronary atherosclerosis
Associated conditions	LV failure; pulmonary HTN; ischemic mitral regurgitation; diabetes mellitus; obstructive pulmonary disease

ANESTHETIC CONSIDERATIONS

(Procedures covered: CABG; LV aneurysmectomy)

PREOPERATIVE

H&P and tests will divide these patients broadly into two groups: (a) high-risk, characterized by poor LV function (cardiac failure; EF < 40%; LVEDP > 18 mmHg; CI < 2.0 L/min/m^2; ventricular dyskinesia; three-vessel disease; occlusion of left main or left main equivalent; valvular disease; recent MI; ventricular aneurysm; VSD; MI in progress; and old age); and (b) low-risk, characterized by good LV function. The type of monitoring chosen will depend on the patient's group.

Respiratory	Hx of smoking or COPD—patient should be encouraged to stop smoking at least 2 wk before surgery. Treat COPD and optimize therapy before surgery. **Tests:** CXR; PFTs; as indicated by H&P.
Cardiovascular	In the preop assessment, the following factors will affect patient management and surgical outcome: • Hx of angina (stable, unstable at rest, and precipitating factors) • Patient's exercise tolerance will provide a clue to LV functions and surgical outcome. • The presence of CHF (Sx: SOB, PND, orthopnea, DOE, pulmonary edema, JVD, 3rd-heart sound). • Recent (< 6 mo) MI, dysrhythmias, HTN, vascular disease (particularly carotid stenosis, aortic disease). • Valvular disease (particularly MR or AS) or the presence of a VSD or LV aneurysm may portend increased risk of periop complications. **Tests:** 12-lead ECG: ✓ ischemia (area involved), LVH, previous MI, dysrhythmias. Exercise stress testing: ✓ exercise tolerance, area of ischemia, maximal HR and BP before ischemia occurs, dysrhythmias. Thallium scan: ✓ component of reversible ischemia. ECHO (may be combined with stress ECHO): ✓ LV function, wall motion abnormalities, valvular disease, VSD. Cardiac catheterization: ✓ extent and location of disease, LV function, valvular pathology, VSD, LVEDP, LV aneurysm.
Postinfarction VSD	The development of a postinfarction VSD is associated with high operative morbidity and mortality because of the difficulty in repairing the lesion due to friable tissue, difficulty in obtaining hemostasis, emergent nature of the condition, and possible pulmonary edema. These patients effectively have poor LV function and should be considered as high-risk patients. They often require support, including IABP, during induction, prebypass, and postbypass.
LV aneurysm	LV aneurysm is usually a late complication of infarction; however, it can occur early, when it usually is associated with cardiac rupture (and high mortality). These patients usually have poor myocardial function and should be anesthetized with full monitoring, including PA catheterization. Postbypass, the LV cavity is reduced in size and compliance. To ensure an adequate CO, maintain adequate preload, a higher than normal HR (A-V pacing if needed), and sinus rhythm, and consider the use of inotropes. LV aneurysms are often associated with dysrhythmias and may require cardiac mapping. Hemostasis is often difficult to obtain, and adequate iv access is a necessity. Treatment usually entails the use of blood and blood products.

Emergency revascularization	Emergency revascularization occurs in the setting of acute MI, often with acute LV failure or after failed PTCA, where the patient may be stable, suffering from acute ischemia and hemodynamically unstable, or even in full cardiac arrest. Factors to consider in these cases are: full stomach (and the need for rapid-sequence induction [p. B-4] in the face of ischemia); the prior use of fibrinolytic agents (with increased risk of hemorrhage); need for inotropes; antianginals; IABP; and dysrhythmias. These patients have a higher morbidity and mortality. In patients who have received fibrinolytic agents, consider postbypass use of antifibrinolytic agents (e.g., aminocaproic acid).
Neurological	Previous stroke or Hx/Sx of carotid artery disease should be documented and evaluated.
Endocrine	Diabetes is common and periop control of blood glucose is important. **Tests:** Blood glucose
Renal	✓ baseline renal function, as CPB places these patients at risk for renal failure. **Tests:** Cr; BUN; electrolytes (particularly K^+)
Hematologic	Patients are often on aspirin or other antiplatelet therapy, which may lead to increased intraop hemorrhage. These agents should be stopped 7–10 d before surgery, if possible. Some patients may be on anticoagulants (usually heparin in the immediate preop period). Heparin should be stopped 6–8 h preop; however, in some patients, heparin infusion is continued into the OR. Other patients may have received thrombolytic agents that put them at increased risk for intraop hemorrhage. **Tests:** Consider Plt count, PTT, if indicated
Laboratory	Hb/Hct; other tests as indicated from H&P. T&C 2–4 U PRBCs.
Premedication	Patients should be instructed to continue all medications (e.g., nitrates, β-blockers; Ca^{++} antagonists, antidysrhythmics, and antihypertensives) before surgery, with the exception of diuretics on the day of surgery. Allaying anxiety may decrease the incidence of periop ischemia and help with the preinduction placement of lines. If necessary, preop sedation may include diazepam (10 mg po) or lorazepam (1–2 mg po) the night before and again 1–2 h before arrival in the OR with the addition of morphine (0.1 mg/kg im) and scopolamine (0.3 mg im). Most often midazolam (1–5 mg) iv immediately prior to OR is used. Severely compromised patients will require less premedication.

INTRAOPERATIVE

Anesthetic technique: GETA. An arterial line should be inserted, using liberal amounts of local anesthetic, before induction. The presence of real-time BP monitoring can be critical in the care of these patients, especially during induction. Although it is helpful to have a CVP line before induction for preload monitoring and drug infusion, it is not essential. This line usually is inserted after the patient is intubated. If infused drugs are necessary before the CVP catheter is in place, they can be administered through a separate peripheral iv.

Induction	Generally, a moderate- to high-dose narcotic technique (e.g., fentanyl 10–100 mcg/kg or sufentanil 2.5–20 mcg/kg), supplemented by etomidate (0.1–0.3 mg/kg) or midazolam (50–350 mcg/kg), is appropriate. As with all cardiac cases, the speed of induction and total drug dose depend on the patient's cardiac function and pathology. Muscle relaxation may be obtained using pancuronium (0.1 mg/kg), given slowly to avoid tachycardia, or vecuronium (possibility of bradycardia, especially if the patient is β-blocked). It is important to avoid the sympathetic response to laryngoscopy. The use of high-dose narcotics (see above), esmolol (100–500 mcg/kg over 1 min, followed by 40–100 mcg/kg/min infusion), SNP (0.5–3 mcg/kg/min), lidocaine (1–2 mg/kg), or a combination of these agents, may decrease or ablate this response. NTG (0.5–2 mcg/kg/min) also may be used during induction if evidence of ischemia occurs.
Maintenance	Usually narcotic (total: fentanyl 10–100 mcg/kg or sufentanil 5–20 mcg/kg) with midazolam (50–350 mcg/kg) for amnesia. Patients with good LV function may benefit from the decreased myocardial O_2 demand associated with the use of volatile agents (2° ↓ contractility). N_2O is generally avoided. Propofol infusion may be used while rewarming and postbypass.

Emergence	Transported to ICU, sedated, intubated, and ventilated. Extubate when able—often < 6 h if lower-dose narcotic technique used (fast-track).	
Blood and fluid requirements	IV: 14 ga × 1–2 NS/LR @ 6–8 mL/kg/h UO 0.5–1 mL/kg/h Warm all fluids. Humidify gases.	
Monitoring	Standard monitors (p. B-1)	Standard monitors and an A-line are placed before induction.
	Arterial line	✓ BP in both arms. Right radial preferred if left IMA graft, because retraction of the sternum may compress the left subclavian.
	CVP or PA catheter	CVP (and/or PA line, if indicated), usually is placed after intubation. In the low-risk/good LV function group, CVP is adequate; in high-risk/poor LV function, a PA catheter is useful for hemodynamic monitoring, weaning from bypass, and vasoactive therapy. Some groups use routine PA catheterization for all patients undergoing CABG surgery.
	ECG	Five-lead monitoring II and V_5 (or area most at risk for ischemia).
	TEE	Will reflect regional wall motion abnormalities, papillary muscle dysfunction, and MR.
Myocardial O_2 Balance	Supply – Coronary blood flow: Perfusion pressure (DBP-LVEDP) Diastolic filling time (HR) Blood viscosity (optimal Hct = 30) Coronary vasoconstriction: Spasm $PaCO_2$ (hypocapnia →constriction) α-sympathetic activity Supply – O_2 delivery: O_2 sat Hct Oxyhemoglobin dissociation curve Demand – O_2 consumption: BP (afterload) Ventricular volume (preload) Wall thickness (↓ subendocardial perfusion) HR Contractility	The balance of myocardial O_2 supply vs demand is important in the management of these patients. The goal of anesthesia is to ensure that this balance remains in equilibrium and that no ischemia occurs, or, if it does, that it is treated promptly. Those patients with poor LV function or complicated disease will benefit from maintenance of contractility (avoid volatile agents) and a high FiO_2, whereas those with good LV function may benefit from mild cardiac depression (↓ demand associated with the addition of low-dose volatile agents). Certain events are associated with **increased risk of intraop ischemia:** intubation, incision, sternotomy, cannulation, tachycardia, ↑ BP or ↓ BP, ventricular fibrillation or distension, inadequate cardioplegia, emboli, spasm, or inadequate revascularization. Care should be taken to avoid these complications and to ablate responses to stimuli.
Detection of ischemia	ECG	ST segment depression or elevation or a new T-wave alteration may suggest ischemia. Monitoring two leads—one lateral (e.g. V_5) and one inferior (e.g., II)—gives the best detection rate.
	PA catheter	Elevations of PCWP may be indicative of ischemia. A new V-wave on the PCWP trace is a better sign of possible ischemia (papillary muscle dysfunction).
	TEE	The appearance of a new regional wall motion abnormality is the most sensitive indicator of ischemia, but it requires constant monitoring.

Cardiovascular Surgery

Treatment of ischemia	Caused by tachycardia: Esmolol (100–500 mcg/kg) ↑ anesthesia Verapamil (2.5–10 mg iv) Caused by ↑ BP: NTG (0.5–4 mcg/kg/min) ↑ anesthesia Caused by ↓ BP: Phenylephrine (0.2–0.75 mcg/kg/min) ↑ preload Caused by ↓ ↓ HR: A-V pacing	While avoidance of ischemia is the goal, when it does occur it should be treated aggressively. Treatment may include inotropic support (e.g., dopamine 1–5 mcg/kg/min, epinephrine 25–150 ng/kg/min or milrinone 0.375–0.75 mcg/kg/min). If LV failure persists despite other therapy, an IABP or VAD may be inserted.
Positioning	✓ and pad pressure points. ✓ eyes.	

POSTOPERATIVE

Complications	Infarction Ischemia Tamponade Dysrhythmias Cardiac failure Coagulopathy Hemorrhage	Postop control of ischemia is important since hemodynamic instability may be associated with inadequate pain relief, awakening and ventilation.
Pain management	Parenteral opioids	Supplement with benzodiazepine for sedation.
Tests	ECG CPK CXR Electrolytes ABG Coag profiles	

Suggested Readings

1. Bondy RJ, Wynands JE, Dorman BH, et al: Anesthesia for coronary artery bypass surgery. In: *Cardiac Anesthesia: Principles and Clinical Practice*, 2nd edition. Estafanous FG, Barash PG, Reves JG, eds. Lippincott Williams & Wilkins, Philadelphia: 2001, 541–56.
2. DiNardo JA, Zvara DA: Anesthesia for myocardial revascularization. In: *Anesthesia for Cardiac Surgery*, 3rd edition. Blackwell Science, Boston: 2008, Ch 4.
3. Moller JT, Cluitmans P, Rasmussen LS, et al: Long-term postoperative cognitive dysfunction in the elderly ISPOCD1 study. International Study of Post-Operative Cognitive Dysfunction. *Lancet* 1998; 351(9119):1888–9.
4. Munsch C: What cardiology trainees should know about coronary artery surgery–and coronary artery surgeons: ischaemic heart disease? *Heart* 2008; 94(2):230–6.
5. Myles PS, McIlroy D: Fast-track cardiac anesthesia: choice of anesthetic agents and techniques. *Semin Cardiothorac Vasc Anesth* 2005; 9(1):5–16.
6. Okum G, Horrow JC: Anesthetic management of myocardial revascularization. In: *A Practical Approach to Cardiac Anesthesia*, 4th edition. Hensley FA, Martin DE, Gravlee GP, eds. Lippincott Williams & Wilkins, Philadelphia: 2008, 289–315.
7. Roach GW, Kanchuger M, Mangano CM, et al: Adverse cerebral outcomes after coronary bypass surgery. Multicenter Study of Perioperative Ischemia Research Group and Ischemia Research and Education Foundation Investigators. *N Engl J Med* 1996; 335(25):1857–63.
8. Rogers WJ, Coggin CJ, Green B, et al: 10-year followup of quality of life in patients randomized to receive medical treatment or coronary artery bypass graft surgery. *Circulation* 1990; 82(5):1647–58.

LEFT VENTRICULAR ANEURYSMECTOMY

SURGICAL CONSIDERATIONS

Description: Extensive MI may → large areas of myocardial necrosis, with subsequent aneurysm formation. LV failure may ensue as a result of continuous LV dilatation or mitral insufficiency 2° annular dilatation or involvement of papillary muscles. Indications for this surgery include worsening CHF and increased dysrhythmias.

Typically, apical dilatation with maintenance of basilar myocardial contractility allows for aneurysm resection and preservation of both myocardial contractility and chamber size to produce an adequate CO. Operation is commenced in the usual manner—by establishing CPB (see p. 336), cross-clamping the aorta, establishing myocardial protection, and then assessing the left ventricle. A thinned, dilated ventricular segment with full-thickness scar formation can be resected and ventricular continuity restored with improvement of ventricular geometry and myocardial energy demands. Coronary bypass can be performed during this same period. Then air is removed from the left side of the heart, the cross-clamp is removed, and coronary perfusion is reestablished. After a sufficient period of resuscitation and return of vigorous contractility, bypass is D/C'd, not infrequently with the assistance of intraaortic balloon pump (IABP) to augment forward output. Decannulation, protamine administration, and closure proceed as described in CPB, p. 336.

Usual preop diagnosis: LV aneurysm with CHF

SUMMARY OF PROCEDURE	
Position	Supine
Incision	Median sternotomy, ± leg incision for saphenous vein harvest if coronary bypass is planned.
Unique considerations	Preparations (ECG leads) should be made for pre- or postop IABP or LV assist device (LVAD)
Antibiotics	Cefazolin 2 g iv prior to incision, then 1 g q 4 h
Surgical time	Aortic cross-clamp: 40–100 min CPB: 70–130 min Total: 3–4 h
EBL	300–400 mL
Postop care	ICU × 1–3 d, intubated 6–24 h; usually requires inotropic support ± mechanical support (LVAD, IABP).
Mortality	5–7%
Morbidity	Overall: 8–10% Requirement for IABP: 10% Respiratory insufficiency: 5% CVA: 2–3%
Pain score	7–10

PATIENT POPULATION CHARACTERISTICS	
Age range	50–70 yr
Male:Female	3:1
Incidence	Uncommon
Etiology	Usually the end result of MI 2° CAD
Associated conditions	Mitral insufficiency; pulmonary HTN; CAD

ANESTHETIC CONSIDERATIONS

See Anesthetic Considerations following Coronary Artery Bypass Graft Surgery, p. 344.

Suggested Readings

1. Mills NL, Everson CT, Hockmuth DR: Technical advances in the treatment of left ventricular aneurysm. *Ann Thorac Surg* 1993; 55:792–800.
2. Ohara K: Current surgical strategy for post-infarction left ventricular aneurysm--from linear aneurysmecomy to Dor's operation. *Ann Thorac Cardiovasc Surg* 2000; 6(5):289–94.
3. Sun B, Gravlee GP: Surgical ventricular restoration and remodeling. In: *A Practical Approach to Cardiac Anesthesia,* 4th edition. FA Hensley, ed. Lippincott Williams & Wilkins, Philadelphia: 2008, Ch 17.

AORTIC VALVE REPLACEMENT

SURGICAL CONSIDERATIONS

Description: Disease of the aortic valve may present as valvular stenosis, insufficiency, or a combination of the two. Valvular disease most commonly occurs as a result of rheumatic disease, but also may occur 2° calcific degeneration (aortic sclerosis) in the elderly. Congenitally bicuspid valves and endocarditis account for most of the remainder. Repair of the aortic valve is rarely possible, and most conditions require valve replacement. The three most commonly used **prostheses** are: porcine bioprostheses, especially in the older patient; mechanical prostheses with the necessity for lifelong anticoagulation; and cryopreserved homografts, which, unfortunately, are expensive and in short supply. The operation, on full CPB, usually is performed through a median sternotomy. After routine bicaval and aortic cannulation, the patient is taken onto full CPB. Left heart drainage is through a pulmonary artery vent, and a left atrial vent usually is inserted through the right superior pulmonary vein. Because of the LV hypertrophy, myocardial protection is of utmost importance. Most centers favor hyperkalemic, hypothermic cardioplegic arrest, augmented by topical cooling, using either a continuous infusion of cold saline into the pericardial well or a cooling jacket. Cardioplegic administration can be achieved either antegrade into the coronary ostia or retrograde via the coronary sinus. Myocardial temperature is monitored continuously.

After the heart is arrested, the aorta is opened to expose the aortic valve. Continuous insufflation of the operative field with CO_2 reduces the amount of dislodged or trapped air. The rheumatic, stenotic valve, including aortic annulus, is frequently heavily calcified, and all Ca^{++} must be débrided to allow the prosthetic valve to be securely seated. This is frequently a tedious and time-consuming procedure, but one which then allows the remainder of the procedure to proceed in a timely fashion. After excision of the valve leaflets and debridement of the annulus, assuring that no particulate debris embolizes into the ventricle or coronary arteries, the annulus is measured to assure a proper match between prosthetic valve and annulus, and an appropriate valve prosthesis is selected. Interrupted sutures are placed through the annulus for its entire circumference and then passed through the sewing ring of the prosthesis. The prosthesis is lowered into the annulus and securely tied in place. Proper sizing and positioning are mandatory to prevent perivalve leaks or impingement on the coronary ostia. Systemic rewarming is initiated during the final stages of the valve implantation and the LV is allowed to fill during aortic closure. With the patient in the head-down position, all remaining air is vented from the left heart and aorta, and the cross-clamp is removed to allow myocardial perfusion. The heart is allowed to recover from this period of ischemia and, after sufficient resuscitation, with continuous venting of air from the aorta, the patient is weaned from CPB. Vasodilators are almost always utilized, as there appears to be excessive vasospasm present in both the coronary and pulmonary circulations after hypothermia. Decannulation and heparin reversal with protamine are then accomplished in the routine manner.

Usual preop diagnosis: Severe AS with syncope, chest pain or CHF; aortic insufficiency with CHF

SUMMARY OF PROCEDURES

	Valve Replacement with Prosthesis	Homograft Valve Replacement
Position	Supine	⇐
Incision	Median sternotomy	⇐
Special instrumentation	TEE; hemodynamic monitoring; CPB	TEE or surface ECHO

Cardiovascular Surgery

SUMMARY OF PROCEDURES (cont'd)

	Valve Replacement with Prosthesis	Homograft Valve Replacement
Unique considerations	ECHO assessment of valve function and regional wall motion intraop	ECHO assessment of annular size and intraop evaluation of valve function after implantation
Antibiotics	Cefazolin 2 g iv prior to incision and 1 g q 4 h	⇐
Surgical time	Aortic cross-clamp: 45 min CPB: 90 min Total: 3 h	60 min 105 min ⇐
EBL	300–400 mL	⇐
Postop care	ICU: 1–3 d, intubated 6–24 h; hypertrophied, noncompliant LV requiring high preload.	⇐
Mortality	5–8%	⇐
Morbidity	Pneumonia: 5–10% Neurological sequela: Transient: 3–7% CVA: 1–2% Permanent: 1–2% Infection: 1%	⇐ ⇐
Pain score	7–10	7–10

PATIENT POPULATION CHARACTERISTICS

Age range	Bicuspid valves – 50–60 yr; rheumatic – 55–80 yr (mean = 58 ± 13 yr)
Male:Female	3:1
Incidence	70–100 cases/yr in tertiary care center
Etiology	Postrheumatic (majority of patients); aortic sclerosis; progressive stenosis of a bicuspid aortic valve; endocarditis
Associated conditions	Poststenotic dilatation of the ascending aorta (may require separate surgical attention); rheumatic mitral valvular involvement; CAD; CHF

ANESTHETIC CONSIDERATIONS

PREOPERATIVE

Respiratory	Respiratory compromise may occur 2° pulmonary congestion (LV failure) and pleural effusion. An effusion, if significant, should be drained prior to surgery, as it may impair oxygenation and, with IPPV, may impair venous return →↓ CO + ↓ myocardial perfusion. **Tests:** CXR
Cardiovascular	**Aortic stenosis (AS):** Sx are those of angina pectoris (if at rest may indicate concurrent CAD), syncope, and CHF (indicates severe disease with 2-yr life expectancy). The ejection murmur of AS is best heard at the 2nd right interspace. ECG shows LVH. Important points in the preop investigations include: • Aortic orifice size: moderate AS = 0.7–0.9 cm^2; critical AS = < 0.5 cm^2 (normal = 2.6–3.5 cm^2) • Aortic valvular gradient: severe = > 70 mmHg • Ejection fraction (EF): ↓ EF indicates evidence of LV failure (normal = > 0.6). • Coronary angiography: associated CAD often demonstrated. AS →↑ LV work (↑ pressure load) → LV concentric hypertrophy →↑ LV diastolic function + ↑ risk for ischemia (MVO_2 + O_2 supply). • Reliance on atrial "kick:" important to maintain NSR. • Sensitivity to changes in SVR:↓ SVR →↓↓ BP →↓ myocardial perfusion + ↓ CO →↓↓↓ BP. • Sensitivity to volume changes: hypovolemia →↓ preload →↓ ↓ CO.

Cardiovascular (cont'd)	• Sensitivity to rate changes: tachycardia →↓ ejection time →↓ myocardial perfusion. • LV wall tension + ↑ duration of systole →↑ MVO_2. • ↑ LVEDP + ↑ wall thickness and tension + ↓ diastolic aortic pressure →↓ O_2 supply. **Aortic regurgitation (AR):** Sx include DOE, orthopnea, PND, palpitations, and (less frequently) angina. Exercise tolerance may remain reasonably good, even with severe chronic AR. Acute AR is very poorly tolerated. The pandiastolic murmur of AR is loudest over the sternum and left lower sternal border. AR → chronic LV volume overload → LV eccentric hypertrophy →massive cardiomegaly →LV failure (CHF) →↑ LVEDP →↑ PA pressure and pulmonary congestion. • Possibility of ischemia: ↑ MVO_2 and ↓ supply (↓ diastolic pressure, ↑ HR). • Sensitivity to rate changes: ↓ HR →↑ AR + ↓ CO. • Sensitivity to changes in SVR: ↑ SVR →↑ regurgitation + ↓ CO. **Tests:** ECG: ✓ hypertrophy, LV strain, ischemia, rhythm. ECHO: ✓ LV function, valve area, regurgitant fraction. Angiography: ✓ LV function, right heart pressure, CAD, valve area, regurgitant fraction.
Hepatic	CHF may result in passive liver congestion with ↓ liver function and possible coagulopathy. **Tests:** LFTs; PT; PTT
Neurological	Syncopal episodes may have resulted in neurologic deficits. These should be well documented.
Renal	Prerenal failure often is associated with AR 2° ↓ CO. **Tests:** BUN; Cr, creatinine clearance, if indicated; electrolytes
Hematologic	**Tests:** Hb/Hct; clotting profile to investigate abnormalities. T&C for 8 U PRBCs.
Laboratory	✓ digitalis level and electrolytes; other tests as indicated from H&P.
Premedication	Beware of oversedation in patients with AS where ↓ BP could be detrimental. Light premedication with an anxiolytic is usually sufficient. Digitalis and diuretics should be continued.

INTRAOPERATIVE

Anesthetic technique: GETA. An arterial line should be inserted, using liberal amounts of local anesthetic, before induction. The presence of real-time BP monitoring can be critical in the care of these patients, especially during induction. Although it is helpful to have a CVP line before induction for preload monitoring and drug infusion, it is not essential. This line usually is inserted after the patient is intubated. If infused drugs are necessary before the CVP catheter is in place, they can be administered through a separate peripheral iv.

Induction	**AS:** Typically, O_2 with moderate- to high-dose narcotic (e.g., fentanyl 10–100 mcg/kg). Avoid sufentanil in AS because of ↓ BP. Etomidate (0.1–0.3 mg/kg), midazolam (50–350 mcg/kg) may be used to supplement the above. Paralysis with vecuronium or pancuronium (0.1 mg/kg, depending on desired HR). Induction is a critical period. CPB and surgeons should be available and ready to proceed. Danger is hypotension with a cycle of ischemia, further hypotension and more ischemia. Hypotension should be treated aggressively with fluid and α-adrenergic agonists (phenylephrine 50–100 mcg iv bolus, infusion 0.1–0.75 mcg/kg/min). Critical AS patients may benefit from the use of phenylephrine as an infusion during induction and prebypass. The avoidance of hypotension is even more critical in the presence of CAD. Drugs causing tachycardia should be avoided. Atrial fibrillation (AF) or SVT should be treated with cardioversion. β-blockers and other negative inotropes are generally contraindicated. Ventricular irritability should be treated early as ventricular fibrillation may be refractory to defibrillation. Beware of vasodilators, including NTG. **AR:** Again, O_2 with moderate- to high-dose narcotic (e.g., fentanyl 10–100 mcg/kg or sufentanil 2.5–10 mcg/kg). Etomidate (0.1–0.3 mg/kg) or benzodiazepines (e.g., midazolam 50–350 mcg/kg) may be used to supplement the opiates. Muscle relaxation with pancuronium (0.1 mg/kg). These patients benefit from fluid augmentation, high normal HR (90 bpm) with afterload reduction (e.g., SNP 0.25–2 mcg/kg/min) to improve forward flow.

Maintenance	Narcotic (e.g., total fentanyl 10–100 mcg/kg). Low–dose volatile agent/air/O_2. Relaxant. (See Anesthetic Considerations for Cardiopulmonary Bypass, pp. 356.) The following table summarizes the goals of intraop management:

Parameter	AS	A
LV preload	↑	Normal-to-↑
HR	Normal-to-slow ↓	Modest ↑
Rhythm	NSR	NSR
Contractility	Maintain	Maintain
SVR	Modest ↑	↓
PVR	Maintain	Maintain

Postbypass	**AS:** Postbypass, patients may be hyperdynamic and require vasodilators for HTN, although inotropes also may be needed. Because of the hypertrophied, noncompliant ventricle, filling pressure may be higher than normally required. **AR:** In the immediate postbypass period, patients with AR may require inotropic support (e.g., dopamine 3–10 mcg/kg/min, dobutamine 5–10 mcg/kg/min; epinephrine 25–100 ng/kg/min) is often needed. Maintain LV filling. Other supportive measures (e.g., IABP) may be necessary.
Emergence	Transport to ICU sedated, intubated (6–24 h), and ventilated. Early extubation may be possible if a lower-dose narcotic technique is used (fast-track).
Blood and fluid requirements	IV: 14 ga × 1–2 NS/LR @ 6–8 mL/kg/h UO 0.5–1 mL/kg/h Warm all fluids. Humidify gases. T&C 2–4 U blood

Monitoring	Standard monitors (p. B-1) Arterial line	Standard monitors and arterial line should be placed before induction.
	CVP line PA catheter	CVP (and/or PA line, if indicated), usually is placed after intubation. CVP may underestimate left-side pressures. In acute AR, PCWP may underestimate true LVEDP.
	ECG	V_5 lead should be monitored for ischemia.
	TEE	TEE may be useful to estimate LV filling and regional wall motion abnormalities.
	Urinary catheter	
Positioning	✓ and pad pressure points. ✓ eyes.	

POSTOPERATIVE

Complications	Hemorrhage Tamponade Cardiac failure Dysrhythmias Ischemia	Inotropic and vasodilator therapy usually is continued into the postop period, and then weaned.
Pain management	Parenteral opioids for pain relief Benzodiazepine for sedation	
Tests	ECG CXR Electrolytes Coag profile HCT	

Cardiovascular Surgery

Suggested Readings

1. Cook DJ, Housmans PR, Rehfeldt KH: Valvular heart disease: replacement and repair. In: *Kaplan's Cardiac Anesthesia,* 5th edition. Kaplan JA, ed. WB Saunders, Philadelphia: 2006, Ch 20.
2. Fann JI, Miller DC, Moore KA, et al: Twenty-year clinical experience with porcine bioprostheses. *Ann Thorac Surg* 1996; 62:1301–12.
3. Frasco PE, de Bruijn NP: Valvular heart disease. In: *Cardiac Anesthesia: Principles and Clinical Practice,* 2nd edition. Estafanous FG, Barash PG, Reves JG, eds. Lippincott Williams & Wilkins, Philadelphia: 2001, 557–84.
4. Murtuza B, Pepper JR, Stanbridge RD, et al: Minimal access aortic valve replacement: is it worth it? *Ann Thorac Surg* 2008; 85(3):1121–31.
5. Tjang YS, van Hees Y, Körfer R, et al: Predictors of mortality after aortic valve replacement. *Eur J Cardiothorac Surg* 2007; 32(3):469–74.

MITRAL VALVE REPAIR OR REPLACEMENT

SURGICAL CONSIDERATIONS

Description: **Mitral valve repair or replacement** is utilized typically for the correction of postrheumatic mitral valvular stenosis or insufficiency, as well as mitral valve prolapse, degenerative mitral insufficiency, or repair after endocarditis. For mitral regurgitation (MR) 2° posterior leaflet abnormalities (myxomatous degeneration, torn chordae) or pure annular dilatation, most valves can be repaired. For severe rheumatic calcific mitral stenosis (MS), mitral valve replacement with preservation of subannular structures may be necessary.

The technique of mitral valve repair or replacement is similar regardless of the mitral valve pathology. After aortic and bicaval venous cannulation, CPB (see p. 336) is established, and the left heart is vented through the PA. After cross-clamping of the aorta, diastolic arrest is accomplished with cardioplegia administered via the aortic root, augmented with topical cooling with either continuous pericardial saline infusion or a cooling jacket. Exposure is accomplished via a vertical incision in the left atrium just posterior to atrial septum. If the left atrium is not large enough, access may be gained via an incision in the right atrium and then incising the atrial septum, with caval snares in place to prevent air entry into the venous cannulae.

After suitable exposure, the atrium, atrial appendage, and mitral valve are carefully inspected, and a decision is made to repair or replace the valve. Repair of regurgitant valves caused primarily by posterior leaflet problems is usually possible. Similarly, annular dilatation 2° LV enlargement is also usually possible by means of a ring annuloplasty. Regurgitation 2° anterior leaflet abnormalities are more problematic, requiring significant expertise, and may be less durable. Preop and postop evaluations are greatly facilitated by use of TEE. Valve replacement can be performed after excising the valve leaflets; or, the leaflets may be preserved in an attempt to maintain the benefits of the subvalvar apparatus to global ventricular performance. After appropriate excision and debridement, the annulus is rimmed with interrupted sutures passed through the sewing ring of the valve prosthesis. The prosthesis is carefully positioned, and the sutures are tied. After filling both the LV and atrium with blood, the atrium is closed, air is evacuated from the left heart, and the cross-clamp is removed to allow coronary perfusion. After a satisfactory period of resuscitation, and after all air has been evacuated from the circulation, CPB may be D/C'd, usually with the assistance of vasodilator agents. TEE may be utilized at this stage to assess adequacy of mitral valve repair.

Variant procedure or approaches: **Mitral commissurotomy** may be done closed (e.g., during pregnancy).

Usual preop diagnosis: Class 3 or 4 CHF 2° mitral insufficiency or mitral stenosis

SUMMARY OF PROCEDURES

	Mitral Valve Replacement/Repair	Closed Commissurotomy
Position	Supine	Right lateral decubitus
Incision	Median sternotomy	Left lateral thoracotomy
Special instrumentation	TEE and epicardial ECHO to assess valve function and regional wall motion; CPB.	Performed without CPB.

SUMMARY OF PROCEDURES (cont'd)

	Mitral Valve Replacement/Repair	Closed Commissurotomy
Unique considerations	Special loading conditions may be used to estimate the amount of MR, which is frequently afterload-dependent.	⇐
Antibiotics	Cefazolin 2 g iv prior to incision, then 1 g q 4 h	⇐
Surgical time	Aortic cross-clamp: 45–150 min CPB: 90–200 min	Total: 2 h Total: 3–4 h
EBL	300–400 mL	200–400 mL
Postop care	ICU × 1–3 d, intubated 6–24 h; vasodilator therapy for reversal of pulmonary HTN and afterload reduction.	⇐
Mortality	5–8%	< 5%
Morbidity	Pneumonia: 10–15% CNS complications: Transient neurologic dysfunction: 5–10% CVA: 1–2% Infection: < 1%	⇐ ⇐ ⇐ ⇐
Pain score	7–10	7–10

PATIENT POPULATION CHARACTERISTICS

Age range	40–75 yr	20–40 yr
Male:Female	1:1	Almost exclusively pregnant females
Etiology	Postrheumatic: majority of cases; increased aging; myxomatous degeneration; ischemic etiologies (increasing)	⇐
Associated conditions	Aortic valvular involvement with rheumatic disease, CAD, pulmonary HTN, and tricuspid regurgitation	⇐

ANESTHETIC CONSIDERATIONS

PREOPERATIVE

Respiratory	Pulmonary congestion, edema, pleural effusions may be present, with an overall restrictive lung pattern. Pleural effusions should be drained before surgery if significant (↓ oxygenation, ↓ venous return with IPPV). ↑ LA volume may compress the left recurrent laryngeal nerve →left vocal cord paralysis (Ortner's syndrome). **Tests:** CXR; PFTs, if indicated
Cardiovascular	**Mitral Stenosis (MS):** Sx include exertional dyspnea and fatigue, progressing to pulmonary edema, atrial fibrillation (AF), and hemoptysis. Embolic events occur in 15% of patients. The opening snap and diastolic murmur of MS are best heard between apex and left sternal border. The ECG may show AF or wide-notched P-waves. It is important to grade the severity of MS by symptomatology and valve area: mild = 1.5–2 cm^2; moderate = 1–1.5 cm^2; and severe = < 1.0 cm^2 (nl = 4–6 cm^2). AF is often the factor precipitating deterioration in these patients. Because of the decreased LV filling, these patients are sensitive to: • Loss of atrial "kick:" maintain NSR. • Volume changes: keep full. • Rate changes: avoid ↑ HR →↓diastolic filling time →↓ CO.

Cardiovascular (cont'd)	Pathophysiology: • MS →↓ LVH filling →↓ CO. • MS →↑ LA pressure →pulmonary edema + ↑ PA pressure →↑ PVR →RV failure + TR + left shift of iv septum →↓ CO →↑ LA pressure →↑ LA volume →AF and thrombi. **Mitral Regurgitation (MR):** May be acute (MI/endocarditis) or chronic (often associated with MS). Chronic Sx include: palpitations, DOE, PND, fatigue, and orthopnea. Acute MR may →sudden ↓↓ CO and pulmonary edema. MR can be classified as mild (< 30% RF), moderate (30–60% RF), or severe (> 60% RF). The pansystolic murmur is loudest at the apex. The ECG may show LA and LV overload. MR patients are sensitive to: • Changes in SVR: ↑ SVR →↑ RF →↓ CO + ↓ BP. ↓ SVR →↓ RF →↑ CO + ↑ BP. • Change in HR: • ↓ HR →acute LA volume overload. Mild ↑ HR→↑ CO Pathophysiology: • Acute MR →↑ ↑ LA pressure →↓ CO + ↓ BP →↑ HR →↑ contractility →↑ O_2 demand. →↑ LV diastolic volume →↑ LVEDP →↑ O_2 demand. → Pulmonary edema. • Chronic MR →↑ LA volume + AF → pulmonary edema → RV failure. → LV volume overload → LVH →↓ CO + LV failure. **Tests:** ECG: ✓ LVH, left and right atrial enlargement, rhythm. ECHO: ✓ RF, valve pressure gradients, LV function, valve pressure gradient and area.
Neurological	The large left atrium and AF may result in thrombus formation, with the possibility of embolism. Neurological deficits should be documented.
Gastrointestinal	Hepatic congestion may → decreased function, which may be reflected in coagulation problems. **Tests:** Consider LFTs; PT; PTT
Renal	↓ CO may lead to renal failure. **Tests:** BUN; Cr; electrolytes
Hematologic	Because of the potential for thromboembolism, these patients may be on anticoagulants, which may be given up to the day before surgery. In the case of Coumadin, anticoagulant effects can be reversed by the use of FFP and vitamin K. **Tests:** Consider PT; PTT
Laboratory	T&C for 2–4 U PRBCs. Hb/Hct; coagulation profile; other tests as indicated from H&P.
Premedication	Premedication with an anxiolytic (e.g., lorazepam 1–2 mg po, midazolam 0.05–0.2 mg/kg im) or an analgesic (e.g., morphine 0.1–0.2 mg/kg); or a combination of these agents may be used, depending on patient status.

INTRAOPERATIVE

Anesthetic technique: GETA. An arterial line should be inserted, using liberal amounts of local anesthetic, before induction. The presence of real-time BP monitoring can be critical in the care of these patients, especially during induction. Although it is helpful to have a CVP line before induction for preload monitoring and drug infusion, it is not essential. This line usually is inserted after the patient is intubated. If infused drugs are necessary before the CVP catheter is in place, they can be administered through a separate peripheral iv.

Induction	Typically, moderate- to high-dose narcotic (fentanyl 10–100 mcg/kg or sufentanil 2.5–20 mcg/kg), supplemental midazolam (50–350 mcg/kg) or etomidate (0.1–0.3 mg/kg). Use pancuronium (MR) or vecuronium (MS) (0.1 mg/kg), depending on the desired HR to facilitate intubation.

Induction (cont'd)

MS: ↓ BP should be treated with fluid, but beware of precipitating pulmonary edema. Occasionally, phenylephrine may be needed to maintain SVR. Tachycardia should be avoided; if it occurs, it should be treated (↑ anesthesia, esmolol if ventricular function is preserved). Sinus rhythm should be maintained. New onset atrial flutter/AF should be treated with defibrillation. Avoid factors that may increase PVR (N_2O, acidosis, hypoxia, hypercarbia).

MR: Maintain or augment preload, depending on response to fluid load. Inotropic agents may be useful to maintain co ntractility. Afterload reduction will improve forward flow. Generally SNP (0.5–4 mcg/kg/min) is used, but NTG (0.5–4 mcg/kg/min) may be more appropriate in patients with ischemia-induced regurgitation. Avoid ↑ PVR caused by N_2O, acidosis, hypoxia, or hypercarbia. IABP may be useful periop in patients with acute MR 2° MI (↓ afterload, ↑ coronary perfusion pressure).

Maintenance

Narcotic (total = fentanyl 10–100 mcg/kg, or sufentanil 5–20 mcg/kg) with benzodiazepine (e.g., midazolam 50–350 mcg/kg) for amnesia; low-dose isoflurane; O_2/air.

The following table summarizes the goals of intraop management:

Parameter	MS	MR
LV preload	Normal-to-↑	Normal →↑
HR	↓	↑
Rhythm	NSR	NSR
Contractility	Maintain	Maintain
SVR	Normal	↓
PVR	Avoid ↑	Avoid ↑

Postbypass

Although patients with MS generally do well after valve replacement, inotropes (e.g., dopamine, dobutamine) occasionally are necessary. This is especially true late in the disease when cardiomyopathy may be present.

Emergence

Transport to ICU, intubated and ventilated 6–24 h. Early extubation is possible if lower-dose narcotic technique is used (fast-track).

Blood and fluid requirements

IV: 14 ga × 1–2
NS/LR @ 6–8 mL/kg/h
Maintain UO 0.5–1 mL/kg/h.
Warm all fluids.
Humidify gases.

Monitoring

Standard monitors (p. B-1) Arterial line CVP line PA catheter Urinary catheter	Standard monitors and an A-line are placed before induction. CVP (and/or PA line, if indicated), usually is placed after intubation. Care should be exercised with PA catheter insertion, because the dilated PA may be susceptible to rupture with the catheter. In MS, PCWP may over estimate the LV filling pressure due to stenosis.
TEE	TEE may help in volume management, regional wall motion abnormalities (postacute MI) and in assessing the success of mitral valve repair. Occasionally, the use of a valve ring during repair may cause systolic anterior motion of the valve leaflet with resultant regurgitation, which may be seen on TEE.

Positioning

✓ and pad pressure points.
✓ eyes.

POSTOPERATIVE

Complications	Hemorrhage Tamponade Cardiac failure Dysrhythmias Conduction defects Atrioventricular disruption	Inotropic support or vasodilator therapy may be needed. IABP for mitral incompetence, especially in the presence of acute MR 2° infarction.
Pain management	Parenteral opioids for pain relief Benzodiazepine for sedation	
Tests	ECG CXR ABG Coag profile Electrolytes	

Suggested Readings

1. Calvinho P, Antunes M: Current surgical management of mitral regurgitation. *Expert Rev Cardiovasc Ther* 2008; 6(4):481–90.
2. Cook DJ, Housmans PR, Rehfeldt KH: Valvular heart disease: replacement and repair. In: *Kaplan's Cardiac Anesthesia,* 5th edition. Kaplan JA, ed. WB Saunders, Philadelphia: 2006, Ch 20.
3. Dunning J, Versteegh M, Fabbri A, et al. Guideline on antiplatelet and anticoagulation management in cardiac surgery. *Eur J Cardiothorac Surg* 2008.
4. Fann JI, Miller DC, Moore KA, et al: Twenty-year clinical experience with porcine bioprostheses. *Ann Thorac Surg* 1996; 62:1301–2.
5. Frasco PE, de Bruijn NP: Valvular heart disease. In: *Cardiac Anesthesia: Principles and Clinical Practice,* 2nd edition. Estafanous FG, Barash PG, Reves JG, eds. Lippincott Williams & Wilkins, Philadelphia: 2001, 557–84.
6. Greco E, Zaballos JM, Alvarez L, et al: Video-assisted mitral surgery through a micro-access: a safe and reliable reality in the current era. *J Heart Valve Dis* 2008; 17(1):48–53.

TRICUSPID VALVE REPAIR

SURGICAL CONSIDERATIONS

Description: Insufficiency of the tricuspid valve is almost always 2° left-sided valvular disease, with tricuspid annular dilatation and resultant valvular insufficiency usually 2° pulmonary HTN. Some congenital conditions (e.g., Ebstein's deformity) may persist into early adulthood, when replacement is usually necessary. Tricuspid repair is normally possible in the absence of primary involvement of tricuspid leaflets. The procedure is usually accomplished on CPB (see p. 336), either with the heart fibrillating or during a brief period of aortic cross-clamping and diastolic arrest. After instituting CPB and snaring the venous cannulae to prevent air entry into the pump circuit, the tricuspid valve is exposed through an incision in the right atrium. In the absence of leaflet involvement by the rheumatic process, repair usually can be accomplished by a simple **annuloplasty.** After atrial closure, evacuation of air, and myocardial resuscitation, the patient is weaned from CPB with vasodilator agents. Temporary pacing wires usually are inserted and passed to the anesthesiologist in case inadvertent injury to the AV node or His bundle causes complete heart block.

Variant procedure or approaches: Tricuspid valve replacement

Usual preop diagnosis: Tricuspid regurgitation, 2° annular dilatation 2° pulmonary HTN and left-side failure

SUMMARY OF PROCEDURE	
Position	Supine
Incision	Median sternotomy

SUMMARY OF PROCEDURE (cont'd)	
Special instrumentation	Intraop ECHO; hemodynamic monitoring; CPB
Antibiotics	Cefazolin 2 g iv prior to incision, then 1 g q 4 h
Surgical time	Aortic cross-clamp: 30–40 min CPB: 70–80 min Total: 3–4 h
EBL	400–800 mL (Long-standing tricuspid regurgitation may → impaired hepatic production of coagulation factors.)
Postop care	ICU × 1–3 d, intubated 6–24 h; vasodilator therapy for pulmonary HTN
Mortality	2–3%
Morbidity	3rd-degree heart block: 10% RV failure: 2–3%
Pain score	7–10

PATIENT POPULATION CHARACTERISTICS	
Age range	50–75 yr
Male:Female	1:1
Incidence	Rare
Etiology	Rheumatic; congenital (Ebstein's anomaly)
Associated conditions	Rheumatic involvement of left-side valves with pulmonary HTN

ANESTHETIC CONSIDERATIONS

PREOPERATIVE

Cardiovascular	**Tricuspid regurgitation (TR)** usually is well tolerated and Sx (↓ CO) may go unnoticed, masked by Sx associated with left-side valvular disease and pulmonary HTN. Occasionally, TR is 2° endocarditis and raises the suspicion of iv drug abuse. TR may be caused by pulmonary HTN → ↑ RV afterload → RV dilation, ↑ RV wall tension → dilation of tricuspid valve annulus and TR. Pathophysiology: • TR →↓ CO 2° ↑ RV size → shift of the intraventricular septum to the left →↓ LV size, ↓ LV compliance → LV underloading due to ↓ LV size and ↓ RV stroke volume. • TR → atrial fibrillation (AF) 2° ↑ right atrial size. In isolated insufficiency, the ↑ in right atrial pressure may result in shunting across a patent foramen ovale (PFO), leading to paradoxical embolization with potentially disastrous consequences. **Tests:** ECG: ✓ AF. ECHO: ✓ relative chamber size, contractility, PFO, valve lesions. Cardiac catheterization: ✓ contractility, CO, pulmonary pressures and their response to vasodilators, other valvular pathology.
Respiratory	Pulmonary HTN (> 25 mmHg mean pressure), pulmonary edema, and effusions may be present. **Tests:** CXR: ✓ pulmonary edema, pleural effusion.
Renal	Chronic venous congestion may → prerenal failure. **Tests:** BUN; Cr; electrolytes
Hepatic	Hepatic congestion may → impaired synthetic function, particularly coag factors. **Tests:** Consider PT; PTT

Hematologic	**Tests:** Hb/Hct; other tests as indicated from H&P and Sx. Consider viral testing (HIV, hepatitis in isolated tricuspid endocarditis or in iv drug abusers). T&C 2–4 U PRBCs.
Laboratory	Other tests as indicated from H&P.
Premedication	Standard premedication (p. B-1) is usually appropriate.

INTRAOPERATIVE

Anesthetic technique: GETA. An arterial line should be inserted, using liberal amounts of local anesthetic, before induction. The presence of real-time BP monitoring can be critical in the care of these patients, especially during induction. Although it is helpful to have a CVP line before induction for preload monitoring and drug infusion, it is not essential. This line usually is inserted after the patient is intubated. If infused drugs are necessary before the CVP catheter is in place, they can be administered through a separate peripheral iv.

Induction	Typically, O_2 and moderate- to high-dose narcotic (fentanyl 10–100 mcg/kg or sufentanil 2.5–20 mcg/kg) with etomidate (0.1–0.3 mg/kg) or midazolam (50–150 mcg/kg). Muscle relaxation is obtained with a nondepolarizing agent (e.g., pancuronium 0.1 mg/kg, vecuronium 0.1 mg/kg).	
Maintenance	The choice of narcotic/benzodiazepine/O_2 or volatile agent and O_2 will be determined by the underlying lesion and ventricular function. Avoid N_2O (pulmonary HTN). Low-dose isoflurane may be used. Benzodiazepines (e.g., midazolam 50–300 mcg/kg, diazepam 0.3–0.5 mg/kg) may be used for amnesia. Exact choice of agents for maintenance depends on underlying lesion, ventricular function, and coexisting disease. Management goals of TR are often those of coexisting valvular problems. The general principles, however, are: (1) Adequate preload (↓ preload →↓ RV stroke volume); (2) HR: normal-to-increased; (3) Contractility: normal. May require inotropic support for ↑ PVR, anesthetic myocardial depression or IPPV. (4) PVR: normal or decreased (high PVR →↓ RV stroke volume). (5) SVR: little effect unless it affects left-side pathology.	
Emergence	To ICU intubated and ventilated × 6–24 h. Early extubation may be possible if a lower-dose narcotic technique is used (fast-track).	
Blood and fluid requirements	IV: 14 ga × 1–2 NS/LR @ 6–8 mL/kg/h UO 0.5–1 mL/kg/h Warm all fluids. Humidify gases. T&C 2–4 U PRBC.	Because of the possibility of PFO and R→L shunt, ensure that all venous lines are clear of air.
Monitoring	Standard monitors (p. B-1) Arterial line CVP or PA catheter Urinary catheter	Standard monitors and an A-line are placed before induction. CVP (and/or PA line, if indicated), usually is placed after intubation. CVP may be a poor indicator of RV or LV filling. The PA catheter may be helpful in the management of fluid balance, CO, and management of pulmonary HTN, but may be difficult to place and will require removal while valve or annular ring is placed.
	TEE	Because RV distention may affect LV filling and stroke volume, TEE may be useful in judging filling and relative LV size.
Pulmonary HTN	↑ PVR can result from: ↓ PaO_2 ↑ $PaCO_2$ ↓ pH N_2O α-agonists	In TR, control of PVR is important because ↑ PVR may result in ↓ CO. Hypoxia, hypercarbia, acidosis, N_2O, or α-agonists may ↑ PVR. PVR may be reduced with hypocarbia, inotropic support with dobutamine (5–10 mcg/kg/min), isoproterenol (10–50 ng/kg/min), or amrinone (loading

Cardiovascular Surgery

Pulmonary HTN (cont'd)	Inadequate anesthesia	0.75 mg/kg, infusion 2–20 mcg/kg/min), and by using pulmonary vasodilators—NTG (1–4 mcg/kg/min), SNP (0.5–4 mcg/kg/min), prostaglandin E_1 (0.05–0.4 mcg/kg/min), or NO (0.1–100 ppm inhaled).
Positioning	✓ and pad pressure points. ✓ eyes.	
Complications	Coagulopathy Hemorrhage RV failure	Coagulopathy 2° prolonged bypass time for multiple valve replacements. RV failure 2° ↑ PVR (previously, RV decompressed by tricuspid incompetence). Rx includes inotropes: dobutamine (5–10 mcg/kg/min), isoproterenol (25–100 ng/kg/min), milrinone (loading 50 mcg/kg, infusion 0.3–0.75 mcg/kg/min), epinephrine (25–100 ng/kg/min), avoidance of factors causing ↑ PVR, and the use of pulmonary vasodilators.

POSTOPERATIVE

Complications	Hemorrhage Coagulopathy Dysrhythmias RV failure Infection Renal impairment Methemoglobinemia	Inotropic support and pulmonary vasodilators will need to be continued. Avoid those factors which ↑ PVR. Measure metHb levels during NO therapy.
Pain management	Parenteral opioids	Supplement with benzodiazepine for sedation.
Tests	ECG Coag profile Renal panel: BUN, Cr ABG Electrolytes	

Suggested Readings

1. Cook DJ, Housmans PR, Rehfeldt KH: Valvular heart disease: replacement and repair. In: *Kaplan's Cardiac Anesthesia*, 5th edition. Kaplan JA, ed. WB Saunders, Philadelphia: 2006, Ch 20.
2. Frasco PE, de Bruijn NP: Valvular heart disease. In: *Cardiac Anesthesia: Principles and Clinical Practice*, 2nd edition. Estafanous FG, Barash PG, Reves JG, eds. Lippincott Williams & Wilkins, Philadelphia: 2001, 557–84.

SEPTAL MYECTOMY/MYOTOMY

SURGICAL CONSIDERATIONS

Description: Patients with asymmetric septal hypertrophy usually present with symptoms 2° LV outflow tract obstruction (LVOTO), increased diastolic dysfunction and stiffness, or a combination of the two, manifested as syncope, CHF, or severe chest pain. The systolic hemodynamic abnormality is caused by the anterior leaflet of the mitral valve being drawn into the LV outflow tract (LVOT), and abutting the asymmetrically hypertrophied intraventricular septum, narrowing the LVOT, and producing a large intracavitary gradient. Additionally, severe mitral insufficiency may result. The most common surgical procedure for asymmetric septal hypertrophy is **septal myectomy/myotomy.** After institution of CPB, aortic cross-clamping, and cardioplegic arrest, the aorta is opened, and visualization of the subvalvar ventricular septum is attained. Bimanual palpation, as well as TEE visualization, can localize the asymmetric hypertrophy. Using the right coronary orifice as a landmark, the ventricular septum is longitudinally incised with two parallel incisions ~1 cm apart, with care being taken to avoid injury of the papillary muscle or mitral valve chordae. A trough of the hypertrophied septum is then excised, alleviating the LVOTO. Removal of a portion of the asymmetrically hypertrophied myopathic septum also usually reduces the systolic anterior motion (SAM) of the anterior mitral leaflet, and reduces the intracavitary gradient and mitral regurgitation (MR). Infrequently, mitral valve replacement may be necessary for persistent MR.

Usual preop diagnosis: Asymmetric septal hypertrophy with CHF, chest pain, and/or syncope

SUMMARY OF PROCEDURE

Position	Supine
Incision	Median sternotomy
Special instrumentation	TEE; hemodynamic monitoring; CPB
Unique considerations	Because of LV hypertrophy, maintenance of adequate preload is essential. Afterload also must be maintained to prevent LVOTO. Temporary pacing wires usually are placed at the start of the procedure.
Antibiotics	Cefazolin 2 g iv prior to incision, then 1 g q 4 h
Surgical time	2.5 h
EBL	150 mL
Postop care	ICU, intubated on ventilator 6–24 h
Mortality	3–4%
Morbidity	Complete heart block: 5% Persistent MR: 5% New aortic insufficiency: 2–5% CVA: < 1% VSD: < 1%
Pain score	6–10

PATIENT POPULATION CHARACTERISTICS

Age range	20–80 yr (mean = 45 yr)
Male:Female	1:1
Incidence	10/yr at Stanford University Medical Center
Etiology	Asymmetric septal hypertrophy

ANESTHETIC CONSIDERATIONS

PREOPERATIVE

Respiratory	Affected only 2° to cardiac failure.
Cardiovascular	Patients with idiopathic hypertrophic subaortic stenosis (IHSS) often present with Sx of syncope, angina pectoris (CAD), CHF, and palpitations. The main feature of IHSS is dynamic LVOTO 2° to septal hypertrophy and a possible venturi effect that draws the anterior mitral valve leaflet into the outflow tract. LVOTO →↑ LV hypertrophy →↓ compliance and

Cardiovascular Surgery

Cardiovascular (cont'd)	↓ diastolic function →↑ LVEDP, making diastolic filling dependent on preload and atrial contraction. Obstruction is worsened by decreased preload or afterload, increased contractility or HR. IHSS also results in ↑ MVO_2 and ↓ coronary perfusion, especially to the septum and subendocardium, which increases the risk of ischemia. Hypertrophy occurs throughout the whole myocardium and may lead to further dysfunction. MR, caused by a venturi suction effect, is often present and is exacerbated by the same conditions that increase LVOTO. (Note that ↓ afterload →↑ MR, unlike the usual [nonventuri-suction] form of MR.) Patients are often on β-blockers or Ca^{++} antagonists. These should be continued to day of surgery. **Tests:** ECG: ✓ Q-waves (indicative of septal hypertrophy); short PR interval with slurred QRS complex; supraventricular tachycardia; LV hypertrophy. ECHO: ✓ septal hypertrophy; MR; LV hypertrophy, myocardial dysfunction. Cardiac catheterization: ✓ LVOT pressure gradient, which may increase with provocation (e.g., Valsalva maneuver); obliteration of the LV cavity; MR; CAD.
Neurological	Document syncope and any neurological deficits.
Laboratory	Hb/Hct; electrolytes; other tests as indicated from H&P.
Premedication	Avoid activation of the sympathetic nervous system since this will cause ↑ HR and ↓ inotropy →↓ CO + ↓ BP. Thus, adequate anxiolysis is essential and can be obtained by premedication with a benzodiazepine (e.g., midazolam 0.05–0.2 mg/kg im, lorazepam 1–2 mg po, or diazepam 5–10 mg po). Avoid ↓ SVR, and maintain β-blockade and Ca^{++} channel blocker therapy.

Cardiovascular Surgery

INTRAOPERATIVE

Anesthetic technique: GETA. An arterial line should be inserted, using liberal amounts of local anesthetic, before induction. The presence of real-time BP monitoring can be critical in the care of these patients, especially during induction. Although it is helpful to have a CVP line before induction for preload monitoring and drug infusion, it is not essential. This line usually is inserted after the patient is intubated. If infused drugs are necessary before the CVP catheter is in place, they can be administered through a separate peripheral iv.

Induction	Typically, moderate- to high-dose narcotic (fentanyl 10–100 mcg/kg; avoid sufentanil due to vasodilation). Supplement with etomidate (0.1–0.3 mg/kg), midazolam (50–350 mcg/kg), or STP (2–4 mg/kg). Ketamine should be avoided due to the activation of the sympathetic nervous system. Introduction of a volatile agent prior to intubation may be helpful. Vecuronium (0.1 mg/kg) for muscle relaxation. Use pancuronium with caution (tachycardia) and avoid d-tubocurarine (↓ BP).	
Maintenance	O_2 and narcotic (total fentanyl 10–100 mcg/kg) + volatile agent. Midazolam (50–350 mcg/kg) can be used for amnesia. The cornerstone of anesthesia for IHSS is to avoid factors which will increase LVOTO: (1) ↓ preload, (2) ↓ afterload, (3) ↑ contractility, (4) loss of NSR, and (5) ↑ HR.	
Emergence	To ICU intubated and ventilated × 6–24 h. Early extubation is possible if a lower-dose narcotic technique is used (fast-track).	
Blood and fluid requirements	IV: 14 ga × 1–2 NS/LR @ 6–8 mL/kg/h Maintain UO 0.5–1 mL/h Warm fluids. Humidify gases.	
Monitoring	Standard monitors (p. B-1) Arterial line PA catheter Urinary catheter	Standard monitors and an A-line are placed before induction. CVP (and/or PA line, if indicated), usually is placed after intubation. A PA catheter is useful for assessment of LV filling (keep high normal PCWP) and for moni-

Monitoring (cont'd)		toring SVR (normal-to-high). A pacing or pace port PA catheter may be useful for conduction problems occurring postop.
	TEE	TEE is useful to judge LV filling, LV contractility, LVOTO, MR, and VSD.
Intraoperative problems	↓ Preload	Rx: volume, phenylephrine
	↓ Afterload	Rx: phenylephrine
	↑ Contractility	Rx: esmolol, halothane
	↑ HR	Rx: esmolol
	Loss of NSR	Rx: cardioversion, verapamil
	Complete heart block	Should have reliable means of pacing available, including temporary ventricular leads.
	VSD	Septum may be damaged, → VSD (diagnosed by TEE). If present, it should be repaired.
Position	✓ and pad pressure points. ✓ eyes.	

POSTOPERATIVE

Complications	Hemorrhage	Dx: from chest tube drainage. Rx with blood and factors as needed. ✓ coag status. May require reexploration.
	Complete heart block	Pacing should be available. Occasionally, inotropes of vasodilators required. β-blockers and Ca^{++} antagonists usually D/C'd.
	Late VSD	Late VSD, indicated by development of a murmur, will require repair.
	Tamponade	Dx: by raising filling pressure, equalization of CVP, and PADP, ↓ CO, ↓ UO, and by ECHO. Rx: re-exploration and drainage.
Pain management	Parenteral opioids	Supplement with benzodiazepine for sedation.
Tests	ECG: ✓ conduction problems. ABG ECHO: ✓ LVOTO; VSD. Coag profile Electrolytes	

Suggested Readings

1. Cook DJ, Housmans PR, Rehfeldt KH : Valvular heart disease: replacement and repair. In: *Kaplan's Cardiac Anesthesia*, 5th edition. Kaplan JA, ed. WB Saunders, Philadelphia: 2006, Ch 20.
2. Frasco PE, de Bruijn NP: Valvular heart disease. In: *Cardiac Anesthesia: Principles and Clinical Practice*, 2nd edition. Estafanous FG, Barash PG, Reves JG, eds. Lippincott Williams & Wilkins, Philadelphia: 2001, 557–84.
3. Maron BJ: Hypertrophic cardiomyopathy: a systematic review. *JAMA* 2002; 287(10):1308–20.
4. Togni M, Billinger M, Cook S, et al: Septal myectomy: cut, coil, or boil? *Eur Heart J* 2008; 29(3):296–8.

PACEMAKER INSERTION

SURGICAL CONSIDERATIONS

Description: Pacemaker insertion may be required for relief of abnormalities of the conduction system. A transvenous pacemaker lead may be placed via the subclavian vein, through the tricuspid valve into the RV (single-chamber pacing); or two leads may be placed, one into the right atrium and the other into the RV (dual-chamber pacing). Typically, 2nd- or 3rd-degree heart block is the diagnostic indication, although sick sinus syndrome (SSS) and other abnormalities also may be found. Access to the subclavian veins usually is attained percutaneously, although a cut-down may be used to expose the cephalic vein in the deltopectoral groove. Passage of a guide wire into the RV may cause frequent premature ventricular beats, which usually subside spontaneously with repositioning of the guide wire or lead. After ventricular and/or atrial lead placement, the pacing lead will have to be tested for sensing threshold, pacing threshold, depolarization amplitude, and lead resistance. After satisfactory placement of the pacing leads, the actual pacemaker generator unit is connected and then placed in a subcutaneous pocket at the site of percutaneous lead placement.

Usual preop diagnosis: Abnormalities of S-A nodal function (SSS) or A-V nodal function (heart block)

SUMMARY OF PROCEDURE

Position	Supine
Incision	Left subclavicular; mostly percutaneous
Special instrumentation	Fluoroscopy with fluoro-table
Unique considerations	Patient usually awake with mild sedation
Antibiotics	Cefazolin 1 g iv prior to incision
Surgical time	1 h
EBL	Minimal
Postop care	PACU → CCU; ECG monitoring × 2–4 h; chest radiograph to document lead configuration.
Mortality	0–1%
Morbidity	Lead displacement: 1–2% Pneumothorax: 1–2%
Pain score	2

PATIENT POPULATION CHARACTERISTICS

Age range	50–80 yr
Male:Female	2:1
Incidence	Infrequent
Etiology	CAD; cardiac valve repair/replacement
Associated conditions	Complete heart block with syncope; SSS; paroxysmal tachycardia; SVT

Table 6.1-4. Five-Position Pacemaker Code (ICHD)

I	II	III	IV	V
Chamber(s) paced	**Chamber(s) sensed**	**Response(s) to sensing**	**Programmability, rate modulation**	**Special tachyarrhythmia functions**
V - Ventricle	V - Ventricle	T - Triggered	P - Simple Programmable (rate and/or output)	B-Bursts
A - Atrium	A - Atrium	I - Inhibited	M -Multiprogrammable	N - Normal rate competition
D - Dual	D - Dual	D - Dual (T + I)	C - Communicating	S - Scanning
O - None	O - None	O - None	R - Rate modulation	
			O - None	E - External

ANESTHETIC CONSIDERATIONS

PREOPERATIVE

The indications for permanent pacemaker insertion are usually bradydysrhythmias (e.g., 3rd-degree heart block, sinus node dysfunction, etc.) or, less commonly, tachycardia (e.g., atrial flutter not responsive to medical therapy). There are many different types of pacemakers, which are classified according to the chamber paced, chamber sensed, response to sensing, programmability, and antitachyrhythmia functions. The anesthesiologist should be aware of the type of pacemaker to be implanted and the means for external control.

Cardiovascular	Evaluate patient for associated disease, including CAD (~50%), HTN (~20%), cardiomyopathy, CHF, valvular defect, and for any symptoms or recent changes related to the conduction problems (syncope, CHF). It is important to know the reason for pacemaker implantation and the patient's escape rhythm. These patients are often on antidysrhythmics, diuretics, cardiac glycosides, and a variety of other cardiovascular agents, which should be continued up to the day of surgery. **Tests:** Exercise tolerance by Hx. ECG: ✓ rate, ischemic changes, rhythm. Other tests as indicated by H&P. ✓ serum digoxin and other antidysrhythmic levels.
Pacemaker	If a permanent pacemaker is already in place, its type and present functional state should be assessed. (Sx of problems include chest pain, palpitations, syncope, and weakness.) If no permanent pacemaker, a temporary transvenous pacemaker should be placed before surgery, except in unusual circumstances. **Tests:** ECG: ✓ Valsalva maneuver or carotid sinus massage—may slow the heart sufficiently to allow the permanent pacemaker to fire and allow assessment of function. A rate lower than the set rate may indicate battery failure. CXR: ✓ lead continuity.
Hematologic	Hct or Hb
Laboratory	✓ K^+ level, which can affect pacing threshold, → loss of pacemaker capture, if low, or ventricular tachycardia, if high. Other tests as indicated from H&P.
Premedication	Standard premedication (p. B-1)

INTRAOPERATIVE

Anesthetic technique: Permanent pacemakers commonly are placed via the transvenous route, requiring only local anesthesia and MAC with sedation. For epicardial pacemaker placement, GETA is required. These patients should be monitored during transport to OR. Care is taken to avoid dislodging temporary pacing electrodes. The function of the temporary pacemaker should be checked prior to induction.

General anesthesia:

Induction	Usually anesthesia can be induced with propofol (1–2 mg/kg) or etomidate (0.2–0.3 mg/kg) in combination with an opiate (e.g., fentanyl 1–2 mcg/kg) to attenuate the response to intubation. Vecuronium (0.1 mg/kg) or rocuronium (1 mg/kg) will provide adequate muscle relaxation.	
Maintenance	Standard maintenance (p. B-2). Avoid excessive hyperventilation (→↓ K^+) and use volatile agents with caution, because they may increase A-V conduction time.	
Emergence	Generally, patient is extubated at the end of the case.	
Blood and fluid requirements	Minimal fluid requirements IV: 16 ga × 1 NS/LR @ 4–6 mL/kg/h	
Monitoring	Standard monitors (p. B-1) Urinary catheter	Rarely, arterial line if patient disease indicates.

Electrocautery interference	Minimize by: • Using bipolar cautery, if possible; • Grounding pad on leg; • Limiting cautery output; • Limiting cautery use.	The use of electrocautery may interfere with pacemaker function and → dysrhythmias or failure of the pacemaker. Monitor ECG and pulse (since electrical activity does not mean CO) for interference. Have a magnet available to convert the pacemaker to asynchronous mode (check that this is possible and will not change the programming of the pacemaker).
Complications	Dysrhythmias Air embolism Cardiac tamponade Hemo/pneumothorax Hemorrhage	Availability of temporary pacing is important because complete heart block or dislodgement of leads may occur. In addition, pharmacologic agents (atropine, 0.5–2 mg; isoproterenol 10–100 ng/kg/min) to increase HR should be available.

POSTOPERATIVE

Complications	Dislodging of electrodes Dysrhythmias Pneumothorax Tamponade
Pain management	Parenteral opioids for pain relief Benzodiazepine for sedation
Tests	ECG CXR Electrolytes

Suggested Readings

1. Luck JC: Arrhythmia, rhythm management devices, and catheter surgical ablation. In: *A Practical Approach to Cardiac Anesthesia,* 4th edition. Hensley FA, Martin DE, Gravlee GP, eds. Lippincott Williams & Wilkins, Philadelphia: 2008, Ch 4.
2. Reynolds DW, Murray CM: New concepts in physiologic cardiac pacing. *Curr Cardiol Rep* 2007; 9(5):351–7.
3. Rosenfeld LE, Elefteriades JA: Surgical and device therapy for cardiac arrhythmias. In: *Cardiac Anesthesia: Principles and Clinical Practice,* 2nd edition. Estafanous FG, Barash PG, Reves JG, eds. Lippincott Williams & Wilkins, Philadelphia: 2001, 617–36.
4. Rozner MA: The patient with a cardiac pacemaker or implanted defibrillator and management during anaesthesia. *Curr Opin Anaesthesiol* 2007; 20(3):261–8.

PERICARDIECTOMY

SURGICAL CONSIDERATIONS

Description: Constrictive pericarditis, either acute or chronic, interferes with ventricular filling, reducing stroke volume and depressing the cardiac index (CI). Although there are many possible etiologies (infectious, nephrogenic, postradiation), the cause remains unknown for a majority of patients. Typically, patients present with a progressive Hx of breathlessness, fatigability, or peripheral or abdominal swelling, often months to years after the inciting event. The Dx may be confirmed by cardiac catheterization, with equalization of end diastolic pressures, although volume loading may be necessary to demonstrate this in the patient under medical management. The differentiation between constrictive pericardial disease and restrictive myocardial disease may be difficult, if not impossible, and may coexist in a single patient. After this Dx has been confirmed, surgical **pericardiectomy** should be undertaken, because the outlook without surgical relief is one of gradual, but persistent deterioration. Although surgical mortality remains in the 10–15% range, long-term relief for survivors is good. Because these patients are usually significantly compromised hemodynamically, intensive monitoring is indicated. Approach may be through a **median sternotomy** or left **anterolateral thoracotomy.** Removal of both visceral and parietal pericardium is essential for relief, but dense adhesions of these layers to underlying muscle may make this dissection very difficult, tedious, and bloody, especially if the visceral pericardium and epicardium are involved in the constrictive process. CPB (see p. 336) may be utilized for hemodynamic instability, but it obviously increases bleeding complications. Complete excision from both ventricular surfaces is mandatory. Most periop difficulties evolve from cardiac failure.

Variant procedure or approaches: A limited **pericardial window,** draining fluid into the left hemithorax, may relieve tamponade, but will be of no benefit for a true constrictive process.

Usual preop diagnosis: Constrictive pericarditis

SUMMARY OF PROCEDURES

	Median Sternotomy	Anterolateral Thoracotomy
Position	Supine	Supine, with elevation of left hemithorax
Incision	Midline	5th interspace
Special instrumentation	TEE; full hemodynamic monitoring; CPB standby	⇐
Antibiotics	Cefazolin 2 g iv prior to incision, then 1 g q 4 h	⇐
Surgical time	2–5 h, depending on tenacity of visceral peel	⇐
Closing considerations	Avoid volume overload and cardiac distention. Chronically depressed hearts may require inotropic or mechanical support (i.e., IABP) postop.	⇐
EBL	100–500 mL	⇐
Postop care	ICU; intubated × 4–6 h. Hemodynamic monitoring. Low CO state may persist postop.	⇐
Mortality	5–15%, predominantly from cardiac failure	⇐
Morbidity	Persistent CHF: 5%	⇐
	Transient phrenic nerve dysfunction: < 1%	
Pain score	7–10	7–10

PATIENT POPULATION CHARACTERISTICS

Age range	10–80 yr (median = 45 yr)
Male:Female	2:1
Incidence	3–4 patients/yr at tertiary referral center
Etiology	Majority unknown. Infectious, radiation, prior cardiac operation, rheumatic pericarditis, amyloid deposition.
Associated conditions	Restrictive myocardial diseases

ANESTHETIC CONSIDERATIONS

PREOPERATIVE

Pericardiectomy is performed most commonly for patients with constrictive pericarditis, whereas pericardial window procedures are used for patients with cardiac tamponade.

Respiratory	Restrictive disease may be present 2° fibrosis (e.g., post-TB) or pleural effusions. This may impair oxygenation and, if the effusions are significant, may ↓ venous return on institution of IPPV → rapid decompensation (↓ CO). Drain prior to surgery. **Tests:** CXR: ✓ active disease, fibrosis, effusions, pericardial calcification. Consider ABG, PFT, as indicated by CXR and Sx and if time permits.
Cardiovascular	Of importance is the presence or absence of a pericardial effusion. A large effusion that develops slowly (chronic pericarditis) may cause minimal Sx. Conversely, a small and rapidly forming effusion may → cardiac tamponade. Although the cardiovascular signs for both tamponade and constriction are similar (pulsus paradoxus, venous HTN, exaggerated venous pulsations, ↓ BP, tachycardia), it is important to differentiate between them because it may affect intraop management. Constrictive pericarditis can be differentiated from cardiac tamponade by ECHO, by pulsus paradoxus (frequent, with tamponade; rare, with constrictive pericarditis). Kussmaul's sign (distention of the jugular veins on inspiration) is rare with tamponade and common with constrictive pericarditis. Electrical alternans is present with tamponade and absent in constrictive pericarditis. Examination of the RV pressure wave form is unchanged in tamponade, but shows a dip and prominent Y descent in constrictive pericarditis. Anesthetic management is influenced by the planned procedure, the underlying process (constriction or tamponade), and its severity. Clues to severity are the physical symptoms and the degree of tachycardia, ↓ BP, and the filling pressure. (Although it is not possible to give exact figures, a HR of >100 bpm, systolic BP < 100 mmHg, and a filling pressure > 15 mmHg are probably significant.) In addition, it is important to assess concurrent cardiac problems: cardiomyopathy, CAD, or valvular disease (especially in constrictive disease associated with TB, radiation therapy, or in rheumatoid diseases, such as lupus). **Tests:** ECG: ✓ low-voltage complexes, electrical alternans. ECHO: ✓ pericardial effusion, calcification of pericardium, valvular lesions, myocardial function.
Gastrointestinal	Chronic hepatic congestion may →↓ synthetic function (↓ procoagulants). Development of ascites may →↑ intra-abdominal pressure. Because of this and the fact that these are sometimes emergency procedures, consider possible full stomach. **Tests:** Consider LFTs; PT; PTT
Renal	Renal failure may cause pericarditis and, conversely, pericarditis may cause renal failure (2° prerenal factors: ↑ venous pressure, ↓ perfusion pressure). This may affect the choice of drugs used for anesthesia that depend on renal clearance (particularly muscle relaxants). **Tests:** BUN; Cr; consider creatinine clearance; electrolytes.
Hematologic	Some renal or hepatic conditions may be associated with coagulation disorders. These include both procoagulant and Plt problems. If possible, any coagulopathy should be corrected before surgery with FFP, Plt, or both. Consult with a hematologist, if necessary. **Tests:** Hb/Hct; PT; PTT; Plt count
Laboratory	Other tests as indicated from H&P.
Premedication	Little or no premedication may be indicated; otherwise, a benzodiazepine (e.g., midazolam 0.05–0.2 mg/kg im) may be used. Consider full-stomach precautions: H_2-antagonists (e.g., ranitidine 50 mg iv), metoclopramide (10 mg iv), antacids (e.g., Na citrate 0.3 M 30 mL po).

INTRAOPERATIVE

Anesthetic technique: GETA. An arterial line should be inserted, using liberal amounts of local anesthetic, before induction. The presence of real-time BP monitoring can be critical in the care of these patients, especially during induction. Although it is helpful to have a CVP line before induction for preload monitoring and drug infusion, it is not essential. This line usually is inserted after the patient is intubated. If infused drugs are necessary before the CVP catheter is in place, they can be administered through a separate peripheral iv. Consider pericardiocentesis or pericardial window under local anesthesia prior to induction, as drainage of even a small amount of fluid may improve the patient's status dramatically. The considerable manipulation of the heart, extensive dissection, blood loss, dysrhythmias, and unrelieved tamponade make pericardiectomy cases a challenge.

Induction	Typically, ketamine (1–2 mg/kg) or etomidate (0.2–0.3 mg/kg) ± narcotic (fentanyl 2–30 mcg/kg), depending on patient status. Consider maintaining spontaneous ventilation in tamponade patients until drained, as institution of IPPV may result in rapid decompensation and cardiac arrest due to ↓ ↓ venous return. Otherwise, succinylcholine (1 mg/kg) with cricoid pressure (full stomach) or vecuronium (0.1 mg/kg) for muscle relaxation. For unstable patients, may prep and drape and have surgeons standing by before induction of anesthesia.	
Maintenance	Narcotic (total fentanyl 5–50 mcg/kg), low-dose volatile agent, midazolam (50–350 mcg/kg), or a combination of these agents in 100% O_2. CO is dependent on maintaining a high preload to ensure adequate cardiac filling, avoiding and treating bradycardia and preserving myocardial contractility. The use of inotropes (dopamine, isoproterenol, or epinephrine) may be necessary; α-agonists should be avoided but, on occasion, may be needed to increase coronary perfusion. These anesthetic-considerations apply to both tamponade and constrictive disease. In patients with acute tamponade, dramatic increases in BP may occur when the pericardium is opened. Aggressive use of vasodilators and additional anesthetic agents may be necessary.	
Emergence	In general, plan for extubation in the OR in the case of pericardial window and transport to ICU for postop ventilation 4–24 h following pericardiectomy.	
Blood and fluid requirements	IV: 14 ga (or 7 Fr) × 1–2 UO: 0.5–1 mL/kg/h Warm fluids and humidify gases. T&C 2–4 U for pericardiectomy.	During pericardiectomy, anticipate rapid blood loss (a major cause of mortality). For this reason, CPB should be available on standby for all pericardiectomy procedures.
Monitoring	Standard monitors (p. B-1) Arterial line CVP line PA catheter TEE Urinary catheter	Standard monitors and an A-line are placed before induction. CVP (and/or PA line, if indicated), usually is placed after intubation. PA catheters aid the management of filling pressures, CO and afterload. TEE may be useful to gauge filling volume and degree of relief of pericardial constriction.
Complications	Cardiac tamponade Dysrhythmias	Intrathoracic pressure associated with IPPV may produce a ↓ ↓ CO in these patients (because of ↓ venous return). Spontaneous ventilation, therefore, is preferred until the tamponade is drained.
	Hemorrhage Coagulopathy Heart failure	Hemorrhage is not usually a problem unless penetrating trauma is the cause of the tamponade. Once constriction is relieved, myocardial function does not return to normal quickly. Inotropes are often needed. Due to extensive dissection and hemorrhage, coagulopathies may develop and should be treated aggressively.
Positioning	✓ and pad pressure points. ✓ eyes.	

POSTOPERATIVE

Complications	Hemorrhage Coagulopathy Ventricular hypofunction Dysrhythmias	Following pericardial window surgery, patients improve with the relief of the tamponade. Post-pericardiectomy patients, however, may have a continuation of intraop dysrhythmias and

Complications (cont'd)	Ischemia	myocardial depression. Inotropes (e.g., dopamine 5–10 mcg/kg/min) may be needed for 24–48 h. Normal cardiac function can take 4–6 wk to return.
Pain management	Parenteral opioids	Supplement with benzodiazepine for sedation.
Tests	ECG CXR ABG Coag profile Electrolytes	

Suggested Readings

1. DiNardo JA, Zvara DA: Pericardial disease. In: *Anesthesia for Cardiac Surgery,* 3rd edition. Blackwell Science, Massachusetts: 2008, Ch 8.
2. Hoit BD: Pericardial disease and pericardial tamponade. *Crit Care Med* 2007; 35(8 Suppl):S355–64.
3. Savage RM, Aronson S, Shanewise JS, et al: Intraoperative echocardiography. In: *Cardiac Anesthesia: Principles and Clinical Practice,* 2nd edition. Estafanous FG, Barash PG, Reves JG, eds. Lippincott Williams & Wilkins, Philadelphia: 2001, 237–94.

CHAPTER

6.2 Minimally Invasive Cardiac Surgery

SURGEON

James I. Fann, MD

ANESTHESIOLOGIST

Lawrence C. Siegel, MD

OFF-PUMP AND MINIMALLY INVASIVE CORONARY ARTERY BYPASS GRAFTING

SURGICAL CONSIDERATIONS

Description: Although coronary artery bypass grafting (CABG) without cardiopulmonary bypass (CPB) was originally proposed more than 5 decades ago, development and advances in CPB resulted in the abandonment of off-pump cardiac surgery by most cardiac centers until the 1990s. The resurgence of off-pump coronary revascularization was due in part to reported adverse effects of CPB, increased comorbidities in an aging population, medical economics, and the development of reliable mechanical stabilization devices (Fig. 6.2-1). From the standpoint of terminology, off-pump coronary artery bypass grafting (OPCAB), applies to all cases of coronary revascularization not using the CPB circuit; and, while it does not refer directly to the surgical approach, most are via conventional median sternotomy. Minimally invasive direct coronary artery bypass grafting (MIDCAB) refers to off-pump coronary revascularization via a small anterolateral thoracotomy incision. Challenges of off-pump coronary revascularization include accurate vascular anastomosis, while minimizing hemodynamic perturbations during the procedure. Interrupting flow to the target artery can → regional ischemia, arrhythmias, and hemodynamic instability; displacing the heart to expose lateral or posterior arteries may → ventricular compression and profound hemodynamic compromise. Pharmacologic interventions to decrease HR and ischemic preconditioning may facilitate the anastomosis. Although not fully defined, ischemic preconditioning results from exposure to transient myocardial ischemia and is an endogenous adaptation that may mitigate the effects of subsequent prolonged myocardial ischemia. Thus, mechanically occluding the coronary artery for a brief period may confer some protection from ischemic injury associated with coronary occlusion during the anastomosis. Important preop considerations include the number and suitability of distal-target coronary arteries, cardiac and pulmonary status, and other medical comorbidities. The presence of cardiomegaly may limit the degree of intraop cardiac manipulation. The perfusionist is present during the procedure so that rapid conversion to conventional on-pump CABG can be achieved if there is hemodynamic compromise, unsuitable distal target, inability

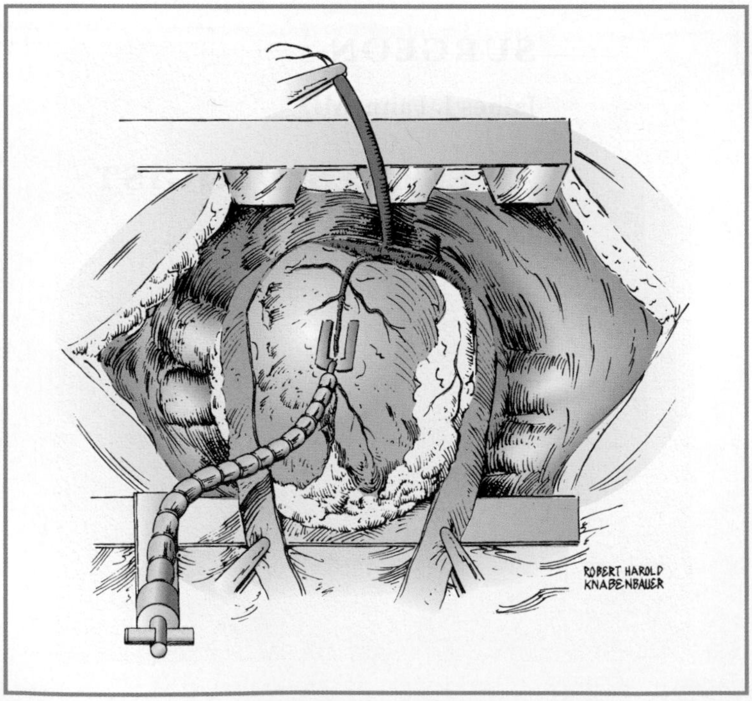

Figure 6.2-1. Manipulation of the heart and placement of a pressure-plate mechanical stabilizer is performed in preparation for OPCAB. (Reproduced with permission from Estafanous FG, Barash PG, Reves JG: *Cardiac Anesthesia: Principles and Clinical Practice,* 2nd edition. Lippincott Williams & Wilkins, Philadelphia: 2001.)

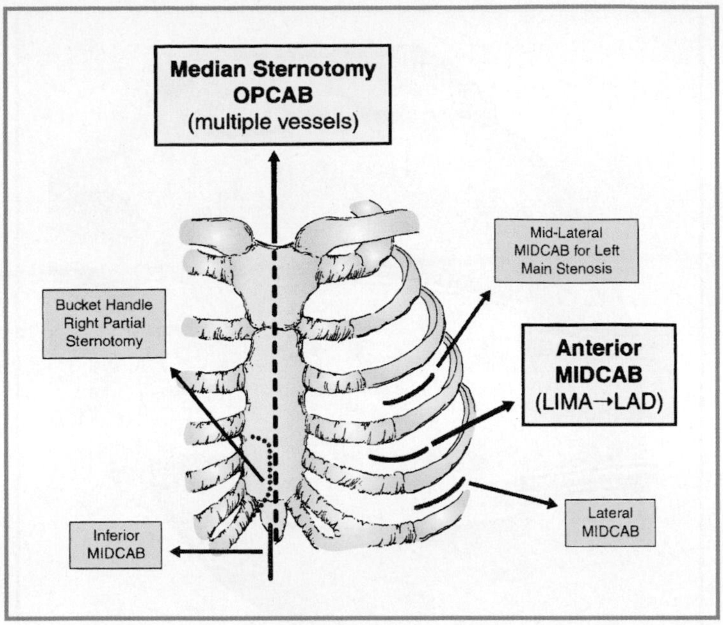

Figure 6.2-2. Incision sites for access to various target coronary arteries in MICAB. (Reproduced with permission from Estafanous FG, Barash PG, Reves JG: *Cardiac Anesthesia: Principles and Clinical Practice,* 2nd edition. Lippincott Williams & Wilkins, Philadelphia: 2001.)

to expose lateral or posterior target vessels, or regional myocardial ischemia. Occasionally, placement of intraaortic balloon pump intraop may facilitate the off-pump approach in a patient with ischemic cardiomyopathy.

For conventional **OPCAB**, a standard median sternotomy is made (Fig. 6.2-2). If the internal mammary artery (IMA) is to be used as a graft, it is harvested in the usual fashion. The patient is partially heparinized, and an intravenous bolus of lidocaine is given. A sternal retractor with attachments for coronary stabilization is placed (Fig. 6.2-1). If vein grafts are used, the proximal anastomoses may be performed at this point or later, after the completion of the distal anastomoses, using a partial side-biting aortic cross-clamp. During the period of partial aortic clamping, BP typically is lowered to reduce potential complications associated with the use of the clamp. The goal of the operation is to establish adequate perfusion of the most critical vascular bed first. Provided it is a target vessel, the LAD artery is often approached first because an IMA graft (or vein graft) can provide immediate perfusion and requires minimal cardiac manipulation to construct the anastomosis. Mechanical coronary artery stabilizers, based on local myocardial compression (Fig. 6.2-1) or vacuum suction (Fig. 6.2-3) and attached to the retractor, provide stable local epicardial motion restraint, thereby facilitating the anastomosis. After stabilization, the artery is occluded (following a period of ischemic preconditioning), and an arteriotomy is made. Equipment that minimizes blood in the operative site includes standard suction attachments, temporary intracoronary shunts, vessel occluders, and "blower-misters" that displace blood by delivering a combination of gas (CO_2) and heparinized saline. The distal anastomosis is then performed. The patient is monitored closely at this point for any signs of myocardial ischemia and/or hemodynamic instability. To expose the lateral and posterior target vessels, manipulation of the heart is necessary and may not be well tolerated. During lateral and posterior pericardial suture placement, the surgeon displaces and compresses the heart, resulting in temporary hemodynamic compromise. Ventilation may need to be decreased temporarily to facilitate this maneuver. Additional exposure techniques include the use of an apical suction device to facilitate cardiac manipulation with potentially less hemodynamic compromise, Trendelenburg position and tilting the operating table to the right, release of right pericardial stay sutures, opening of the right pleura, and incising the right pericardium, and placement of laparotomy sponges. The target vessel is stabilized again, ischemic preconditioning is carried out, and the artery is opened. After construction of the distal anastomosis, the graft is relieved of any residual air before securing the sutures and the proximal anastomosis performed if not already done so as noted earlier. Graft flow is assessed using a Doppler flow probe.

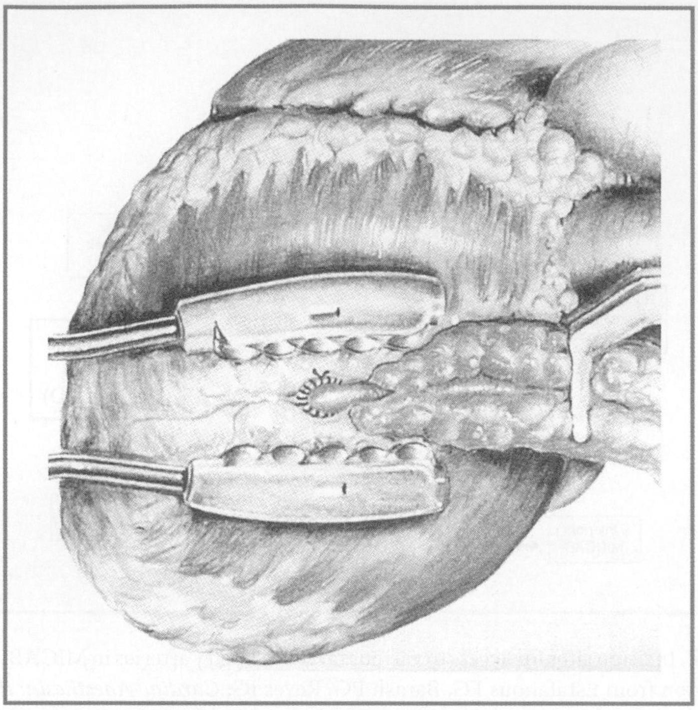

Figure 6.2-3. The Octopus stabilizer (Medtronic, Minneapolis MN) uses a series of suction cups on two fixed arms that adhere to the epicardial surface and reduce myocardial motion at the anastomotic site during OPCAB. (Reproduced with permission from Estafanous FG, Barash PG, Reves JG: *Cardiac Anesthesia: Principles and Clinical Practice,* 2nd edition. Lippincott Williams & Wilkins, Philadelphia: 2001.)

SUMMARY OF PROCEDURE	
Position	Supine (Fig. 6.2-4)
Incision	Median sternotomy (OPCAB); alternatively, limited left anterolateral thoracotomy (MIDCAB) (Fig. 6.2-2)
Antibiotics	Cefazolin 1 g iv
Surgical time	3–4 h
Closing considerations	No special considerations. Patients often can be extubated in OR.
EBL	200–400 mL (consider using Cell-Saver)
Postop care	ICU for cardiac monitoring ± ventilator management; less volume required than with conventional CABG.
Mortality	0–5% (higher with increasing age)
Morbidity	AF: 10–30% Pulmonary insufficiency: 3–5% Reoperation for bleeding: 1–4% Cardiac (e.g., myocardial infarction): 0–4% Mediastinal infection: 1–2% Neurologic (cerebrovascular accident): 1–2% Renal dysfunction: 1–2% IABP use: 0–2%
Pain score	4–6

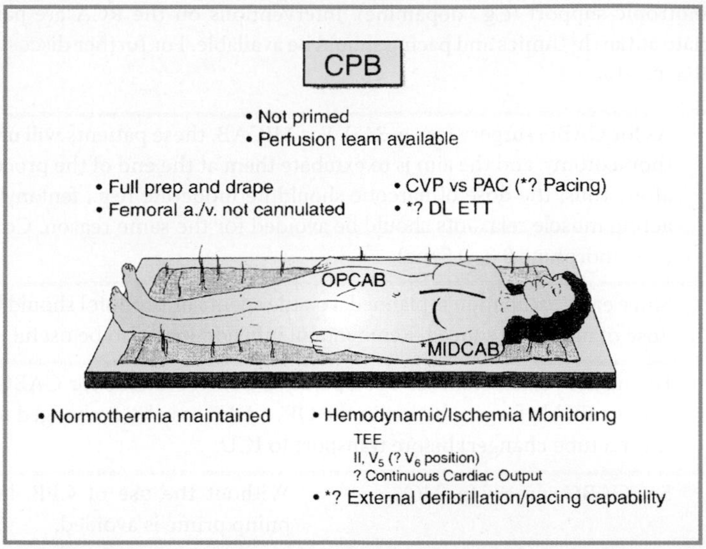

Figure 6.2-4. OR configuration for MICAB. (Reproduced with permission from Estafanous FG, Barash PG, Reves JG: *Cardiac Anesthesia: Principles and Clinical Practice,* 2nd edition. Lippincott Williams & Wilkins, Philadelphia: 2001.)

PATIENT POPULATION CHARACTERISTICS	
Age range	40 to > 90 yr
Male:Female	3:2
Incidence	150,000/yr in the United States.
Etiology	Multifactorial for atherosclerosis
Associated conditions	HTN; diabetes; PVD; COPD; cigarette smoking

ANESTHETIC CONSIDERATIONS FOR MICAB/OPCAB

PREOPERATIVE

Preop assessment is similar to that used for standard CABG patients (see p. 344). Relative contraindications for MICAB include: low EF, morbid obesity, previous cardiac surgery, AF, and COPD. It is important to know the coronary artery anatomy and the planned surgical procedure and sequence. For example, proximal surgical occlusion of a coronary artery with high grade distal disease may be poorly tolerated as compared with severe proximal disease with collateralization.

Premedication	Adequate control of preop anxiety using midazolam (titrated to effect) may reduce periop tachycardia.

INTRAOPERATIVE

Anesthetic technique: GETA. For MICAB, selective lung ventilation with DLT, Univent ETT, or bronchial blocker. Unlike CABG on CPB, the anesthetic demands for OPCABG are somewhat different, as CPB will not be providing hemodynamic support. Positioning of the heart for access to the target vessel, as well as mechanical stabilization of the heart to immobilize the vessel for accurate anastomosis tend to produce hemodynamic compromise. In particular, elevation of the LV apex to allow access to lateral and posterior wall vessels can limit LV filling and obstruct RV outflow tract. Additionally, ↓ TV may be necessary to prevent obstruction of visualization. Snares may be placed around the coronary target vessel to create a dry operative field; however, this may provoke regional ischemia. Many of these changes are assessed by intraop TEE, and they may require resuscitative measures with volume loading, vasoconstriction and inotropic support (e.g., dopamine). Interventions on the RCA are particularly prone to arrhythmias and appropriate antiarrhythmics and pacing should be available. For further discussion, see Intraoperative considerations for CABG, p. 345.

Induction	As for CABG surgery (see p. 345). For MICAB, these patients will undergo a small anterior thoracotomy, and the aim is to extubate them at the end of the procedure or shortly thereafter. Thus, the dose of narcotic should be moderate (e.g., fentanyl 5–15 mcg/kg). Long-acting muscle relaxants should be avoided for the same reason. Consider spinal narcotics (e.g., morphine 0.3–0.5 mg).	
Maintenance	Since early extubation is planned, volatile agents or propofol should be used and the overall dose of narcotic reduced. Remifentanil infusion may also be useful.	
Emergence	For further discussion, see Postoperative Considerations for CABG, p. 347. If the patient is not suitable for extubation in the OR, a DLT may be exchanged for a conventional ETT (over a tube changer) before transport to ICU.	
Blood and fluid requirements	See CABG surgery (p. 346).	Without the use of CPB, hemodilution from the pump prime is avoided.
Monitoring	See CABG surgery (p. 346).	Central venous access. PA catheters are useful for detecting ischemia in patients with poor LV function. If a continuous CO thermodilution catheter is used, consideration must be given to the large delays in data display. ST segment analysis.
	TEE	Useful for detecting ischemia and LV dysfunction. Views may be limited by surgical positioning of the heart within the chest.
Special considerations	Anticoagulation	Heparin should be administered before surgical coronary artery occlusion.
	Ischemic preconditioning Temporary occlusion → ischemia	Prior to occlusion, ischemic preconditioning may be accomplished with surgical manipulation and by pharmacologic means (e.g., isoflurane, sevoflurane). This is a great opportunity to consider how well transient ischemia is tolerated. During grafting, the vessel is temporarily occluded to avoid flooding the field with blood. The myocardium distal to this may become ischemic.
	✓ ECG, TEE.	TEE imaging will be affected by surgical mechanical manipulation of the heart and ECG voltage may be decreased.
	Cardiac positioning →↓ CO	Cardiac output may be markedly reduced by the combination of heart positioning and coronary artery occlusion. Vasoconstriction may be required to maintain adequate blood pressure. Patients poorly responsive to vasoconstrictors may have extremely depressed cardiac output and severe acidosis. Inotropic support or intra-aortic balloon pumping may be necessary.
	Coronary artery shunt	Surgical placement of a coronary artery shunt may be necessary. Treatment of rhythm disorders with pharmacologic agents, pacing, or defibrillation may be required. The capability to institute CPB rapidly should exist. A rest period with the heart returned to the normal position within the chest should be considered following each anastomosis to restore cardiac output and permit resolution of acidosis.

Positioning	✓ and pad pressure points. ✓ eyes.	

POSTOPERATIVE

Complications	See CABG surgery (p. 347). Premature extubation	
Pain management	Same as CABG surgery (p. 347).	Intrathecal narcotics or intercostal blocks (MICAB) placed at the end of surgery may aid in early extubation.
Tests	See CABG surgery (p. 347).	

Suggested Readings – Surgeon's

1. Baumgartner FJ, Gheissari A, Capouya ER, et al: Technical aspects of total revascularization in off-pump coronary bypass via sternotomy approach. *Ann Thorac Surg* 1999; 67:1653–8.
2. Cartier R, Brann S, Dagenais F, et al: Systematic off-pump coronary artery revascularization in multivessel disease: Experience of three hundred cases. *J Thorac Cardiovasc Surg* 2000; 119:221–9.
3. Hannan EL, Wu C, Smith CR, et al: Off-pump versus on-pump coronary artery bypass surgery: rences in short-term outcomes and in long-term mortality and need for subsequent revascularization. *Circulation* 2007 116(10):1145–52.
4. Hirose H, Amano A, Takahashi A: Off-pump coronary artery bypass grafting for elderly patients. *Ann Thorac Surg* 2001; 72:2013–9.
5. Mack M, Bachand D, Acuff T, et al: Improved outcomes in coronary artery bypass grafting with beating-heart techniques. *J Thorac Surg* 2002; 124:598–607.
6. Novitsky D, Bowen TE, Larsen A, et al: Aiming towards complete myocardial revascularization without cardiopulmonary bypass: A systematic approach. *Heart Surg Forum* 2002; 5:214–20.
7. Sabik JF, Gillinov AM, Blackstone EH, et al: Does off-pump coronary surgery reduce morbidity and mortality? *J Thorac Cardiovasc Surg* 2002; 124:698–707.

Suggested Readings – Anesthesiologist's

1. Ankeney JL, Goldstein DJ: Off-pump bypass of the left anterior descending artery: 23- to 34-year follow-up. *J Thorac Cardiovasc Surg* 2007; 133:149–1503.
2. Arom K, Flavin T, Emery R, et al: Safety and efficacy of off-pump coronary artery bypass grafting. *Ann Thorac Surg* 2000; 69:704–10.
3. Diegeler A, Matin M, Kayser S, et al: Angiographic results after minimally invasive coronary bypass grafting using the minimally invasive direct coronary bypass grafting (MIDCAB) approach. *Eur J Cardiothoracic Surg* 1999; 15:680–4.
4. Fukui T, Takanashi S, Hosoda Y, et al: Early and midterm results of of-pump coronary artery bypass grafting. *Ann Thorac Surg* 2007; 83:115–9.
5. Greenspun HG, Adourian UA, Fonger JD, et al: Minimally invasive direct coronary artery bypass (MIDCAB): surgical techniques and anesthetic considerations. *J Cardiothorac Vasc Anesth* 1996; 10(4):507–9.
6. Kessler P, Neidhart G, Bremerich DH, et al: High thoracic epidural anesthesia for coronary artery bypass grafting using two different surgical approaches in conscious patients. *Anesth Analg* 2002; 95:791–7.
7. Motallebzadeh R. Bland JM, Markus HS, et al: Neurocognitive function and cerebral emboli: randomized study of on-pump versus off-pump coronary artery bypass surgery. *Ann Thorac Surg* 2007; 83: 475–82.
8. Nierich AP, Diephuis J, Jansen EWL, et al: Embracing the heart: Perioperative management of patients undergoing off-pump coronary artery bypass grafting using the Octopus tissue stabilizer. *J Cardiothorac Vasc Anesth* 1999; 13:123–9.
9. Place DG, Peragallo RA, Carroll J, et al: Postoperative atrial fibrillation: a comparison of off-pump coronary artery bypass surgery and conventional coronary artery bypass graft surgery. *J Cardiothorac Vasc Anesth* 2002; 16:144–8.
10. Puskas JD, Kilgo PD, Kutner M, et al: Off-pump techniques disproportionately benefit women and narrow the gender disparity in outcomes after coronary artery bypass surgery. *Circulation* 2007; 116 (suppl):I-192–99.
11. Puskas JD, Williams WH, Mahoney EM, et al: Off-pump vs conventional coronary artery bypass grafting: early and 1-year graft patency, cost, and quality-of-life outcomes: a randomized trial. *JAMA* 2004; 291:1841–849.
12. Raja SG, Berg GA: Impact of off-pump coronary artery bypass surgery on systemic inflammation: current best available evidence. *J Card Surg* 2007; 22:445–55.
13. Roosens C, Heerman J, De Somer F, et al: Effects of off-pump coronary surgery on the mechanics of the respiratory system, lung, and chest wall: Comparison with extracorporeal circulation. *Crit Care Med* 2002; 30:2430–7.
14. Sabik JF, Blackstone EH, Lytle BW, et al: Equivalent midterm outcomes after off-pump and on-pump coronary surgery. *J Thorac Cardiovasc Surg* 2004; 127:142–8.

15. Siegel LC, Hennessy MM, Pearl RG: Delayed time response of the continuous cardiac output pulmonary artery catheter. *Anesth Analg* 1996; 83:1173–7.
16. Sisilio E. Marino MR, Juliano G, et al: Comparison of on pump and off pump coronary surgery: risk factors for neurological outcome. *Eur J Cardiothorac Surg* 2007; 31:1076–80.
17. Straka Z, Brucek P, Vanek T, et al: Routine immediate extubation for off-pump coronary artery bypass grafting without thoracic epidural analgesia. *Ann Thorac Surg* 2002; 74:1544–7.
18. Vassiliades TA Jr, Reddy VS, Puskas JD, et al: Long-term results of the endoscopic atraumatic coronary artery bypass. *Ann Thorac Surg* 2007; 83:979–84.
19. Virmani S, Tempe DK: Anaesthesia for off-pump coronary artery surgery. *Ann Card Anaesth* 2007 10(1): 65–71.

PORT-ACCESS CORONARY REVASCULARIZATION

SURGICAL CONSIDERATIONS

Description: Advances in videoscopic technology have led to less invasive approaches in the treatment of many general and thoracic surgical disorders. The development of less invasive surgery has resulted in alternative and novel approaches to cardiac surgery, including port-access cardiac surgery and off-pump coronary revascularization. The port-access approach was developed in the mid-1990s and is used less frequently in the current setting because of its complexity. With the development of robotic (or total endoscopic) techniques, the port-access technology is being employed as a means to achieve cardiopulmonary bypass and cardioplegic arrest. Using a port-access approach, the surgeon can perform cardiac operations (e.g., CABG) and valve surgery in a motionless, bloodless field through smaller chest incisions. This approach typically relies on peripheral CPB (femoral artery and femoral vein cannulation, Fig. 6.2-6). The femoral artery is cannulated with a 19–23 Fr Y-shaped cannula, which permits arterial inflow

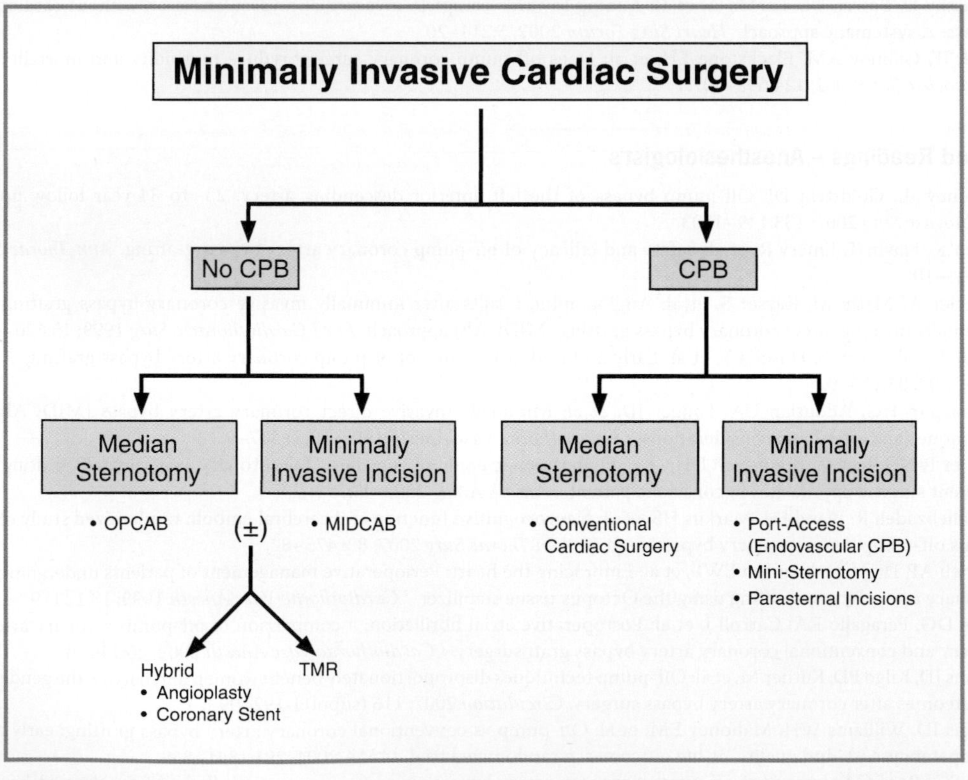

Figure 6.2-5. Variations in coronary artery bypass and valvular heart surgery, with minimally invasive techniques. CPB = cardiopulmonary bypass. OPCAB = off-pump coronary artery bypass. MIDCAB = minimally invasive direct coronary artery bypass. TMR = transmyocardial revascularization. (Redrawn with permission from Estafanous FG, Barash PG, Reves JG: *Cardiac Anesthesia: Principles and Clinical Practice,* 2nd edition. Lippincott Williams & Wilkins, Philadelphia: 2001.)

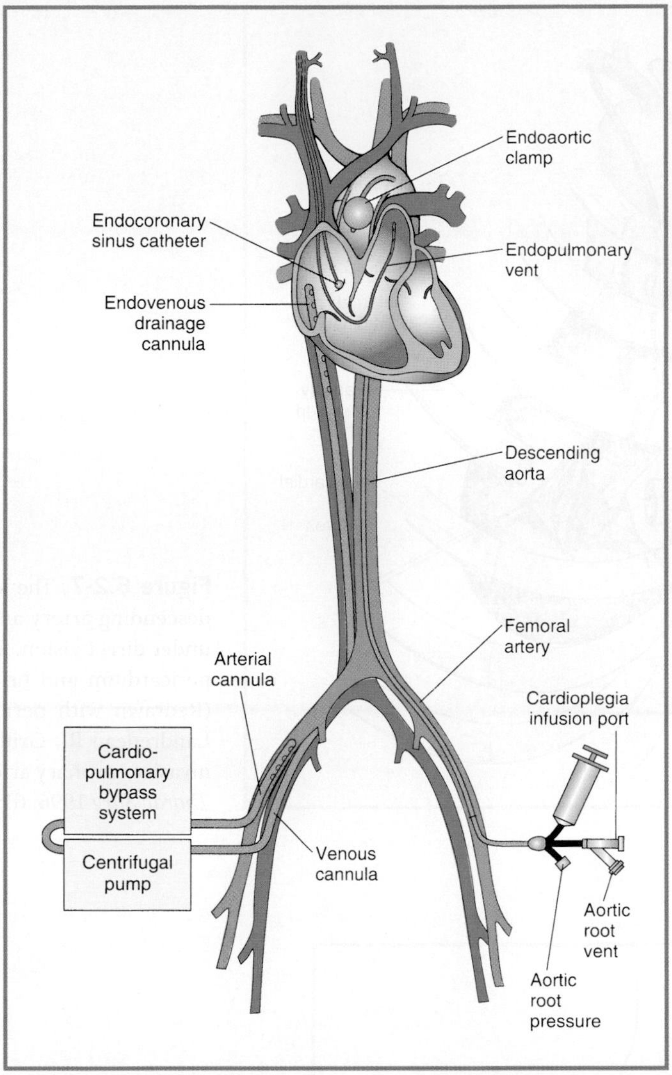

Figure 6.2-6. The port-access cardiopulmonary bypass (CPB) system. Femoro-femoral (fem-fem) CPB is utilized, and a centrifugal pump augments venous drainage. The endoaortic balloon occlusion catheter is inflated in the ascending aorta, and antegrade cardioplegia is delivered through the central lumen. The endopulmonary vent assists in ventricular decompression. (Redrawn with permission from Fann JI, Pompili MF, Stevens JH, et al: Port-access cardiac surgery with cardioplegic arrest. *Ann Thorac Surg* 1997; 63:S35–9.)

and insertion of the endoaortic clamp. Venous drainage is provided by the 22–25 Fr cannula, introduced through a femoral vein. Drainage may be augmented by 20–40%, using vacuum-assisted venous drainage or a centrifugal venous drainage pump placed between the venous cannula and the reservoir. The port-access system includes a 10.5 Fr endoaortic "clamp" (EAC), a triple-lumen catheter with an inflatable balloon at its distal end. This clamp is positioned in the ascending aorta using fluoroscopy and TEE guidance. The lumen used for balloon inflation is connected to a manometer to monitor balloon pressure. Cardioplegic solution is delivered through a central lumen, which also acts as an aortic root vent after cardioplegia delivery. A third lumen serves as an aortic root pressure monitor. Additionally, a percutaneous PA venting catheter, placed via the jugular approach, helps in ventricular decompression. The left internal mammary artery (IMA) is harvested under direct vision (Fig. 6.2-7) or with video-assisted thoracoscopy (VAT) (Fig. 6.2-8). After peripheral CPB is achieved, the EAC provides aortic occlusion and cardioplegic arrest. Exposure of the lateral and posterior aspects of the heart is easily accomplished in the arrested heart, thereby permitting two- and three-vessel coronary revascularization. Notably, if the ascending aorta is accessible, a dual-armed, Y-shaped cannula can be placed directly into the ascending aorta with one arm of the cannula connected to the arterial inflow of the CPB circuit and the other arm as a conduit for introducing the EAC.

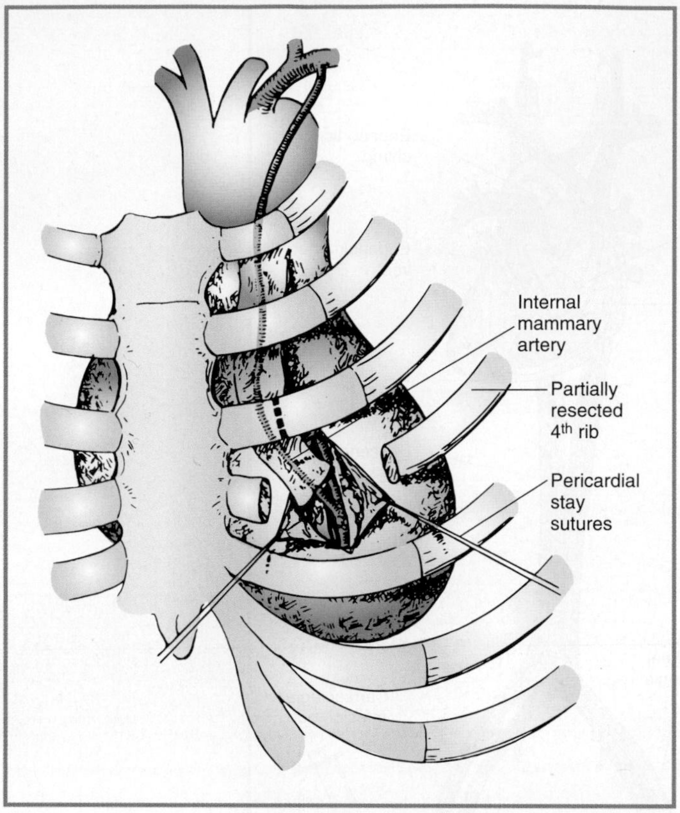

Figure 6.2-7. The left IMA-to-left anterior descending artery anastomosis is performed under direct vision. Stay sutures suspend the pericardium and bring the heart into view. (Redrawn with permission from Acuff TE, Landreneau RJ, Griffith BP, et al: Minimally invasive coronary artery bypass grafting. *Ann Thorac Surg* 1996; 61:135–7.)

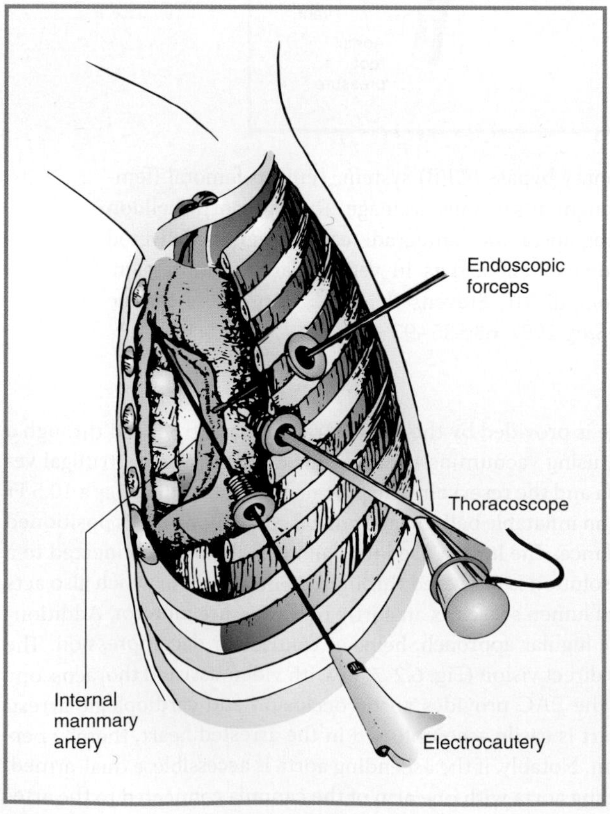

Figure 6.2-8. Dissection and harvesting of the left IMA using a thoracoscopic approach. (Redrawn with permission from Acuff TE, Landreneau RJ, Griffith BP, et al: Minimally invasive coronary artery bypass grafting. *Ann Thorac Surg* 1996; 61:135–7.)

Table 6.2-1. Common Abbreviations Used in Minimally Invasive Cardiac Surgery

Abbreviation	Definition
MICS	Minimally invasive cardiac surgery
MICAB	Minimally invasive coronary artery bypass (includes OPCAB, MIDCAB. port-access, and mini-sternotomy techniques)
OPCAB	Off-pump coronary artery bypass ('beating heart surgery': median sternotomy)
MIDCAB	Minimally invasive direct coronary artery bypass (direct vision, no sternotomy, CPB, or cardioplegia)
MIDCABG	Minimally invasive direct coronary artery bypass graft (same as MIDCAB)
MITACAB	Minimally invasive thoracoscopically assisted coronary artery bypass
VADCAB	Video-assisted direct coronary artery bypass
LAST	Left anterior small thoracotomy
PACAB	Port-access coronary artery bypass (also called Port-CAB, Port-CABG)
TECAB	Totally endoscopic coronary artery bypass grafting

Usual preop diagnosis: CAD

SUMMARY OF PROCEDURE

Position	Supine
Incision	4th interspace, left anterior thoracotomy for CABG; may need to resect 4th rib; may need thoracoscopy for IMA harvest.
Special instrumentation	TEE and fluoroscopy
Unique considerations	CPB used with peripheral femoral cannulation; percutaneous insertion of PA vent and retrograde cardioplegic catheter.
Antibiotics	Cefazolin 1–2 g iv at induction
Surgical time	3–5 h
Closing considerations	Assess chest wall for hemorrhage; chest tube insertion. Bupivacaine for field block.
EBL	250–500 mL
Postop care	ICU monitoring; early extubation; may require inotropic support.
Mortality	1–3%, depending on comorbidities
Morbidity	Arrhythmias (including atrial fibrillation): 10% Conversion to sternotomy: 4% MI: 0–4% Reoperation for bleeding: 3% Stroke: 2% Thrombosis of graft (graft failure): Rare Fem-fem bypass complications (e.g., arterial dissection): Rare
Pain score	1–4

PATIENT POPULATION CHARACTERISTICS

Age range	40–80 yr
Male:Female	3:2
Incidence	< 50,000/yr in the United States.

PATIENT POPULATION CHARACTERISTICS (cont'd)	
Etiology	Multifactorial for atherosclerosis
Associated conditions	LV dysfunction; COPD; PVD; HTN; diabetes mellitus; cigarette smoking

ANESTHETIC CONSIDERATIONS

See Anesthetic Considerations for Port-Access Procedures, p. 385.

Suggested Readings

1. Bonatti J, Schachner T, Bonaros N, et al: Technical challenges in totally endoscopic robotic coronary artery bypass grafting. *J Thorac Cardiovasc Surg* 2006; 131:146–53.
2. Casselman FP, LaMeir M, Jeanmart H, et al: Endoscopic mitral and tricuspid valve surgery after previous cardiac surgery. *Circulation* 2007: 116 (suppl): I-270–5.
3. Dogan S, Graubitz K, Aybek T, et al: How safe is the port access technique in minimally invasive coronary artery bypass grafting? *Ann Thorac Surg* 2002; 74:1537–43.
4. Fann JI, Pompili MF, Stevens JH, et al: Port-access cardiac surgery with cardioplegic arrest. *Ann Thorac Surg* 1997; 63:S35–9.
5. Groh MA, Sutherland SE, Burton HG 3rd, et al: Port-access coronary artery bypass grafting: technique and comparative results. *Ann Thorac Surg* 1999; 68:1506–8.
6. Grossi EA, Groh MA, Lefrak EA, et al: Results of a prospective multicenter study on port-access coronary bypass grafting. *Ann Thorac Surg* 1999; 68:1475–7.
7. Maselli D, Pizio R, Borelli G, et al: Endovascular balloon versus transthoracic aortic clamping for minimally invasive mitral valve surgery: impact on cerebral microemboli. *Interact Cardiovasc Thorac Surg* 2006;5:183–86.
8. Murphy DA, Miller JS, Langford DA, et al: Endoscopic robotic mitral valve surgery. *J Thorac Cardiovasc Surg* 2006; 132:776–81.
9. Stevens JH, Burdon TA, Peters WS, et al: Port-access coronary artery bypass grafting: a proposed surgical method. *J Thorac Cardiovasc Surg* 1996; 111:567–73.
10. Subramanian VA, Patel NU, Patel NC, et al: Robotic assisted multivessel minimally invasive direct coronary artery bypass with port-access stabilization and cardiac positioning: paving the way for outpatient coronary surgery? *Ann Thorac Surg* 2005; 79:1590–6.
11. Walther T, Falk V, Mohr FW: Minimally invasive surgery for valve disease. *Curr Probl Cardiol* 2006; 31:399–437.
12. Woo YJ, Rodriguez E, Atluri P, et al: Minimally invasive, robotic, and off-pump mitral valve surgery. *Semin Thorac Cardiovasc Surg* 2006; 18: 139–47.

Also see Suggested Readings for Port-Access Procedures.

LIMITED THORACOTOMY AND PORT-ACCESS APPROACH TO MITRAL VALVE SURGERY

SURGICAL CONSIDERATIONS

Description: Although the field of mitral valve surgery has seen marked advances in biomaterials and innovative repair techniques since the early 1960s, the **conventional median sternotomy approach** to access and expose the mitral valve has not changed substantially. Because of the progress in video-assisted surgery, a less invasive approach to cardiac surgery has been developed, and various techniques of mitral valve surgery through **limited thoracotomy** or **upper sternotomy** incisions and a **port-access technique** to achieve cardioplegic arrest are now used in the clinical setting.

Limited thoracotomy: The right thoracotomy incision is a less invasive approach (compared to median sternotomy) for mitral valve procedures (Fig. 6.2-9). Utilizing hypothermic fibrillatory or cardioplegic arrest, the mitral valve, annulus, and subvalvular apparatus can be visualized directly and the valve procedure carried out. The addition of video-assisted thoracoscopy (VAT) to mitral valve surgery or using robotic technology has resulted in even smaller incisions for these procedures.

Chitwood, et al. have utilized a **"micro-mitral" approach** to mitral valve replacement, using VAT through a limited thoracotomy. Peripheral cardiopulmonary bypass (fem-fem) is used, and a catheter is placed in the coronary sinus

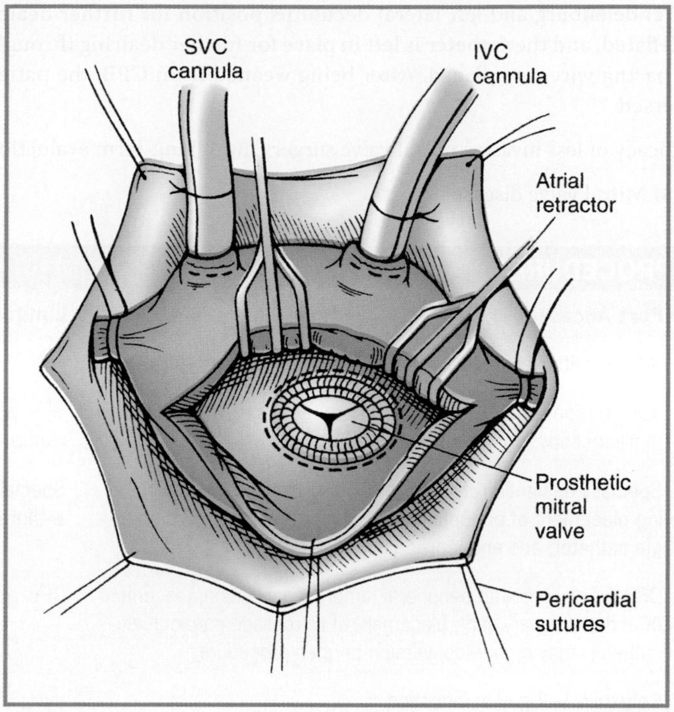

Figure 6.2-9. The right thoracotomy approach with left atriotomy and exposure of the mitral valve area with prosthetic valve in place. (Reproduced with permission from Tribble CG, Killinger WA Jr., Harman PK, et al: Anterolateral thoracotomy as an alternative to repeat median sternotomy for replacement of the mitral valve. *Ann Thorac Surg* 1987; 43:380–2.)

for retrograde cardioplegia delivery. An external aortic cross-clamp is introduced through a separate incision in the chest. After achieving cardioplegic arrest, the mitral valve is replaced with thoracoscopic assistance. Proposed advantages of the micro-mitral approach include the avoidance of a sternotomy, with decreased chest-wall trauma and patient discomfort.

Arom and Emery have described an alternative **partial sternotomy approach** to mitral and aortic valve surgery. The 7-cm partial sternotomy permits aortic and right atrial cannulation for CPB. The external aortic cross-clamp is positioned and a left ventricular vent is placed through the right superior pulmonary vein. Mitral valve exposure is achieved through the dome of the left atrium.

Port-access mitral valve surgery: The port-access system has been used successfully in mitral valve surgery via limited thoracotomy incision using special instrumentation or even less invasive robotic technology. To facilitate dissection and to provide adequate exposure of the left atrium, DLT intubation for OLV is used. Under fluoroscopic and TEE guidance, a retrograde cardioplegia catheter is directed into the coronary sinus via an introducer placed in the jugular vein; a PA-venting catheter is inserted through another jugular vein introducer. A limited right thoracotomy is made, with or without dividing the 4th rib, followed by the placement of a soft-tissue retractor. A separate port is placed in the 6th interspace for introduction of a thoracoscope, if necessary. The pericardium is opened anterior to the phrenic nerve. After systemic heparinization, the femoral artery and vein are cannulated. The endoaortic clamp is introduced through the side limb of the femoral arterial cannula and its tip positioned in the ascending aorta. CPB is initiated and systemic hypothermia achieved. The balloon of the endoaortic clamp is inflated, achieving effective aortic occlusion. Cold blood cardioplegia is delivered using the distal port of the endoaortic clamp; retrograde cardioplegia is administered via the coronary sinus catheter. A left atriotomy is made, and an atrial retractor is placed through a separate port. Valve repair or replacement is carried out using specially designed instruments. Before completion of atriotomy closure, deairing maneuvers are accomplished. These include temporarily discontinuing pulmonary and aortic root venting, inflating the lungs to displace residual air, and increasing the patient's blood volume from the venous reservoir. Also, the patient is placed in a Trendelenburg and left lateral decubitus position for further deairing. The balloon of the endoaortic catheter is deflated, and the catheter is left in place for further deairing through the aortic vent lumen. Temporary ventricular pacing wires are placed. After being weaned from CPB, the patient is decannulated and the anticoagulation reversed.

The overall safety and efficacy of less invasive mitral valve surgery await long-term evaluations and follow-up.

Usual preop diagnosis: Mitral valve disease

SUMMARY OF PROCEDURES

	Port-Access	Limited Thoracotomy
Position	Supine, with right side slightly elevated	⇐
Incision	4th interspace limited right thoracotomy; ports for possible thoracoscopy; port for atrial retractor.	⇐ ± port for aortic cross-clamp
Special instrumentation	Specially designed retractors; TEE and fluoroscopy for guiding placement of endopulmonary vent, retrograde cardioplegia catheter, and endoaortic clamp	Specially designed instruments ± thorascopic instruments
Unique considerations	CPB is achieved with peripheral femoral cannulation; placement of endopulmonary vent; placement of retrograde cardioplegia catheter; may require conversion to open procedure.	CPB via femoral artery and vein
Antibiotics	Cefazolin 1–2 g iv at induction	⇐
Surgical time	3–5 h	⇐
Closing considerations	Assess chest wall for hemorrhage.	⇐
EBL	250–500 mL	⇐
Postop care	ICU monitoring; early extubation; may require inotropic support.	⇐
Mortality	1–6%, depending on comorbidities (lower for mitral valve repairs).	⇐
Morbidity	AF:10–40% Chest-wall hemorrhage: 2–9% Stroke: 1–3% Conversion to sternotomy: 2% Vascular injury: Rare Pneumonia Renal failure	⇐ – – – – ⇐ –
Pain score	1–4	4–7

PATIENT POPULATION CHARACTERISTICS

Age range	40–70 yr
Male:Female	1:1
Incidence	< 20,000/yr in the United States.
Etiology	Myxomatous mitral valve; rheumatic valve disease; endocarditis; ischemic (papillary muscle dysfunction); mitral annular calcification
Associated conditions	Pulmonary HTN; atrial arrhythmias; CAD; aortic valve disease; tricuspid regurgitation

ANESTHETIC CONSIDERATIONS FOR PORT-ACCESS PROCEDURES

PREOPERATIVE

As with all anesthetic procedures, the use of the port-access system should not be attempted without appropriate training. Catheter placement and monitoring relies on TEE and/or fluoroscopy. The evaluation of the patient for port-access cardiac surgery should parallel that of patients having conventional cardiac surgery. (For mitral valve surgery, see p. 354; for CABG surgery, see p. 344.) There are, however, a number of specific conditions which preclude the use of the port-access system:

1. Aortic regurgitation (AR): Although mild-to-moderate AR is not a contraindication, it may make the delivery of antegrade cardioplegia via the endoaortic clamp catheter (EAC) problematic; therefore, insertion of the endocoronary sinus catheter (ESC) is very important. Severe AR is a contraindication.
2. Atherosclerotic disease of the aorta: Perfusion may be associated with embolization of atheromatous plaques (particularly pedunculated lesions).
3. PVD: Femoral bypass may be associated with retrograde arterial dissection. PVD and tortuous femoral and iliac vessels are contraindications to use of femoral arterial cannulation.
4. Thoracic aortic aneurysm/Marfan syndrome: Port-access procedures require passage of the EAC into the thoracic aorta and inflation of the EAC balloon; therefore, aneurysms or a weakened aortic wall are contraindications.
5. Scarring of the pleural cavity (e.g., chest trauma, previous thoracotomy) may make surgical access difficult although the surgical approach may be desirable in the patient with previous median sternotomy.
6. Inability to obtain TEE or fluoroscope imaging, because monitoring and placement of catheters relies on imaging.

Preop evaluation should focus on the underlying pathophysiology (valvular disease vs CAD). In addition, the following aspects should be considered:

Respiratory	OLV is used to facilitate surgical exposure; thus, evaluation of patients with severe lung disease may include CXR, ABG, PFTs (see Thoracic Surgery, pp. 267–332).
Cardiovascular	The vascular system should be evaluated with respect to insertion of the catheters and cannulae for endovascular CPB. Severity of arterial occlusive or atherosclerotic disease should be evaluated (embolization/dissection risk). The possible presence of a persistent left SVC should be considered. **Tests:** CXR; aortography; iliofemoral arteriography; vascular MRI/MRA; vascular ultrasound; TEE
Premedication	As for the underlying condition. Usually, a mild anxiolytic (e.g., midazolam 1–3 mg iv) is sufficient.

INTRAOPERATIVE

Anesthetic technique: GETA (DLT or BB). Anesthetic technique depends on the underlying pathophysiology (e.g., valvular disease vs CAD). Early extubation and postop pain relief can be facilitated by using intrathecal narcotics (e.g., Duramorph 10 mcg/kg intrathecal) injected before induction.

Induction	Typically, induction can be accomplished with etomidate (0.1–0.3 mg/kg) or propofol (0.5–2 mg/kg), with fentanyl (5–20 mcg/kg) and pancuronium or vecuronium (0.1 mg/kg). The overall length of port-access procedures is similar to or slightly longer than conventional approaches, so that a long-acting muscle relaxant can be used. Intubation is accomplished with a DLT, and its placement is checked by auscultation or bronchoscopy. A bronchial blocker or Univent tube may also be used to provide selective lung ventilation.
Maintenance	With the goal of early extubation, it is important to avoid oversedation. The use of volatile agents or a propofol infusion (25–100 mcg/kg/min) before, during, and after CPB will facilitate early extubation. During dissection of the IMA or exposure of the left atrium, OLV is needed.

Emergence	At the end of the procedure, intercostal blocks with ropivacaine or bupivacaine may be placed, and infiltration of the skin incision also is helpful. Extubation in the OR may be appropriate for stable patients. Alternatively, the patient is transported to ICU and ventilated. The DLT may be exchanged for a single-lumen tube when postop mechanical ventilation is required.
Special considerations: Placement/ monitoring of endocardio-pulmonary system	The port-access system consists of CPB with venous drainage via an endovenous drain (EVD) and an aortic or femoral arterial return cannula, which is Y-ed to accept the EAC. These are placed by the surgeon with the aid of fluoroscopy and/or TEE. Additional drainage of the right side of the heart is accomplished via an endopulmonary vent (EPV) placed by the anesthesiologist. Immediately after intubation and before CVP insertion, a TEE exam should be performed to exclude any contraindication to endo-CPB (e.g., severe AR, aortic atheromatous disease, aortic aneurysm); the size of the ascending aorta should be measured (aids the surgeon in inflation of the aortic balloon); and the coronary sinus should be identified to aid placement of the ESC (coronary sinus catheter). The right IJ vein is then cannulated with two sheaths (9 Fr for EPV and 11 Fr for the ESC). Cardioplegia is delivered in an anterograde fashion via the EAC or retrograde via an ESC, also placed by the anesthesiologist (Fig. 6.2-2).
Placement of ESC	The ESC can be placed with fluoroscopy and/or TEE. The coronary sinus is identified on TEE (transverse view of the right atrium or longitudinal bicaval view). Prior to placement, the patient should be partially anticoagulated with 70 U/kg of heparin. The ESC is placed through the 11 Fr sheath. After the tip of the catheter engages the coronary sinus, the catheter is advanced either directly or over a guiding wire until the occlusion balloon is 2–4 cm inside the sinus. Position is confirmed by inflating the balloon and obtaining ventricularization of the pressure tracing. Careful note should be taken of the volume of fluid required to occlude the coronary sinus (1–2 mL) so that overinflation and possible coronary sinus trauma do not occur. Contrast injection will define the correct positioning of the ESC in the coronary sinus. Care should be taken to avoid injecting contrast too quickly, thus pushing the ESC out of the coronary sinus. A time limit (20–30 min) should be set to pass this catheter, as repeated attempts increase the risk of cardiac injury (e.g., cardiac perforation).
Placement of EPV	The EPV (pulmonary vent) is positioned by advancing the catheter, using balloon flotation with pressure monitoring (as with a Swan-Ganz catheter). Fluoroscopy and/or TEE also may be used.
Placement of EVD	The EVD (venous drain) cannula is placed via the femoral vein into the right atrium over a guide wire. Fluoroscopy or TEE is used to ensure that the wire enters the SVC before advancing the EVD into position. The tip of the EVD should be at the SVC/RA junction or just inside the SVC.
Placement of arterial cannula	The aorta may be cannulated with a "Y" cannula with an incising introducer. For femoral arterial cannulation, a guide wire is advanced under fluoroscopy and no resistance to its passage should be felt. The guide wire is advanced into the descending aorta and its intraluminal position confirmed on TEE prior to advancing the aortic return cannulation into its final position. The perfusionist should confirm normal line pressures with a test bolus of fluid and ✓ that normal arterial pulsation is present. These precautions will decrease the likelihood of arterial dissection.
Placement of EAC	The EAC (endoaortic clamp) maybe advanced via the "Y" arterial cannula. For a femoral arterial cannula, the EAC is advanced over a guide wire with imaging into the ascending aorta so that the tip of the catheter is just proximal to the sinotubular ridge (2–3 cm above the aortic valve). Position is confirmed by contrast injection and/or TEE. It is also useful to identify the takeoff of the innominate artery in relation to the balloon. Migration of the balloon proximally or distally can occur and, thus, its position needs to be monitored. Monitoring of the pressure in the aortic root via this catheter should show that the mean aortic root pressure is the same as mean radial artery pressure prior to the initiation of bypass.

Sequence of events during endo-CPB	After initiation of bypass, the anesthesiologist should observe the descending aorta to exclude aortic dissection and open the EPV to allow venting. EPV pressures during bypass should be negative (positive pressures may indicate inadequate decompression of the heart or kinking of the EPV). Once adequate CPB is established and the heart is drained, the EAC balloon can be inflated (balloon pressure = 250–350 mmHg). Occlusion of the aorta is confirmed by a differential between the radial and aortic root pressures and by an aortic root contrast injection. Antegrade cardioplegia is delivered via the EAC with careful monitoring to ensure that the balloon is not displaced distally, thus occluding the innominate artery (see Monitoring of endo-CPB: regional perfusion, below). After cardioplegic arrest, retrograde cardioplegia may be delivered via the ESC, and the left side of the heart may be vented via the EAC. Avoid overventing, high systemic pressures, or high CPB flow, which could displace the EAC toward the aortic valve. Initiation of retrograde cardioplegia should begin with a low flow to avoid displacing the ESC, followed by inflation of the ESC balloon until the pressure in the coronary sinus just starts to rise, indicating coronary sinus occlusion. No further inflation of the balloon should take place. Normal coronary sinus perfusion pressure is < 40 mmHg. After retrograde cardioplegia is delivered, the ESC balloon is deflated. Once the surgery is completed, the EAC balloon is deflated (after deairing procedures, as needed); the heart is reperfused; and the EAC is removed. Prior to weaning from CPB, mobility of the ESC and EPV should be assessed in mitral procedures to ensure that they have not been incorporated in the atrial suture line. Weaning from bypass is routine. The ESC should be removed prior to heparin reversal and the EPV can be replaced with a pulmonary artery catheter, if needed.	
Blood and fluid requirements	As for underlying condition: For mitral valve surgery, see p. 356. For CABG, see p. 346.	
Monitoring	As for underlying condition: For mitral valve surgery, see p. 356. For CABG, see p. 346.	Special monitoring considerations for port-access are discussed below. External defibrillator pads should be placed on all patients.
Positioning	Supine Roll under left chest for CABG and under right chest for mitral valve.	
Monitoring of endo-CPB	Regional perfusion	Distal migration of the EAC (innominate artery occlusion →↓cerebral blood flow) is possible, especially while cardioplegia is being delivered when pressure in the aortic root exceeds that in the systemic arterial system. Monitoring for regional perfusion includes: (1) Right-sided arterial pressure—radial, brachial, or axillary. The pump-induced artifact may be of use if roller heads are being used. (2) Bilateral arterial lines—right-sided, plus a second line in the left radial or in the femoral vessels to allow comparison. (3) TEE—EAC visible in the ascending aorta proximal to the innominate artery. (4) Transcranial or carotid artery Doppler. (5) Fluoroscopy
	Proximal EAC balloon migration	Most likely to occur during aortic root venting when the systemic pressure exceeds aortic root pressure. Monitored by TEE.
	Cardiac decompression	TEE can be useful in monitoring for adequate decompression of the heart.

Cardiovascular Surgery

Monitoring of endo-CPB (cont'd)	EAC balloon pressure	This is usually monitored by the perfusionist and ranges from 250–550 mmHg. Decreases in pressure may be 2° proximal migration of the balloon into a wider area of the ascending aorta, rupture of the balloon, or prolapse into the left ventricle. Loss of balloon occlusion is indicated by blood in the surgical field, return of cardiac activity, cardiac distension, increased root venting, and TEE evidence.
	Aortic root pressure	< 80 mmHg while giving cardioplegia; 0–10 mmHg, during venting. Overventing should be avoided, as should venting when the left side of the heart is open, to avoid drawing air into the aortic root.
	Intracardiac air	TEE is very useful for determining that adequate deairing of the heart has occurred.
Complications of endo-CPB	Retrograde aortic dissection Coronary sinus damage EAC balloon migration	
	EAC balloon rupture	Especially 2° sutures placed in the mitral valve annulus.
	Retained EPV in atrial suture line Chest-wall hemorrhage	It is important that the surgeon ✓ the chest wall before closure.
	Limb ischemia	May follow femoral cannulation.

Cardiovascular Surgery

POSTOPERATIVE

Complications	As for the primary procedure Low CO Chest-wall hemorrhage Problems associated with peripheral cannulation (e.g., dissection, embolization) Perivalvular leak Heart block	See mitral valve surgery (p. 357) or CABG (p. 347).
Pain management	Parenteral narcotics NSAIDs	Pain control is important to facilitate early extubation. Intrathecal narcotics and/or intercostal blocks with wound infiltration may be useful.
Tests	ECG Electrolytes ABG	

Suggested Readings for Port-Access Procedures–Surgeon's

1. Arom KV, Emery RW: Minimally invasive mitral operations (let). *Ann Thorac Surg* 1997; 63:1219–20.
2. Chaney MA, Durazo-Arvizu RA, Fluder EM, et al: Port-access minimally invasive cardiac surgery increases surgical complexity, increases operating room time, and facilitates early postoperative hospital discharge. *Anesthesiology* 2000; 92:1637–45.
3. Chitwood WR, Elbeery JR, Chapman WHH, et al: Video-assisted minimally invasive mitral valve surgery: The "micro-mitral" operation. *J Thorac Cardiovasc Surg* 1997; 113:413–4.
4. Dogan S, Aybek T, Andressen E, et al: Totally endoscopic coronary artery bypass grafting on cardiopulmonary bypass with robotically enhanced telemanipulation: report of forty-five cases. *J Thorac Cardiovasc Surg* 2002; 123:1029–30.
5. Fann JI, Pompili MF, Burdon TA, et al: Minimally invasive mitral valve surgery. *Semin Thorac Cardiovasc Surg* 1997; 9(4):320–30.
6. Glower DD, Siegel LC, Frisshmeyer KJ, et al: Predictors of outcome in a multicenter port-access valve registry. *Ann Thorac Surg* 2000; 70:1054–9.

7. Grossi EA, Galloway AC, LaPietra A, et al: Minimally invasive mitral valve surgery: a 6-year experience with 714 patients. *Ann Thorac Surg* 2002; 74:660–4.
8. Rosengart TK, Feldman T, Borger MA et al. Percutaneous and minimally invasive valve procedures. A scientific statement from the American Heart Association Council on Cardiovascular Surgery and Anesthesia, et al. *Circulation* 2008.
9. Stevens JH, Burdon TA, Peters WS, et al: Port-access coronary artery bypass grafting: A proposed surgical method. *J Thorac Cardiovasc Surg* 1996; 111:567–73.

Suggested Readings for Port-Access Procedures–Anesthesiologist's

1. Applebaum RM, Colvin SB, Galloway AC, et al: The role of transesophageal echocardiography during port-acess minimally invasive cardiac surgery: A new challenge for the echocardiographer. Echocardiography 1999; 16:595–602.
2. Burfeind WR, Glower DD, Davis RD, et al: Mitral surgery after prior cardiac operation: port-access versus sternotomy or thoracotomy. *Ann Thor Surg* 2002; 74:S1323–5.
3. Clements F, Wright S, deBruijn NP: Coronary sinus catheterization made easy for port-access minimally invasive cardiac surgery. *J Cardiothorac Vasc Anesth* 1998; 12:96–101.
4. Glower DD, Komtebedde J, Clements FM, et al: Direct aortic cannulation for port-access mitral or coronary artery bypass grafting. *Ann Thorac Surg* 1999; 68:1878–80.
5. Grocott HP, Stafford-Smith M, Glower DD, et al: Endovascular aortic balloon clamp malposition during minimally invasive cardiac surgery: detection by transcranial Doppler monitoring. *Anesthesiology* 1998; 88:1396–9.
6. Peters WS, Siegel LC, Stevens JH, et al: Closed-chest cardiopulmonary bypass and cardioplegia for less invasive cardiac surgery. *Ann Thorac Surg* 1997; 63:1748–54.
7. Plotkin IM, Collard CD, Aranki SF, et al: Percutaneous coronary sinus cannulation guided by transesophageal echocardiography. *Ann Thorac Surg* 1998; 66:2085–7.
8. Reichenspurner H, Boehm DH, Gulbins H, et al: Three-dimensional video and robot-assisted port-access mitral valve operation. *Ann Thorac Surg* 2000; 69:1176–82.
9. Sagbas E, Caynak B, Duran C, et al: Mid-term results of peripheric cannulation after port-access surgery. *Interact Cardiovasc Thorac Surg* 2007;6:744–7.
10. Siegel LC, StGoar FG, Stevens JH, et al: Monitoring considerations for port-access cardiac surgery. *Circulation* 1997; 96:562–8.
11. Toomasian JM, Peters WS, Siegel LC, et al: Extracorporeal circulation for port-access cardiac surgery. *Perfusion* 1997;12:83–91.

CHAPTER 6.3 Vascular Surgery

SURGEONS

James I. Fann, MD
R. Scott Mitchell, MD
Stephen T. Kee, MD (*Endovascular stent-grafting*)
Michael D. Dake, MD (*Endovascular stent-grafting*)

ANESTHESIOLOGIST

Pieter Van der Starre, MD, PhD

CAROTID ENDARTERECTOMY (VASCULAR)

SURGICAL CONSIDERATIONS

Description: Carotid endarterectomy (CEA) continues to be one of the commonly performed open vascular surgery procedures in the United States, even as carotid stenting is being more frequently employed as an alternative approach. Because of presumed microemboli from stenotic/ulcerated plaques at the carotid bifurcation, CEA has been championed as an effective procedure to reduce the risk of subsequent stroke. The NASCET Collaborators determined, in a prospective, randomized, blinded trial, that CEA is more effective than medical therapy for symptomatic patients with internal carotid artery narrowing between 60% and 90%. Symptoms are usually hemispheric (contralateral, upper or lower extremity paresis or numbness) or retinal (unilateral monocular blindness). Symptoms may be transient (TIA or reversible ischemic neurological deficit [RIND]) or permanent (CVA). The Asymptomatic Carotid Atherosclerosis Study (ACAS) has shown benefit from prophylactic CEA in asymptomatic patients with >60% stenosis of the internal carotid artery. Although some surgeons routinely prefer local anesthesia, most prefer GA with careful hemodynamic monitoring because of the frequent concomitant CAD.

The carotid artery is approached through an oblique neck incision along the anterior border of the sternocleidomastoid muscle. After division of the common facial vein, the carotid sheath is opened and the carotid artery is exposed, avoiding injury to the phrenic, vagus, ansa hypoglossi, and hypoglossal nerves (Fig. 6.3-1). After controlling the internal, external, and common carotid arteries, heparin is administered, and the internal, external, and common carotid arteries are clamped sequentially. To maintain carotid perfusion, an indwelling shunt may be utilized (Fig. 6.3-2 B), at the discretion of the surgeon. An endarterectomy plane is established proximally (Fig. 6.3-2 C), and developed distally into both the external and internal branches, with establishment of a fine tapered end point. After removal of all thrombus, loose smooth-muscle fibers and endothelium, the arteriotomy is closed, with or without a patch, the artery flushed, and flow restored. The incision is closed after meticulous hemostasis has been assured.

Usual preop diagnosis: Carotid artery disease

SUMMARY OF PROCEDURE	
Position	Supine with neck extended and turned away from the side of the lesion
Incision	Anterior to sternocleidomastoid from earlobe to base of neck or curvilinear in a skin crease over the carotid bifurcation
Special instrumentation	EEG monitor; ± shunt
Unique considerations	Capability to measure stump pressure may be needed. This can be accomplished by a high-pressure arterial line passed off the field to a pressure transducer. Avoid ↓BP during carotid cross-clamping. An indwelling shunt may be utilized to restore carotid perfusion. Heparin 5,000–10,000 U 5 min prior to cross-clamping, and protamine may be given after restoration of flow.
Antibiotics	Cefazolin 1 g iv at induction of anesthesia
Surgical time	Carotid cross-clamp: 30 min Total operating time: 90 min
Closing considerations	In order to assess the patient's neurologic status, it is best to be able to awaken and extubate the patient at the conclusion of the procedure. Avoidance of HTN is also critical during this period, because the endarterectomy tissues are thin and friable.
EBL	100–200 mL
Postop care	ICU × 12–24 h; BP control; cardiac monitoring
Mortality	1%
Morbidity	MI: Major cause of postop mortality Cranial nerve injury (recurrent and superior laryngeal nerves): 39% Restenosis Asymptomatic: 9–12%

SUMMARY OF PROCEDURE (cont'd)	
	Symptomatic: < 3% Neurologic complications: < 2% Hemorrhage: 1% False aneurysm: < 0.5%
Pain score	3–5

PATIENT POPULATION CHARACTERISTICS	
Age range	55–80 yr
Male:Female	3:1
Incidence	Second most common vascular surgical procedure (after AAA repair)
Etiology	Arteriosclerosis; fibromuscular dysplasia
Associated conditions	Significant CAD coexists with carotid artery disease in at least 30% of patients, necessitating careful cardiac and hemodynamic monitoring.

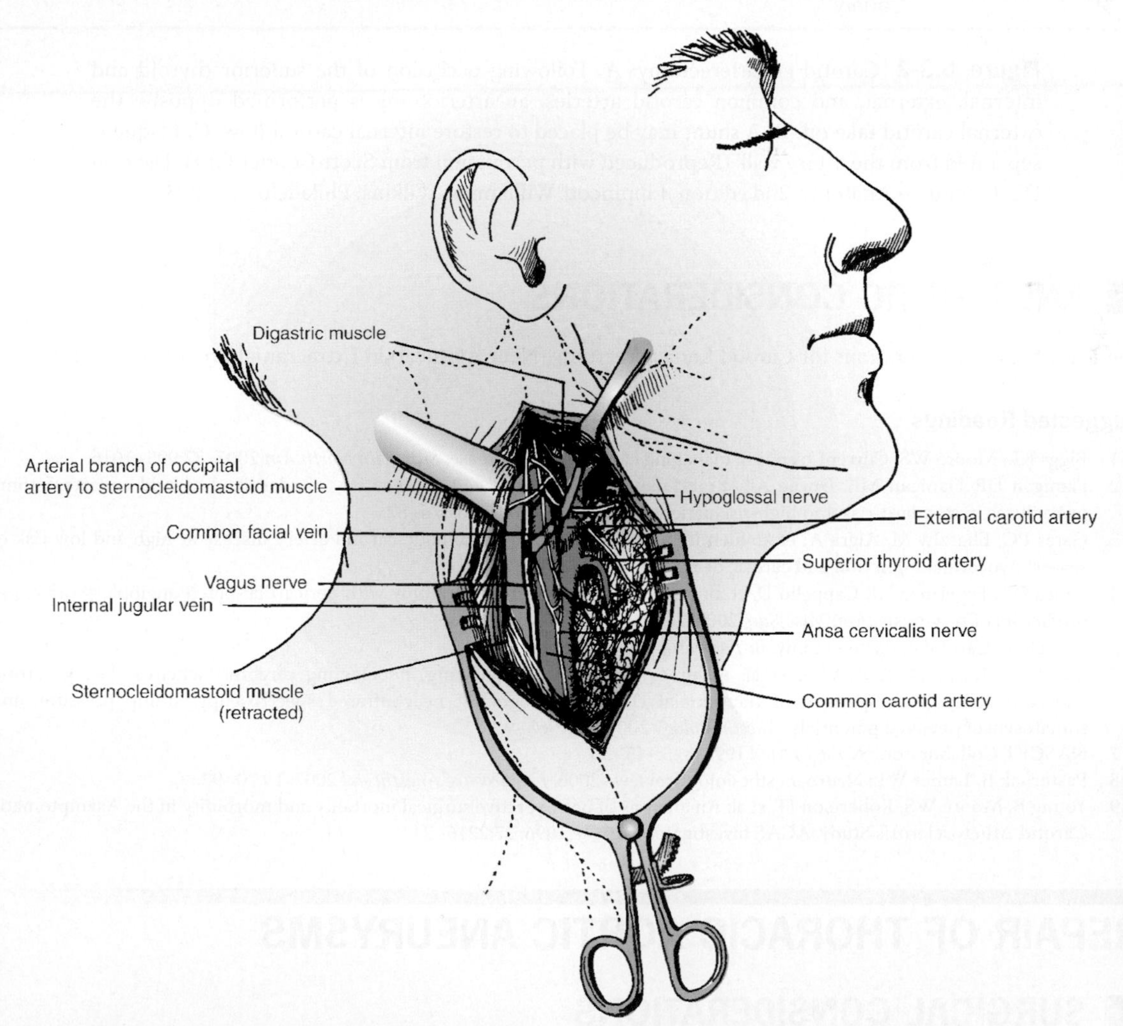

Figure 6.3-1. Exposure of the carotid bifurcation. (Reproduced with permission from Scott-Conner CEH, Dawson DL: *Operative Anatomy,* 2nd edition. Lippincott Williams & Wilkins, Philadelphia, 2003.)

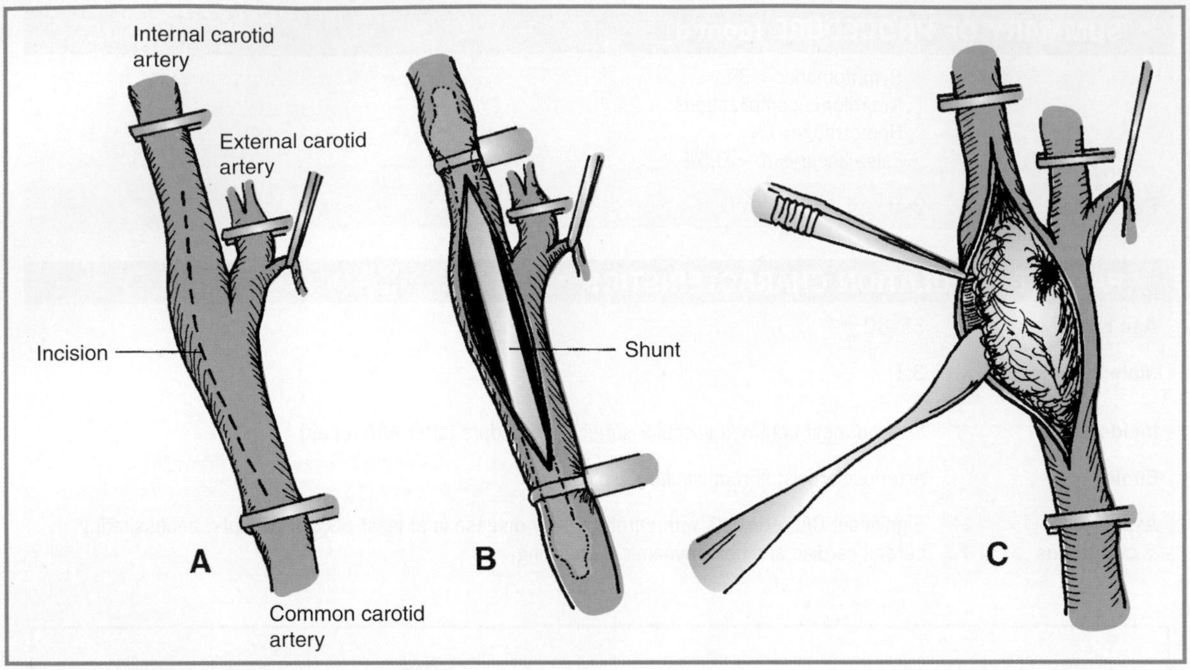

Figure 6.3-2. Carotid endarterectomy: **A.** Following occlusion of the superior thyroid and internal, external, and common carotid arteries, an arteriotomy is performed opposite the external carotid take off. **B.** A shunt may be placed to restore internal carotid flow. **C.** Plaque is separated from the artery wall. (Reproduced with permission from Scott-Conner CEH, Dawson DL: Operative Anatomy, 2nd edition. Lippincott Williams & Wilkins, Philadelphia, 2003.)

ANESTHETIC CONSIDERATIONS

See Anesthetic Considerations for Carotid Endarterectomy (Neurosurgical) in Extracranial Procedures, p. 130.

Suggested Readings

1. Biggs KL, Moore WS: Current trends in managing carotid artery disease. *Surg Clin North Am* 2007; 87:995–1016.
2. Flanigan DP, Flanigan ME, Dorne AL, et al: Long-term results of 442 consecutive, standardized carotid endarterectomy procedures in standard-risk and high-risk patients. *J Vasc Surg* 2007; 46:876–82.
3. Gates PC, Eliasziw M, Algra A, et al: Identifying patients with symptomatic carotid artery disease at high and low risk of severe myocardial infarction and cardiac death. *Stroke* 2002; 33:2413–6.
4. Hines GL, Feuerman M, Cappello D, et al: Results of carotid endarterectomy with pericardial patch angioplasty: rate and predictors of restenosis. *Ann Vasc Surg* 2007; 21:767–71.
5. Howell SJ: Carotid endarterectomy. *Br J Anaesth* 2007; 99:119–31.
6. Moritz S, Kasprzak P, Arlt M, et al: Accuracy of cerebral monitoring in detecting cerebral ischemia during carotid endarterectomy: a comparison of transcranial Doppler sonography, near-infrared spectroscopy, stump pressure, and somatosensory evoked potentials. *Anesthesiology* 2007; 107:563–9.
7. NASCET Collaborators: *N Engl J Med* 1991; 325:445–53.
8. Pasternak JJ, Lanier WL: Neuroanesthesiology review–2006. *J Neurosurg Anesthesiol* 2007; 19:70–92.
9. Young B, Moore WS, Robertson JT, et al: An analysis of perioperative surgical mortality and morbidity in the Asymptomatic Carotid Atherosclerosis Study. ACAS Investigators. *Stroke* 1996; 27:2216–24.

REPAIR OF THORACIC AORTIC ANEURYSMS

SURGICAL CONSIDERATIONS

Description: Repairs of aneurysms of the ascending, transverse arch, and descending thoracic aorta are performed to repair expanding or leaking aneurysms, or prophylactically to prevent rupture. Patients with Sx of rapid expansion or aneurysm leaking may require urgent repair. Each surgical type—ascending, arch, and descending—is considered separately, as follows. Aneurysms of the **ascending aorta** may arise 2° the degenerative changes of atherosclerosis (exacerbated by old age, HTN, tobacco use); from inborn errors of metabolism (Marfan syndrome); or from post-stenotic dilatation and continued expansion of a chronic dissection. Diseases of the entire ascending aorta, including the sinuses of Valsalva, as in Marfan syndrome and annuloaortic ectasia, require replacement of the ascending aorta and aortic root with a composite valved conduit, while acquired diseases limited to the ascending aorta usually allow replacement of the aorta distal to the sinotubular ridge. Repair of the ascending aorta is usually accomplished on full CPB with an aortic cross-clamp placed just proximal to the innominate artery and arterial inflow through the femoral artery. The aneurysmal ascending aorta is replaced with a Dacron tube graft from the sinotubular ridge to the innominate artery. Dilatation of the sinuses of Valsalva mandates replacement with a composite valved conduit sewn proximally to the aortic annulus and distally to a normal caliber ascending aorta, with coronary ostia reimplanted in the side of the tube graft.

Aneurysms of the **aortic arch** are the least common of thoracic aortic aneurysms. Because of the need for concomitant replacement of the arch vessels, however, they are the most complex to repair. Total CPB is utilized, and cerebral protection is accomplished either by CPB perfusion of one or all cerebral vessels, or by profound hypothermic circulatory arrest at 15–18°C. Repair can originate from the aortic annulus and extend distally to the mid descending thoracic aorta at the level of the carina. Routine caval cannulation is accomplished via a median sternotomy, and arterial access is gained via the femoral artery or axillary artery. If circulatory arrest is to be used, the patient is cooled to 15–18°C, the heart is arrested and, with no distal cross-clamp, distal anastomosis is accomplished, followed by implantation of the cerebral vessels attached to an island of aorta. Perfusion is then reinstituted, the graft clamped proximal to the innominate artery, and the proximal anastomosis performed, while the patient is being rewarmed. Alternatively, if one elects to perfuse the cerebral vessels, the innominate and left carotid arteries can be individually cannulated and perfused via a "Y" connection from the femoral arterial perfusion line. If axillary cannulation is used, antegrade cerebral perfusion can be achieved by control of the proximal innominate artery. The necessity for profound hypothermic circulatory arrest is thus avoided. After completion of the distal aortic, arch vessel island and proximal aortic anastomoses, weaning from CPB and subsequent steps proceed in a routine fashion.

Repair of aneurysms of the **descending thoracic aorta** is usually performed for symptomatic and leaking aneurysms, enlarging aneurysms, and aneurysms of sufficient size to warrant prophylactic repair. **Aneurysm repair** is accomplished through a left posterolateral thoracotomy on partial CPB. After entry into the left thorax, venous drainage for CPB may be obtained from the left atrium or the femoral vein, and arterial return is via the femoral artery. If partial bypass without an oxygenator is elected, thus minimizing the amount of heparin necessary, venous access can be gained via the pulmonary veins or left atrium, and arterial return via the femoral artery or distal thoracic aorta. After institution of bypass, the aorta is cross-clamped above and below the aneurysm, the aorta is divided, a tube graft is interposed, and clamps are removed. The patient is weaned from bypass, and the operation is terminated in the routine fashion.

Usual preop diagnosis: Enlarging or symptomatic aortic aneurysm

SUMMARY OF PROCEDURES

	Ascending Aorta	Transverse Arch	Descending Aorta
Position	Supine	⇐	Lateral decubitus with left side up
Incision	Median sternotomy	⇐	Left posterolateral thoracotomy with access to femoral artery and vein
Special instrumentation	CPB, if used.	Complete hemodynamic monitors; CPB	⇐ + DLT; lower extremity BP monitor
Unique considerations	Routine CPB hemodynamic monitoring	If profound hypothermic arrest is utilized, neuroprotective adjuncts, including local hypothermia, barbiturates, and steroids, should be used.	OLV; partial CPB
Antibiotics	Cefazolin 1 g iv	⇐	⇐

SUMMARY OF PROCEDURES (cont'd)

	Ascending Aorta	Transverse Arch	Descending Aorta
Surgical time	Aortic cross-clamp: 40–120 min CPB: 70–150 min Total: 2.5–5 h	Aortic cross-clamp: 75–120 min Circulatory arrest: 30–45 min CPB: 3–4.5 h Total: 4–6 h	Aortic cross-clamp: 25–45 min CPB: 30–60 min Total: 2.5–4.5 h
Closing considerations	Aggressive management of coagulopathy, if a long pump run is necessary.	Aggressive management of coagulopathy	Replacement of DLT with single-lumen tube
EBL	300–400 mL	400–700 mL	200–300 mL
Postop care	ICU, intubated 5–20 h, depending on preop condition	ICU, intubated 6–24 h	ICU, intubated 5–24 h
Mortality	5–10%	10–15%	⇐
Morbidity	Renal failure: 5–10% CVA: 4–6% Respiratory failure: 3–5% MI: 2–5%	— 2–5% 10% ⇐	10–15% 2–4% 10–15% 2–4%
Pain score	7–10	7–10	9–10

PATIENT POPULATION CHARACTERISTICS

Age range	23–80 yr (mean = 55 yr)	50–75 yr	34–79 yr (mean = 65 yr)
Male:Female	3:1	2:1	2.5:1
Incidence	10–30/yr at tertiary center	5–10/yr at tertiary center	10–30/yr at tertiary center
Etiology	Degenerative disease Atherosclerotic disease	⇐ ⇐ Chronic dissections	⇐ ⇐ ⇐
Associated conditions	CHF (50%); angina (30%); HTN (30%); COPD (15%)	Aortic valve disease (30%); COPD (20%); CAD (15%)	HTN (65%); CAD (50%); COPD (30%); CHF (10%)

ANESTHETIC CONSIDERATIONS

PREOPERATIVE

Typically, patients with thoracic aortic aneurysms have atherosclerosis and HTN. A subset of patients will have a connective tissue disorder (e.g., Marfan syndrome). In contrast with thoracic aortic dissections, thoracic aortic aneurysms may be of a more chronic and asymptomatic nature. A ruptured or leaking aneurysm, however, may have a more precipitous presentation.

Cardiovascular	**Arch and ascending aneurysms** (60–70% of aneurysms): commonly associated with HTN, cystic medial necrosis, connective tissue disorder (e.g., Marfan syndrome), atherosclerosis, or syphilis. CHF may occur 2° to dilation of the aortic annulus and aortic incompetence (AR). Aneurysmal compression or intrinsic disease of the coronary arteries may result in myocardial ischemia. **Descending (30%):** usually associated with HTN, cystic medial necrosis, Marfan syndrome, and atherosclerosis.

Cardiovascular (cont'd)	**Tests:** ECG: ✓ for LVH, ischemia. ECHO: ✓ for valvular disease, size and extent of aneurysm, LV function. Angiography: ✓ exact extent of aneurysm (allows planning of procedure and sites for arterial monitoring), coronary artery anatomy, and degree of occlusion.
Respiratory	Recurrent laryngeal nerve palsy may → hoarseness (ascending/arch aneurysms). Tracheal deviation ± stridor or dyspnea may be present 2° tracheal or bronchial compression (✓ CT scan). Hemoptysis or a hemorrhagic pleural effusion suggest an aneurysmal leakage or rupture. The implications include the possibility of compromised oxygenation, risk of massive hemorrhage on thoracotomy, increased intrathoracic pressure, and consequent decreased venous return (especially when IPPV is instituted). **Tests:** CXR: ✓ for widened mediastinum, distortion of trachea and left main bronchus (because it may affect the placement of DLT); MRI/CT with contrast: ✓ anatomic relation of aneurysm to surrounding structures (e.g., trachea/bronchi); others as indicated from H&P.
Neurologic	Any deficit should be well documented as neurologic sequelae (e.g., paraplegia/paraparesia) may occur after surgery.
Renal	Renal problems may occur 2° to AR (↓CO) and heart failure, HTN, or involvement of renal arteries in the aneurysm. **Tests:** BUN; Cr; consider Cr clearance; electrolytes
Gastrointestinal	Descending aneurysms that involve the celiac or superior mesenteric arteries may → bowel ischemia. **Tests:** Consider ABG: ✓ persistent metabolic acidosis (2% bowel ischemia). If indicated by H&P, consider abdominal CT/x-ray: ✓ ileus.
Hematological	If time permits, consider autologous blood donation; pre-existing coagulopathy increases risk of the procedure. **Tests:** PT; PTT; Hct/Hb
Musculoskeletal	✓ Marfanoid appearance; others as indicated from H&P.
Laboratory	Others as indicated from H&P.
Premedication	Pain and anxiety may significantly contribute to HTN and should be treated (e.g., morphine 0.1 mg/kg iv ± midazolam 0.025–0.1 mg/kg iv); but avoid obtundation. Because many of these patients present emergently, consider full-stomach precautions—H_2 antagonists (e.g., ranitidine 5 0 mg iv), metoclopramide (10 mg iv), and antacids (e.g., Na citrate 0.3 M 30 mL po).

INTRAOPERATIVE

Anesthetic technique: The anesthetic management of patients with aortic dissections and aortic aneurysms are similar in many respects. For intraop and postop management of these conditions, see Anesthetic Considerations for Repair of Acute Aortic Dissections and Dissecting Aneurysms, p. 404.

Suggested Readings

1. Cheung AT, Pochettino A, McGarvey ML, et al: Strategies to manage paraplegia risk after endovascular stent repair of descending thoracic aortic aneurysms. *Ann Thorac Surg* 2005; 80:1280–8.
2. Estrera AL, Miller CC III, Huynh TT, et al: Replacement of the ascending and transverse aortic arch: determinants of long-term survival. *Ann Thorac Surg* 2002; 74:1058–65.
3. Estrera AL, Rubenstein FS, Miller CC: Descending thoracic aortic aneurysm: surgical approach and treatment using the adjuncts cerebrospinal fluid drainage and distal aortic perfusion. *Ann Thorac Surg* 2001; 72:481–6.
4. Fann JI: Descending thoracic and thoracoabdominal aortic aneurysms. *Coron Artery Dis* 2002; 13:93–102.
5. Gega A, Rizzo JA, Johnson MH, et al: Straight deep hypothermic arrest: experience in 394 patients supports the effectiveness as a sole means of brain preservation. *Ann Thorac Surg* 2007; 84:759–66.
6. Gleason TG, Benjamin LC: Conventional open repair of descending thoracic aortic aneurysms. *Perspect Vasc Surg Endovasc Ther* 2007; 19:110–21.
7. Hagel C, Ergin MA, Galla JD, et al: Neurologic outcome after ascending aorta-aortic arch operations: effect of brain protection technique in high-risk patients. *J Thorac Cardiovasc Surg* 2001; 121:1107–21.
8. Kahn RA, Stone ME, Moskowitz DM: Anesthetic consideration for descending thoracic aortic aneurysm repair. *Semin Cardiothorac Vasc Anesth* 2007; 11:205–23.
9. Kazui T, Yamashita K, Washiyama N, et al: Aortic arch replacement using selective cerebral perfusion. *Ann Thorac Surg* 2007; 83:S796–8.

10. Okita Y, Ando M, Minatoya K, et al: Early and long-term results of surgery for aneurysms of the thoracic aorta in septuagenarians and octogenarians. *Eur J Cardiothorac Surg* 1999; 16:317–23.
11. Olsson C, Eriksson N, Stahle E, et al: Surgical and long-term mortality in 2634 consecutive patients operated on the proximal thoracic aorta. *Eur J Cardiothorac Surg* 2007; 31:963–9.
12. Pressler BA, McNamara JJ: Thoracic aortic aneurysm. Natural history and treatment. *J Thorac Cardiovasc Surg* 1980; 79:489–98.
13. Stone DH, Brewster DC, Kwolek CJ, et al: Stent-graft versus open-surgical repair of the thoracic aorta: mid-term results. *J Vasc Surg* 2006; 44:1188–97.
14. Svenson LG: Progress in ascending and aortic arch surgery: minimally invasive surgery, blood conservation, and neurologic deficit prevention. *Ann Thora Surg* 2002; 74:1786–8.

ENDOVASCULAR STENT-GRAFTING OF AORTIC ANEURYSMS

SURGICAL CONSIDERATIONS

Description: The standard treatment for descending **thoracic aortic aneurysm** is surgical resection of the aneurysm and replacement with a segment of prosthetic graft material. Although resection of aneurysms often can be performed without the need for extracorporeal circulation, the procedure has a reported mortality rate of up to 50% in emergency cases and 12–15% in elective cases. Transluminal endovascular stent-grafting offers an alternative treatment that is less invasive, less hazardous, and potentially less expensive than standard operative repair.

In the initial workup, all patients have contrast-enhanced spiral CT scans of the thorax, and thoracic aortography to assess the dimensions of the aneurysms. The most important features to consider in evaluating an aortic aneurysm for endovascular stent-graft treatment is the presence of an adequate proximal and distal neck. A minimum neck length of at least 1.5 cm is required to allow secure anchoring of most stent-grafts. The distance from the origins of the left subclavian artery and celiac axis to the aneurysm should be at least 1.5–3 cm to ensure that the stent-graft does not inadvertently block these arteries. In an effort to reduce the incidence of paraplegia, and to limit exclusion of intracostal arteries, the overall length of the stent-graft is kept to a minimum.

Another important anatomic consideration is the size of the proposed conduit vessel (e.g., iliac) to ensure that it is adequate for accommodation of the stent-introducer system, which usually requires at least an 8-mm-diameter vessel. Where the pelvic vessels are less than 8 mm, either a retroperitoneal iliac or retroperitoneal aortic approach is utilized. The stent is the metallic framework to which the graft material is applied. Various balloon-expandable or self-expanding stents are available. For application in the thoracic aorta, stents of 30–40 mm in diameter (mean 35 mm) are required.

Typically, thoracic aortic aneurysm stent-graft procedures are performed in the cath lab (although some may be performed in the OR, depending on equipment availability and local politics), with the patient intubated and under GA. The cath lab is prepared for aortic surgery, with the patient placed on the table in a shallow right decubitus position. The patient's thorax may be prepped and draped for a left thoracotomy. For an approach via the common femoral artery, the groin area is prepped for a femoral artery cutdown. When the iliac arteries are of insufficient size, the left lower abdomen is prepped for a retroperitoneal approach to either the aorta or the common iliac artery. High-quality fluoroscopic equipment is essential to assure accurate placement of the device, and a portable C-arm with digital subtraction capability is moved into position and centered over the thorax. When the iliac vessels are of sufficient size, a cutdown is performed on a femoral artery, the artery is punctured, and a guide wire is advanced into the thoracic aorta. A pigtail catheter is placed and an aortogram is performed. The patient is then anticoagulated with iv heparin (100 IU/kg). A long, stiff guide wire is placed, and the 24 Fr sheath and dilator assembly is advanced over the wire until the sheath tip is proximal to the proximal aneurysm neck. The dilator and guide wire are withdrawn, and the stent-graft is introduced into the sheath from its loading cartridge using the Teflon pusher. The device is pushed through the sheath until the stent-graft approaches the tip of the sheath.

In order to reduce the likelihood of inadvertent downstream deployment of the stent-graft caused by the force of blood flow during initial delivery, the arterial BP may be lowered to a mean of 50–60 mmHg using SNP. Holding the pusher firmly in position, the sheath is rapidly withdrawn, and the stent-graft expands into position. Rapid deployment helps to minimize distal migration of the stent-graft. Immediately following deployment, the SNP is discontinued, allowing the BP to normalize. Repeat aortogram is performed, and any early leakage of contrast into the aneurysm is treated either with balloon angioplasty of the stent-graft or further stent-graft placement. Occasionally a faint, persistent leak of contrast is caused by leakage through the graft material. This typically ceases when the patient's coagulation status returns to normal. Following removal of the delivery sheath, heparin is reversed with protamine sulfate and the arteriotomy is repaired surgically. For stent placement through the retroperitoneal aorta, the procedure has a more extensive surgical component; however, the technique is similar.

The basic concept of **abdominal aortic aneurysm** (AAA) repair via an endovascular route is similar to the preceding section on thoracic aneurysm repair, with some notable exceptions. AAAs commonly arise inferior to the renal arteries, and 80–90% of cases involve either one or both iliac arteries. For this reason, stent-grafts that can accommodate this more complicated anatomy are required. The superior aneurysm neck needs to be of sufficient length (1.5–2 cm) inferior to the most inferior renal artery to provide for stable anchoring. Inferiorly the stent-graft must accommodate either or both iliac arteries. The procedure is performed in a two-stage fashion. Initially an aorta-to-single-iliac-artery device is placed from the infrarenal aortic neck into one of the iliac vessels. A contralateral femoral artery puncture is then performed, and a catheter and guide wire are used to access an open stump of the stent-graft from the contralateral limb. At this stage, a modular section of stent-graft is placed from the aortic component into the contralateral limb; in this way, an aorta-to-bi-iliac graft is placed.

Usual preop diagnosis: Aortic aneurysm

SUMMARY OF PROCEDURES

	Thoracic Aortic Aneurysms	Abdominal Aortic Aneurysms
Position	Supine/slight right decubitus	Supine
Incision	Femoral artery cutdown	Bilateral femoral artery cutdowns
Special instrumentation	Catheters, guide wires, sheaths, dilators and stent-grafts	⇐
Unique considerations	May require adjunctive procedure (e.g., brachial artery catheterization, balloon angioplasty, possible left subclavian-to-common carotid artery bypass procedure); iv heparin 100–300 IU/kg	⇐
Antibiotics	Cefazolin 1 g iv	⇐
Surgical time	1–3 h	⇐
Closing considerations	None	⇐
EBL	Usually minimal; however, can be up to 2–3 U	⇐
Postop care	ICU × 1 d	⇐
Mortality	3–5%	2–3%
Morbidity	Paraplegia: 2–3% Infection: 1% Surgical conversion: < 1%	Acute rupture: < 1% ⇐ ⇐
Pain score	3–4	3–4

PATIENT POPULATION CHARACTERISTICS

Age range	30–90 yr	40–90 yr
Incidence	1/10,000 of the population in the United States.	1/1,000 of the population in the United States.
Etiology	Atherosclerosis; HTN; trauma; aortic dissection; infection	Atherosclerosis; infection
Associated conditions	CAD; aneurysmal disease elsewhere	⇐

Cardiovascular Surgery

ANESTHETIC CONSIDERATIONS

The anesthetic considerations for thoracic and abdominal stent-grafting are similar since the surgical techniques, complications, patient concurrent disease, and stent-graft deployment techniques are similar. Patients may be asymptomatic; most will have coexisting CAD, PVD, and/or cerebrovascular disease.

Suggested Readings

1. Baril D, Kahn R, Ellozy SH, et al: Endovascular abdominal aortic repair: emerging developments and anesthetic considerations. *J Cardiothorac Vasc Anesth* 2007;21:730–42.
2. Makkad B, Pilling S: Management of thoracic aneurysm. *Semin Cardiothorac Vasc Anesth* 2005;9:227–40.
3. Riddell JM, Black JH, Brewster DC, et al: Endovascular abdominal aortic aneurysm repair. *Int Anesthesiol Clin* 2005;43: 79–91.
4. Ruppert V, Leurs LJ, Steckmeier B, et al: Influence of anesthesia type on outcome after endovascular aortic aneurysm repair: an analysis based on EUROSTAR data. *J Vasc Surg* 2006;44:16–21.

PREOPERATIVE

Preop considerations for these patients are the same as for any patient undergoing repair of a descending thoracic aneurysm, abdominal aortic aneurysm, or aortobifemoral aneurysm. Many of these patients, however, are not suitable for conventional repair via a thoracotomy because of respiratory disease (e.g., $FEV_1 < 1$ L, severe COPD, $PaCO_2 > 60$ mmHg), CAD, renal failure, CHF, or a combination of these factors. As such, they generally are at very high risk for periop morbidity and mortality. Before surgery the anesthesiologist should consult with the surgical and radiological teams to decide what will be done should a complication such as penetration or rupture of the aneurysm occur during surgery (typically, an emergency thoracotomy or laparotomy performed in the cath lab).

INTRAOPERATIVE

Anesthetic technique: Usually GETA (OLV may be required for emergency thoracotomy 2° ruptured thoracic aneurysm). Abdominal stent-grafts may be placed under epidural or spinal anesthesia. Rarely, stent-grafting may be carried out with local anesthesia or MAC in patients unable to tolerate GA or epidural. In that case, the patient will come to the OR for removal of the introducer system and repair of the femoral artery.

Induction	Since these patients are typically extubated, the dose of fentanyl (5–10 mcg/kg) is limited to that which will suppress the hypertensive response to intubation, while still allowing for early extubation. The same considerations apply to the use of muscle relaxants (e.g., vecuronium [0.1 mg/kg] or rocuronium [1–1.5 mg/kg]). A DLT or a Univent ETT should be used, unless the team decides that a thoracotomy will not be performed under any circumstance.	
Maintenance	Usually a balanced anesthetic technique of O_2/air/isoflune or sevoflurane, supplemented with fentanyl (or remifentanil infusion) as needed. Hemodynamic control of BP (esmolol, SNP, NTG) and heart rate to avoid myocardial ischemia is important. **Anesthetic management during stent-graft deployment:** During stent-graft deployment, the aorta is momentarily occluded. Formerly, this resulted in a rapid ↑ BP → stent-graft being moved from its intended position. The newer generations of stent-grafts, using thermal or mechanical means for rapid deployment, cause minimal hemodynamic change, eliminating the need for aggressive BP control.	
Emergence	Extubation is desirable, although hypothermia (<34° C) may prevent this. Otherwise, aim for early extubation in the ICU. DLT (if used) may be replaced with a standard ETT at end of procedure if the patient is not extubated in the cath lab. Recovery is usually in the ICU.	
Blood and fluid requirements	IV: 14–16 ga × 1 NS/LR @ 4–8 mL/kg/h PRBC available	Although usually minimal, blood loss can be considerable.

Monitoring	Standard monitors (p. B-1) Arterial line	Arterial line placement should be on the right as the radiologists may require access to the left brachial artery.
	CVP catheter Urinary catheter	CVP monitoring is usually sufficient. Central access for vasoactive drugs may be needed.
	TEE	TEE is used to aid in the identification of the thoracic aneurysm necks, to monitor deployment of the stent-graft and to identify any continued flow of blood into the aneurysmal sac after deployment (endoleak).
	CSF pressure/drainage	CSF drainage → ↓ CSF pressure may be necessary to minimize spinal cord ischemia (anterior spinal artery syndrome).
Positioning	✓ and pad pressure points. ✓ eyes.	Supine ± slight right lateral decubitus
Complications	Hemorrhage	Hemorrhage at the groin site can be considerable and may be concealed.
	Vessel damage	Damage to the vessels (femoral, iliac, or abdominal aorta) during passage of the insertion system can occur with attendant massive hemorrhage.
	Rupture of aorta	Rupture or penetration of the thoracic aneurysm also can occur, necessitating rapid conversion to open thoracotomy.
	Deployment failure/incorrect position	The stent-graft may deploy in an incorrect position or fail to fully deploy. This may require positioning of further stent-grafts, balloon expansion of the stent-graft, or conversion to thoracotomy.
	Hypothermia	Hypothermia can be a problem as a circulating-water warming blanket cannot be used on the operating table (use of fluoroscopy). Much of the patient's body is exposed (upper-body Bair-Hugger usually ok) and a lower-body warming blanket cannot be used as the lower limbs may be ischemic during insertion of the stent-graft.

POSTOPERATIVE

Complications	Aortic perforation/rupture	Requires emergency surgery.
	Migration of grafts	→ loss of distal pulses, mesenteric ischemia, acute renal insufficiency.
	Femoral artery dehiscence	Requires prompt return to OR.
	Distal embolization	✓ pulses; angiography/surgical intervention.
	Paraplegia	✓ reflexes; prompt return to OR.
Pain management	Minimal analgesic requirements	If groin incision, local anesthetic infiltration may be used.
Tests	As indicated by patient condition.	CT scan, angiogram prior to discharge and at regular intervals following discharge.

Suggested Readings

1. Dake MD, Miller DC, Semba CP, et al: Transluminal placement of endovascular stent-grafts for the treatment of descending thoracic aortic aneurysms. *N Engl J Med* 1994: 331(26):1729–34.
2. Fleck T, Hutschala D, Weissl M, et al: Cerebrospinal fluid drainage as a useful treatment option to relieve paraplegia after stent-graft implantation for acute aortic dissection type B. *J Thorac Cardiovasc Surg* 2002; 123: 1003–5.

3. Herold U, Piotrowski J, Baumgart D, et al: Endoluminal stent graft repair for acute and chronic type B aortic dissection and atherosclerotic aneurysm of the thoracic aorta: an interdisciplinary task. *Eur J Cardiothorac Surg* 2002; 22:891–7.
4. Mitchell RS, Dake MD, Semba CP, et al: Endovascular stent-graft repair of thoracic aortic aneurysms. *J Thorac Cardiovasc Surg* 1996; 111(5):1054–62.
5. Mitchell RS: Stent grafts for the thoracic aorta: a new paradigm? *Ann Thorac Surg* 2002; 74:1818–20.
6. Schütz W, Gauss A, Meierhenrich R, et al: Transesophageal echocardiographic guidance of thoracic aortic stent-graft implantation. *J Endovasc Ther* 2002; 9:14–9.
7. Semba CP, Kato N, Kee ST, et al: Acute rupture of the descending thoracic aorta: repair with use of endovascular stent-grafts. *J Vasc Interv Radiol* 1997; 8(3):337–42.

REPAIR OF ACUTE AORTIC DISSECTIONS AND DISSECTING ANEURYSMS

SURGICAL CONSIDERATIONS

Description: Repair of **acute aortic dissection** is performed to prevent life-threatening complications such as hemorrhage, tamponade, and heart failure 2° acute aortic valvular insufficiency and to redirect flow into the true lumen. Emergent repair of acute ascending dissections is generally accepted therapy to prevent rupture of the aortic root with exsanguination or pericardial tamponade. Mortality for acute ascending dissection is estimated at 1% per hour for the first 48 hours. The management of descending thoracic aortic dissections remains controversial, but surgical intervention probably should be recommended only for younger patients, patients with uncontrolled pain or evidence for continued expansion or extravasation, and those with branch-vessel compromise.

Ascending dissections typically produce sharp, tearing retrosternal pain that penetrates straight through to the subscapular area. The presentation, however, is so frequently variable that any patient in extremis, especially with migratory pain or vacillating findings, and even asymptomatic patients with valvular aortic regurgitation (AR), should be considered for the diagnosis. With a suggestive Hx, a new murmur, or a pulse deficit, an enlarged mediastinal shadow on chest radiography should prompt further diagnostic efforts. CT scanning, MRI, and aortography may all be diagnostic, but no diagnostic modality has 100% sensitivity. TEE appears to be highly sensitive in detecting a mobile intimal flap in the ascending or descending aorta. In addition, TEE can provide useful information regarding AR, periaortic hematoma and flow within a false channel. It is usually available at the bedside or in the emergency ward and does not subject the patient to a contrast load.

After the patients are diagnosed, they are transported immediately to the OR. Through a median sternotomy, venous access is gained via the right atrium, and arterial inflow is supplied through a femoral artery or axillary artery. CPB is established, the patient cooled to 18°C, and circulatory support discontinued although antegrade cerebral perfusion may be employed. During a period of circulatory arrest or antegrade cerebral perfusion, the ascending aorta is opened and the tear localized. The repair is carried distally into the arch, if the entire dissection can be resected, and the distal aortic layers are reapproximated with a Teflon felt strip supporting the medial and adventitial layers. The distal graft anastomosis is then completed, the graft clamped, the bypass pump restarted and systemic warming commenced. Proximally, the aortic root is reconstructed, again using Teflon felt to support the medial and adventitial layers and to resuspend the aortic valve, which can be salvaged in approximately 85% of cases. The heart is then cleared of air, and the cross-clamp removed to allow reperfusion of the coronary circulation. After a sufficient period of resuscitation, the patient is weaned from CPB. Aggressive management of an acquired coagulopathy is not unusual prior to chest closure.

Repair of **dissections** involving the **descending thoracic aorta** is accomplished through a left thoracotomy utilizing partial CPB. Venous drainage is usually via the femoral vein, although the pulmonary vein may be used. Arterial access is via the femoral artery. After institution of CPB, the dissected aorta above and below the most damaged area is cross-clamped and the aorta transected. After oversewing patent intercostal arteries, the medial and adventitial layers are buttressed with Teflon felt, and an interposition Dacron graft is sewn into place. After evacuation of air, clamps are removed, and the patient weaned from CPB. Heparin reversal, decannulation, and closure are accomplished in the usual manner.

Usual preop diagnosis: Acute dissection of the aorta (See Fig. 6.3-3 for types of dissection.)

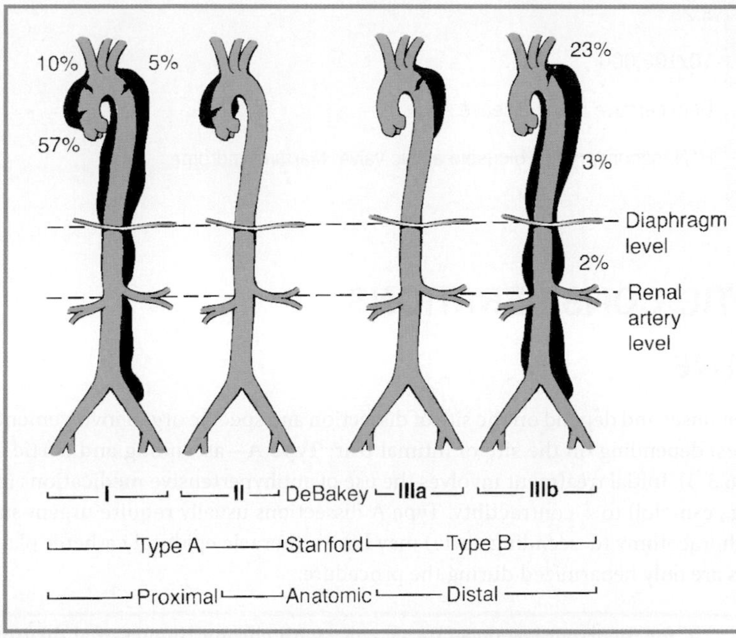

Figure 6.3-3. The three classification systems of aortic dissection and the distribution of the intimal tear.

SUMMARY OF PROCEDURES

	Ascending Aorta	Descending Aorta
Position	Supine	Lateral decubitus, left side up
Incision	Median sternotomy	Left lateral thoracotomy
Unique considerations	Full hemodynamic monitoring, with provisions for circulatory arrest, profound hypothermia, barbiturates and steroids; TEE	DLT; CPB; TEE; lumbar drain
Antibiotics	Cefazolin 1 g iv	⇐
Surgical time	Cross-clamp: 30–50 min Circulatory arrest: 20–30 min CPB: 60–100 min Total: 3–5 h	30–60 min — 35–60 min ⇐
Closing considerations	Aggressively treat coagulopathy (frequently 2° ↓ Plt).	Replace DLT with single-lumen ETT.
EBL	400–800 mL	600–800 mL
Postop care	ICU: 1–2 d, intubated	⇐
Mortality	10–25%	⇐
Morbidity	Bleeding: 3–8% Respiratory insufficiency: 2–5% CVA: 2–4%	Paraplegia: 5% CVA: 1–2% MI: 1–2%
Pain score	7–10	9–10

PATIENT POPULATION CHARACTERISTICS	
Age range	40–70 yr
Male:Female	3:2
Incidence	10/100,000
Etiology	Degenerative aortic disease
Associated conditions	HTN; secondary AR; bicuspid aortic valve; Marfan syndrome

ANESTHETIC CONSIDERATIONS

PREOPERATIVE

Sx are usually of sudden onset and depend on the site of dissection and specific organ involvement. Aortic dissections are divided into 2 types, depending on the site of intimal tear: **Type A**—ascending and aortic arch, and **Type B**—descending aorta (Fig 6.3-3). Initial treatment involves the use of antihypertensive medications (e.g., SNP) to control BP and β-blockers (e.g., esmolol) to ↓ contractility. Type A dissections usually require urgent surgery. Patients presenting electively for thoracotomy (descending aorta) may have a thoracic epidural catheter placed the night before surgery. These patients are only heparinized during the procedure.

Respiratory	✓ for recurrent laryngeal nerve palsy with chronic aneurysmal dilation. Tracheal and left main bronchus compression → difficult intubation, atelectasis; hemoptysis 2° rupture into lung; hemothorax → compromised oxygenation, ↑intrathoracic pressure → ↓ venous return, especially with IPPV. **Tests:** CXR: ✓ for widened mediastinum, tracheal or left main bronchus compression and distortion (affects DLT placement), atelectasis, pleural effusion (or hemothorax 2° rupture).
Cardiovascular	Aortic dissections may be associated with chronic HTN, cystic medial necrosis, or other connective tissue disorder (e.g., Marfan syndrome) and trauma. Dissection may result in cardiac tamponade, acute aortic valve incompetence, acute cardiac failure, angina, MI, or rupture of the aorta. Dissection of major arteries may result in ↓ or absent peripheral pulses, which may affect the placement sites for intraarterial monitoring and central venous access. Pain and anxiety may result in HTN, while rupture or leakage may result in ↓ BP and shock. **Tests:** ECG: ✓ for Sx of LVH, ischemia or infarction, low voltage (tamponade). ECHO: ✓ for site of dissection, valvular competence, LV function, pericardial effusion or tamponade. Angiography: ✓ for site of dissection (Type A or B), valvular function, involvement of coronary and other major arteries, sites of rupture, LV function. CT scan: ✓ site and extent of dissection.
Neurological	Deficits are not uncommon, especially with Type B dissections where the blood supply to the spinal cord may be jeopardized. Document preop exam carefully.
Renal	Renal failure 2° renal artery involvement in dissection, shock, or cardiac failure. UO should be monitored closely during initial medical therapy. **Tests:** UO; BUN; Cr; electrolytes
Gastrointestinal	Compromised blood supply to the bowel or liver may result in ischemia → metabolic acidosis and ↓ liver function. Tests: Consider ABG: ✓ persistent metabolic acidosis; LFTs, if indicated by H&P.
Hematologic	Coagulopathy may be present 2° massive hemorrhage or liver involvement, and can increase risk of the surgery. **Tests:** PT; PTT; Hct/Hb
Laboratory	Other tests as indicated from H&P.

Premedication	Since many of these patients present emergently, consider full-stomach precautions: H_2-antagonists (ranitidine 50 mg iv), metoclopramide (10–20 mg iv), antacids (Na citrate 0.3 M 30 mL po). Alleviate anxiety and pain (e.g., morphine 0.1 mg/kg im, ± midazolam 0.025–0.1 mg/kg iv or 0.05–0.2 mg/kg im), which may worsen HTN, but avoid obtundation.

INTRAOPERATIVE

Anesthetic technique: GETA ± thoracic epidural. Preinduction control of BP and contractility (NTG or SNP to SBP = 105–115 and esmolol to HR = 60–80) is important in preventing extension of the dissection or rupture of the aneurysm. Fluid resuscitation may be necessary prior to induction.

Induction	Control of hypertensive response to laryngoscopy and intubation is important and may be accomplished with moderate-dose narcotic (fentanyl 10–15 mcg/kg or sufentanil 1–2 mcg/kg) and etomidate (0.1–0.3 mg/kg), esmolol (5–10 mg iv bolus), or SNP (25–50 mcg bolus). Pretreatment with lidocaine (1.5 mg/kg) also may be required to further control the hypertensive response to laryngoscopy. Muscle relaxation may be obtained using vecuronium (0.1 mg/kg) or rocuronium (1–2 mg/kg). Remember the possibility of a full stomach in this patient population. Hence, a modified rapid-sequence induction (cricoid pressure with manual ventilation and NMR) may achieve the two goals of relatively rapid induction and intubation and tight control of BP. Usually a left DLT is used in patients with descending lesions to improve surgical access; however, it may be difficult to place due to aneurysmal compression of the trachea and left mainstem bronchus, and it is associated with a small risk of aneurysmal rupture. For these reasons, a right DLT may be preferred. FOB is mandatory to verify ET placement.	
Maintenance	O_2/narcotic/benzodiazepine: low-dose volatile agent (isoflurane [0.3–0.5%] or sevoflurane [0.5–1%]) may be used to control BP (MAP = 60–80), although infusion of vasopressors, vasodilators, or inotropes may be necessary. Control HR (< 80; anesthesia, esmolol) and contractility (β-blockade or inotropes, depending on circumstances). Benzodiazepines may be used for amnesia (midazolam 100 mcg/kg). If thoracic epidural in place, fentanyl (20–30 mcg/kg) or sufentanil (4–6 mcg/kg) may be used. Most Type A aneurysms and ascending/arch aneurysms require hypothermic CPB (see Anesthetic Considerations for Cardiopulmonary Bypass, p. 338). Intraop anesthetic considerations are governed primarily by the site of the aortic pathology. These considerations are discussed below.	
Emergence	Transported to ICU, sedated, intubated, and ventilated × 24–48 h. Following repairs of the descending aorta (thoracotomy incision), weaning from ventilator may be aided by epidural narcotics after documentation of normal spinal cord function and coagulation.	
Blood and fluid requirements	Anticipate large blood loss. IV: 14 ga – 7 Fr × 2 NS/LR @ 6–8 mL/kg/h Warm all fluids. Humidify gases. Cross-match 6–8 U of blood. UO 0.5–1 mL/kg/h	In Type A dissections and arch aneurysms, if possible, avoid iv placement in the left arm or left IJ/subclavian veins because of the possibility of innominate vein ligation. Mannitol (0.25–0.5 g/kg iv) should be given if renal perfusion is compromised by dissection or before cross-clamping. Consider normovolemic hemodilution if the patient is stable and the Hct > 35. After unclamping: furosemide (1 mg/kg), if hemodynamically stable.
Monitoring	Standard monitors (p. B-1). Arterial line CVP, PA catheter (optional) Urinary catheter	Arterial line site is dependent on type of surgery and location of the lesion. Because the right subclavian artery may be compromised in patients with ascending lesions, the left radial or femoral arteries may need to be used. Aortic arch lesions may involve the vascular supply to both upper extremities;

Monitoring (cont'd)		hence, femoral artery catheterization may be necessary. In ascending lesions, two artery lines may be required—right radial (above clamp pressure) and left femoral (below clamp pressure). Consult with surgeon as to best site.
	TEE	TEE is useful to assess cardiac function, regional wall motion abnormalities, valvular pathology, aortic valvular repair (if required as part of a Type A repair). Probe passage may increase compression of the trachea, impeding ventilation. Caution should be used in the presence of aneurysmal compression of the esophagus.
	Temperature	Monitor both core (esophageal/bladder) and tympanic membrane T (as indicative of brain T)—important in deep hypothermic arrest.
	EEG/EP (arch/ascending lesions)	EEG/EP may help in assessing effectiveness of cerebral protection or adequacy of cerebral perfusion.
	SSEPs/MEPs (descending lesions)	SSEPs may detect posterior spinal perfusion problems, while MEPs may detect anterior cord dysfunction. Both EEG and EPs may require expert help to set up, monitor, and interpret.
	Cerebral oximetry	Cerebral oximetry may be helpful in detecting changes in cerebral blood flow after cannulation of the innominate artery.
Complications	Hemorrhage Coagulopathy	Both are common. Hemorrhage should be treated with crystalloid, colloid, or blood products, as indicated.
Ascending lesions	CPB AR Coronary arteries	Usual site of cannulation for CPB is the ascending artery or femoral artery. Aortic valve replacement may be necessary. Patients may have myocardial ischemia 2° coronary artery occlusion; may require CABG or reimplantation of vessels.
	Deep hypothermic arrest	Cerebral protective measures and selective perfusion of cerebral vessels may be required. (See below.)
Arch lesions	CPB Deep hypothermic arrest	Usual site of cannulation for CPB is femoral or axillary artery. Cerebral protection relies on hypothermia (15–18°C) and drugs (methylprednisolone [Solu-Medrol] 1 g, mannitol 0.5 g/kg, STP 15–30 mg/kg) to reduce $CMRO_2$ and neuronal injury. The head is surface cooled (protect eyes and ears from cold injury). EEG may be monitored to ensure absence of brain electrical activity. Monitor tympanic membrane T as an indication of brain T. Avoid hyperglycemia and maintain normal pH and $PaCO_2$ when measured at 37°C (alpha stat). Maintain muscle relaxation.
Descending lesions	Precross-clamping	Mannitol (0.5 g/kg) should be given before clamp application to provide renal protection, even if a shunt is placed. Hypothermia (32–34°C) may protect spinal cord.
	Shunt	A heparin-bonded shunt may be used from the aortic arch to the femoral artery to provide distal perfusion.

Cardiovascular Surgery

Descending lesions (cont'd)	Partial bypass	Partial CPB may be used to provide distal perfusion. In this arrangement, the heart perfuses the head and upper extremities, while CPB is used to perfuse and oxygenate the lower body. Venous drainage is from the femoral vein, PA, or left atrium and returned via the femoral artery. Distal and proximal pressures are altered by controlling cardiac filling, pump flow, and vasodilators.
	Cross-clamping	Application of clamp may → acute HTN with ischemia and LV failure. This may be controlled by partial bypass, shunting or use of vasodilators (SNP 0.5–4 mcg/kg/min, NTG 0.5–4 mcg/kg/min). During cross-clamping, monitor UO and ✓ metabolic acidosis (renal or bowel ischemia) with serial ABGs. Cross-clamp time should be < 30 min to reduce incidence of paraplegia. The surgeons often request that a lumbar CSF drain be inserted to ↓ CSF pressure (to ≤ CVP) and, thus, improve spinal cord blood flow.
	Unclamping	Unclamping may result in severe ↓ BP and myocardial depression. Hypovolemia, acidosis, vasoactive factors, and reactive hyperemia have been implicated as the cause. Prior to unclamping, ensure adequate volume status (PCWP 2–5 mmHg above patient's normal); treat acidosis; have vasopressors available; and the clamp should be released slowly over 1–2 min. Use of partial bypass or a shunt to ensure distal perfusion will mitigate unclamping shock. When hemodynamically stable, give furosemide (1 mg/kg iv). Inotropes (dopamine) may be needed to support circulation.
Positioning	✓ eyes. ✓ and pad pressure points. Arch and ascending: supine, shoulder roll Descending: lateral decubitus, axillary roll, pillow between knees	

POSTOPERATIVE

Complications	Myocardial ischemia, CHF Dysrhythmias Hemorrhage Coagulopathy Renal failure Bowel ischemia Respiratory failure	A DLT may be required in lesions of the descending aorta, if hemorrhage continues from left lung; otherwise, the tube may be replaced at the end of procedure by a single-lumen ETT. BP should be controlled to MAP 60–80 and HR < 100 to decrease the likelihood of repeat dissection, bleeding, or graft dehiscence.
	Paraplegia	Anterior spinal artery syndrome
Pain management	PCA (p. E-4) Epidural (p. E-6)	Thoracic epidural catheter may be used in patients following thoracotomy if coagulation status normal.
Tests	ECG: ischemia, infarction, dysrhythmias CXR: line and ETT placement; pulmonary contusion Coagulation profile Renal: BUN, Cr ABG: Respiratory, gut ischemia CT scan: CNS or spinal neurologic deficits Electrolytes	

Suggested Readings

1. Atkins MD Jr, Black JH 3rd, Cambria RP: Aortic dissection: perspective in the era of stent-graft repair. *J Vasc Surg* (suppl A): 30A–43A.
2. Dong CCJ, MacDonald DB, Janusz MT: Intraoperative spinal cord monitoring during descending thoracic and thoracoabdominal aneurysm surgery. *Ann Thorac Surg* 2002; 74:S1873–6.
3. Dorotta I, Kimball-Jones P, Applegate R: Deep hypothermia and circulatory arrest in adults. *Semin Cardiothorac Vasc Anesth* 2007; 11:66–76.
4. Estrera AL, Miller CC, Goodrick J, et al: Update on outcomes of acute type B aortic dissection. *Ann Thorac Surg* 2007; 83:S842–5.
5. Fann JI, Smith JA, Miller DC, et al: Surgical management of aortic dissection over a 30-year period. *Circulation* 1995; 92(II):113–21.
6. Khan IA, Nair CK: Clinical, diagnostic, and management perspectives of aortic dissection. *Chest* 2002; 122:311–28.
7. Klompas M: Does this patient have an acute thoracic aortic dissection? *JAMA* 2002; 287:2262–72.
8. Knipp BS, Deeb GM, Prager RL, et al: A contemporary analysis of outcomes for operative repair of type A aortic dissection in the United States. *Surgery* 2007; 142:524–8.
9. Kohl BA, McGarvey ML: Anesthesia and neurocerebral monitoring for aortic dissection. *Semin Thorac Cardiovasc Surg* 2005; 17:236–46.
10. Ling E, Arrellano R: Systematic overview of the evidence supporting the use of cerebrospinal fluid drainage in thoracoabdominal aneurysm surgery for prevention of paraplegia. *Anesthesiology* 2000; 93:1115–22.
11. Lips J, de Haan P, de Jager S, et al: The role of transcranial motor evoked potentials in predicting neurologic and histopathologic outcome after experimental spinal cord ischemia. *Anesthesiology* 2002; 97:183–91.
12. Olsson C, Thelin S, Stahle E, et al: Thoracic aortic aneurysm and dissection: increasing prevalence and improved outcomes reported in a nationwide population-based study of more than 14,000 cases from 1987 to 2002. *Circulation* 2006; 114:2611–8.
13. Penco M, Paparoni S, Dagianti A: Usefulness of transesophageal echocardiography in the assessment of aortic dissection. *Am J Cardiol* 2000; 86:53G–56G.
14. Szeto WY, Gleason TG: Operative management of ascending aortic dissections. *Semin Thorac Cardiovasc Surg* 2005;17: 247–55.

REPAIR OF ANEURYSMS OF THE THORACOABDOMINAL AORTA

SURGICAL CONSIDERATIONS

Description: Aneurysms of the thoracoabdominal aorta (TAAA) may occur because of degenerative aortic disease (atherosclerosis), as a consequence of hereditary disorders of metabolism (Marfan syndrome), or as a sequela of chronic aortic dissections. These aneurysms are classified into four types (Fig 6.3-4) that occur with equal frequency: Type I consists of aneurysms that involve most of the descending thoracic and upper abdominal aorta. Type II involves most of the descending thoracic aorta and most or all of the abdominal aorta. Type III involves the distal thoracic and varying segments of the abdominal aorta. Type IV involves most or all of the abdominal aorta, including the origins of the visceral vessels.

Repair of these aneurysms is an extensive, difficult, and demanding procedure, as blood flow to the entire body below the neck is interrupted, with resultant renal and visceral ischemia. Additionally, the blood supply to the spinal cord may arise from lumbar and/or intercostal vessels in the affected aortic segment, producing critical cord ischemia during cross-clamping and postop paraplegia.

Almost all thoracoabdominal aneurysm repairs are performed through a thoracoabdominal incision (Fig. 6.3-5) using the **inclusion technique** (Fig. 6.3-6) as advocated by **Crawford,** et al. After opening the chest, the incision is extended across the costal cartilage onto the abdomen. The diaphragm is radially incised to the aortic hiatus, and the retroperitoneal dissection plane established anterior to the psoas musculature. All intraabdominal contents, as well as the left kidney, are reflected anteriorly (Fig. 6.3-6). Only proximal aortic control is established. After minimal heparinization, OLV is established to allow collapse of the left lung, the proximal aorta at the aneurysm neck is cross-clamped, and the aneurysm is incised. Back-bleeding from patent intercostal, mesenteric, and renal vessels can be

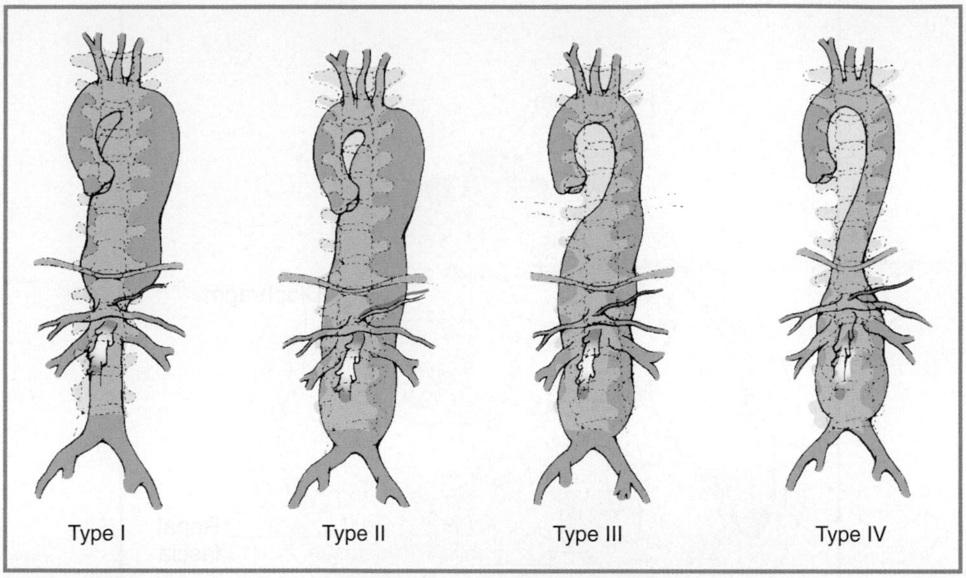

Figure 6.3-4. Crawford's classification of thoracoabdominal aortic aneurysms (TAAA). (Reproduced with permission from Baker RJ, Fischer JE: *Mastery of Surgery,* Vol 2. Lippincott Williams & Wilkins, 2001.)

controlled by balloon catheters; and aggressive blood salvage with autotransfusion devices is mandatory. The repair entails suturing a tube graft proximally to the divided aorta, and then sewing islands of aortic tissue containing intercostal visceral vessels onto appropriate sized holes in the side of the tube graft. This allows reperfusion of important intercostal, celiac axis, superior mesenteric, renal arteries and, finally, the distal aorta or iliac arteries. Because there

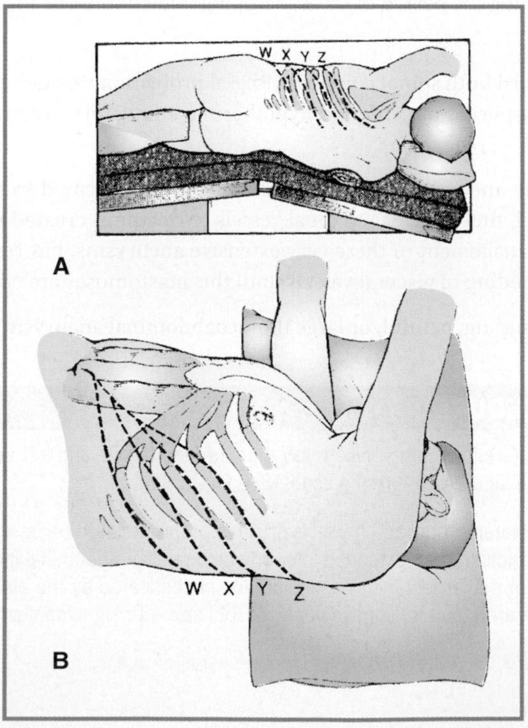

Figure 6.3-5. Lateral (A) and frontal (B) views of the thoracoabdominal incisions used for repair of type IV (W,X), type III (Y,Z), and types I and II (Z) TAAAs. (Reproduced with permission from Baker RJ, Fischer JE: *Mastery of Surgery,* Vol 2. Lippincott Williams & Wilkins, 2001.)

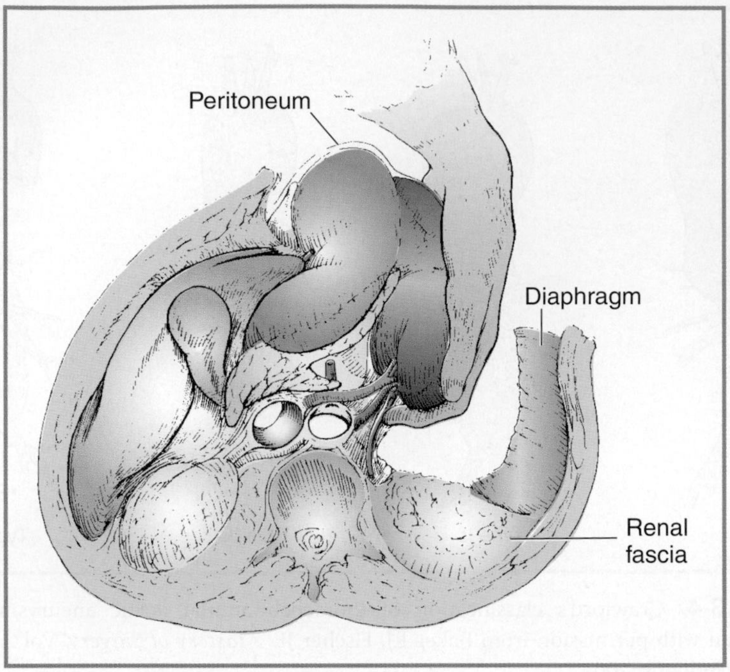

Figure 6.3-6. During the inclusion technique, the anterior renal fascia is opened and the kidney is mobilized, along with the upper abdominal organs (on the left). (Reproduced with permission from Wind GG, Valentine RJ: *Anatomic Exposures in Vascular Surgery*. Williams & Wilkins, Baltimore, 1991.)

is obligate visceral ischemia during the period of cross-clamping (which must be limited to < 60–75 min), the operation must proceed expeditiously.

Alternatively, in an effort to afford both spinal cord and visceral protection through hypothermia, the operation may be performed on CPB during a period of profound hypothermic circulatory arrest, which may exacerbate hemorrhagic complications.

After aortic cross-clamping, the aneurysm is opened and the repair performed from within the aneurysm, sewing on-lay patches of the intercostal, mesenteric, and renal vessels to openings created in the tube graft. This no-clamp technique allows reasonable management of these very extensive aneurysms, but results in an obligatory and ongoing blood loss through back-bleeding of visceral vessels until the anastomoses are complete.

Usual preop diagnosis: Expanding, painful, or large thoracoabdominal aneurysm

SUMMARY OF PROCEDURE

Position	Right lateral decubitus; hips rotated posteriorly to 45° and left arm draped forward over an airplane sling. Axillary roll placed. (See Fig. 6.3-5A.)
Incision	Posterolateral thoracotomy incision, in appropriate interspace, extended across the costal margin to midline, then extended inferiorly as a midline abdominal incision (Fig. 6.3-5). The incision is one of the largest incisions in surgery, necessitated by the absolute need for exposure in this difficult area, and is, unfortunately, associated with significant postop pain.
Special instrumentation	DLT; CPB; NG tube; Cell Saver; rapid-infusion device
Unique considerations	OLV with collapse of left lung necessary for most cases. Cold LR may be injected into renal or visceral arteries for organ preservation. Alternatively, operation can be performed under profound hypothermic circulatory arrest for spinal cord protection in patients with chronic dissections. Frequently, operation is performed with only proximal cross-clamping; so there may be an obligate ongoing blood loss.

SUMMARY OF PROCEDURE (cont'd)

Antibiotics	Cefazolin 1 g iv				
Surgical time	6 h. Proximal aortic cross-clamping until completion of visceral revascularization may extend to 60 min. Longer cross-clamp times may be anticipated in patients with aneurysmal dilation from chronic aortic dissection for which profound hypothermic circulatory arrest may be utilized.				
Closing considerations	OR → ICU, intubated × 24–72 h.				
EBL	Ongoing back-bleeding from visceral and iliac vessels results in substantial volume loss during cross-clamping. Most red-cell volume is salvaged via cardiotomy suckers and returned through cardiopulmonary bypass circuit or via a RBC salvage system (e.g. Cell Saver).				
Postop care	ICU, intubated and ventilated × 24–72 h. Rewarming, hemodynamic monitoring and volume resuscitation are often required in ICU.				
	Aneurysm Group:	**Type I**	**Type II**	**Type III**	**Type IV**
Mortality	Overall: 9%	–	10–25%	–	5%
Morbidity	Paraplegia/spinal cord ischemia	6%	15%	3%	2%
	Other neurological complications	6%	12%	2%	1%
	Renal insufficiency	–	2–5%	–	–
	Respiratory failure	–	10%	–	–
	Hemorrhage	Common	⇐	⇐	⇐
	Graft infection	–	1–6%	–	–
	MI	Rare	⇐	⇐	⇐
	Graft failure	–	Rare	–	–
	False aneurysm	Rare	⇐	⇐	⇐
	Embolization	Rare	⇐	⇐	⇐
	Bowel ischemia	–	2–10%	–	–
	Impotence	Rare	⇐	⇐	⇐
	Ureteral injury	Rare	⇐	⇐	⇐
Pain score	6–10				

PATIENT POPULATION CHARACTERISTICS

Age range	Non-Marfan: 55–75 yr; Marfan: 35–55 yr
Male:Female	3:1
Incidence	< 5 cases/yr in most hospitals, except major referral centers
Etiology	Predominantly atherosclerotic. Patients with Marfan syndrome may present with a progressive dilatation of a chronic dissection.
Associated conditions	HTN (75%); CAD (30%); COPD (30%); renal insufficiency (15%)

ANESTHETIC CONSIDERATIONS

PREOPERATIVE

Sx are usually of sudden onset and depend on the site of dissection and specific organ involvement. Initial treatment involves the use of antihypertensive medications (e.g., SNP) to control BP, and β-blockers (e.g., esmolol) to ↓ contractility. Patients presenting electively for thoracotomy (descending aorta) may have a thoracic epidural catheter placed the night before surgery. These patients are only heparinized during the procedure.

Respiratory	Chronic pulmonary disease is associated with postop morbidity. Preop preparation with bronchodilators, cessation of smoking, incentive spirometry, and chest physiotherapy may decrease the risk of postop problems. **Tests:** CXR: ✓ for distortion of the left mainstem bronchus, which may affect placement of the DLT. May need PFTs, ABG to determine severity of pulmonary disease.
Cardiovascular	CAD is the most frequent cause of periop and late death in elective thoracoabdominal aortic aneurysm repair. It is commonly associated with HTN. **Tests:** ECG: ✓ for LVH and ischemia.
Neurological	Increased risk of spinal cord ischemia with cross-clamping of the aorta; therefore, any preop neurologic deficits should be well documented. The use of CSF drainage and/or deep hypothermic circulatory arrest may be protective in patients with chronic aortic dissections.
Renal	Preop renal dysfunction increases the potential for postop renal problems. Aneurysmal involvement of the renal arteries also may occur. **Tests:** BUN; Cr. Consider creatinine clearance.
Gastrointestinal	Aneurysmal involvement of the inferior mesenteric and superior mesenteric arteries may cause visceral ischemia. **Tests:** Consider abdominal x-ray (ileus) and ABG (metabolic acidosis).
Hematologic	Pre-existing coagulopathy increases risk. Many patients have been on aspirin preop. Excessive alcohol use is associated with anemia, thrombocytopenia, and low production of vitamin K-dependent factors. Rarely, a DIC process may occur within the lumen of the aneurysm. **Tests:** PT; PTT; Plt count; Hct
Laboratory	Electrolytes; radiologic assessment of aneurysm (ultrasonography, CT, and arteriography)
Premedication	Anxiety and pain may contribute to HTN and risk of aneurysmal rupture. Rx: morphine 0.1 mg/kg iv and midazolam 1–5 mg iv. Full-stomach precautions for emergent procedures (e.g., metoclopramide 10 mg iv, ranitidine 50 mg iv, Na citrate 30 mL po).

INTRAOPERATIVE

Anesthetic technique: GETA. The goals of anesthesia for this procedure are: (a) preserve myocardial, renal, pulmonary, CNS and visceral organ function; (b) maintain adequate intravascular volume so that CO is not impaired; (c) control BP so that the transmural pressure across the aneurysm does not increase, which would increase the risk of rupture; and (d) provide good perfusion of other organs. CPB is used to accomplish deep hypothermic circulatory arrest. The rationale for this use is controversial. Deep hypothermic cardiac arrest (DHCA) may confer spinal cord protection and is usually reserved for patients with chronic dissections. Removal of CSF has been proposed as another means of protecting the spinal cord against ischemic injury. CPB also may be used for distal perfusion of organs and afterload protection of the left ventricle. Partial CPB usually is reserved for suprarenal or supraceliac aneurysms to perfuse bowel and kidneys. (See Anesthetic Considerations for Cardiopulmonary Bypass, p. 338, and Repair of Acute Aortic Dissections, p. 404, for more discussion on CPB and DHCA.)

Induction	Prevent hypertensive response to laryngoscopy and intubation with moderate-dose narcotic technique (fentanyl 10–20 mcg/kg or sufentanil 1–2 mcg/kg) in combination with etomidate (0.2–0.3 mg/kg) or propofol (1–2 mg/kg). Esmolol 100–500 mcg/kg over 1 min, NTG 0.5–3 mcg/kg, or lidocaine administered either by topical spray or an iv dose of 1.5 mg/kg also will decrease the cardiovascular response to intubation. Muscle relaxation for intubation may be achieved with vecuronium (beware of ↓ HR) or rocuronium (1 mg/kg). A modified rapid-sequence induction may be necessary in emergent cases. A DLT is mandatory for this procedure; however it may be difficult to position due to distorted anatomy. FOB is mandatory to verify position of DLT.

Maintenance	O_2/air/narcotic, ± low-dose volatile agent. Benzodiazepines may be used for amnesia (e.g., midazolam 100 mcg/kg). When epidural catheter in place, sufentanil (loading dose 25–50 mcg, followed by 4–6 mcg/h) may provide adequate additional analgesia. In hemodynamically unstable patients, scopolamine (400 mcg) provides amnesia. Maintain CO and control of BP at preop levels. These patients may have increased hemodynamic variability on cross-clamping aorta, 2° bleeding, and coexisting disease. Keeping the patient warm may be difficult due to large incision and visceral exposure.	
Emergence	Deferred to ICU. Postop ventilation 24–72 h. DLT may need to be maintained postop 2° to facial, oral, and airway edema.	
Blood and fluid requirements	Anticipate large blood loss. IV: 14 ga or 7 Fr × 2 Rapid infuser Cell Saver T&C 8–10 U PRBCs. Warm fluids and humidify gases. Maintain UO 0.5–1 mL/kg/h.	Large incision and visceral exposure requires administration of large volumes of fluid. Consider use of mannitol or furosemide if concerned about renal function and UO.
Monitoring	Standard monitors (p. B-1) CVP ± PA catheter ± ST segment analysis Arterial line UO	✓ for ↑ PA pressures and PCWP, ↓ in CO, TEE wall motion abnormalities, and changes in SV. Consult with surgeon regarding placement of cross-clamp so arterial line will not be affected.
	TEE	TEE is a good monitor for ventricular filling and myocardial ischemia.
	Core temperature	Monitor core T (esophageal, bladder). Tympanic membrane T (indicative of brain T) is monitored for circulatory arrest cases.
	± EEG, SSEP, MEP	EEG and EPs may be useful in assessment of cerebral protection (SSEP) and spinal cord perfusion problems (MEP ± SSEP).
	± Cerebral oxymetry	In case of the need of DHCA, cerebral oxymetry may be helpful in monitoring cerebral blood flow.
Cross-clamping	Clamping	Application of cross-clamp at supraceliac level probably produces the greatest hemodynamic stress experienced by surgical patients. Application of the clamp may → HTN and ischemia. Preload, afterload, and HR can be controlled with SNP (0.25–5, mcg/kg/min) and esmolol (100–500 mcg/kg/min) infusions. Bolus dose NTG (100 mcg) may be useful to terminate an acute hypertensive episode.
	Unclamping	Ensure adequate volume; replace blood loss. Just before removal of the cross-clamp, filling volumes are allowed to rise gradually, avoiding the occurrence of myocardial ischemia. Dilators are D/C'd. ↓ BP may occur with removal of cross-clamp 2° hypovolemia, reactive hyperemia, acidosis, ↑ K^+, or myocardial dysfunction. BE > -5 should be corrected before unclamping. If necessary, surgeon can reclamp or occlude the aorta.
Positioning	Right axillary roll ✓ and pad pressure points. ✓ eyes.	Right lateral decubitus with hips rotated posteriorly. Left arm placed in airplane sling or supported by pillows.

Complications	Myocardial ischemia HTN Coagulopathy Hemorrhage Hemostasis Hypothermia Other organ ischemia	Coagulopathy due to dilutional and consumptive processes. Hypothermia may exacerbate coagulopathy, cause dysrhythmias, and depress cardiac contractility.

POSTOPERATIVE

Complications	Myocardial ischemia Neurologic deficits 2° cerebral or spinal cord ischemia Renal failure Respiratory failure	BP should be closely controlled postop to decrease bleeding from graft site and raw surfaces.
Pain management	Epidural narcotics (p. C-2)	In selected patients, a thoracic epidural catheter may be placed the night before surgery; otherwise, an epidural is placed only after normal neurologic and coagulation status is determined.
Tests	CXR: line and ETT placement Coagulation profile ABG analysis	

Cardiovascular Surgery

Suggested Readings

1. Cambria RP, Clouse WD, Davison JK, et al: Thoracoabdominal aneurysm repair: results with 337 operations performed over a 15-year interval. *Ann Surg* 2002; 236:471–9.
2. Conrad MF, Crawford RS, Davison JK, et al: Thoracoabdominal aneurysm repair: a 20-year perspective. *Ann Thorac Surg* 2007; 83:S856–61.
3. Coselli JS, Bozinovski J, LeMaire SA: Open surgical repair of 2286 thoracoabdominal aortic aneurysms. *Ann Thorac Surg* 2007; 83:S862–4.
4. Coselli JS, Lemaire SA, Miller CC, et al: Mortality and paraplegia after thoracoabdominal aortic aneurysm repair: A risk factor analysis. *Ann Thorac Surg* 2000; 69:408–14.
5. Dong CCJ, MacDonald DB, Janusz MT: Intraoperative spinal cord monitoring during descending thoracic and thoracoabdominal aneurysm surgery. *Ann Thorac Surg* 2002; 74:S1874–76.
6. Fann JI: Descending thoracic and thoracoabdominal aortic aneurysms. *Coron Artery Dis* 2002; 13:93–102.
7. Jacobs MJ, Mommertz G, Koeppel TA, et al: Surgical repair of thoracoabdominal aortic aneurysms. *J Cardiovasc Surg* 2007; 48:49–58.
8. Kazama S, Masaki Y, Maruyama S, et al: Effect of altering cerebrospinal fluid pressure on spinal cord blood flow. *Ann Thorac Surg* 1994; 58(1):112–5.
9. Levine WC, Lee JJ, Black JH, et al: Thoracoabdominal aneurysm repair: anesthetic management. *Int Anesthesiol Clin* 2005; 43:39–60.
10. Ling E, Arrellano R: Systematic overview of the evidence supporting the use of cerebrospinal fluid drainage in thoracoabdominal aneurysm surgery for prevention of paraplegia. *Anesthesiology* 2000; 93:1115–22.
11. Lips J, de Haan P, de Jager S, et al: The role of transcranial motor evoked potentials in predicting neurologic and histopathologic outcome after experimental spinal cord ischemia. *Anesthesiology* 2002; 97:183–91.

SURGERY OF THE ABDOMINAL AORTA

SURGICAL CONSIDERATIONS

Description: Operations on the abdominal aorta are generally performed for aneurysmal or occlusive diseases. Although **aortic aneurysms** may involve the suprarenal aorta, the majority are infrarenal in origin and may extend into the iliac arteries (Fig. 6.3-7). Most (> 95%) are asymptomatic and are discovered incidentally during investigation

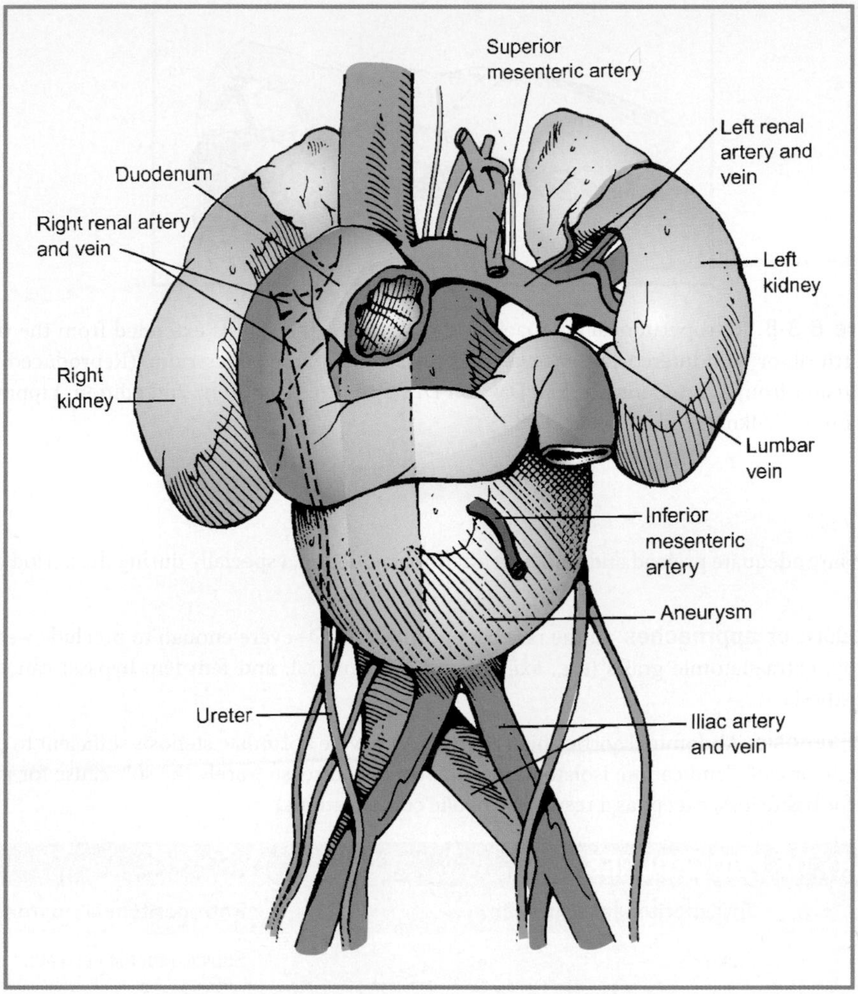

Figure 6.3-7. Aneurysm of the abdominal aorta.

of another medical problem. Because of the associated increased risk for rupture as the aneurysm increases in size, most vascular surgeons recommend prophylactic repair for aneurysms > 5 cm in cross-section dimension. Repair also is indicated for painful aneurysms, those that have been associated with atheroembolism, and when there is documented recent increase in size or evidence of leak or rupture. CAD coexists in 30–40% of these patients and should be assessed preop.

Endovascular stent-grafting of abdominal aortic aneurysm has emerged as an alternative therapeutic approach. The open surgical repair may be either **transperitoneal** or **retroperitoneal** (Fig. 6.3-8). After exposure of the abdominal aorta from the level of the renal vein distally to the iliac arteries, the aorta is cross-clamped, distally at first to prevent atheroembolism, and then proximally. Graft origin is usually from the infrarenal aorta, but may arise from the intramesenteric aorta or even the supraceliac aorta. Graft termination may be to the distal aorta above the bifurcation (tube graft), to the common or external iliac arteries (Y graft), or the femoral arteries. Immediately prior to cross-clamping, vasodilators are increased to reduce afterload, which is significantly increased with application of the aortic cross-clamp. The aorta is then incised, lumbar vessels oversewn, and the aorta transected to allow an interposition graft to be sewn into place. The retroperitoneal approach has many advocates, as it may require less volume intraop, may be associated with less temperature loss, and may result in a shorter period of postop adynamic ileus. In a randomized, prospective study, however, no significant differences could be detected between these two approaches for blood loss or postop recovery time.

Aortoiliac occlusive disease can be a significant cause of lower extremity arterial insufficiency. Although the operative approach may be similar to that for aneurysmal disease, there exists a significant intraop difference in that there are not such profound changes associated with aortic clamping, since there is already some element of increased afterload 2° the occlusive disease. Nevertheless, hemodynamic monitoring is mandatory to allow for rapid volume

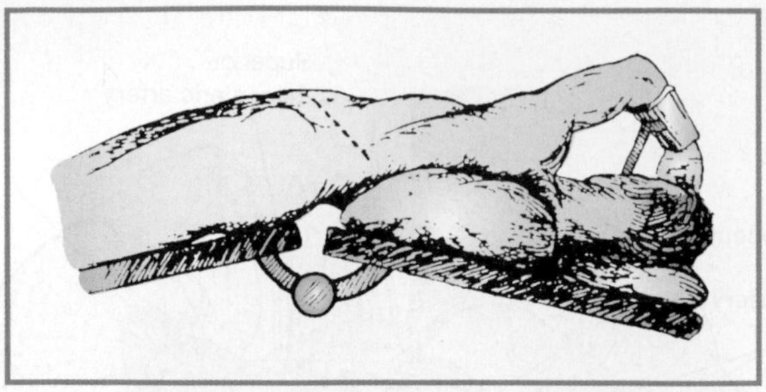

Figure 6.3-8. Retroperitoneal approach to the aorta: the incision is extended from the tip of the 11th rib or 10th intercostal space laterally toward the midhypogastrium. (Reproduced with permission from Scott-Conner CEH, Dawson DL: *Operative Anatomy,* 2nd edition. Lippincott Williams & Wilkins, Philadelphia, 2003.)

shifts, and to assure adequate preload and sufficient afterload reduction, especially during the period of aortic cross-clamping.

Variant procedure or approaches: In the rare patient with COPD severe enough to preclude weaning from the ventilator postop, extraanatomic grafts (e.g., axillofemoral, iliofemoral, and fem-fem bypass) can be constructed under local anesthesia.

Usual preop diagnosis: Abdominal aortic aneurysm (AAA); severe aortoiliac stenosis sufficient to cause debilitating buttock, thigh, or calf claudication; isolated-inflow (aortoiliac) disease (rarely the sole cause for ischemic symptoms at rest or for tissue loss, except as a result of embolic complications)

SUMMARY OF PROCEDURES

	Transperitoneal Approach	Retroperitoneal Approach
Position	Supine	Supine with mild elevation of left flank
Incision	Midline abdominal	Left subcostal, left oblique, along 10th rib toward umbilicus (See Fig. 6.3-8.)
Special instrumentation	Self-retaining retractor; TEE; If suprarenal change: SMA + renal artery perfusion catheters.	⇐
Unique considerations	Will need pharmacologic manipulation to ↓ afterload or ↑ preload coincident with clamping or unclamping of aorta.	⇐ (The retroperitoneal approach is not used for emergency cases.)
Antibiotics	Cefazolin I g iv	⇐
Surgical time	3–5 h	⇐
EBL	500 mL	⇐
Postop care	ICU 8–16 h, often extubated. Requires aggressive volume administration to allow for 3rd-space loss in 1st 12 h postop. Patient comfort and respiratory management markedly improved by epidural catheter for postop analgesia. Careful cardiac monitoring.	⇐
Mortality	2–5% elective; 50% emergent	⇐
Morbidity	MI: 10–15% (3% fatal) Respiratory insufficiency/pneumonia: 5–10% Lower extremity ischemia: 2–5% Renal insufficiency: 2–5% Bowel complications: 3–4%	⇐

SUMMARY OF PROCEDURES (cont'd)

	Transperitoneal Approach	Retroperitoneal Approach
Morbidity (cont'd)	Hemorrhage: 2–4% CVA: < 1% Infection: < 1% Paraplegia: < 0.4%	
Pain score	8–10	7–10

PATIENT POPULATION CHARACTERISTICS

Age range	55 yr +
Male:Female	4:1
Incidence	3% of males > 55 yr; > 5% of patients > 50 yr in a general cardiology clinic; 30–66/1000
Etiology	Atherosclerosis; Marfan syndrome; Ehlers-Danlos syndrome; dissection; infection, including syphilis
Associated conditions	HTN; CAD; COPD; cerebrovascular disease; renal insufficiency

ANESTHETIC CONSIDERATIONS

PREOPERATIVE

Patients presenting for AAA repair are typically older males with multiple coexisting diseases (e.g., CAD, HTN, PVD, COPD). Most commonly these patients are asymptomatic and the Dx is made as an incidental finding during routine exams or other medical procedures; however, some patients may present with severe ↓ BP following aneurysm rupture. These patients require prompt resuscitation (SBP goal: 90–100 mmHg) and emergent aortic cross-clamping. For anesthetic considerations, see Abdominal Trauma: Vascular Injuries (p. 737).

Respiratory	Many patients have COPD and a long Hx of smoking. Preop preparation—including bronchodilators, cessation of smoking, incentive spirometry, and chest physiotherapy—will ↓ risk of postop complications. **Tests:** CXR. May need PFTs and ABG to determine severity of pulmonary disease.
Cardiovascular	CAD is the most common cause of morbidity and mortality in this patient population. HTN increases risk of aneurysmal rupture; hence, preop control of BP is essential. ✓ BP in both arms to determine placement of arterial line intraop (arterial line should be placed in arm with higher BP). **Tests:** Radiologic assessment of aneurysm using ultrasonography, CT, arteriography, and MRI. ECG: ✓ for evidence of ischemia, infarction, and LVH. Stress testing, coronary angiography in case of suspicion of coronary disease.
Renal	Chronic renal insufficiency occurs frequently in this patient population 2° HTN, diabetes mellitus (DM), and atherosclerotic renovascular disease. Hypovolemia 2° radiographic dye studies and bowel prep → renal failure. **Tests:** BUN, Cr; consider creatinine clearance; electrolytes
Hematologic	Preop coagulation disorders should be corrected. Many patients are on aspirin, which should be D/C'd 7 d preop. Alcohol abuse can be associated with anemia, thrombocytopenia, and ↓ vitamin K-dependent factors. **Tests:** PT; PTT; Hct; Plt
Laboratory	Other tests as indicated from H&P.
Premedication	Anxiety and pain may cause HTN and ↑ risk of aneurysmal rupture. Sedatives and analgesics should be used as indicated (p. B-1). Full-stomach precautions for emergent procedures (p. B-4).

INTRAOPERATIVE

Anesthetic technique: GETA or combination of epidural and GA. The goals of anesthesia are to: (a) preserve myocardial, renal, pulmonary, and CNS perfusion; (b) maintain adequate intravascular volume and CO; (c) anticipate the surgical maneuvers that will affect BP and blood volume; and (d) control BP to minimize risk of rupture, while ensuring perfusion of other organs.

Induction	If it is planned to extubate the patient postop, anesthesia should be induced using fentanyl (4–6 mcg/kg) in conjunction with propofol (2 mg/kg) or etomidate (0.2–0.4 mg/kg). If an epidural will be used for postop pain management, decrease intraop i.v. opioid dose. Patients with an epidural typically receive morphine (2–4 mg), hydromorphone (0.2–0.8 mg), fentanyl (150–200 mcg), or sufentanil (50 mcg) in 10 mL into the epidural catheter. Local anesthetics may cause hemodynamic instability after unclamping 2° sympathectomy. Muscle relaxants are chosen to minimize tachycardia or ↓ BP (e.g., vecuronium 0.1 mg/kg or rocuronium 1 mg/kg). Anesthesia is deepened before intubation by mask ventilation with 1% sevoflurane. If there is a hemodynamic response to oral airway insertion, tracheal lidocaine or further anesthetic is given before gentle laryngoscopy and intubation. Etomidate is useful for induction in hemodynamically unstable patients. Full-stomach precautions may be necessary.
Maintenance	O_2/air/narcotic and volatile agent. N_2O can be used, but it may cause bowel distention. Combining epidural and GA offers good abdominal relaxation. Patients receiving epidural local anesthesia may require phenylephrine to treat ↓ BP 2° sympathetic blockade. Epidural catheter placement before systemic anticoagulation is a safe technique. Narcotic epidural analgesia should be given within 1 h of skin incision if morphine 3–8 mg is used. If hydromorphone (0.5–0.8 mg) is given epidurally, it is given within 1 h of abdominal closure. Patient may become hypothermic 2° large incision with visceral exposure and prolonged operation.
Emergence	Normothermic (> 35.5°C) patients who have had uneventful surgery, especially utilizing a retroperitoneal approach, are frequently extubated in the OR, or shortly after arrival in the ICU. Patients with significant cardiac or pulmonary disease generally are left intubated, and weaned from the ventilator in the ICU. Prevention of HTN and tachycardia during emergence may require titration of β-adrenergic-blocking drugs (e.g., esmolol 50–300 mcg/kg/min) and/or vasodilators (e.g., SNP 0.25–2.0 mcg/kg/min) or NTG (0.25–2.0 mcg/kg/min). Epidural morphine (2–4 mg) or hydromorphone (0.5–0.8 mg) is given ~60 min before the end of surgery. It is important to assure full reversal from neuromuscular blockade.

Blood and fluid requirements	Major blood loss iv: 14 ga (or 7 Fr) × 2 4 U PRBC UO 0.5–1 mL/kg/h Warm all fluids. Humidify all gases.	Use of rapid infusion and blood-salvaging devices helpful. Consider acute normovolemic hemodilution. Hemorrhage should be treated with crystalloid, colloid, or blood products as appropriate. Upper-body Bair-Hugger or equivalent.
Monitoring	Standard monitors (p. B-1)	Monitor for cardiac ischemia. Automated ST segment analysis is useful.
	CVP line	The measurement of CVP may be sufficient in patients with good ventricular function and exercise tolerance.
	PA catheter	In patients with recent MI, Hx of CHF, Hx of unstable angina, multisystem disease, or in those presenting emergently (without the benefit of a complete workup) a PA catheter is appropriate.
	TEE	TEE is invaluable for assessing cardiac changes 2° cross-clamping and unclamping the aorta.
	Arterial line Urinary catheter	The arterial line is generally placed in the radial artery of the arm having the higher BP (if difference exists).

Cross-clamping	↑↑ Afterload → HTN ↓ Preload ↑ Filling pressures ± ↓ Spinal cord perfusion ± ↓ Renal perfusion ↓ Perfusion to viscera below the clamp ABGs/electrolytes regularly	Application of aortic cross-clamp causes HTN proximal to the clamp. In a healthy heart, this is well tolerated, with minimal increase in filling pressure. In case of poor left ventricular function, filling pressures generally rise. Control of preload, afterload, and HR can be accomplished with vasodilators and β-blockers. Negative inotropic agents (e.g., β-blockers, inhalational anesthetics) are used cautiously. Occlusion of infrarenal aorta →↓ renal blood flow. Ensure adequate intravascular volume and CO. Administer mannitol (0.25–0.5 g/kg) before clamping to maintain UO.
Aortic unclamping	↓↓ Afterload Volume loading Lactate washout ± Phenylephrine	Immediately before unclamping, D/C dilators and negative inotropic agents. Gradually increase filling pressures (volume loading) to avoid myocardial ischemia. ↓↓ BP may occur with removal of cross-clamp 2° to hypovolemia, reperfusion, or myocardial dysfunction. Reperfusion of lower limbs and washout of lactate does not usually require use of HCO_3. Patients with an epidural sympathetic block often require phenylephrine support during unclamping. The surgeon can reclamp or occlude the aorta if ↓↓ BP persists. If hemodynamically stable with ↓ UO, consider furosemide 20–80 mg.
Positioning	✓ and pad pressure points. ✓ eyes.	
Complications	Myocardial ischemia HTN Hemorrhage Coagulopathy Hypothermia Organ ischemia	Hypothermia may cause dysrhythmias, depress contractility, and exacerbate coagulopathy.

POSTOPERATIVE

Complications	Myocardial ischemia Renal failure Respiratory failure	
Pain management	Epidural narcotics (p. C-1)	
Tests	CXR to ✓ line and ETT placement ABG Coagulation profile BUN; Cr	BP should be closely controlled postop to decrease bleeding from graft site and raw surfaces.

Suggested Readings

1. Adams van der Vliet J, Boll APM: Abdominal aortic aneurysms. *Lancet* 1997; 349:863–6.
2. Arko FR, Lee WA, Hill BB, et al: Aneurysm-related death: primary endpoint analysis for comparison of open and endovascular repair. *J Vasc Surg* 2002; 36:297–304.
3. Boccara G, Jaber S, Eliet J, et al: Monitoring of end-tidal dioxide partial pressure changes during infrarenal aortic cross-clamping: a non-invasive method to predict unclamping hypotension. *Acta Anesthesiol Scand* 2001; 45:188–93.

4. Conrad MF, Crawford RS, Pedraza JD, et al: Long-term durability of open abdominal aortic aneurysm repair. *J Vasc Surg* 2007; 46:669–75.
5. Falk JL, Rackow EC, Blumenberg R, et al: Hemodynamic and metabolic effects of abdominal aortic cross-clamping. *Am J Surg* 1981; 142:174–7.
6. Filinger M. Who should we operate on and how do we decide: predicting rupture and survival in patients with aortic aneurysm. *Semin Vasc Surg* 2007; 20:121–7.
7. Gold MS, DeCrosta D, Rizzuto C, et al: The effect of lumbar epidural and general anesthesia on plasma catecholamines and hemodynamics during abdominal aortic aneurysm repair. *Anesth Analg* 1994; 78(2):225–30.
8. Gooding JM, Archie JP Jr, McDowell H: Hemodynamic response to infrarenal aortic cross-clamping in patients with and without coronary artery disease. *Crit Care Med* 1980; 8:382–5.
9. Nishimori M, Ballantyne JC, Low JHS: Epidural pain relief versus systemic opiod-based pain relief for abdominal aortic surgery (Cochrane reviews). *The Cochrane Library* 2006; 3:1577.
10. Patra P, Chaillou P, Bizouarn P: Intraoperative autotransfusion for repair of unruptured aneurysms of the infrarenal abdominal aorta. *J Cardiovasc Surg* 2000; 41:407–13.
11. Solomon H, Chao AB, Weaver FA, et al: Change in practice patterns of an academic division of vascular surgery. *Arch Surg* 2007; 142:733–6.
12. Sprung J, Abdelmalak B, Gottlieb A, et al: Analysis of risk factors for myocardial infarction and cardiac mortality after major vascular surgery. *Anesthesiology* 2000; 93:129–40.
13. Tang TY, Walsh SR, Fanshawe TR, et al: Comparison of risk-scoring methods in predicting the immediate outcome after elective open abdominal aortic aneurysm surgery. *Eur J Vasc Endovasc Surg* 2007; 34:505–13.
14. Thompson RW, Geraghty PJ, Lee JK: Abdominal aortic aneurysms: basic mechanisms and clinical implications. *Curr Probl Surg* 2002; 39:110–230.
15. Young EL, Holt PJ, Poloniecki JD, et al: Meta-analysis and systematic review of the relationship between surgeon annual caseload and mortality for elective open abdominal aortic aneurysm repairs. *J Vasc Surg* 2007; 46:1287–94.

INFRAINGUINAL ARTERIAL BYPASS

SURGICAL CONSIDERATIONS

Description: Due to the limited durability of distal bypass procedures, surgical bypass to the infrainguinal arteries is indicated only for salvage of the severely ischemic lower extremity, as manifest by gangrene, ischemic ulceration, or ischemic rest pain. Less frequently, it is used to alleviate functional ischemia of claudication, or leg discomfort with exercise. Its use is predicated on the existence of adequate inflow to the level of the groin or femoral artery. Other necessary components include an adequate target vessel, preferably in continuity with runoff into the plantar arch of the foot, and an adequate conduit, preferably autologous saphenous vein. Long-term patency rates of nonautologous conduits to the below-knee arteries are distinctly inferior to that of saphenous vein and should be avoided whenever possible. This population, almost by definition, includes patients with diabetes mellitus (DM), CAD, and cerebrovascular disease, all of which must be assessed preop.

The operative repair usually involves incisions at the groin and distal bypass sites to expose the donor and recipient arteries and to harvest leg or arm venous conduit. The operative approaches are rather similar. An unobstructed inflow source—usually the common femoral, superficial femoral, or deep femoral artery—is exposed in the groin. The target distal artery, usually at the level of the knee or below, can be approached through a medial incision. More distally, the peroneal and anterior tibial arteries can be approached laterally at the midtibial level. At the level of the malleolus, both the dorsalis pedis and posterior tibial arteries can be revascularized. After control of donor and recipient vessels, an anatomic tunnel is created, and the bypass conduit (saphenous vein, prosthetic graft) is passed through its length. After administration of 10,000 U of heparin, the distal anastomosis is constructed first, followed by the proximal anastomosis. A completion arteriogram confirms unobstructed flow. Heparin is then partially reversed and meticulous hemostasis obtained, and the wounds are closed.

Although conventional wisdom has held that the anesthetic and operative risks for patients undergoing distal reconstructions are low, there may be little difference in postop morbidity and mortality when compared with patients undergoing a major inflow procedure within the abdomen.

Usual preop diagnosis: Severe peripheral vascular disease (PVD); CAD; DM; HTN; obstructive PA disease. (These are almost ubiquitous comorbidities.)

SUMMARY OF PROCEDURE

Position	Supine
Incision	Groin, medial knee, ± distal leg incisions; + incision to harvest venous conduit
Antibiotics	Cefazolin 1 g iv at induction of anesthesia
Surgical time	2–5 h
Closing considerations	Optimization of coagulation status
EBL	200–300 mL
Postop care	Possible ICU × 24 h; patients are at risk for myocardial ischemia.
Mortality	2–4%
Morbidity	MI: 5–12% Respiratory insufficiency: 5% Infection: 2–5% Amputation: 2–4% CVA: <1%
Pain score	4–6

PATIENT POPULATION CHARACTERISTICS

Age range	> 55 yr (mean age = > 70 yr)
Male:Female	4:1
Incidence	Claudication fairly common in elderly; however, 75% will remain untreated, but stable, over 2–5 yr, with < 5% requiring amputation.
Etiology	Arteriosclerosis (primarily); chronic embolic disease (rare); vasculitis; popliteal artery entrapment; cystic adventitial disease of popliteal artery
Associated conditions	CAD; cerebrovascular disease; DM; HTN; COPD

ANESTHETIC CONSIDERATIONS

(Procedures covered: infrainguinal arterial bypass; arterial embolectomy; lumbar sympathectomy; venous thrombectomy or vein excision)

PREOPERATIVE

Patients presenting for peripheral vascular surgery may suffer from major systemic diseases, including CAD, HTN, and DM. Three types of occlusive vascular disease have been described: Type 1—isolated to the aortic and iliac bifurcations; is not associated with CAD. Type 2—diffuse pattern involving coronary and cerebral circulations; associated with a higher incidence of DM and HTN. Type 3—involves small vessels, especially of the lower limbs; associated with higher postop morbidity and mortality.

Respiratory	Vascular patients frequently have Hx of smoking and COPD. Preop evaluation of pulmonary function helps to determine whether regional vs GA is appropriate, while providing baseline values for postop comparison. **Tests:** CXR; consider PFTs; ABG

Cardiovascular	Vascular surgery of the lower extremities is often associated with ↑ morbidity and mortality 2° ↑ incidence of CAD and HTN in this patient population. **Tests:** ECG: ✓ for LVH and ischemia; other tests as indicated from H&P.
Neurological	↑ incidence of cerebrovascular disease. Careful neurological assessment is necessary to document existing deficits.
Endocrine	↑ incidence of DM, which may be associated with peripheral and autonomic neuropathies (silent MI, labile BP) and delayed gastric emptying. Insulin requirements for most diabetic patients can be managed by administering one-half the usual a.m. dose of insulin, once a dextrose-containing iv (e.g., D5LR) has been established. Frequent blood glucose measurements should be made periop.
Renal	There is a higher incidence of renal artery disease and renal insufficiency in this patient population. **Tests:** BUN; Cr; consider creatinine clearance; electrolytes; UA
Hematologic	Many patients presenting for this surgery are taking anticoagulant/anti-Plt medications. Inquire as to bleeding or bruising tendency. **Tests:** Hct; Plt; consider PT, PTT.
Laboratory	As indicated from H&P.
Premedication	Continue usual medications up to time of surgery. Anxiety can contribute to HTN and tachycardia. Premedicate conservatively (midazolam 0.5–2 mg iv) for geriatric patients. If ischemic pain is present, a narcotic such as fentanyl (25–50 mcg iv) can be given. Avoid im administration in patients on anticoagulant therapy.

INTRAOPERATIVE

Anesthetic technique: Either regional anesthesia or GETA may be used. For **infrainguinal arterial bypass,** there is evidence that regional anesthesia is superior for promoting graft survival. To date, no study has shown a difference in patient mortality between these anesthetic techniques. **Lumbar sympathectomy** may be accomplished with regional or GA. For **thrombectomy,** GETA with IPPV may reduce the risk of pulmonary emboli.

General anesthesia:

Induction	Hemodynamic stability is important; therefore, a slow, gradual induction is carried out. Preoxygenation is followed by smooth iv induction, using small, incremental doses of fentanyl (1–3 mcg/kg); then STP or propofol is given in divided doses until the patient is asleep. Alternatively, if the LV function is poor, and the depressant effects of STP cannot be tolerated, etomidate (0.2 mg/kg iv) in combination with fentanyl (100–200 mcg) is appropriate. A full dose of muscle relaxant (vecuronium or rocuronium) is given and ventilation is controlled. Muscle relaxation is not necessary during the procedure, but muscle relaxant is given to facilitate intubation. The muscle relaxant is chosen to avoid undesirable effects on HR.
Maintenance	Standard maintenance (p. B-2) with fentanyl (1–2 mcg/kg/h). Continued muscle relaxation is usually unnecessary. These surgical procedures are associated with minimal hemodynamic instability.
Emergence	Tracheal extubation should be based on standard criteria, such as adequacy of ventilation, return of airway reflexes and reversal of muscle relaxation. Control of BP is accomplished with vasodilators (e.g., NTG 0.1–4.0 mcg/kg/min or SNP 0.25–5.0 mcg/kg/min). Esmolol can be given in incremental doses of 10 mg or by infusion (50–200 mcg/kg/min).

Regional anesthesia: Patients presenting for regional anesthesia must have a normal coagulation profile; also, they cannot be on heparin (including low molecular weight), urokinase, or streptokinase. The important goals in regional anesthesia are to achieve hemodynamic stability while establishing an adequate block. An epidural or spinal catheter (multiorifice) is frequently used to infuse local anesthetic for a gradual onset and to prevent an excessively high block. Hemodynamic stability can be improved by infusing 500–1,000 mL of NS/LR before performing the block. The patient may be placed in the lateral decubitus position (with operative side down), which may provide a denser and more prolonged block on that side. Achieving a T8-T10 level is optimal. Overzealous hydration may → CHF in this patient population, when the vasodilation 2° regional sympathectomy dissipates. The use of regional anesthesia in patients who will receive intraop anticoagulation is controversial. We feel it is a relatively safe procedure and have not had a complication with this technique. If blood is aspirated after placement of an epidural, we remove the catheter and then replace it at a different interspace. Patients on minidose heparin should have a normal PTT before use of regional anesthesia.

Spinal	**One-shot spinal:** 1% hyperbaric tetracaine (6–10 mg) or 0.75% bupivacaine (10–15 mg). Add epinephrine 0.2 mg (generally increases duration of block about 50%) or phenylephrine 5 mg (generally increases duration of block about 100%). Do not add vasoconstrictor if patient is diabetic. Large doses of hyperbaric local anesthetic should be avoided as they may cause postop cauda equina syndrome. **Continuous spinal:** A 20-ga catheter is placed via an 18-ga Tuohy needle. 0.5% hyperbaric tetracaine or 0.75% bupivacaine is titrated to desired anesthetic level (T8-T10). Catheters should be redosed every 60–80 min or as soon as BP trends upward. The risk of spinal headache is very low with continuous spinals.	
Epidural	Lidocaine 2% with 1:200,000 epinephrine or 0.5% bupivacaine is used. Titrate to desired anesthetic level (T8-T10).	
Blood and fluid requirements	IV: 14 or 16 ga × 1 NS/LR @ 3–5 mL/kg/h Warm fluids. Humidify gases. Maintain UO 0.5–1 mL/kg/h.	Minimal-to-moderate blood loss. Use forced-air warmer (e.g., Bair-Hugger).
Monitoring	Standard monitors (p. B-1)	
	Arterial line ST-segment analysis	An arterial line is most often used in patients with severe cardiopulmonary disease or brittle diabetics. Blood sampling for ABGs, electrolytes, glucose, and Hct is facilitated by the use of an arterial line.
	± CVP/PA catheters	CVP and PA catheters are not used routinely because large changes in intravascular volumes are uncommon. Patients with poor LV function, recent MI, or severe valvular disease may need PA monitoring.
Positioning	✓ and pad pressure points. ✓ eyes.	Diabetic patients may be at risk of skin ischemia due to poor positioning or inadequate padding of limbs, etc.
Complications	HTN	
	Ischemic reperfusion syndrome (postembolectomy)	Reperfusion of an ischemic limb → ↓ pH, ↑ K+, and release of myoglobin from injured muscle → ATN.
	Hypothermia Hemorrhage	

POSTOPERATIVE

Complications	CHF	Infrainguinal bypass: Avoid overhydration; when epidural sympathectomy fades, these patients are at increased risk for CHF. Maintain normovolemia so that peripheral vasoconstriction (which may limit outflow to the graft) does not occur.
	Hypothermia	Hypothermia causes vasoconstriction and also may limit outflow to the graft.
	Graft occlusion	

Pain management	Epidural/spinal opiates (p. C-1) PCA	Epidural (or spinal) catheter may be used for postop analgesia (p. C-2).
Tests	CXR if central line placed Hct	

Suggested Readings

1. Brumberg RS, Back MR, Armstrong PA, et al: The relative importance of graft surveillance and warfarin therapy in infrainguinal prosthetic bypass failure. *J Vasc Surg* 2007; 46:1160–6.
2. Chung J, Bartelson BB, Hiatt WR, et al: Wound healing and functional outcomes after infrainguinal bypass with reversed saphenous vein for critical limb ischemia. *J Vasc Surg* 2006; 43:1183–90.
3. Damask MC, Weissman C, Barth A, et al: General vs epidural—which is the better anesthetic technique for femoral-popliteal bypass surgery? *Anesth Analg* 1986; 65:539.
4. Darling RC, Reddy BP, Chang BB, et al: Long-term results of revised infrainguinal arterial reconstructions. *J Vasc Surg* 2002; 35:773–8.
5. Denny N, Masters R, Pearson D, et al: Postdural puncture headache after continuous spinal anesthesia. *Anesth Analg* 1987; 66(8):791–4.
6. Rosenfeld BA, Beattie C, Christopherson R, et al: Perioperative Ischemia Randomized Anesthesia Trial Study Group: The effects of different anesthetic regimens on fibrinolysis and the development of postoperative arterial thrombosis. *Anesthesiology* 1993; 79:435–43.
7. Singh N, Sidawy AN, Dezee K, et al: The effects of the type of anesthesia in outcomes of lower extremity infrainguinal bypass. *J Vasc Surg* 2006; 44:964–8.
8. Taylor SM, Cull DL, Kalbaugh CA, et al: Critical analysis of clinical success after surgical bypass for lower-extremity ischemic tissue loss using a standardized definition combining multiple parameters: a new paradigm of outcomes assessment. *J Am Coll Surg* 2007; 204:831–8.

ARTERIAL EMBOLECTOMY

SURGICAL CONSIDERATIONS

Description: The etiology of acute arterial insufficiency is often the result of thromboembolism, which is usually of cardiac origin. Patients at high risk for embolization are those with MI, mitral stenosis, or atrial fibrillation (AF), all of which increase the risk of intracardiac thrombus formation. Noncardiac causes include thoracic and abdominal aortic pathology, such as aneurysms, severe atherosclerotic disease, and paradoxical embolus via a patent foramen ovale (PFO). The emboli usually become lodged at tapering regions and branch sites and most commonly involve the extremities; the cerebrovascular and mesenteric vasculature also may be involved. In the lower extremities, emboli frequently lodge at the iliac, femoral, or popliteal arteries; the common femoral artery is involved in up to 50% of all embolic events. Emboli to the upper extremities typically affect the brachial artery. Because the collateral circulation may not be well developed in patients without underlying peripheral vascular disease, muscle necrosis can appear within 4–6 h after onset, although this time frame is highly variable. Patients are heparinized at time of diagnosis. Therapy directed at the specific etiology is critical to achieve a successful outcome. Revascularization after 8–12 h of ischemia usually is less effective. If the underlying source of the emboli is not adequately treated, recurrence is likely and is associated with poor prognosis. The surgical approach to femoral embolectomy is a groin incision and isolation of the common, superficial, and deep femoral arteries. Both the superficial and deep femoral systems are explored, and small embolectomy catheters are passed into the distal lower extremity. In addition to passage of embolectomy catheters, angioscopy may be helpful. Residual thrombus on intraop arteriogram requires distal surgical exposure and exploration.

Usual preop diagnosis: Peripheral artery embolism

SUMMARY OF PROCEDURE	
Position	Supine
Incision	Limited groin, medial knee, possible distal leg incisions
Antibiotics	Cefazolin 1 g iv

SUMMARY OF PROCEDURE (cont'd)	
Surgical time	Variable, 1–4 h
Closing considerations	Ischemia-reperfusion syndrome with acidosis and hyperkalemia, renal tubular necrosis from myoglobinuria
EBL	100–300 mL
Postop care	May need ICU for cardiac monitoring; monitor metabolic disturbances, neurovascular status, and for compartment syndrome
Mortality	10–40% (~80% cardiac); older age; acute onset →↑ risk.
Morbidity	Arterial reocclusion or thrombosis: 20% Wound hematoma: 10–20% Recurrent emboli: 6–45% (less with anticoagulation) Amputation: 5–10% Metabolic complications: Frequent Compartment syndrome: Occasional
Pain score	4–6

PATIENT POPULATION CHARACTERISTICS	
Age range	30–90 yr
Male:Female	3:2
Incidence	50/100,000 admissions
Etiology	Cardiac origin (AF accounts for 50–75% of patients; less frequent, LV thrombus from MI) or non-cardiac origin (mural thrombus from thoracic or abdominal aortic pathology)
Associated conditions	Rheumatic heart disease and mitral stenosis, mitral or aortic valve prosthesis, CAD and MI, CHF, endocarditis, peripheral vascular and cerebrovascular disease.

ANESTHETIC CONSIDERATIONS

See Anesthetic Considerations following Infrainguinal Arterial Bypass, p. 421.

Suggested Readings

1. Brewster DC: Acute peripheral arterial occlusion. *Cardiol Clin* 1991; 9:497–513.
2. Dregelid EB, Stangeland LB, Eide GE, et al: Patient survival and limb prognosis after arterial embolectomy. *Eur J Vasc Surg* 1987; 1:263–71.
3. Gassage JA, Ali T, Chambers J, et al: Peripheral arterial embolism: prevalence, outcome, and the role of echocardiography in management. *Vasc Endovascular Surg* 2006; 40:280–6.
4. Lau LS, Blanchard DG, Hye RJ: Diagnosis and management of patients with peripheral macroemboli from thoracic aortic pathology. *Ann Vasc Surg* 1997; 11:348–53.
5. Panetta T, Thompson JE, Talkington CM, et al: Arterial embolectomy: a 34-year experience with 400 cases. *Surg Clin North Am* 1986; 66:339–53.
6. Varty K, Johnston JA, Beets G, et al: Arterial embolectomy. A long-term perspective. *J Cardiovasc Surg* 1992; 33: 79–84.

LUMBAR SYMPATHECTOMY

SURGICAL CONSIDERATIONS

Description: The role of open surgical or endoscopic **lumbar sympathectomy** is not well defined. The procedure is used selectively in patients with causalgia, inoperable lower limb ischemia with rest pain or toe gangrene, symptomatic vasospastic disorders (e.g., Raynaud's phenomenon, frostbite), and sometimes as an adjunct to distal

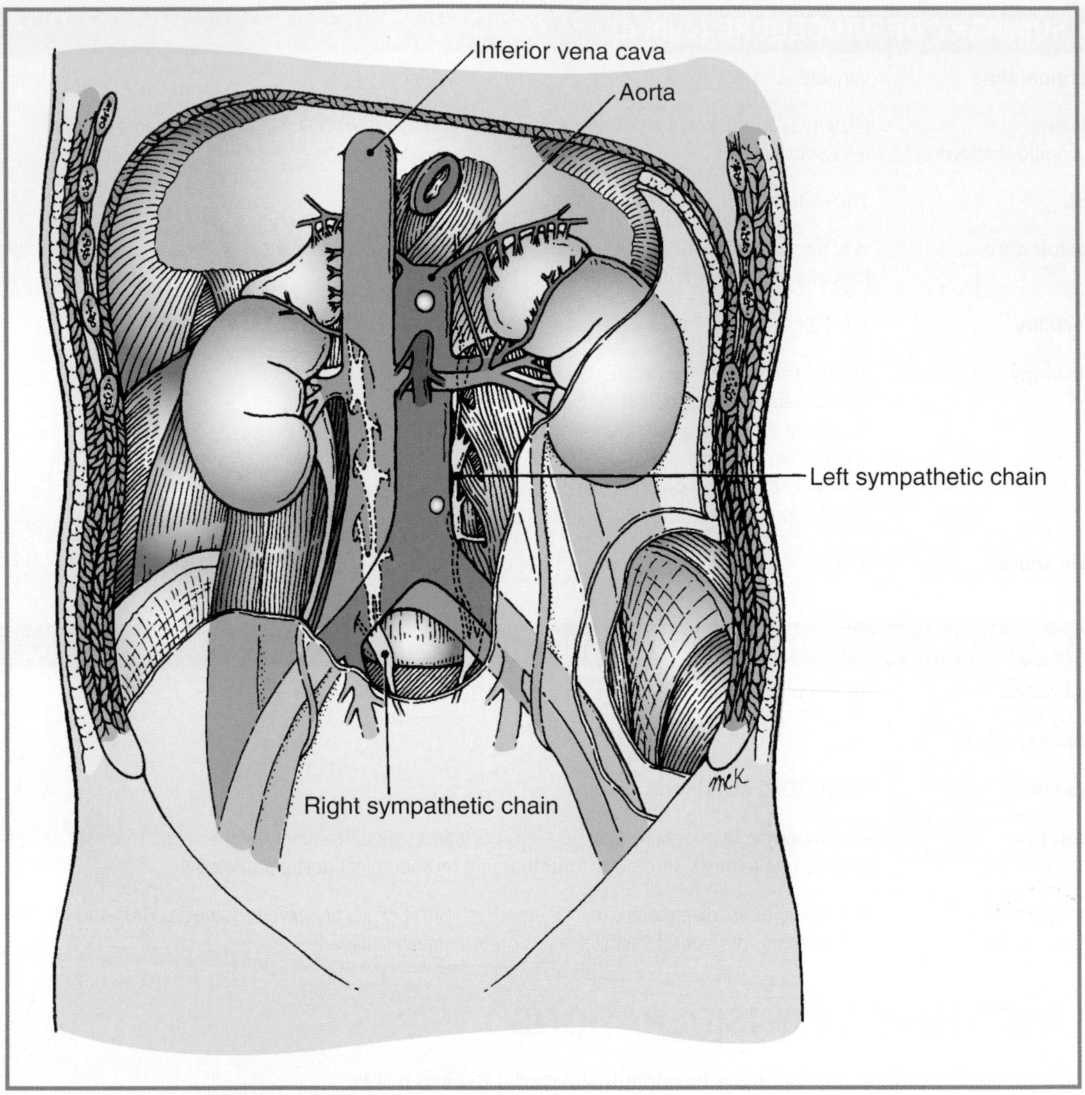

Figure 6.3-9. Surgical anatomy for lumbar sympathectomy. (Reproduced with permission from Scott-Conner CEH, Dawson DL: *Operative Anatomy,* 2nd edition. Lippincott Williams & Wilkins, 2003.)

revascularization procedures. Causalgia responds well to lumbar sympathectomy, especially if performed early in the clinical course. There may be some benefit of the procedure in 50–60% of patients with rest pain or ischemic ulceration. Sympathectomy may increase collateral blood flow and local skin blood flow. Scleroderma with impending 'minor' amputation may benefit from sympathectomy with improved wound healing. Sympathetic denervation involves the division of preganglionic fibers along their segmental origins and resection of corresponding relay ganglia. For most clinical indications, L2 and L3 **ganglionectomy** sufficiently sympathectomizes the lower extremity (Fig. 6.3-9).

The **anterolateral retroperitoneal approach** is the most commonly performed open surgical technique because of the adequate exposure and a relatively well tolerated incision. For this approach, an oblique incision is made through the abdominal musculature, extending from the lateral border of the rectus abdominus to the anterior axillary line. Cephalad and caudad blunt dissection is performed between the transversalis fascia and peritoneum. The dissection is continued in a retroperitoneal fashion. The psoas muscle is identified, with care being taken to leave the ureter and gonadal vessels attached to overlying peritoneum. The sympathetic chain is identified between the psoas muscle and the vertebra (medial to psoas and overlying the transverse process of lumbar vertebra). On the left side, the sympathetic chain is lateral to the abdominal aorta; on the right, the sympathetic chain is beneath the IVC. The sympathetic chain is dissected free from surrounding tissue, clipped proximally and distally, and resected. Hemostasis is achieved and the abdominal wall is closed in layers.

A **posterior approach** is used less often because of significant postop paraspinous muscle spasms. In this approach, a transverse lumbar incision is made, and the paraspinous muscles are partially divided and retracted to expose the vertebra. The sympathetic chain is identified and resected as described. The **anterior/transperitoneal approach** is performed in conjunction with an abdominal aortic or intraperitoneal procedure. Dissection is carried to the psoas muscle; the retroperitoneum is entered and the sympathetic chain is isolated in the groove between the psoas and the vertebra. The sympathetic chain is clipped proximally and distally and resected.

Usual preop diagnosis: Causalgia; inoperable arterial occlusive disease with limb-threatening ischemia causing rest pain, ulceration, or superficial digital gangrene; symptomatic vasospastic disorders (e.g., Raynaud's phenomenon or frostbite)

SUMMARY OF PROCEDURES

	Anterolateral (Flowthow)	Posterior (Royle)	Anterior (Adson)
Position	Supine (flank slightly raised); widen distance between costal margin and iliac crest.	Prone	Supine
Incision	Oblique (lateral edge of rectus to ribs at anterior axillary line)	Posterior transverse over mid-lumbar region	Transverse or midline abdominal
Special instrumentation	Self-retaining retractor	⇐	⇐
Unique considerations	May use frozen section to confirm specimen.	⇐	⇐
Antibiotics	Cefazolin 1g iv	⇐	⇐
Surgical time	2–3 h	3 h	4 h
Closing considerations	Flex table to facilitate abdominal wall closure; occasionally drain is placed.	⇐	⇐
EBL	50–100 mL (unless complicated)	50–100 mL	⇐
Postop care	PACU → ward. (May require cardiac and hemodynamic monitoring in high-risk patients, or if combined with distal revascularization.)	⇐	⇐
Mortality	Minimal	⇐	⇐
Morbidity	Postsympathectomy neuralgia: 50% Sexual derangement—retrograde ejaculation (usually bilateral L1 sympathectomy): 25–50% Wound hematoma: 10% Wound infection: 1–3%	~50% ~25–50% ~10% ~1–3% Paraspinous muscle spasms	⇐ ⇐ ⇐ ⇐
Pain score	5	5	5 (related to primary procedure)

PATIENT POPULATION CHARACTERISTICS

Age range	38–91 yr; younger patients with vasospastic disease; older patients with PVD
Male:Female	2:1

Cardiovascular Surgery

PATIENT POPULATION CHARACTERISTICS (cont'd)	
Incidence	Unknown. Approximately 30 cases/yr at Stanford University Medical Center, mainly for inoperable lower extremity ischemia or as an adjunct to revascularization procedures.
Etiology	PVD (rest pain and tissue loss);vasospastic disorders; causalgia
Associated conditions	PVD (rare); vasospastic disorders (rare)

ANESTHETIC CONSIDERATIONS

See Anesthetic Considerations following Infrainguinal Arterial Bypass, p. 421.

Suggested Readings

1. Abu Rahma AF, Robinson PA: Clinical parameters for predicting response to lumbar sympathectomy in patients with severe lower limb ischemia. *J Cardiovasc Surg* 1990; 31(1):101–6.
2. Bandyk DF, Johnson BL, Kirkpatrick AF, et al: Surgical sympathectomy for reflex sympathetic dystrophic syndromes. *J Vasc Surg* 2002; 35:269–77.
3. Beglaibter N, Berlatzky Y, Zamir O, et al: Retroperitoneoscopic lumbar sympathectomy. *J Vasc Surg* 2002; 35:815–7.
4. Claeys LG: The use of lumbar sympathectomy for peripheral vascular disease. *World J Surg* 1999; 23:981–3.
5. Repelaer van Driel OJ, van Bockel JH, van Schilfgaarde R: Lumbar sympathectomy for severe lower limb ischaemia: results and analysis of factors influencing the outcome. *J Cardiovasc Surg* 1988; 29(3):310–14.
6. Sanni A, Hamid A, Dunning J: Is sympathectomy of benefit in critical left ischaemia not amenable to revascularization? *Interact Cardiovasc Thorac Surg* 2005; 4:478–83.
7. Watarida S, Shiraishi S, Fujimura M, et al: Laparoscopic lumbar sympathectomy for lower-limb disease. *Surg Endosc* 2002; 16:500–3.

VENOUS SURGERY—THROMBECTOMY OR VEIN EXCISION

SURGICAL CONSIDERATIONS

Description: Standard therapy for acute DVT consists of anticoagulation, bed rest, and elevation of the extremity. Endovascular or catheter-directed thrombolysis and thrombectomy systems have been shown to extract large venous thrombus burden. Open surgical thrombectomy for acute iliofemoral DVT remains controversial. **Venous thrombectomy** is recommended for patients with threatened limb loss or venous gangrene caused by massive DVT associated with high compartment pressures and arterial insufficiency (phlegmasia cerulea dolens). Surgical venous thrombectomy requires exposure of the femoral vein via a groin cut-down. The common femoral vein is isolated (located medial or posteromedial to the femoral artery) and controlled proximally and distally. The patient is given iv heparin at this stage, if not already heparinized. A transverse venotomy is followed by extraction of the thrombus, using forceps and Fogarty embolectomy catheters (Fig. 6.3-10). Distal thrombi are expressed through the same incision with the aid of an Esmarch bandage placed on the extremity. After complete removal of the thrombus, the venotomy is closed with nonabsorbable sutures, and flow through the femoral vein is re-established. The femoral incision is closed in layers. A plastic/Silastic drain may or may not be used. The best results of thrombectomy are obtained in young patients with the first episode of proximal (iliofemoral) thrombosis.

Nonsuppurative thrombophlebitis of the superficial veins may develop due to local trauma, prolonged inactivity, fungal infection, or the use of oral contraceptives. Suppurative thrombophlebitis may occur as a complication of iv line placement or iv drug abuse. Underlying varicose veins may predispose to thrombophlebitis. Migratory superficial thrombophlebitis may be associated with chronic ischemia of the extremities in Buerger's disease, or it may develop in patients with a malignancy. Conservative management with hot compresses, nonsteroidal anti-inflammatory medications, and elevation of the extremity is effective in most cases. Rarely, **excision** of the acutely thrombosed greater saphenous vein is indicated to prevent progression of thrombosis to the saphenofemoral junction and into the deep venous system. Vein excision is simply approached by a longitudinal incision directly over the affected vein.

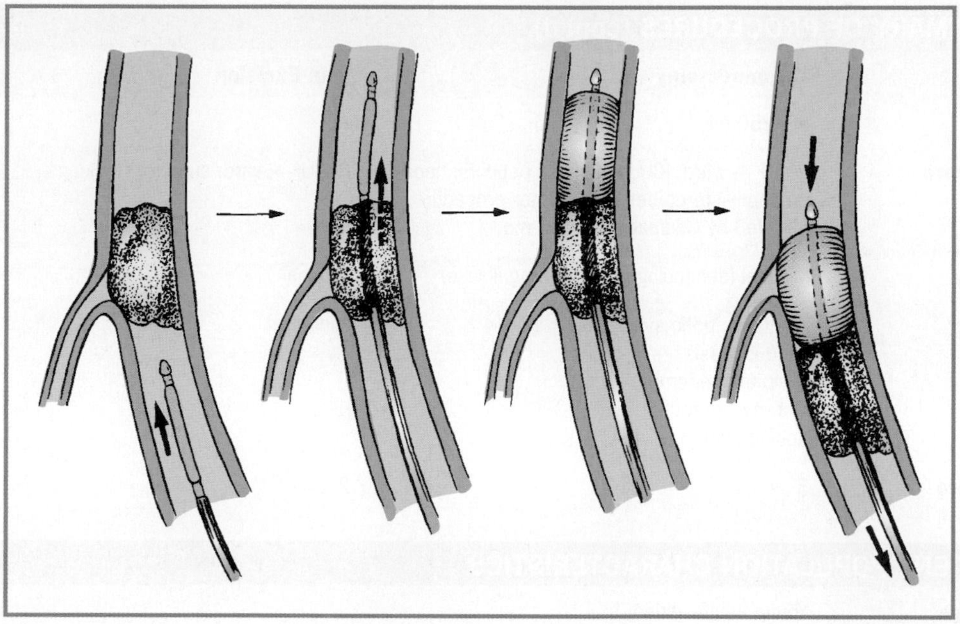

Figure 6.3-10. Fogarty catheter embolectomy with catheter insertion in the distal vessel. (Reproduced with permission from Baker RJ, Fischer JE: *Mastery of Surgery,* Vol 2. Lippincott Williams & Wilkins, 2001.)

The phlebitic vein is dissected from the surrounding tissue, ligated proximally and distally, and removed. The surrounding fibrotic tissue is débrided gently. The wound is irrigated and packed open with moist gauze. Suppurative phlebitis is treated with iv antibiotics and complete excision of the involved vein segment through multiple small incisions.

Usual preop diagnosis: Lower-limb venous thrombosis threatening viability; femoral thrombosis < 10 d; iliac thrombosis < 3 wk; floating thrombi at hip level; acute deep or superficial venous thrombosis; suppurative thrombophlebitis.

SUMMARY OF PROCEDURES

	Thrombectomy	Vein Excision
Position	Supine	⇐
Incision	Ipsilateral longitudinal or oblique groin incision	Multiple small incisions along the course of vein to be excised
Special instrumentation	Fogarty embolectomy catheters; RBC salvage System	None
Unique considerations	IPPV during thrombectomy may decrease chance of PE 2° ↓ venous return → more complete extraction of the thrombus.	None
Antibiotics	Cefazolin 1 g iv. If the patient has septic thrombus, antibiotic is dependent on blood culture.	Dependent on culture of aspirate. Usually a septic patient is on broad-spectrum antibiotics (guided by culture).
Surgical time	2–3 h	1–3 h
Closing considerations	None	Wound packed open for drainage

SUMMARY OF PROCEDURES (cont'd)		
	Thrombectomy	**Vein Excision**
EBL	50–250 mL	⇐
Postop care	PACU → ward; ICU in high-risk patients; heparin administered before and after procedure, followed by Coumadin for 1–6 mo.	PACU → ward; support stockings
Mortality	Minimal (depending on underlying illness)	Minimal
Morbidity	Postthrombotic syndrome: < 10–44% Venous stasis Nonpitting edema Brawny induration Aching pain	Minimal
Pain score	3	2

PATIENT POPULATION CHARACTERISTICS	
Age range	Young adult—elderly
Male:Female	1:2
Incidence	6–7 million in the United States have adverse effects from chronic venous stasis; 500,000 have complications of leg ulceration.
Etiology	Chronic primary varicose veins; defective venous valves; impaired pumping action of muscles in leg; previous iliofemoral thrombophlebitis; obstruction of venous return
Associated conditions	Multifactorial: varicose veins; underlying malignancy; altered coagulation status (hypercoagulability, acquired or congenital); Hx of DVT/thrombophlebitis

ANESTHETIC CONSIDERATIONS

See Anesthetic Considerations following Infrainguinal Arterial Bypass, p. 421.

Suggested Readings

1. Bluckians A, Meier GH 3rd: Treatment of symptomatic lower extremity acute deep venous thrombosis: role of mechanical thrombectomy. *Vascular* 2007; 15:297–303.
2. Gloviczki P, Merrell SW: Surgical treatment of venous disease. *Cardiovasc Glin* 1992; 22(3):81–100.
3. Kim HS, Patra A, Paxton BE, et al: Catheter-directed thrombolysis with percutaneous rheolytic thrombectomy versus thrombolysis along in upper and lower extremity deep vein thrombosis. *Cardiovasc Intervent Radiol* 2006; 29:1003–7.
4. Vedantham S, Vesely TM, Parti N, et al: Lower extremity venous thrombolysis with adjunctive mechanical thrombectomy. *J Vasc Interv Radiol* 2002; 13:1001–8.
5. Wakefield TW: Treatment options for venous thrombosis. *J Vasc Surg* 2000; 31:613–20.

SURGERY FOR PORTAL HYPERTENSION

SURGICAL CONSIDERATIONS

Description: Alcoholic liver disease is the major cause of portal HTN; and end-stage liver disease (ESLD) with cirrhosis is the 10th leading cause of death in the United States (exceeding 23,000/yr). Of patients with portal HTN, 15–20% have variceal hemorrhage during the first yr of diagnosis (additional 5–10 % incidence of bleeding per yr); and the initial episode of variceal hemorrhage is associated with 50% mortality. Portal HTN (>15 mmHg) develops

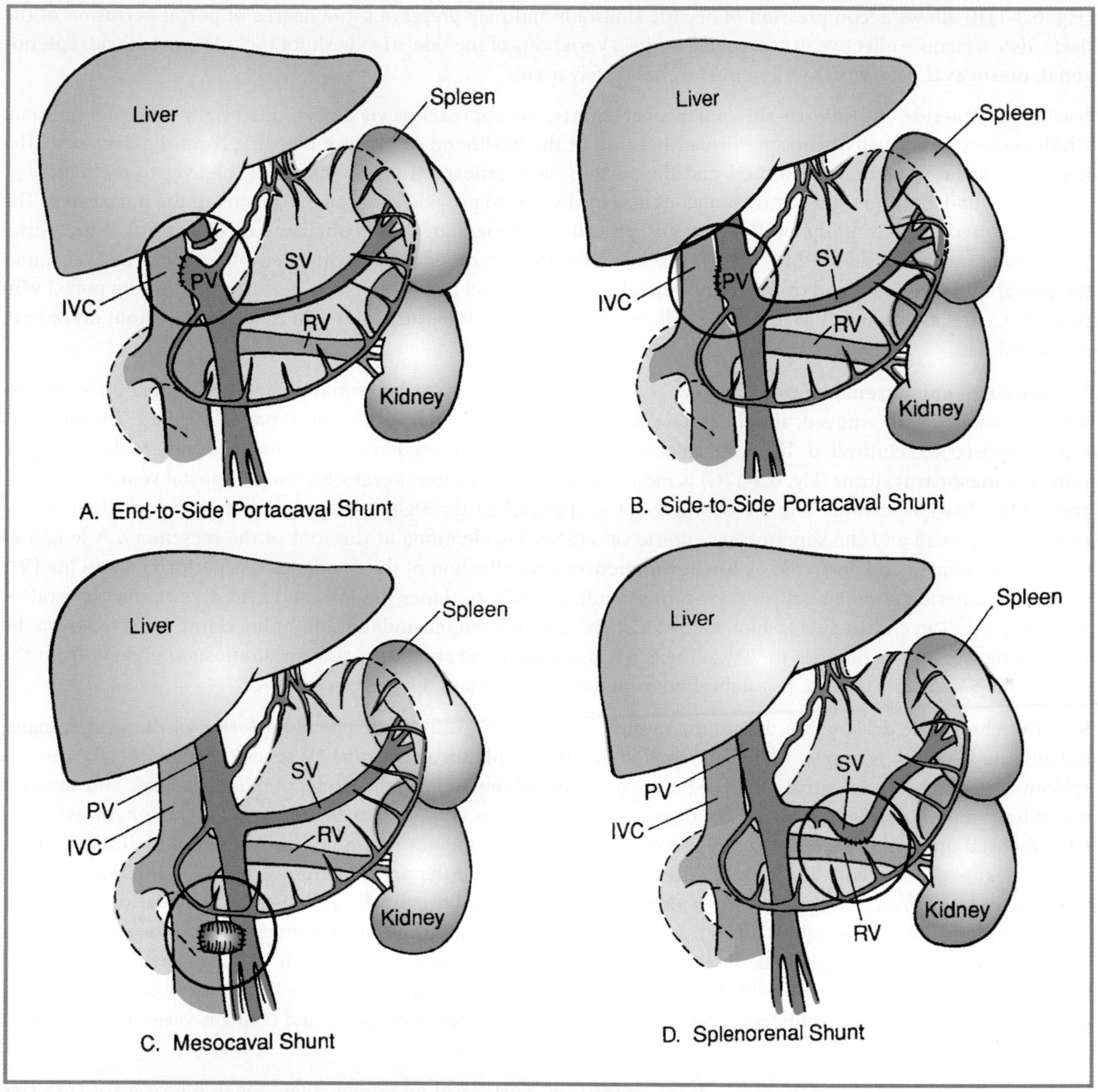

Figure 6.3-11. Types of shunts: **A.** End-to-side portacaval; **B.** side-to-side portacaval; **C.** mesocaval shunt; **D.** distal splenorenal. (Reproduced with permission from Hardy JD: *Hardy's Textbook of Surgery,* 2nd edition. JB Lippincott, 1988.)

when splanchnic venous flow to the right heart becomes impeded. Medical and surgical therapeutic interventions are directed not at portal HTN per se, but at its complications—notably bleeding esophageal varices. Intractable ascites and hypersplenism are less common indications for operative therapy. Presinusoidal portal HTN, unlike sinusoidal or postsinusoidal obstruction, is not associated with severe hepatocellular disease; thus, the prognosis for patients with presinusoidal block is better than for those with sinusoidal or postsinusoidal disease. Surgical approaches can be divided into shunt and nonshunt procedures. **Shunt procedures** can be classified as either **total** (decompression of the portal venous system) or **selective** (decompression of only the varix-bearing area). It should be noted, however, that surgery for portal HTN has been replaced largely by the TIPS procedure (see p. 1462).

SHUNT PROCEDURES

There are two general types of total shunt (**portosystemic shunt**) procedures. The **end-to-side portacaval shunt** (Fig. 6.3-11A) is technically simpler and may be more appropriate in emergency situations. It is associated with immediate control of hemorrhage in the majority of cases. The portacaval shunt, however, does eliminate portal perfusion of the liver and does not decompress the hepatic sinusoids. Alternatively, the **functional side-to-side shunt**

(Fig. 6.3-11B) allows decompression of hepatic sinusoids and may preserve some degree of portal perfusion of the liver. Also, it is more effective in controlling ascites. Variations of the side-to-side shunt include: **portacaval, splenorenal, mesocaval (Clatworthy)**, and **portarenal** (rarely used).

For the **end-to-side** and **side-to-side portacaval shunts,** the approach is via an extended right subcostal incision. **Cholecystectomy** usually is not performed because of the likelihood of profuse bleeding from the liver bed. The hepatoduodenal ligament is identified, and the portal vein is exposed from the hilum of the liver to the pancreas. The gastroduodenal and right gastric branches may be divided to provide additional exposure of the portal vein. The IVC is exposed by incising the peritoneum just beneath the hepatic triad. Proximal and distal control of the portal vein is achieved; and a side-biting clamp is placed on the IVC. In order to perform an end-to-side portacaval shunt, the portal vein is divided and oversewn proximally; the end-to-side anastomosis is performed from the portal vein to the IVC. The alternative is to perform a side-to-side anastomosis of the portal vein to the IVC without division of the portal vein.

The **proximal splenorenal shunt** is approached through a left thoracoabdominal or transabdominal incision. The spleen is isolated and removed, and the distal splenic vein is mobilized from the distal pancreatic bed. The left renal vein is exposed and controlled. The distal splenic vein is then anastomosed in an end-to-side fashion to the mid renal vein. The **mesocaval shunt** (Fig. 6.3-11C) is indicated in cases of ascites, periportal fibrosis, portal vein thrombosis, and Budd-Chiari syndrome. The mesocaval shunt is approached through a vertical midline incision. The colon is retracted cephalad and the superior mesenteric vein (SMV) is identified at the root of the mesentery. A length of the SMV is isolated and encircled. A **Kocher maneuver** (mobilization of the duodenum) is performed and the IVC is exposed anteriorly and laterally. A side-biting clamp partially occludes the IVC and a 14–20 mm dacron graft is anastomosed in an end-to-side fashion to the IVC. The graft is clamped and the side-biting clamp removed from the IVC, thereby restoring flow via the IVC. The SMV is clamped and an end-to-side anastomosis is created from the graft to the SMV. Flow is, thus, re-established from the SMV through the graft to the IVC.

Selective shunts are designed to decompress esophageal varices, while some portal perfusion of the liver is maintained. The hallmark example of this approach is the **distal splenorenal shunt (Warren)** (Fig. 6.3-11D), which is seldom used in emergency situations. The principal feature of this shunt is disconnection of the splenic and superior mesenteric venous drainage systems. The distal splenorenal shunt is approached through a left chevron or extended left subcostal incision. The lesser sac is entered after division of the gastroepiploic vessels and mobilization of the splenic flexure of the colon. The stomach is retracted cephalad and the peritoneum overlying the inferior aspect of the pancreas is incised. The splenic vein is identified and controlled proximally and distally. The inferior mesenteric vein is divided. The splenic vein is divided proximally and the proximal stump is oversewn. Then the splenic vein is mobilized from the pancreatic bed. The left renal vein is identified and 5–7 cm of the vein is isolated. The splenic vein is anastomosed in an end-to-side fashion to the renal vein. The coronary vein is ligated close to its origin. The distal splenorenal shunt decompresses the stomach, distal esophagus, and spleen and controls variceal hemorrhage in 85% of patients.

Variant procedure or approaches: **Total shunt** (e.g., portacaval, proximal splenorenal, mesocaval); **selective shunt** (e.g., **Warren**); **non-shunt procedures** (e.g., **Sugiura, Hassab,** and **esophageal transection with stapling**)

Usual preop diagnosis: Bleeding esophageal varices (as a result of portal HTN); ascites; hypersplenism

SUMMARY OF PROCEDURES (TOTAL AND SELECTIVE SHUNTS)

	Portacaval	Proximal Splenorenal	Mesocaval (Clatworthy)	Distal Splenorenal (Warren)
Position	Supine	Supine ± left flank elevated	Supine	Supine, left side elevated slightly
Incision	Extended right sub- costal—may be lengthened or converted to left thoracoabdominal.	Left thoracoabdominal or left subcostal, or vertical midline	Vertical midline abdominal	Left chevron or left subcostal with midline extension
Special instrumentation	Self-retaining retractor	⇐	⇐	⇐

SUMMARY OF PROCEDURES (TOTAL AND SELECTIVE SHUNTS) (cont'd)				
	Portacaval	**Proximal Splenorenal**	**Mesocaval (Clatworthy)**	**Distal Splenorenal (Warren)**
Unique considerations	May need FFP; consider Cell Saver.	⇐	⇐	⇐
Antibiotics	Cefazolin 1 g iv	⇐	⇐	⇐
Surgical time	4–6 h	⇐	⇐	⇐
Closing considerations	None	⇐	⇐	⇐
EBL	1,000–2,000 mL	⇐	⇐	⇐
Postop care	Patient → ICU; careful fluid management; consider Na+ restriction; may require PA catheter.	⇐	⇐	⇐
Mortality	Emergency: 38% Elective: 3% Child's A: 0–15%* Child's B: 1–43%* Child's C: 6–58%*	5–10%	⇐	1–16%
Morbidity	Late liver failure: 50% Encephalopathy: 32% Child's A: 8%* Child's B: 20%* Child's C: 30%* Early rebleeding: 0–19% Shunt thrombosis: 1–10%	~50% ~32% ~0–19% 20%	⇐ ⇐ ⇐ 9–30% Duodenal obstruction Erosion through bowel wall	– 5–47% (overall) 5% at 2 yr 12% at 3–6 yr 27% at 10 yr – – Loss of selectivity: 60% (@ 2 yr) Recurrent variceal-hem-orrhage (shunt occlusion): 3–19% Portal vein thrombosis: 4–10%
Pain score	6	6	6	6

Note: In addition to the shunt procedure itself, other factors that determine postop morbidity and mortality include: severity of hepatocellular disease, degree of hepatic reserve, and urgency of the procedure. Although the specific numbers may vary, several comparative series have shown no difference in operative mortality rate or long-term survival rate among the various open shunt procedures.

NONSHUNT PROCEDURES

Nonshunt procedures are designed to devascularize the esophagogastric region, thus eliminating acute variceal hemorrhage. Procedures of this type include: **portazygous disconnection; splenectomy; coronary vein ligation;** and **transesophageal** or **transgastric varix ligation**.

The **Sugiura operation,** approached via abdominal and thoracic incisions, includes esophageal transection and devascularization, splenectomy, and pyloromyotomy. This procedure is usually performed in two operative stages, sometimes with a delayed second stage. The **Hassab procedure** involves devascularization of the upper half of the stomach and splenectomy, thus effectively disconnecting the esophageal varices. (This operation has been reserved in some centers for the failures of sclerotherapy.) Finally, **esophageal transection,** using a stapling device, disconnects the varices in the lower esophagus. This is accomplished by placing a row of staples at the esophagus just above the esophagogastric junction. Because portal perfusion of the liver is maintained after the nonshunt procedures, hepatic function is preserved.

SUMMARY OF NONSHUNT PROCEDURES

	Sugiura (Two Stages)	Hassab	Esophageal Transection
Position	Supine, left side elevated	Supine	⇐
Incision	Abdominal stage: midline; thoracic stage: left thoracotomy	Vertical midline	⇐
Special instrumentation	Self-retaining retractor	⇐	⇐
Antibiotics	Cefazolin 1 g iv	⇐	⇐
Surgical time	4–6 h for both stages	4 h	⇐
EBL	1,000–2,000 mL	⇐	⇐
Postop care	ICU; careful hemodynamic monitoring; PA catheterization	⇐	⇐
Mortality	Overall: 5–14% Emergent: 14% (≤ 60%) Elective: 3%	12–38% 10%	10–83%
Morbidity	Recurrent hemorrhage: 2–50% Esophagopleural leak: 6% Encephalopathy: 3% Ascites: 2% Wound infection: 2%	7% – 1–25% 4% –	0–50% 3% 33% 11% 11%
Pain score	6	5	5

PATIENT POPULATION CHARACTERISTICS FOR SHUNT AND NONSHUNT PROCEDURES

Age range	11–72 yr (mean age = 48 yr); depending on etiology: pediatric (e.g., congenital hepatic fibrosis) to adult (e.g., alcoholic liver disease)
Male:Female	2–8:1
Incidence	Rare
Etiology	Alcoholic liver disease (alcoholic hepatitis, chronic alcoholism, cirrhosis); postnecrotic cirrhosis; portal vein thrombosis; splenic vein occlusion; hematologic diseases; hepatic vein occlusion; schistosomiasis; congenital hepatic fibrosis; sarcoidosis; sinusoidal occlusion (vitamin A toxicity, Gaucher's disease); venoocclusive disease
Associated conditions	Alcohol dependency; cirrhosis/liver failure; poor nutritional status; coagulopathy; encephalopathy

ANESTHETIC CONSIDERATIONS

(Procedures covered: shunt and nonshunt procedures for portal HTN surgery)

PREOPERATIVE

Respiratory	Hypoxemia may be present 2° ascites, V/Q mismatch, ↑ R→L pulmonary shunting, atelectasis, pulmonary infections and ↓ pulmonary diffusing capacity. **Tests:** Consider ABG; PFTs, as indicated; CXR

Cardiovascular	Patients presenting with portal HTN often have a hyperdynamic circulatory state with ↑ plasma volume, ↑ CO, and ↓ SVR, with a decreased ability to ↑ SVR or ↑ HR in response to stimuli. Ventricular performance may be abnormal (CHF), especially in patients with alcoholic liver disease. Ascites →↑ intrathoracic pressure, ↓ FRC, ↓ venous return, and ↓ CO. Older patients in this population usually have CAD. **Tests:** ECG. If LV function in question, ECHO or angiography.
Hepatic	The physical manifestations of hepatic disease include palmar erythema, caput medusae, spider angiomas, and gynecomastia. Albumin and other products of liver synthesis (e.g., coagulation factors) may be decreased. Encephalopathy may be present 2° impaired ammonia metabolism. **Tests:** Bilirubin; albumin; PT; SGOT; SGPT; ammonia; alkaline phosphatase
Gastrointestinal	Portal HTN eventually → esophageal and gastric varices. Patients may present emergently with profuse GI bleeding. Ascites occurs in ~80% of patients with portal HTN and splenomegaly is invariably present. As a result of elevated intraabdominal pressure from ascites, and slow gastric emptying, a rapid-sequence induction with full-stomach precautions will be necessary (see p. B-4).
Renal	Portal HTN →↓ GFR and ↓ renal blood flow → renal failure. **Tests:** Consider UA; creatinine clearance as indicated from H&P
Hematologic	These patients are often anemic as a result of poor nutrition, malabsorption, and intestinal tract blood loss. Hypersplenism may be present (Plt count < 50,000 and WBC < 2,000). Synthesis of all coagulation factors is decreased except factor VIII and fibrinogen. A low-grade DIC may be present. T&C for 8–10 U PRBC. **Tests:** CBC; Plt count; PT; PTT; consider DIC screen.
Pharmacologic	The liver is the major site of drug biotransformation; however, the effects of hepatic dysfunction on drug elimination and disposition are inconsistent.
Laboratory	These patients may have significant electrolyte disturbances (e.g., ↓↓ Na^+, ↓ K^+). **Tests:** Electrolytes and others as indicated from H&P.
Premedication	If premedication is appropriate, small doses of anxiolytic, such as midazolam (0.5–1 mg iv), are preferable. Avoid im medications in patients with possible coagulopathy. Full-stomach precautions are necessary. Metoclopramide (10 mg iv) and ranitidine (50 mg iv) may be given 60 min before surgery.

INTRAOPERATIVE

Anesthetic technique: GETA. Preservation of intravascular volume and myocardial stability can be a challenge in these patients.

Induction	Instable patients rapid-sequence induction with propofol (1–2 mg/kg) and succinylcholine (1–2 mg/kg) should be used. Replace blood loss and ensure normovolemia before induction (if possible). Etomidate (0.2 mg/kg) or ketamine (1 mg/kg) may be preferable for induction in hemodynamically unstable patients.
Maintenance	High-dose narcotic technique with fentanyl (50–100 mcg/kg) or sufentanil (10–15 mcg/kg) and low-dose isoflurane. Midazolam (0.1–0.2 mg/kg) often is given in conjunction with the narcotic to ensure amnesia during times of hemodynamic instability when isoflurane cannot be tolerated. N_2O is avoided to prevent bowel distention. Muscle relaxation is needed (e.g., vecuronium 0.1 mg/kg or less, titrated using a nerve stimulator). ***NB:** After drainage of ascitic fluid, there may be a precipitous drop in BP requiring rapid volume replacement ± vasopressor.
Emergence	Generally deferred to ICU due to large fluid shifts and transfusion requirements. Patients who have undergone uneventful and nonemergent surgery may be candidates for extubation.

Blood and fluid requirements	Anticipate large blood loss. IV: 14 ga × 2 or 7 Fr × 2 Rapid infuser RBC salvage device 8–10 U PRBC Warm all fluids. Humidify all gases. Warming blanket	FFP, Plt, and cryoprecipitate should be available to treat coagulopathy. e. g. Bair-Hugger warmer
Monitoring	Standard monitors (p. B-1) Arterial line CVP or PA catheter	Arterial and central pressure monitoring are essential. A PA catheter is useful in this setting because most patients are cirrhotic and may have excessive blood loss and large fluid shifts.
	UO	UO is measured and is helpful as a monitor of renal perfusion. Mannitol (0.25–1 g/kg iv) may be needed to maintain UO.
	Temperature	In these procedures, prevention of hypothermia is important. In patients with large varices, avoid esophageal placement of T probes or stethoscopes.
	ABGs	Serial ABGs to determine adequacy of ventilation and normal acid base status should be done.
	Hct, coags, Ca^{++}	Hct, coagulation, and Ca++ should be measured following replacement of large blood volumes.
	Electrolytes Blood glucose	Electrolytes and glucose also should be monitored. Glucose metabolism in liver disease may be impaired →↓ glucose.
Positioning	✓ and pad pressure points. ✓ eyes.	
Complications	Coagulopathy Hemorrhage Hypothermia	

POSTOPERATIVE

Complications	Coagulopathy Hypothermia Encephalopathy Renal failure	
Pain management	PCA (p. C-3) Parenteral opiates	
Tests	CXR: line placement Hct Electrolytes Glucose	DIC screen, if continued bleeding.

Suggested Readings

1. Gusberg RJ: Selective shunts in selected older cirrhotic patients with variceal hemorrhage. *Am J Surg* 1993; 166(3):274–8.
2. Haberer JP, Schoeffler P, Couderc E, et al: Fentanyl pharmacokinetics in anesthetized patients with cirrhosis. *Br J Anaesth* 1982; 54:1267.
3. Hassab MA: Nonshunt operations in portal hypertension without cirrhosis. *Surg Gynecol Obstet* 1970; 131(4):648–54.
4. Henderson JM: The distal splenoral shunt. *Surg Clin North Am* 1990; 70(2):405–23.

5. Jenkins RL, Gedaly R, Pomposelli JJ, et al: Distal splenorenal shunt: role, indications, and utility in the era of liver transplantation. *Arch Surg* 1999; 134:416–20.
6. Langer B, Taylor BR, Greig PD: Selective or total shunts for variceal bleeding. *Am J Surg* 1990; 160(1):75–9.
7. Orozco H, Mercado MA, Takahashi T, et al: Elective treatment of bleeding varices with the Sugiura operation over 10 years. *Am J Surg* 1992; 163(6):585–9.

ARTERIOVENOUS ACCESS FOR HEMODIALYSIS

SURGICAL CONSIDERATIONS

Description: **Peripheral subcutaneous arteriovenous** (AV) **fistula,** or **prosthetic graft,** is the current procedure of choice for patients requiring permanent hemodialysis access. The blood flow in the autogenous AV fistula increases with time, and the resulting vein wall thickening prevents venous tears and infiltration during dialysis.

The standard AV fistula is usually constructed by anastomosing the cephalic vein to the radial artery at the wrist level (**Brescia-Cimino fistula**) (Fig. 6.3-12). Other locations include the 'snuff box,' or antebrachium. Vascular access using vascular substitutes or prosthetic grafts is performed when there is a lack of suitable veins in patients who have had failed-access procedures, peripheral vein sclerosis, or severe arterial disease involving the upper extremity. Forearm grafts are constructed as a direct communication between the radial or ulnar artery and the antecubital or

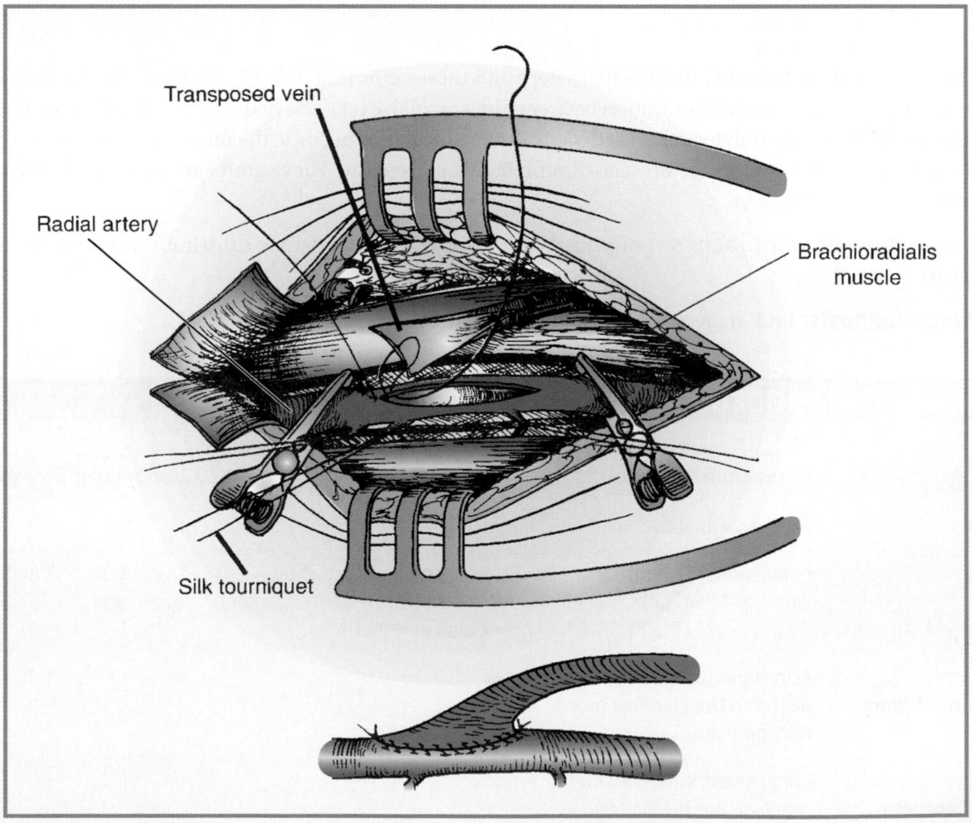

Figure 6.3-12. Brescia-Cimino fistula (side-to-end anastomosis). (Reproduced with permission from Scott-Conner CEH, Dawson DL: *Operative Anatomy,* 2nd edition. Lippincott Williams & Wilkins, Philadelphia, 2003.)

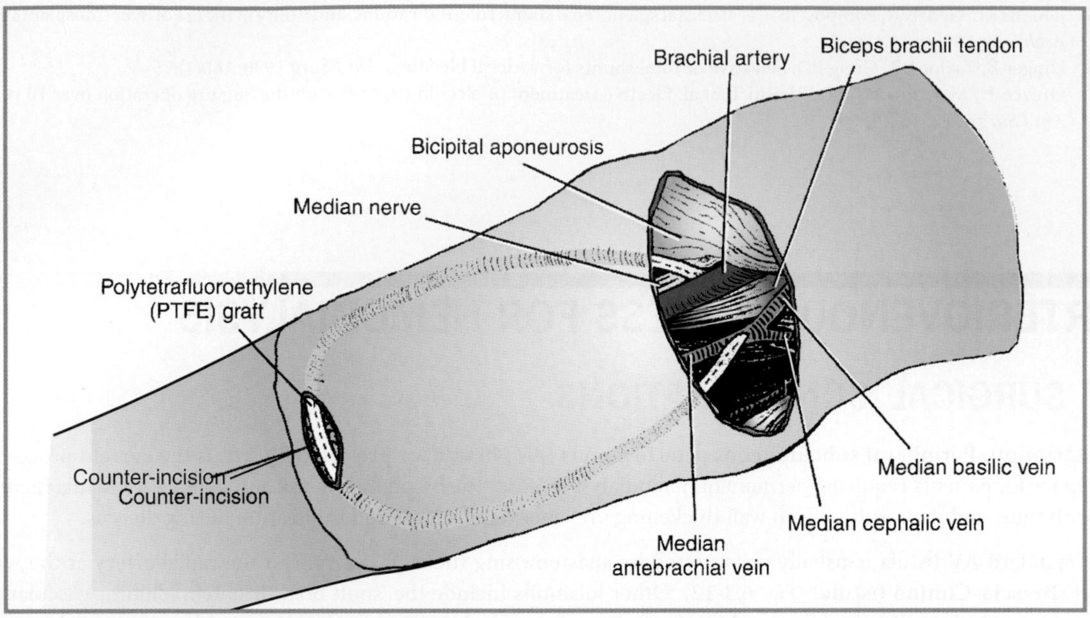

Figure 6.3-13. In arteriovenous hemodialysis access with prosthetic graft, the brachial artery and the median antebrachial, median basilic, and median cephalic veins are exposed via a horizontal incision below the antecubital joint crease. (Reproduced with permission from Scott-Conner CEH, Dawson DL: *Operative Anatomy,* 2nd edition. Lippincott Williams & Wilkins, Philadelphia, 2003.)

brachial vein, or as a 'loop' between the brachial artery and these veins (Fig. 6.3-13). Similarly, an access can be constructed in the upper arm as a communication between the brachial artery above the elbow and the basilic or axillary vein in a straight fashion. The polytetrafluoroethylene (Teflon) graft has become the mainstay for hemodialysis access in patients who are not candidates for Brescia-Cimino fistula placement. These grafts are associated with a primary patency rate of 50–60% at 2–3 yr.

Variant procedure or approaches: **Loop or straight graft,** using vascular substitute in forearm; **upper-arm straight graft**

Usual preop diagnosis: End-stage renal failure requiring graft hemodialysis

SUMMARY OF PROCEDURES

	Forearm AV Fistula	Forearm Loop or Straight Graft	Upper-Arm Straight Graft
Position	Supine, arm abducted	⇐	⇐
Incision	Longitudinal or transverse at wrist, or "snuff box"	Transverse at antecubital fossa and/or at wrist; counter-incision in forearm	Transverse or longitudinal in upper arm
Special instrumentation	Arm/hand table (for arm abduction); Doppler flow probe may be used.	⇐	⇐
Unique considerations	Local anesthesia; consider brachial plexus block (increased incidence of hematoma); heparinization	⇐	⇐
Antibiotics	None	Vancomycin 1 g iv	⇐

SUMMARY OF PROCEDURES (cont'd)			
	Forearm AV Fistula	Forearm Loop or Straight Graft	Upper-Arm Straight Graft
Surgical time	1–2 h	⇐	⇐
Closing considerations	Use of Doppler to ✓ shunt patency	⇐	⇐
EBL	25–50 mL	25–100 mL	⇐
Postop care	Hemodynamic monitoring for poor-risk patients; can be done as outpatient.	⇐	⇐
Mortality	Minimal, depending on associated risk factors	⇐	⇐
Morbidity	Thrombosis: 20% Technical failure: 10–15% Arterial steal: Rare Cardiac failure: Rare Infection: Rare No venous outflow: Rare Seroma: Rare Venous aneurysm: Rare Venous HTN: Rare	8–32% ⇐ ⇐ ⇐ 10% 6% ⇐ ⇐ ⇐	~8–32% ⇐ ⇐ ⇐ ⇐ ~6% ⇐ ⇐ ⇐
Pain score	1	2	2

PATIENT POPULATION CHARACTERISTICS	
Age range	Pediatric and adult population
Male:Female	1:1
Incidence	Hemodialysis access is one of the most commonly performed procedures by vascular surgeons.
Etiology	Glomerulonephritis; diabetes; HTN; pyelonephritis
Associated conditions	Diabetes mellitus; PVD/CAD

ANESTHETIC CONSIDERATIONS

See Anesthetic Considerations following Permanent Vascular Access, p. 441.

Suggested Readings

1. Allon M, Robbin ML: Increasing arteriovenous fistulas in hemodialysis patients: problems and solutions. *Kidney Int* 2002; 62:1109–24.
2. Khosla N, Ahya SN: Improving dialysis access management. *Semin Nephrol* 2002; 22:507–14.
3. Spergel LM, Ravani P Asif A, et al: Autogenous arteriovenous fistula options. *J Nephrol* 2007; 20(3):288–98.

PERMANENT VASCULAR ACCESS

SURGICAL CONSIDERATIONS

Description: Silastic or plastic catheters are placed in patients who require venous access for chronic antibiotic therapy, TPN, chemotherapy, or hemodialysis. **Hickman, Broviac,** and **Groshong catheters** are made of silicone rubber or plastic with a cuff near the skin exit site, which (in theory) serves as a barrier to infection. Access is generally

Cardiovascular Surgery

achieved via subclavian, IJ, or femoral vein puncture. These catheters are available in various sizes and in single- or double-lumen configurations. Larger diameter (13 Fr) Hickman or **Permacath DL** catheters have been introduced for hemodialysis. **Mediport** and **Portacath devices** have a metallic or plastic reservoir connected to the catheters and are intended for complete subcutaneous implantation. These catheters are used in chronically ill patients, particularly those requiring chemotherapy. The implantable access ports have been associated with improved patient comfort and reduced infection rates. Long-term catheter survival is limited by infection. Removal and replacement of the catheter is the only way to eradicate the infection.

Variant procedure or approaches: Two major distinctions: Hickman/Broviac catheters (no reservoir) vs Mediport/Portacath catheters (subcutaneous with reservoir). Subclavian, IJ, or femoral vein puncture is selected, depending on vein status, previous operations, and patient comfort.

Usual preop diagnosis: Chronic antibiotic therapy; TPN; chemotherapy; end-stage renal failure

SUMMARY OF PROCEDURES

	Hickman/Broviac/Groshong	Mediport/Portacath
Position	Supine, slight Trendelenburg	⇐
Incision	Puncture site (subclavian, IJ, or femoral vein); subcutaneous tunnel for passage of catheter. Alternative: cephalic or IJ vein cut-down to achieve access.	Puncture site (subclavian, IJ, or femoral vein); subcutaneous pocket for port. Alternative: cephalic or IJ vein cut-down to achieve access.
Special instrumentation	I.I. or fluoroscope	⇐
Unique considerations	Local anesthesia; may need iv sedation; monitor for ectopy during placement.	⇐
Antibiotics	Cefazolin 1 g iv	⇐
Surgical time	30–90 min	45–90 min
EBL	10–25 mL	25–50 mL
Postop care	CXR in recovery room; may be outpatient.	⇐
Mortality	Minimal	⇐
Morbidity	Catheter thrombosis: 25% Skin exit site infection: 13% Poor flow: 10–13% Catheter sepsis: 5–8% Arterial puncture: 6% Local bleeding: 5% SVC thrombosis: 5% Catheter displacement: 3% Subclavian thrombosis: 2% Pneumothorax 1–2% Failed attempt: 1% Infection: 3–5/1,000 cath days	4% – ~10–13% 2% ~6% – ~5% ~3% ~2% ~1–2% ~1% – Pocket hematoma: 2% Pocket infection: 3% Catheter leakage: 1%
Pain score	1	2

PATIENT POPULATION CHARACTERISTICS

Age range	Pediatrics and adults, 8–80 yr
Male:Female	1:1

■ PATIENT POPULATION CHARACTERISTICS (cont'd)	
Incidence	Depending on underlying disease
Etiology	Access for chemotherapy; infections; hemodialysis; chronic TPN
Associated conditions	Malignancy; chronic illness/infection; renal failure

ANESTHETIC CONSIDERATIONS FOR VASCULAR ACCESS

(Procedures covered: arteriovenous access for hemodialysis; permanent vascular access)

PREOPERATIVE

The patient populations presenting for vascular access surgery are extremely diverse. Patients requiring vascular access for chemotherapy, TPN, and chronic antibiotic therapy frequently can be done with MAC (p. B-3). Also presenting for these procedures are end-stage renal failure patients who need arteriovenous access for hemodialysis (generally involving the upper extremity). These patients return to the OR frequently for revising or replacing of fistulas. They are often ASA III & IV patients who may require GA or an upper extremity block. Anesthetic considerations for the **chronic renal failure patient** are discussed below.

Respiratory	Pulmonary edema may be present from fluid overload. CHF and uremic pleuritis can occur. Pneumonia occurs more frequently in these patients due to depressed immune systems. Hemodialysis contributes to hypoxemia due to V/Q mismatch and hypoventilation. **Tests:** CXR; consider ABG.
Cardiovascular	Often have HTN related to hypervolemia and a disorder of the renin-antiogensin system. May have LVH 2° to HTN. Cardiomyopathy, pericarditis, and pericardial effusion occur with uremia. Hypervolemia and hypoalbuminemia can contribute to CHF. Uremic patients often have defective aortic and carotid body reflex arcs. Ejection murmurs are common. **Tests:** ECG; others as indicated from H&P.
Renal	A comprehensive preop evaluation should include an assessment of renal function and adequacy of recent dialysis therapy. Ascertaining the patient's usual and recent weights is useful. Dialysis is usually advisable shortly before anesthesia and surgery. The symptoms of uremia (Plt dysfunction, electrolyte/fluid abnormalities, CNS, and GI disturbances) improve with dialysis. If a transfusion is needed, it is best done during dialysis so intravascular volume can be controlled. **Tests:** Serum BUN; Cr. If patient produces urine, consider creatinine clearance, UA.
Hematologic	Chronic anemia with Hct ranging from 15–21 g/dL. Normochromic, normocytic anemia present 2° bone marrow depression, lack of erythropoietin, nutritional deficiency, and diminished red-cell survival time. Patients adjust to chronic anemia through ↑CO and ↑2,3-DPG levels. Accumulation of waste products inhibits Plt function. Defects do occur in the coagulation cascade, but PT and PTT are usually normal. **Tests:** CBC; Plt; PT; PTT
Gastrointestinal	Uremic patients commonly have hiccups, anorexia, N/V, and diarrhea. They are very prone to developing GI bleeds. Renal failure causes ↓ gastric emptying. Premedication with metoclopramide (10 mg po) and ranitidine (150 mg po) will ↓ gastric volume and pH.
Nervous system	CNS Sx of uremia range from malaise to Sz to coma. Fatigue and intellectual impairment commonly occur. Peripheral and autonomic neuropathies exist. Peripheral neuropathy presents as itching and paresthesia of the lower extremities. Autonomic dysfunction can cause postural ↓ BP. Document deficits carefully.
Endocrine	Diabetes frequently may be the cause of renal failure, with its attendant problems. **Tests:** Glucose
Immune system	Often impaired. Patients prone to sepsis. Hepatitis and HIV infections from blood products may exist.

Metabolic and biochemical	Accumulation of K^+ urea, parathyroid hormone (hypercalcemia), Mg, aluminum (neurotoxicity), acid metabolites, and phosphate occurs. Knowing hyperkalemia exists is of importance because of the potential for fatal cardiac dysrhythmias. Shift of the oxyhemoglobin curve to the right occurs due to the metabolic acidosis and ↑ 2,3-DPG (improves tissue oxygenation). Hyponatremia is a common electrolyte disturbance in chronic renal failure.
Premedication	If warranted, it is best to use light premedication with sedatives or opioids due to the possibility of exaggerated effects (p. B-1).

INTRAOPERATIVE

Anesthetic technique: GA, upper extremity block, or MAC.

Regional anesthesia: May be advantageous due to decreased number of drug effects. See section on upper extremity blocks (Anesthetic Considerations for Wrist Procedures, p. 914). If the patient was very recently dialyzed, there may be a residual heparin effect. Regional anesthesia is contraindicated if coagulopathy is present.

General anesthesia: The duration of action and elimination of many anesthetic drugs is altered in the patient with renal failure.

Induction	If general anesthesia is indicated, preferably LMA is used. Induction with propofol and low-dose fentanyl (25–50 mcg) is usually well-tolerated. In case of the need for intubation, succinylcholine is indicated if $K^+ < 5.5$ mEq/L. If succinylcholine is contraindicated, cisatracurium (0.1–0.2 mg/kg) is the alternative muscle relaxant of choice, since its elimination is not affected by renal failure. Etomidate (0.2–0.3 mg/kg) is preferred in case of preop hemodynamic instability.	
Maintenance	Inhalation anesthetics (isoflurane, sevoflurane) offer the advantage of not requiring renal elimination. Biotransformation may produce some inorganic fluoride (nephrotoxin); however, this is not an issue in dialysis patients. Opioids can produce an increased magnitude and duration of effect. Increased accumulation of morphine glucuronides → prolonged respiratory depression. Fentanyl and remifentanil are good choices, 2° rapid tissue redistribution (fentanyl) or rapid metabolism (remifentanil). Benzodiazepine dosage should be adjusted, since protein binding in renal insufficiency/failure is reduced.	
Emergence	Prolonged effect of anticholinesterases (e.g., neostigmine and edrophonium) effectively offsets prolongation of blockade. Other factors affecting reversal of nondepolarizers should be taken into account. These include acid-base status, depth of blockade, temperature and use of drugs such as diuretics or antibiotics, which can potentiate blockade.	
Blood and fluid requirements	IV: 18–20 ga × 1 NS @ 1–2 mL/kg/h	IV access may be difficult; avoid iv placement in operated arm. Minimize fluids in renal-failure patients.
Monitoring	Standard monitors (p. B-1)	Avoid BP cuff placement on operated arm.
Positioning	✓ and pad pressure points. ✓ eyes.	
Complications	Local anesthetic toxicity	

POSTOPERATIVE

Complications	Nerve damage Hematoma	These are rare complications of brachial plexus blocks.
Pain management	PO analgesics	

Suggested Readings

1. Bour ES, Weaver AS, Yang HC, et al: Experience with the double lumen Silastic catheter for hemoaccess. *Surg Gynecol Obstet* 1990; 171(1): 33–9.
2. Monk J: Hemodialysis catheters and ports. *Semin Nephrol* 2002; 22:211–20.
3. Murphy GJ, White SA, Nicholson ML: Vascular access for hemodialysis. *Br J Surg* 2000; 87:1300–15.
4. Silberman H, Berne TV, Escandon R: Prospective evaluation of a double-lumen subclavian dialysis catheter for acute vascular access. *Am Surg* 1992; 58:443–5.

VENOUS SURGERY—VEIN STRIPPING AND PERFORATOR LIGATION

SURGICAL CONSIDERATIONS

Description: Chronic venous insufficiency results from static blood flow in the deep, superficial, and perforating veins of the lower extremities. Clinical manifestations include pathologic changes in the skin and subcutaneous tissues, such as pigmentation, dermatitis, induration, and ulceration around the lower portion of the leg. The condition is most commonly caused by defective venous valves and less often by obstruction to the venous return or impaired pumping action of the muscles in the leg. The disorder is sometimes the residual of previous iliofemoral thrombophlebitis. Varicose veins of the primary type, particularly those of long duration, are a common cause of chronic venous insufficiency of milder degrees. Most symptoms respond well to conservative management, which includes compression stockings, elevation of the extremity, and topical treatment of ulcerations. Failure of medical management is an indication for surgical intervention. Split-thickness skin grafting is indicated for large ulcers to accelerate healing and shorten hospitalization time. **Ligation of perforators** is best performed when the ulcer has completely healed. The classic approach of **Linton** is rarely used today. If the quality of the skin overlying the perforators prevents a direct approach, **subfascial ligation** of the perforators may be performed through a short, posterior midline incision. The incompetent greater or lesser saphenous veins are resected only if patency of the deep system is confirmed. Venous ulcers recur in 30% of patients after surgical therapy, and ulcerations persist for prolonged period in 15% of patients. Adjunctive procedures include: **valvuloplasty, vein transposition,** and **venous valve transplant.**

Alternative procedures: Minimally invasive radiofrequency techniques have been used successfully for ablation of varicose veins

Usual preop diagnosis: Chronic deep venous insufficiency

SUMMARY OF PROCEDURE	
Position	Supine
Incision	**Vein stripping:** longitudinal or oblique groin incision and transverse incision at medial malleolus; transverse incision over posterior lower leg for lesser saphenous vein stripping. **Perforator ligation:** longitudinal incision along medial aspect of tibia to posterior medial malleolus
Special instrumentation	Vein stripper
Antibiotics	If patient has an associated venous ulcer, preop antibiotics should be based on culture results; generally, cefazolin 1 g iv, if culture results are not available.
Surgical time	3 h
EBL	50–250 mL
Postop care	PACU → ward; antiembolism stockings and SCDs
Mortality	Minimal

SUMMARY OF PROCEDURE (cont'd)	
Morbidity [5]	Persistence of nonhealing ulcer: 20–53%
Pain score	3

PATIENT POPULATION CHARACTERISTICS	
Age range	Young adult–elderly (generally older adults, although present in younger patients as well)
Male:Female	1:2
Incidence	6–7 million people in the United States have adverse effects from chronic venous stasis;[5] 500,000 have complications of leg ulceration.
Etiology	Chronic primary varicose veins; defective venous valves; impaired pumping action of muscles in leg; previous iliofemoral thrombophlebitis; obstruction of venous return
Associated conditions	Varicose veins; Hx of DVT/thrombophlebitis

ANESTHETIC CONSIDERATIONS

See Anesthetic Considerations following Varicose Vein Stripping, p. 446.

Suggested Readings

1. Roth SM: Endovenous radiofrequency ablation of superficial and perforator veins. *Surg Clin North Am* 2007; 87(5):1267–84.
2. See Suggested Readings for Venous Surgery—Thrombectomy or Vein Excision, p. 430.

VARICOSE VEIN STRIPPING

SURGICAL CONSIDERATIONS

Description: In patients with primary varicose veins, no definite cause has been identified, although age, female sex, pregnancy, obesity, and positive family Hx are predisposing factors. The causes of secondary varicosity include incompetence or obstruction of the deep veins as a result of previous DVT, tumor, trauma, or congenital or acquired arteriovenous fistulas. Usual indications for operative therapy include aching, swelling, heaviness, cramps, itching, cosmesis, stasis dermatitis, pigmentation, burning, and ulcers. Surgical treatment is contraindicated in: pregnant patients; elderly patients who are considered high risk; and patients with arterial insufficiency of the lower extremities, lymphedema, skin infection, or coagulopathy.

There are two principal approaches: the **stab avulsion technique** and **high ligation and stripping**. With **stab avulsion,** the varicosities are marked preop. Small transverse or longitudinal incisions are made directly over these varicosities, which are dissected from the surrounding subcutaneous tissue (with undermining of the skin) and bluntly removed or avulsed. Firm pressure over the region being operated on will achieve hemostasis. After removal of all marked varicosities, sterile dressings are placed and a compression bandage wrapped around the affected leg. The patient is instructed to keep the leg elevated as much as possible while convalescing at home. The chief advantage of the stab avulsion technique is preservation of the saphenous vein when it is not directly involved with varicosities.

If there is valvular incompetence of the saphenous vein, the treatment of choice is **stripping** (**avulsion**) of the incompetent portion of the greater and lesser saphenous veins, together with avulsion of the superficial varicose veins of the thigh and calf. **High ligation and stripping** refers to the removal of the greater saphenous vein from the level of medial malleolus to the saphenofemoral junction. A small transverse incision is made at the level of the ankle and the saphenous vein is dissected free. A longitudinal or oblique incision at the groin permits isolation of the saphenous vein at the saphenofemoral junction. The greater saphenous vein is ligated proximally and distally. After a **venotomy,** a plastic or metallic vein stripper is passed and the vein is removed or stripped in a distal-to-proximal fashion. Sterile dressings are applied, followed by a compressive dressing.

If all varicose veins are removed and the incompetent segment of the saphenous vein is stripped, 85% of the patients will have good-to-excellent results at late follow-up. These procedures can be performed with regional or GA.

Usual preop diagnosis: Varicose veins; symptoms of venous insufficiency; cosmetic considerations

SUMMARY OF PROCEDURES

	Stab Avulsion Technique	High Ligation and Stripping
Position	Supine	⇐
Incision	Varicosities marked preop; short stab incisions made and veins avulsed with small forceps.	Varicosities marked preop; small transverse incision over saphenous vein proximal to medial malleolus; proximal saphenous vein exposed via groin incisions and stripper passed.
Special instrumentation	None	Vein stripper
Unique considerations	May be facilitated by tourniquet.	⇐
Antibiotics	None	⇐
Surgical time	2–3 h	⇐
Closing considerations	Leg compressed with elastic wrap	⇐
EBL	50–250 mL	50–150 mL
Postop care	PACU → ward; support stockings	⇐ + Elevate foot of bed 10°; short periods of ambulation.
Mortality	Minimal	⇐
Morbidity	Recurrence: < 10% Hematoma: Rare Infection: Rare Lymph fistula: Rare Nerve injury: Rare Postop DVT: Rare Femoral artery injury: Nil	⇐ ⇐ ⇐ ⇐ ⇐ 5% Very rare
Pain score	2	2

PATIENT POPULATION CHARACTERISTICS

Age range	Wide range, young adult–elderly (average = 48 yr)
Male:Female	1:3
Incidence	24,000 in the United States.
Etiology	Primary varicose veins: no definite cause (Predisposing factors include age, female sex, pregnancy, obesity, and positive family Hx.) Secondary varicose veins: incompetence or obstruction of the deep veins from DVT, tumor, trauma, or high venous pressures due to congenital or acquired arteriovenous fistulas
Associated conditions	Older age; pregnancy; obesity; DVT; tumor; trauma

ANESTHETIC CONSIDERATIONS

(Procedures covered: vein stripping and perforator ligation; varicose vein stripping)

PREOPERATIVE

Patients presenting for varicose vein surgery are a generally healthy patient population (ASA I & II). Preop considerations and tests, therefore, should be guided by the H&P.

Hematologic	If regional anesthesia planned, check patient's coagulation status. **Tests:** Plt count; Hct
Laboratory	Tests as indicated from H&P.
Premedication	If necessary, standard premedication (p. B-1).

INTRAOPERATIVE

Anesthetic technique: General, regional, or local anesthesia, ± sedation, are all appropriate anesthetic techniques. Choice depends on factors such as extent of surgery, patient physical status, and patient and surgeon preference.

Regional anesthesia:

Spinal	**Single-shot vs continuous:** Patient in sitting or lateral decubitus position (operative site down) for placement of hyperbaric subarachnoid block. Doses of local anesthetic for T10-T12 level: 0.75% bupivacaine in 8% dextrose (7–10 mg); or 0.5% tetracaine in 5% dextrose (10–12 mg). For continuous spinal (multiorifice catheter), titrate local anesthetic to desired surgical level (T12). Large doses of hyperbaric local anesthetic should be avoided as they may cause postop cauda equina syndrome.
Epidural	Patient in sitting or lateral decubitus position for placement of epidural catheter. After locating the epidural space, administer a test dose (e.g., 3 mL of 1.5% lidocaine with 1:200,000 epinephrine) to elucidate whether the catheter is subarachnoid (rapid onset outer block) or intravascular (↑HR, tinnitis, etc.). Titrate local anesthetic until desired surgical level is obtained (3–5 mL at a time) usually < 15 mL.
Local	Requires gentle surgical technique. Surgical field block, plus ilioinguinal and iliohypogastric nerve blocks using 0.5% bupivacaine with 1:200,000 epinephrine. Usually done by surgeon.

General anesthesia:

Induction	LMA/mask vs ETT: Standard induction (p. B-2). LMA or mask GA may be suitable for many patients.
Maintenance	Standard maintenance (p. B-2)
Emergence	No special considerations
Blood and fluid requirements	Minimal blood loss IV: 18 ga × 1 NS/LR @ 5–8 mL/kg/h
Monitoring	Standard monitors (p. B-1)
Positioning	✓ and pad pressure points. ✓ eyes.

POSTOPERATIVE

Complications	Cauda equina syndrome	The diagnosis of cauda equina syndrome (urinary and fecal incontinence, paresis of lower extremities, perineal hypoesthesias) should be sought in the postop period in patients who have received large doses of intrathecal local anesthetic during continuous spinal techniques. ✓ patients for bowel or bladder dysfunction and perineal sensory deficits. If present, consider a neurology consultation and continue followup of the patient's neurologic dysfunction.
	Urinary retention common with regional anesthesia	Patients with urinary retention may require intermittent catheterization until urinary function resumes.
Pain management	PO analgesics: Acetaminophen and codeine (Tylenol #3 1–2 tab q 4–6 h) Oxycodone and acetaminophen (Percocet 1 tab q 6 h)	Regional anesthesia should provide sufficient analgesia postop.

Suggested Readings

1. Hirsch SA, Dillavou E: Options in the management of varicose veins, 2008. *J Cardiovasc Surg (Torino)* 2008; 49(1):19–26.
2. Mackenzie RK, Paisley A, Allan PL, et al: The effect of long saphenous vein stripping on quality of life. *J Vasc Surg* 2002; 35:1197–1203.
3. Merchant RF, DePalma RG, Kabnick LS: Endovascular obliteration of saphenous reflux: A multicenter study. *J Vasc Surg* 2002; 35:1190–6.
4. Vloka JD, Hadzic A, Mulcare R, et al: Femoral and genitofemoral nerve blocks versus spinal anesthesia for outpatients undergoing long saphenous vein stripping surgery. *Anesth Analg* 1997; 84(4):749–52.

CHAPTER

6.4 Heart/Lung Transplantation

SURGEONS

Hari R. Mallidi, MD
Bruce A. Reitz, MD

ANESTHESIOLOGISTS

Lawrence C. Siegel, MD
Linda E. Foppiano, MD

SURGERY FOR HEART TRANSPLANTATION

SURGICAL CONSIDERATIONS

Description: Although heart transplantation has been practiced since 1967, it has had its greatest expansion since the early 1980s with the introduction of cyclosporine and its more recently introduced formulations (e.g., Gengraf). Currently, there are approximately 150 transplant centers and 2,200 heart transplant procedures performed yearly in the United States. Indications for heart transplantation range from hypoplastic left heart syndrome (HLHS) in the neonate to cardiomyopathy and ischemic heart disease in the adult. Recipients usually have end-stage heart disease manifested by CHF and a prognosis of less than 1-yr survival. Many patients are on inotropic drugs or on some type of additional mechanical assist, such as the use of an intraaortic balloon pump (IABP) or an implanted LV-assist device. Current immunosuppressive protocols consist of a combination of cyclosporine with prednisone and mycophenolate mofetil. Immunosuppression begins either immediately preop or perioperatively and will continue throughout the life of the patient. Induction immunosuppression is commenced in the operating room after protamine administration with methylprednisolone 500 mg iv and daclizumab 1 mg/kg iv. Current 1-yr survival averages 85% in most centers with 3-yr survival of approximately 80%, and a median survival approaching 10 years.

In **adult heart transplantation,** following median sternotomy, the pericardium is opened with care being taken to preserve the phrenic nerve. The aorta and vena cava are cannulated, the aorta is cross-clamped, and caval tapes (tourniquets to prevent VAE) are applied. The aorta and PA are then transected. This is followed by an incision through the atria, and the recipient heart is removed. The donor heart is prepared by opening the left atrium through the pulmonary veins, separating the aorta and PA. The donor heart is attached by a long, continuous suture line around the left atrium, followed by separate anastomoses to the inferior and superior vena cavae. Alternatively, the donor right atrium is anastomosed to the recipient right atrium with a single long continuous suture. Next, the PA and aorta are anastomosed to their respective recipient vessels. Multiple deairing maneuvers are followed by aortic unclamping and rewarming and resuscitation of the heart. NSR is established and CPB D/C'd. Heparin is reversed, hemostasis is secured, and the chest is closed in a routine manner. Following chest closure, these patients will often have implanted defibrillators that will be removed. An incision is made to access the pacemaker pocket, and the device is explanted. After hemostasis is established, the pocket is closed. (See pp. 336+ for discussion of CPB.)

Neonatal heart transplantation differs in that the PA is cannulated if the ductus arteriosus is patent. Reconstruction of the aortic arch in the patient with HLHS requires CPB with deep hypothermia (< 18°C) and circulatory arrest. The heart is then excised and the transverse aortic arch is opened beyond the ductus arteriosus to minimize risk of late coarctation. The donor heart is prepared, with special attention given to trimming the transverse aortic tissue for subsequent reconstruction. The left and right atrium, PA, and aorta are sutured in place. The new ascending aorta and right atrium are cannulated and CPB with rewarming is reinstituted. Chest closure is routine. (See Pediatric Transplantation p 1428.)

Pediatric heart transplantation has become common place in the past 10 years. Patients often have had previous cardiac surgery, and re-entry and excision of the native heart are complicated by the presence of adhesions and graft material from previous attempts at palliative/corrective surgery. Patients are often highly sensitized and may require intraoperative plasmapheresis while on cardiopulmonary bypass. Preparation for cardiopulmonary bypass is often similar to the adult heart transplant patient and the implantation procedure is also similar. However, provisions should be made for prolonged cross-clamp times necessary for implantation in the setting of abnormal systemic-cardiac or pulmonary-cardiac connections. (See Pediatric Transplantation p. 1438.)

Usual preop diagnosis: Cardiomyopathy; CAD with ischemic cardiomyopathy; CHD (e.g., HLHS or anomalous left coronary artery); end-stage valvular heart disease

SUMMARY OF PROCEDURES

	Adult Heart Transplantation	Neonatal/Pediatric Heart Transplantation
Position	Supine	⇐
Incision	Median sternotomy	⇐
Special instrumentation	Ascending aortic, SVC, and IVC cannulae	Ascending aortic and right atrial cannulae

SUMMARY OF PROCEDURES (cont'd)

	Adult Heart Transplantation	Neonatal/Pediatric Heart Transplantation
Unique considerations	Due to complete excision of the heart, use of a PA catheter is usually not feasible.	Deep hypothermia with circulatory arrest
Antibiotics	Cefazolin 1–2 g iv	Cefazolin 25–50 mg/kg iv
Surgical time	Cross-clamp: 45–60 min Surgery: 3–4 h	Circulatory arrest: 45–60 min; Cross-clamp: 80 – 100 minutes Surgery: 4–6 h
Closing considerations	Temporary AV pacing wires are occasionally placed. A PA catheter may be advanced, especially with concerns about residual pulmonary HTN and donor right heart function. An isoproterenol infusion is started intraop to keep HR = 100–110 and help improve right heart function and ↓ PVR. Inhaled NO may be used to further ↓ PVR.	Temporary ventricular pacing wire is usually placed. Temporary transthoracic left atrial line may be placed. Extensive aortic suture line requires avoidance of postop hypertensive episodes.
EBL	500–1,500 mL	50–100 mL
Postop care	Cardiac ICU: 1–2 d of assisted ventilation; 2–3 d stay.	Pediatric ICU × 1–2 d of assisted ventilation; 4–5 d stay, with attention to pulmonary care.
Mortality	< 5%	⇐
Morbidity	Early acute rejection episodes from 10–21 d: 50% Infection, particularly pulmonary: 10% Pulmonary HTN with right heart dysfunction: < 10% Dysrhythmias with nodal rhythms: 5% Bleeding: 2–4% Hyperacute rejection: Rare (< 1%) Intracoronary air emboli	⇐ Respiratory problems: 20% Infection: 10% Pulmonary vasospasm with right heart dysfunction: < 10% Bleeding: 2–4%
Pain score	8–10	8–10

PATIENT POPULATION CHARACTERISTICS

Age range	18–75+ yr (average 50–55 yr)	1 d–2 mo (neonatal); 2 mo–18 yr (pediatric)
Male:Female	7:3	1:1
Incidence	2,200/yr (United States)	Rare
Etiology	Cardiomyopathy (50%); CAD with multiple previous infarcts (48%); other (2%)	No apparent correlation with any specific genetic disorder. Cardiomyopathy (49%); CHD (42%); other (7%)
Associated conditions	CHF	Other congenital anomalies

ANESTHETIC CONSIDERATIONS

PREOPERATIVE

Patients scheduled for heart transplantation are terminally ill, typically with CHF, which is associated with a mortality of > 50% in 2 yr. (Studies have shown that patients with severe CHF have a mortality of 50% in 6 mo.) The progression of cardiovascular disease is usually well documented in these patients. A Hx of recent exacerbation of cardiac dysfunction should be sought and all data should be interpreted in light of interval changes.

Respiratory	The presence of pulmonary HTN and ↑PVR may be disclosed by catheterization. The severity of the abnormality and the responsiveness to specific vasodilators must be determined. **Tests:** Right heart catheterization
Cardiovascular	Indicators to consider include: hemodynamic status; LV EF (mortality is rapid in patients with EF < 10% and is worse for patients with EF of 10–20%, as compared with those with EF > 20%); myocardial structure and morphology, symptoms, and functional capacity; neuroendocrine status; serum sodium; and dysrhythmia. Unfortunately, while these measures show trends with mortality, they are not individually strong enough to predict a particular patient's course. Low maximum O_2 consumption (< 10 mL/kg/min) is associated with poor survival. Normal O_2 consumption is 40 mL/kg/min. In practice, however, this measure is too severe, because many patients awaiting heart transplantation have maximum O_2 consumption of 20 mL/kg/min. Dysrhythmia is a major cause of death; unfortunately electrophysiology studies of these patients may not be helpful because dysrhythmia tends to be noninducible. This phenomenon frustrates efforts to select and test antidysrhythmic drug therapy. The effectiveness of past antidysrhythmic therapy should be reviewed. **Tests:** ECG; cardiac catheterization; ECHO
Hematologic	Patients with dilated cardiomyopathy or previous cardiac surgery are frequently treated with anticoagulants to reduce the risk of thrombus formation, although the efficacy of this therapy has not been studied. Hepatic dysfunction may result from RV failure and may reduce synthetic function. Mild hepatic dysfunction and chronic anticoagulation may contribute to postop bleeding. The anticoagulant effect of warfarin should be reversed with FFP. **Tests:** Hct; PT; PTT; fibrinogen; Plts
Endocrine	Neuroendocrine abnormalities are often present in severe CHF cases. The cardiomyopathy produces low CO → compensatory sympathetic activation and renin-angiotensin activity. The result is excessive vasoconstriction with salt and H_2O retention, which further impair myocardial performance. Markedly worse survival is seen in CHF patients with serum sodium < 130. This may indicate the importance of neuroendocrine pathophysiology or may simply be evidence of the severity of the CHF. It may also simply indicate that patients with more severe CHF are treated with more diuretics. When patients are treated with an angiotensin-converting enzyme inhibitor, such as enalapril, the serum sodium is normalized and survival chances are improved because of the slowing of the progression of CHF, not from alteration in the incidence of sudden death. **Tests:** Electrolytes; Cr
Laboratory	Evidence of renal and hepatic dysfunction should be sought by H&P and lab studies. Hypokalemia is generally not treated in view of the K^+ in the graft.
Premedication	Although anxious, these patients are usually well informed and psychologically prepared to undergo heart transplantation. They respond well to the reassurance of the preop visit, and pharmacologic premedication usually is not necessary. O_2 therapy should commence prior to transport of the patient to the OR. Reassuring the family of a patient who suffers from rapidly progressive cardiac dysfunction also is valuable. The patient may be at increased risk for pulmonary aspiration of gastric contents because of the unscheduled nature of the surgery and use of oral cyclosporine immediately preop. Ranitidine (50 mg) and metoclopramide (10 mg) may be administered iv, most efficiently accomplished in the OR.

INTRAOPERATIVE

Anesthetic technique: GETA. After the patient is placed on the operating table, O_2 and noninvasive monitors are applied. Dyspnea (a complication of the supine position) can be treated by raising the back of the table. As infection is a much-feared complication in the immunosuppressed transplant patient, aseptic technique is extremely important. Aseptic technique is used in inserting and securing all vascular catheters. The anesthesia machine should be equipped with a supply of air to control the FiO_2.

Induction	An arterial line for BP and blood gas monitoring should be inserted, using liberal amounts of local anesthetics before induction. There are rare exceptions to this rule, but the presence of real-time BP monitoring can be critical during induction. If infusion drugs (e.g., dopamine) are necessary before insertion of the CVP catheter, they can be infused temporarily through a separate peripheral iv. In patients who have a ↓ EF, it is often helpful to infuse dopamine 3–10 mcg/kg/min during induction to avoid ↓ HR and ↓ CO. Anesthesia is not induced until the team harvesting the graft reports that the donor heart appears to be normal. The patient is denitrogenated (FiO_2 = 1.0), and cricoid pressure is applied just before induction. Induction agents include fentanyl (5–10 mcg/kg) or sufentanil (1–4 mcg/kg). Etomidate (0.1–0.2 mg/kg) is useful in permitting rapid control of the airway and for assuring lack of patient awareness. Midazolam also may be used. Vecuronium (0.15 mg/kg), pancuronium (0.1 mg/kg), or a combination of these two agents should be administered immediately to permit airway control. Care must be taken to avoid bradycardia, which often results in low CO in these patients. Immediate control of the airway is crucial, as hypercarbia and hypoxia must be avoided. The patient can be expected to have a low CO, resulting in a delayed induction of anesthesia, which must be anticipated to avoid anesthetic overdosage. Low CO and a volume-contracted condition make the patient initially very sensitive to anesthetics. Hypotension should be treated promptly with inotropes (bolus and/or infusion). High preload is often necessary, and iv fluid may be administered cautiously to compensate for the vasodilating effect of anesthetic-mediated sympatholysis. Fluid boluses may be poorly tolerated in patients with diminished contractility. Patient should be ventilated by mask and cricoid pressure released only after the airway has been secured with a cuffed ETT. The usual aids for managing the unexpectedly difficult airway should be readily available. Antibiotics are administered, and additional monitors (urinary catheter with thermistor, nasopharyngeal temperature probe, TEE, or esophageal stethoscope) are set up. If there is a delay in the anticipated arrival of the graft, the recipient should be covered and kept warm and skin prep should be delayed. Additional narcotics should be administered only in immediate anticipation of the commencement of surgery.
Maintenance	Typical cumulative anesthetic doses for the entire intraop course are: fentanyl 20–50 mcg/kg or sufentanil 10–15 mcg/kg; midazolam 0.2 mg/kg; vecuronium 0.3 mg/kg or pancuronium 0.2 mg/kg; scopolamine 0.07 mg/kg.
Termination of CPB	Junctional rhythm is common in the denervated transplanted heart. Isoproterenol 10–75 ng/kg/min or epinephrine 50–105 ng/kg/min may be used to achieve a HR of 100–120 bpm. Isoproterenol is also useful in providing inotropic support and pulmonary vasodilation (see below). Atropine and neostigmine do not affect HR. HTN does not produce reflex bradycardia. The graft atrium produces normally conducted P-waves. The graft-conductive tissue contains adrenergic receptors and responds normally to norepinephrine, epinephrine, and isoproterenol. Inotropic support with dopamine (2–10 mcg/kg/min), isoproterenol (10–150 ng/kg/min), and epinephrine (20–100 ng/kg/min) may be necessary, especially if pulmonary HTN promotes RV failure. Inhaled NO (20–40ppm) may provide selective pulmonary vasodilation. A PA catheter may be helpful in guiding the use of inotropes and vasodilators. After termination of CPB, TEE may be of particular value in assessing RV dysfunction, estimating PA pressures and guiding appropriate fluid therapy, pharmacologic support, and mechanical support as necessary. RV failure may be produced by the presence of air in the RCA. Visual inspection may demonstrate this problem, and one should wait for the passage of the air and the resolution of ischemia before terminating CPB. SNP (0.2–2.0 mcg/kg/min) is used for afterload reduction. NO, prostaglandin E_1 (PGE_1) (20–100 ng/kg/min), and NTG (0.2–2.0 mcg/kg/min) may be used for pulmonary vasodilation, especially if a preop catheterization study demonstrates responsiveness of the pulmonary circulation. Isoproterenol infusion (10–100 ng/kg/min) may provide appropriate pulmonary vasodilation, chronotropy, and inotropy. IV fluid and vasodilators must be given with particular care, as the flow produced by the denervated heart is quite sensitive to preload.

Postbypass hemorrhage	Postbypass bleeding is a common problem brought on by the preop use of anticoagulants, the depressed synthetic function of the liver in chronic heart failure, and the trauma of CPB. Following administration of protamine, infusion of Plts, FFP, and RBCs may be necessary. Cryoprecipitate is needed occasionally, especially for patients with previous chest surgery. The use of aprotinin, epsilon amino caproic acid (EACA), or tranexamic acid may be appropriate in some cases.	
Immunosuppression	Methylprednisolone 500 mg is given after bypass is terminated. Daclizumab 1 mg/kg is also administered after administration of protamine, and hemostasis has been secured.	
Diuresis	There may be little urine production, especially if patient received high-dose diuretics preop. Cyclosporine may exacerbate renal dysfunction. Mannitol and furosemide may be needed to induce diuresis.	
Transport	A Jackson-Rees system is used in transporting the patient to the ICU.	
Blood and fluid requirements	Possible severe bleeding IV: 14–16 ga × 1–2 NS/LR @ 4–6 mL/kg/h	Bleeding is often a problem after termination of CPB. A second iv catheter is inserted in patients with previous chest surgery.
Monitoring	Standard monitors (see p. B-1). Arterial line CVP/PA catheter UO	Although it may be helpful to have a triple-lumen CVP line before induction for preload monitoring and infusion of potent infusion drugs, it is not essential. This line is usually inserted after the patient is intubated to avoid patient dyspnea and discomfort. A PA catheter is usually not inserted before bypass since it must be removed during surgery. An 8.5-Fr introducer is used in anticipation that a PA catheter may be necessary to manage right heart failure following the transplantation. In some institutions (not Stanford), the left IJ vein is the preferred site of cannulation, which leaves the right IJ unscarred for repeated postop endomyocardial biopsy of the transplanted heart.
	TEE	TEE is used to optimize fluid therapy, inotropic agents, vasodilators, and chronotropic agents.
Positioning	✓ and pad pressure points. ✓ eyes. Arms padded at sides Chest roll	

POSTOPERATIVE

Complications	RV dysfunction	RV failure may occur in patients with pulmonary HTN and high RV afterload (see pulmonary HTN, below).
	Pulmonary HTN	Maneuvers which exacerbate pulmonary HTN should be avoided. These include hypoxia, hypercarbia, acidosis, and extremes of lung volume. Inhaled NO can be used to treat pulmonary HTN (20–40 ppm inspired concentration); however, it must be used with caution in patients with severe heart failure. Efforts to treat pulmonary HTN with vasodilator therapy may be complicated by impaired V/Q matching with hypoxemia and by systemic ↓ BP producing poor coronary perfusion and RV ischemia. Inotropic support of the RV may be

Complications (cont'd)		necessary. Isoproterenol infusion (10–150 ng/kg/min) is attractive because it combines inotropy, pulmonary vasodilation, and chronotropy.
	Oliguria Drug side effects: • Cyclosporine: HTN, nephrotoxicity, hepatotoxicity • Corticosteroids: glucose intolerance, HTN, obesity, hyperlipidemia, aseptic necrosis of hip, bowel perforation, infection	Preexisting impairment may → chronic ↓ UO state. Other renal problems may be related to cyclosporine toxicity, diuretic toxicity, or CPB. Rx by optimizing hemodynamics. Consider reduction or elimination of nephrotoxins and continuing use of diuretics. Cyclosporine nephrotoxicity occurs in most patients. A functional toxicity with ↓ GFR occurs at low dose and is reversible. Tubular toxicity with morphologic changes occurs at high doses and is generally clinically unimportant and reversible. The most serious damage is vascular interstitial toxicity, which occurs over months at high doses and is not reversible.
Pain management	PCA (see p. C-3) after weaning from mechanical ventilation.	
Tests	Cr Hct	

Suggested Readings

1. Ashary N, Kaye AD, Hegazi AR, et al: Anesthetic considerations in the patient with a heart transplant. *Heart Dis* 2002 4(3):191–8.
2. Baumgartner WA, Reitz BA, Achuff SA, eds: *Heart and Heart-Lung Transplantation.* WB Saunders, Philadelphia: 1990.
3. Bennett LE, Keck BM, Hertz MI, et al: Worldwide thoracic organ transplantation: a report from the UNOS/ISHLT International Registry for Thoracic Organ Transplantation. *Clin Transpl* 2001; 25–40.
4. Boucek RJ, Boucek MM: Pediatric heart transplantation. *Curr Opin Pediatr* 2002; 14:611–19.
5. Cannon DS, Rider AK, Stinson EB, et al: Electrophysiologic studies in the denervated transplanted human heart. II. Response to norepinephrine, isoproterenol and propranolol. *Am J Cardiol* 1975; 36(7):859–66.
6. Cirella VN, Pantuck CB, Lee YJ, et al: Effects of cyclosporine on anesthetic action. *Anesth Analg* 1987; 66(8):703–6.
7. DiNardo JA, Zavara DA: Anesthesia for heart, heart-lung and lung transplantation. In *Anesthesia for Cardiac Surgery*, 3rd edition. Blackwell Science, Boston: 2008; 252–88.
8. Keogh AM, Freund J, Baron DW, et al: Timing of cardiac transplantation in idiopathic dilated cardiomyopathy. *Am J Cardiol* 1988; 61(6):418–22.
9. Kieler-Jensen N, Ricksten SE, Stenqvist O, et al: Inhaled nitric oxide in the elevated pulmonary vascular resistance. *J Heart Lung Transplant* 1994; 13:366–75.
10. Kirklin JK, McGiffin DC, Pinderski LJ, et al: Selection of patients and techniques of heart transplantation. *Surg Clin North Am* 2004; 84(1):257–87.
11. Loh E, Stamler JS, Hare JM, et al: Cardiovascular effects of inhaled nitric oxide in patients with left ventricular dysfunction. *Circulation* 1994; 90:2780–85.
12. Ouseph R, Stoddard MF, Lederer ED: Patent foramen ovale presenting as refractory hypoxemia after heart transplantation. *J Am Soc Echocardiogr* 1997; 10:973–6.
13. Propst J, Siegel L, Feeley T: Aprotinin reduces transfusions during repeat sternotomy for heart transplantation. *Anesthesia Analgesia* 1993; 76(25):5337.
14. Quinlan JJ, et al: Anesthesia for heart, lung, and heart-lung transplantation. In *Kaplan's Cardiac Anesthesia* 5th edition. Kaplan JA, et al., eds. Elsevier Saunders: 2007; 845–66.
15. Schulte-Sasse Y, Hess W, Tarnow J: Pulmonary vascular response to nitrous oxide in patients with normal and high pulmonary vascular resistance. *Anesthesiology* 1982; 57(1):9–13.
16. Shanewise J: Cardiac transplantation. *Anesthesiol Clin North Am* 2004; 22(4):753–65.
17. Thomas Z, et al: Anesthetic management of cardiac transplantation. In: *A Practical Approach to Cardiac Anesthesia*, 4th edition..Hensley Jr FA, et al., eds. Lippincott Williams & Wilkins; 2008, 439–63.
18. Waterman PM, Bjerke R: Rapid-sequence induction technique in patients with severe ventricular dysfunction. *J Cardiothorac Anesth* 1988; 2:602–6.

SURGERY FOR LUNG AND HEART/LUNG TRANSPLANTATION

SURGICAL CONSIDERATIONS

Description: With the availability of cyclosporine, the ability to successfully transplant the heart and both lungs was proven in monkeys and then successfully applied in a patient in March, 1981. Subsequently, single-lung transplantation was successfully performed in 1984 and an en bloc, double-lung transplant in 1986. Clinical lung transplantation of these various types has increased markedly in the last few years, and, currently, approximately 600 single-lung transplants, 800 bilateral lung transplants, and 30 heart/lung transplants are performed in the United States each year.

Current indications for heart/lung transplantation are primarily those of combined heart and lung disease, including Eisenmenger's syndrome due to a congenital heart defect with irreversible pulmonary HTN. Certain types of diffuse lung disease, such as primary pulmonary HTN with significant right heart failure, are also treated in some centers by heart/lung transplantation. Recipients for single-lung transplant usually have end-stage pulmonary disease without significant sepsis. This includes patients with interstitial fibrosis, emphysema, and lymphangioleiomyomatosis. Some patients with pulmonary vascular disease, such as primary pulmonary HTN or pulmonary HTN associated with an ASD, have undergone single-lung transplantation with or without cardiac repair. Bilateral lung transplantation is now performed usually as a sequential single-lung transplant with the major indications being septic lung disease, such as cystic fibrosis, chronic bronchiectasis, severe bullous emphysema, or pulmonary vascular disease with or without cardiac repair. Current immunosuppressive protocols consist of a combination of tacrolimus with prednisone and myophenolate mofetil, with or without early induction therapy, using a cytolytic agent, such as antithymocyte globulin. Immunosuppression may begin preop and continue throughout the life of the patient. Current 1-yr survival rates average 70% for heart/lung transplants and 80% for lung transplants.

Cardiovascular Surgery

Heart/lung transplants usually are performed through a median sternotomy, although occasionally bilateral, transsternal thoracotomy has been used. **Single-lung transplants** (usually left side) and **bilateral sequential lung transplants** use a lateral thoracotomy or transsternal bilateral thoracotomy. Single- and double-lung transplants are greatly facilitated with OLV, which is essential for these procedures. If this type of ventilation is not feasible, a bronchial-blocker must be inserted through the operative field during pneumonectomy and reimplantation. CPB is routinely used for heart/lung transplantation, and is used for either single- or bilateral-lung transplantation, depending on the stability of the patient during OLV and/or clamping of the PA. Patients with severe pulmonary HTN undergoing single- or double-lung transplantation will almost always require CPB to reduce PA pressure during clamping. For combined transplants, the recipient heart is removed as for standard heart transplantation (see Surgery for Heart Transplantation, p. 450). A portion of the PA near the ligamentum arteriosum, however, is left intact in order to preserve the recurrent laryngeal nerve. Next, each recipient lung is excised and the trachea is transected above the carina. For single-lung transplant, usually the left recipient lung is excised, leaving a bronchial stump and vascular pedicles for the PA and veins (left atrium). For bilateral-lung transplants, both recipient lungs are removed, the trachea transected just above the carina, and the main PA and left atrium prepared for subsequent anastomosis.

Implantation of the grafts involves a tracheal anastomosis, aortic and separate SVC and IVC anastomoses for heart/lung transplants, and a bronchial anastomosis with PA and pulmonary venous anastomosis for single-lung transplantation. **Bilateral sequential lung transplants** are performed as if they were single-lung transplants. CPB requires heparinization and protamine reversal. Prior to closure, extensive exploration for potential bleeding sites within the posterior mediastinum is carried out with placement of right and left pleural and mediastinal drainage. Thoracotomies are closed in standard fashion with routine chest tube drainage.

Usual preop diagnosis: End-stage heart and lung disease, such as Eisenmenger's syndrome; cystic fibrosis; primary pulmonary HTN; emphysema; bronchiectasis; lymphangioleiomyomatosis; interstitial pulmonary fibrosis; sarcoidosis; other unusual forms of lung disease

SUMMARY OF PROCEDURES

	Heart/lung Transplantation	Single-Lung Transplantation	Bilateral-Lung Transplantation
Position	Supine	Lateral thoracotomy	Supine
Incision	Median sternotomy, usual; bilateral anterior thoracotomy, occasionally	Posterolateral thoracotomy	Transsternal bilateral thoracotomy
Special instrumentation	Ascending aortic, SVC, and IVC cannulae	Occasional need for BB to be inserted through the operative field.	± Aortic, SVC, and IVC cannulation; occasional need for BB.
Unique considerations	CPB. If recipient has had previous thoracotomies, mediastinal collaterals may cause troublesome bleeding. Some patients with cystic fibrosis have severe bilateral scarring, requiring extensive dissection to remove the recipient lung.	± CPB. Patient may become severely hypoxic or hypercarbic during OLV, requiring CPB. During right thoracotomy, cannulation can be performed through the thorax, but left thoracotomy may require femoral artery and vein cannulation.	CPB. Thoracotomy usually is performed on left side first, with implantation of lung on this side, followed by completion of right side thoracotomy and right-lung transplantation. If patient becomes unstable, cannulation in the thorax is usually possible to facilitate transplantation.
Antibiotics	Continue specific antibiotic regime. Coverage for pseudomonas is suggested in patients with cystic fibrosis.	Cefazolin 2 g iv then 1g q 4 h	⇐ With appropriate coverage for pseudomonas in patients with cystic fibrosis.
Surgical time	4–5 h	2–3 h	5–6 h
Closing considerations	Temporary pacing wire applied and isoproterenol infusion is usually started intraop to keep HR between 100–110, as with a cardiac transplant.	Ventilation with as low an FiO_2 as possible to maintain a PO_2 > 90. Minimize iv fluids.	⇐
EBL	500–2,000 mL	< 500 mL (more if CPB is used)	500–2,000 mL
Postop care	Cardiac ICU: 3–7 d; 1–2 d assisted ventilation	⇐	⇐
Mortality	10–15%	10%	10–15%
Morbidity	Early acute rejection episodes from 10–21 d: 75%	—	—
	Infection, particularly pulmonary: 30–40%	⇐	⇐
	Pulmonary interstitial edema: 20%	Bleeding: 2–4%	⇐
		Bronchial leak or stenosis: 2–4%	⇐
	Return for bleeding: 4–6%		
	Hyperacute rejection: Rare		
Pain score	8–10	8–10	8–10

PATIENT POPULATION CHARACTERISTICS

	Heart/lung Transplantation	Single-Lung Transplantation	Bilateral-Lung Transplantation
Age range	3 mo–55 yr (average 30–40 yr)	1–65 yr	⇐
Male:Female	1:1	⇐	⇐
Incidence	~30/yr (United States) 200/yr (worldwide)	600/yr (United States) 1,000/yr (worldwide)	800/yr (United States) 1,200/yr (worldwide)
Etiology	Eisenmenger's syndrome; CHD; cystic fibrosis; pulmonary HTN; other lung diseases	Acquired chronic lung disease; pulmonary HTN	Cystic fibrosis; interstitial fibrosis; emphysema
Associated conditions	Severe cyanosis and polycythemia; diabetes in patients with cystic fibrosis; sinus infections in patients with cystic fibrosis	Right heart dysfunction; pulmonary valve insufficiency and tricuspid valve insufficiency	Diabetes mellitus; sinus infections in patients with cystic fibrosis

ANESTHETIC CONSIDERATIONS FOR HEART/LUNG TRANSPLANTATION

PREOPERATIVE

Patients scheduled for heart/lung transplantation are terminally ill, although they may still be able to maintain limited activity. Indications include primary pulmonary HTN, Eisenmenger's syndrome, cystic fibrosis, and combined cardiac and pulmonary disease. The standard preanesthetic evaluation is supplemented with considerations particular to these patients. The progression of disease is usually well documented.

Respiratory	Patients with severe pulmonary HTN (80/50 mmHg) have enlarged PAs. Vocal cord dysfunction (Sx: hoarseness, inability to phonate "e") may occur when the left recurrent laryngeal nerve is stretched by an enlarged PA, making these patients at increased risk for pulmonary aspiration. Appropriate precautions to avoid aspiration should be taken (see Induction, below). **Tests:** ABG; cardiac catheterization
Cardiovascular	Hx of recent exacerbation of symptoms should be sought and cardiac catheterization data interpreted in light of interval changes. The severity of pulmonary HTN and the responsiveness to specific vasodilators during catheterization should be reviewed. **Tests:** ECG; cardiac catheterization; ECHO
Neurological	R → L intracardiac shunting may be present in patients with pulmonary HTN, and Hx of embolic episodes should be sought. Extra care should be used to avoid injection of even small quantities of intravenous air.
Hematologic	The medication schedule should be verified with particular attention to the recent use of anticoagulants. **Tests:** Hct; PTT; PT (special tubes required if severe polycythemia present 2° ↓ plasma volume); Plt count; fibrinogen
Laboratory	Evidence of renal and hepatic dysfunction should be sought by H&P and lab studies. Hypokalemia is generally not treated because the heart/lung graft is preserved with K^+ and implantation will reverse hypokalemia.
Premedication	Although anxious, these patients are usually well informed and psychologically prepared. They respond well to the reassurance of the preop visit, and pharmacologic premedication usually is not necessary. O_2 therapy should commence prior to transport of patient to the

Premedication (cont'd)	OR. Patient may be at increased risk for pulmonary aspiration of gastric contents because of the unscheduled nature of the surgery, the use of oral cyclosporine immediately preop and the presence of recurrent laryngeal nerve damage. Ranitidine (50 mg) and metoclopramide (10–20 mg) may be administered iv preop.

INTRAOPERATIVE

Anesthetic technique: GETA. Infection is a much feared complication in the immunosuppressed transplant patient; thus, aseptic technique is important. Aseptic technique is used in inserting and securing all vascular catheters. The anesthesia machine should be equipped with a supply of air to permit control of the FiO_2; and anesthesia is not induced until the team harvesting the graft reports that it appears to be normal to direct inspection.

Induction	In the OR, the patient should be placed on the operating table and O_2 and noninvasive monitors applied. An arterial line for BP and blood gas monitoring should be inserted, using liberal amounts of local anesthetics before induction. There are rare exceptions to this rule, but the presence of real-time BP monitoring can be critical during induction. A patient who is dyspneic in the supine position may be treated by raising the back of the table. Cricoid pressure must be used when the patient is at risk for aspiration of gastric contents. A major goal of anesthetic induction is the avoidance of further increases in PVR by guarding against respiratory acidosis, hypoxia, N_2O, light anesthesia, and extremes of lung volume. When hemodynamically tolerated, fentanyl (5–10 mcg/kg) is useful in blunting the pulmonary vascular response to intubation. Etomidate (0.1–0.2 mg/kg) may be used when hypotension limits administration of narcotics. Vecuronium (0.15 mg/kg), pancuronium (0.1 mg/kg), or a combination of the two, should be administered early to permit rapid airway control. Midazolam and scopolamine produce amnesia. N_2O is not used because it exacerbates pulmonary HTN, reduces FiO_2, and expands intravascular air bubbles. Patient should be ventilated by mask, and cricoid pressure released only after the airway has been secured with a cuffed ETT. Excessive pressure of the cuff on the trachea should be avoided. An ETT of internal diameter of 8.0 mm will facilitate FOB postop.
Maintenance	Typical total anesthetic doses for the *entire* intraop course are: fentanyl 10–50 mcg/kg or sufentanil 10–15 mcg/kg; midazolam 0.2 mg/kg; vecuronium 0.3 mg/kg or pancuronium 0.2 mg/kg; scopolamine 0.07 mg/kg.
Termination of CPB	After tracheal anastomosis is complete, lungs are ventilated with $FiO_2 = 0.21$ at 5 breaths/min and a TV of 6 mL/kg. When bladder temperature reaches 36°C, ventilation is increased to 10 breaths/min and TV of 12 mL/kg. TV should be adjusted to eliminate atelectasis and to achieve a peak inflation pressure of 25–30 cmH_2O with the chest open. The FiO_2 is increased to 0.4 and may be altered in response to pulse oximetry and blood gas data. FiO_2 is limited in the hope of curtailing free radical injury. PEEP may be used to enhance oxygenation and is adjusted with an appreciation of the effect of lung volume on PVR. Hypoxemia must be avoided. Hyperkalemia may be treated with Ca^{++} (e.g., 3–5 mL 10% CaCl q 30 min), glucose (50 g), insulin (10 U), and diuresis. Junctional rhythm is common in the denervated transplanted heart. Epinephrine (50–150 ng/kg/min) or isoproterenol (10–75 ng/kg/min) is used to achieve a HR of 100–120. When sinus rhythm is achieved, it is common to see two P-waves if a biatrial anastomosis has been used. The residual atrial tissue produces nonconducting P-waves. Responses mediated by vagal tone will be seen in the rate of the original atrial tissue and have no clinical importance beyond the ease with which the ECG is interpreted. In the denervated heart, atropine and neostigmine will not affect HR, and HTN will not produce reflex bradycardia. The graft atrium produces normally conducted P-waves. The transplanted heart contains adrenergic receptors and responds normally to norepinephrine, epinephrine, and isoproterenol. The CO of the denervated heart is quite sensitive to preload; thus, iv fluid and vasodilators must be given with particular care. SNP is used for afterload reduction. TEE may be of

Termination of CPB (cont'd)	particular value in assessing RV dysfunction and guiding appropriate fluid therapy, pharmacologic support, and mechanical support as necessary. NO, PGE_1 (20–100 ng/kg/min), isoproterenol, and NTG (0.2–2.0 mcg/kg/min) also may be used for pulmonary vasodilation. Inotropic support with dopamine (2–10 mcg/kg/min), isoproterenol, and epinephrine (20–100 ng/kg/min) may be necessary, especially if pulmonary HTN and RV failure occur.	
Immunosuppression	Methylprednisolone 500 mg iv is given after bypass is terminated.	
Diuresis	There may be little urine production, especially if patient received high-dose diuretics preop. Cyclosporine may exacerbate renal dysfunction. Mannitol and furosemide may be needed to induce diuresis.	
Transport	A sterile, disposable Jackson-Rees system is used in transporting the patient to the ICU.	
Blood and fluid requirements	Anticipate large blood loss. IV: 14–16 ga × 2	Bleeding is often a major problem after termination of CPB. Patients with intracardiac defects are at increased risk for cerebral embolic events. Care must be taken to remove all air bubbles from intravascular lines.
Control of blood loss	Postbypass bleeding is a common problem.	Postbypass bleeding is exacerbated by preop use of anticoagulants, depressed synthetic liver function, trauma of CPB, and/or previous chest therapy.
	Coagulation therapy necessary.	Coagulation therapy may include: protamine (30 mg/kg); Plts; FFP; RBCs; EACA (300 mg/kg); DDAVP; aprotinin (500,000 U/h after loading dose).
	Possible severe bleeding	Severe bleeding prompts further therapy: cryoprecipitate, factor IX concentrate, Feiba VH (factor 8 inhibitor bypassing activity), and/or recombinant factor 7a.
Monitoring	Standard monitors (see p. B-1). Arterial line CVP/PA catheter UO	Typically, invasive monitors are placed prior to induction; however, if patient is very dyspneic in the supine position, it may be advantageous to insert the CVP catheter following anesthetic induction. An introducer permits the rapid insertion of a PA catheter when necessary. In some centers (not Stanford) the left IJ vein is the preferred site of cannulation, leaving the right IJ unscarred for repeated endomyocardial biopsies of the transplanted heart.
	TEE	TEE is used to optimize volume status (LV + RV size), inotropic agents (LV + RV contractility), vasodilators, and chronotropic agents.

POSTOPERATIVE

Complications	Oliguria	Diuresis may be induced with mannitol and furosemide.
	Pulmonary edema	Given the lack of lymphatic drainage in the transplanted lung, pulmonary edema may occur. Diuresis and restriction of iv fluid may be required.
	RV dysfunction	RV failure may occur in patients with pulmonary HTN and high RV afterload (see pulmonary HTN Rx, below).

Cardiovascular Surgery

Complications (cont'd)	Pulmonary HTN	Maneuvers which exacerbate pulmonary HTN should be avoided. These include hypoxia, hypercarbia, acidosis, and extremes of lung volume. NO can be used to treat pulmonary HTN (0.1–100 parts per million inspired concentration); however, it must be used with caution in patients with severe heart failure. Efforts to treat pulmonary HTN with vasodilator therapy may be complicated by impaired V/Q matching with hypoxemia and by systemic hypotension, producing poor right coronary perfusion and RV ischemia. Inotropic support of the RV may be necessary. Isoproterenol is attractive because it combines inotropy, pulmonary vasodilation, and chronotropy.
	Rejection Infection	Monitor rejection Sx with transvenous endomyocardial biopsy and transbronchial biopsy.
	Drug side effects: • Cyclosporine: HTN, nephrotoxicity, hepatotoxicity • Corticosteroids: glucose intolerance, HTN, obesity, hyperlipidemia, aseptic necrosis of hip, bowel perforation, infection • Azathioprine: anemia, thrombocytopenia, leukopenia, hepatotoxicity	Cyclosporine nephrotoxicity occurs in most patients. A functional toxicity with reduced GFR occurs at low dose and is reversible. Tubular toxicity with morphologic changes occurs at high doses and generally is clinically unimportant and reversible. The most serious damage is vascular interstitial toxicity, which occurs over months at high doses and is not reversible.
Pain management	PCA (see p. C-3).	

Cardiovascular Surgery

Suggested Readings

1. Baumgartner WA, Reitz BA, Achuff SA, eds: *Heart and Heart-Lung Transplantation.* WB Saunders, Philadelphia: 1990.
2. Cirella VN, Pantuck CB, Lee YJ, et al: Effects of cyclosporine on anesthetic action. *Anesth Analg* 1987; 66(8):703–6.
3. DiNardo JA, Zavara DA: Anesthesia for heart, heart-lung and lung transplantation. In *Anesthesia for Cardiac Surgery*, 3rd ed. Blackwell Science, Boston: 2008; 252–88.
4. Peterson KL, DeCampli WM, Feeley TW, et al: Blood loss and transfusion requirements in cystic fibrosis patients undergoing heart-lung or lung transplantation. *J Cardiothorac Vast Anesth* 1995; 9:59–62.
5. Propst JW, Siegel LC, Feeley TW: Effect of aprotinin on transfusion requirements during repeat sternotomy for cardiac transplantation surgery. *Transplant Proc* 1994; 26:3719–21.
6. Pucci A, Forbes RD, Berry GJ, et al: Accelerated post-transplant coronary arteriosclerosis in combined heart-lung transplantation. *Transplant Proc* 1991; 23(1P+2):1228–9.
7. Quinlan JJ, et al: Anesthesia for heart, lung, and heart-lung transplantation. In *Kaplan's Cardiac Anesthesia,* 5th edition. Kaplan JA, et al (eds). Elsevier Saunders: 2007.
8. Reitz BA, Wallwork JL, Hunt SA, et al: Heart-lung transplantation: successful therapy for patients with pulmonary vascular disease. *N Engl J Med* 1982; 306(10):557–64.
9. Shaw JH, Kirk AJ, Conacher ID: Anesthesia for patients with transplanted hearts and lungs undergoing non-cardiac surgery. *Br J Anesth* 1991; 67:772–8.
10. Waddell TK, Bennett L, Kennedy R, et al: Heart-lung or lung transplantation for Eisenmenger syndrome. *J Heart Lung Transplant* 2002; 21:731–7.
11. Whyte RI, Robbins RC, Altinger J, et al: Heart-lung transplantation for primary pulmonary hypertension. *Ann Thorac Surg* 1997; 67:937–41.

ANESTHETIC CONSIDERATIONS FOR LUNG TRANSPLANTATION

PREOPERATIVE

The patient presenting for lung transplantation typically has end-stage pulmonary fibrosis or emphysema, although other diseases, such as pulmonary HTN, also may be treated by single-lung transplantation. Double-lung transplantation can be used to treat cystic fibrosis and bronchiectasis. The progression of the disease is usually well documented; however, Hx of recent exacerbation of symptoms should be sought.

Respiratory	Assess the patient's ability to undergo OLV by review of the V/Q scan. If little perfusion of the nonoperative lung is present, anticipate the need for CPB. The extent of the restrictive lung disease and diffusion abnormality must be assessed preop. For example, room-air PaO_2 < 45 mmHg predicts the need for CPB. **Tests:** PFT; V/Q scan; ABG
Airway	Patients with severe pulmonary HTN (80/50 mmHg) have enlarged pulmonary arteries. Vocal cord dysfunction (Sx: hoarseness, inability to phonate "e") may occur when the left recurrent laryngeal nerve is stretched by an enlarged PA, making these patients at increased risk for pulmonary aspiration; therefore, appropriate precautions to avoid aspiration should be taken (see Induction, below).
Cardiovascular	Evidence of RV dysfunction with tricuspid regurgitation should be sought by physical exam, ECHO, and cardiac catheterization. RV ejection fraction (EF) may be estimated with radionuclide ventriculography (normal EF = > 50%). Pulmonary HTN is considered to be severe and may produce RV failure when pressure is > 2/3 of systemic arterial pressure. Note response to specific vasodilators recorded during catheterization. **Tests:** Preview cardiac catheterization data; ECG; mean PAP > 40 mmHg and PVR > 5 mmHg/min/L may predict the need for partial CPB.
Neurological	R→L intracardiac shunting may be present in patients with pulmonary HTN, and Hx of embolic episodes should be sought. Extra care should be used to avoid injection of even small quantities of intravenous air.
Musculoskeletal	Chronic cachexia precludes the procedure.
Hematologic	Polycythemia 2° chronic hypoxemia is common. Autologous blood is collected as CPB is initiated. **Tests:** Hct; coagulation studies require special blood tubes to correct for low plasma volume in patients with severe polycythemia.
Laboratory	Other tests as indicated from H&P.
Premedication	Patients awaiting lung transplantation are generally well informed about the planned perioperative course. These patients respond well to the reassurance of the preop visit, and pharmacologic premedication usually is not necessary. O_2 therapy, with the usual home O_2 regimen, should commence prior to transport to the OR. Patient may be at ↑ risk for pulmonary aspiration of gastric contents because of the unscheduled nature of the surgery, the use of oral cyclosporin immediately before surgery, and the presence of recurrent laryngeal nerve damage. Ranitidine (50 mg) and metoclopramide (10–20 mg) may be administered iv before surgery.

INTRAOPERATIVE

Anesthetic technique: GETA. Typically, OLV through a DLT is required for single-lung transplants. Consider ETT/BB in cystic fibrosis patients with tenacious sputum. Infection is a much feared complication in the immunosuppressed transplant patient; thus, the aseptic technique is important. Aseptic technique is used in inserting and securing all vascular catheters.

Induction	An arterial line for BP and blood gas monitoring should be inserted, using liberal amounts of local anesthetics before induction. There are rare exceptions to this rule, but the presence of real-time BP monitoring can be critical during induction. Typically, fentanyl 5–10 mcg/kg (incremental doses) after invasive monitors placed, ± etomidate 0.1–0.2 mg/kg when rapid control of the airway is desirable; vecuronium 0.15 mg/kg or pancuronium 0.1 mg/kg (avoid succinylcholine 2° ↓ HR); midazolam 0.1 mg/kg or scopolamine 0.005 mg/kg for amnesia. Cricoid pressure must be used when the patient is at risk for aspiration

Induction (cont'd)	because of the unscheduled nature of the surgery, use of preop oral cyclosporin, and possible vocal cord dysfunction associated with stretch injury of the recurrent laryngeal nerve. Avoid further increases in PVR by guarding against hypoxemia, acidosis, hypercarbia, light anesthesia, and extremes of lung volume.	
Maintenance	Typically, narcotic/O_2/air/± isoflurane (in absence of hypoxemia and right heart failure). Typical total anesthetic doses for the entire intraop course: fentanyl 20–50 mcg/kg or sufentanil 10–15 mcg/kg, midazolam 0.2 mg/kg, vecuronium 0.3 mg/kg, or pancuronium 0.2 mg/kg, scopolamine 0.07 mg/kg.	
Emergence	Before closure of the chest, lungs are inflated to 35 cmH_2O to reinflate atelectatic areas and check adequacy of bronchial closure. At the conclusion of surgery, both lumens of the DLT should be suctioned and the tube replaced with a single-lumen 8.0 mm ETT. The patient is transported to the ICU intubated and ventilated.	
Blood and fluid requirements	IV: 14 or 16 ga × 1–2 NS/LR @ 4 mL/kg/h	Patients with intracardiac defects are at increased risk for cerebral embolic events; take care to remove all air bubbles from intravascular lines.
Monitoring	Standard monitors (see p. B-1). Arterial line PA catheter Urinary catheter with thermistor	ECG leads should be covered with tape to insure that electrical contact is not degraded by prep solution or blood. Mixed venous oximetry may be desirable during OLV, and with partial CPB. Be careful of air embolization during catheter insertion. Patients who are profoundly dyspneic (→ high negative intrathoracic pressure) are at high risk for VAE; consider inserting the catheter after GA and IPPV have been instituted. Oxygenation must be watched closely. Blood gases are sampled at 10-min intervals.
	TEE	RV EF measurement may be useful for evaluating RV function (normal EF = 0.5–0.7).
OLV	DLT: 41 Fr (men); 39 Fr (women) Use large TV (12–15 mL/kg) during regular and OLV.	A DLT is inserted in the left mainstem bronchus to permit surgical access. FOB is used to verify proper tube placement. Positioning of the bronchial cuff in the proximal left mainstem bronchus does not interfere with surgical access to the bronchus. The position of the DLT should be verified after the patient is moved to the lateral position. Finally, verify ventilation and proper functioning of the tube, then eliminate volatile anesthetic or vasodilators, which may blunt hypoxic pulmonary vasoconstriction. Apply O_2 with CPAP at 5 cmH_2O to the nondependent lung. Further adjustment of CPAP may enhance oxygenation. The nondependent lung may be reinflated with O_2, if necessary, to achieve adequate oxygenation. If adequate oxygenation cannot be achieved, CPB should be initiated.
	Frequent suctioning	Frequent suctioning is necessary in patients with tenacious secretions.
PA clamping	Improve V/Q mismatch. Improve oxygenation. PAP ↑↑→ RV failure	Clamping of the PA will improve V/Q mismatch and oxygenation; however, severe pulmonary HTN and RV failure may develop. Vasodilators, such as NTG (0.2–2 mcg/kg/min), SNP (0.2–10 mcg/kg/min), PGE_1 (20–100 ng/kg/min) or inhaled NO (20–40 ppm) should be used to treat pulmonary

PA clamping (cont'd)		HTN and ↓ RV afterload; however, care must be taken to avoid systemic hypotension. Inotropic support for the RV may be necessary (dopamine [2–10 mcg/kg/min] or epinephrine [20–100 ng/kg/min]). The right atrial pressure should be monitored for evidence of tricuspid regurgitation associated with RV dilation.
PA unclamping	PIP: 20–25 cmH_2O O_2 sat: 95–100% PEEP: 5–10 mmHg	Temporary unclamping of the PA may be necessary to allow further pharmacologic therapy. If RV failure cannot be controlled pharmacologically, CPB should be initiated. The PA should not be unclamped until ventilation is possible to the transplanted lung. Perfusion without oxygenation of the transplanted lung would produce profound shunt and hypoxemia. TV should be adjusted to eliminate atelectasis and to achieve a PIP of 20–25 cmH_2O with the chest open. The FiO_2 (0.35) is limited in the hope of curtailing free radical injury. PEEP may be used to enhance oxygenation.
Positioning	For single-lung: • Supine to lateral decubitus • Axillary roll • Airplane splint • Avoid arm hyperextension (> 90°). For double-lung: • Supine with arms above head for bilateral subcostal incision ✓ and pad pressure points. ✓ eyes.	Verify correct position of DLT or BB after moving patient to the lateral position. Difficult access to airway after patient positioned. ***NB:** potential for kinking of iv and arterial lines

POSTOPERATIVE

Complications	Pulmonary edema Infection: bacterial, viral, fungal, or protozoan Side effects of immunosuppressive agents: • Corticosteroids: HTN, osteoporosis, glucose intolerance, hyperlipidemia • Azathioprine: anemia, thrombocytopenia, leukopenia	Given the lack of lymphatic drainage in the transplanted lung, pulmonary edema may occur. Diuresis and restriction of iv fluid may be required. Mannitol and furosemide can be used to induce diuresis. Immunosuppression drugs typically include: tacrolimus, myophenolate mofetil, and corticosteroids. Early induction therapy with a cytolytic agent (e.g. antithymocyte globulin) may be used.
Pain management	Epidural narcotics (see p. C-2) Parenteral narcotics (see p. C-2)	Postop analgesia may be provided by infusion of narcotics through an epidural catheter. If CPB is used, the insertion of the epidural catheter should be delayed until normal coagulation function is documented in the ICU.

Suggested Readings

1. Benumof JL, Partridge BL, Salvatierra C, et al: Margin of safety in positioning modern double-lumen endotracheal tubes. *Anesthesiology* 1987; 67(5):729–38.
2. Carere R, Patterson GA, Liu P, et al: Right and left ventricular performance after single and double lung transplantation. The Toronto Lung Transplant Group. *J Thorac Cardiovasc Surg* 1991; 102(1):115–23.
3. Chetham PM: Anesthesia for heart or single or double lung transplantation in the adult patient. *J Card Surg* 2000; 15(3): 167–74.
4. Della Rocca G, Pugliese F, Antonini M, et al: Hemodynamics during inhaled nitric oxide in lung transplant candidates. *Transplant Proc* 1997; 29:3367–70.
5. Dietrich CC, Tobias JD: Intraoperative administration of nitric oxide. *J Intensive Care Med* 2003; 18(3):146–9.
6. DiNardo JA, Zavara DA: Anesthesia for heart, heart-lung and lung transplantation. In: *Anesthesia for Cardiac Surgery*, 3rd edition. Blackwell Science, Boston: 2008; 252–88.
7. Feltracco P, Serra E, Barbieri S, et al: Anesthetic concerns in lung transplantation for severe pulmonary hypertension. *Transplant Proc* 2007; 39(6):1976–80.
8. Hurford WE, Kolker AC, Strauss W: The use of ventilation/perfusion lung scans to predict oxygenation during one-lung anesthesia. *Anesthesiology* 1987; 67(5):841–4.
9. Macdonald P, Mundy J, Rogers P, et al: Successful treatment of life-threatening acute reperfusion injury after lung transplantation with inhaled nitric oxide. *J Thorac Cardiovasc Surg* 1995; 110:861–3.
10. Mair P, Balogh D: Anaesthetic and intensive care considerations for patients undergoing heart or lung transplantation. *Acta Anaesthesiol Scand* 1997; 111:78–9.
11. Marshall SE, Lewiston NJ, Kramer MR, et al: Prospective analysis of serial pulmonary function studies and transbronchial biopsies in single-lung transplant recipients. *Transplant Proc* 1991; 23(1 P+2):1217–19.
12. Maurer JR, Winton TL, Patterson GA, et al: Single-lung transplantation for pulmonary vascular disease. *Transplant Proc* 1991; 23(1 P+2):1211–12.
13. Patterson GA: Indications. Unilateral, bilateral, heart-lung, and lobar transplant procedures. *Clin Chest Med* 1997;18: 225–30.
14. Quinlan JJ, et al: Anesthesia for heart, lung, and heart-lung transplantation. In *Kaplan's Cardiac Anesthesia*, 5th edition. Kaplan JA, et al., eds. Elsevier Saunders: 2007, 845–66.
15. Siegel LC, Brodsky JB: Choice of anesthetic agents for intrathoracic surgery. In: *Thoracic Anesthesia,* 2nd edition. Kaplan JA, ed. Churchill Livingstone, New York: 1991.
16. Smith CM: Patient selection, evaluation, and preoperative management for lung transplant candidates. *Clin Chest Med* 1997; 18:183–97.
17. Thomas Z, et al. Anesthetic management of cardiac transplantation. In: *A Practical Approach to Cardiac Anesthesia*, 4th edition. Hensley Jr FA, et al., eds. Lippincott Williams & Wilkins: 2008, 439–63.
18. Williams EL, Jellish WS, Modica PA, et al: Capnography in a patient after single lung transplantation. *Anesthesiology* 1991; 74(3):621–2.

SECTION

7.0 GENERAL SURGERY

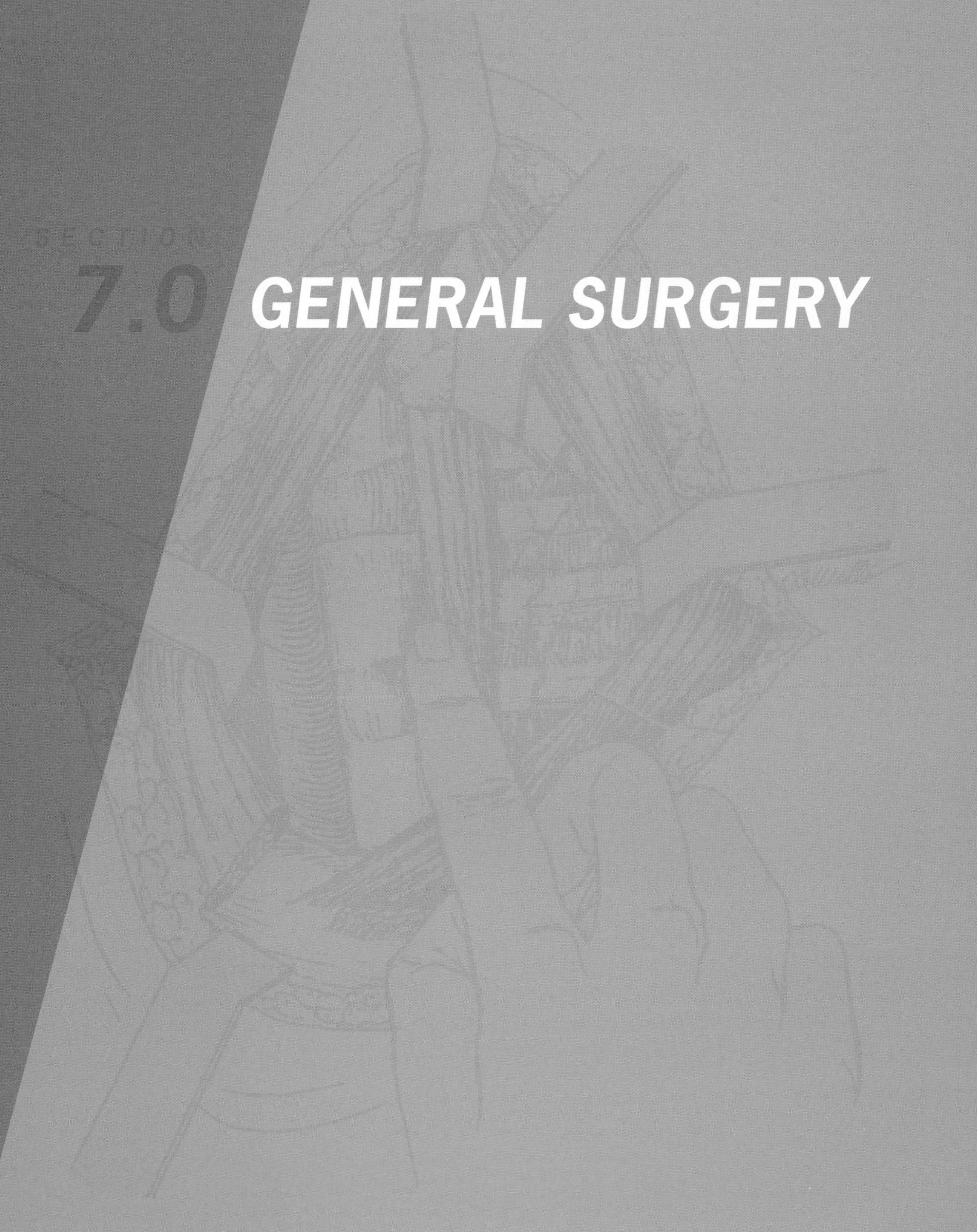

CHAPTER

7.1 Esophageal Surgery

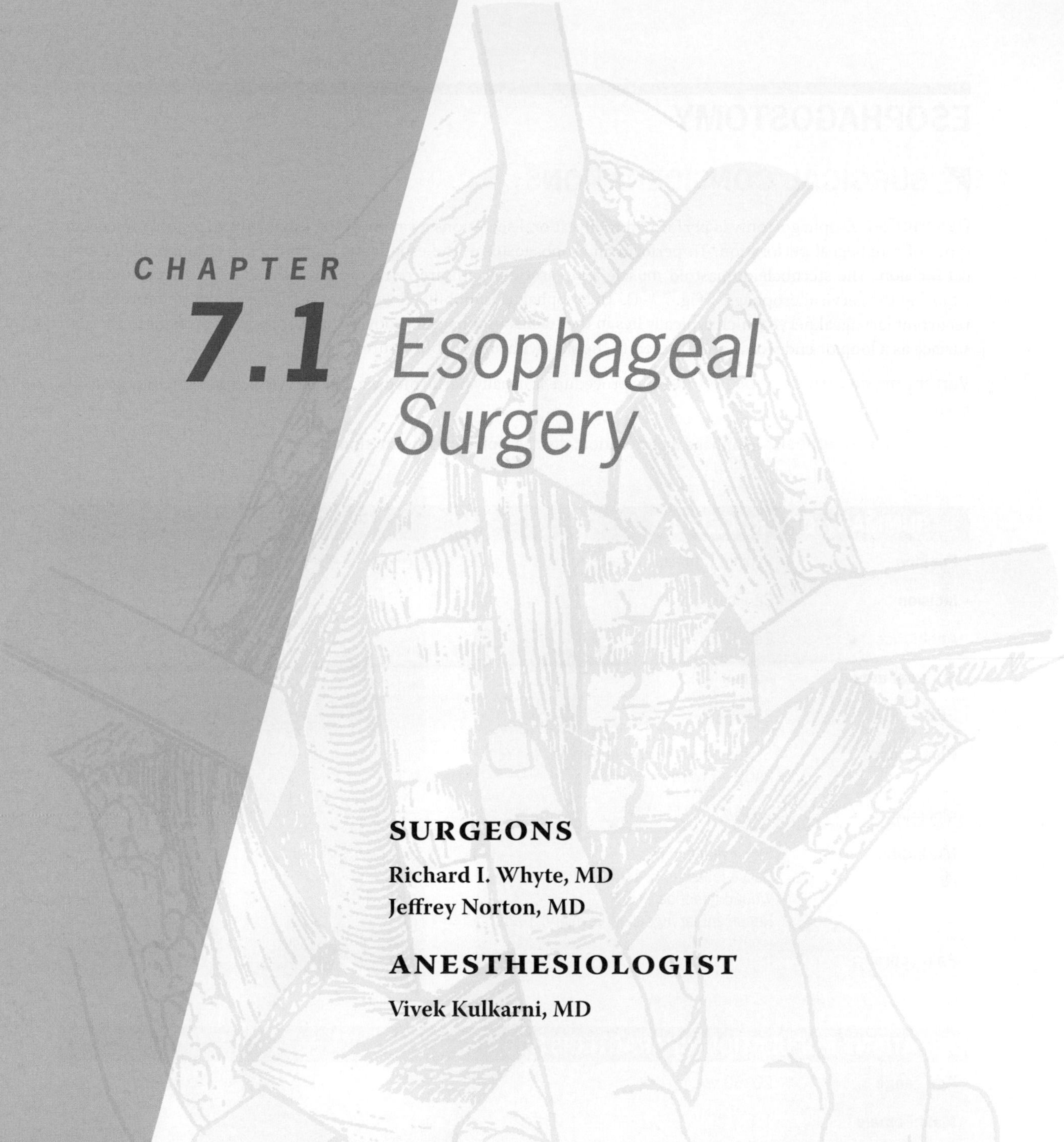

SURGEONS

Richard I. Whyte, MD

Jeffrey Norton, MD

ANESTHESIOLOGIST

Vivek Kulkarni, MD

ESOPHAGOSTOMY

SURGICAL CONSIDERATIONS

Description: Esophagostomy is performed to divert oral secretions away from the esophagus to a stoma in certain types of esophageal perforation. To perform an esophagostomy, the esophagus is approached through a left cervical incision. The sternocleidomastoid muscle and carotid sheath are retracted laterally and the thyroid medially, exposing the cervical esophagus (Fig. 7.1-1). The esophagus is mobilized with care being taken not to injure the left recurrent laryngeal nerve which typically lies in the tracheoesophageal groove. The esophagus is brought to the skin surface as a loop or end stoma and sutured to the skin with absorbable sutures.

Variant procedure or approaches: The procedure is usually performed via a left cervical approach; the right side is an alternative.

Usual preop diagnosis: Esophageal perforation; distal esophageal obstruction

SUMMARY OF PROCEDURE	
Position	Supine, with head rotated to right
Incision	Cervical
Antibiotics	Cefazolin 1 g iv preop
Surgical time	45 min
EBL	25–50 mL
Postop care	Stoma pouch to collect saliva PACU → ward
Mortality	< 0.1%
Morbidity	Skin irritation: 15–20% Saliva leakage: 5–10% Wound infection: < 5% Recurrent laryngeal nerve injury: 1–2%
Pain score	5–7

PATIENT POPULATION CHARACTERISTICS	
Age range	20–60 yr
Male:Female	1:1
Incidence	Not uncommon
Etiology	Surgically created
Associated conditions	Esophageal perforation; pharyngeal cancer

ANESTHETIC CONSIDERATIONS

See Anesthetic Considerations for Esophageal Surgery following Esophagectomy, p. 482.

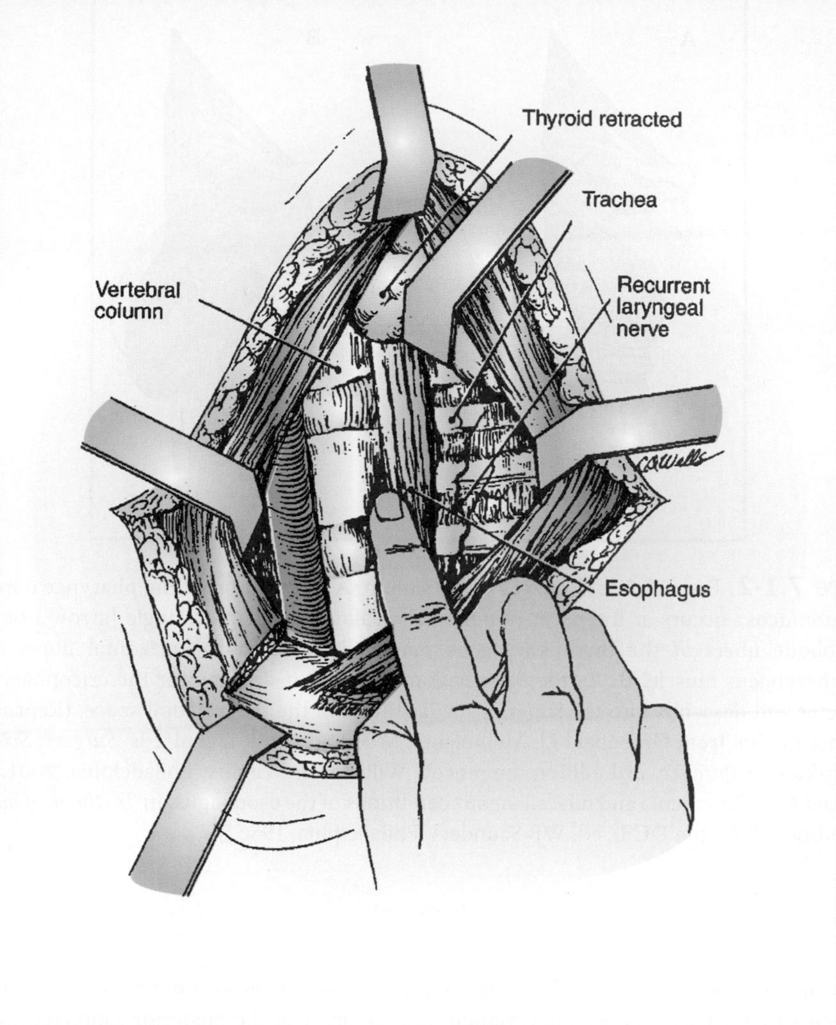

Figure 7.1-1. Surgical anatomy for cervical esophagostomy. (Reproduced with permission from Nora PF, ed: *Operative Surgery Principles and Techniques.* WB Saunders, Philadelphia: 1990.)

Suggested Reading

1. Jones WG, Ginsberg RJ: Esophageal perforations: a continuing challenge. *Ann Thorac Surg* 1992; 53:534.

ESOPHAGEAL DIVERTICULECTOMY

SURGICAL CONSIDERATIONS

Description: Esophageal diverticula are divided into three anatomic types: **pharyngoesophageal (Zenker's), midesophageal,** and **epiphrenic.** Structurally, they are either "true" diverticula—meaning they consist of all three layers of the esophageal wall (mucosa, submucosa, and muscularis)—or "false" diverticula consisting of

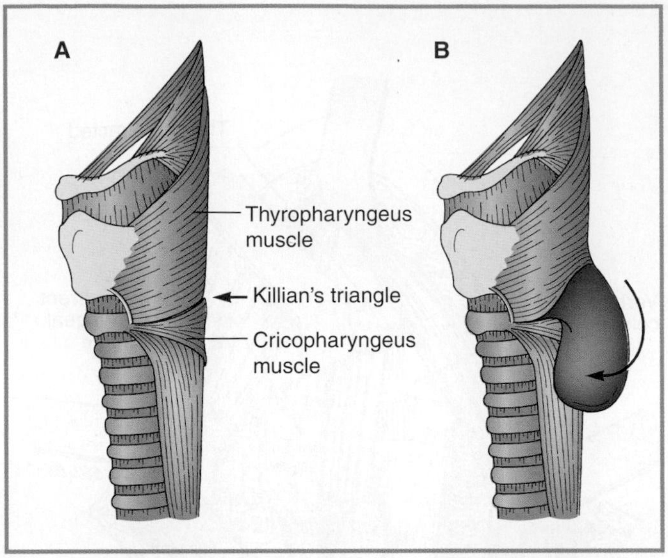

Figure 7.1-2. Formation of Zenker's diverticulum. **A.** Herniation of the pharyngeal mucosa and submucosa occurs at the point of potential weakness (Killian's triangle [arrow]) between the oblique fibers of the thyropharyngeus muscle and the more horizontal fibers of the cricopharyngeus muscle. **B.** As the diverticulum enlarges, it drapes over the cricopharyngeus sphincter and descends into the superior mediastinum in the prevertebral space. (Reproduced with permission from Greenfield LJ, Mulholland, MW, Oldham KT, et al, eds: *Surgery: Scientific Principles and Practice,* 3rd edition. Lippincott Williams & Wilkins, Philadelphia: 2001. After Orringer MB: Diverticula and miscellaneous conditions of the esophagus. In *Textbook of Surgery,* 13th edition. Sabiston DC Jr, ed. WB Saunders, Philadelphia: 1986.)

only mucosa (or mucosa and submucosa). Pharyngoesophageal diverticula account for 60–65% of all cases. These are false diverticula that originate in Killian's triangle, a weak point in the posterior esophagus, just proximal to the transverse fibers of the cricopharyngeal muscle (Fig. 7.1-2). They are associated with incomplete, or discoordinate, upper esophageal sphincter relaxation and the resultant increased hypopharyngeal pressure produces a narrow-mouthed posterior diverticulum. These diverticula frequently present in the seventh decade and are 2–3 times more common in men. Symptoms depend on the stage of the disease. Early on, patients may complain of vague pharyngeal sensations, dysphagia, cough, and excess salivation. Later, more severe symptoms—such as severe (or frequent) dysphagia, regurgitation of food, halitosis, voice changes, aspiration, and odynophagia (painful swallowing)—may occur.

Surgery is the only effective therapy for Zenker's diverticulum. Respiratory complications (aspiration) or nutritional deficiencies (weight loss) may be directly attributable to the diverticulum and should not be contraindications to surgery. Multiple different operative approaches are advocated: diverticulectomy alone, cricopharyngeal myotomy, diverticulectomy with myotomy, and myotomy with suspension of the diverticulum. **Myotomy** alone, which corrects the underlying physiologic abnormality, is up to 78% effective and may be considered for patients with small (< 2 cm) diverticula. **Diverticulectomy** or **suspension** should be added if the diverticulum itself is large or dependant. Both procedures are performed via a left cervical incision (Fig. 7.1-3: inset) and are associated with a low rate of recurrence and complications. The upper esophagus is exposed by retracting the sternocleidomastoid muscle and carotid sheath laterally and the thyroid gland medially. The diverticulum is located in the prevertebral space. Care is taken not to injure the recurrent laryngeal nerve. Following excision of the diverticulum, a cricopharyngeal **myotomy** may be performed, starting on the upper esophagus and extending across the cricopharyngeal muscle near the neck of the diverticulum, and on to the inferior pharyngeal constrictor muscle.

Recent emphasis has been placed on endoscopic treatment of Zenker's diverticulum (**Dohlman procedure**). In this procedure, a modified laryngoscope and endoscopic stapler are used to divide the common wall between diverticulum and true esophageal lumen.

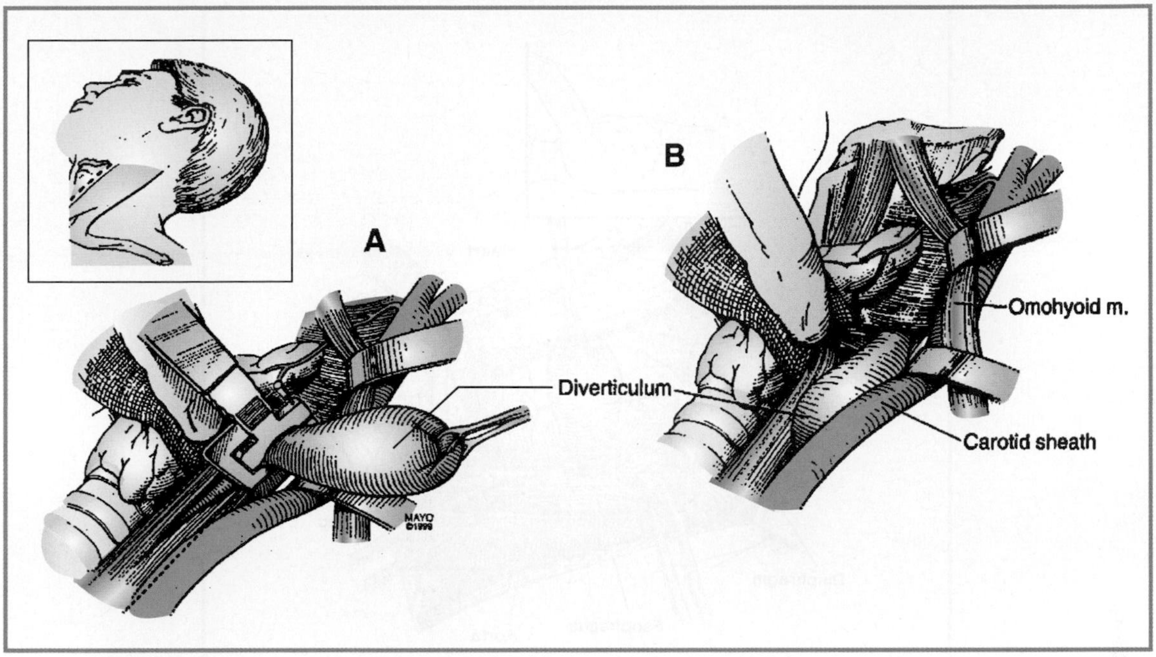

Figure 7.1-3. Zenker's diverticulum approached through a left cervical incision (inset). **A.** The diverticulum is grasped and a cricopharyngeal myotomy is extended onto the upper esophagus. **B.** The base of the diverticulum is stapled and the diverticulum is resected. (Reproduced with permission from Shields TW, LoCicero J III, Ponn RB: *General Thoracic Surgery,* 5th edition. Lippincott Williams & Wilkins, Philadelphia: 2000.)

Midesophageal diverticula, by definition, occur in the middle 3rd of the esophagus. These "true" diverticula typically arise in the setting of mediastinal granulomatous disease whereby a fibrotic reaction around inflamed mediastinal lymph nodes results in traction on the muscular wall of the esophagus. Diverticula usually arise within 4–5 cm of the carina and comprise an estimated 10–17% of all esophageal diverticula. Most midesophageal diverticula are asymptomatic and do not require surgical intervention. In cases that require intervention, because of either regurgitation or development of an esophagobronchial fistula, the approach is through a **right thoracotomy** with excision of the inflammatory mass. Primary closure of the fistula and the interposition of viable tissue should be performed.

Epiphrenic diverticula arise in the distal 10 cm of the esophagus and are thought to be related to an underlying esophageal motility disorder. These false diverticula are most commonly present in the 6th decade. The clinical presentation is variable, with most patients presenting with symptoms related to their underlying dysmotility syndrome: dysphagia, chest pain, or regurgitation. Most patients with epiphrenic diverticula are asymptomatic, and there appears to be no relation between size of the diverticulum and symptoms. Surgery for epiphrenic diverticula typically consists of **diverticulectomy with myotomy** either through a **left thoracotomy** (Fig. 7.1-4) or via laparoscopy. With the transthoracic approach, a low, **left thoracotomy** is used, the esophagus is mobilized and encircled, and the diverticulum is mobilized and excised. A **myotomy** should be performed opposite the diverticulectomy and should extend proximally above the diverticulum and distally onto the stomach. Because there is, by definition, an underlying motility disorder, the myotomy should be carried onto the stomach and a nonobstructing fundoplication may be added to prevent significant postoperative reflux.

Variant procedure or approaches: **Laparoscopic diverticulectomy and myotomy** has gained increasing acceptance, and reported outcomes are similar to those obtained with the open procedure. The surgical approach is similar to that used during laparoscopic fundoplication (see p. 571). Dissection of the diverticula may be facilitated by the passage of a bougie or video endoscope. After the diverticulum is amputated using an endoscopic stapler, a myotomy is performed opposite the diverticula and a partial fundoplication is fashioned.

Usual preop diagnosis: Esophageal diverticulum

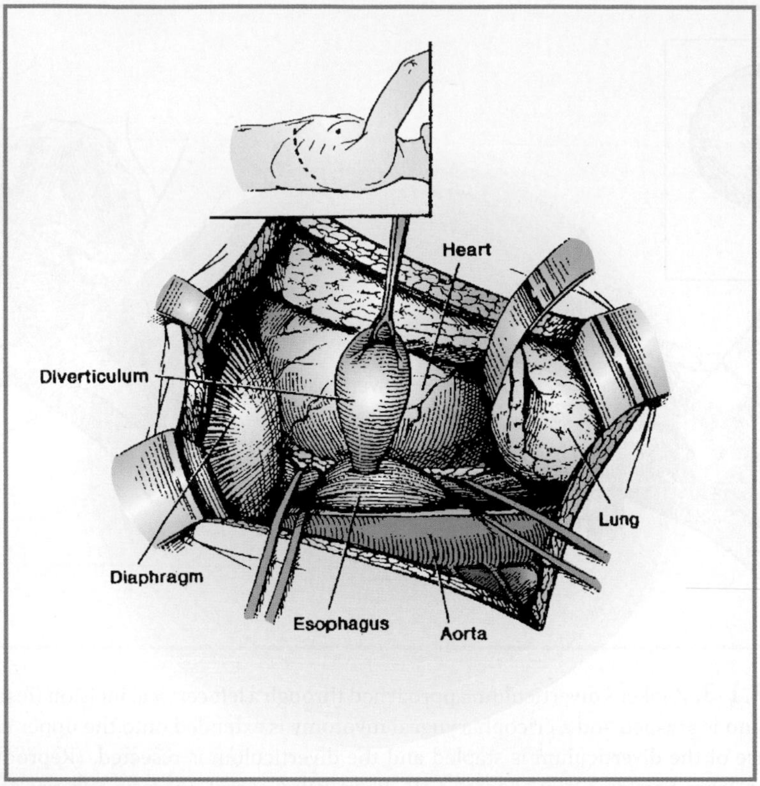

Figure 7.1-4. Epiphrenic diverticulum. Through a left thoracotomy, the diverticulum is mobilized and resected. A contralateral myotomy is then created and extended distally to the stomach to eliminate any functional obstruction secondary to the pre-existent dysmotility. (Reproduced with permission from Shields TW, LoCicero J III, Ponn RB: *General Thoracic Surgery,* 5th edition. Lippincott Williams & Wilkins, Philadelphia: 2000.)

SUMMARY OF PROCEDURES

	Hypopharyngeal	Epiphrenic
Position	Supine	Right lateral decubitus
Incision	Left or right cervical	Left thoracotomy
Special instrumentation	None	Chest retractor
Unique considerations	Care not to injure recurrent laryngeal nerve	10 cm myotomy
Antibiotics	Cefazolin 1 g iv preop	⇐
Surgical time	1–2 h	⇐
Closing considerations	Inspect for perforation	⇐
EBL	50–100 mL	100–200 mL
Postop care	PACU → ward	ICU × 1–2 d

SUMMARY OF PROCEDURES (cont'd)		
	Hypopharyngeal	**Epiphrenic**
Mortality	< 1%	⇐
Morbidity	Recurrent nerve paralysis: < 5% Temporary phonetic problems: < 5% Esophageal stricture: < 3% Esophageal fistula: < 2%	Atelectasis: 5–10% Esophageal perforation: < 2% < 2%
Pain score	6–7	7–9

PATIENT POPULATION CHARACTERISTICS	
Age range	35–90 yr (50% of patients > 70 yr)
Male:Female	2:1
Incidence	Uncommon
Etiology	Uncoordinated cricoesophageal muscle and lower esophageal sphincter; weakness of esophageal wall.
Associated conditions	Cachexia (25–30%); hiatus hernia with or without reflux (25%); chronic pulmonary infection (15–20%); aspiration (30–40%)

ANESTHETIC CONSIDERATIONS

See Anesthetic Considerations for Esophageal Surgery following Esophagectomy, p. 482.

Suggested Readings

1. Deschamps C, Trastek V: Esophageal diverticula. In: *General Thoracic Surgery,* 5th edition. Shields TW, LoCicero J III, Ponn RB, eds. Lippincott Williams & Wilkins, Philadelphia: 2000.
2. Ferreira LE, Simmons DT, Bain TH: Zenker's diverticula: pathophysiology, clinical presentation, and flexible endoscopic management. *Dis Esophagus* 2008;21:1–8.

MANAGEMENT OF ESOPHAGEAL PERFORATION

SURGICAL CONSIDERATIONS

Description: **Esophageal perforation** may be spontaneous, instrumental (iatrogenic), traumatic, or 2° intrinsic esophageal disease. **Spontaneous (or emetogenic) perforation** most commonly occurs in the lower 3rd of the esophagus. **Instrumental perforations** may occur at any level, but are most common just above the cardia and in the cervical esophagus. The level of **traumatic perforation** depends on the location of the penetrating wound. Sx of esophageal perforation at the cricopharyngeal sphincter include neck pain, fever, and crepitations in the substernal and neck areas. Perforation in the mediastinum may result in hydropneumothorax, mediastinitis, fever, and substernal pain. Cervical perforations are managed with antibiotics and drainage in the cervical area. Therapy for intrathoracic perforation generally requires emergent operation. Surgical options include **primary repair, drainage and diversion,** and **esophageal resection.** The optimal choice depends on the nature and duration of the perforation as well as the clinical condition of the patient. Spontaneous perforations are often amenable to primary repair—either through the abdomen or the left chest. Patients suffering from iatrogenic perforation incurred during dilation of a malignant, or nondilatable, stricture may require urgent esophagectomy. Patients with delayed recognition of a perforation may be hemodynamically unstable and may only tolerate drainage and diversion (generally through a cervical esophagostomy).

Variant procedure or approaches: Cervical or right thoracic drainage is indicated when the perforation occurs in the neck or high in the mediastinum.

Usual preop diagnosis: Esophageal perforation

SUMMARY OF PROCEDURES

	Left Thoracotomy	Cervical or Thoracic Drainage
Position	Right lateral decubitus	Supine or right lateral decubitus
Incision	Left thoracotomy	Cervical or right chest
Antibiotics	Zosyn (piperacillin & tazobactom) 3.375 g iv q6h	⇐
VTE prophylaxis	Heparin 5,000 units sq	⇐
Surgical time	2–4 h	1 h
Closing considerations	Chest drain	Cervical or thoracic drain
EBL	100–200 mL	50–100 mL
Postop care	Chest tube to suction; PACU → ward	⇐
Mortality	5–10%	2–5%
Morbidity	Pneumonia: 5–10% Esophageal leak: 2–5% Pericarditis: 1–3%	— 10% —
Pain score	8–10	8–10

PATIENT POPULATION CHARACTERISTICS

Age range	Variable: 20–80 yr
Male:Female	1:1
Incidence	1 in 8,000 admissions
Etiology	Instrumental (endoscopy, dilatation, intubation); traumatic (penetrating, foreign body, caustic agents); intrinsic disease (carcinoma, peptic ulceration); spontaneous
Associated conditions	Esophageal stricture (75%); cancer (25%)

ANESTHETIC CONSIDERATIONS

See Anesthetic Considerations for Esophageal Surgery following Esophagectomy, p. 482.

Suggested Readings

1. Fell SC: Esophageal perforation. In: *Esophageal Surgery.* Pearson FG, Cooper JD, Deslauriers J, et al, eds. Churchill Livingstone, New York: 2002, 615–36.
2. Orringer MB: The mediastinum. In: *Operative Surgery,* 3rd edition. Nora PF, ed. WB Saunders, Philadelphia: 1990, 370–3.
3. Wong AS, Myers JC, Jamieson GG: Esophageal pH profile after laparoscopic total fundoplication compared to anterior fundoplication. *J Gastrointest Surg* 2008; in press.
4. Wu JT, Mattox KL, Wall MJ: Esophageal perforations: new perspectives and treatment paradigms. *J Trauma* 2007;63: 1173–84.

ESOPHAGOMYOTOMY

SURGICAL CONSIDERATIONS

Description: Esophagomyotomy is performed for achalasia and other motility disorders to facilitate esophageal emptying into the stomach. Most authors recommend incising the muscular layer of the distal esophagus and continuing down across the gastroesophageal junction for at least 1 cm (**Heller's myotomy**). The muscle is dissected back from the mucosa so that roughly 180° is exposed (Fig. 7.1-5). The distal esophagus is mobilized either from below the diaphragm or via a left thoracic approach. Care is taken not to injure the vagus nerves.

When approached from the abdomen, the esophagus is exposed by incising the gastroesophageal ligament. The distal esophagus is mobilized and pulled downward to perform the myotomy.

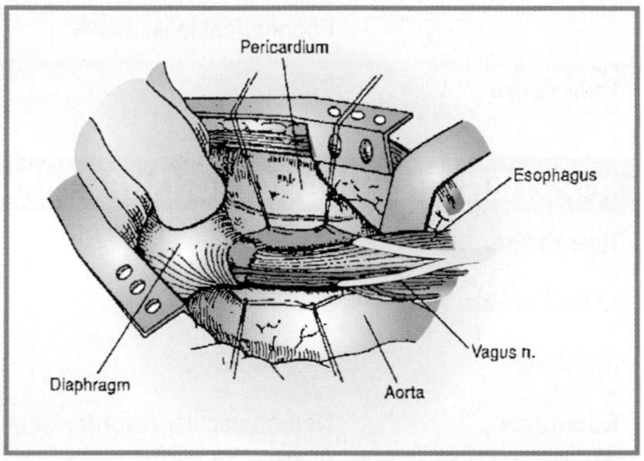

Figure 7.1-5. Surgical anatomy for esophagomyotomy. (Reproduced with permission from Hardy JD: *Hardy's Textbook of Surgery,* 2nd edition. JB Lippincott, Philadelphia: 1988.)

Variant procedure or approaches: The procedure usually is performed through a **left thoracotomy**, but some surgeons prefer a **transabdominal approach.** More recently, laparoscopic or thoracoscopic approaches are being employed to perform esophagomyotomy (see p. 574).

Usual preop diagnosis: Achalasia; diffuse esophageal spasm; nutcracker esophagus

SUMMARY OF PROCEDURES

	Thoracic Approach	Abdominal Approach	Endoscopic Approaches
Position	Right lateral decubitus	Supine	Supine
Incision	Left thoracotomy in 6th interspace	Midline upper abdomen	Multiple small abdominal incisions
Special instrumentation	Chest retractor	Denier retractor	Laparoscopic instrumentation
Unique considerations	Care should be taken to avoid extending gastric myotomy too far to prevent esophageal reflux.	⇐	Legs spread apart (laparoscopic approach)
Antibiotics	Cefazolin 1–2 g iv preop	⇐	⇐
VTE prophylaxis	Heparin 5,000 units sq	⇐	⇐
Surgical time	1–2 h	⇐	⇐
Closing considerations	✓ for perforation. Consider fundoplication to prevent esophageal reflux.	⇐	⇐
EBL	150–200 mL	100–150 mL	50 mL
Postop care	ICU × 1–2 d	PACU → room	⇐
Mortality	< 0.5%	⇐	⇐

SUMMARY OF PROCEDURES (cont'd)			
	Thoracic Approach	**Abdominal Approach**	**Endoscopic Approaches**
Morbidity	Esophagitis: ≤ 20% Transient dysphagia/reflux: 5% Esophageal leak: 1–2%	⇐ ⇐ ⇐	⇐ ⇐ ⇐
Pain score	7–9	6–8	3–4

PATIENT POPULATION CHARACTERISTICS	
Age range	30–50 yr
Male:Female	1:1
Incidence	0.6/100,000
Etiology	Neuromuscular disorder of unknown etiology often characterized by absence of ganglion cells of Auerbach's plexus.
Associated conditions	Predisposition to development of carcinoma (1–20%); pulmonary complications 2° aspiration (5–10%)

ANESTHETIC CONSIDERATIONS

See Anesthetic Considerations for Esophageal Surgery following Esophagectomy, p. 482.

Suggested Readings

1. Ellis FH Jr, Crozier RE, Watkins E Jr: Operation for esophageal achalasia. Results of esophagomyotomy without an antireflex. *J Thorac Cardiovasc Surg* 1984; 88(3):344–51.
2. Pellegrini C, Wetters LA, Palti M, et al: Thorascopic esophagomyotomy. *Ann Surg* 1992; 216:29.
3. Stuart RC, Hennessy TP: Primary motility disorders of the esophagus. *Br J Surg* 1989; 76:111.
4. Zhu ZJ, Chen LQ, Duranceau A: Long-term results of total vs. partial fundoplication after esophagomyotomy for primary esophageal motor disorders. *World J Surg* 2008; 32:401–7.

ESOPHAGOGASTRIC FUNDOPLASTY

SURGICAL CONSIDERATIONS

Description: **Esophagogastric fundoplasty** represents a variety of operations designed to prevent esophageal reflux by wrapping the fundus of the stomach around a 3–4 cm segment of the lower esophagus. This fundal wrapping acts to reinforce the lower esophageal sphincter. Surgery may be performed transabdominally, transthoracically, or laparoscopically, depending on surgeon's preference. The most common approach is the open or laparoscopic **Nissen fundoplication,** wherein the anterior and posterior walls of the stomach are sutured together around the lower esophagus with nonabsorbable sutures (Fig. 7.1-6A). This is accomplished by incising the gastrosplenic ligament and ligating three or four short gastric vessels. Care must be taken not to injure the spleen or vagus nerves during the repair.

Variant procedure or approaches: Modifications of the Nissen fundoplication include the **Toupet procedure,** a posterior partial fundoplication, and the **Hill procedure,** in which the gastroesophageal junction is sutured to the median arcuate ligament of the diaphragm or to the preaortic fascia (Fig. 7.1-6B). Another modification is the **Belsey Mark IV** repair, in which there is a 240° semifundoplication between the stomach and esophagus, making it easier for the patient to overcome the resistance of the wrap. There are proponents of each repair, although the Nissen fundoplication remains the standard to which others are compared. The **laparoscopic approach** is widely used, although the left transthoracic approach provides excellent exposure for either Nissen or Belsey repairs (see p. 574).

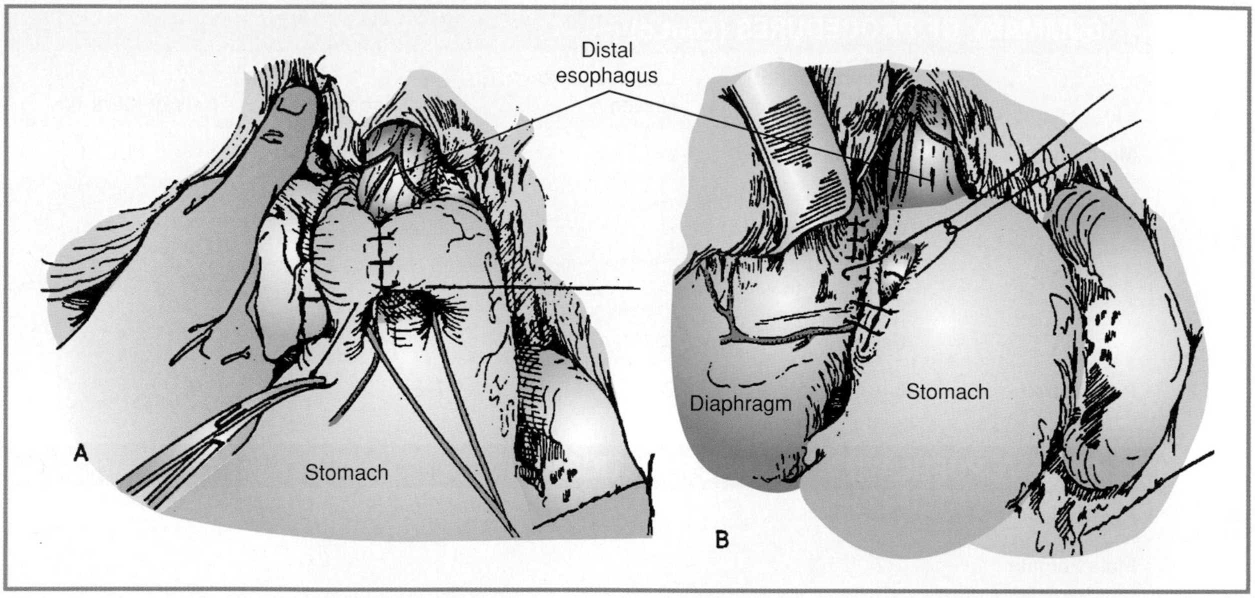

Figure 7.1-6. **A.** Nissen fundoplication may be performed via either the transabdominal or transthoracic approach; **B.** Hill repair is performed through the abdomen. (Reproduced with permission from Hardy JD: *Hardy's Textbook of Surgery,* 2nd edition. JB Lippincott, Philadelphia: 1988.)

Usual preop diagnosis: Sliding hiatus (hiatal) hernia, paraesophageal hiatus hernia, or free reflux

SUMMARY OF PROCEDURES

	Nissen (Toupet) Fundoplication	Laparoscopic Nissen	Hill Procedure	Belsey Mark IV
Position	Supine	Supine, legs apart	⇐	Right lateral decubitus
Incision	Midline abdominal or laparoscopic ports	Laparoscopic ports	Midline abdominal	Left posterolateral thoracotomy
Special instrumentation	#40–50 Hurst dilators; NG tube	Laparoscopic instrumentation	NG tube	Chest retractor; NG tube
Unique considerations	Fundoplication should be loose; parietal cell vagotomy performed if peptic ulcer disease present. Fundoplication may be limited to 180–280° posterior wrap (Toupet)	CO_2 insufflation		⇐ 240° semi-fundoplication
Antibiotics	Cefazolin 1–2 g iv	⇐	⇐	⇐
VTE prophylaxis	Heparin 5,000 units sq		⇐	⇐
Surgical time	1–2 h	⇐	⇐	⇐
Closing considerations	Inspect spleen for bleeding	⇐	⇐	⇐
EBL	100–150 mL	50 mL	100–150 mL	100–200 mL
Postop care	PACU → ward	⇐	⇐	ICU × 1–2 d

SUMMARY OF PROCEDURES (cont'd)	Nissen (Toupet) Fundoplication	Laparoscopic Nissen	Hill Procedure	Belsey Mark IV
Mortality	< 0.5%	⇐	⇐	⇐
Morbidity	Recurrent hernia: 20%	⇐	⇐	⇐
	Gas-bloat syndrome: 10–20%	⇐	< 5%	⇐
	Temporary dysphagia: 5–10%	⇐	5%	2%
	Gastric fistula: < 2%	⇐	⇐	⇐
Pain score	6–8	2–4	7–8	7–9

PATIENT POPULATION CHARACTERISTICS	
Age range	46–60 yr
Male:Female	1:2
Incidence	Not uncommon
Etiology	Esophagogastric reflux (100%); esophageal hiatus hernia (80–90%)
Associated conditions	Diverticulosis of colon (30–35%); cholelithiasis (25–30%)

General Surgery

ANESTHETIC CONSIDERATIONS

See Anesthetic Considerations for Esophageal Surgery following Esophagectomy, p. 482.

Suggested Readings

1. Belsey R: Mark IV repair of hiatal hernia by the transthoracic approach. *World J Surg* 1977; 1(4):475–81.
2. Cuschieri, A: Laparoscopic antireflux surgery and repair of hiatal hernia. *World J Surg* 1993; 17(1):40–5.
3. Wong AS, Myers JC, Jamieson GG: Esophageal pH profile after laparoscopic total fundoplication compared to anterior fundoplication. *J Gastrointest Surg* 2008; in press.

ESOPHAGECTOMY

SURGICAL CONSIDERATIONS

Description: Esophagectomy is most commonly performed for malignant disease of the middle and lower 3rd of the esophagus and gastric cardia. This procedure also may be indicated for intractable benign stricture, **Barrett's esophagus** with high-grade dysplasia, and end-stage achalasia. There are several surgical options for esophageal resection, including the **Ivor Lewis approach,** which involves a laparotomy and right thoracotomy; the transhiatal approach, whereby the esophagus is mobilized through abdominal and neck incisions, and the **left thoracoabdominal approach** (Fig. 7.1-7). Although there are advantages and disadvantages to each, the final result is to use a portion of the stomach to replace the esophagus. In all approaches, the stomach is mobilized while preserving its blood supply from the right gastroepiploic and gastric arteries. The stomach is then transposed into the chest and a gastroesophageal anastomosis is fashioned either in the chest (Ivor Lewis and left chest approaches) or in the neck (transhiatal approach). To avoid delayed gastric emptying, a **pyloroplasty** or **pyloromyotomy** is often added, as is placement of a temporary jejunal feeding tube. Regardless of the surgical technique, patients with larger or locally advanced tumors may have received preoperative chemotherapy or radiation. In these patients, the combination of less distinct tissue planes and radiation-induced inflammation tends to lead to increased bleeding and/or increased insensible fluid losses.

The previously mentioned variants of esophagectomy all involve use of the **stomach** as an esophageal replacement. When the stomach is not available (as with prior resection or caustic injury), the **colon** can be used as an esophageal substitute. Both the left and right colon can be used, with the vascular supply to the grafts based on either the ascending branch of the left colic artery or the right colic artery. Colon interpositions typically have higher complication rates than esophagectomies using gastric conduits.

Usual preop diagnosis: Carcinoma of esophagus or gastroesophageal junction; Barrett's esophagus; benign strictures

SUMMARY OF PROCEDURES

	Ivor Lewis	Transhiatal Esophagectomy	Thoracoabdominal	Total Esophagectomy + Colonic Interposition
Position	Supine and left lateral decubitus	Supine	Right lateral decubitus	Supine and right lateral decubitus
Incision	Midline abdominal + right chest and/or cervical incisions	Cervical and midline abdominal	Thoracoabdominal across costal margin (see Fig. 7.1-8)	Midline + right thoracic and cervical
Unique considerations	DLT	None	DLT	⇐
Antibiotics	Cefoxitin 2 g iv preop	⇐	⇐	⇐
VTE prophylaxis	Heparin 5,000 units sq	⇐	⇐	⇐
Surgical time	3–4 h	4–5 h	3–4 h	5–6 h
Closing considerations	Lung reexpansion	Pneumothorax	Lung reexpansion	Vascular integrity of colonic interposition
EBL	300–800 mL	⇐	⇐	⇐
Postop care	ICU × 1–2 d	⇐	⇐	ICU × 2–3 d
Mortality	5–10%	⇐	⇐	10%
Morbidity	Respiratory complications: 15–20%	⇐	⇐	⇐
	Anastomotic leakage: < 5%	5–10%	< 5%	10%
	Anastomotic stricture: < 5%	⇐	⇐	10%
	Wound infection: < 5%	⇐	⇐	⇐
Pain score	7–9	6–8	7–9	7–9

PATIENT POPULATION CHARACTERISTICS

Age range	4–80 yr
Male:Female	2:1 for carcinoma
Incidence	1–2% of malignant disease
Etiology	Alcohol and tobacco; dietary factors – hot spicy foods; lye burns
Associated conditions	Barrett's esophagus; hiatus hernia; reflux esophagitis; radiation esophagitis; caustic burns

General Surgery

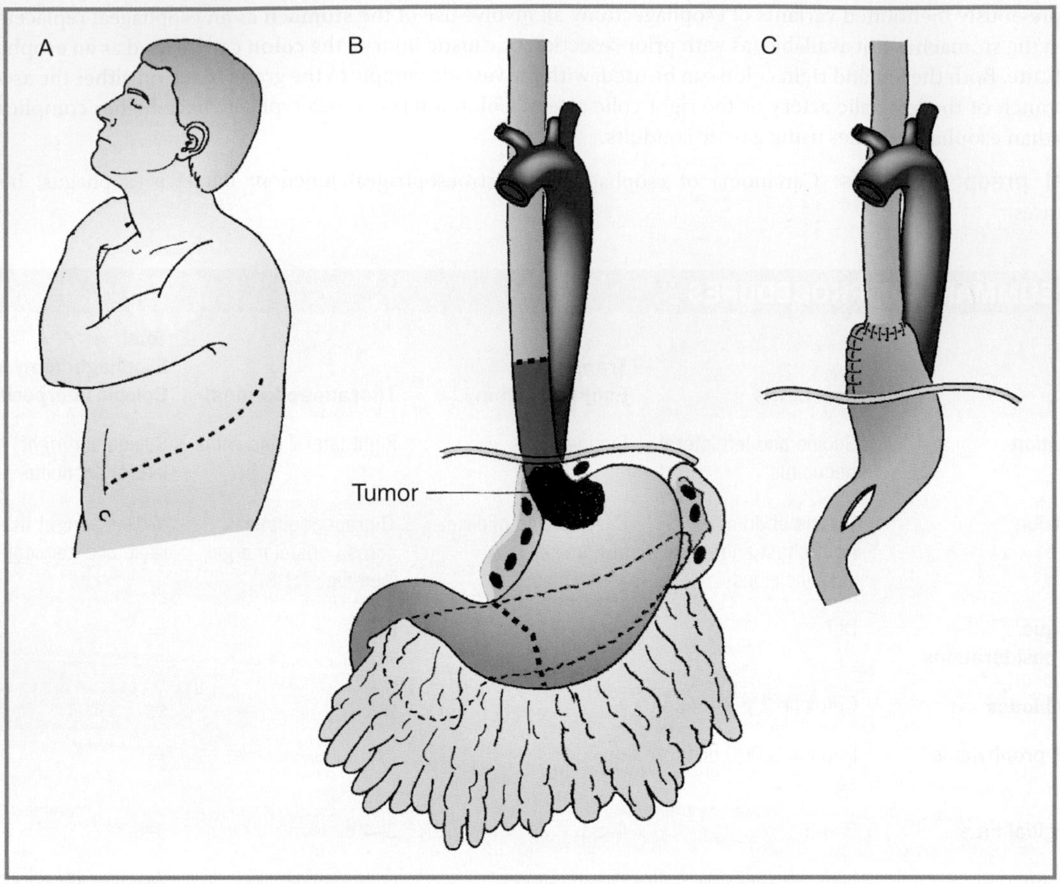

Figure 7.1-7. Standard thoracoabdominal esophagosgastrectomy for carcinomas of the distal esophagus and cardia. **A.** Thoracoabdominal incision. **B.** Tissue to be resected (darker area). **C.** Completed reconstruction after intrathoracic esophagogastric anastomosis and either pyloromyotomy or pyloroplasty to prevent postvagotomy pylorospasm. (Reproduced with permission from Greenfield LJ, Mulholland, MW, Oldham KT, et al, eds: *Surgery: Scientific Principles and Practice,* 3rd edition. Lippincott Williams & Wilkins, Philadelphia: 2001).

Suggested Reading

1. Orringer MB: Resection of the esophagus. In: *General Thoracic Surgery,* 5th edition. Shields TW, LoCicero J III, Ponn RB, eds. Lippincott Williams & Wilkins, Philadelphia: 2000, 1697–722.

ANESTHETIC CONSIDERATIONS FOR ESOPHAGEAL SURGERY

(Procedures covered: esophagostomy; esophageal diverticulectomy; closure of esophageal perforation; esophagomyotomy; esophagogastric fundoplasty; esophagectomy; colonic interposition)

Patients presenting for esophageal surgery typically are those with carcinoma, motility disorders, strictures, hiatal hernia, reflux esophagitis, diverticula, and perforation. Patients tend to be elderly, with a history of tobacco abuse

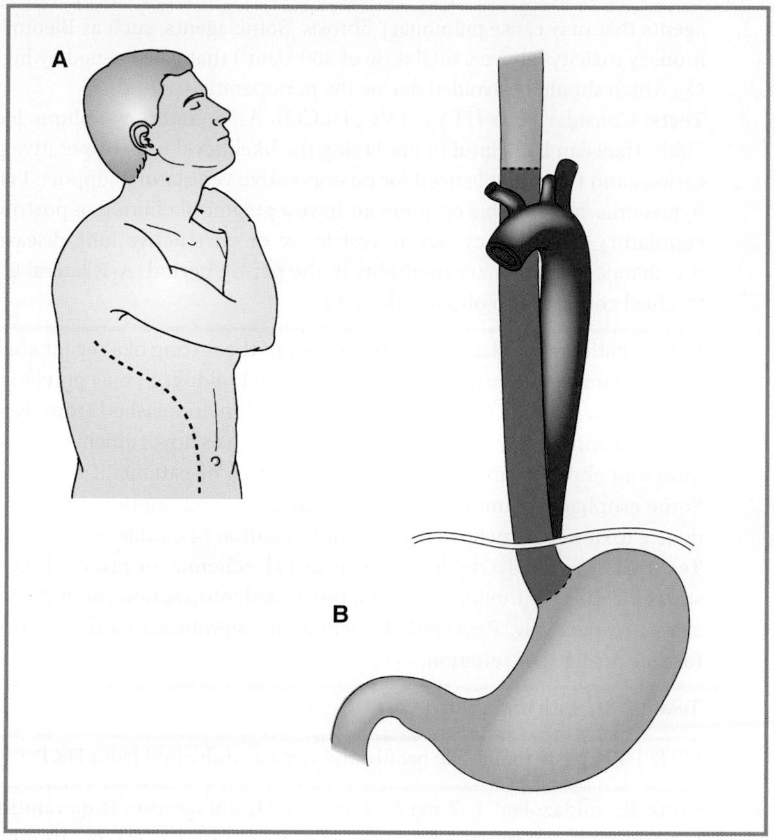

Figure 7.1-8. Standard thoracoabdominal esophagogastrectomy for tumors of the upper and middle 3rd of the thoracic esophagus. **A.** Either a continuous thoracoabdominal incision or separate thoracic and abdominal incisions are used. **B.** Portion of esophagus to be resected (darker area). **C.** Completed reconstruction with high intrathoracic esophagogastric anastomosis and gastric drainage procedure. (Reproduced with permission from Greenfield LJ, Mulholland, MW, Oldham KT, et al, eds: *Surgery: Scientific Principles and Practice,* 3rd edition. Lippincott Williams & Wilkins, Philadelphia: 2001.)

and alcohol consumption, and may have associated cardiopulmonary disease. Obesity and ischemic heart disease are increasingly frequent comorbid conditions. Esophageal disorders such as hiatal hernia, Barrett's esophagus, and carcinoma with incomplete obstruction predispose the patient to recurrent aspiration pneumonitis from intermittent reflux of gastric contents. Patients with esophageal diverticula, stricture, achalasia, and carcinoma with obstruction may present with retained food and oral secretions. Therefore, patients may need to be considered nonfasted.

PREOPERATIVE

Respiratory	Many patients with esophageal cancer have a long history of smoking resulting in COPD. Mediastinal lymphadenopathy and tumors of the upper esophagus may lead to tracheal/bronchial compression or erosion that may be revealed by CT and bronchoscopy. A history of gastric reflux and recurrent aspiration pneumonia → ↓ pulmonary reserve and ↑ risk of regurgitation/aspiration during anesthetic induction. (See Premedication, below.) If thoracotomy is a part of the procedure, the patient should be evaluated to ensure that OLV will be tolerated (see below). Determine if patient has been exposed to radiation and chemotherapeutic

Respiratory (cont'd)	agents that may cause pulmonary fibrosis. Some agents, such as Bleomycin, may cause pulmonary toxicity (above a total dose of 300 U/m^2) that is worsened by high concentrations of O_2, which should be avoided during the perioperative period. **Tests:** Consider PFTs (FEV1, FVC, DLCO), ABG, and flow-volume loops, if indicated by H&P. They can be helpful in predicting the likelihood of perioperative pulmonary complications and the possible need for postoperative ventilatory support. Patients with baseline hypoxemia/hypercarbia on room air have a greater likelihood of postop complications and ventilatory insufficiency. Severe restrictive or obstructive lung disease also will increase the chance of pulmonary morbidity in the periop period. A-P, lateral CXR (if suggestive of tracheal compression obtain MRI/CT).
Cardiovascular	Elderly patients may have coexisting CAD. In the setting of a recent angioplasty/stent, continued management with antiplatelet agents (clopidogrel) may preclude the use of epidural techniques. Patients may be hypovolemic and malnourished from dysphagia or anorexia. Preop chemotherapy treatment with agents such as doxorubicin may cause acute dysrhythmias and chronic cardiomyopathy (seen in 10% of patients if total dose is > 550 mg/m^2). Some esophageal tumors are related to alcohol consumption and chronic abuse may produce a toxic cardiomyopathy. Preop optimization of cardiac status is important. **Tests:** ECG to r/o dysrhythmias, myocardial ischemia, or prior MI. ECHO or dobutamine stress ECHO will provide important functional information about the heart at rest or under stress, respectively. Reversible ischemia and significant cardiomyopathy should prompt further cardiac consultation.
Hematologic	**Tests:** CBC with differential.
Laboratory	PT & PTT, basic metabolic profile and tests as indicated from H&P.
Premedication	Consider midazolam 1–2 mg iv. Consider H_2-antagonists (e.g., ranitidine 50 mg iv), metoclopramide (10 mg iv 1 h preop), and Na citrate (30 mL po 10 min preop) in patients with reflux and partial obstruction. Patients with esophageal motility disorders, strictures/tumors with complete obstruction may not tolerate oral antacids.

INTRAOPERATIVE

Anesthetic technique: GETA (with or without epidural for intraop/postop analgesia). If the patient is clinically hypovolemic, restore intravascular volume before epidural placement and induction of GA. Surgeries involving only a cervical or endoscopic approach typically do not require epidural analgesia. If epidural analgesia is planned, placement and testing of the catheter before anesthetic induction is recommended. This is accomplished by injecting 5–7 mL of 1–2% lidocaine with 1:200,000 epinephrine via the epidural catheter and eliciting a segmental block. If a thoracic or thoracoabdominal approach is performed, placement of a DLT is indicated to provide OLV for optimal surgical conditions. (For additional discussion of DLT placement and OLV, see Anesthetic Considerations in Lobectomy, Pneumonectomy in Thoracic Surgery, p. 275.)

Induction	Patients with esophageal disease are often at risk for pulmonary aspiration; therefore, the trachea should be intubated after rapid-sequence induction with cricoid pressure. In cases with a difficult airway needing a DLT, placement of a single lumen tube should be accomplished (a) with the aid of a bougie, (b) via an LMA, or (c) with FOB. The single lumen tube is then changed to a DLT using a tube exchange catheter.
Maintenance	Standard maintenance (p. B-2), with or without N_2O (for OLV). Alternatively, a combined technique may be used. A local anesthetic (e.g., 2% lidocaine with 1:200,000 epinephrine or 0.25% bupivacaine) can be infused or injected into a thoracic (3–5 mL) or lumbar (5–10 mL) epidural catheter to provide both anesthesia and optimal surgical conditions (contracted bowel and profound muscle relaxation). Continuous infusion of local anesthetic generally provides better hemodynamic stability than hourly bolus injections. To enhance the effect of epidural analgesia, a loading dose of opiates (e.g., hydromorphone 0.4–1 mg [thoracic] or 1–1.5 mg [lumbar]) can be administered early during the surgery and at least 1 h before conclusion of the case. Esophagectomy procedures can cause significant third-space

Maintenance (cont'd)	losses; thus, maintenance of euvolemia with close monitoring of BP and UO. Esophageal procedures involving transient compression of the myocardium (i.e., thoracic approach for esophagomyotomy or esophagectomy) can induce dysrhythmias and/or ↓ BP. Monitoring of BP with an arterial catheter is recommended.	
Emergence	Generally, tracheal extubation should be anticipated at the end of the case. The decision to keep the patient intubated postop depends on cardiopulmonary status and the site and extent of the surgical procedure. Patients with significant intraop fluid shift may develop airway edema that can → airway obstruction if extubated prematurely. This may also occur in operations involving high anastomoses in the neck. For those who may require prolonged postop ventilation, the DLT should be exchanged to a single-lumen ETT before transport to ICU. The use of an airway exchange catheter is safe, and direct laryngoscopy during the exchange prevents inadvertent seepage of blood or silent aspiration. Weaning from mechanical ventilation should begin when the patient is awake and cooperative, able to protect the airway, hemodynamically stable, and has adequate return of pulmonary function (as measured by VC > = 10 mL/kg; MIF of > 30 cmH_2O; rapid, shallow breathing index of ≤ 100 [RR÷TV(L)]; respiratory rate < 25; and ABG that demonstrates adequate gas exchange).	
Blood and fluid requirements	IV: 14–16 ga × 1–2 NS/LR @ 8–12 mL/kg/h Warm fluids Consider T&C for 2–4 U PRBC	Plt, FFP, and cryoprecipitate (if required) should be administered according to lab tests (Plt count, PT, PTT, DIC screen, thromboelastography [TEG]). Maintain euvolemia based on estimates of blood loss, fluid shifts, fluids administered, and HR, BP, UO, base deficit, and invasive monitoring when employed.
Monitoring	Standard monitors (p. B-1) Urinary catheter ± Arterial line ± CVP	CVP cannulation site determined by surgical approach. Attempt to prevent hypothermia during long operations. Consider forced-air warmer, heated humidifier, warming blanket, warming the OR, keeping patient covered until ready for prep, etc.
Positioning	If lateral decubitus position, use axillary roll, airplane arm holder ✓ pressure points, including ears, eyes, and genitals ✓ radial pulses to ensure correct placement of axillary roll (if misplaced, will compromise distal pulses).	Problems that can arise include brachial plexus injuries, damage to soft tissues, ears, eyes, genitals from malpositioning. Check down eye at frequent intervals. Placing the oximeter probe on the down arm may assist in monitoring adequacy of perfusion.
Complications	Hypoxemia	Hypoxemia during OLV most commonly results from luminal obstruction (by blood or pulmonary secretions) of the DLT; ✓ shunting, or malposition of DLT, which can move during surgical manipulation. Rx: suction DLT and ✓ position; PEEP to ventilated lung (but may ↑ shunting); CPAP to nonventilated lung; return to double-lung ventilation. Temporary clamping of the PA (or inflate the balloon of the PA catheter, if available) may be necessary to improve shunting and oxygenation.
	Hypercarbia	Ensure adequate TV and RR.
	Dysrhythmia	✓ for mechanical compression of heart or great vessels. Check K^+

General Surgery

Complications (cont'd)	Hypotension	✓ volume status and cardiac function. Consider neosynephrine for BP support if ↓ BP 2° epidural anesthetic. Maintaining an adequate BP is important for adequate perfusion and hence integrity of a newly formed anastomosis.
	VTE Prophylaxis	See Appendix B

POSTOPERATIVE

Complications	Aspiration Atelectasis Hemorrhage Pneumothorax Hemothorax	For patients at risk for atelectasis or aspiration, recover in the 45° head up or Fowler position (semi sitting) For hemorrhage, ✓ coags; replace factors as necessary. Dx for pneumothorax and hemothorax: wheezing, coughing, dyspnea, ↓ PO_2, ↓ PCO_2. Confirm by CXR. Rx: chest tube drainage as necessary. In emergency (e.g., tension pneumothorax), use needle aspiration. Supportive Rx: O_2, vasopressors, volume, ± ETT and IPPV.
	Hypoxemia Hypoventilation	For hypoxemia and hypoventilation; Rx: adequate analgesia, minimize sedation, supplemental O_2, may require IPPV.
	Recurrent laryngeal nerve injury	For laryngeal nerve injury, Dx: indirect visualization of vocal cords; patient usually will be hoarse.
	Esophageal anastomotic leak	Surgical repair Rx for esophageal anastomotic leak.
	VTE prophylaxis	
	SVT/AFib	Treat underlying cause and correct electrolyte abnormalities. Adenosine (6 mg iv, push and repeat to 12 mg iv) may be used for SVT. Most postop SVTs are 2° catecholamine surge. AFib may resolve spontaneously. Hemodynamically unstable patients will require cardioversion. β-blockers, amiodarone, Ca^{++} channel blockers, and overdrive cardiac pacing are effective in patients with stable AFib.
Pain management	Lumbar-thoracic epidural analgesia: hydromorphone (0.5–1.5 mg load, 0.1–0.3 mg/h infusion) + local anesthetic PCEA (p. C-3).	Patient should recover in ICU or hospital ward that is accustomed to treating side effects of epidural opiates (e.g., respiratory depression, hypotension, breakthrough pain, nausea, pruritus)
	PCA	When an epidural cannot be used, a PCA with an opiate such as fentanyl or morphine/hydromorphone may be used for pain control.
	NSAID	Ketorolac is helpful as adjuvant therapy for postop pain management.
Tests	CBC, basic metabolic profile, ABG CXR (r/o pneumothorax, atelectasis).	

Suggested Readings

1. Al-Rawi OY, Pennefather SH, Page RD, et al: The effect of thoracic epidural bupivacaine and an intravenous adrenalin infusion on gastric tube blood flow during esophagectomy. *Anesth Analg* 2008; 106:884–7.
2. Amar D: Cardiopulmonary complications of esophageal surgery. *Chest Surg Clin N Am* 1997; 7(3):449–56.
3. Cohen E, Neustein SM, Eisenkraft JB: Anesthesia for thoracic surgery. In: *Clinical Anesthesia,* 5th edition. Barash, PG, Cullen BF, Stoelting RK eds. JB Lippincott Williams & Wilkins, Philadelphia: 2006, 813–55.
4. Kahn L, Baxter FJ, Dauphin A, et al: A comparison of thoracic and lumbar epidural techniques for post-thoracoabdominal esophagectomy analgesia. *Can J Anaesth* 1999; 46(5 Pt 1):415–22.

5. Kolker AC: Esophageal surgery. In: *Cardiac, Vascular, and Thoracic Anesthesia.* Youngberg JA, Lake CL, Roizen MF, Wilson RS, eds. Churchill Livingstone, Philadelphia: 2000, 688–702.
6. Kucharczuk JC, Kaiser LR: Esophageal injury, diverticula, and neoplasms. In: *Greenfield's Surgery: Scientific Principles and Practice,* 4th edition. Mulholland MW, Lillemoe KD, et al, eds. Lippincott Williams & Wilkins, Philadelphia: 2006, 691–708.
7. Nagawa H, Kobori O, Muto T: Prediction of pulmonary complications after transthoracic oesophagectomy. *Br J Surg* 1994; 81(6):860–2.
8. Nichols FC, Allen MS, Deschamps C, et al: Ivor Lewis Esophagogastrectomy. *Surg Clin N Am* 2005; 85: 583–92.
9. Orringer MB, Orringer JS: Esophagectomy without thoracotomy: a dangerous operation? *J Thorac Cardiovasc Surg* 1983; 85(1):72–80.
10. Pennefather SH: Anesthesia for Oesophagectomy: *Curr Opin Anaesthesiol* 2007; 20:15–20.
11. Slinger PD, Hickey DR: The interaction between applied PEEP and auto-PEEP during one-lung ventilation. *J Cardiothorac Vasc Anesth* 1998; 12(2):133–6.
12. Smetana GW: Preoperative pulmonary evaluation. *N Eng J Med* 1999; 340(1):937–44.

CHAPTER

7.2 Stomach Surgery

SURGEONS

Sherry M. Wren MD
Myriam J. Curet, MD (*Open operations for morbid obesity*)

ANESTHESIOLOGISTS

Kevin A. Malott, MD
Jay B. Brodsky, MD (*Open operations for morbid obesity*)

GASTRIC RESECTIONS

SURGICAL CONSIDERATIONS

Description: **Total or partial gastrectomy** is performed most commonly for gastric cancers (adenocarcinomas or Gastrointestinal Stromal Tumors GIST), and will include **omentectomy, lymph node dissection,** and occasionally resection of adjacent organs such as the **spleen** or **colon,** depending on the extent of the tumor. Historically there have been other indications for gastrectomy such as ulcer disease, Zollinger-Ellison syndrome and uncontrollable hemorrhagic gastritis, but these operations are rarely if ever performed for those indications in current surgical practice. Occasionally patients who suffer from severe and uncontrollable gastroparesis postgastric surgery may require total gastrectomy.

In a gastric resection, the abdomen is entered through an upper midline incision and the lateral segment of the left lobe of the liver is retracted to the patient's right, exposing the esophagogastric junction. The omentum is taken off of the colon and left attached to the greater curvature of the stomach. The spleen may be removed if involved by tumor or if an unplanned splenic injury occurs. The vessels to the stomach are individually ligated and divided. The short gastric vessels high on the greater curvature are difficult to reach and are a source of potential blood loss. This is also the most likely time that a splenic injury may occur by traction or tearing of the capsule in exposing the short gastric arteries. Currently most surgeons are using various devices to ligate the arteries and these occasionally have a technical failure which can result in blood loss. In the lesser sac, the left gastric artery as it branches from the celiac axis and vein needs to be divided and can be another point of potential unexpected blood loss. A total gastrectomy is performed for more proximal cancers and a partial resection for distal cancers. In all cases of gastric cancer, the antrum and pylorus are resected. One area of potential complication when the stomach is resected is the accidental stapling of the NG tube which remains undetected until too late. To prevent this, the NGT should be pulled back well into the esophagus, preferably with manual confirmation by the surgeon that the tube is no longer present in the stomach.

After completion of the gastric resection, reestablishment of intestinal continuity is performed. In the case of a total gastrectomy, a Roux limb of jejunum will be brought up to the distal esophagus; in partial gastrectomies a Roux limb or loop of jejunum (Billroth II) is connected to the stomach. With a Roux limb the jejunum is divided just beyond the Ligament of Treitz, and the distal end is brought up through a hole in the mesentery of the colon and anastomosed to the esophagus or stomach. Intestinal continuity is established by anastomosing the biliary pancreatic limb of the jejunum to the Roux limb of jejunum, approximately 60 cm distal to the anastomosis with the esophagus. A drain is then placed near the closed end of the duodenum. These anastomosis can either be stapled or handsewn depending on the preference of the surgeon. At completion of the anastomosis a NG tube is advanced across the proximal anastomosis, and the abdomen is irrigated. A number of surgeons will then place a feeding jejunostomy tube into the jejunum which adds a few minutes to the procedure prior to fascial closure. Total gastrectomy traditionally has been associated with a morbidity and mortality out of proportion to the operation's apparent magnitude. This is most likely a consequence of the patient's underlying condition, which often includes advanced malignancy and, almost invariably, some degree of malnutrition. Venous thromboembolism (VTE) is a significant concern in these patients because of their increased hypercoagulable state from the cancer and an operation of greater than one hour in duration. Patients undergoing gastric resection should receive sequential compression devices on the lower extremities and 5000 units of standard Heparin subcutaneously after placement of an epidural catheter. If an epidural catheter is not placed, the patient can receive low molecular weight heparin for VTE prophylaxis.

Variant procedure or approaches: Occasionally a gastric cancer can have extensive local involvement of adjacent organs requiring an **en bloc resection** of the stomach in addition to the colon, spleen, or pancreas. For certain distal gastric cancers a combined gastric resection with a **Whipple procedure (pancreaticoduodenectomy)** may be necessary. The need for en bloc resection of the stomach in combination with other organs increases the complexity of the surgery, risk of blood loss, and postoperative morbidity and mortality. In general, exposure for a **partial gastrectomy** is similar to, but less extensive than that required for a total gastrectomy. The same cancer principles are followed for either a partial or total resection including > 5 cm proximal margin, lymphadenectomy, and omentectomy. A partial gastrectomy is a simpler resection. The blood supply to the distal stomach is divided, and the duodenum is divided just beyond the pylorus. The body of the stomach is divided with a staples (care should be taken to not staple the NG tube) at a level appropriate for the pathology. Reconstruction may be either to the duodenum (**Billroth I**), loop of jejunum (**Billroth II**) (Fig. 7.2-1), or to a **Roux-en-Y loop of jejunum.** The anastomoses may be

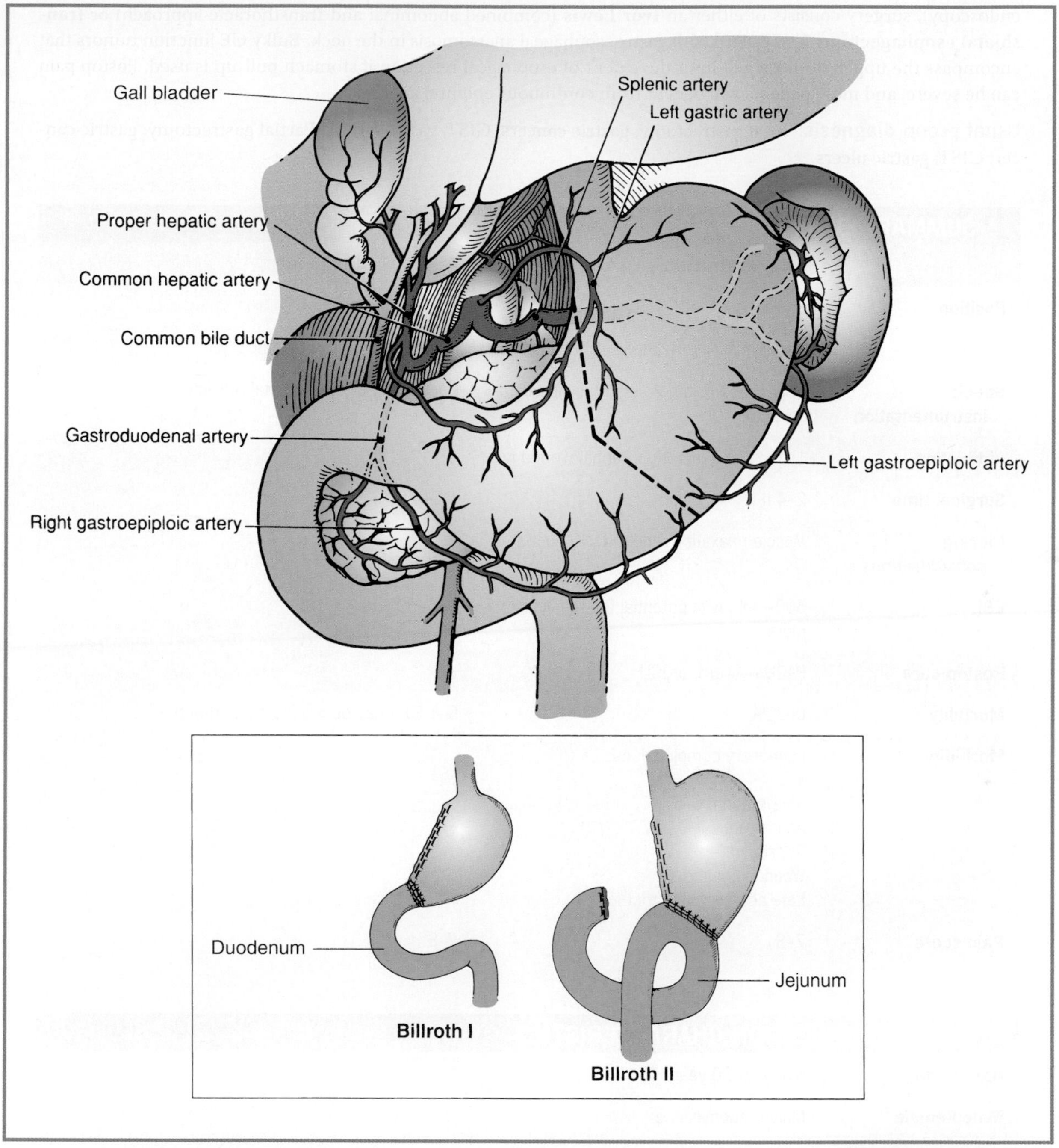

Figure 7.2-1. Anatomy of duodenostomy (Billroth I) and gastrojejunostomy (Billroth II). (Reproduce d with permission from Scott-Conner CEH, Dawson DL: *Operative Anatomy,* 2nd edition. Lippincott Williams & Wilkins, Philadelphia: 2003.)

stapled or sewn; then the abdomen is closed. Like many operations, gastric resections are increasingly performed using minimally invasive techniques. The **laparoscopic approach** has the advantages of diminished postoperative pain and quicker recovery, but the operations have a longer operative time, require a pneumoperitoneum, and reverse Trendelenburg positioning.

Tumors (usually adenocarcinoma) of the gastroesophageal (GE) junction are increasing in frequency and may be of either gastric or esophageal origin. Resection frequently requires a team of thoracic, general, or laparoscopic surgeons. If the tumor is associated with Barrett's esophagus (intestinal metaplasia in the esophagus, seen on endoscopy), surgery consists of either an **Ivor Lewis** (combined abdominal and transthoracic approach) or **transhiatal esophagectomy** (see p. 480) with gastroesophageal anastomosis in the neck. Bulky GE junction tumors that encompass the upper stomach will limit the extent of esophageal resection if stomach pull-up is used. Postop pain can be severe, and most patients will benefit from continuous epidural analgesia.

Usual preop diagnosis: Total gastrectomy: gastric cancers, GIST, gastroparesis; Partial gastrectomy: gastric cancer; GIST, gastric ulcers.

SUMMARY OF PROCEDURES

	Total Gastrectomy	Partial Gastrectomy
Position	Supine	⇐
Incision	Upper midline or bilateral subcostal	Upper midline or right subcostal
Special instrumentation	Upper-hand or other self-retaining costal retractor	Upper-hand or other costal retractor
Antibiotics	1st or 2nd generation Cephalosporin iv	⇐
Surgical time	2–4 h	1.5–2 h
Closing considerations	Muscle relaxation required; NG suction	⇐
EBL	500+ mL, with potential for significantly more	100–500 mL
Postop care	PACU → ward, or ICU	⇐
Mortality	0–22%	0–1.8% (may be > 10% if emergent)
Morbidity	Pulmonary complications: 15%	
	VTE	⇐
	Reoperation: 0–5%	
	Anastomotic leak	⇐
	Sepsis	
	Wound infection	⇐
	Late anastomotic stricture	
Pain score	7–8	7–8

PATIENT POPULATION CHARACTERISTICS

Age range	Mostly > 50 years
Male:Female	Male predominance
Incidence	In the United States, people of Korean, Japanese, Latino, and African American race have a higher incidence than Caucasians.
Etiology	Gastric adenocarcinoma, gastrointestinal stromal tumors associated with: race, age, alcohol and tobacco use, geographic location, and gastric ulcers.
Associated conditions	Weight loss (common); anemia (common); malnutrition (common); VTE

ANESTHETIC CONSIDERATIONS

See Anesthetic Considerations following Operations for Peptic Ulcer Disease, p. 497.

Suggested Readings

1. Adachi Y, Kitano S, Sugimachi K: Surgery for gastric cancer: 10-year experience worldwide. *Gastric Cancer* 2001; 4(4):166–74.
2. Aoki T, Takayama S: Subtotal gastrectomy for gastric cancer. In: *Mastery of Surgery,* 4th edition. Baker RJ, Fischer JE, eds. Lippincott Williams & Wilkins, Philadelphia: 2001, 982–96.
3. Bozzetti F: Principles of surgical radicality in the treatment of gastric cancer. *Surg Oncol Clin N Am* 2001; 10(4):833–54, ix.
4. Brennan MR: Total gastrectomy for carcinoma. In: *Mastery of Surgery,* 4th edition. Baker RJ, Fischer JE, eds. Lippincott Williams & Wilkins, Philadelphia: 2001, 997–1006.
5. Mulholland MW: Gastric neoplasms. In: *Surgery: Scientific Principles and Practice,* 4rd edition. Greenfield LJ, et al, eds. Lippincott Williams & Wilkins, Philadelphia: 2006, 743–55.
6. Soybel DI, Zinner MJ: Stomach and duodenum, operative procedures: In: *Maingot's Abdominal Operations,* Vol. I, 11th edition. Zinner MJ, Ashley SW, eds. McGraw-Hill, New York: 2006, 377–416.

GASTRIC OR DUODENAL PERFORATION

SURGICAL CONSIDERATIONS

Description: Patients who present with gastric or duodenal perforations require emergency surgery since they usually have peritonitis at presentation. The primary reason for perforations that present to the emergency room is ulcer disease most likely from H. pylori infection or from NSAID use. Another cause of gastric perforation is trauma, but that is not in the scope of this section. Simple closure with an omental patch, also called a **Graham's patch,** is the most commonly performed operation. It would be unusual to have a surgeon perform a definitive ulcer operation unless the patient has failed medical treatment regimens aimed at eradication of H. pylori infection along with proton pump inhibitors to suppress acid production.

Duodenal ulcers are almost considered a benign process but gastric ulcer perforation without a history of NSAID use is suspicious of a malignant process. For this reason, surgeons may elect to treat a perforated gastric ulcer by resection. Occasionally in patients who have failed maximal medical management of their peptic ulcer disease and who are not systemically ill at the time of operation, some surgeons may perform **vagotomy and pyloroplasty** or **highly selective vagotomy,** at the time of closure of the perforation.

Many surgeons routinely perform simple closure with **Graham's patch** via a **laparoscopic** approach. This requires a few trocars and a pneumoperitoneum, and can be combined with abdominal washout and irrigation. If an **open approach** is used, an upper midline incision is used. The liver is retracted superiorly and the area of perforation identified. An NG tube will have been placed preop and should remain on suction throughout the case to minimize ongoing leakage from the perforation. Perforation of the stomach may be handled either by resection (see Gastric Resections, p. 490) or by biopsy and simple suture closure. Perforation of the duodenum is usually repaired by simple suture of the site. Omentum often is used to buttress (Graham's patch) the area of closure of the stomach or duodenum. The abdomen is irrigated and closed.

Variant procedure or approaches: In certain patients, **nonoperative management** of perforated ulcer may be appropriate if they have had an upper GI study that shows an ulcer cavity and no extravasation. These patients are treated with NG decompression, antibiotics, and proton pump inhibitors. In general, this has a relatively high likelihood of success if the candidates are chosen well.

Usual preop diagnosis: Free air under diaphragm and peritonitis, perforated peptic ulcer

SUMMARY OF PROCEDURE	
Position	Supine
Incision	Midline or 3–4 trocars for laparoscopic approach
Special instrumentation	Costal retractor or laparoscopic equipment

SUMMARY OF PROCEDURE (cont'd)	
Unique considerations	Patients usually have peritonitis.
Antibiotics	Cefotetan or extended spectrum PCN
Surgical time	1 h
Closing considerations	Muscle relaxation required ; NG suction
EBL	Minimal
Postop care	PACU → ward
Mortality	5–15%, largely dependent on patient population
Morbidity	Pneumonia Intraabdominal abscess Sepsis Wound infection Reperforation
Pain score	7 for open procedure, 3 for laparoscopic

PATIENT POPULATION CHARACTERISTICS	
Age range	Adult, more common in socially disadvantaged populations
Male:Female	Previous heavy male predominance still exists for duodenal ulcer, but there has been a large increase in incidence in gastric perforation in women > 65.
Incidence	Fairly common. Stable incidence, but with change in distribution, especially more elderly women.
Etiology	Peptic ulcer disease (PUD); nonsteroidal medications; malignancy (if gastric)
Associated conditions	Malignancy (if perforation is gastric); nonsteroidal medications; steroid use, especially during pulse therapy; other risk factors for PUD (e.g., alcoholism, smoking, etc.)

ANESTHETIC CONSIDERATIONS

See Anesthetic Considerations following Operations for Peptic Ulcer Disease, p. 497.

Suggested Readings

1. Kasakura Y, Ajani JA, Fujii M, Mochizuki F, Takayama T: Management of perforated gastric carcinoma: a report of 16 cases and review of world literature. *Am Surg* 2002; 68(5):434–40.
2. Mulholland MW: Gastroduodenal Ulceration: In: *Surgery: Scientific Principles and Practice,* 4rd edition. Greenfield LJ, et al, eds. Lippincott Williams & Wilkins, Philadelphia: 2006, 722–35.
3. Sawyers JL: Acute perforation of peptic ulcer. In: *Surgery of the Stomach, Duodenum and Small Intestine.* Scott HW Jr, Sawyers JL, eds. Blackwell Scientific Publications, Boston: 1992, 566–72.
4. Soybel DI, Zinner MJ: Ulcer complications: In: *Maingot's Abdominal Operations,* Vol. I, 11th edition. Zinner MJ, Ashley SW, eds. McGraw-Hill Companies, New York: 2006, 377–416.
5. Svanes C: Trends in perforated peptic ulcer: incidence, etiology, treatment, and prognosis. *World J Surg* 2000; 24(3):277–83.

OPERATIONS FOR PEPTIC ULCER DISEASE

SURGICAL CONSIDERATIONS

These operations are not commonly performed by surgeons and most recently trained general surgeons have never seen or performed an operation for PUD.

Description: Gastric ulcers are commonly associated with advanced age, and patients often have other medical problems, particularly cardiovascular and pulmonary. Two developments have transformed peptic ulcer disease (PUD) from a common surgical problem to a rare surgical emergency (e.g., perforation and bleeding typically in the chronically ill, hospitalized patient). These developments are: (1) inhibitors of gastric acid secretion, and (2) the role of gastric overgrowth by *Helicobacter pylori.* The first antisecretory drugs were H_2-receptor antagonists (e.g., cimetidine, ranitidine); however, proton pump inhibitors (PPIs) have proven to be more effective. The treatment of *H. pylori* consists of 14 d of a PPI, plus antibiotic therapy. The medical management of PUD has so revolutionized the treatment of this disease that few current graduating residents have seen or done the surgical procedures described below. All operations for PUD require exposure of the upper abdomen and may be performed using either an upper midline or a long, right subcostal incision. The choice of surgical procedure depends on a number of considerations, including: whether it is performed as an emergency or electively; the reason for performing the procedure (common factors include bleeding, perforation, intractability, or gastric outlet obstruction); duration of symptoms; condition of the patient; and experience of the surgeon.

Vagotomy and antrectomy (V&A): This is the most extensive of the operations performed for PUD, and generally is reserved for healthy patients with intractable symptoms. The esophageal hiatus is exposed either by taking down the lateral segment of the left lobe of the liver and reflecting it to the patient's right, or by retracting this segment of the liver superiorly to gain exposure. The phrenoesophageal ligament is divided and the anterior and posterior vagus nerves (there may be more than one of each) are identified by feel. Division of all vagal trunks at the esophageal hiatus is performed. The blood supply to the antrum is then divided, usually by dividing the right gastric and gastroepiploic vessels first. The gastrohepatic ligament is divided and the stomach elevated off of its attachments to the transverse colon. The gastric antrum is resected, leaving the duodenum just beyond the pylorus and dividing the stomach just above the junction of the body with the antrum. Reconstruction may be as a **Billroth I** (stomach-to-duodenum) or **Billroth II** (stomach-to-jejunal loop) (Fig. 7.2-1). The anastomosis may be stapled or hand-sewn. Drains are not commonly used if a Billroth I is performed, but may be used in Billroth II because of the concern for a leak from the duodenal stump.

Vagotomy and pyloroplasty (V&P): This is the most commonly performed operation for PUD in the United States and is especially common for emergency operations. It is generally accepted to be simpler and safer to perform than V&A, but not as effective at preventing recurrence of ulcer disease. The abdominal incision and exposure of the hiatus to perform a vagotomy is the same as for V&P. After division of both vagal trunks (Fig. 7.2-2), a longitudinal incision is made through the pylorus. The incision is then sutured together transversely, completing the pyloroplasty.

Parietal cell vagotomy (PCV): This operation requires even more meticulous exposure of the esophageal hiatus than that needed for a truncal vagotomy. The hiatus is exposed as above, and the main vagal trunks supplying the stomach are identified, but not divided. The stomach is retracted downward, and it is often helpful to divide a portion of the gastrocolic omentum to facilitate grasping the stomach. Branches supplying the body of the stomach (Fig. 7.2-2) are individually divided and ligated with fine ligatures. Because the nerve fibers run with the blood vessels to the stomach, this necessarily involves division of the blood supply to the proximal lesser curvature of the stomach.

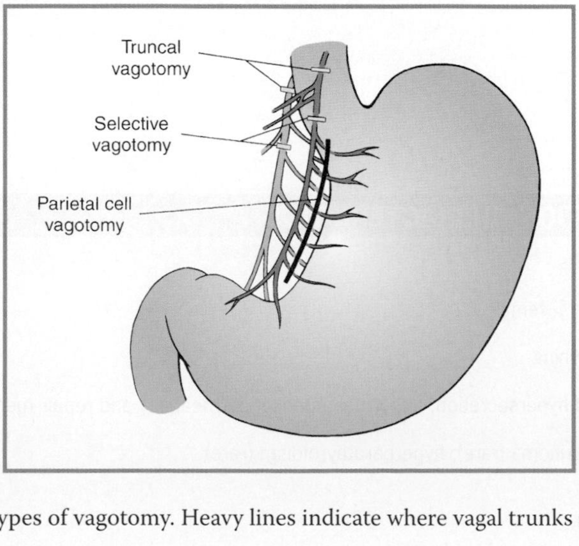

Figure 7.2-2. Types of vagotomy. Heavy lines indicate where vagal trunks are cut.

This dissection is carried to the region of the "crow's foot" of the stomach, which is preserved. By denervating only the acid-producing portion of the stomach, while preserving innervation to the antrum, gastric acidity is diminished without significantly impairing gastric motility or emptying. A pyloroplasty is, therefore, not necessary. The operation is relatively tedious compared to the other procedures, and usually is performed electively or, rarely, urgently if there is a recent perforation and minimal soilage. It can be recommended only for duodenal ulcer disease, not gastric ulcers. Side effects of this operation are generally less than with other ulcer operations.

Variant procedure or approaches: **Laparoscopic approaches** to the treatment of gastroduodenal ulcer are also being used.

Usual preop diagnosis: V&P: complications of duodenal ulcer disease (bleeding, perforation, and gastric outlet obstruction). V&A: duodenal and prepyloric ulcer disease. PCV: isolated duodenal ulcer disease; recent perforation and minimal peritoneal soilage

SUMMARY OF PROCEDURES

	V&P	V&A	PCV
Position	Supine	⇐	⇐
Incision	Midline or long subcostal	⇐	Midline
Special instrumentation	Costal margin retractor	⇐	⇐
Antibiotics	Cefotetan 1 g iv	⇐	Cefazolin 1 g iv
Surgical time	1–2 h	1.5–3 h	1.5–2.5 h
Closing considerations	Muscle relaxation required for closure; NG suction	⇐	⇐
EBL	< 250 mL; greater for emergency surgeries	250–500 mL	< 250 mL
Postop care	PACU → ward	⇐	⇐
Mortality	0–2% (most series include emergencies)	0–1.6% (most series do not include emergencies)	0–0.4%
Morbidity	Dumping and diarrhea: 6–20% Recurrence: 4.9–12.3%	17–27% 0–2%	— 5–15% Impaired gastric emptying: 0.3% Necrosis, lesser curve: < 0.3% PE: rare
Pain score	6	6	6

PATIENT POPULATION CHARACTERISTICS

Age range	Adults
Male:Female	Male > female
Incidence	Declining
Etiology	Acid hypersecretion; abnormal mucosal permeability and repair mechanisms; *H. pylori*
Associated conditions	Gastrinoma (rare); hyperparathyroidism (rare)

ANESTHETIC CONSIDERATIONS

(Procedures covered: gastric resections; oversew gastric/duodenal perforation operations for peptic ulcer disease; duodenotomy)

PREOPERATIVE

Patients presenting for gastric surgery generally comprise two groups: (1) those presenting for emergency surgery following GI bleeding or perforation, and (2) those presenting with gastric carcinoma or elective treatment of PUD (rare). Patients in the first group are often hemodynamically unstable and require rapid preop assessment and appropriate fluid resuscitation. It is prudent to consider full-stomach precautions in both patient groups (see p. B-4).

Respiratory	Patients with GI bleeding are at ↑ risk for aspiration of blood and gastric contents. If this has occurred, patient may have significant respiratory insufficiency (in urgent need of tracheal intubation for "protection" of airway). **Tests:** CXR; consider ABG
Cardiovascular	Hypovolemia may be severe due to N/V, diarrhea, poor po intake, peritonitis, or GI blood loss. Sx include ↓skin turgor, ↑HR, ↓BP, ↓UO. Correct hypovolemia before induction of anesthesia. **Tests:** Orthostatic vital signs; ECG, if indicated from H&P.
Renal	GI fluid loss can lead to renal and electrolyte abnormalities. **Tests:** Consider electrolytes; BUN; Cr.
Hematologic	Misleading ↑Hct 2° GI fluid loss may be present; patients with GI bleeding will likely be anemic and may have a coagulopathy. Correct coagulopathy and anemia before induction, if possible. **Tests:** CBC with Plts, PT/PTT if coagulopathy suspected
Laboratory	Other tests as indicated from H&P
Premedication	Consider midazolam 1–2 mg. Consider H_2-antagonist (ranitidine 50 mg iv slowly), metoclopramide (10 mg iv 1 h preop), and Na citrate (30 mL po 10 min preop). Prophylactic antibiotics should be considered if the patient has been rendered achlorhydric.

INTRAOPERATIVE

Anesthetic technique: GETA ± epidural for postop analgesia (if hemodynamically stable and no coagulopathy). If postop epidural analgesia is planned, insertion of catheter prior to anesthetic induction is helpful to establish correct placement in the epidural space (accomplished by injecting 5–7 mL of 1% lidocaine via the epidural catheter, eliciting a segmental block).

Induction	The patient with gastric disease or upper GI bleeding is often at risk for pulmonary aspiration, and the trachea should be intubated with the patient awake or after rapid-sequence induction with cricoid pressure (see p. B-4). If patient is clinically hypovolemic, restore intravascular volume (colloid, crystalloid, or blood products) before induction, and titrate induction dose of sedative/hypnotic agents.
Maintenance	Standard maintenance (see p. B-2). Balanced anesthesia with inhalational agents and/or propofol infusion, and opiates. Maintain muscle relaxation based on nerve stimulator response. Discuss with surgeon the need for postop NG tube. If not needed, place OG tube to evacuate stomach contents intraop. **Combined epidural/GA:** A local anesthetic (2% lidocaine with 1:200,000 epinephrine) can be injected into a thoracic (3–5 mL) or lumbar (3–6 mL q 60–90 min) epidural catheter to provide both anesthesia and optimal surgical exposure (contracted bowel and profound muscle relaxation). A continuous infusion of local anesthetic (e.g., 2% lidocaine or 0.25% bupivacaine at 3–10 mL/h [lumbar]; 2–5 mL/h [thoracic]), may enhance hemodynamic stability, compared to an intermittent bolus. Be prepared to treat ↓ BP with fluid and vasopressors. GA is administered to supplement regional anes

Maintenance (cont'd)	thesia and for amnesia. Systemic sedatives should be minimized during epidural opiate administration as they increase the likelihood of postop respiratory depression. Treat ↓BP with fluid and vasopressors. If epidural opiates are used for postop analgesia, a loading dose (e.g., hydromorphone 0.6–1.0 mg [lumbar]; 0.4–0.6 mg [thoracic]) may be administered at least 1 h before conclusion of surgery.	
Emergence	The decision to extubate at the end of surgery depends on the patient's underlying cardiopulmonary status and extent of the surgical procedure. Patient should be hemodynamically stable, normothermic, alert, cooperative, and fully reversed from any muscle relaxants and without pulmonary compromise before extubation.	
Blood and fluid requirements	Anticipate large third-space losses IV: 14–16 ga ×1–2 NS/LR @ 8–12 mL/kg/h Fluid warmer	T&C for 4 U PRBC. Plts, FFP, and cryoprecipitate should be administered according to lab tests (Plt count, PT, PTT, DIC screen, thromboelastography). Expect higher fluid requirements if epidural used (2° sympathectomy → vasodilation). Maintaining euvolemia is important goal.
Monitoring	Standard monitors (p. B-1) UO ± Arterial line ± CVP	Consider others as indicated by patient's status. Prevent hypothermia: Use forced air warmer, fluid warmer, and consider warming blanket, warm room temperature, keeping patient covered until ready for prep, etc.
Positioning	✓ and pad pressure points ✓ eyes	
Complications	Acute hemorrhage Hypoxemia	 2° abdominal packs →↓FRC

POSTOPERATIVE

Complications	PONV (see p. B-6) Hemorrhage VTE (see p. B-7) Ileus Hypothermia
Pain management	Epidural analgesics (p. C-2) PCA (p. C-3)
Tests	CXR if CVP placed periop

Suggested Readings

1. Kauffman GL Jr: Duodenal ulcer disease: treatment by surgery, antibiotics, or both. *Adv Surg* 2000; 34:121–35.
2. Nyhus LM: Selective vagotomy, antrectomy, and gastroduodenostomy for the treatment of duodenal ulcer. In: *Mastery of Surgery,* 4th edition. Baker RJ, Fischer JE, eds. Lippincott Williams & Wilkins, Philadelphia: 2001, 921–32.
3. Sawyers JL, Richards WO: Selective vagotomy and pyloroplasty. In: *Mastery of Surgery,* 4th edition. Baker RJ, Fischer JE, eds. Lippincott Williams & Wilkins, Philadelphia: 2001, 933–41.
4. Soybel DI, Zinner MJ: Ulcer complications: In: *Maingot's Abdominal Operations,* Vol. I, 11th edition. Zinner MJ, Ashley SW, eds. McGraw-Hill Companies, New York: 2006, 377–416.
5. Wing TS, Leong HT, Law BKB, et al: Laparoscopic repair for perforated peptic ulcer, a randomized controlled trial. *Ann Surg* 2002; 235(3): 313–9.
6. Zittel TT, Jehle EC, Becker HD: Surgical management of peptic ulcer disease today indication, technique and outcome. *Langenbecks Arch Surg* 2000; 385(2)84–96.

OPEN OPERATIONS FOR MORBID OBESITY

SURGICAL CONSIDERATIONS

Description: Open procedures for morbid obesity have been largely replaced by the laparoscopic approach (see p. 598). In selected patients (e.g., those with previous upper abdominal surgery or BMI > 60 [see p. 502]), however, open procedures may be more appropriate. Open techniques devised to promote weight loss are of two fundamental types: (1) **gastric partitioning procedures,** which work by decreasing the size of the gastric pouch, thereby limiting the amount of food that can be consumed at one time; and (2) **malabsorptive procedures,** which work by bypassing most of the small bowel and creating a state of chronic malabsorption. Of these two general types of procedures, the partitioning procedures are generally less effective at promoting weight loss than are the malabsorptive procedures, but are much more popular because they are associated with far fewer serious side effects.

One partitioning procedure more commonly used in the past is the **vertical banded gastroplasty (VBG).** The abdomen is entered through an upper midline incision, and the esophagogastric junction is exposed either by retracting the liver superiorly or by taking down the ligamentous attachments of the lateral segment of the left lobe of the liver and retracting this down and to the patient's right. The vessels to the lesser curvature are separated for a short distance near the esophagogastric junction, and the posterior attachments of the stomach are separated. A large bougie is passed by the anesthesiologist into the stomach and a circular stapler is used to create a hole in the stomach adjacent to the bougie near the esophagogastric junction. Through this, a special stapler with thick, strong staples is passed and is fired up along the esophagus, creating a pouch of approximately 30 mL in volume (Fig. 7.2-3). This leaves an outlet to the remainder of the stomach of only 1–2 cm, which is reinforced with a band of mesh. An NG tube is placed through the gastroplasty into the distal stomach and the abdomen is closed without drains.

More commonly performed today than the gastroplasty is the **Roux-en-Y gastric bypass** (Fig. 7.2-4). Exposure is similar to that for a VBG. The upper stomach is mobilized and two rows of staples are used to partition the stomach into a small proximal and large distal pouch. A Roux segment of jejunum is then anastomosed to the small proximal pouch to provide drainage of it. An NG tube is placed and the abdomen is closed without drains.

Variant procedure or approaches: An alternative open procedure is the **jejunoileal (JI) bypass** (Fig. 7.2-5), in which the proximal jejunum is anastomosed to the terminal ileum. This procedure has been largely abandoned because of the many associated complications, including cirrhosis, osteoporosis, kidney stones, and intractable diarrhea. Another alternative open procedure is a **sleeve gastrectomy** where a gastric tube is created from the gastroesophageal junction to the pylorus over a 36°F dilator. The remainder of the stomach, based on the greater curvature is resected.

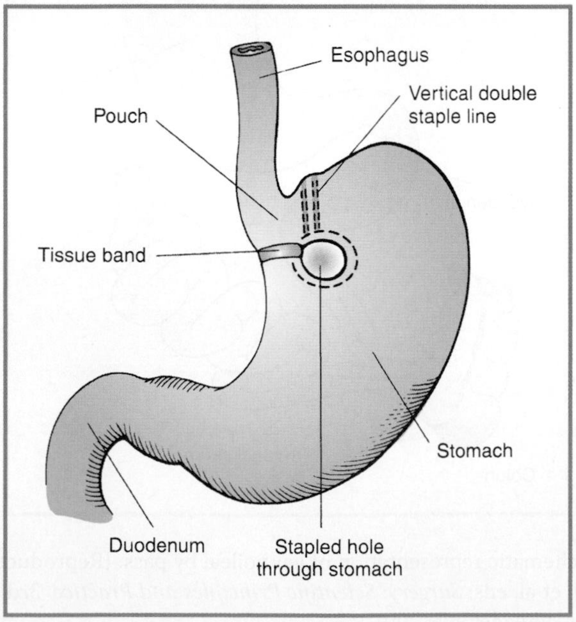

Figure 7.2-3. Vertical banded gastroplasty.

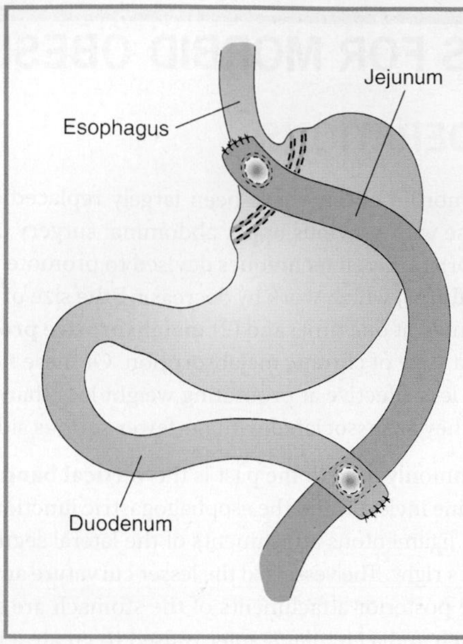

Figure 7.2-4. Proximal Roux-en-Y gastric bypass. (Reproduced with permission from Greenfield LJ, et al, eds: *Surgery: Scientific Principles and Practice,* 3rd edition. Lippincott Williams & Wilkins, Philadelphia: 2001.)

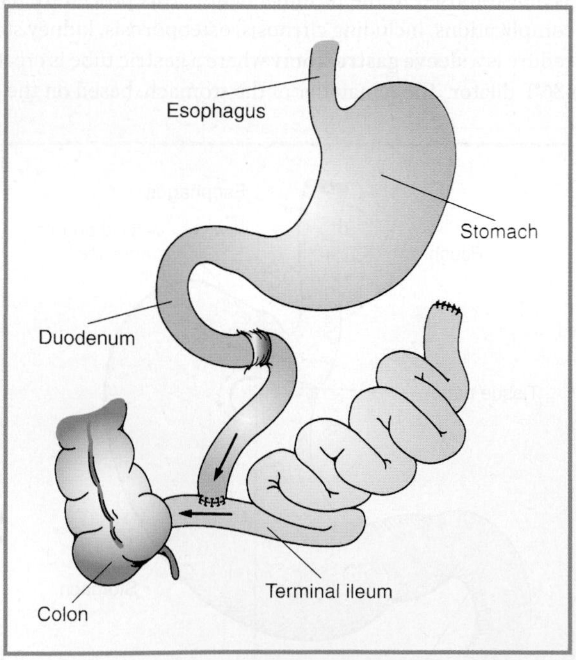

Figure 7.2-5. Schematic representation of jejunoileal by pass. (Reproduced with permission from Greenfield LJ, et al, eds: *Surgery: Scientific Principles and Practice,* 3rd edition. Lippincott Williams & Wilkins, Philadelphia: 2001.)

Usual preop diagnosis: Morbid obesity (> 100 lbs above ideal body weight, 100% over ideal body weight, or BMI > 40), generally in combination with some medical condition felt to be worsened by the obesity (e.g., osteoarthritis, diabetes, respiratory insufficiency, CHF, hypertension, CAD, sleep apnea).

SUMMARY OF PROCEDURE (VGB or Roux-en-Y)

Position	Supine (Fig. 7.2-6)
Incision	Midline
Special instrumentation	Large OR tables; heavy-duty retractors; special stapling devices
Unique considerations	Prophylactic cholecystectomy often advocated. Pneumatic compression boots may not be large enough; heparin (5000 U sc 2 h before surgery, then q 12 h) used commonly. ↑↑aspiration risk + potentially difficult airway
Antibiotics	± Cefoxitin 1 g iv
Surgical time	2–3 h
Closing considerations	Anticipate 30 min closure time; NG suction
EBL	< 500 mL
Postop care	Postop ventilation may be necessary; VTE precautions.
Mortality	0.5–1.6%
Morbidity	Wound infection: 4–8% Anastomotic leak: 3% Dehiscence: 1.6% PE: 1–1.6%
Pain score	7

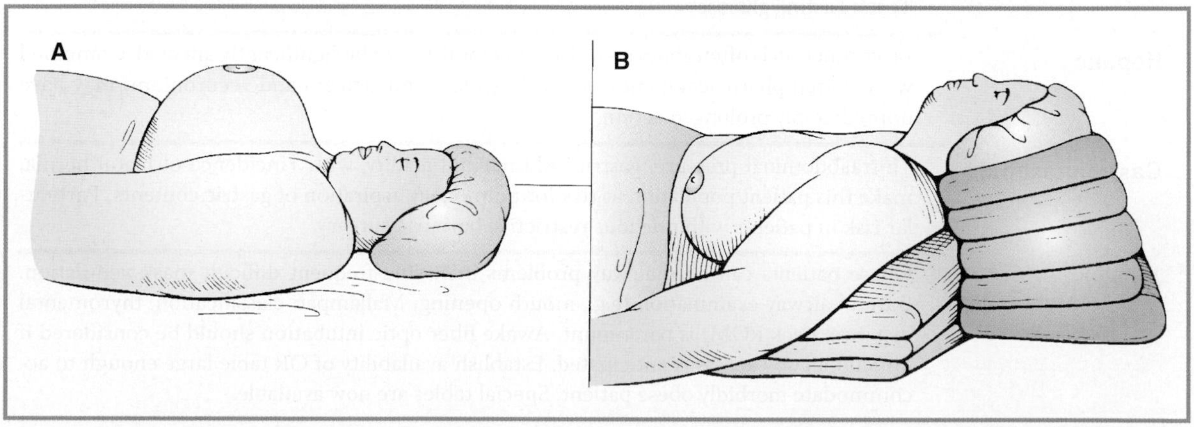

Figure 7.2-6. **(A)** In standard supine position, the atlantooccipital gap of morbidly obese patient is obliterated by fat, and access for laryngoscope is hindered by large breasts. **(B)** By elevating the shoulders and occiput so that head is in the 'sniffing' position, airway access is greatly facilitated.

PATIENT POPULATION CHARACTERISTICS	
Age range	Adult
Male:Female	< 1:1 for disease but 80% of patients who undergo surgery are female
Incidence	~5% of males and ~7% of females in U.S. population considered morbidly obese
Etiology	Multifactorial
Associated conditions	Sleep apnea ± CO_2 retention; CAD/CHF/cardiomyopathy; pulmonary HTN/systemic HTN; diabetes; unusually high risk of DVT and PE; GERD

ANESTHETIC CONSIDERATIONS

PREOPERATIVE

Morbid obesity is variably defined (i.e., >100 lbs over ideal body weight, 2 times ideal body weight, or BMI > 40 [BMI = weight (kg) ÷ height (m)]), and is associated with increased periop mortality/morbidity. Obstructive sleep apnea (OSA) is common in the morbidly obese patient.

Respiratory	Increased O_2 consumption and CO_2 production (e.g., ↑basal metabolic rate). ↓chest-wall compliance (↓20–60%) with normal lung compliance. ↓ERV and FRC; so tidal breathing may fall within the range of closing capacity → V/Q abnormalities. Supine position further ↓FRC → worsening hypoxemia. ↑MV is required to remain normocarbic. There is a normal response to CO_2 unless patient develops the obesity hypoventilation (Pickwickian) syndrome (↑$PaCO_2$, ↓PaO_2, loss of hypercarbic drive, sleep apnea, hypersomnolence, polycythemia, pulmonary HTN, CHF). **Tests:** CXR; PFTs (FVC, FEV_1, $MMEF_{25-75}$ ± bronchodilators; room-air ABG)
Cardiovascular	Blood volume and CO ↑ with increasing weight. HTN is very common (use correct size BP cuff). LV dysfunction may be present; patient unable to increase CO or tolerate ↑ blood volume. Pulmonary HTN may be present in OSA. Obesity is a risk factor for CAD and sudden death. Anticipate problems with vascular access. **Tests:** ECG; others as indicated from H&P. (Patient with SOB may require MUGA scan and ECHO for LV function, as SOB can have a cardiac or pulmonary etiology.)
Endocrine	Glucose intolerance and diabetes mellitus (DM) common. **Tests:** Fasting glucose
Hepatic	Liver function is often abnormal. Drug metabolism can be significantly affected. Combined with altered pharmacokinetics, many drugs (e.g., midazolam and vecuronium) may have unpredictably prolonged action.
Gastrointestinal	↑intraabdominal pressure, gastric volume, and acidity, with ↑incidence of hiatal hernia, make this patient population at risk for pulmonary aspiration of gastric contents. Particular risk in patients with previous restrictive bariatric surgery.
Airway	Obese patients can have airway problems including frequent difficult mask ventilation. Careful airway examination (e.g., mouth opening, Mallampati classification, thyromental distance, neck ROM) is paramount. Awake fiber optic intubation should be considered if difficult airway access is anticipated. Establish availability of OR table large enough to accommodate morbidly obese patient. Special tables are now available.
Hematologic	Polycythemia may occur 2° chronic hypoxemia. **Tests:** CBC
Laboratory	Other tests as indicated from H&P.

Premedication	Sedatives are best avoided for patients with OSA. A small dose of iv midazolam (0.5–1.0 mg) may be appropriate for the especially anxious patient. In the bariatric patient, intramuscular medications can be erroneously injected into adipose tissues. Consider anticholinergics if performing awake fiber optic intubation (glycopyrrolate 0.2 mg iv 30 min preop). Consider full-stomach precautions (p. B-4): metoclopramide (10 mg iv 60 min preop), H_2-antagonist (ranitidine 50 mg iv), and nonparticulate antacid (3 M Na citrate) 30 mL, 10 min prior to induction.

INTRAOPERATIVE

Anesthetic technique: GETA ± epidural for postop analgesia in open surgeries. If using a combined anesthetic approach, placement of an epidural catheter should be accomplished before induction, with the patient in the sitting position. A bilateral sensory block (using 5–7 mL 2% lidocaine) will help confirm correct placement of the catheter within the epidural space. Verification of placement is particularly important in this population since regional anesthesia in the obese patient may be technically more difficult.

Induction	Patients are at risk for aspiration of gastric contents and should be intubated either awake (p. B-4) or after rapid-sequence induction with cricoid pressure. Mask ventilation and ET intubation may be difficult (2° rapid desaturation, head elevated laryngoscopy position, redundant tissue). Following successful intubation and induction of anesthesia, an OG/NG tube should be placed and the stomach contents suctioned. Lipophilic drugs (e.g., STP) will have a greater volume of distribution, necessitating increased dosage.	
Maintenance	Standard maintenance (p. B-2). Obese patients metabolize volatile anesthetics to a greater extent than their nonobese counterparts. **Combined epidural/GA:** A local anesthetic (2% lidocaine with 1:200,000 epinephrine) can be injected into a thoracic (3–5 mL) or lumbar (5–10 mL q 60 min) epidural catheter to provide both anesthesia and improved surgical exposure (contracted bowel and profound muscle relaxation). A continuous infusion of local anesthetic (e.g., 2% lidocaine or 0.25% bupivacaine at 5–10 mL/h [lumbar], 3–5 mL/h [thoracic]) may enhance hemodynamic stability. The dose of local anesthetic given via epidural catheter should be decreased to 75% of normal dose. Be prepared to treat ↓BP with fluid and vasopressors (ephedrine 5–10 mg iv, phenylephrine 50–100 mcg iv). GA is administered to supplement regional anesthesia and for amnesia. Sedative drugs (opiates, benzodiazepines, etc.) should be minimized in the presence of epidural opiates, as they increase the likelihood of postop respiratory depression. If epidural opiates are used for postop analgesia, a loading dose (e.g., hydromorphone 0.6–1.0 mg with lumbar catheter and 0.4–0.6 mg for thoracic) should be administered 1–2 h before end of surgery.	
Emergence	The decision to extubate at the end of open surgery depends on patient's underlying cardiopulmonary status and the extent of the surgical procedure. Patients should be hemodynamically stable, normothermic, alert, cooperative, and fully reversed from any muscle relaxants before extubation. Elective ICU admission for postop care may be appropriate. Following laparoscopic surgery, in contrast, patients typically are extubated and admitted to PACU.	
Blood and fluid requirements	Anticipate large fluid loss. IV: 14–16 ga ×1–2 NS/LR @ 10–15 mL/kg/h T&S for 2 U PRBC. Warm fluids.	Third-space losses greatly exceed blood loss. Guide fluid management by UO, filling pressure. Euvolemia is an important goal.
Monitoring	Standard monitors (p. B-1) UO ± Arterial line	Invasive monitoring as clinically indicated. Arterial line if noninvasive BP unreliable 2° extremity size.

Positioning	Supine position = ↓FRC ✓ and pad pressure points ✓ eyes * **NB:** Avoid Trendelenburg	Supine positioning →↓lung volumes, which may ↑ V/Q mismatch → hypoxemia. This is exacerbated by use of the Trendelenburg position, which usually is not well tolerated by morbidly obese patients.
Complications	Hypoxemia 2° ↓FRC	100% O_2 → absorption atelectasis

POSTOPERATIVE

Complications	Hypoxemia Hypercarbia VTE (see p. B-7) Atelectasis	Recover patient in sitting position to improve ventilatory mechanics. Give supplemental O_2. Verify VTE prophylaxis.
Pain management	Epidural analgesia: hydromorphone (0.6–1.0 mg with lumbar cath and 0.4–0.6 mg for thoracic cath) load then 0.1–0.3 mg/h infusion) PCA (p. C-3)	If epidural is used for postop analgesia, Pain Service management recommended.
Tests	ABG CXR	Others as clinically indicated. CXR for central line placement

General Surgery

Suggested Readings

1. Brodsky JB, Lemmens HJM, Brock-Utne JG, et al: Morbid obesity and tracheal intubation. *Anesth Analg* 2002; 94:732–6.
2. Brodsky JB, Lemmens HJM: Anesthetic drugs and bariatric surgery. *Expert Rev Neurother* 2006; 6(7):1107–13.
3. Brodsky JB, Lemmens HJM: Regional anesthesia and obesity. *Obes Surg* 2007; 17(9):1146–9.
4. Brolin RE: Bariatric surgery and long-term control of morbid obesity. *JAMA* 2002; 288(22):2793–6.
5. Buchwald H, Buchwald JN: Evolution of operative procedures for the management of morbid obesity 1950–2000. *Obes Surg* 2002; 12(5):705–17.
6. Choban PS, Jackson B, Poplawski S, Bistolarides P: Bariatric surgery for morbid obesity: why, who, when, how, where, and then what? *Cleve Clin J Med* 2002; 69(11):897–903.
7. DeMaria EJ: Morbid Obesity. In: *Surgery: Scientific Principles and Practice,* 3rd edition. Greenfield LJ, et al, eds. Lippincott Williams & Wilkins, Philadelphia: 2006, 736–42.
8. Klein S: Medical management of obesity. *Surg Clin North Am* 2001;81(5):1025–38, v.
9. Livingston EH: Obesity and its surgical management. *Am J Surg* 2002; 184(2):103–13.
10. Ogunnaike BO, Jones SB, Jones DB, Provost D, Whitten CW: Anesthetic considerations for bariatric surgery. *Anesth Analg* 2002; 95(6):1793–805.
11. Perilla V, Sollazzi L, Bozza P, et al: The effects of the reverse Trendelenberg position on respiratory mechanics and blood gases in morbidly obese patients during bariatric surgery. *Anesth Analg.* 2000; 91:1520–5.
12. Sachdev M, Miller WC, Ryan T, Jollis JG: Effect of fenfluramine-derivative diet pills on cardiac valves: a meta-analysis of observational studies. *Am Heart J* 2002; 144(6):1065–73.
13. Shenkman Z, Shir Y, Brodsky JB: Perioperative management of the obese patient. *Brit J Anaesth.* 1993;70:340–59.
14. Sugarman HJ, DeMaria EJ: Gastric surgery for morbid obesity. In: *Mastery of Surgery,* 4th edition. Baker RJ, Fischer JE, eds. Lippincott Williams & Wilkins, Philadelphia: 2001, 1026–36.

GASTROSTOMY PLACEMENT

SURGICAL CONSIDERATIONS

Description: A **gastrostomy** is a tube placed through the abdominal wall directly into the stomach. Such tubes can be used for gastric decompression or for feeding, and they may be permanent or temporary. Patients undergoing gastrostomy placement often have neurologic impairment that compromises their ability to handle oral secretions and increases their risk of aspiration. **Percutaneous endoscopic gastrostomy (PEG),** in contrast to the other techniques, most commonly is performed using iv sedation and local anesthesia.

Variant procedure or approaches: The traditional **Stamm gastrostomy** usually is placed at the time of a laparotomy performed for another purpose; or it may be performed through a separate, small laparotomy incision in patients in whom endoscopic placement is not possible for technical reasons. The incision may be upper midline or transverse directly over the stomach. The anterior wall of the stomach is identified, and two purse-string sutures are placed in the stomach around the site where the tube will enter. The gastrostomy tube is introduced through the abdominal wall directly over the intended site of entry into the stomach. A small hole is made in the stomach in the center of the purse-string sutures, the tube is introduced into the stomach, and the purse-strings are tied securely around the tube. The wound is then closed. GA usually is preferred, but the operation may be performed under local anesthesia in thin patients.

The **Janeway gastrostomy,** a technical modification, also requires a laparotomy. The greater curvature of the stomach is identified and a stapler placed across a portion of this, creating a tube that arises from the main body of the stomach. The staple line may be oversewn, and then the end of the tube is brought through the abdominal wall and matured to the skin as a small stoma. This allows for permanent access to the stomach with removal of the tube between feedings and is useful in patients with long-term dependence on gastrostomy access. The Janeway gastrostomy is rarely used, although young patients with neurologic impairment who are expected to need lifetime gastrostomy feeding are good candidates.

For a **PEG,** the stomach is intubated endoscopically and the gastric and abdominal walls punctured under endoscopic guidance. The gastrostomy tube is introduced through the mouth and passed through the stomach and abdominal wall from inside out. In most centers, this has become the most common technique of gastrostomy placement due to its simplicity and because, in many patients, it can be performed under local anesthesia with MAC. Previous gastric operations may make endoscopic placement difficult or dangerous, as may some obstructing lesions of the esophagus or pharynx. To avoid damage to the back wall of the stomach, the anesthesiologist may be asked to inject air forcefully into the stomach.

Usual preop diagnosis: Temporary gastrostomies often are used after major abdominal surgery as an alternative to NG suction. Percutaneous gastrostomies often are placed in patients with advanced malignancy and intestinal obstruction or inadequate oral intake, and in patients with neurologic impairment and difficulty eating.

SUMMARY OF PROCEDURES

	Stamm	Janeway	PEG
Position	Supine	⇐	⇐
Incision	Midline or transverse	⇐	Puncture
Special instrumentation	None	⇐	Endoscope, percutaneous gastrostomy kit
Antibiotics	± Cefazolin 1 g iv	⇐	⇐
Surgical time	45 min	1 h	0.5–1 h
Closing considerations	Muscle relaxation for closure	⇐	None
EBL	Minimal	⇐	⇐
Mortality	Minimal	⇐	⇐
Morbidity	Wound infection: 2.1–9% Hemorrhage: 0.9–1.1% Aspiration pneumonia: 2.2% Failure to function: 2.2%	⇐ ⇐ ⇐ ⇐	– ⇐ 1.6% –
Pain score	4–5	5	1–2

PATIENT POPULATION CHARACTERISTICS	
Age range	All ages, though with peaks in infancy and the elderly
Male:Female	~1:1
Incidence	Common
Etiology	See Preop Diagnosis, above
Associated conditions	Gastrostomy placed at time of laparotomy, when NG drainage is anticipated for prolonged period. For feeding in the neurologically impaired or in those with complex upper digestive difficulties. Advanced malignancy (for either feeding or palliative decompression).

ANESTHETIC CONSIDERATIONS

See Anesthetic Considerations for Ostomy Procedures in Intestinal Surgery, p. 515.

Suggested Readings

1. Jesseph JM: Open gastrostomy. In: *Mastery of Surgery,* 4th edition. Baker RJ, Fischer JE, eds. Lippincott Williams & Wilkins, Philadelphia: 2001, 888–93.
2. Ozmen MN, Akhan O: Percutaneous radiologic gastrostomy. *Eur J Radiol* 2002;43(3):186–95.
3. Pennington C: To PEG or not to PEG. *Clin Med* 2002;2(3):250–5.
4. Ponsky JL: Percutaneous endoscopic gastrostomy. In: *Mastery of Surgery,* 4th edition. Baker RJ, Fischer JE, eds. Lippincott Williams & Wilkins, Philadelphia: 2001, 894–9.

CHAPTER

7.3 Intestinal Surgery

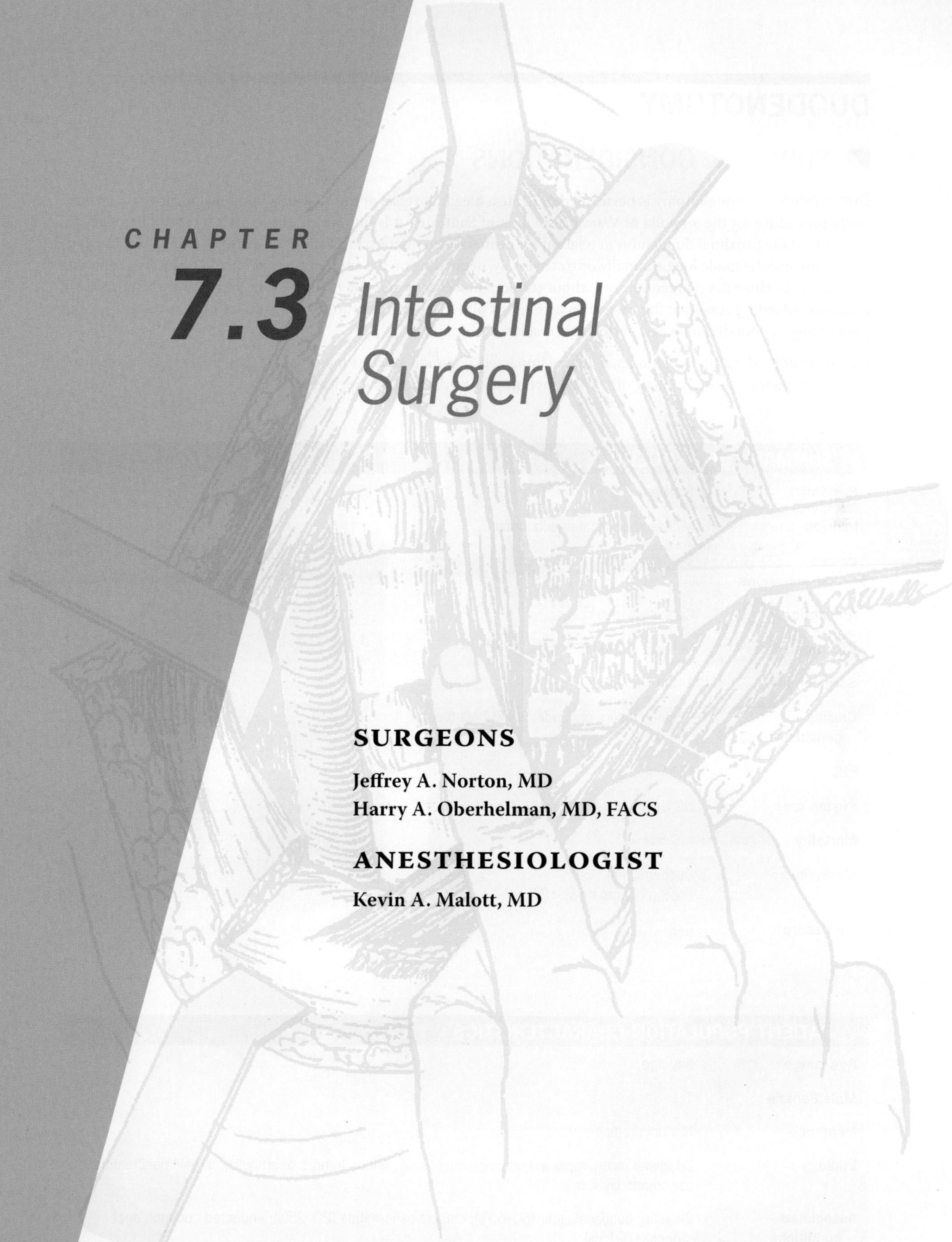

SURGEONS

Jeffrey A. Norton, MD
Harry A. Oberhelman, MD, FACS

ANESTHESIOLOGIST

Kevin A. Malott, MD

DUODENOTOMY

SURGICAL CONSIDERATIONS

Description: A duodenotomy is performed to ligate a bleeding vessel at the base of a duodenal ulcer or to perform some procedure on the ampulla of Vater or the duct of Santorini. It is important, therefore, to be familiar with the anatomy of the proximal duodenum in relation to the major and minor pancreatic duct orifices (Fig. 7.3-1). The duodenotomy may be made longitudinally or transversely, depending on the surgeon's preference. A transverse opening allows one to close the duodenotomy without tension; however, it must be made very accurately for the purpose of exposure. Bleeding vessels at the base of an ulcer must be secured with suture ligatures. Care must be taken to avoid perforating the duodenum when performing a sphincterotomy.

Usual preop diagnosis: Duodenal ulcer; impacted common duct stone; chronic pancreatitis 2° alcoholism, gallstones, pancreatic divisum, or other obstruction of the main pancreatic duct

SUMMARY OF PROCEDURE	
Position	Supine
Incision	Midline abdominal or subcostal
Unique considerations	Magnifying glasses, if operation involves lesser pancreatic sphincter
Antibiotics	Cefoxitin 1 g iv
VTE prophylaxis	Heparin 5,000 units sq
Surgical time	1–2 h
Closing considerations	Secure closure of duodenum without tension
EBL	Minimal
Postop care	NG decompression
Mortality	< 0.5%
Morbidity	Duodenal leak: < 5% Postop pancreatitis: < 3%
Pain score	6–8

PATIENT POPULATION CHARACTERISTICS	
Age range	Any age
Male:Female	1:1
Incidence	Not uncommon
Etiology	Duodenal ulcer; impacted common duct stone; villous tumors of ampulla; chronic pancreatitis, pancreatic divisum
Associated conditions	Bleeding duodenal ulcer (50–60%); chronic pancreatitis (20–25%); impacted common duct stones (10–15%)

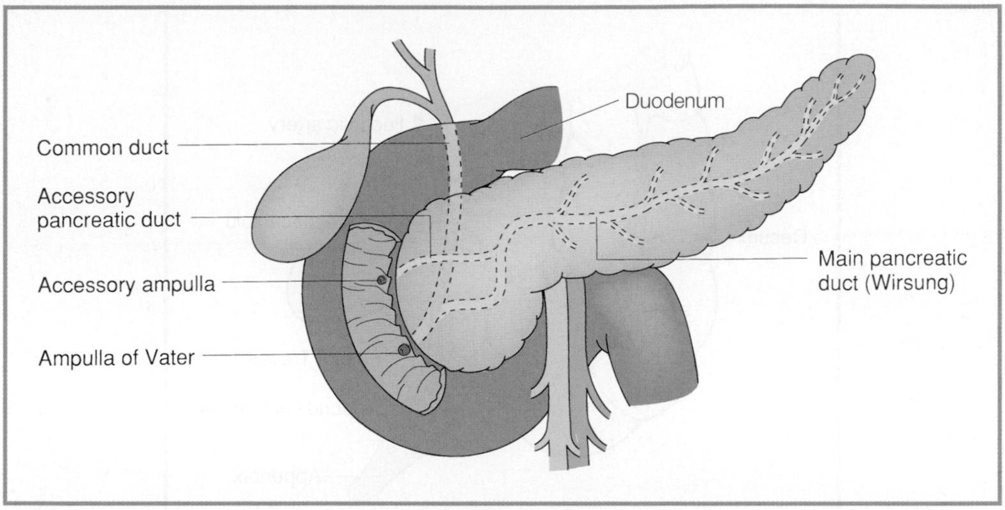

Figure 7.3-1. Anatomy of pancreatic ductal system. In 30% of patients, the accessory duct ends blindly. (Reproduced with permission from Greenfield LJ, Mulholland MW, Oldham KT, et al: *Surgery: Scientific Principles and Practice,* 3rd edition. Lippincott Williams & Wilkins, Philadelphia: 2001.)

ANESTHETIC CONSIDERATIONS

See Anesthetic Considerations following Operations for Peptic Ulcer Disease, Stomach Surgery, p. 515.

Suggested Readings

1. Cisco RM, Norton JA: Surgery for gastrinoma. *Adv Surg* 2007; 41:65–76.
2. Nora PF: *Operative Surgery: Principles and Techniques,* 3rd edition. WB Saunders, Philadelphia: 1990.

OPEN APPENDECTOMY

SURGICAL CONSIDERATIONS

Description: Open appendectomy is performed for appendicitis or suspected appendicitis; however, it has been largely replaced by the laparoscopic approach (see p. 591). The negative laparotomy rate has been reduced by the judicious use of preoperative CT examination. Through a RLQ (**McBurney**) or right paramedian incision, the cecum is exposed and pulled into the wound (Fig 7.3-2). The appendix is then delivered through the wound; and the mesoappendix is clamped, cut, and ligated. The appendix is removed by crushing, ligating, and then transecting the base. The appendiceal stump may be invaginated into the wall of the cecum or left alone. In some instances it may be easier to divide the base of the appendix before delivering the appendix into the wound. The wound should be left open and soft drains used in cases of perforated appendix. In children, the appendix may be inverted and allowed to slough off internally.

Variant procedure or approach: Laparoscopic appendectomy (see p. 592).

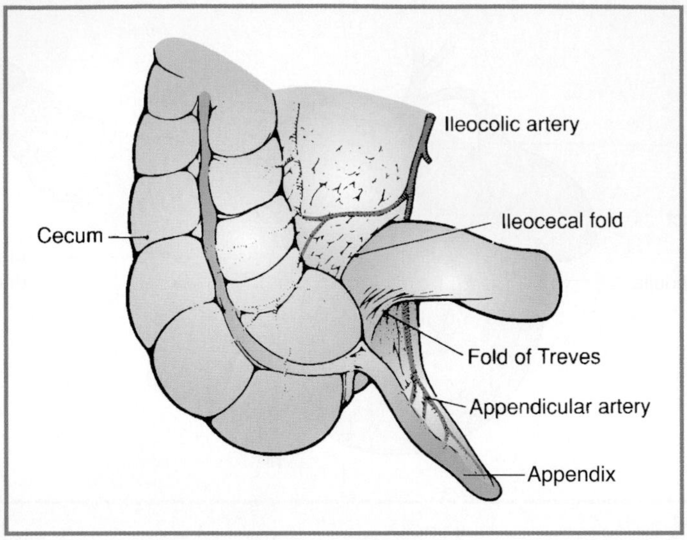

Figure 7.3-2. Relevant anatomy for appendectomy. (Reproduced with permission from Scott-Conner CEH, Dawson DL: *Operative Anatomy,* 2nd edition. Lippincott Williams & Wilkins, Philadelphia: 2003.)

Usual preop diagnosis: Appendicitis

SUMMARY OF PROCEDURE	
Position	Supine
Incision	RLQ (McBurney's) or right paramedian
Unique considerations	Variation in stump closure; NG tube if prolonged ileus expected.
Antibiotics	Cefoxitin 1 g preop
VTE prophylaxis	Heparin 5,000 units sq
Surgical time	1 h
Closing considerations	Skin wound should not be closed when appendix is perforated. Drain in presence of well-defined abscess cavity.
EBL	< 75 mL
Postop care	Wound care when left open
Mortality	Perforated: 2% Nonperforated: < 0.1%
Morbidity	Pelvic, subphrenic, or intraabdominal abscess (perforation): 20% Wound abscess: < 5% Fecal fistula: < 1% Wound hematoma: < 0.5% Ileus: Variable
Pain score	5–7

PATIENT POPULATION CHARACTERISTICS	
Age range	Any age
Male:Female	1:1
Incidence	1/15 persons
Etiology	Obstruction (80–90%); fecaliths (75%); carcinoid tumors (< 5%)
Associated conditions	None

ANESTHETIC CONSIDERATIONS

See Anesthetic Consideration following Excision of Meckel's diverticulum, below p. 512.

Suggested Readings

1. Nguyen NT, Hinojosa MW, Fayad C, et al: Laparoscopic surgery is associated with a lower incidence of venous thromboembolism with a lower incidence of venous thromboembolism compared with open surgery. *Ann Surg* 2007; 246:1021–7.
2. See Suggested Readings following Excision of Meckel's diverticulum, pp. 513–514.

EXCISION OF MECKEL'S DIVERTICULUM

SURGICAL CONSIDERATIONS

Description: Meckel's diverticulum is a true congenital diverticulum, usually arising within 100 cm of the ileocecal valve. It was first described by Meckel in 1809. Excision of a Meckel's diverticulum is indicated for bleeding, obstruction, perforation, inflammation, intussusception, and when there is a palpable mass near the base of the diverticulum. Ectopic mucosa is present in roughly 50% of symptomatic patients, with gastric mucosa the most frequent. After entering the peritoneal cavity, the distal ileum, along with the diverticulum, is delivered into the wound. The diverticulum is excised and the wound is closed in two layers. Following excision of the diverticulum, care must be taken not to narrow the bowel lumen during closure. If a diagnosis can be made preop, a laparoscopic approach may be used (see Laparoscopic Bowel Resection p. 588).

Usual preop diagnosis: Meckel's diverticulum

SUMMARY OF PROCEDURE	
Position	Supine
Incision	Midline abdominal or RLQ (McBurney's)
Antibiotics	Cefoxitin 1–2 g iv
VTE prophylaxis	Heparin 5,000 units sq
Surgical time	1–1.5 h
EBL	< 100 mL
Mortality	< 0.5%

SUMMARY OF PROCEDURE (cont'd)	
Morbidity	Wound infection: 5% Pulmonary complication: < 5% Anastomotic leak: < 1%
Pain score	6–8

PATIENT POPULATION CHARACTERISTICS	
Age range	< 40 yr
Male:Female	3:1
Incidence	0.3–2.5%
Etiology	Congenital
Associated conditions	Exomphalos; esophageal atresia; anorectal atresia; gross malformations of CNS or CV system

ANESTHETIC CONSIDERATIONS

(Procedures covered: open appendectomy; excision of Meckel's diverticulum)

PREOPERATIVE

This patient population is generally fit and healthy, apart from their acutely presenting illness. Full-stomach precautions are appropriate in these patients. Surgery for appendicitis is one of the most common nonobstetric procedures performed on the pregnant patient (~1/1,500 pregnancies). These patients often are more ill at the time of diagnosis, because early symptoms may be attributed to pregnancy, and the gravid uterus may hinder an accurate abdominal exam. Anesthesia management for the gravid appendicitis patient mirrors that of the nongravid patient (full-stomach precautions) with consideration of the maternal physiologic changes of pregnancy and the effects of anesthesia on the fetus and uteroplacental perfusion (See Anesthetic Considerations for Cervical Cerclage, Obstetric Surgery, p. 835.)

Respiratory	Respiratory impairment may occur 2° the acute abdominal pain and splinting. Tachypnea and hyperpnea can be heralding Sx of appendiceal perforation and sepsis. Patients with acute abdomen pain should be treated as if they have full stomachs. Consider administration of metoclopramide (10 mg iv), H_2-antagonist (ranitidine 50 mg iv), and Na citrate 0.3 M 30 mL po. **Tests:** As indicated from H&P.
Cardiovascular	May be dehydrated from fever, emesis, and ↓ oral intake → ↑ HR + ↑ BP (2° pain), or ↓ BP (sepsis, hypovolemia). Assess volume status appropriately and hydrate adequately prior to proceeding with anesthetic induction. **Tests:** ECG, if indicated from H&P.
Gastrointestinal	Patient typically has abdominal pain with N/V. Muscular resistance to palpation of abdominal wall frequently parallels the severity of the inflammatory process. With spreading peritoneal irritation (as with perforation), patient will develop abdominal distension and paralytic ileus. Electrolyte abnormalities are common 2° N/V. **Tests:** Electrolytes

Hematologic	Moderate leukocytosis (10,000–18,000) with moderate left shift. Hemoconcentration is probable if patient is dehydrated. **Tests:** CBC
Laboratory	Other tests as indicated from H&P.
Premedication	Full-stomach precautions (see p. B-4). Consider midazolam 1–2 mg iv. Opiate medications (morphine 0.03–0.15 mg/kg iv) often delayed or minimized until diagnosis made. Opiate analgesics not contraindicated during the evaluation of an acute abdomen including appendicitis.

INTRAOPERATIVE

Anesthetic technique: GETA, with rapid-sequence iv induction, followed by ET intubation (see full-stomach precautions, p. B-4). If systemic sepsis is absent, hydration is adequate, the patient is cooperative, and high abdominal exploration is unlikely, then regional anesthesia may be considered.

Induction	Rapid-sequence induction of anesthesia (see p. B-4). Restore intravascular volume prior to anesthetic induction if patient is clinically hypovolemic.	
Maintenance	Standard maintenance (see p. B-2), without N_2O. Evacuate stomach with OG or NG tube. Maintain muscle relaxation based on nerve stimulator response.	
Emergence	Patient should be extubated awake after return of airway reflexes.	
Blood and fluid requirements	IV: 16–18 ga × 1 NS/LR @ 5–8 mL/kg/h	
Monitoring	Standard monitors (see p. B-1).	Others, as indicated by patient's status.
Positioning	✓ and pad pressure points ✓ eyes	
Complications	Sepsis	

POSTOPERATIVE

Complications	Sepsis (possible with appendiceal rupture)	Adequate antibiotic coverage
	Paralytic ileus	
	Atelectasis PONV (see p. B-6)	Adequate pain control, incentive spirometry, early ambulation
Pain management	PCA (see p. C-4).	
Tests	As indicated clinically.	

Suggested Readings

1. McBurney C: Experience with early operative interference in cases of disease of the vermiform appendix. *NY Med J* 1889; 50:676–84.
2. Meckel JF: Ulcer die divertikel an darmkanal. *Arch Physiol* 1809; 9:421–53.

3. Merritt WT: Anesthesia for gastrointestinal surgery. In: *Principles and Practice of Anesthesiology,* 2nd edition. Longnecker DE, Tinker JH, Edward G, eds. Mosby-Year Book, St. Louis: 1998, 1881–903.
4. Morgan EG, Mikhail MS, Murray MJ: *Clinical Anesthesiology,* 4th edition. Lange Medical Books, Stamford: 2006, 919–20.
5. Rosen MA: Management of anesthesia for the pregnant surgical patient. *Anesthesiology* 1999; 91:1159–63.
6. Way LW, Doherty GM, eds: *Current Surgical Diagnosis Treatment.* Appleton & Lange, Stamford: 1994, 610–13.
7. Zani A, Eatons S, Rees CM, Pierro A. Incidentally detected Meckel diverticulum: to resect or not to resect? *Ann Surg* 2008; 247:276–81.

ENTEROSTOMY

SURGICAL CONSIDERATIONS

Description: Enterostomy is performed for stenting the small intestine with a long tube for feeding purposes, for bypassing small or large bowel obstructions, and following total proctocolectomy. An intestinal tube is either purse-stringed into the small bowel and brought through the abdominal wall or the intestine itself is brought to the exterior and fashioned into a stoma. Different tubes are used for feeding, according to surgeon's preference. After purse-stringing the tube in the bowel, the seromuscular layer of the jejunum is sutured over the tube for a distance of 3–4 cm before exiting through the abdominal wall. The **Brooke ileostomy** is created by bringing a 2-inch segment of ileum through an abdominal wall stab wound. The ileum is folded back on itself and sutured to the skin edge or dermis (Fig. 7.3-3). Some surgeons secure the ileum to the underlying peritoneum and/or fascia, but this is not necessary.

Variant procedure or approaches: There are various intestinal or drainage tubes that may be inserted into the bowel, depending on the function required. For example, certain tubes are used for feeding, while others may be used for drainage or decompression.

Usual preop diagnosis: Intestinal obstruction due to extensive adhesions; following removal of the large intestine (including the rectum); for enteral feedings

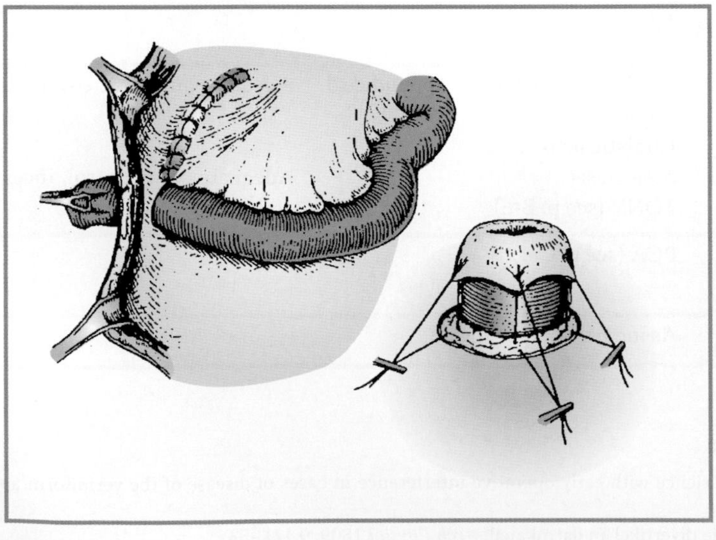

Figure 7.3-3. Brooke ileostomy. (Reproduced with permission from Hardy JD: *Rhoad's Textbook of Surgery,* 5th edition. JB Lippincott, Philadelphia: 1977.)

SUMMARY OF PROCEDURES

	Enterostomy	Ileostomy
Position	Supine	⇐
Incision	Midline abdominal	⇐
Antibiotics	Cefoxitin 1–2 g iv preop	⇐
VTE prophylaxis	Heparin 5,000 units sq	⇐
Surgical time	1–1.5 h	⇐
Closing considerations	Securing tube to abdominal wall	Viable stoma
EBL	< 100 mL	⇐
Postop care	Tube irrigation	Stoma care
Mortality	< 0.5%	⇐
Morbidity	Ileus: 60–70% Wound infection: < 5%	⇐ ⇐ Stoma necrosis: < 2%
Pain score	5–6	5–6

PATIENT POPULATION CHARACTERISTICS

Age range	20–65 yr
Male:Female	1:1
Incidence	Common
Etiology	Intestinal obstruction (60–70%); diseases resulting in total proctocolectomy (10–15%); inability to eat (5–10%)
Associated conditions	Inflammatory bowel disease (IBD); intestinal adhesions; inability to eat orally

ANESTHETIC CONSIDERATIONS FOR OSTOMY PROCEDURES

(Procedures covered: enterostomy; continent ileostomy; gastrostomy; gastrojejunostomy)

PREOPERATIVE

This patient population is very diverse and includes those with IBD, cancer, and those presenting post-CVA and trauma. Thus, the population ranges from the otherwise healthy to the critically ill. Many of these patients will have abnormal protective airway reflexes and are at risk of aspiration of gastric contents.

Respiratory	Patients post-CVA or head trauma may have abnormal laryngeal reflexes and difficulty swallowing, making them prone to aspiration of gastric contents and associated pneumonitis (evaluate gag reflex). Decreased pulmonary reserve and hypoxemia can be seen in patients with pulmonary infections. **Tests:** Consider CXR to r/o pneumonia. Consider ABG.
Cardiovascular	Patients may be hypovolemic 2° chronically poor po intake. **Tests:** ECG; orthostatic vital signs
Musculoskeletal	Patients often sick and debilitated (e.g., post-CVA).

Gastrointestinal	Patients often malnourished and prone to electrolyte abnormalities 2° poor po intake. **Tests:** Electrolytes; BUN; Cr, consider PT/PTT.
Laboratory	CBC with differential; others as indicated from H&P.
Premedication	Depends on patient status. Titrate small doses of benzodiazepines (midazolam 0.25–0.5 mg iv) or opiate (fentanyl 25–50 mcg iv). Consider H_2-antagonists (e.g., ranitidine 50 mg iv, 60 min preop) and metoclopramide (10 mg iv 20 min preop).

INTRAOPERATIVE

Anesthetic technique: GETA is appropriate for most ostomy procedures; MAC with local anesthesia may be appropriate in selected patients.

Induction	Patient may be at risk for pulmonary aspiration. If GA is planned, consider rapid-sequence induction with cricoid pressure. If patient is clinically hypovolemic, restore intravascular volume (colloid, crystalloid, or blood products) prior to induction and titrate induction doses of sedative/hypnotic agents.
Maintenance	**MAC:** Titration of sedatives (e.g., propofol 25–150 mcg/kg/min) and analgesics (fentanyl 25–50 mcg iv). **GA**: Standard maintenance (see p. B-2).
Emergence	Trachea should be extubated after return of protective laryngeal reflexes, if patient at risk for aspiration of gastric contents.
Blood and fluid requirements	Minimal blood loss IV: 16–18 ga × 1 NS/LR @ 5–8 mL/kg/h
Monitoring	Standard monitors (see p. B-1). Others as clinically indicated.
Positioning	✓ and pad pressure points ✓ eyes

POSTOPERATIVE

Complications	Atelectasis Aspiration Hypoxemia Hypercarbia VTE (see appendix p. B-7)
Pain management	PCA (see p. C-3).

Suggested Readings

1. Cingi A, Solmaz A, Attaqllah W, et al: Enterostomy closure site hernias: a clinical and ultrasonographic evaluation. *Hernia* 2008; in press.
2. Zinner MJ, Schwartz SI, Ellis H, eds: *Maingot's Abdominal Operations,* Vol I, 10th edition. Appleton & Lange, Stamford, CT: 1997, 427–51.

CONTINENT ILEOSTOMY POUCH (KOCK)

SURGICAL CONSIDERATIONS

Description: A **Kock pouch** consists of an internal reservoir fashioned from the distal ileum and an intussuscepted nipple valve used to provide continence. Approximately 45 cm of small bowel are required for construction of the

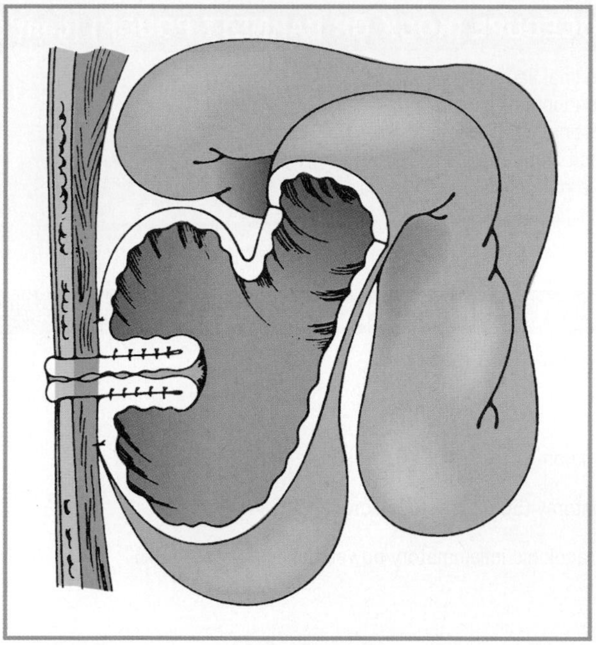

Figure 7.3-4. Continent ileostomy or Kock pouch. (Reproduced with permission from Hardy JD: *Hardy's Textbook of Surgery,* 2nd edition. JB Lippincott, Philadelphia: 1988.)

pouch and valve. After suturing two limbs of the ileum together over a distance of 15 cm, the distal segment is intussuscepted over itself to form the nipple valve. The pouch is then sutured closed and mounted beneath the abdominal wall stoma site (Fig. 7.3-4). The stoma is made flush with the skin for cosmetic reasons and left intubated for 1 month with a special plastic catheter. The pouch remains decompressed for 1 month before intermittent catheterization is initiated. The continent ileostomy reservoir has been modified by **Barnett** to include the construction of an isoperistaltic valve with an intestinal collar around its base to prevent deintussusception and valve prolapse. These procedures are typically performed following a total proctocolectomy or to replace conventional ileostomies.

Usual preop diagnosis: Inflammatory bowel disease; familial polyposis or malfunctioning ileostomies

SUMMARY OF PROCEDURE (KOCK OR BARNETT POUCH)	
Position	Supine
Incision	Midline abdominal
Special instrumentation	GIA or TA staplers
Antibiotics	Usual bowel prep with antibiotics; cefoxitin 1 g iv preop
VTE prophylaxis	Heparin 5,000 units sq
Surgical time	3–4 h
Closing considerations	Valve vascularity
EBL	200–300 mL
Postop care	Maintain pouch decompression
Mortality	< 1%

SUMMARY OF PROCEDURE (KOCK OR BARNETT POUCH) (cont'd)	
Morbidity	Intestinal ileus: 5% Wound infection: < 5% Intestinal obstruction: 2–3% Pouch fistula: 1–3% Valve necrosis: < 0.5%
Pain score	6–8

PATIENT POPULATION CHARACTERISTICS	
Age range	18–80 yr
Male:Female	1:1
Incidence	Common
Etiology	Ileostomy (50%); proctocolectomy (5%)
Associated conditions	Extracolonic inflammatory bowel manifestations (10%)

ANESTHETIC CONSIDERATIONS

See Anesthetic Considerations for Ostomy Procedures, p. 515.

Suggested Readings

1. Barnett WO: Modified techniques for improving the continent ileostomy. *Am Surg* 1984; 50(2):66–9.
2. Becker JM, Stuchni AF: Ulcerative colitis. In: *Surgery: Scientific Principles and Practice,* 3rd edition. Greenfield LJ, Mulholland MW, Oldham KT, et al, eds. Lippincott Williams & Wilkins, Philadelphia: 2001, 1070–89.
3. Little UR, Barboors RN, Shrock TR, et al: The continent ileostomy–long-term durability and patient satisfaction. *J Gastrointest Surg* 1999; 3:625–32.
4. Smith LE: Surgical therapy in ulcerative colitis. *Gastroenterol Clin North Am* 1989; 18:99–110.

SMALL-BOWEL RESECTION WITH ANASTOMOSIS

SURGICAL CONSIDERATIONS

Description: Resection of the small bowel is performed for a number of diseases (listed below). After entering the peritoneal cavity, the involved small bowel is delivered into the wound and the lesion resected between bowel clamps (Fig. 7.3-5). Varying amounts of mesentery are included, depending on the diagnosis. More extensive resections are indicated for malignant disease, including regional lymph nodes. Reanastomosis may be accomplished by various suturing techniques or stapling. The peritoneal cavity may be accessed through vertical or transverse incisions. Operative techniques include **open end-to-end, closed end-to-end, side-to-side,** or **stapled, functional end-to-end anastomoses.**

Variant procedure or approaches: **Laparoscopic small-bowel resections** are being performed more frequently (see p. 588).

Usual preop diagnosis: Intestinal obstruction, complicated by intestinal gangrene due to adhesions, internal hernia, volvulus, intussusception, mesenteric vascular occlusion, Crohn's disease, radiation enteritis, intestinal fistulae, small bowel tumors, and trauma

SUMMARY OF PROCEDURE	
Position	Supine
Incision	Vertical or transverse
Unique considerations	Adequate fluid resuscitation; NG tube

SUMMARY OF PROCEDURE (cont'd)	
Antibiotics	Cefoxitin 1–2 g iv preop
VTE prophylaxis	Heparin 5,000 units sq
Surgical time	1–3 h
EBL	50–100 mL
Postop care	NG or long intestinal tube decompression
Mortality	Varies according to etiology: 1–5%
Morbidity	Atelectasis: < 10% Intestinal ileus: < 10% Wound infection: < 5% Intestinal leak, fistula: < 3%
Pain score	7–9

PATIENT POPULATION CHARACTERISTICS	
Age range	20–90 yr
Male:Female	1:1
Incidence	Common
Etiology	Interference with blood supply (obstruction, strangulated hernia, volvulus, mesenteric thrombosis); trauma; tumors; Crohn's disease
Associated conditions	Multiple, depending on etiology (see Preop diagnosis, above).

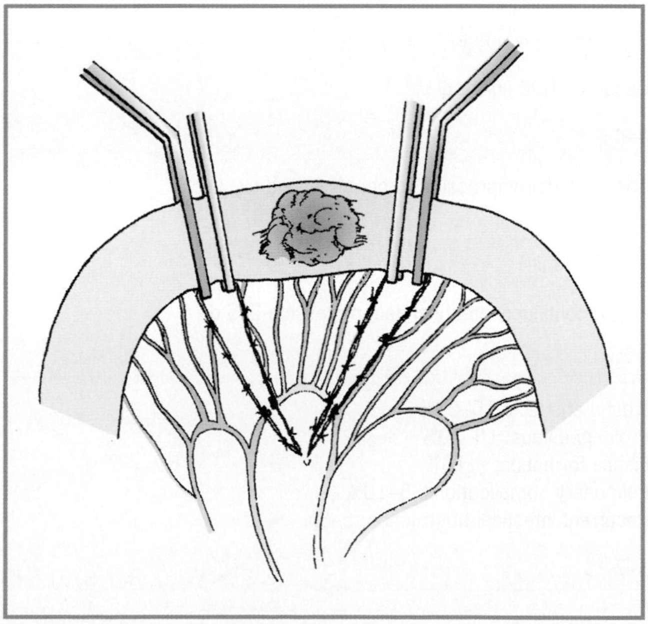

Figure 7.3-5. Block-Potts bowel clamps are applied from the antimesenteric to mesenteric border to avoid twisting. A Kocher clamp is applied on the specimen side, and the bowel is transected with a scalpel. (Reproduced with permission from Baker RJ, Fischer JE, eds: *Mastery of Surgery,* Vol II, 4th edition. Lippincott Williams & Wilkins, Philadelphia: 2001.)

ANESTHETIC CONSIDERATIONS

See Anesthetic Considerations for Intestinal and Peritoneal Procedures, p. 522.

Suggested Readings

1. Chaiyasate K, Jain AK, Cheung LY, et al: Prognostic factors in primary adenocarcinoma of the small intestine. *World J Surg Oncol* 2008; 31:6–12.
2. Zollinger RM Jr, Zollinger RM: *Atlas of Surgical Operations,* 7th edition. MacMillan, New York: 1993.

ENTEROLYSIS

SURGICAL CONSIDERATIONS

Description: Enterolysis consists of separating loops of bowel adhesed to other loops or the abdominal wall by sharp dissection, and by excising adhesive bands. Care must be taken to avoid producing enterotomies. Covering potential adhesion sites with a hyaluronic carboxymethylcellulose membrane may lessen the formation of intraperitoneal adhesions.

Usual preop diagnosis: Intraabdominal adhesions; intestinal obstruction

SUMMARY OF PROCEDURE	
Position	Supine
Incision	Midline abdominal
Special instrumentation	A long intestinal tube may be necessary for decompression and fixation of bowel loop.
Unique considerations	Bowel decompression
Antibiotics	Cefoxitin 1 g iv preop
VTE prophylaxis	Heparin 5,000 units sq
Surgical time	1–4 h
Closing considerations	Adequate decompression to permit wound closure
EBL	150–500 mL
Postop care	PACU; continued intestinal decompression 2–5 d
Mortality	1–3%
Morbidity	Wound abscess: 15–20% Prolonged ileus: 10–20% Fistula formation: < 10% Pulmonary complications: 5–10% Recurrent intestinal obstruction: 5–8%
Pain score	5–7

PATIENT POPULATION CHARACTERISTICS	
Age range	Any age
Male:Female	1:1

PATIENT POPULATION CHARACTERISTICS (cont'd)	
Incidence	Common
Etiology	Previous intraabdominal operative procedure (> 90%); malignant tumors (15–20%); hernias (10–15%); volvulus (5–10%); inflammatory bowel disease (5%); gallstone ileus (< 5%); intussusception (< 5%)

ANESTHETIC CONSIDERATIONS

See Anesthetic Considerations for Intestinal and Peritoneal Procedures, p. 522.

Suggested Readings

1. Aydeniz B, Teppey-Wessels K, Honig A, et al: Laparoscopic enterolysis before adjuvant radiotherapy in a case of endometrial cancer. *Gynecol Oncol* 2004; 92:331–3.
2. Close MB, Christensen NM: Transmesenteric small bowel plication or intraluminal tube stenting. Indications and contraindications. *Am J Surg* 1979; 138(1):89–96.
3. Vrijland WW, Tseng LN, Eijkman HJ, et al: Fewer intraperitoneal adhesions with use of hyaluronic acid-carboxymethylcellulose membrane: a randomized clinical trial. *Ann Surg* 2002; 235:193–9.

CLOSURE OF ENTERIC FISTULAE

SURGICAL CONSIDERATIONS

Description: Enteric fistulae may occur between the bowel and abdominal wall (enterocutaneous), between loops of the intestine (enteroenteric or enterocolic), or between the bowel and bladder or vagina (enterovesical or enterovaginal). Surgical repair is usually reserved for fistulae to the abdominal wall, bladder, and vagina, and consists of excising the fistula and repairing the bowel and the other organ separately. Most fistulae are characterized by the adherence of the two visceral organs with a communication between their lumens.

The organs involved are separated by blunt-sharp dissection and repaired locally after excision of the indurated margins of the defect. In the case of both the small and large intestines, it may be necessary to resect a segment of bowel with the defect and to perform an end-to-end anastomosis. If the repair sites involved lie close together, it is important to interpose tissue, such as the omentum, between the viscera to minimize chance of recurrence. Occasionally, a fistula may be bypassed rather than surgically resected.

Usual preop diagnosis: Enteric fistula

SUMMARY OF PROCEDURE	
Position	Supine
Incision	Midline abdominal
Unique considerations	Preop nutritional support and fistula wound care
Antibiotics	Cefoxitin 1–2 g iv preop
VTE prophylaxis	Heparin 5,000 units sq
Surgical time	2–4 h
Closing considerations	Separation of repairs by interposition of omentum and other tissue
EBL	50–300 mL
Postop care	NG decompression until bowel function returns; TPN support
Mortality	0–5%

SUMMARY OF PROCEDURE (cont'd)	
Morbidity	Ileus: 60–70% Pulmonary complications: 10% Recurrent fistula: 5–10% Wound infection: 5–10%
Pain score	6–8

PATIENT POPULATION CHARACTERISTICS	
Age range	Any age
Male:Female	1:1
Incidence	Common
Etiology	Anastomotic leaks (60–70%); carcinoma (10–15%); Crohn's disease (5–10%); iatrogenic bowel injury (5–10%); perforative diverticulitis (5–10%); radiation enteritis (5%); foreign body perforation (< 5%)
Associated conditions	Malnutrition (30%); inflammatory bowel disease (25%); cancer (15%)

ANESTHETIC CONSIDERATIONS FOR INTESTINAL AND PERITONEAL PROCEDURES

(Procedures covered: small-bowel resection; enterolysis; closure of enteric fistulae; excision of intraabdominal and retroperitoneal tumor; drainage of subphrenic abscess)

PREOPERATIVE

Patients requiring exploratory laparotomy present both electively and emergently for a very wide range of disorders. As a result of their abdominal pathology, these patients are often at high risk for the pulmonary aspiration of gastric contents. Precautions to prevent this are necessary to help assure safe patient outcome (see p. B-4).

Respiratory	Respiratory insufficiency can be present due to intraabdominal pathology (e.g., ascites, large tumor, free blood, bowel distension, pain); ↓ FRC → ↑ A-a gradient and arterial hypoxemia; diaphragmatic impairment and splinting → ↑ respiratory insufficiency. **Tests:** Consider CXR; ABG.
Cardiovascular	Patients for emergency surgery often critically ill and unstable, and should be evaluated for presence of hypovolemia (hypotension, tachycardia) and should receive adequate volume replacement before anesthetic induction. Elective patients may be hypovolemic 2° bowel prep. **Tests:** ECG; consider orthostatic vital signs
Musculoskeletal	Abdominal rigidity may be present; abdominal pain is common.
Gastrointestinal	Diarrhea, vomiting, and prolonged npo status can lead to electrolyte abnormalities. Malnutrition may be present. **Tests:** Electrolytes, consider PT/PTT
Renal	Renal insufficiency/failure may be present, especially in elderly and/or chronically ill patients, and in those who are hypovolemic. **Tests:** Consider BUN; Cr; electrolytes.
Laboratory	CBC with differential; Plt count
Premedication	Standard premedication (see p. B-1). Consider H_2-antagonists (e.g., ranitidine 50 mg iv 1 hr preop), metoclopramide (10 mg iv 30 min preop; although contraindicated in bowel obstruction/perforation), and Na citrate (30 mL po 10 min preop).

INTRAOPERATIVE

Anesthetic technique: GETA ± epidural for postop analgesia. If postop epidural analgesia is planned, placement of catheter prior to anesthetic induction is helpful to establish correct placement in the epidural space (accomplished by injecting 5–7 mL of 2% lidocaine via the epidural catheter, and confirming segmental block).

Induction	The patient with abdominal pathology is often at risk for pulmonary aspiration and the trachea should be intubated with patient awake or after rapid-sequence iv induction with cricoid pressure. (See Rapid-Sequence Induction, p. B-4.) If patient is clinically hypovolemic, restore intravascular volume (colloid, crystalloid, or blood products) prior to induction and titrate induction dose of sedative/hypnotic agents.	
Maintenance	**Balanced anesthesia** without N_2O (see Standard Maintenance Techniques, p. B-2): Maintain neuromuscular blockade based on nerve stimulator response. Place OG or NG tube to evacuate stomach contents. **Combined epidural and GA:** Local anesthetic (2% lidocaine with 1:200,000 epinephrine 5–15 mL initial dose, then 3–5 mL q 60 min) can be injected into the epidural catheter to provide both anesthesia and optimal surgical exposure (contracted bowel and profound muscle relaxation). A continuous infusion of local anesthetic (e.g., 2% lidocaine or 0.25% bupivacaine) at 3–5 mL/h may be used in place of bolus redosing. Be prepared to treat hypotension with fluid and vasopressors. GA is administered to supplement regional anesthesia and for amnesia. If epidural opiates are used for postop analgesia, a loading dose (e.g., hydromorphone 0.5–1.0 mg) should be administered at least 1 h before the conclusion of surgery. Use of systemic analgesics may be minimized during this type of anesthetic with the benefit of decreasing the likelihood of postop respiratory depression.	
Emergence	The decision to extubate at the end of surgery depends on the patient's underlying cardiopulmonary status and the extent of the surgical procedure. Patients should be hemodynamically stable, warm, alert, cooperative, and fully reversed from any muscle relaxants prior to extubation. If the above criteria are not met, consider postop ventilation in ICU setting.	
Blood and fluid requirements	Anticipate large fluid shift. IV: 14–16 ga × 1–2 T&S, consider T&C NS/LR @ 10–15 mL/kg/h Fluid warmer	Plts, FFP, and cryoprecipitate should be administered according to lab tests (Plt count, PT, PTT, DIC screen, thromboelastography [TEG]). Strive to maintain euvolemia based on estimated blood loss and fluid shifts, HR, BP, UO, ABG, and invasive monitors when used.
Monitoring	Standard monitors (see p. B-1). UO ± Arterial line ± CVP/PA catheter ± TEE	Invasive monitors, as indicated by patient's status. Prevent hypothermia: use forced-air warmer; consider warming blanket, warming iv fluids, warm room temperature, keeping patient covered until ready for prep, etc.
Positioning	✓ and pad pressure points ✓ eyes	
Complications	Hemorrhage Sepsis	Acute septic shock may require aggressive hemodynamic support; PA catheter or TEE may help guide management in the unstable patient.

POSTOPERATIVE

Complications	Sepsis Hemodynamic instability Atelectasis Hypoxemia VTE (see p. B-7) Hemorrhage Ileus PONV (see p. B-6)	Pulmonary function abnormalities may persist for 1 wk postop (↓ vital capacity and ↓ FRC).

Pain management	Epidural analgesia (see p. C-2). PCA (see p. C-3).	Patient should be recovered in ICU or ward accustomed to treating the side effects of epidural opiates (e.g., respiratory depression, breakthrough pain, nausea, pruritus).
Tests	CBC; CXR (if central line placed); electrolytes; glucose	Others as directed by intraop course.

Suggested Readings

1. Aguirre A, Fischer JE, Welch CE: The role of surgery and hyperalimentation in the therapy of gastrointestinal-cutaneous fistulae. *Ann Surg* 1974; 180(4):393–401.
2. Becker HP, Willms A, Schwab R: Small bowel fistulas and the open abdomen. *Scand J Surg* 2007; 96:263–71.
3. Merritt WT: Anesthesia for gastrointestinal surgery. In: *Principles and Practice of Anesthesiology,* 2nd edition. Longnecker DE, Tinker JH, Edward G, eds. Mosby-Year Book, St. Louis: 1998, 1881–903.
4. Zinner MJ, Schwartz SI, Ellis H, eds: *Maingot's Abdominal Operations,* 10th edition, Vol. I. Appleton - Lange, Stamford, CT: 1997, 593–616.

CHAPTER

7.4 Colorectal Surgery

SURGEONS

Andrew A. Shelton, MD
Carlos E. Pineda, MD
Mark Lane Welton, MD

ANESTHESIOLOGISTS

Cosmin Guta, MD
Vincent Hsieh, MD

LAPAROSCOPIC COLORECTAL SURGERY

Laparoscopic surgery has changed the face of general surgery with the widespread use of laparoscopic cholecystectomy, appendectomy, and other surgical procedures. Although most colorectal surgery continues to be done in the standard open fashion, laparoscopic techniques are being used more and more for procedures on the colon and rectum. All of the following procedures can be done, and have been done, laparoscopically. Advantages to the patient include smaller incisions, less postop discomfort, and, possibly, a slight decrease in hospital stay, with early return to work and normal activity. Steep positional changes are often used to facilitate retraction of the small bowel out of the operative field. The patient is often placed on a beanbag to prevent movement. The term *laparoscopic-assisted* is more appropriate for colorectal procedures since the colon often is mobilized laparoscopically. A small incision is then made, through which the bowel is exteriorized, the mesentery divided, and an anastomosis created. "Hand-assisted" laparoscopy involves placement of a hand-port through a 5–10 cm incision. The abdominal cavity is then insufflated as in standard laparoscopy, but the surgeon's hand is used alongside the other laparoscopic instruments. An important consideration for any laparoscopic procedure is that the surgeon might need to convert to an open laparotomy. This may occur in a secondary fashion for failure to progress or in an emergent fashion for technical difficulties.

Suggested Readings

1. Bonjer HJ, Hop WC, Neslon H, et al: Laparoscopically assisted vs open colectomy for colon cancer: a meta-analysis. *Arch Surg* 2007; 142(3): 298–303.
2. Dwivedi A, Chahin F, Agrawal S, et al: Laparoscopic colectomy vs. open colectomy for sigmoid diverticular disease. *Dis Colon Rect* 2002; 45(10):1309–14; discussion 1314–5.
3. Gordon PH, Nivatvongs S, eds.: *Principles and Practice of Surgery of Colon, Rectum, and Anus*, 3rd edition. Informa Healthcare, New York: 2006.
4. Ky AJ, Sonoda T, Milsom JW: One-stage laparoscopic restorative proctocolectomy: an alternative to the conventional approach; *Dis Colon Rect* 2002; 45(2):207–11.
5. Scheidbach H, Schneider C, Konradt J, et al: Laparoscopic abdominoperineal resection and anterior resection with curative intent for carcinoma of the rectum. *Surg Endo* 2002; 16(1):7–13.

TOTAL PROCTOCOLECTOMY

SURGICAL CONSIDERATIONS

Description: **A total proctocolectomy** involves the removal of the entire colon, rectum, and anus (Fig. 7.4-1). Indications for this operation include ulcerative colitis (UC), Crohn's disease (CD), and familial adenomatous polyposis (FAP). Inflammatory bowel disease (IBD) can be diagnosed at any age, but there are peaks in diagnosis in the teens and twenties and the sixties and seventies. The most common indication for total proctocolectomy in the setting of UC or CD is intractable symptoms despite maximal medical therapy. Patients are commonly chronically or acutely ill, and may be malnourished or anemic. They are often on high-dose steroids and other immune suppressants, such as 6-mercaptopurine or Imuran. Another important indication for proctocolectomy in patients with UC is the presence of dysplasia or cancer. FAP is an autosomal-dominant disease resulting in hereditary colon cancer. Patients develop hundreds to thousands of adenomatous polyps throughout their colon and rectum, as well as elsewhere in the GI tract. Colorectal cancer is inevitable unless proctocolectomy is performed. This is typically done in the late teens or twenties. In contrast to patients with CD or UC, patients with FAP are usually healthy without other medical comorbidities.

Patients usually are given a preop bowel preparation. The bacterial load of the colon is diminished by mechanical cleansing, which may be accomplished by cathartics, or nonabsorbed lavage solutions. As a result of this preparation, patients are often hypovolemic and hypokalemic. Sequential compression stockings are used for thromboprophylaxis. Patients with CD and UC are at ↑ risk for the development of DVT and are often given subcutaneous heparin. Patients on chronic steroids are given stress-dose steroids before the procedure. Broad-spectrum antibiotics covering gram-negative rods and anaerobes are given prior to the incision.

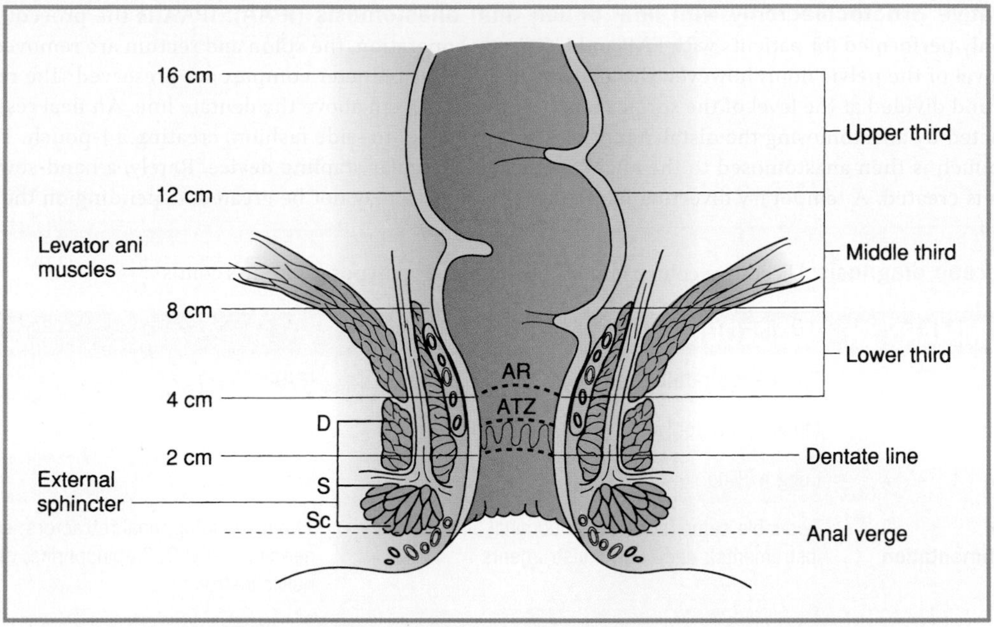

Figure 7.4-1. Anorectal anatomy with important landmarks. Approximate measurements are relative to the anal verge. D = deep; S = superficial; Sc = subcutaneous; AR = anorectal ring; ATZ = anal transition zone. (Reproduced with permission from Yahanda AM, Chang AE: Colorectal cancer. In *Surgery: Scientific Principles and Practice,* 3rd edition. Greenfield LJ, Mulholland MW, Oldham KT, et al, eds. Lippincott Williams & Wilkins, Philadelphia: 2001.)

Total proctocolectomy with end ileostomy, total proctocolectomy with **continent ileostomy (Koch pouch),** and **restorative proctocolectomy** with **ileal pouch anal anastomosis (IPAA)** all involve complete removal of the colon and rectum, down to the level of the pelvic floor or levator ani muscles. They differ in the fate of the anal canal, creation of a stoma, or construction of an anastomosis. The patient is placed in a lithotomy position in padded Allen stirrups. A Foley catheter is placed. The procedure is performed through a midline incision. The abdomen is explored for evidence of unexpected malignancy or, in the case of FAP, for desmoid tumors. The right colon is mobilized first, and then the small bowel mesentery is mobilized to allow for creation of an ileostomy. The transverse colon may be mobilized by separating it from the greater omentum, or the greater omentum may be resected along with the specimen. The sigmoid and descending colon are mobilized, and the splenic flexure is taken down. At this point, the ileum is divided flush with the cecum. The vessels in the colon mesentery are ligated. At this point, the entire abdominal colon has been resected. An avascular fascial envelope surrounds the rectum and its mesentery, the mesorectum. It is possible to circumferentially dissect the rectum down to the level of the pelvic floor without ligating any vessels. There may be significant blood loss if an inadvertent injury to the spleen occurs during mobilization of the splenic flexure. Massive blood loss may occur if the presacral venous plexus is entered during posterior rectal mobilization.

Total proctocolectomy with ileostomy: For patients with CD, elderly patients with UC, or FAP patients with low rectal cancer, complete removal of the colon, rectum, and anus is the procedure of choice. After completing the abdominal mobilization of the colon and rectum, the perineal phase of the operation begins. Ideally, two teams of surgeons participate in the operation simultaneously. The abdominal surgeon can create the ileostomy and close the abdomen, while the perineal surgeon finishes removal of the rectum and anus. A circumferential incision is made at the anal verge and the intersphincteric plane is identified. The dissection proceeds cephalad until the abdominal dissection is encountered, and the specimen is removed. The levator ani muscle, external anal sphincter, and skin are closed. While this is being done, the abdominal surgeon makes a circular incision over the previously marked ileostomy site. A muscle-splitting incision is carried through the rectus fascia. The terminal ileum is then brought through this site. After the fascial and skin are closed, the ileostomy is matured.

Total proctocolectomy with continent ileostomy (Koch pouch): Because of frequent complications and the development of alternative procedures (see below) this procedure has been largely abandoned.

Restorative proctocolectomy with ileal pouch anal anastomosis (IPAA): IPAA is the procedure most commonly performed for patients with FAP and UC. In this operation, the colon and rectum are removed, down to the level of the pelvic floor; however, the anal canal and anal sphincter complex are preserved. The rectum is stapled and divided at the level of the surgical anal canal, ~1–1.5 cm above the dentate line. An ileal reservoir is constructed by anastomosing the distal 30 cm of ileum in a side–to–side fashion, creating a J-pouch. The apex of the pouch is then anastomosed to the anal canal using a circular stapling device. Rarely, a hand-sewn anastomosis is created. A temporary diverting loop ileostomy may or may not be created, depending on the clinical situation.

Usual preop diagnosis: Ulcerative colitis; familial adenomatous polyposis; Crohn's colitis

SUMMARY OF PROCEDURES

	Total Proctocolectomy with End Ileostomy	IPAA
Position	Modified lithotomy	⇐
Incision	Long midline	⇐
Special instrumentation	Two-table setup (separate abdominal and perineal instruments); deep pelvic instruments	Two-table setup; anal retractors; spinal needle; 1:200,000 epinephrine; deep pelvic instruments
Unique considerations	Patients frequently on chronic high-dose corticosteroids	⇐ + Epinephrine solutions injected under the rectal mucosa to facilitate dissection and reduce bleeding.
Antibiotics	Ertapenem 1 g iv or 2nd generation cephalosporin	⇐
Surgical time	3–4 h	⇐
Closing considerations	Ileostomy completed after skin closed (15–30 min).	Temporary ileostomy commonly used, completed after skin closure.
EBL	300–1000 mL (most blood loss during pelvic and perineal dissections)	⇐
Postop care	Transient inability to void common.	Small bowel mesentery lengthened by dissection around duodenum. This frequently necessitates use of postop NG tube. Transient inability to void common.
Mortality	2–5% (older patients and those with underlying medical problems)	⇐
Morbidity	Dyspareunia: 30% Stoma complications: 20% SBO: 10–15% Impotence: 2–4%	5–10% — ⇐ ⇐ Nocturnal incontinence: 20% Poor function: 5% Pelvic sepsis: 0–4%
Pain score	8	8

PATIENT POPULATION CHARACTERISTICS

	Ulcerative Colitis	Familial Adenomatous Polyposis
Age range	3rd–5th decade	2nd–4th decade
Male:Female	1:1	⇐
Incidence	6–10/100,000	100–150 cases/yr

General Surgery

PATIENT POPULATION CHARACTERISTICS (cont'd)		
	Ulcerative Colitis	**Familial Adenomatous Polyposis**
Etiology	Unknown	Genetic
Associated conditions	Cushing's syndrome; anemia; malnutrition; colorectal cancer; sclerosing cholangitis	Colorectal cancer; desmoid tumors; adenomas or cancers of the duodenum and small intestine; brain tumors (Turcot's syndrome); adrenal adenomas; osteomas

ANESTHETIC CONSIDERATIONS

See Anesthetic Considerations for Large Bowel Surgery, p. 534.

Suggested Readings

1. Bertario L, Arrigoni A, Aste H, et al: Recommendations for clinical management of familial adenomatous polyposis. *Tumori* 1997; 83(5):800–3.
2. Ghosh S, Shand A, Ferguson A: Ulcerative colitis. *BMJ* 2000; 320(7242):1119–23.
3. Gordon, PH, Nivatvongs S, eds: *Principles and Practice of Surgery of Colon, Rectum, and Anus,* 3rd edition. Informa Healthcare, New York: 2006.
4. Guy TS, Williams NN, Rosato EF: Crohn's disease of the colon. *Surg Clin North Am* 2001; 81(1):159–68, ix.
5. Litle VR, Barbour S, Schrock TR, et al: The continent ileostomy: long-term durability and patient satisfaction. *J Gastrointest Surg* 1999; 3(6):625–32.
6. Katz JA: Medical and surgical management of severe colitis. *Sem Gastrointest Dis* 2002; 11(1):18–32.
7. King JE, Dozois RR, Lindor NM, et al: Care of patients and their families with familial adenomatous polyposis. *Mayo Clinic Proceedings* 2000; 75(1):57–67.
8. Metcalf AM: Elective and emergent operative management of ulcerative colitis. *Surg Clin North Am* 2007; 87(3):633–41.
9. Michelassi F, Hurst R: Restorative proctocolectomy with J-pouch ileoanal anastomosis. *Arch Surg* 2000; 135(3):347–53.
10. Wolff BG, Garcia-Aguilar J, Roberts PL, et al, eds: *The ASCRS Textbook of Colon and Rectal Surgery*. Springer Science-Business Media, New York: 2007.

SEGMENTAL (PARTIAL) COLECTOMY

SURGICAL CONSIDERATIONS

Description: **Segmental colectomy** involves removal of a portion of the colon (Fig. 7.4-2) with the creation of an anastomosis or a stoma. The most common indications for the operation in the western world are colon cancer and diverticulitis. Less common indications include traumatic perforation, gastrointestinal hemorrhage, ischemic colitis, volvulus, and inflammatory bowel disease (IBD). Both colon cancer and diverticular disease occur most commonly in patients > 50 yr. Patients may have any of the comorbid medical conditions associated with aging, as well as complications related to the disease requiring colon resection. **Free perforation** of the colon can occur from a variety of conditions, including diverticulitis, cancer, and ischemia. Patients may be hypovolemic and have systemic sepsis. Emergent laparotomy should follow a period of resuscitation and administration of antibiotics. The involved segment of bowel is resected, the abdomen is irrigated, and a stoma is created.

Colon cancer is the second most common cancer in the United States with 153,000 new cases diagnosed annually. Patients may be completely asymptomatic with the Dx being made only as the result of a screening exam. Because of the large caliber of the colon and the liquid nature of stool, patients with cancers of the right colon are more likely to present with large cancers and anemia. The caliber of the left colon is smaller, and the stool more solid. Symptoms of obstruction and change in bowel habits predominate for left-sided lesions.

Colonic diverticula occur in up to 60–70% of people > 50 yr in the United States. A colonic diverticulum is a herniation of the mucosa and submucosa through the relative weakening that occurs in the muscular wall of the bowel at the site of penetrating blood vessels. This occurs predominately in the sigmoid colon. Most people with colonic diverticula are completely asymptomatic and will never experience any complications related to

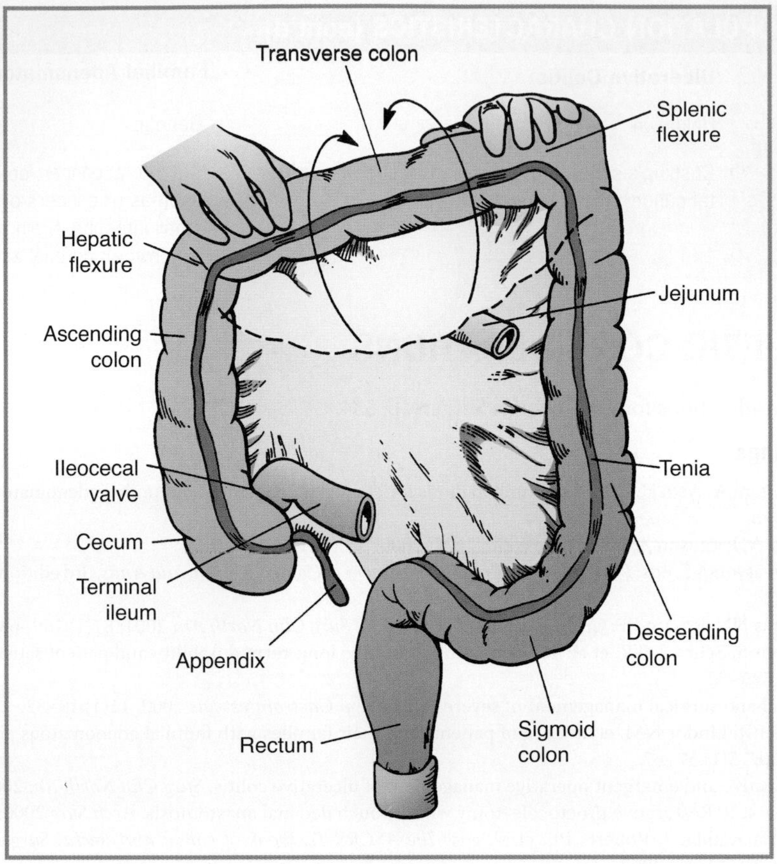

Figure 7.4-2. Anatomy of the colon. (Reproduced with permission from Hardy JD: *Hardy's Textbook of Surgery,* 2nd edition. JB Lippincott, Baltimore: 1988.)

diverticulosis. Diverticulitis occurs when a microscopic or macroscopic perforation of a colonic diverticulum occurs, resulting in a pericolonic inflammatory and infectious process. The severity of the attack depends on the degree of perforation and how well the body is able to wall it off. This ranges from minor inflammation around the sigmoid colon that can be managed with antibiotics, to an intraabdominal or pelvic abscess requiring percutaneous drainage, to free perforation with purulent or feculent peritonitis requiring emergency surgery. Repeated bouts of diverticulitis eventually can result in fibrosis of the colon, stricture formation, and obstruction.

Ideally, surgery on the colon is performed in an elective setting; however, perforation with peritonitis or complete obstruction of the colon may require emergency surgery. Most patients presenting for elective colon resection undergo preop bowel preparation that consists of mechanical cleaning of the colon. As a result, they are frequently hypovolemic and hypokalemic when they come to the OR. The patient is positioned either supine, or in the modified lithotomy position, depending on the segment of colon to be removed. Sequential compression stockings are used for thromboprophylaxis. Intravenous antibiotics covering gram-negative rods and anaerobes should be given prior to the incision with redosing as appropriate for the antibiotic used.

Segmental colectomy: Segmental resection of the colon maybe performed via midline or transverse abdominal incisions, depending on the underlying disease, portion of the colon to be resected, and the surgeon's preference. In general, midline incisions are preferred when: a high-lying splenic flexure must be mobilized, IBD is present, or the extent of the colon resection is not known preop. Transverse incisions are most commonly reserved for resections of the right colon.

The most commonly performed **partial colon resections** are: right hemicolectomy, sigmoid colectomy, left hemicolectomy, and abdominal colectomy with an ileorectal anastomosis. The sequence of steps in a partial colectomy is the same for all parts of the colon. The right colon and left colon are retroperitoneal structures, whereas the transverse colon and sigmoid colon are primarily intraperitoneal. The first step is mobilization of the colon and its mesentery. Care must be taken not to injure the left ureter during mobilization of the sigmoid colon or the duodenum during mobilization of the right colon. Proximal and distal sites for resection are selected and the intervening mesentery is divided. The anastomosis may be hand-sewn or stapled, which is a decision based primarily on the surgeon's preference. There is no clear advantage to either anastomotic technique. Creation of a diverting stoma rather than an anastomosis may be necessary in patients who are hemodynamically unstable, or when intraabdominal conditions, such as inflammation, make an anastomosis unsafe. There may be significant blood loss if an inadvertent injury to the spleen occurs during mobilization of the splenic flexure. Excessive traction of the hepatic flexure can result in difficult-to-control venous bleeding.

Obstruction of the colon most commonly occurs as a result of cancers of the sigmoid colon or repeated bouts of diverticulitis. Patients present with abdominal distention, obstipation, N/V. Patients are treated with NG tube decompression and correction of hypovolemia. An attempt may be made to stent the obstructing lesion endoscopically preop to allow decompression and preparation of the colon. If this is not possible, surgical options include segmental resection with a colostomy, segmental resection with primary anastomosis and an on-table colonic lavage, or subtotal colectomy with an ileorectal anastomosis.

Usual preop diagnosis: Colon cancer; diverticular disease; Crohn's disease; ulcerative colitis; trauma; ischemic colitis; lower GI hemorrhage; intractable constipation; colon volvulus

SUMMARY OF PROCEDURE

Position	Supine or modified lithotomy
Incision	Transverse or vertical midline
Unique considerations	Bowel prep, or underlying disease may → dehydration, electrolyte abnormalities or anemia.
Antibiotics	Ertapenem 1 g iv or 2nd generation cephalosporin
Surgical time	1–3 h
Closing considerations	Colostomy or ileostomy matured after wound is closed (requires 10–20 min).
EBL	100–300 mL (500–2000 mL if splenic injury, loss of major vascular pedicle, or repeat operation for cancer, Crohn's disease)
Postop care	ICU for underlying disease; NG tube for distention or vomiting. Avoid use of long-lasting anticholinergics (e.g., Phenergan).
Mortality	0.5–2% (mostly related to underlying disease)
Morbidity	SBO: 5–10% Wound infection: 4–10% For anastomosis-anastomotic leak: 2–4% Wound dehiscence: 1–2% Bleeding: 1% Splenic injury: 1%
Pain score	8

PATIENT POPULATION CHARACTERISTICS

	Crohn's Disease	**Colon Cancer**	**Trauma**	**Diverticula**
Age range	2nd–4th decade	5th–7th decade	2nd–4th decades	> 40 yr
Male:Female	1:1	1.3:1	3:1	1:1
Incidence	1–6/100,000	30/100,000	1–2/100,000	10/100,000
Etiology	Unknown	Genetic: 5%	Trauma	Western countries: low-fiber diet

PATIENT POPULATION CHARACTERISTICS (cont'd)	Crohn's Disease	Colon Cancer	Trauma	Diverticula
Associated conditions	Malnutrition; anemia; intraabdominal sepsis; intestinal fistulae; perianal disease; nephrolithiasis; sclerosing and ankylosing spondylitis	Iron deficiency; colonic obstruction; colonic perforation	Liver fracture; spleen fracture; rib fracture; closed-head injury; penetration of viscera adjacent to colon injury	Hemorrhoids; chronic constipation

ANESTHETIC CONSIDERATIONS

See Anesthetic Considerations for Large Bowel Surgery, p. 534.

Suggested Readings

1. Blair NP, Germann E: Surgical management of acute sigmoid diverticulitis. *Am J Surg* 2002; 183(5):525–8.
2. Colquhoun PH, Wexner SD: Surgical management of colon cancer. *Curr Gastroenterol Rep* 2002; 4(5):414–9.
3. DeFriend D, Hill J: A review of emergency colonic surgery. *Br J Hosp Med* 1996; 56(7):326–9.
4. Gordon, PH, Nivatvongs S, eds: *Principles and Practice of Surgery of Colon, Rectum, and Anus*, 3rd edition. Informa Healthcare, New York: 2006.
5. Kumar SK, Goldberg RM: Adjuvant chemotherapy for colon cancer. *Curr Oncol Rep* 2001; 3(2):94–101.
6. Lavery IC, Lopez-Kostner F, Pelley RJ, et al: Treatment of colon and rectal cancer. *Surg Clin North Am* 2000; 80(2): 535–69, ix.
7. Maggard MA, Chandler CF, Schmit PJ, et al: Surgical diverticulitis: treatment options. *Am Surgeon* 2001; 67(12):1185–9.
8. Makela J, Kiviniemi H, Laitinen S: Prevalence of perforated sigmoid diverticulitis is increasing. *Dis Colon Rect* 2002; 45(7):955–61.
9. Wolff BG, Garcia-Aguilar J, Roberts PL, et al, eds: *The ASCRS Textbook of Colon and Rectal Surgery*. Springer Science-Business Media, New York: 2007.

STOMA CLOSURE OR PERISTOMAL HERNIA REPAIR

SURGICAL CONSIDERATIONS

Description: A temporary colostomy or ileostomy can be made for a variety of staged procedures. An **end colostomy** is often created after resection of obstructing or perforated lesions of the left colon. A **proximal loop ileostomy or colostomy** is often created to protect a "high-risk" anastomosis, such as a low pelvic colorectal or ileoanal anastomosis. A patient with a permanent stoma may develop a hernia at the stoma site. This may result in complications, such as obstruction or strangulation of the bowel, or problems with appropriate fitting of the stoma appliance. The extent of procedure depends on the type of stoma created.

Closure of loop stoma: Closure of a loop stoma is performed through a circular incision, placed just outside the mucocutaneous junction of the stoma and the skin. The proximal and distal ends of the bowel are separated from the subcutaneous tissue and anterior fascia, and then the posterior fascia. The bowel is cleaned of adherent skin, and the previously opened antimesenteric border of the bowel is simply closed with sutures. Alternatively, the previously exteriorized portion of bowel is resected and the two ends are anastomosed with sutures or staples. On rare occasions, it is necessary to extend the incision transversely through the abdominal wall to safely affect an anastomosis. The fascia is closed in the standard fashion.

Closure of end stoma: Closure of an end stoma usually requires a midline abdominal incision. After entering the peritoneal cavity, the stoma is freed from the abdominal wall. Adhesions are lysed and the dysfunctional distal bowel is identified. It may be necessary to mobilize the proximal bowel to provide a tension-free anastomosis. An anastomosis can then be created using either hand-sewn or stapled techniques.

Paracolostomy hernia repair: The abdomen may be entered via a midline or a peristomal incision. The stoma is freed from the abdominal wall and hernia sac. The stoma is then moved to an alternate site and the defect in the abdominal wall is closed. Alternatively, the stoma may be left in its original site and the fascia closed around the bowel. When performed laparoscopically, transfascial sutures and tackers are used to hold the mesh in place. These may cause significant postop pain.

Usual preop diagnosis: Stomal stenosis; retraction; parastomal hernia; fistula

SUMMARY OF PROCEDURES

	Closure of Loop Stoma	Closure of End Stoma	Repair of Parastomal Hernia
Position	Supine	Supine or modified lithotomy*	Supine
Incision	Circumstomal	Midline or transverse abdominal	Midline or circumstomal
Special instrumentation	Anastomotic staplers	Endoscope for closure of Hartmann's procedure	Prosthetic mesh
Antibiotics**	Ertapenem 1 g iv or 2nd generation cephalosporin	⇐	⇐
Surgical time	1–1.5 h	1–3 h	⇐
Closing considerations	Requires only a few fascial sutures; skin may be left open.	None	Stoma matured after abdomen closed.
EBL	< 100 mL	100–500 mL	< 100 mL
Mortality	1%	2–4%	1 %
Morbidity	Anastomotic leak SBO Wound infection	⇐ ⇐ ⇐	Recurrent hernia Peristomal infection Stomal ischemia
Pain score	5	8	6

*The modified lithotomy position is used for closure of a Hartmann's procedure when an endoscope or stapling device may need to be passed through the anus.

**Bowel prep consists of mechanical cleaning of the colon, accomplished with cathartics or lavage solutions, as well as oral antibiotics. A commonly used regimen is: neomycin 1 g po and erythromycin base 1 g po given at 1 PM, 2 PM and 10 PM on the night before surgery.

PATIENT POPULATION CHARACTERISTICS

Age range	Variable
Male:Female	1:1
Incidence	Not uncommon
Etiology	Protection or avoiding an insecure anastomosis; traumatic injuries to the colon; complete colonic obstruction; colonic infections, such as diverticulitis; inflammatory processes, such as Crohn's disease or ulcerative colitis; after-emergency resection for ischemic colitis
Associated conditions	Multiple trauma; inflammatory bowel disease (IBD); colon cancer; gut ischemia

Suggested Readings

1. Amin SN, Memon MA, Armitage NC, et al: Defunctioning loop ileostomy and stapled side-to-side closure has low morbidity. *Ann Royal Coll Surgeons England* 2001; 83(4):246–9.
2. Doberneck RC: Revision and closure of the colostomy. *Surg Clin North Am* 1991; 71(1):193–201.
3. Edwards DP, Chisholm EM, Donaldson DR: Closure of transverse loop colostomy and loop ileostomy. *Ann Royal Coll Surgeons England* 1998; 80(1): 33–5.
4. Ghorra SG, Rzeczycki TP, Natarajan R, et al: Colostomy closure: impact of preoperative risk factors on morbidity. *Am Surgeon* 1999; 65(3):266–9.

5. Gordon, PH, Nivatvongs S, eds: *Principles and Practice of Surgery of Colon, Rectum, and Anus*, 3rd Edition. Informa Healthcare, New York: 2006.
6. Israelsson LA: Parastomal hernias. *Surg Clin North Am* 2008; 88(1): 113–25.
7. Londono-Schimmer EE, Leong AP, Phillips RK: Life table analysis of stomal complications following colostomy. *Dis Colon Rect* 1994; 37(9): 916–20.

ANESTHETIC CONSIDERATIONS FOR LARGE BOWEL SURGERY

(Procedures covered: total proctocolectomy; partial colectomy with anastomosis; colostomy; stoma closure and peristomal hernia repair)

PREOPERATIVE

Patients presenting for this group of surgical procedures have in common an increased risk for pulmonary aspiration. In addition, patients with bowel obstruction must be treated urgently as the obstruction may rapidly progress to bowel necrosis, perforation, and septic shock. Patients with IBD (e.g., ulcerative colitis or Crohn's disease) may have extracolonic manifestations of the disease (e.g., ankylosing spondylitis, liver disease, anemia), requiring modification of their anesthetic plan.

Respiratory	Patients may have respiratory insufficiency 2° pulmonary metastases (colon cancer) or acute abdominal process (e.g., pain, splinting, sepsis, metabolic acidosis) and bowel distention limiting diaphragmatic excursion (↓ TV, ↓ FRC). Arthritis associated with IBD → ↓ neck ROM → difficult intubation. **Tests:** Consider CXR, ABG
Cardiovascular	Hemodynamic instability 2° sepsis or pain (↑ HR, ↓ BP). Hypovolemia 2° poor po intake, vomiting, diarrhea, and bowel prep. Should restore intravascular volume and hemodynamic stability before induction of anesthesia. **Tests:** Orthostatic VS; ECG
Renal	Electrolyte abnormalities (hypokalemic hypochloremic metabolic alkalosis 2° vomiting or NG suctioning, hyperchloremic metabolic acidosis from diarrhea) are common and may be worsened by bowel prep. **Tests:** Electrolytes
Gastrointestinal	A NG tube is usually in place and the stomach should be emptied before induction of anesthesia. IBD may be associated with impaired liver function and altered drug metabolism.
Hematologic	Hemoconcentration due to GI fluid loss; anemia due to acute/chronic GI bleeding **Tests:** CBC with Plt
Laboratory	Other tests as indicated from H&P
Premedication	Standard premedication (p. B-1) is usually appropriate. For aspiration prophylaxis, ranitidine 50 mg iv 1 h before induction, followed by Na citrate (30 mL, 0.3 M po) 10 min before induction, will significantly decrease the acidity of gastric contents. Metoclopramide is contraindicated in patients with bowel obstruction or perforation. Patients with IBD on chronic steroid therapy should receive their usual daily dose of steroids throughout the periop period and may require full stress-dose steroids. (Glucocorticoid-dependent, critically ill patients requiring vasopressors should be tested for adrenocortical insufficiency and started on 100 mg iv hydrocortisone immediately.)

INTRAOPERATIVE

Anesthetic technique: GETA ± epidural for postop analgesia. Thoracic epidural is associated with improved postop pain control, earlier return of bowel function, intake of food, and out-of-bed mobilization. Placement of the catheter before anesthetic induction is helpful to establish correct placement in the epidural space (accomplished by injecting 5–7 mL of 1% lidocaine via the epidural catheter with development of a segmental block).

Induction	The patient with an acute abdominal process is at risk for pulmonary aspiration; trachea should be intubated with patient awake or after rapid-sequence induction with cricoid pressure (p. B-4). A NG tube does not interfere with cricoid pressure and may be left in place, or removed immediately prior to induction after suctioning as may obscure airway anatomy during laryngoscopy. If patient is clinically hypovolemic, restore intravascular volume (colloid, crystalloid, or blood products) before induction and titrate induction dose of sedative/hypnotic agents.	
Maintenance	Standard maintenance (p. B-2) without N_2O. **Combined epidural/GA:** local anesthetic (1.5–2% lidocaine with 1:200,000 epinephrine (5–10 mL q 60–90 min) can be injected into the epidural catheter to provide both anesthesia and optimal surgical exposure (contracted bowel and profound muscle relaxation). A continuous infusion of local anesthetic (e.g., 0.25% or 0.125% bupivacaine at 4–8 mL/h may enhance hemodynamic stability compared to bolus technique. A loading dose of epidural opiate (e.g., hydromorphone 0.4–0.8 mg) should be administered at least 1 h before conclusion of surgery for optimal results. Patients receiving epidural opiates should be monitored for development of delayed postop respiratory depression and systemic sedatives (e.g., opiates, benzodiazepines) should be minimized.	
Emergence	The decision to extubate at the end of surgery depends on the patient's underlying cardiopulmonary status and extent of surgical procedure. Patient should be hemodynamically stable, warm, alert, and cooperative, and fully reversed from any muscle relaxants before extubation, and have adequate return of pulmonary function (as measured by VC of 15 mL/kg, MIF of -25 cmH_2O, RR < 25, and ABG that approaches patient's baseline).	
Blood and fluid requirements	Anticipate large 3rd-space losses. IV: 14–16 ga × 1 NS/LR @ 10–15 mL/kg/h Warm fluids Consider T&S or T&C	Plt, FFP, and cryoprecipitate should be administered according to lab tests (Plt count, PT, PTT, DIC screen). NS preferable to LR for fluid replacement in patients with metabolic alkalosis. Maintain euvolemia based on EBL, and estimates of fluid shifts, UO, HR, BP, base deficit, lab studies, and invasive monitoring when used.
Monitoring	Standard monitors (p. B-1) UO ± Arterial line ± CVP Temperature	Arterial line and CVP, as indicated by patient's status. Hypothermia may delay healing and predispose patients to wound infections. Avoid hypothermia with forced-air warmer(s), warming blanket, warming room temperature, keeping patient covered until ready for prep.
Positioning	✓ and pad pressure points ✓ eyes	
Complications	Septic shock	Hemodynamic instability 2° sepsis, hemorrhage, especially during manipulation of necrotic bowel.

POSTOPERATIVE

Complications	Hypoxemia Hemodynamic instability Sepsis VTE (see Appendix B) PONV (see Appendix B)	Patients with metabolic alkalosis receiving opiates are especially prone to hypoxemia/hypoventilation. Patients may have considerable 3rd-space losses that require invasive monitoring, ICU admission, vasopressors.

Pain management	Epidural analgesia (p. C-2) PCA (p. C-3)
Tests	CBC; CXR (if central line placed); electrolytes; glucose

Suggested Readings

1. Brown CJ, Buie W: Perioperative stress dose steroids: do they make a difference? *J Am Coll Surg* 2001; 193(6):678–86.
2. Carli F, Mayo N, Klubien K, et al: Epidural analgesia enhances functional exercise capacity and health-related quality of life after colonic surgery: Results of a randomized trial. *Anesthesiology* 2002; 97(3):540–9.
3. Carli F, Trudel J, Belliveau P: The effect of intraoperative thoracic epidural anesthesia and postoperative analgesia on bowel function after colorectal surgery: A prospective, randomized trial. *Dis Colon Rect* 2001; 44(8):1083–9.
4. Kurz A, Sessler D, Lenhardt R: Perioperative normothermia to reduce the incidence of surgical-wound infection and shorten hospitalization. *New Eng J Med* 1996; 334(19):1209–15.

OPERATIONS FOR RECTAL PROLAPSE

SURGICAL CONSIDERATIONS

Description: Rectal prolapse (procidentia) is intussusception of the full thickness of the rectal wall beyond the anal canal. It must be distinguished from rectal mucosal prolapse, caused by elongation of the mucosal attachments to the underlying sphincter muscle, and internal intussusception, where the upper rectum folds into the lower rectum, but does not descend through the sphincter mechanism. Rectal mucosal prolapse is treated as part of the spectrum of hemorrhoidal disease, and mild-to-moderate intussusception does not benefit from surgery. Procidentia is associated frequently with anal incontinence. The surgical approaches to procidentia are determined by patient age, concurrent medical disease, sphincter function, and operative Hx.

Surgical treatment of procidentia may be undertaken through an abdominal or a perineal approach. The **abdominal approaches** have a lower recurrence rate and, because they do not diminish the capacity of the rectal reservoir, are generally preferable for maintaining fecal continence. **Rectopexy** is an abdominal approach in which the rectum is mobilized in the posterior plane from the sacral promontory to the levator muscles. The rectum is then pulled cephalad and sutured to the presacral fascia with multiple nonabsorbable sutures. Many surgeons routinely perform **sigmoid resection** along with rectopexy. They believe that removal of the redundant sigmoid further diminishes the chance of late recurrence and may alleviate constipation. The rectum also may be suspended by use of a sling attached to the rectum and secured to the presacral fascia. A number of approaches have been described, the most popular being the **Ripstein procedure. Sling procedures** have equivalent recurrence rates, but higher complication rates. As in rectopexy, the rectum is mobilized along the presacral plane down to the level of the levators. A band of Marlex mesh is sewn to the presacral fascia at the sacral promontory, upward traction is placed on the rectum, and the mesh is sutured to the rectum.

In patients with significant comorbidities, prolapse may be repaired via a **perineal approach.** The most common of these is **perineal rectosigmoidectomy** (or **Altemeier procedure**). The prolapsed rectum is withdrawn through the anal canal to its full extent, and a circumferential incision is made in the outer tube of the prolapsed bowel just proximal to the dentate line. This exposes the inner tube of prolapsed bowel and mesentery. Redundant bowel is mobilized from the distal end, up to the point that no additional bowel can be delivered into the operative field. The redundant bowel is transected and a primary anastomosis is fashioned between the cut ends of the inner and outer bowel. Prior to anastomosis, the levator muscles are often approximated in the midline in an effort to aid continence. When the volume of prolapsed tissue is small or a previous abdominal approach makes blood supply to the rectum questionable, the **Delorme procedure** often is performed. During this procedure, the mucosa is stripped off the prolapsed rectum, and the prolapsed rectal muscle is foreshortened by plication until it resides above the sphincters.

Usual preop diagnosis: Full-thickness rectal prolapse (procidentia)

SUMMARY OF PROCEDURES

	Rectopexy	Rectopexy with Sigmoid Resection	Perineal Rectosigmoidectomy	Delorme Procedure
Position	Lithotomy	⇐	Prone jackknife; lithotomy	⇐
Incision	Low transverse; low midline	⇐	No external incision	⇐
Special instrumentation	Deep pelvic instruments; mesh if sling planned	Deep pelvic instruments	Hip-roll for jackknife position; anastomosis may be created with EEA stapler	Hip roll for jackknife position
Unique considerations	Presacral venous plexus bleeding may occur; bowel prep may cause dehydration or hypokalemia.	⇐	Epinephrine solutions may be used to diminish bleeding; bowel prep may cause dehydration or hypokalemia.	⇐
Antibiotics	Ertapenem 1 g iv or 2nd generation cephalosporin	⇐	⇐	⇐
Surgical time	1–2 h	⇐	⇐	⇐
EBL	< 100 mL; more if reoperation	100–300 mL; more if reoperation	100–200 mL	100 mL
Postop care	No rectal probes or medications	⇐	⇐	⇐
Mortality	0–2%	0–4%	1–4%	0–1%
Morbidity	Rectal stricture (with sling): 5–10%	—	—	—
	Recurrent prolapse: 2–8%	2–5%	20–40%	5–10%
	Pelvic infection: 5%	—	—	—
		Anastomotic leak: 2–4%	—	—
Pain score	7	7	2	2

PATIENT POPULATION CHARACTERISTICS

Age range	Women: peak incidence in 6th–7th decade; men: evenly distributed through age range
Male:Female	1:4
Incidence	Unknown
Etiology	Decreased pelvic muscular support; congenital deficiency of rectal support; pudendal neuropathy; chronic constipation and straining; multiparity; myelomeningocele; spina bifida; cystic fibrosis (children); acute parasitic diarrheal illness (children)
Associated conditions	Fecal incontinence; urinary stress incontinence; rectocele; cystocele

ANESTHETIC CONSIDERATIONS

See Anesthetic Considerations following Operations for Fecal Incontinence, p. 546.

Suggested Readings

1. Gordon, PH, Nivatvongs S, eds: *Principles and Practice of Surgery of Colon, Rectum, and Anus*, 3rd edition. Informa Healthcare, New York: 2006.
2. Hayashi S, Masuda H, Hayashi I, et al: Simple technique for repair of complete rectal prolapse using a circular stapler with Thiersch procedure. *Eur J Surg* 2002; 168(2):124–7.
3. Kariv Y, Delaney CP, Casillas S, et al: Long-term outcome after laparoscopic and open surgery for rectal prolapse: a case-control study. *Surg Endosc* 2006; 20(1): 35–42.
4. Lechaux JP, Atienza P, Goasguen N, et al: Prosthetic rectopexy to the pelvic floor and sigmoidectomy for rectal prolapse. *Am J Surg* 2001; 182:465–9.
5. Liberman H, Hughes C, Dippolito A, et al: Evaluation and outcome of the Delorme procedure in the treatment of rectal outlet obstruction. *Dis Colon Rectum* 2000; 43(2):188–92.
6. Schultz I, Mellgren A, Dolk A, et al: Long-term results and functional outcome after Ripstein rectopexy. *Dis Colon Rectum* 2000; 43: 35–43.
7. Solomon MJ, Young CJ, Eyers AA, et al: Randomized clinical trial of laparoscopic versus open abdominal rectopexy for rectal prolapse. *Br J Surg* 2002; 89(1):35–9.
8. Zbar AP, Takashima S, Hasegawa T, et al: Perineal rectosigmoidectomy (Altemeier's procedure): a review of physiology, technique and outcome. *Tech Coloproctol* 2002; 6(2):109–16.

RECTAL SURGERY

SURGICAL CONSIDERATIONS

Description: Many lesions within the distal two-thirds of the rectum can be excised through a **transanal approach.** The most common benign tumors treated by local excision are adenomas. Lesions such as carcinoid tumor, endometrioma, and solitary rectal ulcer also may be locally excised. **Transanal excision** of benign lesions may be performed in the submucosal plane, whereas suspected malignancies are excised by removing the entire thickness of the rectal wall. A full antibiotic and mechanical bowel prep is given. Transanal excision usually is performed in the prone jackknife position, although the lithotomy position may be used when the lesion is located on the posterior rectal wall. A local anal block, usually 0.25% bupivacaine with 1:200,000 epinephrine, is performed to relax the sphincter mechanism and minimize sphincter injury, aid in hemostasis, and diminish postop pain. An anoscope is inserted into the anal canal. Stay sutures may be placed adjacent to the area of resection. On occasion, lesions may be prolapsed all the way through the anus and excised outside of the body. Generally, the dissection starts at the distal end of the lesion and proceeds proximally. The proctotomy may be closed with running or interrupted sutures. These sutures are then grasped and used for further traction. When the specimen is removed, a few final sutures are needed to close the proximal-most incision. **Rigid proctoscopy** is performed to confirm preservation of an adequate lumen.

Variant procedure or approaches: The **transsacral (Kraske) approach** to rectal tumors offers wider exposure than the transanal approach, but is more painful and has a substantially greater likelihood of complications (wound infection, fecal fistula, incontinence). A transsacral approach may be advantageous when the lesion is located behind the rectum (retrorectal tumors) and when resection of the lower sacrum or coccyx is anticipated. Transsacral resection generally is performed in the prone jackknife position. An incision is made from the posterior commissure of the anus to the base of the sacrum. The sphincter muscles are spared, but the levator muscles are divided to expose the posterior wall of the rectum. The coccyx may be disarticulated and removed to improve exposure. It is also possible to remove the lower sacral segments through this approach, but increasing morbidity accrues as the sacral nerve roots are sacrificed. For a posterior-wall lesion, the posterior wall of the rectum is opened and the lesion, along with a full-thickness disc of rectal wall, is excised. If the lesion is on the anterior wall, two proctotomy incisions are necessary. The proctotomy incisions are closed with standard anastomotic techniques. The levator muscles are reapproximated and the skin is closed. A drain may be placed within the retrorectal space before closing. The transsacral approach may be combined with an abdominal approach (**abdominal-transsacral resection**) in some cases of low rectal cancer.

The **transsphincteric (Mason) approach** to rectal lesions also gives wider exposure than does the transanal approach, but at the expense of a substantially greater risk of fecal incontinence. Transsphincteric excision is performed with the patient in the prone jackknife position. An incision is made at the posterior commissure of the anus and is extended along the lateral border of the coccyx and sacrum. The external sphincter, internal sphincter and levator ani muscles are sequentially transected in the posterior midline. As each muscle is cut, the cut edges are tagged with sutures to facilitate accurate reapproximation. The rectal wall is incised and the lesion is excised. The proctotomy incision is closed via standard anastomotic suturing techniques, and the individual components of the sphincter muscle are reapproximated with interrupted sutures. The overlying skin is closed in a standard fashion.

Transanal endoscopic microsurgery involves the use of a resectoscope, 4 cm in diameter, that is inserted in the rectum. An airtight faceplate is placed and the rectum insufflated. The plate is exchanged for an adapter with working ports, through which instruments are placed and the resection is done similarly to the transanal approach described above.

Usual preop diagnosis: Villous adenoma; tubular adenoma; adenocarcinoma; carcinoid tumor; endometrioma; solitary rectal ulcer; retrorectal tumors (in decreasing frequency)

SUMMARY OF PROCEDURES

	Transanal Excision	Transsacral Excision	Transsphincteric Excision	Transanal Endoscopic Microsurgery
Position	Prone jackknife or lithotomy	Prone jackknife	⇐	Prone jackknife, lithotomy, or lateral decubitus
Incision	Intrarectal	Anus-to-lateral sacral wall	⇐	Intrarectal
Special instrumentation	Rigid proctoscope; headlight and/or fiber optic retractors; Foley catheter	Gigli or power saw if sacral resection contemplated; headlight and/or fiber optic retractors; Foley catheter	Headlight and/or fiber optic retractors; Foley catheter	Proctoscope (40 mm diameter), removable faceplate, optical stereoscope, light cord, pressure transducer, laparoscopic camera, insufflator, instruments (5 mm diameter), 'Martin arm' to hold equipment
Unique considerations	Bowel prep may → dehydration and hypokalemia.	⇐	⇐	⇐
Antibiotics	Ertapenem 1 g iv or 2nd generation cephalosporin	⇐	⇐	⇐
Surgical time	15–120 min	1–2 h	⇐	⇐
EBL	< 100 mL	< 100 mL (500 mL if sacral resection)	⇐	⇐
Postop care	No rectal temperatures, suppositories, or enemas	⇐	⇐	⇐
Mortality	0–2%	⇐	⇐	0.3–2%
Morbidity	Tumor recurrence: 5–50% Urinary retention: 10–20%	50% ⇐	5–50% ⇐	4–20% ⇐

SUMMARY OF PROCEDURES (cont'd)	Transanal Excision	Transsacral Excision	Transsphincteric Excision	Transanal Endoscopic Microsurgery
Morbidity (cont'd)	Bleeding: 2–5% Pelvic sepsis: 0–4% Ureteral injury: <; 1% (minimized by use of Foley)	⇐ ⇐ ⇐ Fecal fistula: 10–30% Fecal incontinence: 5–10%	⇐ ⇐ ⇐ 10–40%	2% 0.8% Intraperitoneal entry: 1–4% 2%
Pain score	3	7	7	3

PATIENT POPULATION CHARACTERISTICS	
Age range	Rectal adenomas: 5th–7th decades; rectal adenocarcinoma: 6th–9th decades; endometrioma: 2nd–4th decades; solitary rectal ulcer syndrome: 4th–8th decades; carcinoid tumors: 5th–8th decades
Male: Female	1:1
Incidence	Varies with disease; not uncommon
Etiology	Varies with disease
Associated conditions	Preexisting anorectal pathology, such as fecal incontinence, may require concurrent treatment

ANESTHETIC CONSIDERATIONS

See Anesthetic Considerations following Operations for Fecal Incontinence, p. 546.

Suggested Readings

1. Bleday R, Breen E, Giacco GG, et al: Prospective evaluation of local excision for small rectal cancers. *Dis Colon Rectum* 1997; 40(4): 388–92.
2. Cataldo PA: Transanal endoscopic microsurgery. *Surg Clin North Am* 2006; 86(4): 915–25.
3. Chapuis P, Bokey L, Fahrer M, et al: Mobilization of the rectum: anatomic concepts and the bookshelf revisited. *Dis Colon Rect;* 2002; 45(1): 1–9.
4. Glimelius BL: The role of preoperative and postoperative radiotherapy in rectal cancer. *Clin Colorect Can* 2002; 2(2): 82–92.
5. Gould TH, Grace K, Thorne G, et al: Effect of thoracic epidural anaesthesia on colonic blood flow. *Brit J Anaesth* 2002; 89(3):446–51.
6. Kapiteijn E, van de Velde CJ: Developments and quality assurance in rectal cancer surgery. *Euro J Cancer* 2002; 38(7): 919–36.
7. Moore HG, Guillem JG: Local therapy for rectal cancer. *Surg Clin North Am* 2002; 82(5):967–81.
8. Visser BC, Varma MG, Welton ML, et al: Local therapy for rectal cancer. *Surg Oncol* 2001; 10(1–2):61–9.
9. Wolff BG, Garcia-Aguilar J, Roberts PL, et al, eds: *The ASCRS Textbook of Colon and Rectal Surgery*. Springer Science-Business Media, New York: 2007.

ANAL FISTULOTOMY/FISTULECTOMY/FISTULA PLUG

SURGICAL CONSIDERATIONS

Description: The majority of perianal fistulae are 2° infection in the anal glands within the rectal wall that communicates with crypts located at the dentate line (cryptoglandular fistula). Fistulae also may be the result of trauma, Crohn's disease, inflammatory processes within the peritoneal cavity, neoplasms, or as a consequence of radiation therapy. The ultimate treatment of fistula-in-ano is determined by the etiology and the anatomic course of the fistula. The principle behind treatment of cryptoglandular fistulae is to ablate the offending gland and lay open the tract. Fistulae that track above the majority of the sphincter mechanism must be treated by procedures that either do not cut the overlying sphincter, cut the sphincter and repair it, or cut the sphincter very gradually (**seton,** see below). A fistula may be treated at the time of drainage of a perianal abscess or as a separate, elective operation. The route of a fistula tract is best determined by exploration at the time of operation. Although local anesthesia is acceptable for most fistulae, a few fistula operations require regional or general anesthesia because the ultimate route and depth of the fistula is unknown. Special consideration is given to fistulae that arise in the setting of Crohn's disease. Poor wound healing and the importance of sphincter function in patients with chronic diarrhea dictate that only the most superficial fistulae are laid open. The primary goal is palliation; specifically, abscess drainage and recurrence prevention. This is often accomplished by placing a Silastic Seton (a ligature around sphincter muscles) around the fistula tract and leaving it in place indefinitely. In the absence of active Crohn's disease in the rectum and anus, attempts at fistula cure may be undertaken.

Variant procedure or approaches: **Fistulotomy** involves cutting all tissues superficial to a fistula so that the fistula tract is brought to the skin level. The opened, fibrotic fistula wall is often sewn to the skin edge (marsupialized). **Fistulectomy** involves excision of the entire fistula tract. When conventional fistulotomy would cause incontinence, a **Seton** may be used. Other approaches that may be used to avoid fecal incontinence are **complete fistulotomy with immediate reconstruction** of the sphincter and excision of the internal opening by an **endorectal advancement flap** technique.

The fistula plug involves the use of a bioabsorbable xenograft made of lyophilized porcine intestinal submucosa that is reconstituted in saline and placed in the fistula tract. This method may be preferred for fistulae that would require transection of a significant portion of the anal sphincters such that the surgeon is concerned about the impact on continence. It is used for both cryptoglandular fistulas and Crohn's disease-related fistulas.

Usual preop diagnosis: Fistula-in-ano

SUMMARY OF PROCEDURES

	Fistulotomy or Fistulectomy	Fistulotomy with Seton	Endorectal Advancement Flap	Fistula Plug
Position	Prone jackknife; rarely lithotomy	⇐	Prone jackknife	⇐
Incision	Perianal	⇐	⇐	None
Antibiotics	None	None	Ertapenem 1 g iv or 2nd generation cephalosporin	None
Surgical time	10–30 min	⇐	60–90 min	5–10 min
EBL	< 50 mL	⇐	⇐	Negligible
Mortality	Minimal	⇐	⇐	⇐
Morbidity	Fecal incontinence: 0–30% Nonhealing, or recurrent fistula: 5%	10–30% 10–20%. (This procedure used only in complex fistulae, so complication rate appears higher.)	0–10% 10–40%. (This procedure used only in complex fistulae, so complication rate appears higher.)	0% 25–50%
Pain score	6	6	6	0–1

PATIENT POPULATION CHARACTERISTICS

Age range	2nd–7th decades
Male:Female	2:1

PATIENT POPULATION CHARACTERISTICS (cont'd)	
Incidence	Common
Etiology	Infection within anal glands located at dentate line (cryptoglandular fistula); trauma; Crohn's disease; inflammatory processes within the peritoneal cavity; neoplasms; consequence of radiation therapy

ANESTHETIC CONSIDERATIONS

See Anesthetic Considerations following Operations for Fecal Incontinence, p. 546.

Suggested Readings

1. Bailey HR, Snyder MJ, eds: *Ambulatory Anorectal Surgery*. Springer-Verlag, New York: 2000.
2. Champagne BJ, O'Connor LM, Ferguson M, et al: Efficacy of anal fistula plug in closure of cryptoglandular fistulas: long-term follow-up. *Dis Colon Rectum* 2006; 49(12): 1817–21.
3. Garcia-Aguilar J, Davey CS, Le CT, et al: Patient satisfaction after surgical treatment for fistula-in-ano. *Dis Colon Rectum* 2000; 43:1206–12.
4. Gordon, PH, Nivatvongs S, eds: *Principles and Practice of Surgery of Colon, Rectum, and Anus*, 3rd Edition. Informa Healthcare, New York: 2006.
5. Ho YH, et al: Marsupialization of fistulotomy wounds improves healing (RCT). *Br J Surg* 1998; 85:105–7.
6. Knoefel WT, Hosch SB, Hoyer B, et al: The initial approach to anorectal abscesses: fistulotomy is safe and reduces the chance of recurrence. *Dig Surg* 2000; 17(3):274–8.
7. Ortiz H, Marzo J: Endorectal flap advancement repair and fistulectomy for high trans-sphincteric and suprasphincteric fistulas. *Br J Surg* 2000; 87(12):1680–3.
8. Zimmerman DD, Briel JW, Gosselink MP, et al: Anocutaneous advancement flap repair of transsphincteric fistulas. *Dis Colon Rectum* 2001; 44: 1474–80.

HEMORRHOIDECTOMY/STAPLED HEMORRHOIDOPEXY

SURGICAL CONSIDERATIONS

Description: Hemorrhoids are normally occurring vascular tissues located in discrete aggregations known as hemorrhoidal cushions within the distal rectum and anus. Thought to play a role in the fine control of enteric continence, they are only treated if they cause a symptom that persists after conservative therapy. Hemorrhoids may bleed, prolapse, and cause mucous drainage, itching, or pain (when thrombosed). The primary pathophysiologic event in the development of symptomatic hemorrhoids is thought to be mucosal prolapse 2° degeneration of the fibroelastic tissue that tethers vascular cushions and overlying mucosa to the submucosa. Many modern treatments diminish prolapse by fixing the mucosa to the submucosa with scar tissue. Hemorrhoids are classified as internal (when above the dentate line) or external (when below). Internal hemorrhoids are further classified by symptoms: I–bleed; II–bleed, prolapse, and spontaneously reduce; III–bleed, prolapse, and require manual reduction; IV–bleed, prolapse, and cannot be reduced. The most common symptom from external hemorrhoids is severe pain caused by thrombosis. Surgical treatment involves excision of the thrombosed hemorrhoid, often under local anesthetic, in the office. Internal hemorrhoids may be treated by nonexcisional or excisional techniques. Nonexcisional techniques generally are used in the office or outpatient clinic. They do not require an anesthetic because their use is limited to the insensate tissues above the dentate line. Nonexcisional treatments include **rubber-band ligation, infrared coagulation, sclerotherapy,** and **cryotherapy.**

Surgical hemorrhoidectomy may be performed in the lithotomy or prone jackknife position. An anoscope is placed in the anal canal and a hemorrhoid column is grasped and tented up into the lumen. A suture is placed at the internal apex of the complex. An incision is started at the external apex of the hemorrhoidal complex and a plane is developed deep to the hemorrhoidal tissue and superficial to the sphincter muscles. When the internal sphincter is identified, the dissection proceeds in the avascular space along its luminal surface. The dissection is continued up into the rectum to the transfixing suture. Lateral incisions along the redundant tissue are completed to excise the hemorrhoid. Care is taken to leave healthy bridges of mucosa between adjacent hemorrhoidal columns. Hemostasis is obtained with cautery and the mucosal defect may be closed with a running, absorbable suture. It also is acceptable to leave the mucosal wound open. The procedure is repeated over the other enlarged, symptomatic hemorrhoidal complexes, removing redundant tissue and leaving long, vertical scars to prevent further mucosal prolapse.

Variant procedure or approaches: The **Whitehead hemorrhoidectomy (circumferential hemorrhoidectomy)** and **Lord procedure (sphincter stretch)** have been largely abandoned. **Lasers** have not been shown to improve results in the treatment of hemorrhoids.

Rubber-band ligation requires no anesthesia because the band is placed on the insensate, distal rectal mucosa. An anoscope is inserted into the anal canal to visualize a hemorrhoid column. The most proximal area of redundant mucosa is grasped with a clamp and pulled into the barrel of the ligation gun. A rubber band is placed on the base of the tented-up hemorrhoid tissue. The encompassed tissue sloughs over 4–7 d, and a scar is formed between the mucosa and the underlying muscle.

Stapled hemorrhoidopexy is used for the correction of mucosal hemorrhoidal prolapse. This procedure is performed in the same position and under the same anesthesia as a conventional hemorrhoidectomy. A circular anal dilator is anchored to the skin with heavy sutures, an obturator is passed and a purse-string is created with absorbable 2-0 suture 3 to 4 cm above the dentate line. The stapler head is passed above the purse-string, and the sutures are pulled while the stapler is closed. In women, the vaginal wall must be examined to ensure that it has not been incorporated. The stapler is fired, cutting the incorporated mucosal prolapse, pulling the internal and external hemorrhoids proximally. Thus the hemorrhoids themselves are not removed. Hemostasis is obtained with sutures as needed. Cautery should be used with caution, because of the staples. This procedure is associated with a higher rate of disease recurrence and cost.

Usual preop diagnosis: Symptomatic hemorrhoids; bleeding, and/or prolapse

SUMMARY OF PROCEDURE

	Surgical Hemorrhoidectomy	Stapled Hemorrhoidopexy
Position	Prone jackknife, lithotomy or left lateral decubitus	Prone jackknife, lithotomy
Incision	Series of vertical incisions from anal verge to top of hemorrhoid columns	None
Special instrumentation	Headlight or lighted anoscope; operating anoscope	Circular anal dilator, obturator, stapler
Antibiotics	None	None
Surgical time	30–90 min	10–20 min
EBL	< 100 mL	100 mL
Postop care	Sitz baths, oral fluids, fiber supplements	
Mortality	Rare	
Morbidity	Urinary retention: 15–30% Incontinence: 1–6% Bleeding: 2–5% Stricture: 2–5% Infection: 1–2%	
Pain score	9	5

PATIENT POPULATION CHARACTERISTICS

Age range	Peak prevalence 45–65 yr
Male:Female	1:1
Incidence	Prevalence 75/1000

PATIENT POPULATION CHARACTERISTICS (cont'd)	
Etiology	Low-fiber diet; genetic; pregnancy
Associated conditions	Constipation

ANESTHETIC CONSIDERATIONS

See Anesthetic Considerations following Operations for Fecal Incontinence p. 546.

Suggested Readings

1. Bailey HR, Snyder MJ, eds: *Ambulatory Anorectal Surgery*. Springer-Verlag, New York: 2000.
2. Corman ML, Gravie JF, Hager T, et al: Stapled haemorrhoidopexy: a consensus position paper by an international working party - indications, contra-indications and technique. *Colorectal Dis* 2003; 5(4): 304–10.
3. Gencosmanoglu R, et al: Hemorrhoidectomy: open or closed technique technique (RCT)? *Dis Colon Rectum* 2002; 45:70–5.
4. Hussein AM: Ligation-anopexy for treatment of advanced hemorrhoidal disease. *Dis Colon Rectum* 2001; 44:1887–90.
5. Khan S, Pawlak SE, et al: Surgical treatment of hemorrhoids: prospective, randomized trial comparing closed excisional hemorrhoidectomy and the Harmonic Scalpel technique of excisional hemorrhoidectomy. *Dis Colon Rectum* 2001; 44: 845–9.
6. Konsten J, Baeten CG: Hemorrhoidectomy vs. Lord's method: 17-year follow-up. *Dis Colon Rectum* 2000; 43:503–6.
7. Moore BA, Fleshner PR: Rubber band ligation for hemorrhoidal disease can be safely performed in select HIV-positive patients. *Dis Colon Rectum* 2001; 44:1079–82.
8. Shao WJ, Li GC, Zhang GH, et al: Systematic review and meta-analysis of randomized controlled trials comparing stapled haemorrhoidopexy with conventional haemorrhoidectomy. *Br J Surg* 2008;95(2):147–60.
9. Wolff BG, Garcia-Aguilar J, Roberts PL, et al, eds: *The ASCRS Textbook of Colon and Rectal Surgery*, Springer Science-Business Media, New York: 2007.

OPERATIONS FOR FECAL INCONTINENCE

SURGICAL CONSIDERATIONS

Description: In the majority of patients, fecal incontinence is caused by a combination of pudendal neuropathy and atrophy of pelvic floor muscles. Only when an anatomic defect in the sphincter mechanism can be identified is surgery likely to be beneficial. **Sphincteroplasty** is performed in the prone jackknife position after a full mechanical bowel prep. An incision is made at the anal verge, centered over the area of injured sphincter, and extended sufficiently around the anus to reach the retracted, cut edges of the sphincter. The anoderm and rectal mucosa are dissected off of the internal surface of the sphincter. The external surface of the sphincter mechanism is then dissected free to the level of the pelvic diaphragm. Care must be taken not to injure the inferior hemorrhoidal nerves during dissection around the posterior-lateral sphincter. The fibrotic portion linking the two ends of sphincter is cut, and the ends are overlapped and secured in place with two layers of interrupted horizontal mattress sutures. In women with obstetric injuries, the transverse perineal muscles are reapproximated. The skin may be reapproximated at the anal verge and along the reconstructed perineum or left open. The remainder of the skin is closed as completely as possible.

Variant procedure or approaches: The surgical options for patients without anatomic defects in their sphincters are generally unsuccessful. The **posterior anoplasty of Parks** was designed to passively enhance continence by increasing the normally occurring angle between the rectum and the anal canal, and to increase the mechanical efficiency of weak sphincter muscle by shortening the fiber length. Lack of efficacy has limited its use, although some surgeons still perform it in the setting of continued incontinence after abdominal repair of rectal prolapse. The operation is performed in the prone jackknife position after a standard bowel prep. A hemispherical incision is placed at the level of the intersphincteric groove over the posterior half of the anus. The plane between the internal and external anal sphincters is identified and developed proximally to above the puborectalis musculus. The puborectalis fibers are "reefed," or pulled together, as far as possible with nonabsorbable suture. The external sphincter is plicated together in the midline with a series of nonabsorbable sutures that start at the deep external sphincter and progress to the subcutaneous sphincter. Skin is closed with absorbable sutures.

The **Thiersch operation (pinch graft)** has a high complication rate and should be considered primarily in debilitated patients with symptomatic rectal prolapse or fecal incontinence. As originally described, the anal canal was encircled with a silver wire, which served as a passive obstacle to prolapse or defecation. In more recent years, an elastic sheet of Dacron-impregnated Silastic mesh has been used. Two small incisions are made on opposite sides of the anal verge. A pathway around the anal canal is created by blunt dissection and a 1.5-cm wide piece of mesh is led around the anal canal. The ends of the mesh are overlapped in one of the incisions and either sutured or stapled together at an appropriate level of tension. The wounds are irrigated with antibiotic solution, and the incisions are closed.

Usual preop diagnosis: Fecal (enteric) incontinence

SUMMARY OF PROCEDURES

	Overlapping Sphincteroplasty	Parks Repair	Modified Thiersch Procedure
Position	Prone jackknife	⇐	Prone jackknife or lithotomy
Incision	Circumanal	⇐	2 small incisions lateral to the anus
Special instrumentation	Headlight	⇐	Headlight; Silastic mesh
Unique considerations	Urinary catheter preop; standard bowel prep	⇐	None
Antibiotics	Ertapenem 1 g iv or 2nd generation cephalosporin	⇐	⇐
Surgical time	1–2 h	1 h	30–45 min
EBL	< 100 mL	⇐	⇐
Postop care	Early: Sitz baths Late: fiber supplement, stool softener	⇐ ⇐	⇐ ⇐
Mortality	Rare	⇐	⇐
Morbidity	Unimproved incontinence: 20% Improved, but minor incontinence: 30% Prolonged wound healing: 20% Infection: 1–2%	60–80% — — —	20% Erosion of prosthesis: 30–60% Obstructed defecation: 20–40% Infection
Pain score	8	7	6

PATIENT POPULATION CHARACTERISTICS

Age range	Bimodal: 3rd–5th decades for obstetric injury, fistulotomy, and perineal trauma; 6th–8th decades for pudendal neuropathy/pelvic floor atrophy
Male:Female	1:4
Incidence	Not uncommon
Etiology	Pudendal neuropathy; pelvic floor atrophy; obstetric injury; injury during anal surgery (fistulotomy, sphincterotomy, hemorrhoidectomy); perineal trauma; neurologic disease; congenital anomalies
Associated conditions	Urinary incontinence; chronic constipation; multiparity

ANESTHETIC CONSIDERATIONS

(Procedures covered: excision or repair of rectal prolapse; rectal surgery; anal fistulotomy/fistulectomy; anal sphincterotomy/sphincteroplasty; hemorrhoidectomy; operations for fecal incontinence)

PREOPERATIVE

Respiratory	A careful evaluation of patient's respiratory status is important. If patient has ↓ reserve, the lithotomy position may be better tolerated than the prone or jackknife positions. **Tests:** As indicated from H&P.
Musculoskeletal	Pain is likely to be present at the surgical site and should be considered when positioning patient for anesthetic induction (e.g., if patient has pain while sitting, perform regional anesthesia in the lateral decubitus position). Evaluate bony landmarks if regional anesthetic is planned.
Hematologic	Patients rarely anemic from chronic GI bleeding **Tests:** CBC
Laboratory	Other tests as indicated from H&P.
Premedication	Standard premedication (p. B-1)

INTRAOPERATIVE

Anesthetic technique: MAC, GA, spinal, or epidural techniques may be used.

General anesthesia:

Induction	**General (LMA vs ETT):** Standard induction (p. B-2). Procedures done in the prone or jackknife position may require ET intubation for airway control if regional anesthesia is not performed.
Maintenance	Standard maintenance (p. B-2)
Emergence	No special considerations

Regional anesthesia:

Spinal	Patient in either sitting, lateral decubitus, prone, or jackknife position for placement of a subarachnoid block. Doses of local anesthetics should be adequate to provide a high lumbar level (L1-2) of sensory anesthesia (e.g., tetracaine 10–14 mg; bupivacaine 8–12 mg). Patients should remain in relative head-up position with hyperbaric solution and in head-down position with hypobaric solutions to limit cephalad spread of block.
Epidural	Patient in sitting or lateral decubitus position for placement of epidural catheter. A test dose (e.g., 3 mL of 1.5% lidocaine with 1:200,000 epinephrine) is administered and the patient is observed for the development of a subarachnoid block or symptoms of an intravascular injection. Titrate 2% lidocaine with epinephrine (3–5 mL at a time) until the desired level (usually L1-2 adequate) is obtained.
MAC	Should be performed only on selected patients who are highly motivated and with surgeons experienced in performing procedure with infiltration of local anesthesia (usually 2% lidocaine with 1:200,000 epinephrine and 0.5% bupivacaine mixture). Perirectal injection of local anesthetic is quite painful and very short-acting agents (e.g., propofol 30–50 mg, remifentanil 25–100 mcg, ketamine 20–50 mg, or alfentanil 250–750 mcg) should be administered to minimize patient discomfort during the injection. As drug effect will vary widely in patients, they should be carefully titrated to desired level of sedation. Deep sedation and apnea must be avoided, especially in patients in prone or jackknife positions. A bed must be immediately available to turn patients supine and the anesthesiologist should always be prepared to administer GA if necessary.

Blood and fluid requirements	IV: 16–20 ga × 1 (depending on scope of rectal procedure NS/LR @ 5–8 mL/kg/h	Blood products rarely needed.
Monitoring	Standard monitors (p. B-1)	Others as clinically indicated.
Positioning	✓ and pad pressure points ✓ eyes	Chest support or bolsters to optimize ventilation in the jackknife position; care in positioning the patient's extremities and genitals after turning into jackknife position. Avoid pressure on eyes and ears after turning patient.
Complications	Peroneal nerve injury	Lithotomy position can → damage to peroneal nerve, resulting in foot drop. Laryngospasm may occur if inadequate depth of anesthesia during anal dilation.

POSTOPERATIVE

Complications	Urinary retention. Cauda equina syndrome Poor wound healing Atelectasis	Catheterize until return of urinary function. Cauda equina syndrome is characterized by varying degrees of urinary/fecal incontinence, sensory loss in the perineal area, and lower extremity motor weakness.
Pain management	PCA (p. C-3) Epidural analgesia (p. C-2)	PO analgesics may be suitable: acetaminophen and codeine (Tylenol #3 1–2 tab q 4–6 h) or oxycodone and acetaminophen (Percocet 1 tab q 6 h).
Tests	As indicated by patient status.	

Suggested Readings

1. Bachoo P, Brazelli M, et al: Surgery for faecal incontinence in adults. *Cochrane Database Syst Rev* (2):CD001757.
2. Bailey HR, Snyder MJ, eds: *Ambulatory Anorectal Surgery*: Springer-Verlag, New York: 2000.
3. Barisic G, Krivokapic Z, Marković V, et al: The role of overlapping sphincteroplasty in traumatic fecal incontinence. *Acta Chir Iugosl* 2000; 47(4 Suppl 1):37–41.
4. Bernard C: Epidural and spinal anesthesia. In *Clinical Anesthesia,* 3rd edition. Barash PG, Cullen BF, Stoelting RK, eds. Lippincott-Raven, Philadelphia: 1997, 645–65.
5. Gordon, PH, Nivatvongs S, eds: *Principles and Practice of Surgery of Colon, Rectum, and Anus,* 3rd Edition. Informa Healthcare, New York: 2000.
6. Malouf AJ, Norton CS, Engel AF, et al: Long-term results of overlapping anterior anal-sphincter repair for obstetric trauma. *Lancet* 2000; 355(9200):260–5.
7. Matsuoka H, Mavrantonis C, Wexner SD, et al: Postanal repair for fecal incontinence–is it worthwhile? *Dis Colon Rectum* 2000; 43(11): 1561–7.
8. Rigler ML, Drasner K, Krejcie TC, et al: Cauda equina syndrome after continuous spinal anesthesia. *Anesth Analg* 1991; 72(3):275–81.
9. Wolff BG, Garcia-Aguilar J, Roberts PL, et al, eds: *The ASCRS Textbook of Colon and Rectal Surgery.* Springer Science-Business Media, New York: 2007.
10. Wong WD, Congliosi SM, Spencer MP, et al: The safety and efficacy of the artificial bowel sphincter for fecal incontinence: results from a multicenter cohort study. *Dis Colon Rectum* 2002; 45(9):1139–53.

CHAPTER

7.5 Hepatic Surgery

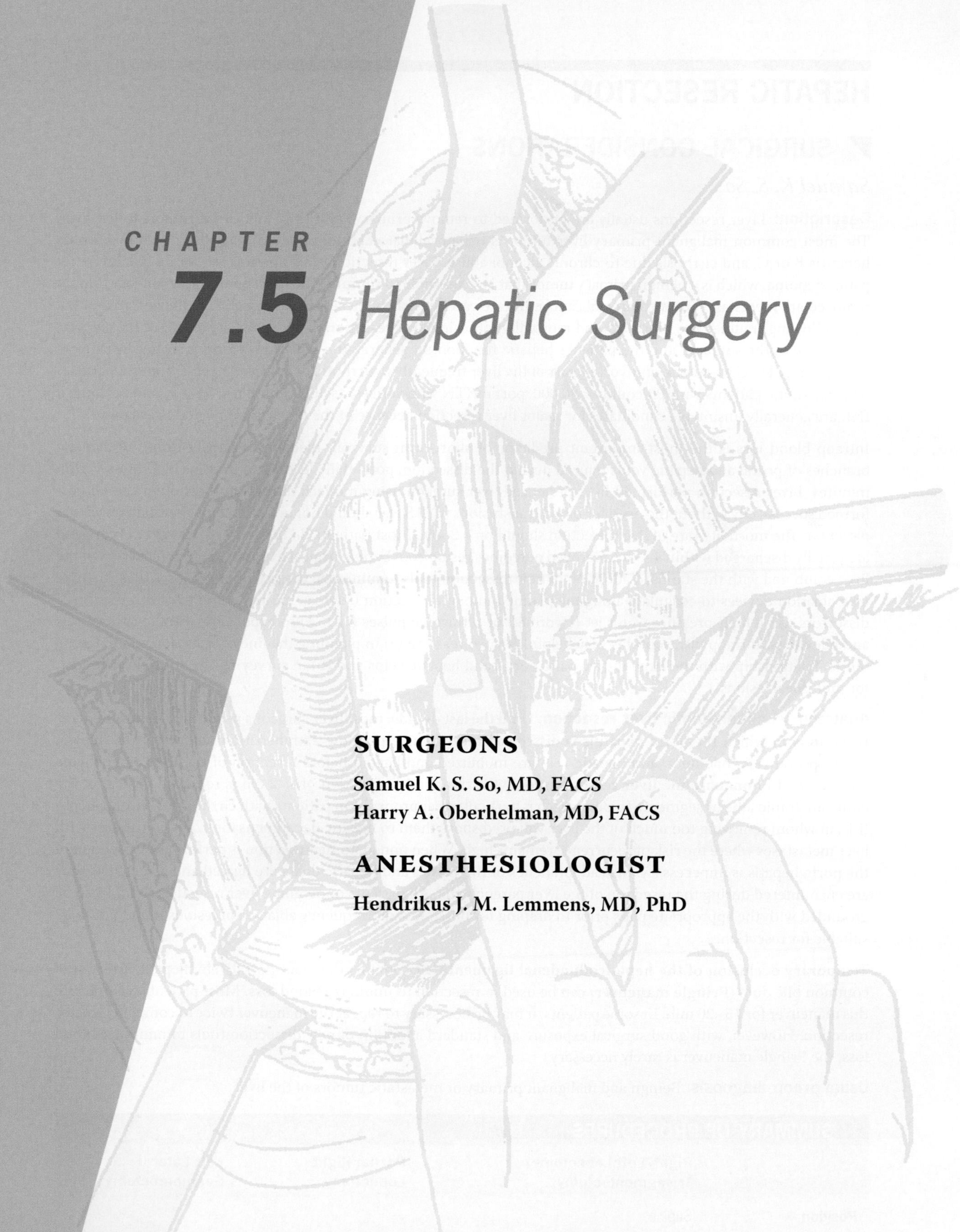

SURGEONS

Samuel K. S. So, MD, FACS

Harry A. Oberhelman, MD, FACS

ANESTHESIOLOGIST

Hendrikus J. M. Lemmens, MD, PhD

HEPATIC RESECTION

SURGICAL CONSIDERATIONS

Samuel K. S. So

Description: Liver resections usually are performed to remove primary tumors or metastatic tumors to the liver. The most common malignant primary liver tumor is hepatocellular carcinoma (HCC), usually caused by chronic hepatitis B or C, and cirrhosis due to chronic alcohol abuse. Liver resection is also performed for an enlarging hepatic adenoma, which is a benign primary tumor that is susceptible to rupture. The most common secondary tumors removed are metastases from colorectal cancer. In rare cases, it may be necessary to resect a devitalized area of the liver following trauma. The mortality and morbidity following liver resection depends on the extent of the surgery, experience of the surgeon, and the patient's hepatic function. In general, the risk of resection is higher in patients with primary HCC where the uninvolved part of the liver frequently is cirrhotic or diseased from chronic hepatitis B or C. Cirrhotic patients with Plt counts < 80,000, portal HTN with varices, ascites, albumin < 3.5 g/L, and prolonged INR are generally unsuitable candidates for major liver resection because of the high risk of postop liver failure.

Intraop blood loss is the most important predictor of short-term survival. Bleeding is largely from intrahepatic branches of portal and hepatic veins injured during the dissection, potentially leading to massive blood loss within minutes. Liver resection performed by experienced liver surgeon using modern dissection tools often can be performed successfully without the need for blood transfusions (Cell Saver should not be used when operating on cancer patients). The mortality rate of liver resection should be < 2–5%. Most patients do not require postop ICU care and are usually discharged within 4–5 d. Improved outcomes result from better surgical exposure and mobilization of the liver combined with the standard adoption of new dissection tools to minimize the risk of blood loss. These include new ablation devices to coagulate along the planned line of a resection (such as InLine) combined with the use of dissectors using high-pressure water jet (Hydrojet) or ultrasonic pulses (CUSA) to expose the intrahepatic vessels and bile ducts. Intraop ultrasound is very helpful for two reasons: (a) in planning the line of resection and mapping out its relationship with the large intrahepatic portal and hepatic veins and (b) in surveying the entire liver to look for multifocal lesions.

Anatomic vs nonanatomic liver resection: Until the last decade, most liver surgeons performed **anatomic liver resections** in which the porta hepatitis is dissected and the corresponding extrahepatic branches of the hepatic artery, portal vein, bile duct, and hepatic vein are mobilized and ligated before resection of the liver parenchyma (Fig. 7.5-1). In **nonanatomic liver resections**, only the tumor with a margin of 1–2 cm is removed instead of the entire anatomic lobe or segment. This approach is particularly appropriate in patients with cirrhosis or chronic hepatitis, in whom removing too much of the liver will predispose them to hepatic decompensation, and in patients with liver metastases where the risk of recurrence remains high. When nonanatomic resection is performed, dissection of the porta hepatis is unnecessary. Instead, branches of the vessels and hepatic ducts are ligated and resected as they are encountered during the resection of the liver parenchyma. All patients undergoing liver resection should also be grounded with the appropriate pads prior to draping for possible radiofrequency ablation of lesions found not to be suitable for resection.

Temporary occlusion of the hepaticoduodenal ligament that contains the main portal vein, hepatic artery, and common bile duct (**Pringle maneuver**) can be used in resection to minimize blood loss. Most patients will tolerate this maneuver for 15–20 min. In some patients, it may be necessary to repeat the maneuver twice to complete a major resection. However, with good surgical exposure and standard adoption of new dissection tools to minimize blood loss, the Pringle maneuver is rarely necessary.

Usual preop diagnosis: Benign and malignant primary or metastatic tumors of the liver

SUMMARY OF PROCEDURES

	Right/Left Lobectomy/ Trisegmentectomy	Partial Right Lobectomy	Left Lateral Segmentectomy
Position	Supine	⇐	⇐
Incision	Upper midline, extending to right subcostal (Lexus incision)	⇐	Upper midline

SUMMARY OF PROCEDURES (cont'd)

	Right/Left Lobectomy/ Trisegmentectomy	Partial Right Lobectomy	Left Lateral Segmentectomy
Special instrumentation	Thompson liver retractor; InLine, Helix Hydro-jet or CUSA; TissueLink dissecting sealer; argon beam laser; tumor ablation device; intraop ultrasound	⇐	⇐
Unique considerations	Maintain normal core Temp. Most intrahepatic bleeding can be controlled temporarily by compression. Note the duration of Pringle maneuver, if applied. Give mannitol furosemide for hemoglobinuria associated with extensive radiofrequency ablation of the liver to reduce the risk of postoperative acute tubular necrosis	⇐	⇐
Antibiotics	Vancomycin/cefazolin 1 g iv preop	⇐	⇐
Surgical time	3–8 h	4–6 h	< 3 h
Closing considerations	Secure meticulous hemostasis; place two perihepatic Jackson Pratt flat bulb suction drains.	⇐	⇐
EBL	Variable (50–800 mL)	100–500 mL	100–300 mL
Postop care	PACU → ward	⇐	⇐
Mortality	< 2–5%	⇐	< 1%
Morbidity	Ascites: 20–30% Wound infection: 5–10% Liver failure: < 5% Bile leak: < 5% Postop bleeding: < 2–5%	10–20% ⇐ ⇐ < 2–5% ⇐	< 10% ⇐ < 2% ⇐ ⇐
Pain score	7–8	7–8	7

PATIENT POPULATION CHARACTERISTICS

Age range	19–85 yr
Male:Female	4:1 in primary HCC 2:1 in liver metastases
Incidence	Metastatic colorectal cancer is the most common disease treated with liver resection in the United States. The incidence of primary HCC is rising 2° the prevalence of chronic hepatitis C; however, because of delayed Dx and associated hepatitis C cirrhosis, many are not suitable resection candidates. Primary HCC is a common cancer in Asian Americans because of the high incidence of chronic hepatitis B. Many young Asians (30–50 yr) with HCC 2° chronic hepatitis B may not have cirrhosis.
Associated conditions	Cirrhosis; chronic hepatitis; and, rarely, hemochromatosis; Hx of colorectal surgery in patients with liver metastases

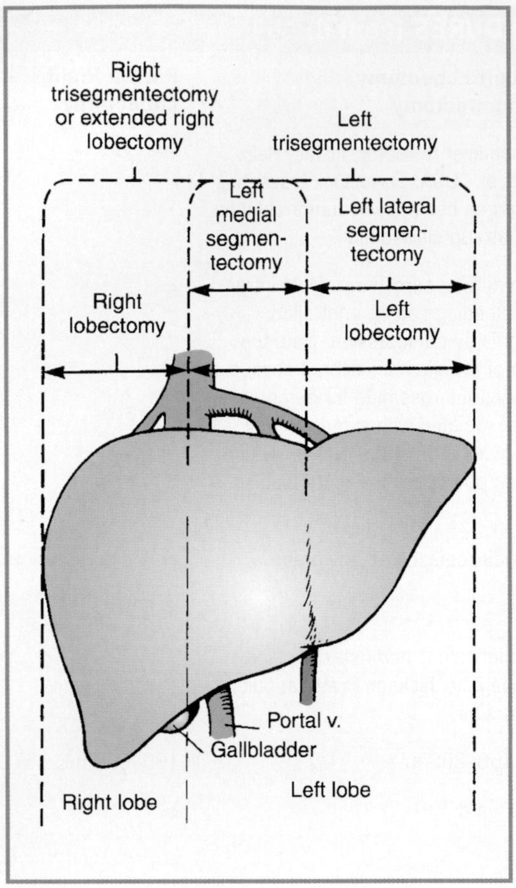

Figure 7.5-1. Types of liver resection. (Reproduced with permission from Hardy JD: *Hardy's Textbook of Surgery,* 2nd edition. JB Lippincott, Philadelphia: 1988.)

ANESTHETIC CONSIDERATIONS

See Anesthetic Considerations following Hepatorrhaphy, p. 553.

Suggested Readings

1. D'angelica M, Fung Y: The liver. In *Sabiston's Textbook of Surgery,* 18th edition. Townsend CM, et al, eds. Sanders Elsevier, Philadelphia: 2007, 1463–523.
2. Delman KA, Curley SA: Hepatic neoplasms. In *Greenfield's Surgery: Scientific Principles and Practice,* 4th edition. Mulholland MW, et al, eds. Lippincott Williams & Wilkens, Philadelphia: 2006, 956–77.
3. Jarnegan WR: Liver and portal venous system. In *Current Surgical Diagnosis and Treatment,* 12th edition. Doherty GM, ed. McGraw-Hill Medical, New York: 2006, 539–72.

HEPATORRHAPHY

SURGICAL CONSIDERATIONS

Harry A. Oberhelman

Description: Although most liver lacerations have stopped bleeding by the time a surgeon sees them, others require suturing or partial liver resection to control bleeding. Various techniques are available to control hemorrhage, including packing, suturing, inflow occlusion, and resection. Small lacerations that have stopped bleeding require no specific therapy other than possible drainage. Lacerations that continue to bleed usually can be sutured and drained. Extensive tears of the liver that are actively bleeding may require temporary occlusion of the porta hepatis, containing the hepatic artery, portal vein, and bile duct (**Pringle maneuver**) to excise deviated parenchyma and control bleeding with sutures, clips, coagulators, etc. Occasionally, the hepatic vein draining the involved lobe will require clamping to control back-bleeding. When the bleeding cannot be controlled, it is expedient to pack the wound, drain the abdomen, and close. The pack can be removed without much risk of rebleeding within 48–72 h.

Usual preop diagnosis: Trauma with CT evidence of hepatic laceration

SUMMARY OF PROCEDURE	
Position	Supine
Incision	Midline abdominal
Special instrumentation	Denier retractor
Antibiotics	Cefazolin I g iv
Surgical time	1–2 h
EBL	~300–2000 mL
Mortality	1–2%
Morbidity	Continued bleeding: 2–3% Biliary fistula Perihepatic abscess Intrahepatic hematoma Arterioportal fistula Hepatic and renal failure
Pain score	7–9

PATIENT POPULATION CHARACTERISTICS	
Age range	Variable
Male:Female	1:1
Incidence	Rare
Etiology	Trauma (blunt vs penetrating); surgical; hepatic adenomas; needle biopsies of liver

ANESTHETIC CONSIDERATIONS FOR HEPATIC PROCEDURES

(Procedures covered: hepatic resection; hepatorrhaphy)

PREOPERATIVE

Patients presenting for hepatic surgery may have primary or metastatic tumors from GI and other sources. Liver function may be entirely normal in these patients. HCC is seen commonly in males > 50 yr, and is associated with chronic active hepatitis B and cirrhosis. The preop considerations listed below describe patients without cirrhosis. (See Preoperative Considerations for Surgery for Portal Hypertension, p. 434) for evaluation of patients with cirrhosis).

Respiratory	Respiratory function is typically normal; however, patients with ascites may have respiratory compromise. **Tests:** CXR; others as clinically indicated.
Cardiovascular	Patients may be hypovolemic, and volume status should be carefully assessed before induction of anesthesia (skin turgor, UO, orthostatic BP, HR, etc). Tumors may surround major vascular structures and impede venous return. Consider evaluation with CT/MRI scan.

Hepatic	Liver resection can be indicated for hemangiomas, hydatid cysts, and tumors. It is important to determine the size of the tumor and involvement of vascular structures preop so as to be adequately prepared for major intraop blood and fluid losses. **Tests:** LFTs; albumin; ultrasound/CT/MRI
Hematologic	The liver produces all clotting factors except VIII, and the degree of hepatic insufficiency determines the extent of any coagulopathy. T&C 4 U PRBCs. **Tests:** CBC; PT; PTT; Plt count; others as indicated from H&P.
Laboratory	* Tests as indicated from H&P. **NB:** For elective cases, if abnormal LFTs are present on preop labs, it is important to perform a complete medical workup. This can include reviewing old lab data, hepatitis serology, and an abdominal ultrasound to r/o cholestatic causes of liver dysfunction. Surgery and anesthesia in the presence of acute hepatitis is associated with a high mortality.
Premedication	Consider midazolam 1–2 mg iv (see B-1). Consider administering vitamin K (e.g., 10 mg iv/sc) if PT is prolonged. Beneficial results from vitamin K usually occur within 24 h. Consider FFP for rapid correction of PT.

INTRAOPERATIVE

Anesthetic technique: GETA. For major liver resections, the surgeon may attempt to reduce blood loss by applying intermittent vascular inflow occlusion or total vascular exclusion. As the result of ischemia induced by vascular occlusion and the loss of liver mass during resection, liver function may be significantly abnormal in the postop period. Coagulation abnormalities may exist; consequently, an epidural catheter for postop pain relief may be associated with ↑ risk of hematoma formation.

Induction	Standard induction (see B-2). Restore intravascular volume before induction. Trauma patients or those with ascites require rapid-sequence induction (see B-5) with cricoid pressure until intubation has been confirmed. If patient is hemodynamically unstable, consider etomidate (0.2–0.4 mg/kg) or ketamine (1–3 mg/kg) in place of propofol.	
Maintenance	Standard maintenance (p. B-2); N_2O can be used if bowel distention will not impede surgical exposure/closure. If total vascular occlusion is used, elevate CVP to at least 12 mmHg by rapid fluid administration before cross-clamping. Have Neo-Synephrine and epinephrine infusions ready to treat ↓ BP. After major resections, significant hemodynamic changes occur. CO and HR increase, and systemic vascular resistance decreases.	
Emergence	For major hepatic resections, the patient will be best cared for in an ICU. After major blood loss, consider keeping the patient mechanically ventilated.	
Blood and fluid requirements	Anticipate large blood loss. IV: 14–16 ga × 2 NS/LR @ 10–20 mL/kg/h Fluid warmer Humidify gases Consider utilizing rapid-transfusion device.	Blood loss can be significant; keep at least 2 U PRBC ahead. Lobectomies often are associated with more blood loss than wedge resections. Massive transfusions may be required and appropriate blood products should be available (e.g., 2 FFPs + 6 Plt per 10 U PRBC). If procedure does not involve cancer, blood salvage devices may be used.
Control of blood loss	Surgical control Pringle maneuver Total vascular exclusion	Surgical occlusion of the main blood vessels entering the hilar area (Pringle maneuver), or total vascular occlusion. Total vascular exclusion is accomplished by complete occlusion of liver inflow and outflow.
Monitoring	Standard monitors (see B-1) UO CVP Arterial line ± TEE	Others as clinically indicated. If the extent of the resection is not known at the beginning of surgery, appropriate monitoring (CVP, arterial line, additional iv's) should be established prior to beginning resection. Forced-air warmer.

General Surgery

Positioning	✓ and pad pressure points ✓ eyes	
Complications	Massive hemorrhage	Ensure adequate vascular access. Consider rapid-transfusion device.

POSTOPERATIVE

Complications	✓ liver function Hemorrhage Electrolyte imbalance Hypoglycemia Hypothermia, shivering DIC	Patients with normal liver function preop may have significant postop impairment of liver function 2° loss of liver mass or ischemic injury induced by vascular occlusion.
	Pulmonary insufficiency	> 90% of patients will develop some form of respiratory complication (atelectasis, effusion, pneumonia).
Pain management	PCA (see C-3)	Patient should be recovered in ICU or hospital ward that is accustomed to treating the side effects of opiates (e.g., respiratory depression, breakthrough pain, nausea, pruritus).
Tests	ABG; CXR; others as clinically indicated.	

Suggested Readings

1. Kaufman BS, Roccoforte JD: Anesthesia and the liver. In *Clinical Anesthesia*, 5th edition. Barash PG, Cullen BF, Stoelting RK, eds, Lippincott Williams & Wilkins, Philadelphia: 2006, 1072–111.
2. Niemann CU, Roberts JP, Ascher NL, et al: Intraoperative hemodynamics and liver function in adult to adult living liver donors. *Liver Transpl* 2002; 8:1126–32.
3. Redai I, Emond J, Brentjens T: Anesthetic considerations during liver surgery. *Surg Clin North Am* 2004; 84(2):401–11.
4. Suman A, Carey W: Assessing the risk of surgery in patients with liver disease. *Cleve Clin J Med* 2006; 73(4):398–404.

CHAPTER

7.6 Biliary Tract Surgery

SURGEON

C. Andrew Bonham, MD

ANESTHESIOLOGIST

Hendrikus J.M. Lemmens, MD, PhD

OPEN CHOLECYSTECTOMY AND COMMON BILE DUCT EXPLORATION

SURGICAL CONSIDERATIONS

Description: With the advent of laparoscopic cholecystectomy, the traditional **open cholecystectomy** has become a rarity and is generally reserved for gallbladders that are expected to be difficult to remove due to inflammation, previous operations and adhesions, or because of other medical problems, such as coagulopathy or cirrhosis. In most institutions, fewer than 10% of cholecystectomies will be begun as open procedures, and perhaps 5% of laparoscopic cholecystectomies will be converted to open cholecystectomies during the course of the operation due to technical difficulties, complications, or unexpected findings. Because of its rarity, the open cholecystectomy may be a more challenging operation for both surgeon and anesthesiologist than it was in previous decades. A small number of open cholecystectomies are performed in an urgent fashion following a complication of an attempted laparoscopic cholecystectomy and may be associated with significant instability from hemorrhage or sepsis related to an iatrogenic injury of abdominal or retroperitoneal structures.

The technical aspects of **open cholecystectomy** have not changed since its original description over 100 years ago. The operation can be performed through a right subcostal **(Kocher)**, paramedian, or midline incision. Upward traction is applied to the liver or gallbladder, whereas downward traction on the duodenum exposes the region of the cystic duct and artery and common duct. Adequate exposure is critical to performing a safe operation. Depending on local conditions and the surgeon's preference, the gallbladder may be removed from the top down, excising the gallbladder from the liver bed and isolating the cystic duct and artery as the final stage of the operation. The cystic duct and artery may be isolated and divided first, and the gallbladder removed retrograde from the gallbladder bed as the final step of the procedure. The anatomy of the biliary tree is quite variable, with the classic anatomy present in only 30% of patients, and few surgeons always remove the gallbladder in exactly the same way every time. (Fig. 7.6-1 shows exposure of the gallbladder.)

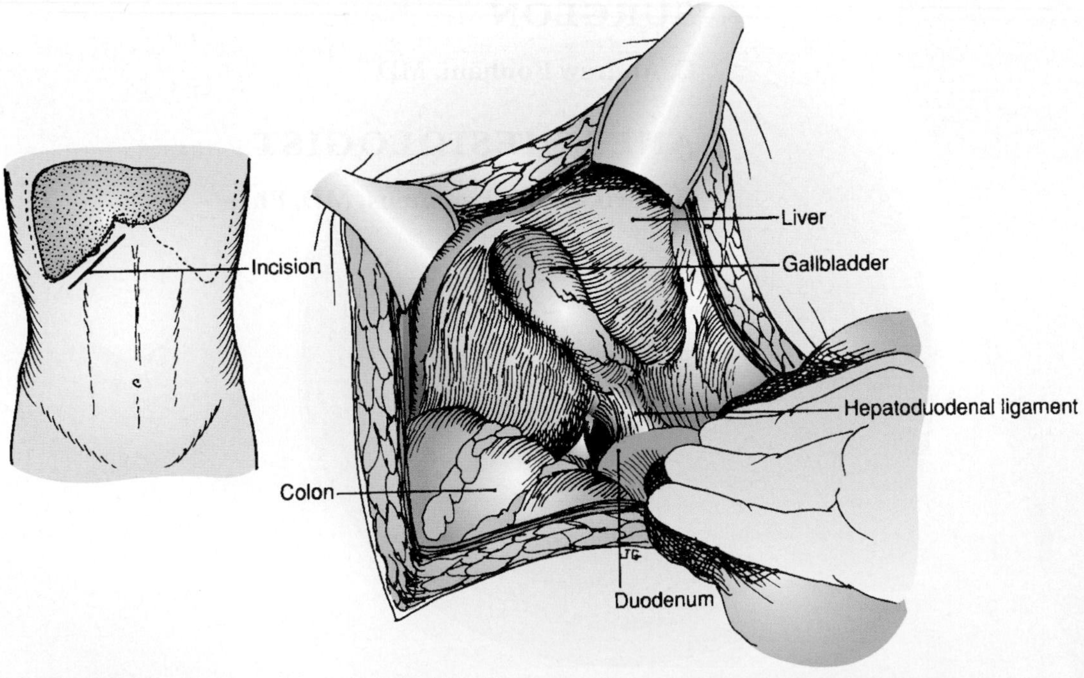

Figure 7.6-1. Incision and exposure of the gallbladder. (Reproduced with permission from Scott-Conner CEH, Dawson DL: *Operative Anatomy,* 2nd edition. Lippincott Williams & Wilkins, Philadelphia: 2002.)

Cholangiography may be performed at the discretion of the surgeon. Some surgeons perform it in all patients and others perform it only in patients in whom there is some clinical evidence of choledocholithiasis. The cystic duct is opened and a catheter placed into the duct and secured with a ligature, tie, or special cholangiogram clamp. Dye is injected into the biliary tree via the catheter, and x-rays are taken. If stones are found, a **common duct exploration** may be performed. Alternatively, an **endoscopic retrograde cholangiogram** (ERCP) with stone extraction may be carried out postoperatively. Cholangiography usually adds 10–15 min to the procedure.

Choledochotomy, or **"common duct exploration,"** is the opening and exploration of the common duct for the purpose of extracting stones. Once commonly performed, it is a procedure reserved chiefly for patients who have failed management of common duct stones with endoscopic (ERCP) or laparoscopic techniques. Common duct stones are visualized by operative cholangiography to determine number of stones, position, and the anatomy of the duct. Ducts smaller than 5 mm in diameter are at greater risk of injury with common duct exploration and should be managed endoscopically. An extensive **Kocher maneuver** is performed to allow exposure and palpation of the entire duct, including the intrapancreatic portion. A longitudinal incision is made in the duct and exploration is carried out through this incision. The duct may be irrigated with NS, balloon catheters may be passed, and various instruments introduced to grasp, remove, or crush retained stones. The duct may be biopsied by this approach and **choledochoscopy**—the direct visualization of the duct's interior using a small flexible scope—can be performed. Rarely, an impacted stone may require electrohydraulic or laser lithotripsy through the choledochoscope, adding considerable time to the operation in centers equipped to perform the procedure. The choledochotomy is closed over a T-tube to allow decompression of the edematous duct and later extraction of stones missed at the initial exploration. In the past, **transduodenal sphincteroplasty** was utilized for stones impacted near the sphincter of Oddi, but this procedure has largely been replaced by endoscopic or percutaneous techniques at specialized centers. It is reserved for highly unusual cases, such as a patient with a previous **Billroth II gastrectomy**. Depending on the complexity of the findings, a common duct exploration can be expected to add from 30 min to over 1 h to the cholecystectomy. In general, the mortality of patients undergoing common duct exploration is ~2–5 times that of a simple cholecystectomy. This difference can be explained by the fact that patients undergoing common duct exploration tend to be older and sicker or suffering from concomitant cholangitis—the opening of the duct itself is not necessarily a significant physiologic insult.

Variant procedure or approaches: Cholecystectomy remains the mainstay of treatment for symptomatic biliary stone disease. **Nonsurgical treatment of cholelithiasis,** particularly by oral dissolution and/or **lithotripsy**, has very limited usefulness and is rarely used in clinical practice. **Tube cholecystostomy** can be performed as an open procedure or percutaneously. It is generally reserved as a temporary measure in patients too ill to tolerate a more extensive procedure.

Usual preop diagnosis: Symptomatic cholelithiasis; acute cholecystitis; chronic cholecystitis; biliary dyskinesia; gallbladder polyps or carcinoma; choledocholithiasis

SUMMARY OF PROCEDURES

	Cholecystectomy	Cholecystectomy/Common Duct Exploration
Position	Supine	⇐
Incision	Right subcostal or midline	Right subcostal and/or midline
Special instrumentation	Costal margin retractor; cholangiocatheter	Choledochotomy instruments; choledochoscope
Unique considerations	Requires intraop x-ray for cholangiogram.	May include choledochoscopy
Antibiotics	Ampicillin, piperacillin, or mezlocillin, 1–3 g iv; gentamicin; or cefotetan 1–2 g iv	⇐
Surgical time	45–90 min	1–2.5 h
Closing considerations	Muscle relaxation	⇐
EBL	Minimal to 250 mL	⇐
Postop care	PACU → ward	⇐

■ SUMMARY OF PROCEDURES (cont'd)

	Cholecystectomy	Cholecystectomy/Common Duct Exploration
Mortality	0.1% under 50 yr; 0.5% over 50 yr	0–1.5% under 60 yr; 5% in advanced age
Morbidity	Postop bile leak: 0–9% Pancreatitis: 0–4.6% Bile duct injury: 0–0.25% Cardiac and respiratory complications: Rare, but leading cause of death Hemorrhage: Rare	⇐ 2–5%
Pain score	6	6–7

■ PATIENT POPULATION CHARACTERISTICS

Age range	Mostly adult; increases with age
Male:Female	1:2–3
Incidence	600,000/yr in the United States; ≥ 90% performed laparoscopically
Etiology	See Associated Conditions (below).
Associated conditions	Ileal disease; cirrhosis; hemolytic disorders; choledocholithiasis; cholangitis or active pancreatitis

ANESTHETIC CONSIDERATIONS

See Anesthetic Considerations for Biliary Tract Surgery, p. 565.

Suggested Readings

1. Blumgart LH: Stones in the common bile duct–clinical features and open surgical approaches and techniques. In *Surgery of the Liver, Biliary Tract, and Pancreas,* 4th edition. Blumgart LH, ed. Saunders Elsevier, Philadelphia: 2007, 528–47.
2. Fried GM, Feldman LS, Klassen DR: Cholecystectomy and common bile duct exploration. In *ACS Surgery: Principles and Practice 2006.* Souba WW, Fink MP, Jurkovich GJ, et al., eds. WebMD, New York: 2006, 651–72.
3. Gertsch P: The technique of cholecystectomy. In *Surgery of the Liver, Biliary Tract, and Pancreas,* 4th edition. Blumgart LH, ed. Saunders Elsevier, Philadelphia: 2007, 496–505.
4. Matthews BD, Strasberg SM: Management of common duct stones. In *Current Surgical Therapy,* 9th edition. Cameron JL, ed. Mosby Elsevier, Philadelphia: 2008, 412–17.
5. Nagle AP, Soper NJ, Hines JR: Cholecystectomy (open and laparoscopic). In *Maingotis Abdominal Operations,* 11th edition. Zinner MJ, Ashley SW, eds. McGraw Hill Medical, New York: 2007, 847–63.
6. Zemon H, Ponsky TA: Acute cholecystitis. In *Current Surgical Therapy,* 9th edition. Cameron JL, ed. Mosby Elsevier, Philadelphia: 2008, 408–12.

BILIARY DRAINAGE PROCEDURES

SURGICAL CONSIDERATIONS

Description: Biliary drainage procedures may be performed for malignant and nonmalignant indications, and the type of drainage procedure performed depends on factors such as the nature of the biliary obstruction, the patient's overall condition and prognosis, the need for other surgical procedures, and institutional expertise. Most drainage procedures of the biliary tree are performed with **endoscopic** and/or **transhepatic techniques**. These techniques allow concomitant treatment of biliary stone disease, decompression of obstructive jaundice, relief of cholangitis and delineation of the anatomy of the biliary tree. There remain a significant number of patients, however, for whom a traditional surgical procedure is the most appropriate. With the advent of laparoscopic cholecystectomy, surgical bile duct injuries have become the most common reason for surgical biliary drainage procedures. In general, the complexity of the different operations that may be performed and the morbidity attendant to these has more to do with the indications for operation than with the procedure that is performed.

All of these operations are performed under GA through an upper midline or right subcostal incision. Self-retaining retractors are used to retract the liver superiorly to expose the region of the porta hepatis. If the gallbladder will not be used for the bypass procedure (**cholecystojejunostomy**), then it usually is removed as the first step in the procedure (see **Open Cholecystectomy**, p. 558). If the patient has had previous upper right quadrant surgery, the complexity and duration of the procedure and blood loss may increase significantly. Any associated hepatic cirrhosis may make the procedure particularly demanding. Most patients undergoing surgical biliary drainage procedures have had several nonsurgical instrumentations of the bile duct prior to presenting to surgery. Indwelling stents result in colonization of the biliary tract with any number of bacterial or fungal organisms from which the patient may have already suffered bouts of cholangitis. It is not unusual for the patient to develop bacteremia during the operation while these stents are being manipulated.

Transduodenal sphincteroplasty for benign obstruction of the ampulla of Vater or for extensive choledocholithiasis has largely been abandoned in favor of the more well-tolerated and less invasive **endoscopic sphincterotomy.** It remains the treatment of choice for rare cases of early ampullary carcinoma. Endoscopic sphincterotomy and/or placement of an internal stent is the most commonly performed technique for opening the ampulla, and usually is performed by gastroenterologists outside of the OR with iv sedation. **Open sphincteroplasty** is usually reserved for patients in whom endoscopic retrograde cholangiopancreatogram (ERCP) has been unsuccessful or in whom a laparotomy is required for other reasons. For these open procedures, the second portion of duodenum is incised over the region of the ampulla, and the ampulla is cannulated. A longitudinal incision is made over the course of the ampulla, and the mucosa of the ampulla is sutured to the mucosa of the duodenum with fine interrupted sutures with care being taken not to compromise the pancreatic duct. The duodenum is closed with suture, a small closed suction drain is placed, and the wound is closed. A postop stay of 5–7 d can be expected.

Cholecystojejunostomy usually is performed as palliation for malignant obstruction of the distal bile duct. Its advantage is that it does not require dissection of the portal triad, but the long-term results are poor as biliary obstruction typically recurs as the malignancy advances. The abdomen is opened as described above, and the region of the porta hepatis examined to ensure that the cystic duct is not imminently compromised by tumor. The jejunum is then brought up to the gallbladder, usually bypassing the jejunum through the transverse mesocolon. The anastomosis may be performed either to an intact loop of jejunum (**loop cholecystojejunostomy**) or to a Roux-en-Y loop of jejunum (**Roux-en-Y cholecystojejunostomy**), and is carried out with one or two layers of sutures, depending on surgeon's preference. If a Roux-en-Y is created, a second jejunojejunal anastomosis must be performed. This procedure has largely been replaced by transhepatic and endoscopic techniques.

Choledochoduodenostomy is an archaic procedure in which the bile duct is incised longitudinally and anastomosed directly to the adjacent duodenum. This was performed historically in patients with gallstones impacted at the ampulla. However, loss of the normal sphincter mechanism at the ampulla allows reflux of duodenal contents directly into the bile duct. Patients may suffer from repeated episodes of cholangitis or obstructive jaundice from debris occluding the anastomosis. Secondary biliary cirrhosis may occur, and the author has seen one case proceed to liver transplantation in which a cast of the biliary tree comprised of fibrous food material was extracted from the choledochoduodenal anastomosis. **Roux-en-y choledochojejunostomy or hepaticojejunostomy** remains the gold standard by which all other biliary drainage procedures are measured. An anastomosis is fashioned between the common bile duct, common hepatic duct, or even the lobar or segmental bile ducts and a Roux-en-Y loop of jejunum. This is often a relatively demanding operation because it requires dissection deep in the porta hepatis to gain access to the bile duct. Furthermore, many patients have had previous surgery in the porta hepatis with extensive formation of adhesions. Long-term results are more reliable, however, and thus surgical drainage is preferred to less invasive procedures for benign disease. Exposure of the biliary tree is the same as for the above procedures. The gallbladder is always removed (if it is still present). The bile duct is dissected free from the surrounding structures in the porta hepatic and traced proximally into the liver to healthy tissue above the level of obstruction.

Variant procedure or approaches: Endoscopic or transhepatic placement of temporary or permanent **biliary stents** is an increasingly common alternative to surgical drainage in patients with incurable pancreatic or biliary tract disease.

Usual preop diagnosis: Transduodenal sphincteroplasty: extensive choledocholithiasis, often after failed attempt at ERCP; rarely, malignant disease. Cholecystojejunostomy: malignant obstruction of the distal common bile duct, usually due to pancreatic cancer. Choledochojejunostomy or hepaticojejunostomy: benign strictures of the distal bile duct; longstanding stone disease; pancreatitis; iatrogenic injury; Oriental cholangiohepatitis; after resection of some tumors of the pancreas or bile duct.

PATIENT POPULATION CHARACTERISTICS	
Age range	5th–7th decade; may be younger for repair of laparoscopic cholecystectomy injuries
Male:Female	1.1:2.1
Incidence	Procedure-related incidence not available, but clearly declining in favor of techniques by interventional gastroenterology and radiology.
Etiology	See Usual Preop Diagnosis, above.
Associated conditions	Jaundice (very common); fat-soluble vitamin deficiencies; malignancy, especially pancreatic (common); malnutrition (common)

ANESTHETIC CONSIDERATIONS

See Anesthetic Considerations for Biliary Tract Surgery, p. 565.

Suggested Readings

1. Baker MS, Lillemoe KD: Benign biliary strictures. In *Current Surgical Therapy,* 9th edition. Cameron JL, ed. Mosby Elsevier, Philadelphia: 2008, 420–5.
2. Blumgart LH, DíAngelica M, Jarnagin WR: Biliary-enteric anastomosis. In *Surgery of the Liver, Biliary Tract, and Pancreas,* 4th edition. Blumgart LH, ed. Saunders Elsevier, Philadelphia: 2007, 455–74.
3. Jarnagin WR, Blumgart LH: Biliary stricture and fistula. In *Surgery of the Liver, Biliary Tract, and Pancreas,* 4th edition. Blumgart LH, ed. Saunders Elsevier, Philadelphia: 2007, 628–81.
4. Melton GB, Lillemoe KD: Choledochal cyst and biliary strictures. In *Maingotís Abdominal Operations,* 11th edition. Zinner MJ, Ashley SW, eds. McGraw Hill Medical, New York: 2007, 889–920.
5. Taylor BR, Langer B: Procedures for benign and malignant biliary tract disease. In *ACS Surgery: Principles and Practice 2006.* Souba WW, Fink MP, Jurkovich GJ, et al., eds. , New York: 2006, 673–87.

EXCISION OF BILE DUCT TUMOR

SURGICAL CONSIDERATIONS

Description: Primary tumors (cholangiocarcinomas) of the extrahepatic bile ducts, including the hepatic bifurcation (Klatskin tumors) are uncommon malignancies, with the only curative treatment for them being surgical excision. Such tumors are usually classified as being proximal bile duct tumors, involving the hepatic bifurcation and above; middle bile duct tumors, involving the midportion of the common hepatic and common bile duct; and distal bile duct tumors, which involve the distal bile duct, including the intrapancreatic or intraduodenal portion of the bile duct (Fig. 7.6-1). The gallbladder usually will be removed in any such operation.

Distal bile duct tumors, which carry a significantly higher cure rate than either proximal bile duct or pancreatic tumors, may be treated by **pancreaticoduodenectomy**. (See p. 618 for discussion of this operation.)

Mid-bile duct tumors usually are excised by removing a generous portion of the mid bile duct, resecting the ducts up to the hepatic bifurcation, and sometimes performing a pancreaticoduodenectomy. Biliary drainage usually is established by anastomosing the proximal bile duct to a Roux loop of jejunum. For proximal bile duct tumors, most of the extrahepatic bile ducts are excised and biliary drainage is established by anastomosis of the right and left hepatic ducts or even multiple segmental ducts to a Roux loop of jejunum. These are often technically demanding operations with the potential for major blood loss. It may be necessary to perform a major hepatic resection at the same time, and the possibility of this should always be assumed when an operation of this sort is carried out. Often, a transhepatic catheter will have been placed radiographically preoperatively to provide relief of jaundice and to facilitate identification of the bile ducts. Colonization of the biliary tract with enteric bacteria or yeast is common, and may result in bacteremia during surgical manipulation. Prolonged cholestasis may lead to fat soluble vitamin deficiencies, in particular Vitamin K deficiency, which may cause coagulopathy. Long-standing biliary obstruction may cause moderate atrophy and portal venous compromise.

Surgical exposure for any of these operations usually is achieved through a long midline or transverse subcostal incision with midline extension and the use of self-retaining retractors. The liver and gallbladder are retracted superiorly while downward traction is placed on the duodenum. If the gallbladder is still in place, a cholecystectomy is performed (see p. 558). For proximal bile duct tumors and mid bile duct tumors not requiring pancreaticoduodenectomy, the bile duct is divided distally, just above the duodenum, and the pancreatic portion of the bile duct is oversewn. The bile duct is then resected proximally to the level of the bifurcation of the hepatic ducts. A Roux-en-Y loop of jejunum is anastomosed to the hepatic ducts to establish biliary drainage. Drains are placed and most surgeons place a NG tube for such cases.

Variant procedure or approaches: **Endoscopic** or **transhepatic stenting** of areas of stricture often is used as a palliative alternative to surgical excision. These are usually performed radiographically and do not require GA. They may be used as an alternative to resection or in preparation for surgery.

Usual preop diagnosis: Cholangiocarcinoma (common); benign strictures of the bile ducts (infrequent); sclerosing cholangitis (rare)

SUMMARY OF PROCEDURE

Position	Supine
Incision	Midline or subcostal
Special instrumentation	Costal retractor
Unique considerations	Many cases prove unresectable at operation. Intraoperative radiation therapy may be used.
Antibiotics	Ampicillin, piperacillin, or mezlocillin, 1–3 g iv, ± gentamicin; or cefotetan 1–2 g iv; Diflucan 200 mg iv; antibiotics may be adjusted based on preoperative bile cultures
Surgical time	3–8 h
Closing considerations	Muscle relaxation required for closure; NG suction.
EBL	500–5000 mL, depending on need for liver resection and presence of portal HTN.
Postop care	ICU postoperatively
Mortality	5–10%
Morbidity	Sepsis; hemorrhage; anastomotic leakage; wound infection; liver failure; VTE
Pain score	7–8

PATIENT POPULATION CHARACTERISTICS

Age range	50–70
Male:Female	Male > female
Incidence	4500 cases of bile duct cancer/yr in the United States.
Etiology	Multifactorial
Associated conditions	Ulcerative colitis; sclerosing cholangitis; typhoid carrier state; Clonorchis sinensis; choledochal cyst; Caroli's disease; gallstones

ANESTHETIC CONSIDERATIONS

See Anesthetic Considerations for Biliary Tract Surgery, p. 565.

Suggested Readings

1. Cunningham SC, Schulick RD: Bile duct cancer. In *Current Surgical Therapy*, 9th edition. Cameron JL, ed. Mosby Elsevier, Philadelphia: 2008, 442–7.

2. Jarnagin WR, DíAngelica M, Blumgart LH: Intrahepatic and extrahepatic biliary cancer. In *Surgery of the Liver, Biliary Tract, and Pancreas,* 4th edition. Blumgart LH, ed. Saunders Elsevier, Philadelphia: 2007, 782–826.
3. Taylor BR, Langer B: Procedures for benign and malignant biliary tract disease. In *ACS Surgery: Principles and Practice 2006.* Souba WW, Fink MP, Jurkovich GJ, et al, eds. WebMD, New York: 2006, 673–87.
4. Whang EE, Zinner MJ: Cancer of the gallbladder and bile ducts. In *Maingotis Abdominal Operations,* 11th edition. Zinner MJ, Ashley SW, eds. McGraw Hill Medical, New York: 2007, 921–35.

CHOLEDOCHAL CYST EXCISION OR ANASTOMOSIS

SURGICAL CONSIDERATIONS

Description: This rare congenital anomaly includes various types of dilatation of the biliary tree, and patients may present with cystolithiasis, cholangitis, pancreatitis or, rarely, malignancy. Adults with long-standing obstructive jaundice from a choledochal cyst may present with secondary biliary cirrhosis. Although four types of cysts are commonly recognized, the vast majority consist of fusiform dilatation of much or most of the extrahepatic biliary tree. While the traditional description of choledochal cyst is that of an infant with a palpable abdominal mass and jaundice or cholangitis, this is a relatively rare presentation today. Today, many cysts are found in adults undergoing evaluation for symptoms thought to be due to gallbladder disease. These patients may present with biliary colic, pancreatitis, or cholangitis. Recommended treatment consists of **excision of the cyst** when technically safe. **Cyst-enteric bypass,** usually to a Roux loop of jejunum, is almost never performed today because of the small, but real risk of developing malignancy in these cysts. Only in an elderly patient under unusual technical circumstances would this be appropriate.

The operation is performed through a midline or right subcostal incision. The liver is retracted superiorly and the duodenum inferiorly, exposing the biliary tree. The gallbladder is excised, along with as much of the cyst as possible. Intraoperative cholangiogram demonstrates the transition from cyst to normal biliary tract. The duct is divided as distally as possible, just above the duodenum, and the cyst reflected superiorly. The entire cyst should be excised to prevent the development of malignancy in the remnant. This not infrequently requires excision to the hepatic bifurcation; and an anastomosis is performed at this level, often between the common orifice of the right and left hepatic ducts and a Roux loop of jejunum. Diffuse involvement of the intrahepatic bile ducts (Caroliís disease) may require liver resection or transplantation.

Reoperative cases are increasingly common; most follow a cyst-enteric bypass. These cases may be significantly more difficult than first-time operations.

Variant procedure or approaches: There is an increasing tendency among gastroenterologists to perform **endoscopic sphincterotomy** in these patients, rather than to refer them for surgical resection, particularly in older patients. It remains to be seen if these patients will develop cancer in the retained cysts.

Usual preop diagnosis: Choledochal cyst, the most common type involving fusiform enlargement of the entire extrahepatic biliary tree

SUMMARY OF PROCEDURE	
Position	Supine
Incision	Midline or right subcostal
Special instrumentation	Costal retractor
Antibiotics	Ampicillin, piperacillin, or mezlocillin, 1–3 g iv, ± gentamicin; or cefotetan 1–2 g iv
Surgical time	2–4 h
Closing considerations	NG suction

General Surgery

SUMMARY OF PROCEDURE (cont'd)	
EBL	250 mL, with potentially greater blood loss in re-operations
Postop care	PACU
Mortality	Very rare
Morbidity	Anastomotic leak Wound infection Pulmonary complications Pancreatitis
Pain score	5–7

PATIENT POPULATION CHARACTERISTICS	
Age range	Classically, 60% < 10 yr of age, although this may be changing; also adults of all ages
Male:Female	1:3
Incidence	Rare in the United States; more common in Japan
Etiology	Unclear
Associated conditions	Jaundice; pancreatitis; malignancy within the cyst

Suggested Readings

1. Locke JE, Lipsett PA: Cystic disorders of the bile ducts. In *Current Surgical Therapy,* 9th edition. Cameron JL, ed. Mosby Elsevier, Philadelphia: 2008, 430–7.
2. Melton GB, Lillemoe KD: Choledochal cyst and biliary strictures. In *Maingot's Abdominal Operations,* 11th edition. Zinner MJ, Ashley SW, eds. McGraw Hill Medical, New York: 2007, 889–920.
3. Nagorney DM: Bile duct cysts in adults. In *Surgery of the Liver, Biliary Tract, and Pancreas,* 4th edition. Blumgart LH, ed. Saunders Elsevier, Philadelphia: 2007, 991–1004.
4. Nagorney DM, Sarmiento JM: Surgical management of cystic disease of the liver. In *Surgery of the Liver, Biliary Tract, and Pancreas,* 4th edition. Blumgart LH, ed. Saunders Elsevier, Philadelphia: 2007, 1021–33.

ANESTHETIC CONSIDERATIONS FOR BILIARY TRACT SURGERY

(Procedures covered: open cholecystectomy; cholangiography; choledochotomy; biliary drainage procedures; transduodenal sphincterotomy or sphincteroplasty; cholecystojejunostomy; excision of bile duct tumor; choledochal cyst excision/anastomosis)

PREOPERATIVE

Patients presenting for biliary tract surgery are an extremely diverse group, ranging from the otherwise healthy to the extremely ill. With the increasing popularity of laparoscopic surgery, open cholecystectomies will be performed rarely, or when it is not possible to complete the laparoscopic procedure. Cirrhosis, even of a mild degree, substantially increases the risk of cholecystectomy, with hemorrhage being the greatest danger. Patients with bile duct tumors are usually jaundiced at presentation and have undergone transhepatic and/or endoscopic studies for diagnostic purposes. Often an external transhepatic biliary drain may be present and jaundice may have been relieved in this way. Rarely, a hepatic resection may be performed as part of the procedure. Prior operation or the presence of portal HTN may substantially increase the duration, complexity, and blood loss of the procedure.

Respiratory	Pain 2° an acute abdominal process may impair respiratory function (↓ FRC, hypoventilation, atelectasis). For patients undergoing laparoscopic cholecystectomy, intraabdominal CO_2 insufflation may → atelectasis, ↓ FRC, ↑ PIP, and ↑ $PaCO_2$. Studies comparing patients undergoing open vs laparoscopic cholecystectomy reveal that respiratory function is less impaired and function is recovered more quickly in those undergoing laparoscopic cholecystectomy. Tachypnea, hyperpnea, and acute respiratory alkalosis can be signs of sepsis, or due solely to pain associated with inflammation of the gallbladder. **Tests:** Consider CXR and others as indicated from H&P.
Cardiovascular	Patients may be dehydrated from fever, vomiting, and decreased oral intake; assess hemodynamic status by evaluating BP and HR in the supine and standing positions. Fluid resuscitate if patient shows Sx of orthostatic ↓ SBP until hemodynamic status improves. Patients undergoing laparoscopic cholecystectomy may experience hemodynamic compromise 2° positioning (reverse Trendelenburg → excessive intraabdominal pressure with subsequent impairment of venous return). Epigastric discomfort is common with biliary tract disease and can mimic symptoms of myocardial ischemia. **Tests:** ECG; others as indicated from H&P.
Renal	In patients with obstructive jaundice, preop administration of bile salts po may prevent renal insufficiency following surgery. **Tests:** UA and others as indicated from H&P.
Gastrointestinal	Patients with peritonitis will exhibit guarding and may develop abdominal distention and paralytic ileus. Therefore, full-stomach precautions are warranted. Laparoscopic approach is contraindicated in these patients. Ensure adequate hydration and consider administration of lactulose or bile salts. **Tests:** Bilirubin; AST (SGOT); ALT (SGPT); alkaline phosphatase; albumin
Hematologic	Leukocytosis is often present with a moderate left shift. ✓ coags. Administer vitamin K as needed (10 mg iv/sc). **Tests:** CBC, with differential and Plt
Laboratory	Other tests as indicated from H&P.
Premedication	Meperidine (0.5–0.6 mg/kg iv) is thought to cause less sphincter of Oddi spasm than other opiates. Sphincter spasm can interfere with intraop cholangiograms and cause pain; reverse opiate-induced spasm with naloxone in 40 mcg increments. Atropine (0.4–0.6 mg im or iv) or glycopyrrolate (0.2–0.3 mg im or iv) may help decrease spasm of the sphincter and can be given in combination with the opiate. Parenteral vitamin K is indicated if PT is prolonged (10 mg/d po or im for 3 d). Administer H_2-antagonists (ranitidine 50 mg iv); metoclopramide (10–20 mg iv) may be given if patient is at risk for gastric aspiration.

INTRAOPERATIVE

Anesthetic technique: GETA. In patients at risk for aspiration, ET intubation should be accomplished following a rapid-sequence iv induction (see p. B-4).

Induction	Standard induction (see p. B-2) if no aspiration risk. In patients at risk of aspiration, a rapid-sequence induction should be performed (see p. B-4).	
Maintenance	Standard maintenance (see p. B-2). Muscle relaxants facilitate surgery and are indicated.	
Emergence	If there is a risk for aspiration of gastric contents, patient should be extubated awake after return of protective airway reflexes; otherwise, no special considerations.	
Blood and fluid requirements	Minimal blood loss	Blood products usually not required. Anticipate that patient maybe dehydrated and require generous iv hydration (e.g., 10–15 mL/kg) before anesthetic induction.

General Surgery

Blood and fluid requirements (cont'd)	Possible 3rd-space loss IV: 16–18 ga × 1–2 NS/LR @ 5–8 mL/kg/h	IV size and number according to risk of significant blood loss.
Monitoring	Standard monitors (see p. B-1).	Others as clinically indicated.
Positioning	✓ and pad pressure points ✓ eyes	A steep, reverse Trendelenburg position may be required, causing cardiorespiratory impairment: venous return →↓ CO
Complications	Atelectasis 2° surgical retraction ↓BP	These complications are unique to laparoscopic procedures.

POSTOPERATIVE

Complications	Ventilatory impairment Pneumothorax Atelectasis PONV VTE Subcutaneous emphysema	Monitor patients for hypoxemia in the postop period. Administer supplemental O_2, and consider a portable CXR to aid in the diagnosis. See p. B-1 See p. B-2
Pain management	PCA (See p. C-3) Shoulder pain	Intercostal nerve blocks, intrapleural analgesia, or epidural analgesia are also useful techniques. Prolonged PCA meperidine is associated with ↑ normeperidine → CNS disorder, seizures. 2° subdiaphragmatic gas trapping

General Surgery

Suggested Readings

1. Marco AP, Yeo CJ, Rock P: Anesthesia for a patient undergoing laparoscopic cholecystectomy. *Anesthesiology* 1990; 73(6):1268–70.
2. Nakeeb A, Ahrendt SA, Pitt HA: Calculous biliary disease. In *Greenfield's Surgery: Scientific Principles and Practice,* 3rd edition. Mulholland MW, Lillemore KD, Doherty GM, et al, eds. Lippincott Williams & Wilkins, Philadelphia: 2006, 978–98.
3. Pain JA, Cahill CJ, Gilbert JM, et al: Prevention of post-operative renal dysfunction in patients with obstructive jaundice: a multicenter study of bile salts and lactulose. *Br J Surg* 1991; 78:467–9.

CHAPTER

7.7 Laparoscopic General Surgery

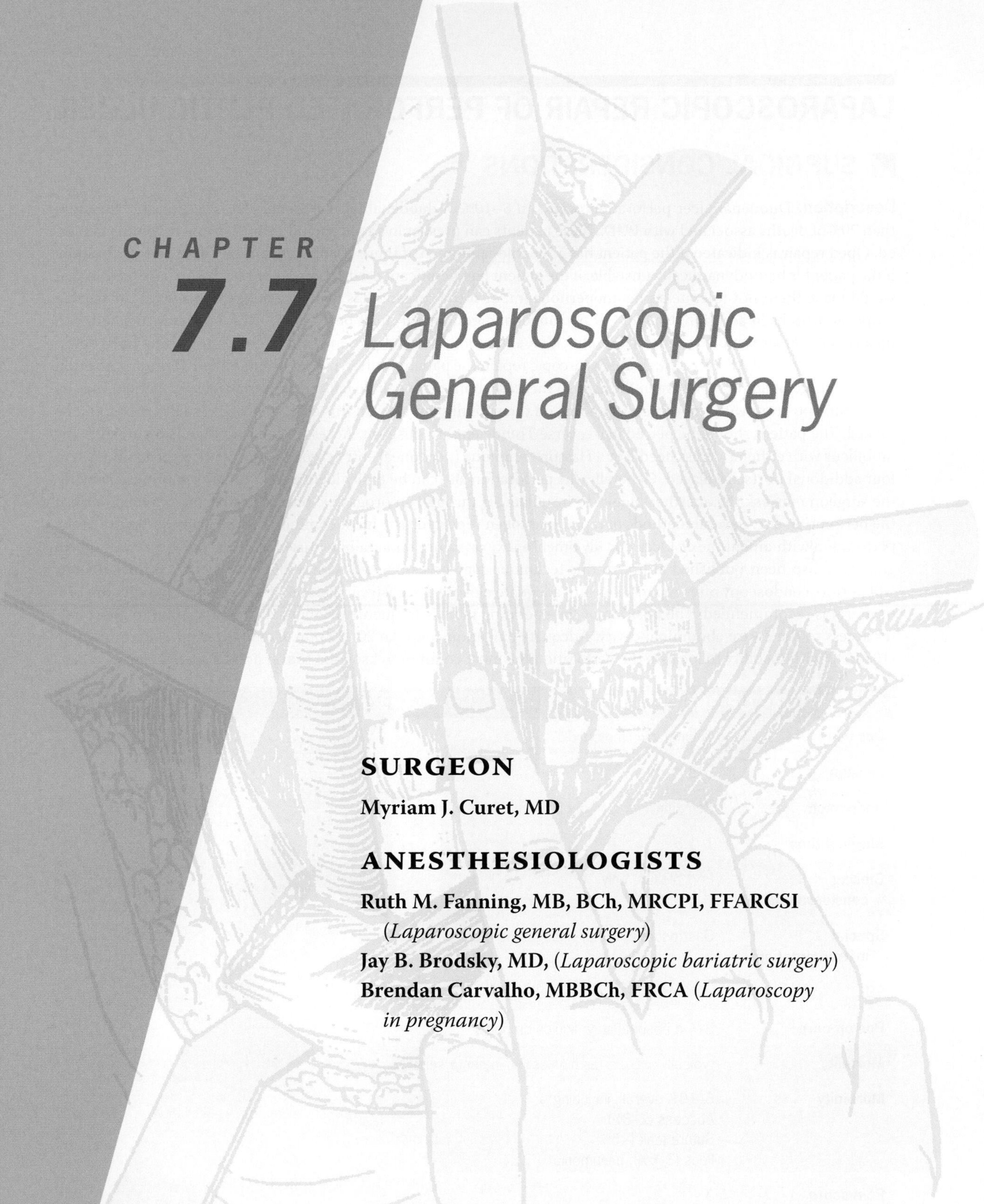

SURGEON

Myriam J. Curet, MD

ANESTHESIOLOGISTS

Ruth M. Fanning, MB, BCh, MRCPI, FFARCSI (*Laparoscopic general surgery*)

Jay B. Brodsky, MD, (*Laparoscopic bariatric surgery*)

Brendan Carvalho, MBBCh, FRCA (*Laparoscopy in pregnancy*)

LAPAROSCOPIC REPAIR OF PERFORATED PEPTIC ULCER

SURGICAL CONSIDERATIONS

Description: Duodenal ulcer perforation occurs in 5–10% of duodenal ulcer patients and is responsible for more than 70% of deaths associated with PUD. These patients can present in shock and often are extremely volume depleted. Open repair is indicated if the patient has a "hostile" abdomen, if there is simultaneous bleeding and perforation, if the patient is hemodynamically unstable, if the patient has significant cardiovascular or respiratory risk factors that would make them not tolerate a pneumoperitoneum, or if the surgeon has inadequate experience with the laparoscopic approach. In addition, trained OR personnel and equipment must be available. Risk factors associated with unsuccessful laparoscopic repair include shock on admission, delayed presentation (>24 h), underlying comorbidities, age > 70 yr, and ASA III to iv. For laparoscopic repair, the patient is often placed in a modified lithotomy position with the surgeon standing between the legs. In this case, both arms can be left out. Alternatively, the patient may be in a supine position with the surgeon standing on the patient's left side. In this case, the patient's left arm should be tucked. The patient should be placed in a reverse Trendelenburg position. Access to the abdomen is obtained at the umbilicus with either a Veress needle or a Hasson technique (peritoneal entry through a ~1 cm skin incision). Two to four additional ports are placed. Generally, the perforation site can be easily identified by laparoscopy. Occasionally, the surgeon may ask the anesthesiologist to insufflate air through an orogastric or nasogastric tube to help localize the perforation site. Several methods of repair have been reported. The most common involves suture closure of the perforation with omentopexy. Occasionally omentopexy or suture repair alone is used. Reports of closure with fibrin glue have also been published although this technique may be associated with a higher leak rate. Some surgeons will perform endoscopy after repair to ensure adequate closure. Extensive irrigation of the peritoneal cavity (6–10 L or more) is recommended. The position of the operating table is frequently changed during irrigation to allow better access to the entire abdominal cavity. Adequate irrigation can take 20–30 min. Conversion rates are quite high (10–15%) with inability to localize the perforation the most common reason for conversion to open surgery.

SUMMARY OF PROCEDURE	
Position	Supine, low lithotomy
Incision	3–5 ports
Antibiotics	Cefoxitin 1–2 g iv preop
Surgical time	1–1.5 h
Closing considerations	Port closure only
Special instrumentation	Gastroscope; oro or nasogastric tube
EBL	< 75 mL
Postop care	2–4 d hospital stay; liquids on pod 1
Mortality	typically < 0.1% (as high as 3% in some series)
Morbidity	6–10% overall, including: Abscess (2–8%) Suture leak (~5%) Ileus (3–6%); pneumonia
Pain score	3

PATIENT POPULATION CHARACTERISTICS	
Age range	40–60 yr
Male:Female	May be slightly more common in males

PATIENT POPULATION CHARACTERISTICS (cont'd)	
Incidence	~10% lifetime risk for perforation
Etiology	May be related to H. pylori infection; NSAID use; stress; corticosteroid use
Associated conditions	gastrinoma; MEN type 1; COPD; CRF; up to 20% may be in shock at the time of admission

ANESTHETIC CONSIDERATIONS

See Anesthetic Considerations following Laparoscopic Cholecystectomy, p. 577.

Suggested Readings

1. Lunevicius R, Morkevicius M: Management strategies, early results, benefits, and risk factors of laparoscopic repair of perforated peptic ulcer. *World J Surg* 2005; 29(10):1299–310.
2. Sanabria AE, Morales CH, Villegas MI: Laparoscopic repair for perforated peptic ulcer disease. *Cochrane Database Syst Rev 2005*; 4:CD004778.

LAPAROSCOPIC ESOPHAGEAL FUNDOPLICATION

SURGICAL CONSIDERATIONS

Description: Approximately 40% of Americans suffer from heartburn, and most cases are treated medically. Indications for **esophageal fundoplication** (to ↑ lower esophageal sphincter pressure) include complications of GERD, such as stricture, respiratory problems, esophageal ulcerations, and Barrett's esophagus (a premalignant condition). Other indications include failure of medical management or an unwillingness to submit to a lifetime of medication. Most patients with GERD are treated laparoscopically; those undergoing laparoscopic fundoplication have the benefits of a minimally invasive approach—decreased pain, earlier return of GI function, earlier ambulation, earlier discharge, quicker return to normal activities, decreased incidence of wound infections and hernias. The most common fundoplication is the **Nissen (360°) wrap;** and its variations include the Rossetti modification, a **Toupet** (270° posterior) wrap, and the **Dor** (anterior) wrap. Before surgery, patients with GERD should have documented esophageal hyperacidity (by either pH probe or by esophagitis revealed on upper endoscopy), and also should have a hypotensive sphincter (demonstrated on manometry). Typically, they will have been treated with proton pump inhibitors (e.g., lansoprazole) and sometimes with prokinetic agents (e.g., metoclopramide). The patient is placed supine in a low lithotomy position, with the surgeon standing between the legs. The abdomen is entered ~2 cm above the umbilicus with either a closed (**Veress needle:** blind placement) or open (**Hasson trocar:** direct visual placement through small skin incision) technique. A total of five trocars are inserted—two in the LUQ, two in the RUQ, and one at the umbilicus. The stomach should be decompressed either with a OG tube or with a gastroscope. The liver is elevated with a liver retractor, and the gastroesophageal (GE) junction and both diaphragmatic crura are dissected out. The hiatus should be closed with one or two sutures. The esophagus is encircled (Fig. 7.7-1 A), and the vagal nerves are identified and preserved. The short gastrics are then taken down to decrease tension on the wrap. The fundus is brought in through the retroesophageal window (Fig. 7.7-2). An esophageal dilator (56–60 Fr) generally is placed (often by the anesthesiologist) to calibrate the wrap. Passage of the dilator is possibly the most hazardous part of the procedure, because it may cause perforation of the esophagus at the GE junction. As the dilator approaches the stomach, it is important to watch the junction on the video monitors to ensure that the dilator is not being held at an angle that will risk perforation. The anesthesiologist should stop passing the dilator immediately if any resistance is felt. The dilator is withdrawn. An NG tube may be placed at this time.

Variant procedure or approaches: **Open surgery** (see Esophageal Surgery, p. 478) may be indicated if the patient has had previous gastric surgery or if there is a complication with an ongoing laparoscopic procedure. In the **Rossetti modification,** the short gastrics are not taken down, which decreases operative time. The **Dor fundoplication** is an anterior hemifundoplication in which the fundus is wrapped and sutured to the left and right sides of the esophagus and to the left and right crura, but anteriorly. A Dor fundoplication is often used in combination with a Heller myotomy for treatment of achalasia. A **Toupet procedure** (Fig. 7.7-1 B) is a posterior hemifundoplication

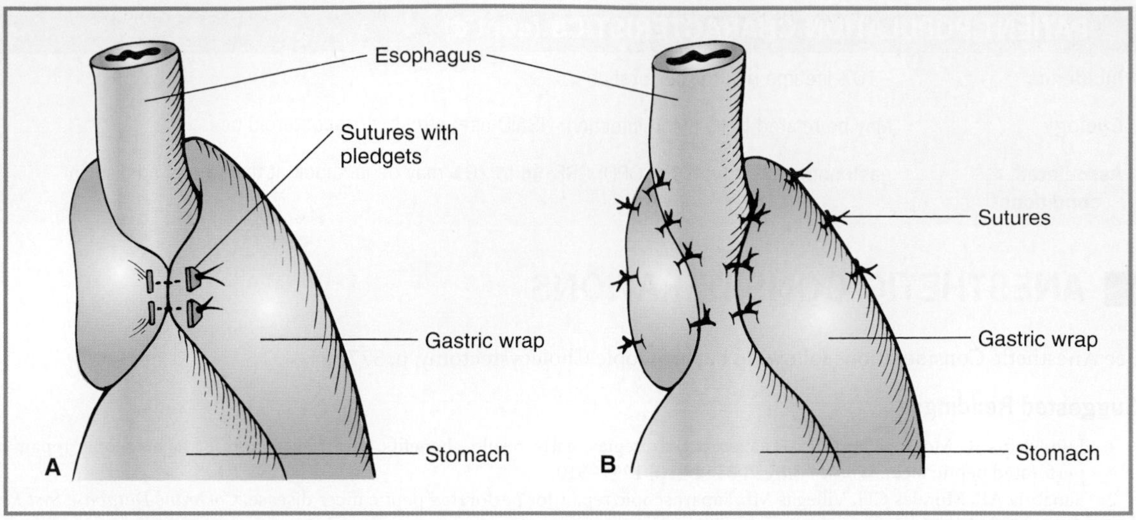

Figure 7.7-1. **(A)** Nissen fundoplication. **(B)** Partial fundoplication (Toupet procedure).

in which the two walls of the fundus do not actually meet. The stomach is sewn to the left and right walls of the esophagus and then are anchored to the right and left crura. In the past, these procedures were performed commonly in patients with a high risk of postop dysphagia (e.g., those who have impaired esophageal peristalsis or a preop stricture). Now, because of their higher failure rate, they are seldom performed except in patients with severe esophageal dysmotility, such as patients with scleroderma. These procedures are identical to the Nissen fundoplication except for the wrap itself.

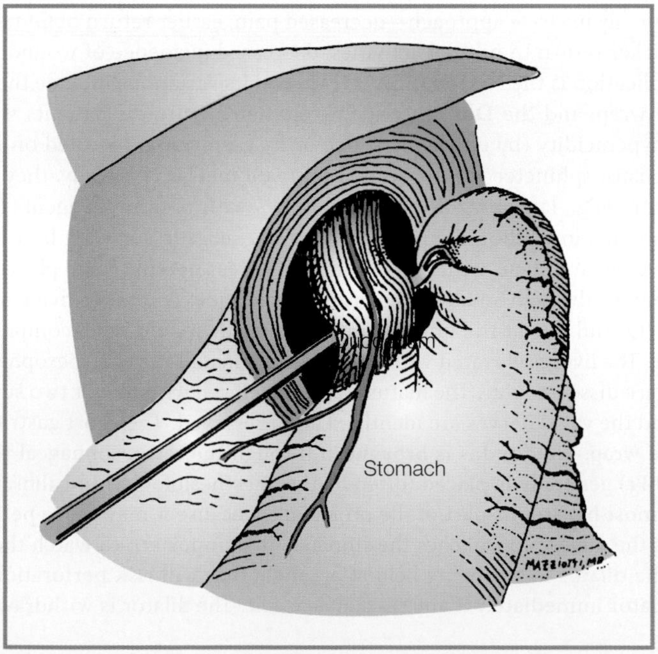

Figure 7.7-2. Gastric fundus is pulled posteriorly and to the right of the esophagus, with the fundus itself used as a retractor, reaching from right to left behind the esophagus to grasp the fundus and retract it back to the right side behind the esophagus. Placing caudad traction on the wrapped fundus, the GE junction and distal esophagus can be brought further into the abdominal cavity. (Reproduced with permission from Baker RJ, Fischer JE: *Mastery of Surgery*, Lippincott Williams & Wilkins, Philadelphia: 2001.)

Usual preop diagnosis: GERD, with or without esophagitis, esophageal stricture, or Barrett's esophagus

SUMMARY OF PROCEDURE	
Position	Supine low lithotomy
Incision	Five ports, upper abdomen
Special instrumentation	Harmonic Scalpel; bipolar cautery or endoscope. Esophageal dilators should be available.
Antibiotics	Cefazolin 1 g iv
Surgical time	1.5–2.5 h
Closing considerations	Port closures only; muscle relaxation may be needed for fascial closure
EBL	< 75 mL
Postop care	1–2 d hospital stay; liquids on pod 1
Mortality	< 0.1%
Morbidity	Overall: 8% Atelectasis: common Esophageal or gastric perforation: rare (most commonly associated with passage of NG tube or esophageal dilator) Hemorrhage from short gastrics or splenic tear Pneumothorax (does not usually require treatment) Postop dysphagia
Pain score	4

PATIENT POPULATION CHARACTERISTICS	
Age range	All ages (indcidence ↑ with age). May be performed in infants; next peak occurs in adulthood; rare in children and adolescents.
Male:Female	1:1
Incidence	1% (increasing significantly over past 5 yr)
Etiology	Unknown
Associated conditions	Aspiration risk; reactive airway disease; occasionally, respiratory problems associated with chronic aspiration

ANESTHETIC CONSIDERATIONS

See Anesthetic Considerations following Laparoscopic Cholecystectomy, p. 577.

Suggested Readings

1. Bammer T,m Hinder RA, Klaus A, et al: Fve-to eight-year outcome of the first laparoscopic Nissen fundoplications. *J Gastrointest Surg* 2001; 5(1):42–8.
2. Champion JK, McKernan JB: Laparoscopic Toupet fundoplication. In *Surgical Laparoscopy,* 2nd edition. Zucker KA, ed. Lippincott Williams & Wilkins, Philadelphia: 2001, 401–8.
3. Cowgill SM, Gillman R, Kraemer E, et al: Ten year follow up after laparoscopic Nissen fundoplication for gastroesophageal reflux disease. *Am Surg* 2007; 73(8):748–53.
4. Dallemagne B: Laparoscopic Nissen fundoplication. In *Atlas of Laparoscopic Surgery.* Ballantyne GH, ed. WB Saunders, Philadelphia: 2000, 92–101.
5. Hughes SG, Chekan EG, Ali A, et al: Unusual complications following laparoscopic Nissen fundoplication. *Surg Laparosc Endosc Percutan Tech* 1999; 9(2): 143–7.
6. Zucker KA: Laparoscopic Nissen fundoplication technique. In *Surgical Laparoscopy,* 2nd edition. Lippincott Williams & Wilkins, Philadelphia: 2001, 375–400.

LAPAROSCOPIC HELLER'S MYOTOMY ± ANTIREFLUX PROCEDURE

SURGICAL CONSIDERATIONS

Description: Laparoscopic and thoracoscopic esophageal myotomies have become much more common over the last 5 yr as confidence in laparoscopic esophageal surgery—particularly antireflux surgery—has increased. These procedures are performed for achalasia, an uncommon condition in which the lower esophageal sphincter fails to relax with swallowing, and in which the body of the esophagus is aperistaltic and dilates. Patients typically complain of dysphagia with chest pain and may experience regurgitation. The etiology of this condition remains unknown.

Treatment options consist of pneumatic dilation, botulinum toxin injection of the lower esophageal sphincter, or surgical myotomy. **Pneumatic dilation** remains the most common procedure performed for achalasia, and is effective in ~60% of patients. Many gastroenterologists are reluctant to perform this procedure, however, because of the risk of esophageal perforation, which is generally considered to be ~3–5%, but may be as high as 10%. **Botulinum toxin injection** is a newer technique that is effective to some degree in most patients, but the duration of its effectiveness is short. Most patients require retreatment within 1.5 yr, and the efficacy of retreatment may diminish over time. In many centers, **surgical myotomy (Heller's operation)** has become the procedure of choice for the treatment of achalasia.

The patient is positioned as for a laparoscopic antireflux procedure—supine in the lithotomy position with reverse Trendelenburg. The abdomen is usually entered with a Veress needle (blind) or Hasson trocar (direct vision) at the umbilicus, and five laparoscopic ports are placed across the upper abdomen—two beneath the left costal margin, two beneath the right costal margin, and one in the midline either at the umbilicus or midway between the umbilicus and the xiphoid. The liver is elevated, and the ligamentous attachments anterior to the esophagus are divided. The esophagus is not usually encircled; and, as hiatal hernias are uncommon with achalasia, crural repair is seldom necessary.

The myotomy is begun at the gastroesophageal junction using monopolar cautery, bipolar scissors, or a Harmonic Scalpel (ultrasonic cutting/coagulation). It is carried proximally until normal musculature is encountered. Some surgeons perform intraop esophagoscopy to ensure that the myotomy has been carried proximally enough and that there has not been a mucosal perforation. Generally, a myotomy of 5–8 cm is adequate, although sometimes a longer myotomy may be necessary. Some surgeons then perform a very loose, partial fundoplication to prevent reflux. This can be performed as an anterior or posterior fundoplication, bringing the fundus either anterior (Dor fundoplication–our preference) or posterior (Toupet fundoplication) to the esophagus. The stomach is secured to the esophageal wall and crural with sutures, and an NG tube may be passed. The ports are removed and port closure carried out.

Variant procedure or approaches: Although most of these procedures are being performed laparoscopically, they also can be performed by thoracoscopy or thoracotomy. If a thoracoscopy or thoracotomy is performed, a DLT is placed to allow collapse of the left lung.

Usual preop diagnosis: Achalasia required

SUMMARY OF PROCEDURE

Position	Supine lithotomy, reverse Trendelenburg
Incision	Five ports, upper abdomen
Special instrumentation	Laparoscopic instrumentation ± gastroscope
Antibiotics	Cefazolin 1 g iv
Surgical time	1.5–2 h
Closing considerations	None
EBL	Minimal
Postop care	2-d hospital stay; liquids on pod 1

SUMMARY OF PROCEDURE (cont'd)	
Mortality	Rare
Morbidity	Insignificant atelectasis: Common Esophageal or gastric perforation: Rare Pneumothorax (does not usually require treatment) Gastroesophageal reflux: > 15%
Pain score	4

PATIENT POPULATION CHARACTERISTICS	
Age range	20–40 yr
Male:Female	1:1
Incidence	Uncommon but not rare
Etiology	Unknown
Associated conditions	None. Chagas' disease may produce identical esophageal findings.

ANESTHETIC CONSIDERATIONS

See Anesthetic Considerations following Laparoscopic Cholecystectomy, p. 577.

Suggested Readings

1. Bonavina L. Minimally invasive surgery for esophageal achalasia. *World J Gastroenterol* 2006; 12(37):5291–5.
2. Bonatti H, Hinder RA, Dlocker J, et al: Long-term results of laparoscopic Heller myotomy with partial fundoplication for the treatment of achalaisa. *Am J Surg* 2005; 190(6):874–8.
3. Jeansonne LO, White BC, Pilger KE, et al: Ten-year follow-up of laparoscopic Heller myotomy for achalasia shows durability. *Surg Endosc* 2007; 21(9):1498–1502.
4. Sharp KW, Khaitan L, Scholz S, et al: 100 minimally invasive Heller myotomies: lessons learned. *Ann Surg* 2002; 235(5):631–9.

LAPAROSCOPIC CHOLECYSTECTOMY, ± COMMON DUCT EXPLORATION

SURGICAL CONSIDERATIONS

Description: This operation typically is performed for symptomatic gallstones or acute cholecystitis. A laparoscopic approach is preferred over an open cholecystectomy because of its minimally invasive nature, which allows earlier recovery and return to normal activities. Laparoscopic cholecystectomy may be contraindicated for patients with uncorrectable coagulopathy, severe COPD, or severe cardiac disease (unable to tolerate ↑ intraabdominal pressure). In addition, patients with prior abdominal surgery or with acute cholecystitis are at a higher risk for conversion to open surgery. The operation begins with access to the abdominal cavity at the umbilicus, either with a Veress needle (closed technique: blind placement) or a **Hasson trocar** (open technique: ↓ risk of vascular, bowel, and bladder injury). If a **Veress needle** is to be used, the patient will need an OG tube and a Foley catheter to decompress the stomach and bladder before proceeding. CO_2 is insufflated to an intraabdominal pressure of 15 mmHg. If the patient develops ventilatory or hemodynamic problems, consider decreasing the intraabdominal pressure to 10–12 mmHg. A total of four trocars are used—one at the umbilicus and three in the RUQ. The patient is placed in a reverse Trendelenburg position and rotated to the left to move the stomach, duodenum, and transverse colon away from the operative field.

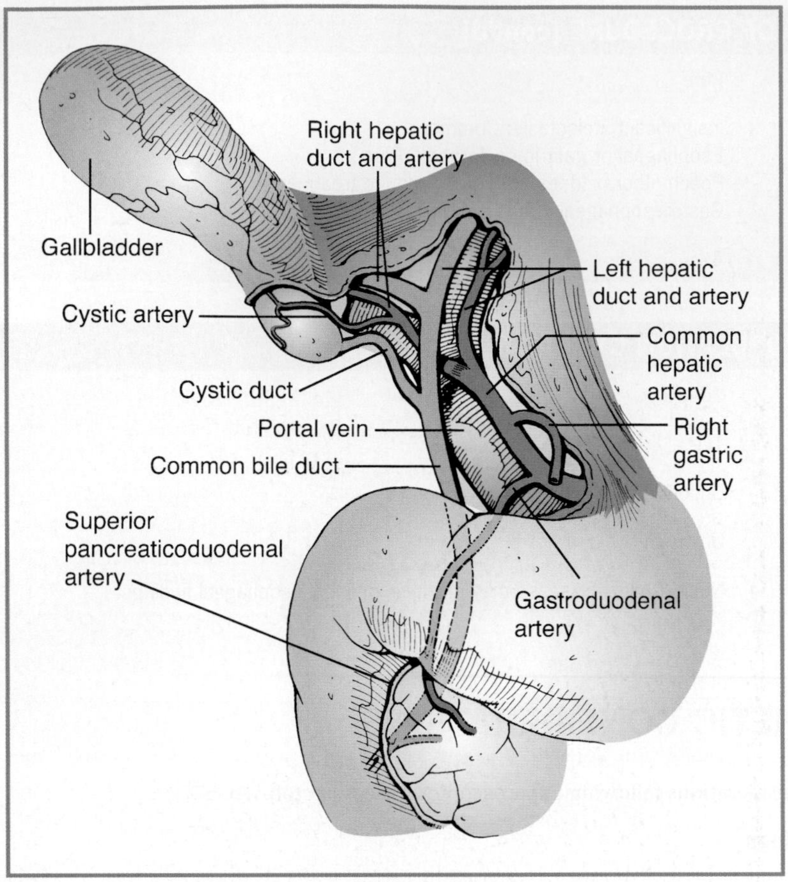

Figure 7.7-3. Surgical anatomy for laparoscopic cholecystectomy and common duct exploration.

The cystic artery and cystic duct (with hepatic duct = triangle of Calot) are clipped and cut (Fig. 7.7-3). The gallbladder is then dissected off the liver with monopolar cautery, placed in a bag, and brought out, usually through the umbilical cord site. Hemostasis is then achieved, the area is irrigated with NS, and the 10 mm trocar sites are closed. The rate of conversion to an open operation is ~5% for elective gallbladder surgery and ~10% for acute cholecystitis. Should this occur, the operation is then converted to an open cholecystectomy (see p. 558).

Cholangiography can be added easily to the laparoscopic cholecystectomy. A clip is placed high on the cystic duct; then a small incision is made in the duct just beneath the clip. A cholangiocatheter may be introduced and dye injected into the biliary tree. X-rays—either fluoroscopy or, more commonly, hard copy—are used to assess the biliary anatomy and to look for stones within the ductal system. Cholangiography carries few risks, generally adds about 10–15 min to the procedure, and can be used to identify the important anatomy ~85% of the time. Some surgeons perform it routinely during all cholecystectomies; others perform it selectively and only if there is evidence that the patient has had common duct stones or if the anatomy is in question.

In rare circumstances, **laparoscopic common duct exploration** may be carried out to treat common duct stones. A number of techniques have been used, most employing a thin fiber optic choledochoscope passed through the cystic duct into the common duct. This procedure is performed in only a relatively few centers. More commonly, **endoscopic retrograde cholangiopancreatography (ERCP)** will be used, either preop or postop to demonstrate the presence or absence of stones and to remove any stones that are found.

Variant procedure or approaches: **Open cholecystectomy** (p. 558) remains the major alternative to laparoscopic cholecystectomy, either because the cholecystectomy is predicted to be technically difficult or because of the illness of the patient. Approximately 5% or less of laparoscopic cholecystectomies are converted to open cholecystectomy intraop because of difficulties with the procedure. **ERCP** remains the most common means of treating choledocholithiasis in the industrialized world with laparoscopic techniques used in a relatively small number of centers and by a small number of surgeons. **Open common duct exploration** is occasionally necessary for stones not retrievable by ERCP (generally < 5%).

Usual preop diagnosis: Acute or chronic cholecystitis, usually with cholelithiasis, with or without choledocholithiasis

SUMMARY OF PROCEDURE	
Position	Supine
Incision	For upper abdominal ports
Special instrumentation	Routine laparoscopic instruments. May require fluoroscopy and choledochoscopes for cholangiography, common duct exploration; OG tube
Antibiotics	Cefazolin 1 g iv
Surgical time	0.5–2 h; may be longer for common duct exploration.
Closing considerations	Muscular relaxation helpful for closure of umbilical port site
EBL	Minimal
Postop care	Usual discharge within 24 h
Mortality	< 1/1000
Morbidity	Bile leak: 1% Common duct injury: 0.5% Hemorrhage (requiring transfusion) Infection Injury to bowel Major vascular injury: Uncommon
Pain score	3

PATIENT POPULATION CHARACTERISTICS	
Age range	Typically adult, increasing with age
Male:Female	Female > Male
Incidence	Common
Etiology	Stone disease. Risk factors = female gender, age, parity, obesity.
Associated conditions	Hemolytic anemia for pigmented stones

ANESTHETIC CONSIDERATIONS

(Procedures covered: repair of perforated peptic ulcer; laparoscopic esophageal fundoplication; laparoscopic Heller's myotomy and antireflux surgery; laparoscopic cholecystectomy)

PREOPERATIVE: LAPAROSCOPIC FUNDOPLICATION/HELLER'S MYOTOMY

In general, this patient population is healthy, with the exception of those with a perforated peptic ulcer or GERD. GERD patients often present with intractable heartburn, which is the reason for undergoing these surgical procedures.

Respiratory	Patients undergoing laparoscopic fundoplication may have a history of gastroesophageal reflux resulting in aspiration, particularly when recumbent. Recurrent aspiration may result in a number of respiratory complications including bronchospasm, pneumonia, and chronic pneumonitis. A prolonged history of reflux may give rise to premalignant Barrett's esophagus which may result in stricture formation and weakness of the esophageal wall. Patients with

Respiratory (cont'd)	achalasia may also present for laparoscopic fundoplication. Achalasia may result in severe regurgitation and aspiration. Pulmonary physiological changes include both restrictive and obstructive lung defects, and broncho-alveolar injury. A detailed history and physical examination may reveal cyanosis, wheezing, and rhonchi. Pulmonary function tests findings: ↓ FCV, ↓ FEV_1, ↑↓ FEV_1/FVC, ↓ FRC, ↓ TLC, and ↓ DLCO. **Tests:** Consider PA & lateral CXR. Consider baseline arterial blood gases, and pulmonary function tests if compromised pulmonary function is suspected.
Cardiovascular	Patients with both reflux and achalasia may present with chest pain. Typically the pain of reflux is sharp and substernal. Chest pain in achalasia may radiate to the neck, back and arms, and may be difficult to differentiate from pain of cardiac or vascular origin. Differentiation should be made before surgery both by careful history taking and appropriate tests. In patients with a long history of aspiration, who may have coexisting obstructive airways disease leading to parenchymal lung disease, cor pulmonale or right heart failure may result. Typical physical findings include elevated neck veins, hepatojugular reflux, right ventricular 3rd heart sound and dependent edema. **Tests:** ECG (r/o MI as cause of pain), exercise or chemical stress testing. If severe pulmonary dysfunction consider echocardiography. Other tests as indicated from H&P.
Laboratory	Patients with severe inflammation and erosion may suffer from an iron deficient anemia. In such patients consider CBC. Otherwise laboratory tests as indicated from H&P.
Premedication	These patients are at risk for aspiration and should be treated with full-stomach precautions. H_2 antagonists and continue proton pump inhibitors. Metoclopramide may be administered to aid gastric emptying. Na citrate 30 mL po immediately before induction.

PREOPERATIVE: LAPAROSCOPIC CHOLECYSTECTOMY

The preop evaluation of patients undergoing open cholecystectomy is discussed under Anesthetic Considerations for Biliary Tract Surgery, p. 565. Laparoscopic cholecystectomy is being performed much more commonly than the open procedure and can be accomplished quickly and safely, even in very sick patients.

Respiratory	Patients presenting for laparoscopic cholecystectomy may present electively or acutely. Increasingly, cholecystectomy is performed in patients with acute cholecystitis. This presents more challenges to the anesthesiologist than in the elective setting. Patients presenting acutely may experience severe abdominal pain, leading to diaphragmatic splinting and basal lung atelectasis. On examination, the patient may exhibit shallow, rapid breathing, and be cyanosed as a result of poor respiratory effort and increased metabolic demands. Adequate pain relief and respiratory exercises in conjunction with supplemental oxygen preoperatively may help to optimize the patient prior to surgery. During the procedure, intraabdominal CO_2 insufflation → atelectasis, ↓ FRC, ↑ PIP, ↑ $PaCO_2$ and ↓ PaO_2; therefore, laparoscopic procedures may be contraindicated in patients with severe respiratory or cardiovascular disease. Postop respiratory function, however, is less impaired (e.g., ↓ FRC 30% vs. 50%) and is recovered more quickly (24 h vs. 72 h) in patients undergoing laparoscopic cholecystectomy then in the open procedure.
Systemic	Patients presenting for laparoscopic cholecystectomy with acute cholecystitis may have evidence of mild to moderate sepsis. They may be febrile, tachycardic and hypotensive, and need appropriate resuscitation prior to surgery. Elderly patients may exhibit an acute confusional state.
Laboratory	CBC. Consider T & S in patients with recurrent and chronic gall bladder disease. They may have liver adhesions. During the acute inflammatory stage vascularity may occur → bleeding.
Premedication	See Anesthetic Considerations for Biliary Tract Surgery, p. 566.

INTRAOPERATIVE

Anesthetic technique: GETA

Induction	**Laparoscopic fundoplication** and **Heller's myotomy:** Given the patient's risk for aspiration, the trachea should be intubated after rapid-sequence induction with cricoid pressure (p. B-4). Additional iv access may be required if the arms are inaccessible. **Laparoscopic cholecystectomy:** Standard induction (p. B-2). In acutely unwell patients, despite resuscitation, patients may be more susceptible to the effects of anesthesia, and positive pressure ventilation. Consider additional iv access, invasive arterial pressure monitoring, and central access in labile patients. Etomidate may be a useful induction agent in this setting. Ensuring optimal venous return and right heart filling, through adequate fluid resuscitation and ventilatory strategies to minimize the effect of positive pressure ventilation will be beneficial.	
Maintenance	Standard maintenance (p. B-2). Continue muscle relaxation. Intra-abdominal CO_2 insufflation will →↑ intraabdominal pressure, which will predispose to passive regurgitation of gastric contents. In addition, intraabdominal pressure > 15 mmHg → ↓ venous return + ↑ SVR → ↓ CO. Controlled ventilation will minimize the possibility of hypercarbia from absorbed CO_2. N_2O can diffuse into CO_2 containing intraabdominal space and ↑ distension, as well as risk of explosion.	
Emergence	Given the high incidence of PONV, prophylactic antiemetic rx (e.g., odansetron 4 mg iv) recommended and should be given 30–60 min before the end of the case (p. B-2).	
Blood and fluid requirements	iv: 16–18 ga × 1 NS/LR @ 8–12 mL/kg/h Fluid warmer	Blood loss should be minimal, although assessment may be difficult 2° concealed bleeding. Consider retroperitoneal bleeding.
Monitoring	Standard monitors (p. B-1) Urinary catheter NG tube	Others as clinically indicated. Prevent hypothermia (forced-air warmer, warming blanket, warm OR, etc.)
Positioning	✓ and pad pressure points ✓ eyes	Initially in Trendelenburg position (↑ venous return, ↓ lung volumes, potential for mainstem intubation) for trocar placement; then reverse Trendelenburg (↓ venous return, ↑ lung volumes) during subsequent portions of the surgical procedure. Maintain adequate MAP to ensure cerebral perfusion in reverse Trendelenburg.
Complications	Respiratory: Pneumoperitoneum Hypercarbia/hypoxemia Pneumothorax Pneumomediastinum Endobronchial intubation	Pneumoperitoneum with CO_2 allows the surgeon to operate laparoscopically. This creates cephalad displacement of the diaphragm with ↓ FRC, ↓ pulmonary compliance, and atelectasis. This can manifest as ↑ PIP, ↓ PO_2 and ↑ PCO_2. Ventilation should be controlled during the operation to minimize the effects of pneumoperitoneum and hypercarbia. An increase in MV is appropriate. Pneumothorax can occur 2° retroperitoneal dissection of insufflated CO_2. Pneumothorax will manifest as ↓ PO_2, ↑ PIP, hemodynamic instability (↑ HR, ↓ BP), and possibly subcutaneous emphysema. The position of the ETT may change with altered patient position → endobronchial intubation.
	Cardiovascular: ↓BP Hemorrhage Dysrhythmias	↓ BP can occur 2° patient positioning (reverse Trendelenburg) and from ↓ venous return 2° pneumoperitoneum (↑ intraabdominal pressure > 15 mmHg). Hemorrhage can result from inadvertent injury to blood vessels (during trocar placement). Vascular injection of CO_2 (air embolism) can cause

General Surgery

Complications (cont'd)		↓ BP, dysrhythmias, and even cardiovascular collapse. If cardiopulmonary compromise occurs, the pneumoperitoneum can be released to allow for differential diagnosis and treatment.
	Visceral injury	Injury to the viscera may necessitate an open procedure or may go undiagnosed and → other postop complications, depending on the organ that is injured. At all times, be prepared to convert to an open procedure.
	Hypothermia	2° dry gas insufflation
	Subcutaneous emphysema	Dx: Sudden ↑ $ETCO_2$ + subcutaneous crepitation (abdomen/chest wall). Rx: Stop insufflation of CO_2, D/C N_2O, ↑ ventilation. Prevention: Keep CO_2 insufflation pressure < 12 mmHg.

POSTOPERATIVE

Complications	PONV (common)	
	Shoulder pain	From pneumoperitoneum; usually self-limited (p. B-2).
	Respiratory	Respiratory complications can be seen in the postoperative period as well. Typical post operative complications are secondary to pneumoperitoneum but mainly to pain. Adequate pain relief is essential to ensure good respiratory efforts. In the pre-emergence period, lung recruitment measures may help to offset potential respiratory problems. Bronchodilators may also be used in patients with coexisting bronchospasm. Early in the postoperative period, starting in the PACU incentive spirometry may be beneficial particularly in obese patients.
Pain management	PCA (see p. C-3). Oxycodone/hydrocodone in combination with acetaminophen	Shoulder pain responds to ketorolac (15–30 mg iv), or other NSAIDs such as Diclofenac provided there are no contraindications.
Tests	As indicated from H&P.	

Suggested Readings

1. Callery MP, Strasberg SM, Soper NJ: Complications of laparoscopic general surgery. *Gastrointest Endosc Clin N Am* 1996; 6(2):423–44.
2. Cunningham AJ, Nolan C: Anesthesia for minimally invasive surgery. In: *Clinical Anesthesia,* 5th edition, Barash PG, Cullen BF, Stoelting, RK, eds. Lippincott Williams & Wilkens, Philadelphia: 2006, 1061–71.
3. Feteiha MS, Curet MJ: Laparoscopic cholecystectomy. In: *Surgical Laparoscopy,* 2nd edition. Zucker KA, ed. Lippincott Williams & Wilkins, Philadelphia: 2001, 121–32.
4. Gadacz TR: Update on laparoscopic cholecystectomy, including a clinical pathway. *Surg Clin North Am* 2000; 80:1127–50.
5. Gurbuz AT, Peetz ME: The acute abdomen in the pregnant patient. Is there a role for laparoscopy? *Surg Endosc* 1997; 11(2):98–102.
6. Hein HA: Hemodynamic changes during laparoscopic cholecystectomy in patients with severe cardiac disease. *J Clin Anesth* 1997; 9(4):261–5.
7. Keus F, Broeders IA, van Laarhoven J: Gallstone disease: Surgical aspects of symptomatic and acute cholecystitis. *Best Pract Res Clin Gastroenterol* 2006; 20(6):1031–51.
8. Keus F, d Jong JA, Gooszen HG, et al: Laparoscopic versus open cholecystectomy for patients with symptomatic cholecystolithiasis. *Cochrane Database Syst Rev* 2006; 18(4):CD006231.
9. Nakeeb A, Ahrendt SA, Pitt HA: Calculous biliary disease. In: *Greenfield's Surgery,* 4th edition. Greenfield LJ, Mulholland MW, Lillemone MB, Dohersy GM, eds. Lippincott Williams & Wilkins, Philadelphia: 2006, 978–98.

LAPAROSCOPIC SPLENECTOMY

SURGICAL CONSIDERATIONS

Description: Laparoscopic-assisted splenectomy is best suited for normal or slightly enlarged spleens (e.g., idiopathic thrombocytopenic purpura [ITP]). Laparoscopic splenectomy usually is contraindicated in patients who have cancer, large hilar lymph nodes, or portal hypertension. At present, the only absolute contraindication to the procedure is massive splenomegaly, with spleens > 30 cm in the longitudinal axis. There is a high conversion rate (to open surgery) if the size of the spleen is between 20–30 cm. Sometimes a hand-assisted approach may be helpful for spleens in this size range. Conversion rates are higher in patients with perisplenitis and morbid myeloproliferative disorders. For the procedure, patients should be placed on a beanbag in a 45° lateral decubitus position or a full lateral decubitus position. The advantage of the 45° right lateral decubitus position is that it is easy to rotate the table and place the patient in a supine position if there is an urgent need for conversion. With the 45° lateral decubitus or the full lateral decubitus position, the kidney rest should be elevated and the OR table should be flexed to increase the area between the costal margin and the superior iliac crest. All pressure points should be padded, and the patient should be secured firmly to the table. The first trocar site is generally in the LUQ. Access can be with a closed (Veress needle or Optiview trocar) or open (Hasson trocar) approach. The initial approach may be to the hilum, short gastrics, or inferior pole. Most surgeons use the Harmonic Scalpel to take down the various ligaments and to dissect out the hilum, which generally is stapled with an endo GIA. The short gastrics are taken down either with the Harmonic Scalpel or are stapled. The lateral and superior attachments are taken down last. The spleen is then placed in a bag. Removal of the spleen can be done in several ways. Some surgeons remove it with a morselizer placed through one of the trocar sites. Others enlarge one trocar site slightly and remove the spleen in chunks. For very large spleens, some surgeons make a Pfannenstiel incision and extract it through the pelvis.

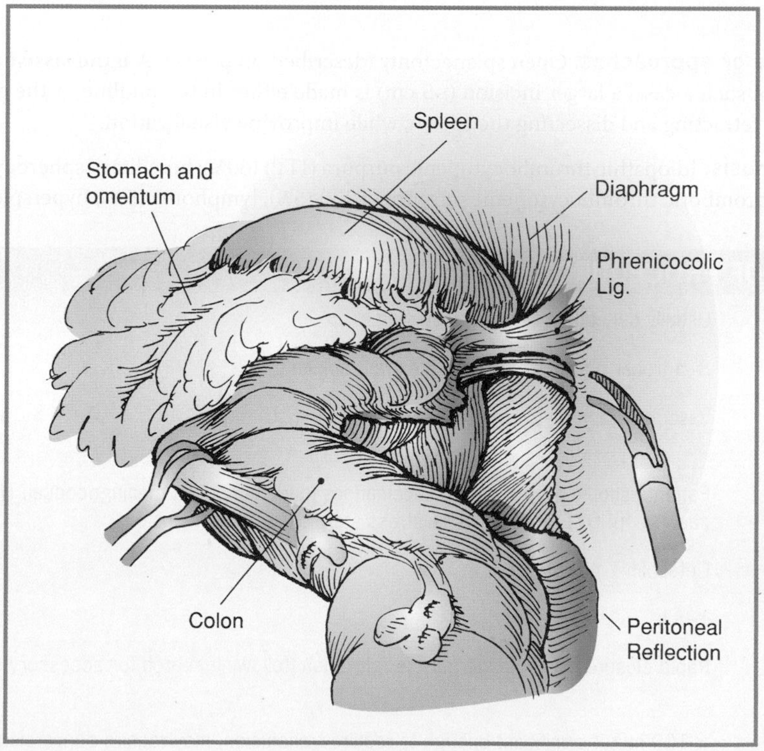

Figure 7.7-4. Anatomy of the spleen. (Reproduced with permission from Wind GG: The spleen. In *Applied Laparoscopic Anatomy: Abdomen and Pelvis.* Williams & Wilkins, Baltimore: 1997.)

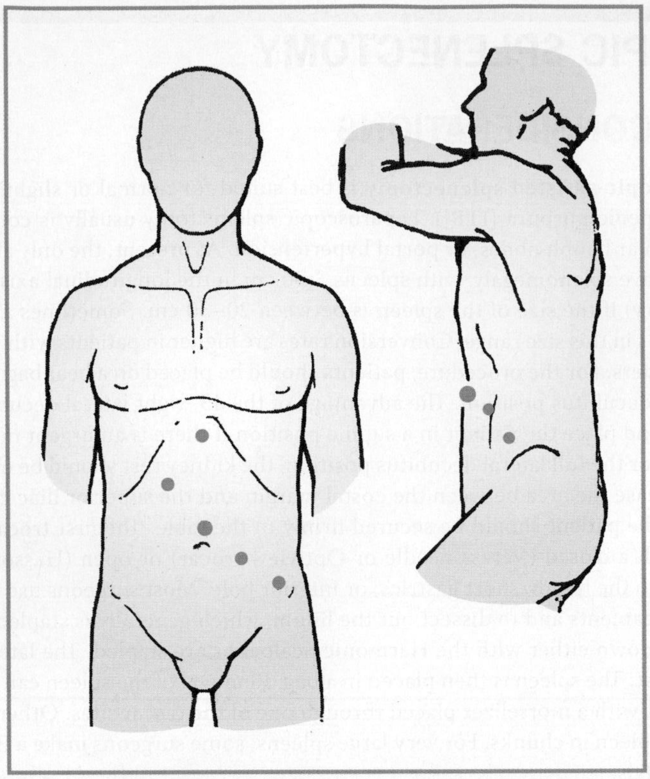

Figure 7.7-5. Trocar location for splenectomy. (Reproduced with permission from Scott-Conner CEH, Dawson DL: *Operative Anatomy,* 2nd ed. Lippincott Williams & Wilkins, Philadelphia: 2003.)

Variant procedure or approaches: Open splenectomy (described on p. 631). **A hand-assist device** can be used for larger spleens. In such a case, a larger incision (~5 cm) is made either in the midline or the pelvis and a hand is inserted to assist in retracting and dissecting the spleen, while improving visualization.

Usual preop diagnosis: Idiopathic thrombocytopenic purpura (ITP) (60%); hereditary spherocytosis (10%); hemolytic anemia (5%); thrombotic thrombocytopenic purpura (TTP) (5%); lymphoma (5%); hypersplenism (5%)

SUMMARY OF PROCEDURE	
Position	Usually decubitus, flexed or beanbag
Incision	3–5 trocar ports; 1 enlarged to extract spleen
Special instrumentation	Vascular staplers; Harmonic Scalpel; bipolar instruments
Unique considerations	Patients should have received vaccinations (pneumococcal, meningococcal, *Haemophilus influenzae*) preop. DVT prophylaxis; ± stress steroids; ± Plt transfusion.
Antibiotics	Cefazolin 1 g iv preop
Surgical time	1–3 h
Closing considerations	Rapid closure not requiring muscle relaxation (following search for accessory spleen)
EBL	< 100 mL; if significant enough to require transfusion, may require conversion to laparotomy.
Postop care	PACU → ward. Generally begin liquids pod 1 and discharge pod 2.
Mortality	0.1 % (predominately related to underlying disease)

SUMMARY OF PROCEDURE (cont'd)	
Morbidity	5% Hemorrhage Pulmonary complications Injury to pancreas, stomach or splenic flexure of colon
Pain score	5–6

PATIENT POPULATION CHARACTERISTICS	
Age range	All ages; more common in adults
Male:Female	1:1
Incidence	Uncommon
Etiology	Hematologic disorders (e.g., ITP, TTP); hemolytic anemia, tumor of the spleen (e.g., Hodgkin's disease); hypersplenism
Associated conditions	Steroid dependence; neutropenia; thrombocytopenia; hemolytic anemias

ANESTHETIC CONSIDERATIONS

PREOPERATIVE

Patients present for laparoscopic splenectomy with a variety of diseases, including ITP, lymphomatous disease (Hodgkin's and non-Hodgkin's), autoimmune hemolytic anemia, TTP, hereditary spherocytosis, Evans' syndrome, hairy-cell leukemia, hypersplenism 2° portal HTN, sarcoidosis, polycythemia vera, and myelofibrosis. Open splenectomy is usually reserved for traumatic laceration of the spleen. Previous upper abdominal surgery does not absolutely mitigate against the laparoscopic procedure. Laparoscopic cases tend to take longer than open splenectomies. Patients who have been treated with chemotherapeutic drugs will require careful preop exam to evaluate for potentially toxic side effects. See Anesthetic Considerations for (open) Splenectomy, p. 627. Patients should receive pneumococcal, meningococcal, and H. influenza vaccinations at least 1 wk preop.

Respiratory	Patients who present with splenomegaly may have a degree of left lower-lobe atelectasis, which should be evaluated by physical examination. As intraabdominal CO_2 insufflation → further atelectasis, ↓ FRC, ↑ PIP, ↑ $PaCO_2$ and ↓ PaO_2; therefore, laparoscopic procedures may be contraindicated in patients with severe respiratory disease. **Tests:** Consider P/A & lateral CXR; ABG; PFTs, if clinically indicated.
Cardiovascular	Cardiovascular changes caused by the pneumoperitoneum include ↓ venous return → ↓ CO and ↑ SVR. Decreased blood flow to the splanchnic and renal circulations (→ ↓ UO) may result from high intraabdominal pressures.
Hematologic	Cytopenias are very common. **Tests:** CBC with differential & Plt count. In view of potential bleeding, a type and screen should be performed. Consider cross matching in patients with coexisting disease. It may be difficult to cross match patients as they may exhibit antibodies, extra time should be allotted for cross matching preoperatively
Hepatic	Consider presence of coexisting hepatic dysfunction due to primary disease and/or therapy for it. **Tests:** Hepatinc panel, PT/PTT
Laboratory	As indicated from H&P.
Premedication	Standard premedication (p. B-1).

INTRAOPERATIVE

Anesthetic technique: GETA

Induction	Standard induction (p. B-2). In patients with coexisting liver disease, modify medication choice and dosage accordingly.	
Maintenance	Standard maintenance (p. B-2)	
Emergence	No special considerations. Prophylactic antiemetics are appropriate.	
Blood and fluid requirements	iv: 18–16 ga × 1 NS/LR @ 8–12 mL/kg/h Fluid warmer	Blood loss should be < 1 U. If Plt transfusion is necessary, it should be given after ligation of splenic vessels (↓ sequestration). Be prepared to obtain more iv access if bleeding is excessive. Consider extra iv access if arms inaccessible at the start of the case.
Monitoring	Standard monitors (p. B-1). Urinary catheter NG tube	Others as indicated by patient status. Prevent hypothermia (forced-air warmer, heated and humidified inspired gases, warming blanket, warm OR, etc.).
Positioning	✓ and pad pressure points ✓ eyes	Careful positioning and padding of patient is essential.
General Considerations		If the spleen is large (> 20 cm), there is a higher rate of conversion to an open procedure. In particular, intraoperative pain will be greater; hence, analgesic requirements will be higher.
Complications	Respiratory: Cardiovascular: ↓ BP Hemorrhage Dysrhythm Visceral injury Hypothermia Subcutaneous emphysema Bleeding	The complications of laparoscopy are discussed in Anesthetic Considerations for Laparoscopic Cholecystectomy, p. 577. Typically, when blood loss > 750–1000 mL, convert to open splenectomy. Plt transfusion may be necessary.

POSTOPERATIVE

Complications	Shoulder pain PONV Atelectasis	2° pneumoperitoneum; usually self-limited. Ketorolac (30 mg iv) or other NSAIDs effective. See p. B-2. Usually left lower lobe
Pain management	PCA (p. C-3). A multimodal approach to analgesia is useful in these patients. Be cautious with NSAIDs in patients with coexisting bone marrow disease.	
Tests	As indicated by patient status.	

Suggested Readings

1. Farab RR: Comparison of laparoscopic and open splenectomy in children with hematologic disorders. *J Pediatr* 1997; 131(1):41–6.
2. Fraker, DL: Splenic disorders. In *Greenfield's Surgery,* 4th edition, Greenfield LJ, Mulholland MW, Oldham KT, et al, eds. Lippincott Williams & Wilkins, Philadelphia: 2006, 1222–50.
3. Grahn SW, Alvarez J, Kirkwood K: Trends in laparoscopic splenectomy for massive splenomegaly. *Arch Surg* 2006; 141(8):755–62.
4. Katkhouda N, Mavor E: Laparoscopic splenectomy. *Surg Clin North Am* 2000; 80:1285–98.
5. Pace DE, Chiasson PM, Schlachta CM, et al: Laparoscopic splenectomy for idiopathic thrombocytopenic purpura. *Surg Endosc* 2003; 17(1):95–8.

6. Park AE: Lateral approach to laparoscopic splenectomy. In *Surgical Laparoscopy,* 2nd edition. Zucker KA, ed. Lippincott Williams & Wilkins, Philadelphia: 2001, 625–34.
7. Rescoria RJ: Laparoscopic splenectomy. *Semin Pediatr Surg* 2002; 11(4):226–32.
8. Sampath S, Meneghetti At, MacFarlane JK, et al: An 18-year review of open and laparoscopic splenectomy for idiopathic thrombocytopenic purpura. *Am J Surg* 2007; 193(5): 580–58.

LAPAROSCOPIC ADRENALECTOMY

SURGICAL CONSIDERATIONS

Description: **Laparoscopic adrenalectomy** typically is performed for a variety of adrenal problems, such as Conn's disease, functioning adenoma, pheochromocytoma, Cushing's disease, hyperplasia, virilizing or feminizing tumors, and an enlarging, nonfunctioning adenoma. Contraindications to laparoscopic surgery include invasive malignancy, malignant pheochromocytoma, and coagulopathy that cannot be corrected. Urologists generally use a retroperitoneal approach, while other surgeons use a transabdominal approach. The patient should be on a beanbag in the full lateral decubitus position (Fig. 7.7-6). The kidney rest should be elevated and the table should be flexed to open up the area between the costal margin and iliac crest. A left adrenalectomy is typically easier than a right adrenalectomy. On the left side, three trocars are required along the costal margin. Surgery begins by immobilizing the spleen and the colon laterally, which allows the spleen to fall away completely from the adrenal gland. The adrenal is then seen behind the hilum of the spleen. Care should be taken to minimize manipulation of a pheochromocytoma, to prevent sudden, unexpected HTN during the operation. In general, most surgeons prefer to clip and cut the adrenal vein first. After the adrenal is completely mobilized, it is removed through one of the port sites. For a right-sided approach, four trocars generally are required along the costal margin. The 4th trocar is used to retract the liver. The first step on the right side is to mobilize the lateral attachments of the liver to expose the adrenal. An enlarged right adrenal may be difficult to mobilize enough to see the adrenal vein, because the right adrenal vein empties directly into the IVC. Most surgeons recommend using an endo GIA stapler to divide the right adrenal vein.

Variant procedure or approaches: Open procedure (p. 668) or retroperitoneal approach

Usual preop diagnosis: Indeterminate adrenal mass (nonfunctional adenoma); also can be performed for functional adenomas, rarely for pheochromocytoma. Contraindicated for known carcinoma.

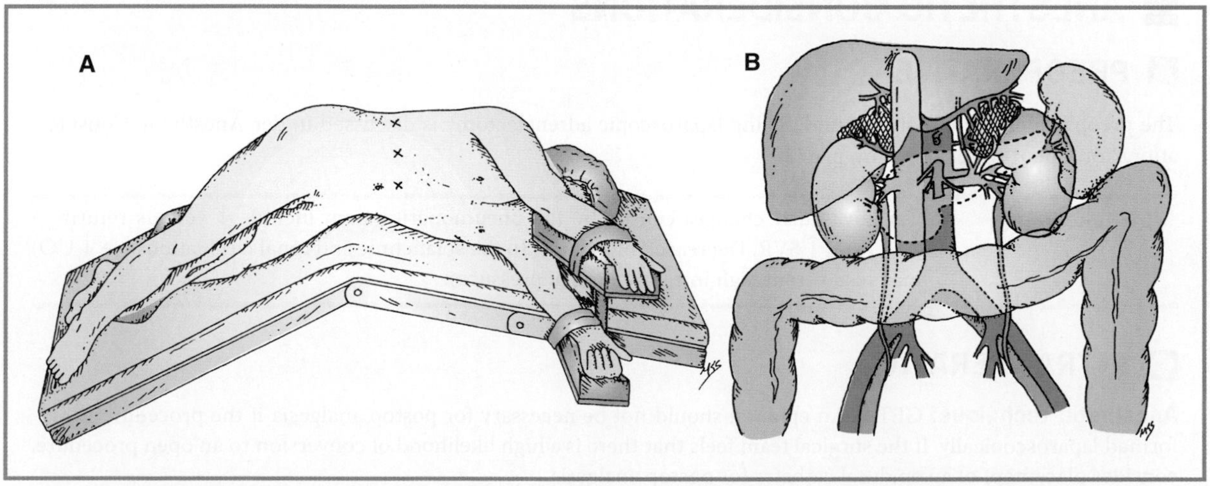

Figure 7.7-6. Laparoscopic adrenalectomy. **(A)** Patient positioning and port locations. **(B)** Anatomic relationships of adrenals (sutured) to adjunct and overlying structures. (Reproduced with permission from Scott-Conner CEH, Dawson DL: *Operative Anatomy,* 2nd ed. Lippincott Williams & Wilkins, Philadelphia: 2003.)

SUMMARY OF PROCEDURE	
Position	Lateral decubitus. A patient with bilateral disease may need repositioning between sides; or surgeon may use a supine approach.
Incision	3 ports on left side; 4 ports on right side
Antibiotics	Cefazolin 1 g iv
Surgical time	1–2 h
Closing considerations	Brief closure; muscle relaxation helpful for fascial repair
EBL	< 75 mL, although occasionally significant blood loss may occur.
Postop care	Patient usually discharged on pod 1 or 2, depending on BP control.
Mortality	< 0.1%
Morbidity	Hemorrhage/hematoma Injury to pancreas or kidney UTI DVT
Pain score	4

PATIENT POPULATION CHARACTERISTICS	
Age range	All ages
Male:Female	1:1
Incidence	Varies with underlying disorder
Etiology	Pheochromocytoma (25%); nonfunctioning adenomas, aldosteronoma (21%); cortisol-producing adenoma (15%); Cushing's disease (8%)
Associated conditions	Depending on function of tumor (e.g., HTN for aldosteronoma, Cushing's disease)

ANESTHETIC CONSIDERATIONS

PREOPERATIVE

The preop evaluation of patients undergoing laparoscopic adrenalectomy is discussed under Anesthetic Considerations for (open) Adrenalectomy, p. 672.

Cardiovascular	Cardiovascular changes caused by the pneumoperitoneum include ↓ venous return → ↓ CO and ↑ SVR. Decreased blood flow to the splanchnic and renal circulations (→ ↓ UO) may result from high intra-abdominal pressures.

INTRAOPERATIVE

Anesthetic technique: GETA. An epidural should not be necessary for postop analgesia if the procedure is performed laparoscopically. If the surgical team feels that there is a high likelihood of conversion to an open procedure, consider placement of an epidural catheter for postop analgesia.

Induction	See induction under (open) Adrenalectomy, p. 673.
Maintenance	See maintenance under (open) Adrenalectomy, p. 673.

Emergence	See emergence under (open) Adrenalectomy, p. 674. Case is likely to take longer if performed laparoscopically, but usually has a less painful postop course. Prophylactic antiemetics are appropriate.	
Blood and fluid requirements	iv: 16–14 ga × 1 NS/LR @10–15 mL/kg/h	Warming techniques important (forced-air warmers, fluid warmers, humidified inspired gases, etc.).
Monitoring	Standard monitors (p. B-1). UO Arterial line ± PA catheter TEE	 A PA catheter is useful in the management of patients with pheochromocytoma. TEE may be needed to evaluate cardiac function and filling.
Positioning	✓ and pad pressure points ✓ eyes	Careful support and padding of extremities and torso is very important.
Complications: laparoscopic	Respiratory: Pneumoperitoneum Hypercarbia/hypoxemia Pneumothorax Pneumomediastinum Endobronchial intubation Cardiovascular: ↓ BP Hemorrhage Dysrhythmias Visceral injury Subcutaneous emphysema Hypothermia	The complications of laparoscopy are discussed in Anesthetic Considerations for Laparoscopic Cholecystectomy, p. 579.
Complications: endocrine	Pheochromocytoma: BP lability Myocardial dysfunction Conn's syndrome: CHF 2° hypervolemia ↓ BP Electrolyte disturbances Hyperglycemia Cushing's syndrome: ↓ BP Acute adrenal insufficiency	Rx: intraop HTN with SNP or phentolamine (2.5–5 mg q 5 min); ↑ HR with esmolol; ↓ BP with phenylephrine or dopamine. (See Anesthetic Considerations for Adrenalectomy, p. 673.) See Anesthetic Considerations for Adrenalectomy, p. 673. Continue replacement steroids. (See Anesthetic Considerations for Adrenalectomy, p. 673.)

POSTOPERATIVE

Complications	PONV Shoulder pain	See p. B-2. Consider ketorolac 30 mg iv.
Pain management	PCA (p. B-4).	See Anesthetic Considerations for Adrenalectomy, p. 674.
Tests	As indicated	

Suggested Readings

1. Area MJ, Gagner M: Laparoscopic management of adrenal lesions. In *Surgical Laparoscopy,* 2nd edition. Zucker KA, ed. Lippincott Williams & Wilkins, Philadelphia: 2001, 635–42.

2. Ciriac J, Weizman D, Urback DR: Laparoscopic adrenalectomy for the management of benign and malignant adrenal tumors. *Expert Rev Med Devices* 2006; 3(6):777–86.
3. Hasan R, Harold KL, Matthews BD, et al: Outcomes for laparoscopic bilateral adrenalectomy. *J Laparoendosc Adv Surg Tech A* 2000; 12(4):233–6.
4. Horgan S, Sinan M, Helton WS, et al: Use of laparoscopic techniques improves outcome from adrenalectomy. *Am J Surg* 1997; 173:371–4.
5. Lodin M, Priitera A, Giannone G: Laparoscopic adrenalectomy: kers to success: correct surgical indications, adequate preoperative perparation, surgical team experience. *Surg Laprosc Endosc Percutan Tech* 2007; 17(5):392–5.
6. Olson JA: Adrenal gland. In *Greenfield's Surgery,* 4th edition, Greenfield LJ, Mulholland MW, Oldham KT, et al, eds. Lippincott Williams & Wilkins, Philadelphia: 2006, 1334–53.
7. Raeburn CD, McIntyre RC Jr: Laparoscopic approach to adrenal and endocrine pancreatic tumors. *Surg Clin North Am* 2000; 80:1427–42.

LAPAROSCOPIC BOWEL RESECTION

SURGICAL CONSIDERATIONS

Description: The surgical community has not uniformly embraced **laparoscopic bowel surgery.** It is technically very difficult because the surgeon has to maneuver in several quadrants during the operation. In benign diseases (e.g., ulcerative colitis, Crohn's disease, diverticular disease, and polyps) there are clear advantages to a laparoscopic approach to bowel resection, including decreased pain, earlier return of GI function, earlier ambulation, and earlier discharge from the hospital. Although these advantages also apply to the patient with cancer, there are still reservations about whether cure and survival rates are the same. Preliminary data from several ongoing multicenter trials indicate

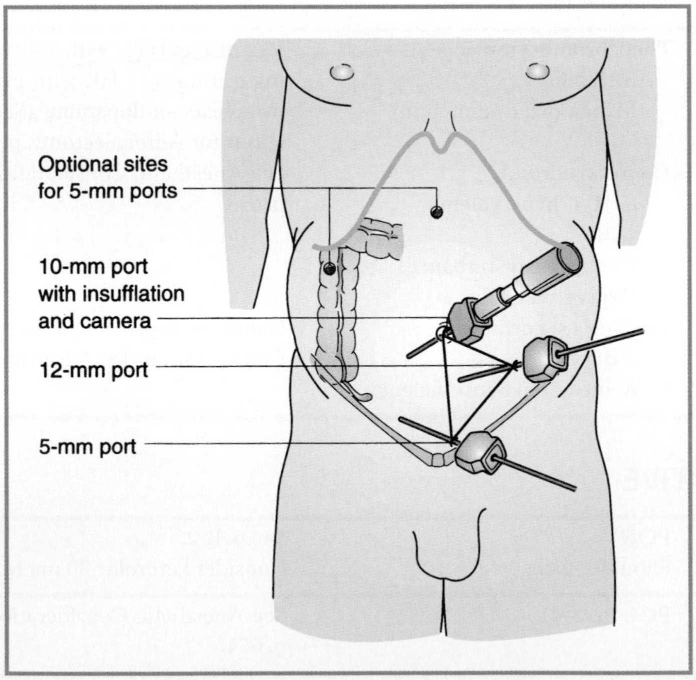

Figure 7.7-7. Trocar placement for a right colectomy. The general principle is to place the camera port so that the surgeon's visual axis is parallel to the telescope, and to place the working ports so that the operative site is at the apex of an isosceles triangle. (Reproduced with permission from Greenfield LJ, Mulholland MW, Oldham KT, et al, eds: *Surgery: Scientific Principles and Practice,* 2nd ed Lippincott-Raven Publishers, Philadelphia: 1997.)

that the length of the specimen and the number of lymph nodes removed are the same with both approaches. Data regarding staging and survival indicate similar outcomes are similar with laparoscopic or open approaches.

For a left-sided colon resection, the patient is placed in a low lithotomy position, while in other bowel resections, a supine position is used. The patient's arms should be tucked to improve access to all four quadrants. Generally, four to five ports are required, one in each quadrant. For a **laparoscopic-assisted approach,** one of these ports will be enlarged slightly for removal of the specimen. Very often the operating table will need to be tilted or rotated throughout the course of the procedure to help move the small intestines away from the surgical dissection site. The procedure typically begins with localization of the pathology. This may require an intraop sigmoidoscopy if the lesion has not already been marked on colonoscopy or if it is not grossly apparent. The involved section of the intestine is then mobilized. Often, division of the mesentery is done intracorporeally. Occasionally, surgeons will exteriorize the bowel and do extracorporeal division of the mesentery and extracorporeal division of the bowel. For right-sided lesions, the anastomosis typically is done extracorporeally; however, for left-sided lesions, once the bowel is removed, the extraction site will be closed. The pneumoperitoneum will be reinsufflated and the anastomosis will be performed intracorporeally with an end-to-end stapler placed through the anus.

Unipolar and bipolar cautery, the Harmonic Scalpel, and many different surgical staplers may be used during these procedures. These generally require longer operative times than the corresponding open procedures but, typically, they are associated with shorter hospitalization stays and earlier return to work than traditional laparotomy.

Variant procedure or approaches: Open surgery (see p. 518), laparoscopic-assisted, or totally laparoscopic procedures. Some surgeons also have recommended a hand-assisted procedure where a pneumoperitoneum is still used, but the port site of extraction is enlarged at the beginning of the operation. The surgeon's hand can be placed through a special sleeve that maintains pneumoperitoneum, but also allows the surgeon to retract and dissect manually. Occasionally, the specimen is removed via the anus or through a vaginotomy.

Usual preop diagnosis: Intestinal obstruction; inflammatory conditions (e.g., diverticulitis, bleeding, neoplasms); cancer (controversial)

SUMMARY OF PROCEDURE

Position	Usually supine; sometimes lithotomy for left-sided procedures
Incision	4–5 trocar sites, one in each quadrant. One site will be enlarged for specimen removal and/or anastomosis in laparoscopic-assisted procedures.
Special instrumentation	Harmonic Scalpel, various laparoscopic stapling instruments
Unique considerations	The operating table will be moved quite frequently to help with visualization.
Antibiotics	Cefotetan 1 g iv preop
Surgical time	1.5–2 h (small bowel resection); 3–4 h (colonic resection). Surgical times will ↑ in the presence of acute inflammation and as the bowel resection becomes more extensive.
Closing considerations	Usually requires closure of several port sites; muscle relaxation helpful.
EBL	< 200 mL
Postop care	NG tube seldom used. Most patients begin regular diet within 48 h; discharge, generally 3–4 d.
Mortality	< 0.1%
Morbidity	< 5% (similar in magnitude to those seen with open operations) Complications include: Hemorrhage Infection Anastomotic leak Intestinal obstruction
Pain score	6–7

PATIENT POPULATION CHARACTERISTICS	
Age range	All ages (increases with age)
Male:Female	1:1
Incidence	Varies with disease process.
Etiology	Diverticulitis; polyps; inflammatory bowel disease (IBD)
Associated conditions	None

ANESTHETIC CONSIDERATIONS

PREOPERATIVE

For respiratory, cardiovascular, musculoskeletal, gastrointestinal, and renal considerations, see Anesthetic Considerations for Intestinal and Peritoneal Procedures, p. 627.

Additional considerations	Laparoscopic bowel resection is performed for both malignant and benign disease. Patients presenting may have a long history of inflammatory bowel disease such as ulcerative colitis or Crohn's disease. Typically they have received medical therapy, surgical treatments or both. Medical therapies include 5-aminosalicylic acid compounds and immunosuppressants, such as corticosteroids and methotrexate. Side effects of medical therapies include interstitial nephritis, pancreatitis, pleuropericarditis (5-aminosalicylic acids) immunosuppression, truncal obesity, diabetes, and hypertension (corticosteroids). Patients who have had previous surgery or severe disease may have adhesions making the impending laparoscopic surgery more technically challenging. Inflammatory bowel disease is associated with a number of coexisting conditions including arthritis, uveitis, biliary stasis which may impact upon anesthetic management.
Tests	CBC, Renal panel, T&S. Others as per history and physical exam
Premedication	Standard premedication (p. B-2). If patient is at risk for a full stomach, administration of metoclopramide (10 mg iv) and H_2 blocker (ranitidine 50 mg iv), as well as Na citrate 0.3 M 30 mL po. Metoclopramide should not be used in patients with bowel obstructions or perforations.

INTRAOPERATIVE

Anesthetic technique: GETA

Induction	Standard induction (p. B-2). Standard rapid-sequence induction if at risk for aspiration (p. B-4).	
Maintenance	Standard maintenance (p. B-2).	
Emergence	No special considerations unless the patient is at risk for aspiration; extubation should then occur after the patient is fully awake and has protective airway reflexes.	
Blood and fluid requirements	IV: 16–18 ga × 1 NS/LR @ 8–12 mL/kg/h Fluid warmer	Blood loss should be < 1 U.
Monitoring	Standard monitors (p. B-1). Urinary catheter NG tube to decompress the stomach	Others as indicated by patient status. Prevent hypothermia (forced-air warmer, warming blanket, warm room, etc).
Positioning	✓ and pad pressure points ✓ eyes	

General Surgery

Complications	Respiratory: Pneumoperitoneum Hypercarbia/hypoxemia Pneumothorax Pneumomediastinum Endobronchial intubation Cardiovascular: ↓ BP Dysrhythmias Hemorrhage Visceral injury Hypothermia Subcutaneous emphysema	These complications (associated with the preperitoneal approach), as well as the general complications of laparoscopy, are discussed in Anesthetic Considerations for Laparoscopic Cholecystectomy, p. 577.

POSTOPERATIVE

Complications	PONV Shoulder pain	See p. B-2. Ketorolac (30 mg iv) or other NSAIDS.
Pain management	PCA (p. C-3).	
Tests	As indicated by patient status.	

Suggested Readings

1. Ballantyne GH, ed: *Atlas of Laparoscopic Surgery.* WB Saunders, Philadelphia: 2000, 300–404.
2. COST (Clinical Outcomes of Surgical Therapy Study Group): A comparison of laparoscopically assisted and open colectomy for colon cancer. *N Engl J Med* 2004; 350(20):2050–9.
3. Fleshman JW, Sargent DJ, Green E, et al: Laparoscopic colectomy for cancer is not interior to open surgery based on 5-year data from the COST Study Group trial. *Ann Surg* 2007; 246(4):655–64.
4. Hinojosa MW, Murrell ZA, Konyalian VR: Comparison of laparoscopic vs open sigmoid colectomy for benign and malignant disease at academic medical centers. *J Gastrointest Surg* 2007; 11(11):1423–30.
5. Milsom JW, Hammerhofer KA, Bohn B, et al: Prospective randomized trial comparing laparoscopic vs. conventional surgery for refractory ileocolic Crohn's disease. *Dis Colon Rectum* 2001; 44(1):1–8.
6. Wexner SD: Laparoscopic colectomy in diverticular and Crohn's disease. *Surg Clin North Am* 2000; 80:1299–1320.
7. Wichmann MW, Meyer G, Angele MK, et al: Recent advances in minimally invasive colorectal cancer surgery. *Onkologie* 2002; 25(4):318–23.

LAPAROSCOPIC APPENDECTOMY

SURGICAL CONSIDERATIONS

Description: **Appendectomy** generally is performed for suspected appendicitis. The patient is placed in the supine position with the left arm tucked. An OG tube should be inserted to decompress the stomach. Access is obtained at the umbilicus, either through a closed (**Veress needle**) technique or open (**Hasson trocar**) technique. If a Veress needle is used, a Foley catheter should be inserted. Two additional trocars are inserted—one suprapubic and the other in the LLQ. The port in the LLQ is a 10/12 mm trocar to allow passage of an endo GIA stapler. Occasionally, a 4th trocar may be placed in the RUQ to help with mobilization and retraction. The table will then be rotated to the left side and the surgeon may ask for it to be placed in Trendelenburg or reverse Trendelenburg position, depending on the location of the cecum. The base of the cecum is identified and the appendix is mobilized (Fig. 7.7-8B). This may require dissection of the peritoneal edge along the right gutter. After the appendix is mobilized, a window is created in the mesoappendix, and the base of the appendix is stapled with an endo GIA. The mesoappendix is then stapled with a vascular-cartridge endo GIA. The appendix generally is placed in a bag prior to delivering it or it may

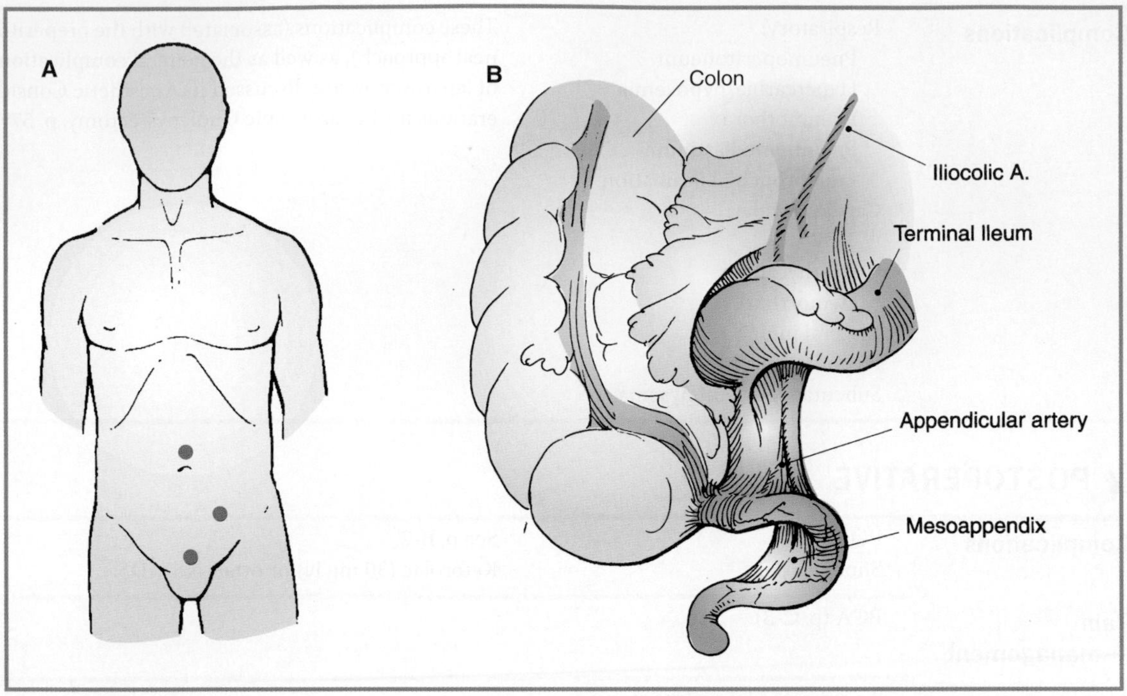

Figure 7.7-8. Setup and initial view for laparoscopic appendectomy. **(A)** Reproduced with permission from Scott-Conner CEH, Dawson DL: *Operative Anatomy,* 2nd edition. Lippincott Williams & Wilkins, Philadelphia: 2003. **(B)** Reproduced with permission from Wind GG: The spleen. In *Applied Laparoscopic Anatomy: Abdomen and Pelvis.* Williams & Wilkins, Baltimore: 1997.

be brought directly through the 10/12-mm trocar. The umbilical fascia is closed and the skin is loosely approximated. When unexpected pathology is identified, it can be dealt with by laparoscopy or by laparotomy, with incision placement dependent on findings.

Variant procedure or approaches: **Open appendectomy** (see p. 509) via RLQ or midline incision

Usual preop diagnosis: **Acute abdomen;** possible acute appendicitis

SUMMARY OF PROCEDURE	
Position	Supine
Incision	3–4 ports (see Fig. 7.7-8A)
Antibiotics	Cefazolin 1 g iv preop
Surgical time	60–90 min
Closing considerations	Muscular relaxation helpful for umbilical closure; NG tube if prolonged ileus suspected.
EBL	< 75 mL
Postop care	Patients are hospitalized for varying lengths of time, depending on their need for antibiotics. Many with simple acute appendicitis can go home within 24 h.
Mortality	Perforated: 2–5% (nonperforated: < 0 .1%); increased in elderly patients and infants.
Morbidity	Overall: 3% if nonperforated; 20–50% with perforation Intraabdominal abscess Hematoma Ileus

SUMMARY OF PROCEDURE (cont'd)	
Morbidity (cont'd)	Risk of intraabdominal abscess, mostly dependent on pathology (e.g., early acute inflammation vs perforation) Hemorrhage Infection Stump leak: exceedingly rare Conversion to open procedure: dependent on pathology and experience of surgeon
Pain score	4

PATIENT POPULATION CHARACTERISTICS	
Age range	All ages; commonly, 19–25 yr
Male:Female	1:1
Incidence	Common (7%)
Etiology	Acute appendicitis; etiology unknown
Associated conditions	Consider other pelvic pathology in women of childbearing age.

ANESTHETIC CONSIDERATIONS

PREOPERATIVE

This patient population is generally fit and healthy, apart from their acutely presenting illness. Full-stomach precautions (see p. B-4) are appropriate in these patients.

Respiratory	Respiratory impairment can occur 2° acute abdominal pain and splinting. Tachypnea and hyperpnea can be heralding Sx of appendiceal perforation and sepsis. Patients with acute abdomen should be treated as if they have full stomachs. **Tests:** As indicated from H&P.
Cardiovascular	Cardiovascular changes caused by the pneumoperitoneum include ↓ venous return → ↓ CO and ↑ SVR. Decreased blood flow to the splanchnic and renal circulations (→ ↓ UO) may result from high intraabdominal pressures. May be dehydrated from fever, emesis, and decreased oral intake. Assess volume status with VS and hydrate adequately before anesthetic induction. **Tests:** ECG, if indicated from H&P.
Gastrointestinal	Patient typically has abdominal pain with N/V. Muscular resistance to palpation of abdominal wall frequently parallels the severity of the inflammatory process. With spreading peritoneal irritation (as with perforation), patient will develop abdominal distension and paralytic ileus. **Tests:** Renal panel, consider pregnancy test
Hematologic	Moderate leukocytosis (10,000–18,000) with left shift. Hemoconcentration likely if patient dehydrated. **Tests:** CBC
Laboratory	Others as indicated from H&P.
Premedication	Patients with acute appendicitis should be treated as if they have full stomachs. Consider administration of metoclopramide (10 mg iv) and H_2 blocker (ranitidine 50 mg iv), as well as Na citrate 0.3 M 30 mL po. Opiate premedication (morphine 0.08–0.15 mg/kg im) is indicated after patient is scheduled for surgery if patient in pain. Acertain if patient received opiates during ED eval and management.

INTRAOPERATIVE

Anesthetic technique: GETA, with rapid-sequence iv induction.

Induction	Preoxygenate patient and have an assistant apply cricoid pressure. Etomidate 0.1–0.4 mg/kg or propofol 1.5–3 mg/kg + succinylcholine 1.5 mg/kg, for intubation.	
Maintenance	Standard maintenance (p. B-2), without N_2O.	
Emergence	Extubate when the patient is awake and with active laryngeal protective reflexes.	
Blood and fluid requirements	IV: 16–18 ga × 1 NS/LR @ 5–8 mL/kg/h	
Monitoring	Standard monitors (p. B-1). Urinary catheter NG tube	Others as indicated by patient status. Prevent hypothermia (forced-air warmer, warming blanket, warm room, etc.)
Positioning	✓ and pad pressure points ✓ eyes Secure or tuck arms	Trendelenburg position with elevation of the right side of the abdomen improves surgical exposure.
Complications	Respiratory: Pneumoperitoneum Hypercarbia/hypoxemia Pneumothorax Pneumomediastinum Endobronchial intubation Cardiovascular: Hypotension Dysrhythmias Visceral injury Hypothermia Subcutaneous emphysema	These complications (associated with the preperitoneal approach), as well as the general complications of laparoscopy, are discussed in Anesthetic Considerations for Lap Cholecystectomy, p. 577.

POSTOPERATIVE

Complications	PONV Urinary retention	See p. B-2. Straight catheterization of the bladder
Pain management	PCA (p. C-3). Oral analgesics Ketorolac	 Acetaminophen po q 6 h or Percocet – 2 po q 6 h 30 mg iv
Tests	As indicated by patient status.	

Suggested Readings

1. Bennett J, Boddy A, Rhode M: Choice of approach for appendicectomy: a meta-analysis of open versus laparoscopic appendicectomy. *Surg Laparosc Endosc Percutan Tech* 2007; 17(4):245–55.
2. Caushaj PF: Laparoscopic appendectomy. In *Atlas of Laparoscopic Surgery*. Ballantyne GH, ed. WB Saunders, Philadelphia: 2000, 300–7.
3. Chiarugi M: Laparoscopic compared with open appendectomy for acute appendicitis: a prospective study. *Eur J Surg* 1996; 162(5):385–90.
4. Fogli L, Brulatti M, Boschi S, et al: Laparoscopic appendectomy for acute and recurrent appendicitis: retrospective analysis of a single-group 5-year experience. *J Laparosc Adv Surg Tech A* 2002; 12(2): 107–10.
5. Kumar R, Erian M, Sirrot S, et al: Laparoscopic appendectomy in modern gynecology. *J Am Assoc Gynecol Laparosc* 2002; 9(3):252–63.
6. Laine S: Laparoscopic appendectomy—is it worthwhile? A prospective, randomized study in young women. *Surg Endosc* 1997; 11(2):95–7.

LAPAROSCOPIC INGUINAL HERNIA REPAIR

SURGICAL CONSIDERATIONS

Description: **Laparoscopic hernia repair** is clearly preferred in patients with recurrent or bilateral hernias. In patients with first-time unilateral hernias, there are no clear advantages in terms of operative time, postop pain, time to discharge, or time to return to normal activities, compared with tension-free open repair (see p. 636). There are three types of laparoscopic hernia repairs. The first, **ONLAY,** generally has been discarded because of high recurrence rates. The other two are the **totally extraperitoneal** (**TEP**) and the **transabdominal preperitoneal** (**TAPP**) techniques. Of these, the TEP is somewhat more difficult to learn, but is associated with lower recurrence rates and complications than is the TAPP. For both the TEP and the TAPP, the patient is placed in the supine position with both arms tucked. Some surgeons insert a Foley, but many do not. A small incision is made at the umbilicus. For a **TEP,** this incision only goes to the preperitoneal space, and a balloon is then used for dissection. Two additional ports are placed in the midline—one suprapubic and one halfway between the umbilicus and the suprapubic port. Further dissection is required to identify the hernia defects, which are then reduced. The cord structures are completely freed and any cord lipomas are dissected. Mesh is placed to cover the entire area and is tacked to Cooper's ligament. For a **TAPP** repair, the umbilical incision extends into the abdomen. Two additional ports are placed at the level of the iliac crest—one in the RLQ and one in the LLQ. A peritoneal flap over the hernia defect is created and the preperitoneal space is entered. The rest of the dissection and the placement of the mesh are the same as with the TEP repair. At the end of the TAPP procedure, the peritoneal flap is placed over the mesh and tacked into place to prevent exposure of the bowel to the mesh.

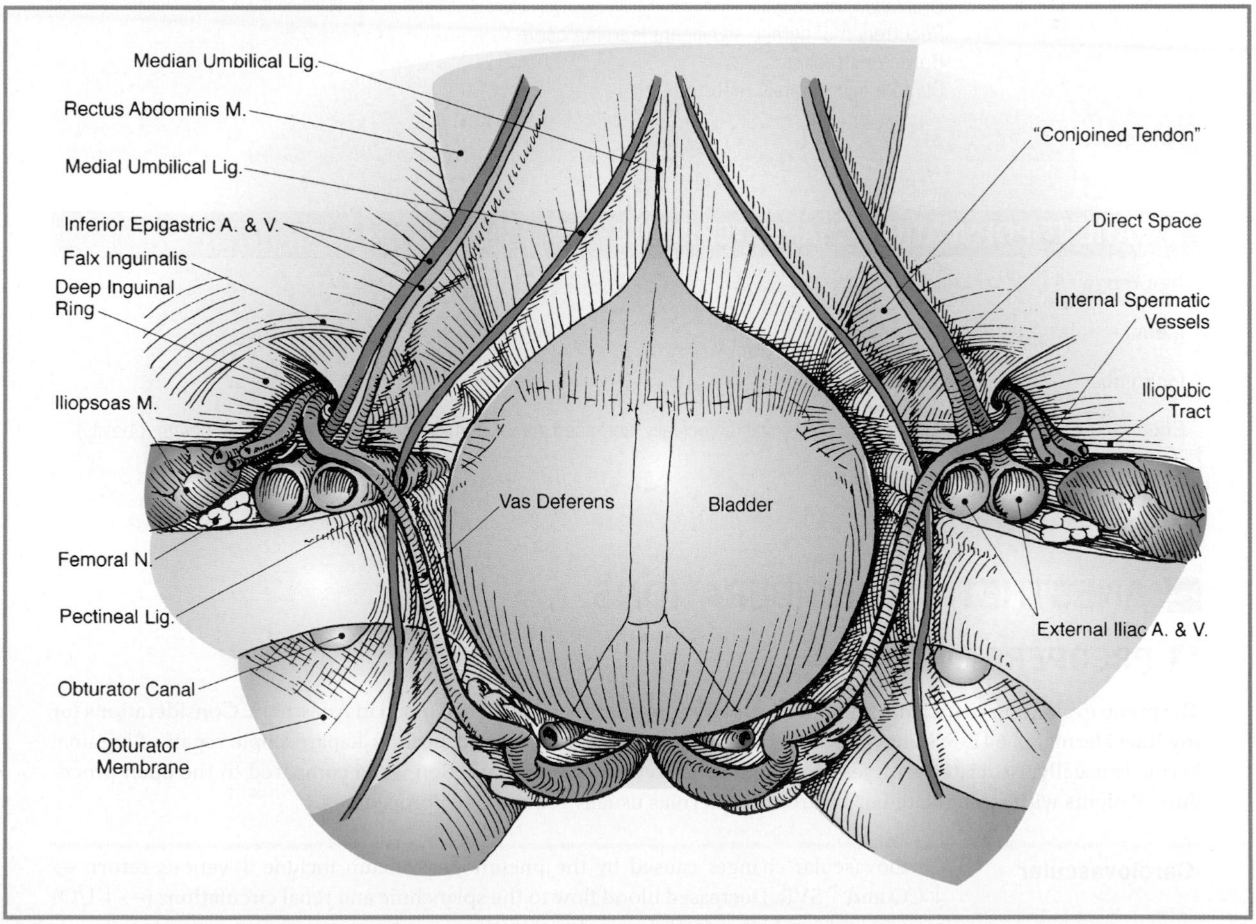

Figure 7.7-9. The inguinal region. (Reproduced with permission from Wind GG: The inguinal region. In *Applied Laparoscopic Anatomy: Abdomen and Pelvis.* Williams & Wilkins, Baltimore: 1997.)

Variant Procedure or approaches: **Open hernia repair** (see Inguinal Herniorrhaphy, p. 636).

Usual preop diagnosis: Inguinal hernia

SUMMARY OF PROCEDURE	
Position	Supine, arms tucked
Incision	3 ports—1 at the umbilicus; 2 either in the midline or RLQ or LLQ, depending on the laparoscopic approach.
Special instrumentation	Balloon dissector for TEP repair
Antibiotics	Cefazolin 1 g iv preop
Surgical time	1–2 h
Closing considerations	Minimal time; muscle relaxation may be helpful.
EBL	< 50 mL
Postop care	1–2 h in PACU/holding area → home
Mortality	< 0.1%
Morbidity	2% Orchialgia, neuralgia Recurrence of hernia: significant learning curve Bowel obstruction Bladder injury: rarely reported
Pain score	3–4

PATIENT POPULATION CHARACTERISTICS	
Age range	Mostly adults
Male:Female	Male > Female
Incidence	Common
Etiology	Most hernias congenital; chronically increased intraabdominal pressure (e.g., chronic cough, obesity)
Associated conditions	None important

ANESTHETIC CONSIDERATIONS

PREOPERATIVE

The preop evaluation of patients undergoing laparoscopic hernia repair is discussed in Anesthetic Considerations for Inguinal Hernia, p. 641. Patients presenting for this procedure are generally healthy. Laparoscopic repair of inguinal hernia is usually associated with less pain and earlier return to preop function when compared to the open procedure. Patients with strangulated or incarcerated hernias usually require open procedures.

Cardiovascular	Cardiovascular changes caused by the pneumoperitoneum include ↓ venous return → ↓ CO and ↑ SVR. Decreased blood flow to the splanchnic and renal circulations (→ ↓ UO) may result from high intraabdominal pressures.
Laboratory	Hb/Hct (healthy patients); otherwise, as indicated from H&P.
Premedication	Standard premedication (p. B-2).

INTRAOPERATIVE

Anesthetic technique: GETA

Induction	Standard induction (p. B-2)	
Maintenance	Standard maintenance (p. B-2)	
Emergence	No special considerations except to minimize coughing on emergence. Consider 1 mg/kg iv lidocaine.	
Blood and fluid requirements	iv: 18 ga × 1 NS/LR @ 5–8 mL/kg/h	Blood loss should be minimal.
Monitoring	Standard monitors (p. B-1). Urinary catheter NG tube	Others as indicated by patient status. Prevent hypothermia (forced-air warmer, heated and humidified gases, warming blanket, warm OR, etc.).
Positioning	✓ and pad pressure points ✓ eyes	Careful positioning and padding of the patient is essential.
Complications	Hemorrhage from trocar insertion. Subcutaneous emphysema	These complications (associated with the preperitoneal approach), as well as the general complications of laparoscopy, are discussed in Anesthetic Considerations for Laparoscopic Cholecystectomy, p. 577.

POSTOPERATIVE

Complications	PONV (see B-6) Urinary retention	Ondansetron (4 mg iv) Straight catheterization of the bladder
Pain management	Oral opiates Ketorolac	Tylenol #3 – 2 po q 6 h or Percocet – 2 po q 6 h. 15–30 mg iv
Tests	As indicated by patient status.	

Suggested Readings

1. Cooper SS: Laparoscopic inguinal hernia repair: is the enthusiasm justified? *Am Surg* 1997; 63(l):103–6.
2. Corbitt J: Laparoscopic transabdominal preperitoneal patch hernia repair. In *Atlas of Laparoscopic Surgery.* Ballantyne GH, ed. WB Saunders, Philadelphia: 2000, 502–15.
3. Crawford DL, Philips EH: Totally extraperitoneal laparoscopic herniorrhaphy. In *Surgical Laparoscopy,* 2nd edition. Zucker KA, ed. Lippincott Williams & Wilkins, Philadelphia: 2001, 571–84.
4. Cunningham AJ: Laparoscopic surgery—anesthetic implications. *Surg Endosc* 1994; 8(11):1272–84.
5. Kozal R, Lange PM, Kosir M, et al: A prospective, randomized study of open vs laparoscopic inguinal hernia repair. *Arch Surg* 1997; 132:292–5.
6. Liem MS: Comparison of conventional anterior surgery and laparoscopic surgery for inguinal-hernia repair. *N Engl J Med* 1997;336(22):1541–7.
7. Matthews RD, Anthony T, Kim LT, et al: Factors associated with postoperative compilations and hernia recurrence for patients undergoing inguinal hernia repair: a report from the VA Cooperative Hernia Study Group. *Am J Surg* 2007; 194(5):611–7.
8. Neumayer L, Giobbie-Hurder A, Jonasson O, et al. Open mesh versus laparoscopic mesh repair of inguinal hernia. *N Engl J Med* 2004; 350(18):1819–27.

LAPAROSCOPIC BARIATRIC SURGERY

SURGICAL CONSIDERATIONS

Description: Morbid obesity is increasing worldwide. Many patients have associated comorbidities including HTN, diabetes, and sleep apnea, which they have been unable to correct by dieting and exercise. Surgical treatment results

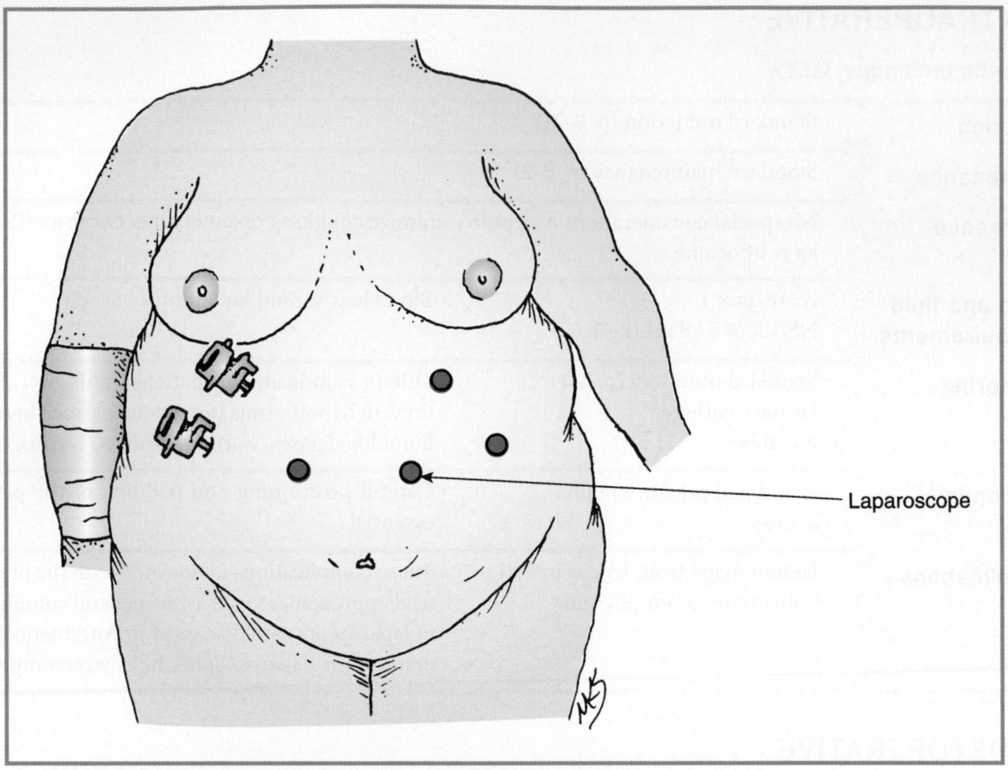

Figure 7.7-10. Patient position and trocar position for bariatric laparoscopic surgery. (Reproduced with permission from Scott-Connors CEH, Dawson, DL: *Operative Anatomy,* Lippincott Williams & Wilkins, Philadelphia: 2003.)

in weight loss of approximately 2/3–3/4 of excess body weight, usually with consequent correction of comorbidities. Operations for morbid obesity are classified as restrictive, such as the **adjustable gastric banding** and **vertical banded gastroplasty;** malabsorptive, such as a **jejunoileal bypass;** or a combination, such as the **Roux-en-Y gastric bypass.** The 1991 NIH consensus statement identified the Roux-en-Y bypass as the best surgical treatment for morbid obesity. In general, this operation is approached laparoscopically in most patients because of the decreased pain, earlier ambulation, earlier discharge from the hospital, quicker return to regular activity, and decreased wound complication rates, when compared with an open approach. Open approaches are undertaken in patients with previous upper abdominal surgery; patients who may not tolerate an increased intra-abdominal pressure (e.g., CHF, severe CAD, severe pulmonary disease); patients undergoing revision bariatric surgery, and, occasionally, in patients who fall into a super morbidly obese group (BMI > 60 kg/m^2). Surgery is indicated in patients with a BMI of 35–40 kg/m^2, if they have associated comorbidities, or > 40 kg/m^2, if they have no associated comorbidities.

In these procedures, the patient generally is placed in RT-HELP position. Some surgeons prefer a split-leg table, with the surgeon standing between the legs. For a laparoscopic Roux-en-Y bypass, the first incision is made in the midline, approximately halfway between the umbilicus and the xyphoid; 4–5 additional ports are then placed in the LUQ and the midline. Most surgeons begin by performing a jejunojejunostomy. During this time, the patient is placed in a reverse Trendelenburg position to drop the small intestines into the pelvis. The omentum is placed in the upper abdomen and the ligament of Treitz is identified. The jejunum is divided with an endo GIA stapler ~20 cm from the ligament of Treitz. A Roux limb of 100 cm is then measured. (Occasionally, this Roux limb may be 150 cm, if the patient's BMI is > 50 kg/m^2.) The jejunojejunostomy is created with a stapler and the enterotomy is closed. Some surgeons prefer a **retrocolic approach,** wherein a passage is made through the transverse mesocolon. Other surgeons prefer an **antecolic approach,** in which the omentum is divided to allow for a place where the Roux limb can pass without tension. At this point, the liver retractor is placed and the gastric pouch is created. Before stomach stapling, everything in the stomach, including temperature probes, OG tubes, and calibrating tubes, should be removed. The gastric pouch is then stapled and cut. Often a calibrating tube is placed after the first two staple firings to help maintain the size of the pouch and the anastomosis. Some surgeons hand sew the gastrojejunostomy and some staple it with a linear stapler. Some surgeons staple the anastomosis and place the anvil of the end-to-end anastomotic stapler through the mouth (rarely done). Other surgeons place the anvil through a separate gastrotomy prior to complete division of the pouch. At the end, the gastrojejunostomy typically is tested by inflating air into the gastric pouch, either through an OG tube, the sizing tube, or a gastroscope. Generally, the NG or OG tube is removed at the end of the procedure. Often, at this point, surgeons will close the defect of the transverse mesocolon.

Variant procedure or approaches: Open bypass (see p. 499).

Usual preop diagnosis: Morbid obesity (100 lb above ideal body weight or 100% over ideal body weight), generally in combination with a medical condition(s) felt to be worsened by the obesity (e.g., osteoarthritis, diabetes, respiratory insufficiency, CHF, hypertension, sleep apnea), BMI > 40 kg/m^2, or BMI > 35 kg/m^2 if associated comorbidities present.

SUMMARY OF PROCEDURE	
Position	Supine or split leg (see Fig. 7.2-6 in Open Operations for Morbid Obesity, p. 501 for suggested positioning.)
Incision	Five to six port sites
Unique considerations	Patients are at high risk for aspiration, and airway management may be difficult. Patients are at high risk for thromboembolic events and VTE prophylaxis is critical (p. B-2).
Antibiotics	Cefoxitin 1 g iv
Surgical time	2–4 h
Closing considerations	Typically, fascial defects are not closed.
EBL	< 50 mL
Postop care	Most patients receive an upper GI study the next day. Clear liquids are begun if the study is normal, and most patients are discharged within 48 h.
Mortality	< 1%
Morbidity	Overall: 10% Stricture: 10% Leak: 1–2% VTE Pneumonia Hemorrhage Hernia Obstruction Infection
Pain score	5–6

PATIENT POPULATION CHARACTERISTICS	
Age Range	Generally, between 18–60 yr
Male:Female	Female > Male
Incidence	5%
Etiology	Genetic; environmental
Associated conditions	Sleep apnea; HTN; diabetes; GERD, osteoarthritis

ANESTHETIC CONSIDERATIONS

PREOPERATIVE

Obesity is associated with many chronic medical problems. A moderately overweight patient probably carries no excess health risks, especially while still young. However, morbidity and mortality rise sharply with increasing age and BMI. Medical comorbidities must be optimized before elective bariatric surgery. Evaluate any patient who has had previous bariatric surgery for metabolic changes that can include protein, vitamin, iron and calcium deficiencies.

Review a list of all current medications the patient is taking, including nonprescription appetite suppressors and diet drugs. Many of these drugs can have important side effects. For example, the combination of phentermine and fenfluramine ("phen-fen"), which is no longer prescribed in the United States, is associated with persistent, serious, heart and lung problems. Another weight loss medication, sibutramine, works in the brain by inhibiting the reuptake of norepinephrine, serotonin, and dopamine, producing a feeling of "anorexia," which limits food intake. Sibutramine has been implicated as a cause of dysrhythmias and hypertension. Orlistat blocks digestion and absorption of dietary fat by binding lipases in the gastrointestinal tract and can cause deficiencies in fat-soluble vitamins (A, D, E, K). A reduction in vitamin K levels can increase the anticoagulation effects of Coumadin.

Respiratory	Adipose tissue is metabolically active. Oxygen consumption and CO_2 production rise with increasing weight 2° ↑ metabolic demands. The work of breathing is increased, while respiratory muscle performance is impaired. Mass loading of the thoracic and abdominal walls causes abnormalities in both lung volume and gas exchange, especially when the patient is supine. The increased total respiratory resistance and decreased compliance associated with extreme obesity result in shallow, rapid breathing. Decreased FRC 2°↓ ERV →↓ TLC. Airways close during normal ventilation→ ↑pulmonary shunt → hypoxemia. These changes increase in direct proportion with increasing BMI. General anesthesia further reduces FRC. Preop PFTs show a restrictive breathing pattern. For symptomatic patients, an ABG obtained while the patient breathes room air is useful to establish a baseline. Younger obese patients have an increased ventilatory response to hypoxia and a relatively decreased response to hypercapnia. Their arterial blood sample often demonstrates alveolar hyperventilation ($PaCO_2$ 30–35 mm Hg) and relative hypoxemia (PaO_2 70–90 mm Hg) while breathing air. With increasing age, sensitivity to CO_2 decreases, so that $PaCO_2$ rises and PaO_2 falls further. Preop assessment of a patient's face, neck, and upper airway is required because mask ventilation and tracheal intubation can be a challenge in some obese patients. A review of the patient's previous anesthetic records will reveal whether airway problems had been encountered during previous surgical procedures. **Tests:** As indicated from H&P
Cardiovascular	Cardiac output rises proportionally with increased weight. ↑ CO and normal PVR → ↑ BP. Mild to moderate hypertension is seen in most morbidly obese patients. The increased left ventricular wall stress caused by increased stroke volume and the resultant ventricular dilation leads to cardiac hypertrophy. Left ventricular dysfunction is often present in young, asymptomatic patients. Even normotensive patients have increased pre-load and after-load, ↑ PAP, and elevated right and left ventricular stroke work. Because these patients are often not physically active, they may appear to be asymptomatic even in the presence of significant cardiovascular disease. Signs of pulmonary HTN (exertional dyspnea, fatigue, syncope) should be sought and TEE obtained in symptomatic patients. RV failure is common in older patients. A medical consultation with a cardiologist may be indicated before bariatric surgery. The ECG may show increased rate, changes in QRS voltage, left QRS axis shift, slowed conduction, and evidence of ischemia or previous myocardial infarction. Polycythemia suggests chronic hypoxemia. **Tests:** ECG and others as indicated from H&P.
Obstructive Sleep Apnea (OSA) Syndrome	Many obese patients maintain a normal $PaCO_2$ during the day, but have CO_2 retention, sleep disturbances, intermittent airway obstruction with hypoxemia, pulmonary hypertension, and cardiac dysrhythmias at night. OSA syndrome is characterized by frequent episodes of apnea (> 10 sec cessation of airflow, despite continuous respiratory effort against a closed airway) and hypopnea (50% reduction in airflow or reduction associated with a decrease of SpO_2 > 4%). OSA is frequently undiagnosed in patients scheduled for bariatric surgery. OSA occurs more often in patients with large fat necks and high Mallampati (III and

General Surgery

Obstructive Sleep Apnea (OSA) Syndrome (cont'd)	IV) scores. The patient may not be aware of symptoms, so it is important to interview the patient's sleeping partner. If OSA is present, the partner will describe loud snoring followed by silence as airflow ceases with obstruction, then gasping or choking as the patient awakes and airflow restarts. A definitive diagnosis of OSA can only be confirmed by polysomnography in a sleep laboratory. Because of fragmented sleep patterns, OSA patients may complain of daytime sleepiness and headaches. Chronic sleep apnea leads to secondary polycythemia, hypoxemia, and hypercapnia, all of which increase the risk of cardiac and cerebral vascular disease. Patients with a history of snoring or OSA are often difficult to ventilate by mask, and their tracheas may be more difficult to intubate than those of similar weight patients without OSA. OSA patients who use CPAP devices at home should be instructed to bring them to the hospital to use following surgery. A patient known or even suspected of having OSA should be continuously monitored by pulse oximetry in the postop period, even following a completely uneventful operation.
Obesity Hypoventilation Syndrome	A small number of patients have obesity hypoventilation syndrome (OHS), characterized by somnolence, cardiac enlargement, polycythemia, hypoxemia, and hypercapnia. OHS patients tend to be older, super obese (BMI > 50 kg/m^2), and have more restricted pulmonary function than other patients with OSA. Hypoventilation that is central and independent of intrinsic lung disease is probably caused by the respiratory center's progressive desensitization to hypercapnia from nocturnal sleep disturbances. In the most severe form of OHS, the "Pickwickian Syndrome," hypersomnolence, hypoxia, hypercapnia, pulmonary hypertension, right ventricular enlargement, and hypervolemia occur. These patients rely on a hypoxic ventilatory drive and may hypoventilate or even become apneic following emergence from general anesthesia after being given 100% O_2 to breathe.
Gastrointestinal	It is widely believed that morbidly obese patients are at greater risk for acid aspiration during induction of general anesthesia. Recently this belief has been challenged. One study reported that fasting obese patients actually had a lower incidence of high-volume, low-pH gastric fluid than lean patients while another found no differences in gastric volume or pH between lean and moderately obese surgical patients. Obese patients without GERD symptoms have relatively normal gastroesophageal sphincter tone. Obese patients at special risk for gastric acid aspiration may be those with diabetes and gastroparesis. Nonalcoholic steatohepatitis (NASH, "fatty hepatitis"), with or without liver dysfunction, is extremely common. Histologic abnormalities are present in the livers of as many as 90% of morbidly obese patients. Preop liver function tests should be obtained, but they often do not reflect the actual severity of liver dysfunction. Alanine aminotransferase (ALT) is the most frequently elevated liver enzyme. Liver clearance of many anesthetic agents is usually not altered with NASH.
Renal	There is ↑ RBF and ↑ GFR associated with obesity. Renal clearance of drugs may be greater than in the normal weight patient. The most common renal abnormality seen is proteinuria. **Tests:** As indicated from H&P
Premedication	Sedative drugs should be avoided. For the very anxious patient small amounts of midazolam (1–2 mg, iv) can be given. If a fiberoptic airway intubation is planned, atropine or glycopyrrolate will decrease oral secretions. Most medications for chronic HTN are continued before surgery. An exception is the ACE inhibitors, which should be stopped preop, because they can cause ↓↓BP following induction of anesthesia. Diabetic medications (insulin, oral hypoglycemics) are usually withheld on the morning of surgery, but blood sugar levels must be closely monitored in the perioperative period. Antibiotics and heparin (VTE prophylaxis) are usually administered before surgery at the surgeon's request. For protection against acid aspiration an H_2-receptor antagonist can be given the night before and again on the morning of surgery along with 30 mL of nonparticulate antacid to increase gastric fluid pH and decrease gastric fluid volume.

INTRAOPERATIVE

Anesthetic Technique: Despite conflicting evidence that morbidly obese patients are at greater risk for acid aspiration, it remains prudent to establish a secure airway as quickly and safely as possible. Patients cannot tolerate the supine position and should be preoxygenated in the reverse Trendelenburg position (RTP) until SPO_2 is 100% for several min. With apneic patients expect rapid desaturation, because FRC is reduced and O_2 reserves are limited. Preoxygenation in RTP can increase O_2 reserves, but may cause pooling of blood and →↓ BP. Drug dosing by monitoring clinical endpoints (HR, BP, degree of sedation) may be more important than empirical dosing based on patient weight formulae. In obese patients, highly lipophilic drugs have a significantly larger volume of distribution compared to that in nonobese patients, as a result loading doses are usually increased. Because lipophilic drug elimination half-lives are longer, maintenance dosing should be decreased to reflect IBW. Non- or weakly lipophilic drugs are given based on IBW.

Tracheal intubation is necessary for controlled ventilation and airway protection. High Mallampati score and large neck circumference are the most reliable predictors of potential intubation difficulties. If a problem is anticipated preop, an "awake intubation" with a fiberoptic bronchoscope is recommended. Appropriate nerve blocks and topical anesthesia to the airway are applied, and sedative drugs are kept to a minimum. It is important that the patient breathes supplemental O_2 during the intubation procedure. Successful direct laryngoscopy requires proper patient position. The patient must be placed with the head, upper body and shoulders significantly elevated ("stacked" or "ramped") so that the ear is level with the sternum (head elevated laryngoscopy position, H.E.LP.) (see Fig. 7.2-6). When a morbidly obese patient is in this position, the endoscopist's view during direct laryngoscopy is significantly improved.

Induction	For most patients a rapid sequence induction with propofol (1.5–2.5 mg/kg TBW) and succinylcholine (1 mg/kg TBW), combined with cricoid pressure (~10 lb), is the best means for securing the airway. Bag and mask ventilation is often difficult 2° upper airway obstruction and ↓ pulmonary compliance. Gastric insufflation during ineffective mask ventilation will further increase the risk of regurgitation and acid aspiration. A 2nd person experienced with airway management, preferably another anesthesiologist, must always be present to assist when difficulty is anticipated. Aids for difficult intubation, including a short laryngoscope handle, a variety of laryngoscope blades, special laryngoscopy equipment (Bullard laryngoscope, Wu laryngoscope) a gum elastic bougie, a light-wand, and equipment for cricothyroidotomy and transtracheal jet ventilation should be available. A Pro-Seal LMA or intubating LMA can serve as a 'bridge' until an endotracheal tube is placed when difficulty is encountered.
Maintenance	Patients should be ventilated with an FiO_2 of 0.5–1.0 and a tidal volume 12–15 mL/kg IBW, preferably in the RTP. Larger tidal volumes will only marginally improve oxygenation, while producing hypocapnia and potentially causing lung trauma. PEEP superimposed upon a large tidal volume can actually worsen hypoxemia by ↓CO cardiac output, which in turn will ↓ O_2 delivery. Placement of subdiaphragmatic packs or retractors or changing to lithotomy or Trendelenburg positions will also impair ventilation. Our maintenance technique consists of an iv infusion of remifentanil, supplemented with small amounts of fentanyl and/or dexmedetomidine infusion. The patient is ventilated with an inhalational anesthetic (isoflurane, sevoflurane or desflurane) with a FiO_2 of 50–100% O_2. All inhalational anesthetics, including isoflurane, are rapidly eliminated. With appropriate timing there are no clinical differences in the recovery time after general anesthesia with any inhalational anesthetic agent. N_2O can be used because it does not dilate the bowel during laparoscopic bariatric surgery, but its role is limited due to the high oxygen demand of many patients. The anesthesiologist is usually responsible for proper placement of the gastric tube to decompress the stomach and to help size the gastric pouch. The anesthesiologist may be asked to help perform leak tests for anastomotic integrity, either by insufflation of the gastric tube or placement of saline or dye down the tube. It is extremely important that the gastric tube and anything else in the esophagus (such as a temperature probe or TEE probe) be completely withdrawn before the gastric pouch is stapled. Heat loss may be exaggerated by the CO_2 pneumoperitoneum and by cold irrigating fluids. Warming blankets and other devices should be employed intraop, and warmed iv and irrigating fluids are occasionally needed if there is a significant drop in temperature.

Maintenance (cont'd)	Loss of pneumoperitoneum may indicate incomplete paralysis. Because nondepolarizing muscle relaxants are hydrophilic, there is limited distribution to adipose tissue and no clinical advantage between any of the commonly used agents. Neuromuscular recovery time is similar in obese and nonobese patients with atracurium, vecuronium or rocuronium. Relaxants should be administered in incremental doses based on IBW, and neuromuscular blockade must be completely reversed before extubation of the trachea.	
Emergence	The inhalation agent is discontinued several min before surgery is completed, but the remifentanil infusion is continued until the very end of the procedure. After the remifentanil is stopped, the patient is awake and the trachea can be extubated within 3 min. If hemodynamically stable, the patient's airway should be extubated with the upper body elevated 30–45°. Then, the patient should be transferred from the OR in that position. Postop admission to an ICU and/or mechanical ventilation is rarely needed. Factors that may necessitate ventilatory support include extremes of age, super obesity, coexisting cardiac disease or pulmonary disease and CO_2 retention, fever or infection, and an uncooperative or extremely anxious patient. The need for postop admission to an ICU is relatively common after open bariatric procedures, but rare after laparoscopic surgery.	
Blood and Fluid Requirements	iv: 16–18 × 1 NS/LR @ 8–12 mL/kg/h Fluid warmer	Intraop fluid requirements are usually greater than would be anticipated in a normal weight patient. Several liters of crystalloid should be given during a laparoscopic bariatric operation. It is essential that adequate amounts of iv fluid be given to reduce postop renal failure, and to avoid other rare but serious complications such as rhabdomyolysis.
Monitoring	± CVP Standard monitors (p. B-1)	Noninvasive cuff pressure may be inaccurate if the anatomy of the upper arm doesn't allow a proper fit. Cuff pressures can be obtained from the wrist or ankle. Because venous access is often limited, a central line can be helpful for postop needs. Note that the length of a standard iv catheter placed percutaneously in the neck of a very large patient may not be long enough to reach an intrathoracic location.
Positioning	RTP ✓ and pad pressure points ✓ eyes SCD's	In the supine position FRC is ↓↓ → V/Q mismatch + ↑ O_2 consumption, ↑ CO, and ↑ PAP. A left lateral tilt will prevent inferior vena cava compression in the supine patient. The Trendelenburg and lithotomy positions further decrease lung volumes. If possible, the patient should always be in the reverse Trendelenburg position (RTP) during surgery because in this position the diaphragm is "unloaded" and FRC is maximized.
CO_2 Pneumoperitoneum	↑ PIP + ↓ TV ↑ $ETCO_2$ + $PaCO_2$ ↑ HR + ↑ MAP	The physiologic effects of the CO_2 pneumoperitoneum are usually well tolerated by the patient and require no intervention. Maintaining the patient in the RTP minimizes the restriction of respiratory mechanics from the CO_2 insufflation. All changes return to normal once the pneumoperitoneum is relieved. However, complications can occur.
Complications	Hypoxemia Massive gas embolism Pneumothorax Pneumomediastinum	The pneumoperitoneum can displace the diaphragm cephalad, causing the position of the endotracheal tube to change. Occasionally the endotracheal tube's tip can enter a bronchus, so always consider tube displacement in the differential diagnosis of hypoxemia during laparoscopy.

POSTOPERATIVE

Position and Oxygenation	Semirecumbent and RTP	Maximize oxygenation by allowing the diaphragm to fall and FRC to increase. Patients can become hypoxemic if supplemental O_2 is withheld in the immediate recovery period. Restoration of normal pulmonary function after open abdominal surgery may take several days.
	CPAP/BiPAP	In theory, CPAP could distend the gastric pouch, but its use following bariatric surgery has not been associated with anastomotic leaks.
Complications	Venous thromboembolism	VTE prophylaxis should always be considered in the postop, even for patients with epidural catheters. A vena cava umbrella is occasionally placed preop in older and high-risk patients. Early ambulation must be encouraged.
	PONV	Multimodal intraop prophylaxis with several antiemetic agents will reduce but not eliminate PONV. Dexamethasone (4–8 mg) should be part of the therapeutic regimen (see p. B-2).
Pain Management	PCA	PCA with opioid dose based on IBW is usually satisfactory. Avoid large amounts of opioids, which can depress ventilation. The use of nonopioid analgesic adjuncts should be instituted early. Dexmedetomidine, which has no respiratory depressant effects, is a useful alternative or supplement to opioids. Nonsteroidal anti-inflammatory drugs are helpful initially, but should be discontinued within a day or two to avoid the potential complication of gastric ulceration.
Tests	As indicated by patient status	

Suggested Readings

1. Altermatt FR, Munoz HR, Delfino AE, et al: Pre-oxygenation in the obese patient: effects of position on tolerance to apnoea. *Br J Anaesth* 2005; 95:706–9.
2. Arain SR, Barth CD, Shankar H, et al: Choice of volatile anesthetic for the morbidly obese patient: sevoflurane or desflurane. *J Clin Anesth* 2005; 17:413–9.
3. Brodsky JB: Positioning the morbidly obese patient for anesthesia. *Obes Surg* 2002; 12:751–8.
4. Brodsky JB, Lemmens HJM, Collins JS, et al: Nitrous oxide and laparoscopic bariatric surgery. *Obes Surg* 2005; 15:494–6.
5. Frappier J, Guenoun T, Journois D, et al: Airway management using the intubating laryngeal mask airway for the morbidly obese patient. *Anesth Analg* 2003; 96:1510–5.
6. Helling TS, Willoughby TL, Maxfield DM, et al: Determinants of the need for intensive care and prolonged mechanical ventilation in patients undergoing bariatric surgery. *Obes Surg* 2004; 14:1036–41.
7. Holte K, Klarskov B, Christensen DS, et al: Liberal versus restrictive fluid administration to improve recovery after laparoscopic cholecystectomy. A randomize, double-blind study. *Ann Surg* 2004; 240:892–9.
8. Huerta S, DeShields S, Shpiner R, et al: Safety and efficacy of postoperative continuous positive airway pressure to prevent pulmonary complications after Roux-en-Y gastric bypass. *J Gastrointest Surg* 2002; 6:354–8.
9. Juvin P, Vadam C, Malek L, et al: Postoperative recovery after desflurane, propofol, or isoflurane anesthesia among morbidly obese patients: a prospective, randomized study. *Anesth Analg* 2000; 91:714–9.
10. Lemmens HJM, Brodsky JB: The dose of succinylcholine in morbid obesity. *Anesth Analg* 2006; 102:438–42.
11. McCarty TM, Arnold DT, Lamont JP, et al: Optimizing outcomes in bariatric surgery. Outpatient laparoscopic gastric bypass. *Ann Surg* 2005; 242:494–501.
12. Nguyen NT and Wolfe BM: The physiologic effects of pneumoperitoneum in the morbidly obese. *Ann Surg* 2005; 241:219–26.
13. Ogunnaike BO, Jones SB, Jones DB, et al: Anesthetic considerations for bariatric surgery. *Anesth Analg* 2002; 95:1793–1805.
14. Perilli V, Sollazzi L, Bozza P, et al: The effects of the reverse Trendelenburg position on respiratory mechanics and blood gases in morbidly obese patients during bariatric surgery. *Anesth Analg* 2000: 91:1520–5.

ANESTHESIA FOR LAPAROSCOPY IN PREGNANCY

ANESTHETIC CONSIDERATIONS

PREOPERATIVE

Approximately 0.75–2% of pregnant woman require nonobstetric surgery, and 10–20% of those will require intraabdominal surgery (diagnostic or therapeutic), most commonly for cholecystectomy, appendectomy, trauma or gynecological indications. If surgery cannot be avoided, it is best carried out in the 2nd trimester. Warn patients about possible fetal loss (3–12% in 1st trimester) and premature labor (5–8% in 2nd and 25–40% in 3rd trimesters). Anesthesia and surgery are associated with increased spontaneous abortion, growth retardation, and perinatal mortality; however, no increase in congenital abnormalities has been found. Rates of fetal loss, premature labor, and maternal mortality are higher among sicker patients. It is unclear whether adverse outcomes after surgery relate to the disease process itself, disturbances in nutrition, the surgical procedure, exposure to radiation, or drugs. No correlation has been found between outcome and any specific anesthetic technique or agent (including N_2O).

Laparoscopy is the procedure of choice for many surgeries in nonpregnant patients; however, its use in pregnancy remains controversial, although significant experience now supports its safety and efficacy. Advantages of laparoscopy include more rapid recovery, shorter hospital stays, less postop narcotic use (→↓ fetal depression) and lower risk of wound infection. No differences in fetal outcome or incidence of preterm labor have been found. Risks of laparoscopy include difficult surgical access and potential uterine injury with Veress needles or trocars. Current recommendations suggest an open technique (e.g., Hasson cannula) for obtaining laparoscope access.

Note that acute appendicitis and cholecystitis often present with advanced or complicated disease because of difficulty diagnosing the "acute abdomen" and a reluctance to use radiation-based diagnostic tests in pregnancy.

Respiratory	Pregnant patients have ↑ MV with respiratory alkalosis ($PaCO_2$ = 32–34 mmHg) and are subject to the rapid onset of hypoxemia if ventilation is compromised due to alterations lung and metabolic functions including a 20% ↓ in FRC and a 20% ↑ in O_2 consumption. Uptake of and sensitivity to inhalational anesthetics is enhanced (↓ FRC, ↓ MAC, and hyperventilation). During laparoscopy, peritoneal insufflation and head-down positioning may further compromise lung function (↓ FRC and ↓ lung compliance). Mucosal capillary engorgement in upper airways may necessitate a smaller ETT and mandates careful airway suctioning to avoid bleeding. Airway management is more difficult in this patient population. **Tests:** As indicated from H&P.
Cardiovascular	Pregnancy →↑ CO, ↓ MAP, ↑ HR, ↑ blood volume, and ↓ oncotic pressure → ↑ risk of pulmonary edema. Supine hypotensive syndrome: To minimize aortocaval compression and → ↓↓ BP (> 20 wk gestation), the supine position should be modified by the use of a left lateral pelvic tilt to displace the uterus. Moderate abdominal insufflation pressures (8–12 mmHg) should be used to minimize further caval compression and ↓ uterine blood flow. **Tests:** As indicated from H&P.
Hematologic	WBC count is elevated during pregnancy (8000–12,000/mm) and may delay diagnosis of concurrent infections (e.g., appendicitis). Iron deficiency anemia often is superimposed on the dilutional anemia of pregnancy (Hct 33%). Pregnant patients are hypercoagulable, and antiembolic compression devices should be used. **Tests:** Hb/Hct. T&S if significant blood loss is anticipated. Coag studies and Plt count if + PIH.
Gastrointestinal	Emergency surgery, ↓ gastric motility, ↑ GERD, ↑ intragastric pressure and gastric hyperacidity →↑ risk of aspiration pneumonitis. All pregnant patients (> 16–20 weeks) should be considered to have full stomachs and should receive a nonparticulate antacid (e.g., 0.3 M Na citrate 30 mL) immediately before GA, as well as iv metoclopramide 10 mg and ranitidine 50 mg 30–60 min before surgery.

Renal	Pregnancy →↑ renal blood flow and creatinine clearance and ↓ serum creatinine and ↓ BUN. Dependent edema results from increased water and sodium retention and ↓ oncotic pressure. **Tests:** As indicated from H&P.
Laboratory	Others tests as indicated from H&P.
Premedication	Full-stomach precautions (see Gastrointestinal, above); midazolam (1–2 mg) given as appropriate to decrease anxiety.

INTRAOPERATIVE

Anesthetic technique: After 16 wk gestation, anticipate ↑ risks of aspiration and difficult intubation. Plan ahead for management of a difficult airway (see pp. 581–582). GA is the preferred technique, because laparoscopy and abdominal surgery are poorly tolerated under regional anesthesia. A lead shield should be used to protect the fetus during fluoroscopy. Obtain preop obstetric consultation with baseline fetal heart rate (FHR) and uterine contraction readings. After ~24 wk gestation, consider continuous monitoring of FHR during surgery (transvaginal Doppler) and develop a management plan for evaluation and action if a nonreassuring trace develops.

General anesthesia: If difficult intubation is anticipated, an awake fiber-optic intubation (p. B-4) is recommended. In any event, emergency airway management equipment (e.g., LMA, transtracheal jet ventilator), must be immediately accessible in the OR. Communication with the surgeon and obstetrician regarding maternal and fetal condition is essential.

Induction	Tilt table or elevate left hip to displace uterus. Standard rapid-sequence induction with cricoid pressure (p. B-5) as appropriate. To optimize intubation, place patient in maximal "sniff" position with elevation of shoulders if necessary (obese patients) (Fig. 7.2-6, p. 501). If tracheal intubation is unsuccessful, follow the difficult intubation/ventilation drill (p. B-5). After ETT is secured, pass OG tube and decompress stomach to minimize injury from the Veress needle or trocar.	
Maintenance	0.8–1% isoflurane or 1.5–2.0% sevoflurane in air/O_2 (50%) mixture. Avoid N_2O → distention of bowel, PONV. Administer an opioid (e.g. fentanyl 50–200 μg iv) and/or midazolam (1–2 mg) to ↓ volatile requirements and ↓ maternal awareness. Administer muscle relaxants (e.g., vecuronium 0.1 mg/kg). Control ventilation, avoiding hypocapnia (PCO_2 < 30 mmHg) → ↓ umbilical blood flow, and hypercapnia (PCO_2 > 36 mmHg) → fetal acidosis. Maintain $ETCO_2$ or $PaCO_2$ at 32–36 mmHg by ↑ MV. Use low insufflation cut-off pressure (8–12 mmHg, not 15 mmHg as for nonpregnant patient).	
Emergence	Reverse muscle relaxation with neostigmine 0.05 mg/kg and glycopyrrolate 0.01 mg/kg or atropine 0.02 mg/kg. Anticholinergics (glycopyrrolate/atropine) given before neostigmine may minimize possible ↑ uterine tone 2° neostigmine. Delay extubation until patient is fully awake and muscle strength has returned to normal. O_2 by mask and transport in the lateral position. Metoclopramide (10 mg iv) and/or ondansetron (4 mg iv) may be needed for PONV.	
Blood and fluid requirements	iv: 16–18 ga × 1 NS/LR 4–6 ml/kg/h	Laparoscopy is associated with minimal blood loss; however, inadvertent vascular injury may occur.
Monitoring	Standard monitors (see B-1) ± Arterial line (major surgery)	Maternal and neonatal outcome good, and severe acidosis absent when maternal ventilation controlled by $PaCO_2$ or $ETCO_2$ measurement.
	FHR monitor	Continuous FHR monitoring may be appropriate after 24 wk gestation.
	Uterine contraction monitor	Uterine contraction monitoring is usually not possible intraop; however, ✓ preop and postop. Maternal and neonatal outcome good, and severe acidosis absent when maternal ventilation controlled by $PaCO_2$ or $ETCO_2$ measurement. Clinical experience indicates no long-term adverse neonatal effects.

Positioning	✓ and pad pressure points ✓ eyes	Changes in position have marked effects on respiration (↓ compliance/↑ pressure, hypoxemia) and hemodynamics. Head-up position + GA + peritoneal insufflation → 50% ↓ CO in the nonpregnant patient and even greater decrease in late pregnancy. **Position changes should be gradual** to minimize adverse effects.
	± left uterine displacement	If > 20 wk gestation, left uterine displacement to avoid aortocaval compression.
CO_2 peritoneum: Maternal effects	↓ ventilation	Impairs ventilation → hypoxemia and respiratory acidosis.
	↓ BP	↓ venous return → ↓ BP.
	Reflux	↑ GI reflux (↑ abdominal pressure)
	CO_2 absorption	Absorption of CO_2 →↑ MAP & ↑ SVR.
CO_2 peritoneum Fetal effects	↓ uterine blood flow	Up to 60% in animal studies → fetal hypoxia.
	↑ preterm labor	2° ↑ abdominal pressure
	Fetal acidosis	2° absorbed CO_2
	Fetal ↑ HR/↑ BP	
Complications	Uterine injury	
	Bowel/organ injury	
	Venous air embolism	Dx: ↓ $ETCO_2$ hypoxemia, hypotension. Rx: 100% O_2, stop insufflation immediately, volume and pressors, attempt CVP air aspiration.
	Thromboembolism/PE	Prevention: Pneumatic compression devices. Rx: Supportive
	Pneumothorax	Dx: ↑ Airway pressure, ↓ breath sounds, and hyperresonance. Rx: 100% O_2, stop insufflation, tube thoracostomy.

POSTOPERATIVE

Pain management	Standard pain management (p. C-2)	Minimize NSAIDS (e.g., ibuprofen) → pulmonary and CV fetal effects (closure of ductus venosus).
Tests	HCT/CBC Others as indicated by operative course.	

Suggested Readings

1. ACOG Committee Opinion Number 284, August 2003: Nonobsteric surgery in pregnancy. *Obstet Gynecol* 2003; 102:431.
2. Cohen-Kerem R, Railton C, Oren D, et al: Pregnancy outcome following non-obstetric surgical intervention. *Am J Surg* 2005; 190:467–73.
3. Curet MJ: Special problems in laparoscopic surgery. *Surg Clin North Am* 2000; 80(4):1093–110.
4. Czeizel AE, Pataki T, Rockenbauer M: Reproductive outcome after exposure to surgery under anesthesia during pregnancy. *Arch Gynecol Obstet* 1998; 261(4):193–9.
5. Fatum M, Rojansky N: Laparoscopic Surgery during Pregnancy. *Obstet Gynecol Survey* 2001; 56(1):50–9.
6. Levinson G: Anesthesia for surgery during pregnancy. In *Shnider and Levinson's Anesthesia for Obstetrics,* 4rh ed. Hughes SC, Levinson G, Rosen MA, eds. Lippincott Williams & Wilkins, Philadelphia: 2002, 249–65.
7. Naughton NN, Cohen SE: Nonobstetric surgery during pregnancy. In *Obstetric Anesthesia: Principles and Practice,* 2nd edition. Chestnut DH, ed. CV Mosby, St. Louis: 2004: 255–72.
8. SAGES Guidelines for laparoscopic surgery during pregnancy. *Surg Endosc* 1998; 12:189–90.
9. Steinbrook RA, Bhavani-Shankar K: Hemodynamics during laparoscopic surgery in pregnancy. *Anesth Analg* 2001; 93: 1570–1.
10. Steinbrook RA, Brooks DC, Datta S: Laparoscopic cholecystectomy during pregnancy. Review of anesthetic management, surgical considerations. *Surg Endosc* 1996; 10:511–5.

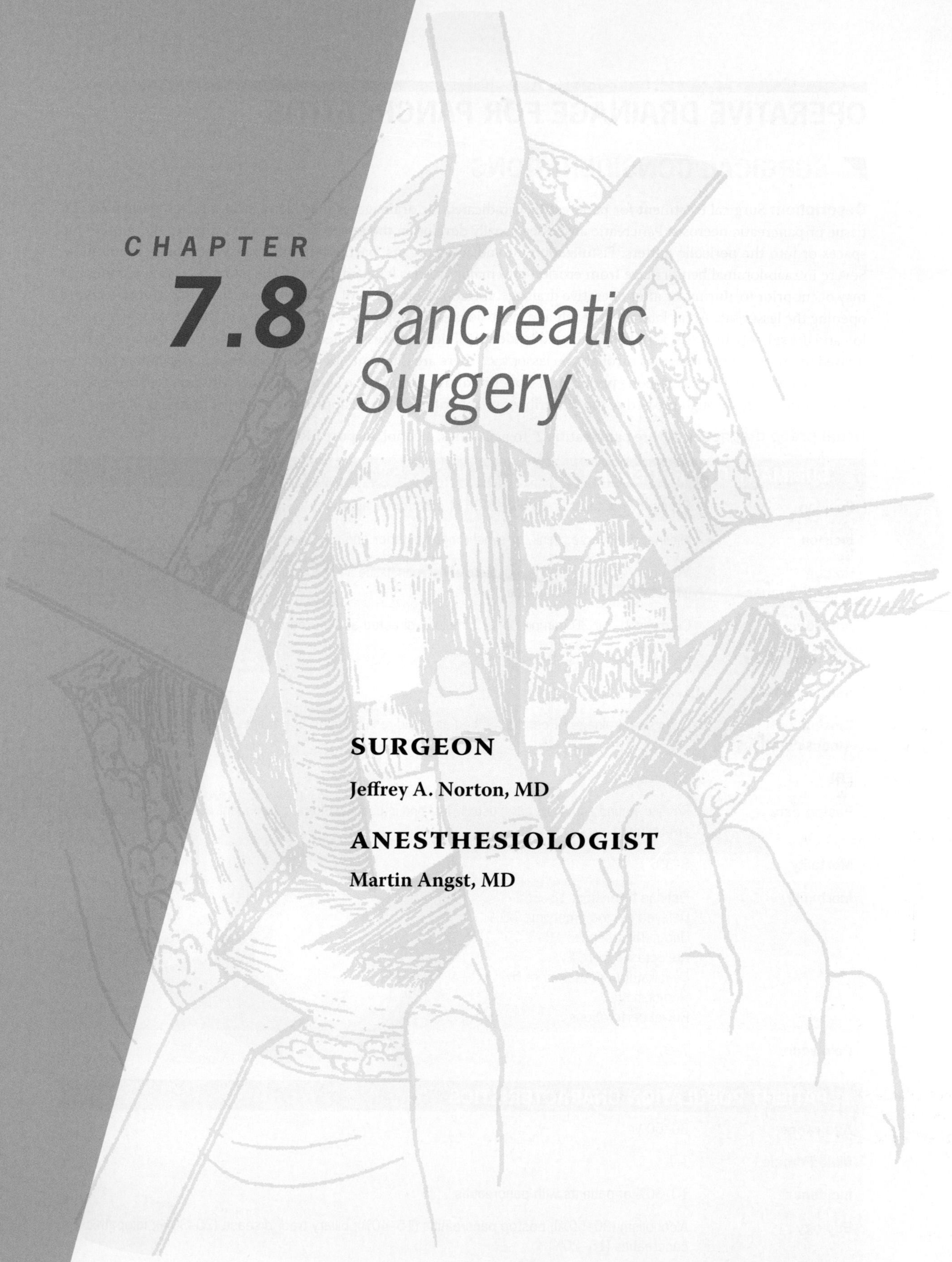

CHAPTER

7.8 Pancreatic Surgery

SURGEON

Jeffrey A. Norton, MD

ANESTHESIOLOGIST

Martin Angst, MD

OPERATIVE DRAINAGE FOR PANCREATITIS

SURGICAL CONSIDERATIONS

Description: Surgical treatment for pancreatitis is indicated for drainage or debridement of infected peripancreatic tissue or pancreatic necrosis. Pancreatic abscesses usually develop in the lesser sac, but may spread to the subphrenic spaces or into the pericolic gutters. Fistulization into adjacent organs, particularly the transverse colon, is common. Severe intraabdominal hemorrhage from erosion into major arteries lying adjacent to the pancreas is uncommon, but may occur prior to, during, or after operative drainage. Intraop, exploration of the peritoneal cavity is performed before opening the lesser sac. Areas lateral to the left and right sides of the colon, as well as the base of the transverse mesocolon and the subhepatic areas, should be palpated to identify fluid or abscess collections. The gastrocolic ligament is then incised to approach the pancreas through the lesser sac. There are different operative approaches, depending on location of involved tissue and surgeon's preference. Upper midline or transverse abdominal incisions are used most often. Posterior drainage through the bed of the 12th rib, or retroperitoneal lateral approaches, may be used (Fig. 7.8-1).

Usual preop diagnosis: Severe pancreatitis 2° to gallstones, alcohol, or post ERCP

SUMMARY OF PROCEDURE

Position	Supine or rotated slightly (Fig. 7.8-1) for posterior approach
Incision	Midline, transverse, flank, or synchronous anterior and posterior
Unique considerations	Must perform adequate debridement of necrotic tissue and provide adequate drainage of abdomen; NG tube; jejunal feeding tube
Antibiotics	Cefoxitin 1–2 g 30 min preop, or antibiotic directed at cultured organisms
VTE prophylaxis	Heparin 5000 units sq
Surgical time	1–2 h
Closing considerations	Adequate drainage of pancreatic bed and fluid resuscitation of patient
EBL	300–750 mL
Postop care	Routine wound and drain care; usually ICU and intubated; often, subsequent operative procedures are required.
Mortality	8–30%
Morbidity	Fistulae formation: 18–55% Delayed gastric emptying: 50% Unremitting sepsis: 10–30% Atelectasis: 5–10% Respiratory deterioration: 5% Hemorrhage Bowel perforations
Pain score	7–9

PATIENT POPULATION CHARACTERISTICS

Age range	30–60 yr
Male:Female	1:1
Incidence	10–30% of patients with pancreatitis
Etiology	Alcoholism (30–50%); postop pancreatitis (15–40%); biliary tract disease (20–30%); idiopathic pancreatitis (15–20%)
Associated conditions	Malnutrition; glucose intolerance; multiorgan dysfunction

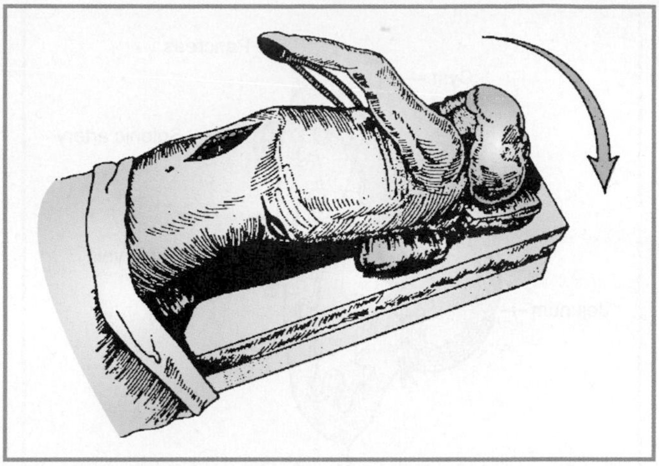

Figure 7.8-1. Incision for anterior and posterior drainage in pancreatitis. Note that bed or table is rotated until patient is almost supine. (Reproduced with permission from Berne TV, Donovan AJ: Synchronous anterior and posterior drainage of pancreatic abscess. *Arch Surg* 1981; 116:527–33. Copyright 1981, American Medical Association.)

ANESTHETIC CONSIDERATIONS

See Anesthetic Considerations for Pancreatic Surgery, p. 619.

Suggested Readings

1. Berne TV: Pancreatic abscesses. *Probl Gen Surg* 1984; 1:569–82.
2. Bradley EL: Fifteen-year experience with open drainage for infected pancreatic necrosis. *Surg Gynecol Obstet* 1993; 177(3): 215–22.
3. Feranandez-del Castillo C, Rattner DW, Makary MA, et al: Debridement and closed packing for the treatment of necrotizing pancreatitis. *Ann Surg* 1998; 228:676–84.
4. Gotzinger P, Sautner T, Kriwanek S, et al: Surgical treatment for severe acute pancreatitis: Extent and surgical control of necrosis determine outcome. *World J Surg* 2002; 474–8.
5. Shinzeki M, Ueda T, Takeyama Y, et al: Prediction of early death in severe acute pancreatitis. *J Gastroenteral* 2008; 43:152–8.
6. Villazon A, Villazon O, Terrazas F, et al: Retroperitoneal drainage in the management of the septic phase of severe acute pancreatitis. *World J Surg* 1991; 15:103–8.

DRAINAGE OF PANCREATIC PSEUDOCYST

SURGICAL CONSIDERATIONS

Description: Internal drainage of a pancreatic pseudocyst may be accomplished by anastomosing the cyst to the stomach, duodenum, or other small bowel via a Roux-en-Y loop of jejunum. The procedure of choice for internal decompression depends on the location of the pseudocyst in relation to the portion of the GI tract that will provide maximal dependent drainage of the cyst. Operation is reserved for patients with refractory symptoms. At operation, the abdomen is entered via a midline incision. The pseudocyst is localized by palpation with or without intraoperative ultrasound. If the pseudocyst lies behind the stomach (or duodenum), it is approached anteriorly, through the posterior wall of the stomach (or duodenum). A portion of the posterior wall is excised, allowing entry into the cyst cavity, which is then drained. An anastomosis is created between the cyst and stomach (or duodenum). The anterior wall of the stomach (or duodenum) is then closed. If the cyst presents inferior to the stomach, it is anastomosed in a

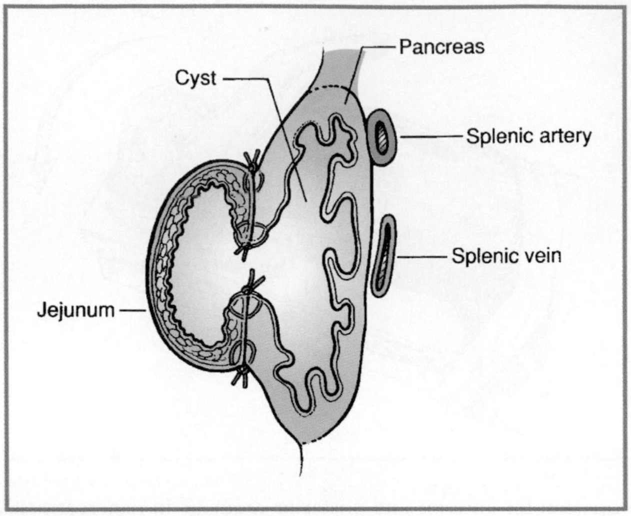

Figure 7.8-2. Roux-en-Y drainage of a pseudocyst. (Reproduced with permission from Scott-Conner CEH, Dawson DL: *Operative Anatomy,* 2nd edition. Lippincott Williams & Wilkins, Philadelphia: 2003.)

similar fashion to a Roux-en-Y loop of jejunum (Fig. 7.8-2). Drains are placed; external drainage is sometimes necessary, especially in the setting of infection. Spontaneous resolution of pancreatic pseudocyst may be expected in most patients. If infection of the pseudocyst occurs with clinical signs of sepsis, percutaneous drainage under CT guidance can be performed, although subsequent operative drainage is often necessary.

Usual preop diagnosis: Pancreatic pseudocyst 2° to acute pancreatitis refractory to medical management

SUMMARY OF PROCEDURE	
Position	Supine
Incision	Midline abdominal or transverse
Unique considerations	Location of pseudocyst in relation to GI tract; NG tube
Antibiotics	Cefoxitin 1 g iv 30 min preop
VTE prophylaxis	Heparin 5000 units sq
Surgical time	1–2 h
Closing considerations	Adequate drainage
EBL	100–300 mL
Postop care	NG decompression
Mortality	5–10%
Morbidity	Bleeding: 5–7% Sepsis: < 5% Recurrence: 2–3%
Pain score	6–8

PATIENT POPULATION CHARACTERISTICS	
Age range	15–80 yr
Male:Female	1:1

PATIENT POPULATION CHARACTERISTICS (cont'd)	
Incidence	Rare
Etiology	Acute pancreatitis; trauma
Associated conditions	Acute pancreatitis: 90%; gallstones; alcohol use; chronic pain

ANESTHETIC CONSIDERATIONS

See Anesthetic Considerations for Pancreatic Surgery, p. 619.

Suggested Readings

1. Barthlet M, Lamblin G, Gasmi M, et al: Clinical usefulness of a treatment algorithm for pancreatic pseudocysts. *Gastrointest ENdosc* 2008; 67:245–52.
2. Neff R: Pancreatic pseudocysts and fluid collections. *Surg Clin North Am* 2001; 81(2):399–403.
3. Vitas GJ, San MG: Selected management of pancreatic pseudocysts: operative versus expectant management. *Surgery* 1992; 11(2):123–30.
4. Warshaw AL, Rattner DW: Timing of surgical drainage for pancreatic pseudocyst: clinical and chemical criteria. *Ann Surg* 1985; 202(6):720–4.
5. Yeo CJ, Bastidas JA, Lynch-Nyhan A, et al: The natural history of pancreatic pseudocysts documented by CT. *Surg Gyn Obstet* 1990; 170:411.

LONGITUDINAL PANCREATICOJEJUNOSTOMY

SURGICAL CONSIDERATIONS

Description: **Pancreaticojejunostomy,** as described by **Puestow,** consists of a longitudinal opening of the pancreatic duct, which is then anastomosed to a Roux-en-Y loop of jejunum (Fig. 7.8-3). This approach is necessary to ensure adequate drainage of a duct with multiple strictures and dilatations. Through a midline or transverse abdominal incision, the pancreas is exposed by mobilizing the duodenum (**Kocher maneuver**), exposing the head of the pancreas, and opening the lesser sac to visualize the body and tail. The pancreatic duct may be aspirated to identify its location and intraoperative ultrasound is commonly used, then it is incised longitudinally. A Roux-en-Y loop of jejunum is then brought up to the pancreas and anastomosed to the opened duct. A drain is left along the anastomosis; and the wound is closed in the usual fashion.

Variant procedure or approaches: A **Whipple resection (pancreaticoduodenectomy;** see p. 618) is an alternative surgical treatment for chronic pancreatitis confined to the head of the gland. Rarely, subtotal pancreatectomy is indicated.

Usual preop diagnosis: Abdominal pain with chronic pancreatitis and dilated pancreatic duct (chain of lakes)

SUMMARY OF PROCEDURE	
Position	Supine
Incision	Midline abdominal or transverse
Antibiotics	Cefoxitin 1 g iv
VTE prophylaxis	Heparin 5000 units sq
Surgical time	2–3 h
Closing considerations	Adequate drainage
EBL	300–400 mL
Postop care	Monitor for glucose intolerance

SUMMARY OF PROCEDURE (cont'd)	
Mortality	1–4%
Morbidity	Failure to relieve pain: 25–50% Pancreatic leak: 5–10% Wound infection: 5%
Pain score	6–8

PATIENT POPULATION CHARACTERISTICS	
Age range	17–72 yr
Male:Female	2.5:1
Etiology	Alcoholism; biliary tract disease; idiopathic; trauma; familial pancreatitis
Associated conditions	Biliary tract disease (25–50%); hyperparathyroidism (< 5%); chronic pain; narcotic dependency

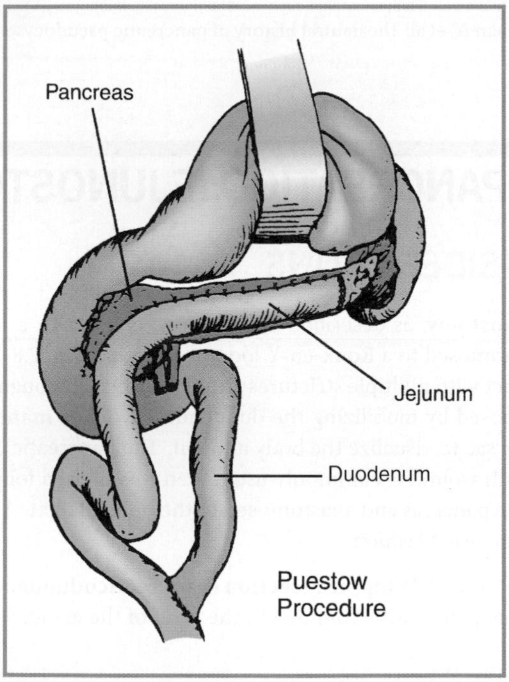

Figure 7.8-3. Operative management of chronic pancreatitis with onlay Roux-en-Y pancreaticojejunostomy (Puestow). (Reproduced with permission from Hardy JD: *Hardy's Textbook of Surgery.* JB Lippincott, Philadelphia: 1988.)

ANESTHETIC CONSIDERATIONS

See Anesthetic Considerations for Pancreatic Surgery, p. 619.

Suggested Readings

1. Harrison JL, Prinz RA: Surgical management of chronic pancreatitis: pancreatic duct drainage. *Adv Surg* 1999; 32:1.
2. Howard VM, Zhaug Z: Pancreaticodenectomy (Whipple resection) in the treatment of chronic pancreatitis. *World J Surg* 1990; 14:77–82.
3. Nealon WH, Aatin S: Analysis of success in preventing recurrent acute exacerbations in chronic pancreatitis. *Ann Surg* 2001; 233:793–800.
4. Puestow CB, Gillesby WJ: Retrograde surgical drainage of the pancreas for chronic relapsing pancreatitis. *Arch Surg* 1958; 76:898–907.

PANCREATECTOMY

SURGICAL CONSIDERATIONS

Description: **Distal pancreatectomy** is performed for tumors in the distal half of the pancreas (Fig. 7.8-4). The lesser sac is opened by dividing the gastro-colic ligament. After entering the lesser sac, the gastrosplenic ligament is divided, ligating the short gastric vessels and the left gastroepiploic vessel. The peritoneum is incised along the inferior surface of the pancreas, with care being taken to avoid injury to the middle colic vessels. Following mobilization of the spleen, the splenic artery is ligated near its origin. The inferior mesenteric vein is ligated sometimes at the inferior border of the pancreas, and the splenic vein is ligated at the proposed point of transection. The transected pancreas (Fig. 7.8-5) is usually stapled and drained, although some surgeons suture the cut end and ligate the duct. The spleen may be preserved when operating for benign disease.

Variant procedure or approaches: **Subtotal pancreatectomy** usually implies resecting the pancreas from the mesenteric vessels distally, leaving the head and uncinate process intact. This procedure may be performed for tumor or chronic pancreatitis. **Child's procedure** (near-total pancreatectomy) consists of removing the entire pancreas except a rim of tissue along the lesser curvature of the duodenum (Fig. 7.8-6); preserving the duodenum makes it unnecessary to reconstruct the bile duct. This procedure is usually reserved for patients with chronic pancreatitis.

Usual preop diagnosis: Carcinoma of pancreas; islet cell tumors; cystic neoplasms; chronic pancreatitis

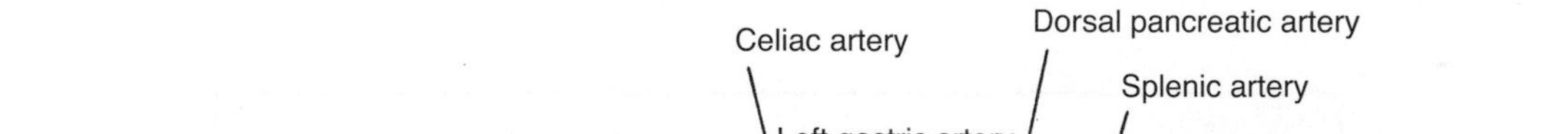

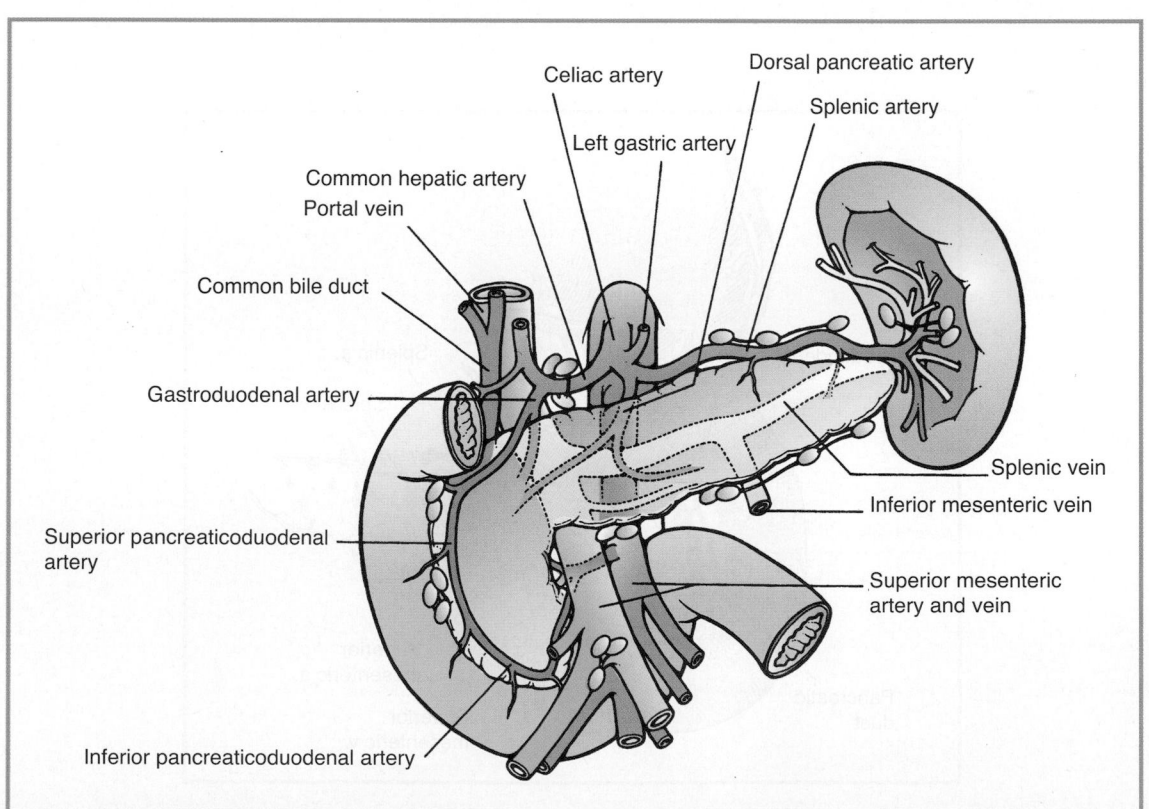

Figure 7.8-4. Pancreatic anatomy. (Reproduced with permission from Scott-Conner CEH, Dawson DL: *Operative Anatomy,* 2nd edition. Lippincott Williams & Wilkins, Philadelphia: 2003.)

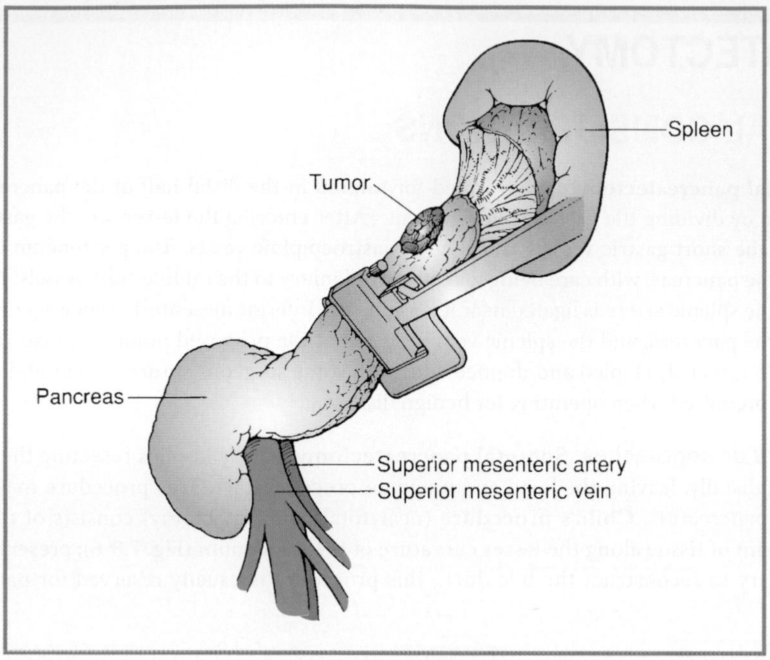

Figure 7.8-5. Resection of distal pancreas. (Reproduced with permission from Scott-Conner CEH, Dawson DL: *Operative Anatomy,* 2nd edition. Lippincott Williams & Wilkins, Philadelphia: 2003.)

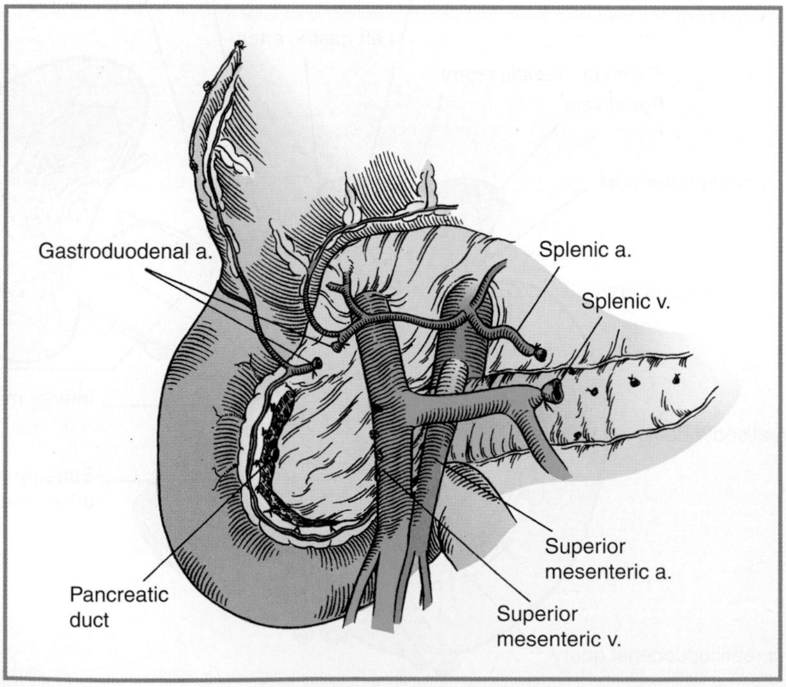

Figure 7.8-6. Near-total pancreatectomy. Shown is the operative field at the conclusion of the procedure. (Reproduced with permission from Baker RJ, Fischer JE: *Mastery of Surgery,* 4th edition. Lippincott Williams & Wilkins, Philadelphia: 1997.)

SUMMARY OF PROCEDURES

	Distal Pancreatectomy	Subtotal Pancreatectomy	Child's Procedure
Position	Supine	⇐	⇐
Incision	Midline abdominal or transverse	⇐	⇐
Unique considerations	NG tube	⇐	Preservation of vasculature of duodenum
Antibiotics	Cefoxitin 1–2 g iv	⇐	⇐
VTE prophylaxis	Heparin 5000 units sq	⇐	⇐
Surgical time	2–3 h	⇐	3–4 h
Closing considerations	Adequate drainage	⇐	⇐
EBL	300–500 mL	500–750 mL	500–1000 mL
Postop care	NG decompression; PACU	⇐	⇐
Mortality	< 5%	⇐	⇐
Morbidity	Diabetes: 5% Wound infection: 5% Pancreatic fistula: < 5% Common bile duct injury Hemorrhage Duodenal necrosis Pancreatic leakage Pancreatic insufficiency	⇐ ⇐ ⇐ ⇐ ⇐ ⇐ ⇐ ⇐	⇐ ⇐ 90% ⇐ ⇐ ⇐ ⇐ ⇐
Pain score	6–8	6–8	6–8

PATIENT POPULATION CHARACTERISTICS

Age range	30–60 yr
Male:Female	1:1
Incidence	~26,000/yr in the United States.
Etiology	Adenocarcinoma; chronic pancreatitis; islet cell tumors
Associated conditions	Alcoholism and biliary tract disease with chronic pancreatitis (90%); other endocrine disorders (3–5%)

ANESTHETIC CONSIDERATIONS

See Anesthetic Considerations for Pancreatic Surgery, p. 619.

Suggested Readings

1. Samuel I, Joehl RJ: Chronic pancreatitis. In *Surgery: Scientific Principles and Practice,* 4th edition. Mulholland MW, et al., eds. Lippincott Williams & Wilkins, Philadelphia: 2006, 849–60.
2. Sohn TA, Campbell KA, Pitt MA, et al: Quality of life and long-term survival after surgery for chronic pancreatitis. *J Gastrointest Surg* 2000; 4:355–64.

WHIPPLE RESECTION

SURGICAL CONSIDERATIONS

Description: A **Whipple resection** consists of a **pancreaticoduodenectomy,** followed by a **pancreaticojejunostomy**, a **hepaticojejunostomy** and a **gastrojejunostomy** (Fig. 7.8-7). On entering the peritoneal cavity, the resectability of the pancreatic tumor is determined. Contraindications to standard resection include: liver or peritoneal metastases; involvement of the superior mesenteric vessels; infiltration by tumor into root of the mesentery; and extension into the porta hepatis, with involvement of the hepatic artery. If the tumor is deemed resectable, further mobilization of the head of the pancreas is performed. The common duct is transected above the cystic duct entry and the gall bladder is removed. After the superior mesenteric vein is freed from the pancreas, the latter is transected, with care being taken not to injure the splenic vein. The duodenum is transected 2 cm distal to the pylorus, or the stomach proximal

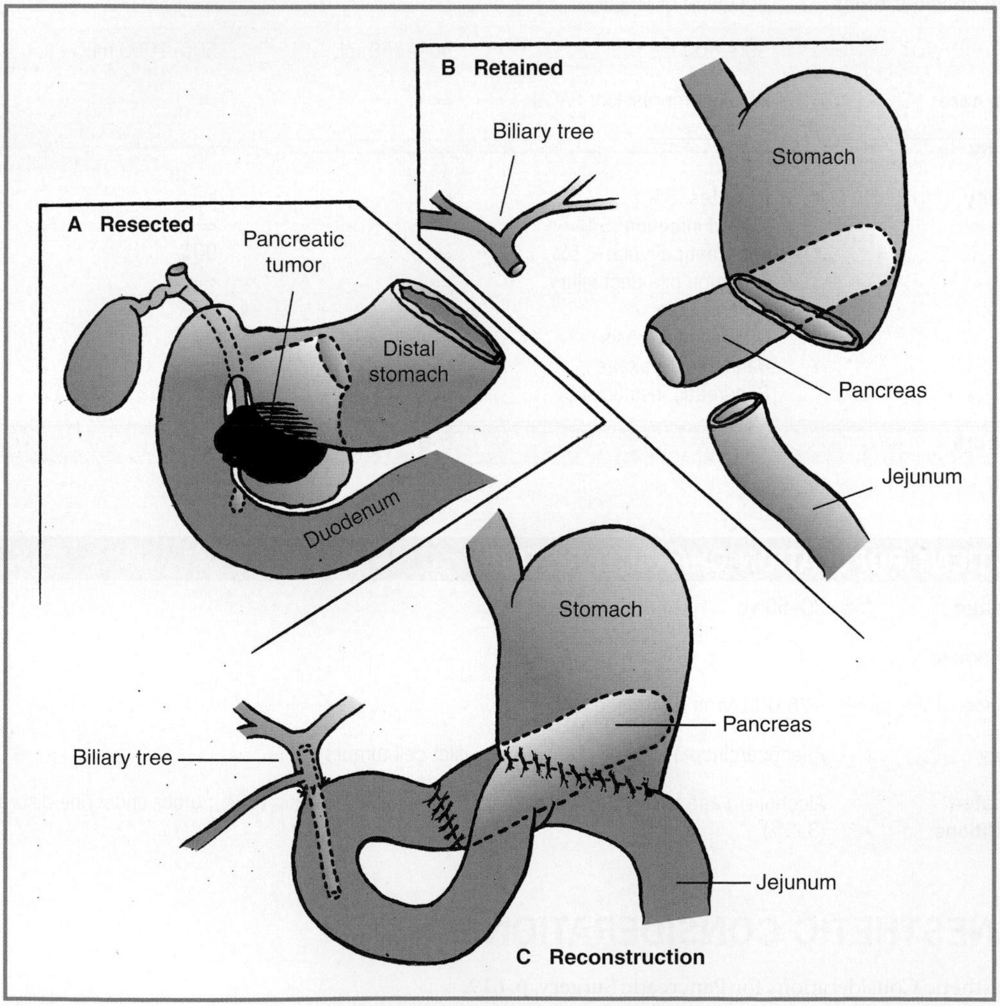

Figure 7.8-7. Standard pancreaticoduodenectomy. **(A)** Structures resected, including distal stomach, entire duodenum, head and neck of pancreas with tumor, gallbladder, and distal extrahepatic biliary tree. **(B)** Structures retained, including proximal stomach, body and tail of pancreas, proximal biliary tree, and jejunum distal to ligament of Treitz. **(C)** Reconstruction: proximal pancreaticojejunostomy, hepaticojejunostomy over T tube, and distal gastrojejunostomy. (Reproduced with permission from Hardy JD: *Hardy's Textbook of Surgery,* 2nd edition. JB Lippincott, Philadelphia: 1988.)

to the pylorus if involved by tumor. The jejunum is transected beyond the ligament of Treitz and the specimen is removed by severing the vascular connections with the mesenteric vessels. Reconstitution is achieved by anastomosing the pancreatic stump, bile duct, and duodenum into the jejunum. Drains are placed adjacent to the pancreatic anastomosis.

Variant procedure or approaches: There are several variants that consist of extensions of the Whipple procedure: **total pancreatectomy; regional pancreatectomy,** involving resection and reconstruction of the retropancreatic superior mesenteric vein and/or artery; and the pylorus-preserving **pancreaticoduodenectomy** as described above. In addition, the distal pancreatic stump may be anastomosed to the posterior wall of the stomach.

Usual preop diagnosis: Carcinoma of the pancreas; malignant cystadenomas; chronic pancreatitis

SUMMARY OF PROCEDURES

	Whipple	Total Pancreatectomy	Regional Pancreatectomy
Position	Supine	⇐	⇐
Incision	Midline abdominal or transverse (chevron)	⇐	⇐
Unique considerations	Large-bore iv lines	⇐	⇐
Antibiotics	Cefoxitin 1–2 g iv	⇐	⇐
VTE prophylaxis	Heparin 5000 units sq		
Surgical time	4–5 h	4–6 h	5–6 h
Closing considerations	Adequate drainage	⇐	⇐
EBL	500–750 mL	750–1000 mL	750–1500 mL
Postop care	NG decompression; PACU/ICU	NG decompression; diabetes management	
Mortality	5–10%	12%	15%
Morbidity	Delayed gastric emptying: 25% Pancreatic fistula: 10–20% Sepsis: 5–15% Hemorrhage: 5% MI: 1–3% Biliary fistula: < 2%	⇐ NA 5% < 5% ⇐ < 1 %	⇐ 10–20% 25% 5% < 5% < 2%
Pain score	7–9	7–9	7–9

PATIENT POPULATION CHARACTERISTICS (FOR CANCER OF PANCREAS)

Age range	40–80 yr
Male:Female	1:1
Incidence	10th most common cancer in the United States. (~33,000/yr)
Etiology	Familial and genetic factors (p16, K-vas); tobacco; diabetes; alcohol; diet; pancreatitis
Associated conditions	See Etiology, above.

ANESTHETIC CONSIDERATIONS FOR PANCREATIC SURGERY

(Procedures covered: drainage for pancreatitis; drainage of pancreatic pseudocyst; pancreaticojejunostomy; pancreatectomy; Whipple resection)

General Surgery

PREOPERATIVE

Patients presenting for pancreatic surgery can be divided into four groups: (a) those with acute pancreatitis, who failed medical treatment and may be extremely ill, presenting for operative excision or drainage of necrotic or infected foci; (b) patients with adenocarcinoma of the pancreas; (c) patients with neuroendocrine active (60–70%) or inactive islet cell tumors (mainly insulinoma and gastrinoma; rarely VIP-oma and glucagonoma); and (d) patients suffering from the sequelae of chronic pancreatitis (e.g., pseudocyst or abscess).

Respiratory	Respiratory compromise—such as pleural effusions, atelectasis, and ARDS, progressing to respiratory failure, may occur in up to 50% of patients with acute pancreatitis. Postop mechanical ventilation may be needed for these patients **Tests:** Consider CXR; ABG; others as indicated from H&P.
Cardiovascular	Patients with acute pancreatitis may suffer from severe intravascular volume depletion 2° plasma exudation and in severe cases 2° hemorrhage (erosion of blood vessels). Aggressive volume resuscitation with crystalloids, colloids, and blood products may be required during surgery. Hypocalcemia is often present (arrhythmias and ↓ myocardial contractility). Serum K^+ may be elevated (2° acidosis or renal failure associated with acute pancreatitis) or decreased (2° watery diarrhea associated with gastrinoma, VIP-oma, prolonged NG suction), and should be corrected before surgery. Hypokalemia resistant to K^+ replacement may point to ↓ Mg^{++} and warrants replacement. **Tests:** ECG; electrolytes; others as indicated from H&P.
Gastrointestinal	Jaundice and abdominal pain are common presenting Sx in this group of patients. The presence of ileus (common in acute pancreatitis) or intestinal obstruction should mandate full-stomach precautions and rapid-sequence induction. Electrolyte abnormalities are common and may be 2° metabolic acidosis (↑ K^+ 2° acute pancreatitis) or alkalosis and intestinal losses (↓ K^+ and ↓ Mg^{++} 2° diarrhea, NG suction). Acute pancreatitis is associated with ↓ Ca^{++} (omental fat saponification) and ↑ Na^+ (dehydration). Gastrinoma (Zollinger-Ellison syndrome) is associated with diarrhea, severe peptic ulcer, and GERD. VIP-oma often causes massive watery diarrhea (up to 20 L). Electrolyte abnormalities should be treated preop. **Tests:** Electrolytes; glucose; LFTs; others as indicated from H&P.
Renal	Patients should be evaluated for renal insufficiency predominantly 2° dehydration, with anesthetic plan adjusted accordingly. **Tests:** BUN; creatinine; others as indicated from H&P.
Endocrine	Many patients with acute pancreatitis have diabetes 2° loss of islet cells. Endocrine tumors of the pancreas are linked (10–30%) with multiple endocrine syndrome type I (MEN I), featuring adenoma of the pituitary, parathyroid, and/or pancreas. Endocrine tumors also can secrete parathyroid hormone-related peptide, growth hormone-RH, and corticotrophin-RH and adrenocorticotropin, and may be associated with ↑ Ca^{++}, acromegaly, and Cushing's syndrome. Insulinoma is the most common endocrine tumor of the pancreas and can result in severe hypoglycemia, necessitating frequent periop blood glucose measurements (up to every 15 min has been suggested). Surgical manipulation of the insulinoma may result in massive release of insulin. VIP-oma is associated with mild diabetes and ↑ Ca^{++}. **Tests:** Electrolytes; glucose; others as indicated from H&P.
Hematologic	Hct may be falsely elevated, 2° hemoconcentration, or low, 2° hemorrhage. Coagulopathy may be present (DIC). **Tests:** CBC with differential; Plt; consider PT, PTT, fibrinogen.
Laboratory	Other tests as indicated from H&P.
Premedication	Consider midazolam 1–2 mg. Note: full-stomach precautions in patients with intestinal obstruction (see p. B-4): ranitidine (50 mg iv 30–60 min preop) and 0.3 M Na citrate (30 mL po 10 min preop).

INTRAOPERATIVE

Anesthetic technique: GETA ± epidural for postop analgesia. If postop epidural analgesia is planned, establishing correct catheter placement in the epidural space can be accomplished by injecting 1–2% lidocaine (50–100 mg) via the catheter to elicit a segmental block. The use of epidural anesthetic techniques for postoperative pain management in patients undergoing major, non-vascular abdominal surgery has been shown to provide superior pain control compared with IV-PCA. However, adequate pain control can be achieved with the use of IV-PCA.

Induction	The patient with bowel obstruction or ileus is at risk for pulmonary aspiration, and rapid-sequence induction with cricoid pressure is indicated (see p. B-4). If the patient is clinically hypovolemic, restore intravascular volume (colloid, crystalloid, or blood products) prior to induction and titrate induction dose of sedative/hypnotic agents. Etomidate (0.2–0.4 mg/kg iv) or ketamine (1–3 mg/kg iv) may provide better hemodynamic stability during induction of anesthesia. Both thiopental and propofol are associated with a significant reduction of SVR.
Maintenance	Standard maintenance (see p. B-2). **Combined epidural/GA:** The epidural catheter ideally is placed at the level of a dermatome corresponding to the surgical site (generally mid-to-low thoracic spine). This allows the use of both lipophilic and hydrophilic drugs at the lowest possible dose and adds flexibility to the anesthesiologist's drug selection while also minimizing the likelihood of side effects. A continuous infusion (after an initial bolus) is the preferred mode of administering local anesthetics via the epidural catheter because satisfactory analgesia can be achieved without major fluctuations in BP. Lower concentrations (e.g., bupivacaine 0.125–0.25%) are used to provide supplemental analgesia, while higher concentrations (e.g., bupivacaine 0.5%) generally provide optimal surgical conditions (i.e., a complete sensory and motor block). The infusion rate is contingent on the desired segmental spread, but often ranges between 5–10 mL/h. Lipophilic opioids can effectively be given by continuous infusion (e.g., fentanyl 2 mcg/mL) and offer the advantage of limited segmental spread. Longer-acting hydrophilic opioids (e.g., hydromorphone 0.4–0.6 mg or morphine 2–3 mg for epidural placement at the lower thoracic spine) can be injected as a bolus along with an initial bolus dose of local anesthetics. However, hydrophilic opioids tend to spread rostrally within the intrathecal space and may cause sedation and respiratory depression if dosed too aggressively. Vulnerable patients include the elderly, patients with obstructive airway disease, and patients suffering from obesity. The use of epidural local anesthetics is associated with sympatholysis and ↓ BP has to be anticipated. Critical ↓ BP is treated with fluids and/or vasopressors (e.g., ephedrine 5–10 mg iv). In patients undergoing a surgical procedure with a significant risk for major bleeding it is prudent to delay administration of epidural local anesthetics until the critical part of surgery has been completed. Systemic sedatives (e.g., opiates and benzodiazepines) should be minimized as they increase the likelihood of postop respiratory depression. **Low-dose ketamine:** If the placement of an epidural catheter is not an option, the use of a low-dose ketamine iv infusion may be considered as an adjuvant analgesic regimen (0.5 mg/kg bolus before surgical incision, followed by an infusion of 0.2 mg/kg/hr that is stopped 30 min before the end of surgery). Low-dose ketamine provides opioid-sparing effects (30–50%), reduces the incidence of opioid-mediated side effects, decreases postop wound hyperalgesia, and may decrease development of chronic pain after surgery. The risk for occurrence of psychomimetic side effects appears to be low in patients undergoing general anesthesia. **Gabapentin:** Single dose administration of 600–1200 mg gabapentin po before surgery should be considered as an adjuvant analgesic regimen in patients who are not eligible for an epidural anesthetic technique. Gabapentin provides opioid-sparing effects (30–50%), reduces postoperative pain (30–50%) and lowers the incidence of opioid-mediated side effects. Gabapentin can cause postoperative sedation. However, available data suggest that pronounced sedation only occurs in a small fraction of patients.
Emergence	The decision to extubate a patient at the end of surgery depends on the patient's underlying cardiopulmonary status. Patients undergoing extensive surgery with major fluid shifts may

Emergence (cont'd)	require prolonged intubation until sufficient reduction of soft tissue edema (compromised airway) is achieved.	
Blood and fluid requirements	Anticipate large fluid loss IV: 14–16 ga × 2 NS/LR ~6–10 mL/kg/h Warm fluids ± Humidify inhaled gases	Blood loss can be significant, and blood products should be immediately available. Adequate large-bore IV access is mandatory. Procedures tend to be long and extensive, leading to hypothermia and large 3rd-space fluid loss. If procedure does not involve cancer or infection, cell-saving devices can be utilized. Intraoperative fluid management should be titrated to a patient's particular needs (adequate peripheral perfusion, urine output > 0.5 mL/kg/min, no base deficit). Overly generous intraoperative fluid administration may be associated with increased postoperative morbidity (e.g., delayed recovery of bowel function) and extended hospital stay.
Monitoring	Standard monitors (see p. B-1) UO Arterial line ± CVP or PA catheter	Most pancreatic surgery is associated with major fluid shifts and fluid loss. Availability of an infusion device assisting rapid delivery of intravenous fluids at body temperature is advised. Invasive monitoring is usually required. In patients with cardiopulmonary compromise, a PA catheter may prove helpful for intraop cardiovascular and fluid management. Use forced-air warmer to maintain normothermia.
Positioning	✓ and pad pressure points ✓ eyes	
Complications	Hypocalcemia Hypovolemia Severe hypoglycemia Sepsis	Release of pancreatic lipase → omental fat saponification. Extensive 3rd-spacing, major hemorrhage during pancreatic dissection. Uncontrolled insulin release from insulinoma Manipulation of infected tissue → cardiovascular instability, respiratory deterioration, DIC.

POSTOPERATIVE

Complications	Hyperglycemia Electrolyte imbalance Hypovolemia Hypothermia Hypocalcemia PONV (see p. B-6) VTE (see p. B-7)	Total pancreatectomy is associated with a brittle diabetes that can be very difficult to control. Subtotal resections lead to variable hyperglycemia.
Pain management	Continuous epidural analgesia (see p. C-2). PCA (see p. C-3).	Patient should be recovered in an ICU or hospital ward that is accustomed to treating the side effects of epidural opiates (e.g., arterial hypotension, respiratory depression, breakthrough pain, nausea, pruritus). Postop pain control with an epidural rather than a PCA regimen is superior in patients undergoing major abdominal surgery. Particularly in high-risk patients, an epidural regimen may reduce the incidence of respiratory failure. The improvement of other major clinical outcomes (e.g., cardiovascular) has not yet been demonstrated convincingly in patients undergoing nonvascular abdominal surgery.

Tests	CXR (if CVP placed); ABG; Hct	Electrolytes; Ca^{++}; glucose; Plts—as indicated for postop management.

Suggested Readings

1. Aldridge MC: Islet cell tumours: surgical treatment. *Hosp Med* 2000; 61:830–3.
2. Angst MS, Ramaswamy B, Riley ET, et al: Lumbar epidural morphine in humans and supraspinal analgesia to experimental heat pain. *Anesthesiology* 2000; 92:312–24.
3. Bell RF, Dahl JB, Moore RA, et al: Perioperative ketamine for acute postoperative pain. *Cochrane Database Syst Rev* 2006; 25:CD004603.
4. De Kock M, Lavand'homme P, Waterloos H: Balanced analgesia in the perioperative period: is there a place for ketamine? *Pain* 2001; 92:373–80.
5. Ginosar Y, Columb MO, Cohen SE, et al: The site of action of epidural fentanyl infusions in the presence of local anesthetics: a minimum local analgesic concentration infusion study in nulliparous labor. *Anesth Analg* 2003; 97:1439–45.
6. KY, Gan TJ, Habib AS: Gabapentin and postoperative pain–a systematic review of randomized controlled trials. *Pain* 2006; 126:91–101.
7. Longmire WP Jr: Cancer of the pancreas: palliative operation, Whipple procedure, or total pancreatectomy. *World J Surg* 1984; 8(6):872–9.
8. Merritt WT: Anesthesia for gastrointestinal surgery. In *Principles and Practice of Anesthesiology.* Longnecker DE, Tinker JH, Morgan GE, eds. Mosby-Year Book Inc, St Louis: 1998, 1881–903.
9. Moossa AR, Scott MH, Lavelle-Jones M: The place of total and extended total pancreatectomy in pancreatic cancer. *World J Surg* 1984; 8(6):895–9.
10. Murakami Y, Uemura K, Hayashidani Y, et al. No mortality after 150 consecutive pancreaticoduodenectomies with duct to mucosa pancreaticogastrostomy. *J Surg Oncol* 2008;97:205–9.
11. Nakeeb A, Lillemoe KD, Yeo CJ, et al: Neoplasms of the exocrine pancreas. In *Surgery: Scientific Principles and Practice*, 4th edition. Mulholland MW, et al., eds. Lippincott Williams & Wilkins, Philadelphia: 2006, 861–79.
12. Nisanevich V, Felsenstein I, Almogy G, et al: Effect of intraoperative fluid management on outcome after intraabdominal surgery. *Anesthesiology* 2005; 103:25–32.
13. Park WY, Thompson JS, Lee KK: Effect of epidural anesthesia and analgesia on perioperative outcome: a randomized, controlled Veterans Affairs cooperative study. *Ann Surg* 2001; 234:560–9.
14. Rigg JR, Jamrozik K, Myles PS, et al: Epidural anaesthesia and analgesia and outcome of major surgery: a randomized trial. *Lancet* 2002; 359:1276–82.
15. Rigg JR, Jamrozik K, Myles PS, et al:.Epidural anaesthesia and analgesia and outcome of major surgery: a randomized trial. *Lancet* 2002; 359, 1276–82.
16. Taheri S, Meeran K: Islet cell tumours: diagnosis and medical management. *Hosp Med* 2000; 61:824–9.
17. Tiippana EM, Hamunen K, Kontinen VK, et al: Do surgical patients benefit from perioperative gabapentin/pregabalin? A systematic review of efficacy and safety. *Anesth Analg* 2007; 104:1545–56.

CHAPTER

7.9 Peritoneal Surgery

SURGEONS

Jeffrey A. Norton, MD
Harry A. Oberhelman, MD, FACS

ANESTHESIOLOGIST

Martin Angst, MD

EXPLORATORY OR STAGING LAPAROTOMY

SURGICAL CONSIDERATIONS

Description: Exploratory laparotomy is indicated primarily in patients suffering abdominal trauma or other acute abdominal catastrophes. It is important that a thorough and systematic intraabdominal examination be carried out to prevent missing significant injuries (e.g., ruptured duodenum or transected pancreas). Any active bleeding should be controlled prior to a systematic examination. Other indications for laparotomy include certain patients with fever of undetermined origin or those in whom a specific diagnosis cannot be made, or for staging of selected patients with Hodgkin's disease. A **staging laparotomy** (Fig. 7.9-1) consists of **splenectomy, wedge** and **needle biopsies** of both lobes of the liver, and biopsies of the periaortic, celiac, mesenteric, and portahepatic lymph nodes. In young women, suturing (pexing) the ovaries in the midline protects them from radiation. Indications for staging in Hodgkin's disease and lymphomas vary from institution to institution, but PET /CT scans have limited their use.

Basically, the procedure begins with a midline abdominal incision; then the abdomen is explored, and both needle and wedge biopsies of the liver may be performed. The spleen may be removed by incising the lateral peritoneal attachment and delivering the spleen into the wound. The short gastric vessels are cut and ligated and the splenic vessels exposed. These are cut individually and ligated, and the spleen is removed. Paraaortic nodes are exposed through a left paraaortic incision in the retroperitoneum, and removed for biopsy. Lymph channels are clipped to prevent lymphatic leakage. The nodes dissected extend to the inferior margin of the duodenum. It may be necessary to cross the aorta and biopsy any enlarged nodes on the right side. More recently, laparoscopy is being performed for staging of certain intraabdominal malignancies (e.g., pancreatic cancer); however, its use has decreased with improved multiphasic CT scans.

Usual preop diagnosis: Abdominal trauma; Hodgkin's disease or other lymphomas

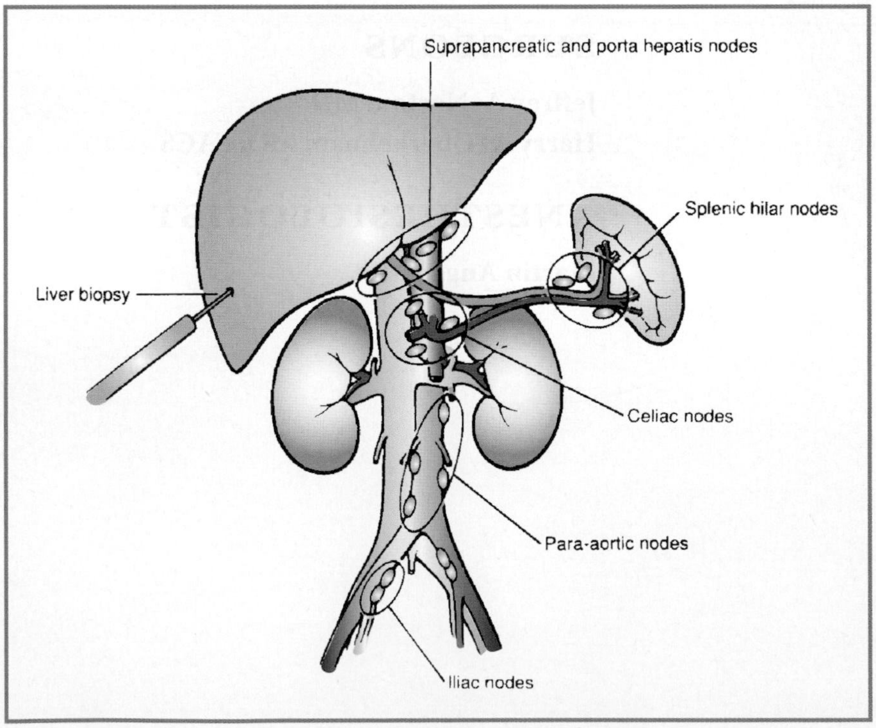

Figure 7.9-1. Staging laparotomy. (Reproduced with permission from Scott-Conner C.E.H., Dawson DL: *Operative Anatomy,* 2nd edition. Lippincott Williams & Wilkins, Philadelphia: 2003.)

SUMMARY OF PROCEDURES

	Staging Laparotomy	Exploratory Laparotomy
Position	Supine	⇐
Incision	Midline abdominal	⇐ or transverse
Special instrumentation	Abdominal retractor	⇐
Unique considerations	Ovarian pexy	Careful monitoring of VS in trauma patients
Antibiotics	Cefoxitin 1 g iv	Cefazolin iv 1 g; 1–2 g iv in trauma patients
VTE prophylaxis	Heparin 5000 units sq	⇐
Surgical time	1.5–2 h	Variable, 1–2 h+
Closing considerations	Splenic bed hemostasis	Hemostasis
EBL	100–200 mL	Variable, 200–500 mL
Postop care	NG decompression; PACU → ward	ICU for trauma patients
Mortality	< 1%	2–5%
Morbidity	Prolonged ileus: 10–15% Pulmonary complications: 5–10% Wound infection: 2–3% Small bowel obstruction: 1% Intraperitoneal bleeding: < 1%	⇐ Atelectasis: 5–10% Wound infection: 5–10% Hemorrhage: 1–3% Pneumonia: < 1%
Pain score	6–8	6–8

PATIENT POPULATION CHARACTERISTICS

Age range	15–60 yr	15–75 yr
Male:Female	1:1.5	1:1
Incidence	Common	⇐
Etiology	Unknown	Trauma
Associated conditions	Hodgkin's disease (95%); lymphoma (5%)	Other visceral or vascular injuries in trauma

ANESTHETIC CONSIDERATIONS

(Procedures covered: exploratory/staging laparotomy that is not trauma-related; splenectomy)

PREOPERATIVE

Typically, nongynecologic patients presenting for **staging laparotomy** (which may include **splenectomy**) have Hodgkin's disease or other lymphomatous disorder. Apart from the primary disease, these patients are typically in reasonably good health and will not have had radiation or chemotherapy before the staging laparotomy. Patients presenting for **splenectomy** may be divided into two less healthy groups: (a) trauma patients (whose management is described in Trauma Surgery, p. 737) and (b) a more complex group with myeloproliferative disorders and other varieties of hypersplenism. The periop management of these two groups is more complicated. The latter group may have received chemotherapy and/or radiation therapy, which may affect a variety of organ systems. It is incumbent upon the anesthesiologist to be aware of the periop implications of these adjunctive treatments. The actual extent of a staging or exploratory laparotomy can vary substantially. A good understanding of the surgeon's plan and its inherent risks (e.g., removing tumor in close proximity to a major blood vessel) is crucial for providing adequate anesthesia care.

Respiratory	Patients who have splenomegaly may have a degree of left lower lobe atelectasis and compromised ventilation 2° intraabdominal pathology: ↓ FRC → ↑ A-a gradient + ↓ PaO_2. This should be evaluated by physical exam. Some may have been treated with chemotherapeutic agents (e.g., bleomycin at a total dose > 200 mg/m²) that cause pulmonary pathology including fibrosis. Toxic drug effects are potentiated by smoking, XRT, and high FiO_2. **Tests:** CXR, PFT, and ABG as clinically indicated
Cardiovascular	Patients with systemic disease requiring splenectomy may be chronically ill and have ↓ cardiovascular reserve. Patients who have received certain chemotherapeutic agents (e.g., doxorubicin at a dose > 550 mg/m²) may suffer from cardiotoxic side effects that can be worsened by XRT. Manifestations include CHF and dysrhythmias. **Tests:** ECG, ECHO, and stress test as clinically indicated.
Neurological	Patients may have neurological deficits from receiving certain chemotherapeutic agents (e.g., peripheral neuropathies caused by vinblastine and cisplatin or CNS pathology caused by 5-fluorouracil and mithramycin). Evidence of neurologic dysfunction should be documented in the preop evaluation.
Hematologic	Patients are likely to present with splenomegaly 2° hematologic disease (e.g., Hodgkin's disease, non-Hodgkin's lymphoma, chronic leukemia, myeloid metaplasia, thrombotic thrombocytopenic purpura, idiopathic autoimmune hemolytic anemia, and sickle cell disease). Cytopenia is very common. Myelosuppression should be anticipated in all patients receiving active chemotherapy. **Tests:** CBC
Hepatic	Some chemotherapeutic agents (e.g., methotrexate and mithramycin) may be hepatotoxic. Evaluation of LFTs should be considered in patients at risk. **Tests:** LFTs including INR
Renal	Some chemotherapeutic drugs (e.g., methotrexate and cisplatin) are nephrotoxic and patients may present with impaired renal function. **Tests:** BUN, creatinine and electrolytes
Laboratory	Other tests as indicated from H&P
Premedication	Consider midazolam 1–2 mg iv. In patients with suspected gastrointestinal stasis the use of a H_2-antagonists (e.g., ranitidine 50 mg iv) and metoclopramide (10 mg iv) 1 h preop, and Na citrate (30 mL po) 10 min preop may be used to minimize the risk of pulmonary aspiration. Metoclopramide is contraindicated in patients with bowel obstruction or perforation. A supplemental intravenous steroid dose (e.g., 25–100 mg hydrocortisone) may be required in patients receiving preop steroids as part of their chemotherapeutic regimen.

INTRAOPERATIVE

Anesthetic technique: GETA ± epidural for postop analgesia. If postop epidural analgesia is planned, placement of catheter prior to anesthetic induction is helpful to establish correct placement in the epidural space (accomplished by injecting 1–2% lidocaine (50–100 mg) via the epidural catheter to elicit a segmental block). The use of epidural anesthetic techniques for postoperative pain control in patients undergoing major, nonvascular abdominal surgery has been shown to provide superior pain control compared with IV-PCA. However, adequate pain control can be achieved with the use of IV-PCA.

General Surgery

Induction	Standard induction (see p. B-2) except in patients at risk for pulmonary aspiration, who require a rapid-sequence induction (see p. B-4).	
Maintenance	Standard maintenance (see p. B-2). High inspired O_2 concentrations (>30%) may aggravate chemotherapy-induced (e.g., bleomycin) lung injuries. Combined epidural/GA: the epidural catheter ideally is placed at a level corresponding to the surgical site (generally, low thoracic). This allows the use of both lipophilic and hydrophilic drugs at the lowest possible dose, adds flexibility to the anesthesiologist's choice of agents, and minimizes the likelihood of side effects. A continuous infusion (after an initial bolus dose) is the preferred mode of administering epidural local anesthetics because satisfactory analgesia can be achieved without major fluctuations in BP. Lower concentrations of bupivacaine (0.125–0.25%) can be infused to provide supplemental analgesia, whereas higher concentrations (0.5%) may improve surgical conditions (complete motor block). The infusion rate is contingent on the desired segmental spread, but often ranges between 4–8 mL/h. Longer-acting hydrophilic opioids (e.g., hydromorphone 0.4–0.6 mg or morphine 2–3 mg for an epidural placement at the lower thoracic spine) can be injected as a bolus along with the initial bolus dose of a local anesthetic. However, hydrophilic opioids tend to spread rostrally within the intrathecal space and may cause sedation and respiratory depression if dosed too aggressively. Vulnerable patients include the elderly, patients with obstructive airway disease and patients suffering from obesity. The use of epidural local anesthetics is associated with sympatholysis and ↓ BP has to be anticipated. Critical ↓ BP is treated with fluids iv and/or vasopressors (e.g., ephedrine 5–10 mg iv). In patients undergoing a surgical procedure with a significant risk for major bleeding, it is prudent to delay administration of epidural local anesthetics until the critical part of surgery has been completed. Systemic sedatives (e.g., opiates and benzodiazepines) should be minimized as they increase the likelihood of postop respiratory depression. **Low-dose ketamine:** If the placement of an epidural catheter is not an option, the use of a low-dose ketamine iv infusion may be considered as an adjuvant analgesic regimen (0.5 mg/kg bolus before surgical incision, followed by an infusion of 0.2 mg/kg/h that is stopped 30 min before the end of surgery). Low-dose ketamine provides opioid-sparing effects (30–50%), decreases the incidence of opioid-mediated side effects, reduces wound hyperalgesia, and may decrease the development of chronic pain after surgery. The risk for the occurrence of psychomimetic side effects appears to be low in patients undergoing general anesthesia. **Gabapentin:** Single dose administration of 600–1200 mg gabapentin po before surgery should be considered as an adjuvant analgesic regimen in patients who are not eligible for an epidural anesthetic technique. Gabapentin provides opioid-sparing effects (30–50%), reduces postop pain (30–50%) and lowers the incidence of opioid-mediated side effects. Gabapentin can cause postop sedation. However, available data suggests that pronounced sedation only occurs in a small fraction of patients.	
Emergence	Most patients can be extubated at the end of surgery. Patients undergoing extensive surgery with major fluid shifts may require prolonged intubation until cardiovascular stability and sufficient reduction of soft-tissue edema (compromised airway) is achieved.	
Blood and fluid requirements	IV: 14–16 ga × 1–2	Potential for major blood loss. In patients with difficult iv access, postinduction placement of additional access is prudent. In splenectomy patients, Plt transfusions should be given after ligation of splenic vessels (↓ sequestration).
	NS/LR @ 6–10 mL/kg/h T&C for PRBC Warm iv fluids Airway humidifier	Intraoperative fluid therapy should be titrated to a patient's particular needs (adequate peripheral perfusion, urine output > 0.5mL/kg/h, no base deficit). Overly generous intraoperative fluid administration may be associated with postoperative morbidity (e.g., delayed recovery of bowel function) and extended hospital stay.

Monitoring	Standard monitors (see p. B-1). ± Arterial line ± CVP UO	Others as indicated by patient's status. To prevent hypothermia during long operations, use warming blanket(s), consider heated humidifier and warming room temperature. Place an arterial line in patients with hemodynamic instability or those at risk for significant intraop bleeding. Consider CVP for guiding fluid management, particularly in patients with concomitant cardiovascular disease. Monitoring UO is mandatory.
Positioning	✓ and pad pressure points ✓ eyes	
Complications	Unexpected bleeding	Plt transfusion may be necessary.

POSTOPERATIVE

Complications	Bleeding Atelectasis (usually left lower lobe) PONV (see p. B-6) VTE (see p. B-7)	Patient should be recovered in ICU or hospital ward that is accustomed to treating side effects of epidural local anesthetics and opiates (e.g., arterial hypotension, respiratory depression, breakthrough pain, nausea, pruritus).
Pain management	Epidural analgesia PCA (see p. C-3).	Epidural analgesia provides superior postop pain control, compared to other analgesic modalities. In high-risk patients, epidural analgesia may ↓ incidence of respiratory complications, but beneficial effects on other systems have not yet been demonstrated in patients undergoing nonvascular abdominal surgery.
Tests	CXR, if CVP placed perioperatively CBC and Plt count	

Suggested Readings

1. Angst MS, Ramaswamy B, Riley ET, et al: Lumbar epidural morphine in humans and supraspinal analgesia to experimental heat pain. *Anesthesiology* 2000;92:312–24.
2. Bell RF, Dahl JB, Moore RA, et al: Perioperative ketamine for acute postoperative pain. *Cochrane Database Syst Rev* 2006: CD004603.
3. Brown CJ, Buie WD: Perioperative stress dose steroids: do they make a difference? *J Am Coll Surg* 2001; 193:678–86.
4. DeKock M, Lavand'homme P, Waterloos H: Balanced analgesia in the perioperative period: is there a place for ketamine? *Pain* 2001; 92(3):373–80.
5. Ginosar Y, Columb MO, Cohen SE, et al: The site of action of epidural fentanyl infusions in the presence of local anesthetics: a minimum local analgesic concentration infusion study in nulliparous labor. *Anesth Analg* 2003;97:1439–45.
6. Ho KY, Gan TJ, Habib AS: Gabapentin and postoperative pain–a systematic review of randomized controlled trials. *Pain* 2006;126:91–101.
7. Nisanevich V, Felsenstein I, Almogy G, et al: Effect of intraoperative fluid management on outcome after intraabdominal surgery. *Anesthesiology* 2005;103:25–32.
8. Park WY, Thompson JS, Lee KK: Effect of epidural anesthesia and analgesia on perioperative outcome: a randomized, controlled Veterans Affairs cooperative study. *Ann Surg* 2001; 234:560–9.
9. Rigg JR, Jamrozik K, Myles PS, et al: Epidural anaesthesia and analgesia and outcome of major surgery: a randomised trial. *Lancet* 2002; 359:1276–82.
10. Rigg JR, Jamrozik K, Myles PS, et al: Epidural anaesthesia and analgesia and outcome of major surgery: a randomized trial. *Lancet.* 2002; 359:1276–82.
11. Tiippana EM, Hamunen K, Kontinen VK, et al: Do surgical patients benefit from perioperative gabapentin/pregabalin? A systematic review of efficacy and safety. *Anesth Analg* 2007;104:1545–56.
12. White R, Winston C, Gonen M, et al: Current utility of staging laparoscopy for pancreatic and peripancreatic neoplasms. *J Am Coll Surg* 2008; 206:445–50.

SPLENECTOMY

SURGICAL CONSIDERATIONS

Description: Through a midline abdominal or left subcostal incision, the spleen is mobilized by dividing the lateral peritoneal attachments while the spleen is retracted medially. (Relevant anatomy is shown in Fig. 7.9-2.) Once the spleen is delivered into the operative wound, the short gastric vessels are clamped, cut, and ligated. The splenic artery and vein are then exposed with care being taken not to injure the tail of the pancreas. By keeping the splenic hilum between the operator's fingers and thumb, inadvertent bleeding can he controlled easily. Accessory spleens (incidence, 15–30%) also should be looked for if the splenectomy is being done for a hematologic disorder. They are found along the cephalad and caudad edges of the pancreas behind the stomach and in the area of the gastrohepatic ligament, greater omentum, and the splenic hilum. All patients undergoing splenectomy should receive polyvalent pneumococcal and H-influenza vaccines. Children may also require vaccination against meningococcus.

Variant procedure or approaches: Following trauma, efforts at splenic salvage (**splenorrhaphy**) may be made, if possible, to preserve all or part of the spleen. This may be accomplished by the use of local hemostatic techniques (electrocoagulation, argon beam coagulator, Surgicel or Gelfoam soaked in thrombin, microfibrillar collagen, and the use of fine sutures or mattress sutures with Teflon felt pledgets). Recently, splenectomy has been performed laparoscopically if the spleen is near normal size (see Laparoscopic Splenectomy, p. 581).

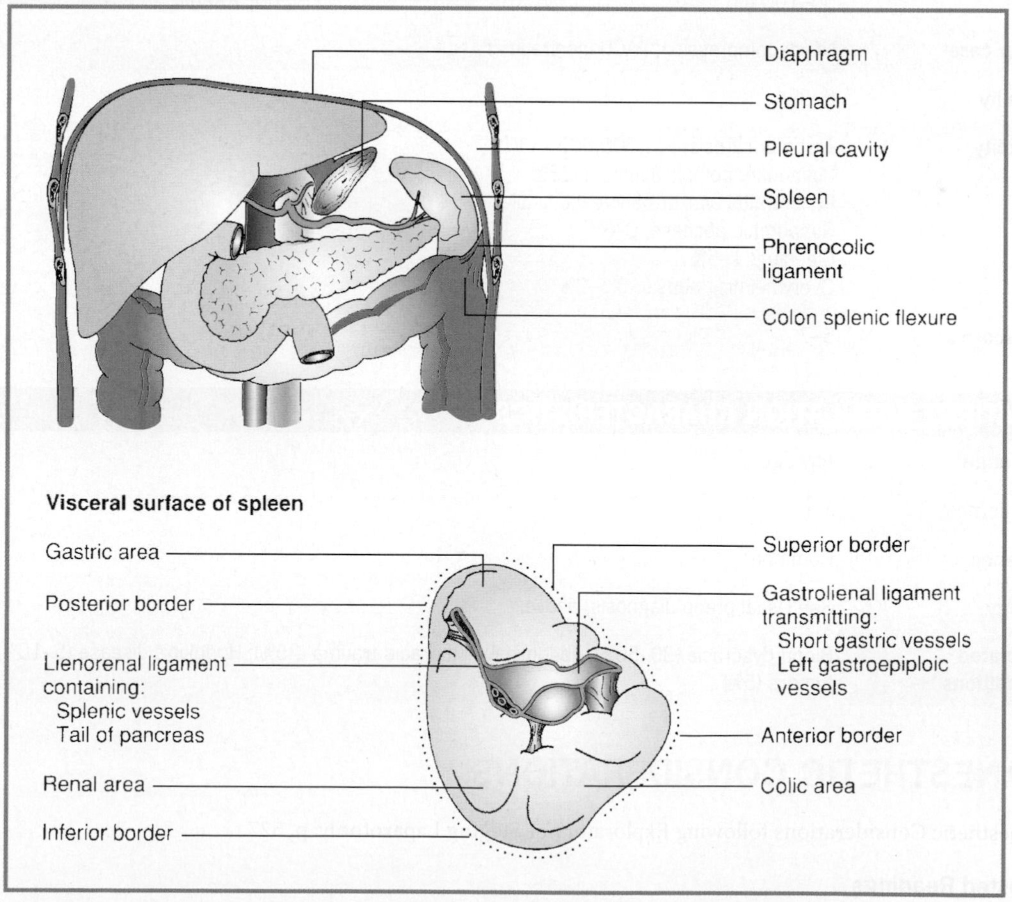

Figure 7.9-2. Anatomic relation of the spleen to the liver, diaphragm, pancreas, colon, and kidney. The stomach is sectioned to illustrate the anatomic relations in situ. (Reproduced with permission from Greenfield LJ, Mulholland MW, Oldham KT, et al., eds: *Surgery: Scientific Principles and Practice,* 3rd edition. Lippincott Williams & Wilkins, Philadelphia: 2001.)

Usual preop diagnosis: Staging laparotomy results; trauma; immune thrombocytopenic purpura; hereditary spherocytosis; other hereditary hemolytic anemia types; or a variety of myeloproliferative disorders

SUMMARY OF PROCEDURES

	Splenectomy	Splenorrhaphy
Position	Supine	⇐
Incision	Midline or left subcostal	⇐
Special instrumentation	Suitable abdominal retractors	⇐
Unique considerations	Potential for major blood loss during procedure; avoid splenic laceration and damage to tail of pancreas.	⇐
Antibiotics	Cefoxitin 1 g iv	⇐
VTE prophylaxis	Heparin 5000 units sq	⇐
Surgical time	1–2 h	1–2 h
Closing considerations	Adequate hemostasis	⇐
EBL	50–100 mL	200–500 mL
Postop care	NG decompression; PACU (nontrauma)	⇐
Mortality	0–3%	⇐
Morbidity	Thrombocytosis: > 1,000,000 → VTE Pulmonary complications: 3–23% Pancreatitis and/or pancreatic fistula: 1–8% Subphrenic abscess: 0–6% Bleeding: 1–5% Overwhelming sepsis: 0.3–2%	⇐
Pain score	5–7	5–7

PATIENT POPULATION CHARACTERISTICS

Age range	Any age
Male:Female	1:1
Incidence	Common
Etiology	See Usual preop diagnosis, above.
Associated conditions	Blood dyscrasia (30–50%); abdominal or thoracic trauma (25%); Hodgkin's disease (5–10%); tumors (5%)

ANESTHETIC CONSIDERATIONS

See Anesthetic Considerations following Exploratory or Staging Laparotomy, p. 527.

Suggested Readings

1. Brunt LM, Langer JC, Quasebarth MA, et al: Comparative analysis of laparoscopy versus open splenectomy. *Am J Surg* 1996; 172:596–601.
2. Davidson RN, Wall RA: Prevention and management of infection in patients without a spleen. *Clin Microbiol Infect* 2001; 12:657–60.

General Surgery

3. Feliciano DV, Bitondo CG, Mattox KL, et al: A four-year experience with splenectomy versus splenorrhaphy. *Ann Surg* 1985; 201(5):568–75.
4. Fraker DL: Splenic disorders. In *Greenfield's Surgery, Scientific Principles and Practice,* 4th edition. Mulholland MW, Lillemore KD, Doherty GM, et al., eds. Lippincott Williams & Wilkens, Philadelphia: 2006, 1222–50.
5. Nurden AT, Nurden P. Increasing the platelet count in chronic ITP. *Lancet* 2008; 371:362–4.

EXCISION OF INTRAABDOMINAL, RETROPERITONEAL TUMORS

SURGICAL CONSIDERATIONS

Description: Intraabdominal and retroperitoneal tumors, other than those of visceral origin, consist primarily of sarcomas (liposarcoma, fibrous histiocytomas, mesenteric fibromas, and gastrointestinal stromal tumors). They are usually approached through a long midline incision for adequate exposure and to assess their resectability. Resection of such lesions may require excision of adjacent or involved small bowel or large intestine or other involved abdominal viscera. Care must be taken not to injure the ureters or major vessels, particularly at the root of the mesentery to the small bowel. It may be prudent to have ureteral stents placed to avoid injury to the ureters. If residual microscopic tumor remains, IORT may be indicated. In certain tumors, the patient may still benefit from "tumor debulking" (removing as much tumor as possible and treating the remaining tumor with radiation and/or chemotherapy). Operative approaches are dictated by location of tumor. Although most operative approaches are transabdominal, some retroperitoneal tumors may be approached retroperitoneally via oblique incision on either side of the abdomen. Some require thoracoabdominal incisions.

Usual preop diagnosis: Intraabdominal or peritoneal tumor

SUMMARY OF PROCEDURE	
Position	Supine
Incision	Midline abdominal or transverse
Unique considerations	Availability of blood
Antibiotics	Cefoxitin 1–2 g iv preop
VTE prophylaxis	Heparin 5000 units sq
Surgical time	3–4 h
Closing considerations	Hemostasis
EBL	300–1000 mL
Mortality	1–3%
Morbidity	Respiratory problems: 5–10% Wound infection: 2–4% Hemorrhage: 1–3%
Pain score	8–10

PATIENT POPULATION CHARACTERISTICS	
Age range	Variable, 20–75 yr
Male:Female	1:1

PATIENT POPULATION CHARACTERISTICS (cont'd)	
Incidence	Common
Etiology	Unknown
Associated conditions	Partial bowel obstruction (10–15%); hydronephrosis (10–15%)

ANESTHETIC CONSIDERATIONS

See Anesthetic Considerations for Intestinal and Peritoneal Procedures, p. 522, and for Exploratory or Staging Laparotomy, p. 627.

Suggested Readings

1. Sabel MS: Sarcomas of bone and soft tissue. In *Greenfield's Surgery, Scientific Principles and Practice,* 4th edition. Mulholland MW, Lillemore KD, Doherty GM, et al., eds. Lippincott Williams & Wilkens, Philadelphia: 2006, 2151–76.
2. Shukla PJ, Bareto SG, Shrikhande SV: Retroperitoneal sarcoma. *Br J Surg* 2007; 94:1057–8.

DRAINAGE OF SUBPHRENIC ABSCESS

SURGICAL CONSIDERATIONS

Description: Abscesses may occur in subphrenic spaces, including the right subphrenic, right subhepatic, left subphrenic, lesser sac, or bare area of the liver (Fig. 7.9-3), following peritonitis, abdominal surgery or trauma. It is

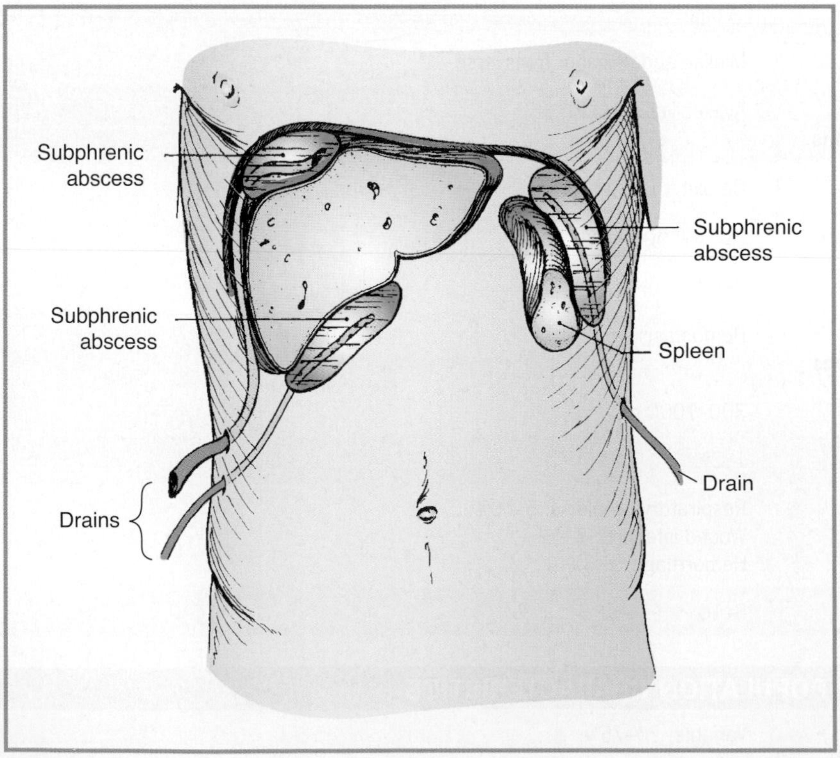

Figure 7.9-3. Anatomy of subphrenic abscess. (Reproduced with permission from Baker RJ, Fischer JE: *Mastery of Surgery,* Vol. I. Lippincott Williams & Wilkins, Philadelphia: 2001.)

General Surgery

important to know the anatomy of these spaces for making a correct diagnosis and for treatment. Most commonly abscesses are drained by interventional radiology (85%), but some may require an open surgical approach.

Drainage is accomplished by a **posterior** or **anterior extraperitoneal approach** or by a **transpleural approach,** depending on location of the abscess. Lesser sac abscesses are best approached by an **anterior transperitoneal route.** Abscesses in the bare area of the liver are drained posteriorly. After the abscess is localized, the cavity is entered by finger dissection and drained. Loculations are broken up and the cavity thoroughly irrigated with NS or a suitable antibiotic solution. Appropriate drains are placed and the wound is closed in a conventional manner. Cultures are routinely obtained.

Variant procedure or approaches: **Percutaneous approaches** have become more popular as experience is gained by interventional radiologists. This technique should be reserved for unilocular collections, where sterile cavities are not penetrated and a safe route is available.

Usual preop diagnosis: Subphrenic abscess

SUMMARY OF PROCEDURES

	Subphrenic Abscess Drainage	Percutaneous Approach
Position	Supine or lateral decubitus, right or left	⇐
Incision	Subcostal or oblique abdominal	None
Special instrumentation	Drainage tubes	Special catheters; CT guidance
Antibiotics	Zosyn (Piperacillin & Tazobactam) 3.375 g q6h	⇐
VTE prophylaxis	Heparin 5000 units sq	⇐
Surgical time	1–1½ h	⇐
EBL	50–100 mL	10–25 mL
Postop care	Maintain patency of the drainage tubes	⇐
Mortality	< 5%	⇐
Morbidity	Inadequate drainage: 5–10% Pulmonary complications: 5–10% Bowel perforation: < 2%	⇐
Pain score	7–9	4–5

PATIENT POPULATION CHARACTERISTICS

Age range	Variable, 15–80 yr
Male:Female	1:1
Incidence	Common
Etiology	Postop (70–80%); peritonitis (25–30%); trauma (5–10%)
Associated conditions	See Etiology, above.

ANESTHETIC CONSIDERATIONS

See Anesthetic Considerations for Intestinal and Peritoneal Procedures, p. 522.

Suggested Readings

1. Baker RJ, Fischer JE: *Mastery of Surgery,* 4th edition. Lippincott Williams & Wilkins, Philadelphia: 2001, 1075–80.
2. Doherty GM, Way LW: Peritoneal cavity. In *Current Surgical Diagnosis and Treatment,* 12th edition. Doherty GM, ed. McGraw-Hill, New York: 2005, 493–507.
3. Goulet CJ: Endoscopic transgastric drainage of subphrenic abscess. *Gastrointest Endosc* 2007; 65:733–5.

INGUINAL HERNIORRHAPHY

SURGICAL CONSIDERATIONS

Description: Groin hernias are defects in the transverse abdominis layer, where a direct hernia comes through the posterior wall of the inguinal canal and an indirect hernia comes through the internal inguinal ring (Fig. 7.9-4). Direct hernias are medial to the inferior epigastric artery and vein, whereas indirect hernias are lateral to these vessels. Surgical approach can be either anterior or posterior. In general, an **anterior approach** (Bassini, McVay's, Shouldice, or mesh repair) is used for primary repair of an indirect or direct inguinal hernia. The **Bassini repair** consists of ligation of the hernia sac and suturing the conjoint tendon to the shelving edge of Poupart's ligament. **McVay's repair** sutures the conjoint tendon to Cooper's ligament and usually is reserved for femoral inguinal hernias. **Shouldice** emphasizes the closing of the transverse fascia and transversus abdominal muscle layers. Currently, the interposing of Marlex mesh or insertion of a Marlex plug between the conjoint tendon, the internal oblique muscle, and the inguinal ligament is commonly used. Other modifications are indicated in special situations.

A **posterior approach** is used by some surgeons for the repair of femoral hernias and recurrent inguinal hernias and for treating incarcerated and strangulated hernias. The **posterior preperitoneal approach** is normally performed by suturing the transversus abdominis arch on the superior aspect of the hernia defect to Cooper's ligament and the iliopubic tract on the inferior aspect of the defect.

The **laparoscopic approach** is indicated for the repair of recurrent or bilateral inguinal hernias and utilizes a **preperitoneal patch repair** and results in less postop pain and an earlier return to normal physical activity (see Laparoscopic Inguinal Hernia Repair, p. 595).

Usual preop diagnosis: Groin pain or lump

SUMMARY OF PROCEDURE

Position	Supine
Incision	Oblique or transverse
Unique considerations	Avoid damage to nerve structure and spermatic cord. Avoid interfering with blood supply to testes.
Antibiotics	Cefazolin 1 gm iv preop
Surgical time	1–1.5 h
Postop care	PACU → room
EBL	25–50 mL
Mortality	3/100,000
Morbidity	Wound abscess: < 3% Wound hematoma: < 2%
Pain score	4–5

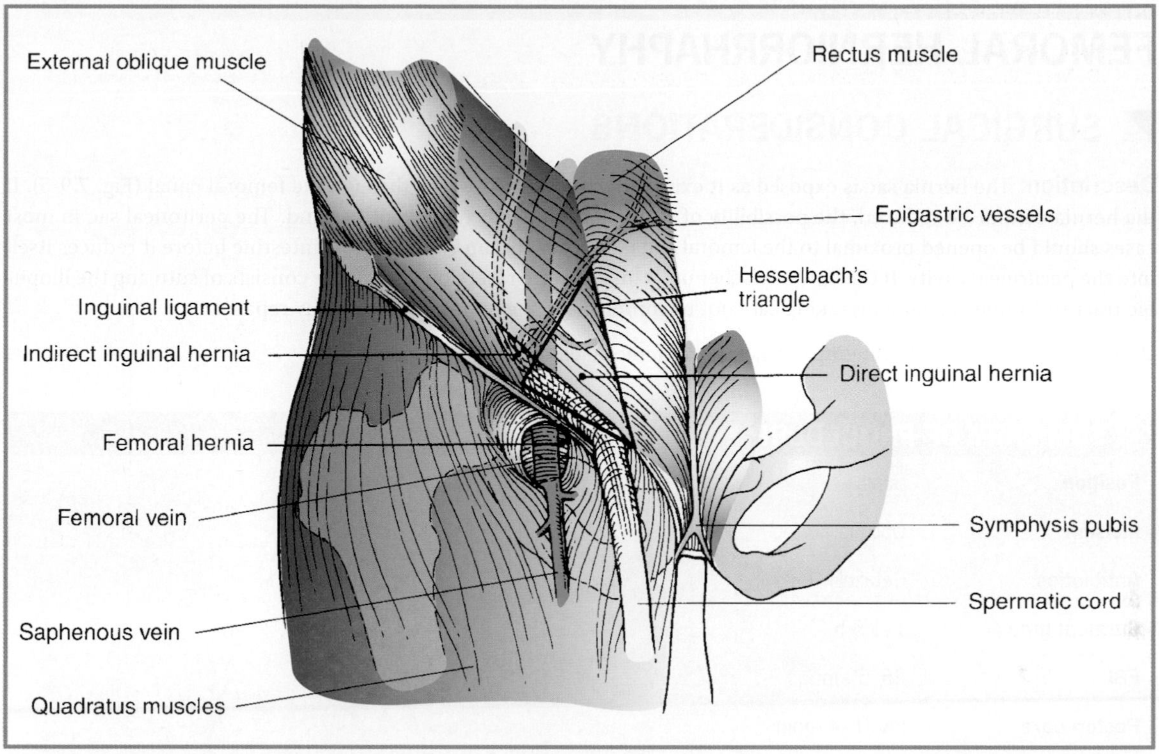

Figure 7.9-4. Inguinal anatomy. (Reproduced with permission from Scott-Conner CEH, Dawson DL: *Operative Anatomy,* 2nd edition. Lippincott Williams & Wilkins, Philadelphia: 2003.)

PATIENT POPULATION CHARACTERISTICS	
Age range	1–90 yr
Male:Female	85:15
Incidence	15/1000
Etiology	Congenital variants; reduced collagen synthesis in adults
Associated conditions	Chronic cough; urinary retention; chronic constipation

ANESTHETIC CONSIDERATIONS

See Anesthetic Considerations following Repair of Abdominal Dehiscence, p. 641.

Suggested Readings

1. Gray SH, Hawn MT, Itani KM: Surgical progress in inguinal and ventral hernia repair. *Surg Clin North Am* 2008; 88:17–26.
2. Hallen M, Bergenfelz A, Westerdahl J: Laparoscopic extraperitoneal inguinal hernia repair versus open mesh repair: long-term follow-up of a randomized control trial. *Surgery* 2008; 143:313–7.
3. Javid PF, Brooks DC: Hernias. In *Maingot's Abdominal Operations,* 11th edition. Zinner MJ, Ashley JS, eds. McGraw Hill, New York: 2007, 105–40.
4. Read RC: Preperitoneal herniorrhaphy: a historical review. *World J Surg* 1989; 13(5):532–40.
5. Richards AT, Quinn TH, Fitzgibbons RJ: Abdominal wall hernias. In *Greenfield's Surgery: Scientific Principles and Practice,* 4th edition. Mulholland MW, Lillemore KD, Doherty GM, et al., eds. Lippincott Williams & Wilkins, Philadelphia: 2006, 1172–209.
6. Suzuki S, Furui S, Okinaga K, et al: Differentiation of femoral vs inguinal hernia: CT findings. *AJR* 2007; 189:78–83.

FEMORAL HERNIORRHAPHY

SURGICAL CONSIDERATIONS

Description: The hernia sac is exposed as it exits the preperitoneal space through the femoral canal (Fig. 7.9-5). If the hernia cannot be reduced, the possibility of strangulation needs to be kept in mind. The peritoneal sac in most cases should be opened proximal to the femoral canal in order to gain control of the intestine before it reduces itself into the peritoneal cavity. If the bowel is ischemic, it may require resection. The repair consists of suturing the iliopubic tract to Cooper's ligament, taking care not to compromise the femoral vein (McVay repair).

Usual preop diagnosis: Bulging of tissues over femoral canal

SUMMARY OF PROCEDURE	
Position	Supine
Incision	Oblique
Antibiotics	Cefazolin 1 g iv
Surgical time	1–1.5 h
EBL	25–50 mL
Postop care	PACU → room
Mortality	< 1% (6–20%, if strangulated)
Morbidity	Recurrence: 6%
Pain score	5–6

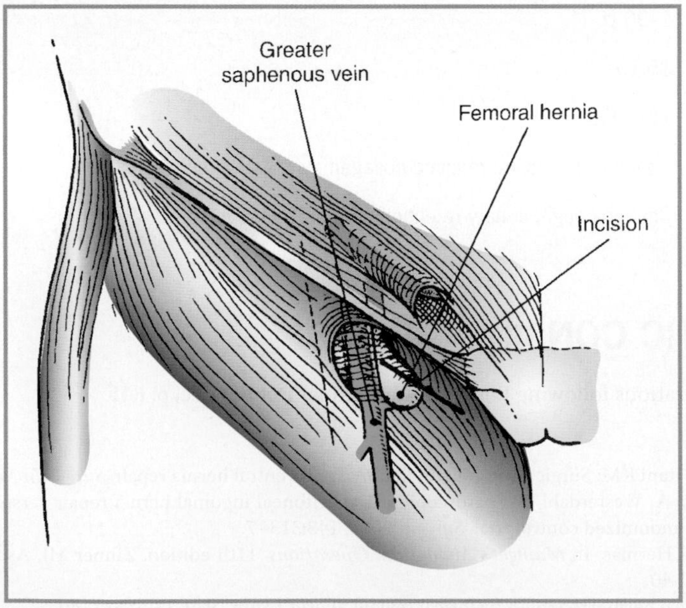

Figure 7.9-5. Femoral hernia repair. (Reproduced with permission from Scott-Conner CEH, Dawson DL: *Operative Anatomy,* 2nd edition. Lippincott Williams & Wilkins, Philadelphia: 2003.)

PATIENT POPULATION CHARACTERISTICS	
Age range	Adults; rare in children
Male:Female	1:4
Incidence	1.5% of all groin hernias
Etiology	Failure of preformed peritoneal sac to obliterate; muscle atrophy in older age group

ANESTHETIC CONSIDERATIONS

See Anesthetic Considerations following Repair of Abdominal Dehiscence, p. 641.

Suggested Readings

1. Javid PF, Brooks DC: Hernias. In *Maingot's Abdominal Operations,* 11th edition. Zinner MJ, Ashley JS, eds. McGraw Hill, New York: 2007, 105–40.
2. Richards AT, Quinn TH, Fitzgibbons RJ: Abdominal wall hernias. In *Greenfield's Surgery: Scientific Principles and Practice,* 4th edition. Mulholland MW, Lillemore KD, Doherty GM, et al, eds. Lippincott Williams & Wilkins, Philadelphia: 2006, 1172–209.
3. Suzuki S, Furui S, Okinaga K, et al: Differentiation of femoral vs inguinal hernia: CT findings. *AJR* 2007;189:78–83.

REPAIR OF INCISIONAL HERNIA

SURGICAL CONSIDERATIONS

Description: Incisional hernias can occur after any abdominal incision, but are most common following midline incisions. Factors leading to herniation are: wound infection, trauma, inadequate suturing, and ischemia. Following skin incision, the skin edges and subcutaneous fat are retracted and the dissection is carried down to the hernia defect. The redundant hernia sac is excised and the fascia is freed up on both sides of the wound. Primary closure is preferred, if possible.

Variant procedure or approaches: In addition to primary repair, the latter may be reinforced by an onlay mesh prosthesis, or the prosthesis may be used to fill the hernial defect or placed behind the muscle layer. In the repair of incisional hernias, laparoscopic tacking of mesh is gaining in popularity.

Usual preop diagnosis: Incisional hernia

SUMMARY OF PROCEDURE	
Position	Supine
Incision	Vertical or transverse
Special instrumentation	Mesh prosthesis (when indicated)
Antibiotics	Cefoxitin 1 g iv
VTE prophylaxis	Heparin 5000 units sq
Surgical time	1–2 h
Closing considerations	Retention sutures
EBL	100–200 mL

SUMMARY OF PROCEDURE (cont'd)	
Postop care	NG decompression; abdominal binder; PACU → ward
Mortality	< 1%
Morbidity	Ileus: 5–10% Respiratory complications: 5–10% Wound infection: 1–2%
Pain score	5–6

PATIENT POPULATION CHARACTERISTICS	
Age range	20–70 yr
Male:Female	1:1
Incidence	3–5% of midline abdominal incisions
Etiology	Wound infection; trauma; inadequate suturing; weak tissues
Associated conditions	Obesity; malnutrition

ANESTHETIC CONSIDERATIONS

See Anesthetic Considerations following Repair of Abdominal Dehiscence, p. 641.

Suggested Readings

1. Condon RE: Ventral abdominal hernia. In *Mastery of Surgery,* Vol II, 4th edition, Baker RJ, Fischer JE, eds. Lippincott Williams & Wilkins, Philadelphia: 2001, 1983–8.
2. Gray SH, Hawn MT, Itani KM: Surgical progress in inguinal and ventral hernia repair. *Surg Clin North Am* 2008; 88:17–26.
3. Javid PF, Brooks DC: Hernias. In *Maingot's Abdominal Operations,* 11th edition. Zinner MJ, Ashley JS, eds. McGraw Hill, New York: 2007, 105–40.
4. Liberman HA, Rosenthal RJ, Phillips EH: Laparoscopic ventral and incisional hernia repair: a simplified method of mesh placement. *J Am Coll Surg* 2002; 194:93–5.
5. Richards AT, Quinn TH, Fitzgibbons RJ: Abdominal wall hernias. In *Greenfield's Surgery: Scientific Principles and Practice,* 4th edition. Mulholland MW, Lillemore KD, Doherty GM, et al., eds. Lippincott Williams & Wilkins, Philadelphia: 2006, 1172–209.

REPAIR OF ABDOMINAL DEHISCENCE

SURGICAL CONSIDERATIONS

Description: Dehiscence implies a "splitting apart" or "bursting open" of the abdominal wall fascia. A complete dehiscence is a separation of all layers of the abdominal wall and often is associated with an extrusion of abdominal viscera. If incomplete, the separation of fascial and muscular layers results in an incisional hernia or an obstruction of a herniated loop of intestine. The earliest sign of a wound dehiscence is the presence of serosanguineous drainage from the wound. Minimal disruptions may be treated conservatively with occlusive dressings and an abdominal binder. Major dehiscence requires operative repair using retention sutures.

Variant procedure or approaches: Variations in the type of closure depend on surgeon's preference. Interrupted, nonabsorbable sutures and skin bridges are often used.

Usual preop diagnosis: Wound dehiscence

SUMMARY OF PROCEDURE	
Position	Supine
Incision	Closure of previous incision
Unique considerations	Adequate muscle relaxation essential
Antibiotics	Cefoxitin 1–2 g iv
VTE prophylaxis	Heparin 5000 units sq
Surgical time	1–2 h
EBL	50–100 mL
Postop care	Abdominal binder to relieve tension on suture line; PACU → ward
Mortality	5–10%
Morbidity	Recurrent incisional hernia: 5–10% Wound infection: < 5% Wound ischemia: 1–2%
Pain score	4–5

PATIENT POPULATION CHARACTERISTICS	
Age range	25–90 yr
Male:Female	1:1
Incidence	1.3% in patients < 45 yr 5.4% in patients > 45 yr
Etiology	Wound infection; excessive coughing or sneezing; excessive abdominal distention; weak tissue; poor nutrition; hematoma formation; poor surgical technique with tissue ischemia
Associated conditions	Malnutrition (25–30%); ascites (20–25%); hypoproteinemia (20%); chronic anemia (5–10%); vitamin C deficiency (< 5%)

ANESTHETIC CONSIDERATIONS

Procedures covered: inguinal herniorrhaphy; femoral herniorrhaphy; incisional hernia repair; repair of abdominal dehiscence

PREOPERATIVE

Predisposing factors for hernia often include increased abdominal pressure 2° chronic cough, bladder outlet obstruction, constipation, pregnancy, vomiting, ↑BMI, and acute or chronic muscular effort. These factors should ideally be managed preop to avoid postop recurrence. The patient population may range from premature infants to the elderly, who have the potential for presenting with multiple medical problems.

Musculoskeletal	Pain is likely to be present in area of hernia; evaluate bony landmarks if regional anesthesia is planned.
Gastrointestinal	Hernias may become incarcerated, obstructed, or strangulated, requiring emergency surgery. Fluid and electrolyte imbalance is likely. **Tests:** Electrolytes, if indicated from H&P
Hematologic	For regional anesthesia, ✓ patient's coagulation status, if indicated from H&P. **Tests:** As indicated from H&P

Laboratory	Other tests as indicated from H&P
Premedication	If necessary, standard premedication (see p. B-2).

INTRAOPERATIVE

Anesthetic technique: GA, regional, or local anesthesia ± iv sedation (MAC) may all be appropriate anesthetic techniques for uncomplicated cases (e.g., without incarceration or obstruction). Choice depends on factors such as site of incision, patient physical status, and preference of both patient and surgeon. Profound muscle relaxation may be necessary to facilitate exploration and repair.

Regional anesthesia:

Spinal	**Single-shot vs continuous:** Patient in sitting or lateral decubitus position (operative site down) for placement of hyperbaric subarachnoid block. Doses of local anesthetics are as follows for T4-T6 level: 0.75% bupivacaine in 8.25% dextrose (10–15 mg); 0.5% tetracaine in 5% dextrose (12–16 mg). Consider adding fentanyl (10–20 mcg).
Epidural	Patient in sitting or lateral decubitus position for placement of epidural catheter. After locating the epidural space, administer a test dose (e.g., 3 mL of 1.5% lidocaine with 1:200,000 epinephrine) to determine whether the catheter is subarachnoid or intravascular. Titrate local anesthetic (e.g., 1–2% lidocaine or 0.5% bupivacaine or ropivacaine) until desired surgical level is obtained (5–7 mL at a time), usually 20 mL. Consider adding fentanyl (25–100 mcg).
Local	Requires gentle surgical technique. Surgical field block, plus ilioinguinal and iliohypogastric nerve blocks, using 0.5% bupivacaine with 1:200,000 epinephrine. Usually performed by surgeon.

General anesthesia:

Induction	**LMA vs ETT:** Standard induction (see p. B-2). LMA may be suitable for the patient who presents with a simple chronic hernia. If there is obstruction, incarceration, or strangulation, however, a rapid-sequence induction (see p. B-5) with ET intubation is indicated. GETA also may be indicated in the patient with wound dehiscence.	
Maintenance	Standard maintenance (see p. B-3). Muscle relaxants may be necessary to facilitate surgical repair.	
Emergence	Consider extubating the trachea while patient is still anesthetized to prevent coughing and straining. Patients who are at risk for pulmonary aspiration and require awake intubation or rapid-sequence induction (see p. B-4) are not candidates for deep extubation.	
Blood and fluid requirements	Minimal blood loss IV: 16–18 ga × 1 NS/LR @ 5–8 mL/kg/h	
Monitoring	Standard monitoring (see p. B-2).	
Positioning	✓ and pad pressure points ✓ eyes	
Complications	↓↓ HR + ↓ BP	Vagal reflex evoked by bowel traction.

General Surgery

POSTOPERATIVE

Complications	PDPH after neuraxial block Urinary retention, common with regional anesthesia Wound dehiscence with coughing/straining	Patients with urinary retention may require intermittent catheterization until urinary function resumes.
Pain management	PO analgesics: Acetaminophen and codeine (Tylenol #3 1–2 tab q 4–6 h) or oxycodone and acetaminophen (Percocet 1 tab q 6 h)	Surgical field block or regional anesthesia should provide sufficient analgesia postop.

Suggested Readings

1. Abbott DE, Dumanian GA, Halverson AL: Management of laparotomy wound dehiscence. *Am Surg* 2007; 73:1224–7.
2. Cousins MJ, Bridenbaugh PO, eds: *Neural Blockade Pain Management,* 3rd edition. Lippincott-Raven Publishers, Philadelphia: 1998.
3. Ellis H: Incisions, closures and management of the wound. In: *Maingot's Abdominal Operations,* Vol. I, 10th edition. Zinner MJ, ed. Appleton & Lange, Stamford, CT: 1997, 395–426.
4. Horlocker TT, McGregor DG, Matsushige DK, et al: A retrospective review of 4767 consecutive spinal anesthetics: central nervous system complications. Perioperative Outcomes Group. *Anesth Analg* 1997; 84(3):578–84.

CHAPTER

7.10 Breast Surgery

SURGEONS

Irene L. Wapnir, MD, FACS
Jennifer L. De la Pena, MD
Stefanie S. Jeffrey, MD, FACS

ANESTHESIOLOGIST

Lindsey Vokach-Brodsky, MB, ChB, FFARCSI

BREAST BIOPSY

SURGICAL CONSIDERATIONS

Description: **Breast biopsy,** or **lumpectomy,** is the surgical removal of breast tissue for histopathological examination. Many biopsies are done percutaneously as office procedures. Two approaches are used: **fine-needle aspiration cytology** and **core needle biopsy.** Ultrasound-guided biopsies, mammographically guided, stereotactic-core biopsies, and MRI-guided biopsies are used as preop diagnostic procedures. **Open breast biopsies** are performed primarily in the OR for palpable or nonpalpable abnormalities. **Palpable lesions** include masses, nodules, or areas of asymmetric breast thickening. Breast pathology can manifest as skin changes—specifically, edema, redness, brawny discoloration, or ulceration—mandating biopsy of the involved skin and underlying breast tissue. The term **excisional biopsy** usually is applied to benign entities and implies the complete removal of the lesion in question (e.g., excision of a fibroadenoma). The term **lumpectomy** is used to characterize cancerous lesions that are removed with a rim of normal breast tissue to achieve tumor-free margins.

Another common reason for excisional biopsy is the occurrence of bloody or pathological **nipple discharge.** The underlying cause of this abnormality is, in most instances, a benign intraductal papilloma or, infrequently, carcinoma. **Ductoscopy** may be used to explore breast ducts that produce abnormal discharge fluid. The ductoscope is a 0.9-mm fiber optic microendoscope. It is inserted into the duct(s) following progressive dilatation with lacrimal probes. After the intraductal lesion is visually identified, the surgeon injects methylene blue to further guide the duct excision and breast biopsy.

Nonpalpable lesions are usually discovered on routine screening mammography. Microcalcifications, masses, densities, and architectural distortion fall into the category of potentially malignant lesions. Similarly, ultrasound can identify complex cystic or solid masses and MRI areas of abnormal enhancement. In all these instances, the breast usually feels and looks normal. Typically, the radiologist places a percutaneous hook-wire in close proximity to the lesion, using local anesthesia. The surgeon uses this guide to identify the area of abnormality; therefore, these procedures are referred to as **wire localization, needle localization,** or **hook-wire localization** breast biopsies. In the OR, the surgeon removes the breast tissue surrounding the wire and confirms the removal of the wire and target lesion on specimen radiography and/or ultrasound.

Breast biopsies, or lumpectomies, are usually done under local anesthesia with iv sedation. In some cases, breast biopsies or lumpectomies are done under general anesthesia, either because of the size of the lesion, patient preference, or concerns of implant injury for patients who have subglandular implants. Alternatively, regional or paravertebral blocks may be used.

Usual preop diagnosis: Breast mass; nipple discharge; atypical hyperplasia; known in-situ cancer; mammographic, sonographic, or MRI abnormalities

SUMMARY OF PROCEDURES

	Breast Biopsy/Lumpectomy	Wire Localization Breast Biopsy
Position	Supine with ipsilateral arm abducted. Table may be banked to center breast.	⇐
Incision	Over the breast mass, circumareolar, along the inframammary fold or radial	⇐ Plus, incision may or may not incorporate skin entry site of wire.
Special instrumentation	Ductoscope; ultrasound	⇐
Antibiotics	Cefazolin 1 gm iv (optional)	⇐
Surgical time	0.5–1 h	1–1.5 h, depending on time needed to get results of specimen radiograph.
Closing considerations	Steri-Strips, gauze, or transparent bandage	⇐ Plus, specimen radiograph result must be obtained before completion of operation.
EBL	< 25 mL	⇐

SUMMARY OF PROCEDURES (cont'd)	Breast Biopsy/Lumpectomy	Wire Localization Breast Biopsy
Postop care	PACU → home	⇐
Mortality	Minimal	⇐
Morbidity	Seroma: very common Ecchymosis or hematoma: < 10% Infection: 1–2%	⇐ ⇐ ⇐ Wire cut traverses or migrates into chest. Target lesion is missed (2° misplacement or dislodging of wire)
Pain score	2–5	2–5

PATIENT POPULATION CHARACTERISTICS		
Age range	18–90 yr	25–90 yr
Male:Female	Mainly female	⇐
Incidence	Common	⇐
Etiology	Unknown	⇐

ANESTHETIC CONSIDERATIONS

See Anesthetic Considerations for Breast Biopsy and Sentinel Lymph Node Biopsy, p. 649.

SENTINEL LYMPH NODE BIOPSY

SURGICAL CONSIDERATIONS

Description: Sentinel lymph node biopsy is a technique applied to patients with small, invasive breast cancers who do not have clinically pathologic lymph nodes. The sentinel lymph node is the first node to drain afferent lymphatics from the particular region of the breast where the cancer is located. The sentinel node is commonly located in the axilla, but may be situated in the internal mammary chain or other extra-axillary sites. Because the sentinel lymph node is the first to drain the lymphatics from a breast cancer, it is the most likely lymph node to harbor metastatic tumor. Early studies suggest that absence of tumor metastasis on histological examination of sentinel nodes accurately predicts the histological status of nonsentinel nodes. The goal of this approach is to avoid conventional Level I and Level II axillary node dissection in node-negative patients. The technique has been validated in several large institutional and multicenter studies. Results from large, randomized trials show an overall accuracy of sentinel node resection of 97%. Failure to identify a sentinel node by the above-described techniques or palpation of axillary contents mandates proceeding to an axillary lymphadenectomy. **Completion axillary dissection** is currently recommended for patients outside clinical trials with tumor-positive sentinel nodes with a metastasis greater than 0.2 mm.

Two types of agents have been principally tested for lymphatic mapping and sentinel node identification procedures: **blue vital dyes** (1% isosulfan blue or methylene blue) and **99^m-technetium-labeled sulfur colloid (TSC)** (unfiltered or filtered). Methylene blue can be used in lieu of isosulfan blue, a change precipitated by national shortages of the dye. Differences and controversy exist regarding ideal injection sites of these agents—peritumoral or around biopsy cavity, dermal, subareolar, or in combination. The first method instills 3–5 mL of isosulfan blue subareolar or at 3, 6, 9, and 12 o'clock surrounding the lesion. The breast is massaged and the axilla is incised 3–7 min later, inferior to the hair-bearing area a few cms inferior to the axillary skin fold, depending on the distance of the tumor to the axilla. Typically, blue afferent lymphatics and blue nodes are identified below the clavipectoral fascia. The

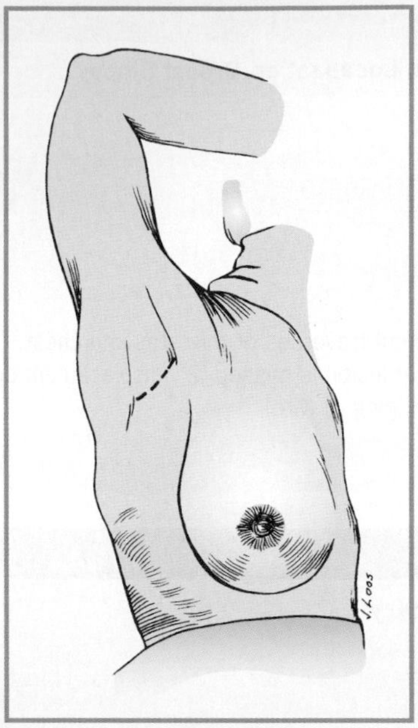

Figure 7.10-1. Arm may be draped into field and positioned on arm board at 90° or suspended over head, as shown. Incision site for lymph node biopsy is indicated by dotted line. (Reproduced with permission from Baker RJ, Fischer JE: *Mastery of Surgery,* 4th edition. Lippincott Williams & Wilkins, 2001.)

surgeon should inform the anesthesiologist when injecting the dye, because a transient drop in the pulse oximeter reading of 2–5% is frequently seen. Patients may retain a bluish hue for a few hours or longer and will excrete blue-tinged urine, stool, or emesis. Allergic reactions, consisting of "blue hives" to full-blown, life-threatening anaphylactic shock, have been reported following the injection of isosulfan blue. Methylene blue has a lower incidence of allergic reactions, but can cause skin necrosis if injected undiluted intradermally.

Sentinel nodes can also be identified using **TSC** (~1 mCi). This agent can be injected in nuclear medicine the day of or the day before the operative procedure. The tracer has very low radioactivity and is safe to handle with no special protection required in handling specimens. Postinjection **lymphoscintigraphy** is considered optional. After induction of GA or regional anesthesia, the operative field (chest and lymph node-bearing areas) is surveyed with a hand-held gamma probe (a slim rod, similar to a Geiger counter). The "hot" spot(s), denoting accumulated tracer in lymph nodes, are identified and an incision is made in the overlying skin. It is customary to have a pathologist examine the sentinel node intraop using touch-prep cytology or frozen section. The purpose is to identify node-positive cases and proceed with standard axillary dissection during the course of the same operation.

Combination of blue dye and TSC yield the highest sentinel node identification rates. Whenever the sentinel node cannot be identified, a conventional axillary dissection should be performed.

Usual preop diagnosis: Invasive breast cancer

SUMMARY OF PROCEDURE

Position	Supine
Incision	Small transverse incision
Special instrumentation	Hand-held gamma-detection probe
Unique considerations	Radiation exposure negligible. Avoid BP cuff or iv in ipsilateral arm. Possible need to avoid muscle relaxants. Isosulfan blue vital dye → allergic reaction (1–2/100).
Antibiotics	Cefazolin 1 gm iv (optional)
Surgical time	10–30 min, up to 1.5 h for axillary lymph node dissections
EBL	Minimal
Postop care	PACU → home
Mortality	Rare
Morbidity	Discoloration of urine and stool up to 48 h Permanent tattooing of skin with blue dye Transient blue staining of skin Allergic dye or radioisotope reaction: ~1–2% Anaphylaxis 1/2,000 Large intravascular doses associated with idiopathic encephalitis; may be related to concurrent SSRI use.
Pain score	2–5

PATIENT POPULATION CHARACTERISTICS	
Age range	25–85 yr
Incidence	~1/8 American women will develop breast cancer.
Etiology	Unknown in most cases; familial history may be related to genetic mutation (BRCA I & 2).

ANESTHETIC CONSIDERATIONS FOR BREAST BIOPSY AND SENTINEL LYMPH NODE BIOPSY

PREOPERATIVE

Breast masses may vary in size and depth, which will, in part, determine what type of anesthetic is most suitable for the procedure in these generally healthy patients. Typically, excisional biopsies can be accomplished with iv sedation and local anesthesia; however, patient wishes must be considered in the anesthetic plan. The suitability of local versus GA may be best addressed by preoperative discussion with the surgical team.

Psychosocial	Patients are likely to be very anxious concerning the possibility of breast malignancy, and should be counseled and premedicated appropriately.
Laboratory	CBC; other tests as indicated from H&P.
Premedication	Consider midazolam 1–2 mg iv

INTRAOPERATIVE

Anesthetic technique: GA or local anesthesia + iv sedation are both appropriate techniques. Choice of anesthetic technique depends on the size and depth of lesion and the wishes of the patient. Surgery is typically done on an outpatient basis.

MAC	Propofol infusion (25–100 mcg/kg/min), combination of analgesics (e.g., fentanyl/remifentanil) and anxiolytics (e.g., midazolam), titrated to effect, are most commonly used. The surgeon may choose to add Na bicarbonate to 1% lidocaine (1:10) to reduce injection pain. The anesthesiologist may give remifentanil 0.5–1 mcg/kg 90 sec before initial injection of local anesthetic into the skin.	
Induction	Standard induction (see p. B-2). Mask or LMA anesthetic may be appropriate.	
Maintenance	Standard maintenance (see p. B-3). Muscle relaxants are not necessary for surgical procedure.	
Emergence	No special considerations	
Blood and fluid requirements	Minimal blood loss IV: 18–20 ga × 1 NS/LR @ 3–5 mL/kg/h	
Monitoring	Standard monitors (see p. B-1). Maintain verbal contact with patient if MAC.	Other monitors as clinically indicated. Isosulfan blue vital dye → artifactual ↓ O_2 sat as low as 92–94%.
Positioning	✓ and pad pressure points ✓ eyes	
Complications	Inadequate analgesia Isosulfan dye reaction	May have to supplement surgical field block with local anesthetic or convert to GA. Pruritus, localized swelling, blue hives. Rx: diphenhydramine (10–50 mg iv). ↓ BP may require epinephrine.

POSTOPERATIVE

Complications	No specific complications anticipated.	Inform patients that urine, emesis, or stool may be blue for 24–48 h.
Pain management	PO analgesics (see p. C-2)	
Tests	As clinically indicated.	

Suggested Readings

1. Albertini JJ, Lyman GH, Cox C, et al: Lymphatic mapping and sentinel node biopsy in the patient with breast cancer. *JAMA* 1996; 276:1818–22.
2. Alex JC, Krag DN: The gamma-probe guided resection of radiolabeled primary lymph nodes. *Surg Oncol Clin N Am* 1996; 5:33–41.
3. Bland KI, Copeland EM, eds: *The Breast: Comprehensive Management of Benign and Malignant Diseases,* 3rd edition. WB Saunders, Philadelphia: 2003.
4. Dooley WC: Routine operative breast endoscopy for bloody nipple discharge. *Ann Surg Oncol* 2002; 9(9):920–3.
5. Freire AR, White PF: Monitored anesthesia care. In *Anesthesia,* 6th edition. Miller RD, ed. Churchill Livingstone, New York: 2005, 2609–11.
6. Greene FL, Page DL, Fleming ID, et al. AJCC staging for breast cancer. In *AJCC Cancer Staging Manual,* 6th edition. Springer-Verlay, New York: 2002, 225–8.
7. Harris JR, Lippman ME, Morrow M, Hellman S, eds: *Diseases of the Breast,* 3rd edition. Lippincott Williams & Wilkins, Philadelphia: 2004.
8. Krag D, Weaver D, Ashikaga T, et al: The sentinel node in breast cancer: A multicenter study. *N Eng J Med* 1998; 339:941–6.
9. Krag DN, Anderson SJ, Julian TB, et al: Technical outcomes of sentinel-lymph node resection and conventional axillary lymph node dissection in patients with clinically node negative breast cancer: results from the NSABP B-32 randomised phase III trial. *Lancet Oncol* 2007; 8(10):881–8.
10. Montgomery LL, Thurne AC, VanZee KJ, et al: Isosulfan blue dye reactions during sentinel lymph node mapping for breast cancer. *Anesth Analg* 2002; 95:385–8.
11. Simmons R, Thevarajah S, Brennan MB, et al. Methylene blue dye as an alternative to isosulfan blue dye for sentinel lymph node localization. *Annals of Surgical Oncology* 2003; 10(3)242–7.
12. Sweet G, Standifird MD: Methylene blue- associated encephalopathy. *J Am Coll Surg* 2007; 204(3):454–8.
13. Vokach-Brodsky L, Jeffrey SS, Lemmens HJM, et al: Isosulfan blue affects pulse oximetry. *Anesthesiology* 2000; 93:102–3.

BREAST-CONSERVING SURGERY AND MASTECTOMY ± RECONSTRUCTION

SURGICAL CONSIDERATIONS

Description: The treatment of invasive breast cancer has evolved greatly in the last 30 years. The **radical mastectomy,** which removes the breast, the underlying pectoral muscles, and the axillary lymph nodes, has been replaced by the **modified radical mastectomy** or **lumpectomy (partial mastectomy)** with lymphatic mapping/sentinel node biopsy and/or **axillary dissection.** Modified radical mastectomy entails removal of the breast and axillary lymph nodes. Lumpectomy or re-excision lumpectomy and axillary nodal staging are normally done through separate incisions. Postop adjuvant radiation therapy is routinely recommended in breast-conserving surgery and is administered following the completion of adjuvant chemotherapy.

In an **axillary dissection,** Levels I and II lymph nodes are removed. These nodes lie behind and lateral to the edge of the pectoralis minor muscle. The Level III, or highest group of axillary lymph nodes, are medial to the pectoralis minor muscle. For prognostic and treatment purposes, no advantage can be shown in removing Level III lymph nodes. As part of the axillary dissection, the surgeon preserves the thoracodorsal nerve (innervates the latissimus dorsi muscle) and the long thoracic nerve (innervates the serratus anterior muscle), as well as the blood and nerve supply to the pectoral muscles. The intercostobrachial nerves (sensory to the upper arm) course through the axillary contents. Preservation of some or all of these nerves usually can be accomplished, avoiding the occurrence of permanent dysesthesias.

A **total mastectomy** (also known as a **simple mastectomy**) removes only breast tissue. It is done mainly for treatment of extensive duct carcinoma in situ or for prophylaxis in high-risk patients.

Immediate breast reconstruction is an option for most women undergoing mastectomy. Postop chest radiation may be a relative, but not absolute, contraindication to immediate reconstruction. Two approaches are commonly used: (a) **prosthetic reconstruction** with a temporary tissue expander or a saline-filled implant placed behind the pectoral muscles and (b) **autologous myocutaneous flaps** (see Breast Reconstruction, p. 1129). Truly excellent cosmetic results are possible with mastectomy techniques that preserve much of the breast skin (skin-sparing, areolar-sparing, or nipple-sparing mastectomies). The latter are usually performed through smaller incisions therefore requiring more operative time.

Usual preop diagnosis: Invasive or in situ breast cancer, high-risk patients

SUMMARY OF PROCEDURES

	Modified Radical Mastectomy	Total Mastectomy	Lumpectomy, Axillary Lymph Node Dissection
Position	Supine with ipsilateral arm abducted and prepped on field. May require repositioning (latissimus dorsi reconstruction).	⇐	⇐
Incision	Elliptical oblique or elliptical transverse to include nipple/areola and previous biopsy; periareolar, or "tennis-racquet."	⇐	Incision over breast mass or previous biopsy site. Separate transverse or oblique incision in axilla.
Unique considerations	Avoid iv and BP cuff on ipsilateral arm	⇐	⇐
Antibiotics	Cefazolin 1 gm iv (optional)	⇐	⇐
Surgical time	1.5–3 h (+ 1–7 h, if immediate breast reconstruction performed)	1–2 h (+ 1–7 h, if immediate breast reconstruction performed)	1–3 h
Closing considerations	Gauze bandage over incision	⇐	⇐
EBL	150–500 mL, depending on whether scalpel or electrocautery is used.	⇐	25–100 mL
Postop care	PACU → 2 d hospitalization	PACU → 1–2 d hospitalization or occasionally → home	PACU → home
Mortality	Rare	⇐	⇐
Morbidity	Lymphedema: 5–30% (depending on extent of axillary dissection) Seroma: 25% Infection: 2–10% Flap necrosis: < 5% Hematoma: < 5% Injury to axillary neurovascular structures: Rare Pneumothorax: Rare (may occur with attempts to obtain hemostasis of intercostal perforating vessels)	⇐ ⇐ ⇐ ⇐ ⇐ ⇐	⇐ ⇐ ⇐ < 10% ⇐
Pain score	4–8	4–6	4–8

General Surgery

PATIENT POPULATION CHARACTERISTICS	
Age range	20–90 yr (generally > 40 yr)
Incidence	Over their lifetime, ~1/8 of American women develop breast cancer. In 2007, according to American Cancer Society estimates, there were 178,480 invasive cancers and 60,000 carcinomas in situ.
Etiology	Unknown in most cases; familial Hx may be related to genetic mutation (BRCA 1 & 2).

ANESTHETIC CONSIDERATIONS

PREOPERATIVE

Patients often have no other underlying medical problems. Some consideration, however, should be given to the anesthetic implications of metastatic spread to bone, brain, liver, lung, etc.

Respiratory	Respiratory compromise can be present if patient has received XRT to the thorax as part of treatment. **Tests:** CXR (✓ for pleural effusion and rib or vertebral lesions). If patient shows any signs of respiratory compromise, obtain room air ABG. Consider PFTs (FVC, FEV_1, $MMEF_{25\text{-}75}$) if CXR or ABG abnormal. This will help predict pulmonary reserve and patient tolerance to GA.
Cardiovascular	Chemotherapeutic agents (e.g., doxorubicin at doses > 550 mg/m^2) may cause severe cardiomyopathies. If patient was exposed to this type of drug, cardiac dysfunction may be present, and a cardiac consultation or cardiac imaging may be helpful to evaluate ventricular function. **Tests:** Consider ECHO or MUGA scan; ECG.
Neurological	Breast cancer often metastasizes to the CNS and can present with focal neurologic deficits, ↑ ICP, or altered mental status. If patient has altered mental status, full workup should proceed without delay; postpone surgery until cause is found. **Tests:** CT/MRI scan should be recommended, if indicated from H&P.
Hematologic	Patient may be anemic 2° chronic disease or chemotherapeutic agents. **Tests:** CBC, with differential and Plt count
Laboratory	Routine lab exam; other tests as indicated from H&P.
Premedication	Consider midazolam 1–2 mg iv.

INTRAOPERATIVE

Anesthetic technique: GETA or GA with LMA. Regional anesthesia (paravertebral block [PVB]) in breast surgery is associated with less PONV, less postop pain, earlier discharge from the hospital, and less chronic incisional pain.

General anesthesia:

Induction	Standard induction (see p. B-2)
Maintenance	Standard maintenance (see p. B-2). The use of muscle relaxants during axillary dissection should be avoided to permit surgical identification of nerves by nerve stimulator or if electrocautery is used in the axilla.
Emergence	Pressure dressings may be applied with the patient anesthetized and "sitting up" at the end of the procedure. Discuss with surgeons whether they intend to apply this type of dressing, to enable appropriate timing of emergence. Consider PONV prophylaxis (see p. B-6).

Regional anesthesia: Unilateral multiple-level PVB provides satisfactory anesthesia for modified radical mastectomy and lumpectomy with axillary lymph node dissection. A block from T1-T6 is required. Suitable local anesthetics

General Surgery

(4–5 mL/level) are 0.5% bupivacaine or 0.5% ropivacaine with 1:400,000 epinephrine. Sedation is useful during block placement and is continued intraop. (See Anesthetic Considerations for Breast Biopsy, p. 649.) PVB is contraindicated for the following reasons: (a) patient refusal, (b) local anesthetic allergy, (c) pathology or previous surgery → anatomic distortion of paravertebral space, and/or (d) infection at sites of injection.

Blood and fluid requirements	Minimal-to-moderate blood loss IV: 16–18 ga × 1 (avoid operative side) NS/LR @ 3–5 mL/kg/h	
Monitoring	Standard monitors (see p. B-1).	Others as indicated by patient status. BP cuff on arm opposite surgical site.
Positioning	✓ and pad pressure points ✓ eyes	
Complications	Pneumothorax	Deep surgical exploration may cause inadvertent pneumothorax; monitor patient for Sx (e.g., ↑ PIP, ↓ $PaCO_2$, asymmetric breath sounds, hyperresonance to percussion over the affected side, hemodynamic instability). Dx: CXR. Rx: Chest tube and ↑ FiO_2.
Complications 2° PVB	Inadequate block (10%) Pleural puncture May result in pneumothorax. Horner's syndrome Inadvertent epidural spread of local anesthetic	

POSTOPERATIVE

Complications	Pneumothorax Psychological trauma PONV (see p. B-6)	If index of suspicion for pneumothorax is high, maintain oxygenation (100% FiO_2) and ventilation; inform surgeons of the likelihood of the Dx. If patient is hemodynamically unstable (suggesting a tension pneumothorax), place a 14-ga iv catheter in the second intercostal space, while the surgeons set up for placement of a chest tube. If patient is hemodynamically stable and not hypoxemic, a portable CXR may aid in diagnosis.
Pain management	PCA (see p. C-3). PO analgesics (see p. C-2).	
Tests	Postop portable CXR, if pneumothorax is a consideration.	

Suggested Readings

1. Greengrass RA, O'Brien F, Lyerly K, et al: Paravertebral block for breast cancer surgery. *Can J Anaesth* 1996; 143(8):858–61.
2. Greengrass RA: Regional anesthesia for ambulatory surgery. *Anesth Clin North Am* 2000; 18(2):858–61.
3. Harris JR, Lippman ME, Morrow M, Hellman S, eds: *Diseases of the Breast,* 3rd edition. Lippincott Williams & Wilkins, Philadelphia: 2004.
4. Hunt KK, Baldwin BJ, Strom EA, et al: Feasibility of postmastectomy radiation after TRAM flap reconstruction. *Ann Surg Oncol* 1997; 4:377–84.
5. Kairaluoma P, Bachmann M, Rosenberg P, et al: Preincisional paravertebral block reduces the prevalence of chronic pain after breast surgery. *Anesth Analg* 2006; 103(3):703–8.
6. Karmakar MK: Thoracic paravertebral block. *Anesthesiology* 2001; 95:771–80.
7. Klein SM, Bergh A, Steele SM, et al: Thoracic paravertebral block for breast surgery. *Anesth Analg* 2000; 90:1402–5.
8. Sacchini V, Pinotti JA, Barros AC, et al: Nipple sparing mastectomy for breast cancer and risk reduction: oncologic or technical problem? *J Am Coll* Surg 2006; 203(5):704–14.
9. Singletary SE: Skin-sparing mastectomy with immediate reconstruction: the MD Anderson Cancer Center experience. *Ann Surg Oncol* 1996; 3:411–16.

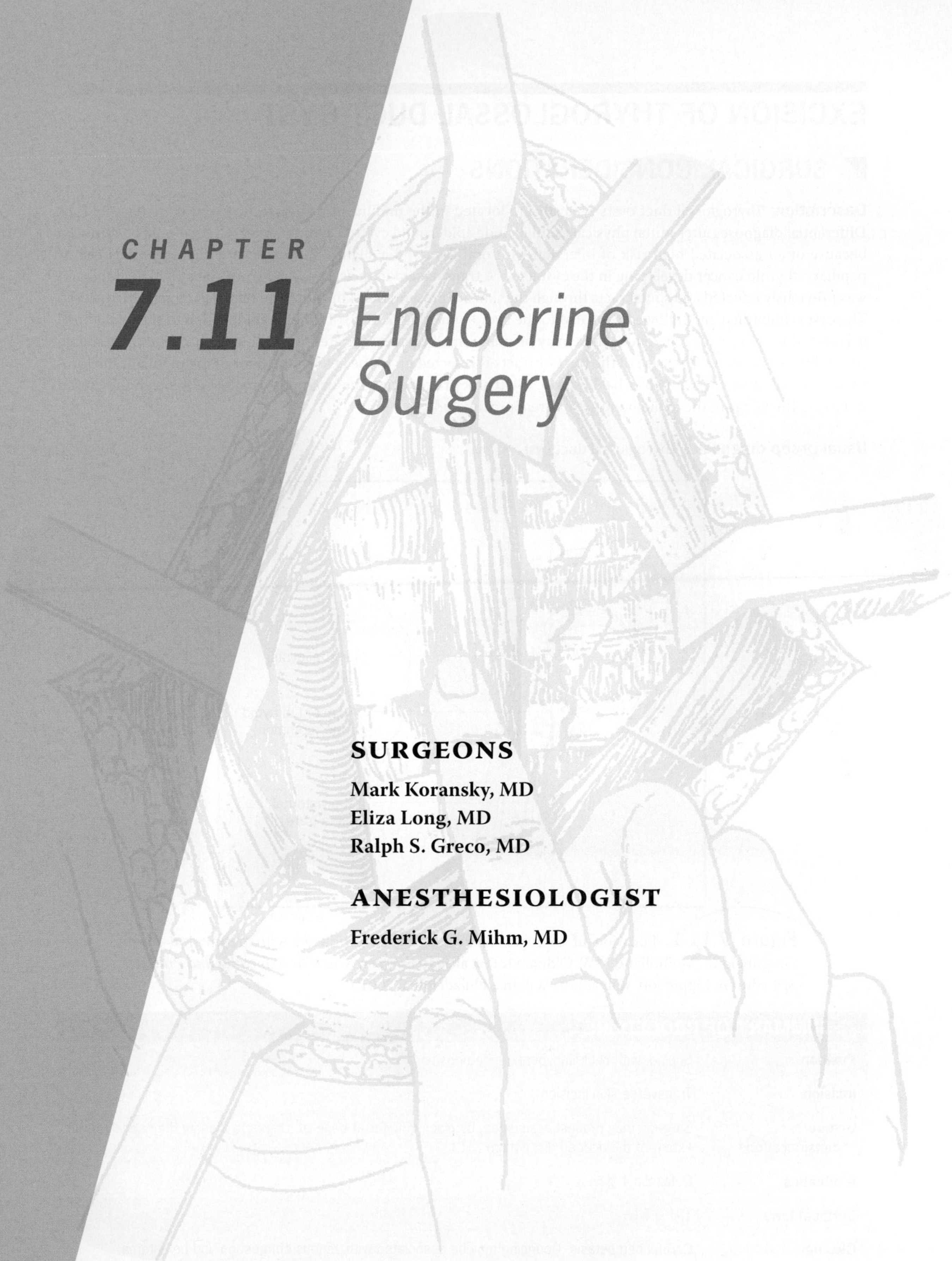

CHAPTER

7.11 Endocrine Surgery

SURGEONS

Mark Koransky, MD
Eliza Long, MD
Ralph S. Greco, MD

ANESTHESIOLOGIST

Frederick G. Mihm, MD

EXCISION OF THYROGLOSSAL DUCT CYST

SURGICAL CONSIDERATIONS

Description: Thyroglossal duct cysts typically are located in the midline at or below the hyoid bone (Fig. 7.11-1). Differential diagnoses after initial physical exam include epidermoid cysts or lymph nodes. Cysts should be removed because of an associated high risk of infection with oral flora and a slight (< 1%) risk of either squamous-cell or papillary-thyroid cancer developing in the cyst itself. A transverse skin incision is made over the cyst; and, if the cyst was previously infected and sinus tracts through the skin are present, the skin should be removed along with the cyst. The cyst is identified and followed cephalad to the hyoid bone (Fig. 7.11-2). Then, the midportion of the hyoid bone is resected to minimize recurrence. There may be many small tracts associated with the cyst that tend to attenuate beyond the hyoid bone. The base of the tract or tracts is resected up to the level of the floor of the mouth at the foramen cecum and ligated with absorbable suture (**Sistrunk procedure**). The wound is irrigated copiously and closed in layers. The wings of the hyoid bone are not reapproximated.

Usual preop diagnosis: Thyroglossal duct cyst

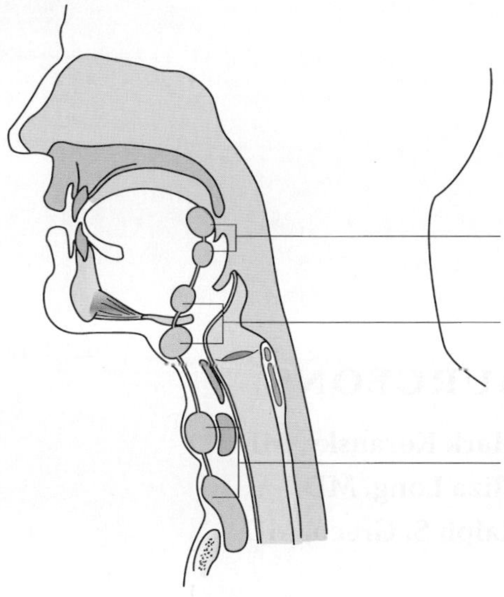

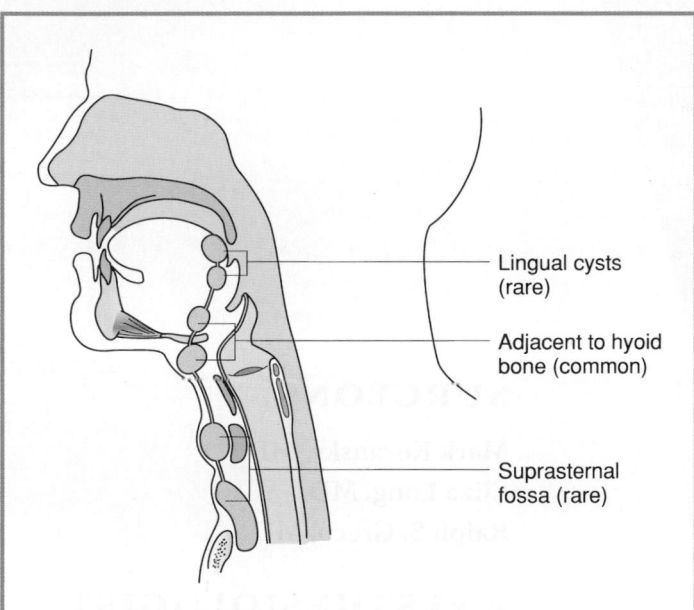

Figure 7.11-1. Location of thyroglossal duct cysts. (Reproduced with permission from Greenfield LJ, Mulholland MW, Oldham KT, et al., eds: *Surgery: Scientific Principles and Practice* 3rd edition. Lippincott Williams & Wilkins, Philadelphia: 2001.)

SUMMARY OF PROCEDURE	
Position	Supine, with neck in hyperextended position
Incision	Transverse skin incision
Unique considerations	Surgeon may request assistance, by placing finger at base of tongue to identify the cephalad extent of the needed dissection.
Antibiotics	Cefazolin 1 g iv
Surgical time	1–1.5 h
Closing considerations	Careful hemostasis. Coughing may be associated with venous congestion and hematoma formation.
EBL	5–10 mL

■ SUMMARY OF PROCEDURE (cont'd)	
Mortality	< 0.1%
Morbidity	Bleeding: < 5% Infection: < 5%
Pain score	3–4

■ PATIENT POPULATION CHARACTERISTICS	
Age range	6 mo–30 yr (40% present at < 10 yr)
Male:Female	1:1
Incidence	~ 1:3000
Etiology	Persistence of undifferentiated epithelial cells in area of hyoid bone that later become squamous-cell epithelium or glandular tissue

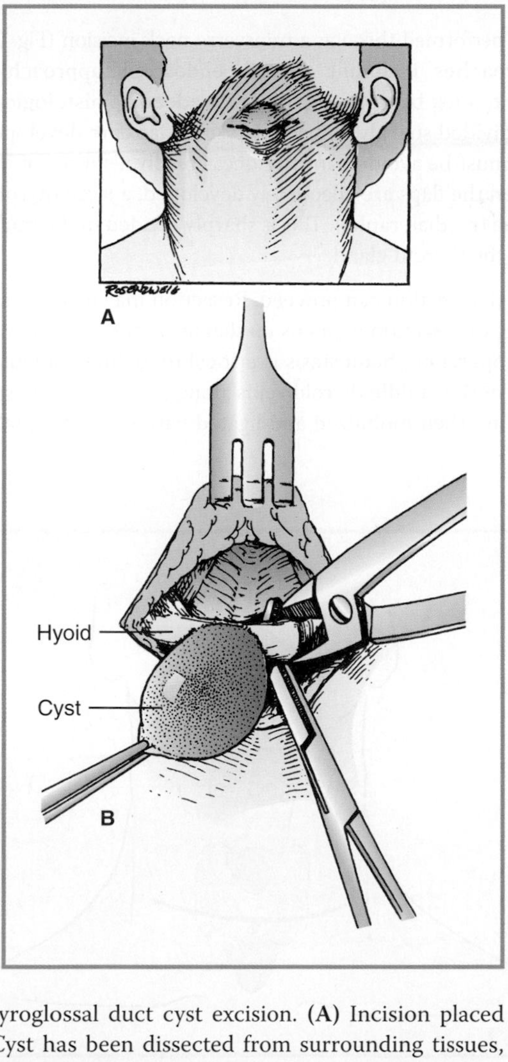

Figure 7.11-2. Thyroglossal duct cyst excision. **(A)** Incision placed over presenting cyst; no skin excised. **(B)** Cyst has been dissected from surrounding tissues, and hyoid is exposed after division of sternohyoid and thyrohyoid muscles at insertion. The bone is encircled with a short right-angle clamp 1 cm from its midpoint, where it is divided with a bone cutter or cautery. (Reproduced with permission from Baker RJ, Fischer JE: *Mastery of Surgery,* 4th edition. Lippincott Williams & Wilkins, Philadelphia: 2001.)

ANESTHETIC CONSIDERATIONS

See Anesthetic Considerations following Thyroidectomy, p. 660.

Suggested Readings

1. Gauger PG: Thyroid gland. In *Greenfield's Surgery, Scientific Principles and Practice*, 4th edtion. Mulholland MW, Lillemore KD, Doherty GM et al., eds. Lippincott Williams & Wilkins, Philadelphia: 2006, 1289–309.
2. Organ GM, Organ CH: Thyroid gland and surgery of the thyroglossal duct: exercise in applied embryology. *World J Surg* 2000; 24(8):886–90.
3. Tracy TF Jr, Muratore CS. Management of common head and neck masses. *Semin Pediatr Surg* 2007; 16(1):3–13.

THYROIDECTOMY

SURGICAL CONSIDERATIONS

Description: **Thyroidectomy** is performed through a transverse neck incision (Fig. 7.11-3) (**Kocher**), usually 6–8 cm long. **Minimally invasive approaches**, including a totally endoscopic approach, have been described, but they remain controversial, as the gland must be removed intact for adequate histological analysis. In the traditional approach, the platysma muscle is divided sharply and subplatysmal flaps are developed superiorly and inferiorly. The two large anterior jugular veins must be avoided and are occasionally a source of blood loss, although rarely of any hemodynamic significance. When the flaps are adequately developed, a large thyroid retractor may be placed to expose the midline prethyroid fascia (median raphe). This is sharply divided in the midline, exposing the strap muscles, which can then be mobilized off the thyroid gland.

After the thyroid gland is exposed, resection can proceed. Resection may be total, subtotal (lobe + isthmus ± partial remaining lobe), or lobar. Degree of resection depends on diagnosis and may be modified based on operative findings. During this portion of the operation, hemostasis is critical to maintain adequate visualization. Resection of a lobe usually begins with ligation of the middle thyroid veins along the midlateral aspects of the thyroid (Fig. 7.11-4). The superior and inferior poles are then mobilized and ligated with care being taken to identify the superior and

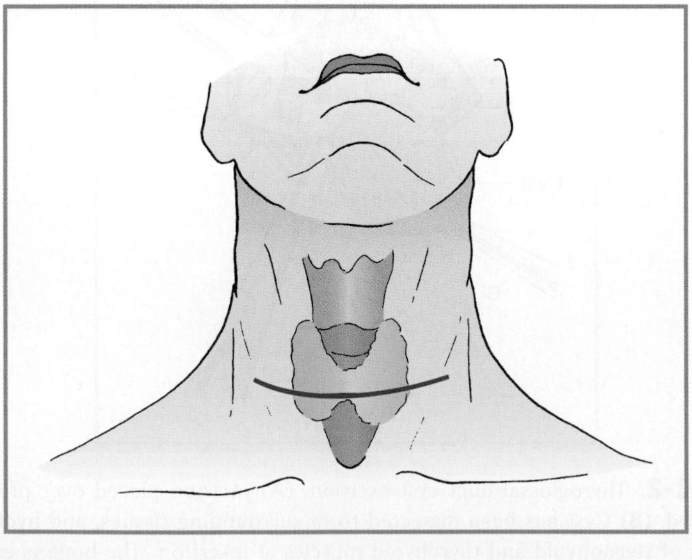

Figure 7.11-3. Transverse incision at base of neck for thyroidectomy. (Reproduced with permission from Baker RJ, Fischer JE: *Mastery of Surgery*, 4th edition. Lippincott Williams & Wilkins, Philadelphia: 2001.)

General Surgery

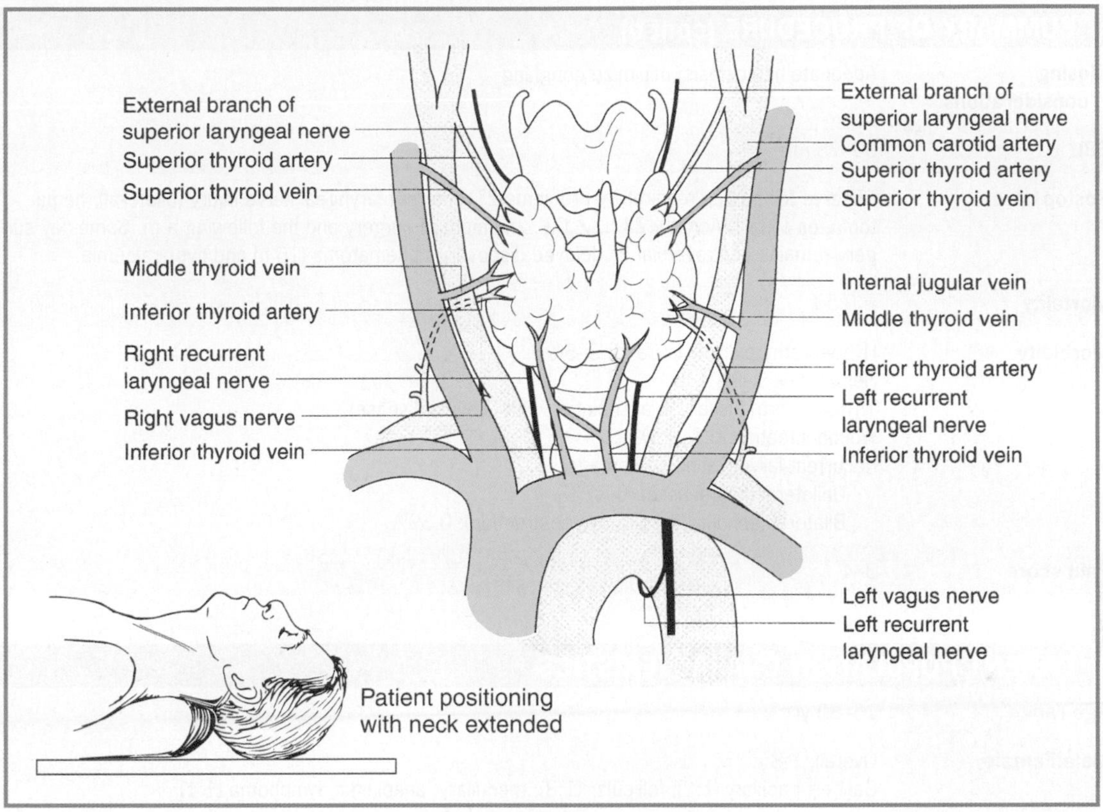

Figure 7.11-4. Vascular relationships to the thyroid gland. (Reproduced with permission from Greenfield LJ, Mulholland MW, Oldham KT, et al., eds: *Surgery: Scientific Principles and Practice*. Lippincott Williams & Wilkins, Philadelphia: 2001.) Inset shows patient positioning with neck extended.

inferior parathyroid glands. When the lateral aspects of the thyroid are mobilized, the medial portions may be dissected. Special care must be taken medially along the tracheal-esophageal groove to prevent damage to the recurrent laryngeal nerve, especially in reoperation. As soon as the gland is mobilized to the degree that it is only adherent to the trachea, it may be fully resected using a knife to prevent cautery injury to the trachea. Any enlarged or suspicious lymph nodes should be excised and sent for pathological examination. After excision, hemostasis is secured. Closure involves the use of absorbable sutures to repair the midline fascia and the platysma. The skin may be closed with running monofilament suture or staples. The use of drains remains controversial and has not been shown to decrease the rate of hematoma formation.

Usual preop diagnosis: FNA findings of definite/suspicious/inconclusive for malignancy; goiter; thyroid cancer (papillary, follicular, medullary, anaplastic); thyroid nodule; hyperthyroidism; Grave's disease

SUMMARY OF PROCEDURE

Position	Supine with head elevated to 30° and neck extended (see Fig. 7.11-4, inset)
Incision	Transverse cervical
Unique considerations	Patients with uncontrolled hyperthyroidism are at ↑ risk for developing thyroid storm during surgery. Hyperthyroidism may be controlled preop with either ß-adrenergic blockade or propylthiouracil. Preop iatrogenic hypothyroidism may be associated with ↓ BP and circulatory collapse during induction of anesthesia.
Antibiotics	None routinely used
Surgical time	1–2 h

SUMMARY OF PROCEDURE (cont'd)	
Closing considerations	Adequate hemostasis; minimize coughing
EBL	50–75 mL
Postop care	Observe for postop respiratory problems 2° recurrent laryngeal nerve injury (bilateral), hematoma, or ↓ Ca^{++}. Admit × 24 h. ✓ Ca^{++} the night of surgery and the following a.m. Same-day surgery remains controversial 2° delayed discovery of hematoma (16 h) and hypocalcemia.
Mortality	< 0.5%
Morbidity	Hypoparathyroidism (↓ Ca^{++}): 3–5% Hematoma: 1–2% Thyroid storm (usually in association with Graves' disease) Wound infection: 0.2–0.5% Recurrent laryngeal nerve damage Unilateral (hoarseness): 0.77% Bilateral (aphonia, respiratory obstruction): 0.39%
Pain score	3–4

PATIENT POPULATION CHARACTERISTICS	
Age range	15–80 yr
Male:Female	Overall: 1:8 Cancer: papillary (1:2); follicular (1:3); medullary; anaplastic; lymphoma (1:1)
Incidence	Cancer (Uncommon) Benign (Relatively common)
Etiology	Cancer (50%): papillary (80%); follicular (10%); medullary (5%); anaplastic (1%); lymphoma (1%) Benign lesions (50%): nontoxic goiter (20%); thyrotoxicosis (10%); thyroiditis (5%); benign nodules (5%); other (10%)
Associated conditions	Other endocrine disorders (e.g., pheochromocytoma in association with medullary thyroid carcinoma in patients with MEN 2A and 2B)

ANESTHETIC CONSIDERATIONS

(Procedures covered: excision of thyroglossal duct cyst; thyroidectomy)

PREOPERATIVE

Hyperthyroidism may be 2° Graves' disease (common), toxic multinodular goiter, thyroid adenomas, TSH-secreting tumor (rare), or overdosage of thyroid hormone. Common Sx are fatigue, sweating, intolerance to heat, ↑ appetite, ↑ HR, ↑ BP, ↑ pulse pressure, ↑ T, weight loss or gain, thyroid goiter, and exophthalmos. Some older patients exhibit apathetic thyrotoxicosis, which is often mistaken for hypothyroidism. CHF and AF are common with these patients. Hypothyroidism may be iatrogenic or 2° autoimmune thyroiditis. Common Sx are intolerance to cold, anorexia, fatigue, weight gain or loss, constipation, ↓ HR, ↓ pulse pressure, ↓ DTR, ↓ T, ↓ mentation. Patients presenting for thyroidectomy usually are made euthyroid before surgery and may be taking one or more of the following medications: propylthiouracil, methimazole, potassium iodide, glucocorticoids, or ß-blockers. An important aspect of the preop visit is to ensure that the patient is in a physiologically euthyroid state (✓ T, HR, pulse pressure, reflexes).

General:

Respiratory	Beware of tracheal compression with large goiters, → tracheal deviation, stridor. **Tests:** CXR; consider preop CT scan of neck to evaluate possible tracheal involvement, especially in patients with large goiters.

Endocrine	<table><tr><th></th><th>T4</th><th>T3ru</th><th>T3</th><th>TSH</th></tr><tr><td>Hyperthyroid</td><td>↑</td><td>↑</td><td>↑</td><td>Normal or ↓</td></tr><tr><td>1° hypothyroid</td><td>↓</td><td>↓</td><td>↓ or normal</td><td>↑</td></tr><tr><td>2° hypothyroid</td><td>↓</td><td>↓</td><td>↓</td><td>↓</td></tr></table> **Tests:** Thyroid function; Ca^{++}; Mg^{++}; phosphate; alkaline phosphatase; glucose

Hyperthyroidism:

Respiratory	↑ BMR →↑ VO_2 → rapid desaturation on induction.
Cardiovascular	↑ HR, AF (10–40% incidence), palpitations, CHF. A normal resting HR is helpful in determining whether the patient is ready for surgery. If the situation calls for it (e.g., emergency surgery), the patient can be treated with ß-blockers to blunt the sympathomimetic effects of the hyperthyroid state. ß-blocker therapy can be problematic in patients with CHF (titrate while monitoring filling pressures and CO). **Tests:** ECG; consider preoperative ECHO for evaluation of LV function.
Neurological	Warm, moist skin, nervousness, anxiety (may require generous sedation), tremor, ↑DTRs.
Musculoskeletal	Higher incidence of myasthenia gravis and skeletal muscle weakness (↑ sensitivity to muscle relaxants), clubbing of the fingers, weight loss, myopathy **Tests:** CK, urine myoglobin
Hematologic	Mild anemia, thrombocytopenia **Tests:** CBC
Gastrointestinal	Weight loss and diarrhea **Tests:** As indicated from H&P.
Laboratory	Other tests as indicated from H&P.
Premedication	Midazolam 1–2 mg iv. Continue antithyroid medications preop. Hyperthyroid patients must be made euthyroid before **elective** surgery and may be on the following drugs: propylthiouracil, methimazole, potassium iodide, ß-blockers, and glucocorticoids.
Thyroid storm	A life-threatening exacerbation of hyperthyroidism occurring during periods of stress, which is manifested by hyperthermia (> 40°C), tachycardia, widened pulse pressure, anxiety, altered mental state → psychosis → coma, and myopathy (rhabdomyolysis in 50%; severe in 4%). (Thyroid storm has been mistaken intraop for malignant hyperthermia, sepsis, anaphylaxis, and other hypermetabolic reactions, e.g., neuroleptic malignant syndrome.) Thyroid storm is most often associated with Graves' disease that has been incompletely treated prior to surgery. **General Rx:** ↑ FiO_2; fluid resuscitation; electrolyte replacement/correction (↑Ca^{++}); cooling blankets; acetaminophen; maintain diuresis (**maintain euvolemia**) if rhabdomyolysis; treat precipitating event (infection, CHF, DKA, pregnancy). **Specific Rx:** propylthiouracil (block synthesis) (200–250 mg po q 4 h); sodium iodide (block release) (1–2.5 g iv); steroids (mechanism unclear)—hydrocortisone (100 mg iv q 8 h), or dexamethasone (4 mg iv q 24 h); ß-blockers (use with caution in patients with reactive airway disease, AV block, or CHF)—propranolol (20–120 mg po q h or 0.25–1.0 mg iv q 5 min), and/or esmolol (50–300 mcg/kg/min). Note: Block synthesis **BEFORE** (1 h is adequate) giving iodides to block release, otherwise "iodine escape" will occur later.

Hypothyroidism:

Respiratory	Beware of tracheal compression with large goiters → tracheal deviation, stridor. ↓ ventilatory response to ↑ CO_2 and ↓ O_2 (caution with opioids and sedatives). **Tests:** CXR; consider preop CT scan of neck to evaluate possible tracheal involvement, especially in patients with large goiters.

Cardiovascular	Bradydysrhythmias, diastolic HTN, pericardial effusions, ECG → ↓voltage, ST-T wave Δ's, ↑QT, occasional VT (torsades de pointe—pause-dependent). This type of VT is treated with $MgSO_4$, cardioversion; then isoproterenol or pacing to shorten QT. Thyroid replacement must be weighed against the risk of precipitating myocardial ischemia in patients with known CAD. Diastolic dysfunction, ↓ LV compliance → **cautious** volume expansion. **Tests:** ECG; consider preoperative ECHO for evaluation of LV systolic/diastolic function, pericardial effusion/tamponade.
Endocrine	Addison's disease occurs in 5–10% of patients with severe hypothyroidism; some patients may receive a 'stress dose' of steroids (hydrocortisone 100 mg iv q 8 h × 3) in the periop period. **Tests:** Cortisol stimulation test
Neurological	↓ BMR → slow mentation and movement, cold intolerance, ↓ reflexes with "hangup" (delayed relaxation phase)
Musculoskeletal	Arthralgias and myalgias
Renal	Impaired renal function 2° amyloidosis, urinary retention, oliguria. (50% incidence of ↓ Na^+) **Tests:** Consider BUN; Cr; Na^+
Hematologic	Coagulation abnormalities, anemia **Tests:** CBC
Gastrointestinal	GI bleeding, constipation, ileus **Tests:** As indicated from H&P.
Laboratory	Other tests as indicated from H&P.
Premedication	Midazolam 1–2 mg iv. (None in the patient who is clinically hypothyroid and requires emergent surgery.) Hypothyroid patients can safely undergo anesthesia/surgery if they have mild-to-moderate disease. Clinically hypothyroid patients (↓ HR, ↓ T, ↓ pulse pressure, ↓ DTRs) should be given thyroid replacement before elective surgery.
Myxedema comma	Severe hypothyroidism constituting a medical emergency, with mortality of > 50%. Manifestations include stupor or coma, hypothermia (which correlates inversely with mortality), hypoventilation with hypoxemia, bradycardia (HR 50–60), hypotension, apathy, hoarseness, and hyponatremia. **Supportive measures:** early intubation and mechanical ventilation; treat ↓ BP with **cautious** volume expansion (risk of pulmonary edema), inotropes (risk of arrhythmias), pacing (carefully, 60–70 b/min) and r/o pericardial effusion, passive rewarming only, especially if ↓ BP (active warming for T < 30°C); correct ↓ Na^+ carefully (risk of Central Pontine Myelinolysis); correct ↓ glucose. **Specific Rx:** L-thyroxine (T_4) (200–500 mcg iv loading dose, 100–300 mcg iv the next day); or tri-iodothyronine (T_3) (20–50 mcg iv q 6–12 h); hydrocortisone (100–300 mg iv q d). T_4 onset is slow (6 h after iv administration) and has to be converted peripherally (slowed in hypothyroid state) to biologically active T_3. Also, T_4 may be converted in some critically ill patients to biologically inactive rT_3 ("reverse T_3"). ↓ TSH level is the earliest sign of response.

INTRAOPERATIVE

Anesthetic technique: Normally, GETA; infrequently, under local anesthesia. For inadequately treated hyperthyroid patients, it is important to establish an adequate depth of anesthesia to prevent an exaggerated sympathetic response to surgical stimulation. Avoid agents that stimulate the sympathetic nervous system (e.g., ketamine, pancuronium, meperidine). Hypothyroidism may be associated with ↑ sensitivity to anesthetic agents and muscle relaxants.

Induction	Standard induction for euthyroid patients (p. B-2). If the patient has airway compromise 2° a large thyroid goiter, consider an awake fiber optic intubation (p. B-5).

Maintenance	Standard maintenance (p. B-2). Maintain muscle relaxation. Use nerve stimulation to guide relaxant dosing.	
Emergence	Airway obstruction 2° recurrent laryngeal nerve damage, tracheomalacia (especially in patients with large destructive goiters), or hematoma can occur. Consider visualizing vocal cord function before extubation.	
Blood and fluid	Minimal blood loss IV: 18 ga × 1 NS/LR @ 5–8 mL/kg/h Head-up position	Slight head-up position can help make for a bloodless surgical field without substantially increasing the risk of VAE.
Monitoring	Standard monitors (p. B-1).	+ others as indicated by patient's status. **Maintain normothermia,** especially in hypothyroid patients.
Positioning	✓ pad pressure points ✓ eyes	Supine, with head slightly hyperextended, allows for surgical exploration of the neck.
Complications	Cardiorespiratory depression	In hypothyroid patients, marked ↓ BP and ↓ RR may occur with minimal anesthetic doses.

POSTOPERATIVE

Complications	Recurrent laryngeal nerve damage	Bilateral: patient will be unable to speak and will require reintubation. CPAP may temporize situation and make re-intubation less emergent. Unilateral: characterized by hoarseness.
	Tracheomalacia or hematoma with airway compromise	Acute airway obstruction may occur immediately postop, and rapid reintubation may be lifesaving. If airway compromise is 2° hematoma, reopen incision and drain remaining blood; if patient still requires artificial airway, consider CPAP or awake re-intubation.
	Acute hypoparathyroid state (hypocalcemia)	Acute hypocalcemia can present as laryngeal stridor (24–48 h postop), although it most often presents with tingling in the fingertips and in the lips. If untreated and severe, this can progress to tetany and seizures. Administering 1 amp Ca^{++} gluconate given iv over 20 min usually alleviates symptoms. Rx: measure Ca^{++}; replace if necessary. CPAP is effective for airway compromise.
	Thyroid storm	Can mimic MH (see Rx above).
Pain management	PCA morphine (see p. C-3)	
Tests	Vocal cord function	Ability to phonate "e" implies continued vocal cord function.

Suggested Readings

1. Abbas G, Dubner S, Heller KS: Re-operation for bleeding after thyroidectomy and parathyroidectomy. *Head Neck* 2001; 23(7):544–6.
2. Arora N, Dhar P, Fahey TJ 3rd: Seminars: local and regional anesthesia for thyroid surgery. *J Surg Oncol* 2006; 94(8): 708–13.
3. Bhattacharyya N, Fried MP: Assessment of the morbidity and complications of total thyroidectomy. *Arch Otolaryngol Head Neck Surg* 2002; 128(4):389–92.
4. Farling PA: Thyroid disease. *Br J Anaesth* 2000; 85:15–28.
5. Fitzgibbons SC, Brams DM, Wei JP: The treatment of thyroid cancer. *Am Surg* 2008; 74(5):389–99.
6. Gauger PG: Thyroid gland. In: *Greenfield's Surgery: Scientific Principles and Practice,* 4th edition. Mulholland MW, Lillemore KD, Doherty GM et al., eds. Lippincott Williams & Wilkins, Philadelphia: 2006, 1289–311.

7. Gaz, RD: Hyperthyroidism. In: *Current Surgical Therapy,* 7th edition. Cameron JL, ed. Mosby Inc, St. Louis: 2001, 653–7.
8. Kearney T, Dang C: Diabetic and endocrine emergencies. *Postgrad Med J* 2007; 83(976):79–86.
9. Miccoli P: Minimally invasive surgery for thyroid and parathyroid diseases. *Surg Enclose* 2002; 16(1):3–6.
10. Schwartz JJ, Rosenbaum SH: Anesthesia and the endocrine system. In: *Clinical Anesthesia,* 5th edition. Barash PG, Cullen BF, Stoelting RK, eds. Lippincott Williams & Wilkins, Philadelphia: 2006, 1129–51.
11. Zeiger, MA: Nontoxic goiter. In: *Current Surgical Therapy,* 7th edition. Cameron JL, eds. Mosby Inc, St. Louis: 2001, 642–4.

PARATHYROIDECTOMY

SURGICAL CONSIDERATIONS

Description: The traditional approach for primary hyperparathyroidism requires **four-gland visualization** with removal of any abnormally large glands. Newer methods of localization and confirmation of adenomas have ushered in an era of minimally invasive parathyroid surgery, using either a **minimally invasive approach,** with a small skin incision and focused operative dissection, or an **endoscopic technique,** with trocar ports and CO_2 insufflation. The minimally invasive approach is aided by the preop localization studies described below. If localization is unsuccessful at identifying the correct gland than the minimally invasive approach is converted to the standard incision and all four glands are explored until the diseased gland is identified.

For the standard open operation, an incision in the lower neck (Fig. 7.11-5) is made and the platysma is divided. Flaps are created below the platysma superiorly and inferiorly to allow increased working space and expose the prethyroid fascia. The midline between the strap muscles is identified and divided, exposing the thyroid gland. The superior parathyroids are located behind the upper pole, in association with the superior thyroid artery, which often must be taken to locate the parathyroid. The inferior glands are located near the junction of the inferior thyroid artery and the recurrent laryngeal nerve (Fig. 7.11-6). Hemostasis is crucial to maintain adequate visualization in the surgical field. For the traditional approach, all four glands are located, and biopsies are sent for confirmation of parathyroid tissue. Abnormal glands are removed. If four-gland hyperplasia is found, which may occur with multiple endocrine neoplasia (MEN) 1 or 2A (secondary or tertiary hyperparathyroidism), then all four glands are removed and some tissue is saved for reimplantation in the forearm.

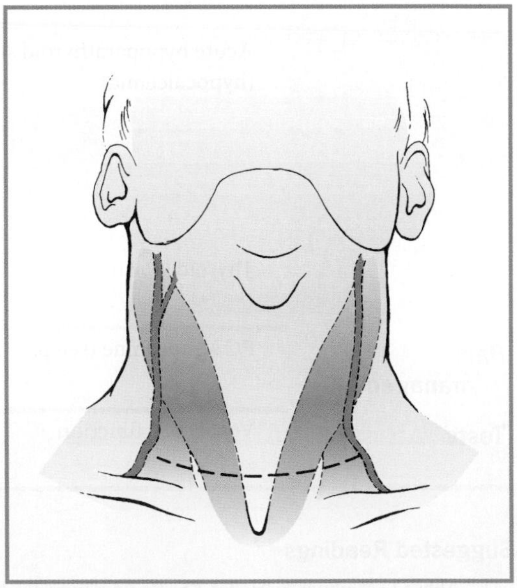

Figure 7.11-5. Skin incision for parathyroid exploration, made 1–2 finger-breadths superior to sternal notch, as far lateral as the external jugular veins on both sides. (Reproduced with permission from Baker RJ, Fischer JE: *Mastery of Surgery,* 4th edition. Lippincott Williams & Wilkins, Philadelphia: 2001.)

With preop localization studies, dissection may be limited to the area of suspicion, and the abnormal gland or glands removed. Confirmation of successful resection may be made by observing a 50% decrease in the parathormone level, 5 min after removal, as compared with the preop level. This very sensitive assay is rapidly becoming the standard of care in the treatment of primary hyperparathyroidism. The addition of preop methylene blue or radioactive tracers may lend additional assurances that the parathyroid tissue has been identified. If the parathyroid adenoma cannot be found, the surgeon should investigate other areas of the neck, including the retroesophageal space, carotid sheath, posterior triangle, and below the thyroid. Unilateral thyroid lobectomy may be performed when three normal glands have been found and the fourth gland is missing, as the adenoma may be in the thyroid substance. Mediastinal exploration should not be done on primary exploration.

General Surgery

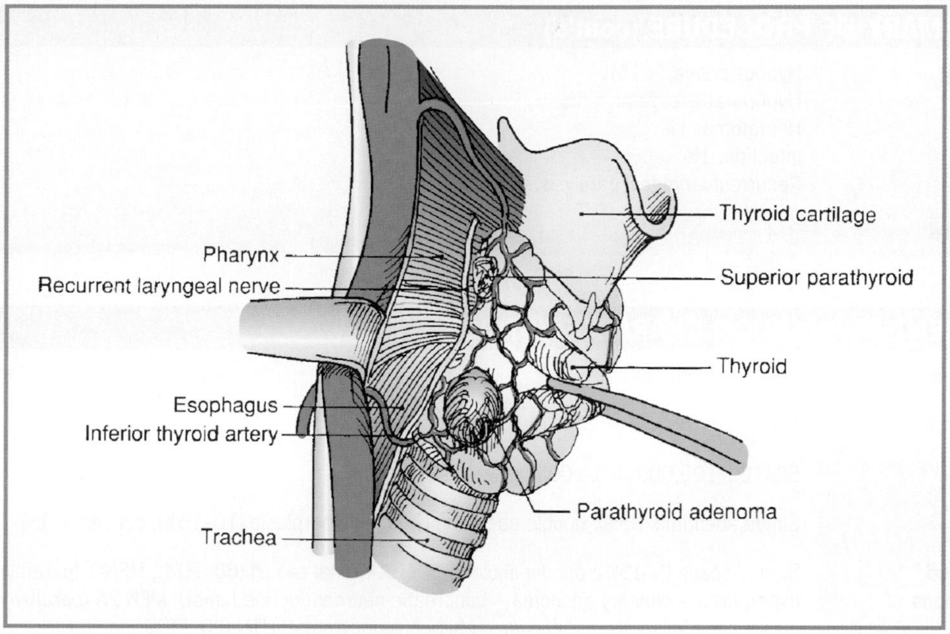

Figure 7.11-6. Identification of upper parathyroid gland on right side. (Reproduced with permission from Scott-Conner CEH, Dawson DL: *Operative Anatomy,* 2nd edition. Lippincott Williams & Wilkins, Philadelphia: 2003).

Variant procedure or approaches: Initial studies of the endoscopic approach have suggested morbidity and rates of cure similar to those of standard procedures, with better cosmetic results. Larger series of randomized trials need to be completed before this approach can be applied broadly.

Usual preop diagnosis: Parathyroid adenoma (multiple in 2–3% of cases); hyperparathyroidism (secondary or tertiary); parathyroid carcinoma

SUMMARY OF PROCEDURE

Position	Supine; shoulder roll; reverse Trendelenburg or 30° tilt; head rest (gel donut)
Incision	Transverse cervical (4–8 cm) (see Fig. 7.11-5)
Unique considerations	Methylene blue (7.5 mg/kg in 500 mL of NS) may be administered in the preop holding area 30 min before surgery → spurious ↓ SpO_2. Radioactive technetium sestamibi (20 mCi) may be administered 60–90 min before operation. Methylene blue and radioactive tracers may be used independently or simultaneously to aid in identification of parathyroid tissue.
Antibiotics	Cefotetan 1 g iv preop
Surgical time	1–2 h
Closing considerations	Coughing may be associated with venous congestion and hematoma formation.
EBL	25–50 mL
Postop care	Monitor serum Ca^{++} (nl = 8.5–10.5 mg% total Ca; 1–1.3 mM ionized Ca^{++}). Patients typically admitted for 24 h observation to ✓ serum ✓ Ca^{++} levels and monitor for hematoma/airway compromise.
Mortality	< 0.5%

SUMMARY OF PROCEDURE (cont'd)	
Morbidity	Hypocalcemia: < 15% Hypoparathyroidism: < 5% Hematoma: 1% Infection: 1% Recurrent laryngeal paralysis: < 1%
Pain score	3–4

PATIENT POPULATION CHARACTERISTICS	
Age range	Increases with age
Male:Female	4:1
Incidence	50–100/100,000 (1.5/100 in elderly)
Etiology	Single adenoma (85%); double adenoma (2–3%); hyperplasia (10–15%); cancer (< 1%)
Associated conditions	Bone disease (5–15%); duodenal ulcer (5–10%); renal calculi (60–70%); MEN-1 (parathyroid + hyperplasia + pituitary adenoma + pancreatic neuroendocrine tumor); MEN-2A (parathyroid hyperplasia + medullary thyroid cancer + pheochromocytoma); HTN (20–50%)

ANESTHETIC CONSIDERATIONS

PREOPERATIVE

These patients typically present with hypercalcemia (hyperparathyroidism), which must be controlled before surgery. Although 25–50% of cases are asymptomatic, many will present with a variety of Sx, including fatigue, muscle weakness, depression, anorexia, nausea, constipation, abdominal and bone pain, HTN, renal stones, and polydipsia. Differential diagnosis for the hypercalcemic patient includes: metastatic disease, multiple myeloma, milk-alkali syndrome, vitamin D intoxication, sarcoidosis, hyperthyroidism, thiazide diuretics, adrenal insufficiency, Paget's disease, immobilization, or an exogenous parathyroid hormone-producing tumor.

Respiratory	Hyperparathyroidism is associated with ↓ clearance of secretions from the tracheobronchial tree → postop atelectasis. Avoid respiratory or metabolic acidosis, which will ↑ the free fraction of Ca → hypercalcemia (↑ BP, ↑ muscle weakness, ↑ HR). **Tests:** As indicated from H&P.
Cardiovascular	HTN (usually resolves with treatment; if severe or episodic, r/o pheochromocytoma); ECG may show tachycardia with ↓ PR and ↓ QT intervals. Patients may be hypovolemic (2° anorexia, N/V, and polyuria) and have ↑ sensitivity to digitalis + resistance to catecholamines. ↓ BP may result from polyuria → hypovolemia. **Preop management** includes correction of intravascular volume and electrolyte abnormalities. Preop treatment of hypercalcemia includes aggressive expansion of intravascular volume, followed by diuresis (**maintain** euvolemia), to ↑ renal Ca^{++} excretion, usually accomplished with iv NS, and then furosemide. Calcium channel blockers (verapamil, nifedipine, diltiazem) can be used. Hypophosphatemia can impair myocardial contractility and should be corrected; hemodialysis or peritoneal dialysis can be used to lower dangerously elevated serum Ca^{++} levels. Mithramycin, plicamycin, calcitonin, bisphosphonates, cisplatin, or steroids are not useful for acute Rx of ↑ Ca^{++} (too slow). **Tests:** ECG; electrolytes; others as indicated from H&P.
Neurological	Patient may present with seizures, hyporeflexia, mental status changes (somnolence, depression, memory loss, psychosis, coma), or peripheral neuropathy. Significant improvement often follows correction of hypercalcemia.

Musculoskeletal	These patients may have muscle atrophy and weakness, osteopenia, arthralgia, pathologic fractures (careful laryngoscopy and positioning), osteitis fibrosa cystica. Response to NMBs may be enhanced 2° ↑ Ca^{++} → muscle weakness.
Hematologic	Patients also tend to be hypophosphatemic and may show signs of hemolysis, Plt dysfunction, impaired ventricular contractility, and leukocyte dysfunction. **Tests:** CBC with Plt count, PO_4^{-2}
Endocrine	Primary hyperparathyroidism is most commonly due to benign parathyroid adenoma (90%), or hyperplasia (9%) and rarely carcinoma. It may be associated with MEN syndrome. MEN-1 consists of tumors of the parathyroid, pancreatic islets, and pituitary. MEN-2 includes pheochromocytoma, mucosal neuromas, parathyroid tumors, and medullary thyroid carcinoma. *NB: **Anesthetizing a patient with an unrecognized pheochromocytoma could result in a fatality.** **Tests:** As indicated from H&P.
Renal	Patients may have renal dysfunction 2° nephrolithiasis, nephrocalcinosis, renal tubular disorders, and glomerular disorders. Polyuria 2° ↑ Ca^{++} → electrolyte disturbances. **Tests:** Cr; BUN; electrolytes
Gastrointestinal	These patients may have constipation, anorexia, N/V, epigastric pain.
Laboratory	Symptoms not related as well to absolute Ca^{++} level but to rate of change. Serum Ca^{++} < 12 mg/dL: likely asymptomatic; 12–14 mg/dL: mild symptoms; >16 mg/dL: life-threatening. Albumin (↑ albumin by 1 g/dL will ↑ total serum Ca^{++} by 0.8 mg/dL); electrolytes; Mg^{++}; phosphate (usually low).
Premedication	All medications to lower hypercalcemia should be continued unless Ca^{++} levels have normalized. If patient has been treated with steroids in the preop period, administer a stress dose (hydrocortisone 100 mg iv q 8 h × 24 h) before induction of anesthesia and continue into the early postop period. Standard premedications (p. B-1) are usually appropriate in this patient group, unless patient has mental status changes.

INTRAOPERATIVE

Anesthetic technique: GETA, with head slightly hyperextended, allows for surgical exploration of the neck. Cervical plexus blocks may be appropriate in selected patients; however, phrenic nerve block → respiratory compromise.

Induction	Standard induction (p. B-2). If patient is clinically hypovolemic, restore intravascular olume before induction and titrate induction dose of sedative/hypnotic agents.	
Maintenance	Standard maintenance (p. B-2), with muscle relaxant titrated to effect, using peripheral nerve stimulator. Avoid hyperventilation or hypoventilation (acidosis will ↑ Ca^{++} levels, while alkalosis will ↓ Ca^{++} levels). Maintain adequate hydration and UO throughout the procedure.	
Emergence	No special considerations (see postop complications, below).	
Blood and fluid requirements	Minimal blood loss IV: 18 ga × 1 NS @ 5–8 mL/kg/h	Avoid Ca^{++}-containing iv solution (e.g., LR), use Normosol, NS.
Monitoring	Standard monitors (p. B-1)	Others as indicated by patient status.
Positioning	✓ and pad all pressure points ✓ eyes	Patients should be positioned carefully as they tend to be osteopenic and are prone to pathologic bone fractures. Slight head-up position may ↓ blood loss and improve surgical visibility without significantly ↑ risk of VAE.
Complications	Hypocalcemia	See postop complications (below).

POSTOPERATIVE

Complications	Hypocalcemia Hypocalcemic tetany Seizure Laryngospasm	Hypocalcemia may occur in the immediate postop period. Sx include paresthesias, muscle spasm, tetany, laryngospasm, bronchospasm, and apnea. Rx: includes 10–20 mL Ca^{++} gluconate 10% over 10 min. Follow levels and repeat therapy until the clinical signs of hypocalcemia are controlled. CPAP is effective for airway obstruction.
	Recurrent laryngeal nerve injury Hypophosphatemia Laryngeal edema 2° surgical trauma Stridor Hematoma with airway compromise	Recurrent laryngeal nerve dysfunction can be monitored by having the patient vocalize the letter "e." Unilateral vocal cord dysfunction results in hoarseness, while bilateral vocal cord dysfunction results in aphonia. CPAP is effective for airway obstruction.
	Pneumothorax	Dx: pleuritic chest pain, dyspnea, ↑ RR, ↓ breath sounds, ↑ resonance, hypoxemia; ✓ CXR. Rx: O_2; chest tube and reintubation as necessary.
Pain management	PCA (p. C-3)	
Tests	Serial measurements of: Ca^{++} Phosphate Mg^{++} Others as clinically indicated CXR to rule out pneumothorax	The lowest Ca^{++} level usually is seen after 4–5 d postop. Follow clinical Sx of hypocalcemia: Trousseau's sign (carpopedal spasm in response to application of a BP cuff at a pressure > SBP for 3 min); Chvostek's sign (contracture of the facial muscles produced by tapping on the facial nerve).

General Surgery

Suggested Readings

1. Abbas G, Dubner S, Heller KS: Re-operation for bleeding after thyroidectomy and parathyroidectomy. *Head Neck* 2001; 23(7):544–6.
2. Carling T, Udelsman R. Focused Approach to Parathyroidectomy. *World J Surg* 2008; Apr 5:[Epub ahead of print]
3. Doherty GM: Parathyroid gland. In *Greenfield's Surgery: Scientific Principles and Practice,* 4th edition. Mulholland MW, Lillemore KD, Doherty GM, eds. Lippincott Williams & Wilkins, 2006: 1310–33.
4. Gauger PG, Thompson NW: Persistent or recurrent hyperparathyroidism. In *Current Surgical Therapy,* 7th edition. Cameron JL, eds. Mosby Inc, St. Louis: 2001, 668–71.
5. Miccoli P: Minimally invasive surgery for thyroid and parathyroid diseases. *Surg Endosc* 2002; 16(l):3–6.
6. Mihai R, Farndon JR: Parathyroid disease and calcium metabolism. *Br J Anaesth* 2000; 85:29–43.
7. Schwartz JJ, Rosenbaum SH: Anesthesia and the endocrine system. In *Clinical Anesthesia,* 5th edition. Barash PG, Cullen BF, Stoelting RK, eds. Lippincott Williams & Wilkins, Philadelphia: 2006, 1129–51.
8. Stalberg P, Delbridge L, van Heerden J et al: Minimally invasive parathyroidectomy and thyroidectomy--current concepts. *Surgeon* 2007; 5(5):301–8.

ADRENALECTOMY

SURGICAL CONSIDERATIONS

Description: Adrenalectomy can be performed via a number of different approaches, each with its own merits. Traditionally, the adrenal glands have been removed with an open incision through either the transperitoneal or extraperitoneal (flank) approach (Fig. 7.11-8). With some exceptions (see below), laparoscopic approaches are becoming the favored methods. Indication in malignant disease or metastasis remains controversial and is currently being evaluated. Relative contraindications include large adrenal adenocarcinomas (> 5 cm),

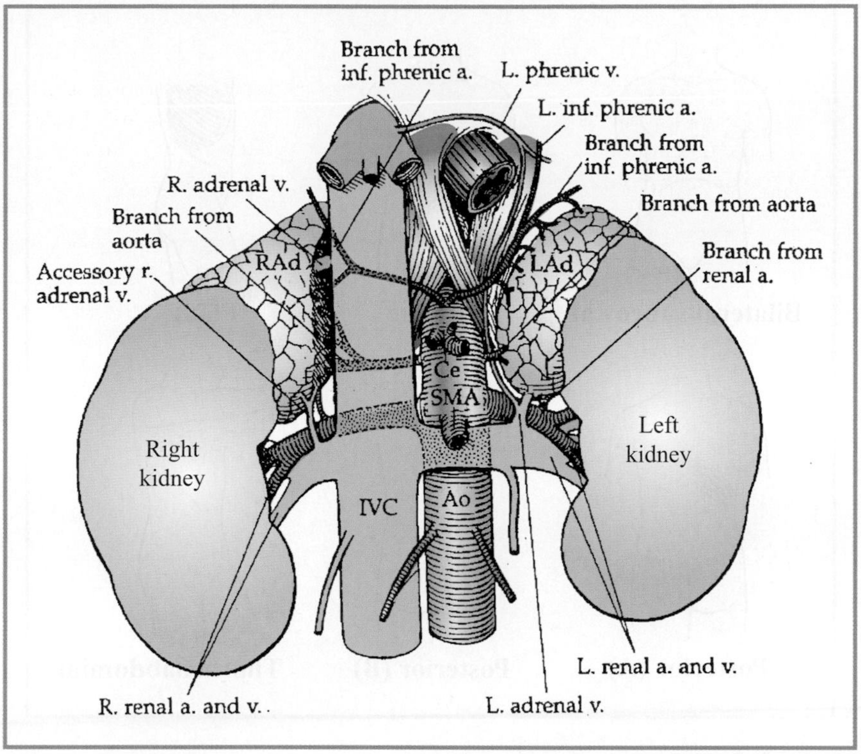

Figure 7.11-7. Anatomic relationships of the adrenal glands. Note the origins of the three main arteries: inferior phrenic, aortic, and renal branches. Note also the single draining veins (except for a small accessory right adrenal vein): the right-located superior and medial, and the left-found inferior and medial. (Ao = aorta; Ce = celiac; LAd = left adrenal gland; RAd = right adrenal gland.) (Reproduced with permission from Baker RJ, Fischer JE: *Mastery of Surgery,* 4th edition. Lippincott Williams & Wilkins, Philadelphia: 2001.)

malignant pheochromocytoma, invasive adrenal mass, large adrenal mass (> 8–10 cm), or other contraindications to abdominal laparoscopic surgery (e.g., multiple previous abdominal surgeries). Each approach is discussed individually, but their basic principles remain the same. The anatomy of the retroperitoneum is shown in Fig. 7.11-7.

Open transperitoneal approach: This approach allows for easy access to both adrenals and is preferred for large tumors. A midline or bilateral subcostal incision (Fig. 7.11-8) is used, with the patient in the supine position. The left adrenal is accessed by incising the lateral peritoneal attachments of the spleen. The spleen and tail of the pancreas are rotated medially, exposing Gerota's fascia, which is then incised at the upper pole of the kidney, exposing the adrenal gland. A combination of blunt and sharp dissection is used to mobilize the gland and expose the adrenal vein, which is ligated between ties, and the gland is removed. The right gland is exposed by retracting the liver cephalad and depressing the hepatic flexure inferiorly. The peritoneum is then incised lateral to the duodenum and the inferior vena cava (IVC) is exposed. The right kidney is pulled down and the right adrenal vein entering the IVC is identified. The adrenal vein is ligated and the gland is removed.

Open extraperitoneal approach (flank): Before the advent of laparoscopic surgery, this approach was favored to minimize pain and improve postop recovery of adrenalectomy through use of smaller incision size and by remaining extraperitoneal. In general, this approach is best used for unilateral, smaller tumors. The patient is placed in the prone jackknife position and a dorsal curved flank incision is made, exposing the 12th rib. The rib is resected and Gerota's fascia is identified and incised, and the adrenal gland is resected.

Laparoscopic anterior transperitoneal approach: This approach may be used for bilateral adrenalectomy with the patient in the supine position. The surgical plan is similar to that of the transabdominal open approach, but is associated with longer operating times and additional trocar sites for placement of more retractors to mobilize the intraabdominal organs.

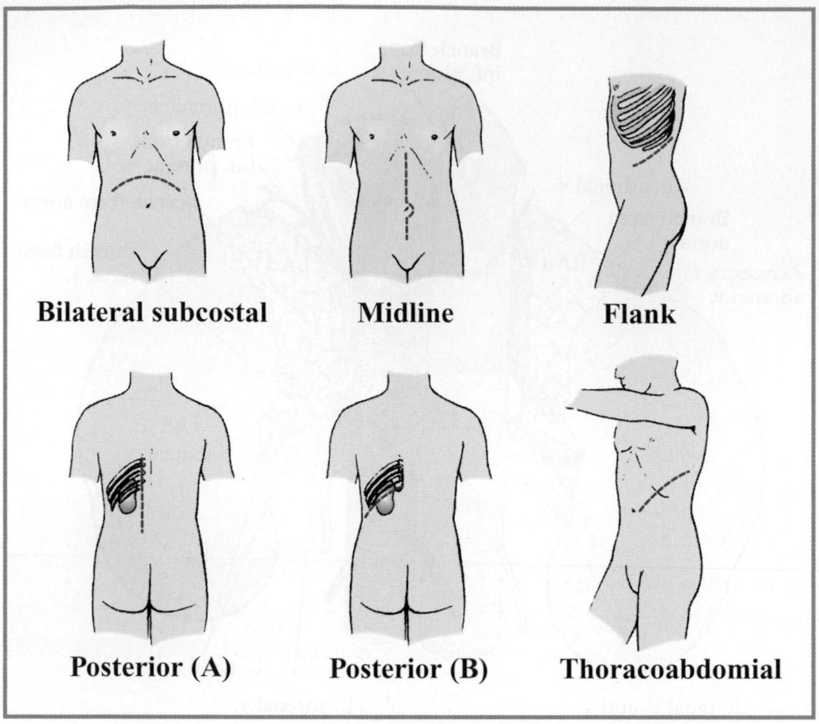

Figure 7.11-8. Potential incisions for adrenalectomy. (Reproduced with permission from Baker RJ, Fischer JE: *Mastery of Surgery,* 4th edition. Lippincott Williams & Wilkins, Philadelphia: 2001.)

Laparoscopic lateral transperitoneal approach: This is the preferred approach for adrenalectomy in most centers. The patient is positioned in the lateral decubitus position with the operative site up, and is immobilized with a carefully placed beanbag to minimize nerve compression injuries. The patient is prepped for either an open or laparoscopic approach (so that conversion to an open procedure may be done swiftly, if necessary). If both adrenal glands are to be removed, the right is done first, because there is a slightly higher risk of converting to an open procedure because of the proximity of the adrenal vein to the IVC.

For **right adrenalectomy,** pneumoperitoneum (15 mmHg) is established, with a Veress needle placed in the midclavicular line below the right costal margin. A 5 mm liver retractor is placed, as are two operating trocar sites (usually a 5 mm and a 10 mm or 12 mm port) (Fig. 7.11-9). The liver is retracted cephalad and the retroperitoneum incised with hook cautery. The right renal vein is dissected out carefully and ligated with clips. Dissection of the gland then proceeds from medial to lateral and inferior to superior. The gland is removed through a laparoscopic retrieval bag.

The **left adrenal gland** is approached in a similar fashion, with the Veress needle being placed in the left midclavicular line just below the costal margin. After placement of additional trocars, the peritoneum lateral to the spleen and the splenorenal ligament are incised. With the patient in the decubitus position, gravity will help pull the spleen medially, exposing the anterior surface of the kidney (Fig. 7.11-10). The inferior and medial edges of the gland are dissected first, and the left adrenal vein is identified. After the vein is clipped, the remainder of the gland may be dissected free and the gland removed as above.

Usual preop diagnosis: Hyperaldosteronism; hypercortisolism; pheochromocytoma; metastatic tumor; metastasis; lymphoma; angiomyolipoma; adrenal adenoma; adenocarcinoma

SUMMARY OF PROCEDURES

	Open Adrenalectomy	Laparoscopic Adrenalectomy
Position	Transperitoneal: supine; extraperitoneal: prone jackknife	Transperitoneal anterior: supine; transperitoneal lateral: decubitus

■ **SUMMARY OF PROCEDURES (cont'd)**

	Open Adrenalectomy	Laparoscopic Adrenalectomy
Incision	Transperitoneal: midline or bilateral subcostal (Fig. 7.11-8); extraperitoneal: dorsal flank oblique or curved posterior	Transperitoneal anterior: 4–5 trocar incisions (Fig. 7.11-9); transperitoneal lateral: 3–4 trocar incisions
Special instrumentation	Transperitoneal: Denier or Bookwalter retractor; extraperitoneal: none	Transabdominal anterior/lateral: video set-up
Unique considerations	BP monitoring essential for pheochromocytoma patients	⇐
Antibiotics	None	⇐
Surgical time	1–2 h	1–3 h
Closing considerations	Hemostasis; hemodynamic stability	⇐
EBL	100–250 mL	⇐
Postop care	Continue monitoring BP; PACU → ward; ± ICU, based on hemodynamic stability	⇐
Mortality	< 0.5%	⇐
Morbidity	Overall: 1–12% Bleeding: < 10% Pancreatic fistula: < 1% DVT: 0.8% PE: 0.5% Renovascular HTN: < 1% Peroneal nerve palsy: < 1% Venous thrombosis with embolism (Cushing's): 2%	⇐ ⇐ ⇐ ⇐ ⇐ ⇐ ⇐ ⇐
Pain score	6–8	5–6

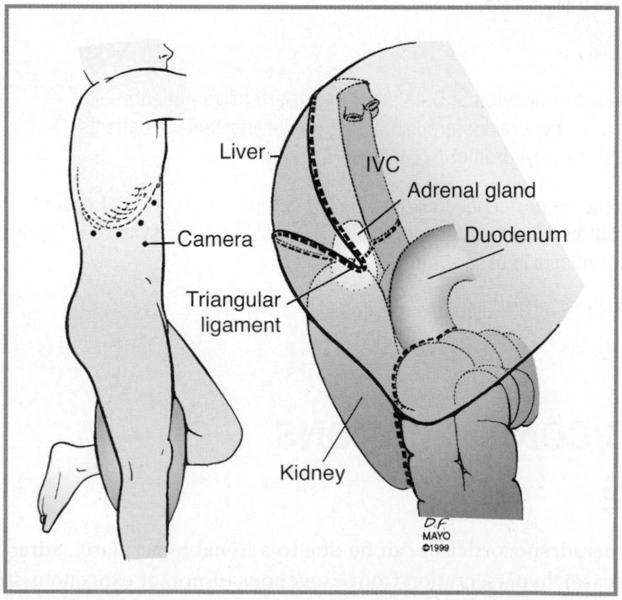

Figure 7.11-9. Port placement for laparoscopic right adrenalectomy. Relevant anatomy is displayed through the right lobe of the liver. (Reproduced with permission from Baker RJ, Fischer JE: *Mastery of Surgery,* 4th edition. Lippincott Williams & Wilkins, Philadelphia: 2001.)

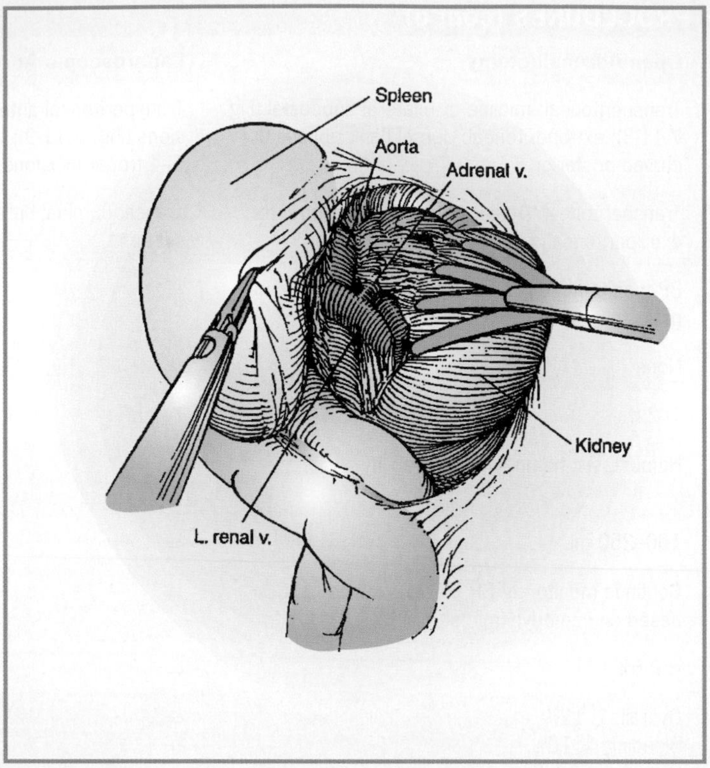

Figure 7.11-10. Exposure of left adrenal after mobilization of the spleen. (Reproduced with permission from Baker RJ, Fischer JE: *Mastery of Surgery,* 4th edition. Lippincott Williams & Wilkins, Philadelphia: 2001.)

PATIENT POPULATION CHARACTERISTICS	
Age range	13–75 yr
Male:Female	1:2.8
Incidence	Pheochromocytoma: 0.4–2% of all hypertensive patients Primary hyperaldosteronism: ~4% of all hypertensive patients Cushing's syndrome: 6/1 million
Etiology	Adenoma or adenocarcinoma (90%); ectopic ACTH (15% of patients with Cushing's); Cushing's syndrome (hyperadrenocorticism) (10–15%); Conn's syndrome (hyperaldosteronism). Idiopathic hyperplasia is usually treated medically.
Associated conditions	HTN (75–80%); diabetes mellitus (10–15%)

ANESTHETIC CONSIDERATIONS

PREOPERATIVE

Cushing's syndrome: Hyperadrenocorticism can be due to adrenal hyperplasia, adrenal carcinoma, pituitary hypersecretion (Cushing's disease), hypersecretion from exogenous tumor, or exogenous steroid administration (most common). Adrenalectomy is the traditional treatment for hyperadrenocorticism 2° adrenal carcinoma. These typically moon-faced patients present with one or more of the following: HTN 2° glucocorticoids, renin (usually not severe); renal calculi; osteoporosis; glucose intolerance; personality changes; and myopathy. In addition, a fragile vasculature predisposes these patients to easy bruising and difficult vascular access.

Respiratory	Patient may be obese with all attendant problems of morbid obesity (see Preoperative Considerations in Operations for Morbid Obesity, p. 502). **Tests:** As indicated from H&P.
Cardiovascular	HTN, hypervolemia, dysrhythmias 2° hypokalemia **Tests:** ECG; orthostatic vital signs; consider ECHO or MUGA scan, to evaluate LV function, if indicated from H&P.
Renal	Excess steroid production → Na^+ retention, K^+ excretion and glucose intolerance (hyperglycemia). **Tests:** UA; creatinine; glucose; urine concentrations of catecholamine metabolites; others as appropriate
Neurological	Psychiatric changes, headache
Musculoskeletal	Striae, muscular wasting, buffalo hump, truncal obesity, thin skin, easy bruisability, osteopenia (compression fractures), weakness
Hematologic	Polycythemia
Laboratory	Tests as indicated from H&P.
Premedication	Midazolam (1–2 mg iv), consider withhold if morbidly obese

Conn's syndrome: Hyperaldosteronism can be primary (Conn's syndrome–adrenal adenoma or hyperplasia) or secondary (caused by excess renin secretion related to renal dysfunction). These patients are typically hypokalemic and alkalotic → muscle weakness, paresthesias, tetany and polyuria. They may also be hypervolemic → CHF, hypernatremic and hypertensive (diastolic).

Respiratory	Respiratory muscle weakness. **Tests:** As indicated from H&P.
Cardiovascular	HTN, dysrhythmias, T wave, + U wave **Tests:** ECG; orthostatic vital signs; consider ECHO or MUGA scan, to evaluate LV function, if indicated from H&P.
Renal	Renal HTN, polyuria, polydipsia, K^+, Na^+. Correction of hypokalemia requires > 24 h supplemental K infusion (e.g., 5–20 mEq/h). **Tests:** UA; creatinine; glucose; urine concentrations of catecholamine metabolites; others as appropriate
Musculoskeletal	Conn's syndrome: muscle weakness, tetany, sensitivity to muscle relaxants, osteoporosis
Laboratory	Tests as indicated from H&P.
Premedication	Spironolactone often given to inhibit excess aldosterone effects. Midazolam (1–2 mg iv); hydrocortisone 100 mg q 8 h.

INTRAOPERATIVE

Anesthetic technique: GETA (± epidural for postop analgesia). If postop epidural analgesia is planned, placement of catheter prior to anesthetic induction is helpful in establishing correct placement in the epidural space and assuring a bilateral block (accomplished by placing 5–7 mL of 1% lidocaine via the epidural and eliciting a segmental block). Epidurals cannot be used for a posterior approach since they are in the operative field.

Induction	Gentle iv induction (titration to effect with STP or etomidate) and muscle relaxation (vecuronium 0.1 mg/kg). Patient should be adequately anesthetized prior to any stimulation. Unopposed parasympathetic response to laryngoscopy may → bradycardia/asystole.

Maintenance	Volatile anesthetic (isoflurane), opiate, muscle relaxant. N_2O may cause bowel distention and is best avoided. Local anesthetic (2% lidocaine 3–5 mL q 60 min) can be injected into the epidural catheter to provide both anesthesia and optimal surgical exposure (contracted bowel and profound muscle relaxation). A continuous infusion of local anesthetic (e.g., 2% lidocaine or 0.25% bupivacaine) at 3–5 mL/h may enhance hemodynamic stability. Some anesthesiologists will not use the epidural catheter intraop because chemical "sympathectomy" is more difficult to reverse. If epidural opiates are used for postop analgesia, a loading dose (e.g., hydromorphone 0.4–1.0 mg) should be administered at least 1 hour before the conclusion of surgery. Systemic sedatives (droperidol, opiates, benzodiazepines, etc.) should be minimized during this type of anesthetic as they increase the likelihood of postop respiratory depression.	
Emergence	Depends on ease of the surgical procedure and the hemodynamic stability of the patient intraop. If patient is hemodynamically unstable, hypothermic, or has a large 3rd-space fluid requirement, consider postop ventilation.	
Blood and fluid requirements	Anticipate large fluid loss. IV: 14–16 ga × 2 NS/LR @ 10–15 mL/kg/h Warm all fluids. ± Cell Saver	As blood loss can be significant, blood should be immediately available. If procedure does not involve cancer, cell-saving devices can be utilized. Guide fluid management by EBL, known volume deficits, UO, and filling pressures/CO if available.
Monitoring	Standard monitors (p. B-1) UO	Others as clinically indicated. Forced air warmer useful for maintaining body temperature.
Complications	Labile HTN	Surgical manipulation of the adrenal may cause ↑↑ BP and dysrhythmias. Rx: Alert surgeon and control BP with esmolol/SNP.
Positioning	✓ and pad pressure points ✓ eyes	Strict attention to patient positioning, padding and taping are important in patients with glucocorticoid excess because of osteopenia and thin, easily traumatized skin.

POSTOPERATIVE

Complications	Pneumothorax Hypoglycemia	Dx: pleuritic chest pain, dyspnea, ↑ RR, ↓ breath sounds, hypoxemia. ✓ CXR. Rx: O_2; chest tube and reintubation as necessary.
	Hypoadrenocorticism after tumor resection Cushing's syndrome: Hypoventilation 2° to obesity (hypoxemia, hypercarbia) HTN	Consider glucocorticoid and mineralocorticoid replacement—hydrocortisone 100 mg q 8 h.
Pain management	Epidural analgesia (p. C-1). PCA (p. C-3)	Patient should be recovered in an ICU or ward accustomed to treating the side effects of epidural opiates (e.g., respiratory depression, breakthrough pain, nausea, pruritus).
Tests	CXR; ECG; electrolytes; glucose	

ANESTHETIC CONSIDERATIONS FOR PHEOCHROMOCYTOMA

Pheochromocytoma: Tumors of chromaffin tissue origin release massive amounts of catecholamines (norepinephrine > epinephrine) and are responsible for the patient's clinical presentation. The tumor is usually found unilaterally in one of the adrenal glands, but also can be found anywhere in the body that chromaffin tissue arises (e.g., urinary bladder, sympathetic chain). There is an increased incidence of pheochromocytoma in certain diseases (multiple-endocrine neoplasia II, neurofibromatosis, tuberous sclerosis, Sturge-Weber syndrome, von Hippel-Lindau disease).

These patients require extensive preoperative preparation, consisting of α-blockade (phenoxybenzamine 40–400 mg/d × 2 wk) and should ideally be monitored closely by the anesthesiologist who is to provide the intraoperative management. In contrast to its use in essential HTN, ß-blockade is not indicated to control hypertension in patients with pheochromocytoma and is dangerous when used alone. When used alone, ß-blockade may cause serious hypertension, ↓ CO, intense vasoconstriction → CHF, organ ischemia, and shock (unopposed α-agonism). Patients with tachydysrhythmias may require some ß-blockade only after institution of the α-blockers to control reflex tachycardia. Titration of adrenergic blockade may take 2–4 wk prior to surgical removal of the tumor and should be titrated to relief of all episodic symptoms (HAs, sweating, palpitations) and control of blood pressure. Inadequate preop preparation will increase the perioperative morbidity of patients with pheochromocytomas. The adequacy of medical therapy is assessed by the absence of symptoms of catecholamine excess, BP in the normal range. "Resetting" of autoregulation, including cardiac "recovery" from catecholamine-induced myocarditis and organ recovery from ischemia, may be an important process that prepares the patient to tolerate the surgery and post-tumor removal period. It is anticipated that some degree of postural hypotension will be observed during titration of phenoxybenzamine. At a minimum, a BP of = 160/90 (usually much better than this can be achieved) on two measurements in the 36 hours preceding surgery, SBP dropping by > 15% on standing, but not less than an absolute BP of 80/45; no ST-T wave changes, and resolution of episodic symptoms, for 2 weeks prior to surgery is the goal. There is no rush to surgery.

Respiratory	Cardiogenic pulmonary edema
Cardiovascular	Paroxysmal/continuous HTN, tachydysrhythmias, orthostatic hypotension, hypovolemia, myocardial dysfunction, cardiomyopathy, ventricular ectopy, ↓ intravascular volume, ↓ sensitivity of α and β (cardiac)-receptors to normal levels of catecholamines, CHF, acute myocarditis. **Tests:** ECG; ± CK/TP enzymes, orthostatic vital signs; ECHO to evaluate LV function and mitral valve
Renal	HTN from excess catecholamine state may damage kidneys; hyperglycemia. **Tests:** UA; creatinine; glucose; urine concentrations of catecholamine metabolites; others as appropriate
Neurological	Sx include: Tremulousness, headache, anxiety, nervousness, personality changes, psychosis (rare), paresthesia in arms, hypertensive retinopathy, dilated pupils.
Musculoskeletal	Weight loss, weakness, fatigue
Hematologic	Polycythemia 2° hemoconcentration (common) or tumor erythropoietin production (rare)
Laboratory	Tests as indicated from H&P.
Premedication	Midazolam (0.025–0.05 mg/kg iv). Preop steroid replacement if bilateral adrenalectomy is contemplated.

Anesthetic technique: GETA: Consider establishing invasive hemodynamic monitoring (arterial and PA lines) PRIOR to induction (this is not difficult, can be done safely, and provides all hemodynamic information to the anesthesiologist from the start; and also lets the anesthesiologist pay attention to the patient at the start of the surgery, rather than being distracted with placing invasive lines after induction) using iv fentanyl (50–200 mcg) and generous local anesthesia. Femoral arterial pressure monitoring is preferred over radial artery, because of the concern over monitoring "central" arterial pressures in a patient who may experience high catecholamine levels during surgery with intense vasoconstriction. If postop epidural analgesia is planned (open surgical procedures), placement of catheter prior to anesthetic induction is helpful in establishing correct placement in the epidural space and assuring a bilateral block (accomplished by placing 5–7 mL of 2% lidocaine **without epinephrine)** via the epidural and eliciting a segmental block. Consider administering epidural narcotic (Dilaudid 0.4–1.0 mg) prior to skin incision. Epidurals cannot be used for a posterior approach since they are in the operative field. Epidurals are not indicated for laparoscopic procedures. Epidurals block neurally mediated sympathetic responses and may → ↓ tumor release of catecholamines, but do not block catecholamine release resulting from direct surgical manipulation of tumor. Local anesthetic-induced sympathetic block after tumor resection may compound ↓ BP at this important stage in the operation.

Induction	Gentle iv induction (titration to effect with propofol) and muscle relaxation (vecuronium 0.1 mg/kg). Deep mask GA prior to laryngoscopy. Consider double DL with LTA spray (4% lidocaine).	
Maintenance	Volatile anesthetic (isoflurane), opiate, muscle relaxant. Systemic sedatives (opiates, benzodiazepines, etc.) should be minimized during this type of anesthetic as they increase the likelihood of postop respiratory depression. **Intraop HTN Rx:** 1. Na nitroprusside 0.5–3.0 mcg/kg/min ± esmolol 50–300 mcg/kg/min 2. Fenoldopam 0.1–1 .5 mcg/kg/min 3. Nitroglycerin 0.5–10 mcg/kg/min The surgeon may need to stop manipulating the tumor in order to control BP. Lidocaine may be needed for ventricular ectopy (especially with epinephrine-secreting tumors). **Hypotension (after tumor removal) Rx:** 1. anticipation → fluid loading prior to tumor removal 2. fluid resuscitation based on PA pressures, TEE, stroke volume response 3. inotropes (epinephrine) if ↓ CO 4. vasopressor (phenylephrine, NE,) if ↓ MAP with normal/ ↑ CO Good communication with surgical team is very important, especially when the ↑↑ adrenal gland is being mobilized, and when the tumor veins are being ligated.	
Emergence	Depends on ease of the surgical procedure and the hemodynamic stability of the patient after tumor removal. If patient is hemodynamically unstable, hypothermic, or has a large 3rd-space fluid requirement, consider postop ventilation, as with any other surgical case. Most cases done laparoscopically can be extubated.	
Blood and fluid requirements	Prepare for large fluid loss (unusual). IV: 14–16 ga × 2 NS/LR @ 10–15 mL/kg/h Warm all fluids. ± Cell Saver	As blood loss can be significant, blood should be immediately available. If procedure does not involve cancer, cell-saving devices can be utilized. Guide fluid management by UO, filling pressures, CO, TEE.
Monitoring	Standard monitors (p. B-1) UO Arterial line (femoral artery) CVP/±PA catheter ± TEE	Others as clinically indicated (e.g., PA catheter for patients with pheochromocytoma). Forced air warmer useful for maintaining body temperature. The use of TEE may be helpful in establishing fluid status and other hemodynamic parameters.
Complications	↑↑↑ BP and dysrhythmias	Surgical manipulation of the adrenal will cause ↑↑ BP ± dysrhythmias. Rx: Alert surgeon and control BP with SNP/fenoldopam/TNG ± esmolol.
	↓↓ BP (postexcision – most dangerous part of anesthetic)	↓↓ BP common after removal of tumor. May be severe and life-threatening. Rx: anticipate event; fluids, phenylephrine or epinephrine infusions depending on need for inotropic support.
Positioning	✓ and pad pressure points ✓ eyes	

POSTOPERATIVE

Complications	Pneumothorax Hypoglycemia	Dx: pleuritic chest pain, dyspnea, ↑ RR, ↓ breath sounds, hypoxemia. ✓ CXR. Rx: O_2; chest tube and reintubation as necessary.
	Hypoadrenocorticism after tumor resection (usually only with bilateral tumors)	Consider glucocorticoid and mineralocorticoid replacement → hydrocortisone 100 mg q 8 h.
	HTN Hypotension Myocardial dysfunction Pulmonary edema	Patient may have other cause for HTN. Continue vasopressor/inotropes, fluids as indicated. Patient should be recovered in ICU overnight.
Pain management	Epidural analgesia (p. C-2). PCA (p. C-3)	Patient should be recovered in an ICU or ward accustomed to treating the side effects of epidural opiates (e.g., respiratory depression, breakthrough pain, nausea, pruritus).
Tests	CXR; ECG; electrolytes; glucose	

Suggested Readings

1. Brunt, LM: Laparoscopic adrenalectomy. In: *Current Surgical Therapy,* 7th edition. Cameron JL, eds. Mosby Inc., St. Louis: 2001, 1460–7.
2. Cooper ZA, Mihm FG: Blood pressure control with fenoldopam during excision of a pheochromocytoma *Anesthesiology* 1999; 91(2):558–60.
3. Kebebew E, Siperstein AE, Clark OH et al: Results of laparoscopic adrenalectomy for suspected and unsuspected malignant adrenal neoplasms. *Arch Surg* 2002; 137(8):948–53.
4. Mihm FG: Pheochromocytoma: decreased perioperative mortality *Anesth Clin North Am* 1998; 16(3):645–62.
5. Olson JA: Adrenal gland. In: *Greenfield's Surgery, Scientific Principles and Practice,* 4th edition. Mulholland MW, Lillemore ED, Doherty GM eds. Lippincott Williams & Wilkins, Philadelphia: 2006, 1334–53.
6. Prys-Roberts C: Phaeochromocytoma—recent progress in its management. *Br J Anaesth* 2000; 85:44–57.
7. Schwartz JJ, Rosenbaum SH: Anesthesia and the endocrine system. In: *Clinical Anesthesia,* 5th edition. Barash PG, Cullen BF, Stoelting RK, eds. Lippincott Williams & Wilkins, Philadelphia: 2006, 1129–51.
8. Sieber FE: Evaluation of the patient with endocrine disease and diabetes mellitus. In: *Principles and Practice of Anesthesiology,* 2nd edition. Longnecker DE, Tinker JH, Morgan GE Jr, eds. Mosby-Year Book, St Louis: 1998, 303–22.
9. Smith CD, Weber CJ, Amerson JR: Laparoscopic adrenalectomy: New gold standard. *World J Surg* 1999; 23(4):389–96.
10. Witteles RM, Kaplan EL, Roizen MF: Safe and cost-effective preoperative preparation of patients with pheochromocytoma. *Anesth Analg* 2000; 91:302–4.

CHAPTER

7.12 Liver/Kidney/Pancreas Transplantation

SURGEONS

Stephan Busque, MD, MSc, FRCSC (*Kidney, pancreas transplantation*)

Marc L. Melcher, MD, PhD (*Kidney, pancreas transplantation*)

Dev M. Desai, MD, PhD (*Liver transplantation*)

Carlos O. Esquivel, MD, PhD (*Liver transplantation*)

ANESTHESIOLOGISTS

Timothy Angelotti, MD, PhD (*Kidney, pancreas transplantation, multiorgan procurement*)

Hendrikus J.M. Lemmens, MD, PhD (*Liver transplantation*)

KIDNEY TRANSPLANTATION—CADAVERIC AND LIVE-DONOR

SURGICAL CONSIDERATIONS

Description: Kidney transplantation offers patients with end-stage renal disease (ESRD) freedom from dialysis. The source of the renal graft may be a cadaveric donor, a relative (e.g., parent, sibling) or a genetically unrelated, but emotionally related individual (e.g., spouse).

After induction of anesthesia, a 3-way Foley catheter is placed into the bladder. The kidney allograft is placed in the extraperitoneal iliac fossa. A curvilinear incision is made in the right or left lower quadrant. The retroperitoneal space is developed by retracting the peritoneum medially and cephalad exposing the iliac vessels. A self-retaining retractor is usually placed to maintain exposure. The external iliac artery and vein are identified and surrounding lymphatics are ligated and divided. Several centimeters of the vessels are mobilized. The external iliac vein is clamped first and the renal-vein-to-iliac-vein anastomosis is performed. Then the external iliac-artery-to-renal-artery anastomosis is performed and the clamps are released (Fig. 7.12-1). The patient should be euvolemic at this point; mannitol and/or furosemide can be given. The bladder is filled with an antibiotic irrigation solution to facilitate the implantation of the ureter. The spatulated ureter is anastomosed to the mucosa of the bladder. The detrusor muscle is then re-approximated over 3–4 cm of ureter to create an anti-reflux valve. The wound is closed, normally leaving native kidneys intact.

Variant procedure or approaches: Cadaveric or live-donor transplantation

Usual preop diagnosis: ESRD

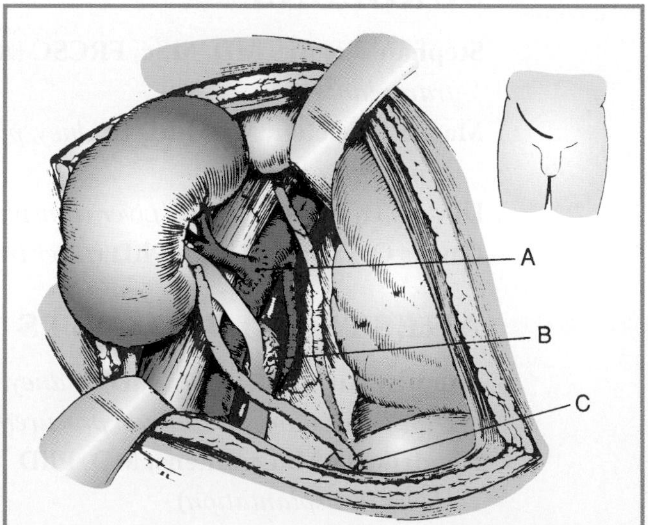

Figure 7.12-1. Kidney transplantation, showing anastomoses of: (A) renal artery to external iliac artery; (B) renal vein to iliac vein; and (C) ureter to bladder. To increase exposure of bladder for a ureteroneocystostomy, antibiotic solution is used to fill the bladder. Lower quadrant curvilinear incision is shown in inset. (Reproduced with permission from Hardy JD: *Hardy's Textbook of Surgery,* 2nd edition. JB Lippincott, Philadelphia: 1988.)

SUMMARY OF PROCEDURES

	Cadaveric Kidney	Live-Donor Kidney
Position	Supine	⇐
Incision	Lower quadrant curvilinear (Fig. 7.12-1 inset)	⇐
Special instrumentation	Self-retaining retractor; vascular instruments; CVP; Foley catheter (3-way)	⇐
Unique considerations	CVP 10–12 mmHg; mannitol 12.5–25 g; intraop immunosuppression before reperfusion (steroids, antilymphocyte preparation); potassium-free iv fluid; protection of shunt or fistula important.	⇐
Antibiotics	Cefazolin 1 g iv, 1 h preop	Cefazolin 1 g iv, 1 h preop
Surgical time	1.5–3 h	2–3 h
EBL	250 mL	⇐
Postop care	Replace UO mL/mL with i.v. fluids; may have delayed graft function 2° prolonged cold storage; ICU selectively	Fluid replacement; delayed graft function unlikely; ICU selectively
Mortality	1–2%	⇐
Morbidity	Lymph or serous leak/stenosis: 3–5%	⇐
	Postop bleeding: 3–5%	1–2%
	MI: 2–3%	⇐
	Ureteral leak/stenosis: 2–3%	⇐
	Wound infection: 2–3%	⇐
	Arterial thrombosis: 1–2%	⇐
	Venous thrombosis: 1–2%	⇐
	Wound hematoma: 1–2%	⇐
	Other infectious complications: 15–40%	⇐
Pain score	5	5

PATIENT POPULATION CHARACTERISTICS

Age range	3–70 yr
Male:Female	1:1
Incidence	60/1,000,000
Etiology	Glomerulonephritis (15%); HTN (20%); diabetes mellitus (45%); polycystic disease and others (20%)
Associated conditions	CAD (40%); HTN (25%); uremic and/or diabetic neuropathy (25%); hyperparathyroidism (15–20%)

ANESTHETIC CONSIDERATIONS

See Anesthetic Considerations following Cadaveric Kidney/Pancreas Transplantation, p. 684.

Suggested Readings

1. Flye MW, ed: *Atlas of Organ Transplantation.* WB Saunders, Philadelphia: 1995.
2. Kahan BD, Ponticelli C: *Principles and Practice of Renal Transplantation.* Martin Dunitz, Ltd., London: 2000.
3. Morris PJ: *Kidney Transplantation.* WB Saunders, Philadelphia: 2001.
4. Morris PJ: Renal transplantation: a quarter century. *Semin Nephrol* 1997; 17:188–95.
5. Odorico JS, Sollinger HW: Technical and immunosuppressive advances in transplantation for insulin-dependent diabetes mellitus. *World J Surg* 2002; 26:194–211.

CADAVERIC KIDNEY/PANCREAS TRANSPLANTATION

SURGICAL CONSIDERATIONS

Description: **Pancreas transplantation:** Combined kidney and pancreas transplantation not only provides renal replacement for the Type I diabetes patient with end-stage renal disease (ESRD), but also controls diabetes. Over eighty percent or more of pancreas transplants are performed in combination with kidney transplantation from the same donor (**simultaneous kidney/pancreas transplant [SPK]**). Pancreas transplantation also can be performed for patients who have already received a kidney transplant (**pancreas after kidney [PAK]**). Less commonly, pancreas transplantation is done for patients with brittle diabetes or with impending complications while they still enjoy normal or near-normal kidney function. Immunosuppression regimen for pancreas transplantation is generally more aggressive than that used for kidney transplantation, and induction therapy with antilymphocyte preparation (ATG, IL-2 blockers, OKT3) is commonly used. The pancreas transplant is placed in the right iliac fossa and the kidney transplant is placed in the left iliac fossa. This can be done through a transperitoneal lower midline incision or through two separate extraperitoneal lower-quadrant incisions in the same manner as kidney transplantation. The graft is first prepared on the back table. For arterial in-flow, a Y-graft is fashioned using the donor iliac artery bifurcation. The portal vein coming off the pancreatic graft is anastomosed to the external iliac vein. The Y extension vascular graft is then anastomosed to the recipient external or common iliac artery. The donor duodenum is anastomosed to a loop of small bowel or to the urinary bladder to drain the exocrine secretions (Fig. 7.12-2 A). With pancreas transplantation, there may be significant blood loss if the graft mesenteric vessels are not occluded properly. After the pancreas is implanted, the kidney transplant is placed into the opposite iliac fossa (as described in Kidney Transplantation, p. 680).

Variant procedure or approaches: The pancreas may be placed in the upper abdomen with the portal vein anastomosed to the superior mesenteric vein. The exocrine secretions are bowel-drained. This more physiologic approach, however, is associated with a higher technical failure rate and requires a long upper midline incision (Fig. 7.12-10). Pancreatic islet cells may be infused via a radiological **portal vein approach,** a procedure that is usually performed in the radiology/angio suite.

Usual preop diagnosis: ESRD 2° diabetes mellitus (DM)

SUMMARY OF PROCEDURE	
Position	Supine; cushion heels
Incision	Midline or bilateral lower quadrant
Special instrumentation	Thompson retractor; vascular instruments; Foley catheter; NG tube; CVP; arterial line
Unique considerations	Do not correct hyperglycemia < 300 mg/dl. Maintain adequate hydration, CVP 10–12 mmHg; mannitol 0.25–0.5 g/kg on unclamping; intraop immunosuppression before reperfusion (125–250 mg methylprednisolone, monoclonal or polyclonal preparation [e.g., ATG, Zenepax, OKT3, Simulect]).
Antibiotics	Piperacillin (Zosyn) 3.375 g iv q 6 h × 5 d; fluconazole 200–400 mg (nl creatine clearance)
Surgical time	4–6 h
EBL	250–500 mL
Postop care	ICU × 1–2 d, hourly monitoring of glucose; serum glucose should decline by 50 mg/dl each h and remain < 200 mg/dl.
Mortality	2%
Morbidity	Thrombosis of graft: 5–10% Postop bleeding: 5–10% Wound infection: 2–6%

SUMMARY OF PROCEDURE (cont'd)	
Morbidity (cont'd)	Pancreatitis: 2–4% Anastomotic leak: 1%
Pain score	7

PATIENT POPULATION CHARACTERISTICS	
Age range	15–55 yr
Male:Female	1:1
Incidence	15–20% of all patients with ESRD
Etiology	Type I diabetes
Associated conditions	Retinopathy (100%); uremic and/or diabetic neuropathy (50%); CAD (25–50%); gastropathy (25%); hyperparathyroidism (15–20%)

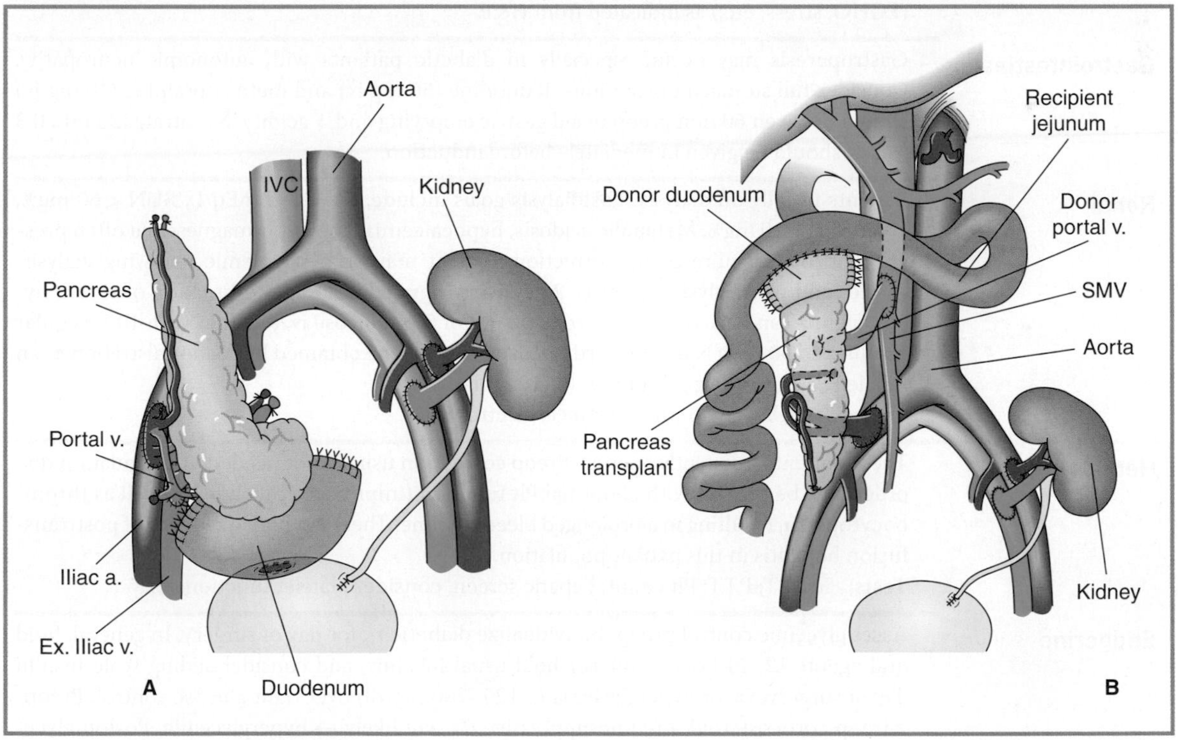

Figure 7.12-2. **(A)** SPK transplantation, with drainage of pancreatic exocrine secretions into the bladder. Note that portal vein drains into iliac vein (systemic venous [SV] drainage). In normal individuals, 50% of secreted insulin is extracted from the circulation in the first pass through the liver. Transplant recipients with SV have peripheral insulin levels 2-2½ × higher than normal. **(B)** SPK transplantation with drainage of pancreatic exocrine secretions into the proximal jejunum (enteric drainage [ED]). This technique has been adopted for SPK by most transplant centers in the U.S. For solitary pancreas transplantation, most centers still utilize ED to allow monitoring of the urinary amylase. Note that donor portal vein drains into the recipient superior mesenteric vein (portal venous [PV] drainage) preventing peripheral hyperinsulinemia. Most centers continue to place the pancreas in the pelvis, combining ED and SV, which requires enteric anastomosis to a more distal segment of jejunum or ilium. (Reproduced with permission from Greenfield LJ, et al, eds: *Surgery: Scientific Principles and Practice,* 3rd edition. Lippincott Williams & Wilkins, Philadelphia: 2001.)

ANESTHETIC CONSIDERATIONS FOR KIDNEY AND KIDNEY/PANCREAS TRANSPLANTATION

PREOPERATIVE

Typically, patients presenting for renal transplantation fall into two patient populations: (1) the young and relatively healthy (following dialysis), or (2) an older, more chronically ill group. Rarely, patients will present for transplant surgery without adequate preparation (e.g., ↑K^+, ↓pH, hypervolemia). Patients presenting for pancreas transplantation are usually severe diabetics with many of the associated problems, such as CAD, autonomic neuropathy, gastroparesis, and stiff-joint syndrome (difficult intubation).

Respiratory	Pleuritis and pleural effusions may occur in this patient population. Increased susceptibility to infection is common in the patient with chronic uremia.
Cardiovascular	Pericarditis (acute or constrictive), HTN, CHF, dysrhythmias, pericardial effusion are common, especially in the undialyzed patient. Diabetes, a common cause of ESRD, is often associated with PVD, CAD, and autonomic neuropathy. **Tests:** ECG (rhythm, CAD, electrolyte abnormalities, pericarditis, LVH). Other tests (ECHO, stress, etc.) as indicated from H&P.
Gastrointestinal	Gastroparesis may occur, especially in diabetic patients with autonomic neuropathy. Consider full stomach precautions. Ranitidine (50 mg iv) and metoclopramide (10 mg iv) should be given 60 min preop to aid gastric emptying and ↓ acidity. Na citrate (30 mL, 0.3 M po) should be given immediately before induction.
Renal	Patients usually on dialysis. Postdialysis goals include: K^+ = 4–5 mEq/L, BUN < 60 mg%, creatinine < 10 mg%. Metabolic acidosis, hypocalcemia, and hypermagnesemia often present, and may require preop correction. Patient may be hypovolemic following dialysis; ✓ pre- and postdialysis weight (> 2 kg loss is significant). Rapid correction of severe hyperkalemia can be achieved by giving 50 mL of 50% glucose iv, together with 10 U regular insulin and 50 mEq NaHCO. Further correction can be obtained by coadministration of an inhaled β-agonist (e.g., albuterol) (5–10 puffs). **Tests:** Cr; BUN; creatinine clearance; electrolytes
Hematologic	These patients frequently anemic. Preop correction usually not needed. A coagulation disorder may be present with abnormal Plt function (improved by dialysis) as well as thrombocytopenia, resulting in a prolonged bleeding time. There is a high incidence of posttransfusion hepatitis in this patient population. **Tests:** Hct; PT; PTT; Plt count; hepatic screen, consider platelet function assay.
Endocrine	Asses glycemic control preop. Individualize diabetic rx for day of surgery. In general, hold oral agents 12–24 hours, and ↓or hold usual insulins, and consider sliding scale insulin day of surgery. Favor hyperglycemia (≥ 120–200 mg/dl) over tight glucose control. Preop/intraop corticosteroid immunosuppressive Rx will likely → hyperglycemia. Postop glycemic management complex and dynamic. **Tests:** Serial glucose levels
Neurologic	Peripheral neuropathy may occur and specific deficits should be documented. Autonomic neuropathy can → cardiac problems (e.g., orthostatic hypotension, ↑HR, or ↓HR), silent MI, and GI problems.
Premedication	Consider midazolam 1–2 mg iv.

INTRAOPERATIVE

Anesthetic technique: GETA favored. Spinal, epidural, or combined spinal-epidural anesthesia may be considered for renal transplantation, if coagulation and platelet function acceptable. Avoidance of hypotension after organ(s) transplanted an important consideration which may limit effectiveness of RA techniques.

Induction	Rapid-sequence induction (see p. B-4). ET intubation is aided by succinylcholine (1 mg/kg), if K^+ < 5.5 mEq/L; otherwise, use cisatracurium (0.2–0.5 mg/kg) or rocuronium (1.2 mg/kg). Fentanyl (2–5 mcg/kg) may be used to suppress the cardiovascular response to intubation.	
Maintenance	Standard maintenance (see p. B-2). Maintain muscle relaxation with cisatracurium or rocuronium, titrated to effect using a nerve stimulator. Avoid meperidine (accumulation of normeperidine → CNS toxicity). Anticipate prolonged drug effects, and avoid agents that are primarily excreted by the kidney.	
Emergence	Usually extubated in the OR after protective laryngeal reflexes have returned. Ensure adequate reversal of NMB's drugs. Pancreatic transplant patients (e.g., brittle diabetics, hemodynamically unstable) are sent to the ICU for close glycemic management.	
Blood and fluid requirements	IV: 14–16 ga × 1 NS/colloid to keep CVP = 10–15 mmHg Warm fluids	Preop fluid status is highly variable (hypo→ hypervolemia). Give fluids to maintain CVP 10–15 mmHg. Important to maintain adequate vascular volume and BP. Mannitol (0.25–1 g/kg), furosemide (5–20 mg), and low-dose dopamine are often given with reperfusion of the kidney.
Monitoring	Standard monitors (see p. B-1). Arterial line CVP/PA line	Arterial pressure is often monitored. Avoid the side of AV fistulae. Axillary artery is a useful alternative. CVP is essential and a PA line is needed occasionally (severe cardiac disease). CVP is kept at 10–15 mmHg, especially after the new kidney is reperfused, to ensure adequate renal blood flow.
	Hct, K+, and glucose	In pancreatic transplant patients, glucose should be checked q 30 min and then q 10 min for the first h following reperfusion. Keep glucose < 300 mg/dl prior to reperfusion, but do not fully correct to < 150 mg/dl.
	Neuromuscular	Monitor neuromuscular block to avoid excessive use of neuromuscular relaxants; anticipate prolonged effects.
Positioning	✓ and pad pressure points ✓ eyes Protect/pad AV fistulas	Pressure on AV fistula may lead to thrombosis. Carefully pad and protect.
Complications	Disruption of renal anastomoses Hemorrhage Low UO Reperfusion injury (pancreas transplant)	Bucking or coughing during emergence, due to inadequate neuromuscular blockade, may → forceful tugging on transplanted kidney. This "popping" of kidney may → disruption of venous and arterial anastomoses and possible ischemic damage requiring urgent surgical revision.

POSTOPERATIVE

Complications	Fluid overload and CHF Femoral neuropathy Hemorrhage Electrolyte abnormalities	Monitor UO. Dialysis may be needed until renal function returns. Sudden cardiac arrest can complicate pancreatic transplantation (due to autonomic neuropathy).
	Hypo/hyperglycemia	Especially dynamic in pancreas tx
	PONV	see p. B-6
	VTE	see p. B-7

Pain management	PCA (see p. C-3) Epidural	Anticipate prolonged effect of some opiates. Strive to avoid hypotension.
Tests	Hct Electrolytes Cr, BUN Amylase Glucose	A rise in amylase and blood glucose may indicate failure of the pancreatic transplant.

Suggested Readings

1. Hadimioglu N. Ertug Z. Bigat Z. Yilmaz M. Yegin A: A randomized study comparing combined spinal epidural or general anesthesia for renal transplant surgery. *Transplant Proc* 2005; 37(5):2020–2.
2. Halpern H. Miyoshi E. Kataoka LM. Khouri Fo RA. Miranda SB. Marumo CK. Omati O. Genzini T. Miranda MP. Anesthesia for pancreas transplantation alone or simultaneous with kidney. *Transplant Proc* 2004; 36(10):3105–6.
3. Lemmens, HJM. Kidney transplantation: recent developments and recommendations for anesthetic management. *Anesthesiol Clin North Am* 2004; 22(4):651–62.

LIVE-DONOR NEPHRECTOMY—LAPAROSCOPIC AND OPEN

SURGICAL CONSIDERATIONS

Description: Use of a kidney donated by a healthy genetically or emotionally related donor greatly increases the number and quality of kidneys available for transplantation. Kidney transplantation from living donors is associated with a better patient and graft survival rate. **A laparoscopic (LSC) approach** for kidney donation was introduced in 1995 as an alternative that would reduce postop pain, wound morbidity, and recovery time associated with open nephrectomy. Now the LSC approach is the procedure of choice for more than 75% of the live kidney donations in the United States. Initial concerns regarding ureteral complications and longer warm ischemic time have mostly subsided with the improvement of the surgical technique and greater experience. The left kidney is preferred for the LSC approach, as the renal vein is longer. Some centers use the LSC approach for the right kidney with comparable results.

The patient is positioned in lateral decubitus over a cushioned beanbag, the kidney rest is slightly elevated, and pillows and an axillary roll are used to prevent compression injuries. Three or four ports are used. The pneumoperitoneum is kept < 15 mmHg to avoid decreased perfusion to the kidney. Aggressive hydration and intermittent use of IV mannitol help improve kidney perfusion. On the left side, the descending colon and spleen are mobilized medially; the renal vessels are exposed; the adrenal, lumbar, and gonadal veins are clipped and divided; the ureter is mobilized en bloc, along with the gonadal vein, down to the pelvic inlet. The artery is freed from surrounding lymphatic and neural tissue as it comes off the aorta (Fig. 7.12-3). Gerota's fascia is mobilized to completely free the kidney. The ureter is transected distally. A 6-cm suprapubic incision is made, the peritoneum is exposed in the midline, and an 18-mm port is used to insert a 15-mm Endocatch retrieval bag. The kidney is placed in the bag as it continues to be perfused, avoiding warm ischemia. The patient is fully heparinized. An endo GIA vascular stapler is used to staple and transect the artery close to the aorta and the vein close to the vena cava. An endo TA vascular stapler can also be used. It may add safety and vessel length. The retrieval bag is brought to the suprapubic incision and gently extracted. The kidney is immediately immersed in the cold slush solution, and the staple lines are cut off the renal artery and vein. The kidney is perfused with preservation solution in the usual manner. The heparin is reversed with protamine, the suprapubic incision is closed, and homeostasis is verified before extracting the ports. For a right nephrectomy, the right colon and duodenum are mobilized medially and the liver is retracted upward. The remainder of the operation is as described for the left kidney. The surgeon's hand may be inserted in the abdomen to help with the stapling of the vessels and kidney retrieval.

The **hand-assisted laparoscopic donor nephrectomy** is similar to the pure laparoscopic approach described earlier; however, a midline 8–10-cm incision is made at the level of the umbilicus or infra-umbilical to position a device (e.g.,

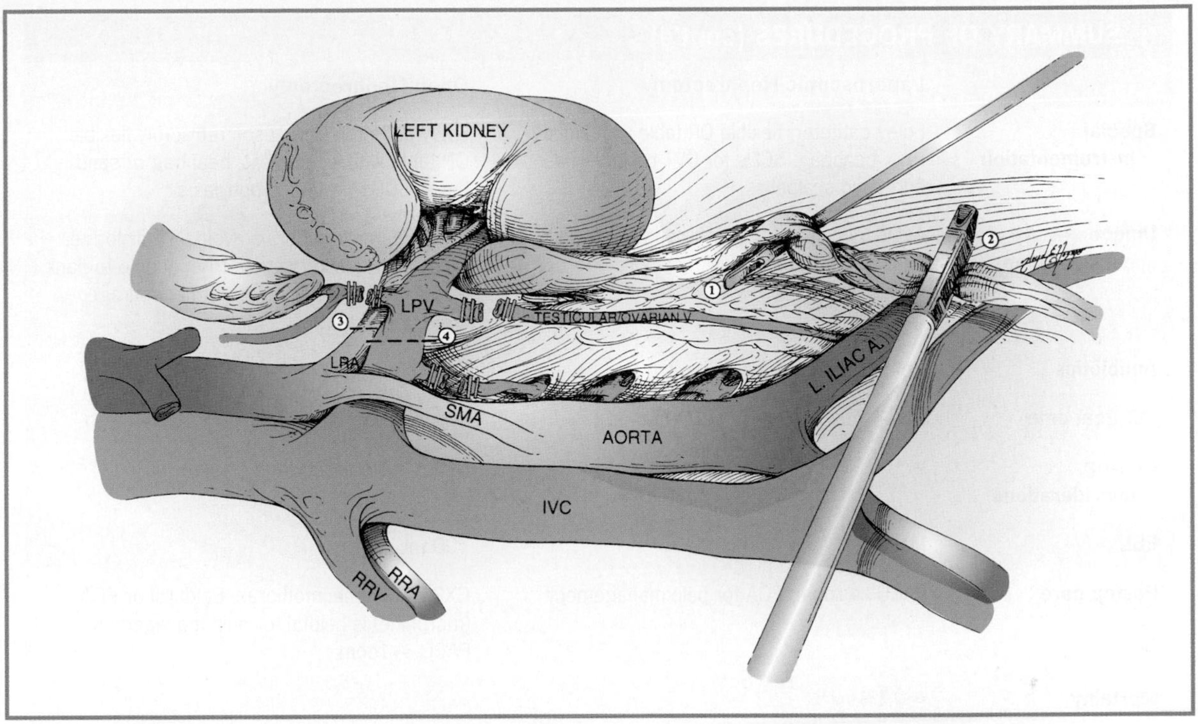

Figure 7.12-3. Anatomy for laparoscopic live-donor nephrectomy. (Reproduced with permission from Cho ES, Flowers JL: Laparoscopic live-donor nephrectomy. In *Surgical Laparoscopy,* 2nd edition. Zuker KA, ed. Lippincott Williams & Wilkins, Philadelphia: 2001.)

Gelport, Lapdisc) that allows the surgeon to put one hand inside the abdomen without losing the pneumoperitoneum. The hand is used to help with retraction and exposure to the kidney. The warm ischemia time (clamping of the renal artery to perfusion) is reduced 50%. Operative time also may be reduced. This approach requires a longer abdominal incision and could be associated with slightly more wound complications than the pure laparoscopic approach. The hand-assisted approach has gained popularity over the years and it is now the preferred technique of a majority of Transplant Centers in the United States.

In **open nephrectomy,** the **donor/patient** is placed in a lateral decubitus position on a flexible OR table with a kidney rest. A beanbag or sandbags are also helpful for positioning. An incision is made from the rectus muscle, angling slightly cephalic to cross into the flank just below the tip of the 12th rib. The retroperitoneum is exposed using a Thompson retractor. The kidney is then mobilized and the ureter is transected. A clamp is placed across the renal artery at the aorta and the renal vein at the IVC. Just before clamping the renal artery, furosemide and/or mannitol may be given to stimulate diuresis. It is important to keep the vascular volume expanded in these patients before kidney removal. The kidney is removed and taken to the back table where it is flushed with a cold preservation solution. It is then transported into the recipient room for reimplantation. Some surgeons use a full dose of heparin (75 U/kg) before clamping and use protamine afterwards. Smaller incisions and muscle-sparing incisions are now used to improve postop recovery.

Usual preop diagnosis: Donor nephrectomy

SUMMARY OF PROCEDURES

	Laparoscopic Nephrectomy	Open Nephrectomy
Position	Lateral decubitus	⇐
Incision	3–4 ports; retrieval incision, Pfannenstiel's or vertical suprapubic	Flank; may require 12th rib resection

SUMMARY OF PROCEDURES (cont'd)

	Laparoscopic Nephrectomy	Open Nephrectomy
Special instrumentation	Foley catheter; flexible OR table with kidney rest; beanbag; SCDs for DVT prophylaxis; harmonic scalpel	Foley catheter; Thompson retractor; flexible OR table with kidney rest; beanbag or sandbags; SCDs for DVT prophylaxis
Unique considerations	Avoid ETT dislodgement when turning patient from supine to flank position; vigorous hydration.	Possible pneumothorax; avoid ETT dislodgement when turning patient from supine to flank position. Vigorous hydration to encourage urine production.
Antibiotics	Cefazolin 1 g iv	Cefazolin 1 g, iv
Surgical time	2.5–4.5 h	2–2.5 h
Closing considerations	–	Delfex table to facilitate closure
EBL	Minimal	100 mL
Postop care	PACU → room; PCA for pain management	CXR to r/o pneumothorax. Epidural or PCA (morphine) is helpful for pain management. PACU → room.
Mortality	< 0.1%	⇐
Morbidity	Ileus: 2–5% Urinary retention: 2–5% Wound infection: 1–2% Bleeding: 0.1–0.5%	5–10% 5–10% 1–3% Pneumothorax: 1%
Pain score	3–5	7

PATIENT POPULATION CHARACTERISTICS

Age range	18–70 yr
Male:Female	1:1
Incidence	Up to 50% of all kidney transplants at some centers
Etiology	N/A
Associated conditions	Good health is mandatory for renal donation.

ANESTHETIC CONSIDERATIONS

See Anesthetic Considerations following Kidney Transplant Nephrectomy, p. 690.

KIDNEY TRANSPLANT NEPHRECTOMY

SURGICAL CONSIDERATIONS

Description: With improvements in graft survival and immunosuppressive therapy, the necessity of removing a kidney transplant graft for uncontrolled rejection has decreased significantly. This operation is divided into categories: **early nephrectomy,** performed during the first month post-transplant, and **late nephrectomy,** thereafter. **Early transplant nephrectomy** may be required for primary nonfunction, vascular thrombosis, and, rarely, refractory rejection. In these cases, an **extracapsular approach,** through the original transplant incision, is used. The kidney is freed up from the surrounding adhesion to obtain vascular control of the renal artery and renal vein. These structures are clamped and oversewn individually. The ureter is ligated as close as possible to the bladder and excised completely, with primary repair of the bladder. A suction drain is used if minimal oozing or lymph drainage is present. **Late transplant nephrectomy** is performed most commonly for acute, irreversible rejection with failure of the renal allograft. Most of these patients have returned to dialysis and the immunosuppressive medications are stopped. Chronic infection and HTN associated with nonfunctional grafts are also an indication for surgical removal of the kidney allograft. It may be a difficult operation, as intense inflammatory adhesions are present between the renal capsule and the surrounding tissue. In the setting of acute late rejection, the graft is usually swollen and enlarged. Hematuria may be present, and the graft is friable. Spontaneous rupture and hemorrhage have been reported. The surgical approach is through the same incision as the implantation. In contrast to early transplant nephrectomy, extracapsular dissection may not be possible with late nephrectomy. To avoid injury to extrarenal structures, such as the iliac vessels, an **intracapsular approach** may be preferred. The kidney is mobilized gently from within the capsule toward the hilum. The capsule is reopened on the medial side to have access to the renal vessel high in the hilum. When the hilum is sufficiently mobilized, a strong vascular clamp is applied high in the hilum of the kidney away from the iliac vessels. After clamping the hilum en bloc, confirmation of distal pulses is obtained; then the kidney is excised over the vascular clamp. A running suture is used over the clamp, which is then released, and hemostasis is obtained. The ureter is identified and excised as close as possible to the bladder. The intracapsular dissection of the kidney may be associated with significant bleeding, as the kidney may fracture. This step should be done expeditiously to avoid excessive bleeding. The patient must have good vascular access for fluid resuscitation. Blood must be available for transfusion. After hemostasis is obtained, a low-pressure suction drain may be placed before closing.

Usual preop diagnosis: Transplant rejection

SUMMARY OF PROCEDURE	
Position	Supine
Incision	Previous incision used for kidney transplant
Instrumentation	Self-retaining retractor; vascular instruments
Unique considerations	Large-bore vascular access; PRBCs available; stress dose of steroids, if chronic usage; protection of shunt or fistula
Antibiotics	Cefazolin 1 g iv
Surgical time	1–2.5 hr
EBL	200–1000 mL
Postop care	PCA for pain management → PACU → room
Mortality	1–3%
Morbidity	Overall: 3–5% Wound infection: 3–5% Abscess formation: 1–2% Exsanguinating hemorrhage: < 1%
Pain score	5

PATIENT POPULATION CHARACTERISTICS	
Age range	3–75 yr
Male:Female	1:1
Incidence	60/1,000,000
Etiology	Failed kidney transplant
Associated conditions	CAD (40%); HTN (25%); uremic and/or diabetic neuropathy (25%); hyperparathyroidism (15–20%)

ANESTHETIC CONSIDERATIONS FOR LIVE-DONOR AND POSTTRANSPLANTATION NEPHRECTOMY

PREOPERATIVE

In order to be a live donor, one must be in good health with bilaterally functional kidneys. Diabetes, HIV infection, liver disease, and malignancy are all contraindications to kidney donations.

Cardiovascular	Assess for HTN and CAD
Renal	Normal bilateral renal function is required. **Tests:** IVP; Cr, creatinine clearance
Fluid status	Adequate hydration is important and UO should be >1.5 mL/kg/h. Various regimes are used to ensure adequate hydration, usually with iv fluid starting the night before.
Premedication	Consider midazolam 1–2 mg iv. Organ donors are making a great sacrifice and should be treated with special care. Standard premedication (see p. B-1).

INTRAOPERATIVE

Anesthetic technique: GETA ± epidural for postop pain management. Epidurals are not necessary for most laparoscopic donor nephrectomies.

Induction	Standard induction (see p. B-2).	
Maintenance	Standard maintenance (see p. B-2). Avoid long-acting, renally excreted drugs. Ventilate to maintain normocapnia to avoid possible renal artery vasoconstriction. Use of an epidural with local anesthetic and/or narcotic may aid both intraop and postop pain relief, but ↓BP should be avoided.	
Emergence	Routine extubation in OR	
Blood and fluid requirements	IV: 14–16 ga ×2 NS/LR @ 6–8 mL/h Warm fluids UO ≥ 1.5 mL/kg/h	Aim for a minimum of 1.5 mL/kg/h UO. Mannitol (0.25–1 g/kg) given iv once kidney is being manipulated, and if UO decreases. Consider dopamine infusion to ↑ BP as needed. Limit use of direct vasoconstrictors.
Monitoring	Standard monitors (see p. B-1).	CVP or invasive arterial monitoring are rarely required. Lower extremity NIBP measurements on the same side as implant will be inaccurate during period of iliac vessel clamping.
Positioning	✓ and pad pressure points ✓ eyes	
Complications	Hemorrhage Pneumothorax	Because the vessels are tied close to the aorta and IVC, the possibility of severe hemorrhage exists. Pneumothorax is always possible, especially when the 12th rib is resected.

POSTOPERATIVE

Complications	Pneumothorax/pulmonary problems Hemorrhage Infection PONV (see p. B-6) Electrolyte abnormalities VTE (see p. B-7) Ileus

Pain management	Epidural narcotics (see p. C-2). Avoid hypotension. PCA (see p. C-3).
Tests	CXR Hct. electrolytes, BUN/Cr

Suggested Readings

1. Kahan BD, Ponticelli C: *Principles and Practice of Renal Transplantation.* Martin Dunitz, Ltd., London: 2000.
2. Morris PJ: *Kidney Transplantation.* WB Saunders, Philadelphia: 2001.
3. Odorico JS, Sollinger HW: Technical immunosuppressive advances in transplantation for insulin-dependent diabetes mellitus. *World J Surg* 2002; 26:194–211.
4. Lemmens HJM: Kidney transplantation: recent developments and recommendations for anesthetic management. *Anesth Clin North Am* 2004; 22(4):651–62.
5. Sener M. Torgay A. Akpek E. Colak T. Karakayali H. Arslan G. Haberal M: Regional versus general anesthesia for donor nephrectomy: effects on graft function. *Transplant Proc* 2004; 36(10):2954–8.

LIVER TRANSPLANTATION

SURGICAL CONSIDERATIONS

Description: Liver transplantation is the treatment of choice for patients with acute and chronic end-stage liver disease (ESLD). Patients with ESLD, besides intrinsic liver dysfunction, also may have other organ system dysfunction, including hepatorenal and hepatopulmonary syndrome resulting in oliguria and hypoxia, respectively. Patients with alcohol-mediated cirrhosis and Wilson's disease are at risk for significant cardiomyopathy, while those with fulminant hepatic failure may have significantly elevated intracranial pressures. These additional comorbidities present an added level of complexity to the anesthetic and surgical management of the liver transplant recipient. The liver transplant operation can be divided into three stages: **(1) hepatectomy; (2) anhepatic phase,** which involves the implantation of the liver; and **(3) postrevascularization,** which includes hemostasis and reconstruction of the hepatic artery and common bile duct.[16] There are many variations in the technical aspects of the liver transplant operation that may result in physiologic changes during anesthesia. The anesthesiologist must be aware of these technical variations to optimize the intraoperative management of the liver transplant recipient. Examples of these variations include: cross-clamping of the vena cava during the implantation of the liver, which results in impairment of the systemic venous return, with possibility of profound hypotension; utilization of the venovenous bypass, which may be associated with thrombus or air embolism, and/or fibrinolysis; and the use of a "cutdown liver," which may result in significant bleeding from the cut surface following revascularization.

The **hepatectomy** may be a formidable task in patients with severe portal hypertension (HTN), coagulopathy, and previous surgery in the upper abdomen. In such circumstances, blood loss is significant and may be minimized by placing the patient on venovenous bypass or by creating a temporary portocaval shunt to relieve the portal HTN. Table 7.12-1 lists factors that may be associated with significant blood loss during the transplant operation. The hepatectomy is usually much easier in patients with acute fulminant hepatitis, primary biliary cirrhosis, or inborn

Table 7.12-1. Contributing Factors Associated with Increased Blood Loss in Liver Transplantation

1. Severe coagulopathy	7. Retransplantation
2. Severe portal HTN	8. Transfusion reaction
3. Portal or splenic vein thrombosis	9. Venous bypass-induced fibrinolysis
4. Previous surgery in the RUQ	10. Primary graft nonfunction
5. Renal failure	11. Intraop vascular complications
6. Uncontrolled sepsis	

errors of metabolism than in patients with shrunken cirrhotic livers, such as in postnecrotic cirrhosis from hepatitis B or C, alpha-1 antitrypsin deficiency, or Wilson's disease, among others. The subcostal incision usually extends from the left midclavicular line across the midline to just medial of the right 12th floating rib, along with a vertical midline extension from the xiphoid process to the transverse incision. This provides wide exposure to the upper abdomen.

The hepatectomy usually begins with manual exploration of the abdomen to ensure that there are no occult malignancies, abscesses, or other abdominal processes that may contraindicate proceeding with the transplant. The liver is then mobilized by freeing the falciform and left cardinal ligaments, followed by entering the lesser sac through the division of the gastrohepatic ligament. The mobilization of the liver and the subsequent dissection of the portahepatis may be significantly complicated and a tedious process due to large, thin-walled varices that require careful dissection and ligation. The dissection of the portahepatis begins with identification and ligation of the hepatic artery, followed by the common bile duct. The portal vein is carefully dissected from its bifurcation into left and right branches, proximally to its emergence from behind the pancreas. If the degree of portal HTN is severe—such that mobilization of the liver may result in significant blood loss—or the patient is hemodynamically unstable—then portal vein mobilization may be performed early so that a temporary portocaval shunt or venous bypass may be instituted to allow decompression of the varices and enhance venous return to the heart.

After the portal dissection is complete, the right lobe of the liver is mobilized. The infrahepatic vena cava is carefully dissected to prevent injury to the right renal and adrenal veins, followed by mobilization of the suprahepatic vena cava. The liver can be removed easily by cross-clamping and dividing the supra- or infrahepatic vena cava, with or without the use of venous bypass. Alternatively, the recipient vena cava may be left in situ (piggy-back technique) by further mobilization of the liver with division of the short hepatic veins that run from the anterior surface of the vena cava directly into the posterior aspect of the liver. To gain access to the short hepatic veins, the liver must be lifted and rotated to the left. This maneuver may result in partial occlusion of the inferior vena cava, which may impair venous return causing a temporary drop in blood pressure. The piggyback technique, where the recipient vena cava is left in situ, has the advantage that venous return is not compromised during the anhepatic phase and thus precludes the need for venous bypass.

The **anhepatic phase** may be associated with significant hemodynamic changes, depending on the technique used for vascular control. This stage of the operation consists of implantation of the liver allograft, with or without venous bypass. The use of venous bypass is particularly helpful in coagulopathic patients with severe portal HTN. In these high-risk patients, the goal of the venous bypass system is to relieve the portal HTN by "bypassing" the liver.[13] Cannulas, placed in the femoral and portal veins, draw the blood out of the systemic and splanchnic venous systems into a Biomedicus pump that delivers the blood into the axillary or jugular vein, maintaining the venous return (Fig. 7.12-4). This system allows the interruption of the vena cava with mild-to-moderate hemodynamic changes, depending on the blood flow rate through the system. The benefits and potential complications of the venous bypass system are listed in Table 7.12-2.

Wound complications and nerve injuries may be prevented by introducing the bypass cannulas percutaneously, rather than approaching the vessels through a surgical incision. A subclavian or IJ line may be placed preop, and can be easily and rapidly exchanged during the operation to bypass cannulas using the **Seldinger technique.** If lines are placed preoperatively for the specific purpose of venous bypass, a confirmatory CXR should be performed to ensure that the 15 Fr or larger bypass cannula will lie in the appropriate vessel when placed later in the operation. This also obviates the need for a CXR when the bypass cannula is placed later, when the patient may be unstable. Because of the potential complications, several transplant teams have opted not to use venous bypass. In these cases, vascular control is obtained by placing vascular clamps across the supra- and infrahepatic vena cava or the confluence of the hepatic veins (piggy-back technique) and the portal vein. The splanchnic venous return is interrupted during the anhepatic phase while the systemic venous return is either interrupted in the case of formal cross-clamping of the supra- and infra-hepatic vena cava or mildly diminished in the case of the piggy-back technique which can lead to significant hypotension unless preventive measures, as reviewed in Anesthetic Considerations (p. 699), are taken (Fig. 7.12-5).

In a **standard orthotopic liver transplant,** with or without venous bypass, the recipient's vena cava is removed, leaving two cuffs—one just below the diaphragm and the other above the entry of the renal veins. A cadaveric donor liver comes with the corresponding segment of the vena cava that is used for restoring the continuity of the recipient's vena cava. The first vascular anastomosis consists of an end-to-end anastomosis of the allograft suprahepatic vena cava and the cuff of the recipient's infradiaphragmatic vena cava. This is followed by the reconstruction of the infrahepatic vena cava with an end-to-end anastomosis. Immediately prior to completion of the infrahepatic vena

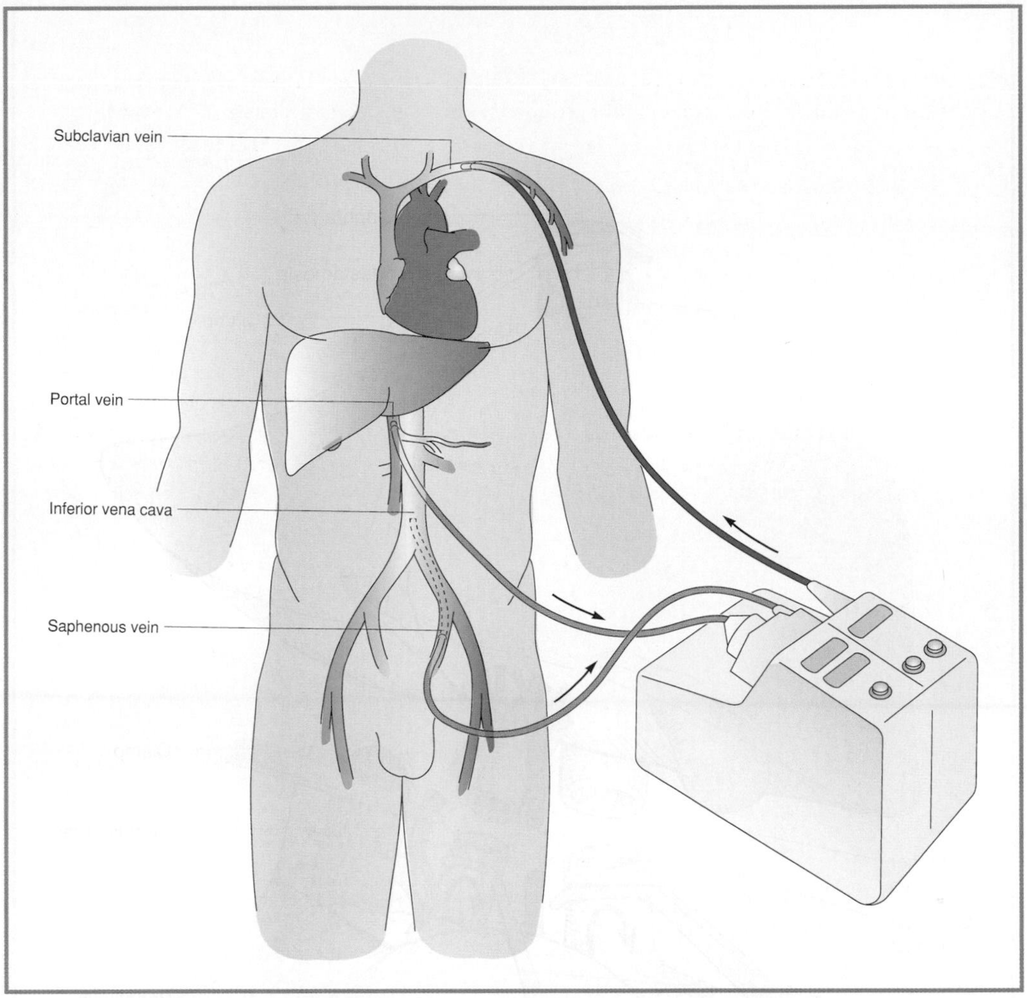

Figure 7.12-4. Setup for venovenous bypass during hepatic transplantation. Cannulas are placed into the portal vein to decompress the splanchnic bed and inferior vena cava (through the greater saphenous vein) to decompress the lower extremities and kidneys during the anhepatic phase of the transplant. A centrifugal pump is used to deliver bypassed blood to the central circulation by means of a cannula passed into the axillary vein. Cannulas also may be placed percutaneously directly into the femoral and subclavian veins. (Reproduced with permission from Greenfield LJ, et al, eds: *Surgery: Scientific Principles and Practice*, 3rd edition. Lippincott Williams & Wilkins, Philadelphia: 2001.)

Table 7.12-2. Benefits and Potential Complications of the Venovenous Bypass System

Benefits	Complication
Improved hemodynamics during anhepatic phase	PE
↓ blood loss	Air embolism
May improve perioperative renal function.*	Brachial plexus injury Wound seroma/infection Vascular injury

*In a prospective randomized trial comparing venovenous bypass with no bypass, no difference was found in the periop renal function between the two groups.[5]

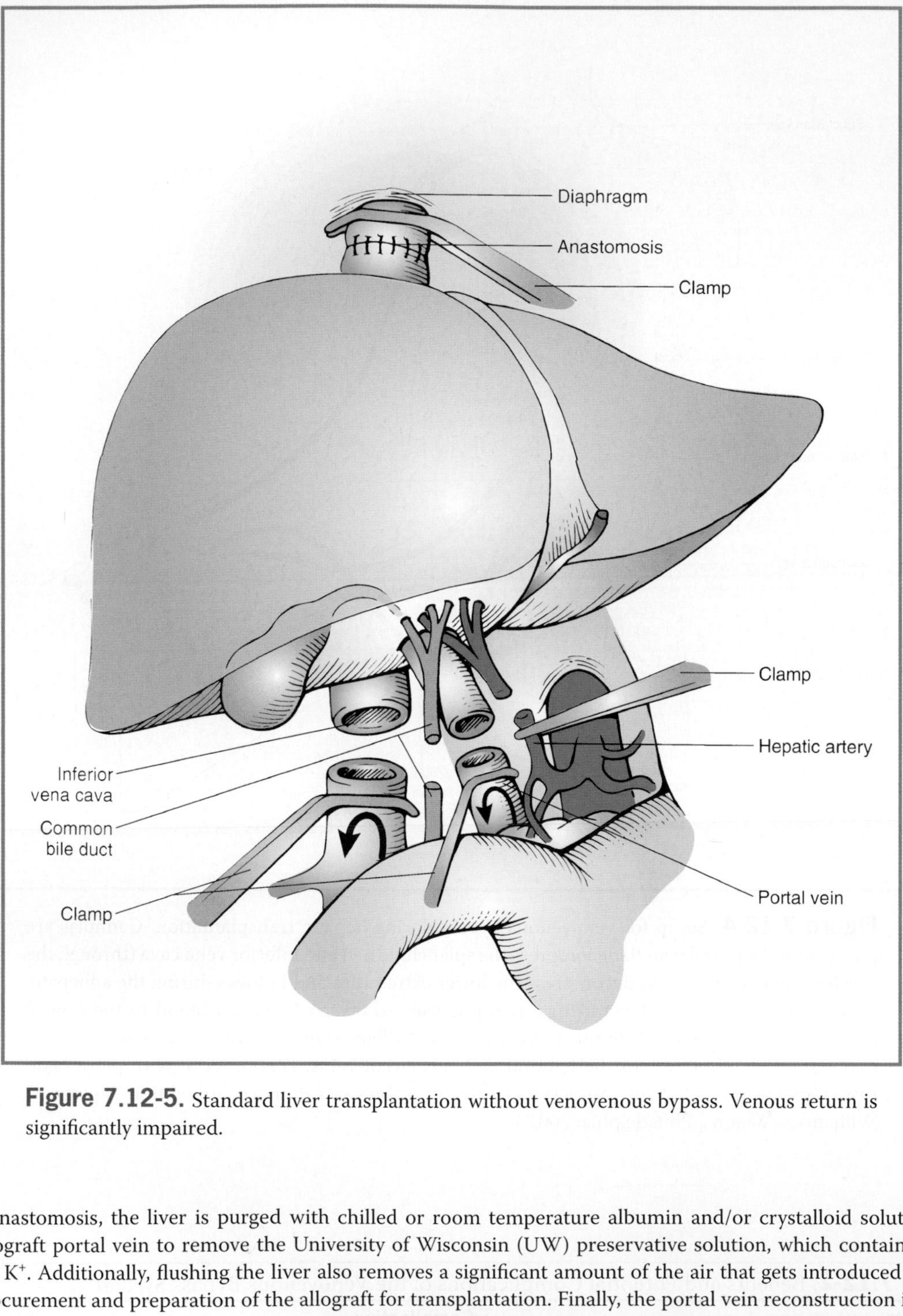

Figure 7.12-5. Standard liver transplantation without venovenous bypass. Venous return is significantly impaired.

caval anastomosis, the liver is purged with chilled or room temperature albumin and/or crystalloid solution via the allograft portal vein to remove the University of Wisconsin (UW) preservative solution, which contains ~145 mEq/L K^+. Additionally, flushing the liver also removes a significant amount of the air that gets introduced during the procurement and preparation of the allograft for transplantation. Finally, the portal vein reconstruction is completed with an end-to-end anastomosis. At this point, the clamps are removed, ending the anhepatic phase of the operation.

Venous bypass is not necessary when the **piggyback technique of liver transplantation** is utilized, because the diseased liver is separated from the vena cava (systemic venous return remains unimpaired), and vascular control is obtained by placing a clamp across the confluence of the hepatic veins as they join the vena cava (Fig. 7.12-6). A temporary portocaval shunt may be created to minimize bleeding in cases with severe portal HTN. The first anastomosis is between the suprahepatic vena cava of the liver allograft and the cuff created from the hepatic veins. The infrahepatic vena cava of the liver allograft is ligated, and the portal vein reconstruction is then completed. The clamps are then removed and the liver is revascularized.

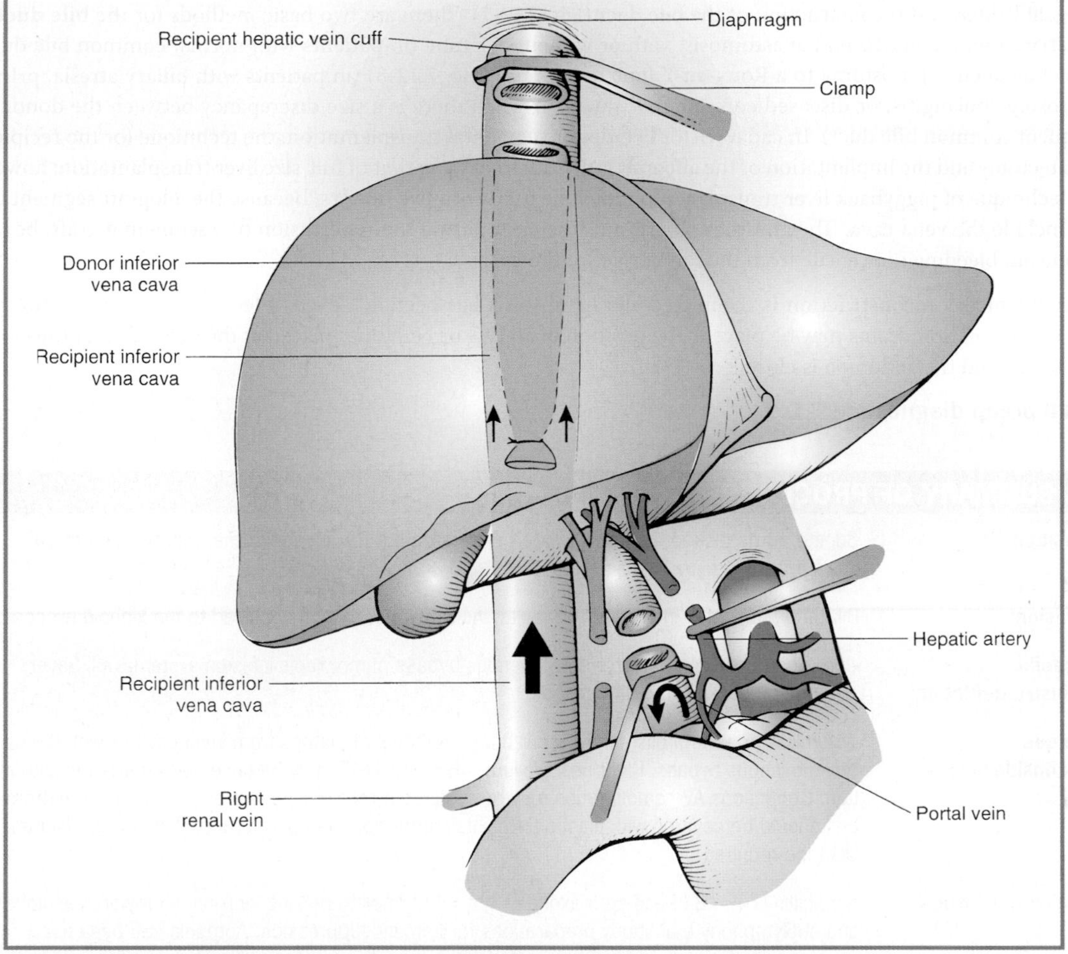

Figure 7.12-6. Piggyback liver transplantation. Note that the recipient's vena cava is left intact and systemic venous return is unimpaired.

The **postrevascularization stage** of the transplant begins with the removal of the vascular clamps. The reperfusion of the liver may be the most critical part of the operation. Despite flushing the liver to remove the high K^+-containing organ preservation solution, hyperkalemia may be troublesome following liver reperfusion, particularly with livers that sustained significant injury during preservation and reperfusion. Additionally, massive air embolism is an immediate concern following revascularization, as it may quickly lead to cardiac arrest. It is also during this stage that the patient may experience pulmonary HTN, which can lead to right heart failure and severe systemic hypotension. Pulmonary hypertension and right heart failure must be treated aggressively with inotropic agents; otherwise, the liver is subjected to high outflow resistance resulting in congestion and worsening of the allograft preservation injury. The cause of this phenomenon is not well understood; fortunately, it is seen in very few patients. Another reperfusion phenomenon is that of systemic hypotension secondary to peripheral vasodilation. This may be due to the release of systemic inflammatory mediators, which include kinins, cytokines, and free radicals from the liver allograft. Reperfusion of the liver also can have dramatic effects on coagulation, such as fibrinolysis resulting in severe hemorrhage or hypercoagulation that can result in venous thrombosis and massive pulmonary embolism with cardiovascular collapse.

Immediately prior to revascularization, the patient is usually given methylprednisolone (250–1000 mg) as part of the immunosuppressive regimen, as well as an adjunct to counteract the systemic effects of ischemia-reperfusion injury of the liver. At this point, all of the vascular anastomoses, the retroperitoneum, and the liver (especially the cut surface in segmental or reduced-size grafts) are inspected for surgical bleeding.

The hepatic artery reconstruction is performed after stabilization of the patient following revascularization of the liver. After the hepatic arterial anastomosis is completed, it is important to maintain adequate arterial BP (MAP > 65 mmHg) to prevent hepatic artery thrombosis. This is especially critical in pediatric transplant recipients, where the hepatic artery diameter ranges from 1–3 mm. The last part of the procedure involves hemostasis, removal of the gallbladder, and reconstruction of the bile duct (Fig. 7.12-7). There are two basic methods for the **bile duct reconstruction:** an end-to-end anastomosis, with or without a T tube (in patients with normal common bile ducts), or a choledochojejunostomy to a Roux-en-Y limb of jejunum (Fig. 7.12-8) (in patients with biliary atresia, primary sclerosing cholangitis, or diseased common bile ducts, or when there is a size discrepancy between the donor and recipient common bile duct). In cadaveric or live-donor segmental transplantation, the technique for the recipient's hepatectomy and the implantation of the allograft is not different from that of full-size liver transplantation; however, the technique of piggyback liver transplantation must be used with live donors, because the allograft segment does not include the vena cava. The anesthesiologist must be alert during the reperfusion of a segmental graft, because significant bleeding may ensue from the raw surface of the liver.

After the biliary reconstruction is completed and hemostasis has been achieved, a feeding jejunostomy tube and 2–3 closed-suction drains may be placed. The position of an OG or NG tube (placed at the beginning of the case) is confirmed and the abdomen is closed.

Usual preop diagnosis: ESLD

SUMMARY OF PROCEDURE

Position	Supine; arms tucked. Left arm and left groin area out for access to the axillary and femoral veins if venous bypass is anticipated.
Incision	Bilateral subcostal, in children; in adults, incision must extend cephalad to the xiphoid process.
Special instrumentation	Upper hand or Thompson retractor; venous bypass pump; rapid-infusion system; Cell Saver; argon beam coagulator, ultrasound.
Unique considerations	Thrombus or air embolism may occur during removal of clamps from vena cava or with the use of venovenous bypass. Right heart failure, ↓BP, and ↓SVR may be observed after revascularization. Continuous AV hemofiltration may be required if renal failure is present. Head and extremities should be covered with plastic to maintain core body temperature, particularly in children. OG tube required.
Antibiotics/drugs	Ampicillin (1 g q 8 h) and ceftriaxone (1 g q 24 h) prior to making incision. Methylprednisolone and antilymphocyte antibody preparations for immunosuppression. Aprotinin had been used occasionally during the hepatectomy and anhepatic phase in patients with severe coagulopathy and fibrinolysis (venous thrombus formation and pulmonary embolism can be seen with aprotinin use); however, its use is now contraindicated due to multiple reports of increased renal failure and mortality in cardiac surgery patients, although this has not been reported in liver transplant recipients.[19, 20] Just recently, the manufacturer, Bayer, has removed aprotinin from clinical use.[21]
Surgical time	4–12 h
EBL	6 U average blood loss (range 0–100 U)
Postop care	ICU: 1–2 d. HTN commonly seen.
Mortality	10% at 1 yr
Rejection	20–50% during first yr
Morbidity	Infectious complications: 20–50% Biliary stenosis or leaks: 5–15% Retransplantation: 6–14% Primary graft nonfunction: 2–5% Hepatic artery thrombosis: 0–6% Portal vein thrombosis: 1–4%
Pain score	7–8

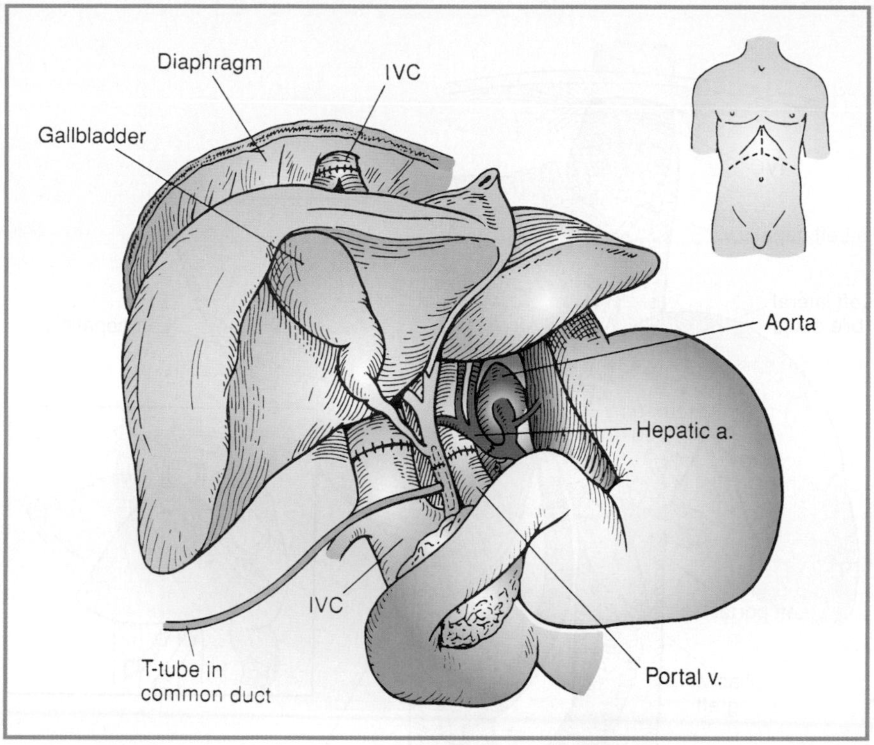

Figure 7.12-7. Liver transplantation. Anastomoses—including suprahepatic and infrahepatic IVC, portal vein, hepatic artery, and common bile duct—are complete as shown here. Roux-en-Y loop of small intestine is an alternative biliary drainage conduit. Inset shows a chevron incision with midline extension. (Reproduced with permission from Hardy JD: *Hardy's Textbook of Surgery*, 2nd edition. JB Lippincott, Philadelphia: 1988.)

PATIENT POPULATION CHARACTERISTICS	
Age range	Neonate-70 yr
Male:Female	1:1
Incidence	10/million/yr (15% pediatrics)
Etiology	Adult: hepatitis C cirrhosis; alcoholic cirrhosis; primary biliary cirrhosis; primary sclerosing cholangitis; hepatitis B cirrhosis; hepatocellular carcinoma. Pediatric: biliary atresia; inborn errors of metabolism, hepatoblastoma.
Associated conditions	Coagulopathy; hypoalbuminemia; ascites; cardiomyopathy (in alcoholic patients, hemochromatosis, and Wilson's disease); hepatorenal syndrome; hepatopulmonary syndrome, GI bleed, hepatic encephalopathy, and hypoglycemia in acute fulminant hepatitis.

ANESTHETIC CONSIDERATIONS

PREOPERATIVE

Patients needing liver transplantation represent a formidable challenge to the anesthesiologist. Frequently, these patients present for surgery with multiorgan system failure.

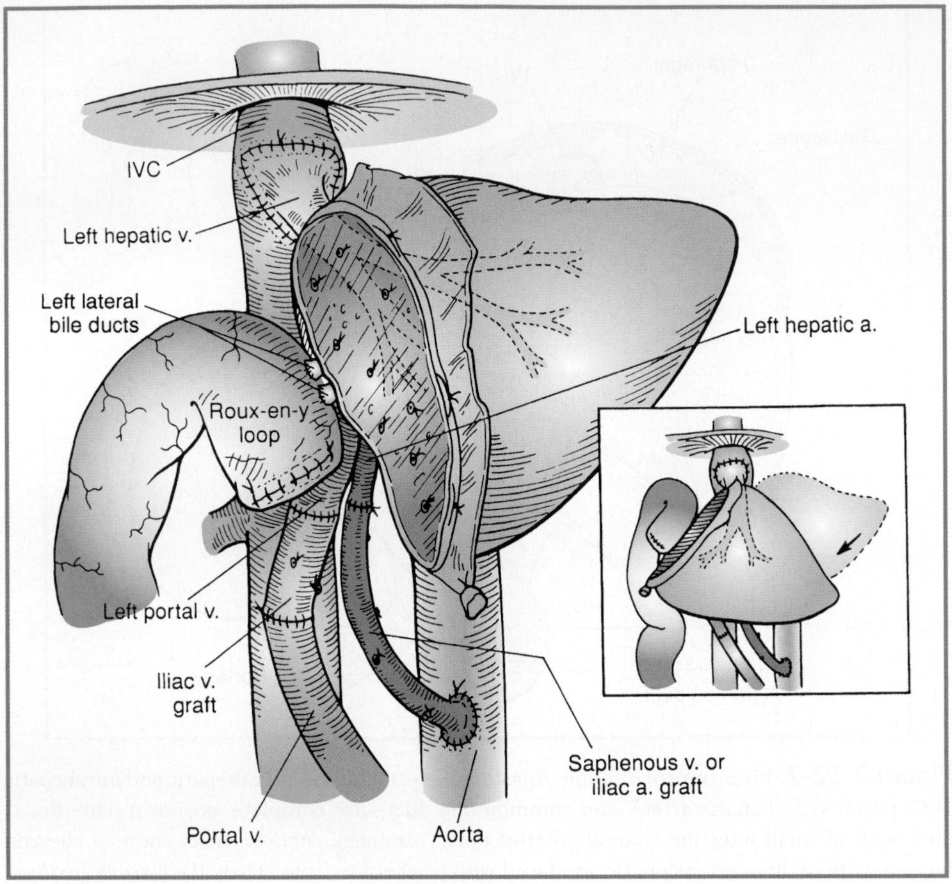

Figure 7.12-8. Liver transplantation (child) using left lateral segment from an adult liver. The hepatic artery and portal vein are extended with donor iliac artery and vein, respectively. The final position of the graft is shown (inset). A Roux-en-Y loop of small intestine is used to drain the bile duct(s). The IVC is left intact. The cut surface of the liver can bleed excessively if the central venous pressure is too high. (Reproduced with permission from Broelsch CE, et al: Liver transplantation in children from living related donors: surgical techniques and results. Ann Surg 1991; 214(4):432.)

Respiratory	Patients are often hypoxic because of ascites, pleural effusions, atelectasis, V/Q mismatch, pulmonary AV shunting, or hepatopulmonary syndrome. As a result, they are usually tachypneic and have a respiratory alkalosis. Evidence of pulmonary infection is usually a contraindication to surgery, but ARDS that may occur with hepatic failure is not. **Tests:** ABG; PFT, as indicated. CXR: ✓infection, effusions, atelectasis.
Cardiovascular	These patients demonstrate a hyperdynamic state with ↑plasma volume, ↑CO, and ↓SVR 2° arteriolar vasodilation in the splanchnic circulation, with intense vasoconstriction in other vascular territories (e.g., renal, brain, muscle, spleen). The SVR usually is not responsive to α-agents. AV fistulae may occur across the pulmonary circulation, so that precautions to prevent air embolism are important. Ejection fraction (EF) is usually high (> 60%), but some patients have cirrhotic cardiomyopathy → ↓contractility 2° ↓β-receptors, alterations in myocardial cell membrane properties, and ↑myocardial depressant substances. This cardiac dysfunction, however, usually is masked by a reduction in afterload. Pericardial effusions may be present, and should be drained at surgery. Many of these patients will have dysrhythmias, HTN, pulmonary HTN (very high risk), valvular disease, cardiomyopathy (alcoholic disease, hemochromatosis, Wilson's disease), and CAD. These patients will require appropriate preop consultation and workup. **Tests:** ECG; stress ECHO: ✓EF, contractility, pulmonary HTN, wall motion abnormalities, valve problems. If abnormal, right- and left-heart catheterization with coronary artery angiography should be performed.

Neurological	Patients are often encephalopathic and may be in hepatic coma; however, other organic causes of coma should be ruled out. In fulminant hepatic failure, ↑ICP is common, accounting for 40% of mortality (herniation), and may require prompt treatment (mannitol, hyperventilation, etc.). **Tests:** Continuous ICP monitoring in fulminant hepatic failure
Hepatic	Hepatitis serology and the cause of hepatic failure should be determined. Vascular abnormalities, previous RUQ surgery or portal-vein decompressive surgery places the patient in a high-risk group. Albumin is usually low, with consequent low plasma oncotic pressure → edema, ascites. The magnitude and duration of drug effects may be unpredictable, but, generally, these patients have ↑sensitivity to all drugs and their actions are prolonged. **Tests:** Bilirubin; PT; ammonia level; SGOT; SGPT; albumin
Gastrointestinal	Portal HTN, esophageal varices, and coagulopathies ↑ risk of GI hemorrhage. Gastric emptying is often slow and, together with the emergent nature of this surgery, warrants rapid-sequence induction (see p. B-4). H_2-antagonists are indicated preop.
Renal	Renal function ↓, especially in fulminant hepatic failure (hepatorenal syndrome). The kidneys often recover after transplantation, but simultaneous kidney transplantation may be justified. These patients are often hypervolemic, hyponatremic, and possibly hypokalemic. Ca^{++} is usually normal. Metabolic alkalosis may be present. Consider preop dialysis and intraop continuous AV hemofiltration. Mannitol (0.5–1 g/kg) may be used intraop to maintain renal function. **Tests:** BUN; Cr, creatinine clearance; electrolytes; ABG
Endocrine	Patients often glucose-intolerant or frankly diabetic, although acute hypoglycemia may be seen in acute hepatic failure. Hyperaldosteronism may be present. **Tests:** Glucose; electrolytes
Hematologic	These patients are often anemic 2° either blood loss or malabsorption. Coagulation is impaired because of ↓ hepatic synthetic function (all factors except VIII and fibrinogen are ↓), abnormal fibrinogen production,↓/impaired Plt, fibrinolysis, and low-grade DIC. **Tests:** PT; PTT; Plt count; bleeding time; fibrinogen; fibrin-split products (FSP); TEG
Premedication	Low doses of benzodiazepines may be used judiciously, but often nothing is given prior to surgery. Usually good preop evaluation and discussion suffice. Intramuscular injection should be avoided. Full-stomach precautions are justified. Metoclopramide 10 mg iv, ranitidine 50 mg iv and Na citrate 0.3 M 30 mL po should be given prior to surgery.

INTRAOPERATIVE

Anesthetic technique: GETA. These patients are extremely complex to manage because of the hemodynamic instability, massive blood loss, coagulopathy, and metabolic problems. It is convenient to divide the operation into three stages: preanhepatic, anhepatic and neohepatic (discussed later).

Induction	Often, a narcotic (e.g., fentanyl 2–5 mcg/kg) is given just before induction; and rapid-sequence induction is preferred. STP (3–5 mg/kg) or etomidate (0.3 mg/kg) with succinylcholine (1–2 mg/kg), together with cricoid pressure.
Maintenance	Standard maintenance (see p. B-2) with fentanyl 10–50 mcg/kg. A benzodiazepine (e.g., midazolam 0.1–0.3 mcg/kg or scopolamine) often is given to ensure amnesia during periods of hemodynamic instability when the volatile agent may need to be off. N_2O is avoided because of bowel distention and possible air embolism. Ventilation with $FiO_2 > 0.5$ and $PaCO_2 = \sim35$ mmHg. Occasionally, PEEP (5 cm H_2O) is added. Antibiotics and immunosuppressants should be given per surgeon's direction. Muscle relaxation usually is maintained with vecuronium.
Preanhepatic phase	The **preanhepatic phase** starts at skin incision and ends with removal of the recipient liver. Pleural and pericardial effusions are drained, which may improve oxygenation. Hyperglycemia is common during this period. A drop in filling pressures may be 2° hemorrhage or

Preanhepatic phase (cont'd)	vascular compression. Hemorrhage can be severe 2° portal HTN. Coagulation problems usually increase during this stage, although fibrinolysis is not usually a problem. Blood loss replacement is accomplished with blood (PRBC) and FFP. Cryoprecipitate and Plts are given as needed, but a hypercoagulable state should be avoided, particularly if venovenous bypass is contemplated. Hemodynamic instability is not uncommon during the hepatic vascular dissection 2° manipulation of the liver and ↓ venous return. Venovenous bypass relieves most of the complications of portal and IVC cross-clamping (↓ venous return, low CO, tachycardia, acidosis, ↓ renal function, intestinal swelling.) Blood is pumped from the femoral vein and the portal system (either portal vein or inferior mesenteric) via a centrifugal pump to the left axillary or subclavian vein. Generally, no heparin is used, but heparin-bonded cannulas and tubing are used. Bypass flow need to be at least 1 L/min to avoid possible thromboembolism. Bypass flow depends on venous inflow and is drawn into the pump by negative pressure. Low flows may be caused by hypovolemia or obstructed cannulae. Complications include unexpected decannulation, thromboembolism, and air embolism, all of which may need rapid termination of bypass and treatment of ↓ BP; fibrinolysis is seen with prolonged venovenous bypass. Massive blood transfusion is associated with ↓ Ca^{++}, and replacement is usually needed (± 500 mg/1000 mL of blood/FFP/plasmalyte mixture). If hyperkalemia occurs, it should be treated aggressively. Metabolic acidosis > 5 mEq/L should be treated with bicarbonate or THAM acetate (tris-hydroxymethyl aminomethane) to avoid a rapid increase in sodium. Typical loading dose: mL of 0.3M THAM = lean body weight [kg] x base deficit [mmol/L]. Occasionally, inotropic support is needed, but α-adrenergic agents should be avoided because of ↓ renal and peripheral perfusion. UO needs to be maintained by ensuring adequate intravascular volume; occasionally mannitol may be needed.
Anhepatic phase	The **anhepatic phase** begins with clamping of the hepatic vessels and vena cava and removal of the liver; it ends with the reperfusion of the donor liver. Problems during this period include hemorrhage, increasing coagulopathy and fibrinolysis, acidosis, hypothermia, and ↓ renal function. The hemodynamic instability associated with clamping of the hepatic vessels and the congestion of the bowel that occurs can be decreased by venovenous bypass (see the previous text). Care should be taken to maintain intravascular volume, while avoiding volume overload, because this would worsen fluid overloading on reperfusion. At the completion of vena caval anastomoses, the liver is flushed via the portal vein to remove air, preservation fluid, and metabolites. Reperfusion may take place after completion of the portal vein anastomosis or after both portal vein and hepatic artery anastomoses are completed. As in the preanhepatic phase, acidosis, ↓ Ca^{++}, glucose, coagulation, and other electrolyte abnormalities should be treated. Fibrinolysis usually starts in this period, but is not usually treated unless severe, because of the potential for embolism during venovenous bypass.
Neohepatic phase	The **neohepatic phase** begins with the unclamping of the portal vein, hepatic artery, and vena cava and reperfusion of the donor liver. Preparation for this phase is important because this may be a period of great hemodynamic instability. Before removal of the clamps, acidosis should be corrected, ionized Ca^{++} should be normal, and K^+ should be < 4.5 mEq/L. $CaCl_2$, $NaHCO_3$, and epinephrine should be readily available. Fluid overload prior to declamping should be avoided. High venous filling pressures decrease hepatic perfusion, especially prior to hepatic artery anastomosis. Declamping can be attended by ↓BP, ↓HR, dysrhythmias, hypothermia, lactic acidosis, coagulopathy, hyperglycemia, and thromboembolism.
Reperfusion syndrome	**The "reperfusion syndrome"** (which can occur in this phase) is characterized by ↓HR, ↓BP (30% of patients develop MAP < 70% of baseline), conduction defects, and ↓SVR in the face of acutely ↑RV filling pressures. Cause unknown. A rapid ↑K^+ can → cardiac arrest. (Rx: ensure normal pH and electrolytes prior to unclamping; rapid therapy when it occurs.) ↓BP and ↓ HR are treated with epinephrine (10 μg increments), whereas $CaCl_2$ and $NaHCO_3$ are used to correct hyperkalemia and acidosis. Pulmonary edema may occur as a result of fluid overload and can be treated with diuretics, inotropes, and phlebotomy. A

General Surgery

Reperfusion syndrome (cont.)	high venous pressure will cause graft congestion and should be avoided. Reperfusion is associated with severe coagulopathy due to fibrinolysis (usually primary), release of heparin, and hypothermia. As liver function returns, there should be an improvement in coagulation, acid-base status (metabolic alkalosis may occur), ↓lactic acidosis, return of glucose to normal, and bile production. Hypokalemia may occur 2° uptake by the liver. Graft failure is associated with coagulopathy, ↑lactic acid, citrate intoxication, hyperglycemia, and ↓ bile formation.	
Emergence	Extubation is deferred. These patients are generally ventilated postop in ICU until stable and able to be weaned from ventilatory support. Apart from the usual tests, monitor hepatic function. Also ensure immunosuppression provided, infection controlled, analgesia adequate (usually fentanyl), and peptic ulcer prophylaxis given (ranitidine preferred).	
Blood and fluid requirements	Massive blood loss IV: 10 Fr × 2 Plasmalyte A or Normosol UO > 1 mL/kg/h Warm all fluids Humidify gases Rapid-infusion system Cell Saver 20 U PRBC 20 U FFP 20 U PLT	Generally, iv's are placed in the right antecubital fossa, left or right IJ or EJ. The left arm is avoided because the axillary or left subclavian vein may be used for venovenous bypass. Plasmalyte A or Normosol are preferred (absence of glucose, Ca^{++}, and lower Na^+ content) over NS or LR. Hypernatremia may occur due to administration of $NaHCO_3$. The ability to infuse up to 1.5 L/min of blood should be available. Usually a mixture of Normosol (250 mL), PRBC (1 U), and FFP (1 U) is used, yielding Hct = 26–30%. Actual blood loss estimation is extremely difficult, and usually replacement is judged by hemodynamic status, UO, and S_vO_2. Cell Savers are used to conserve blood. Anticoagulation is achieved with citrate solution to avoid heparin contamination, and cells are washed with Normosol/Plasmalyte A. Discontinue use before biliary reconstruction (infection) or in neoplasms, hepatitis B, or spontaneous bacterial peritonitis.
Monitoring	Standard monitors (see p. B-1). ECG (5-lead) Temp-bladder	Include 5-lead ECG and bladder T. (These patients sustain significant heat loss.) A full-time anesthesia technologist and lab/blood bank runner are useful. Lab and blood bank should be notified of the expected transplant. An automated data acquisition system also is useful, because there are times during the case when record keeping may not be kept up to date in favor of providing patient care.
	ETN_2 Arterial line(s)	One or two arterial lines are placed at the outset—one in the right radial, for ongoing lab and blood gas sampling; another line, in the right femoral artery is utilized for continuous pressure measurement.
	PA catheter/S_vO_2/CO	A PA catheter is essential for management of hemodynamics in these patients, because of the rapid changes in VS. A catheter capable of measuring mixed-venous O_2 sat is very useful, because it gives early clues to impending decompensation. Coagulopathy complicates the placement of central lines, and the use of ultrasound-guidance is recommended.
	TEE	TEE is useful to monitor cardiac filling and function and to diagnose problems such as PE or air embolism. Care needs to be taken in placing the TEE because many of these patients have esophageal varices.

Monitoring (cont'd)	ICP	ICP should be measured in patients with fulminant hepatic failure if ↑ICP is a concern.
	Laboratory	ABG, acid base status, electrolyte, lactate, osmolality, Ca^{++}, PT, PTT, Plt, Hct—all should be monitored on a regular basis (hourly or half-hourly; occasionally, more frequently).
	Thromboelastograph (TEG)	TEG is useful for monitoring coagulation (see the subsequent discussion of coagulation management).
Coagulation management	PT PTT Plt counts Fibrinogen FSP	Patients are prone to a variety of coagulopathies (↓Plt, ↓coagulation factors, DIC, fibrinolysis, etc.) because of preop factors, massive hemorrhage, anhepatic period, and reperfusion of the new liver; therefore, monitoring and treatment are necessary. Also, states of hypercoagulopathy need to be avoided because of unheparinized venovenous bypass.
	TEG	While PT, PTT, Plt counts, fibrinogen, and FSP may provide relevant information, they may not reflect the true coagulability of patient's blood, and tend to take considerable time to perform. Thus, in some centers, TEG has gained in popularity. It measures whole blood coagulability, not specific factors. TEG works by measuring viscoelastic properties of blood as it forms clot (fibrin connections) between a rotating cuvette and a spindle. Characteristic patterns are formed by the various coagulopathies with the common types shown in Fig. 7.12-9. Evaluation of the TEG leads to more rational transfusion therapy, reducing the number of U of blood/blood products used. Comparing specimens of native whole blood vs blood mixed with EACA or protamine can guide pharmacologic therapy of coagulopathies. Table 7.12-3 gives specific recommendations.
Positioning	✓and pad pressure points ✓eyes	Table and arm boards should be very well padded. Head should be placed on a foam rest. Particular care should be taken to pad the retractor supports where they may impinge on the arms and on the radial nerve as it curls around the humerus.
Temperature control	Warming blanket Humidifier	Patient's arms, head, and legs should be wrapped in plastic to protect against heat loss. Plastic drapes and the use of a cesarian section-type drape to protect the ECG electrodes and direct fluid flow off the table are useful to prevent the patient from lying in a pool of fluid. A warming blanket under the patient and over the lower legs is very useful.
Complications	Coagulopathy Hemorrhage Air embolism RV failure Metabolic acidosis	

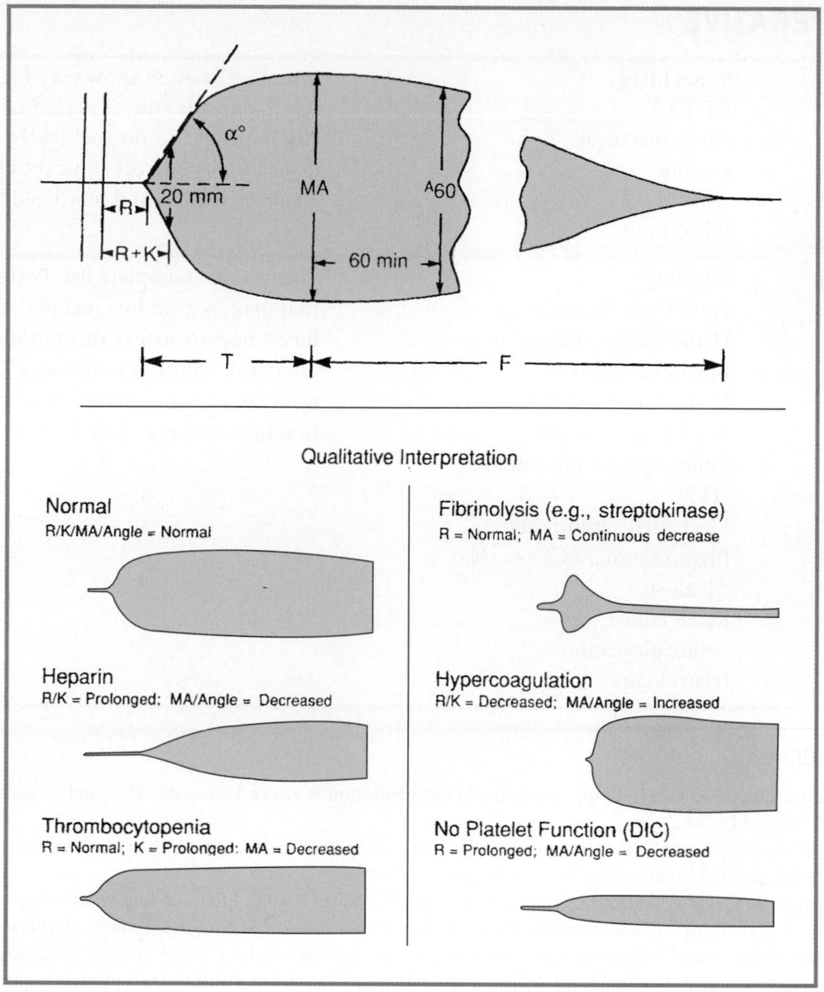

Figure 7.12-9. Variables and normal values measured by TEG: R = reaction time, 6–8 min R + k = coagulation time, 10–12 min α = clot formation rate, > 50° MA = maximum amplitude, 50–70 mm A_{60}= amplitude 60 min after MA A_{60}/MA-100 = whole blood clot lysis index, > 85% F = whole blood clot lysis time, > 300 min (Reproduced with permission from Kang YG, et al: Intraoperative changes in blood coagulation and thromboelastographic monitoring in liver transplantation. *Anesth Analg* 1985; 64:891.)

Table 7-12-3. Coagulation Therapy Guided by TEG Monitoring[6]

1. Maintenance fluid
RBC: FFP: Plasmalyte A = 300:200:250 mL
2. Replacement therapy
a. FFP (2 U) for prolonged reaction time (R > 15 min)
b. Plt (10 U) for small MA (MA < 40 mm)
c. Cryoprecipitate (6–12 U) for persistent slow-clot formation rate (α < 40°) with normal MA
3. Pharmacologic therapy
a. Compare coagulability of whole blood, blood treated with protamine sulfate, and blood treated with epsilon aminocaproic acid.
b. Epsilon aminocaproic acid (1 g) for severe fibrinolysis(F < 60 min)
c. Protamine sulfate (50 mg) for severe heparin effect
d. Heparin (1000–2,000 U) for hypercoagulable state

POSTOPERATIVE

Monitoring of hepatic function	Serial LFTs PT, PTT Ammonia level Lactate TEG Bile output	Initial LFTs often show very high liver enzymes, which subside over a period of days. PT generally improves to normal levels, while lactic acidosis usually corrects quickly. Often a metabolic alkalosis follows and may need HCl treatment.
Complications	Bleeding Partial vein thrombosis Hepatic artery thrombosis Biliary tract leaks Primary nonfunction Rejection Infection Pulmonary complication HTN Electrolyte abnormalities (hypokalemia, ↓Ca++, ↑Na) Alkalosis Renal failure Peptic ulceration Neurologic	This is not a complete list. Feared complications that may → graft loss include portal vein thrombosis, hepatic artery thrombosis, bile leaks, and rejection. These are attended by ↑LFTs, lactic acidosis, coagulopathy, hypoglycemia, ↓renal function, and poor bile formation.

General Surgery

Suggested Readings

1. Adachi T: Anesthetic principles in living-donor liver transplantation at Kyoto University Hospital: experiences of 760 cases. *J Anesth* 2003; 17(2):116–24.
2. Casavilla A, Gordon RD, Starzl TE: Techniques of liver transplantation. In *Surgery of the Liver and Biliary Tract.* Blumgart LH, Fong Y, eds. Churchill Livingstone, New York: 2000, 2155–80.
3. Grande L, Rimola A, Cugat E, Alvarez L, Garcia-Valdecasas JC, Taura P, et al: Effect of venovenous bypass on perioperative renal function in liver transplantation: results of a randomized controlled trial. *Hepatology* 1996; 23:1418–28.
4. Merritt WT: Metabolism and liver transplantation: review of perioperative issues. *Liver Transpl* 2000; 6(4 Suppl 1):S76–84.
5. Nakazato PZ, Concepcion W, Bry W, Limm W, Tokunaga Y, Itasaka H, et al: Total abdominal evisceration: an en bloc technique for abdominal organ harvesting. *Surgery* 1992; 111:37–47.
6. Ozaki CF, Katz SM, Monsour HP, et al: Surgical complications of liver transplantation. *Surg Clin North Am* 1994; 74(5):1155–67.
7. Shaw BW, Martin DJ, Marquez JM, Kang YG, Bugbee AC, Iwatsuki S, et al: Venous bypass in clinical liver transplantation. *Ann Surg* 1984; 200:524–34.
8. Starzl TE, Demetris AJ: Liver transplantation: a 31-year perspective, Part III. *Curr Probl Surg* 1990; 27:181–240.
9. Starzl TE, Iwatsuki S, Esquivel CO, Todo S, Kam I, Lynch S, et al: Refinements in the surgical technique of liver transplantation. *Semin Liver Dis* 1985; 5:349–59.
10. Steadman RH: Anesthesia for liver transplant surgery. *Anesthiol Clin North Am* 2004; 22(4):687–711.
11. Warnaar N, Mallett SV, de Boer MT, Rolando N, Burroughs AK, Nijsten MW, Slooff MJ, Rolles K, Porte RJ. The impact of aprotinin on renal function after liver transplantation: an analysis of 1,043 patients. *Am J Transplant.* 2007; 7(10):2378–87.
12. Washburn WK, Lewis WD, Jenkins RL: Percutaneous venovenous bypass in orthotopic liver transplantation. *Live Transpl Surg* 1995; 1(6):377–82.

LIVING-DONOR LIVER TRANSPLANTATION

SURGICAL CONSIDERATIONS

Description: The success of deceased donor liver transplantation has resulted in an ever-increasing number of patients with end stage liver disease (ESLD) waiting for transplantation; however, the number of deceased donors has remained relatively constant. Consequently, the waiting time to receive an organ has increased significantly, and ~15% of patients will die while waiting. The success of **living-donor renal transplantation,** coupled with the experience in adult-to-pediatric living-donor liver transplantation, as well as advances in surgical and postsurgical care of patients undergoing major liver resections, has lead to the implementation of adult-to-adult living-donor liver transplantation. This provides a potentially larger source of healthy livers for transplantation.

Potential liver donors undergo extensive medical and psychosocial evaluation to ensure psychological as well as physical fitness to undergo a major surgical procedure with no medical benefits to the donor. Donors must have full blood typing to ensure compatibility with the recipient, and then fill out an extensive medical questionnaire, followed by a complete physical exam and screening lab tests. Any evidence of diabetes, HTN, or renal, pulmonary, cardiovascular, or hepatic abnormalities usually is a contraindication to donation. After the potential donor is medically and psychosocially cleared, they undergo a detailed imaging study of the liver; and, if there are no anatomical contraindications, then an elective living-donor transplant is scheduled.

The donor and recipient operations usually are conducted simultaneously to minimize the ischemic injury to the donor liver segment. The donor operation, however, is initiated first, with the recipient operation started only after the donor liver has been directly examined and no barriers to proceeding are found. The donor operation is similar to either a right or left hepatic lobectomy, although there are some differences that can have a significant impact on anesthetic management, as detailed later.

The donor may elect to have an epidural catheter for postop analgesia, and this usually is placed before surgery. A vertical midline incision is made from the xiphoid to just above the umbilicus and extended transversely to the right anterior axillary line. Occasionally, bisubcostal incisions are required. Following exploration of the abdomen, intraoperative ultrasound may be performed to map the hepatic venous anatomy so the plane of dissection can be delineated. Additionally, an intraoperative cholangiogram is performed via the cystic duct (a cholecystectomy is performed in a right or left hepatic lobectomy) or the common bile duct, to define the biliary anatomy. After this is performed, the corresponding portal vein and hepatic artery are isolated. Unlike in a hepatic lobectomy for tumor, the venous and arterial inflow to the liver segment is not ligated; thus, the transaction of the liver parenchyma may result in significant hemorrhage. Next, the respective lobe of the liver is mobilized from its attachments, and the liver is dissected from the retrohepatic vena cava, with ligation of the short-hepatic veins. This maneuver can cause transient hypotension secondary to torque and compression of the IVC and hepatic veins, as well as potential bleeding from the vena cava itself. Next, the hepatic vein is isolated, and the liver is then divided, which can be a slow and tedious process. After the parenchyma is divided, the liver segment is ready to be removed. Heparin (80–100 U/kg) is given to prevent intrahepatic clot formation. Following heparinization, the hepatic artery and portal vein are ligated and divided, followed by the hepatic vein. The donated hepatic lobe is immediately placed in ice and flushed with Viaspan or other organ preservation solution. After the donated liver segment is flushed, the recipient's hepatic vein stump is oversewn and the abdomen and cut surface of the remaining liver are inspected for hemostasis and bile leak. Closed drains are placed, after which the abdomen is closed. Essentially, the same procedure is followed for a left lateral segmentectomy (adult-to-child), except that the extent of liver resection is about 25%, compared with 40% or 60% for a left or right hepatic lobectomy, respectively.

Usual preop diagnosis: Healthy, living liver donor

SUMMARY OF PROCEDURE

Position	Supine; arms tucked
Incision	Vertical midline with a right and/or left subcostal extension, depending on liver segment being utilized
Special instrumentation	Retractor; ultrasonic or hydrojet dissection/aspirator; irrigating bipolar cautery; argon beam coagulator; Cell Saver; rapid-infusion system
Unique considerations	Intraop cholangiogram and/or ultrasound. Hemodilution immediately before surgery, with removal of 1 U whole blood if Hct ≥ 40. Patients also may have donated 1–2 U of autologous blood. Heparin (80–100 U/kg)
Antibiotics	Ampicillin 1 g and ceftriaxone 1 g iv before skin incision
Surgical time	3–5 hr
EBL	250–500 mL
Postop care	ICU overnight or surgical floor. Hospital stay 5–7 d.

SUMMARY OF PROCEDURE (cont'd)	
Mortality	14 deaths reported world-wide (as of December 2006) following ~1,500 donor operations.
Morbidity	Infectious complications: 3% Biliary leak: 1% Reoperation: 3–5% Acute hepatic failure: < 0.1%
Pain score	7–9

PATIENT POPULATION CHARACTERISTICS	
Age range	18–55 yr
Male:Female	1:1
Incidence	Uncommon

ANESTHETIC CONSIDERATIONS

See Anesthesia for Hepatic Resection, p. 553.

Suggested Readings

1. Barr ML, Belghiti J, Villamil FG, Pomfret EA, Sutherland DS, Gruessner RW, Langnas AN, Delmonico FL. A report of the Vancouver Forum on the care of the live organ donor: lung, liver, pancreas and intestine data and medical guidelines. *Transplantation* 2006; 81:1373–85.
2. Broelsch CE, Emond JC, Whitington F, et al: Application of reduced size liver transplants as split grafts, auxiliary orthotopic grafts and living related segmental transplants. *Ann Surg* 1990; 212:368–75.
3. Everhart JE, Lombardero M, Detre KM, et al: Increased waiting time for liver transplantation results in higher mortality. *Transplantation* 1997; 64(9):1300–6.
4. Singer PA, Siegler M, Whitington PF, et al: Ethics of liver transplantation with living donors. *N Eng J Med* 1989; 321:620–2.
5. Strong RW, Lynch SV: Live related donors in liver transplantation. In *Surgery of the Liver and Biliary Tract.* Blumgart LH, Fong Y, eds. Churchill Livingstone, New York: 2000, 2129–40.

General Surgery

MULTIORGAN PROCUREMENT

SURGICAL CONSIDERATIONS

Description: The families of brain-dead patients may allow donation of the patient's functioning organs—which may include, but is not limited to, heart, lungs, liver, kidneys, pancreas, and small intestine. The process of organ procurement can be chaotic, with multiple operative teams and technicians working simultaneously. Moreover, brain-dead patients tend to be hemodynamically unstable, sometimes requiring multiple pressors, and the possibility of acute decompensation is ever present.

The donor patient's chest and abdomen are opened in the midline from sternal notch to pubis (Fig. 7.12-10). The chest is opened with a sternal saw and generally an extra-large Balfour retractor is used to widely retract the abdomen. The aorta and IVC are dissected first to allow rapid placement of a flush line in the event that the patient experiences a cardiovascular collapse. Following this, the liver vasculature is identified in the hepatoduodenal ligament and is dissected out. This part of the procedure generally takes about 1.5 h. In cases where the pancreas is procured, an additional 45–60 min is required for mobilization of the pancreas. During pancreas procurement, a Betadine/amphotericin B solution is administered through an NG tube into the stomach and duodenum. A total of about 300–500 mL of the Betadine solution is passed in two divided aliquots. After the heart, liver, pancreas, and kidneys have been mobilized, the supraceliac aorta just below the diaphragm is dissected for placement of the aortic cross-clamp. Immediately before cross-clamping, 30,000 U of heparin (300 U/kg) is given systemically, with the α-antagonist phentolamine in some cases. The supraceliac aorta is then clamped and the organs are perfused with

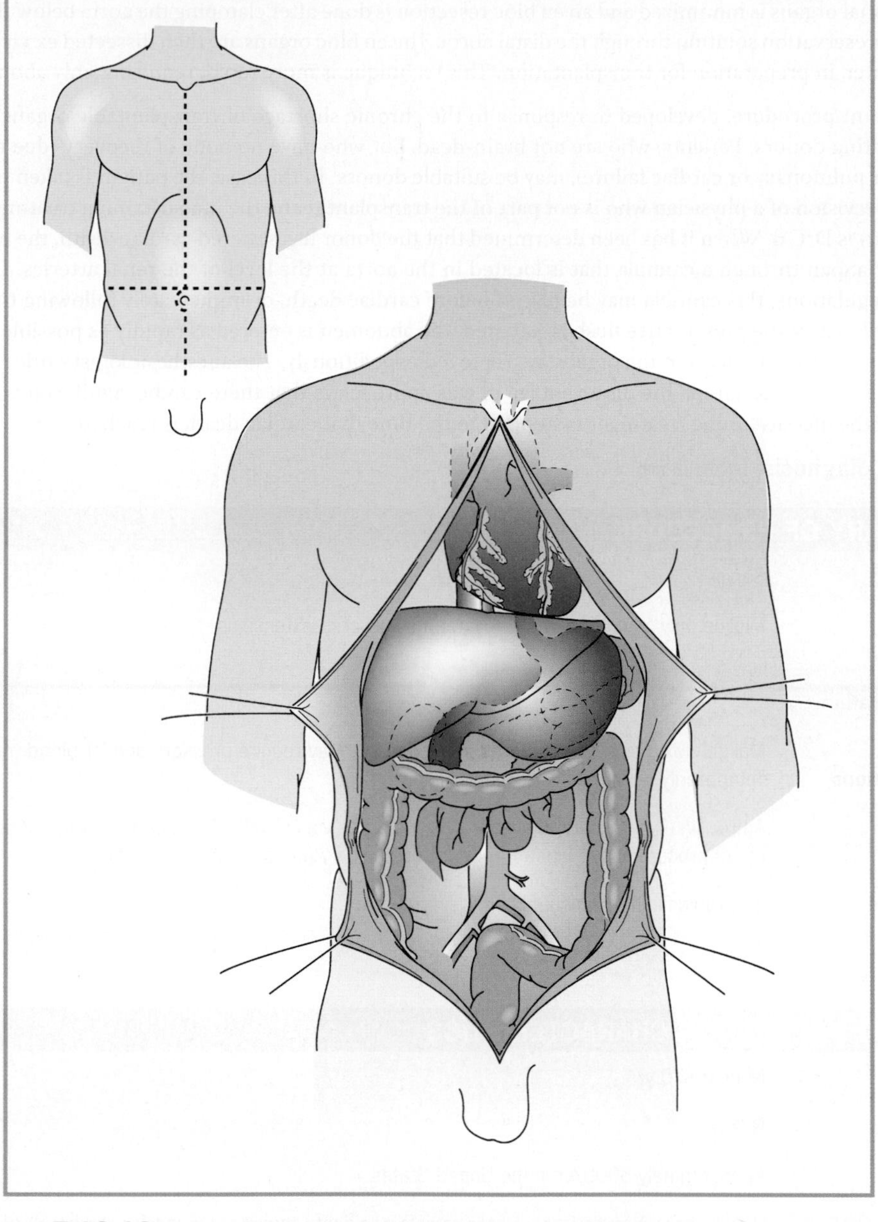

Figure 7.12-10. A complete midline incision, from suprasternal notch to pubis, is made for multiple organ procurement; and the sternum is split. If necessary, cruciate abdominal incisions are added to facilitate exposure of the intraabdominal organs. (Reproduced with permission from Greenfield LJ, et al, eds: *Surgery: Scientific Principles and Practice,* 3rd edition. Lippincott Williams & Wilkins, Philadelphia: 2001.)

Viaspan, a hyperosmotic and hyperkalemic solution containing insulin, glucose, and reducing agents. At this point, the ventilator can be turned off, except in cases where the lungs are being procured. In this case, the lungs must be inflated with 100% O_2 just before removal. The heart is the first organ to be removed, followed by the lungs.

If the lungs are procured, an extra 20–30 min of perfusion time is required. After removal of the heart and/or lungs, the liver can be removed, followed by the pancreas, small intestines, and kidneys. After the organs are removed, spleen and lymph nodes for tissue typing are obtained from the abdominal and thoracic cavities; and, because of the possible need for vascular reconstruction in the recipients, bilateral iliac veins and arteries are removed. The total time for multiorgan procurement is ~4 h, although the anesthesia time typically ends with aortic cross-clamping.

Variant procedures: During the **"rapid-flush" technique** used by some procurement teams, the dissection of individual abdominal organs is minimized and an en bloc resection is done after clamping the aorta below the diaphragm and flushing preservation solution through the distal aorta. The en bloc organs are then dissected ex vivo, often at the transplant center, in preparation for transplantation. This technique is more rapid, requiring only about 1.5 h.

A second variant procedure, developed in response to the chronic shortage of transplantable organs, is the use of non-heart-beating donors. Patients, who are not brain-dead, but who have no hope of recovery (due to irreversible brain injury or pulmonary or cardiac failure), may be suitable donors. In this case, the patient is taken to the OR and, under the supervision of a physician who is not part of the transplant team, the life-sustaining treatment (e.g., pressors, ventilator) is D/C'd. When it has been determined that the donor has suffered cardiac death, the body is rapidly cooled with ViaSpan through a cannula that is located in the aorta at the level of the renal arteries. Depending on the regional regulations, this cannula may be placed before cardiac death, or immediately following the declaration of cardiac death. After the preservative flush is initiated, the abdomen is entered as rapidly as possible and the peritoneal cavity is packed with ice and the organs are removed expeditiously. The anesthesiologist's role is ended when cardiac death has been declared. The disadvantage of this approach is that there can be significant warm ischemia from the time the life-sustaining treatment is stopped to the time that cardiac death is reached.

Usual preop diagnosis: Brain death

SUMMARY OF PROCEDURE	
Position	Supine
Incision	Midline only, neck to pubis, ± bilateral transverse extensions
Special instrumentation	Chest and abdominal retractors
Unique considerations	Maintain oxygenation and BP as if live patient. May require pressors and/or blood transfusion. Temporarily deflate lungs for sternal sawing.
Antibiotics	Ampicillin (1 g iv), ceftriaxone (1 g iv); Betadine via NG tube for pancreas (with duodenal segment) procurement. Heparin, relative. (Betadine/Amphotericin in B solution)
Surgical time	4 h; rapid flush technique: 1.5 h
EBL	200 mL

PATIENT POPULATION CHARACTERISTICS	
Age range	Neonate-70 yr
Male:Female	N/A
Incidence	Approximately 5000/yr in the United States.
Etiology	Usually head trauma (e.g., motor vehicle accidents, gunshot wounds to the head) or intracranial bleeding
Associated conditions	Vasomotor instability; diabetes insipidus (DI); intracranial HTN

ANESTHETIC CONSIDERATIONS

PREOPERATIVE

In general, organ donors are previously healthy individuals who have suffered catastrophic, irreversible brain injury of known etiology, most commonly due to blunt head trauma, penetrating head injury, or intracranial hemorrhage. A declaration of brain death by physicians not participating in the organ procurement must be documented. This documentation, together with certification of death and familial consent, should be verified by the anesthesiologist before organ procurement. The United Network for Organ Sharing (UNOS) has produced *The Critical Pathway for the Organ Donor* to facilitate the administrative aspects of organ procurement (http://www.unos.org/resources/donorManagement.asp). There should be no evidence of disease or trauma involving the organs targeted for donation and, in general, the patient should be hemodynamically stable with minimal inotropic requirements. After brain death has been declared, it is important to shift the emphasis away from cerebral resuscitation efforts and to focus instead on the maintenance of adequate tissue perfusion and oxygenation. Brain death is frequently followed by a series of pathophysiological events that may complicate the management of these patients.

Recently, Donation after Cardiac Death (DCD) has been instituted at many medical centers, where a non-brain dead patient is brought to the operating room for withdrawal of life support and subsequent removal of organs for transplant. Although the ethics of such organ donation had been debated, the ASA and other organizations have developed protocols to separate the teams caring for the patient during the withdrawal of life support and the operating room team responsible for organ retrieval. However, in most institutions, an anesthesiologist is present in the operating room as a member of the latter team. After withdrawal of life support has been initiated and the patient meets criteria for cessation of cardio-pulmonary function, organ removal is initiated as quickly as possible to limit warm ischemia time and possible damage to the organs to be removed. DCD patients often do not have as serious pathophysiological alterations as patients who meet brain death criteria.

Respiratory	Pulmonary dysfunction following brain death has many possible etiologies: aspiration, atelectasis, pneumonia, and pulmonary edema. In addition, trauma may cause pulmonary dysfunction related to contusion, pneumothorax, or hemothorax. Meticulous pulmonary toilet is essential to prevent atelectasis and pneumonia. Maintenance of adequate oxygenation is requisite to ensure preservation of other organs for transplantation. Use mechanical ventilation with TVs of 10–12 mL/kg and a minute ventilation that maintains $PaCO_2$ 30–35 mmHg and pH 7.35–7.45. The FiO_2 should ensure a PaO_2 75–150 mmHg and arterial saturation > 95%. PEEP usually is applied at 3–5 cmH_2O and should not exceed 7.5 cmH_2O because of the deleterious effects on CO and regional blood flow, and possible barotrauma. The FiO_2 generally should be increased to 100% before transport to the OR. An important exception is in the case of heart-lung or lung retrieval, where it is important to maintain FiO_2 < 40% to minimize possible effects of O_2 toxicity. Ideally, PIP should be < 30 cmH_2O to minimize possible barotrauma to the lungs. **Tests:** Frequent ABGs, including immediate preop period. Proper position of the ETT should be confirmed preop.
Cardiovascular	Hypotension should be anticipated in all organ donors. This results most commonly from neurogenic shock (derangement of descending vasomotor control → progressive ↓SVR and venous pooling) and hypovolemia. Hypovolemia is usually the result of dehydration therapy for cerebral edema, hemorrhage, DI, or osmotic diuresis 2° hyperglycemia. Hypothermia, LV dysfunction, and endocrine abnormalities also can contribute to ↓BP. Fluid resuscitation with crystalloid, colloid, and PRBCs to maintain Hct > 30% should be initiated preop. Hemodynamic goals are: (1) CVP 10–12 cmH_2O (6–8 cmH_2O if lungs are to be procured); (2) MAP between 60–100 mmHg; (3) SBP > 100 mmHg; (4) PCWP ≤ 12 mmHg; (5) SVR 800–1200 dynes/second × cm^{-5} (or 800–1200 woods units); and (6) UO > 1 mL/kg/h. Donors are often placed on inotropic therapy to maintain these parameters; however, following adequate volume resuscitation, preop inotropic therapy often may be gradually decreased or D/C'd. If inotropic therapy remains necessary, typically it would consist of dopamine (2–10 mcg/kg/min), followed by dobutamine (3–15 mcg/kg/min) or epinephrine (0.1–1.0 mcg/kg/min), then norepinephrine. The latter 3 agents may be combined with dopamine (2–3 mcg/kg/min) in an attempt to augment or preserve renal, mesenteric, and coronary arterial blood flow. It should be noted that brain death may be accompanied initially by a transient hypertensive crisis that may require short-term treatment with SNP and/or esmolol. ECG abnormalities are common in patients with intracranial injury and are of no pathologic consequence. Atrial and ventricular dysrhythmias and various degrees of conduction block occur frequently in organ donors; the etiology may be electrolyte imbalance, ABG disturbance, ↑ICP, loss of the vagal motor nucleus, inotropic therapy, hypothermia, or myocardial contusions or ischemia. Antidysrhythmic therapy should follow the usual guidelines except for ↓HR, which is resistant to atropine in this setting. Bradycardia, if accompanied by ↓BP, should be treated with isoproterenol, dopamine, epinephrine, or temporary cardiac pacing. **Tests:** ECG; ECHO (to assess wall motion abnormalities) and possibly coronary angiography (if CAD is suspected).

Neurological	Diabetes insipidus (DI) frequently occurs in brain-dead donors; it is likely the result of destruction of the hypothalamic-pituitary axis. Untreated, it may cause marked hypovolemia and electrolyte disturbances (↑Na^+, ↑Mg^{++}, ↓K^+, ↓PO^-_4, ↓Ca^{++}). Therapy with iv vasopressin (titrated from 2 mcg/kg/min) or DDAVP (titrated from 0.3 mcg/kg/min) often is initiated to maintain UO < 1.5–3 mL/kg/h. Many believe that the benefits of minimizing electrolyte imbalance, fluid shifts, and reduction of core T outweigh the risks of vasopressin or desmopressin therapy, including coronary and renal vasoconstriction and possible organ ischemia or uneven distribution of the preservation solutions during flushing. It may be prudent, however, to D/C vasopressin or DDAVP infusions for at least 1 h prior to aortic cross-clamping and infusion of preservation solutions. Thermoregulation is abnormal in brain-dead donors due to hypothalamic dysfunction; and core T should be monitored (bladder, or esophageal). Aggressive warming techniques may have to be employed early to maintain a core T > 34–35°C, as there are numerous undesirable consequences of significant hypothermia (< 32°C) in the organ donor (e.g., cardiac dysrhythmia, cardiac instability, ↓GFR and cold diuresis, a left shift in the oxyhemoglobin dissociation curve, and pancreatitis). While other endocrine or metabolic disturbances may exist as a result of destruction of the hypothalamic-pituitary axis, currently there is no consistent recommendation for any other hormonal replacement therapy. **Tests:** Serum electrolytes and osmolality every 4 h
Hematologic	Donors may be anemic from hemodilution and/or hemorrhage. To ensure adequate tissue O_2 delivery, PRBCs are transfused to maintain Hct > 30. Some donors may exhibit a coagulopathy; clinically significant bleeding should be treated with clotting factors and Plts. Persistent or severe primary fibrinolysis or DIC may require rapid transfer of the donor to the OR for organ retrieval. Administration of epsilon-aminocaproic acid to treat fibrinolysis is avoided for fear of microvascular thrombosis in the donor organs. **Tests:** Hb/Hct; PT; PTT; Plt count; DIC screen as clinically indicated.
Other	The role of oxygen-free radicals, with regard to reperfusion injury, has prompted the suggested use of mannitol and steroids (and other compounds) as scavengers.

INTRAOPERATIVE

Anesthetic technique: Although anesthesia is unnecessary in brain-dead organ donors, both visceral and somatic reflexes can lead to physiologic responses during the procedure. The goals of intraop management with regard to respiratory, cardiovascular, hematologic, and neurologic status are identical to those discussed under preop considerations earlier.

Induction	Settings for mechanical ventilation parallel those of the ICU, although it may be advisable to begin with an FiO_2 of 100% until the first ABG result is obtained. The exception is when procurement of the lungs or heart-lungs is anticipated; then FiO_2 should not exceed 40%. To eliminate reflex neuromuscular activity and to facilitate surgical retraction, a long-acting neuromuscular blocking agent, such as pancuronium or pipecuronium (0.15 mg/kg), should be given at the beginning of the procedure and supplemented as necessary.
Maintenance	Reflex hypertensive responses to surgical stimulation occur frequently and may → excessive intraop blood loss and damage to donor kidneys; management should include the weaning of vasopressors and the initiation of vasodilator therapy with isoflurane, SNP, or NTG. Anesthetic care continues until the proximal aortic cross-clamp is applied. D/C all monitoring and supportive therapy at this point. The notable exception is the case of heart-lung or lung procurement; in this situation, all monitoring except FiO_2 should cease with proximal aortic cross-clamping. All supportive care is terminated, with the exception of mechanical ventilation of the lungs at 4 breaths/min or as directed by the transplant team, and suctioning of the ETT after cessation of mechanical ventilation just prior to removal of the tube. Extubation marks the termination of anesthetic care of the heart-lung or lung donor.

Blood and fluid requirements	IV: 14–16 ga × 1–2 NS/LR @ 2–4 mL/kg/h	Significant 3rd-space losses may require large volumes of crystalloid, colloid (up to 1 L) and PRBCs (not uncommon to transfuse 2 or more U to maintain Hct > 30). Central venous access is necessary for monitoring and for vasoactive drug delivery.
Monitoring	Standard monitors (see p. B-1). Art line CVP line UO	If a PA catheter is in place, it may be used or removed based on concerns of catheter-related, right-side endocardial lesions. Rarely is insertion of a PA catheter warranted in these operations. ABG, Hb/Hct, serum electrolytes, and glucose should be monitored hourly; for operations involving procurement of lungs or heart-lungs, ABGs should be obtained at least every 30 min.
Complications	Hypotension	Most commonly 2° hypovolemia and neurogenic shock (loss of descending vasomotor control). Ensure adequate volume repletion as described previously, then institute or increase inotropic/vasopressor therapy as previously outlined.
	Dysrhythmias	Multiple possible etiologies as described previously. Standard treatment and diagnosis should be employed, with the exception of bradycardia, which is atropine-resistant and should be treated with isoproterenol, dopamine, epinephrine, or transvenous pacing.
	Cardiac arrest	CPR should be instituted in an effort to maintain the viability of the liver, kidneys, and other abdominal viscera intended for transplantation. Procurement of the liver and kidneys should proceed rapidly to aortic cross-clamping at the diaphragm and administration of cold preservation fluid into the aorta and portal vein. This series of events will undoubtedly preclude use of the heart and lungs for transplantation.
	Oliguria	Ensure adequate volume replacement and BP as outlined, then add dopamine (2–3 mcg/kg/min), if not previously instituted to promote renal vasodilation and to increase renal blood flow, glomerular filtration rate, and UO. If these measures are ineffective at restoring adequate UO (> 1 mL/kg/h), then furosemide or mannitol may be used, after consultation with the transplant team.
	Diabetes insipidus (DI)	Fluid and electrolyte therapy as determined by filling pressures and hourly serum electrolyte values. Adjustment of vasopressin or DDAVP infusion to maintain UO < 1.5–3.0 mL/kg/h; initiation of this infusion should be done in consultation with the transplant team. As previously discussed, it may be advisable to D/C vasopressin or DDAVP at least 1 h before aortic cross-clamping.
	Coagulopathy	Transfuse Plt, FFP, and cryoprecipitate as necessary for clinical bleeding in the setting of abnormal coagulation studies. Avoid EACA due to risk of microvascular thrombosis in the donor organs.
	Hyperglycemia	Avoid dextrose-containing solutions, which may aggravate existing hyperglycemia and contribute to osmotic diuresis and electrolyte abnormalities.

Complications (cont'd)	Hypothermia	Early aggressive attempts to minimize intraop heat loss are essential and include warming the OR, use of a forced-air warming blanket, insulating exposed areas warming all fluids, and using heated, humidified inspired gases.
Special considerations	Heart-lung procurement	Division of the mediastinal pleura and tracheal dissection with manipulation of each lung outside the mediastinum may result in ↓↓BP and may cause problems with oxygenation and ventilation. Adequate intravascular volume is essential, and inotropic therapy may be required during this period. Problems with ventilation and oxygenation must be communicated immediately to the transplant team. Following aortic cross-clamping and infusion of cardioplegia solution, the lung preservation fluid will be infused via the right and left PAs. During this period, the lungs should be ventilated manually with 4 bpm, or as otherwise directed by the transplant team. It is prudent early on in the procurement procedure to verify the position of the ETT with the transplant surgeon to ensure that the tube does not contribute to mucosal injury at the site of the anticipated suture line.
	Organ preservation	Therapy aimed at improving organ preservation may require several pharmacologic manipulations, as directed by the transplant team. Agents commonly used during organ procurement include dopamine (2–3 mcg/kg/min), furosemide, mannitol, allopurinol (free-radical scavenger), chlorpromazine and phentolamine (vasodilators), heparin (prevents microvascular thrombosis and promotes reperfusion), and PGE_1 (vasodilator, membrane stabilizer, antiplatelet effect). Systemic infusion of PGE_1 prior to aortic cross-clamping (commonly used in heart-lung or lung procurement) will lead to predictable and profound ↓BP; efforts at volume resuscitation toward optimal CVP should continue until the aortic cross-clamp is applied. If heparin is to be administered iv, a catheter should be used after verifying the ability to freely aspirate blood. Methylprednisolone (30 mg/kg) is commonly administered at least 2 h before organ retrieval in an effort to protect the heart and kidneys from ischemic injury.

Suggested Readings

1. Mandell MS and Hendrickse A. Donation after cardiac death. *Curr Opin Organ Transplant* 2007; 12:298–302.
2. Phillips MG, ed: *Organ Procurement, Preservation and Distribution in Transplantation.* William Byrd Press, Richmond, VA: 1991.
3. Powner DJ, Kellum JA, Darby JM: Abnormalities in fluids, electrolytes, and metabolism of organ donors. *Prog Transplant* 2000; 10(2):88–94.
4. Report of a National Conference on Donation after Cardiac Death. *Am J Transplant* 2006; 6:281–91.
5. Robertson KM, Cook DR: Perioperative management of the multiorgan donor. *Anesth Analg* 1990; 70(5):546–56.
6. Salter DR, Dyke CM: Cardiopulmonary dysfunction after brain death. In *Anesthesia for Organ Transplantation.* Fabian JA, ed. JB Lippincott, Philadelphia: 1992, 81–94.

CHAPTER

7.13 Trauma Surgery

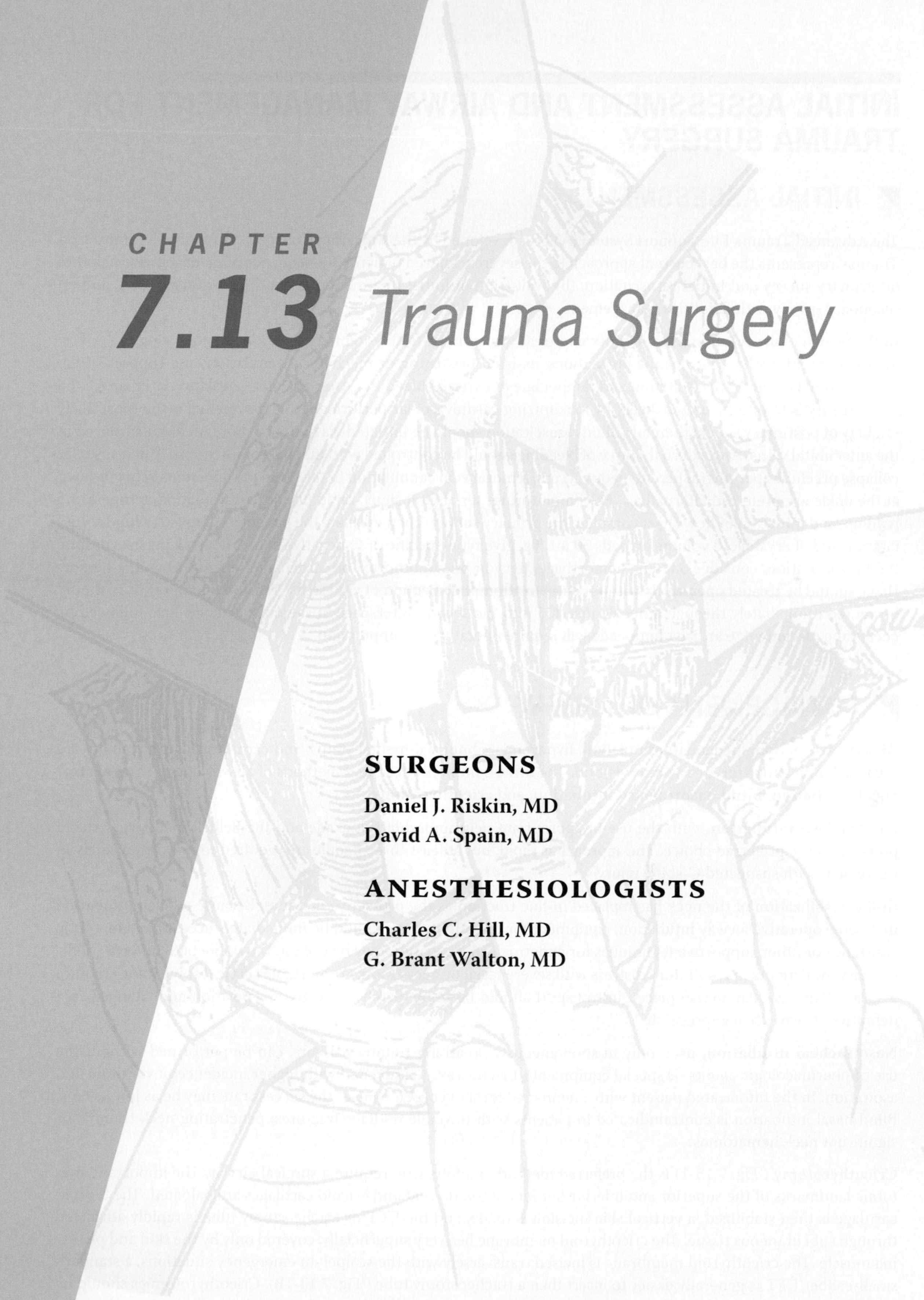

SURGEONS

Daniel J. Riskin, MD
David A. Spain, MD

ANESTHESIOLOGISTS

Charles C. Hill, MD
G. Brant Walton, MD

INITIAL ASSESSMENT AND AIRWAY MANAGEMENT FOR TRAUMA SURGERY

INITIAL ASSESSMENT

The Advanced Trauma Life-Support System (ATLS), developed by the American College of Surgeons Committee on Trauma, represents the best current approach to the severely injured patient. The sequence of management includes: (a) primary survey and initial resuscitation, (b) evaluation of initial treatment and continued resuscitation, and (c) secondary survey with definitive management.

In the primary survey, attempt to identify and treat immediate life-threatening conditions by following the ABCs: **airway control,** with cervical spine precautions; assisted **breathing** or mechanical ventilation; and support of the **circulation** via volume resuscitation and tamponade of external bleeding. After alveolar ventilation is ensured, the next priority is to optimize O_2 delivery by maximizing cardiovascular performance. Hypovolemia is the most likely etiology of postinjury shock; therefore, fluid resuscitation should be initiated via two large-bore iv cannulas placed in the antecubital veins. Any external source of bleeding should be controlled with manual compression. When vascular collapse precludes peripheral percutaneous access, femoral vein cannulation in the groin or saphenous vein cutdown at the ankle are preferred alternatives. ECG monitoring, serial vital signs, rapid physical examination, temperature reading, and initiation of flow sheet complete the primary survey. Then evaluate the patient's response to fluid resuscitation and, if crystalloid volume exceeds 50 mL/kg, give type-specific or O negative blood. If shock persists despite fluid resuscitation, consider ongoing hemorrhage, tension pneumothorax, or cardiac tamponade. Ongoing hemorrhage should be treated operatively without delay to attempt correction of vital signs. Tension pneumothorax should be vented immediately through a needle inserted into the second interspace in the midclavicular line, followed by chest tube placement. Cardiac tamponade will require operative decompression.

MANAGEMENT OF AIRWAY

Airway obstruction, inadequate ventilation, hypoxemia, abnormal mental status, and cardiovascular instability are the usual indications for airway intervention. The three commonly accepted methods of airway control are: **orotracheal intubation, blind nasotracheal intubation,** and **cricothyrotomy**.

Oraltracheal intubation, with the use of appropriate neuromuscular blockade and the Sellick maneuver cricoid pressure, is the preferred choice. The approach is rapid, but at least three people are required to perform it safely in the patient with suspected C-spine injury.

In-line stabilization of the neck has replaced in-line traction as the protective measure. Because a failed intubation may force operative airway intubation, equipment for cricothyrotomy should be immediately accessible. Fiberoptic assistance or other supportive techniques for endotracheal intubation may be used in the stable patient with a difficult airway. Patients in respiratory distress with severe facial or neck trauma or unstable cervical spine injury require a surgical airway. An airway placed in transport should be immediately evaluated for position and changed to a definitive airway when appropriate.

Nasotracheal intubation, used only in spontaneously breathing trauma patients, can be performed without the use of pharmacologic agents or special equipment. It is, however, associated with higher incidence of vomiting and aspiration. In the intoxicated patient with a depressed level of consciousness, the success rate may be as low as 65%. Blind nasal intubation is contraindicated in patients with unstable midface fractures, penetrating neck trauma, or significant neck hematomas.

Cricothyrotomy (Fig. 7.13-1) is the preferred method in adults who require a surgical airway. The important anatomic landmarks of the superior and inferior borders of the thyroid and cricoid cartilages are palpated. The thyroid cartilage is then stabilized, a vertical skin incision is made, and the ETT or tracheostomy tube is rapidly advanced through subcutaneous tissue. The cricothyroid membrane lies very superficially, covered only by the skin and platysma muscle. The cricothyroid membrane is incised transversely with the scalpel. In emergency situations, a standard small-caliber ETT is generally easier to insert than a tracheostomy tube (Fig. 7.13-1B). Cricothyrotomies should be converted to tracheotomies within 72 h after the initial injury, provided the patient's condition permits.

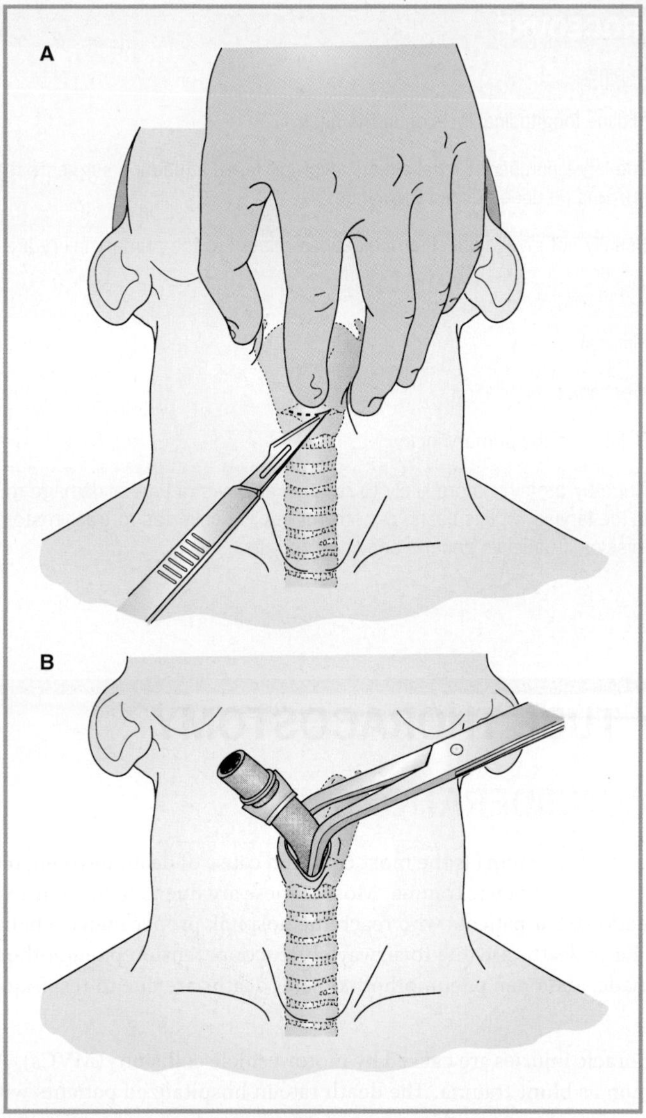

Figure 7.13-1. Cricothyrotomy (vertical skin incision not shown). **(A)** Identification of the cricothyroid membrane by palpation and incision of the membrane transversely. **(B)** Insertion of a tracheostomy tube or ETT through the cricothyroid membrane, which is spread with a tracheal dilator. (Redrawn with permission from Greenfield LJ, Mulholland MW, Oldham KT, et al., eds: *Surgery: Scientific Principles and Practice,* 2nd edition. Lippincott Williams & Wilkins, Philadelphia: 1997.)

A **tracheostomy** is indicated for patients requiring surgical airway in less dramatic situations or if a cricothyrotomy cannot be performed due to direct laryngeal injury. A tracheostomy can be accomplished through the same incision, extended caudally, if laryngeal injury is found (see p. 714). On rare occasions, the injury is in the distal cervical or proximal intrathoracic trachea. In such cases, it may be necessary to intubate the distal end of the airway through the wound. A subsequent median sternotomy may be required to expose the injury. Right thoracotomy provides access to the distal intrathoracic trachea (see Chest Trauma, p. 723).

Usual preop diagnosis: Airway compromise

SUMMARY OF PROCEDURE	
Position	Supine
Incision	Midline longitudinal incision in the neck
Unique considerations	The large number of legal claims involving failed intubation suggests that surgical cricothyrotomy remains an underutilized technique.
Antibiotics	Usually not given until clear indications related to the primary injury are apparent.
Surgical time	2 min
EBL	Minimal
Postop care	Mechanical ventilation
Mortality	Related to the primary injury
Morbidity	Cricothyrotomy is more likely to result in airway stricture or damage to more proximal structures in the larynx. On this basis, cricothyrotomy is converted to tracheostomy within 48–72 h of admission if patient's general condition permits.
Pain score	3

EMERGENCY TUBE THORACOSTOMY

SURGICAL CONSIDERATIONS

Description: In the United States, trauma is the most common cause of death in young people; 25% of these deaths (~16,000 per year) are the result of thoracic trauma. Most of these are due to lethal injuries at the scene (e.g., cardiac rupture, free aortic transection). For patients who reach the hospital, proper management is crucial, because many deaths can be prevented. Early deaths are due to airway obstruction, tension pneumothorax, massive hemothorax, flail chest, cardiac tamponade, and open pneumothorax. Later deaths are due to respiratory failure, sepsis, and unrecognized injuries.

Eighty percent of blunt thoracic injuries are caused by motor vehicle collisions (MVCs). Penetrating injuries to the chest are almost as common as blunt trauma. The death rate in hospitalized patients with isolated chest injury is 4–8%; this increases to 10–15% when one other organ system is involved and to 35% if multiple additional organs are injured. Eighty-five percent of chest injuries do not require thoracotomy, and the patient can be managed with relatively simple measures, such as airway control, tube thoracostomy, and pain management. Blunt trauma can induce injury by three distinctive mechanisms: direct blow, deceleration injury, and compression injury. Rib fracture is the most common sign of blunt thoracic trauma. Fracture of the upper ribs (1st–3rd), clavicle, or scapula implies high-energy impact and is associated with a higher likelihood of major vascular injury.

Life-threatening injuries caused by penetrating trauma are distinctly different from those caused by blunt trauma. In penetrating chest injuries, pneumothorax is almost always present and hemothorax is present in 80% of cases. Hypovolemia from intrathoracic hemorrhage is second only to rib fractures as a sequela of thoracic trauma.

Tension pneumothorax may be caused by blunt or penetrating trauma. Venous return to the heart is impaired by the increased intrathoracic pressure and compression of the vena cava → ↓ BP and distended neck veins. Loss of lung volume on the ipsilateral side and subsequent compression of the contralateral side leads to impaired ventilation and hypoxia. The diagnosis of tension pneumothorax is made clinically. The presence of respiratory distress and absent or diminished breath sounds warrant immediate needle decompression (14–16-ga catheter through the 2nd intercostal space, midclavicular line), followed by subsequent tube thoracostomy. Treatment should not be delayed for radiographic confirmation. Because sequelae of thoracic injuries interfere with air exchange, treatment must take high priority, just after securing the airway, obtaining iv access, and beginning fluid resuscitation. In the hemodynamically stable patient, however, suspicion of a pneumothorax should be confirmed by x-ray. On the CXR, a 20% loss of lung dimension corresponds to ~50% loss of lung volume. A small, simple pneumothorax (< 10%) with no respiratory compromise may be observed. These patients require close observation in the hospital

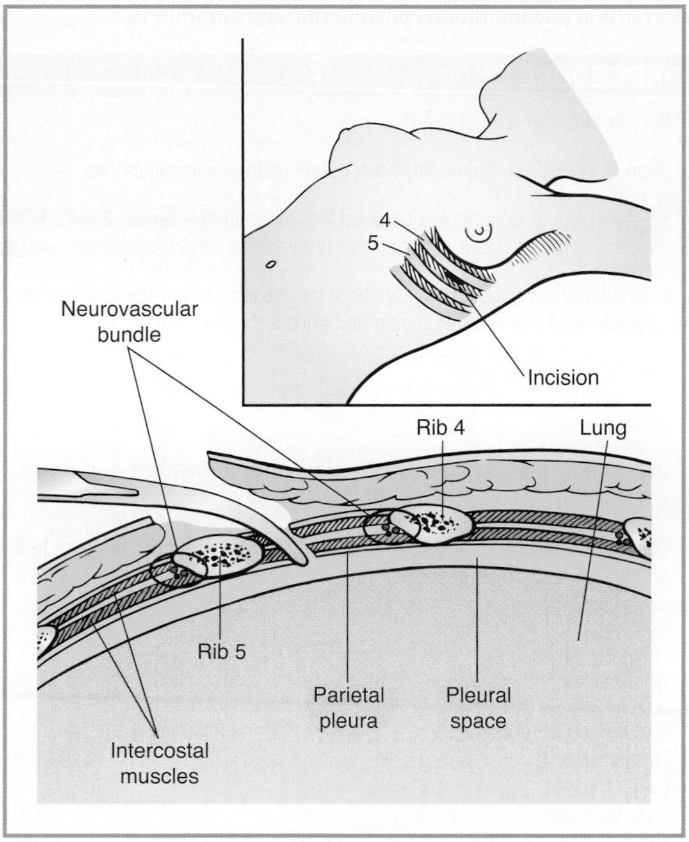

Figure 7.13-2. Tube thoracostomy. Incision through 4th or 5th interspace at anterior axillary line. Forceps are used to tunnel over the superior edge of the rib and to bluntly enter the pleural space.

and a repeat CXR in 4–6 h. Tube thoracostomy should be performed for a large pneumothorax (> 10%), for patients with respiratory compromise or multiple injuries, or when it is not possible to adequately monitor the patient (e.g., during extended transport).

As much as 40% of the circulating blood volume can accumulate in a **hemothorax**. The most frequent sources of bleeding are the intercostal and internal mammary vessels. Some degree of hemothorax is present in almost every patient with chest injury. A supine CXR may miss up to 1 L of blood. Although an upright CXR is more sensitive, this is generally impractical in a multiple-trauma patient (whose spine often has not been fully evaluated). Following chest tube placement, blood loss > 1200–1500 mL or an ongoing loss of 250 mL/h for 4 h suggest the need for surgical intervention.

Simple pneumothorax without associated hemothorax can be treated with a 20–22 Fr chest tube placed in the 4th intercostal space in the midaxillary line or in the 5th intercostal space in the anterior axillary line. Hemothorax and tension pneumothorax require a large-bore, 38–40 Fr chest tube placed in the midaxillary line through the 5th intercostal space (Fig. 7.13-2). A 20-mL syringe with 1% lidocaine can be used not only to provide local anesthesia, but also to locate the upper edge of the rib in the obese patient. A generous 3-cm incision should be made one interspace below the targeted level. The subcutaneous tissues are dissected bluntly, creating a tunnel that is directed upwards. The pleural space should be entered just above the upper edge of the rib to avoid injury to the intercostal neurovascular bundle, located just below the lower edge of the rib. After the pleural space has been entered bluntly, it should be explored with the operator's finger swept around to ensure proper location and to free potential adhesions. The chest tube should be inserted and advanced in the posterior and superior direction. The tube then should be connected to a suction/collection system under 20 cm of water-negative pressure, preferably through an autotransfusion device. CXR should immediately follow chest tube placement to evaluate decompression and assess for other injuries. If the pleural space still contains blood, another chest tube could be inserted or video-assisted thoracoscopy (VAT) could be considered if major vascular injury is not suspected.

Usual preop diagnosis: Tension pneumothorax; pneumothorax; hemothorax

SUMMARY OF PROCEDURE	
Position	Supine with arm abducted 90°
Incision	3 cm in interspace below 5th intercostal space in midaxillary line
Special instrumentation	38–40 Fr chest tube should be used in most patients. Small, 20–22 Fr tube reserved for simple pneumothorax in stable patients. Autotransfusion device should be available in ER.
Unique considerations	In tension pneumothorax, a large-bore needle inserted in the 2nd intercostal space of the mid-clavicular line can relieve tension and save a patient's life.
Antibiotics	Cefazolin 1 g iv
Surgical time	5 min
EBL	Minimal from tube placement. Variable amounts drained out, depending on extent of hemothorax and associated injuries.
Postop care	Chest tube may be removed after at least 48 h, when there is no air leak from lung and < 100–150 mL of fluid drainage per 24 h.
Mortality	Isolated chest injury: 4–8% When one other organ system is involved: 10–15% When two or more organ systems involved: > 35%
Morbidity	Clotted hemothorax Empyema Lung abscess Lung contusion
Pain score	5

EMERGENCY DEPARTMENT THORACOTOMY

SURGICAL CONSIDERATIONS

Description: Rarely, emergency department thoracotomy may offer the only chance of survival in highly selected trauma patients. Its use should be restricted largely to patients who show signs of life in the emergency department (ED) but lose such signs shortly thereafter. The usual indications are: (a) massive exsanguination in the left chest, usually due to cardiac, vascular, or pulmonary injuries and (b) pericardial tamponade. For patients with penetrating cardiac injuries who show signs of life in the ED, survival may be as high as 15%. For blunt trauma in this setting, survival is < 1%, regardless of presentation. With either mechanism, functional survival is almost unprecedented if the patient arrives without vital signs and unreactive pupils.

A **left anterolateral thoracotomy** is the preferred approach since pericardiotomy, open cardiac massage, and aortic occlusion are best achieved by this means. This incision can be extended easily across the sternum and into the right chest to improve exposure and to control massive blood loss and/or air embolism from the right lung. The entire chest is prepped liberally, and left anterolateral thoracotomy is performed rapidly in the 5th intercostal space using a large-blade scalpel. Heavy scissors can be used to quickly divide the intercostal muscles and to cut across the sternum. If pericardial tamponade is encountered, the pericardium is opened longitudinally, anterior to the phrenic nerve. Blood and clot are evacuated and bleeding sites controlled with gentle digital pressure. Large, full-thickness lacerations that extend into the chambers may be controlled by inserting a Foley catheter, inflating the balloon, and pulling it snug against the myocardium. The open end of the Foley can be clamped or used as an infusion line for resuscitation. During ED thoracotomy, placement of clamps on the atria or ventricles should be avoided as they may extend the laceration. Attempts to repair cardiac lacerations should be delayed until resuscitative measures have been completed. In the nonbeating heart, suturing is performed prior to defibrillation. If coronary or systemic air embolism is present, the appropriate hilum is cross-clamped and air is aspirated from the left ventricle through the elevated apex. Cardiac arrest is an indication for immediate internal massage. The two-hand method is preferred, and internal defibrillation should be instituted. If internal defibrillation does not restore proper cardiac activity, cross-clamping of the aorta will improve coronary perfusion. To cross-clamp the aorta, the left lung is retracted anteriorly and superiorly, and the posterior pleura is dissected under direct vision. Despite proper exposure and an NG tube in the esophagus, cross-clamping the aorta in the ED is difficult.

Usual preop diagnosis: Penetrating chest trauma with cardiac arrest and recent recorded signs of life

SUMMARY OF PROCEDURE	
Position	Supine
Incision	Left anterolateral thoracotomy. Extension of incision across sternum could be considered for improved exposure.
Special instrumentation	ED thoracotomy tray; internal defibrillator paddles; suction device; Foley catheter; rapid-infusion device; O(-) blood
Unique considerations	Airway should be secured first. NG tube should be placed if possible. Typically, patients are not anesthetized for this procedure.
Antibiotics	Cefazolin 1 g iv
Surgical time	10 min
EBL	1–2 L
Postop care	ICU
Mortality	Blunt trauma: 98% All penetrating chest injuries requiring ED thoracotomy: 85% Penetrating cardiac injury: 50%
Morbidity	Arrhythmias Acute MI
Pain score	10

EXPLORATORY SURGERY FOR NECK TRAUMA

SURGICAL CONSIDERATIONS

Description: The cervical region contains a greater variety of vital structures than any other region of the body (Fig. 7.13-3). The cardiovascular, respiratory, digestive, endocrine, and CNS systems are all represented in the neck; injury to any of these can be fatal.

Injuries to the neck may result from blunt or penetrating trauma. In blunt trauma, < 5% of cases will have C-spine injuries. Because the consequences are so grave, however, all patients should be evaluated for C-spine injuries (H&P, x-rays, CT), and full spinal precautions should be maintained until the C-spine is cleared. Blunt airway injuries can be devastating and present significant management difficulties; however, the majority of blunt neck trauma consists of minor soft-tissue injuries that can be managed nonoperatively.

Penetrating neck trauma is defined as penetration of the platysma muscle. For these injuries, the neck is usually divided into three horizontal zones (Fig. 7.13-3, inset). Zone I extends from the sternal notch to the cricoid cartilage. Penetrating injuries in this area are associated with a high mortality. Zone II extends from the cricoid cartilage to the angle of the mandible. Because this is the most exposed region of the neck, injuries can be evaluated and explored relatively easily. Zone III extends from the angle of the mandible to the base of the skull. Because of anatomic constraints, injuries to Zones I and III can be difficult to identify and repair. In patients with a Zone I injury, iv access should be established in the contralateral upper extremity because of the possible injury to the ipsilateral internal jugular vein or subclavian vein.

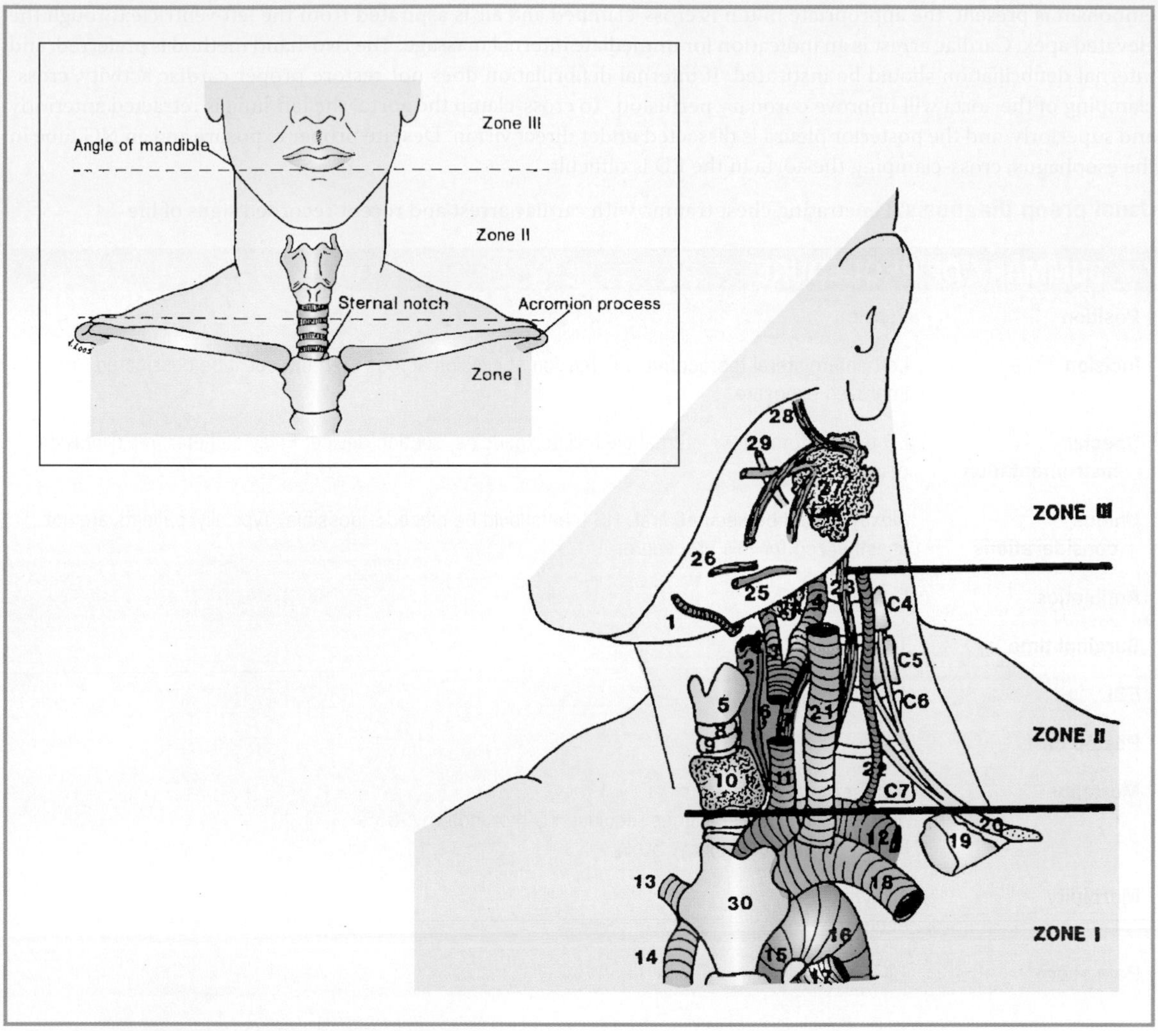

Figure 7.13-3. Cervical structures contained in Zones I, II and III: (1) facial artery; (2) esophagus; (3) internal carotid artery; (4) external carotid artery; (5) thyroid cartilage; (6) sympathetic trunk; (7) vagus nerve; (8) cricothyroid membrane; (9) cricoid cartilage; (10) thyroid cartilage; (11) common carotid artery; (12) subclavian artery; (13) right innominate vein; (14) SVC; (15) ascending aorta; (16) descending aorta; (17) PA; (18) subclavian vein; (19) clavicle; (20) brachial plexus; (21) IJ vein; (22) vertebral artery; (23) phrenic nerve; (24) submandibular gland; (25) lingual artery; (26) hypoglossal nerve; (27) parotid gland and duct; (28) facial nerve and its branches; (29) maxillary artery; (30) sternal manubrium. The thoracic duct is not shown in this figure. (Adapted with permission from Ordog GJ, et al. *J Trauma* 1985; 25:238). (Inset reproduced with permission from Baker RJ, Fischer JE: *Mastery of Surgery.* Lippincott Williams & Wilkins, Philadelphia: 2001.)

Until recently, evaluation and management of stable patients with neck injuries that penetrated the platysma depended on location of injury. Injuries to Zones I and III were evaluated radiographically, whereas injuries to Zone II were indications for mandatory exploration. With the increased availability of CT and arteriography, however, a selective exploration strategy is now favored. Evaluation of the larynx, pharynx, trachea, and esophagus should be performed if Sx are present; however, a penetrating neck wound should never be probed or explored locally, as this may dislodge a clot and precipitate significant hemorrhage or air embolus.

Management of hemodynamically unstable or symptomatic patients with penetrating neck injuries should be limited to applying direct pressure, protecting the airway, establishing iv access, and obtaining a CXR. Exploration and definitive management of the injury in the OR should follow as soon as possible. In stable patients with penetrating injuries and no indications for exploration, CT is generally the first diagnostic test.

A **median sternotomy incision** may be used for patients with right-neck Zone I injuries or if injuries to the mediastinum involving the innominate artery or right subclavian artery are suspected. Exposure of injuries to the proximal left subclavian artery is extremely difficult via median sternotomy. In this case, a left anterior thoracotomy is preferred. The chest and left arm should be prepped and draped so as to allow arm manipulation.

Usual preop diagnosis: Penetrating neck injury

SUMMARY OF PROCEDURE	
Position	Supine with head turned away from side of exploration and neck extended. If both sides of neck require exploration, head should be in midposition. It is helpful to clear the C-spine before exploration.
Incision	Sternocleidomastoid anterior border
Unique considerations	Monitor BP and HR carefully during carotid sinus manipulation.
Antibiotics	Cefazolin 1 g iv. If pharyngoesophageal injury: ampicillin 1 g and gentamicin 80 mg iv.
Surgical time	1 h
Closing considerations	Wound requires drainage, especially in Zone I exploration and if esophagus or airway was violated.
EBL	Variable
Postop care	ICU 12–24 h for neurologic and airway monitoring. After carotid injury repair, angiography should be considered.
Mortality	1%
Morbidity	Hemorrhage: acute from injuries; delayed from pseudoaneurysms Airway injury: acute loss of airway; delayed tracheal stenosis Damage to neural or vascular structures Esophageal fistula
Pain score	4

PATIENT POPULATION CHARACTERISTICS	
Age range	Typically young adult
Etiology	Typically male
Incidence	5–10% of all trauma involves neck structures.
Associated conditions	Intrathoracic injuries; spinal cord injuries; recurrent laryngeal nerve injury; phrenic nerve injuries; thoracic duct injury

ANESTHETIC CONSIDERATIONS FOR NECK TRAUMA SURGERY

PREOPERATIVE

Patients with neck injuries often present unique challenges for ET intubation. Extensive internal damage may be present despite minimal external signs. High-velocity deceleration events, or "clothesline" injuries, are often associated with airway compromise. Vascular injuries, particularly involving the carotid artery, can markedly distort internal anatomy and prevent visualization of laryngeal structures or passage of an ETT. Known or suspected C-spine injuries will restrict optimal positioning of the head and neck for laryngoscopy. Facial or dental injuries may impede access for laryngoscopy because of limited mouth opening or the presence of blood in the oropharynx. The use of alternative methods to secure the airway (e.g., fiber optic bronchoscopy) or a surgical approach may be the safest option. Equipment for a surgical airway should be available prior to attempting ET intubation.

Airway	Preop assessment of the airway and nature and extent of the cervical injury is crucial. Stridor and hoarseness may be present with laryngeal injury or compression of the trachea. Assess patient's ability to talk as a part of the airway evaluation. C-spine injury (though not common with penetrating neck injuries) should be evaluated by x-ray or CT scan. Airway injury can be associated with subcutaneous emphysema or pneumothorax. The extent of mouth opening, dental injuries, and any distortion of internal and external structures due to tissue swelling or hematoma should be determined before induction. The CXR or CT should be examined carefully for evidence of tracheal deviation compression or pneumothorax. **Tests:** x-ray; CT scan; ABG
Cardiovascular	The patient should be evaluated for the extent of blood loss (BP, HR, capillary refill, peripheral pulse, skin condition). In addition to vascular injuries, associated facial and dental injuries may result in significant occult blood loss accumulated in the stomach. Venous lacerations can allow air embolism.
Neurological	Deficits associated with acute compromise of cerebral arterial blood flow should be evaluated on physical exam. Damage to the recurrent laryngeal nerve can occur, resulting in changes in voice and ↑ aspiration risk. C-spine injuries should be assessed by physical exam (neck pain, neurologic examination) and radiologic studies (lateral C-spine x-rays [including C-7] CT scan, MRI).
Premedication	Full-stomach precautions (see p. B-4).

INTRAOPERATIVE

Anesthetic technique: GETA

Induction	The induction technique will depend on the associated injuries and physical exam. In the hypovolemic patient, induction doses of STP or propofol should be reduced by 50–75% to minimize ↓↓ BP. Consider etomidate (0.2–0.3 mg/kg) or ketamine (0.5–1 mg/kg iv) as alternative induction agents. A rapid-sequence iv induction with cricoid pressure is usually required. In the presence of a vascular injury, the cough reflex and the BP response to intubation should be suppressed (e.g., remifentanil 1 mcg/kg iv), in addition to induction agents, to prevent expansion of the hematoma. A wide range of ETT sizes (5.0–8.0 mm) should be available. If C-spine injury is suspected, in-line stabilization of the patient's head and neck should be provided by an assistant. In the presence of an unstable C-spine, cricoid pressure should be avoided to prevent further injury. If a difficult intubation is anticipated, fiber optic intubation (see p. B-5) or an awake surgical airway (cricothyrotomy or tracheotomy) should be considered. In patients with penetrating neck injuries; "blind" intubation techniques should be avoided.
Maintenance	Standard maintenance (p. B-2) is usually appropriate for the normotensive neck-trauma patient. In cases of vascular injury, careful control of BP in the low normal range is advantageous. When nerve testing is anticipated, either no muscle relaxation or a short-acting agent (e.g., mivacurium) should be used.
Emergence	Postop intubation and mechanical ventilation is prudent in patients with residual neurological deficits or oropharyngeal swelling. BP control at low normal levels and slight elevation of the head of the bed (10–20°) will help to resolve tissue edema. Awake extubation is the goal in patients with minimal distortion of the airway at the conclusion of the procedure.

Blood and fluid requirements	IV: 14–16 ga × 2 NS/LR @ 4–6 mL/kg/h	Blood transfusion may be necessary with vascular injuries.
Monitoring	Standard monitors (see p. B-1). ± Arterial line	Invasive monitoring may be indicated for patients with major vascular injuries; however, the placement should not delay the start of emergency surgery.
Positioning	✓ and pad pressure points ✓ eyes	With suspected or known C-spine injuries, stabilization of the head and neck in the neutral position is required.
Complications	Awareness Hypothermia	

POSTOPERATIVE

Complications	Hemorrhage Hematoma Airway compromise	BP control at low normal levels (SNP infusion, labetalol, NTG) and elevation of the head of the bed (10–20°) will help minimize tissue edema and hematoma formation, which could lead to airway compromise.
Pain management	See p. C-1.	
Tests	As indicated.	

Suggested Readings

1. Dutton RP, McCunn M: Anesthesia for trauma. In: *Miller's Anesthesia,* 6th edition, Vol 2. Miller RD, et al., eds. Churchill Livingstone, New York: 2005, 2451–95.
2. Kendall JL, Anglin D, Demetriades D: Penetrating neck trauma. In: *Emerg Med Clin North Am: Contemporary Issues in Trauma.* Eckstein M, Chan D, eds. WB Saunders, Philadelphia: 1998, 85–106.
3. Wisner D, Blaisdell FW: Neck injuries. In: *Scientific American Surgery,* Vol 1. Scientific American, New York: 1998.

CHEST TRAUMA: PERICARDIAL WINDOW, RELEASE OF TAMPONADE, REPAIR OF CARDIAC LACERATION

SURGICAL CONSIDERATIONS

Description: Cardiac contusions may occur in patients with blunt chest trauma. The degree of injury varies from localized contusion to cardiac rupture, but most are clinically insignificant if the patient survives to the hospital. Autopsy studies of victims of immediately fatal accidents show that as many as 65% have rupture of one or more cardiac chambers and 45% have pericardial lacerations. Most of the patients with cardiac rupture die at the scene; however, survivors are reported if vital signs are present during transport. Early clinical findings in cardiac contusion are most commonly dysrhythmias, but occasionally patients can develop cardiac failure. The initial ECG in the ED is the most sensitive diagnostic test. The most common abnormalities are atrial arrhythmias and right bundle branch block. Serial cardiac monitoring is indicated only if the initial ECG is abnormal. Serum enzymes are not helpful. Management is symptomatic. Arrhythmias should be treated in the standard fashion and are not a contraindication to surgery. Pericardial lacerations from stab wounds tend to seal and cause tamponade, present in 80–90% of patients with stab wounds to the heart. Accumulation of 150 mL of blood in the pericardium may impair preload and cause shock. **Beck's triad** of distended neck veins, muffled heart sounds, and ↓ BP is present in only 30% of patients with tamponade. Pulsus paradoxus is even less reliable. The diagnostic test of choice is ultrasound, performed in the ED as part of the focused assessment by sonography for trauma (FAST) exam.

Treatment of penetrating cardiac injuries has gradually changed from initial management by **pericardiocentesis** to prompt **thoracotomy** and **pericardial decompression.** Pericardiocentesis, with ultrasound guidance, may be used to stabilize a patient until sternotomy or thoracotomy can be performed. A subxiphoid pericardial window is an option, but is best performed in the OR.

Gunshot wounds (GSWs) can produce extensive myocardial damage, multiple perforations, and massive bleeding into the pleural space. Hemothorax, shock, and exsanguination occur in nearly all cases of cardiac GSWs. Pericardial tamponade is often absent. Hemodynamically stable patients with penetrating injuries close to the heart should have ECG evaluation in the ED only if equipment is immediately available. The presence of pericardial fluid should be evaluated with a FAST scan. If a hemopericardium is confirmed, blood should be evacuated and injury treated in the OR.

Patients who are stable enough to be transported to the OR have excellent prognosis with reported survival of 97% for stab wounds and 71% for GSWs. In contrast, patients who require ED thoracotomy have only a 15% survival rate for penetrating injuries.

Subxiphoid pericardial window under local or GA: The entire chest is prepped for potential sternotomy. A vertical midline incision is made over the xiphoid process and upper epigastrium. The xiphoid is elevated or excised, allowing access to the pericardiophrenic membrane and anterior mediastinum. The pericardium is opened between two stay sutures and inspected for the presence of blood. If blood is found, definitive repair should follow without delay. With the use of FAST scanning, this operation is rarely indicated as a diagnostic procedure.

Median sternotomy provides excellent exposure to the heart, great vessels, and pulmonary hila. This approach is ideal for anterior injuries and for the unstable patient, but is less well suited for posterior injuries and left subclavian injuries.

Left anterior/anterolateral thoracotomy in the 5th intercostal space can be used in the stable patient or in the newly unstable ED patient with penetrating injury. The pericardium is opened anterior to the phrenic nerve and tamponade is relieved. The bleeding heart is controlled with digital occlusion and the laceration is closed with mattress sutures, with care being taken not to occlude coronary flow. Small coronary branches can be ligated, whereas others should be repaired and may even require CPB.

Usual preop diagnosis: Cardiac laceration

SUMMARY OF PROCEDURE

Position	Supine, L arm abducted 90°
Incision	Median sternotomy or left anterior or anterolateral thoracotomy in 5th intercostal space. (See Fig. 7.13-4.) Further exposure may be obtained by transsternal extension into the R chest.
Special instrumentation	Rapid-infusion device; active rewarming system; internal defibrillator
Unique considerations	Massive blood loss is expected upon opening pericardium and during repair of laceration. Large-bore peripheral lower extremity iv and central venous access are recommended for monitoring of volume replacement. A Foley catheter can be used to occlude laceration and as access for infusion. Arrhythmias are common.
Antibiotics	Cefazolin 1 g iv
Surgical time	45 min
Closing considerations	Hypothermia and coagulopathy contribute to mortality.
EBL	1–2 L
Postop care	ICU
Mortality	Without tamponade: ~90% With tamponade: ~30%

SUMMARY OF PROCEDURE (cont'd)	
Morbidity	Overall: 85% Pulmonary complications Acute MI Arrhythmias Intracardiac shunts Ventricular aneurysms Valvular lesions Retained foreign bodies
Pain score	8

PATIENT POPULATION CHARACTERISTICS	
Age range	Usually young adult
Etiology	GSWs, stab wounds, blunt trauma
Associated conditions	Hemothorax; pneumothorax; great-vessel injury; lung contusion

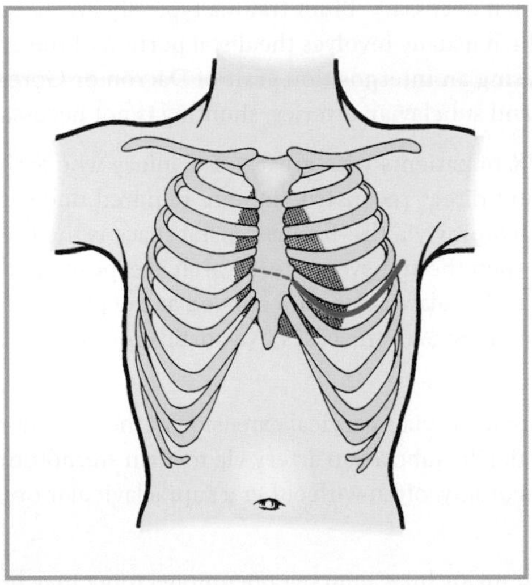

Figure 7.13-4. Incision (dashed/solid line) for ED thoracotomy: made immediately below the nipple, extending from sternum as far laterally as possible. (Reproduced with permission from Baker RJ, Fischer JE: *Mastery of Surgery.* Lippincott Williams & Wilkins, Philadelphia: 2001.)

ANESTHETIC CONSIDERATIONS

See Anesthetic Considerations for Chest Trauma, p. 729.

CHEST TRAUMA: REPAIR OF GREAT VESSELS

SURGICAL CONSIDERATIONS

Description: Thoracic great vessel injury accounts for 8–9% of all vascular injuries seen in the trauma center. The subclavian artery and descending thoracic aorta are the vessels injured most often (21% of cases), followed by PA (16%), subclavian vein (13%), vena cava (11%), and innominate artery and pulmonary veins (9%).

Rupture of the thoracic aorta is the most lethal injury following blunt chest trauma and causes up to 50% of fatalities in MVCs. Proposed mechanism of injury is a deceleration force causing flexion or torsion of the aortic arch and subsequent disruption of the aortic wall at the ligamentum arteriosum immediately distal to the left subclavian artery. Survival of the patient depends on retention of the hematoma by the adventitial layer of the aorta. The mechanism of injury and the mediastinal silhouette on CXR are the two most sensitive markers for an injured thoracic aorta. Depressed left mainstem bronchus, apical capping, and a deviated trachea or esophagus (NG tube) seen on CXR may be suggestive of aortic injury. CT angiogram of the chest has high sensitivity and is the preferred modality of evaluation in most trauma centers as a screening test. Arteriography is the gold standard for evaluating aortic injuries and may also allow therapeutic intervention.

Smaller dissections in blunt trauma may be managed in the ICU with tight blood pressure control. Injuries requiring operative intervention are traditionally managed with thoracotomy and graft interposition. Newer endovascular techniques are increasingly used as an adjunct to surgery or for definitive repair. Investigation of these techniques is ongoing.

Ascending aorta: Rupture requires median sternotomy, CPB and repair with a Dacron graft. Penetrating injury to the anterior aspect of the aorta can be repaired primarily; if there is additional posterior injury, CPB is required for successful repair.

Aortic arch: Complete exposure of the great vessels is required; median sternotomy with extension to the neck and division of the innominate vein may be utilized. Complex injuries may require CPB.

Innominate artery, right carotid artery: Approach is via a median sternotomy with right cervical extension and division of the innominate vein, if necessary. Blunt trauma typically involves the proximal innominate artery, in contrast to penetrating trauma, which usually involves the distal portion of the artery near the carotid or subclavian bifurcation. Injuries are repaired using an interposition graft of Dacron or Gore-Tex. Because cerebral perfusion is maintained through the L carotid and subclavian arteries, shunting is not necessary.

Descending thoracic aorta: 97% of patients with great-vessel injury who arrive alive at the hospital will have an injury at the isthmus. Clamping and direct reconstruction are required under temporary bypass shunt or pump-assisted shunt. Posterolateral thoracotomy via the 4th intercostal space is the preferred access. Distal control of the descending aorta is obtained first; then the transverse aortic arch is exposed and umbilical tape is applied between L carotid and L subclavian arteries. Vascular clamps are applied at the proximal aorta, distal aorta, and subclavian artery. Graft interposition is utilized in 85% of the cases. An aortic cross-clamp time of < 30 min minimizes the incidence of paraplegia.

Subclavian artery or vein: Approach is via a cervical extension of the median sternotomy for right-sided injuries. Exposure of injuries to the proximal, left, subclavian artery via median sternotomy is usually inadequate. In patients with such injuries, a high left thoracotomy, often with either a supraclavicular or trap-door incision, is needed. Graft interposition is often necessary.

Pulmonary artery and veins: In major hilar injury, a pneumonectomy may be necessary, despite high mortality. Cross-clamping of the hilum prevents air embolus and hemorrhage. Simultaneous cross-clamping of the vessels and bronchus may reduce mortality in those patients requiring pneumonectomy. Fluid administration should be kept to a minimum to prevent right heart failure.

Thoracic vena cava: Intrathoracic IVC injury may cause hemopericardium and tamponade. Repair often is performed through the R atrium. SVC repair often is performed via a lateral venorrhaphy.

Usual preop diagnosis: Thoracic great vessel injury

SUMMARY OF PROCEDURE

Position	Supine
Incision	Anterolateral thoracotomy is preferred as it provides access to the descending aorta for cross-clamping, good access to heart, and may be extended across sternum into right chest.
Special instrumentation	Intraop blood recovery device; rapid-infusion device; graft materials for any vessels larger than 5 mm. CPB may be necessary.
Unique considerations	Use of vasodilators (SNP) prevents cardiac strain during cross-clamping of the aorta. Large amount of fluid is required to prevent hypotension after clamp removal.

SUMMARY OF PROCEDURE (cont'd)	
Antibiotics	Cefazolin 1 g iv
Surgical time	1–3 h
EBL	≥ 1 –2 L
Postop care	ICU. Careful hemodynamic monitoring is critical since underlying pulmonary contusion may be worsened by inappropriate fluid administration. PA catheter may be necessary to optimize hemodynamic parameters, particularly in older patients. Coagulation studies must be carefully monitored and corrected with appropriate blood products.
Mortality	In general, mortality is associated with multisystem trauma and usually 2° concomitant head injury, infection, respiratory insufficiency, and renal insufficiency. Pulmonary artery or vein, suprahepatic IVC, or SVC injury: > 70% Ascending thoracic aorta, aortic arch (in patients with stable vital signs on arrival): 50% Blunt injury to the descending thoracic aorta: 5–25% Subclavian artery injury: 5%
Morbidity	Paraplegia: ~8% (with descending aortic injuries)
Pain score	10

PATIENT POPULATION CHARACTERISTICS	
Age range	Typically young adult
Incidence	Thoracic great vessel injury accounts for 8–9% of all vascular injuries seen in the trauma center.
Etiology	Blunt trauma from MVC; penetrating trauma from stab wounds or GSWs
Associated conditions	Pneumothorax; hemothorax; head injury

ANESTHETIC CONSIDERATIONS

See Anesthetic Considerations for Chest Trauma, p. 729.

CHEST TRAUMA: PNEUMONECTOMY, LOBECTOMY, REPAIR OF TRACHEOBRONCHIAL INJURY

SURGICAL CONSIDERATIONS

Description: Penetrating injuries to the chest can be divided into high- and low-velocity injuries. All stab wounds are classified as low-velocity injuries. GSWs may be considered low- or high-velocity injuries, depending on energy of the bullet. The majority of GSWs seen in the ED are low-velocity; however, higher velocity injuries are being seen with increased frequency. The extent of tissue destruction in high-velocity injuries is related to blast effect, tumbling, and fragmentation of the missile, as well as secondary missiles, such as bone fragments. Patients with such injuries are more likely to require thoracotomy and pulmonary resection. In general, pulmonary resection is required in 1% of stab wounds and 2% of GSWs. The indications for early operation are continued shock, prolonged bleeding, a larger air leak with inability to oxygenate or ventilate the patient, and suspected concomitant injuries to the vital intrathoracic structures. In most patients with stab wounds or low-velocity GSWs, bleeding from the lung tissue stops spontaneously after evacuation of the hemothorax and re-expansion of the lung. Only 5–10% of such patients will require thoracotomy to control bleeding as compared to a thoracotomy rate of 70% for high-velocity injuries. Pulmonary contusion is a frequent sequela of GSWs or blunt trauma to the chest. Pulmonary contusion occurs in

75% of patients with flail chest but also can occur following blunt trauma without rib fracture. Alveolar rupture with fluid transudation and extravasation of blood are early findings.

The incidence of tracheobronchial injuries reported in the autopsy series from MVC is 1%. Mechanisms of injury include rapid deceleration, direct blow, or sudden increase of intratracheal pressure against a closed glottis. The most common injury is transverse rupture, occurring in 74%, followed by longitudinal rupture in 18%, and complex in the remaining 8%. Approximately 80% of cases with tracheal rupture occur within 2.5 cm of the carina. Patients with injury to the airway may present with severe dyspnea and with massive subcutaneous emphysema. About 90% of these patients will have an abnormal CXR, showing pneumothorax, pneumomediastinum, subcutaneous emphysema, or pleural effusion.

Tracheobronchoscopy should be performed in all patients with suspected tracheobronchial injuries to establish the diagnosis and plan operative treatment.

Parenchymal lacerations are repaired by the simplest method available to stop bleeding or air leak. If pulmonary resection is required, formal segmental resection is not necessary. A stapling device should be used to preserve as much lung tissue as possible.

Anatomic pulmonary resections are indicated when bronchial injury repair is not feasible or may lead to complete lobar collapse. **Pneumonectomy** may be required for major hilar injuries but is associated with a mortality rate of 75%. **Primary repair of tracheobronchial injuries** should be performed as soon as possible. Transverse rupture may require the placement of a sterile tracheal tube into the distal trachea through the operative field. After posterior sutures are placed, an orotracheal tube is advanced beyond the area of injury. **Main-stem bronchial repair** is performed under one-lung ventilation. High-frequency jet ventilation may be required to maintain oxygenation. Occasionally, total CPB is necessary for repair of complex airway injuries. Before closing, the suture line is pressure-tested and evaluated by fiberoptic bronchoscopy.

Usual preop diagnosis: Tracheobronchial injury; penetrating/blunt chest trauma

SUMMARY OF PROCEDURE

Position	Supine, with neck extended for proximal tracheal injury, or lateral decubitus
Incision	Transverse cervical for almost all proximal tracheal injuries Right posterolateral thoracotomy in 5th intercostal space for thoracic trachea and right bronchial wounds. Left posterolateral thoracotomy for L bronchial injury
Special instrumentation	Fiber optic bronchoscope, intrabronchial tube, jet ventilator/oscillator
Unique considerations	In patients with lobar resection or after pneumonectomy, PEEP may result in bronchopleural fistula
Antibiotics	Cefazolin 1 g iv
Surgical time	2–3 h
EBL	Variable
Postop care	ICU (typically)
Mortality	Pneumonectomy for trauma: 75% Penetrating tracheobronchial injuries: ~15%
Morbidity	Bronchopleural fistula: 10% Empyema: 5% Hemothorax: 2–5% Pneumothorax ARDS (depends on extent of injuries)
Pain score	Cervical approach: 5–7 Thoracic approach: 8–10

ANESTHETIC CONSIDERATIONS FOR CHEST TRAUMA SURGERY

Blunt and penetrating chest trauma may present as hemopericardium, hemo/pneumothorax, blunt cardiac injury, airway injuries, pulmonary contusion with or without associated flail-chest syndrome, and diaphragmatic injury. Hemopericardium may rapidly progress to pericardial tamponade, requiring immediate pericardiocentesis or pericardial window, followed by surgical exploration and repair of the cardiac or vascular laceration. These patients typically present in shock (↓↓ BP) with distended neck veins (↑↑ venous pressure) and distant heart sounds (Beck's triad) without evidence of tension pneumothorax. Hemothorax may present as respiratory failure, shock and absent breath sounds over the affected hemithorax. Blunt cardiac trauma may present with findings ranging from isolated ECG changes to cardiac rupture. The right ventricle and interventricular septum are most commonly affected. Arrhythmias and ventricular dysfunction are frequently observed. Intrathoracic tracheobronchial injuries are less frequent than upper airway injuries, although they are associated with a high mortality and usually require operative intervention. Pulmonary contusion often presents with hypoxia and tachypnea; hemoptysis may also be present. Large flail-chest defects may require mechanical ventilation. VATS has emerged as the leading diagnostic tool for detection of diaphragmatic injury. Preoperatively, and particularly during the induction of GA, the patient's intravascular volume must be expanded and myocardial contractility, HR, and SVR maintained. Inotropes and antiarrhythmic drugs may be required if hemodynamic instability occurs and does not respond to iv fluid administration. CPB is usually not required.

PREOPERATIVE

Respiratory	Associated injuries, such as hemothorax and/or pneumothorax, may be present, requiring thoracostomy tube placement. Fractures of the first or second rib should prompt a detailed search for associated intrathoracic injuries. A widened mediastinum, apical pleural capping, or fracture of the first or second rib often occurs with injury to the great vessels. Multiple rib fractures are often associated with pulmonary contusions, which may not be apparent on the initial CXR, but can progressively impair oxygenation. With tamponade, spontaneous respiration is preferred over PPV (→↓ venous return + ↓ CO). Significant intrathoracic tracheobronchial disruption may require rigid bronchoscopy or a surgical airway. **Tests:** CXR (PA +lateral views). Upright inspiratory films best delineate chest structures; expiratory films enhance visualization of pneumothorax, but are difficult to obtain in multiple-trauma patients; ABG; Chest CT if the patient's condition permits.
Cardiovascular	BP and HR should be followed and responses to fluid resuscitation noted. With adequate resuscitation, the EJ veins should appear full. CO can be significantly reduced despite normal BP measurements. Pulsus paradoxus may be present, with decreases in SBP of 10–12 mmHg during inspiration. Preop, intravascular volume should be restored, especially in the setting of suspected severe RV dysfunction, and myocardial contractility supported with inotropes as necessary. Correction of metabolic acidosis with iv bicarbonate may be indicated (e.g., 1 mEq/kg, then ✓ ABG). Myocardial contusion also can occur and can be associated with atrial or ventricular arrhythmias, RBBB, and RV failure, because the right heart is substernal and most directly involved in blunt trauma to the sternum. Supportive therapy with antiarrhythmics (e.g., lidocaine 1–2 mg/min) and inotropes (dopamine or epinephrine) may be required. Electrolyte abnormalities should be corrected. Substantial intravascular access should be obtained, with strong consideration given to the need for invasive monitoring (arterial line, CVP, etc.). **Tests:** ABG, serial ECGs with myocardial contusion. FAST-scan is the test of choice for detection of pericardial effusions. TTE or TEE may definitively diagnose cardiac tamponade, significant hemothorax and major aortic injuries.
Neurological	↓ BP and ↓ CO may compromise cerebral perfusion. Associated head injury also can contribute to alterations in mental status. Pupil size and reactivity should be noted. Glasgow Coma Scale score ≤ 8 indicates significant brain injury.
Musculoskeletal	Known or suspected C-spine fractures require intubation precautions, with laryngoscopy performed while an assistant provides in-line stabilization of the patient's head in the neutral position. **Tests:** Lateral C-spine x-rays, including C-7; CT; MRI

INTRAOPERATIVE

***Anesthetic technique:** GETA with full-stomach precautions (see p. B-4). **NB:** In the patient with an unstable C-spine, cricoid pressure (~10 lb) may cause spinal cord injury, and consideration should be given to the establishment of a surgical airway under local anesthesia.

Induction	GETA is required for exploration through a median sternotomy or left thoracotomy. In the latter case, a DLT or BB is desirable. If a difficult airway is anticipated, a single-lumen ETT may be placed initially with a DLT placed with an airway exchange catheter. Rapid-sequence induction with ketamine (0.5–2.0 mg/kg) and succinylcholine is attractive because higher doses of ketamine are usually associated with ↑ HR, ↑ BP and ↑ CO. Careful consideration should be given to the catecholamine-depleted trauma patient, in whom the direct myocardial depressant effects of ketamine may be unmasked. Etomidate (0.2–0.6 mg/kg) is a useful alternative for patients with head injuries. Inotropic agents (ephedrine, dopamine, epinephrine) should be immediately available to treat ↓ BP. Agents which tend to decrease SVR, such as inhalational anesthetics and narcotics, should be introduced with caution. The potential for sudden and substantial blood loss exists and PRBCs (cross-matched, type-specific or O neg) should be available in the OR prior to induction.	
Maintenance	Initially, low-dose inhalational agents and low-dose narcotics may be used, as tolerated. ↓ BP may require dopamine infusion (1–10 mcg/kg/min). Muscle relaxation and PPV are used. N_2O should be avoided if there will be a need for one-lung ventilation or there is associated pulmonary contusion. If the patient is hypotensive and acidotic, scopolamine (0.2–0.4 mg iv) will ↓ risk of recall. As cardiac and vascular injuries are repaired, BP and CO often will improve, permitting increased depth of anesthesia and decreased inotropic support. Indicators of improved tissue perfusion should be followed, such as resolution of lactic acidosis, central or mixed venous oxygen saturation, and improved urine output.	
Emergence	Trauma patients often require prolonged intubation; however, hemodynamically stable patients with limited injuries may be extubated awake. Patients who received significant blood replacement (> 50% of blood volume), those requiring inotropic support, intoxicated patients and those with head injuries should remain intubated and mechanically ventilated postop. Consideration for continued mechanical ventilation should be given to those patients with large pulmonary contusions and/or flail-chest segments.	
Blood and fluid requirements	Be prepared for large blood loss. IV: 14 ga × 2 Fluid warmer Rapid-infusion device Airway humidifier T&C PRBCs	Large blood losses occur occasionally, depending on the severity of the injury. Crystalloid and/or blood products should be infused to maintain BP and CVP (full jugular veins).
Monitoring	Standard monitors (see p. B-1). Arterial line CVP ± PA catheter	ECG should be observed for changes associated with myocardial contusion (atrial/ventricular dysrhythmias, RBBB, ST-T wave changes). CVP monitoring can be useful in guiding fluid management. With release of tamponade, CVP rapidly drops toward normal, and CO and BP will markedly improve.
	± TEE	Will provide excellent monitor of LVEDV and SVR, as well as RVSP.
Positioning	✓ and pad pressure points ✓ eyes ± C-spine: neutral position	Axillary roll, if lateral decubitus position; chest roll if median sternotomy.
Complications	Hypothermia	Hypothermia → dysrhythmias + ↓ CO → acidosis. Rx: warm OR, warm iv fluids, humidify gases, and use patient warming devices.
	Awareness	May be unavoidable in unstable patients. Rx: Consider scopolamine 0.2–0.4 mg iv.

General Surgery

Complications (cont'd)	Renal failure	Usually 2° ↓ renal perfusion (prerenal). Rx: Restore CO with volume and inotropes.
	Coagulopathy	Most commonly 2° dilutional thrombocytopenia. DIC may require replacement therapy with Plts, FFP and cryoprecipitate. Massive transfusion may benefit from a 1:1 ratio of PRBC to FFP. Maintain nl Ca^{++} (1.05–1.3 mM/L).

POSTOPERATIVE

Complications	Hypotension Arrhythmias	Cardiogenic shock may be 2° prolonged ↓ BP or cardiac contusion. Neurogenic shock may be seen with associated spinal cord injuries. Hemodynamic instability with atrial/ventricular dysrhythmias may occur. Treatment with inotropic infusions (dopamine 5–10 mcg/kg/min or epinephrine 50–200 ng/kg/min) and antiarrhythmics.
	Hypothermia	Active warming of iv fluids and warming blanket should be continued in ICU or PACU if hypothermia persists. If neurologic injury is present, consideration should be given to mild hypothermia.
	ARDS	Interstitial and alveolar edema → progressively worsening pulmonary function requiring prolonged mechanical ventilation. Institution of lung protective ventilation strategies should be considered.
	Coagulopathy Renal failure	Based on clinical assessment and laboratory data (PT, Plt count, fibrinogen); transfusion of Plts, FFP, and/or cryoprecipitate may be indicated.
	VTE	See p. B-7.
Pain management	PCA (p. C-3) or parenteral narcotics Epidural (p. C-2)	Epidural infusions of narcotic and/or low dose local anesthetics can be effective in patients without coagulopathy. Continuous epidural anesthesia will also be beneficial in the setting of multiple rib fractures.

ABDOMINAL TRAUMA: DAMAGE CONTROL

SURGICAL CONSIDERATIONS

Description: The incidence of abdominal injuries requiring laparotomy approaches 25% for penetrating and 5–8% for blunt abdominal trauma. In blunt trauma, liver and spleen injuries occur with an incidence of ~50%. In penetrating trauma, the most common injuries are small bowel (29%), liver (28%), colon (23%), and stomach (13%). Many preventable deaths in trauma patients are related to shock from unrecognized intraabdominal hemorrhage caused by solid organ injury.

Victims of severe multisystem trauma are particularly susceptible to development of a fatal coagulopathic state 2° hypothermia, acidosis, dilution, and consumption. Replacement of two or more blood volumes with NS or PRBCs will decrease the level of coagulation factors to 15%. Because of delays in obtaining coagulation profile results, coagulation factors should be replaced empirically in the setting of a large transfusion requirement (e.g., 1 U FFP/1.5 U PRBC). Metabolic acidosis affects both the circulatory system and coagulation, → ↓ CO and triggering DIC. Chances of salvaging a patient with pH < 7.0 approach zero. To stop this self-perpetuating downward cycle, the concept of "Damage Control" has evolved. This involves rapid laparotomy to control hemorrhage and GI spillage, followed by temporary closure of the abdomen and subsequent exploration after the patient has been warmed and stabilized. With the use of this technique, ~40% of critically injured patients can be saved from otherwise fatal injuries.

With the patient on a heated operating table, the patient is prepped from the thighs to the neck and draped, and the abdomen is entered through a midline incision. This critical moment can be associated with significant blood loss and may require rapid blood transfusion. Four-quadrant packing with laparotomy pads is performed in the abdominal cavity, and manual compression of the subdiaphragmatic aorta may be instituted if packing alone does not control the hemorrhage. If necessary, the operation is stopped and blood/fluid resuscitation is performed. After consultation with the anesthesiologist, the surgeon proceeds with the sequential unpacking of each of the four quadrants and identifying injuries. Vascular injuries are controlled with clamping and ligation or shunting, bowel injuries are stapled across, but no attempt is made for primary repair. Liver and retroperitoneal injuries are controlled with packing alone. When damage control is performed, the abdomen is closed with a running skin suture, if appropriate; otherwise, a temporary vacuum dressing is used. PIP should be monitored during closure, as patients may develop abdominal compartment syndrome (↑↑ intra-abdominal pressure → ↑ PIP, ↓ UO, normal filling pressures). The patient is then transported to ICU and actively warmed and resuscitated. Reoperation should be performed at 24–48 h when the patient is rewarmed and acidosis and coagulopathy have resolved. Definitive repair of the injured organs should be completed.

Usual preop diagnosis: Intra-abdominal trauma and hemorrhage

SUMMARY OF PROCEDURE

Position	Supine
Incision	Midline abdominal
Special instrumentation	Fluid-warming, rapid-infusion device
Unique considerations	Autotransfusion device (e.g., Cell Saver) may be of use if no contamination of abdominal cavity.
Antibiotics	Cefotetan 1 g iv
Surgical time	45–90 min
Closing considerations	Even temporary closure may not be possible because of severe bowel edema. A silo made from a plastic iv bag may be used to cover the bowel. Monitor PIP and UO during abdominal wall closure, because abdominal compartment syndrome may develop.
EBL	Average transfusion requirement: 12 L crystalloids, 20 U PRBCs, 10–15 U FFP, 6 U Plts
Postop care	ICU; patient remains intubated. Active rewarming is of primary importance.
Mortality	70%
Morbidity	Intraabdominal abscesses: 30% Fistulas: 10%
Pain score	10

PATIENT POPULATION CHARACTERISTICS

Age range	Typically young adult
Male:Female	9:1
Incidence	25% for penetrating and 5% for blunt abdominal trauma
Etiology	MVC; penetrating injury (e.g., GSW or stab wound)
Associated conditions	Chest trauma; closed head trauma; pelvic fracture

ANESTHETIC CONSIDERATIONS

See Anesthetic Considerations for Abdominal Trauma Surgery, p. 737.

ABDOMINAL TRAUMA: HEPATIC AND SPLENIC INJURIES

SURGICAL CONSIDERATIONS

Description: The liver is the most commonly injured organ in patients with penetrating trauma, while the spleen is the most commonly injured organ with blunt trauma. Approximately 30% of all patients requiring laparotomy for trauma will have hepatic injuries. The majority of injuries can be managed nonoperatively unless other injuries mandate laparotomy. Thus, most liver injuries that require operation are complex (grades IV-V), with large blood loss and high mortality (up to 30%).

Several maneuvers can be used to facilitate **repair of liver injuries: Manual compression** temporarily controls bleeding and allows time for volume resuscitation. **Portal triad occlusion** (**Pringle maneuver**) (Fig. 7.13-5) decreases blood loss and identifies the patient who might benefit from selective hepatic artery ligation. Perihepatic

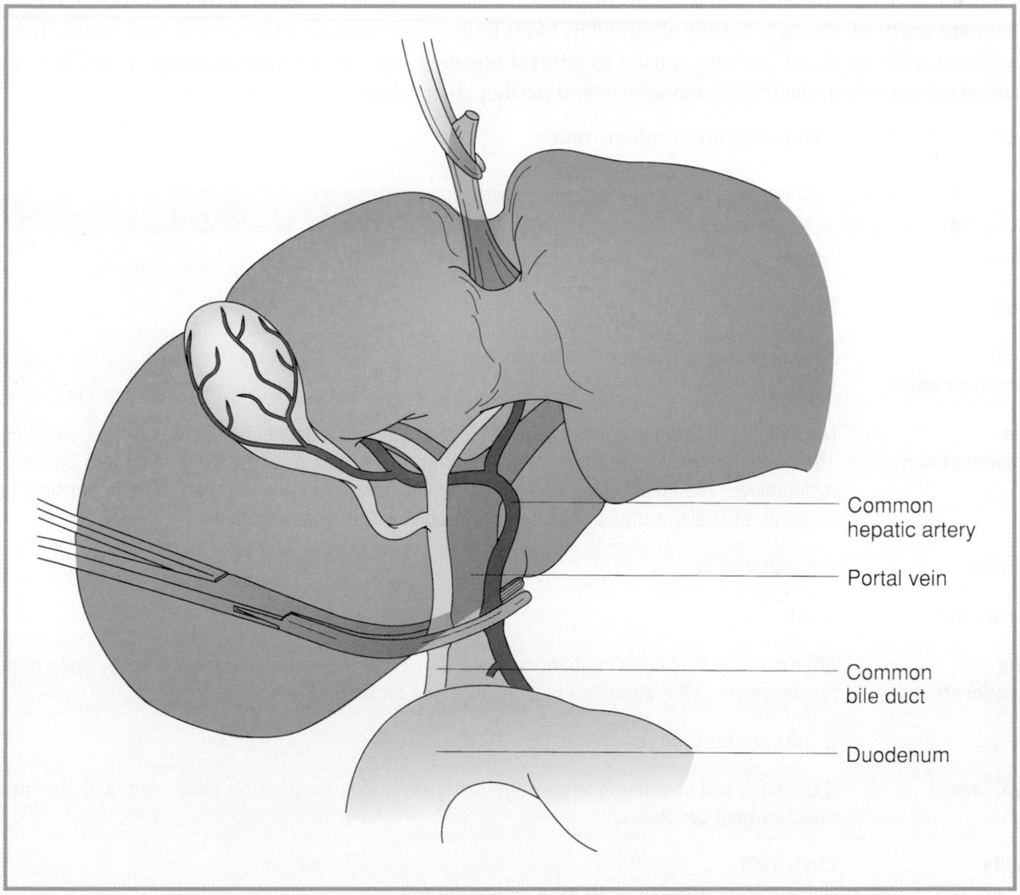

Figure 7.13-5. Pringle maneuver compression of the portal triad structures with a noncrushing vascular clamp for hepatic inflow control. (Reproduced with permission from Greenfield LJ, Mulholland MW, Oldham KT, et al., eds: *Surgery: Scientific Principles and Practice,* 3rd edition. Lippincott Williams & Wilkins, Philadelphia: 2001.)

packing and planned reexploration is a life-saving maneuver and should be used early for patients with severe injuries, before they become hypothermic, coagulopathic, and acidotic. Extensive liver mobilization, parenchymal disruption (i.e., finger fracturing), and atriocaval shunts are rarely indicated. Hepatic angiogram and embolization in the immediate or early postop phase may be very useful for patients with severe injuries. At reexploration, intrahepatic omental packing may be used for obliterating dead space. Closed suction drains should be used in all patients.

Portal triad (portal vein, hepatic artery, common bile duct) injuries, although rare, are associated with extremely high mortality. Isolated portal vein injuries are associated with a 70% mortality. The portal vein should be repaired if possible; however, ligation can be tolerated. Careful volume resuscitation should follow portal vein ligation to avoid ↓ BP 2° fluid sequestration in the splanchnic bed. Simple ligation of the hepatic artery, preferably proximal to the gastroduodenal artery, is recommended for most major hepatic artery injuries. Shock and transfusion-related coagulopathy occurring in the immediate postop period are responsible for 80% of the deaths in liver injury patients. Control of hemorrhage remains the critical component in the successful management of liver injuries.

More than 90% of splenic injuries are caused by blunt trauma. Approximately 75–80% of these patients can be managed nonoperatively. Of the remaining patients, most will require splenectomy, because usually only grade IV (active intraperitoneal bleeding) or V (shattered/avulsed injuries) require operation. Massive bleeding from the LUQ is probably caused by splenic injury. For severe injuries, the spleen is delivered into the wound by blunt dissection. The spleen is removed by cross-clamping the hilum and dividing the short gastric vessels. The LUQ is packed and reinspected for hemostasis once better resuscitation is provided. The splenic salvage rate in the pediatric population approaches 90%.

In a patient with massive **intraabdominal hemorrhage,** sudden cardiovascular collapse is predictable when the abdomen is opened. Laparotomy with manual compression of the aorta at the aortic hiatus is recommended. Access for subsequent aortic clamping is rapidly obtained by blunt finger dissection of the lesser sac. After removing all clots and free blood, four-quadrant packing is used to control bleeding. Significant liver bleeding should be controlled with manual compression, the Pringle maneuver, and perihepatic packing.

Usual preop diagnosis: Hepatic injury; splenic injury

SUMMARY OF PROCEDURE

Position	Supine
Incision	Midline abdominal
Special instrumentation	Active rewarming device; Cell Saver
Unique considerations	Most emergency laparotomies require close cooperation between anesthesiologist and surgeon. The procedure may need to be interrupted for fluid or blood resuscitation if patient becomes hypotensive. The entire chest and abdomen, including both groins, need to be accessible to the surgeon; ECG electrodes are placed preferably on the patient's back.
Antibiotics	Cefazolin 1 g iv
Surgical time	1–2 h
Closing considerations	After massive fluid resuscitation, concern over compartment syndrome may preclude primary fascial closure. The abdomen may be left open for later closure.
EBL	2–10 L (transfusion requirement 6–20 U)
Postop care	ICU: shock and coagulopathy management; monitoring for possible rebleeding and abdominal compartment syndrome.
Mortality	Liver: 10% Spleen: 10% (usually due to associated injuries)
Morbidity	Liver: perihepatic abscess: 10% Spleen: septic complications: 7%
Pain score	8–10

■ PATIENT POPULATION CHARACTERISTICS	
Age range	Any age
Male:Female	3:1
Incidence	Liver: 30% of patients requiring laparotomy for trauma Spleen: 10% of patients requiring laparotomy for trauma
Etiology	Liver: penetrating wound (80%) with gunshot wounds responsible for 60% and stab wounds for 40% Spleen: blunt trauma (90%), mostly due to MVC
Associated conditions	Liver: isolated hepatic injury (30%); injury to one or two other organs (50%), with diaphragm, major vascular structures, stomach, lung, and colon being most common.

ANESTHETIC CONSIDERATIONS

See Anesthetic Conditions for Abdominal Trauma Surgery, p. 737.

ABDOMINAL TRAUMA: VASCULAR INJURIES

SURGICAL CONSIDERATIONS

Description: Penetrating trauma is the most common cause of abdominal vascular injuries: IVC/hepatic veins, 36%; celiac/mesenteric vessels, 30%; iliac vessels, 11%; and aorta, portal/splenic, and renal vessels, each 5%. Patients with gunshot wounds to the abdomen have ~25% incidence of major vascular injury; however, only ~10% of patients with penetrating stab wounds will have vascular injuries. Patients sustaining blunt abdominal trauma who require laparotomy have a 5–10% incidence of vascular injury.

Initial resuscitation of the patient with abdominal vascular injuries depends on the patient's condition. Multiple large-bore catheters should be inserted in the upper extremities or, if necessary, central venous access should be obtained. Because of the probable intraabdominal venous injury, lower-extremity venous access is not indicated. Blood replacement during resuscitation is done preferably with type-specific blood. It is a good practice to have 2 U of O neg blood available immediately in the ED in case there is no time for a limited cross-match. Efforts to limit hypothermia should start as soon as the patient arrives (use of warmed fluids and high-flow blood warmers and covering the patient with warm blankets or a forced-air warming blanket).

Injuries to the abdominal vessels can be grouped into four regions, which require different surgical approaches:

Midline supramesocolic hemorrhage or hematoma (superior to the transverse mesocolon) is usually 2° injury to the suprarenal aorta, celiac axis, proximal superior mesenteric artery, or proximal renal artery. Proximal aortic control should be obtained at the hiatus by either aortic compression or manually by entering the lesser sac and digitally splitting the muscle fibers of the crura. Once this is done, direct access to the vessels is achieved through medial visceral rotation of all left-sided viscera. Injuries to the aorta are then repaired directly or with the appropriate graft. An injured celiac axis probably can be ligated safely if the remaining visceral vessels are intact. Superior mesenteric artery injuries must be repaired, usually with a jump graft. Repair of the superior mesenteric vein is preferred, but the vein may be ligated if complex injuries are present. These patients require substantial fluid resuscitation postop and are at high risk for abdominal compartment syndrome. Injuries to the IVC or right side of the aorta can be exposed by **duodenal mobilization (Kocher maneuver).**

Midline inframesocolic hemorrhage or hematoma results from infrarenal aorta or IVC injury. Exposure is obtained by incising posterior peritoneum in the midline after displacement of the small bowel and cephalic retraction of the transverse mesocolon. A proximal aortic clamp is then placed just below the left renal vein, with a distal clamp near the aortic bifurcation. The defect is repaired primarily, using patch aortoplasty, end-to-end anastomosis, or a graft. If the aorta is intact and an inframesocolic hematoma seems to be more extensive on the right side, or if there is active bleeding coming through the base of the mesentery, then injury to the IVC should be suspected. Access to the infrahepatic IVC is preferably obtained by mobilization of the R colon and duodenum. Proximal and distal controls are best obtained by either digital compression or two sponge sticks. The injury is then repaired directly. Blind clamping should be avoided, but occasionally, with good exposure, a **Satinsky clamp** can be placed. In young patients with exsanguinating hemorrhage, the infrarenal IVC can be ligated, providing time for appropriate fluid management. These patients require significant fluid postop and will likely have chronic venous insufficiency.

Lateral perirenal hematoma or hemorrhage suggests injury to the renal vessels or kidney. In patients with blunt abdominal trauma who have a negative abdominal CT, IVP, or arteriogram, surgery is not required. A penetrating injury usually requires surgical exploration. Vascular control of the ipsilateral renal artery is obtained before the hematoma is entered. If there is active bleeding from the kidney or overlying retroperitoneum, then the kidney is exposed via a lateral incision, and a vascular clamp is applied to the renal vessel. This usually is followed by nephrectomy (after palpation and a one-shot IVP to verify function of a normal contralateral kidney). If the contralateral kidney is missing or nonfunctional, then back-table salvage surgery and autotransplantation of the injured kidney should be attempted. Only 30–40% of kidneys with arterial injuries can be salvaged.

Lateral pelvic hematoma or hemorrhage indicates injury to the iliac vessels. Pelvic hematoma 2° blunt trauma and pelvic fracture should not be explored. Primary control of bleeding is by angiography/embolization and possibly external fixation of the pelvis. This need should be recognized and arranged early in the resuscitative period. For penetrating injuries, vascular control is obtained at the aortic bifurcation proximally and close to the inguinal ligament distally. The internal iliac artery is best visualized by elevating common and external iliac arteries on vascular tapes. Unilateral internal iliac artery injuries can be ligated. Common or external iliac artery injuries can be repaired or a graft can be inserted. Grafts may be used even in the presence of GI contamination, provided the abdomen is thoroughly irrigated and the retroperitoneum is closed over the graft. A temporary intravascular shunt should be used in patients requiring damage control surgery. Injuries to the iliac veins are treated with lateral venorrhaphy or ligation.

Usual preop diagnosis: Abdominal vascular injury

SUMMARY OF PROCEDURE

Position	Supine, with left arm abducted 90°
Incision	Midline abdominal
Special instrumentation	Autotransfusion device (e.g., Cell Saver); thoracotomy tray; aortic compressor
Unique considerations	Prevent heat loss and warm all infusions and irrigation solutions. Ventilator warming should be used for cold patients. For the patient requiring massive transfusion, ratio of 1 U FFP:1.5 U PRBCs useful. After prolonged aortic cross-clamp, prophylactic administration of $NaHCO_3$ (1–2 mEq/kg) may be indicated to prevent 'washout' acidosis.
Antibiotics	Cefazolin 1 g iv
Surgical time	Variable
Closing considerations	Once vascular injuries are repaired, hepatic injuries are controlled with packing, bowel injuries are closed with staplers, and the abdominal wall is closed temporarily.
EBL	5–10 L
Postop care	ICU; Patients after infrarenal vena cava ligation require volume expansion and prevention of lower extremity venous pooling. Elastic wraps and lower-extremity elevation should be maintained for at least 1 wk. Similarly, after superior mesenteric vein ligation, splanchnic hypervolemia requires vigorous fluid resuscitation and lasts ~3 d.
Mortality	Combined injury to the suprarenal aorta and IVC: 100% Aorta: 60% Infrarenal abdominal aorta: 50% Superior mesenteric artery: 40–80% Iliac artery: 40% Iliac vein: 30%

SUMMARY OF PROCEDURE (cont'd)	
Mortality (cont'd)	Infrarenal vena cava: 30% Superior mesenteric vein: 20% Renal artery: 15%
Morbidity	Abdominal compartment syndrome (↑↑ abdominal pressure → ↑ PIP + ↓ UO) Acute renal failure Intraabdominal infection Fistula
Pain score	8–10

PATIENT POPULATION CHARACTERISTICS	
Age range	Typically young adult
Male:Female	Male > female
Incidence	15% of patients with abdominal trauma
Etiology	10% of penetrating stab wounds and 25% of gunshot wounds to the abdomen will cause a major vascular injury.
Associated conditions	Multiple vascular injuries; hollow viscus perforation; fecal contamination

ANESTHETIC CONSIDERATIONS FOR ABDOMINAL TRAUMA SURGERY

Abdominal injuries range from relatively simple penetrating injuries (e.g., a stab wound) to severe blunt trauma (e.g., liver lacerations and pelvic fractures) and are often associated with massive hemorrhage. Head injuries and spinal fractures may complicate management plans. The ability to provide rapid, aggressive volume replacement is often the key to survival. Coagulopathy (DIC) and hypothermia present additional challenges.

PREOPERATIVE

Respiratory	Associated injuries, such as hemothorax and/or pneumothorax, may be present, requiring thoracostomy tube placement. A widened mediastinum, apical pleural capping, or fracture of the 1st or 2nd rib often occurs with serious vascular injuries. Multiple rib fractures suggest possible pulmonary contusions, which may not be evident on initial CXR, but can progressively impair oxygenation and ventilation. **Tests:** CXR (PA +lateral views); ABG
Cardiovascular	BP and HR should be followed and responses to fluid resuscitation noted. Tachycardia can maintain an adequate BP with reduced pulse pressure, despite 25–30% loss of blood volume. Attempt to quantify overt blood loss (e.g., scalp lacerations, open fracture sites). Blunt chest trauma (e.g., steering wheel contact) may result in myocardial contusion with various dysrhythmias, most often premature ventricular or atrial complexes. **Tests:** Serial Hct; ECG in patients > 50 yrs of age or with blunt chest trauma.
Neurological	Seek physical evidence of open or closed head injuries, such as palpable depressions of the skull or scalp lacerations, abrasions, or contusions. Pupil size and reactivity should be noted. Intubation in the ER is necessary for patients who are unable to protect their airway, require hyperventilation or are combative and unable to cooperate with medical staff for exam and treatment. In general, any patient with a Glasgow Coma Scale (GCS) ≤ 8 (no spontaneous eye opening, inappropriate or incomprehensible speech and only reflexive motor responses) requires intubation. Motor and/or sensory deficits may reflect spinal cord injury and may be associated with neurogenic ("spinal") shock, particularly with upper thoracic or cervical cord injuries.

Neurological (cont'd)	**Tests:** C-spine x-rays (lateral view, including C7), is a good screening exam: ✓ for altered vertical alignment and unequal disk interspaces. CT scan or MRI of head: ✓ for gross asymmetry, hemorrhage, or midline shift.
Musculoskeletal	Known or suspected C-spine injuries require intubation precautions. In urgent cases, intubation without neck extension is achieved with an assistant providing in-line stabilization of the head in the neutral position. If time permits, awake, blind, or fiber optic intubation may be attempted. Basilar skull fractures contraindicate nasal ET or NG tubes. Pelvic and femur fractures may represent sources of significant (> 1000 mL) occult blood loss. **Tests:** Radiographs of C-spine (see above), skull, extremities
Hematologic	Depending on estimations of prior, ongoing, and anticipated surgical blood losses, preop T&C may be desired. O neg or type-specific blood should be available until the T&C is complete. **Tests:** Serial Hct; T&C; ✓ Ca^{++} and K^+ following massive transfusions.
Laboratory	Other tests as indicated from H&P or suspected injuries, including electrolytes, liver panel, toxicology screen, blood alcohol level.
Premedication	Premedication is rarely useful due to the urgency of the procedures and the need to have an alert, responsive patient for serial evaluations of mental status or abdominal pain. Sedative premedication should be avoided in patients who are hemodynamically unstable and those with probable head injuries. Virtually all patients are considered to have full stomachs, and any compromise of the ability to protect the airway is inappropriate. Na citrate (30 mL po) may be administered to alert patients at risk for aspiration; however, ranitidine and metoclopramide may not reach effective levels in the short interval before induction.

INTRAOPERATIVE

Anesthetic technique: GETA with full-stomach precautions (p. B-4)

Induction	Before induction, a variety of laryngoscope blades (e.g., Miller 1 and 2, Mac 3 and 4) and ETTs with stylets (6.0, 7.0, and 8.0 mm) should be ready. LMA may be useful for providing temporary airway control without C-spine manipulation if direct laryngoscopy is difficult. LMA may be used as a conduit for ET intubation (fiber optic or fast-track LMA). A size 7.0 mm ETT will pass through a #4 LMA. Equipment for emergent cricothyrotomy (a 14-ga iv catheter + adapter) and jet ventilation should be in OR. Most often, preoxygenation is followed by a rapid-sequence iv induction with cricoid pressure (Sellick's maneuver) using Propofol (1–2.5 mg/kg) and succinylcholine (1.0–1.5 mg/kg). If hypotension is present or a concern, alternate induction agents (e.g., ketamine 0.5–2.0 mg/kg iv or etomidate 0.1–0.3 mg/kg iv) may be used. Verify any meds already administered in ED and field. Axial head and neck stabilization is necessary if C-spine injury is present or suspected. Some trauma patients are intubated in the ED. Verify ETT placement by auscultation and $ETCO_2$ monitoring. Very low $ETCO_2$ values may be obtained in patients with markedly reduced CO. Ventilation with 100% O_2 and paralysis with muscle relaxant (such as rocuronium or vecuronium) is appropriate. Ongoing fluid resuscitation should be continued during this time. Consider sending lab studies/ABG at this point and ensuring availability of blood products.
Maintenance	Titrate O_2/air, muscle relaxants, narcotics, and volatile agents. Avoid N_2O in the presence of pneumothorax, pneumocephalus, bowel distention, or prolonged procedures. Shorter-acting agents (e.g., volatile agents, remifentanil, rocuronium), carefully titrated, may be preferred in patients with head injuries to facilitate early postop assessment of neurologic status. If ↓ BP precludes use of volatile anesthetics and opiates, consider low-dose scopolamine (0.1–0.3 mg iv) or ketamine (0.25 mg/kg/15–30 min) for amnesia. Use forced-air warming blanket(s) and warmed IV fluids, and consider elevated OR temperatures, and warmed irrigation fluids (surgical field, bladder) to maintain normothermia.

Emergence	Prior to extubation, patient should be awake and able to protect his/her airway, and should be hemodynamically stable and spontaneously ventilating with ease through the ETT. Consider postop mechanical ventilation and ICU care for trauma patients with the following conditions: elderly with rib fractures, significant pulmonary compromise/trauma, ongoing acidosis, hemodynamic instability ongoing or anticipated significant fluid and blood product resuscitation, coagulopathies, intoxication or neurological impairment.	
Blood and fluid requirements	Anticipate large blood loss IV: 14–16 ga × 2 or 7–9 Fr × 2 NS/LR variable depending on blood loss Fluid warmers Rapid-infusion device T&C PRBCs, ± other blood products	Large blood losses may have already occurred and continue to occur, depending on the mechanism of injury (e.g., liver lacerations, major vascular injury, pelvic fractures). Determine prior fluid administration in field and ED. Early determination of availability of blood products advised. Crystalloid, colloid and blood products should be given to re-establish euvolemia based injuries, EBL, and clinical assessment, which may include: BP, HR, CVP/PCWP, UO, Hct, ABG, TEE, etc. With massive transfusion, Plts and FFP will be needed. In general, 2–4 U FFP and 6 U of Plts should be transfused after ~10 U of PRBCs (1 blood volume in a 70-kg person) have been given. Postop hypothermia is best minimized by warming all iv and irrigating fluids, maintaining OR temperature @ 78–80°F, humidifying inspired gases, and use of forced air and circulating water warming blankets. Frequent assessment of Hct/Hgb, Plts, coags, Ca^{++}, and ABG essential in managing significant ongoing hemorrhage and resuscitation.
Monitoring	Standard monitors (see B-1). Urinary catheter	Monitor patient during transport to OR and apply standard monitoring as soon as patient enters the OR.
	± Arterial line	Arterial line useful in unstable patient or when frequent lab sampling anticipated.
	± CVP line ± PA catheter ± TEE	CVP line or PA catheter may be useful if vasoactive infusions needed or if ventricular dysfunction apparent. Placement of additional monitoring should be accomplished without delaying the surgical control of hemorrhage or without interrupting aggressive volume resuscitation.
Positioning	✓ and pad pressure points ✓ eyes	If C-spine has not been cleared by both radiographically and clinically, neck should remain immobilized intraop and postop.
Complications	Hypothermia	Preexisting hypothermia common in trauma patient. Measures to manage hypothermia early are key and include: warm OR, use of forced air warming and warm IV fluids.
	Awareness	May be unavoidable in unstable or hypotensive patients. Rx: Consider scopolamine 0.2–0.4 mg iv or midazolam 1–2 mg iv in such situations.
	Coagulopathy	Causes include dilutional, hypothermia and brain injury. Assess status and treat early.
	Aspiration	Assume full stomach; aspiration may have occurred prior to OR
	Airway trauma	Sources include trauma or subsequent AW management

POSTOPERATIVE

Complications	Hypothermia	Active warming of fluids and blood products and forced-air warming blankets and warm room temperatures should be continued in PACU/ICU if hypothermia persists.
	Atelectasis, V/Q mismatch	Pulmonary compliance may decrease with large volumes of fluid replacement. Pulmonary contusions may aggravate this problem and severely compromise oxygenation and ventilation, requiring high-inspired O_2 concentration, high PIP, and PEEP.
	Coagulopathy	Causes include dilutional, hypothermic, brain injury, and development of SIRS/Sepsis.
	VTE	See p. B-7.
Pain management	PCA or parenteral narcotics epidural narcotic (see p. C-3, C-2)	Patients with rib fractures benefit from epidural narcotic and/or low-dose local anesthetic infusions.
Tests	Hb/Hct CXR	PT/PTT, Plt counts, if unexplained bleeding postop Fibrinogen, fibrin split products, if DIC suspected

PEDIATRIC TRAUMA

AIRWAY AND VASCULAR ACCESS

Description: Children younger than 15 yr are victims in about 25% of all trauma occurring in the United States. This incidence translates to ~200,000 hospitalizations and 10,000 deaths annually. Another 10,000–12,000 children sustain permanent impairment as a result of their injuries. According to the National Pediatric Trauma Registry, 40% of all pediatric injuries occur as a result of MVC and 35% are injuries sustained at home. Falls remain the most common cause of severe injury in infants and toddlers, whereas bicycle accidents cause most of the injuries in older pediatric groups. The majority of pediatric injuries that occur are 2° blunt trauma, and infants < 2 yr of age are known to have higher mortality rates for the same level of injury compared to older children.

The same sequence of primary survey, resuscitation, secondary survey, and definitive care should be followed as in adults. Confirmation of a patent airway is the essential first step. The best method for restoring airway patency is the **jaw thrust maneuver** and removal of any debris from the mouth. The most common reason for intubation in the pediatric trauma patient is loss of consciousness or as part of resuscitation from shock. Only 2% of children sustaining trauma will present with complete mechanical obstruction to the airway. In the rare child who presents with acute airway obstruction, **needle cricothyrotomy** is the preferred method of securing the airway until definitive airway control can be achieved. This technique of ventilation uses the principle of jet insufflation as defined in the adult. **Surgical cricothyrotomy** in children results in a high incidence of subglottic stenosis, but it is still a viable option in children > 10 if needle cricothyrotomy fails to be effective.

Because infants are obligatory nasal and diaphragmatic breathers, fractures and soft-tissue injuries that occlude the nostrils may actually obstruct the airway. Because air swallowed by the infant or insufflated into the stomach may cause acute gastric distention and restrict diaphragmatic excursion, the stomach should be decompressed with an OG tube.

Once the airway is secured and breathing is assured, attention should be given to the circulation. In the noncrying child, the SBP should be ~80 + their age in years ×2. Children may compensate for as much as 25% of circulating volume blood loss without a change in BP. Poor peripheral perfusion, decreased level of consciousness and ↓ UO are suggestive of hypovolemia. IV access must be obtained rapidly to begin crystalloid resuscitation in any child with impending signs of shock. If the peripheral iv access is difficult to obtain, as is often the case, saphenous vein cutdown at the saphenofemoral junction should be performed. In infants, if iv access cannot be obtained within 2 min,

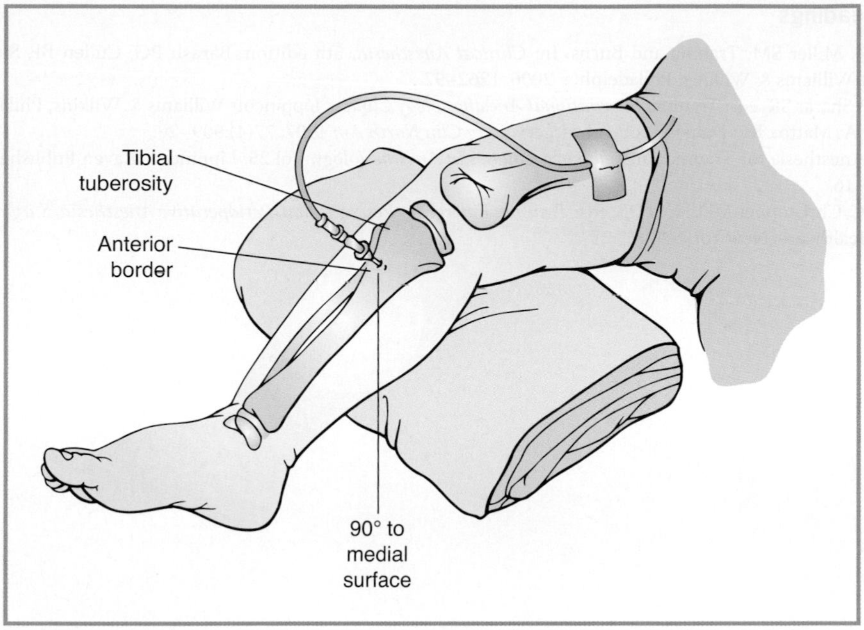

Figure 7.13-6. Intraosseous infusion. (Reproduced with permission from *Textbook of Pediatric Life Support.* American Heart Association, 1994.)

intraosseous access should be attempted (see below and Fig. 7.13-6). After iv access has been obtained, as many as three boluses of crystalloid, using a volume of 20 mL/kg, can be given. If the hypovolemic shock state has not been reversed after the 2nd bolus, and other causes of shock—such as spinal injury, cardiac tamponade, or pneumothorax—are excluded, blood (10 mL/kg) should be administered without delay.

Another important problem in the management of pediatric trauma is related to a high ratio of body surface area to body mass and a lack of substantial subcutaneous tissue. A small infant who is hypothermic may be refractory to therapy; therefore, every attempt should be made to prevent heat loss, and all iv fluids should be warmed.

Needle cricothyrotomy: With the head in neutral position (which may require placement of towels under the shoulders), the neck should be prepped from the jaw to the chest. The neck is protected by in-line immobilization. The cricothyroid membrane should be identified, and the thyroid cartilage immobilized with the surgeon's left hand. The cricothyroid membrane is punctured perpendicularly with a 14–16-ga iv catheter over a needle. The needle is then redirected caudally, the catheter slid off into the trachea, and jet insufflation initiated. Placement of a permanent airway should follow.

Saphenous cutdown: The groin should be prepped and draped and a curvilinear incision made 1–2 cm below and parallel to the inguinal ligament. The saphenous vein is identified at the saphenofemoral junction medial to the femoral artery. Two ligatures are passed underneath; the distal ligature is tied and used to apply tension to the vein. The vein is punctured with a scalpel blade (No. 11) and cut, creating a small flap. Tension applied to the proximal ligature reduces backbleeding during cannulation. A catheter is then introduced, the proximal ligature is tied, and the distal ligature is used to secure the catheter in place.

Intraosseous infusion: After skin preparation, an incision is made 2 cm distal to the tibial tuberosity on the flattened medial aspect of the tibia. An 18–20-ga spinal needle (with obturator) can be used in children < 18 months of age. Older patients may require use of a 13–16 bone marrow biopsy needle. Pressure and rotational motion are applied in a direction perpendicular to the bone until a decrease in resistance is felt. Position of the needle can be confirmed by bone marrow or blood aspiration. This route can be used for rapid fluid infusion and most resuscitation medications can be given this way. Interosseus infusion, however, is only an emergency maneuver and should be used to restore circulating volume to the level that enables more permanent iv access.

Usual preop diagnosis: Airway obstruction; hypovolemic shock; hypovolemic shock with difficult iv access

Suggested Readings

1. Capan LM, Miller SM: Trauma and Burns. In: *Clinical Anesthesia,* 5th edition. Barash PG, Cullen BF, Stoelting RK, eds. Lippincott Williams & Wilkins, Philadelphia: 2006, 1262–97.
2. Dutton RP, Sharar SR, eds: Trauma. *International Anesthesiology Clinics,*. Lippincott Williams & Wilkins, Philadelphia: 2002.
3. Hirshberg A, Mattox KL: Damage control surgery. *Surg Clin North Am* 1997; 77(4):909–20.
4. Karlin A: Anesthesia for Trauma. In: *Reference Courses in Anesthesiology,* Vol 25. Lippincott-Raven Publishers, Philadelphia: 1997, 107–16.
5. Wilson WC, Christopher MD, Hoyt DB, eds: *Trauma: Emergency Resuscitation, Perioperative Anesthesia, Surgical Management.* Informa Healthcare, New York: 2007.

SECTION

8.0 OBSTETRIC/ GYNECOLOGIC SURGERY

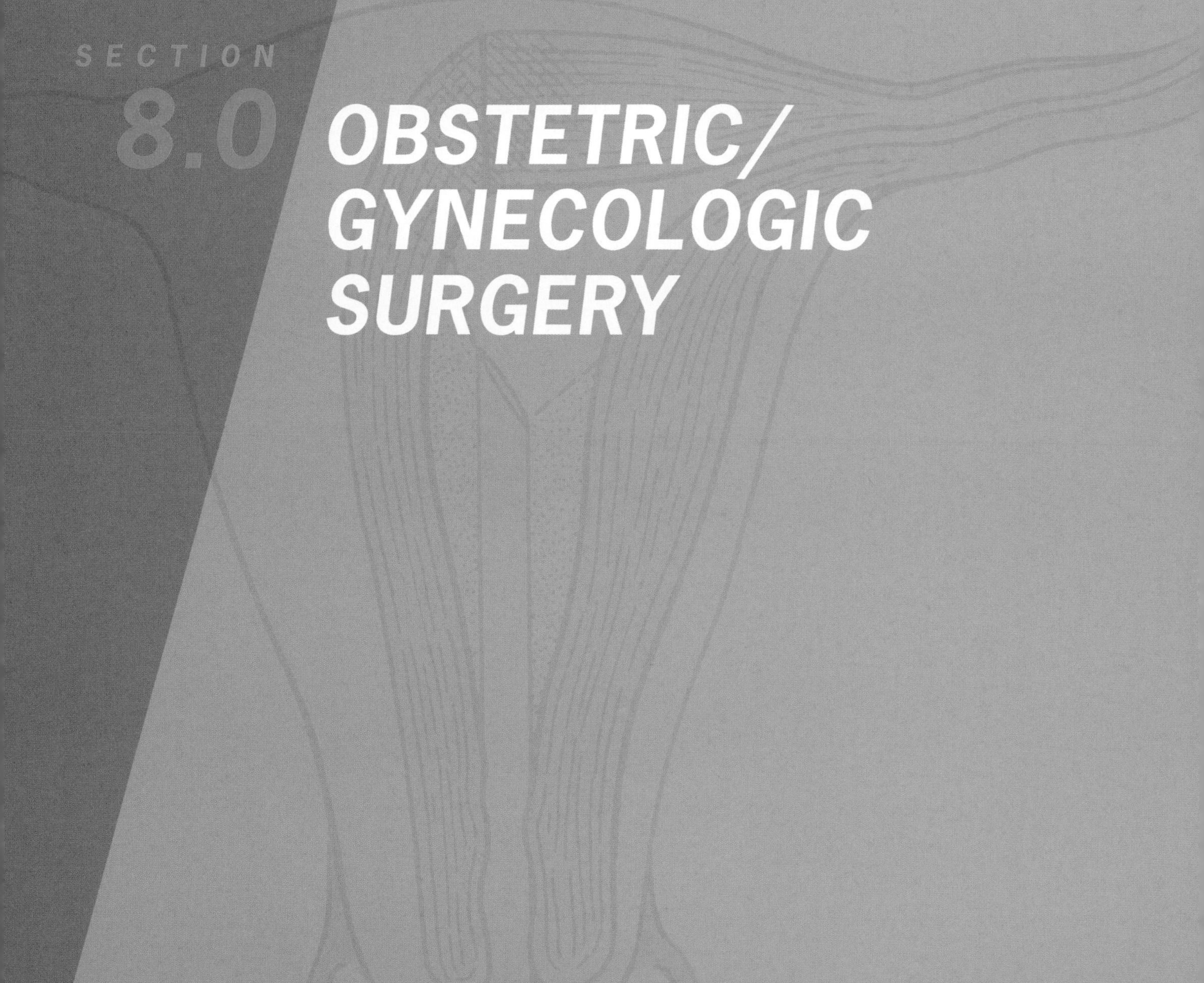

CHAPTER

8.1 Gynecologic Oncology

SURGEONS

O.W. Stephanie Yap, MD
Amreen Husain, MD
Daniel S. Kapp, MD, PhD
Nelson N. Teng, MD, PhD

ANESTHESIOLOGIST

Cliff Schmiesing, MD

STAGING LAPAROTOMY FOR OVARIAN, FALLOPIAN TUBE, AND PRIMARY PERITONEAL CANCER

SURGICAL CONSIDERATIONS

Description: Ovarian carcinoma has the highest mortality rate of all gynecologic malignancies, because it is usually discovered in advanced stages with a pelvic mass, omental caking, and ascites being common findings at presentation. Surgery is used for staging as well as therapy. Studies have demonstrated an inverse relationship between postop residual tumor mass and survival; therefore, the goals of surgery are: accurate staging and optimal tumor debulking (< 1 cm residual disease). The standard procedure consists of a meticulous exploration of the abdominopelvic cavity, abdominopelvic cytology, multiple random and targeted biopsies, **total abdominal hysterectomy (TAH), bilateral salpingo-oophorectomy (BSO), pelvic** and **paraaortic lymph node dissection, infracolic omentectomy, appendectomy,** and additional cytoreductive procedures. After access to the abdomen is obtained through a midline abdominal incision, cytologic washings of the pelvis, pericolic gutters, lesser sac, and hemidiaphragms are done. The

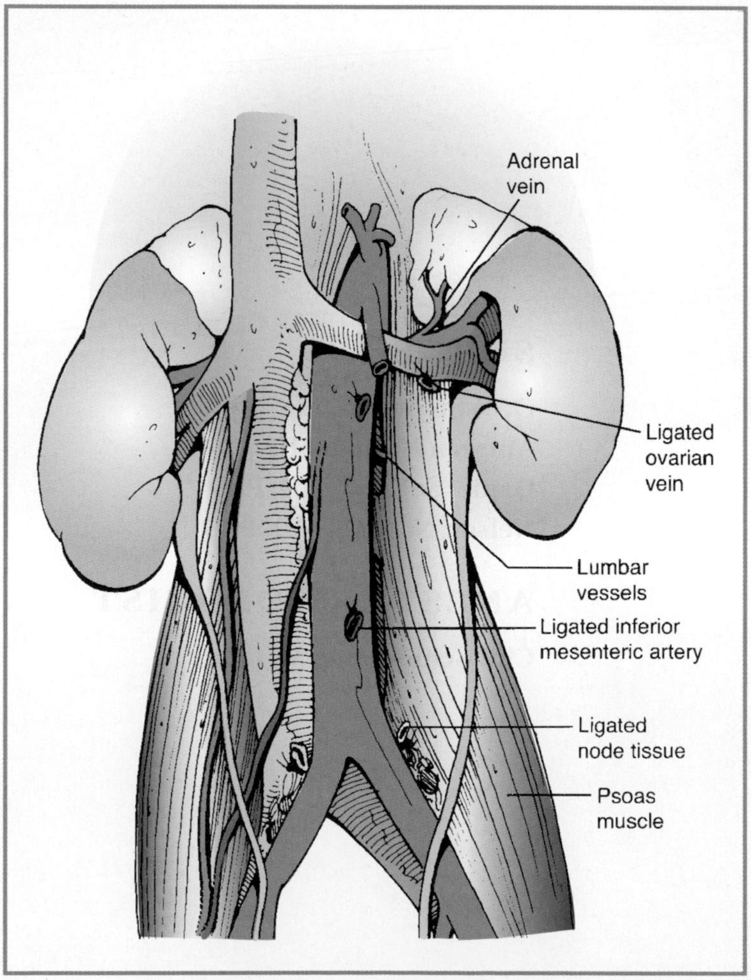

Figure 8.1-1. Aortic node dissection in staging laparotomy for ovarian cancer. In this case, both right and left node dissections have occurred, leaving the kidney, renal hilum, and psoas muscle exposed. Because the dissection is infrarenal and anterior to the lumbar vessels, there is residual fatty and nodal tissue at the posterior limit of the dissection.

peritoneal cavity is carefully explored. A TAH/BSO is performed by ligating and transecting the round, infundibulopelvic, broad, cardinal, and uterosacral ligaments on both sides. The specimen is cut away from the vagina and the cuff closed. The pelvic and paraaortic lymph nodes are dissected in a manner similar to that described under **Radical Hysterectomy,** p. 776. All residual tumor is removed, using sharp dissection and/or CUSA and/or argon beam coagulator (ABC), and then an appendectomy is usually performed. The omentum is clamped, transected, and ligated along its attachment to the transverse colon. A **bowel resection** with possible **colostomy** formation may be necessary to achieve optimal cytoreductive surgery (see **Pelvic Exenteration,** p. 767). Next, the peritoneal cavity is irrigated copiously. Targeted and random biopsies of bladder, cul-de-sac of Douglas, pericolic gutters, hemidiaphragms, small bowel, large bowel, and anterior abdominal wall are performed. A peritoneal port may be placed subcutaneously for use in future intraperitoneal chemotherapy. A less extensive surgical procedure may be appropriate if a large volume of unresectable tumor is discovered. Surgery in these cases must be individualized.

In some Stage I lesions, a **unilateral salpingo-oophorectomy** is sufficient therapy. The decision to use this approach depends on cell type, age, reproductive status, and extent of disease. Generally, biopsies**, a retroperitoneal lymph node dissection,** omentectomy**,** and appendectomy also are performed. Approximately 25% of patients undergoing cytoreductive surgery for advanced stages of ovarian carcinoma require bowel resection with either primary reanastomosis or colostomy. **A splenectomy** is not routinely done unless the spleen is involved with tumor. Some patients with unresectable disease and bowel obstruction will require a **gastrostomy tube** placement at this time.

Usual preop diagnosis: Ovarian cancer/pelvic mass

SUMMARY OF PROCEDURE

Position	Supine
Incision	Midline or paramedian abdominal
Special instrumentation	CUSA, Vital View (suction-irrigation device combined with light source) helpful; laparoscopic biopsy forceps (laparoscope, laparoscopic instruments for evaluation of upper abdomen through lower vertical abdominal incision); Argon beam coagulator (ABC); TA, GIA, EEA stapling devices.
Unique considerations	Removal of large amounts of ascites may → fluid shifts and intravascular volume depletion intraop and postop.
Antibiotics	Cefotetan 2 g iv; further doses as indicated by large EBL, duration of surgery.
Surgical time	1–4 h; 4–5 h, including splenectomy and bowel surgery for more advanced stages
Closing considerations	NG tube placement by anesthesiologist (in select cases with extensive bowel involvement or bowel procedures); peritoneal or central venous access for subsequent chemotherapy
EBL	500–1000 mL; 250–500 mL for Stage I lesions; > 1000 mL for more advanced stages
Postop care	Extensive peritoneal raw surfaces → intraperitoneal fluid 3rd-spacing. Patients require good hydration to maintain intravascular volume. Central hemodynamic monitoring and ICU admission are useful in selected patients. Use SCDs and mini-dose heparin for VTE prophylaxis.
Mortality	1–2/1000
Morbidity	Postop fever: 14–19% Wound infection: < 5% Wound dehiscence: 0.3–3% PE: 1–2% Ureteral injury: < 1% Vaginal vault prolapse: Rare
Pain score	7–8

PATIENT POPULATION CHARACTERISTICS

Age range	All age groups; most common, 50–59 yr
Incidence	15/100,000 (26,700+ new cases/yr); 1.4% lifetime risk of ovarian cancer

PATIENT POPULATION CHARACTERISTICS (cont'd)

Etiology	Unknown
Predisposing factors	Family Hx of ovarian carcinoma; personal or family Hx of breast cancer (BRCA gene mutations); ↑age at first pregnancy; gonadal dysgenesis; exposure to radiation; environmental factors
Associated conditions	Familial cancer syndromes (e.g., endometrial, colon, breast); Peutz-Jeghers syndrome—5% of cases develop gonadal stromal tumor; XY gonadal dysgenesis—gonadoblastomas; multiple nevoid basal cell carcinoma (Gorlin's syndrome); ataxia telangiectasia (hereditary, progressive cerebellar lack of muscular coordination associated with recurrent pulmonary infections and ocular and cutaneous telangiectasias)

ANESTHETIC CONSIDERATIONS

PREOPERATIVE

Ovarian carcinoma is usually diagnosed at a relatively late stage and, therefore, the patient may have malignant ascites and pleural effusion, and large tumor mass. Surgery is indicated for resection of localized tumor and for staging of distant and local metastases. Additional procedures, including bowel resection or lymph node dissection, may be performed at the same time.

Respiratory	Significant ascites and pleural fluid may produce respiratory compromise. The presence of dyspnea, orthopnea, tachypnea, or other chest findings need to be investigated. Underlying lung diseases, such as asthma, also may be exacerbated by the abdominal distension/ascites. **Tests:** Consider CXR; others as indicated from H&P.
Cardiovascular	An ECHO or other studies may be requested to evaluate cardiac function. Exercise tolerance should be evaluated in every patient and any preexisting cardiac disease explored in the preop visit. Irreversible, dose-dependent cardiotoxicity may result from doxorubicin chemotherapy. **Tests:** Consider ECG, others as indicated from H&P.
Gastrointestinal	Patient should have adequate preop iv hydration if given a bowel prep overnight. Opiate use may cause ↓GI motility. May be malnourished.
Neurological	Not usually significant. Taxol and cisplatin may → peripheral neuropathy.
Hematologic	Bone marrow suppression common following chemotherapy. Carboplatin, commonly used for ovarian cancer, often induces thrombocytopenia. **Tests:** CBC
Laboratory	CBC, hepatic function, PT/PTT, T & S or T & cross
Premedication	Consider midazolam 1–2 mg iv

INTRAOPERATIVE

Anesthetic technique: GETA ± epidural analgesia. Typically, a balanced anesthetic with inhalational agents and/or propofol infusion (25–200 mcg/kg/min) and narcotics. An epidural catheter may be placed for postop pain management and also may be used intraop to ↓ anesthetic requirements.

Induction	Standard induction (see p. B-2), though consider full stomach precautions if ascites present.
Maintenance	Standard maintenance (p. B-2). Continue muscle relaxation based on nerve stimulator response. Epidural 2% lidocaine with epinephrine 1:200,000 (~3–5 mL/h) if catheter is placed preop. Consider NG/OG tube. Patients with combined regional/GA may require increased fluids due to vasodilation and ↓BP.

Emergence	The patient may be extubated at the conclusion of surgery, unless hemodynamically unstable and/or requiring continued vigorous fluid resuscitation. Reverse muscle relaxant with neostigmine 0.07 mg/kg and glycopyrrolate 0.01 mg/kg, and give supplemental O_2 after extubation. Consider postop ICU bed for unstable patients or those requiring invasive monitoring for fluid management.	
Blood and fluid requirements	Significant blood loss possible IV: 16–18 ga × 2 NS/LR at 4–6 mL/kg/h 5% albumin 6% hetastarch	Blood loss may be > 1 L. Order T & S or T & cross preop. 5% albumin or 6% hetastarch are useful for rapid volume replacement if Hct is acceptable. If large volumes of ascites are removed, significant ↓BP may develop. Third-space losses may be significant (≥10–15 mL/kg/h). Consider alternating NS and LR to avoid development of a nonanion gap hyperchloremic acidosis 2° NS. Warm fluids. Strive to maintain euvolemia based on clinical data: BP, HR, ABG, UO, EBL, and fluid shift estimates, ± CVP, etc.
Monitoring	Standard monitors (p. B-1) ± Arterial catheter ± CVP catheter Foley catheter	Arterial and CVP catheters indicated for extensive surgery and/or patients with significant comorbidities (CHF, CAD, COPD, renal failure, etc).
Positioning	✓ and pad pressure points, especially important for longer surgeries ✓ eyes Antiembolism stockings and SCDs	
Complications	Hypothermia	Hypothermia likely to develop. Warm all IV fluids. Heating blanket on bed and forced-air warming blanket should be used.
	Coagulopathy	Preop malnutrition and/or significant blood loss may → coagulopathy

POSTOPERATIVE

Complications	Hemorrhage VTE Ascites/pleural effusion Respiratory insufficiency PONV	 See p. B-7 See p. B-6
Pain management	PCA Epidural	See PCA and epidural narcotic recommendations on pages C-2 and C-3. Epidural may ↓pain, PONV, and risk of VTE.

Suggested Readings

1. Copeland LJ: Epithelial ovarian cancer. In *Clinical Gynecologic Oncology.* DiSaia PJ, Creasman WT, eds. CV Mosby, St Louis: 2007; 289–350.
2. Creasman WT, Van Nagell J, Gershenson DM: Gynecologic Oncology. In *Barek & Novak's Gynecology.* Barek JS, ed., 14th edition. Lippincott, Williams, & Wilkins, Philadelphia: 2007, 1373–488.
3. Curtin JP, Malik R, Venkataraman ES, et al: Stage IV ovarian cancer: impact of surgical debulking. *Gynecol Oncol* 1997; 64:9.
4. Morrow CP, Curtin JP: Surgery for ovarian neoplasia. In *Gynecologic Cancer Surgery.* Churchill Livingstone, New York: 1996, 627–716.
5. Ozols RF, Rubin SC, Thomas G, Robboy S: Epithelial ovarian cancer. In *Principles and Practice of Gynecologic Oncology, 3rd edition.* Hoskins WJ, Perez CA, Young RC, Barakat RR, Markman B, eds: Lippincott Williams & Wilkins, Philadelphia: 2004, 981–1058.
6. Wheeless CR Jr: Staging of gynecologic oncology patients with exploratory laparotomy. In *Atlas of Pelvic Surgery,* 3rd edition. Lippincott, Williams & Wilkins, Baltimore: 1997, 380–1.

INTERVAL, SECOND-LOOK/REASSESSMENT, AND SECONDARY CYTOREDUCTIVE LAPAROTOMY FOR OVARIAN CANCER

SURGICAL CONSIDERATIONS

Description: The clinical evaluation of an ovarian cancer patient's response to chemotherapy may be unreliable because tumor that may defy detection by noninvasive methods can be present in the abdominopelvic cavity. Historically, surgery in the form of **'second-look' laparotomy** was undertaken to determine whether a patient was surgically and pathologically free of disease, after an appropriate number of treatment cycles with platinum-based (CDDP or carboplatin) chemotherapy. However, 50% of patients with negative second-look surgeries ultimately recur, and the number of second-look surgeries has decreased significantly in favor of non-invasive evaluation including the use of tumor markers (CA-125) and imaging techniques (CT, MRI, PET). Select patients will benefit from second-look surgery to guide further therapy. Intraabdominal assessment may be performed in conjunction with placement of an intraperitoneal port. Second-look procedures also may be done laparoscopically (see p. 626).

In patients where neoadjuvant chemotherapy was utilized or when optimal debulking could not be performed at initial surgery, an interval (after 3–6 cycles of chemotherapy) or secondary debulking laparotomy is done to achieve optimal cytoreduction. The surgery involves methodical and meticulous exploration of all of the abdomen and pelvis, multiple cytologies and biopsies, lysis of adhesions, and resection of the residual tumor, as well as the pelvic and periaortic lymph nodes (if not done at time of first surgery). Patients may also be candidates for secondary or tertiary cytoreductive surgical procedures, particularly if isolated recurrences are found in the setting of longer disease-free intervals.

Usual preop diagnosis: Ovarian carcinoma

SUMMARY OF PROCEDURE	
Position	Supine
Incision	Midline or paramedian vertical abdominal
Antibiotics	Cefotetan 2 g iv, then q 12 h × 2 doses
Surgical time	2–3 h
Closing considerations	Placement of permanent central venous or intraperitoneal access
EBL	350–700 mL
Postop care	PACU → ward
Mortality	1–2/1000
Morbidity	Postop fever: 14–19% Wound infection: < 5% Wound dehiscence: 0.3–3% PE: 1–2% Incisional hernia: 0.5–1% Ureteral injury: 0.5–1%
Pain score	7–8

PATIENT POPULATION CHARACTERISTICS	
Age range	All ages; most common, 50–59 yr
Incidence	15/100,000; 26,700+ new cases/yr; 1.4% lifetime risk of ovarian cancer

PATIENT POPULATION CHARACTERISTICS (cont'd)

Etiology	Risk factors include: positive family Hx; nulliparity; ↑age at first pregnancy; gonadal dysgenesis; exposure to radiation; environmental factors.
Associated conditions	Familial cancer syndromes (e.g., endometrial, colon, breast); Peutz-Jeghers syndrome (5% of cases develop gonadal stromal tumor); XY gonadal dysgenesis (gonadoblastomas); multiple, nevoid basal-cell carcinoma (Gorlin's syndrome); ataxia telangiectasia

ANESTHETIC CONSIDERATIONS

PREOPERATIVE

Patients having a second-look laparotomy have undergone surgical resection of a tumor with lymph node biopsy, usually followed by chemotherapy and/or radiation therapy. Depending on the type of adjunctive treatment given, the patient may come to surgery in poor physical condition from malnutrition or toxicity from chemotherapy (see Table 8.1-1). Vascular access may be difficult to obtain due to sclerosis or thrombosis of peripheral veins.

Respiratory	Pulmonary function may be impaired by several chemotherapeutic drugs, most commonly bleomycin. Patients often have a Hickman catheter or other central line already in place, which can be used for induction of anesthesia. Obtain preop CXR to assess the presence of lung injury if prior chemo given. Patients who have dyspnea at rest or with mild exertion, or who have known pulmonary fibrosis, should be evaluated by PFTs, including FVC, FEV_1, $MMEF_{25-75}$, and ABGs. Patients who have received bleomycin should not receive O_2 > 39% intraop, but arterial O_2 saturation ideally should be kept ≥ 93%. The pulmonary toxicity of bleomycin is dose-related with a much higher incidence occurring if > 200 mg/m^2. Combination chemotherapy with vincristine or cisplatin also increases pulmonary toxicity. Postop mechanical ventilation may be necessary. **Tests:** Consider CXR; others as indicated from H&P.
Cardiovascular	Cardiotoxicity is seen with several antineoplastic agents, especially daunorubicin and doxorubicin. The cardiomyopathy produced by these drugs occurs in two forms: (1) acute—ST-T wave changes and dysrhythmias, which are transient and usually not a serious problem; and (2) chronic—a dose-related toxicity manifested by CHF. Total doses of doxorubicin as low as 250 U can cause myocardial damage, but is more common at doses > 400 U. Cardiac

Table 8.1-1. Toxicities of Selected Antineoplastic Chemotherapeutic Agents

Agent	Toxic Effects
Vincristine, vinblastine	Neuropathies, SIADH, myelosuppression
Cyclophosphamide	Prolonged neuromuscular block
Mechlorethamine	Prolonged neuromuscular block
Bleomycin	Pulmonary fibrosis
Doxorubicin, daunorubicin	Cardiotoxicity, GI upset, myelosuppression
Methotrexate	Myelosuppression, GI upset, stomatitis, pulmonary infiltrates
Fluorouracil	Myelosuppression, hepatic and GI alterations, nervous system dysfunction
Mercaptopurine	Myelosuppression
Thioguanine	Myelosuppression
Actinomycin D	Myelosuppression, GI upset, stomatitis
Mitomycin	Myelosuppression, GI upset
Cisplatin, carboplatin	Peripheral neuropathy, GI upset, electrolyte disturbances, nephrotoxicity myelosuppression
Paclitaxel	Myelosuppression, peripheral neuropathy, GI upset, arthralgia/myalgias, mucositis
Docetaxel	Myelosuppression, peripheral neuropathy, malaise, maculopapular rash, GI upset

Cardiovascular (cont'd)	irradiation, or combination chemotherapy with cyclophosphamide, increases the risk of cardiac toxicity. Patients who have received cardiotoxic drugs are usually followed by serial ECHOs or MUGA scans, and the results of these tests should be reviewed preop. Patients with CHF or ECG changes should have a cardiology consultation preop to optimize their medical condition. **Tests:** ECG; others as indicated from H&P.
Neurological	Peripheral neuropathies are produced by vincristine, cyclophosphamide, Taxol (paclitaxel), 5-fluorouracil and several other drugs. Vincristine can also → SIADH. Other CNS effects include N/V, Seizure, and cerebellar dysfunction. A preop neurologic exam useful for patients with evidence of neurotoxicity. Document presence of neurologic deficits preop for subsequent comparisons.
Endocrine	Corticosteroids (e.g. prednisone) are commonly used with chemotherapeutic agents, as treatment for pulmonary fibrosis and other complications of chemotherapy. The use of steroids for several weeks suppresses the endogenous secretion of the adrenal cortex, which may take up to 6 mo to recover fully. Hydrocortisone 100 mg iv, preop with an additional 2–3 subsequent doses q 8 h will provide adequate "stress dose" coverage perioperatively. The dose is tapered rapidly over 2 or 3 d postop. **Tests:** As indicated by the H&P.
Renal	Many chemotherapeutic drugs have renal toxicity; therefore, a preop set of renal function tests is mandatory. Patients with impaired renal function should be given appropriate dosages of medications (e.g., antibiotics), which depend on renal excretion. **Tests:** Renal function tests
Musculoskeletal	Vincristine produces a neurotoxicity manifested by numbness and tingling in the extremities, weakness, foot drop, loss of reflexes, ataxia, and muscle pains. Muscle weakness in the arms and legs indicates that the drug should be stopped. Muscle weakness may also involve the larynx and extraocular eye muscles. Reduced amounts of NMBs should be used intraop and a nerve stimulator used to follow twitches.
Gastrointestinal	Consider hydration overnight if given a bowel prep or if there is significant N/V. **Tests:** Consider serum electrolytes, if indicated from H&P.
Hematologic	Bone marrow suppression is a very common side effect of antineoplastic drugs. The toxicity usually produces a reversible drop in leukocytes, erythrocytes, and platelets, with a nadir 10–14 d posttreatment. Patients with a total neutrophil count of < 1,000 should be kept in isolation until counts improve. A low Plt count (< 75,000) is an indication for Plt transfusion preop. Regional anesthesia in patients with thrombocytopenia needs to be considered carefully due to ↑ risk of bleeding complications. It is useful to ✓PT/PTT preop when in doubt about the coag status of a patient. Consider preop transfusion of Plts and/or RBCs if lab values are below acceptable limits (Plt < 75,000, Hct < 25%). **Tests:** Hemogram, WBC, Plt, PT/PTT
Laboratory	LFTs if indicated by H&P.
Premedication	Consider midazolam 1–2 mg iv. Stress-dose hydrocortisone (100 mg iv) if indicated.

INTRAOPERATIVE

Anesthetic technique: GETA usually indicated. Combined GETA/epidural or spinal are also excellent choices. Consider surgery under regional anesthesia in patients with severe bleomycin pulmonary toxicity.

General anesthesia:

Induction	Standard induction (see p. B-2). Consider renal function and surgery duration when deciding on agents.
Maintenance	Standard maintenance: see Anesthetic Considerations for Staging Laparotomy, p. 627. An epidural may be used to reduce GA requirements (p. B-2). Consider NGT/OGT.

Emergence	Extubate when patient is responsive and neuromuscular block is fully reversed. In patients with borderline pulmonary function, extubation may be delayed until patient is in the PACU or ICU, and after ABG is checked while the patient breathes spontaneously. Consider PONV prophylaxis (see p. B-6).	

Regional anesthesia:

Epidural	2% lidocaine ± epinephrine 1:200,000 (10–20 mL) or 0.25% bupivacaine (10–20 mL) initially; then at ~3–5 mL/h. Narcotics, such as morphine (2–4 mg) or hydromorphone (0.3–0.6 mg), may be given in the epidural for postop pain control.	
Blood and fluid requirements	IV: 16–18 ga × 1–2 NS/LR at 7–10 mL/kg/h Keep UO > 0.5 mL/kg/h Consider PRBC for Hct < 27%	Excessive use of NS can lead to hyperchloremic metabolic acidosis; therefore, alternating NS and LR solutions makes sense when giving large volumes of iv fluids.
	5% albumin 6% hetastarch	5% albumin or 6% hetastarch may be used as volume replacement, although no proven advantages over crystalloid solutions.
	FFP/Plt	Consider FFP and Plt if evidence of coagulopathy (↑PT, ↑PTT, ↓Plt).
Monitoring	Standard monitors (see p. B-1). ± Arterial line ± CVP catheter Foley catheter	Consider Arterial and CVP catheters for patients with compromised cardiac or pulmonary function or patients having extensive surgical procedures.
Positioning	✓and pad pressure points ✓eyes Anti-embolism stockings and SCD	It is useful to maintain access to at least one arm for blood drawing and additional iv access.
Complications	Hypothermia	Warm fluids; keep heating pad on bed; use forced-air warmer
	Bleeding	✓PT; PTT, Plts periodically if large blood loss

POSTOPERATIVE

Complications	Bleeding PONV (see p. B-6) Infection Respiratory insufficiency VTE (see p. B-7)	
Pain management	PCA (see p. C-3). Epidural/spinal narcotics (see p. C-2).	Surgeons may infiltrate wound edges with 0.25% bupivacaine in those patients without epidurals. Consider iv ketorolac (30 mg)
Tests	CXR ABG	As indicated by postop clinical findings.

Suggested Readings

1. Chabner BA, Ryan DP, Paz-Ares S, et al: Antineoplastic agents. In *Goodman and Gilman's: The Pharmacologic Basis of Therapeutics,* 10th edition. Hardman JG, Limbird LE, Gilman AG, eds. McGraw Hill, New York: 2001, 1389–459.
2. Creasman WT, Van Nagell J, Gershenson DM: Gynecologic Oncology. In *Barek & Novak's Gynecology.* Barek JS, ed., 14th edition. Lippincott Williams, & Wilkins, Philadelphia: 2007, 1373–488.
3. DiSaia PJ, Creasman WT: Epithelial ovarian cancer. In *Clinical Gynecologic Oncology.* DiSaia PJ, Creasman WT, eds. CV Mosby, St. Louis: 2002, 289–350.
4. Ozols RF, Rubin SC, Thomas G, Robboy S: Epithelial ovarian cancer. In Principles and Practice of Gynecologic Oncology, 3rd edition. Hoskins WJ, Perez CA, Young RC, Barakat RR, Markman B, eds: Lippincott, Williams & Wilkins, Philadelphia: 2004, 981–1058.

RADICAL VULVECTOMY

SURGICAL CONSIDERATIONS

Description: Historically, invasive vulvar carcinoma has been treated with en bloc dissection of the inguinal-femoral region and the vulva. The surgery involves bilateral excision of lymphatic and areolar tissue in the inguinal and femoral regions, combined with removal of the entire vulva between the labia-crural folds, from the perineal body to the upper margin of mons pubis (Fig 8.1-2). A large surgical wound is created and, if 1° closure without tension is not possible, a skin or myocutaneous graft may be necessary. Deep pelvic nodes are almost never involved with metastases when the superficial and deep groin nodes are free of disease; therefore, a **pelvic lymphadenectomy** is no longer routinely performed. If presence of tumor is documented in the groin nodes, particularly in Cloquet's sentinel nodes (the most cephalad, deep inguinal nodes), a **deep pelvic lymphadenectomy** may be performed. **Postop radiation therapy,** however, is widely used instead of a pelvic lymph node dissection to minimize operative morbidity and confer a survival advantage.

A skin incision in the shape of a bull's head (Fig 8.1-2) allows access to the inguinal-femoral region. (The incision ideally should extend 2+ cm beyond the tumor margin.) The inguinal ligament and rectus fascia should be cleared bilaterally of all nodal tissues, and the fossae ovalis on both sides identified. The lateral aspect of the femoral sheath is incised along the sartorius muscle, with care being taken not to injure the femoral nerve or vessels, and the cribriform fascia is cleaned off the femoral artery. The external pudendal artery, which marks the entrance of the saphenous vein into the fossa ovalis, should be identified and ligated. The proximal and distal segments of the saphenous vein should be ligated and excised as the fibrofatty, lymph-bearing tissue of the femoral sheath is resected. Cloquet's nodes at the femoral ring beneath the inguinal ligaments on both sides should be resected and submitted for frozen-section pathology evaluation. The deep inguinal lymphatic chain is removed on both sides by opening the inguinal canal from the external inguinal ring. The vulvar incision is carried down through the labia-crural folds. The internal pudendal vessels at the posterior lateral margin of the vulvar incision are identified as they emerge from Alcock's canal, and then they are ligated and incised.

Use of electrocautery in this portion of the procedure usually tends to decrease operative blood loss. The dissection is continued along the periosteum of the symphysis at the level of the fascia of the deep muscles of the urogenital diaphragm. The bulbocavernosus, ischiocavernosus, and superficial transverse perinei muscles are removed. A circumferential vaginal incision, excluding the urethral meatus, is then performed and the vulva is removed. The incisions overlying the groin node dissections should be closed with minimal tension after placement of closed-suction

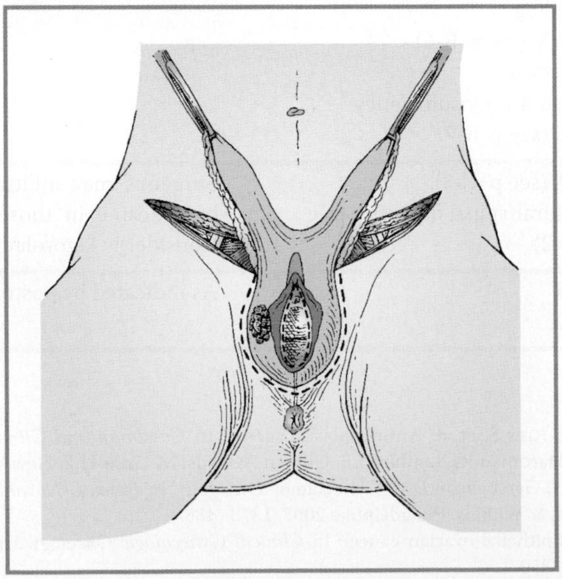

Figure 8.1-2. En bloc radical vulvectomy incisions shown; bilateral inguinal lymphadenectomy is complete. (Reproduced with permission from Rock JA, Thompson JD: *TeLinde's Operative Gynecology,* 8th edition. Lippincott Williams & Wilkins, 1997.)

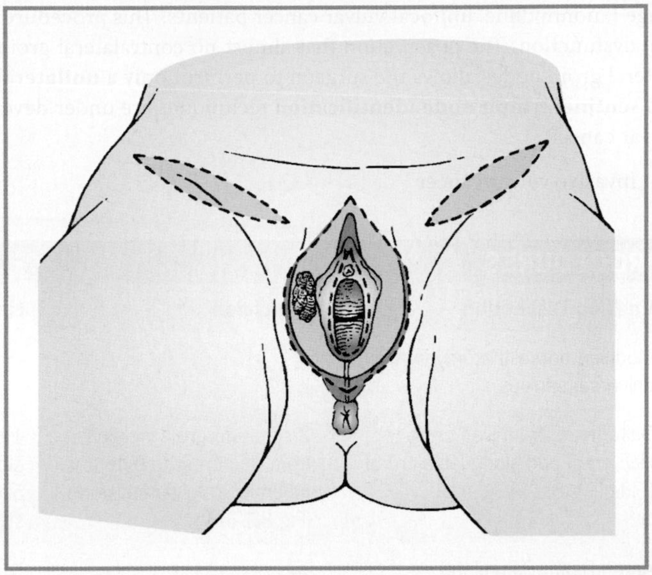

Figure 8.1-3. 3-incision radical vulvectomy and bilateral inguinofemeral lympha- denectomy. (Produced with permission from Rock JA, Thompson JD: *TeLinde's Operative Gynecology,* 8th edition. Lippincott Williams & Wilkins, 1997.)

Jackson-Pratt drains. The vulvar surgical wound is closed by slightly undermining the skin of the edges of the incision and suturing them to the vaginal mucosa. A **vulvar reconstruction,** using myocutaneous flaps, also can be performed at this time (see Pelvic Exenteration, p. 767).

Variant procedure or approaches: In 1962, Byran and associates popularized a **3-incision technique** first described by Kehrer in 1918. This 3-incision technique, with separate vulva and groin incisions, is the most common approach (Fig 8.1-3). This operative approach has led to a significant decrease in wound infection and breakdown, apparently without increasing tumor recurrence in the inguinal dermal bridge above the symphysis pubis. Another variant is the **hemivulvectomy** (Fig 8.1-4), in which unilateral radical hemivulvectomy and groin node dissection are

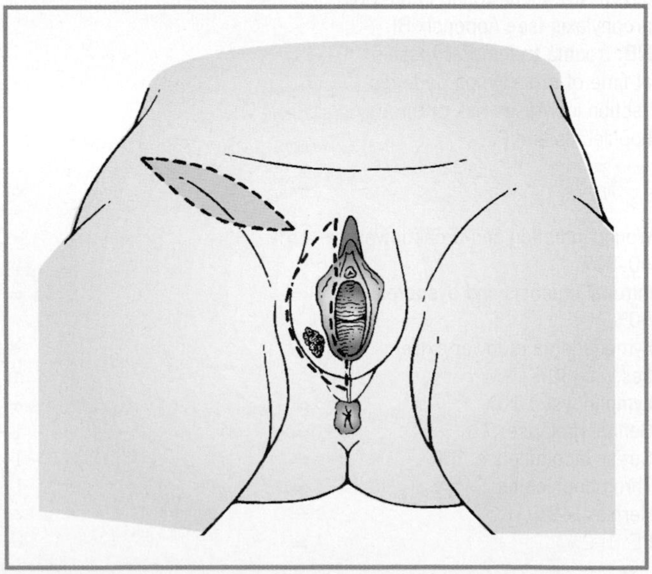

Figure 8.1-4. Unilateral lymphadenectomy for a well lateralized lesion. (Produced with permission from Rock JA, Thompson JD: *TeLinde's Operative Gynecology,* 8th edition, Lippincott Williams & Wilkins, 1997.)

performed in selected stage I, nonmidline, unifocal vulvar cancer patients. This procedure will minimize morbidity, disfigurement, and sexual dysfunction. The observation that almost no contralateral groin metastases occur in the absence of positive ipsilateral groin nodes allows the surgeon to perform only a **unilateral groin node dissection.** **Lymphatic mapping** and **sentinel lymph node identification** techniques are under development for the management of patients with vulvar cancer.

Usual preop diagnosis: Invasive vulvar cancer

SUMMARY OF PROCEDURES

	En Bloc Dissection	3-Incision	Hemivulvectomy
Position	Modified dorsolithotomy in Allen universal stirrups	⇐	⇐
Incision	Bull's head, from iliac crest to iliac crest and along labia-crural folds (Fig 8.1-2)	2 separate groin incisions from iliac crest to pubic tubercle; 1 vulvar incision (Fig 8.1-3)	1 or 2 separate groin incisions from iliac crest to pubic tubercle; vulvar incision (Fig 8.1-4)
Special instrumentation	Argon Beam Coagulator	⇐	⇐
Unique considerations	Two-team approach to minimize surgical time. Preop bowel prep and constipating medications (e.g., Lomotil) to ↓postop bowel movements.	⇐	⇐
Antibiotics	Cefotetan 2 g iv; then 2 g iv q 12 h × 72 h	⇐	⇐
Surgical time	3–4 h	⇐	2–3 h
Closing considerations	Possible skin graft; vulvar and groin suction drains	⇐	⇐
EBL	500–1000 mL	⇐	250–1000 mL
Postop care	PACU or ICU, if necessary; aggressive local wound care. VTE prophylaxis (see Appendix B). **NB:** trauma to femoral vessels at time of groin lymph node dissection increases risk of thrombophlebitis and PE.	⇐	⇐
Mortality	1–2%	⇐	⇐
Morbidity	Wound infection and breakdown: 40–80%	15%	< 15%
	Introital stenosis and dyspareunia: 50%	⇐	⇐
	Lymphedema of lower extremities: 25–30%	⇐	< 25% (if deep groin nodes not dissected)
	Lymphocysts: 10%	⇐	⇐
	Genital prolapse: 7%	⇐	1–2%
	Stress incontinence: 5%	⇐	1–2%
	Thrombophlebitis: 3–5%	⇐	1–2%
	Hernia: 1–2%	⇐	⇐
	PE: 1–2%	⇐	⇐
Pain score	8	8	7

PATIENT POPULATION CHARACTERISTICS	
Age range	Median = 70 yr
Incidence	2.5/100,000; 3–5% of female genital malignancies
Etiology	Exact etiology unknown; risk factors include vulvar dystrophies; granulomatous disease of vulva; Bowen's disease; condyloma acuminata
Associated conditions	Diabetes; obesity; HTN; arteriosclerosis; nulliparity; positive serology for syphilis; cervical malignancy; human papilloma virus infection

ANESTHETIC CONSIDERATIONS

PREOPERATIVE

Patients with vulvar carcinoma are usually elderly. Consider and evaluate coexisting medical conditions, including HTN, CAD, and diabetes. Radical vulvectomy is performed for invasive tumor that has not metastasized to distant sites.

Respiratory	The presence of lung disease and smoking Hx should be discussed with the patient preop. Consider CXR and PFTs for patients with significant respiratory disease. **Tests:** Others as indicated from H&P.
Cardiovascular	There is an increased incidence of HTN and atherosclerosis in these patients. A cardiology consultation is indicated for angina, recent MI, CHF, or heart murmurs. Review recent ECG for patients > 50. **Tests:** ECG; others as indicated from H&P.
Renal	In old age, creatinine clearance is decreased 2° ↓renal mass, but serum creatinine remains unchanged because of decreased muscle mass. **Tests:** Serum creatine; others as indicated from H&P.
Gastrointestinal	Patients should have iv hydration preop if given bowel prep overnight.
Neurological	Document a neurological exam if Hx of stroke, Sz, or other neurologic disease. Hx of peripheral neuropathy or autonomic dysfunction should be assessed in diabetic patients. **Tests:** As indicated from H&P.
Endocrine	Diabetes, obesity, and hypothyroidism are common in this patient population. **Tests:** Fasting blood sugar; thyroid function; others as indicated from H&P.
Hematologic	Chronic anemia may be present. **Tests:** Hb/Hct; Plt count
Laboratory	LFTs, if indicated.
Premedication	Consider midazolam iv 1–2 mg

INTRAOPERATIVE

Anesthetic technique: GETA or regional anesthesia, alone or in combination.

General anesthesia:

Induction	Standard induction (see p. B-2)
Maintenance	Standard maintenance (see p. B-2)
Emergence	No special considerations

Regional anesthesia:

Epidural	2% lidocaine ± epinephrine 1:200,000 (10–20 mL) or 0.5% bupivacaine (10–20 mL) are used; then at ~3–5 mL/h. Narcotics such as morphine (2–4 mg) in the epidural for postop pain control.	
Spinal	Tetracaine (12 mg) or bupivacaine (12–15 mg), preservative-free morphine (0.1–0.2 mg) → T8 sensory level.	
Blood and fluid requirements	IV: 16–18 ga × 2 NS/LR at 6–8 mL/kg/h Warm iv fluids UO > 0.5 mL/kg/h	Occasionally, femoral vessels may be injured, requiring rapid blood replacement. Consider PRBCs for Hct < 21% in healthy patients and < 25–30% in patients with cardiac or pulmonary disease.
Monitoring	Standard monitors (p. B-1) ± Arterial line ± CVP line Foley catheter	Invasive monitors indicated for patients in poor condition or with cardiovascular or respiratory disease. An arterial catheter is useful for drawing labs in surgery to check Hct, coags, glucose, or ABGs.
Positioning	✓ and pad pressure points ✓ eyes Antiembolism stockings and SCD	

POSTOPERATIVE

Complications	Hypothermia Bleeding PONV VTE	 See p. B-6 See p. B-7
Pain management	PCA (p. C-3) Epidural or spinal narcotics (p. C-2)	Incisions may be left open to granulate in, or be covered with skin grafts. Epidural analgesia allows earlier ambulation with less sedation in elderly patients.
Tests	Tests as indicated from postop clinical findings	

Obstetric/Gynecologic Surgery

Suggested Readings

1. Burke TW, Eifel P, McGuire W, Wilkinson EJ: Vulva. In *Principles and Practice of Gynecologic Oncology,* 3rd edition. Hoskins WJ, Perez CA, Young RC, eds. Lippincott Williams & Wilkins, Philadelphia: 2000, 775–810.
2. Burke TW, Levenback C, Coleman RC, et al: Surgical therapy of T1 and T2 vulvar carcinoma: further experience with radical wide excision and selective inguinal lymphadenectomy. *Gynecol Oncol* 1995; 57:215–20.
3. DiSaia PJ, Creasman WT: Invasive cancer of the vulva. In *Clinical Gynecologic Oncology.* DiSaia PJ, Creasman WT, eds. CV Mosby, St. Louis: 2002, 211–39.
4. Eifel P, Levenback C: Surgery for vulvar cancer. In *American Cancer Society Atlas of Clinical Oncology, Cancer of the Female Lower Genital Tract.* BC Decker, Hamilton: 2001, 203–16.
5. Hoffman MS: Malignancies of the vulva. In *TeLinde's Operative Gynecology.* Rock JA, Jones HW, eds. Lippincott Williams & Wilkins, Philadelphia: 2003, 1293–1350.
6. Holschneider CH: Vulvar Cancer. In *Barek & Novak's Gynecology.* Barek JS, ed., 14th edition. Lippincott Williams & Wilkins, Philadelphia: 2007, 1549–88.
7. Siller BS, et al: T2/3 vulva cancer: A case-controlled study of triple incision versus en bloc radical vulvectomy and inguinal lymphadenectomy. *Gynecol Oncol* 1995; 57:335.
8. Wheeless CR Jr: Radical vulvectomy with bilateral inguinal lymph node dissection. In *Atlas of Pelvic Surgery.* Williams & Wilkins, Baltimore: 1997, 405–11.

CONIZATION OF THE CERVIX

SURGICAL CONSIDERATIONS

Description: Conization of the cervix can be used for both diagnostic and therapeutic purposes. It is performed in cases of biopsy-proven dysplasia with unsatisfactory colposcopy (inadequate visualization of the endocervical canal) or following endocervical curettage showing dysplasia or atypical glandular epithelial cells (Fig 8.1-5). Persistent abnormal cytology associated with normal colposcopy, colposcopic suspicion of invasion, and/or cervical biopsy showing microinvasive cancer is also an indication for this procedure. The surgery consists of the annular removal of a cone-shaped wedge of tissue from the cervix with a scalpel. With the advent of the LEEP (loop electrosurgical excision procedure), most cone biopsies are done under local paracervical/intracervical block in an office setting and do not require the services of an anesthesiologist.

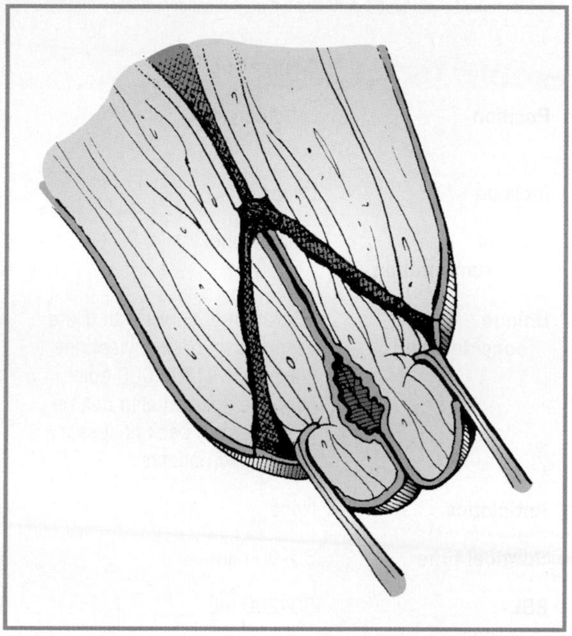

Figure 8.1-5. Cut across endocervix to complete cone excision.

Variant procedure or approaches: In selected patients, a **laser** is used in place of the scalpel. This procedure can be performed under local anesthesia with less blood loss, but operative time is usually longer. The thermal effect of the laser at the cone margins, although usually minimal, may interfere with pathologic interpretation. In pregnant patients, a **shallower cone** is done to minimize complications. Approximately 1% of women with cervical carcinoma are pregnant at the time of diagnosis, and 1/1240 pregnancies is complicated by cervical cancer. Recognition and therapy of preinvasive cervical lesions during pregnancy, therefore, are of

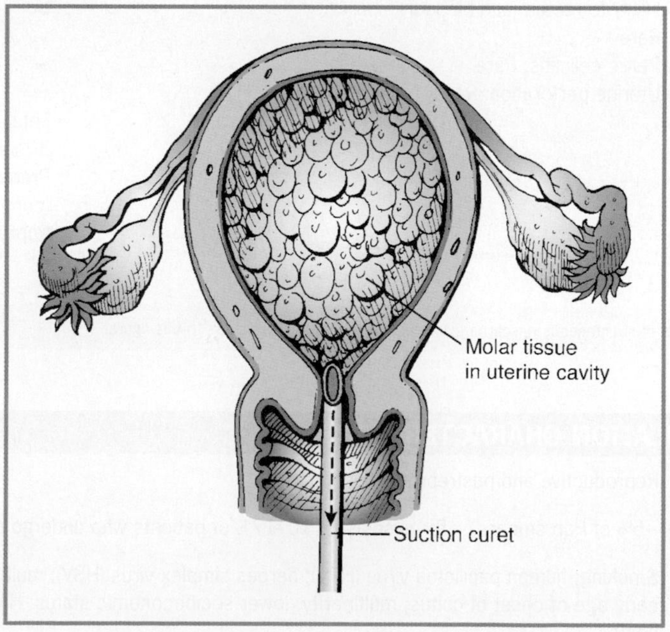

Figure 8.1-6. Suction curettage of a molar pregnancy.

paramount importance. Because of the increased vascularity of the pregnant uterus and cervix, conization is usually associated with increased blood loss and morbidity.

Usual preop diagnosis: Cervical dysplasia

SUMMARY OF PROCEDURES

	Conization	Laser Conization	Shallow Cone In Pregnancy
Position	Lithotomy	⇐	Lithotomy; with left lateral tilt in 3rd trimester
Incision	Cervical	⇐	⇐
Special instrumentation	Colposcope	CO_2 laser; protective eye wear; colposcope	Colposcope
Unique considerations	Infiltration of cervix with dilute vasopressin or phenylephrine solution. A 1:200,000 epinephrine solution also can be used. Vaginal pack necessary in selected patients.	⇐	Phenylephrine, vasopressin, or epinephrine should not be used during pregnancy. Liberal use of hemostatic sutures should be made.
Antibiotics	None	⇐	⇐
Surgical time	30–60 min	30–90 min	⇐
EBL	50–200 mL	50 mL	100–350 mL
Postop care	Monitor for postop bleeding	⇐	⇐
Mortality	< 0.01%	⇐	⇐
Morbidity	Hemorrhage: 5–10% Cervical incompetence: 2–3% Cervical stenosis: 2–3% Dysmenorrhea: Rare Infertility: Rare Injury to rectum and bladder: Rare Pelvic cellulitis: Rare Uterine perforation: Rare	⇐ ⇐ ⇐ ⇐ ⇐ ⇐ ⇐ ⇐	10–15% ⇐ ⇐ ⇐ ⇐ ⇐ ⇐ ⇐ Fetal loss: 10–15% (up to 30% in 1st trimester)* Premature labor: 5–10% (controversial) Rupture of membrane: 2–5%
Pain score	3	3	3

*The naturally higher incidence of spontaneous miscarriages in the 1st trimester contributes to this figure.

PATIENT POPULATION CHARACTERISTICS

Age range	Reproductive and postreproductive years
Incidence	~5% of Pap smears (+ for dysplasia); 10–17% of patients who undergo colposcopic exams
Etiology and predisposing factors	Smoking; human papilloma virus (HPV); herpes simplex virus (HSV); multiple sexual partners; early age of onset of coitus; multiparity; lower socioeconomic status; HIV; immunocompromised hosts

ANESTHETIC CONSIDERATIONS

PREOPERATIVE

Conization is done for diagnosis and treatment of cervical lesions. Occasionally it is necessary to perform the procedure during pregnancy, which increases the risk of bleeding complications. The effect of anesthetic agents on the fetus (especially 1st trimester) also needs to be considered when choosing anesthetic technique (see p. 835).

Respiratory	Not usually a problem, unless there is Hx of lung disease or smoking.
Cardiovascular	These patients are generally young and, therefore, less likely to have significant heart disease.
Neurological	Usually not significant, unless there is Hx of seizure disorder or other neurologic illness.
Hematologic	Consider hemogram
Laboratory	Consider pregnancy test
Premedication	Consider midazolam 1–2 mg iv (Though generally held if pregnant). Na citrate 30 mL po should be given 30 min prior to induction in all pregnant patients.

INTRAOPERATIVE

Anesthetic technique: Usually a local or MAC anesthetic; occasionally, GETA or spinal. Pregnancy makes it desirable to perform the procedure under local or regional anesthesia if appropriate.

General anesthesia:

Induction	Standard induction (p. B-2). If pregnant patient, rapid-sequence induction (p. B-4) with cricoid pressure is appropriate.
Maintenance	Standard maintenance (p. B-2)
Emergence	No special issues

Regional anesthesia: Both spinal and epidural techniques are acceptable, and may be preferred for pregnant patients who cannot tolerate local anesthesia. Prehydration with 1000 mL LR before block is recommended. Treat ↓BP with ephedrine 5–10 mg iv, or Neo-Synephrine 50–100 mcg, titrated to effect.

Blood and fluid requirements	Minimal blood loss IV: 18–20 ga × 1 NS/LR at 2–4 mL/kg/h	
Monitoring	Standard monitors (see p. B-1). Fetal monitoring may be indicated for pregnancies > 16 wk	Monitor for fetal distress or onset of labor. Mg^{++} or terbutaline may be necessary to suppress a sudden onset of premature labor. Consult with obstetrician on the need for these tocolytic agents. Consider having L & D nursing staff in OR if fetal monitoring used.
Positioning	✓ and pad pressure points ✓ eyes Left uterine displacement	***NB** peroneal nerve compression at lateral fibular head → foot drop. Left uterine displacement with a wedge under mattress should be used for pregnant patients (after ~20 wk).

Complications	Laser eye damage Fire Premature labor	If a laser is used, eye protection is required for the patient and all OR personnel; be alert for fire hazards when using a laser.

POSTOPERATIVE

Complications	Peroneal nerve injury (2° lithotomy position)	Nerve injury manifested as foot drop and loss of sensation over dorsum of foot.
	PONV	See p. B-6.
	Premature labor	Tocolytic agents (e.g., terbutaline, magnesium) may be needed, consult obstetrician.
	Bleeding	
Pain management	Oral analgesics	Consider acetaminophen or Vicodin.

Suggested Readings

1. Copeland LJ, Landon MB: Malignant disease in pregnancy. In *Obstetrics. Normal and Problem Pregnancies.* Gabbe SG, Niebyl JR, Simpson JL, eds. Churchill Livingstone, New York: 2002, 1255–81.
2. DiSaia PJ, Creasman WT: Cancer in pregnancy. In *Clinical Gynecologic Oncology,* DiSaia PJ, Creasman WT, eds. CV Mosby, St. Louis: 2000, 439–72.
3. Duggan BD, Felix JC, Muderspach LI, et al: Cold-knife conization versus conization by the loop electrosurgical excision procedure: a randomized, prospective study. *Am J Obstet Gynecol* 1999; 180:276–82.
4. Hoffman MS: Cervical conization. In *Gynecologic Surgery.* Mann WJ, Stovall TG, eds. Churchill Livingstone, New York: 1996, 265–83.
5. Kristensen GB: The outcome of pregnancy and preterm delivery after conization of the cervix. *Arch Gynecol* 1985; 236:127.
6. Matseoane S, Williams SB, Navarro C, et al: Diagnostic value in the conization of the uterine cervix. Management of cervical neoplasia: a review of 756 consecutive patients. *Gynecol Oncol* 1992; 47:287.
7. Mazze RI, Kallen B: Reproductive outcome after anesthesia and operation during pregnancy: a registry study of 5405 cases. *Am J Obstet Gynecol* 1989; 161(5):1178–85.

ANESTHETIC CONSIDERATIONS FOR LASER THERAPY TO VULVA, VAGINA, CERVIX

PREOPERATIVE

Laser therapy is indicated for preinvasive lesions of the vulva, vagina, or cervix. It destroys tissues by the selective application of light energy focused into a beam. Vaporized tissues tend to heal without scarring, and blood loss is minimal due to the cauterizing effect of the laser. Many gynecological laser procedures are done with local anesthesia in the clinic setting and do not require the services of an anesthesiologist.

Respiratory	Not significant, unless there is underlying lung disease.
Cardiovascular	In elderly patients, exercise tolerance should be assessed. **Tests:** ECG if > 50 yr
Hematologic	**Tests:** Hct
Laboratory	Consider pregnancy test in young women
Premedication	Consider midazolam 1–2 mg iv

INTRAOPERATIVE

Anesthetic technique: Usually MAC; GETA/LMA or regional technique may be used. Sedation with propofol, midazolam, and fentanyl in small doses usually is effective.

General anesthesia:

Induction	Standard induction (see p. B-2)	
Maintenance	Standard maintenance (see p. B-2). Muscle relaxation not necessary. A technique with relatively rapid emergence (e.g., propofol and/or sevoflurane/desflurane/N_2O combinations) is useful for outpatient surgery.	
Emergence	Limit opiates	

Regional anesthesia: Spinal or epidural anesthesia may be used with a sensory level to T10. Provide supplemental O_2 if iv sedation given.

Spinal	A T10 sensory level is desirable; bupivacaine 10–12 mg can be used. Small-diameter spinal needles (e.g., 26-ga Quincke or 25-ga Sprotte needles) minimize chance of postdural puncture headache (PDPH).	
Epidural	2% lidocaine, ± epinephrine 1:200,000 (10–15 mL), or 0.5% bupivacaine (10–15 mL) is used; redose as needed with 3–5 mL. Narcotics, such as morphine (4 mg) or hydromorphone (0.5 mg), may be given in the epidural for postop pain control.	
Blood and fluid requirements	Minimal blood loss IV: 18 ga × 1 NS/LR at 2–4 mL/kg/h	Consider prehydrating patient if using neuraxial block.
Monitoring	Standard monitors (see p. B-1).	
Positioning	✓ and pad pressure points ✓ eyes	
Complications	Eye injury OR fires Aerosolization of viral particles	Goggles should be worn by both patient and all OR personnel during laser use to prevent injury to eyes from light. If the patient is asleep, cover eyes with saline-soaked gauze. Whenever laser is in use, be prepared for fires: know where fire extinguisher is located, and watch for improper handling of lasers. Vaporization of condyloma may produce aerosolization of viral particles; therefore, appropriate ventilation is suggested to disperse smoke.

POSTOPERATIVE

Complications	PONV PDPH	See p. B-6 PDPH may require epidural blood patch for treatment.
Pain management	Oral analgesics	e.g., acetaminophen 325–650 mg or Vicodin 1–2 tabs.

Suggested Readings

1. Addis IB, Hatch KD, Berek JS: Intraepithelial disease of the cervix, vagina, and vulva. In *Barek & Novak's Gynecology.* Barek JS, ed., 14th edition. Lippincott Williams & Wilkins, Philadelphia: 2007, 561–600.
2. McKenzie AL, Carruth JA: Lasers in surgery and medicine. *Phys Med Biol* 1984; 29(6):619–41.

SUCTION CURETTAGE FOR GESTATIONAL TROPHOBLASTIC DISEASE

SURGICAL CONSIDERATIONS

Description: **Suction curettage** is the most efficient method of evacuating a gestational trophoblastic neoplasm (mole). The procedure involves dilation of the cervix by instruments or by laminaria tents, followed by insertion of suction cannula of appropriate diameter into the uterine cavity. Standard negative pressures used are in the range of 30–70 mmHg. IV oxytocin—to maintain uterine contraction and minimize blood loss—is started after a moderate amount of tissue has been removed. Suction curettage is followed by gentle, sharp curettage of the uterus to ensure adequate evacuation. Paracervical injection of dilute vasopressin solution or 1% Xylocaine with 1:200,000 epinephrine may decrease operative blood loss (in cases not complicated by thyrotoxicosis or HTN).

Variant procedure or approaches: Evacuation of a mole > 16 wk gestation size is associated with a significant risk of trophoblastic embolization and cardiorespiratory embarrassment (2° pulmonary HTN/edema, cyanosis, ↓CO, ↓BP, right heart failure). Central hemodynamic monitoring with TEE or a PA catheter is useful in the management of cardiovascular changes associated with trophoblastic embolization and to prevent inadvertent fluid overload. In general, earlier diagnosis of molar pregnancies has decreased the incidence of complications such as HTN and thyroxicosis.

Usual preop diagnosis: Gestational trophoblastic disease (GTD)

SUMMARY OF PROCEDURES

	Small Mole < 16 Weeks' Size	Large Mole > 16 Weeks' Size
Position	Lithotomy	⇐
Incision	None	⇐
Special instrumentation	Suction evacuation kit	⇐
Unique considerations	If mole > 12 wk size, laparotomy setup should be readily available. Oxytocin drip. In some cases, thyrotoxicosis may be present, requiring control with β-blockers.	⇐ ± central hemodynamic monitoring with TEE or PA catheter; avoid overzealous use of crystalloids and blood transfusions. Preop ABG.
Antibiotics	Cefotetan 2 g iv	⇐
Surgical time	30–60 min	⇐
EBL	200–400 mL	⇐
Postop care	Outpatient (usually)	ICU admission in selected cases
Mortality	Rare	⇐
Morbidity	Trophoblastic embolization: 2.6% Excessive bleeding: 2% Infection: < 2% Uterine perforation: < 1%	11–27% 10% ⇐ 1–2% Acute pulmonary edema: 2–11%
Pain score	3	3

PATIENT POPULATION CHARACTERISTICS

Age range	Reproductive age group
Incidence	1/1200 deliveries in the United States

Obstetric/Gynecologic Surgery

PATIENT POPULATION CHARACTERISTICS (cont'd)	
Etiology	Genetics: androgenous (all chromosomes in true moles are paternal in origin); nutritional deficiency: protein, folic acid, carotene (vitamin A)
Associated conditions	Lower socioeconomic status; Asian, Hispanic populations; hyperemesis gravidarum (2° ↑ levels of HCG); preeclampsia in 1st trimester; thyrotoxicosis (because of its analogy to TSH molecule, ↑ levels of HCG can bind TSH receptors and cause thyrotoxicosis); prior GTD (incidence ↑ to 0.6–2.0%)

ANESTHETIC CONSIDERATIONS

PREOPERATIVE

Some 80% of cases are diagnosed at 12–18 wk of development. Most patients have an unusually large uterus for the length of the pregnancy and vaginal bleeding is common. Trophoblastic disease is classified by the degree of invasiveness; **retained mole** is the most common type, and the least invasive; **invasive mole** involves the wall of the uterus; and **metastatic mole** involves more distant sites. Chemotherapy with methotrexate and actinomycin D usually is given postop for invasive or metastatic disease. (See Table 8.1-1 for toxicities of chemotherapeutic agents.)

Respiratory	Pulmonary edema may complicate preeclampsia, which occurs in 25% of patients with GTD. If respiratory distress is present, it also may be 2° embolization of tumor to lungs. Avoid overhydration → pulmonary complications in patients with large moles. **Tests:** Consider preop ABG if pulmonary function impaired, and in patients at high risk of developing trophoblastic embolization. Others as indicated by H&P.
Cardiovascular	Dehydration and/or ↓ blood volume may exist due to hyperemesis and vaginal bleeding. Adequate hydration should be given preop if patient shows Sx of hypovolemia (e.g., tachycardia, orthostatic ↓ BP, low UO). Preeclampsia also may complicate this disease and can be diagnosed by HTN, proteinuria, and edema. If the patient has preeclampsia, invasive monitoring of BP may be advisable. Also, if patient is receiving Mg^{++} therapy, a serum level should be ✓'d preop. Mg^{++} therapy may inhibit myocardial contractility in high doses. Ca^{++} is the preferred antidote for myocardial depression. $MgSO_4$ → uterine atony →↑blood loss.
Neurological	Sz prophylaxis with Mg^{++} is indicated for women with severe preeclampsia. If Sz occurs a small dose of STP (50–100 mg) or midazolam (1–2 mg) should be given iv and respiration assisted with supplemental O_2 by mask. The trachea should be intubated for airway protection in patients with full stomachs and in those who are difficult to ventilate by mask.
Musculoskeletal	✓reflexes if patient has received Mg^{++}. Reduce amount of muscle relaxant to compensate for the effects of Mg^{++} on muscle strength.
Hematologic	Anemia may be masked by hypovolemia. Rh– patients with Rh+ partners should receive 300 mcg of Rh immune globulin (RhoGAM) within 72 h postop to ↓ possibility of Rh isoimmunization in future pregnancies. **Tests:** CBC; ✓Plt in preeclamptics. If patient has received chemotherapy recently, ✓HCT; complete blood count (WBC, Plt).
Endocrine	Hyperthyroidism occurs in 5% of women with hydatidiform moles and is 2° the thyroid-stimulating effects of HCG. **Tests:** Thyroid function tests should be ✓'d preop in women with Sx of hyperthyroidism, and managed before surgery.
Laboratory	Serum HCG level; consider thyroid function tests; LFTs; PT; PTT; Plt count; Mg^{++} level; UA—as indicated from H&P.
Premedication	Consider midazolam 1–2 mg iv. A nonparticulate antacid (Na citrate 30 mL 0.3 M) should be given po just before induction.

INTRAOPERATIVE

Anesthetic technique: Usually GETA, although may be carried out under spinal or epidural anesthesia.

General anesthesia:

Induction	A rapid-sequence induction (p. B-4) with cricoid pressure should be used.
Maintenance	Standard maintenance (p. B-2). Control BP, if preeclamptic, with labetalol, hydralazine, or SNP. Try to keep DBP at 90–100 mmHg.
Emergence	Extubate when fully awake and protective airway reflexes have returned. Consider PONV prophylaxis. Give supplemental O_2.

Regional anesthesia:

Spinal	A T8 sensory level is desirable; bupivacaine (10–12 mg) may be used.	
Epidural	Use 2% lidocaine ± epinephrine 1:200,000 (10–20 mL) or 0.25% bupivacaine (10–15 mL)	
Blood and fluid requirements	Possible large blood loss IV: 16–18 ga × 1 NS/LR at 2–4 mL/kg/h	One large-volume iv line should be placed and blood readily available. The usual causes of bleeding are uterine perforation, cervical laceration, or uterine atony.
Control of bleeding	Oxytocin (30 U/L) infusion	Oxytocin is begun about halfway through procedure at 30–60 drops/min (consult obstetrician). Large oxytocin boluses may →↓BP.
	↑% volatile anesthetic may → ↓uterine tone	Try to keep anesthetic <1 MAC to prevent uterine relaxation.
	Ergonovine maleate 0.2 mg im	Ergonovine may be given for severe bleeding. Since this drug can cause HTN, it is contraindicated in cases of preeclampsia with elevated BP.
Monitoring	Standard monitors (p. B-1) ± Arterial catheter ± CVP/PA catheter Foley catheter	An arterial catheter and CVP are indicated in cases of thyrotoxicosis, preeclampsia, or significant hemorrhage. The use of vasodilators, such as SNP, is also an indication for invasive monitors.
Positioning	✓ and pad pressure points ✓ eyes	* **NB:** peroneal nerve compression at lateral fibular head → foot drop. Lifting the legs may cause the level of spinal or epidural anesthesia to move cranially if performed too quickly after the block.
Complications	Embolization of trophoblastic material	Embolization may occur, especially if > 16 wk gestation. Significant respiratory and cardiac compromise may occur, requiring postop ventilation and PEEP, hemodynamic support, ICU.

POSTOPERATIVE

Complications	Bleeding	Continue oxytocin infusion. Significant hemorrhage should be evaluated by surgeons for possible perforation, laceration, or atony.
	PONV	Consider PONV prophylaxis with odansetron 4 mg.
	HTN	BP should be monitored closely in preeclamptics. Consider ICU admission if unstable.

Complications (cont'd)	↓ BP	Consider trophoblastic embolization and manage aggressively.
	Peroneal nerve injury (2° to lithotomy position)	Nerve injury manifested as foot drop and loss of sensation over dorsum of foot.
Pain management	Oral analgesics	Acetaminophen (325–650 mg po). Vicodin, or ketorolac (15–30 mg iv). Patients receiving Mg^{++} for preeclampsia may require less opiates for pain control. This may be 2° NMDA receptor antagonism.

Suggested Readings

1. Berkowitz RS, Goldstein DP: Gestational Trophoblastic Disease. In *Barek & Novak's Gynecology*. Barek JS, ed., 14th edition. Lippincott Williams & Wilkins, Philadelphia: 2007, 1601–38.
2. Berkowitz RS, Goldstein DP: Gestational trophoblastic disease. In *Principles and Practice of Gynecologic Oncology*, 3rd edition. Hoskins WJ, Perez CA, Young RC, Barakat RR, Markman B, eds: Lippincott Williams & Wilkins, Philadelphia: 2004, 1117–38.
3. Berkowitz RS, Goldstein DP: Presentation and management of molar pregnancy. In *Gestational Trophoblastic Disease.* Hancock BW, Newlands ES, Berkowitz RS, eds. Chapman and Hall, London: 1997, 127.
4. Burger RA, Creasman WT: Gestational trophoblastic neoplasia. In *Clinical Gynecologic Oncology.* DiSaia PJ, Creasman WT, eds. CV Mosby, St. Louis: 2000, 185–210.
5. Guido RS, Stovall DW: Dilation and curettage and hysteroscopy. In *Gynecologic Surgery.* Mann WJ, Stovall TG, eds. Churchill Livingstone, New York: 1996: 225–63.

PELVIC EXENTERATION

SURGICAL CONSIDERATIONS

Description: **Pelvic exenteration** was introduced by Brunschwig as an ultraradical surgical approach for advanced and radioresistant cervical cancer. Although advanced vaginal and vulvar carcinoma occasionally have been treated with this procedure, its most important role is in the management of centrally recurrent, surgically resectable, radioresistant cervical carcinoma. **Total pelvic exenteration** involves **en bloc resection** of all pelvic tissues, including uterus, cervix, vagina, bladder, and rectum. Involvement of the distal vagina may require resection of vulva and groin nodes. The goal of this procedure is curative with removal of all cancer tissue and reconstruction of appropriate diversions for the urine and stool, if the colon cannot be reanastomosed to the rectum. It is rare for cervical and vaginal cancer to involve the lower 5 cm of the rectum and anus. It is, therefore, often possible to mobilize the descending colon and anastomose it primarily to the distal rectum. Otherwise, an **end colostomy** is created. A continent or incontinent urinary diversion, **omental pelvic carpet** or **sling** and **gracilis myocutaneous flaps** for vaginal and perineal reconstruction are performed. A **rectus abdominis muscle flap** also can be used for vaginal reconstruction. This type of flap yields excellent aesthetic and functional results. In cases where an omental sling (shown in (Fig. 8.1-7) cannot be developed, an absorbable synthetic mesh is sutured to the pelvic peritoneum to create a pelvic lid (like a hammock) to keep the small bowel off the denuded pelvic peritoneum, thus decreasing the possibility of small-bowel obstruction. In general, an additional 2–3 h of surgical time and an additional 300 mL of EBL are expected when a vaginal reconstruction is undertaken. An exploratory laparotomy is needed prior to initiation of the exenterative procedure to exclude spread of disease outside the pelvis and/or extension to pelvic sidewalls and pelvic lymph nodes, all of which are absolute contraindications to this procedure.

Resectability is evaluated by examination of pelvic and paraaortic lymph nodes, liver, hemidiaphragms, and peritoneal surfaces of the upper abdomen and pelvic wall. Washings are obtained for cytology. Evaluation of lymph nodes is then performed and all suspicious nodes are submitted for frozen-section pathologic examination. The pararectal, paravesical, and presacral spaces are then developed. If the patient is found to be inoperable, CUSA can be used to decrease the tumor burden. Consideration also should be given to IORT, which may provide an adjunctive treatment to radical surgery in the setting of: (1) recurrent disease close to the pelvic sidewalls; and (2)

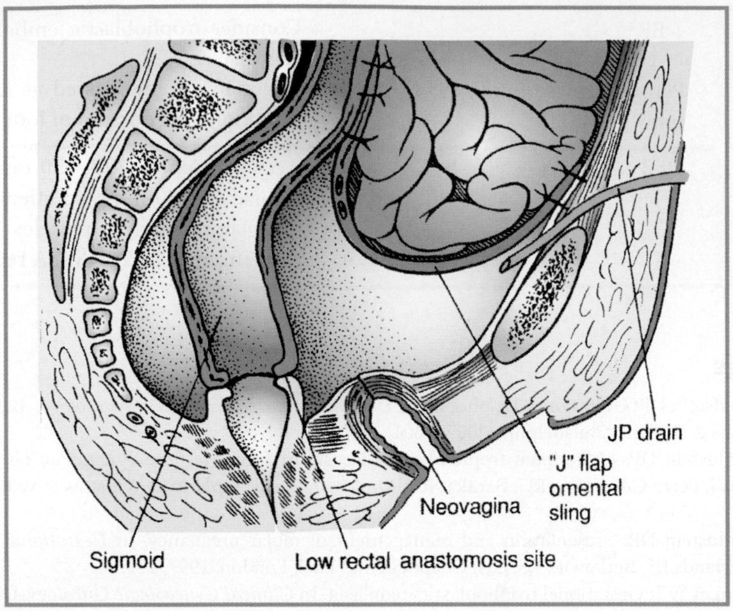

Figure 8.1-7. Sagittal section of the pelvis after a total pelvic exenteration. Note that all the reproductive organs, along with their supporting structures, the rectum and the bladder, have been resected. Drains can be placed through separate stab incisions in the abdomen. The small bowel is kept away from the operative site by a pelvic lid. The urinary and fecal diversions are not diagrammed. (Reproduced with permission from Wheeless CR: *Atlas of Pelvic Surgery*. Lea & Febiger: 1988.)

microscopically positive surgical margins or 'close' resection margins. If the patient is deemed operable, the space of Retzius is developed. The round ligaments are then transected close to the pelvic sidewall bilaterally; and the infundibulopelvic ligaments also are ligated and transected. The ureters are divided as close to the bladder as possible. The superior hemorrhoidal vessel is ligated and transected; and the colon is transected at the appropriate level. The anterior divisions of the internal iliac artery on both sides are ligated and divided; and the web of tissue is clamped close to the pelvic sidewall, transected, and suture-ligated. Following this, sharp dissection can be done to free up the specimen from the low attachments to the levator muscles. In larger tumors, the levator muscle is partially removed with the specimen to provide adequate margins. From a combined perineal and abdominal approach, the distal vagina, urethra, and perineum (± rectum) can be resected. The specimen is handed off the field, hemostasis is achieved, and the bladder is reconstructed with a continent urinary diversion using an ileocolonic segment, ileal loop, or transverse colon conduit. An ileal loop or other urinary conduit is performed, a colostomy or low rectal anastomosis is done, vaginal reconstruction is undertaken, and the pelvic floor is covered. (Fig. 8.1-7 and 8.1-8 show the completed exenteration.)

Variant procedure or approaches: **Anterior pelvic exenteration** is technically similar to a total pelvic exenteration, except the rectum is left intact. **Posterior pelvic exenteration** involves preservation of bladder. Posterior exenteration has proved more useful in cancer of vulva or vagina than in cervical cancer. Anterior and posterior exenterations are used in selective cases because of the increased risk of an incomplete tumor resection and multiple complications and malfunctioning of the preserved organ.

Usual preop diagnosis: Recurrent cervical carcinoma following radiotherapy

SUMMARY OF PROCEDURE

Position	Modified dorsolithotomy with Allen stirrups
Incision	Midline longitudinal, perineal
Special instrumentation	Vital View, ABC may be helpful; EEA, GIA, TA staplers; Robo-retractor or similar devices

SUMMARY OF PROCEDURE (cont'd)	
Unique considerations	Full and thorough mechanical and antibiotic intestinal prep. NG tube placement intraop. SCD and minidose heparin intraop for VTE prophylaxis. Preop PFTs. Consider preop Greenfield IVC filter placement to avoid PE for high-risk patients. Consider intraop radiation of tumor bed and/or of resection margins. Abort case if extrapelvic metastases and/or tumor extension to pelvic sidewalls noted.
Antibiotics	Cefotetan 2 g iv preop and continue q 12 h for 3 days. Alternatively, a combination of ampicillin (1 g), gentamicin (80 mg), and metronidazole (500 mg) may be given.
Surgical time	8–12 h (2-team approach); 5–10 h (for anterior and posterior exenteration)
Closing considerations	Abdominal drains; colostomy; ureteral stents; urostomy; intraop radiation therapy. Triple-lumen central line placement. Copious irrigation of the operative sites.
EBL	1200–4000 mL
Postop care	ICU: 2–3 d. Correction of electrolyte imbalance. Extensive peritoneal raw surfaces → intraperitoneal fluid 3rd-spacing. Patients require good hydration to maintain intravascular volume. SCDs and heparin VTE prophylaxis. Consider concentrated albumin infusion to maintain intravascular volume. Early and aggressive use of TPN is important. Maintain Hct in the low 30s, as concentrated blood may → sludging and contribute to flap necrosis and wound breakdown. Remove ureteral stents 1–2 wk postop, when the edema at the ureterointestinal site has subsided.
Mortality	5–11%
Morbidity	Intraop hemorrhage requiring a median of 5 U PRBC Infectious: Nonspecific: 25% Flap necrosis: 20% Pelvic cellulitis: 19% Pyelonephritis: 17% Wound infection: 6% Sepsis: 3% Psychiatric: Confusion: 24% Intestinal: Ileus: 18% GI fistula: 13% Stoma breakdown: 3% Small bowel obstruction: 5% Renal: Ureteral fistulae: 14% Failure: 5% Cardiovascular: CHF: 8% Venous thrombosis: 3–7% DIC: 3% Dysrrhythmia: 3% MI: 3% Pulmonary: Pneumonia: 3% PE: 2% Neurologic: CVA: 2% Spinal cord infarction: < 2%
Pain score	7–8

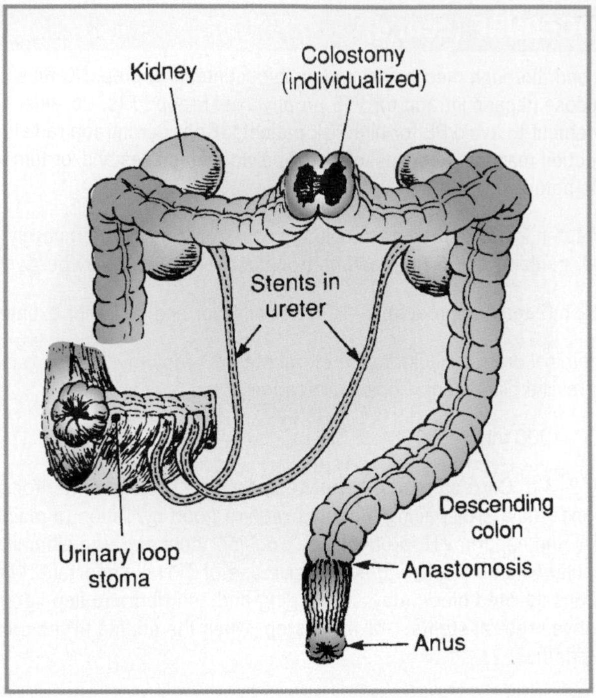

Figure 8.1-8. Conceptual drawing shows the urinary and fecal diversions after a total pelvic exenteration. (Reproduced with permission from Wheeless CR: *Atlas of Pelvic Surgery.* Williams & Wilkins: 1997.)

PATIENT POPULATION CHARACTERISTICS

Age range	All age groups
Incidence	1.5–17% of cervical cancers treated with radiation therapy (depending on stage and cell type)
Associated conditions	Advanced or recurrent gynecologic malignancies; radiation injury

ANESTHETIC CONSIDERATIONS

PREOPERATIVE

This procedure is performed for recurrent rectal, cervical, or other gynecologic cancers and involves removal of all pelvic organs. Occasionally, the bladder or rectum is preserved, if not involved with tumor. Most patients have undergone preop radiation or chemotherapy.

Respiratory	Usually not significant unless there is Hx of smoking or lung disease. Ask about prior chemotherapy. (See Anesthetic Considerations for Second-Look/Reassessment Laparotomy for Ovarian Cancer, p. 751.) **Tests:** Consider CXR; others as indicated from H&P.
Cardiovascular	Exercise tolerance should be assessed. Underlying CAD or CHF should be medically optimized preoperatively. Any exposure to cardiotoxic chemotherapy should be investigated and may require further tests, such as an ECHO. **Tests:** Consider ECG; others as indicated from H&P.
Neurological	Any Hx of stroke, Sz, carotid artery disease, or other neurologic disease should be evaluated and documented.
Endocrine	Any endocrine disease, such as diabetes, should be optimized in consultation with the patient's primary care physician or endocrinologist. Ask about recent corticosteroid use. **Tests:** Fasting blood sugar in the diabetic; others as indicated from H&P.

Obstetric/Gynecologic Surgery

Gastrointestinal	Patients should have iv hydration if given a bowel prep.
Hematologic	Many patients will be anemic from chronic disease and malnutrition. Consider preop transfusion PRBC to ↑ Hct > 30%. **Tests:** CBC, PT, PTT
Laboratory	LFTs
Premedication	Consider midazolam 1–2 mg iv. Detailed explanation about the procedure and the potential for postop events including intubation and mechanical ventilation worthwhile.

INTRAOPERATIVE

Anesthetic technique: GETA ± supplemental epidural anesthesia.

General anesthesia:

Induction	Standard induction (p. B-2), unless otherwise indicated by patient condition. Keep in mind possibility surgery could be significantly shortened if metastatic tumor found during initial ex lap.	
Maintenance	Balanced anesthetic technique based on comorbidities, use of concomitant epidural anesthesia and likelihood of needing ICU postop. Epidural anesthetic or epidural narcotic (morphine or hydromorphone) can be given to reduce anesthetic requirements when using inhalation agents.	
Emergence	If patient is hemodynamically stable, with favorable oxygenation and pulmonary function, normothermic, and responsive at the end of surgery, extubation may be appropriate. Any patient who is unstable, hypothermic, has high-oxygen requirements, significant edema of the face or airway, or ongoing excessive fluid requirements should be admitted to ICU and remain intubated. Due to the large fluid shifts and significant complication rates, postop monitoring in the ICU is appropriate.	
Epidural	Consider epidural for intraop and/or postop use: 2% lidocaine (10–15 mL), with or without hydromorphone (0.3–0.8 mg), may be given in the epidural for postop pain control. Intraop use may ↑ hemodynamic instability in setting of ↑ bleeding and fluid shifts. Post op efficacy may be limited if patient remains intubated > 1 day.	
Ventilation	5–7 cm H_2O PEEP may help prevent atelectasis.	✓ABGs during surgery. Adjust ventilation to keep normocarbic. Give HCO_3 for metabolic acidosis when pH < 7.20 and treat underlying cause.
Blood and fluid requirements	Potential large blood loss IV: 14–16 ga × 2 NS/LR at 10–15 mL/kg/h Colloid solutions	Renal ultrafiltration improved by NS/LR, bowel edema ↑'d. LR useful when acidosis occurs. NS is better when giving blood products or when metabolic alkalosis is present. Rapid-infuser should be available. Strive to maintain euvolemia based on BP, HR, UO, ABG, invasive monitoring (CVP, CO, art line tracing), and estimates of ongoing EBL and fluid shifts.
	Hetastarch Consider PRBCs when Hct < 30% Maintain UO of 0.5–1 mL/kg/h.	Use of 6% hetastarch should be limited to 1,000 mL due to potential coagulopathy with larger volumes. Dopamine 2–3 mcg/kg/min may be used to maintain UO.
	Ionized Ca^{++}	Measure ionized Ca^{++} and K^+ after rapid administration of blood products; replace Ca^{++} as necessary.
	FFP/Plt	Plt or FFP for coagulation abnormalities. Monitor values during case periodically.

Monitoring	Standard monitors (see p. B-1). ± Arterial line Consider CVP/PA catheter Foley catheter	Invasive hemodynamic monitoring with arterial and PA catheters usually helpful in these cases which are of very long duration, and associated with major bleeding, fluid shifts, ICU postop, and potential need for vasoactive infusions.
	± TEE	TEE allows intraop assessment of myocardial function and may be appropriate in selected patients.
Positioning	✓ and pad pressure points ✓ eyes Antiembolism stockings and SCD	* **NB:** peroneal nerve compression at lateral fibular head → foot drop.
Complications	Hypothermia	Use forced air and fluid warmers and monitor temperature.
	VTE	See Appendix B.
	Coagulopathy	
	Trauma to kidney	Watch for hematuria or ↓UO.
	Bleeding	Monitor hemoglobin and coagulation status periodically during long surgery. Keep adequate reserve blood products available.
	Peripheral nerve injury	Prolonged surgery, carefully pad, secure, and monitor all extremities.

POSTOPERATIVE

Complications	Bleeding	✓Hct and coags periodically. Be prepared for continued increased fluid requirements for 24 h postop.
	Fluid overload Hypothermia	Maintain euvolemia, if significant fluid gain occurs, consider ICU postop ventilation.
	PONV	If extubated. See p. B-6.
	VTE	See p. B-7.
	Peripheral nerve injury	For prolonged surgery, carefully pad, secure, and monitor all extremities.
Pain management	Epidural or iv opiates	See p. C-2.
Tests	CBC, chemistry panel, coags, ABG	Others as indicated from postoperative course. Patient will likely need ongoing critical care/ICU management.

Suggested Readings

1. Burke TW, Morley GW: Pelvic exenteration. In *Te Linde's Operative Gynecology.* Rock JA, Jones HW, eds., 9th edition. Lippincott Williams & Wilkins, Philadelphia: 2003, 1523–36.
2. Eisenkop SM, Nalick RH, Teng NH: Modified posterior exenteration for ovarian cancer. *Obstet Gynecol* 1991; 78:879–85.
3. Gemignani M, Alektiar KM, Leitao M, et al: Radical surgical resection and high-dose intraoperative radiation therapy (HDR-IORT) in patients with recurrent gynecologic cancers. *Int J Radiat Oncol Biol Phys* 2001; 50:687–94.
4. Husain A, Curtin J, Brown C, et al: Continent urinary diversion and low-rectal anastomosis in patients undergoing exenterative procedures for recurrent gynecologic malignancies. *Gynecol Oncol* 2000; 78:208–11.
5. Numa F, Ogata H, Suminami Y, Tsunaga N, et al: Pelvic exenteration for the treatment of gynecological malignancies. *Arch Gynecol Obstet* 1997; 259:133–8.
6. Ramirez PT, Modesitt SC, Morris M, et al: Functional outcomes and complications of continent urinary diversions in patients with gynecologic malignancies. *Gynecol Oncol* 2002; 85:285–91.
7. Stehman FB, Perez CA, Kurman RJ, Thigpen JT: Uterine cervix. In: *Principles and Practice of Gynecologic Oncology*, 3rd edition. Hoskins WJ, Perez CA, Young RC, Barakat RR, Markman B, eds: Lippincott Williams & Wilkins, Philadelphia: 2004, 841–918.
8. Wheeless CR Jr: Total pelvic exenteration. In *Atlas of Pelvic Surgery.* Williams & Wilkins, Baltimore: 1997, 447–57.

EXPLORATORY LAPAROTOMY, HYSTERECTOMY/BSO FOR UTERINE CANCER

SURGICAL CONSIDERATION

Description: Currently, endometrial cancer is the most common gynecologic malignancy in the United States. The first step in the management of this cancer is an **exploratory laparotomy,** concurrent with a **hysterectomy.** The objective, aside from 1° therapy, is to obtain as much surgical and pathological staging data as feasible for determination of adjuvant postop therapy. Careful exploration is carried out for evidence of omental, liver, peritoneal, and adnexal metastases. Aortic and pelvic areas are palpated for metastases, and suspicious nodes are removed. In patients with low grade histology and no or minimal suspected invasion, complete lymph node dissection remains an area of controversy and treatment is generally individualized based on clinicopathologic factors. In patients with more extensive disease, a pelvic and periaortic lymph nodes dissection is performed. The lymph node sampling may be omitted in the treatment of some uterine sarcomas. A **total hysterectomy** with **BSO** is then performed in the usual manner (see discussion of TAH/BSO in Staging Laparotomy for Ovarian Cancer, p. 746).

Variant procedure or approaches: A combined **laparoscopically assisted vaginal hysterectomy and BSO,** as well as laparoscopic pelvic and paraaortic node sampling, is appropriate in selected patients and is being performed with increasing frequency. The GOG conducted a randomized prospective study evaluating exploratory laparotomy with open staging versus laparoscopic staging (GOG LAP2) to compare outcomes and safety. Although results of this large prospective study are currently pending, retrospective studies have reported similar outcomes. The benefits of this approach are shorter hospital stay and convalescence and decreased postop pain. Adhesions of variable severity may be present from prior surgery or radiation. Care should be taken to avoid possible bowel injury at time of trocar insertion. Patient needs to be in steep Trendelenburg position for duration of the procedure; and both arms should be tucked in at the patient's sides. Because argon is a heavy gas, prolonged use of the endoscopic ABC in a patient in steep Trendelenburg can → significant facial and neck subcutaneous emphysema. As with the open technique, the lymph nodes being removed are in the immediate proximity of the great pelvic vessels. The surgeon and anesthesiologist should be mindful of the potential for severe hemorrhage if these vessels are injured.

Usual preop diagnosis: Endometrial carcinoma

SUMMARY OF PROCEDURES

	Open Technique	Laparoscopic Technique
Position	Supine	Modified dorsolithotomy in Allen stirrups
Incision	Midline longitudinal abdominal/transverse	Vertical infraumbilical and multiple small transverse incisions
Special instrumentation	None	Videolaparoscopy equipment. Endoscopic GIA staplers, endoscopic ABC, endoscopic vascular clips, and CO_2 laser
Unique considerations	None	Mechanical bowel preop; steep Trendelenburg
Antibiotics	Cefotetan 2 g iv	⇐
Surgical time	2–4 h	2–3 h
Closing considerations	NG tube placement	Release the pneumoperitoneum completely. Closure of fascia at trocar sites ≥ 10 mm diameter
EBL	400–750 mL	100–500 mL
Postop care	Consider using SCDs and minidose heparin for DVT prophylaxis.	Begin early ambulation and feeding. Patients generally can be discharged on POD 1 or 2.

SUMMARY OF PROCEDURE (cont'd)	Open Technique	Laparoscopic Technique
Mortality	0.1%	⇐
Morbidity	Hemorrhage requiring transfusion: 15% Thrombophlebitis: 7% UTI: 7% Paralytic ileus: 2–5% Wound infection: 3% PE: 1–2% Pelvic infection: 1.5% Wound dehiscence: 1% Bowel injuries: < 1% Urinary tract injuries: < 1%	0.3–3% ⇐ ⇐ 1–2% Rare ⇐ ⇐ N/A 1.1% 0.3–3% Trocar site herniation: 0.5–2% Trocar site tumor: 1.6% (estimated)
Pain score	7	2–3

PATIENT POPULATION CHARACTERISTICS	
Age range	Reproductive and postreproductive ages (average = 61 yr)
Incidence	70–80/100,000
Etiology	Exposure to unopposed endogenous or exogenous estrogen; ↑ extraglandular conversion of androstenedione to estrone; sequential oral contraceptive pills; exposure to radiation (sarcomas)
Associated conditions	Obesity; diabetes; HTN; nulliparity; late menopause; early menarche; family Hx; Stein-Leventhal syndrome; chronic anovulation; ovarian and colon cancer; granulosa cell ovarian tumors; arthritis; hypothyroidism

ANESTHETIC CONSIDERATIONS

PREOPERATIVE

Endometrial cancer usually is diagnosed in postmenopausal women who present with vaginal bleeding. Exploratory laparotomy and TAH/BSO are commonly performed for removal of the primary tumor as well as staging of metastatic disease. Occasionally, preop radiation therapy may be in progress, with consequent systemic effects.

Respiratory	✓for Hx of lung disease or smoking. **Tests:** Others as indicated from H&P.
Cardiovascular	Hx of CAD, HTN, or CHF Sx (e.g., angina, dyspnea, or peripheral edema) should be investigated. Assess patient's exercise tolerance and current medications. Tests such as an exercise treadmill or ECHO may be indicated if patient has significant angina or CHF. **Tests:** Patients > 50 yr should have a preop ECG.
Neurological	Seldom a significant problem unless there is Hx of cerebrovascular disease, Sz, or other neurologic disease.
Endocrine	Inquire about the presence of endocrine diseases, such as diabetes and hypothyroidism, which have been associated with this tumor. If the patient has received corticosteroids within the previous 6 mo, a supplemental dose of hydrocortisone (100 mg iv q 12 h × 2 d) should be considered. **Tests:** Consider tests if indicated from H&P.
Neuromuscular	Osteoarthritis and osteoporosis common in this patient population. Ask about NSAID usage.

Hematologic	If vaginal bleeding has been profuse or of long duration, significant anemia may occur. Consider preop iron supplements if there are several days until surgery. **Tests:** CBC	
Laboratory	LFTs	
Premedication	Consider anxiolytic, such as midazolam 1–2 mg iv. Discuss anesthetic plan and options for postop pain management with patient.	

INTRAOPERATIVE

Anesthetic technique: GETA ± epidural or spinal analgesia/anesthesia. In unusual circumstances (e.g., severe lung disease), surgery may be done under spinal or epidural anesthesia only.

General anesthesia:

Induction	Standard induction (p. B-2)	
Maintenance	Standard maintenance (p. B-1).	
Emergence	Reverse muscle relaxant with neostigmine (0.07 mg/kg with glycopyrrolate 0.01 mg/kg). Provide supplemental O_2 until patient is fully recovered from anesthesia. Consider PONV prophylaxis (e.g., ondansetron 4 mg iv).	

Regional anesthesia:

Epidural	2% lidocaine (10–20 mL), ± epinephrine 1:200,000, or 0.25% bupivacaine (15–20 mL) is used; then at ~3–5 mL/h. Narcotics, such as morphine (2–4 mg) or hydromorphone (0.3–0.6 mg), may be given in the epidural for postop pain control.	
Spinal	Tetracaine (12–14 mg) ± preservative-free morphine (0.3–0.5 mg). Sensory level ~T5.	
Blood and fluid requirements	IV: 16–18 ga × 1 NS/LR at 4–6 mL/kg/h Consider PRBC for Hct < 25%	Crystalloid is used for volume replacement. If anemia is present preop, it may be necessary to give PRBCs to keep Hct > 25%.
Monitoring	Standard monitors (p. B-1) Foley catheter ± Arterial line, CVP NG tube	Direct monitoring of arterial pressure is indicated in patients with CAD, severe HTN, or lung disease. Consider art line and/or CVP if significant comorbidities exist.
Positioning	✓ and pad pressure points ✓ eyes Antiembolism stockings and SCD	
Complications	Hypothermia Trauma or obstruction of ureter	Warm iv fluids; use forced-air warmer. Heating pad on OR table. Watch for hematuria or ↓ UO.

POSTOPERATIVE

Complications	PONV VTE Hypothermia Bleeding	See p. B-6 See p. B-7
Pain management	PCA (p. C-3) Epidural/spinal narcotics (p. C-2)	Ketorolac (30 mg im/iv) is useful for breakthrough pain. A multimodal approach—including local anesthetics, NSAIDs or acetaminophen, or even low-dose (0.1–0.2 mg/kg/h) ketamine—in the OR may provide analgesia and ↓ PONV.

Suggested Readings

1. Barakat RR, Grigsby PW, Sabbatini P, Zaino RJ: Corpus: epithelial tumors. In: *Principles and Practice of Gynecologic Oncology*, 3rd edition. Hoskins WJ, Perez CA, Young RC, et al., eds: Lippincott Williams & Wilkins, Philadelphia: 2004, 919–60.
2. Dicker RC, Greenspan JR, Straus LT, et al: Complications of abdominal and vaginal hysterectomy among women of reproductive age in the United States. The Collaborative Review of Sterilization. *Am J Obstet Gynecol* 1982; 144(7):841–8.
3. DiSaia PJ, Creasman WT: Adenocarcinoma of the uterus. In *Clinical Gynecologic Oncology.* DiSaia PJ, Creasman WT, eds. CV Mosby, St. Louis: 2002, 137–71.
4. Edraki B, Schwartz PE. Operative laparoscopy and the gynecologic oncologist. Commentary and review. *Cancer* 1995; 76:1987–91.
5. Liu CY: Complications of laparoscopic hysterectomy: prevention, recognition and management. In *Laparoscopic Hysterectomy and Pelvic Floor Reconstruction.* Liu CY, ed. Blackwell Science, Cambridge: 1996; 277–96.
6. Mohan DS, Samuels MA, Selim MA, et al: Long-term outcomes of therapeutic pelvic lymphadenectomy for Stage I endometrial adenocarcinomas. *Gynecol Oncol* 1998; 70:165.
7. Orr JW, Holloway RW, Orr PF, et al: Surgical staging of uterine cancer: An analysis of perioperative morbidity. *Gynecol Oncol* 1991; 42:209.
8. Stovall TG: Vaginal, abdominal, and laparoscopic-assisted hysterectomy. In *Gynecologic Surgery.* Mann WJ, Stovall TG, eds. Churchill Livingstone, New York: 1996, 403–44.

RADICAL HYSTERECTOMY

SURGICAL CONSIDERATIONS

Description: **Radical hysterectomy** is the preferred mode of therapy for young women with Stage IA, IB, or nonbulky IIA cervical carcinoma, who want to preserve ovarian function. It is also appropriate with Stage II endometrial and Stage I vaginal carcinoma. The operation involves the removal of the uterus, along with the upper vagina and all the parametrial tissues to the pelvic sidewall. A pelvic and paraaortic **lymph node dissection** usually is performed at the beginning of the procedure. Suspicious nodes are submitted for pathological frozen-section evaluation. The paravesical and pararectal spaces are then developed, with the 'web' of tissue between these two spaces being palpated carefully (Fig. 8.1-9). If parametrial tumor extension is noted and/or the lymph nodes are positive on frozen section, the hysterectomy may be aborted. The radical hysterectomy is performed after the pararectal and paravesical spaces have been developed. The uterine arteries are divided at their origin from the anterior division of the internal iliac artery. The ureters are dissected free of the parametrial tissues, which are then transected close to the pelvic sidewall. Next, the rectovaginal space is developed (Fig. 8.1-10). The uterosacral ligaments are transected between their uterine and sacral attachments. The upper third of the vagina is cross-clamped and divided in such a manner as to provide a 3 cm margin, and the specimen is delivered en bloc. Note that, during this procedure, the ureters and bladder are dissected free and left intact.

In reproductive-age women, who may require postop radiotherapy, ovarian function is preserved by performing an **oophoropexy.** This is accomplished by severing the uteroovarian ligament and mobilizing the ovarian vessels as they course through the infundibulopelvic ligament. The ovaries are then sutured outside the radiation therapy field and marked with metal clips for future identification.

Variant procedure or approaches: **Stallworthy, Dolstad, Novak, Rutledge, Wertheim,** and other surgeons have proposed several modifications in an effort to reduce the incidence of ureteral and bladder fistulae. These approaches include preservation of blood supply to the terminal 2 cm of the pelvic ureter by widely displacing ureters (not dissecting them from their fascial beds) and limiting parametrial dissection to the proximal 1/3 or 1/2.

Usual preop diagnosis: Stage IA, IB, or nonbulky IIA cervical carcinoma; Stage II endometrial or Stage I vaginal carcinoma (less common)

SUMMARY OF PROCEDURE	
Position	Supine/modified lithotomy
Incision	Midline longitudinal or low transverse abdominal (Maylard/Cherney)
Special instrumentation	ABC, Vital View (suction, irrigation, and light source combined in 1 instrument) helpful

SUMMARY OF PROCEDURE (cont'd)	
Unique considerations	Abort case if positive paraaortic lymph nodes found on frozen section, or if obvious parametrial involvement noted. Consider intraop radiation therapy (investigational), if patient is inoperable.
Antibiotics	Cefotetan 2 g iv; then q 12 h × 2 doses
Surgical time	3–6 h
Closing considerations	Vaginal and abdominal drains; NG tube placement; suprapubic bladder catheter placement; oophoropexy; copious irrigation
EBL	500–1500 mL
Postop care	Transient ileus very common. Advance diet slowly. Transient bladder dysfunction very common; therefore, continued bladder drainage for 1+ wk may be necessary. Consider using SCDs and minidose heparin for DVT prophylaxis.
Mortality	0.3–2.0%
Morbidity	Paralytic ileus: 3–11% Pelvic lymphocyst: 6.4% Intraop hemorrhage: 5.6% Thrombophlebitis: 5% Pneumonia: 1.5–4% Wound infection: 3.5% Vesical injury: 2–3.5% Pelvic infection: 2.2% PE: 2.2% Vesical fistulae: 1.8% Small bowel obstruction: 1.5% Ureteral fistulae: 1.1% Ureteral injury: 1.1% Wound dehiscence: 1% Postop lymphedema: < 1% Rectal injury: < 1% Pelvic urinoma: Rare
Pain score	8

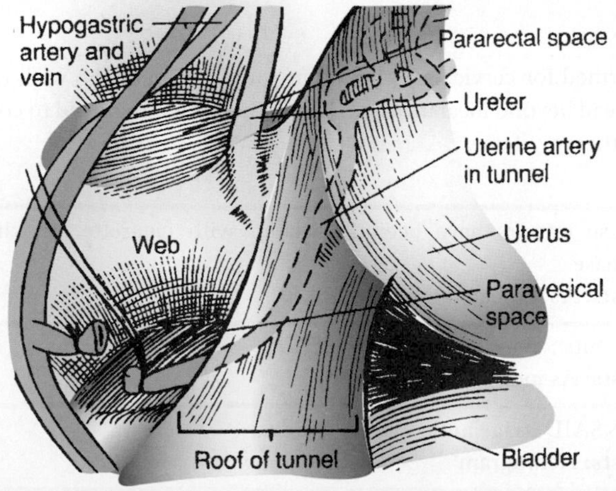

Figure 8.1-9. View of parametrial area, showing positions of ureter and uterine artery to web, hypergastric vessels, paravesical, and pararectal spaces. (Reproduced with permission from Wheeless CR: *Atlas of Pelvic Surgery.* Williams & Wilkins: 1997.)

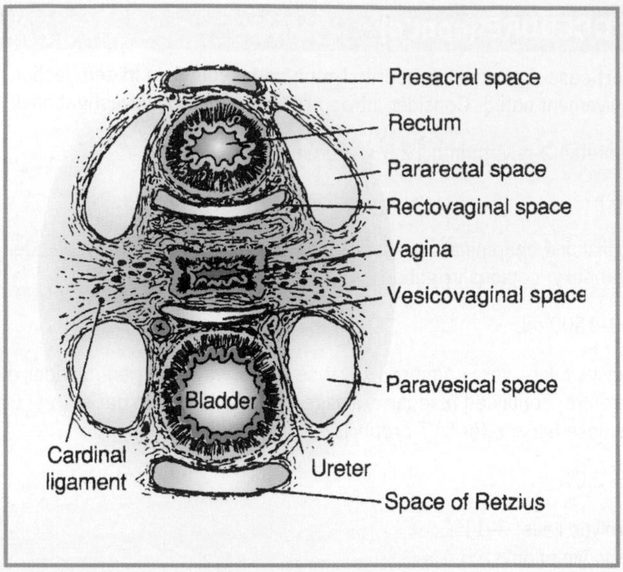

Figure 8.1-10. Schematic diagram of a cut in the anteroposterior plane with positions of all spaces in relation to pelvic organs. (Reproduced with permission from Wheeless CR: *Atlas of Pelvic Surgery.* Williams & Wilkins, 1997.)

PATIENT POPULATION CHARACTERISTICS	
Age range	Reproductive and postreproductive years
Incidence	10/100,000
Etiology	Human papilloma virus (HPV), subtypes 16, 18 (most common), and others
Associated conditions	Smoking; venereal warts; genital herpes; multiple sexual partners; early-age onset of coitus; multiparity; lower socioeconomic status; HIV infection

ANESTHETIC CONSIDERATIONS

PREOPERATIVE

This surgery usually is performed for cervical carcinoma in young women who wish to preserve ovarian function, and whose tumor has not spread beyond local invasion. Lymph nodes are removed to confer a therapeutic advantage and to plan postop adjuvant therapy, if any.

Respiratory	These tumors have been associated with cigarette smoking. ✓ for preexisting lung disease. **Tests:** As indicated from H&P
Cardiovascular	Patients > 50 yr need a preop ECG. **Tests:** As indicated fro m H&P
Hematologic	✓ NSAID usage in the previous week. **Tests:** Hemogram
Laboratory	Renal panel if age ≥ 65 yr, HTN, renal disease, DM
Premedication	Consider midazolam 1–2 mg iv

INTRAOPERATIVE

Anesthetic technique: GETA ± epidural or spinal analgesia for postop pain control.

Induction	Standard induction (p. B-2)	
Maintenance	Standard maintenance (p. B-2)	
Emergence	No special considerations	
Blood and fluid requirements	500–1500 mL IV: 16–18 ga × 1–2 NS/LR at 6–8 mL/kg/h Maintain UO > 0.5 mL/kg/h Warm iv fluids	Good iv access is necessary to deal with potential for bleeding. A lymph node dissection will ↑ 3rd space losses and should be accounted for in fluid management. Fluid requirements generally are increased by a functioning epidural catheter 2° vasodilation. Maintain euvolemia based on HR, BP, UO, invasive monitoring, ABG, and estimates of ongoing blood loss and fluid shifts.
Monitoring	Standard monitors (p. B-1) Foley catheter ± CVP catheter ± Arterial catheter	Invasive monitoring is indicated for patients with underlying cardiopulmonary disease, advanced age, or in cases of large anticipated or unanticipated blood loss.
Positioning	✓ and pad pressure points ✓ eyes Antiembolism stockings and SCD	
Complications	Injury to ureters Hypothermia	Watch for hematuria or ↓ UO. Warm iv fluids; use forced-air warmer.

POSTOPERATIVE

Complications	Atelectasis Hypothermia Bleeding VTE PONV	Give supplemental O_2 postop. Encourage use of incentive spirometer. See p. B-6 See p. B-7
Pain management	PCA (p. C-3) Epidural or spinal narcotics (p. C-2)	Consider ketorolac 15–30 mg im/iv q 8 h for breakthrough pain.

Suggested Readings

1. DiSaia PJ, Creasman WT: Invasive cervical cancer. In *Clinical Gynecologic Oncology.* DiSaia PJ, Creasman WT, eds. CV Mosby, St. Louis: 2002, 53–111.
2. Mann WJ: Radical hysterectomy. In *Gynecologic Surgery.* Mann WJ, Stovall TG, eds. Churchill Livingstone, New York: 1996, 481–512.
3. Nguyan HN, Donato DM, et al: Radical hysterectomy for invasive cervical cancer: a 25-year prospective experience with the Miami technique. *Cancer* 1993; 71:1422.
4. Stehman FB, Perez CA, Kurman RJ, Thigpen JT: Uterine cervix. In: *Principles and Practice of Gynecologic Oncology,* 3rd edition. Hoskins WJ, Perez CA, Young RC, Barakat RR, Markman B, eds: Lippincott Williams & Wilkins, Philadelphia: 2004, 841–918.

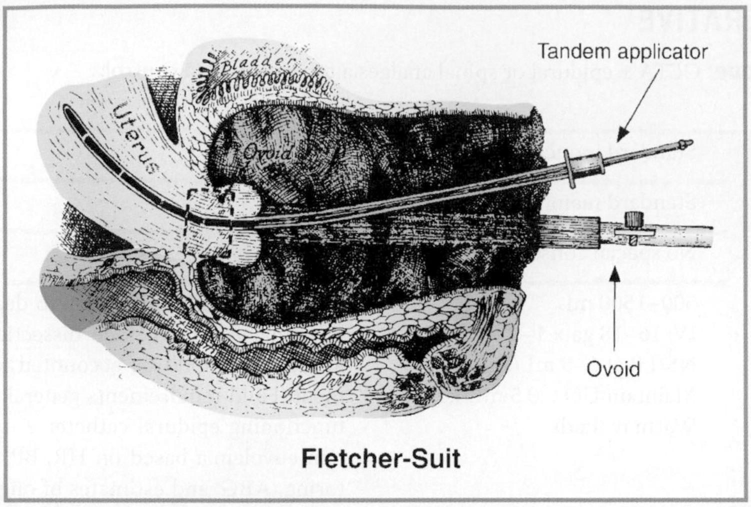

Figure 8.1-11. 'Fletcher-Suit.' The tandem and ovoid applicators are packed into the vagina, leaving the maximum distance between the bladder and radium sources. (Reproduced with permission from Wheeless CR: *Atlas of Pelvic Surgery.* Williams & Wilkins, 1997.)

INTERSTITIAL PERINEAL IMPLANTS

SURGICAL CONSIDERATIONS

Description: **Radiotherapy** is the treatment of choice for International Federation of Gynecology and Obstetrics (FIGO) Stage IIB-IVA carcinoma of the cervix; Stage I, II, III, and IVA vaginal cancers; selected vulvar cancers; and pelvic recurrences of gynecologic cancers. Often, **external-beam therapy** is combined with **brachytherapy,** either in the form of **intracavitary insertion** or as an **interstitial perineal template implant.** Intracavitary radiotherapy utilizes devices such as **Fletcher-Suit** tandem and ovoid applicators (Fig. 8.1-11) or cylinders that are fitted into the vagina and provide a therapeutic boost to the vaginal apex region after external beam irradiation. In general, these devices do not require a laparotomy or laparoscopy for guidance. For selected patients with distorted anatomy and/or bulky tumors, interstitial implants provide superior dose distribution and better local tumor control. The two most widely used systems are the **Martinez Universal Perineal Interstitial Template (MUPIT)** and the **Syed-Neblett applicator.** These systems have similar efficacy and both are performed in the OR with the patient under local or GA. A **laparotomy** is frequently performed at the time of interstitial implant placement to accurately guide the needles into their target tissues and to avoid radiation injury to bowel and/or other pelvic organs not involved with tumor. To minimize postop patient discomfort, some centers use **laparoscopy** instead of laparotomy for needle guidance. A two-team approach is used: a gynecologic oncology team performs the laparotomy or laparoscopy and guides the needles from above; a radiation oncology team inserts the implants from below. The implants are afterloaded with the appropriate radiation sources when the patient has returned to her shielded room. If a hysterectomy has been done previously, an omental pelvic carpet, or a pelvic lid made of delayed, absorbable mesh, is performed to provide additional space between the radiation source and bowel.

Usual preop diagnosis: Cervical, vaginal, vulvar carcinomas; pelvic recurrence of gynecologic malignancies

SUMMARY OF PROCEDURES

	Laparotomy-Guided	Laparoscopy-Guided
Position	Modified dorsolithotomy; Allen stirrups	⇐
Incision	Midline longitudinal abdominal	Vertical infraumbilical and multiple small transverse incisions at the pubic hairline

SUMMARY OF PROCEDURE (cont'd)

	Laparotomy-Guided	Laparoscopy-Guided
Special instrumentation	Syed-Neblett or MUPIT systems, or modifications thereof	⇐+ videolaparoscopy equipment, preferably with a 3-chip camera
Unique considerations	MRI and/or CT scans + information from physical exam are used to preplan implant with a computer dosimetry program. Patients require thorough preop mechanical and antibiotic bowel prep. Preop epidural placement or postop PCA (see p. C-3) may prove helpful for pain control. Foley catheter needs to be inserted through an opening at the top of the clear plastic template prior to implant positioning.	⇐+ Adhesions of variable severity may be present from prior surgery or radiation. Care should be taken to avoid possible bowel injury at time of trocar insertion. Patient needs to be in steep Trendelenburg position for duration of procedure.
Antibiotics	Cefotetan 2 g iv; then q 12 h × 3 doses	⇐
Surgical time	1.5–3 h	⇐
EBL	150–350 mL	Minimal
Closing considerations	Suture template to perineum. Perform rectal exam and adjust any needles that are too close to, or have protruded through, the rectal mucosa. Pack any space between template and perineum with Vaseline gauze. Obtain A-P and lateral orthogonal localization films with the patient in the supine bed-rest position. Insert Hypaque dye into Foley catheter balloon before localization films. Consider insertion of a large Foley into the rectum, and attach to a drainage bag. Consider NG tube placement.	⇐+ Release the pneumoperitoneum completely. Consider insertion of 1 L heparinized LR to cause the bowel to float and remain mobile, thus minimizing the risk of radiation injury.
Postop care	Patient is confined to bed while interstitial implants are in place. SCDs and minidose heparin for DVT prophylaxis. Vigorous use of incentive spirometry. Consider constipating medications (e.g., Lomotil). Patient must be placed in a shielded room. Visitors and medical personnel should interact with patient from behind a lead shield until radiation sources have been removed.	⇐
Mortality	0.1–0.3%	⇐
Morbidity	Hemorrhagic proctitis with diarrhea and tenesmus: 7–18%	⇐
	Radiation cystitis: 7–10%	⇐
	Cervical necrosis: 5–6%	⇐
	Rectovaginal fistula: < 5%	⇐
	Vesicovaginal fistula: < 5%	⇐
	Vaginal vault necrosis: 3–5%	⇐
	Rectal fibrosis: 2–5%	⇐
	Pelvic infection: 2–3%	⇐
Pain score	8–9	8–9

PATIENT POPULATION CHARACTERISTICS

Age range	Reproductive and postreproductive yr; childhood—rare
Etiology	Cervical, vaginal, or vulvar carcinomas; pelvic recurrence of gynecologic malignancies

Obstetric/Gynecologic Surgery

ANESTHETIC CONSIDERATIONS

PREOPERATIVE

Radiation implants are used for palliation or cure in cervical, endometrial, and ovarian cancer. The implants concentrate the radiation close to the site of the tumor and may be supplemented by external beam radiation. The unusual tolerance of the uterus and vagina to radiation permits large doses to be given, and accounts for the success in treating cervical lesions. The sigmoid, rectum, and large bowel are much more sensitive to radiation injury, limiting the dose of radiation that may be given to the pelvis.

Respiratory	Usually not significant unless underlying lung disease is present.
Cardiovascular	Many patients with pelvic tumors are elderly and prone to cardiovascular disease. **Tests:** ECG if age ≥ 50; others as indicated from H&P.
Hematologic	**Tests:** CBC, consider PT/PTT if at risk for coagulopathy
Laboratory	Renal panel
Premedication	Consider midazolam 1–2 mg iv

INTRAOPERATIVE

Anesthetic technique: Regional or GA, depending on site involved. A postop epidural is useful for pain management.

Induction	Standard induction (see p. B-2).
Maintenance	Standard maintenance (see p. B-2).
Emergence	Consider PONV prophylaxis (see p. B-6)
Blood and fluid requirements	Small blood loss IV: 18–20 ga × 1 NS/LR at 2–4 mL/kg/h
Monitoring	Standard monitors (see p. B-1).
Positioning	May be necessary to keep patient motionless during implant insertion. ✓and pad pressure points. ✓eyes. Antiembolism stockings and SCD.

POSTOPERATIVE

Pain management	Epidural narcotics (see p. C-2). PCA (see p. C-3).	Consider ketorolac 15–30 mg im/iv q 6 h for breakthrough pain. Implants are associated with significant discomfort.

Suggested Readings

1. DiSaia PJ: Radiation therapy in gynecology. In *Obstetrics and Gynecology,* 8th edition. Scott JR, DiSaia PJ, Hammond CB, Spellacy WN, eds. Lippincott-Raven, Philadelphia: 1999, 909–26.
2. Edraki B, Teng NN, Kapp DS, O'Hanlan KA: Laparoscopically assisted interstitial perineal implantation and pelvic lid construction: description of an effective and minimally invasive method (abstract). *Gynecol Oncol* 1995; 56:133.
3. Hughes-Davies L, Silver B, Kapp DS: Parametrial interstitial brachytherapy for advanced or recurrent pelvic malignancy: the Harvard/Stanford experience. *Gynecol Oncol* 1995; 58:24–7.
4. Monk BJ, Walker JL, Tewari K, Ramsinghani NS, Syed AM, DiSaia PJ: Open interstitial brachytherapy for the treatment of local-regional recurrences of uterine corpus and cervix cancer after primary surgery. *Gynecol Oncol* 1994; 52:222–8.

5. Paley PJ, Koh WJ, Stelzer KS, et al: A new technique for performing Syed template interstitial implants for anterior vaginal tumors using an open retropubic approach. *Gynecol Oncol* 1999; 73:121–5.
6. Perez CA, Hall EJ, Purdy JA, Williamson J: Biologic and physical aspects of radiation oncology. In: *Principles and Practice of Gynecologic Oncology,* 3rd edition. Hoskins WJ, Perez CA, Young RC, Barakat RR, Markman B, eds: Lippincott Williams & Wilkins, Philadelphia: 2004, 327–402.
7. Syed AM, Puthawala AA, Abdelaziz NN, et al: Long-term results of low-dose-rate interstitial-intracavitary brachytherapy in the treatment of carcinoma of the cervix. *Int J Radiat Oncol Biol Phys* 2002: 54(1):67–78.

LAPAROSCOPIC SURGERY IN GYNECOLOGIC ONCOLOGY

SURGICAL CONSIDERATIONS

Description: With the advent of minimally invasive laparoscopic techniques and instrumentation, the role of laparoscopic procedures in gynecologic cancer treatment continues to be actively defined. The potential advantages of a laparoscopic approach include a shorter hospital stay, better pain control, faster recovery time, ↓ morbidity, and cosmetically appealing smaller incision. There is an acceptable complication rate; however, questions with regard to safety of use in malignant diseases, ↑ operative time, and cost remain to be studied. The authors believe that there is a role for laparoscopy in select situations, such as:

- Second-look evaluation for ovarian cancer;
- Assessment of adnexal masses and diagnosis of ovarian cancer;
- Laparoscopic lymphadenectomy with laparoscopically assisted vaginal hysterectomy or laparoscopic hysterectomy in staging of endometrial cancer;
- Laparoscopically assisted radical vaginal hysterectomy or laparoscopic radical hysterectomy with lymphadenectomy in early-stage cervical cancer; and
- Laparoscopically assisted application of interstitial brachytherapy implants.

Details of each of these procedures are beyond the scope of this section; however, common principles of laparoscopic techniques (e.g., adhesiolysis, biopsies, oophorectomy, omentectomy) apply (see discussion in Laparoscopic Procedures for Gynecologic Surgery, p. 854). The patient is placed in the dorsal lithotomy position, with the buttocks extended over the edge of the table to allow for instrument manipulation, and may need to be placed in steep Trendelenburg position during surgery. Various techniques are used for entry into the abdominal cavity, but the open laparoscopic technique is favored by many and may ↓ risk of vascular or visceral injuries. Other incision-related complications include dehiscence and hernia.

Usual preop diagnosis: Ovarian tumor and other gynecological cancers/tumors

SUMMARY OF PROCEDURE	
Position	Dorsal lithotomy; legs in Allen universal stirrups; steep Trendelenburg
Incisions	Intraumbilical; bilateral suprapubic; midline suprapubic
Special instrumentation	CO_2 laser; bipolar Kleppinger forceps; suction irrigator; may require Harmonic Scalpel; various laparoscopic stapling instruments
Unique considerations	Extended operative time and period of abdominal insufflation for radical procedures. Possible rapid need for laparotomy. Extensive use of electrocautery, ABC, CO_2 laser
Antibiotics	Cefazolin 1 g or cefotetan 2 g iv
Surgical time	1.5–5 h
Closing considerations	Quicker than with laparotomy; but fascia of all 10- to 12-mm ports need to be closed. Five mm trocar sites can be closed in a subcuticular fashion.
EBL	50–1500 mL, depending on extent of procedure

SUMMARY OF PROCEDURE (cont'd)	
Postop care	Clear liquid diet; ambulate POD 1
Mortality	4.4/100,000
Morbidity	Overall complication rate: 0.2–10.3% Conversion to laparotomy: 2.1–7% Port-site metastasis: < 1% Subcutaneous emphysema: 0.3–2% Pneumomediastinum: 0.26% Brachial plexus neuropathy: 0.16% Incisional hernia: 0.06–1% Visceral injury: 0.06–0.5% Major vascular injury: 0.04–0.08% Bladder/ureteral injury: 0.02–1.7% Gas embolism: 0.0014% Wound infection: Uncommon
Pain score	3–4

PATIENT POPULATION CHARACTERISTICS	
Age range	Reproductive and postreproductive yr
Incidence	Depends on primary disease
Etiology	Numerous, depending on primary disease (see appropriate sections earlier in this chapter).
Associated conditions	See specific procedures in this chapter.

ANESTHETIC CONSIDERATIONS

See Anesthetic Considerations for Laparoscopic Hysterectomy, p. 854.

Suggested Readings

1. Canis M, Dauplat J, Pomel C, et al: Laparoscopic radical hysterectomy for cervical cancer. Results from about 41 cases (IGCS abstract). *Int J Gynecol Cancer* 1997; 7:3.
2. Canis M, Rabischong B, Houlle C, et al: Laparoscopic management of adnexal masses: a gold standard? *Curr Opin Obstet Gynecol* 2002; 14:423–8.
3. Dargent DF: Laparoscopic surgery in gynecologic oncology. *Surg Clin North Am* 2001; 81:949–64.
4. Husain A, Chi DS, Prasad M, et al: The role of laparoscopy in second-look evaluations for ovarian cancer. *Gynecol Oncol* 2001; 80:44–7.
5. Joshi GP: Complications of laparoscopy. *Anesthesiol Clin North Am* 2001; 19:89–105.
6. Magrina JF: Complications of laparoscopic surgery. *Clin Obstet Gynecol* 2002; 45:469–80.
7. Magrina JF, Mutone NF, Weaver AL, et al: Laparoscopic lymphadenectomy and vaginal or laparoscopic hysterectomy with bilateral salpingo-oophorectomy for endometrial cancer: morbidity and survival. *Am J Obstet Gynecol* 1999; 181:376–81.
8. Munro MG: Laparoscopic access: complications, technologies, and techniques. *Curr Opin Obstet Gynecol* 2002; 14:365–74.
9. Pasic R, Hilgers R, Levine R: The role of laparoscopy in the management of gynecologic malignancies. *J Surg Oncol* 2000; 75:60–71.

CHAPTER

8.2 Gynecology/ Infertility Surgery

SURGEONS

Bertha Chen, MD
Eva D. Littman, MD (*Infertility surgery*)
Amin A. Milki, MD (*Infertility surgery*)
Lynn M. Westphal, MD (*Infertility surgery*)

ANESTHESIOLOGIST

Cliff Schmiesing, MD

DILATATION AND CURETTAGE (D&C)

SURGICAL CONSIDERATIONS

Description: During dilatation and curettage (D&C), the endometrial lining of the uterus and coexisting lesions (myoma, polyp) are removed. This procedure is performed to diagnose and treat bleeding from uterine and cervical lesions, to complete an incomplete or missed spontaneous abortion, or to treat cervical stenosis. It is used infrequently as a method for pregnancy termination. A D&C is performed less frequently with the advent of the office endometrial biopsy and medical management of bleeding problems.

With the patient in the dorsal lithotomy position, the surgeon initially performs a bimanual examination under anesthesia to obtain information about both the presence of adnexal pathology and anatomic detail of the uterus. A speculum is inserted into the vagina, and the cervix is grasped with a clamp. The cervix is pulled gently toward the operator, who then uses a uterine probe to delineate the length of the uterus and the angulation between the cervical canal and uterus. The uterine cavity is reached by dilating the cervical canal with progressively larger dilators (Hegar's or Pratt) to an 8- to 9-mm diameter. A ureteral stone forceps is often used at this stage to remove existing polyps; and a curette is used to systematically remove the endometrial lining (Fig. 8.2-1).

Usual preop diagnosis: Uncontrolled uterine bleeding refractory to hormonal treatment in young women; abnormal uterine bleeding; incomplete, missed, or induced abortion; pregnancy termination; cervical stenosis causing dysmenorrhea or obstruction of menstrual flow.

SUMMARY OF PROCEDURE	
Position	Dorsal lithotomy with stirrups
Incision	None
Special instrumentation	To prevent peroneal nerve injury, the area of the leg leaning against the stirrup should be well cushioned.
Unique considerations	Following induction, perineum is positioned at the very end of the table to ensure optimum exposure. During the cervical dilatation, a vasovagal response can occur, with subsequent bradycardia and ↓BP. Uterine perforations will often manifest as severe postop pain.
Antibiotics	None
Surgical time	5–15 min
EBL	50–100 mL
Mortality	Minimal
Morbidity	Postop fever: 1.7% Uterine perforation: 0.63% Severe immediate postop bleeding (caused by either uterine artery perforation or cervical injury): < 1%
Pain score	3–5

PATIENT POPULATION CHARACTERISTICS	
Age range	20–80 yr
Incidence	> 1/50 females
Etiology	Dysfunctional uterine bleeding
Associated conditions	Obesity; HTN

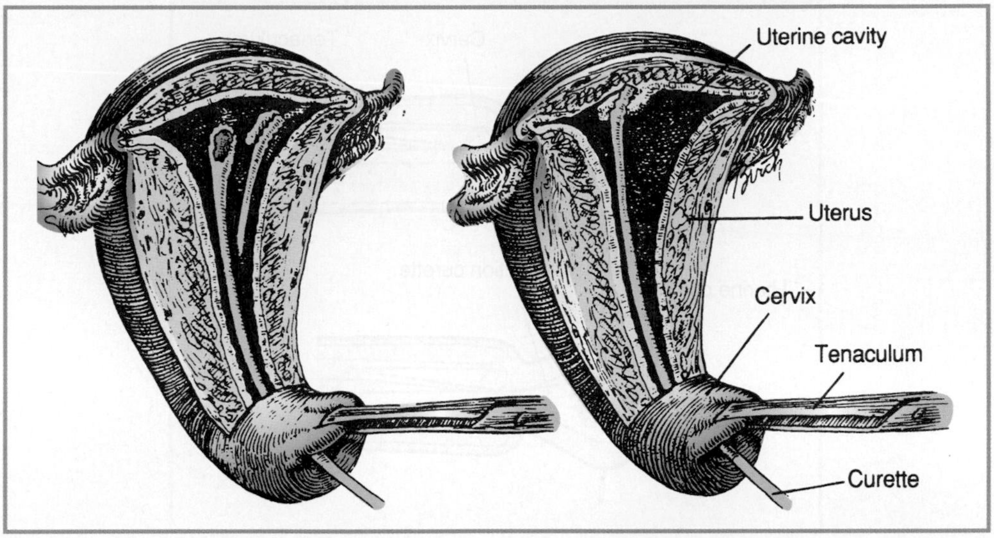

Figure 8.2-1. Curettage of endometrial lining. (Reproduced with permission from Rock JA, Thompson JD, eds: *TeLinde's Operative Gynecology*, 8th edition. Lippincott Williams & Wilkins, 1997.)

ANESTHETIC CONSIDERATIONS

See Anesthetic Considerations following Therapeutic Abortion, Dilatation, and Evacuation, p. 789.

Suggested Readings

1. Bulter WJ: Normal and abnormal uterine bleeding. In *TeLinde's Operative Gynecology*, 9th edition. Rock JA, Jones HW, eds. Lippincott Williams & Wilkins, Philadelphia: 2003, 457–82.
2. Mackenzie IZ, Bibby JG: Critical assessment of dilatation and curettage in 1029 women. *Lancet* 1978; 2(8089):566–8.
3. Stovall TG: Early pregnancy loss and ectopic pregnancy: In *Berek & Novak's Gynecology*, 14th.edition. Berek JS, ed. Lippincott Williams & Wilkins, Philadelphia, 2007, 601–36.

THERAPEUTIC ABORTION, DILATATION, AND EVACUATION (D&E)

SURGICAL CONSIDERATIONS

Description: Therapeutic abortion (TAB) is the elective termination of a pregnancy prior to viability (usually considered to be 24 wk). In 1982, 1,574,000 legal abortions were performed in the United States, a ratio of 426 abortions per 1,000 live births. **Suction curettage** is the most efficient method to terminate pregnancies during the first trimester (< 12 wk), and the great majority of abortions are performed this way. Few (< 5%) of first trimester abortions in the United States are performed with a sharp curette. Increased operative time and blood loss is seen with this method, resulting in its being practiced mainly in locations where a suction apparatus is not available. Suction curettage for a spontaneous abortion is performed in a manner identical to a regular TAB, except that a cervical dilatation might not be needed and the blood loss is usually 2–3 times greater. Very early termination (< 4 wk following LMP) can be performed without anesthesia via medical termination.

The **TAB procedure** consists of a standard cervical dilatation (required for gestations > 6 wk), followed by vacuum aspiration of the uterine contents, using a plastic suction curette (Fig. 8.2-2). Alternatively, the cervical canal can be

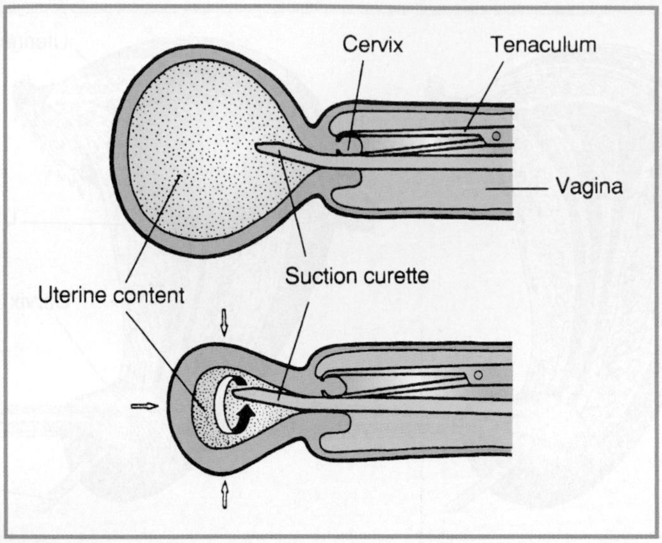

Figure 8.2-2. Uterine aspiration. Top—uterus at beginning of procedure; bottom—at conclusion of procedure. (Reproduced with permission from Rock JA, Thompson JD, eds: *TeLinde's Operative Gynecology,* 8th edition. Lippincott Williams & Wilkins, 1997.)

dilated > 6 hr prior to the operation with laminaria or synthetic osmotic dilators which, after insertion, swell to provide dilatation. A sharp curette often is used at the very end to gently verify the emptiness of the cavity, followed by reaspiration. Due to the risk of missing the pregnancy, most physicians wait until 7–8 wk following the LMP before performing the operation. Ergonovine maleate (0.2 mg im) and oxytocin (Pitocin) 20–30 U/1000 mL iv is often used during the procedure to reduce bleeding, although the efficacy of oxytocin has been questioned. The procedure is performed under either local with or without iv sedation or GA; it is generally felt that local is safer. Regardless of the method used, the obtained product of conception (POC) is sent for histological examination to exclude the presence of trophoblastic neoplasm or ectopic pregnancy.

Variant procedure: Dilatation and evacuation (D&E) remains the safest method for mid-trimester pregnancy termination. It is performed similarly to first-trimester suction curettage with the addition of using large-ring forceps to grasp and remove fetal parts intermittently. This procedure is often performed under GA.

Usual preop diagnosis: Pregnancy (viable or nonviable): 52% within 8 wk estimated gestational age; 90% within 12 wk estimated gestational age.

SUMMARY OF PROCEDURES

	1st-Trimester Suction Curettage OR 2nd-Trimester D&E
Position	Dorsal lithotomy with patient in Allen stirrups. Following induction, perineum positioned at end of table to ensure optimum exposure.
Incision	None
Special instrumentation	Suction; + large-ring forceps for 2nd trimester D&E
Unique considerations	To prevent peroneal nerve injury, the area of the leg leaning against stirrup should be well cushioned. During cervical dilatation, a vasovagal reaction can occur → ↓HR + ↓BP. During injection of lidocaine for paracervical block, seizures may occur if > 12 mL of 1% solution are injected. Uterine perforations often will cause excessive postop pain.
Antibiotics	Doxycycline 100 mg iv

SUMMARY OF PROCEDURE (cont'd)

Surgical time	5–15 min; 15–45 min (2nd trimester D&E)			
EBL	No. wk gestation: 1–4 – 10 mL 5–8 – 10–30 mL 9–10 – 30–80 mL 11–12 – 80–200 mL 13–14 – 200–400 mL 300–500 mL (2nd trimester D&E)			
Postop care	PACU			
Mortality	0–3.1/100,000; 13/100,000 (2nd trimester D&E)			
Morbidity	Mild infection	1/216	for 2nd trimester D&E:	
	Resuctioned day of surgery	1/553	T > 38° for > l d	13.4/1,000
	Resuctioned subsequently	1/596	Cervical injury	11.6/1,000
	Cervical stenosis causing amenorrhea	1/6,071	Cervical tear	10/1,000
			Retained POC	9/1,000
	Cervical incompetence	1/9,444	Hemorrhage	7.1/1,000
	Underestimation of gestational age	1/15,454	UTI	1.8/1,000
	Convulsive Sz (after local anesthesia)	1/25,086		
Complications requiring hospitalization	Incomplete abortion	1/3,617	for 2nd trimester: D&E:	
	Sepsis	1/4,722	Endometritis	8.5/1,000
	Uterine perforation	1/10,625	Uterine perforation	3.2/1,000
	Vaginal bleeding	1/14,166	Need for laparotomy	2.1/1,000
	Inability to complete	1/28,333	Need for blood transfusion	1.9/1,000
	Coexisting tubal pregnancy	1/42,500		
	Total	1/1,405		
Pain score	5			

PATIENT POPULATION CHARACTERISTICS

Age range	15–45 yr
Incidence	Abortions: 21.3/1000 women age 15–44 yr in the United States. (2000)
Etiology	Desire for pregnancy termination

ANESTHETIC CONSIDERATIONS FOR D&C, TAB, D&E

PREOPERATIVE

These are among the most common procedures performed in gynecology. Patients presenting for these procedures are generally healthy; however, bleeding and sepsis may alter ASA status.

Cardiovascular	Hemodynamic status may be impaired 2° preop uterine bleeding, and patient may be septic from retained uterine products. ✓BP and HR. **Tests:** As indicated from H&P.
Laboratory	Hb/Hct; Consider T & S/T & cross; other tests as indicated from H&P.
Premedication	Consider midazolam 1–2 mg iv

INTRAOPERATIVE

Anesthetic technique: Local/MAC, regional, or GA all may be appropriate. In the younger patient population, spinal anesthesia may be less desirable because of increased incidence of postdural puncture headache (PDPH).

Local anesthesia: Some obstetricians/gynecologists perform these procedures under local anesthesia. Paracervical block has the potential for inadvertent iv administration, with consequent toxic reaction.

Regional anesthesia: A T10 sensory level is sufficient to provide anesthesia for procedures on the uterus.

Spinal	0.75% bupivacaine 7.5–12 mg in 8.25% dextrose. (See Anesthetic Considerations for Cesarean Section, p. 819.) If spinal anesthesia is indicated, a pencil-point spinal needle (e.g., Whitacre or Sprotte) should be used to decrease the incidence of PDPH.
Epidural	1.5–2.0% lidocaine with epinephrine 5 mcg/mL, 15–20 mL; supplement with 5 mL as needed. Supplemental iv sedation. (See Anesthetic Considerations for Cesarean Section, p. 819.)
CSE	**Combined spinal/epidural (CSE):** An alternative technique combining the rapid onset and density of spinal anesthesia with the flexibility of continuous epidural anesthesia. Apply monitors, administer fluid, and position patient as for spinal or epidural. The most common technique is the needle-through-needle. After the epidural space is located with a standard 17 ga Tuohy needle, insert a 4" 26- to 27-ga pencil-point spinal needle through it to administer 0.6 mL of spinal bupivacaine (0.75%) ± fentanyl 10 mcg and morphine sulfate 0.1–0.2 mg. Secure the epidural catheter and use if needed (a test dose is advisable).

Obstetric/Gynecologic Surgery

General anesthesia:

Induction	Standard induction (see p. B-2).	
Maintenance	Standard maintenance (see p. B-2) used commonly, although frequently done by mask with O_2/N_2O + volatile anesthetic and spontaneous ventilation. May also use propofol infusion (50–200 mcg/kg/min), with N_2O, without volatile anesthetic. A small amount of opiate may be used.	
Emergence	Be ready with suction in the event of vomiting on emergence.	
Blood and fluid requirements	Minimal blood loss IV: 18 ga × 1 (unless hypovolemic) NS/LR at 2 mL/kg/h	Usual replacement of maintenance fluids and overnight deficit with crystalloid to restore euvolemia. Blood replacement rarely indicated.
Control of blood loss	Oxytocin (Pitocin) 20–30 U/L iv Methylergonovine maleate (0.2 mg) im	Oxytocin causes uterine contraction, with a consequent decrease in blood loss. Rapid iv bolus may lead to hypotension. 20–30 U Oxytocin is usually diluted in 1 L of crystalloid and then infused. Methylergonovine maleate also causes uterine contraction and is usually given im. Side effects include HTN, myocardial ischemia and dysrhythmias, especially if given iv.
Monitoring	Standard monitors (p. B-1)	
Positioning	✓ hip, leg, hand position ✓ and pad pressure points ✓ eyes Shoulder abducted < 90°	Lithotomy position may worsen pulmonary function. Rarely, hemodynamic changes can occur on elevation of the legs into the stirrups, as this increases venous return to the heart. Problems with hypotension on lowering legs postop are more common.

Vagal stimulation	Bradycardia	When the cervix is grasped and dilated, the patient may have excessive vagal stimulation, which can be treated by prompt cessation of stimulation and with atropine (0.4 mg iv), if indicated.
Complications	Nerve injury	Common peroneal nerve palsy (e.g., foot drop) is possible if pressure on the nerve over the fibula is not prevented by adequate padding or positioning. Hyperflexion of the hip joint can cause femoral and lateral femoral cutaneous nerve palsy. Obturator and saphenous nerve injury are also complications of the lithotomy position.
	Finger trauma	Take care to ensure safety of patient's fingers when manipulating foot of the bed. Avoid finger injury by placing patient's arms on arm boards or by wrapping her hands.

POSTOPERATIVE

Complications	PONV (see p. B-6)	
	Uterine perforation with severe abdominal pain (rare)	
	Severe hemorrhage, necessitating blood transfusion (rare)	Severe postop bleeding may be caused by uterine atony, retained POCs, uterine perforation, or cervical injury.
Pain management	IV opiates	Oral pain medications may be satisfactory. With extreme pain consider uterine perforation.
Tests	Hb/Hct, if hemorrhage	

Suggested Readings

1. Courtney, MA: Neurologic sequelae of childbirth and regional anesthesia. In *Manual of Obstetric Anesthesia.* Churchill Livingstone, New York: 1992.
2. Grimes DA: Management of abortion. In *TeLinde's Operative Gynecology,* 9th edition. Rock JA, Jones HW, eds. Lippincott Williams & Wilkins, Philadelphia: 2003, 483–506.
3. Hakim-Elahi E: Complications of first-trimester abortion: a report of 170,000 cases. *Obstet Gynecol* 1990; 76(1):129–35.
4. Nakata DA, Stoelting RK: Positioning. *In Patient Safety in Anesthetic Practice.* Morell RC, Eichhorn JH, eds. Churchill Livingstone, New York: 1997, 293–318.
5. Stovall TG: Early pregnancy loss and ectopic pregnancy: In *Berek & Novak's Gynecology,* 14th edition.. Berek JS, ed. Lippincott Williams & Wilkins, Philadelphia, 2007, 601–36.

HYSTEROSCOPY

SURGICAL CONSIDERATIONS

Description: **Hysteroscopy** is a procedure in which the endometrial cavity can be examined, allowing for direct visualization of lesions. The procedure is used primarily to investigate abnormal uterine bleeding, often caused by intra-uterine submucous myoma and polyps. After the diagnosis, these lesions can be removed through the operative hysteroscope using a variety of techniques.

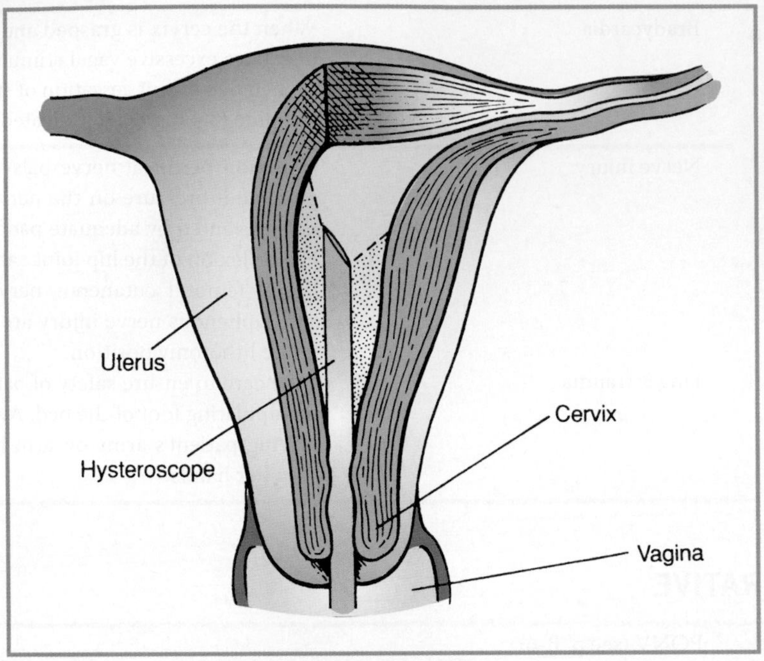

Figure 8.2-3. Hysteroscopy. (Reproduced with permission from Baggish MS, Barbot S, Valle RF: *Diagnostic & Operative Hysteroscopy.* Year Book Medical Pub, 1989.)

Variant procedure or approaches: **Diagnostic hysteroscopies** can be performed under both GA and local anesthesia with iv sedation, whereas **operative hysteroscopies** are usually performed under GA. An examination under anesthesia is performed, followed by the insertion of open speculum and the attachment of a tenaculum to the cervix. The cervical canal is dilated until the hysteroscope can be introduced with its sheath (Fig. 8.2-3). A distention medium—usually a low-viscosity fluid—is then used to provide visualization of the uterine cavity. In the past, other media, such as CO_2 gas and Hyskon, were used frequently to distend the uterus; however, these have been replaced by low-viscosity fluids, due to the ease of its use and safety concerns about Hyskon. It has been recommended that no more than 300 mL of this solution be infused, to avoid these potentially serious complications. The most commonly used low-viscosity fluids are NS, sorbitol 3%/mannitol 0.5%, and mannitol 5% solutions. NS is most commonly used for diagnostic hysteroscopies, while the other nonconductive fluids are used for operative hysteroscopies. Certain bipolar operative hysteroscopies also allow the use of NS.

The distension medium is delivered to the hysteroscope by means of gravity or by a pump. Most systems use gravity, whereby the fluid is delivered via a wide-bore tubing and the maximum intrauterine pressure (IUP) is determined by the height of the fluid container above the uterus. The maximum IUP is thus limited by gravity, making this system relatively safe. The lowest IUP necessary to provide adequate visualization should be used to decrease the rate of absorption of the distention medium. A video camera is usually attached to the hysteroscope to allow for easier visualization. During operative cases, an accompanying laparoscope is sometimes introduced from the abdomen to evaluate the progress of the hysteroscopy and to safeguard against uterine perforation and potential bowel injury.

Usual preop diagnosis: Abnormal uterine bleeding; infertility; recurrent pregnancy loss

SUMMARY OF PROCEDURE

Position	Dorsal lithotomy (Allen stirrups)
Incision	None

SUMMARY OF PROCEDURE (cont'd)	
Special instrumentation	Fluid pump; laser; electrocautery equipment
Unique considerations	Accelerated fluid absorption with prolonged procedures or with resections may → pulmonary edema. Laparoscopy may accompany this procedure.
Surgical time	15 min to 2 h
Antibiotics	Cefazolin 1 g iv
EBL	0–100 mL
Postop care	Excessive postop bleeding can be controlled by using a 5 mL Foley balloon catheter in the uterus for several h.
Mortality	Minimal
Morbidity	Pleural effusion can be seen with use of low-viscosity medium.
Pain score	3–5

PATIENT POPULATION CHARACTERISTICS	
Age range	20–80 yr
Incidence	> 1/50
Etiology	Unexplained uterine bleeding; infertility
Associated conditions	Obesity

ANESTHETIC CONSIDERATIONS

PREOPERATIVE

Hysteroscopy may be performed for diagnostics or treatment of intrauterine pathology.

Cardiovascular	As patient may be undergoing hysteroscopy for uterine bleeding, consider hypovolemia and anemia. ✓BP, HR and Orthostatic VS. **Tests:** As indicated from H&P.
Laboratory	Hb/Hct if bleeding Hx. Other tests as indicated from H&P; consider pregnancy testing.
Premedication	Consider midazolam 1–2 mg iv.

INTRAOPERATIVE

Anesthetic technique: Local, regional, or GA may be used. In the younger patient population, spinal anesthesia may be less desirable because of increased incidence of postdural puncture headache (PDPH). If spinal anesthesia is indicated, pencil point spinal needles (e.g., Sprotte or Whitacre) should be used to decrease the incidence of PDPH.

Local anesthesia: Some procedures may be done under local, usually with supplemental iv sedation, especially if they are diagnostic. Paracervical block has the potential for an inadvertent intravenous administration, with consequent toxic reaction.

Regional anesthesia: A T10 sensory level is sufficient to provide anesthesia for these procedures.

Spinal	0.75% bupivacaine 7.5–10 mg in 8.25% dextrose. (See Anesthetic Considerations for Cesarean Section, p. 819.)
Epidural	1.5–2.0% lidocaine with epinephrine 5 mcg/mL, 15–20 mL; redose with 3–5 mL as needed. Supplemental iv sedation. (See Anesthetic Considerations for Cesarean Section, p. 819.)
CSE	**Combined spinal/epidural (CSE):** An alternative technique combining the rapid onset and density of spinal anesthesia with the flexibility of continuous epidural anesthesia. Apply monitors, administer fluid, and position patient as for spinal or epidural. The most common technique is the needle-through-needle. After the epidural space is located with a standard 17-ga Tuohy needle, insert a 4" 26- to 27-ga pencil-point spinal needle through it to administer 7.5–10 mg of spinal bupivacaine (0.75%) ± fentanyl 10 mcg and morphine sulfate 0.1–0.2 mg. Secure the epidural catheter and use if needed (a test dose is advisable).

General anesthesia:

Induction	Standard induction (see p. B-2). LMA if appropriate	
Maintenance	Standard maintenance (see p. B-2).	
Emergence	Standard emergence	
Blood and fluid requirements	Minimal blood loss IV: 18–20 ga × 1 (unless hypovolemic) NS/LR at 2–4 mL/kg/h	
Positioning	✓ hip, leg, and hand positions ✓ and pad pressure points ✓ eyes Shoulder abduction < 90°	Lithotomy position can be deleterious to pulmonary function, as it may impair respiratory mechanics. Rarely, hemodynamic changes occur on elevation of legs into the stirrups, as this increases venous return to the heart. Problems with hypotension on lowering legs postop are common. Common peroneal nerve palsy is possible if pressure on the nerve over the fibula is not prevented by adequate padding or positioning. Hyperflexion of hip joint can cause femoral and lateral femoral cutaneous nerve palsy. Obturator and saphenous nerve injury are also complications of the lithotomy position.
Monitoring	Standard monitors (see p. B-1).	
Surgical stimulation	When cervix is grasped and dilated, patient may have excessive vagal nerve stimulation.	Rx: prompt cessation of stimulation by surgeons and treatment with atropine, if indicated.
Complications	Pulmonary and cerebral edema (2° hypotonic fluid overload) Coagulopathy Air embolism Anaphylactoid reactions	Air embolism can occur with the use of gas distention media: thus, most institutions currently use low-viscosity fluids for distension. Low-viscosity media can be grouped, based on their tonicity and electrolyte content: (1) hypotonic, electrolyte-free media that may cause hypotonic fluid overload; and (2) isotonic, electrolyte-containing media that may cause isotonic fluid overload. It is important to monitor the volume of fluid used during the

Complications (cont'd)		procedure. It is not uncommon to use 10–20 L of distention fluid during an operative hysteroscopy. Monitor for fluid balance. Adjust iv fluid to maintain euvolemia.
	Finger injury (2° positioning)	When manipulating the foot of the bed, avoid finger injury by placing patient's arms on arm boards or by wrapping her hands.

POSTOPERATIVE

Complications	PONV (see p. B-6) Fluid overload/pulmonary edema from excessive fluid absorption	
Pain management	Small dose of titrated opiate	Patients usually tolerate oral pain medications.
Tests	Consider CXR and ABG. Serum electrolytes	For patient with respiratory compromise

Suggested Readings

1. Baggish MS: Operative hysteroscopy. In *TeLinde's Operative Gynecology*, 9th edition. Rock JA, Jones HW, eds. Lippincott Williams & Wilkins, Philadelphia: 2003, 483–506.
2. Cooper JM, Brady RM: Intraoperative and early postoperative complications of operative hysteroscopy. *Obstet Gynecol Clin North Am* 2000; 27(2):247–66.
3. Nakata DA, Stoelting RK: Positioning. In *Patient Safety in Anesthetic Practice.* Morell RC, Eichhorn JH, eds. Churchill Livingstone, New York: 1997, 293–318.
4. Stovall TG: Hysteroscopy. In *Berek & Novak's Gynecology,* 14th edition. Berek JS, ed. Lippincott Williams & Wilkins, Philadelphia, 2007, 601–36.

PELVIC LAPAROTOMY

SURGICAL CONSIDERATIONS

Description: Laparotomy and its variants are all common gynecological procedures. Laparotomy is most frequently performed via a Pfannenstiel's incision, which permits good pelvic exposure. A vertical incision is used in oncological surgery or in the presence of a large uterus. A knife or Bovie is used to cut through the skin and underlying tissue until the rectus fascia is reached. The fascia is nicked, and then sharply incised bilaterally 2–4" with scissors or electrocautery (Bovie). The rectus muscle is separated sharply in the midline down to the pubis and the peritoneum is entered. The peritoneal incision is then extended vertically or transversely. The pelvis and entire abdominal cavity are explored first by palpation. Then the bowels usually are packed in a cephalad direction with surgical laparotomy sponges (laps) to prevent them from falling back into the pelvis. Good muscle relaxation is important during this stage to ensure optimal packing. A self-retaining retractor frequently is used to keep the laps in place and to enhance exposure. After the desired operation has been performed, the retractor and packs are removed. During the peritoneal closure, abdominal muscle relaxation is again critical to minimize tension on this layer and risk of bowel injury with the needle. The rectus fascia, the subcutaneous tissue, and the skin are closed in succession.

Variant procedures: Myomectomies are performed to remove myomata that are causing pain, abnormal bleeding, or infertility. Myomata are heavily vascularized at the base, and the surgeon has several ways to minimize this bleeding. A clamp can be placed across the uterine vasculature to minimize blood flow to the uterus. A common alternative is the use of a vasoconstrictor, such as diluted epinephrine (1:200,000) or vasopressin solution (1–5 U/10 mL NS). The solution (2–10 mL) is injected around the myoma prior to incising the uterus, which invariably →↑HR (epi) or ↓HR (vasopressin) and ↑BP. Gonadotropin releasing hormone (Gn-RH) agonists may be used for a few months prior to the operation to render the patient hypoestrogenic and, thus, decrease the vascularity of the myomata. After the myomata have been removed, the uterine defects are closed with several layers of suture, and the uterine serosa is closed.

Ovarian cystectomies are performed to alleviate related pain and to diagnose the identity of asymptomatic cysts. Small, single-functional ovarian cysts are found at different stages in a woman's menstrual cycle. At times, these cysts can increase in size and quantity, which may cause severe pain. The ovary also can contain various nonfunctional cysts (e.g., tumors) which have to be removed, even if asymptomatic, to exclude malignancy. After the pelvic structures are well visualized, the cystic ovary is stabilized with instruments or surgical laps. Sharp or blunt dissection is used to shell out the cyst intact. If there is any suspicion about the nature of the cyst, an intraop frozen section is obtained. The ovary is then reapproximated and the abdomen closed. If the cyst is large and little healthy ovarian stroma remains, an **oophorectomy** is performed.

Ectopic pregnancies are usually medical emergencies. Increasingly, **laparoscopy** is being used to treat this condition (see p. 849), although laparotomies for ectopic pregnancies are still widely performed. The abdomen is entered, and the pregnancy located quickly. An attempt is made to control the bleeding with the surgeon's hand, a clamp, or suture. Frequently, large amounts of blood in the pelvis are suctioned and the ectopic pregnancy is removed via a **partial tubal resection, salpingostomy,** or **salpingectomy;** then the abdomen is closed. A **D&C** is often performed at the end to prevent late bleeding from the pregnancy-induced endometrial proliferation (see p. 786).

In **abdominal colpopexy** (fixation of vagina), the patient is placed in the lithotomy position, usually with Allen stirrups, to perform an examination under anesthesia, as well as to insert a vaginal pack needed to identify the vaginal apex. A urethral catheter is inserted prior to staging the laparotomy. A rectus fascia graft is obtained during the opening of the abdomen (a synthetic graft can be used instead). The bowel is packed and the defect is examined from the abdominal perspective. Frequently there is an accompanying enterocele which must be closed initially (see **Moschowitz procedure,** later). The peritoneum over the vaginal apex is then entered and the neighboring rectum and bladder are dissected a distance away from the vaginal apex. The peritoneum over the sacrum is incised and the cephalad end of the graft is sutured to the anterior sacral ligament of the third vertebrae. Severe bleeding can occur if there is injury to the middle sacral artery. The caudal end of the graft is attached to the vaginal apex, with the surgeon frequently using a vaginal hand to place these last sutures. The peritoneum and abdomen are closed, and the patient's legs are elevated to the dorsal lithotomy position for a high-posterior **colporrhaphy** (repair of vagina).

The **Moschowitz procedure** is used to reduce enteroceles via an abdominal approach. The abdomen is entered in the usual fashion, the uterus held up with a traction suture, the bowel packed, and the patient placed in the Trendelenburg position. Multiple concentric purse-string sutures are used to close the defect in the pouch of Douglas and the abdomen is closed.

The **presacral neurectomy** is an operation performed for women with severe chronic midline pelvic pain. Usually the patient has a history of prior surgeries to diagnose and treat the problem. A laparotomy is initially performed with packing of the bowels. The rectosigmoid is brought over to the left to make a vertical, posterior, parietal, peritoneal incision over the sacral area. The anatomy is examined closely and the presacral nerves are obliterated or excised; then the peritoneum and abdomen are closed. Severe bleeding can be seen intraop from the hemorrhoidal and sacral veins, but usually can be controlled with pressure.

Usual preop diagnosis: Myomata (pelvic pain, hypermenorrhea, infertility); ovarian cysts and pelvic pain with undiagnosed ovarian mass; ectopic pregnancy; vaginal vault prolapse; enterocele; presacral neurectomy (chronic pelvic pain)

SUMMARY OF PROCEDURE

Position	Supine or lithotomy
Incision	Pfannenstiel's or low midline abdominal
Unique considerations	Muscle relaxation is important during bowel packing and abdominal closure. Vasoconstrictor substances for controlling myomata bleeding (1:200,000 epinephrine and 1–5 U vasopressin/10 mL NS) are often used and can alter BP and HR.
Antibiotics	1–2 g iv cefoxitin or cefotetan

SUMMARY OF PROCEDURE (cont'd)	
Surgical time	45 min–4 h Abdominal colpopexy: 4–5 h
EBL	150–1000 mL (maximum related to procedure)
Postop care	PACU
Mortality	Minimal
Morbidity	Gastric dilatation: 3% Thrombophlebitis: 3% PE: 2% Ureteral stenosis: 1%
Pain score	8

PATIENT POPULATION CHARACTERISTICS

	Myomectomy	Ovarian Cystectomy, Oophorectomy	Ectopic Pregnancy	Abdominal Colpopexy, Moschowitz	Presacral Neurectomy
Age range	20–45 yr	20–85 yr	15–45 yr	40–80 yr	20–50 yr
Incidence	> 1/5 females	⇐	1/100 females	1/500 females	⇐
Etiology	Congenital	Endometriosis Anovulation Adenoma	Preexisting tubal disease	Multiparous Obesity Chronic cough	Endometriosis
Associated conditions	Menorrhagia	Endometriosis	Pelvic adhesions	Pelvic relaxation	Endometriosis

ANESTHETIC CONSIDERATIONS

See Anesthetic Considerations following Infertility Operations, p. 800.

Suggested Readings

1. Berek JS, ed: *Berek & Novak's Gynecology.* Lippincott Williams & Wilkins, Philadelphia, 2007.
2. Rock JA, Jones HW, eds: *TeLinde's Operative Gynecology.* 14th edition. Lippincott Williams & Wilkins, Philadelphia: 2003.

TRANSVAGINAL OOCYTE RETRIEVAL (TVOR)

SURGICAL CONSIDERATIONS

Description: Transvaginal oocyte retrieval (TVOR) is performed on patients who have undergone ovarian stimulation using ovulation-inducing agents. This procedure is performed 35–36 h after the patient has been injected with human chorionic gonadotropin (HCG) to induce oocyte maturation. It is very important for the success of the procedure that retrieval be performed within this time period. If a retrieval is performed too late, ovulation will have occurred and oocyte retrieval will no longer be possible.

In the procedure room, the patient is placed in the dorsal lithotomy position, and moderate to heavy iv sedation is started at this time. A sterile speculum is inserted into the vagina and a vaginal prep is performed. After the prep, the speculum is removed and an ultrasound probe with a 16-ga needle on a needle guide is placed into the patient's vagina. One of the ovaries is identified and entered by inserting the needle through the vaginal fornix. Patients may experience a combination of pain and pressure at this point of the procedure. After the needle is in the ovary, the surgeon will then proceed with sequential aspiration of the ovarian follicles. It is important that the patient remain relaxed and motionless during this part of the procedure, as movement may prevent aspiration of oocytes and increase the risk of injury to the surrounding organs and vessels. After retrieval is completed in the first ovary, the needle is withdrawn; the other ovary is identified, and a second puncture is made through the vaginal fornix. Depending on the number of follicles present, the entire procedure may last anywhere from 10–30 min. After all of the follicles have been aspirated, the needle and ultrasound probe are removed from the vagina. A sterile speculum is then reintroduced into the vagina and the vaginal wall and cervix are inspected for hemostasis. It is possible that a few minutes of applied pressure using sterile gauze are needed to obtain adequate hemostasis. Subsequently, the patient is taken to the recovery room and discharged to home after a recovery period of 30–60 min.

SUMMARY OF PROCEDURE	
Position	Dorsal lithotomy
Incision	Vaginal punctures (usually 2)
Special instrumentation	Ultrasound probe with needle guide, 16- to 17-ga needle
Unique considerations	Requires complete relaxation/sedation to prevent injury and loss of oocyte during follicle aspiration.
Antibiotics	Cefotetan of cefazolin 1 g iv prior to procedure
Procedure time	Setup: 5–10 min Procedure: 10–30 min (depending on # of follicles)
Postop care	PACU→ Home
Morbidity	Bleeding: rare infection: rare
Pain Score	1–3 (abdominal cramping)

PATIENT POPULATION CHARACTERISTICS	
Age Range	18–50 yr (rare after age 43)
Incidence	It is estimated that at least 14% of American couples of reproductive age who desire pregnancy are unable to conceive within 1 yr.
Etiology	A male factor is responsible for 35%; pelvic factor, 25%; ovulatory factor, 20%; cervical factor, 10%; and 10% are unexplained.
Associated conditions	Thyroid disorders; polycystic ovarian syndrome; endometriosis; depression

ANESTHETIC CONSIDERATIONS

PREOPERATIVE

This is generally a healthy patient population. Little is required beyond routine tests, unless otherwise indicated.

Laboratory	Tests as indicated from H&P
Premedication	Consider midazolam 1–2 mg iv

INTRAOPERATIVE

Anesthetic technique: Moderate to heavy iv sedation or, rarely, local or regional anesthesia and GA have been used. Intravenous sedation (hypnotic agent, ± benzodiazepine, ± a narcotic analgesic), however, is the most commonly used and the safest technique for IVF. The most stimulating parts of the procedure occur when the vaginal fornix is pierced on each side and when the ovarian follicles are entered for aspiration of the eggs.

MAC	Propofol infusion (25–200 mcg/kg/min), ± midazolam (1–2 mg iv) and ± fentanyl titrated to achieve the desired combination of moderate to heavy sedation and analgesia (see p. B-3).
Blood and fluid requirements	Minimal blood loss IV: 18–20 ga × 1
Monitoring	Standard monitors (p. B-1)
Positioning	✓ hip, leg, and hand positions ✓ and pad pressure points

POSTOPERATIVE

Complications	PONV (p. B-6) Bleeding: rare	PONV rare with propofol based-TIVA. Minimal post op pain →limit intraop opiates.
Pain management	Pain: usually minimal	Oral analgesics are usually sufficient or small doses fentanyl (25–50 mcg iv).

Suggested Readings

1. Burney RO, Schust DJ, Yao MW: Infertility: In *Berek & Novak's Gynecology*, 14th edition. Berek JS, ed. Lippincott Williams & Wilkins, Philadelphia, 2007, 1185–276.
2. Hadimioglu N, Titiz TA, Dosemeci L, Erman M: Comparison of various sedation regimens for transvaginal oocyte retrieval. *Fertility and Sterility* 2002; 78(3):648–9.
3. Meniru GI: *Cambridge Guide to Infertility Management and Assisted Reproduction.* Cambridge University Press, Cambridge: 2001, 130–1.

INFERTILITY OPERATIONS/ASSISTED REPRODUCTIVE TECHNOLOGIES

SURGICAL CONSIDERATIONS

Description: These operations all deal with reproductive problems. The general trend is to avoid laparotomies and to perform operations using outpatient laparoscopy and hysteroscopy techniques whenever possible.

Fimbrioplasty is used to repair distal fallopian tubal occlusion—a common cause for infertility—which is usually a consequence of pelvic inflammatory disease (PID). The operation may be performed by **pelvic laparotomy** or **laparoscopy** (see p. 795). If done by laparotomy, a urethral catheter is inserted to empty the bladder, followed by the insertion of a transcervical uterine catheter for chromopertubation (dye injection). The abdomen is opened and the pelvic structures are exposed. During the operation, microsurgical techniques are followed closely to minimize trauma. Meticulous hemostasis is important. A wound protector is often used instead of self-retaining retractors. The peritoneum and pelvic structures are kept moist with intermittent irrigation. Salpingolysis and ovariolysis may be performed microsurgically. After the adnexae have been freed, they are elevated by loosely packing the pouch of Douglas with insulated pads (plastic sheathed covered laps). Chromopertubation is then performed and, if occlusion is present, a new stoma is created using microsurgical instruments and sutures. The abdomen is then closed.

Tubal reanastomosis, performed to restore fertility, is very similar to fimbrioplasty, with microsurgical techniques followed diligently. After the tubal segments have been freed slightly from their underlying mesosalpinx, the occluded ends are cut and chromopertubation is performed to ensure patency. After patency has been established, anastomosis is performed in two layers. The mesosalpinx is reapproximated to the tubal serosa and the abdomen closed.

The uterus is embryologically formed by the fusion of two paramesonephric tubes. At times, the fusion is incomplete and a septated uterus or bicornuate uterus is formed. The malformed uterus is associated with an increased risk for miscarriages and preterm labor. **Metroplasty** is used to correct this condition. The **Strassmann procedure** (extremely rare) for bicornuate uteri uses a standard pelvic laparotomy. Following uterine exposure, an incision is made on the medial side of each hemicorpus and carried down until the uterine cavity is entered. The edges are reapproximated to form a single uterus. Septated uteri are usually repaired via a hysteroscopic approach (see Hysteroscopy, p. 791) with scissors or laser.

Proximal tubal cannulation is a procedure in which proximal tubal occlusion can be repaired through either fluoroscopic or hysteroscopic approach. The hysteroscopic approach, usually performed under GA, allows the surgeon to insert a small cannula to restore tube patency. This procedure is often done with laparoscopy to follow the progress of the cannulization and to visualize the chromopertubation (see Hysteroscopy, p. 791, and Laparoscopy, p. 846).

Gamete intrafallopian transfer (GIFT), **zygote intrafallopian transfer** (ZIFT), and **tubal embryo transfer** (TET) are methods of **advanced reproductive technology (ART), but are seldom used**. Couples who have undergone extensive infertility workups and treatment without success may become candidates for GIFT, ZIFT, or TET procedures. Ovarian follicles are stimulated to grow with the help of gonadotropins. These follicles are then punctured with a needle transvaginally to 'harvest' the eggs. These eggs can be mixed with semen and placed directly into the distal end of the fallopian tube (GIFT) using laparoscopic techniques and a small tubal catheter (see Laparoscopy, p. 846). In the ZIFT and TET procedures, the semen and eggs are allowed to incubate 1–2 days in vitro; embryos form and are transferred to the fallopian tubes in a manner similar to the GIFT procedure. Most patients undergoing ART procedures utilize conventional in vitro fertilization (IVF) and do not need laparoscopy.

Usual preop diagnosis: Infertility; history of multiple spontaneous abortion and preterm labor

SUMMARY OF PROCEDURE

(For summaries of specific procedures, see Laparoscopy, p. 846; Hysteroscopy, p. 791; or Pelvic Laparotomy, p 795.)

PATIENT POPULATION CHARACTERISTICS

Age range	18–50 yr
Incidence	1/20 women
Etiology	PID; endometriosis; idiopathic
Associated conditions	Obesity

ANESTHETIC CONSIDERATIONS

(Procedures covered: pelvic laparotomy for myomectomy; ovarian cystectomy; oophorectomy; ectopic pregnancy removal; abdominal colpopexy; Moschowitz enterocele repair; presacral neurectomy; infertility operations)

PREOPERATIVE

This is generally a healthy patient population; however, this procedure can be performed for a wide variety of pathologic conditions.

Cardiovascular	Patients undergoing myomectomy and, especially, ectopic pregnancy removal, may have had a significant amount of preop bleeding; therefore, assess for hypovolemia. Preexisting comorbidities and preop status will vary considerably. Assess as appropriate. **Tests:** As indicated from H&P.

Laboratory	Hb/Hct. Patients with ectopic pregnancy may have urine/serum pregnancy tests, as well as pelvic ultrasound.
Premedication	Patients with ruptured ectopic pregnancies may come to the OR urgently, and should be treated as for full stomach. This includes premedication with a nonparticulate antacid, Na citrate 30 mL po, metoclopramide 10 mg iv, and ranitidine 50 mg iv.

INTRAOPERATIVE

Anesthetic technique: GETA is indicated for patients undergoing laparoscopic surgery and in patients presenting for emergency surgery. Regional anesthesia is best avoided in hemodynamically unstable patients (i.e., ectopic pregnancies), and for laparoscopy where breathing difficulty may develop 2° to pneumoperitoneum and Trendelenburg position. Regional anesthesia may be suitable for simple laparotomies. In the younger patient population, spinal anesthesia is less desirable because of an increased incidence of postdural puncture headache (PDPH). If spinal anesthesia is indicated, a pencil-point needle (e.g., Whitacre, Sprotte) should be used in order to decrease the incidence of PDPH.

General anesthesia:

Induction	Standard induction (see p. B-2) In a patient with a ruptured ectopic pregnancy, bleeding and hemodynamic instability, consider ketamine 1–2 mg/kg or etomidate 0.1–0.4 mg/kg. These patients are generally considered unfasted and would require rapid-sequence induction (see p. B-4). Use OGT/NGT to decompress stomach after induction for laparoscopic surgery
Maintenance	Standard maintenance (see p. B-2). Consider PONV prophylaxis.
Emergence	Standard emergence

Regional anesthesia: A T4-6 sensory level is recommended for pelvic/lower abdominal surgery.

Spinal	0.75% bupivacaine 12–14 mg in 8.25% dextrose. (See Anesthetic Considerations for Cesarean Section, p. 819.)	
Epidural	1.5–2.0% lidocaine with epinephrine 5 mcg/mL, 15–20 mL; redose with 3–5 mL as needed. Supplemental iv sedation. (See Anesthetic Considerations for Cesarean Section, p. 819.)	
CSE	**Combined spinal/epidural (CSE):** An alternative technique combining the rapid onset and density of spinal anesthesia with the flexibility of continuous epidural anesthesia. Apply monitors, administer fluid, and position patient as for spinal or epidural. The most common technique is the needle-through-needle. After the epidural space is located with a standard 17-ga Tuohy needle, insert a 4" 26- to 27-ga pencil-point spinal needle through it to administer 12–14 mL of spinal bupivacaine (0.75%) ± fentanyl 10 mcg and morphine sulfate 0.1–0.2 mg. Secure the epidural catheter and use if needed (a test dose is advisable).	
Blood and fluid requirements	Blood loss will vary by procedure. Generally limited unless ruptured ectopic pregnancy or vascular complication of laparoscopy. IV: 16–18 ga × 1–2 NS/LR at 4–7 mL/kg/h	Maintain euvolemia, UO ≥0.5 cc/kg/h
Control of blood loss	Epinephrine Vasopressin	During myomectomies, surgeons may inject vasopressors into the area surrounding myomata prior to excision. This can cause HTN and cardiac and either brady- or tachydysrhythmia.

Monitoring	Standard monitors (see p. B-1) ±Foley catheter ± Arterial catheter	Patients with ectopic pregnancies may need intra-arterial monitoring if major hemorrhage occurs.
Positioning	✓and pad pressure points ✓eyes	During abdominal colpopexy, patient is placed intermittently in both the lithotomy and supine positions. (See p. 789 for concerns regarding the lithotomy position.)
Complications	Pneumoperitoneum ↑$PaCO_2$, ↓PaO_2 ETT migration	Pneumoperitoneum with CO_2 and steep Trendelenburg position cause cephalad displacement of diaphragm with ↓FRC, ↓pulmonary compliance, and ↑airway closure/atelectasis. Hypercarbia and hypoxia, due to respiratory compromise, can result unless ventilation is controlled during GA. Check for endobronchial migration of ETT upon assumption of Trendelenburg position.
	Pneumothorax	Pneumothorax due to retroperitoneal dissection of insufflated gas into the mediastinum can cause hypoxemia, ↑airway pressure, subcutaneous emphysema, and ↓BP.
	↓BP	↓BP can result from ↓venous return caused by pneumoperitoneum.
	Hemorrhage Dysrhythmias Peripheral nerve injury	Hemorrhage can result from blood vessel injury or rapid reversal of head-down position.
	Venous CO_2 embolism	Unintended intravascular injection of CO_2 gas can →↓BP and dysrhythmias.

POSTOPERATIVE

Complications	PONV (see p. B-6) Anemia Shoulder pain
Pain Management	PCA (see p. C-3)
Tests	Hb/Hct if hemorrhage occurs.

ANESTHETIC CONSIDERATIONS FOR ASSISTED REPRODUCTIVE TECHNOLOGIES (ART)

PREOPERATIVE

This is generally a fit, healthy patient population. Little is required beyond routine tests, unless otherwise indicated.

Laboratory	Tests as indicated from H&P.
Premedication	Standard premedication (see p. B-1).

INTRAOPERATIVE

Anesthetic technique: Conscious sedation, local anesthesia, regional (e.g., spinal and epidural) and GA all have been employed for ART. The standard in vitro fertilization (IVF) technique consists of transvaginal egg retrieval and embryo transfer (not laparoscopic technique), and one study suggests higher pregnancy and delivery rates if conscious sedation or epidural anesthesia is used as opposed to GA. Laparoscopy is only performed for GIFT, ZIFT, or TET, but not for in vitro fertilization. For TVOR, use moderate → heavy iv sedation. For laparoscopic procedures, breathing difficulty can develop due to pneumoperitoneum and Trendelenburg position. Therefore, GETA with controlled ventilation is most commonly used. If GA is used, isoflurane-N_2O vs propofol-N_2O is controversial. No difference in pregnancy rates with the use of isoflurane, propofol, N_2O, or midazolam has been demonstrated.

Induction	Standard induction (see p. B-2). Avoidance of succinylcholine may decrease postop myalgia.	
Maintenance	Standard maintenance (see p. B-2). N_2O does not appear to adversely affect success of fertilization.	
Emergence	No special considerations	
Blood and fluid requirements	Minimal blood loss IV: 18 ga × 1 NS/LR at 2 mL/kg/h	Blood loss minimal, unless trauma to vasculature. Rarely, trauma to blood vessels or organs following laparoscopy may necessitate laparotomy.
Monitoring	Standard monitors (p. B-1)	
Positioning	✓and pad pressure points ✓eyes	
Complications	Ventilatory	Pneumoperitoneum with CO_2 and steep Trendelenburg position cause cephalad displacement of diaphragm with ↓FRC, ↓pulmonary compliance, and ↑airway closure/atelectasis. Hypercarbia and hypoxia, due to respiratory compromise, can result unless ventilation is controlled during GA. Check for endobronchial migration of ETT upon assumption of Trendelenburg position.
	Pneumothorax	Pneumothorax due to retroperitoneal dissection of insufflated gas into the mediastinum can cause hypoxemia, ↑airway pressure, subcutaneous emphysema and ↓BP.
	Cardiovascular	↓BP may result from ↓venous return 2° pneumoperitoneum.
	Hemorrhage	Hemorrhage may result from blood vessel injury or rapid reversal of head-down position.
	Venous CO_2 embolism Dysrhythmias	Unintended intravascular injection of CO_2 gas → ↓BP and dysrhythmias.
	Nerve injury Bowel injury	Use of Trendelenburg position incurs risk of nerve injury. Hyperextension of arm may result in brachial plexus injury, and careful padding of vulnerable points is necessary.

POSTOPERATIVE

Complications	Shoulder pain	Postop pain may be referred to the shoulder, due to irritation of diaphragm by residual pneumoperitoneum or bleeding.
Pain management	Oral analgesics are usually sufficient.	

Suggested Readings

1. Beilin Y, Bodian C, Eisenkraft J, et al: The use of propofol, nitrous oxide, or isoflurane does not affect the reproductive success rate following gamete intrafallopian transfer (GIFT). *Anesthesiology* 1999; 90:36–41.
2. Burney RO, Schust DJ, Yao MW: Infertility: In *Berek & Novak's Gynecology,* 14th edition.. Berek JS, ed. Lippincott Williams & Wilkins, Philadelphia, 2007, 1185–276.
3. Gonen O, Shulman A, Ghetler Y, Shapiro A, Judekin R, Beyth Y, Ben-Nun I. The impact of different types of anesthesia or *in vitro* fertilization-embryo transfer treatment outcome. *J Assist Reprod Genet* 1995; 12(10): 678–82.
4. Meniru GI: *Cambridge Guide to Infertility Management and Assisted Reproduction.* Cambridge University Press, Cambridge: 2001, 130–1.
5. Rock JA, Jones HW, eds: *TeLinde's Operative Gynecology,* 8th edition. Lippincott-Raven, Philadelphia: 2003.
6. Tanbo T: Assisted fertilization in infertile women with patent tubes: a comparison of *in vitro* fertilization, gamete intrafallopian transfer and tubal embryo stage transfer. *Hum Reprod* 1990; 5:266–70.

HYSTERECTOMY—VAGINAL OR TOTAL ABDOMINAL

SURGICAL CONSIDERATIONS

Description: After cesarean section (C-section), **hysterectomy** is the most commonly performed operation in the United States (650,000/year). Two approaches are possible: vaginal and abdominal. The **vaginal approach,** performed with the patient in a dorsal lithotomy position, is preferred, because it offers significantly less morbidity and mortality. Its use is limited by situations in which pelvic bony architecture, uterine size, pelvic adhesions, or the presence of gynecological cancers requires an **abdominal approach.** The approach may be changed in the OR, where a pelvic examination under anesthesia will determine the true uterine size, degree of prolapse, and the presence of pelvic pathology. A laparoscopy may be performed at the outset of surgery to evaluate the pelvis and free up adhesions that would have made a vaginal approach initially unsafe. In patients ≥ 45 years, **bilateral salpingo-oophorectomy** (BSO) is often performed in addition to the hysterectomy to provide ovarian cancer prophylaxis. Pelvic relaxation syndrome is the most frequent preop diagnosis in patients having a vaginal hysterectomy. Pelvic relaxation includes one or more of the following: prolapse of the uterus; intestine into the pouch of Douglas (enterocele); bladder into the anterior vaginal wall (cystocele); urethra into the anterior vaginal wall (urethrocele); and rectum into the posterior vaginal wall (rectocele). In these cases, the hysterectomy is often accompanied by an anterior/posterior colporrhaphy, bladder neck suspension, and perineoplasty.

Variant approaches: **Abdominal hysterectomy** is performed through a Pfannenstiel's or midline incision, depending on the uterine size and the need to perform a lymph node dissection for cancer. A Pfannenstiel's incision often can be improved with two types of muscle-splitting steps: the **Maylard,** in which the rectus muscles are cut, or a **Cherney rectus muscle detachment** performed at the pubic insertion. After entering the abdomen, a self-retaining retractor is placed and the round, ovarian, and broad ligaments are clamped, cut, and tied, in that order. The uterine vessels are identified and ligated, followed by the creation of a bladder flap and, finally, the cutting and ligation of the uterosacral and cardinal ligaments. The vagina is entered and the cervix removed. Then the vaginal cuff is closed in a way to incorporate the uterosacral ligaments for support. The visceral peritoneum is reapproximated, the retractor removed, and the abdominal layers closed.

In a **vaginal hysterectomy,** the cervix is retracted, a paracervical incision is made, and the anterior and posterior cul de sacs are entered (Fig. 8.2-4). The uterosacral and cardinal ligaments and the uterine vessels are cut and ligated. With steady downward traction, the broad ligament is ligated in a step-wise manner until either the ovarian or infundibulopelvic ligament is reached, and one of the two is ligated, depending on whether the ovaries are to be removed or not. After the uterus has been removed, the peritoneum is reapproximated, followed by the closing of the vaginal cuff, which often includes the uterosacral and cardinal ligaments for support. A vaginal pack often is left in place. Frequently, laparoscopy is being combined with vaginal hysterectomy to evaluate the pelvis for unrecognized disease and to ensure prophylactic adnexectomy in women ages ≥ 40–45 yr.

Usual preop diagnosis: Uterine myoma; pelvic relaxation syndrome; pelvic pain 2° endometriosis or adhesions; uncontrolled uterine bleeding/dysmenorrhea; endometrial hyperplasia; gynecological cancers

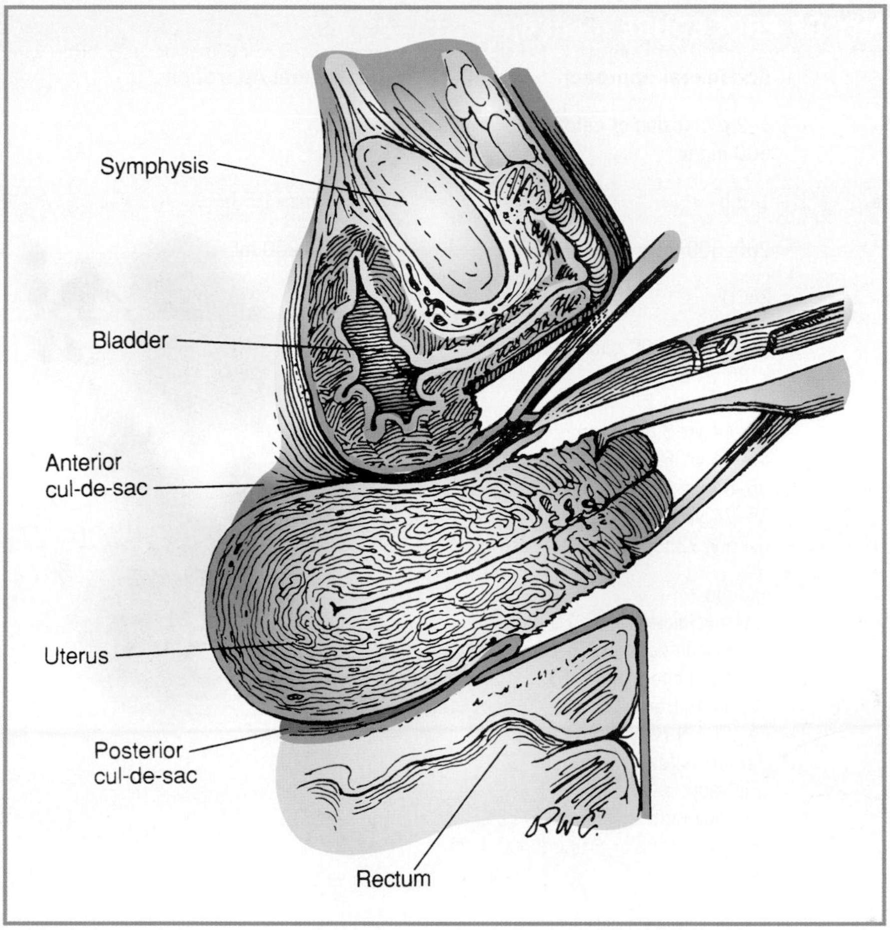

Figure 8.2-4. Surgical anatomy for vaginal hysterectomy. (Reproduced with permission from Rock JA, Thompson JD, eds: *TeLinde's Operative Gynecology,* 8th edition. Lippincott Williams & Wilkins, 1997.)

SUMMARY OF PROCEDURES

	Abdominal Approach	Vaginal Approach
Position	Supine	Lithotomy. Following induction, position patient so that the perineum is at the end of operating table to ensure optimum surgical exposure.
Incision	Pfannenstiel's or low midline. The Pfannenstiel's incision can be extended with a Maylard muscle-splitting procedure or a Cherney rectus muscle detachment at pubic insertion.	Pericervical vaginal
Special instrumentation	None	Stirrups
Unique considerations	None	To prevent peroneal nerve injury, the area of leg leaning against stirrup should be well cushioned. Often, vasoconstriction agents (1:200,000 epinephrine and vasopressin) are used to cut down perioperative vaginal cuff bleeding.

SUMMARY OF PROCEDURE (cont'd)

	Abdominal Approach	Vaginal Approach
Antibiotics	1–2 g cefoxitin or cefotetan + clindamycin 600 mg iv	⇐
Surgical time	1–2 h	45 min–1.5 h
EBL	200–300 mL	100–200 mL
Postop care	PACU	⇐
Mortality	Overall (10,000 patients): 14.6 < 25 yr: 8.9 25–34 yr: 4.7 35–44 yr: 3.8 45–54 yr: 6.5 55–64 yr: 41.3 65–74 yr: 93.0 > 75 yr: 255.8	20 0 0.9 0.5 2.7 1.9 18.3 56.8
Morbidity	Infection: Unexplained fever: 10–20% Pelvic infection: 3.2–10% Wound infection: 4–8% Urinary tract: 1.1–5% Femoral nerve injury: 11.6% Hemorrhage: Intraop: 1–2% Requiring transfusion: 2–12% Unintended major procedures: 1.7% Injury: Bladder: 1–2% Bowel: 0.1–0.5% Ureter: 0.1–0.5% Vesicovaginal fistula: 0.1–0.2% Thromboembolic events: 0.4–1.3%	⇐ 5–8% 3.9–10% – 1.7–5% – ⇐ 0.7–2–5% 2–8.3% 5.1% ⇐ 0.5–1.5% 0.1–0.8% 0.05–0.1% ⇐ 0.62–1.7%
Pain score	5–8	4–6

PATIENT POPULATION CHARACTERISTICS

Age range	30–80 yr
Incidence	> 1/5 females; 650,000/yr in the United States.
Etiology	Uterine myomata; endometriosis; uterine prolapse; uterine cancer
Associated conditions	Stress urinary incontinence; obesity

ANESTHETIC CONSIDERATIONS

PREOPERATIVE

Although many patients presenting for this procedure are otherwise healthy, others may have metastatic cancer.

Respiratory	CXR may be indicated to r/o pleural effusion or other lung pathology in cancer patients. Additionally, ABG, ± PFTs, may be indicated preop in patients with significant pulmonary involvement. **Tests:** As indicated from H&P.

Obstetric/Gynecologic Surgery

Cardiovascular	Patient may have blood loss from the primary problem. Bowel prep may cause dehydration and electrolyte abnormalities. **Tests:** As indicated from H&P.
Hematologic	Hb/Hct. Patients with Hx of easy bruising or bleeding should have coagulation parameters evaluated (PT, PTT, Plt).
Laboratory	Other tests as indicated from H&P.
Premedication	Consider midazolam 1–2 mg iv

INTRAOPERATIVE

Anesthetic technique: GA is commonly used; however, spinal, epidural, or combined spinal–epidural (CSE) anesthesia is appropriate for adequately hydrated patients who are undergoing simple hysterectomy through a Pfannenstiel's incision or vaginal hysterectomy. In the younger patient population, spinal anesthesia may be less desirable because of the increased incidence of postdural puncture headache (PDPH) in using this technique. If spinal anesthetic is indicated, a pencil–point needle (e.g., Sprotte or Whitacre) should be used to decrease the incidence of PDPH.

General anesthesia:

Induction	Standard induction (see p. B-2).
Maintenance	Standard maintenance (see p. B-2). Muscle relaxation is necessary if the procedure is performed abdominally. These patients have a high incidence of PONV; consider prophylaxis (see p. B-6).
Emergence	Standard emergence

Regional anesthesia: A T4-6 sensory level is sufficient to provide anesthesia for procedures on the uterus.

Spinal	0.75% bupivacaine 10–15 mg in 8.25% dextrose. (See Anesthetic Considerations for Cesarean Section, p. 819) Supplement with iv sedation.
Epidural	1.5–2.0% lidocaine with epinephrine 5 mcg/mL, 15–20 mL; supplement with 3–5 mL as needed. Supplemental iv sedation. (See Anesthetic Considerations for Cesarean Section, p. 819.) Supplement with iv sedation.
CSE	**Combined spinal/epidural (CSE):** An alternative technique combining the rapid onset and density of spinal anesthesia with the flexibility of continuous epidural anesthesia. Apply monitors, administer fluid, and position patient as for spinal or epidural. The most common technique is the needle-through-needle. After the epidural space is located with a standard 17-ga Tuohy needle, insert a 4" 26- to 27-ga pencil-point spinal needle through it to administer 0.6 mL of spinal bupivacaine (0.75%) ± fentanyl 10 mcg and morphine sulfate 0.1–0.2 mg. Secure the epidural catheter and use if needed (a test dose is advisable).
Blood and fluid requirements	Consider ↑blood loss in cancer patients, prior XRT, prior abdominal surgery IV: 18 ga × 1–2 Warm fluids Type & screen/cross patients at ↑risk of bleeding
Control of blood loss	**Vaginal hysterectomy:** Moderate blood loss NS/LR at 4–5 mL/kg/h **Abdominal hysterectomy:** Moderate-to-heavy blood loss NS/LR at 6–10 mL/kg/h

Monitoring	**Vaginal hysterectomy:** Standard monitors (see p. B-1) ± Foley catheter **Abdominal hysterectomy:** Standard monitors (see p. B-1) Foley catheter ± Arterial line ± CVP line	Consider in patients with anticipated ↑blood loss or major medical comorbidities.
Positioning	✓and pad pressure points. Shoulder abduction < 90°	The lithotomy position has several considerations for safety. (See p. 789 for details.)
Complications	**Vaginal hysterectomy:** Cervical stimulation Epinephrine/vasopressin injection **Abdominal hysterectomy:** Blood loss Epinephrine/vasopressin injection	Vagal stimulation and ↓↓HR may occur with cervical /peritoneal manipulation. Surgeon may inject epinephrine or vasopressin to decrease local bleeding →HTN and brady or tachydysrhythmias.

POSTOPERATIVE

Complications	PONV (see p. B-6) VTE (see p. B-7) Anemia	
Pain management	Epidural opiates (p. C-2) PCA (p. C-3)	If catheter to be used postop.
Tests	Hct CXR (if CVP catheter placed intraop)	CXR to evaluate central line placement and rule out pneumothorax.

Suggested Readings

1. Carley ME, McIntire D, Carley JM, Schaffer J: Incidence, risk factors and morbidity of unintended bladder or ureter injury during hysterectomy. *Int Urogynecol J Pelvic Floor Dysfunct* 2002; 13(1): 18–21.
2. Clough TF: Perioperative morbidity of hysterectomy for benign gynaecological disease. *J Obstet Gynaecol* 2001; 21(5):504–6.
3. Davies A, Hart R, Magos A, Hadad E, Morris R: Hysterectomy: surgical route and complications. *Eur J Obstet Gynecol Reprod Biol* 2002; 104(2):148–51.
4. Jones HW: Hysterectomy. In *TeLinde's Operative Gynecology*, 9th edition. Rock JA, Jones HW, eds. Lippincott Williams & Wilkins, Philadelphia: 2003, 799–828.
5. Stovall TG: Hysterectomy. In *Berek & Novak's Gynecology*, 14th edition. Berek JS, ed. Lippincott Williams & Wilkins, Philadelphia, 2007, 601–36.

ANTERIOR AND POSTERIOR COLPORRHAPHY, ENTEROCELE REPAIR, VAGINAL SACROSPINOUS SUSPENSION

SURGICAL CONSIDERATIONS

Description: Cystocele (Fig. 8.2-5A) and rectocele (Fig. 8.2-5B) are prolapses (relaxations) of the anterior and posterior vaginal wall, respectively. They occur 2° multiparity and congenital weakening of pelvic tissue. The term *pelvic relaxation syndrome* includes the often coexisting anatomical 'relaxations' (e.g., enterocele [Fig. 8.2-5C] and uterine

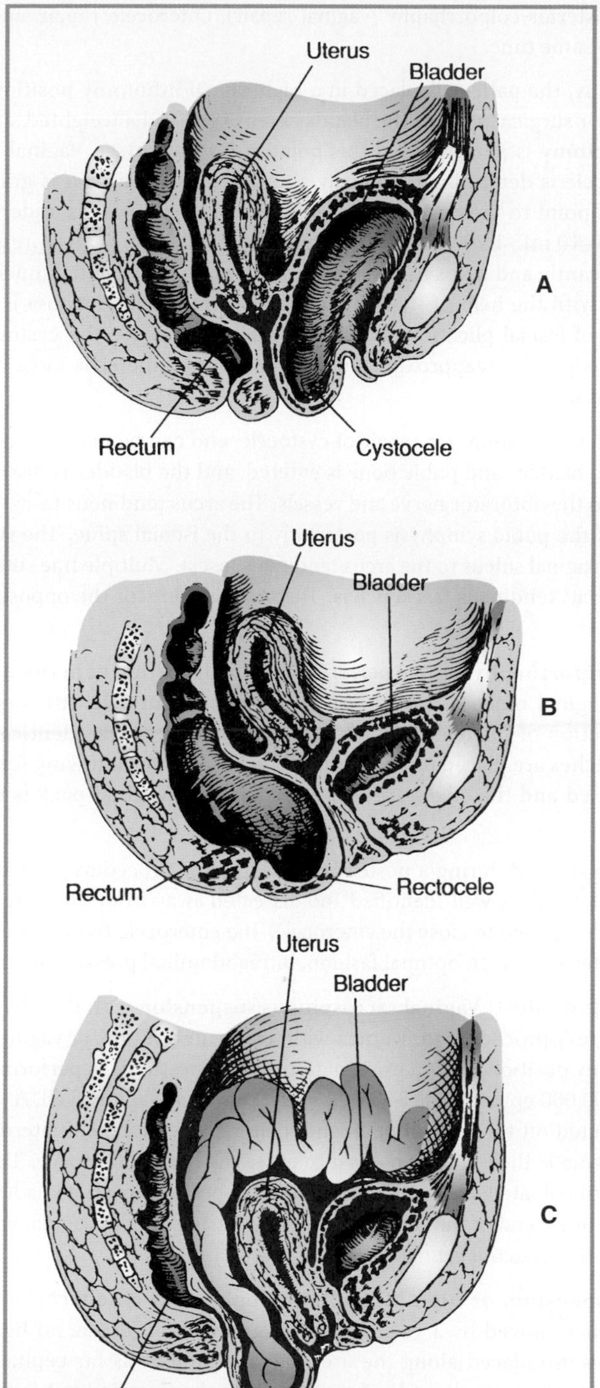

Figure 8.2-5. (**A**) Anatomy of cystocele. (**B**) Anatomy of rectocele. (**C**) Anatomy of enterocele. (Reproduced with permission from Pernoll ML, ed: *Current Obstetrics and Gynecological Diagnosis and Treatment.* Appleton & Lange: 1991.)

prolapse). Cystoceles are often symptomatic due to bladder protrusion past the introitus during straining. Often this relaxation will allow the bladder neck to lose its important anatomical relationship to the urethra and the rest of the bladder. The result can be bothersome stress urinary incontinence for the patient (see Operations for Stress Urinary Incontinence, p. 812). The rectocele often is experienced as a vaginal bulge during straining, and tends to cause incomplete evacuation of stool. The goal of the colporrhaphy is to restore the original anatomy. Due to the frequent coexisting relaxations, a posterior colporrhaphy (vaginal repair), enterocele repair, and vaginal hysterectomy are frequently performed at the same time.

In an **anterior colporrhaphy,** the patient is placed in a high-dorsal lithotomy position with the perineum at the end of the operating table for surgical access. The bladder is emptied and a weighted speculum is inserted into the vagina. A **vaginal hysterectomy** is performed at this point, if indicated (see Vaginal Hysterectomy, p. 804). The extent of the urethrocystocele is determined manually and the vaginal mucosa is grasped at its cephalic border with two clamps. From this point to the external urethral meatus, the mucosa is undermined with a vasoconstrictive solution (epinephrine 5–10 mL, 1:200,000), phenylephrine (1:200,000), or vasopressin (1–5 U/10 mL NS). This decreases blood loss significantly and helps to determine the depth of the vaginal mucosa. The mucosa is cut over this undermined area and, with the help of sharp and blunt dissection; the mucosa is dissected laterally from its underlying fascia. A series of fascial plication sutures are placed to reduce the cystourethrocele. The redundant mucosa is excised and the edges are reapproximated. A suprapubic catheter is most often inserted at the end to prevent bladder overdistention.

Paravaginal repair is another procedure for repair of cystocele, and can be performed via the abdomen or the vagina. The space between the bladder and pubic bone is entered, and the bladder is dissected off the pelvic sidewall, taking care to avoid injury to the obturator nerve and vessels. The arcus tendineus fascia pelvis is visualized, running from the inferior margin of the pubic symphysis posteriorly to the ischial spine. The surgeon places a hand in the vagina to elevate the lateral vaginal sulcus to the arcus tendineus fascia. Multiple fine sutures are placed to secure the paravaginal tissues to the arcus tendineus fascia pelvis. The same is done for the opposite pelvic sidewall if bilateral defects are present.

If necessary, a **posterior colporrhaphy** may be performed. A small portion of perineum posterior to the introitus is removed initially. The vaginal mucosa over the rectocele is undermined with vasoconstrictor fluid prior to incision, followed by dissection of the overlying mucosa in a manner nearly identical to anterior colporrhaphy. One or several layers of stitches are placed to plicate the pararectal fascia, allowing for reduction of the rectocele. Redundant mucosa is excised and the edges are reapproximated. A vaginal pack is usually placed to minimize bleeding.

An **enterocele** often is first noticed during a posterior colporrhaphy procedure, and is repaired prior to finishing the posterior repair. The enterocele is well-identified and dissected away from the surrounding tissue. Two or more parallel purse-string stitches are used to close the enterocele. The enterocele tissue distal to the purse-string closure is excised. To reduce the enterocele in an optimal fashion, intraabdominal pressure has to be at a minimum.

Variant procedure or approaches: **Vaginal sacrospinous suspension** with the Miya hook is an elegant alternative to the abdominal colpopexy procedure for women with severe uterine and/or vaginal vault prolapse. The patient is placed in a dorsal lithotomy position, and an examination under anesthesia is performed. A vasoconstrictive solution is injected (usually 1:200,000 epinephrine 3–5 mL) in the posterior vaginal wall. A vertical incision is made and the mucosa is bluntly dissected off the rectum in an anterolateral direction. An enterocele, if found, is repaired at this time. The pararectal tissue is then bluntly pierced to enter the pararectal space. The anatomy surrounding the sacrospinous ligament is well palpated and, with the help of the special Miya hook, a large suture is placed into the sacrospinous ligament. The other end of the suture is placed at the apex of the vagina, which, after tying, is pulled in a lateral cephalad direction. The mucosa is finally closed.

Uterosacral ligament suspension, or **high McCall's culdoplasty,** is an alternate procedure for vaginal apex support. After the uterus is removed by a vaginal hysterectomy, the uterosacral ligaments are identified. Two separate permanent sutures are placed along the uterosacral ligament as far cephalad (toward the sacrum) as possible. The same is done on the opposite side. A cystoscopy is then carried out with all four stitches placed on tension in order to r/o ureteral obstruction due to ligation or kinking of the ureters. The stitches are replaced if obstruction is observed. After ureteral patency has been confirmed, these stitches are sutured to the fibromuscular layer of the vaginal cuff and tied, to bring the apex as cephalad as possible. The vaginal cuff is closed with absorbable sutures.

The **Le Fort procedure** is now a rare operation and is performed in very elderly women with complete prolapse of the uterus and/or vagina who do not desire to remain sexually active. With the patient in a dorsal lithotomy position, a rectangular strip from the anterior and posterior vaginal wall is removed initially, followed by closure of the margins each to the other. The result is a near-complete closure of the vagina.

Usual preop diagnosis: Symptomatic cystocele; symptomatic uterine prolapse; enterocele; rectocele causing severe constipation; dyspareunia

SUMMARY OF PROCEDURE		
Position	Dorsal lithotomy	
Incision	Vaginal mucosal; peritoneum for enterocele repair	
Unique considerations	To prevent peroneal nerve injury, the area of the leg leaning against the stirrup should be well cushioned. Putting the legs in a high position increases venous return to the heart. Infiltration with epinephrine and vasopressin often is used to reduce intraop bleeding. This causes changes in CO, HR, and BP. Low intraabdominal pressure (good muscle relaxation) is needed during the enterocele reduction.	
Antibiotics	Cefoxitin or cefotetan 1–2 gm iv	
Surgical time	45 min (anterior colporrhaphy) 30 min (posterior colporrhaphy/enterocele repair) 45 min (uterosacral ligament suspension) 1 h (paravaginal repair)	
Closing considerations	Suprapubic catheter (anterior colporrhaphy); vaginal pack (enterocele repair)	
EBL	20–500 mL	
Postop care	PACU	
Mortality	1%	
Morbidity	**Anterior colporrhaphy** Delayed voiding 1–7 d: 30% Foul vaginal discharge: 14% Bacteriuria: 13% Pyrexia (>100.4F): 11% Atelectasis: 3% Delayed voiding > 7 d: 0.6% Need for blood transfusion: 0.6% Urethrovaginal fistula: 0.4% Acute gastric dilatation: 0.2% **Uterosacral ligament suspension** Ureteral obstruction Perirectal abscess due to stitch in rectum	**Vaginal sacrospinous suspension (Miya hook)** Bleeding in gluteal and pudendal vessels Pararectal burning pain = 2 mo Sciatic pain (indicating misplaced sutures, which must be removed) Peritoneal tear (during Miya hook insertion) **Paravaginal repair** Obturator vessel laceration Obturator nerve injury Ureteral obstruction Bladder laceration
Pain score	5–8	

PATIENT POPULATION CHARACTERISTICS	
Age range	40–80 yr
Incidence	> 1/5 women
Etiology	Multiparous state; obesity; chronic cough; previous pelvic surgery
Associated conditions	Pelvic relaxation syndrome

ANESTHETIC CONSIDERATIONS

See Anesthetic Considerations following Operations for Stress Urinary Incontinence, p. 814.

Suggested Readings

1. Richter HE, Varner RE: Pelvic organ prolapse. In *Berek & Novak's Gynecology,* 14th edition. Berek JS, ed. Lippincott Williams & Wilkins, Philadelphia, 2007, 601–36.

2. Zimmerman CS, Shull B, Grody MHT, et al: Surgery for correction of defects in pelvic support and pelvic fistulas. In *TeLinde's Operative Gynecology,* 9th edition. Rock JA, Jones HW, eds. Lippincott Williams & Wilkins, Philadelphia: 2003, 925–1160.

OPERATIONS FOR STRESS URINARY INCONTINENCE

SURGICAL CONSIDERATIONS

Description: Stress urinary incontinence is a common condition affecting mostly older and multiparous women. It is a disorder of the musculofascial support to the bladder neck and pelvic floor. These patients usually have extensive preop workup to exclude urge incontinence and many have been treated with pelvic floor exercises (Kegel) prior to surgery. Two surgical approaches exist: **abdominal suspension** procedures and **suspension by the vaginal route.** Ongoing controversy exists concerning which approach is best. Patient positioning is crucial for all vaginal surgery.

Vaginal approaches: The **Kelly urethral plication** often has been used as the primary surgical treatment, especially when other vaginal surgery is to be performed. The patient initially is placed in a high-dorsal lithotomy position with the perineum at the end of the operating table for surgical exposure. The bladder is emptied and a weighted speculum is inserted into the vagina. The extent of the cystourethrocele is determined and the vaginal mucosa is grasped at its cephalic border with two clamps. From this point to the external urethral meatus, the mucosa usually is undermined with 5–10 mL of a vasoconstrictive solution (epinephrine 1:200,000, phenylephrine 1:200,000, or vasopressin 1–5 U/10 mL NS). This decreases blood loss significantly and helps to determine the depth of the mucosa. With the help of sharp and blunt dissection, the mucosa is freed laterally from its underlying adherent fascia. A series of vertical mattress sutures are placed in the mobilized paraurethral and paravesicle fascia to reduce the cystourethrocele and elevate the posterior urethra to a high-retropubic position. The redundant mucosa is excised and the edges are reapproximated. A suprapubic catheter is often inserted at the end of the surgery to prevent bladder overdistention.

Two anterior vesicle neck suspension techniques—Stamey and modified **Pereyra**—are very similar procedures wherein the vaginal mucosa is incised and dissected off the underlying paraurethral fascia, much the same way as in the Kelly plication. Instead of using a layer of mattress sutures, both suspension methods use two lateral sutures that suspend the vesicle neck on each side (see Fig. 9-21, p. 899). The ends of the sutures are tied over the rectus fascia to provide support. The Stamey method uses a small Dacron cuff to prevent the suture from tearing through the paravesicle fascia, while in the modified Pereyra method, the posterior loop is attached firmly to the pubourethral ligament. One or two small suprapubic abdominal incisions must be made to allow for the tying of the sutures. Specialized long needles are used to help the placement of these sutures, and a cystoscope often is used to verify their placement. Perforation of the bladder is a common complication found upon cystoscopy. Finally, a suprapubic catheter is placed at the end of the operation.

Abdominal approaches: The **Marshall-Marchetti-Krantz (M-M-K)** and **Burch** (urethropexy) are probably the most common abdominal suspension procedures. The patient is placed in the frog-leg position with a urethral catheter in place. A Pfannenstiel's incision is used to enter the space of Retzius, which lies between the parietal peritoneum and the rectus fascia under the pubic bone. Blunt dissection is used to open and extend this space. The surgeon then inserts two fingers into the vagina to raise the anterior vagina and bladder neck. This enables the surgeon to place two or more sutures in the tissue just lateral to the urethra and attach them to Cooper's ligament (Burch) or to the periosteum of the posterior pelvic bone (M-M-K).

The **urethral sling procedure** was once reserved for women with low urethral pressure and/or for whom other incontinence operations had failed. It is now also used as primary treatment for stress urinary incontinence. The goal of the sling procedure is to produce extrinsic compression of the urethrovesical junction with the help of a strip anchored to the rectus fascia or pubic bone (see Fig. 9-21, p. 899). With the patient in the dorsal lithotomy position, a urethral catheter is placed and the vaginal mucosa incised and dissected off the underlying paravesicle and paraurethral fascia, similar to the Kelly plication. The retropubic space is entered through a Pfannenstiel's incision and a strip of rectus fascia, is obtained. The strip is then brought through the vagina, around the urethra, and back to the abdomen, where it is fastened to the rectus fascia, creating a sling under the urethra at the junction of the bladder neck. The vaginal and abdominal incisions are closed, and a suprapubic catheter is placed. If donor fascia lata or synthetic material is used, a small (~2") horizontal incision is made above the pubic bone for attachment of the sling.

Tension-free vaginal tape (TVT) is a new 'sling' type procedure for treatment of stress urinary incontinence. A Prolene mesh sling is used to support the urethra, although it is not attached to the fascia. The Prolene is woven in such a way that the sling cannot slide out over time. Fibroblasts grow into the sling to anchor it throughout the endopelvic fascia and around the dependent surface of the urethra. Placement of the sling material is through a vaginal incision similar to that of the Kelly plication. The TVT curved needle is introduced from the vagina through the space of Retzius on each side of the urethra, and is brought out to the abdomen above the pubic bone. The sling mesh is attached to the ends of each needle; thus, when both needles are pulled through the abdominal sites, the mesh will rest under the urethra. A cystoscopy is done before pulling the mesh through to verify that neither needle is in the bladder or the urethra. The mesh is then adjusted so that the urethra is resting on the sling, under no tension.

Usual preop diagnosis: Stress urinary incontinence; intrinsic sphincter deficiency

SUMMARY OF PROCEDURES

	Kelly Plication	M-M-K/Burch	Urethral Sling
Position	Dorsal lithotomy	Frog-leg	⇐
Incision	Vaginal mucosa	Pfannenstiel's	Vaginal
Unique considerations	Cushion area of leg against stirrup to prevent peroneal injury. Epinephrine (1:200,000) or vasopressin are often infiltrated to reduce intraop bleeding for vaginal approaches. Injections may cause ↑BP and tachydysrhythmias (epi) or bradydysrhythmias (vasopressin). The urethral catheter is frequently removed and reinserted during surgery.	⇐	⇐
Antibiotics	Cefoxitin 1–2 g iv	⇐	⇐
Surgical time	1 h	⇐	⇐
Closing considerations	Suprapubic catheter	⇐	⇐
EBL	50 mL	100–200 mL	50–100 mL
Postop care	Inpatient	⇐	± outpatient
Mortality	Minimal	⇐	⇐
Morbidity	Detrusor instability: Rare (due to vaginal approach) Enterocele: Rare Incisional hernia: Rare Osteitis pubis: Rare Voiding difficulties: Rare Wound infection: Rare	14% 15% 0.09% ⇐ 2% 8.7%	⇐ N/A Rare ⇐ ~40% Rare Prolonged catheter time: > 50% Outlet obstruction: 10–20% Urethral perforation: 7% Bladder perforation: 1%
Pain score	4–6	6–8	4–6

PATIENT POPULATION CHARACTERISTICS	
Age range	40–80 yr
Incidence	>1/5 women
Etiology	Multiparous state; obesity; chronic cough
Associated conditions	Other components of pelvic relaxation syndrome (rectocele, uterine prolapse, enterocele)

ANESTHETIC CONSIDERATIONS

(Procedures covered: anterior and posterior colporrhaphy; enterocele repair; vaginal sacrospinous suspension; operations for stress urinary incontinence)

PREOPERATIVE

This is usually an older patient population, past child-bearing age. Assess for medical comorbidities.

Laboratory	Hb/Hct, as indicated from H&P.
Premedication	Consider midazolam 1–2 mg iv

INTRAOPERATIVE

Anesthetic technique: Regional or GA may be used.

Regional anesthesia: A T10 sensory level is sufficient to provide anesthesia for procedures using a perineal approach, but a T4 level is recommended for abdominal/combined approaches.

Spinal	0.75% bupivacaine 10–15 mg in 8.25% dextrose. (See Anesthetic Considerations for Cesarean Section, p. 819.)
Epidural	1.5–2.0% lidocaine with epinephrine 5 mcg/mL, 15–20 mL; supplement with 3–5 mL as needed. Supplemental iv sedation. (See Anesthetic Considerations for Cesarean Section, p. 819.) Spinal may provide better perineal block.
CSE	**Combined spinal/epidural (CSE):** An alternative technique combining the rapid onset and density of spinal anesthesia with the flexibility of continuous epidural anesthesia. Apply monitors, administer fluid, and position patient as for spinal or epidural. The most common technique is the needle-through-needle. After the epidural space is located with a standard 17-ga Tuohy needle, insert a 4" 26- to 27-ga pencil-point spinal needle through it to administer 0.6 mL of spinal bupivacaine (0.75%) ± fentanyl 10 mcg and morphine sulfate 0.1–0.2 mg. Secure the epidural catheter and use if needed (a test dose is advisable).

General anesthesia:

Induction	Standard induction (see p. B-2).
Maintenance	Standard maintenance (see p. B-2).
Emergence	No special considerations
Blood and fluid requirements	Normally minimal blood loss IV: 18–20 ga × 1 NS/LR at 2–4 mL/kg/h

Control of blood loss	Epinephrine, vasopressin, phenylephrine used by surgeons.	Surgeons may inject vasopressors into the submucosa to minimize blood loss, which may cause ↑ BP and tachydysrhythmias (epi) or bradydysrhythmias (phenylephrine/vasopressin).
Monitoring	Standard monitors (p. B-1)	Although bladder catheterization prior to incision is normal, the catheter is not left in place throughout surgery in those patients undergoing anterior and posterior colporrhaphy, enterocele repair, and Kelly urethral plication. Suprapubic bladder catheters are placed toward the end of surgery in these procedures, as well as in the Stamey, Pereyra, and urethral sling procedures.
Positioning	✓ and pad pressure points ✓ eyes	See p. 789 for concerns regarding the lithotomy position.

POSTOPERATIVE

Complications	PONV (see p. B-6)
Pain management	IV opiates, ketorolac Usually rapid conversion to po pain medications
Tests	None indicated

Suggested Readings

1. Nygaard I, Menefee SA, Wall LL: Lower urinary tract disorders. In *Berek & Novak's Gynecology,* 14th edition. Berek JS, ed. Lippincott Williams & Wilkins, Philadelphia, 2007, 601–36.
2. Pereyra AJ, et al: Pubourethral supports in perspective: modified Pereyra procedure for urinary incontinence. *Obstet Gynecol* 1982; 59(5):643–8.
3. Richter HE, Varner RE: Pelvic organ prolapse. In: *Berek & Novak's Gynecology,* 14th edition. Berek JS, ed. Lippincott Williams & Wilkins, Philadelphia, 2007, 601–36.
4. Ross BK, Chaduck HS, Mancuso JS, Benedetti C: Sprotte needle for obstetric anesthesia: Decreased incidence of post dural puncture headache. *Reg Anesth* 1992; 17:29–33.
5. Wall LL: Urinary stress incontinence. In *TeLinde's Operative Gynecology,* 9th edition.. Rock JA, Jones HW, eds. Lippincott Williams & Wilkins, Philadelphia: 2003, 1033–80.

CHAPTER

8.3 Obstetric Surgery

SURGEONS

M. Mark Taslimi, MD
Yasser El-Sayed, MD

ANESTHESIOLOGISTS

Brendan Carvalho, MBBCh, FRCA
Lee Coleman, MD

CESAREAN SECTION—LOWER SEGMENT AND CLASSIC

SURGICAL CONSIDERATIONS

Description: Cesarean section (C-section) is the delivery of the fetus through a horizontal or, more commonly, through a vertical incision in the lower uterine segment. The skin incision is made either as a Pfannenstiel's (transverse in the crease above the pubis), a Maylard (in extremely obese patients), or vertical midline from umbilicus to pubis. The peritoneal cavity is entered as in any laparotomy. A retractor is placed inferiorly and the reflection of visceral peritoneum from the bladder dome to the anterior lower segment of the uterus (bladder flap) is incised and displaced inferiorly, along with the bladder. The uterus is entered sharply and the incision extended with digital pressure and/or bandage scissors. The fetal head is elevated out of the pelvis and delivered through the uterine incision. In cases of nonvertex lie, the infant's breech or foot is grasped and brought out of the incision. After the delivery of the fetus, the cord is double-clamped and cut, and cord blood is obtained for analysis. The placenta is removed manually and the uterine cavity cleared of all debris and clots. The uterine incision is closed with a running, interlocking stitch, followed by a 2nd imbricating layer. The bladder flap and parietal peritoneum do not require closure. Finally, the fascia is closed and the skin reapproximated with staples. **Classic C-section** usually involves a fundal vertical uterine incision (Fig. 8.3-1). Patients with a history of prior classical C-section should be delivered abdominally via a repeat C-section, because their risk of uterine rupture with labor and vaginal delivery is ~12%.

Usual preop diagnosis: Failure to progress in labor; elective repeat C-section; fetal distress; malpresentation

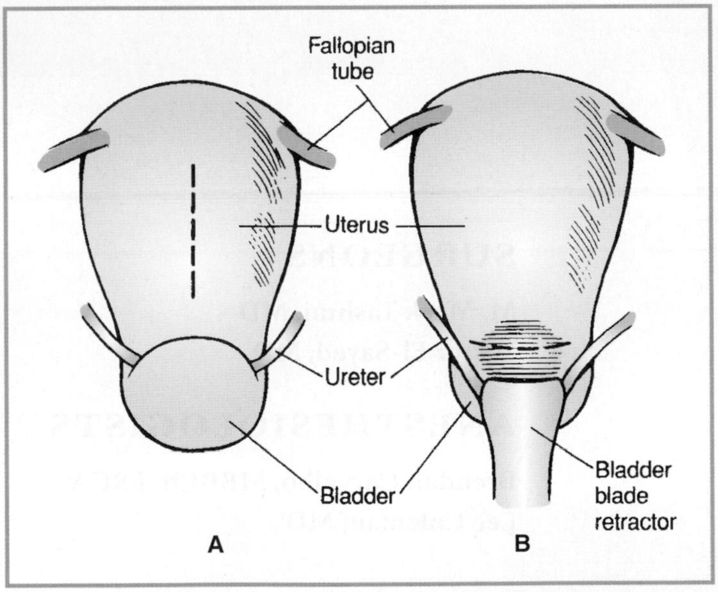

Figure 8.3-1. Typical C-section incisions. **A:** Classic incision, in upper uterine segment. **B:** Low transverse incision.

SUMMARY OF PROCEDURES

	Lower-Segment C-Section	Classic C-Section
Position	Supine with left lateral tilt. (In obese patients, the pannus may be lifted superiorly by tape or towel clips.)	⇐
Incision	Skin: transverse low abdominal (Pfannenstiel's) or repeat vertical. Uterus: transverse (Kerr) or low vertical (for premature infants or nonvertex lie)	Skin: Pfannenstiel's or, more commonly, vertical midline. Uterus: vertical fundal

SUMMARY OF PROCEDURE (cont'd)		
	Lower-Segment C-Section	**Classic C-Section**
Special instrumentation	Bladder blade retractor; small ring forceps; bandage scissors; suction bulb; DeLee suction trap (if meconium)	⇐
Unique considerations	✓ fetal heart tones before procedure. If for CPD: vaginal exam within last 15 min before procedure. If for fetal distress: continuous monitoring until skin incision.	⇐
Antibiotics	If in labor or membranes ruptured: continue prophylactic antibiotics or cefazolin 1–2 gm iv (prior to incision or 30 minutes prior to delivery)	⇐
Surgical time	20–90 min	40–90 min
Closing considerations	Low transverse: closed in 2 layers. Low vertical: 2 layers; may require additional operative time for control of incision bleeding or repair of incision extension into cervix.	3-layer closure requires additional time.
EBL	750–1,000 mL	1,000–2,000 mL
Postop care	Observation for bleeding and ↓ BP	Special attention to VS needed due to additional blood loss.
Mortality	< 0.1%	⇐
Morbidity	Infection: Not in labor: < 5% In labor/ruptured membranes: 50% (antibiotics reduce incidence to 15%) Small-bowel obstruction (SBO): Rare	 ⇐ ⇐ ⇐
Pain Score	4	7

PATIENT POPULATION CHARACTERISTICS	
Age range	14–45 yr
Incidence	10–30%
Etiology	Failure to progress (30%); repeat C-section (30%); fetal anomaly/other (20%); abnormal presentation (10%); fetal distress (10%)
Associated conditions	Preeclampsia/eclampsia; DIC; hemolysis, elevated liver enzyme, low Plt count (HELLP) syndrome; obstetrical hemorrhage/shock; chorioamnionitis

ANESTHETIC CONSIDERATIONS

(Procedures covered: C-section; emergent obstetrical hysterectomy; repair of uterine rupture)

PREOPERATIVE

In general, patients are young and healthy, although the pregnant patient has undergone profound physiologic changes that affect the conduct of anesthesia. Patients present for emergency C-section for nonreassuring fetal heart rate tracing and/or hemorrhage (placenta previa, abruptio placenta, and, rarely, uterine rupture).

Respiratory	The pregnant patient has a compensated respiratory alkalosis (PCO_2 = 32–34), ↑ minute ventilation (MV) (↑ 50%), and ↓ FRC (↓ 20%). ↑ O_2 consumption (↑ 20%) with ↓ FRC results in rapid onset of hypoxemia if ventilation is compromised. Small airway closure due to elevation of diaphragm (exaggerated by obesity and supine position) can → shunting

Obstetric/Gynecologic Surgery

Respiratory (cont'd)	and ↓ PaO_2. ↑ MV and ↓ FRC enhance uptake of inhalational anesthetics. Mucosal capillary engorgement in upper airways may necessitate a smaller ETT and mandates careful airway suctioning to avoid bleeding. **Tests:** As indicated from H&P.
Cardiovascular	Typically, there is a ↓ SVR (↓ 15%), ↓ diastolic pressure and ↓ MAP (↓ 15%) with ↑ HR (↑ 20%) and ↑ CO (↑ 30–40%, higher in multi-fetal pregnancy, higher in labor). Use left lateral tilt to minimize aortocaval compression and supine hypotension. Immediately postpartum, 600–800 mL blood enters the central circulation, due to placental transfusion, with further ↑ in CO. **Tests:** As indicated from H&P.
Hematologic	These patients have ↑ red cell mass (↑ 300–400 mL), ↑ plasma volume (↑ 1,200–1,300 mL), ↑ blood volume (↑ 1,500–1,600 mL), ↑ more with multifetal pregnancy. WBC count may ↑ to 15,000/mm^3. Iron deficiency anemia often is superimposed on the dilutional anemia of pregnancy (Hct 33%). The typical blood loss of 500–800 mL is usually well tolerated. Excessive blood loss is possible with multiple gestation, previous C-section, PIH, placenta previa, abruptio placenta, prolonged labor, and uterine atony. Repeat C-section associated with placenta previa poses high risk for hemorrhage because of placenta accreta. **Tests:** Hgb/Hct
Gastrointestinal	Abnormalities, including ↓ gastric motility (after onset of labor), gastroesophageal reflux, raised intragastric pressure, and gastric hyperacidity, predisposes to aspiration pneumonitis. All parturients should be considered to have full stomachs and should receive clear antacid (e.g., 0.3 M Na citrate 30 mL) immediately prior to general or regional anesthesia. Administer iv metoclopramide 10 mg and ranitidine 50 mg before emergent C-section. Before elective C-section, parturients at high risk for aspiration (e.g., planned or potential GA, difficult airway, or any patient with esophageal reflux or obesity) should receive an H_2-blocker (e.g., ranitidine 150 mg po) the night before and the morning of surgery.
Hepatic	Liver enzymes can be mildly elevated and plasma protein concentration is diminished (↑ unbound drug levels). **Tests:** As indicated from H&P
Renal	These patients have ↑ renal blood flow (↑ 50%), ↑ GFR, and ↑ creatinine clearance, and ↓ serum creatinine and ↓ BUN. Dependent edema results from increased water and Na^+ retention 2° resetting of the osmotic threshold for thirst and vasopressin secretions. **Tests:** As indicated from H&P.
Laboratory	T&S maternal blood if risk factors for blood loss are present (e.g., third C-section). Crossmatch unnecessary unless significant blood loss is anticipated. Routine autologous blood donation is not recommended. Coagulation studies and Plt count recommended with PIH, abruptio placenta, heavy maternal bleeding. BUN; Cr; UA; fasting blood glucose; others as indicated from H&P.
Premedication	Agents to decrease risk of aspiration pneumonitis include a clear antacid (e.g., Na citrate 30 mL po), ranitidine 50 mg iv and metoclopramide 10 mg iv. Sedatives are not routinely administered. In extremely anxious patients, however, 0.5–1.0 mg midazolam iv is an excellent anxiolytic, without apparent effect on maternal memory or alertness or neonatal condition.

SPECIAL CONSIDERATIONS

Pregnancy-induced hypertension (PIH)	PIH is characterized by generalized vasoconstriction with relative intravascular volume depletion and, occasionally, diffuse capillary leak. There may be ↑ risk of hypotension with regional anesthesia. Cautious hydration prior to regional anesthesia is necessary to prevent hypotension or pulmonary edema. Hepatic dysfunction may be present (HELLP syndrome). Epidural, spinal, and combined spinal-epidural (CSE) are all considered safe

Pregnancy-induced hypertension (PIH) (cont'd)	techniques in PIH. Cardiovascular stability is better with regional than GA, provided intravascular volume is adequate. Abnormal coagulation (↓ Plt count or dysfunctional Plt) contraindicates regional anesthesia. If GA is necessary, control BP with small doses of labetalol (5–20 mg iv over 3–5 min) and/or low doses of a short-acting opioid (e.g., fentanyl 50–100 mcg) prior to induction to blunt hypertensive response to laryngoscopy. There is a potential for difficult intubation in PIH due to airway edema; therefore, a small ETT (6.0 mm) should be available. $MgSO_4$ potentiates neuromuscular blocking agents; avoid defasciculating dose of muscle relaxant before induction, use smaller than normal doses of nondepolarizing agents, and monitor neuromuscular function. **Tests:** PT; PTT; Plt; TEG or bleeding time; LFTs
Eclampsia	Treat eclamptic Sz with adequate oxygenation and a small dose of STP (50–100 mg) or diazepam (5 mg). Intubate if necessary to protect airway. Initiate $MgSO_4$ therapy (loading dose: 4–6 g iv over 20–30 min; then infuse @ 1–2 g/h).
Massive maternal hemorrhage: • Placenta previa • Abruptio placenta • Ruptured uterus	Insert 2 large-bore iv catheters (14–16 ga). Assure immediate availability of cross-matched blood. Rapidly restore intravascular volume with crystalloid, colloid, or both. Induction of GA with ketamine (1–1.5 mg/kg) is preferred in hypovolemic patients. DIC can follow abruptio placenta or amniotic fluid embolism. Dilutional thrombocytopenia following massive blood loss might require Plt transfusion. Uterine atony is treated with oxytocin 20–40 U/L in NS @ rate sufficient to control atony (risk of ↓ BP with boluses); methylergonovine, 0.2 mg im (risk of HTN); or 15-methyl prostaglandin F_2-alpha, 0.25 mg im or intramyometrially (risk of pulmonary HTN, bronchospasm). Uterine artery embolization is often effective in controlling continued postpartum bleeding and may be considered before surgical artery ligation or hysterectomy. Emergency hysterectomy, however, may be the only solution to continued bleeding. Induction of GA may be necessary if massive bleeding occurs during regional anesthesia.
Diabetes	Diabetic patients have an increased propensity to ↓ BP following regional anesthesia, with the fetus becoming more acidotic than normal as a result. Determine blood glucose hourly and maintain at 80–100 mg/dL. Insulin requirements decrease drastically after delivery, and insulin dosage must be reduced to prevent maternal hypoglycemia. **Tests:** Fasting blood glucose; UA
Response to anesthetic drugs	In pregnant patients, MAC is ↓ 40% for inhaled agents; combined with more rapid uptake, this predisposes to anesthetic overdose. Sensitivity to local anesthetics also is increased. Epidural space capacity is decreased 2° engorgement of epidural veins; this decreases requirements for local anesthetics and increases possibility of intravascular injection of drugs. Increased sensitivity to nondepolarizing muscle relaxants (especially in patients receiving $MgSO_4$) mandates careful monitoring and use of reduced doses. Decreased protein binding may increase toxicity of highly protein-bound drugs such as bupivacaine.

INTRAOPERATIVE

Anesthetic technique: General considerations involve primarily the choice of anesthetic. Compared with regional anesthesia, the risks of aspiration and difficult intubation with GA increase maternal morbidity and mortality. Anesthetic choice in specific circumstances depends on maternal and fetal conditions and degree of urgency. Properly conducted GA or regional anesthesia probably are equally safe for the fetus.

Spinal anesthesia is preferred for elective or semielective C-section (unless patient has an existing epidural) when no contraindications to regional anesthesia exist (e.g., patient refusal, coagulopathy, active neurological disease, hypovolemia, sepsis). With the use of a pencil-point needles (e.g., Sprotte, Whitacre), the risk of headache is low (1–2%). Advantages of spinal over epidural anesthesia include: technical ease, rapid onset of block, and more solid anesthesia, and less shivering. ↓ BP, however, is more common with spinal anesthesia. Fluid loading (1–1.5 L crystalloid/500 mL colloid), leg wrapping (e.g., compression stockings), and vasopressors reduce the incidence and severity of ↓ BP, but do not eliminate it. Pressors (e.g., ephedrine [5–10 mg], phenylephrine [50–100 mcg], and atropine [0.4 mg iv]) should be used as appropriate to treat ↓ BP and ↓ HR. Ephedrine, even in large doses, may not reverse severe ↓ BP, and may ↑ fetal acidosis. Consider using epinephrine (50–100 mcg iv) if other pressors/fluids are unsuccessful.

General anesthesia normally is used when regional anesthesia is contraindicated or when there is inadequate time to institute regional blockade. Obstetric emergencies for which rapid induction of GA may be indicated include: severe maternal hemorrhage, prolapsed umbilical cord, severe fetal bradycardia, severe persistent fetal decelerations, or the need for intrauterine manipulation. Less dire situations often permit the performance of a "quick spinal" or extension of a functioning epidural block with an agent having a rapid onset (e.g., 15–20 mL 3% 2-chloroprocaine or 2% lidocaine with epinephrine). Continuous monitoring of the fetal heart rate (FHR) in the OR may allow use of regional anesthesia if the FHR tracing is reassuring. Constant communication with the obstetrician regarding maternal and fetal condition is essential. Although situations exist in which a GA is preferable to regional, the risks must be weighed against the benefits for patients with greater potential for complications. If difficult intubation is anticipated, rapid-sequence induction of GA should not be undertaken. Alternative approaches include awake intubation, spinal anesthesia, or local infiltration by the obstetrician. Sometimes, a nonreassuring FHR pattern is diagnosed as "fetal distress" and the fetus is delivered immediately. Fetal distress is an imprecise and nonspecific term with little positive predictive value. The severity of any FHR abnormality should be considered when the urgency of delivery and type of anesthesia are determined. C-section performed for a nonreassuring FHR pattern does not necessarily preclude the use of regional anesthesia.

Regional anesthesia:

Epidural	Apply monitors, fluid load, and place the patient in the sitting or lateral decubitus position. A 3 mL test dose of 1.5–2% lidocaine (45–60 mg) with 1:200,000 epinephrine (15–20 mcg) is given through the epidural needle or catheter to exclude intravascular injection (Sx: tachycardia, palpitations, dizziness, tinnitus, new taste in mouth) or subarachnoid placement (motor/sensory block in lower extremities). After 3–5 min, inject 15–20 mL 2% (300–400 mg) lidocaine with 1:200,000 epinephrine (75–100 mcg) incrementally over 5 min. Sodium bicarbonate, 1 mEq/10 mL lidocaine, hastens onset of block, but increases risk of ↓ BP. Bupivacaine, levobupivacaine, or ropivacaine 0.5%, 15–20 mL (75–100 mg), with or without epinephrine 1:200,000 and/or fentanyl (50–75 mcg), or 3% 2-chloroprocaine, 15–20 mL (450–600 mg) can also be used. To ensure a T4 level of anesthesia throughout surgery, additional local anesthetic often is needed. If a functioning epidural catheter is in place and an urgent C-section becomes necessary, 15–20 mL 3% 2-chloroprocaine (450–600 mg) or 2% lidocaine with epinephrine should produce adequate surgical anesthesia within 5–10 min. Tilt table or use left hip elevation. Administer O_2 by mask or nasal cannula, and check FHR prior to abdominal prep. Monitor BP every min until stable, then every 3–5 min. Treat ↓ 20% in BP or SBP < 95–100 mmHg with further uterine displacement, additional fluids, and ephedrine 5–10 mg or phenylephrine 50–100 mcg iv. For inadequate anesthesia, give additional epidural local anesthetic, 50–100 mcg fentanyl iv or epidurally, 50% N_2O/O_2, ketamine 5–10 mg iv and/or infiltrate with local anesthetic. The patient must remain conscious to avoid risk of aspiration. If anesthesia is still inadequate, induce GA (see below). After delivery of infant and placenta, rapidly infuse oxytocin 20–30 U/L. Observe for excessive blood loss. Chest pain, mild oxyhemoglobin desaturation, and SOB after delivery may be due to irritation of diaphragm by blood or packs, too high or inadequate level of anesthesia, or venous air or amniotic fluid embolization. S-T segment changes on ECG occur, but do not usually signify myocardial ischemia.
Spinal	Apply monitors, administer fluid, and position as for epidural anesthesia. Metoclopramide 10 mg iv, 5–10 min prior to block decreases intraop N/V. Insert 24–25-ga pencil-point needle and verify free flow of CSF. In urgent situations, a larger pencil-point needle (e.g., 22-ga Sprotte) is easier and faster to place with minimal increase in headache. Inject hyperbaric 0.75% spinal bupivacaine 11.25–12.0 mg (1.5–1.6 mL) ± fentanyl 10–15 mcg and preservative-free morphine 0.1–0.2 mg, and position the patient with left uterine displacement. Monitor and treat ↓ BP as for epidural. Adjust operating table position to insure a T4 level of anesthesia. If anesthesia is inadequate and time permits, consider repeating block with CSE, repeat spinal (caution with dosing), or placement of an epidural catheter. Treat persistent inadequate anesthesia as for epidural. Induce GA if other measures fail.

Combined spinal-epidural (CSE)	An alternative technique combining the rapid onset and density of spinal anesthesia with the flexibility of continuous epidural anesthesia (e.g., if necessary to extend the duration or intensity of the block). Apply monitors, administer fluid, and position as for spinal/epidural. The most common technique is the needle-through-needle. When the epidural space is located with a 17-ga Tuohy needle, insert a 26–27 ga pencil-point spinal needle through it and administer 11.25–12 mg of spinal bupivacaine. Secure the epidural catheter and use if needed. (An epidural test dose is advisable.)

General anesthesia:

Induction	Tilt table or use left hip displacement and administer 500–750 mL dextrose-free crystalloid before induction. Preoxygenation for 3 min is optimal; however, 4 maximal inspiratory breaths in 30 sec is a satisfactory substitute in an emergency. Place patient in maximal "sniff" position with elevation of shoulders, if necessary, to optimize position for intubation. After patient is prepped and draped and obstetric team is ready to begin, perform rapid-sequence induction with cricoid pressure. Administer STP 4–5 mg/kg or propofol 2–3 mg/kg (or ketamine 1–1.5 mg/kg in hypovolemic patients) and succinylcholine 1–1.5 mg/kg to induce GA and facilitate intubation. Inflate cuff of ETT and verify tracheal placement by $ETCO_2$ waveform and auscultation of bilateral breath sounds.
Failed intubation	If tracheal intubation is unsuccessful, monitor O_2 sat and mask ventilate, maintaining cricoid pressure. Summon experienced help and quickly decide whether surgery must proceed. The risks of continuing with mask GA and cricoid pressure must be weighed against the risk of allowing the mother to awaken. If mask ventilation is impossible, quickly attempt ventilation with an LMA. If this succeeds, either continue to use throughout the case or place an ETT (6 mm ID) through LMA blindly or with FOL; alternatively, use an intubating LMA. A Pro-seal LMA has been used in this situation and may negate the necessity for ET intubation. If LMA fails to allow ventilation, attempt emergency transtracheal ventilation using a 12–14 ga iv catheter and appropriate tubing to connect to a high-pressure O_2 source (e.g. jet ventilator). If these measures are unsuccessful, an emergency cricothyrotomy or tracheostomy should be performed by experienced personnel. **Planning for a failed intubation must occur before it actually happens.** A difficult-intubation tray, including equipment for emergency jet ventilation, must be immediately accessible in or very near the delivery room.
Maintenance	50% N_2O/O_2 with isoflurane or sevoflurane (limit MAC < 1.5 to prevent uterine atony). Control ventilation, avoiding extreme hypocapnia (PCO_2 < 30 mmHg), which decreases umbilical blood flow. After delivery, substitute an opioid (e.g., fentanyl 50–100 mcg) for volatile agent and increase concentration of N_2O to 70%. Administer small doses of muscle relaxants (e.g., vecuronium 2–3 mg) as needed. Reverse with neostigmine 0.05 mg/kg and glycopyrrolate 0.01 mg/kg or atropine 0.02 mg/kg. Midazolam (1–2 mg), given after delivery, helps avoid maternal awareness, which occasionally occurs with this anesthetic technique.
Emergence	Delay extubation until patient is fully awake and muscle strength has returned to normal.

Blood and fluid requirements	Moderate blood loss IV: 16–18 ga × 1 NS/LR 1–3 L typical replacement	Infuse 1–2 L dextrose-free crystalloid (± colloid 500 mL) immediately prior to regional anesthesia. Typical blood loss = 500–800 mL. A rapid-fluid infuser and blood warmer should be available in the event that large-volume blood transfusion is required.
Monitoring	Standard monitors (see p. B-1) FHR monitor ±CVP or PA catheter ±arterial line	Arterial BP monitoring via automated BP device, or arterial line for severe or labile HTN. CVP useful in PIH for oliguric patients unresponsive to fluid challenges. Occasionally, a PA catheter is indicated (e.g., for pulmonary edema, unresponsive oliguria).
Positioning	Left uterine displacement (blanket under right hip and/or table tilt)	Minimizes aortocaval compression.

Complications	Amniotic fluid embolism	Rare cause of hemodynamic instability, hypoxemia, and DIC. Often fatal. Rx: supportive: 100% O_2, PEEP, and vasopressors. Correct Plt, clotting factors, and metabolic disturbances. CPB has been used successfully.

POSTOPERATIVE

Complications	VTE	DX: pleuritic chest pain, cough, hypoxemia, ↑ RR, ↑ HR, ↑ A-a gradient. Rx: supportive: 100% O_2, volume expansion, and vasopressors. See p. B-7.
	Postpartum hemorrhage	See Anesthetic Considerations for Removal of Retained Placenta, p. 825.
Pain management	**Epidural:** 4–5 mg preservative-free morphine in 10 mL after delivery. **Intrathecal:** Morphine (preservative-free) 0.1–0.2 mg given with spinal local anesthetic. Chloroprocaine interferes with analgesia from epidural opioids	Common side effects include: pruritus 70%, nausea 30–40%, and, rarely, respiratory depression. Nalbuphine (5–10 mg) and naloxone (0.1–0.4 mg) are used for reversal of these side effects. Metoclopramide (10 mg iv) and/or ondansetron (4 mg iv) may be needed for persistent nausea. Risk of delayed respiratory depression in healthy patients is small; however, adequately trained nursing staff and a protocol for treatment of complications are mandatory if intraspinal opioids are used. These patients should not routinely receive sedatives or other systemic opioids for 12 h, and close monitoring of RR every hour and level of consciousness is necessary. Pulse oximetry is recommended in high-risk patients.
	Parenteral opioids: iv or im opioids or PCA instituted in recovery room. **Oral analgesics:** NSAIDs (e.g., ibuprofen), acetaminophen ±codeine (or equivalent oral narcotics), after the patient can tolerate oral medication.	
Tests	As indicated	

Suggested Readings

1. Carvalho B, Roland LM, Chu LF, et al: Single-dose, extended-release epidural morphine (DepoDur) compared to conventional epidural morphine for post-cesarean pain. *Anesth Analg* 2007; 105(1):176–83.
2. Chadwick HS: An analysis of obstetric anesthesia cases from the American Society of Anesthesiologists closed claims project database. *Int J Obstet Anesth* 1996; 5:258–63.
3. Cunningham FG, MacDonald PC, Gant NF, et al., eds: Cesarean delivery and postpartum hysterectomy. In: *Williams Obstetrics*, 22nd edition., Appleton & Lange, Stamford: 2005, 587–606.
4. Ezri T, Szmuk P, Evron S, et al: Difficult airway in obstetric anesthesia: a review. *Obstet Gynecol Surv* 2001; 56(10):631–41.
5. Hawkins JL, Koonin LM, Palmer SK, et al: Anesthesia-related deaths during obstetric delivery in the United States, 1979–1990. *Anesthesiology* 1997; 86:277–84.
6. Macarthur A, Riley ET: Obstetric anesthesia controversies: vasopressor choice for postspinal hypotension during cesarean delivery. *Int Aneshtesiol Clin* 2007; 45(1):115–32.
7. McLintic AJ, Pringle SD, Lilley S, et al: Electrocardiographic changes during cesarean section under regional anesthesia. *Anesth Analg* 1992; 74(1):51–6.
8. Mercier FJ, Riley ET, Frederickson WL, et al: Phenylephrine added to prophylactic infusion during spinal anesthesia for elective cesarean section. *Anesthesiology* 2001; 95(3):668–74.
9. Morgan PJ, Halpern SH, Tarshis J: The effects of an increase of central blood volume before spinal anesthesia for cesarean delivery: a qualitative review. *Anesth Analg* 2001; 92(4):997–1005.
10. Richardson MG: Regional anesthesia for obstetrics. *Anesthesiol Clin North America* 2000;18(2):383–406.
11. Vedantham S, Goodwin SC, McLucas B, et al: Uterine artery embolization: an underused method of controlling pelvic hemorrhage. *Am J Obstet Gynecol* 1997; 176(4):938–48.

MEDICAL AND SURGICAL MANAGEMENT OF POSTPARTUM HEMORRHAGE

SURGICAL CONSIDERATIONS

Description: The most common indication for **postpartum uterine devascularization and hysterectomy** is **intractable postpartum hemorrhage (PPH)**. PPH is clinically defined as any uncompensated postpartum blood loss → tissue hypoperfusion. There are four major causes of PPH: retained products of conception (POC), laceration of the genital tract, uterine atony, and coagulopathies. Inherited coagulopathies include von Willebrand's disease, hemophilia, and factor XI deficiency. Acquired coagulopathies are most often related to thrombocytopenia 2° preeclampsia/eclampsia, hypofibrinogenemia 2° long-standing fetal demise, placental abruption, and DIC related to massive blood loss.

Postpartum blood loss can be reduced by prophylactic use of oxytocin, methylergonovine, or prostaglandins and these same agents are used as the first line of treatment for PPH. A concentrated oxytocin infusion (e.g., 80–100 U in 500 mL over 30 min) may be used. Methylergonovine should be given im only (0.2 mg q 2–4 h up to 1 mg), since iv infusion has been reported to cause acute HTN, stroke, and Sz. Ergot derivatives are contraindicated in patients with Hx of HTN, asthma, Raynaud's syndrome, or migraine. $PGF_{2\alpha}$ (Hemabate) may be injected im (intramyometrial) at a dose of 0.25 mg, up to a total of 2 mg. Misoprostol, an inexpensive PGE, may be given rectally (up to 800 mcg).

Simultaneously, the surgeon should explore the cause of PPH and apply a specific treatment. If PPH is not controlled with treatment of uterine atony, and after volume replacement and correction of any coagulopathy, temporizing measures should be applied while preparing the patient for definitive invasive treatments. Temporizing measures include packing of uterine cavity with a long gauze and use of balloon tamponade. Extensive experience on non-pneumatic anti-shock garment (ASG) on non-pregnant patients is applied to post partum patients with remarkable success in temporizing hypovolemic shock from abdominal and pelvic bleeding. ASG can be applied quickly and results in an immediate 1,500–2,000 mL autotransfusion. ASG should not be used with fetus in situ or thoracic site of hemorrhage. After stabilization, patient should be transferred to Radiology for uterine artery embolization under fluoroscopic control where uterine arteries are selected and absorbable Gelfoam pledgets are introduced. Treatment may be repeated until bleeding is stopped. In known cases of placenta accreta, in anticipation of PPH, catheters have been placed in uterine arteries before C-section.

If selective embolization is not available, or fails to stop hemorrhage, more invasive surgical intervention should be employed, including uterine compression sutures, iliac artery ligation, **uterine devascularization**, and **hysterectomy**. The decision for surgical intervention is made when other options (i.e., medical, interventional radiology) have not been successful in decreasing the hemorrhage. Volume and coagulation factor replacement should continue while proceeding with surgery.

The technique for an **emergent obstetrical hysterectomy** is largely similar to a hysterectomy for other indications. Of note is the engorged and prominent nature of the vessels supplying the gravid uterus. The edematous tissues surrounding the uterus are very friable and may bleed profusely if improperly manipulated. A **supracervical** or **total hysterectomy** may be performed. Through a midline or Pfannenstiel's incision, the uterus is elevated out of the abdominal cavity. The round ligaments are clamped, transected, and ligated; and the anterior leaf of the broad ligament is incised bilaterally from the transected round ligaments to the vesicouterine reflection. The posterior leaf of the broad ligament adjacent to the uterus is entered at a level just below that of the fallopian tubes and uteroovarian ligaments. These are then clamped, transected, and ligated. Next, incision of the posterior leaf of the broad ligament toward the cardinal ligaments is performed. With gentle blunt dissection, the bladder and attached vesicouterine peritoneal flap are dissected off the lower uterine segment. The ascending uterine arteries and veins are identified bilaterally, then clamped, transected, and ligated. If a **subtotal hysterectomy** is planned, the body of the uterus is amputated at this level, and the cervical stump is closed with interrupted sutures. If a total hysterectomy is planned, dissection of the bladder off the cervix is continued until the cervicovaginal margin is identified. The cardinal and uterosacral ligaments are clamped, transected, and ligated, with clamps placed as close to the cervix as possible without including cervical tissue. After the level of the lateral vaginal fornix is reached, a clamp is swung below the cervix, across the lateral vaginal fornix. The cervix is then amputated off the vaginal cuff. Throughout the procedure, it is vital to clamp and ligate any bleeding vessels and to take extra care to avoid damage to the ureter or bladder. Following removal of the uterus and cervix, the vaginal cuff angles are sutured to the ipsilateral cardinal ligament stumps, and the vaginal cuff is closed with a running locked stitch. The abdominal wall is closed in layers.

Usual preop diagnosis: Intractable postpartum bleeding; rupture of gravid uterus

SUMMARY OF PROCEDURE

Position	Supine, with left lateral tilt
Incision	Pfannenstiel's or midline longitudinal
Unique considerations	Monitoring of coagulation parameters and correction of DIC. Consider central venous hemodynamic monitoring. Pediatrics team present, if indicated.
Antibiotics	Cefazolin 1 g iv q 8 h; total 3 doses
Surgical time	2–3 h
Closing considerations	Subcutaneous intraperitoneal drains, if indicated.
EBL	3,000–4,000 mL
Postop care	ICU if blood loss severe; patient may require continued intubation and mechanical ventilatory support. Monitor for infectious morbidity and acute renal failure.
Mortality	< 1%
Morbidity	Hemorrhage Postop febrile morbidity DIC Wound infection Sheehan's syndrome Bladder injury Intraperitoneal bleeding requiring reoperation Vesicovaginal fistula Ureterovaginal fistula Transfusion-related complications
Pain score	7

PATIENT POPULATION CHARACTERISTICS

Age range	Reproductive age
Incidence	0.11% of obstetric patients
Etiology	Unknown
Associated conditions	Placenta accreta; uterine atony nonresponsive to medical or other surgical intervention; extension of cervical tear to lower uterine segment; placenta previa; uterine rupture; uterine inversion

ANESTHETIC CONSIDERATIONS

See Anesthetic Considerations following Cesarean Section, p. 819.

Suggested Readings

1. AbdRabbo SA: Stepwise uterine devascularization: a novel technique for management of uncontrolled postpartum hemorrhage with preservation of the uterus. *Am J Obstet Gynecol* 1994; 171:694–700.
2. B-Lynch C, Coker A, Lawal AH, et al: The B-Lynch surgical technique for the control of massive postpartum haemorrhage: an alternative to hysterectomy? Five cases reported. *Br J Obstet Gynecol* 1997; 104:372–5.
3. Bukowski R, Hankins GDV: Managing postpartum hemorrhage. *Contemporary* OB/GYN 2001; 9:92–105.
4. Cho JH, Jun HS, Lee CN: Hemostatic suturing technique for uterine bleeding during cesarean delivery. *Obstet Gynecol* 2000; 96(1):129–31.
5. Cunningham FG, MacDonald PC, Gant NF, et al: Cesarean delivery and cesarean hysterectomy. In *Williams Obstetrics*, 22nd edition. Appleton & Lange, Stamford: 2005.
6. Hansch E, Chitkara U, McAlpine J, et al: Pelvic arterial embolization for control of obstetric hemorrhage: a five-year experience. *Am J Obstet Gynecol* 1999; 180(6):1454–60.

7. Hensleigh PA: Anti-shock garment provides resuscitation and haemostasis for obstetric haemorrhage. *BJOG* 2002; 109(12):1377–84.
8. Mousa H, Walkinshaw S: Major postpartum hemorrhage. *Curr Opin Obstet Gynecol* 2001; 13(6):595–603.
9. Oyelese Y, Scorza W, Mastrolia R, et al: Postpartum hemorrhage. *Obstet Gynecol Clin North Am* 2007; 34(3):421–41.
10. Tamizian O, Arulkumaraqn S: The surgical management of postpartum hemorrhage. *Curr Opin Obstet Gynecol* 2001; 13(2):127–31.

REPAIR OF UTERINE RUPTURE

SURGICAL CONSIDERATIONS

Description: **Rupture of the gravid uterus** is considered a true obstetric emergency and can be catastrophic, with significant maternal and fetal mortality. The classic symptoms are "shearing" pain, cessation of uterine contractions, loss of fetal heart tones, and the onset of vaginal bleeding. Unfortunately, these warning symptoms occur only in a minority of uterine rupture cases. Extrusion of the placenta through the uterine rupture may result in late decelerations due to uteroplacental insufficiency. Extrusion of the umbilical cord may be manifested by recurrent variable decelerations. Suprapubic pain as the only symptom has not been associated with uterine rupture. Causes of **uterine rupture** include breakdown of a previous uterine scar, obstructed labor, or uterine trauma. In cases where the uterine rupture occurs at the site of a prior uterine scar, the clinical course is usually less severe and the blood loss less than in cases of primary rupture of an intact uterus. The incidence of uterine rupture at the site of the old scar is 0.5% for lower-uterine transverse C-sections, and 12% for classic C-sections.

Total abdominal hysterectomy (see p. 804), or **supracervical hysterectomy** (p. 825), is the definitive therapy; however, depending on the clinical situation and the patient's wishes for future fertility, a **uterine repair** may be undertaken. This consists of a 2- to 3-layered closure of the defect, using synthetic absorbable sutures. A transverse abdominal incision is made ~3 cm above the symphysis pubis and carried to the anterior rectus fascia. The fascia is incised and the muscles of the anterior abdominal wall separated sharply and bluntly from the midline. The peritoneum is elevated and entered sharply. Because of the emergent nature of this condition and the possible massive blood loss associated with rupture of a gravid uterus, the anesthesiologist must act quickly. Prompt O_2 administration, together with aggressive iv fluid resuscitation, is indicated. Serious consideration should be given to the use of unmatched O(-) or type-specific blood until cross-matched blood becomes available. Intraop hypogastric or uterine artery ligation may help minimize blood loss. Patient's coagulation parameters must be monitored, because hypoxia and massive blood loss are associated with DIC.

Usual preop diagnosis: Uterine rupture

SUMMARY OF PROCEDURE

Position	Supine with left-lateral tilt
Incision	Pfannenstiel's (low, transverse abdominal) or midline longitudinal
Unique considerations	Pediatrics team present for infant resuscitation, if necessary. Thorough surgical exploration of the urinary tract (bladder and ureters), because ~10% of cases are associated with bladder lacerations. Cell Saver may be helpful.
Antibiotics	Cefazolin 1 gm iv q 8 h × 3 doses
Surgical time	1–2 h
EBL	500–3,000 mL
Postop care	ICU if blood loss severe; continued intubation and mechanical ventilatory support if aggressive fluid resuscitation results in pulmonary edema. Acute renal failure may occur 2° hypoxic and hypovolemic renal injury at time of acute uterine rupture with massive bleeding; monitor UO and serial renal function tests.
Mortality	Fetal : 35–45% Maternal: 5%

SUMMARY OF PROCEDURE (cont'd)	
Morbidity	Blood transfusion > 5 U: 58% Postop wound infection: 33% Pelvic abscess: 8% Repeat uterine rupture with subsequent pregnancies: 5%
Pain score	6

PATIENT POPULATION CHARACTERISTICS	
Age range	Reproductive age
Incidence	1/1,400 deliveries
Etiology	Prior uterine surgery; grand multiparity; obesity; manual removal of placenta; injury from tools of abortion; direct or indirect violence; oxytocin use; intraamniotic or vaginal prostaglandins; breech extractions; internal or external version; forceps rotation; shoulder dystocia; fundal pressure; neglect (cephalopelvic disproportion, etc.); congenital uterine anomaly; cornual pregnancy; gestational trophoblastic neoplasia; placenta percreta; abruptio placenta

ANESTHETIC CONSIDERATIONS

See Anesthetic Considerations following Cesarean Section. p. 819.

Suggested Readings

1. Chazotte C, Cohen WR: Catastrophic complications of previous cesarean section. *Am J Obstet Gynecol* 1990; 163(3):738–42.
2. Cunningham FG, MacDonald PC, Gant NF, et al: Surgical sterilization. In *Williams Obstetrics*, 22nd edition. Appleton & Lange, Stamford: 2005.
3. Eden RD, Parker RT, Gall SA: Rupture of the pregnant uterus: a 53-year review. *Obstet Gynecol* 1986; 68(5):671–74.
4. Kaczmarczyk M, Sparen P, Terry P, et al: Risk factors for uterine rupture and neonatal consequences of uterine rupture: a population-based study of successive pregnancies in Sweden. *BJOG* 2007; 114(10):1208–14.
5. Plauche WC, VonAlmen W, Muller R: Catastrophic uterine rupture. *Obstet Gynecol* 1984; 64(6):792–97.
6. Sawyer MM, Lipshitz J, Anderson GD, et al: Third-trimester uterine rupture associated with vaginal prostaglandin E_2. *Am J Obstet Gynecol* 1981; 140(6):710–11.
7. Walsh C, Baxi L: Rupture of the primigravid uterus: a review of the literature. *Obstet Gynec Surv* 2007; 62(5):327–34.

Obstetric/Gynecologic Surgery

POSTPARTUM TUBAL LIGATION

SURGICAL CONSIDERATIONS

Description: **Postpartum tubal ligation (PPTL)** is female surgical sterilization performed at the time of cesarean section (C-section) after delivery of the infant and repair of the uterine incision or within the first several days after a vaginal delivery. Although PPTL can be performed immediately postpartum, problems in the neonate may not be immediately evident, and a delay in surgery may be appropriate. If performed after a vaginal delivery, a small infraumbilical incision is made in the skin and carried down through the parietal peritoneum. The fallopian tubes are identified and brought out of the incision. It is important to identify the fimbriated end of the tube to ensure that the structure ligated is not the round ligament. A midsegment portion of the tube over an avascular portion of mesosalpinx is selected and tubal patency is disrupted by a variety of methods (**Pomeroy, Parkland, Irving, Uchida,** etc.). The Pomeroy, or a modification of it, is the most common technique used. The segment of tube grasped is ligated with absorbable suture and the knuckle of tube formed is excised. The cut ends of the tubes should be hemostatic before replacing the tubes into the abdomen. The wound is closed in layers in the usual fashion.

The consent for sterilization requires special consideration. The procedure is strictly elective and voluntary and must be considered permanent, even though reversal may be possible. Some patients will eventually regret the decision to undergo permanent sterilization. The risk of sterilization failure and an increased risk of ectopic pregnancy in case of failure must be reviewed. The full range of alternatives to PPTL, including an interval sterilization procedure (sterilization performed remote from pregnancy) must also be considered.

Usual preop diagnosis: Desire for permanent sterilization

SUMMARY OF PROCEDURE	
Position	Supine; steep Trendelenburg often required to allow bowel to fall away for exposure.
Incision	Infraumbilical
Special instrumentation	Small Richardson and Army/Navy retractors; Babcock clamps; vein retractor
Unique considerations	A special consent form for sterilization must be signed by the patient in advance of the surgery. The bladder must be drained prior to the procedure.
Antibiotics	None recommended
Surgical time	15–25 min (Uchida technique may ↑ operative time)
EBL	10 mL
Postop care	Routine postpartum care after recovery from anesthesia
Mortality	3/100,000
Morbidity	Hemorrhage Infection Incidental damage to bowel or bladder
Pain score	3

PATIENT POPULATION CHARACTERISTICS	
Age range	Reproductive age
Incidence	The most common contraceptive procedure in the United States.

ANESTHETIC CONSIDERATIONS

PREOPERATIVE

Optimal timing of tubal ligation is controversial. The patient with a functioning epidural catheter may benefit from having surgery immediately after delivery. Many surgeons, however, favor waiting 8–24 h, when adequate assessment of the neonate should be complete and risk of maternal hemorrhage lessened. Alternatively, the epidural catheter can be left in place and reinjected later (successful epidural reactivation within 24 h is possible in > 92% of patients). Because pulmonary aspiration remains a theoretical risk, initiation of GA or spinal anesthesia often is delayed 8–24 h until the acute GI changes of pregnancy have regressed. There is no benefit to delaying surgery beyond this time. Shorter hospital stays after vaginal delivery are encouraging more tubal ligations during the first 12 h after delivery. It is unknown whether this will affect morbidity or mortality.

Respiratory	FRC returns to normal almost immediately after delivery. Laryngeal edema may persist in preeclamptic and postpartum patients after protracted expulsive efforts during labor → requirement for a small ETT. **Tests:** As indicated from H&P.
Cardiovascular	The physiologic changes of pregnancy return to normal at varying intervals after delivery. For example, risk of aortocaval compression disappears immediately. Blood volume returns to pre-pregnant values over several days. Postpartum hemorrhage can occur without warning. **Tests:** As indicated from H&P.

Gastrointestinal	Postpartum patients continue to be at risk for acid aspiration, although it is not known exactly when normal GI function returns. If elective PPTL is planned within 8 h of delivery, patient should have no oral intake of solid foods during labor and the postpartum period. Precautions for prevention of acid aspiration should be followed as discussed in Cesarean Section, p. 820.
Neurological	Local anesthetic requirements for spinal anesthesia remain decreased after delivery but are greater than for pregnant patients.
Laboratory	Hct; other tests as indicated from H&P.
Premedication	Precautions should be taken to ↓ risk of aspiration pneumonitis, as discussed in Cesarean Section, p. 820.

INTRAOPERATIVE

Anesthetic technique: Spinal anesthesia is preferred, if a functioning epidural catheter is not in place. Epidural catheters frequently become dislodged after a patient becomes ambulatory. GA is acceptable if patient has a strong preference or if contraindications to regional anesthesia exist. These patients may be at risk for aspiration of gastric contents at least 8–24 h postdelivery.

Regional anesthesia:

Spinal	For technique and monitoring for spinal anesthesia, see Cesarean Section, p. 822. Hyperbaric bupivacaine (7.5–12 mg) ± fentanyl (10–25 mcg). With the patient supine, adjust position of the operating table to obtain a T6 level of anesthesia. Sedate patient as necessary with small doses of iv midazolam 0.5–1.0 mg or opioid.
Epidural	A 3 mL epidural test dose, followed after 3–5 min by 15–20 mL of 1.5–2% lidocaine with 1:200,000 epinephrine injected incrementally. Additional local anesthetic as needed to ensure adequate level of anesthesia.

General anesthesia:

Induction	Rapid-sequence induction with STP (4–5 mg/kg) or propofol (1.5–2 mg/kg) and succinylcholine (1 mg/kg) for ET intubation.	
Maintenance	Standard maintenance (p. B-2)	
Emergence	Extubation should be delayed until patient is fully awake and protective airway reflexes have returned.	
Blood and fluid requirements	Minimal blood loss IV: 18 ga × 1 NS/LR @ 2–4 mL/kg/h	1–1.5 L dextrose-free crystalloid immediately prior to regional anesthesia
Monitoring	Standard monitors (p. B-1)	
Positioning	✓ and pad pressure points ✓ eyes	
Complications	None specific	

POSTOPERATIVE

Complications	Minimal bleeding

Obstetric/Gynecologic Surgery

Pain management	**Intraspinal opioids** 10–25 mcg fentanyl **Parenteral opioids:** IV or im opioids (e.g., morphine 2–4 mg iv up to 20 mg), or meperidine 10–20 mg iv q 10–15 min, titrated to RR and patient's level of pain and instituted in the recovery room.	Intrathecal fentanyl 10–25 mcg, given with spinal local anesthetic, enhances intraop anesthesia, particularly with low doses of bupivacaine, and provides several h postop analgesia.
Tests	None routinely indicated.	

Suggested Readings

1. Abouleish El: Postpartum tubal ligation requires more bupivacaine for spinal anesthesia than does cesarean section. *Anesth Analg* 1986; 65(8):897–900.
2. American College of Obstetricians and Gynecologists: ACOG Committee Opinion, Committee on Ethics: Sterilization of women, including those with mental disabilities. No 371, 2007 (replaces No 63, 1988, No 73, 1989, and No 216 1999). *Obstet Gynecol* 2007;110(1):217–20.
3. American College of Obstetricians and Gynecologists: ACOG Committee Opinion, Committee on Obstetrics, Maternal and Fetal Sterilization: Postpartum tubal sterilization. No 105, 1992. *Int J Gynaecol Obstet* 1992; 39(3):244.
4. American College of Obstetricians and Gynecologists: ACOG technical bulletin. Benefits and Risks of Sterilization. No 46, 2003 (replaces No 222, 1996 and No 113, 1988). *Obstet Gynecol* 2003; 102(3):647–58.
5. Bucklin BA: Postpartum tubal ligation: timing and other anesthetic considerations. *Clin Obstet Gynecol* 2003; 46(3)657–66.
6. Cunningham FG, MacDonald PC, Grant NF, et al., eds: Surgical sterilization. In *Williams Obstetrics*, 22nd edition. Appleton & Lange, Stamford: 2005.
7. Goodman EJ, Dumas SD: The rate of successful reactivation of labor epidural catheters for postpartum tubal ligation surgery. Reg *Anesth Pain Med* 1998; 23(3):258–61.
8. Hampl KF, Schneider MC, Pargger H, et al: A similar incidence of transient neurologic symptoms after spinal anesthesia with 2 percent and 5 percent lidocaine. *Anesth Analg* 1996; 83:1051–54.
9. Hughes SC, Levinson G, Rosen MA, et al., eds: *Shnider and Levinson's Anesthesia for Obstetrics*, 4th edition. Lippincott Williams & Wilkins, Philadelphia: 2002.
10. Practice Guidelines for Obstetrical Anesthesia: A report by the American Society of Anesthesiologists' Task Force on Obstetrical Anesthesia. *Anesthesiology* 1999; 90:600–11.
11. Viscomi CM, Rathmell JP: Labor epidural reactivation or spinal anesthesia for delayed postpartum tubal ligation: a cost comparison. *Anesthesiology* 1994; 81:A1160.
12. Wheeless CR Jr: *Atlas of Pelvic Surgery*, 2nd edition. Lea & Febiger, Philadelphia: 1988, 282–8.

REPAIR OF VAGINAL/CERVICAL LACERATIONS

SURGICAL CONSIDERATIONS

Description: Vaginal and cervical lacerations may occur 2° trauma of spontaneous and operative vaginal delivery. Adequate repair requires optimal surgical assistance, exposure, and patient comfort. Repair may be performed in a birthing bed, or may require patient positioning, lighting, anesthesia, or monitoring capabilities available only in an OR. Vaginal and cervical lacerations can extend into the perineum, rectum, urethra, bladder, lower uterine segment, broad ligament, or peritoneal cavity.

Lacerations of the lower vagina generally are easy to identify and repair. Small, superficial lacerations that do not bleed often do not need repair, whereas larger ones should be approximated. Deep lacerations may cause profuse bleeding; if it persists despite placement of multiple stitches, brief tamponade may be adequate to achieve hemostasis or vaginal packing may be required. Lacerations involving the perineum are classified as follows: First degree—involves break in mucosa and skin. Second degree—involves deeper tissue (bulbocavernosus and levator ani fascia and muscle). Third degree—involves anal sphincter. Fourth degree—extends into rectal mucosa. First- and second-degree lacerations are repaired in layers with continuous or interrupted stitches. The skin usually is closed with a subcuticular stitch. When the anal sphincter is lacerated, it often retracts. The ends are grasped with Allis clamps and approximated with multiple stitches. When the laceration extends into the rectum, the rectal mucosa usually is closed in two layers, with the second layer imbricating the first. With periurethral lacerations, a catheter may need to be placed in the urethra to prevent passing a stitch through it. A laceration involving the urethra or bladder should be closed in multiple layers, followed by bladder drainage for several days.

Lacerations of the upper vagina are often difficult to visualize. Uterine bleeding and the umbilical cord of an undelivered placenta can obscure the field, and it can be difficult to determine if bleeding is vaginal or uterine. It is helpful to deliver the placenta and control uterine bleeding before proceeding. After visualization is adequate, it is important to place the first stitch above the apex of the laceration to control bleeding from vessels that may have retracted. Again, vaginal packing may be required if oozing of blood persists.

Superficial **lacerations of the cervix** occur with most deliveries but usually do not require treatment. Deep lacerations can cause significant blood loss, especially when they involve larger branches from the uterine artery or extend into the lower uterine segment. Again, the first stitch must be placed above the apex of the laceration to control bleeding from vessels that may have retracted. A **laparotomy** may be necessary if a laceration extends into the lower uterine segment or broad ligament and is causing significant bleeding that cannot be controlled otherwise. Alternatively, uterine artery embolization may be considered.

Usual preop diagnosis: Vaginal or cervical laceration

SUMMARY OF PROCEDURE	
Position	Dorsal lithotomy
Incision	None (unless exploratory laparotomy is performed)
Special instrumentation	Right-angle retractors; ring forceps; Allis clamps; Gelpi retractor; vaginal packing
Antibiotics	May be used for lacerations involving entry into the peritoneal cavity or the rectal mucosa.
Surgical time	10–45 min (possibly longer if exploratory laparotomy is performed)
EBL	Variable. Possible need for transfusion. Areas that persistently ooze after repeated placement of suture may be managed with vaginal packing.
Postop care	PACU → ward
Mortality	Rare
Morbidity	Hemorrhage Hematoma Infection Rectovaginal fistula Vesicovaginal fistula
Pain score	3

PATIENT POPULATION CHARACTERISTICS	
Age range	Reproductive age
Incidence	Not uncommon
Etiology	Trauma 2° spontaneous or operative vaginal delivery (98%); other vaginal/pelvic trauma (2%)
Associated conditions	Major blood loss possible; with non-obstetric etiology, the possibility of sexual assault needs to be explored.

ANESTHETIC CONSIDERATIONS

PREOPERATIVE

Vaginal and cervical lacerations may go undetected until considerable blood loss has occurred. Patients should be examined carefully for Sx of hypovolemia with appropriate volume resuscitation prior to anesthesia.

Obstetric/Gynecologic Surgery

Respiratory	FRC returns to normal almost immediately after delivery. **Tests:** As indicated from H&P.
Cardiovascular	The physiologic changes of pregnancy return to normal at varying intervals after delivery. For example, risk of aortocaval compression disappears immediately. Blood volume returns to pre-pregnant values over several days. Postpartum hemorrhage can occur without warning. Ensure adequate fluid resuscitation prior to induction of GA or regional anesthesia. **Tests:** As indicated from H&P.
Gastrointestinal	Postpartum patients continue to be at risk for acid aspiration, although it is not known exactly when normal GI function returns. Precautions for prevention of acid aspiration should be followed as discussed in Cesarean Section, p. 820.
Neurological	Local anesthetic requirements for spinal anesthesia remain decreased after delivery.
Laboratory	Hct; other tests as indicated from H&P.
Premedication	Precautions should be taken to ↓ risk of aspiration pneumonitis, as discussed in Cesarean Section, p. 820.

INTRAOPERATIVE

Anesthetic technique: In many patients, a functioning epidural catheter will be in place, and supplemental doses of anesthetic may be given to provide adequate analgesia for the surgery. If no epidural is placed and the patient is hemodynamically stable, a spinal anesthetic may be satisfactory. Occasionally, GA may be required.

Regional anesthesia:

Epidural	Supplemental doses of local anesthetic (2-chloroprocaine or 1.5–2% lidocaine 10–15 mL) injected incrementally with patient in sitting position (if tolerated) to promote perineal anesthesia.
Spinal	Hyperbaric bupivacaine 0.75% 7.5–10 mg with patient in sitting position, if tolerated. 24–25 ga pencil-point needle (e.g. Sprotte or Whitacre) to ↓ incidence of spinal headache. Anesthesia to T10 is usually adequate. Repair of more extensive lacerations may require a higher level and, consequently, a higher dose of anesthetic.
Combined spinal-epidural (CSE)	An alternative technique combining the rapid onset and density of spinal anesthesia with the flexibility of continuous epidural anesthesia (e.g., if necessary to extend the duration or intensity of the block). Apply monitors, administer fluid, and position as for spinal/epidural. The most common technique is the needle-through-needle. When the epidural space is located with a 17-ga Tuohy needle, insert a 26–27 ga pencil-point spinal needle through the Tuohy needle and administer 7.5–10 mg of spinal bupivacaine. Secure the epidural catheter and use if needed. (An epidural test dose is advisable.)

General anesthesia:

Induction	Rapid-sequence induction (see p. B-4) with STP (4–5 mg/kg) or propofol (2–3 mg/kg) and succinylcholine (1 mg/kg) for ET intubation. If significant blood loss, ketamine 1.5 mg/kg is preferred for induction.	
Maintenance	Standard maintenance (see p. B-2).	
Emergence	Extubation should be delayed until patient is fully awake and protective airway reflexes have returned.	
Blood and fluid requirements	IV: 16–18 ga × 1 NS/LR @ 2–4 mL/kg/h	1–1.5 L dextrose-free crystalloid immediately prior to regional anesthesia. Blood loss may be extensive until laceration is repaired.

Monitoring	Standard monitors (see p. B-1)	
Complications	Bleeding	
Positioning	✓ and pad pressure points ✓ eyes	* **NB:** peroneal nerve compression at lateral fibular head → foot drop.

POSTOPERATIVE

Complications	Bleeding Peroneal nerve injury (2° lithotomy position)	 Nerve injury manifests as foot drop and loss of sensation over dorsum of foot.
Pain management	**Intraspinal opioids:** 10 mcg fentanyl **Parenteral opioids:** iv or im opioids (e.g., morphine 2–4 mg iv analgesia up to 20 mg, or meperidine 10–20 mg iv q 10–15 min up to 100 mg) instituted in the recovery room.	Intrathecal fentanyl given with spinal local anesthetic enhances intraop anesthesia and provides 3–4 h postop analgesia.
Tests	Hct	

Suggested Readings

1. American College of Obstetricians and Gynecologists: ACOG Educational Bulletin: Postpartum hemorrhage. No 76, 2006 (replaces No 243, 1998 and No 143, 1990). *Obstet Gynecol* 2006;108(4):1039–47.
2. Cunningham FG, MacDonald PC, Grant NF, eds: Obstetrical hemorrhage. In *Williams Obstetrics,* 22nd edition. Appleton & Lange, Stamford: 2005.
3. Golan A, David MP: Repair of birth injuries. In *Operative Perinatology: Invasive Obstetric Techniques.* Iffy L, Charles D, eds. MacMillan, New York: 1984, 730–50.
4. Zuspan P, Quilligan EJ, eds: *Douglas-Stromme: Operative Obstetrics,* 5th edition. Appleton & Lange, New York: 1988.

CERVICAL CERCLAGE-ELECTIVE AND EMERGENT

SURGICAL CONSIDERATIONS

Description: Cervical cerclage is the reinforcement of the cervix to prevent premature cervical dilation in a patient with an incompetent cervix. With cervical incompetence, there is painless dilation of the cervix in the midtrimester of pregnancy. The membranes bulge through the cervix and rupture, followed by delivery of a severely premature infant.

An **elective cerclage** is performed prophylactically before pregnancy or usually after the first trimester of pregnancy on a patient with a Hx of cervical incompetence. If cerclage is performed before pregnancy, it may need to be removed because of spontaneous abortion or fetal anomalies. It generally is performed between 14–16 wk gestation, but may be performed as early as 10 wk gestation. An **emergent (rescue) cerclage** is performed in a patient who presents in the second trimester with painless cervical dilation and/or effacement. Ultrasound is performed before the procedure to confirm viability and to r/o major congenital anomalies. An emergent cerclage should not be performed if there is advanced cervical dilation or any evidence of infection, contractions, or uterine bleeding.

There are two types of cerclage procedures generally performed: the McDonald and the Shirodkar. The **McDonald cerclage** is technically easier, and the one most commonly performed. A purse-string stitch with nonabsorbable monofilament suture is placed high around the cervix near the level of the internal os and tied at the twelve o'clock position. The end of the suture is cut long to facilitate removal. The cerclage is removed electively at term or earlier if there is rupture of membranes, persistent contractions, bleeding, or evidence of infection. The **Shirodkar cerclage** involves incising the cervix transversely, anteriorly, and posteriorly, and advancing the bladder off the cervix. A nonabsorbable monofilament suture is placed submucosally between the incisions, and the mucosa is closed, burying the stitch. A Shirodkar cerclage may be left for future pregnancies if abdominal delivery is performed. If the cervix cannot be adequately accessed through the vagina, cerclage may be attempted through laparotomy or laparoscopy.

Usual preop diagnosis: Cervical incompetence

SUMMARY OF PROCEDURE

Position	Dorsal lithotomy, with use of cane stirrups. Left lateral pelvic tilt (if performed during pregnancy); Trendelenburg
Incision	None with McDonald cerclage; transverse cervical with Shirodkar cerclage
Special instrumentation	Right-angle retractors; monofilament, nonabsorbable stitch
Unique considerations	For emergent cerclage, when prolapsing membranes are present, they may be reduced by filling the bladder and/or possibly removing amniotic fluid transabdominally.
Antibiotics	None recommended.
Surgical time	30 min–1 h (may be longer for Shirodkar cerclage)
EBL	25–50 mL (may be higher with the Shirodkar cerclage)
Postop care	PACU → ward; tocolysis with indomethacin or other agent can be considered.
Mortality	Rare
Morbidity	Morbidity is increased for emergent cerclage, especially when performed later in 2nd trimester. The McDonald cerclage is associated with less trauma and bleeding than the Shirodkar cerclage. Cervical trauma Rupture of membranes Chorioamnionitis Preterm labor Spontaneous abortion
Pain score	McDonald—2; Shirodkar—3

PATIENT POPULATION CHARACTERISTICS

Age range	Reproductive age
Incidence	Not uncommon
Etiology	Cervical trauma from previous vaginal delivery; cervical trauma at time of previous D&C; previous treatment for cervical dysplasia (laser therapy, cryotherapy, loop electrosurgical excision procedure [LEEP]/large loop excision of transitional zone [LLETZ], cone biopsy); congenital anomalies; idiopathic

ANESTHETIC CONSIDERATIONS

PREOPERATIVE

This is a generally fit and healthy patient population. Little will need to be done other than routine tests, unless otherwise indicated. Cerclage is usually performed between 14–24 wk of pregnancy. When performed after 20 wk, relevant physiologic changes are as discussed under Cesarean Section, p. 819. Patient may receive drugs such as β-sympathomimetics (e.g., terbutaline), nifedipine, or indomethacin to decrease uterine irritability.

Laboratory	Hct; other tests as indicated from H&P.
Premedication	None usually. If >18 wks gestation, precautions should be taken to decrease risk of aspiration pneumonitis, as discussed in Cesarean Section, p. 820.

INTRAOPERATIVE

Anesthetic technique: Drug exposure during the critical period of organogenesis (15–56 d) should be minimized, although no particular anesthetic techniques or agents have proven teratogenic in humans. Through an action on vitamin B_{12}, N_2O inhibits methionine synthase, which is involved in thymidine and methionine synthesis. This may explain why N_2O is teratogenic in rodents. There is no evidence, however, that N_2O is teratogenic when used for cervical cerclage or other operations in humans. Large, retrospective analysis has shown no increase in congenital abnormalities following surgery under anesthesia. Avoid diazepam during the period of organogenesis (may → cleft lip). Ensure adequate uteroplacental perfusion and fetal oxygenation by maintaining normal maternal BP and oxyhemoglobin saturation. Use left uterine displacement after 20 wk gestation. Maternal hyperventilation and IPPV may diminish uteroplacental and umbilical blood flow. Monitoring FHR may permit optimization of fetal well-being by adjustment of anesthetic technique or patient position. Spinal anesthesia is ideal as it minimizes fetal drug exposure and provides good operating conditions. Risk of headache is low with the use of small gauge pencil-point needles (e.g., Sprotte, Whitacre). Epidural anesthesia is an appropriate alternative for this procedure. GA may be used if regional anesthesia is contraindicated.

Regional anesthesia:

Spinal	Hyperbaric bupivacaine 7–10 mg ± fentanyl 10–15 mcg. Position patient to obtain T8 block. Monitor BP every min until stable, then every 3–5 min. Treat >20% ↓ in BP or SBP < 95–100 mmHg with additional fluids and ephedrine 5–10 mg iv.

General anesthesia:

Induction	Standard induction (see p. B-2). If > 18 wk gestation, rapid-sequence induction is indicated (see p. B-4).	
Maintenance	Standard maintenance (p. B-2). If < 15–18 wk gestation, use of LMA or mask anesthesia with O_2/N_2O/volatile agent/opioid is appropriate. If > 18 wk gestation, ET intubation will be necessary.	
Emergence	If > 18 wk gestation, extubate patient when fully awake and protective airway reflexes have returned.	
Blood and fluid requirements	Minimal blood loss IV: 18 ga × 1 NS/LR @ 4 mL/kg/h	1–1.5 L dextrose-free crystalloid immediately prior to regional anesthesia
Monitoring	Standard monitors (see p. B-1) ±FHR monitor	Consider FHR monitoring for viable fetuses and in earlier gestation, as the FHR may indicate inadequate placental perfusion and can guide BP management.
Positioning	Left uterine displacement, if > 20 wk gestation ✓ and pad pressure points ✓ eyes	Left uterine displacement with a wedge under mattress should be used for pregnant patients. * **NB:** peroneal nerve compression at lateral fibular head → foot drop.

POSTOPERATIVE

Complications	Preterm labor Maternal dysrhythmias Hypotension	Observe for preterm labor in recovery area. Tocolytic agents β-adrenergic agents) given to inhibit uterine contractions can cause maternal dysrhythmias or ↓ BP.
	Peroneal nerve injury	Nerve injury manifests as foot drop and loss of sensation over dorsum of foot.

Pain management	**Intraspinal opioids:** 10–15 mcg fentanyl **Parenteral opioids:** iv or im opioids (e.g., morphine 2–4 mg iv up to 20 mg or meperidine 10–20 mg q 15 min up to 100 mg) instituted in the recovery room. **Oral analgesics:** NSAIDS (e.g., ibuprofen), acetaminophen ± codeine (or equivalent oral narcotics), once patient can tolerate oral medication.	Intrathecal fentanyl given with spinal improves intraop analgesia and provides short-period postop analgesia. Risk of delayed respiration depression minimal in healthy patients.

Suggested Readings

1. Aboujaoude R, Maloof P, Alvarez M, et al: A novel method for laparoscopic abdominal cerclage utilizing minimally invasive hydrodissection: a case report. *J Reprod Med* 2007; 52(5):428–30.
2. Aldridge LM, Tunstall ME: Nitrous oxide and the fetus. A review and the results of a retrospective study of 175 cases of anaesthesia for insertion of a Shirodkar suture. *Br J Anaesth* 1986; 58(12):1348–56.
3. American College of Obstetricians and Gynecologists: *Cervical Cerclage, Prophylactic. ACOG Criteria, Set 17.* American College of Obstetricians and Gynecologists, Washington: 1996.
4. American College of Obstetricians and Gynecologists: *Cervical Cerclage, Therapeutic. ACOG Criteria, Set 18.* American College of Obstetricians and Gynecologists, Washington: 1996.
5. American College of Obstetricians and Gynecologists: Cervical insufficiency. ACOG Practice Bulletin No 48. *Int J Gynecol Obstet* 2004; 85:81–9.
6. Barmat L, Glaser G, Davis G, et al: Da Vinci-assisted abdominal cerclage. *Fertil Steril* 2007; 88(5):1437.
7. Crawford IS, Lewis M: Nitrous oxide in early human pregnancy. *Anaesthesia* 1986; 41(9):900–5.
8. Czeizel AE, Pataki T, Rockenbauer M: Reproductive outcome after exposure to surgery under anesthesia during pregnancy. *Arch Gynecol Obstet* 1998; 261(4):193–9.
9. Gilstrap LC, Cunningham FG, Vandorsten JP, eds. Operative procedures on the Cervix. In *Operative Obstetrics.* McGraw-Hill, New York: 2002:503–22.
10. Goodman S: Anesthesia for nonobstetric surgery in the pregnant patient. *Semin Perinatol* 2002; 26(2):136–45.
11. Levinson G: Anesthesia for surgery during pregnancy. In Hughes SC, Levinson G, Rosen MA, eds. *Shnider and Levinson's Anesthesia for Obstetrics*, 4th ed. Lippincott Williams & Wilkins, Philadelphia: 2002.
12. Mazze RI, Kallen B: Reproductive outcome after anesthesia and operation during pregnancy: a registry study of 5405 cases. *Am J Obstet Gynecol* 1989; 161(5):1178–85.
13. Naughton NN, Cohen SE: Non-obstetric surgery during pregnancy. In Chestnut D, ed. *Obstetric Anesthesia: Principles and Practice*, 3rd ed. Mosby, St. Louis: 2004.
14. Rosen MA: Management of anesthesia for the pregnant surgical patient. *Anesthesiology* 1999; 91:1159–63.
15. Safra MJ, Oakley GP Jr: Association between cleft lip with or without cleft palate and prenatal exposure to diazepam. *Lancet* 1975; 2(7933):478–84.

REMOVAL OF RETAINED PLACENTA

SURGICAL CONSIDERATIONS

Description: In most deliveries, the placenta is easily removed with gentle cord traction and uterine massage. If, after 30 min, the placenta remains undelivered, **manual removal,** following either parenteral analgesia or GA, must be initiated. NTG (100–200 mcg iv or 0.4 mg sublingually) may induce uterine relaxation during manual removal. A possible alternative to manual removal involves injection of 10 mL of oxytocin (10 U/mL) into the umbilical vein; however, the success of this procedure is unpredictable. A retained placental fragment may cause immediate or late postpartum hemorrhage. An ultrasound evaluation of the uterus may help in the detection of a retained fragment. If retained products are found, **curettage** is recommended. Frequently, the retained product will already have been flushed out of the uterus by brisk bleeding. In such cases, iv oxytocin, rectal misoprostol, im prostaglandins or methylergonovine may be administered to contract the uterus prior to curettage.

Bleeding from a retained placenta or fragment is frequently brisk, so the anesthesiologist must be ready to administer iv fluids and O_2, and to correct any coagulopathy. Cross-matched blood must be available. Placenta accreta, if extensive, can cause profuse bleeding at delivery, and a hysterectomy is often necessary.

Oxytocin 20–40 U in 1,000 mL of LR should be administered at a rate sufficient to maintain uterine tone after manual removal of the placenta or after sharp/suction curettage of a retained placental fragment.

Usual preop diagnosis: Retained placenta

SUMMARY OF PROCEDURE	
Position	Dorsal lithotomy
Incision	None
Special instrumentation	Banjo curette/suction cannula
Unique considerations	IV fluids; use of blood and blood products, as needed; monitoring of VS
Antibiotics	Cefazolin 1 g iv q 8 h; 3 total doses
Surgical time	30 min
EBL	300–900 mL
Postop care	PACU → ward. Monitor for infection and further bleeding.
Mortality	Rare
Morbidity	Hemorrhage Endometritis Uterine perforation 2° curettage Asherman's syndrome Transfusion-related morbidity (hepatitis, HIV, transfusion reactions)
Pain score	5

PATIENT POPULATION CHARACTERISTICS	
Age range	Reproductive age
Incidence	0.25–0.8% of vaginal deliveries
Etiology	Unknown
Associated conditions	Placenta accreta; avulsed cotyledon; succenturiate lobe

ANESTHETIC CONSIDERATIONS

PREOPERATIVE

The degree of urgency associated with these patients may vary dramatically. Some patients may be hemodynamically unstable as a result of continued bleeding in the postpartum period; others may have a retained placenta with minimal bleeding. Patient's volume status should be carefully assessed.

Respiratory	FRC returns to normal almost immediately after delivery. **Tests:** As indicated from H&P.
Cardiovascular	Restore intravascular volume prior to institution of analgesia or anesthesia. Extension of existing lumbar epidural blockade may aggravate hypovolemia and should proceed with caution. Consider possibility of placenta accreta (placental villi are attached to myometrium).
Gastrointestinal	Postpartum patients continue to be at risk for acid aspiration, although it is not known exactly when normal GI function returns. Precautions for prevention of acid aspiration should be followed as discussed in Cesarean Section, p. 820.

Neurological	Local anesthetic requirements for neuraxial anesthesia remain decreased after delivery.
Hematologic	Coagulopathy can develop with retained placenta if bleeding is severe and persistent. **Tests:** Hct, PT, PTT, Plt, FSP, as indicated.
Laboratory	Other tests as indicated from H&P. T&C for 2 U+ if time permits. Emergency transfusion with Type O(-) or type-specific blood may be necessary.
Premedication	Precaution should be taken to decrease risk of aspiration, as discussed in Cesarean Section, p. 820.

INTRAOPERATIVE

Anesthetic technique: Anesthesia for the removal of a retained placenta may vary from MAC to GA performed as an emergency. In the multiparous patient, MAC may be sufficient to enable the obstetrician to empty the uterus. If better analgesia and additional uterine relaxation are needed, however, then GA may be required. The incidence of retained placenta is about 1%. If intravascular volume has been restored and an existing epidural catheter is in place, the block can be extended to provide adequate anesthesia. Initiating spinal anesthesia is also an option if intravascular volume status is adequate, there is no active bleeding, and uterine relaxation is not required. Small doses of opioids and midazolam sometimes provide sufficient analgesia and sedation to allow removal of a retained placenta without compromising maternal safety. If this proves inadequate or hemorrhage is severe, however, GA with ET intubation is required. Anecdotal experience indicates that NTG in 100–200 mcg iv boluses or sublingual NTG 400 mcg provides uterine relaxation and delivery of a retained placenta in normovolemic patients receiving iv analgesia.

Regional anesthesia:

Spinal	For technique and monitoring of spinal anesthesia, see Cesarean Section, p. 822. Hyperbaric bupivacaine 8–10 mg; adjust the position of operating table to obtain T8 level of anesthesia.
Epidural	For technique and monitoring, see Cesarean Section, p. 822. Administer increments of 3% 2-chloroprocaine or 2% lidocaine with 1:200,000 epinephrine and bicarbonate until block level adequate. Additional local anesthetic as needed to ensure adequate level of anesthesia.
MAC	Titrate small doses of opioids (e.g., fentanyl 25–50 mcg) and midazolam 0.5–1.0 mg or ketamine 0.1 mg/kg. Sedation and analgesia should be titrated carefully, due to the potential risk of pulmonary aspiration in the parturient with an unprotected airway. Ensure patient is awake and responsive throughout. Consider NTG 100–200 mcg iv for uterine relaxation, repeated as necessary to obtain the desired effect. Transient ↓ BP may follow vasodilation due to NTG, and should be treated with volume and pressors if necessary.

General anesthesia:

Induction	Preoxygenation, rapid-sequence induction with cricoid pressure (see p. B-4), and hydration, as discussed in Cesarean Section (p. 823). Ketamine (1 mg/kg) is preferred for induction of hypotensive patient; but, in larger doses (> 1.5 mg/kg), it theoretically may increase uterine tone and make removal of placenta more difficult. Anesthesia with N_2O/O_2 + opioid (but no volatile agent) often permits delivery of the placenta.	
Maintenance	If uterine relaxation is necessary, administer volatile agent (> 1 MAC) or NTG (see above) until uterine tone decreases.	
Emergence	Extubation should be delayed until patient is fully awake and protective airway reflexes have returned.	
Blood and fluid requirements	Anticipate large blood loss IV: 16–18 ga × 1–2 NS/LR @ 6–8 mL/kg/h	Infuse crystalloid solution (1–1.5L) to maintain BP prior to regional anesthesia. Treat ↓ BP with fluids and ephedrine, and by decreasing concentration of volatile agent. Surgery is usually brief; additional muscle relaxation not usually necessary.

Monitoring	Standard monitors (see p. B-1)	
Complications	Bleeding	Uterine atony: Rectal misoprostol, concentrated oxytocin infusion, 277–1667 mU/min. (50–300 U in 500 mL 1/2 normal saline over 3 h), uterine massage, ± methylergonovine 0.2 mg im (may →↑ BP), or $PGF_{2\alpha}$ (Hemabate) 250 mcg iv/im/intrauterine (may → cardiovascular collapse/bronchospasm).
Positioning	✓ and pad pressure points ✓ eyes	***NB:** peroneal nerve compression at lateral fibular head → foot drop.

POSTOPERATIVE

Complications	Peroneal nerve injury (2° lithotomy position) Bleeding	Nerve injury manifested as foot drop and loss of sensation over dorsum of foot. See uterine atony, above.
Pain management	IV or im opioids, titrated to effect, as usual, instituted in recovery room.	
Tests	Hct	

Suggested Readings

1. Chedraui P, Insuasti D: Intravenous nitroglycerin in the management of retained placenta. *Gynecol Obstet Invest* 2003; 56(2):61–4.
2. Clark SL: Placenta previa and abruptio placentae. In *Maternal-Fetal Medicine: Principles and Practice,* 5th edition. Creasy RK, Resnik R, eds. WB Saunders, Philadelphia: 2003.
3. Cunningham FG, MacDonald PC, Gant NF, eds: Obstetrical hemorrhage. In *Williams Obstetrics,* 22nd edition. Appleton & Lange, Stamford: 2005.
4. Decherney AH, Pernoll ML, ed: *Current Obstetric and Gynecologic Diagnosis and Treatment,* 9th edition. Appleton & Lange, Stamford: 2006.
5. Desimone CA, Norris MC, Leighton BL: Intravenous nitroglycerin aids manual extraction of a retained placenta [Letter]. *Anesthesiology* 1990; 73(4):787.
6. Gilstrap LC, Cunningham FG, Vandorsten JP: *Operative Obstetrics.* New York: McGraw-Hill, 2002: 397–419.
7. Hughes SC, Levinson G, Rosen MA, et al., eds: *Shnider and Levinson's Anesthesia for Obstetrics,* 4th edition. Lippincott Williams & Wilkins, Philadelphia: 2002.
8. Jha S, Chiu J, Yeo I: Intravenous nitroglycerine versus general anaesthesia for placental extraction–a sequential comparison. *Med Sci Monit* 2003; 9(7):CS63–6.
9. O'Grady JP, Gimovsky ML, McIlhargie, eds: *Operative Obstetrics.* Williams & Wilkins, Baltimore: 2002, 503–4.
10. Owen J, Hauth JC: Concentrated oxytocin plus low-dose prostaglandin E2 compared with prostaglandin E2 vaginal suppositories for second-trimester pregnancy termination. *Obstet Gynecol* 1996;88:110–3.
11. Practice Guidelines for Obstetrical Anesthesia: An updated report by the American Society of Anesthesiologists' Task Force on Obstetrical Anesthesia. *Anesthesiology* 2007; 106(4)843–63.
12. Riley ET, Flanagan B, Cohen SE, et al: Intravenous nitroglycerin: a potent uterine relaxant for emergency obstetrical procedures. Report of 3 cases and review of literature. *Int J Obstet Anesth* 1996; 5:264–8.

MANAGEMENT OF UTERINE INVERSION

SURGICAL CONSIDERATIONS

Description: Uterine inversion is associated with fundal implantation of the placenta whereby a thinning of the uterine wall, together with placental separation, causes an invagination of the myometrium, resulting in inversion. Vigorous fundal pressure or cord traction also can contribute to uterine inversion, which can be complete or incomplete. **Complete inversion** results in the inverted fundus extending beyond the cervix and appearing at the vaginal introitus, whereas in an **incompletely inverted uterus,** the fundus does not extend beyond the external cervical os. Uterine inversion can cause hemorrhage and shock out of proportion to observed bleeding, and must be managed as an obstetrical emergency. An anesthesiologist must be called to the delivery room as soon as a diagnosis of uterine inversion is made. The ready availability of GA is paramount. IV access with two infusion systems and appropriate fluid resuscitation must be initiated emergently. Blood and blood products should be available for administration as indicated.

Frequently, **uterine replacement** can be accomplished with iv tocolytics, such as terbutaline, $MgSO_4$, and, more recently, NTG; however, GA with a volatile agent may be necessary. Three primary methods for uterine replacement are the Johnson, Huntington and Haultain procedures. Normally, the **Johnson method** is attempted first. Persistent pressure applied to the fundus is used to elevate the uterus into the vagina. The placenta, if attached, is not removed until iv resuscitation has been initiated, and iv tocolytics (or anesthesia) have been administered. Oxytocin is given when the uterus has been replaced. Laparotomy must be performed if uterine replacement with the Johnson method is unsuccessful. The **Huntington procedure** involves grasping the round ligaments and applying upward traction on them, while an assistant exerts upward pressure on the uterus via a hand in the vagina. If the inverted uterus is trapped below the cervical ring, the **Haultain procedure** is used. This procedure involves making a longitudinal fundal incision posteriorly to allow easier reinversion of the fundus. Hydrostatic and laparoscopic reduction of uterine inversion have also been described.

Usual preop diagnosis: Uterine inversion

SUMMARY OF PROCEDURES

	Manual Reinversion	Huntington/Haultain
Position	Dorsal lithotomy	Supine
Incision	None	Pfannenstiel's or midline longitudinal
Unique considerations	Prompt O_2 and iv fluid resuscitation; use of blood and blood products as necessary.	⇐
Antibiotics	Cefazolin 1 g iv q 8 h; total 3 doses	⇐
Surgical time	30 min	1–2 h
EBL	150–4,000 mL	⇐
Postop care	±ICU. ARDS may necessitate mechanical ventilation. Monitor for acute renal failure 2° hypoxia and hypovolemia.	⇐
Mortality	Rare	⇐
Morbidity	Febrile morbidity Clinical shock Infectious morbidity from blood transfusion	⇐ ⇐ ⇐
Pain score	5	7

PATIENT POPULATION CHARACTERISTICS

Age range	Reproductive age
Incidence	1/2,000–6,000 deliveries
Etiology	Unknown
Associated conditions	Fundal implantation of the placenta; primiparity; intrapartum oxytocin; placenta accreta; therapy of preeclampsia with $MgSO_4$; macrosomic fetus

ANESTHETIC CONSIDERATIONS

PREOPERATIVE

These patients often present in shock out of proportion to blood loss; and immediate resuscitation may be necessary. Since patient condition will improve as soon as the uterus is replaced, however, surgical treatment should not be delayed.

Respiratory	FRC returns to normal almost immediately after delivery. **Tests:** As indicated from H&P.
Cardiovascular	Massive hemorrhage and pain usual with complete inversion. Prior to induction, insert large-bore iv and rapidly infuse fluids, including colloid, to treat ↓ BP. Blood transfusion may be necessary, although is seldom available until after surgery.
Gastrointestinal	Postpartum patients continue to be at risk for acid aspiration, although it is not known exactly when normal GI function returns. Precautions for prevention of acid aspiration should be followed as discussed in Cesarean Section, p. 820.
Neurological	Local anesthetic requirements for neuraxial anesthesia remain decreased after delivery.
Laboratory	Hct; Plt; other tests as indicated from H&P. T&C for 2 U; keep 2 U ahead.
Premedication	Na citrate 30 mL po within 30 min of induction. If time permits, other agents to decrease risk of aspiration pneumonitis, as discussed in Cesarean Section, p. 820.

INTRAOPERATIVE

Anesthetic technique: Attempted uterine replacement and induction of anesthesia should not await intravascular volume replacement. Bleeding usually stops when uterus is replaced. IV NTG (50–200 mcg) is very effective in providing uterine relaxation to facilitate replacement, and can be given immediately in the patient's room. Other tocolytics, such as terbutaline or Mg^{++}, also may help. **Do not give oxytocin before uterine replacement.** Sometimes, however, GETA is required, often with increasing concentrations of volatile agents to facilitate uterine replacement. If regional anesthesia (e.g., epidural or spinal) was used for delivery, replacement of uterus may be accomplished with little further anesthetic intervention, with or without NTG. If regional anesthesia was not used for delivery, iv analgesia with small doses of fentanyl (25–50 mcg iv) occasionally allows reduction.

Induction	Rapid-sequence induction (see p. B-4) with ketamine (1.0 mg/kg) preferred. Higher dose may adversely increase uterine tone.	
Maintenance	Halothane, isoflurane and sevoflurane are all effective uterine relaxants, but sevoflurane is most rapidly eliminated. ↓ BP should be treated with fluids + vasopressors.	
Emergence	Extubation should be delayed until patient is fully awake and protective airway reflexes have returned.	
Blood and fluid requirements	Significant blood loss IV: 16–18 ga × 1 or 2	Possible continued blood loss after reduction of uterus due to uterine atony.
Monitoring	Standard monitors (see p. B-1)	Arterial line may be useful, if time allows.
Positioning	✓ and pad pressure points ✓ eyes	
Complications	Uterine atony Massive blood loss	Rx:↓ volatile anesthetic concentrations. Oxytocin infusion, uterine massage, ±methylergonovine 0.2 mg im (may ↑ BP), $PGF_{2\alpha}$ (Hemabate) 250 mcg iv/im/intrauterine (may → cardiovascular collapse/bronchospasm)

POSTOPERATIVE

Complications	Bleeding
Pain management	Parenteral opioids, titrated to effect, as usual, instituted in recovery room.
Tests	Hct

Suggested Readings

1. American College of Obstetricians and Gynecologists: ACOG practice bulletin: postpartum hemorrhage. No 76, 2006 (replaces No 243, 1998 and No 143, 1990). *Obstet Gynecol* 2006; 108(4)1039–47.
2. Bowes W: Clinical aspects of normal and abnormal labor. In *Maternal-Fetal Medicine: Principles and Practice,* 5th edition. Creasy RK, Resnik R, Bralow L, eds. WB Saunders, Philadelphia: 2003.
3. Cunningham FG, MacDonald PC, Gant NF, eds: *Williams Obstetrics,* 22nd edition. Appleton & Lange, Stamford: 2005.
4. Hostetler DR, Bosworth MF: Uterine inversion: a life threatening obstetric emergency. *J Am Board Fam Pract* 2000; 13(2): 120–3.
5. Hughes SC, Levinson G, Rosen MA, et al., eds: *Shnider and Levinson's Anesthesia for Obstetrics,* 4th edition. Lippincott Williams & Wilkins, Philadelphia: 2002.
6. Riley ET, Flanagan B, Cohen SE, et al: Intravenous nitroglycerin: a potent relaxant for emergency obstetrical procedures. Review of literature and reports of 3 cases. *Int J Obstet Anesth* 1996; 5:264–8.
7. Tan KH, Luddin NS: Hydrostatic reduction of acute uterine inversion. *Int J Gynaecol Obstet* 2005; 1:63–4.
8. Vijayaraghavan R, Sujutha Y: Acute postpartum uterine inversion with haemorrhagic shock: laparoscopic reduction: a new method of management? *BJOG* 2006; 9:1100–2.

CHAPTER

8.4 Laparoscopic Procedures for Gynecologic Surgery

SURGEON

Camran R. Nezhat, MD

ANESTHESIOLOGIST

Cliff Schmiesing, MD

LAPAROSCOPIC SURGERY FOR ENDOMETRIOSIS

SURGICAL CONSIDERATIONS

Description: There are numerous theories about the etiology of endometriosis, including: (a) the peritoneal cavity is seeded with endometrial cells via the fallopian tubes during menses; (b) totipotential cells in the peritoneal cavity are transformed by hormonal exposure into endometrial cells; (c) endometrial cells are transported intravascularly or via lymphatics to ectopic sites, where they respond to hormonal stimuli (this theory has been used to explain the presence of endometriosis in the brain and pleura); (d) decreased cytotoxic response of the immune system suggests that it is a failure of natural killer-cell activity to eliminate ectopic endometrial cells; and (e) it is an inherited disorder, because the incidence of endometriosis is higher in first-degree relatives. Intervention usually is indicated for intractable pain, infertility, or impaired function of the gastrointestinal (GI) or genitourinary (GU) tracts. GU endometriosis may range from superficial involvement of peritoneum overlying the ureters and bladder to frankly invasive endometriosis penetrating through to bladder mucosa. Scarring and fibrosis can → ureteral obstruction and hydronephrosis with renal insufficiency. Patients with GI endometriosis may have thickening of the rectovaginal septum, suggesting obliteration of the posterior cul-de-sac or rectosigmoid involvement. Adhesions may make rectovaginal examination difficult or painful. Pelvic structures may be immobile, suggesting adhesions are fixing bowel or bladder to the uterus. Sigmoidoscopy should be performed to r/o malignancy and to determine whether endometriosis has penetrated through to the bowel mucosa.

Two treatment approaches can be taken. **Hysterectomy** and **bilateral salpingo-oophorectomy** (**BSO**) may be indicated for patients with severe symptoms who have not responded to medical or conservative surgical treatment and who do not desire fertility (see **laparoscopic hysterectomy**, p. 852). **Bilateral oophorectomy** might be necessary to eliminate the estrogen that sustains and stimulates the ectopic endometrium. Conservative surgery is indicated for women who desire pregnancy and whose disease is responsible for their symptoms of pain or infertility. Although seldom curative, surgery improves fertility and offers at least temporary pain relief. **Laparoscopy** (Fig. 8.4-1) is the most appropriate surgical technique for the diagnosis and treatment of endometriosis. Data from animal and clinical studies suggest that laparoscopic surgery is more effective for adhesiolysis, causes fewer de novo adhesions than laparotomy and reduces impairment of tuboovarian function. Special consideration must be given to the patient's past Hx of abdominal or pelvic surgery, pelvic inflammatory disease (PID) and endometriosis, as this will affect the choice of surgical approach. Ovarian endometriosis is common and can be challenging to diagnose and treat. It can be divided into Type I (primary endometriomas or small cysts measuring > 3 cm on the ovarian surface) or Type II (secondary endometriomas, usually functional [e.g., follicular] in origin, which become enlarged to > 3 cm). Regardless of classification, it is critical to remove all endometriotic lesions to prevent exacerbation and recurrence.

Bladder endometriosis: If the lesions are superficial, **hydrodissection** and **vaporization** are adequate for removal. Using hydrodissection, the areolar tissue between the serosa and muscularis beneath the implants is dissected. The lesion is circumscribed with a laser and fluid is injected into the resulting defect. The lesion is grasped with forceps and dissected with the laser. Traction allows the small blood vessels supplying the surrounding tissue to be coagulated as the lesion is resected. Frequent irrigation is necessary to remove char, ascertain the depth of vaporization, and ensure that the lesion does not involve the muscularis and mucosa. Endometriosis extending to the muscularis but without mucosal involvement can be treated laparoscopically, and any residual or deeper lesions may be treated successfully with hormonal therapy. When endometriosis involves **full bladder-wall thickness,** the lesion is excised and the bladder reconstructed in one layer. Simultaneous cystoscopy is performed and bilateral ureteral catheters are inserted. The bladder dome is held near the midline with the grasping forceps and the endometriotic nodule is excised 5 mm beyond the lesions. An incision is made with the CO_2 laser, using the suction-irrigating probe as a backstop. The specimen is removed from the abdominal cavity with a long grasping forceps. The lesion is regrasped and removed with the laparoscope as one unit. CO_2 distends the bladder cavity, allowing excellent observation of its interior. After again identifying the ureters and examining the bladder mucosa, the bladder is closed. Cystoscopy is performed to identify possible leaks. The duration of laparoscopic segmental cystectomy is ~35 min. Patients are discharged the following day and instructed to take trimethoprim and sulfamethoxazole for 2 wk. The Foley catheter is removed 7–14 d later, and cystograms are made.

GI/GU endometriosis: In a patient with no Hx of pelvic surgery, the **direct-trocar insertion method** may be used with an intraumbilical incision. The incision is made within the umbilicus because this is the anatomical area closest to the fascia and peritoneum and involves the least risk of injury to retroperitoneal structures. Once the incision is made, the trocar is placed through the skin incision. Using an intraumbilical incision and inserting the trocar at 90° facilitates access to the abdominal cavity and decreases the risk of aortocaval injury. This technique of direct-trocar insertion may

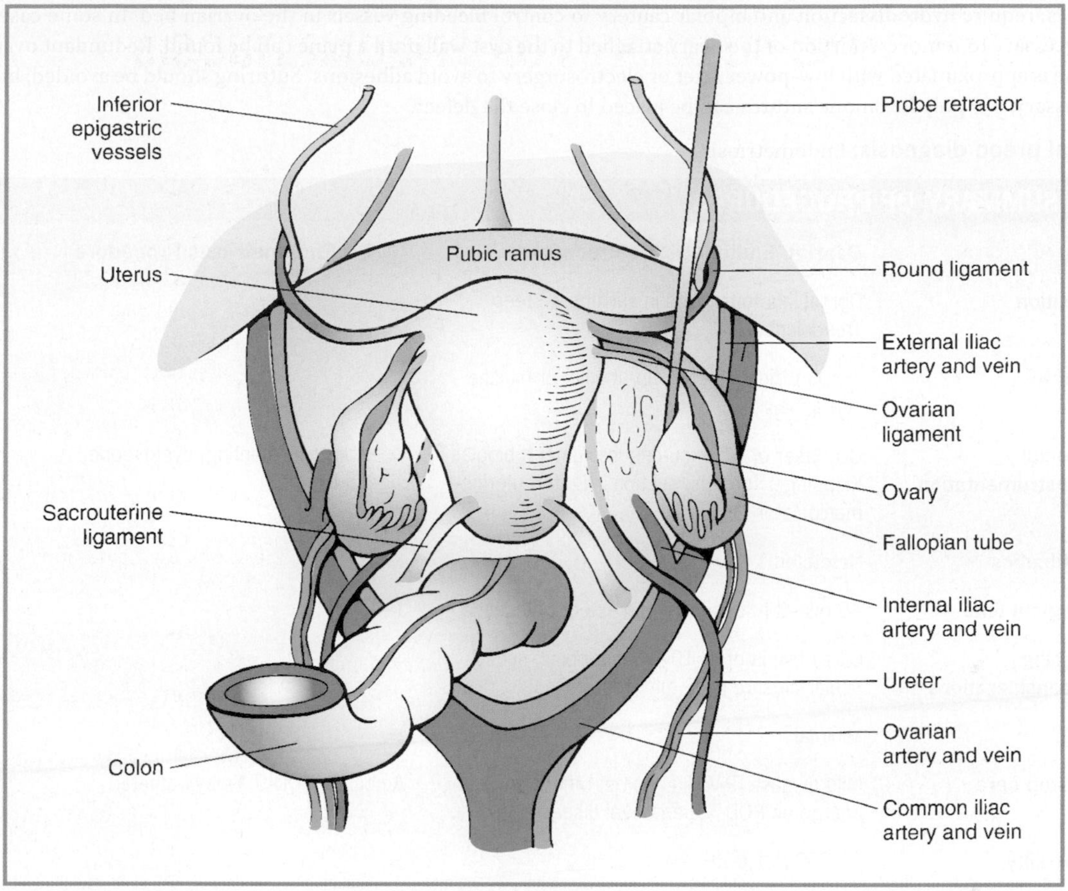

Figure 8.4-1. Laparoscopic view of the female pelvis.

not be recommended for patients who have had prior laparotomy or laparoscopy that revealed adhesive disease. After insufflation of the abdomen with CO_2, assessment of intraabdominal and pelvic structures is made. A second skin incision is made 2–3 cm above the symphysis. A Foley catheter should be in place throughout the procedure to allow continuous drainage of the bladder, thereby reducing the likelihood of trocar injury to the bladder. A 5-mm trocar is placed under direct visualization with attention to peritoneal vessels and bladder. Two lateral ports are placed in a similar fashion, taking care to avoid the inferior epigastric vessels. The suction irrigator, a blunt grasper, and the bipolar cautery are placed into the trocars. Filmy adhesions of the bowel or omentum to the anterior abdominal wall or uterus are lysed using CO_2 laser, bipolar cautery, monopolar scissors, or hydrodissection. Treatment of peritoneal endometriosis ranges from laser ablation of superficial peritoneal implants to excision and dissection of deeply embedded, fibrotic areas. Scarring from endometriosis that has penetrated the peritoneum to involve deeper structures destroys normal surgical planes and distorts anatomical relationships. Identification of structures and landmarks is critical before attempting to treat the peritoneal disease. During laparoscopy, normal anatomic relationships along the pelvic sidewall may appear distorted. Because scarring from endometriosis may change these relationships, patients are at risk for accidental ureteral or vascular injury at the time of surgery. Identification of ureters and blood vessels is critical prior to treatment of pelvic sidewall disease. Although different modalities have been used, hydrodissection and high-power superpulse or ultrapulse CO_2 lasers are the best options for endometriosis treatment. Because the CO_2 laser does not penetrate water, this fluid backstop allows the surgeon to work on selected tissue with a greater safety margin.

Ovarian endometriosis: A Type I endometrioma of < 2 cm is vaporized using laser or bipolar coagulation. Larger Type I lesions may require excision using scissors or biopsy forceps. For Type IIA endometriomas, the procedure begins with lysis of periovarian adhesions using laser or monopolar scissors. The ovarian cortex is evaluated, the endometrioma cyst is identified, the cyst wall is perforated (using laser or scissors), and an irrigation device is inserted to assess cyst contents and wall. Suspicious areas are biopsied and sent for frozen-section analysis. A plane is developed between the cyst wall and ovary by grasping the wall and separating it from ovarian stroma, using traction and countertraction. Difficult areas where endometriosis has embedded through the cyst wall, disrupting the planes, require hydrodissection and bipolar cautery to control bleeding vessels in the ovarian bed. In some cases, it is necessary to remove a portion of the ovary attached to the cyst wall until a plane can be found. Redundant ovarian tissue is approximated with low-power laser or electrosurgery to avoid adhesions. Suturing should be avoided; but, if necessary, 4-0 polydioxanone sutures can be placed to close the defect.

Usual preop diagnosis: Endometriosis

SUMMARY OF PROCEDURES

	Ovarian Endometriosis Procedure	GI/GU Endometriosis Procedure
Position	Dorsal lithotomy, legs in stirrups ± steep Trendelenburg	⇐
Incision	Intraumbilical; lateral suprapubic; or midline suprapubic	⇐
Special instrumentation	CO_2 laser or other cutting instrument; bipolar Kleppinger forceps; suction irrigator, uterine manipulator	⇐ ± Ureteral stenting, cystoscope, sigmoidoscope
Antibiotics	Cefotetan 1 g iv	⇐
Surgical time	45 min–3 h, depending on extent of disease	1–4 h
Closing considerations	Close fascia of all 10–12 mm ports; subcuticular closure for 5 mm trocar sites	⇐
EBL	Minimal	⇐
Postop care	Mild disease: PACU → home; otherwise, discharge on POD 1 (peritoneal disease).	Ambulate POD 0; Foley catheter.
Mortality	0.08–0.2/1,000	⇐
Morbidity	Overall complication rate: 2.5% Conversion to laparotomy: 0.42% VAE (CO_2 embolism) Peroneal nerve damage Vascular damage Bowel injury: Rare Urinary tract injury: Rare	Urinary tract injury
Pain score	4–8	4–8

PATIENT POPULATION CHARACTERISTICS

Age range	Reproductive age	20s–40s
Incidence	10–15% of all reproductive age women/25% of all gynecologic laparotomies	1–11% of women with known endometriosis
Etiology	Numerous theories (see above).	Extensive disseminated endometriosis
Associated conditions	Infertility; pelvic pain; bladder or bowel symptoms; HTN (2° to urinary tract involvement); GI tract involvement (3–7%)	Pelvic pain; GI or GU symptoms

ANESTHETIC CONSIDERATIONS

See Anesthetic Considerations following Laparoscopic Hysterectomy, p. 854.

Suggested Reading

1. Berker B, Nezhat C, Nezhat F, et al: Laparoscopic treatment of endometriosis. In *Nezhat's Operative Gynecologic Laporoscopy and Hysteroscopy*. Nezhat C, Nezhat F, eds. Cambridge University Press, New York: 2008, 263–303.

LAPAROSCOPIC SURGERY FOR ECTOPIC PREGNANCY

SURGICAL CONSIDERATIONS

Description: Ectopic pregnancy is defined as a pregnancy occurring outside the uterus. The majority of ectopic pregnancies occur in the fallopian tubes (95–97%); the remainder occurs in the cornua (2–4%), ovary (0.1%), cervix (0.1%), or abdomen (0.03%). Ectopic pregnancy remains a leading cause of maternal morbidity and mortality. Predisposing factors include Hx of tubal ligation or other tubal surgery, pelvic inflammatory disease (PID), IUD use and Hx of in vitro fertilization (IVF) or other treatments for infertility. Other associations include developmental anomalies of the Müllerian system, intrauterine polyps, or myomas.

Patients present with lower quadrant pain, vaginal bleeding, and an ↑ β-hCG. Shoulder pain from subdiaphragmatic intraperitoneal blood is a less frequent finding. Treatment options for an asymptomatic ectopic gestation include operative laparoscopy or a trial of medical management with intramuscular methotrexate. In cases where the size of the ectopic pregnancy is too large for conservative medical management (> 3.5 cm), and the patient is hemodynamically stable, operative management is essential. Hypotension or an acute abdomen in the presence of a positive β-hCG value are strongly suggestive of rupture and require expeditious surgical intervention.

Access to the abdomen is obtained in the usual fashion (e.g., through a Veress needle or direct-trocar insertion, followed by insufflation and insertion of accessory trocars). Ruptured tubal pregnancies can be treated endoscopically if the bleeding has ceased or can be controlled. Actively bleeding vessels are identified and cauterized, and forced irrigation is used to dislodge clots and trophoblastic tissue. Depending on their size, the products of conception (POCs) are removed through either a 5 or 10 mm trocar sleeve or placed into an endoscopic bag for removal; or a minilaparotomy can be performed. Copious irrigation should follow to ensure hemostasis and identify and remove any remaining trophoblastic tissue. Trophoblast is invasive, and residual tissue may implant into bowel, bladder, peritoneum, or other abdominal structures and cause significant future morbidity.

For an unruptured ectopic pregnancy, the tube is identified and stabilized using laparoscopic forceps. To minimize bleeding, 5–7 mL of a solution of 50 U vasopressin in 100 mL NS is injected into the mesosalpinx just below the ectopic pregnancy and over the antimesenteric surface of the tubal segment containing the gestation. Intravascular injection of vasopressin solution can precipitate acute arterial HTN, bradycardia, or even death; therefore, care must be taken to avoid such injection. A linear incision is made over the thinnest portion of the tube. The pregnancy usually protrudes through the incision, and forceful irrigation will dislodge the gestation from its implantation site. Oozing from the tube is common, but usually ceases spontaneously.

In a ruptured tubal or isthmic pregnancy, resection of the tubal segment containing the gestation is preferable to salpingostomy. **Segmental tubal resection** is performed with bipolar electrosurgery, laser (KTP, argon, Nd:YAG, or CO_2), sutures, or stapling devices. Similarly, **total salpingectomy** can be performed by progressive coagulation and cutting the mesosalpinx, which is separated from the uterus using bipolar coagulation and scissors or laser. The isolated tube segment containing the ectopic pregnancy is removed intact or in sectioned parts through the 10-mm trocar sleeve. At the completion of the procedure, the abdomen is irrigated and inspected and incisions are closed in the usual fashion.

Usual preop diagnosis: Ectopic pregnancy

SUMMARY OF PROCEDURE	
Position	Dorsal lithotomy, legs in Allen universal stirrups, steep Trendelenburg
Incision	Intraumbilical, lateral suprapubic, midline suprapubic
Special instrumentation	CO_2 laser; laparoscopic instrumentation, uterine manipulator
Unique considerations	Intraperitoneal hemorrhage and hemodynamic instability are potential risks. Patient should be cross-matched for 2 U PRBCs.
Antibiotics	Cefotetan 1 g iv
Surgical time	45 min–2 h

SUMMARY OF PROCEDURE (cont'd)	
Closing considerations	Fascia of 10–12 mm trocar sites closed in layers. Smaller 5 mm ports closed in a subcuticular fashion.
EBL	100 mL, severe hemorrhage, if ruptured.
Postop care	The patient may be admitted overnight for observation. Quantitative β-hCG should be followed until undetectable, to r/o the possibility of retained trophoblastic tissue.
Mortality	5/1000. For any laparoscopy: 0.08–0.2/1,000
Morbidity	Overall complication rate: 2.5% Hemorrhage and need for transfusion Conversion to laparotomy: 4.2/1,000 Air embolism: Rare Unintended puncture of a viscus: Rare Puncture of a major vessel: Rare Insufflation of incorrect site: Rare
Pain score	3–5

PATIENT POPULATION CHARACTERISTICS	
Age range	Reproductive-age females
Incidence	1/100 pregnancies
Etiology	Distorted tubal or uterine anatomy
Associated conditions	Hx of PID; endometriosis; tubal damage; IUD; IVF

ANESTHETIC CONSIDERATIONS

See Anesthetic Considerations following Laparoscopic Hysterectomy, p. 854.

Suggested Readings

1. Farquar CM: Ectopic Pregnancy. *Lancet* 2006; 366:583–91.
2. Querleu D, Chapron C: Complications of gynecologic laparoscopic surgery. *Curr Opin Obstet Gynecol* 1995; 7:257–61.
3. Tedesco M, Curet, M: Laparoscopy in the Pregnant Patient. In *Nezhat's Operative Gynecologic Laporoscopy and Hysteroscopy*, 3rd edition. Nezhat C, Nezhat F eds. Cambridge University Press, New York: 2008, 499–508.

LAPAROSCOPIC MYOMECTOMY

SURGICAL CONSIDERATIONS

Description: Uterine myomata or fibroids are the most common uterine neoplasm, affecting ~20–25% of women of reproductive age. Their growth is influenced by many factors, such as estrogen acting alone or synergistically with growth hormone and human placental lactogen in pregnancy. The severity of symptoms depends on the number, size, and location of the tumors. Symptoms may include constipation, pelvic or abdominal pressure, urinary frequency and, most commonly, menorrhagia. Although leiomyomata are seldom the cause of infertility, there is a link between fibroids, fetal wastage, and premature delivery. Patients present with profound anemia from menorrhagia or menometrorrhagia, the usual indications for surgery. Other indications include rapidly changing size, ureteral compression, hydroureter, or hydronephrosis and size > 12 wk. Size, number, and location are the primary factors that will determine surgical approach to myomata.

The simplest approach is a combination of **laparoscopy** and **minilaparotomy** for removal of myomas. This approach limits operative time. Three major objectives of laparoscopic myomectomy are: minimizing blood loss, which can be severe; minimizing postop adhesion formation; and maintaining uterine-wall integrity. Preop treatment with GnRH analogues to shrink fibroids has been shown to decrease the size of the myoma and reduce the need for transfusion. Although myomectomy is performed to preserve fertility, postop adhesion formation often jeopardizes this goal. This can be minimized by using a single, vertical, anterior midline uterine incision.

The abdomen is entered in the usual fashion for laparoscopy (e.g., through Veress needle or direct trocar insertion, followed by insufflation and insertion of accessory trocars). To reduce blood loss in pedunculated myomas, diluted vasopressin (3–5 mL) is injected into the base of the stalk where it joins the uterine wall. IV vasopressin can cause ↑ BP, myocardial ischemia, dysrhythmias, or cardiac arrest, and should be avoided. The pedicle is coagulated with the bipolar forceps and cut with CO_2 laser or scissors. For subserosal or intramural myomas, diluted vasopressin is injected between the myometrium and the myoma pseudocapsule. An incision is made on the serosa overlying the myoma using the CO_2 laser or monopolar needle. As the incision is made, the myometrium is retracted away from graspers to expose the tumor. Vessels are coagulated prior to cutting. After the myoma is removed, the myoma bed is irrigated with LR, and bleeding points are coagulated again. After closure, the serosa is irrigated with LR. An adhesion barrier may be placed over the incision site to prevent future adhesion formation. Uteroperitoneal fistulae may follow laparoscopic myomectomy, because meticulous laparoscopic approximation of all layers of the myometrium is impossible. The use of electrocoagulation for hemostasis inside the uterine defect also may increase this risk.

Removal of the specimen is frequently the most challenging aspect of the operation. The myoma can be removed either by **morcellation of the specimen** or by extending the suprapubic incision. Alternatively, **posterior culdotomy** may be performed and the myoma removed via the vagina. A retractor is placed in the vagina and the laser is used to cut along the tented vaginal mucosa. After the myoma is removed, the incision can be closed using laparoscopic suturing. Minilaparotomy or culdotomy facilitate removal but increase postop wound complication risks, such as infection or hernia formation. After myoma removal, the abdomen and pelvis are irrigated, the patient is taken out of the Trendelenburg position, and any fluid that might have tracked into the upper abdomen is suctioned. The ports are closed in the usual fashion.

Usual preop diagnosis: Uterine myoma, fibroids

SUMMARY OF PROCEDURE

Position	Dorsal lithotomy; steep Trendelenburg to move bowel out of operating field
Incisions	Infraumbilical, 5 mm lateral and 5–12 mm midline suprapubic; minilaparotomy via extension of suprapubic incision or posterior culdotomy for removal of large myomata
Special instrumentation	CO_2 laser; laparoscopic instrumentation, uterine manipulator
Unique considerations	For large myomata: pretreatment with GnRH analogues (3–6 mo). Intraop injection of dilute vasopressin (1 IU in 100 mL LR) into myometrium to ↓ bleeding.
Antibiotics	Cefotetan 1 g iv
Surgical time	1–3 h
Closing considerations	Close fascia of all 10–12 mm ports; 5 mm ports are closed in a subcuticular fashion. Fascial closure essential in minilaparotomy. Posterior culdotomy requires laparoscopic suturing or vaginal closure.
EBL	100–600 mL
Postop care	1–2 d hospital stay; early ambulation; clear liquids POD 0; gradually advance diet after discharge home.
Mortality	0.08–0.2/1,000
Morbidity	Rates: 1.3–5.9/100 Peroneal nerve damage from positioning Severe bleeding with possible need for transfusion Uteroperitoneal fistulae Infertility GI/GU injury Air embolism

SUMMARY OF PROCEDURE (cont'd)	
	Puncture of a major vessel Insufflation in the wrong place Need for emergent laparotomy Uterine rupture in pregnancy: 2% Adhesion formation
Pain score	4–6

PATIENT POPULATION CHARACTERISTICS	
Age range	Reproductive-age women; myomas shrink in postmenopausal women and are less symptomatic.
Incidence	20–25% of all women
Etiology	Benign transformation and proliferation of a single smooth-muscle cell
Associated conditions	Menorrhagia; anemia; ureteral obstruction; pelvic pain or pressure

ANESTHETIC CONSIDERATIONS

See Anesthetic Considerations following Laparoscopic Hysterectomy, p. 854.

Suggested readings

1. Glaser MH: Minimally invasive approaches to myomectomy. In *Nezhat's Operative Gynecologic Laporoscopy and Hysteroscopy*, 3rd edition. Nezhat C, Nezhat F eds. Cambridge University Press, New York: 2008, 316–33.
2. Querleu D, Chapron C: Complications of gynecologic laparoscopic surgery. *Curr Opin Obstet Gynecol* 1995; 7:257–61.

LAPAROSCOPIC HYSTERECTOMY

SURGICAL CONSIDERATIONS

Description: Hysterectomy is the second most common gynecologic operation, after cesarean section. The indications for **hysterectomy ± salpingo-oophorectomy** include: leiomyomata (38%); malignancy (15%); ovarian tumors (10%); abnormal bleeding (13%); adenomyosis (9%); pelvic pain or adhesions (5%); endometriosis (3%); and uterine prolapse (1%). Other less common indications include parametrial disease, pelvic infection, and complications of pregnancy and delivery. Selection of surgical approach to hysterectomy requires consideration of the patient's age, medical Hx, Hx of prior pelvic surgery, the presence or possibility of adhesions or endometriosis, uterine size, adnexal pathology, and the presence or amount of uterine prolapse.

Laparoscopic hysterectomy offers the advantages of excellent visibility and exposure. There is shorter recovery time, rapid return of bowel function, less pain, and a lower wound complication rate. The disadvantages are higher cost and the level of surgical expertise required. The most commonly performed procedure is the **laparoscopically assisted vaginal hysterectomy** (LAVH), in which hysterectomy is begun by laparoscopy, but four or more steps are performed vaginally. Variants include: **total laparoscopic hysterectomy** (TLH), in which all steps are performed laparoscopically; **subtotal laparoscopic hysterectomy** (SLH), a supracervical hysterectomy; and **vaginally assisted laparoscopic hysterectomy** (VALH), in which four steps are completed laparoscopically and the procedure is completed vaginally. Combinations are usually performed, depending on findings at surgery. A mechanical and antibiotic bowel preparation is advised. Consultation with a urologist, bowel surgeon, and oncologist are sought as necessary.

Access to the abdomen is obtained in the usual fashion (e.g., through a Veress needle or direct-trocar insertion, followed by insufflation and insertion of accessory trocars). Diagnostic laparoscopy is performed, adhesions lysed, and any endometriosis treated. The course of the ureters is noted through the peritoneum until they are no longer visible at the level of the cardinal ligaments. When ureters cannot be identified clearly because of severe scarring or endometriosis, they are dissected retroperitoneally, and the dissection proceeds as for a radical hysterectomy. At the cardinal ligaments, the peritoneum is opened above or below the ureter and hydrodissection is performed to lift the peritoneum off the ureter without damaging it. Routine hysterectomy using hydrodissection to identify tissue planes and limit blood loss can be performed following identification of the ureters.

If the ovaries are to be spared, the uteroovarian ligament, proximal tube and mesosalpinx are cauterized and cut progressively, and the posterior leaf of the broad ligament is opened with hydrodissection. The bladder is dissected free from the cervix and uterus; and, if bladder trauma is suspected, 5 mL of indigo carmine injected iv (possible ↑ BP) may help identify the site of perforation. Next, the uterine vessels are identified, noted to be free of ureter, desiccated, and cut. At the level of the cardinal ligaments, the ureters and descending branches of the uterine artery are close to one another and the cervix; therefore, cardinal ligament dissection and cautery must be precise to prevent bleeding and ureteral injury. A small uterus can be removed easily through the vagina. In benign disease, a large uterus can be morcellated and then removed segmentally through the vagina. Pneumoperitoneum will be lost during this procedure, and care must be taken to keep instruments free of bowel or other abdominal structures as this occurs.

If the procedure is to be completed entirely laparoscopically, pneumoperitoneum can be maintained by placing a glove containing two 4" × 4" sponges in the vagina. The vaginal wall is cut circumferentially, and the uterus is pulled to mid vagina, but not removed, to preserve the pneumoperitoneum. Alternatively, the uterus may be morcellated and removed through a 10-mm suprapubic port or placed in a laparoscopic specimen bag. The suprapubic incision also may be extended into a minilaparotomy incision for specimen removal. The vaginal cuff is closed transversely using laparoscopic sutures, and any coexisting cystocele or enterocele is repaired. After the uterus is removed and the vaginal cuff closed, the pelvic and abdominal cavities are reevaluated, irrigated, and cleared of blood and debris. The skin and fascia are closed in the usual fashion.

Variant procedure: In patients with severe rectovaginal and vesical endometriosis, the retroperitoneal space is entered using hydrodissection, and the external iliac vessels, hypogastric artery, and ureter are identified. In cases where extensive dissection and resultant blood loss is anticipated, coagulation or ligation of the hypogastric artery with laparoscopic clips may be performed. Endometriosis of the rectum, rectovaginal septum, and uterosacral ligaments is treated by vaporization, excision, or a combination of these. Sigmoidoscopy with concurrent laparoscopic visualization of the pelvis may be necessary to r/o the presence of incidental enterotomy. Cystoscopy with ureteral stenting also may be indicated to identify anatomy. (Treatment of bladder and bowel endometriosis have been described in Laparoscopic Surgery for Endometriosis, p. 846.) After the ureter is identified along its course and entry into the bladder, the uterine vessels are retracted medially and separated from the ureter using a CO_2 laser. The uterus is retracted medially and the ureter laterally as the cardinal and uterosacral ligaments are cauterized and cut with the ureter under direct visualization. After these vascular pedicles have been ligated and all endometriosis treated, the hysterectomy and specimen removal proceed as described above.

Robotic Assistance: With the advent of robotic-assisted surgery all of the above procedures can be performed with three-dimensional visualization, improved magnification and 90° articulation of the robotic arm. With this set up, the surgeon sits at a console and two or three assistants are at the side of the patient. The only major difference is location and size of trocars used for the robotic arms as well as possible increased operative time. Patient positioning is not different from standard laparoscopy.

Usual preop diagnosis: Leiomyomata; malignancy; ovarian tumors; abnormal bleeding; adenomyosis; pelvic pain or adhesions; endometriosis; uterine prolapse; parametrial disease; pelvic infection; complications of pregnancy and delivery

SUMMARY OF PROCEDURE

Position	Dorsal lithotomy; legs in Allen universal stirrups; steep Trendelenburg
Incisions	Intraumbilical; bilateral suprapubic; midline suprapubic (5 or 10 mm)
Special instrumentation	CO_2 laser; laparoscopic instruments, uterine manipulator
Unique considerations	Extensive ureterolysis and treatment of endometriosis may require addition of cystoscopy, ureteral stent placement, and/or sigmoidoscopy.
Antibiotics	Cefotetan 1 g iv

SUMMARY OF PROCEDURE (cont'd)	
Surgical time	2–6 h. Operative time is increased in cases of extensive adhesiolysis or endometriosis.
Closing considerations	Close fascia of all 10–12 mm ports; 5 mm trocar sites closed in a subcuticular fashion. Mini-laparotomy closure if needed.
EBL	100–800 mL, depending on anatomy and difficulty of dissection
Postop care	Clear liquid diet; ambulate POD 1
Mortality	0.08–0.2/1,000
Morbidity	Overall complication rate: 2.5% Conversion to laparotomy: 4.2/1,000 Air embolism: Rare Peroneal nerve damage from positioning: Rare Unintended puncture of a viscous: Rare Puncture of a major vessel: Rare Insufflation of incorrect site: Rare Urinary and ureteral trauma, including fistulae: 1.6%
Pain score	6–9

PATIENT POPULATION CHARACTERISTICS	
Age range	30s–70s
Incidence	20% of women < 40 yr; 37% of women < age 65
Etiology	See Associated Conditions.
Associated conditions	Myomata; abnormal uterine bleeding; adenomyosis; malignancy; pelvic pain; endometriosis

Suggested Readings

1. Advincula A, Falcone T: Minimally invasive gynecologic surgery: the evolving role of robotics. In *Nezhat's Operative Gynecologic Laporoscopy and Hysteroscopy*, 3rd edition. Nezhat C, Nezhat F eds. Cambridge University Press, New York: 2008, 567–76.
2. Lanfranco AR, Castellanos AE, Desai JP, et al: Robotic surgery: a current perspective. *Ann Surg* 2004; 239(1):14–21.
3. Nezhat F, Yadav J: Laparoscopy and Hysterectomy. In *Nezhat's Operative Gynecologic Laporoscopy and Hysteroscopy*, 3rd edition. Nezhat C, Nezhat F eds. Cambridge University Press, New York: 2008, 341–62.
4. Querleu D, Chapron C: Complications of gynecologic laparoscopic surgery. *Curr Opin Obstet Gynecol* 1995; 7:257–61.
5. Rock JA, Jones JW, eds: *TeLinde's Operative Gynecology*. 10th edition. Lippincott-Williams and Wilkens, Philadelphia: 2008.

ANESTHETIC CONSIDERATIONS

(Procedures covered: laparoscopic surgery for endometriosis, ectopic pregnancy, myomectomy, hysterectomy)

PREOPERATIVE

Respiratory	There can be intraop respiratory compromise from ↑ intra-abdominal pressure 2° CO_2 insufflation; however, patients without significant respiratory disease tolerate the insufflation quite well. **Tests:** As indicated from H&P.
Cardiovascular	Insufflation of the abdomen (typically with pressures of 14–22 mmHg) →↑ SVR and ↓ venous return. ↑ $PaCO_2$ →↑ dysrhythmias. These are usually well tolerated in the otherwise healthy patient. **Tests:** As indicated from H&P.

Gastrointestinal	Patients often have a mechanical bowel prep the night before. Check for Sx of dehydration (↓ skin turgor, orthostatic ↓ BP, ↑ HR, etc.) and hypokalemia (e.g., weakness, flattened T waves, dysrhythmias, etc.). The combination of ↑ intra-abdominal pressure + Trendelenburg position →↑ aspiration risk. **Test:** Electrolytes
Hematologic	These patients often are having surgery for abnormal uterine bleeding → consider anemia. **Test:** Hct
Laboratory	Other tests as indicated from H&P.
Premedication	Consider midazolam 1–3 mg iv

INTRAOPERATIVE

Anesthetic technique:GETA

Induction	Standard induction (see p. B-2). Rapid sequence induction (see p. B-4) usually is indicated for patients with an ectopic pregnancy. OGT/NGT to decompress stomach prior to surgery start.	
Maintenance	Standard maintenance (see p. B-2). Muscle relaxation helpful for initial trocar insertions and may be helpful throughout procedure.	
Emergence	Standard emergence	
Blood and fluid requirements	Usually minimal blood loss IV: 18 ga × 1 NS/LR @ 2–6 mL/kg/h	Before induction, these patients may need extra fluid 2° dehydration if given mechanical bowel preparation. During surgery, large volumes of fluid are sometimes given intra-abdominally for irrigation and hydrodissection → fluid overload; therefore, carefully account for all fluids, and titrate iv fluids to maintain euvolemia.
Monitoring	Standard monitors (see p. B-1). Foley catheter	
Positioning	✓ and pad pressure points ✓ eyes	See Neuropathies, below.
Complications	Bradydysrhythmias	Attributed to peritoneal or fallopian-tube stimulation. Rx: stop surgery; deflate pneumoperitoneum; administer atropine 0.5 mg or glycopyrrolate 0.4–0.6 mg.
	Bleeding	Vascular puncture a rare risk with trocar insertion.
	Hypothermia	2° the large volume of fluid and CO_2 infused into the abdomen and lithotomy position. Consider warming iv fluids and use of forced-air warming device.
	Extra-abdominal insufflation	Occasionally, the insufflating gas can enter a vein, hollow viscera, subcutaneous tissue, thorax, mediastinum, or pericardium. Fortunately, since the gas is usually CO_2, small volumes are absorbed quickly and usually do not cause major physiologic compromise; however, large volumes may → cardiopulmonary collapse (e.g., 2° pneumothorax, VAE). Subcutaneous air can compromise the airway in some cases. ✓ airway before extubation.

Complications (cont'd)	Neuropathies	These can be long cases, with the patient in lithotomy position. Make sure the pressure points are padded well and, if the arms are out, relieve stress on the brachial plexus.
	Fluid overload	✓ fluid volume entering and exiting the abdomen. Fluid absorption → fluid overload → CHF, edema.

POSTOPERATIVE

Complications	PONV VTE Hypothermia	↑↑ Risk for PONV. See p. B-6. See p. B-7.
Pain management	Consider ketorolac 15–30 mg and LA into surgical wounds	Patients may complain of shoulder pain due to diaphragmatic irritation.

Suggested Readings

1. Gerges FJ, Kanazi GE, Jabbour-Kohoury SI: Anesthesia for laparoscopy–a review. *J Clin Anesth* 2006; 18(1): 67–78.
2. Goulson DT: Anesthesia for outpatient gynecologic surgery. *Curr Opin Anaesthesiol* 2007; 20(3): 195–200.

SECTION

9.0 UROLOGY

SURGEONS

Harcharan S. Gill, MD
Benjamin Chung, MD

ANESTHESIOLOGISTS

Steven A. Deem, MD
Ronald G. Pearl, MD, PhD

DIAGNOSTIC TRANSURETHRAL (ENDOSCOPIC) PROCEDURES

SURGICAL CONSIDERATIONS

Description: Many urologic diseases are diagnosed and evaluated endoscopically through the urethra with the use of specialized instruments, such as cystoscopes and resectoscopes. With the patient in a lithotomy position, the cystoscope is introduced into the urethra and advanced under direct vision all the way into the bladder (Figs 9-1, 9-2), allowing inspection of the urethra (**urethroscopy**) and bladder (**cystoscopy**). If pathology is noted, a biopsy can be obtained easily through the cystoscope. It is also possible to introduce a small catheter into the ureteral orifice and advance it up to the kidney for radiologic evaluation (**retrograde pyelography**) to collect a urine specimen or to bypass areas of obstruction. If the upper urinary tract needs to be visualized, a ureteroscope is introduced through the urethra into the bladder and through the ureteral orifice into the ureter and advanced up to the kidney, allowing inspection of the ureter (**ureteroscopy**) and intrarenal collecting system (**nephroscopy**). These procedures often precede a major surgical operation.

Usual preop diagnosis: Hematuria; hydronephrosis; benign prostatic hypertrophy; cancer of the urethra, prostate, bladder, ureter, and renal pelvis; urinary tract stones; strictures; ureteropelvic junction obstruction; hemorrhagic or interstitial cystitis

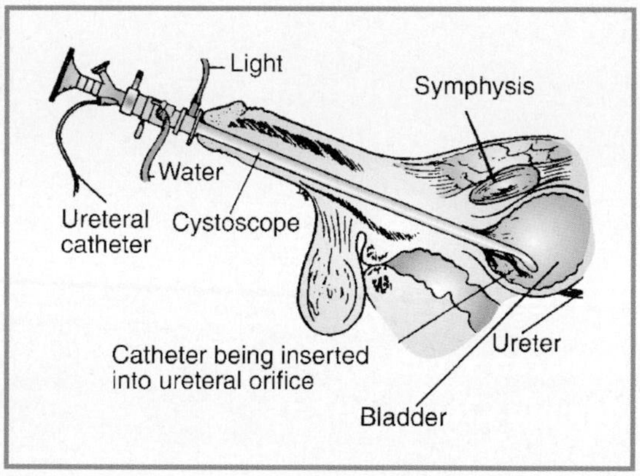

Figure 9-1. Cystoscope introduced into bladder via urethra (male anatomy). (Reproduced with permission from Hardy JD: *Textbook of Surgery.* JB Lippincott, 1988.)

SUMMARY OF PROCEDURES

	Urethroscopy/Cystoscopy	**Ureteroscopy/Nephroscopy**
Position	Lithotomy	⇐
Incision	None	⇐
Special instrumentation	Cystoscope	Ureteroscope
Unique considerations	Use of x-ray and fluoroscopy	⇐
Antibiotics	Gentamicin 80 mg iv, slowly	⇐
Surgical time	15 min	45 min
EBL	None	⇐

SUMMARY OF PROCEDURES (cont'd)		
	Urethroscopy/Cystoscopy	**Ureteroscopy/Nephroscopy**
Postop care	PACU → home	⇐
Mortality	Minimal	⇐
Morbidity	Infection: 5%	⇐ Ureteral perforation: < 5%
Pain score	1	1

PATIENT POPULATION CHARACTERISTICS		
Age range	All ages	⇐
Male:Female	1:1	⇐
Incidence	30% of all urologic procedures	⇐
Etiology	Hematuria Urethral and bladder tumors Stones Urethral strictures	⇐ ⇐ ⇐ ⇐ Ureteropelvic junction obstruction
Associated conditions	Prostatic hypertrophy Cystitis	Hydronephrosis ⇐

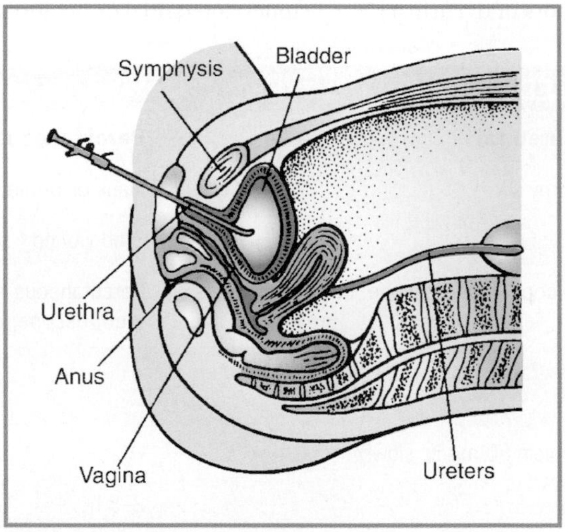

Figure 9-2. Cystoscope introduced into bladder (female anatomy). (Reproduced with permission from Govan DE: *Roche Manual of Urologic Procedures.* Hoffmann-LaRoche, 1976.)

ANESTHETIC CONSIDERATIONS

See Anesthetic Considerations following Therapeutic Transurethral Procedures (Except TURP), p. 861.

Suggested Readings

1. Bagley, DH: Ureteroscopy. In *Smith's Textbook of Endourology,* Vol 1, 1st edition. Smith AD, Badlani G, Bagley D, et al, eds. Quality Medical Publications, St. Louis: 2000, 369–513.
2. Wein AJ et al: Basics of urologic surgery. In: *Campbell-Walsh Urology,* 9th edition. WB Saunders, Philadelphia: 2006.

THERAPEUTIC TRANSURETHRAL PROCEDURES (EXCEPT TURP)

SURGICAL CONSIDERATIONS

Description: Therapeutic transurethral procedures, the most common urologic operations, require the use of specialized instruments, such as cystoscopes and resectoscopes. Because of continuously improving instrumentation and fiber optics, the range and complexity of these operations are widening, and more operations are being done transurethrally now than ever before. These operations are: **transurethral resection (TUR)** of any urethral, prostatic or bladder pathology; **fulguration** of bleeding vessels; **instillation of chemicals,** such as oxychlorosene (Chlorpactin) and formalin, into the bladder; **extraction** of stones; and **incision and dilation** of strictures.

With the patient in the lithotomy position, the cystoscope or resectoscope is introduced into the urethra and advanced under direct vision into the bladder, allowing inspection of the urethra and bladder (Figs 9-1 and 9-2). The pathology is identified. If it is a tumor, it is resected piecemeal with the electrode of the resectoscope, using the cutting current and cauterizing the base of the tumor with the coagulating current. If the pathology is a stone, it is extracted with special forceps or a stone basket. Large stones have to be fragmented, prior to extraction, with a mechanical lithotrite, electrohydraulic probe, ultrasound lithotrite or laser (Holmium or pulsed-dye). Chemicals can be instilled through the cystoscope to control interstitial and hemorrhagic cystitis. Bleeding vessels can be coagulated with the electrode. Strictures of the urethra can be dilated or incised with an endoscopic knife. Strictures of the ureter also can be treated endoscopically by dilatation with a balloon catheter or by incision with electrocautery. Balloon catheters with attached cutting electro-wires (Acucise) often are used. A temporary ureteral stent is placed at the end of most endoscopic ureteral surgeries.

Variant procedure or approaches: Occasionally, access to the intrarenal collecting system (renal pelvis and calyces) and upper ureter is easier and more appropriately done by a **percutaneous nephrostomy** than a transurethral procedure. The patient is placed in a prone or flank position, a percutaneous stab wound is made at the costovertebral angle, and a tube is introduced into the kidney under fluoroscopic control.

Usual preop diagnosis: Tumors of the urinary tract; stones; interstitial or hemorrhagic cystitis; strictures

SUMMARY OF PROCEDURES

	Transurethral	Percutaneous
Position	Lithotomy	Flank or prone
Incision	None	Stab wound
Special instrumentation	Cystoscope; resectoscope; catheters; stents	Percutaneous nephrostomy kit; nephroscope; urethroscope; catheters; stents
Unique considerations	Use of x-rays, fluoroscopy, and electrocautery	⇐
Antibiotics	Gentamicin 80 mg iv, slowly	⇐
Surgical time	1 h	2–3 h
EBL	100 mL	500 mL
Postop care	Irrigation of tubes and catheters to clear clots and prevent obstruction	⇐
Mortality	< 1%	⇐
Morbidity	Bleeding: 10% Infection: 5% Perforation: 2% Retained stones: 2%	⇐ ⇐ ⇐ ⇐
Pain score	1	3

PATIENT POPULATION CHARACTERISTICS		
Age range	All ages	⇐
Male:Female	1:1	⇐
Incidence	10% of urologic diseases involve these procedures	⇐
Etiology	Urethral and bladder tumors; bladder and ureteral stones; interstitial cystitis; hemorrhagic cystitis; urethral stricture	Kidney stones; upper ureteral stones; ureteropelvic junction obstruction

ANESTHETIC CONSIDERATIONS FOR TRANSURETHRAL PROCEDURES (EXCEPT TURP)

PREOPERATIVE

Patients of all ages may present for ureteral stone extraction. Paraplegics and quadriplegics have a predilection for nephrolithiasis and may present for repeated cystoscopies. Bladder tumors usually are seen in older patients, who may present for cystoscopy or TUR. These patients may have preexisting medical problems, including CAD, CHF, PVD, cerebrovascular diseases, COPD, and/or renal impairment. Preop evaluation should be directed toward the detection and treatment of these conditions prior to anesthesia.

Neurological	Paraplegics and quadriplegics may present for repeated cystoscopies and stone extractions. Note Hx of autonomic hyperreflexia; Sx may include flushing, headache, and nasal stuffiness, associated with voiding or noxious stimuli below the level of spinal cord injury (see below).
Musculoskeletal	Contractures and pressure sores may make positioning difficult in paraplegics or quadriplegics.
Laboratory	Tests as indicated from H&P.
Premedication	Sedation prn anxiety (e.g., lorazepam 1–2 mg po 1–2 h before surgery; midazolam 1–2 mg iv in preop area).

INTRAOPERATIVE

Anesthetic technique: Spinal, continuous lumbar epidural, and GA are acceptable, with the choice dependent on type and length of procedure, age, coexisting disease, and patient preference. Simpler transurethral procedures (e.g., cystoscopy) are amenable to topical anesthesia, while longer and more complex procedures (e.g., ureteral stone extraction) will require regional or GA (see discussion below regarding autonomic hyperreflexia). Note that many of these procedures are done on an outpatient basis and the anesthetic should be planned accordingly. For regional anesthesia, a sacral block is required for urethral procedures (T9-T10 level for procedures involving the bladder and as high as T8 for procedures involving the ureters).

Regional anesthesia:

Topical	2% lidocaine jelly
Spinal	0.75% bupivacaine 10–12 mg. For shorter procedures (< 1 h), consider low-dose bupivacaine (0.75%, 7.5 mg); mepivacaine (1.5%, 45 mg); or procaine (10%, 100–150 mg). Lidocaine may be used, but the incidence of transient neurologic symptoms may be as high as 30% for procedures performed in the lithotomy position.

Lumbar epidural	1.5–2.0% lidocaine with epinephrine 5 mcg/mL, 15–25 mL; supplement with 5–10 mL boluses as needed. Supplemental iv sedation.

General anesthesia:

Induction	Standard induction (see p. B-2). ET intubation may not be necessary for shorter procedures; consider LMA. Succinylcholine should be avoided in paralyzed (e.g., paraplegic, quadriplegic) patients 2° ↑ K^+→ VF or asystole.	
Maintenance	Pure inhalation anesthetic (e.g., N_2O, sevoflurane/desflurane) for short cases. IV technique (e.g., propofol 100–200 mcg/kg/min; supplement with N_2O ± volatile anesthetic ± narcotic). Muscle relaxation not essential. Narcotics unnecessary, because postop pain is usually minimal.	
Emergence	No specific considerations	
Blood and fluid requirements	Usually minimal blood loss IV: 18 ga × 1 NS/LR @ 2–4 mL/kg/h	
Monitoring	Standard monitors (see p. B-1).	
Positioning	✓ and pad pressure points. ✓ eyes.	* **NB:** In lithotomy position, peroneal nerve compression at lateral fibular head → foot drop.
Complications	Anticipate ↓ BP upon returning from lithotomy position. Autonomic hyperreflexia (**AH**): • Severe HTN • Bradycardia • Dysrhythmias • Cardiac arrest	Rx: volume (200–500 mL NS/LR) or ephedrine (5 mg iv) may be necessary. Patients with spinal cord injury level above T10 are at risk for autonomic hyperreflexia (**AH**) associated with stimulation below the level of transection. Transection levels below T5 may be associated with less severe manifestations. AH can be prevented by GA, spinal, or epidural anesthesia. If AH occurs intraop, it should be treated by deepening the level of anesthesia, and iv antihypertensive agents (e.g., SNP 0.5–5 mcg/kg/min; labetalol 5–10 mg iv; phentolamine 2–5 mg iv), if necessary.

POSTOPERATIVE

Complications	Peroneal nerve injury 2° lithotomy position Fever/bacteremia Bladder perforation	Peroneal nerve injury manifested as foot drop with loss of sensation over dorsum of foot. Seek neurology consultation. Bladder perforation may present as shoulder pain in the awake patient, but may go unnoticed in a patient under GA. Sx include unexplained HTN, tachycardia, ↓ BP (rare).
Pain management	Pain usually mild	Rx: morphine 2–4 mg iv q 10–15 min prn, fentanyl 25–50 mcg iv, ketorolac 15–30 mg im or iv

Suggested Readings

1. Amzallog M: Autonomic hyperreflexia. *Int Clin Anesth* 1993; 31:87–102.
2. Hambly PR, Martin B: Anesthesia for chronic spinal cord lesions. *Anesthesia* 1998; 53:273–89.
3. Mebust WK: Transurethral surgery. In *Campbell-Walsh Urology*, 9th edition. WB Saunders, Philadelphia: 2006.

TRANSURETHRAL RESECTION OF THE PROSTATE (TURP)

SURGICAL CONSIDERATIONS

Description: **TURP** is one of the most common urologic operations, performed to relieve bladder outlet obstruction by an enlarging prostate gland. It is often preceded by **cystoscopy,** which is used to evaluate the size of the prostate gland and to rule out any other pathology, such as bladder tumor or stone. The operation is performed with the resectoscope, a specialized instrument having an electrode capable of transmitting both cutting and coagulating currents. Resectoscopes are either single inflow only, or continuous flow with an inflow and outflow system. The latter allows the surgeon to maintain low pressure in the bladder and prostatic fossa and thus limiting fluid absorption. Two different electrical options are available. The traditional resectoscope is a monopolar system, and this requires a grounding pad and possible interference with electric devices, such as pace makers. Bipolar resectoscopes have both the active and return electrode fitted in the resectoscope and do not cause any electrical interference with cardiac electrical devices.

The resectoscope is introduced into the bladder (Fig. 9-3) and the tissue protruding into the prostatic urethra is resected in small pieces called "chips." Bleeding vessels are coagulated with the coagulating current. The resection is performed with continuous irrigation using an isotonic solution, such as sorbitol 2.7% with mannitol 0.54% in monopolar resectoscopes and normal saline in bipolar resectoscopes. After the obstructing prostatic tissues are completely resected and bleeding vessels coagulated, the chips are irrigated from the bladder and the resectoscope is removed. An indwelling Foley catheter is introduced into the bladder. The time of transurethral resection should not exceed 2 h, because excessive absorption of the irrigating fluid may → dilutional hyponatremia, confusion, seizures, and heart failure. However, this is less of an issue with a continuous flow bipolar resectoscope where saline is used as an irrigant. Although fluid absorption can occur, hyponatremia does not occur with the use of saline. The size of the enlarged prostate or adenoma, therefore, needs to be carefully assessed preop to determine if it is possible to complete the resection within 2 h. If not, an **open prostatectomy** is performed. This variant approach is discussed under Open Prostate Operations, p. 867.

Variant procedure or approaches: A number of techniques have been developed to avoid the morbidity of TURP. These are either **vaporization** (electrocautery or laser) or **thermocoagulation** of the prostate (laser, microwave, radiofrequency). The following techniques are available and approved:

TUVP: Transurethral vaporization of the prostate with a standard resectoscope using a roller ball electrode at 275–300 watts setting.

Laser Ablation: Laser coagulation of the prostate is done with Nd:YAG or Ho:YAG laser through a standard cystoscope. This procedure has been largely replaced by laser ablation with the KTP laser (PVP, green light laser) or diode laser. This wavelength allows vaporization of the prostate tissue with minimal blood loss. This is currently the most popular minimally invasive technique used for treatment of BPH. It can also be done on patients while on anticoagulation or with bleeding disorders. All personnel in the OR, including the patient, must wear protective glasses to protect the eyes from inadvertent exposure from a break in the laser fiber.

TUNA: Transurethral needle ablation of the prostate is done with a special disposable device connected to a radiofrequency generator.

TUMT: Transurethral microwave thermotherapy is done with a catheter that has a microwave antenna attached to it. A microwave generator is needed for this procedure.

All of the above have several advantages over TURP, including shorter surgical time, no blood loss, reduced risk of fluid absorption, and all can be done as outpatient procedures.

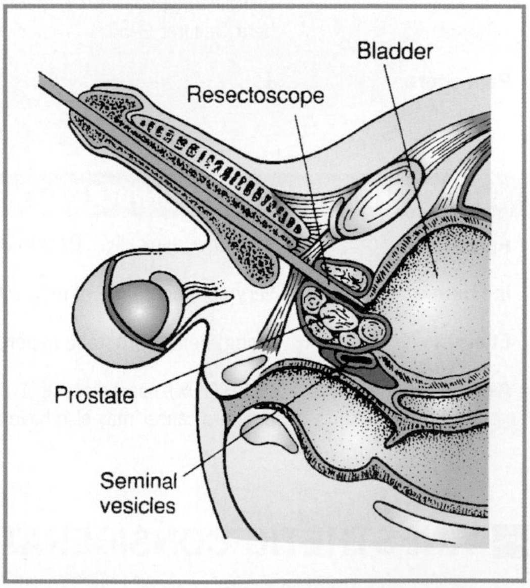

Figure 9-3. Transurethral resection of prostate using a resectoscope. (Reproduced with permission from Govan DE: *Roche Manual of Urologic Procedures.* Hoffmann-LaRoche, 1976.)

Usual preop diagnosis: Benign prostatic hypertrophy; prostate cancer

SUMMARY OF PROCEDURES

	TURP	Thermotherapy
Position	Lithotomy	⇐
Incision	None	⇐
Special instrumentation	Cystoscope; resectoscope; catheters; electrocautery	Cystoscope; resectoscope; catheters; electrocautery (standby); laser equipment
Unique considerations	During resection, the patient should be absolutely still, because any movement may lead to perforation or injury to the external sphincter, → postop incontinence.	During laser resection, the patient and all personnel should wear protective eyeglasses.
Antibiotics	Gentamicin 80 mg iv, slowly	⇐
Surgical time	1–2 h (not to exceed 2 h)	1 h
EBL	500 mL	None
Postop care	Irrigation of the Foley catheter to clear it of clots and keep it from being blocked. Determination of serum Na^+	⇐
Mortality	< 1%	⇐
Morbidity	Significant intraop bleeding: 10% Intraop perforation and fluid extravasation which may require placement of retropubic drain: <0.5% Postop bleeding, which may necessitate a return to OR for fulguration of bleeding vessels: <5% Absorption of irrigating fluid, which may → dilutional hyponatremia, mental confusion, and heart failure: 2–5%	Prolonged catheterization: 10% Postop bleeding: 1%
Pain score	1	1

PATIENT POPULATION CHARACTERISTICS

Age range	49–90 yr; typically, 70s and 80s
Incidence	Very common; 90% of men will develop benign hypertrophy; 20% may need surgical intervention.
Etiology	Aging; benign prostatic hypertrophy; prostate cancer
Associated conditions	COPD (10%); heart disease (10%); HTN (10%); diabetes mellitus (DM) (5%); DIC (1–2% of patients with prostate cancer may also have a low-grade, subclinical DIC, which becomes clinically manifest postop).

ANESTHETIC CONSIDERATIONS

PREOPERATIVE

Patients presenting for prostate surgery are generally elderly and may have preexisting medical problems, including CAD, CHF, PVD, cerebrovascular disease, COPD, and renal impairment. Preop evaluation should be directed toward the detection and treatment of these conditions before anesthesia.

Respiratory	COPD common in this age group. Patients with > 50 pack/year smoking Hx, or with any respiratory Sx, may need PFTs. For dyspnea with moderate exercise, ✓ VC, FEV_1, MMEF. If VC < 80%, FEV_1 < 60%, or MMEF < 40% predicted, ✓ ABG. If ABG and PFT markedly abnormal, consider postponing surgery until patient's respiratory condition has been optimized. **Tests:** PFT; CXR; ABG, as indicated from H&P.
Cardiovascular	HTN, CAD common in this age group. Assess exercise tolerance by H&P (e.g., should be able to climb a flight of stairs without difficulty or SOB). **Tests:** ECG; others as indicated from H&P.
Neurological	Cerebrovascular disease, Alzheimer's, and other neurologic problems may be present in this age group. Assess mental status to guide evaluation of any intraop or postop changes.
Renal	Anticipate renal impairment 2° chronic obstruction. **Tests:** BUN; Cr; electrolytes. If ↑ BUN and ↑ Cr, ✓ creatinine clearance (nl = 95–140 mL/min).
Musculoskeletal	Various arthritides in this age group may cause problems with positioning for regional anesthesia and surgery.
Endocrine	Increased incidence of DM.
Hematologic	Moderate blood loss expected with larger glands. If gland < 80 g, no T&C necessary. **Test:** Hct
Laboratory	Other tests as indicated from H&P.
Premedication	Continue commonly used drugs (e.g., digitalis, β-blockers, NTG) to prevent cardiovascular problems. Sedation prn anxiety (e.g., lorazepam 1–2 mg po 1–2 h before surgery).

INTRAOPERATIVE

Anesthetic technique: Regional or GA. Choice of technique depends on the coexisting disease and the patient's preference. Regional anesthesia may hold some advantage over GA for TURP in that it allows evaluation of mental status and, thus, earlier detection of TURP syndrome. The incidence of postdural puncture headache is very low in this age group (< 1%). A T9 level is optimal. Continuous lumbar epidural anesthesia has no advantage over spinal anesthesia for TURP, because a sacral block may be less reliable, the procedure is relatively short and supplemental doses are usually not necessary.

Regional anesthesia:

Spinal	0.75% bupivacaine, 12 mg in 7.5% dextrose solution (1.6 mL)

General anesthesia:

Induction	Standard induction (see p. B-2).	
Maintenance	Standard maintenance (see p. B-2). Muscle relaxation is not mandatory, although patient movement during the procedure must be avoided.	
Emergence	Postop pain is usually not significant. Anticipate ↓ BP when legs are repositioned from lithotomy. Avoid stress on lumbar spine by slowly and simultaneously bringing legs together and returning to supine position.	
Blood and fluid requirements	Moderate blood loss (TURP) Minimal blood loss (thermotherapy)	Blood loss can be large (TURP) if venous sinuses are entered; it also can be difficult to quantify because of irrigant. To flush away blood and tissue and to promote

Blood and fluid requirements (cont'd)	IV: 16–18 ga × 1 NS/LR @ 2–4 mL/kg/h	visibility during TURP (or thermotherapy), continuous irrigation is used. For monopolar procedures, irrigating fluid must be nonelectrolytic to prevent dispersion of current, but near iso-osmotic to prevent hemolysis. For these reasons, sorbitol (2.7%) with mannitol (0.54%) or glycine (1.5%) is added to distilled water to produce solutions that are nearly isotonic.
Monitoring	Standard monitors (see p. B-1).	Regional anesthesia allows monitoring of mental status. Invasive monitoring, if indicated from H&P.
TURP syndrome	Intravascular volume overload Hyponatremia Hypotonicity 2° absorption of irrigant Symptoms include: • N/V • Visual disturbances • Mental status changes • Coma • Sz • HTN • Angina • Cardiovascular collapse	Factors that influence the absorption of irrigant include: surgical technique (TURP or thermotherapy); hydrostatic pressure of irrigant (height of bag); number of venous sinuses opened; peripheral venous pressure; duration of surgery; and experience of the surgeon. Resections should optimally be limited to 1 h or less. Some CNS manifestations are 2° glycine and its metabolites. Rx may include observation, diuresis (e.g., furosemide 5– 20 mg iv), and administration of hypertonic saline (e.g., 100 mL of 3% saline over 1–2 h). Serum sodium < 120 is associated with more severe symptoms, and the goal of therapy is to restore sodium to > 120. In milder cases, observation and water restriction may be sufficient.
Positioning	✓ and pad pressure points. ✓ eyes.	***NB:** In lithotomy position, peroneal nerve compression at lateral fibular head → foot drop.
Complications	Bladder perforation TURP syndrome	Bladder perforation may produce shoulder pain in the awake patient. Bladder perforation (and TURP syndrome) may go unnoticed under GA; Sx: ↑ BP, ↑ HR (occasionally ↓ BP).

POSTOPERATIVE

Complications	TURP syndrome Bladder perforation Fever/bacteremia/sepsis Hypothermia	See discussion of TURP syndrome, above.
Pain management	Minimal postop pain	Rx: Morphine 1–4 mg iv prn until comfortable.
Tests	Hct; electrolytes Blood cultures if febrile	Consider serum osmolarity, CXR, ECG in TURP syndrome

Suggested Readings

1. Abrams PH, Shah PJ, Bryning K, et al: Blood loss during transurethral resection of the prostate. *Anaesthesia* 1982; 37(1): 71–3.
2. Hanson RA, Zornow MH, Conlin MJ, et al: Laser resection of the prostate: implications for anesthesia. *Anesth Analg* 2007; 105(2): 475–9.
3. Jensen V: The TURP syndrome. *Can J Anaesth* 1991; 38(1):90–6.
4. Malhotra V: Transurethral resection of the prostate. *Anesthesiol Clin North Am* 2000; 18(4):883–97.
5. Mebust WK: Transurethral surgery. In *Campbell-Walsh Urology*, 9th edition. WB Saunders, Philadelphia: 2006.

OPEN PROSTATE OPERATIONS

SURGICAL CONSIDERATIONS

Description: Open (in contrast to transurethral or endoscopic) operations on the prostate gland are common. They include: **simple prostatectomy, radical prostatectomy,** and are done through either a midline extraperitoneal incision, which extends from the umbilicus to the symphysis pubis, or through a Pfannenstiel's incision (Fig. 9-4, inset).

Simple prostatectomy: When the benign prostatic hypertrophy or adenoma is too large to be resected transurethrally, it is removed by a simple prostatectomy. The prostate gland is exposed through a retropubic approach (Fig. 9-4A) and the anterior capsule is incised, exposing the adenoma—the central part of the prostate which is excised, "shelled" out by blunt dissection (Fig. 9-4B), leaving behind the peripheral prostate and all the associated structures. A Foley catheter is left indwelling in the urethra, and the incision in the prostate capsule is closed. In a **suprapubic prostatectomy,** the incision is made in the bladder and the adenoma shelled from within the bladder.

Radical prostatectomy: The term **radical prostatectomy** is used because the entire prostate, both seminal vesicals and pelvic nodes, are removed. It is used to differentiate this cancer operation from a simple prostatectomy (used for benign prostatic hypertrophy). Radical prostatectomy can be achieved through a **retropubic** or **perineal approach,** the choice being a matter of training, expertise, and surgeon's preference. In radical prostatectomy, all of the prostate gland is removed, together with the bladder neck, the seminal vesicles, and the ampullae of the vas deferens. A **limited pelvic lymphadenectomy** (Fig. 9-5) also is performed. After the prostate gland and its associated structures are removed, the bladder neck is reduced to 1 cm diameter and anastomosed to the membranous urethra over an indwelling Foley catheter. Most of the blood loss occurs during control of the dorsal vein complex. In early stage cancers, which nowadays comprise 90% of patients, a nerve sparing procedure is done. This involves preserving

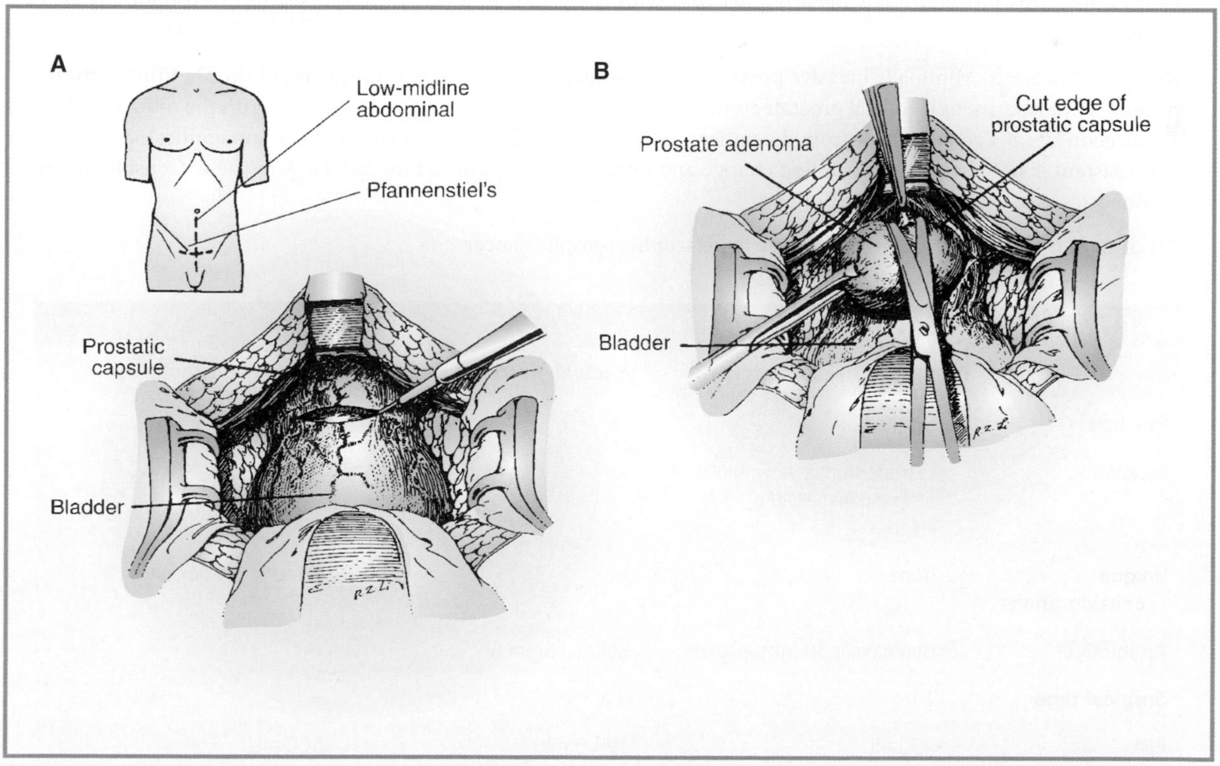

Figure 9.4. Retropubic prostatectomy: **A:** A transverse capsulotomy is made between heavy hemostatic stay sutures. **B:** The cleavage plane between the adenoma and the surgical capsule is developed with scissors. (Reproduced with permission from Fowler JE: *Urologic Surgery.* Little & Brown, 1990.)

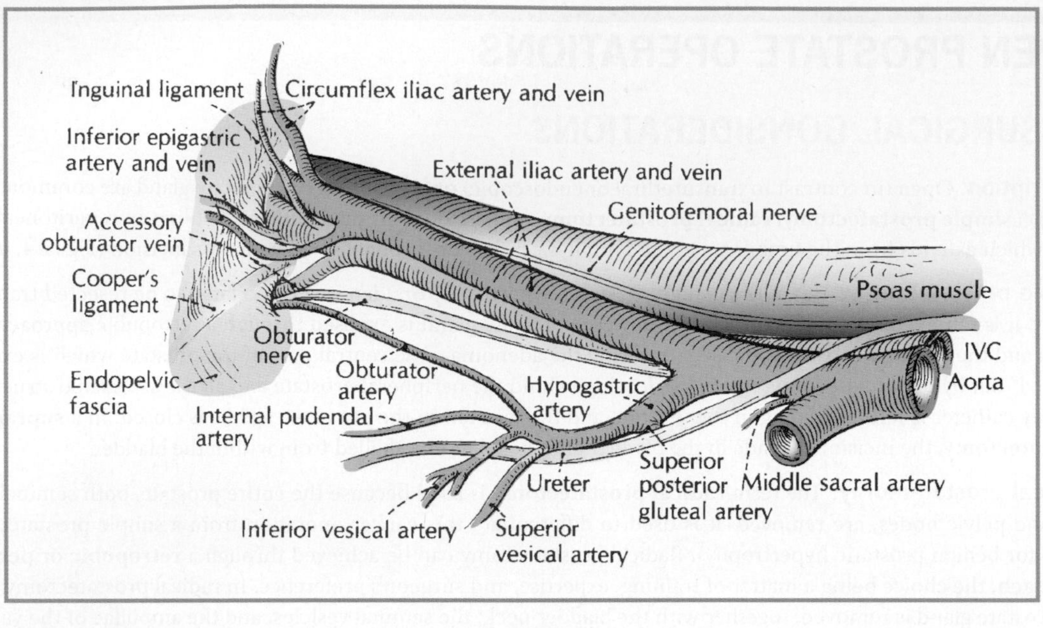

Figure 9-5. Right lateral pelvic wall. Anatomy of pelvic blood vessels and nerves encountered in a pelvic lymph node dissection. (Reproduced with permission from Graham SD Jr: *Glenn's Urologic Surgery.* Lippincott Williams & Wilkins, 1998.)

potency by preserving the nerves to the corpora cavernosa. More recently, radical prostatectomy is being done by laparoscopy. This procedure has been popularized with the use of robots. Please see section of robotic urologic surgery.

Variant approach: Minimally invasive prostate cancer surgery has expanded with the use of the **Da Vinci Robotic system**. Most laparoscopic radical prostatectomies are done with the assistance of the robot. With the robotic system the surgeon sits at a console away from the patient and has a three-dimensional view with 10× magnification. A bedside assistant is necessary for instrument change and retraction. See page 902 for special Anesthetic Considerations for Robotic-Assisted Laparoscopic Surgery.

Usual preop diagnosis: Benign prostatic hypertrophy; prostate cancer

SUMMARY OF PROCEDURES

	Simple Prostatectomy	Radical–Retropubic	Radical–Perineal
Position	Supine	⇐	Lithotomy
Incision	Extraperitoneal, low midline, or Pfannenstiel's (Fig. 9-4A, inset)	⇐	Perineal (Fig. 9-6)
Unique considerations	None	⇐	Extreme hip flexion
Antibiotics	Gentamicin 80 mg iv, slowly	Keflex 1Gram IV	⇐
Surgical time	1 h	3 h	⇐
EBL	500 mL	1,500 mL	500 mL
Postop care	Irrigate catheter to clear blood clots and prevent obstruction; frequently, if urine is bloody.	⇐	⇐

Urology

SUMMARY OF PROCEDURES (cont'd)

	Simple Prostatectomy	Radical–Retropubic	Radical–Perineal
Mortality	<1%	⇐	⇐
Morbidity	Bleeding: 2% DVT: 2% Infection: 2% PE: 1%	⇐ ⇐ ⇐ ⇐ Impotence: Non nerve-sparing: 100% Nerve-sparing: 20–50% Lymphocele: 4%	⇐ ⇐ ⇐ ⇐
Pain score	8	8	6

PATIENT POPULATION CHARACTERISTICS

Age range	40–80 yr
Incidence	20% of men will develop symptomatic benign prostatic hypertrophy; 9% will develop clinically evident prostate cancer.
Etiology	Aging
Associated conditions	COPD (10%); CAD (10%); HTN (10%); diabetes mellitus (5%); renal failure (1%)

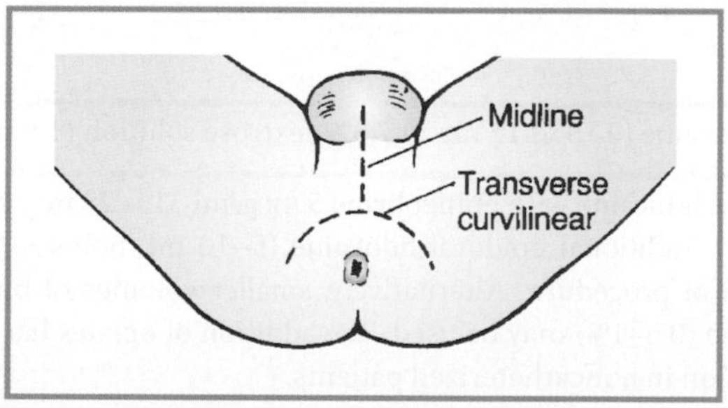

Figure 9-6. Perineal incisions.

ANESTHETIC CONSIDERATIONS

PREOPERATIVE

Patients presenting for prostate surgery are generally elderly and may have preexisting medical problems, including CAD, CHF, PVD, cerebrovascular disease, COPD, and renal impairment. Preop evaluation should be directed toward the detection and treatment of these conditions prior to anesthesia.

Respiratory	COPD common in this age group. Patients with Hx of > 50 pack-year smoking, or with respiratory Sx, may require PFTs. For dyspnea with moderate exercise, check VC, FEV_1, MMEF. If VC < 80%, FEV_1 < 60%, or MMEF < 40% predicted, ✓ ABG. If ABG and PFT are markedly abnormal, consider postponing surgery until patient's respiratory condition has been optimized. **Tests:** PFT; CXR; ABG, as indicated from H&P.
Cardiovascular	HTN, CAD common in this age group. Assess exercise tolerance by H&P (e.g., should be able to climb a flight of stairs without difficulty or SOB). **Tests:** ECG; others as indicated from H&P.

Neurological	Cerebrovascular disease, Alzheimer's, and other neurologic problems may be present in this age group. Assess mental status to guide evaluation of any intraop or postop changes.
Renal	Anticipate renal impairment 2° chronic obstruction. **Tests:** Cr
Musculoskeletal	Various arthritides may cause problems with positioning for regional anesthesia and surgery.
Endocrine	Increased incidence of diabetes mellitus.
Hematologic	Moderate blood loss expected with larger glands. For glands < 30 g, no T&C necessary; for glands 30–80 g, T&C 2 U PRBCs; for glands > 80 g, T&C 4 U PRBCs. **Tests:** Hct
Laboratory	Other tests as indicated from H&P.
Premedication	Continue commonly used drugs (e.g., digitalis, β-blockers, diuretics, NTG) to prevent cardiovascular complications. Sedation prn anxiety (e.g., lorazepam 1–2 mg po on call to OR).

INTRAOPERATIVE

Anesthetic technique: Regional (spinal, continuous spinal, continuous lumbar epidural), GA, or combined techniques are acceptable. If regional anesthesia used, optimal block level is T8-T10 (depending on incision site). Advantages of regional anesthesia include potential for lower intraop blood loss, possible lower incidence of DVT postop, and faster return of bowel function. Disadvantages include positioning considerations (see below).

Regional anesthesia:

Spinal	Bupivacaine (0.75%) 12 mg in 7.5% dextrose solution (1.6 mL)
Epidural	1.5–2% lidocaine with epinephrine 5 mcg/mL, 15–25 mL, supplemental iv sedation as necessary. Additional epidural lidocaine (5–10 mL boluses) may be needed, depending on length of procedure. Alternatively, smaller volumes of bupivacaine (0.25–0.5%) or ropivacaine (0.5–1%) may be used. The addition of opiates has been associated with ↑ urinary retention in noncatheterized patients.

General anesthesia:

Induction	Standard induction (see p. B-2).	
Maintenance	Standard maintenance (see p. B-2).	
Emergence	No special considerations	
Blood and fluid requirements	Moderate-to-large blood loss IV: 14–16 ga × 1–2 NS/LR @ 4–6 mL/kg/h	Additional requirements dependent on type of anesthesia. Regional techniques are associated with higher fluid requirement because of sympathectomy and systemic vasodilation; they also may be associated with lower blood loss than GA.
Monitoring	Standard monitors (see p. B-1). Depending on underlying disease: ± CVP ± Arterial line	Some patients require CVP to aid in assessment of volume status. Arterial line is often useful for continuous BP monitoring and frequent blood draws. Patients at particularly high risk (e.g., Hx of preexisting cardiopulmonary disease) should probably have both.

Urology

Positioning	Anticipate ↓ BP on return from lithotomy position. ✓ and pad pressure points. ✓ eyes.	Rx: volume (200–500 mL NS/LR) or ephedrine (5 mg iv) may be necessary. Elderly patients with arthritis or respiratory impairment may not tolerate the extreme positioning associated with perineal prostatectomy for extended periods of time, thus precluding the use of regional anesthesia. *(A combined technique with GA maybe considered.) * **NB:** In lithotomy position, peroneal nerve compression at lateral fibular head → foot drop.
Complications	Indigo carmine reaction Hemorrhage Hypothermia VAE	Indigo carmine → false ↓ O_2 sat ± ↑ BP; rare allergic reaction → rash + bronchoconstriction + ↓ BP.

POSTOPERATIVE

Complications	Peroneal nerve injury 2° lithotomy position DVT	Manifested by foot drop with loss of sensation on dorsum of foot. Seek neurology consultation. Incidence of DVT less with regional than GA. Sx: variable, with pain and tenderness over involved area.
Pain management	Significant postop pain. Rx: morphine 0.1–0.3 mg/kg iv in incremental doses (e.g., 2–4 mg q 10–15 min prn).	Consider epidural infusion of dilute local anesthestics/opiates or PCA (see p. C-3).
Tests	Hct	

Suggested Readings

1. Donald JR: The effect of anaesthesia, hypotension, and epidural analgesia on blood loss in surgery for pelvic floor repair. *Br J Anaesth* 1969; 41(2):155–66.
2. Eastham JA, Scardino PT: Radical prostatectomy. In *Campbell-Walsh Urology*, 9th edition. WB Saunders, Philadelphia: 2006.
3. Gibbons RP: Radical perineal prostatectomy. In *Campbell-Walsh Urology*, 9th edition. WB Saunders, Philadelphia: 2006.
4. Hendolin H, Mattila MA, Poikolainen E: The effect of lumbar epidural analgesia on the development of deep-vein thrombosis of the legs after open prostatectomy. *Acta Chir Scand* 1981; 147(6):425–9.
5. Nelson JB: Debate: open radical prostatectomy vs. laparoscopic vs. robotic. *Urol Oncol* 2007; 25(6): 490–3.
6. Oesterling JE: Retropubic and suprapubic prostatectomy. In *Campbell-Walsh Urology*, 9th edition. WB Saunders, Philadelphia: 2006.
7. Whalley DG, Berrigan MJ: Anesthesia for radical prostatectomy, cystectomy, nephrectomy, pheochromocytoma, and laparoscopic procedures. *Anesthesiol Clin North Am* 2000; 18(4):899–917.

NEPHRECTOMY

SURGICAL CONSIDERATIONS

Description: Nephrectomies fall into three basic groups: simple, partial, and radical. (Surgical anatomy is shown in Fig. 9-7.)

Simple nephrectomy, performed for benign conditions, is the surgical excision of the kidney and a small segment of proximal ureter. The dorsal approach is well suited for this operation, and begins with an incision extending from

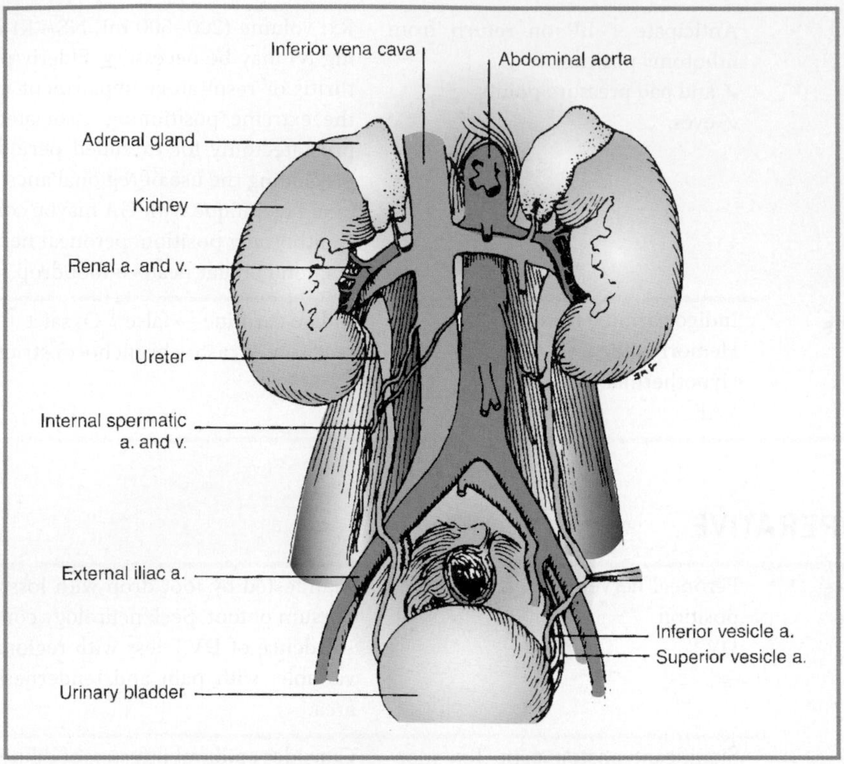

Figure 9-7. Surgical anatomy of the urinary tract. (Reproduced with permission from Hardy JD: *Textbook of Surgery.* JB Lippincott, 1988.)

the 12th rib to the iliac crest along the lateral edge of the sacrospinalis muscle and quadratus lumborum muscle. The dorsolumbar fascia is opened, exposing Gerota's fascia and the perinephric fat (Fig. 9-8). The kidney is mobilized until the hilum is exposed. The artery and vein are tied, suture-ligated, and transected. The ureter is followed distally as far as possible, tied, and transected. The kidney is delivered out of the incision, which is then closed by approximating the dorsolumbar fascia and the fascia of the sacrospinalis muscle.

Usual preop diagnosis: Chronic hydronephrosis; hypoplastic kidney; renovascular HTN; double collecting system

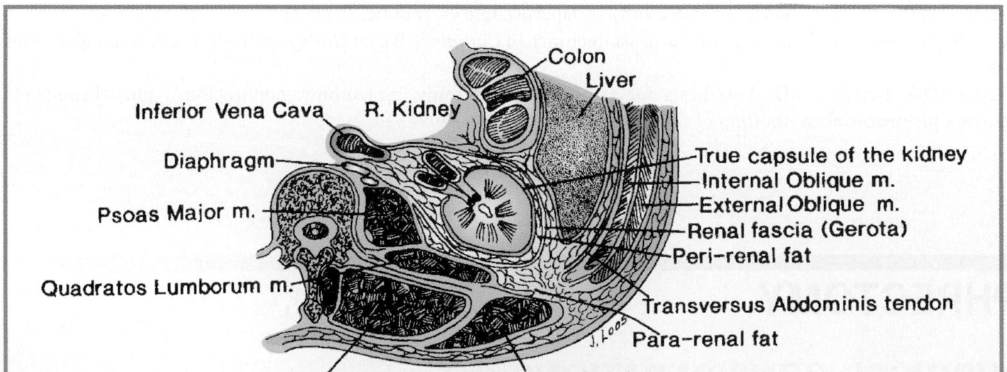

Figure 9-8. Transverse section showing the relation of the renal fascias to the right kidney. (Reproduced with permission from Baker RJ, Fischer JE: *Mastery of Surgery,* 4th edition. Lippincott Williams & Wilkins, 2001.)

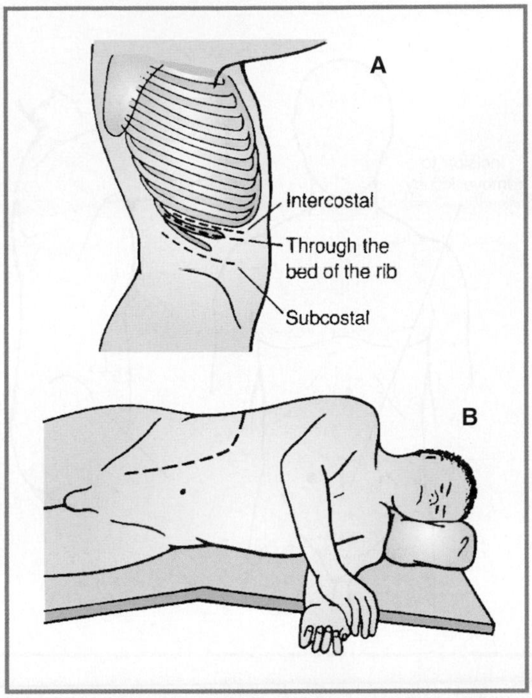

Figure 9-9. **A:** Flank incisions. **B:** Subcostal transabdominal incision.

Partial nephrectomy is the surgical excision of the segment of the kidney harboring the pathology. It is performed for small renal-cell carcinomas and benign tumors of the kidney, such as angiomyolipomas, and for duplicated collecting systems with a diseased moiety. If the partial nephrectomy is being done for renal-cell carcinoma, it may be accompanied with a **regional lymphadenectomy.** The flank approach (Fig. 9-9A) is well suited for this operation and begins with an incision over the 12th or 11th rib, or in between, and extends anteriorly over the external and internal oblique muscles, which are transected. The transversalis muscle and fascia are opened, exposing Gerota's fascia. The renal capsule is exposed at the planned site of resection. Control of the renal vessels is advised for control of bleeding, if excessive. Incision in the renal parenchyma is made by sharp and blunt dissection, suture-ligating all bleeders. If the collecting system is opened, it should be closed with absorbable sutures. After complete hemostasis, Gelfoam, thrombin, Floseal, or perinephric fat is used to cover the raw surface of the kidney.

Usual preop diagnosis: Renal-cell carcinoma; double collecting system

Radical nephrectomy is the surgical excision of the kidney with its surrounding perinephric fat and Gerota's fascia and the proximal 2/3 of the ureter, accompanied by paracaval or para-aortic **lymphadenectomy.** It is performed for renal-cell carcinoma. Early control of renal vessels is advised before excessive manipulation of the tumor to minimize blood loss and hematogenous spread. Transabdominal or flank approaches (Fig. 9-9A, B) are best suited for this operation. Surgery in patients with renal vein or inferior vena cava involvement is more complex and prone to more intraoperative complications, including blood loss. When the tumor thrombus involves a large segment of the vena cava or is in the right atrium, a team approach with cardiac surgeons is used. Often patients have to be put on cardiopulmonary bypass under hypothermia.

Laparoscopic simple or radical nephrectomy: A pneumoperitoneum is created by insufflating CO_2 to a pressure of 14–16 mmHG. Three to four trochars are inserted as necessary (Fig. 9-10). Typically, the patient is placed in a flank position as in an open radical nephrectomy. This procedure can be either **transperitoneal** or **retroperitoneal,** depending on the surgeon's preference or experience. The transperitoneal approach may be modified by using a hand-assistance device through one of the ports (**hand-assisted laparoscopic nephrectomy**). Most radical nephrectomies can be done by an experienced laparoscopic surgeon.

Usual preop diagnosis: Renal-cell carcinoma, nonfunctioning kidney 2° infection or obstruction; kidney donation

Nephroureterectomy is a radical nephrectomy with ureter resection, including the ureteral orifice and a cuff of bladder wall around it. It is accompanied by a regional lymphadenectomy, since it is performed for a cancerous condition. The approach is either **transabdominal** or **extraperitoneal** through an extended flank incision, starting at

Urology

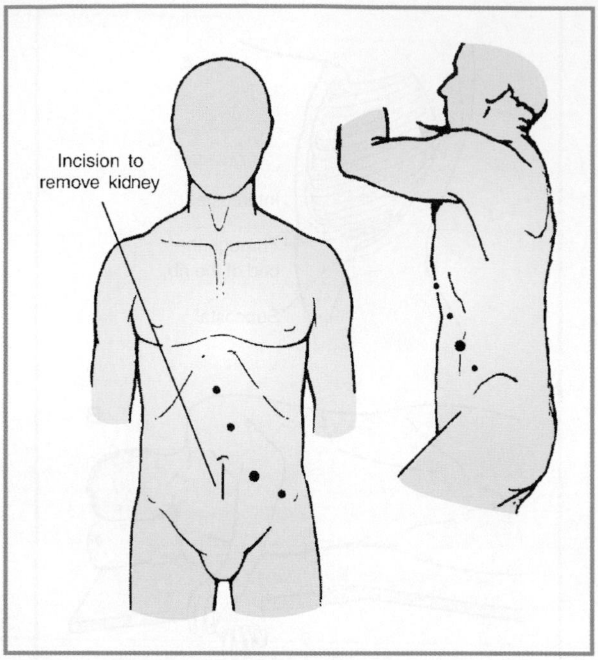

Figure 9-10. Incision and placement of trocars in laparoscopic nephrectomy. (Reproduced with permission from Scott-Conner CEH, Dawson DL: *Operative Anatomy,* 2nd edition. Lippincott Williams & Wilkins, 2003.)

the tip of the 11th rib and curving caudally along the lateral edge of the rectus abdominis muscle down to the pubic bone (Fig. 9-9B). Some surgeons prefer two separate incisions: a flank incision for the radical nephrectomy part and a lower abdominal incision for the ureterectomy. This procedure can be done by laparoscopy with a lower midline incision made to remove the specimen.

Usual preop diagnosis: Transitional-cell carcinoma of the renal collecting system or ureter

SUMMARY OF PROCEDURES

	Simple Nephrectomy	Partial Nephrectomy	Radical Nephrectomy	Laparoscopic Nephrectomy or Nephroureterectomy
Position	Flank or prone	Flank	Supine or flank	Flank
Incision	Flank (Fig. 9-9A) or dorsal along paraspinous muscles	Flank (Fig. 9-9A)	Midline or subcostal transabdominal (Fig. 9-9B) or flank; subcostal or intercostal or through bed of 11th or 12th rib (Fig. 9-9A)	3–4 ports (Fig. 9-10)
Unique considerations	None	⇐	If tumor involves renal vein and/or IVC, clamp IVC.	Risk of emergent conversion to open case
Antibiotics	None	⇐	⇐	⇐
Surgical time	2–3 h	3–4 h	⇐	⇐
Closing considerations	Chest tube may be required if pleura opened with flank incision.	⇐	⇐	A small incision is made at the end of the case to remove the specimen.

SUMMARY OF PROCEDURES (cont'd)

	Simple Nephrectomy	Partial Nephrectomy	Radical Nephrectomy	Laparoscopic Nephrectomy or Nephroureterectomy
EBL	500 mL	1,200 mL	500 mL	300 mL
Mortality	< 1%	⇐	1%	⇐
Morbidity	Prolonged ileus: 5% Pneumothorax 2° unrecognized pleural perforation: 2%	⇐	⇐	Vascular injury requiring conversion to open case
Pain score	10	10	10	4

PATIENT POPULATION CHARACTERISTICS

Age range	All ages	⇐	⇐	⇐
Male:Female	1:1	⇐	⇐	⇐
Incidence	<1%	⇐	⇐	⇐
Etiology	Double collecting system; chronic hydronephrosis; hypoplastic kidney; renovascular HTN	Localized renal-cell carcinoma	Wilms' tumor (8% of all childhood malignancies); transitional cell carcinoma (7% of all kidney tumors); renal-cell carcinoma (3% of adult malignancies)	
Associated conditions	HTN if nephrectomy is used for renovascular HTN.			

ANESTHETIC CONSIDERATIONS

See Anesthetic Considerations following Operations on the Renal Pelvis and Upper Ureter, p. 877.

Suggested Readings

1. Cadeddu JA, Ono Y, Clayman RV: Laparoscopic nephrectomy for renal cell cancer. Evaluation of efficacy and safety: a multicenter experience. *Urology* 1998; 52:773–7.
2. Coleman DL: Control of postoperative pain: non-narcotic and narcotic alternatives and their effect on pulmonary function. *Chest* 1987; 92(3):520–8.
3. Conacher ID, Soomro NA, Rix D: Anaesthesia for laparoscopic urological surgery. *Br J Anaesth* 2004; 93(6): 859–64.
4. Novic AC, Streem SB: Surgery of the kidney. In *Campbell-Walsh Urology*, 9th edition. WB Saunders, Philadelphia: 2006.

OPERATIONS ON THE RENAL PELVIS AND UPPER URETER

SURGICAL CONSIDERATIONS

Description: Operations on the renal pelvis and upper ureter are becoming less common because of the increasing use of endoscopic and percutaneous procedures. The basic surgical approach is the same as that for nephrectomy (see p. 871). Specific procedures include the following:

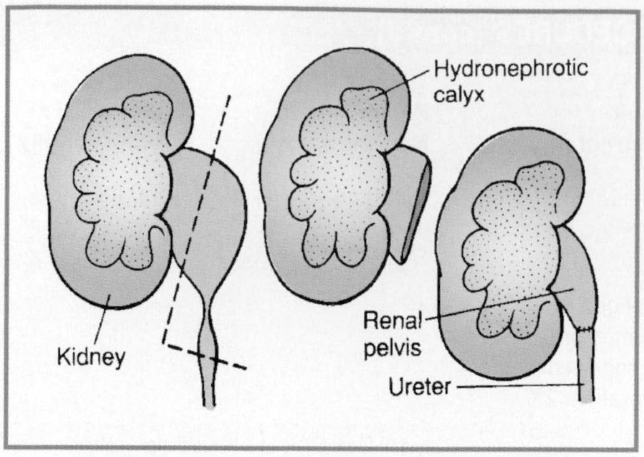

Figure 9-11. Dismembered pyeloplasty.

Pyeloplasty is the surgical correction of congenital ureteropelvic junction stenosis to relieve obstruction. The most commonly used is the **dismembered pyeloplasty,** or **Anderson-Heinz pyeloplasty,** wherein the diseased ureteropelvic junction is excised, the redundant renal pelvis is reduced, and an anastomosis is established between the renal pelvis and ureter (Fig. 9-11).

Usual preop diagnosis: Ureteropelvic junction obstruction

Pyelolithotomy and ureterolithotomy are used to remove calculi from the renal pelvis or ureter. The upper ureter and renal pelvis are exposed, usually through a flank approach, the calculus is palpated and an incision is made in the ureter or renal pelvis over the calculus, which is then delivered. The incision is closed with fine, absorbable sutures.

Usual preop diagnosis: Renal pelvic or ureteral stone

Transureteroureterostomy is the transposition of one ureter across the midline and anastomosing it to the other ureter (Fig 9-12). This operation is performed whenever the distal ureter is traumatized or diseased, and the proximal ureter is not long enough to reimplant into the bladder. The recipient ureter should be normal.

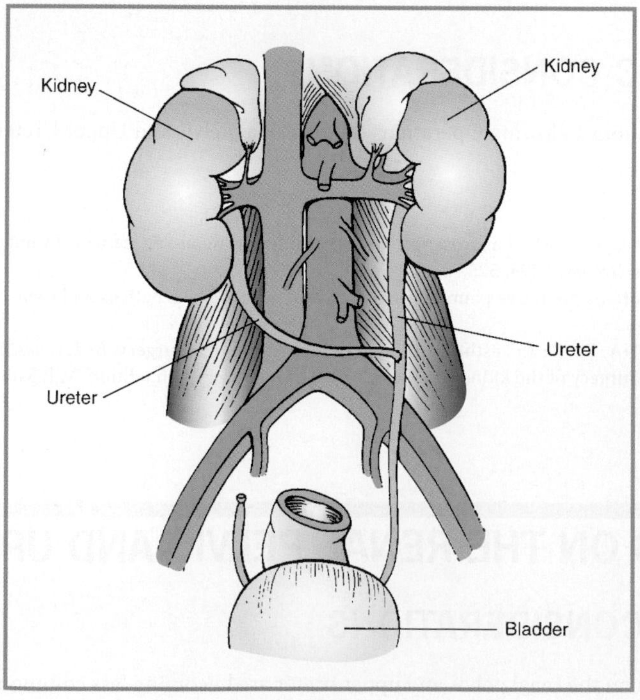

Figure 9-12. Transureteroureterostomy.

Usual preop diagnosis: Traumatic loss of distal ureter; distal ureteral tumor requiring distal ureterectomy

SUMMARY OF PROCEDURES

	Pyeloplasty	Pyelolithotomy/ Ureterolithotomy	Transureteroureterostomy
Position	Flank or prone	⇐	Supine
Incision	Flank (Fig. 9-9A) or dorsal	⇐	Midline abdominal (Fig. 9-9A, inset)
Antibiotics	None	⇐	⇐
Surgical time	3 h	1–2 h	3 h
EBL	Minimal	⇐	⇐
Mortality	< 1%	⇐	⇐
Morbidity	Urinary leakage: 5% Infection: 2%	⇐ ⇐	⇐ ⇐
Pain score	10	10	10

PATIENT POPULATION CHARACTERISTICS

Age range	All ages	⇐	⇐
Male:Female	1:1	⇐	⇐
Incidence	Rare	Extremely rare	⇐
Etiology	Ureteropelvic junction obstruction: 80% (of causes of dilated collecting system in the newborn)	Renal pelvic and upper ureteral stone	Traumatic loss of lower ureter; lower ureteral tumor
Associated conditions	Renal failure: 1%		

ANESTHETIC CONSIDERATIONS

(Procedures covered: nephrectomy and operations on the renal pelvis and upper ureter)

PREOPERATIVE

Patients presenting for nephrectomy and operations on the renal pelvis and upper ureter may be of any age, depending upon the etiology of the abnormality. Many patients may have renal insufficiency 2° the underlying problem or from renovascular HTN. Elderly patients frequently have preexisting medical problems, including CAD, CHF, PVD, cerebrovascular disease, COPD, and renal impairment. Preop evaluation should be directed toward the detection and treatment of these conditions prior to anesthesia.

Respiratory	Increased postop pulmonary complications because of location of incision (nonlaparoscopic). If Hx of pulmonary disease (e.g., asthma, COPD), consider postop respiratory therapy. **Tests:** As indicated from H&P.
Cardiovascular	Consider possibility of renal HTN.

Hematologic	Polycythemia may be seen in association with polycystic kidney disease, renal-cell carcinoma. Consider preop blood donation for autologous transfusion. **Tests:** Hct	
Laboratory	Electrolytes; BUN; Cr; other tests as indicated from H&P.	
Premedication	Standard premedication (see p. B-1).	

INTRAOPERATIVE

Anesthetic technique: GA is recommended for these procedures; technique depends on underlying disease. Regional techniques (spinal or epidural) may be alternatives for some open procedures, but are less than optimal because of awkward positioning that may → patient discomfort and pain resulting from diaphragmatic stimulation. Consider combined technique with regional opiates.

Induction	Standard induction (see p. B-2).	
Maintenance	Standard maintenance (see p. B-1). If intraperitoneal or laparoscopic approach is used, consider limiting N_2O to avoid distention of bowel and interference with operative field.	
Emergence	No specific considerations	
Blood and fluid requirements	Mild-to-moderate blood loss IV: 14–16 ga × 1 NS/LR @ 6–8 mL/kg/h Warm all fluids.	Intraperitoneal approach associated with higher fluid requirements (8–10 mL/kg/h). When renal vessels are to be cross- clamped, mannitol (0.5 g/kg) is often given prior to occlusion (20 min maximum).
Monitoring	Standard monitors (see p. B-1). Urinary catheter Arterial line (partial nephrectomy) ± CVP line	Invasive monitoring if indicated from H&P. CVP line useful for partial nephrectomy in patients with solitary kidneys (↑↑ blood loss).
Positioning	Use axillary roll if lateral. Avoid stretching brachial plexus – limit abduction to 90°. If prone, repeatedly ✓ eyes and pressure points. Assure free excursion of abdomen.	The lateral position with kidney rest and table flexion may →↓ BP, possibly 2° vena cava obstruction. Moderate iv volume administration and gradual assumption of the position are recommended to avoid this complication.
Complications	Pneumothorax ↓ BP with positioning (see above). Indigo carmine →↑ BP, ↑ SVR Methylene blue →↓ BP	Sx of pneumothorax include: ↑ RR, ↑ PIP, hypoxemia, hypercarbia. If in doubt, ✓ CXR.

POSTOPERATIVE

Complications	Postnephrectomy syndrome Eye injury (if prone) Brachial plexus injury (if lateral) Pneumothorax Atelectasis Pneumonia	Postnephrectomy syndrome 2° retractor injury. L1 nerve root damage with resulting pain, dysesthesia, and sensory loss in L1 dermatome distribution.
Pain management	Morphine 0.1–0.3 mg/kg iv in incremental doses Consider epidural narcotic	Postop analgesia critical to minimize pulmonary complications. PCA. See p. C-3.

Tests	Hct CXR	Others dependent on operative course, coexisting disease.

Suggested Reading

1. Franke JJ, Smith JA: Surgery of the ureter. In *Campbell-Walsh Urology*, 9th edition. WB Saunders, Philadelphia: 2006.

CYSTECTOMY

SURGICAL CONSIDERATIONS

Description: Open (in contrast to transurethral or endoscopic) bladder operations (cystectomies) account for 15–20% of all urological procedures. They are grouped as simple, partial, and radical procedures.

Simple cystectomy is performed for benign conditions of the bladder, such as severe hemorrhagic cystitis, radiation cystitis, and contracted bladder. It involves the removal of the bladder only. The operation is performed through a lower abdominal incision. The peritoneal reflections are incised down to the pouch of Douglas; the vasa deferentia and superior vesical arteries are identified, cross-clamped, transected, and tied. The ureters are identified, separated from the surrounding tissues, cross-clamped near the bladder, transected, and tied. The bladder is bluntly separated from the anterior rectal wall all the way to the apex of the prostate. The lateral pedicles of the bladder are cross-clamped, cut, and tied. The endopelvic fascia is incised, separating the prostate from the lateral pelvic wall. The puboprostatic ligaments are transected and the dorsal vein of the penis is suture-ligated. The tied dorsal vein and urethra are incised just distal to the apex of the prostate. The specimen is delivered out of the incision and hemostasis secured with electrocautery. An ileal conduit is then performed (see below).

Partial cystectomy is the excision of only the part of the bladder containing the pathology. This is not a commonly performed operation and is reserved for tumors located in the dome of the bladder of older patients who are poor surgical risks for major operations, such as radical cystectomy. The operation is preceded by a cystoscopy to identify the site of pathology. Beginning with a lower abdominal incision, the dome and lateral walls of the bladder are separated from the surrounding tissues, which are covered by wet packs to minimize contamination. An incision is made in the dome of the bladder at least 2 cm away from the pathology. The inside of the bladder is inspected and the pathology identified. The incision in the bladder is continued around, and at least 2 cm away from, the pathology, until the latter is completely excised. Bleeders in the wall of the bladder are electrocoagulated. The bladder wall is then closed in two layers—a through-and-through layer and an inverting layer—using absorbable material. Wet packs are removed, a drain is left in the region, and the abdominal incision is closed.

Radical cystectomy (or **radical cystoprostatectomy**) is performed for treatment of invasive bladder cancer. It encompasses the removal of the bladder and the lower ureters, the prostate gland, and seminal vesicles in men (Fig. 9-13A), and the uterus, ovaries, and anterior vaginal wall in women (Fig. 9-13B). Accompanied by a **pelvic lymphadenectomy,** it is performed in the supine position, except when a concomitant **urethrectomy** is required, wherein a lithotomy position is used.

Following cystectomy, whether radical or simple, some form of **urinary diversion** is required. This can be accomplished with either a standard ileal conduit or a bladder substitution. The **ileal conduit** is constructed from 6–8 inches of terminal ileum isolated, with its blood supply, from the small intestine. The continuity of the small intestine is accomplished by a simple anastomosis. The ureters are implanted into the proximal end of the conduit and the distal end is brought through the abdominal wall as a stoma (Fig. 9-14). **Bladder substitution** is a more complex operation wherein a longer segment of bowel is isolated, with its blood supply, and fashioned into a pouch. The ureters are implanted in the pouch and the most dependent part of the pouch is connected to the membranous urethra, avoiding a stoma (Fig. 9-15). Not all patients undergoing cystectomies are candidates for bladder substitution. For example, patients who require a urethrectomy are not candidates because of the need to remove the urethra.

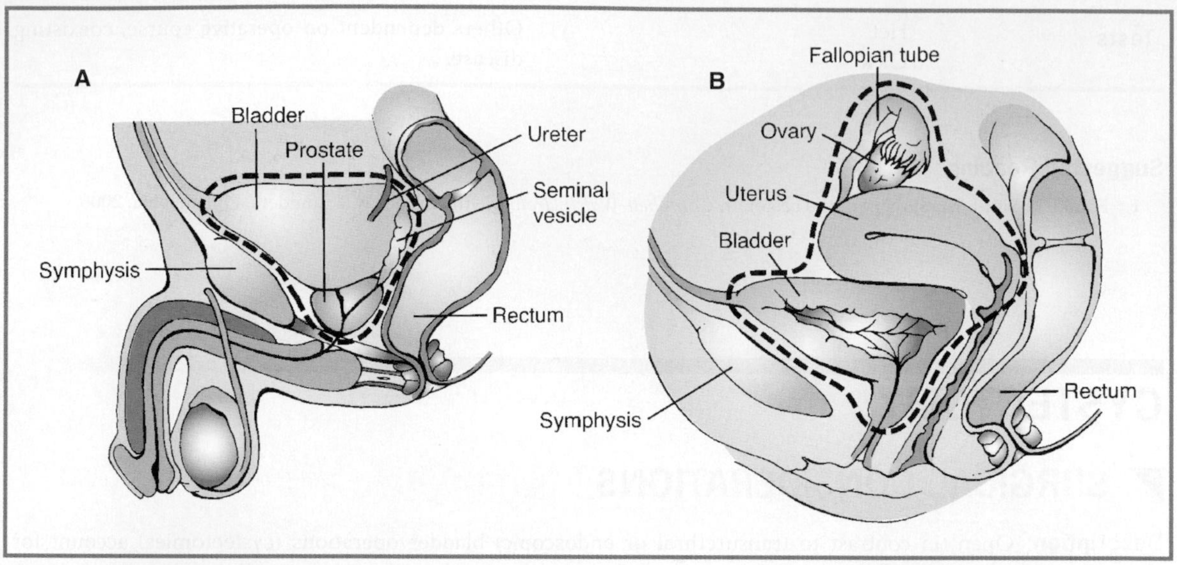

Figure 9-13. Anatomy of the pelvis with tissue to be excised outlined by dashed line: (**A**) male; (**B**) female.

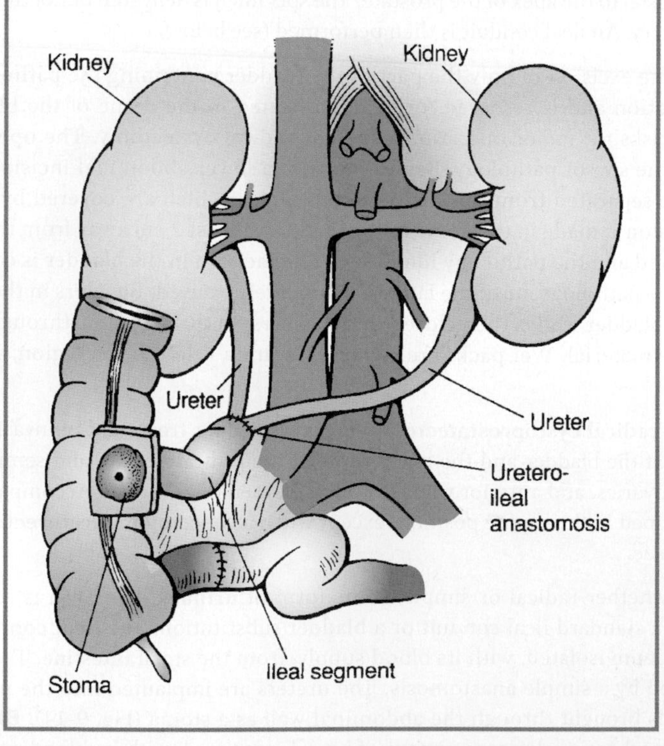

Figure 9-14. Ileal conduit: A segment of ileum is isolated from terminal ileum and continuity of the bowel is reestablished with an end-to-end anastomosis. Ureters are joined to the proximal end of the ileal segment and the distal end is brought out to the skin as a stoma.

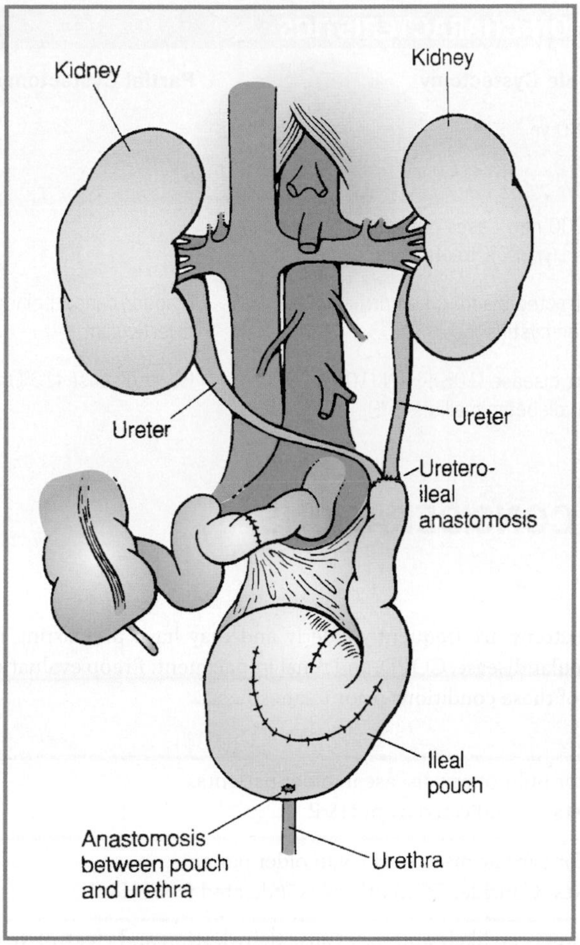

Figure 9-15. Bladder substitution: A segment of ileum is fashioned into a pouch and anastomosed to the urethra. The ureters are joined to the proximal, nondetubularized segment.

Usual preop diagnosis: Bladder cancer; contracted bladder; hemorrhagic cystitis; radiation cystitis; bladder diverticulum

SUMMARY OF PROCEDURES

	Simple Cystectomy	Partial Cystectomy	Radical Cystectomy
Position	Supine	⇐	Supine or lithotomy
Incision	Transperitoneal, midline	⇐	⇐
Antibiotics	Cefotetan or ceftriaxone 1 g	⇐	⇐
Surgical time	4 h	2 h	6 h
EBL	1,000 mL	Minimal	1,500 mL
Postop care	Care of the stoma	Catheter care	Care of the stoma
Mortality	1%	< 1%	2%
Morbidity	Prolonged ileus: 5% Infection: 2%	– – Hematuria: 5%	5% 2%
Pain score	10	10	10

PATIENT POPULATION CHARACTERISTICS

	Simple Cystectomy	Partial Cystectomy	Radical Cystectomy
Age range	40–80 yr	⇐	⇐
Male:Female	3:1	⇐	⇐
Incidence	60,000 new cases of bladder cancer diagnosed/yr; 20% treated with cystectomy.	⇐	⇐
Etiology	Contracted bladder; hemorrhagic and radiation cystitis	Bladder cancer; bladder diverticulum	⇐
Associated conditions	Heart disease (10%); HTN (10%); COPD (5%); diabetes mellitus (5%)	Heart disease (10%)	⇐

ANESTHETIC CONSIDERATIONS

PREOPERATIVE

Patients presenting for cystectomy are frequently elderly and may have preexisting medical problems, including CAD, CHF, PVD, cerebrovascular disease, COPD, and renal impairment. Preop evaluation should be directed toward the detection and treatment of these conditions prior to anesthesia.

Respiratory	✓ for pulmonary disease in older patients. **Tests:** As indicated from H&P.
Cardiovascular	✓ for cardiac disease, HTN in older patients. **Tests:** Consider ECG; others as indicated from H&P.
Gastrointestinal	Bowel prep likely and may cause dehydration and electrolyte disturbances. **Tests:** Electrolytes, if indicated.
Hematologic	T&C for 2–4 U PRBC. **Tests:** Hct
Laboratory	Other tests as indicated from H&P.
Premedication	Sedation prn anxiety in adults (e.g., lorazepam 1–2 mg po 1–2 h preop; midazolam 1–2 mg iv in preop area).

INTRAOPERATIVE

Anesthetic technique: Spinal, continuous lumbar epidural, or GA are acceptable, with choice dependent on length of procedure, coexisting disease, and patient preference. A combined technique using GA and regional anesthesia may be preferable. A T4 sensory level is recommended, because peritoneal stimulation is likely during this procedure.

Regional anesthesia:

Spinal	0.75% bupivacaine 12–15 mg in 7.5% dextrose; hyperbaric tetracaine 10–15 mg with 200 mcg epinephrine for procedures > 3 h.
Epidural	1.5–2% lidocaine with epinephrine 5 mcg/mL, 15–25 mL; supplement with 5–10 mL as needed. Supplemental iv sedation (e.g., midazolam 1 mg iv prn; fentanyl 50 mcg iv prn). Bupivacaine (0.25–0.5%), levobupivacaine (0.25–0.5%), or ropivacaine (0.5–0.75%), with or without sufentanil or fentanyl, may also be used. The addition of opiates has been associated with ↑ urinary retention in noncatheterized patients.

General anesthesia:

Induction	Standard induction (see p. B-2). These patients may be significantly dehydrated and require volume replacement before induction.	
Maintenance	Standard maintenance (see p. B-2).	
Emergence	No specific considerations	
Blood and fluid requirements	Significant blood loss possible IV: 16 ga × 1 NS/LR @ 6–10 mL/kg/h Warm fluids. Humidify gases.	Blood loss may be less with regional than GA.
Monitoring	Standard monitors (see p. B-1). Arterial line CVP line	Consider PA catheter in patients with cardiopulmonary disease. UO as measure of volume status may be lost during procedure.
Complications	Major blood loss 3rd-space losses Hypothermia	

POSTOPERATIVE

Complications	Hypothermia	
Pain management	Morphine 0.1–0.3 mg/kg iv in incremental doses Consider epidural narcotics or PCA.	See p. 1548.
Tests	Hct	Others as indicated by intraop course.

Suggested Readings

1. Marshall FF: Surgery of the bladder. In *Campbell-Walsh Urology*, 9th edition. WB Saunders, Philadelphia: 2006.
2. Whalley DG, Berrigan MJ: Anesthesia for radical prostatectomy, cystectomy, nephrectomy, pheochromocytoma, and laparoscopic procedures. *Anesthesiol Clin North Am* 2000; 18(4):899–917.

OPEN BLADDER OPERATIONS (OTHER THAN CYSTECTOMY)

SURGICAL CONSIDERATIONS

Description: Open bladder operations include:

Augmentation cystoplasty (or **enterocystoplasty**): Small, contracted bladders can be enlarged and their size and capacity augmented with a segment of intestine. The bladder is opened widely, anteroposteriorly, or from side-to-side, or with a cruciate incision. A segment of intestine— small bowel, cecum, or colon—is isolated from the intestinal tract, detubularized, and added onto the bladder.

Variant procedure: The antrum of the stomach can also be used (**gastrocystoplasty**).

Usual preop diagnosis: Contracted bladder from chronic cystitis

Repair of vesicovaginal or enterovesical fistulas: The communication between the vagina and bladder or bladder and bowel is identified and excised, and the edges freshened until normal, noninflamed tissues are exposed. The openings in the bladder and in the vagina or bowel are closed, and omentum is interposed in between to promote healing and prevent recurrence. With enterovesical fistulas, often the diseased segment of the intestine is excised and an **end-to-end anastomosis** of the intestine is performed.

Variant procedure: Transvaginal repair of vesicovaginal fistula (see Vaginal Operations, p. 898).

Usual preop diagnosis: Vesicovaginal or enterovesical fistula

Ureteral reimplantation, performed to correct vesicoureteral reflux, is more commonly used in the pediatric group than in adults. In adults, it is performed mainly for lower ureteral injuries, iatrogenic or traumatic. The lower ureter is identified and dissected proximally until adequate length is obtained. The bladder is opened and a 2–3 cm submucosal tunnel is created in or near the trigone, and the ureter is brought into the tunnel and fixed with sutures. If there is a large gap between the ureter and the bladder, a **psoas hitch procedure** is necessary. The bladder is mobilized and stitched to the psoas muscle in order to reach the ureter. In children, if the ureter is dilated, its diameter is reduced by imbrication before reimplantation. In adults, a nonrefluxing implantation is usually not necessary if the operation is being performed for ureteral injury.

Usual preop diagnosis: Vesicoureteral reflux; lower ureteral injuries

SUMMARY OF PROCEDURES

	Augmentation Cystoplasty	Repair of Fistulas	Ureteral Reimplantation
Position	Supine	Supine or lithotomy	Supine
Incision	Low abdominal	⇐	⇐
Antibiotics	Gentamicin 80 mg iv, slowly	⇐	⇐
Surgical time	4 h	3 h	⇐
EBL	Minimal	⇐	⇐
Postop care	Care of catheters and stents	⇐	⇐
Mortality	< 1%	⇐	⇐
Morbidity	Infections: 5% Urinary leakage: 1%	⇐ ⇐	⇐ ⇐
Pain score	10	10	10

PATIENT POPULATION CHARACTERISTICS

Age range	All ages	⇐	⇐
Male:Female	1:4	⇐	⇐
Incidence	Rare	⇐	⇐
Etiology	Contracted bladders from chronic cystitis	Traumatic fistulas; vesicovaginal; regional enteritis; diverticulitis; colon cancer	Vesicoureteral reflux; injury to lower ureters

ANESTHETIC CONSIDERATIONS

PREOPERATIVE

Patients presenting for open bladder operations may be of any age, depending on the etiology of the abnormality. Elderly patients frequently have pre-existing medical problems, including CAD, CHF, PVD, cerebrovascular disease, COPD, and renal impairment. Preop evaluation should be directed toward the detection and treatment of these conditions prior to anesthesia.

Respiratory	✓ for pulmonary disease in elderly patients. **Tests:** As indicated from H&P.
Cardiovascular	✓ for of cardiac disease in elderly patients. **Tests:** Consider ECG; others, if indicated from H&P.
Neurological	Paraplegics and quadriplegics may present for operations on the bladder and urinary tract. Obtain Hx of autonomic hyperreflexia (AH). Sx are: flushing, HA, nasal stuffiness, and HTN associated with voiding or noxious stimuli below level of transection.
Laboratory	Other tests as indicated from H&P.
Premedication	Sedation prn anxiety (e.g., lorazepam 1–2 mg po 1–2 h before surgery; midazolam 1–2 mg iv in preop area).

INTRAOPERATIVE

Anesthetic technique: Spinal, continuous lumbar epidural, or GA are acceptable, with choice dependent on length of procedure, coexisting disease, and patient preference. A combined technique using light GA with regional anesthesia is also acceptable. A T10 sensory level is sufficient to provide anesthesia for procedures on the bladder, but a T4 level is recommended if the peritoneum is opened. (See Anesthetic Considerations for Transurethral Procedures [except TURP)] p. 861, for patients with AH.)

Regional anesthesia:

Spinal	0.75% bupivacaine 10–12 mg. For shorter procedures (< 1 hr), consider low dose bupivacaine (0.75%, 7.5 mg); mepivacaine (1.5%, 45 mg); or procaine (10%, 100–150 mg). Lidocaine may be used, but the incidence of transient neurologic symptoms is significant (30%).
Epidural	1.5–2% lidocaine with epinephrine 5 mcg/mL, 15–25 mL; supplement with 5–10 mL as needed. Supplemental iv sedation. Bupivacaine (0.25), levobupivacaine (0.25–0.5%), or ropivacaine (0.5–0.75%), with or without sufentanil or fentanyl, may also be used. The addition of opiates has been associated with ↑ urinary retention in noncatheterized patients.

General anesthesia:

Induction	Standard induction (see p. B-2).	
Maintenance	Standard maintenance (see p. B-2). Consider limiting N_2O for long intraperitoneal procedures to minimize bowel distention.	
Emergence	No specific considerations	
Blood and fluid requirements	Minimal-to-moderate blood loss IV: 16–18 ga × 1 NS/LR @ 2–4 mL/kg/h Warm fluids. Humidify gases for lengthy procedures.	Intraperitoneal procedures have considerably higher requirements (e.g., NS/LR @ 6–10 mL/kg/h).
Monitoring	Standard monitors (see p. B-1) for simpler procedures. ± Arterial/CVP lines	UO as a measure of volume status may be lost during the procedure. Consider arterial line, CVP for longer, more complex procedures.
Positioning	✓ and pad pressure points. ✓ eyes.	* **NB:** In lithotomy position, peroneal nerve compression at lateral fibular head → foot drop.
Complications	AH in spinal cord injured patients	See discussion in Anesthetic Considerations for Transurethral Procedures, p. 862.

POSTOPERATIVE

Complications	Hypothermia Fever, bacteremia	
Pain management	Morphine 0.1–0.3 mg/kg in incremental doses. Consider epidural narcotics or PCA.	See p. C-3.
Tests	Hct Blood cultures if febrile	Others as indicated by intraop course.

Suggested Reading

1. Marshall FF: Surgery of the bladder. In *Campbell-Walsh Urology*, 9th edition. WB Saunders, Philadelphia: 2006.

INGUINAL OPERATIONS

SURGICAL CONSIDERATIONS

Description: Inguinal operations are very common, and are usually performed on an outpatient basis. Groin dissection, however, may necessitate inpatient care.

Inguinal herniorrhaphy: A 3″ inguinal incision is made, starting 1″ medial to the anterior-superior iliac spine, and ending at the pubic tubercle. The external oblique aponeurosis is excised, opening the external inguinal ring. The spermatic cord and the hernial sac are freed off the inguinal canal; then the hernial sac is dissected off the spermatic cord and followed proximally into the internal inguinal ring, where it is suture-ligated and excised. The floor of the inguinal canal is strengthened by approximating the conjoined tendon to the reflected part of the inguinal ligament. Modifications include laparoscopic repair and use of surgical mesh. Please see section 7.9 for details.

Usual preop diagnosis: Inguinal hernia (See Figs 9-16 and 9-17 for details of anatomic relationships.)

Orchiopexy is performed through the same incision as used in herniorrhaphy. After the inguinal canal is exposed, a search for the undescended testis begins. The testis and cord are dissected free from all surrounding tissue until adequate length is obtained to bring the testis down to the scrotum. Next, a pouch is created in the wall of the scrotum by incising the scrotal skin and dissecting it off dartos fascia. The testis is brought down into the pouch and fixed to the dartos fascia with sutures, and the incisions are closed. Often a **herniorrhaphy** is performed at the same time.

Unusual preop diagnosis: Undescended testis.

Radical orchiectomy is performed through a herniorrhaphy incision (described above). The spermatic cord is freed and cross-clamped at the internal inguinal ring, transected, and suture-ligated. The testis, with its tunica vaginalis, is then delivered through the incision by blunt and sharp dissection and the inguinal incision is closed. Sometimes, a testicular prosthesis is inserted and fixed in the scrotum before the inguinal incision is closed.

Usual preop diagnosis: Testicular cancer

Ligation of spermatic vein is performed through a small, transverse incision 1–2″ above the internal inguinal ring. Muscles are split and peritoneum reflected medially to expose the spermatic vessels; the vein is identified and ligated. This operation can also be done through a scrotal incision.

Usual preop diagnosis: Varicocele causing infertility

Groin dissection, or **inguinofemoral lymphadenectomy** (lymph node dissection), is the most critical of the inguinal operations. It is performed through either an inguinal incision (Fig. 9-17, inset) curved distally over the femoral

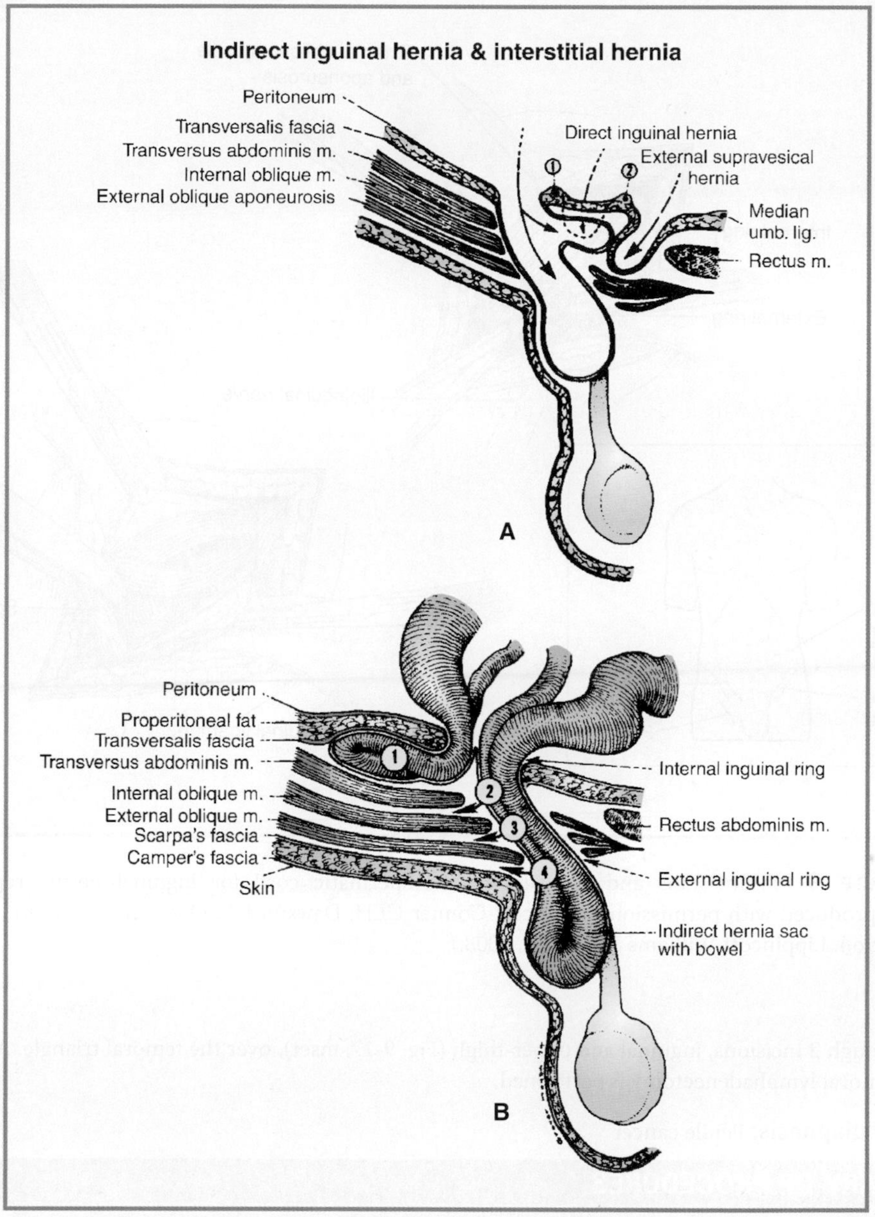

Figure 9-16. **A:** Relationships of four groin hernias in one patient. Indirect inguinal hernia with intraparietal diverticulum, direct hernia, and external supravesical hernia. 1 = lateral umbilical ligament; 2 = medial umbilical ligament. Arrows indicate different sites of origin of each hernia. (Reproduced with permission from Skandalakis JE, Gray SW, Burns WB, et al: Internal and external supravesical hernia. *Am Surg* 1976; 42:142.) **B:** Diagram of intraparietal hernia. The sac, entering at the internal ring may pass into any one or more spaces between layers of the abdominal wall. 1, properitoneal; 2 and 3, interstitial; 4, superficial. An indirect hernia also may be present. (Reproduced with permission form Skandalakis JE, Gray SW, Akin JT Jr: The surgical anatomy of hernial rings. *Surg Clin North Am* 1974; 54:1227.)

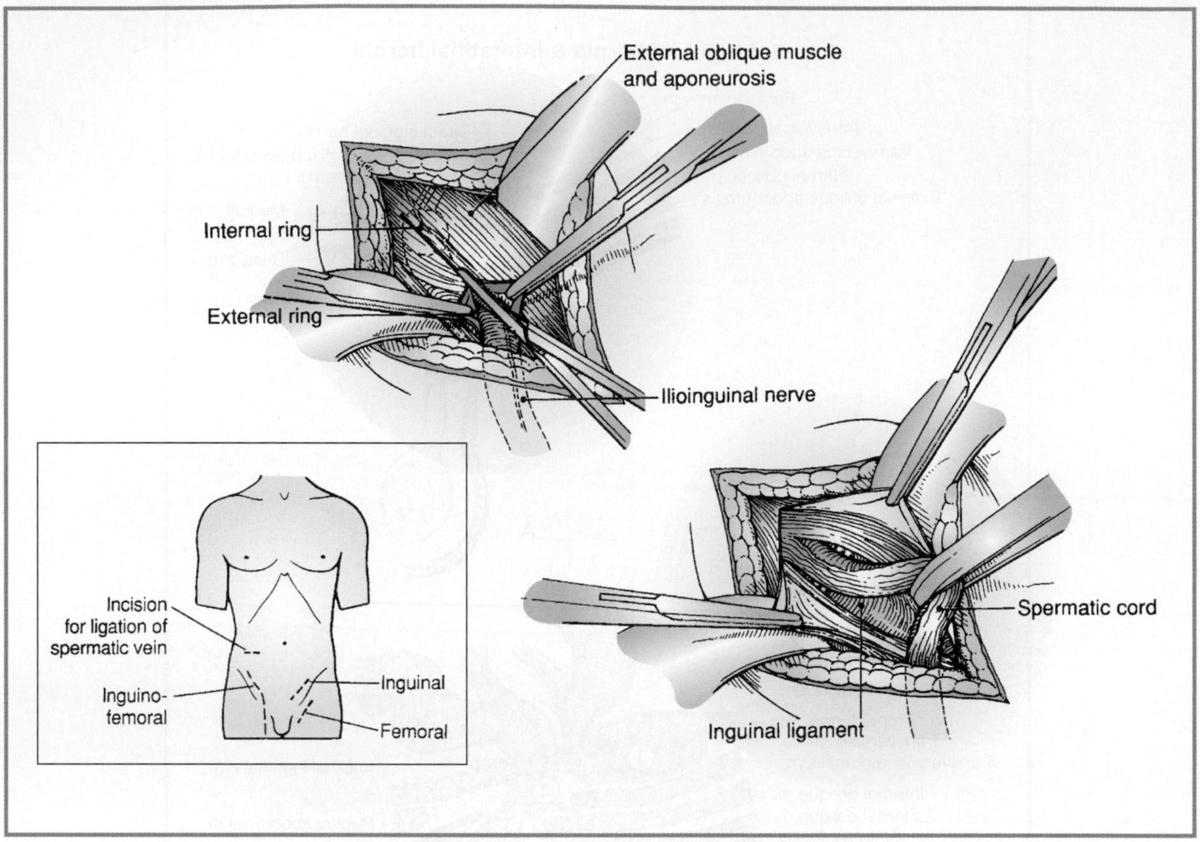

Figure 9-17. Incisions and exposure of the spermatic cord for inguinal hernia repair. (Reproduced with permission from Scott-Conner CEH, Dawson DL: *Operative Anatomy,* 2nd edition. Lippincott Williams & Wilkins, 2003.)

vessels or through 2 incisions, inguinal and upper-thigh (Fig. 9-17, inset), over the femoral triangle. A complete inguinal and femoral lymphadenectomy is performed.

Usual preop diagnosis: Penile cancer

SUMMARY OF PROCEDURES

	Herniorrhaphy, Orchiopexy, Orchiectomy	Ligation of Spermatic Vein	Groin Dissection
Position	Supine	⇐	⇐
Incision	Inguinal (Fig. 9-17, inset)	Transverse groin (Fig. 9-17, inset)	Inguinal and upper thigh (Fig. 9-17, inset)
Antibiotics	None	⇐	⇐
Surgical time	1 h	⇐	3 h
EBL	Minimal	⇐	200 mL
Postop care	PACU → home	⇐	PACU → ward; leg elevation
Mortality	< 1%	⇐	⇐
Morbidity	Wound infection: 2%	⇐	⇐
Pain score	7	5	7

■ PATIENT POPULATION CHARACTERISTICS			
Age range	All ages	Young adults	Middle age
Incidence	Hernia: 5% of population Undescended testis: 0.8% of male children Testis cancer: 6/100,000	1% of young men	Extremely rare, < 1% of all males
Etiology	Unknown; congenital	Varicocele	Penile cancer (very rare)

ANESTHETIC CONSIDERATIONS

PREOPERATIVE

Typically, patients presenting for inguinal operations are healthy, with most returning home on the day of surgery. The most common inguinal operation is herniorrhaphy. In these patients, consider causes of increased intraabdominal pressure during H&P. (Pediatric inguinal operations are discussed in Pediatric General Surgery, p. 1305.) A hernia may strangulate → acute abdomen.

Respiratory	Chronic cough is a common precipitating factor.
Gastrointestinal	Constipation may be a precipitating factor.
Laboratory	Tests as indicated from H&P.
Premedication	Sedation for adults prn anxiety (e.g., lorazepam 1–2 mg po 1–2 h before surgery; midazolam 1–2 mg iv in preop area).

INTRAOPERATIVE

Anesthetic technique: Local anesthesia (with sedation), spinal, epidural, or GA are acceptable techniques with the choice dependent on patient age and coexisting disease, type and length of procedure, and patient preference. Local anesthesia is acceptable for simple herniorrhaphy, although discomfort may be elicited if the peritoneum is manipulated. If a spinal or epidural anesthetic is chosen, a T6 level should be sought. Most inguinal procedures are done on an outpatient basis, and the anesthetic should be planned appropriately.

Regional anesthesia:

Spinal	0.75% bupivacaine 10–12 mg. For shorter procedures (< 1 h), consider low-dose bupivacaine (0.75%, 7.5 mg); mepivicaine (1.5%, 45 mg); or procaine (10%, 100–150 mg). Lidocaine may be used, but the incidence of transient neurologic symptoms is significant.
Epidural	1.5–2.0% lidocaine with epinephrine 5 mcg/mL, 15–25 mL; supplement with 5 10 mL as needed. Supplemental iv sedation with local or regional technique in adults; e.g., midazolam (1–2 mg iv), fentanyl (25–50 mcg iv prn anxiety or discomfort); or propofol infusion (25–50 mcg/kg/min).

General anesthesia:

Induction	Standard induction (see p. B-2). ET intubation and/or controlled ventilation may not be needed for shorter cases; consider LMA.
Maintenance	Standard maintenance (see p. B-2); consider propofol infusion (100–200 mcg/kg/min). Muscle relaxation usually not required.
Emergence	No specific considerations

Blood and fluid requirements	Usually minimal blood loss IV: 18 ga × 1 NS/LR @ 1–2 mL/kg/h	Minimize NS/LR to avoid postop urinary retention after herniorrhaphy.
Monitoring	Standard monitors (see p. B-1).	

POSTOPERATIVE

Complications	PONV Failure to void	May delay discharge from PACU → home.
Pain management	Local anesthesia Ketorolac 30 mg im or iv in adults ± morphine 2–4 mg iv or fentanyl 25-50 mcg iv	Instillation (2 min) or infiltration of wound with 0.25% bupivacaine or ilioinguinal nerve block provides prolonged postop analgesia and decreases need for narcotics in outpatients. This can be used in both adult and pediatric patients.

Suggested Readings

1. Casey WF, Rice LJ, Hannallah RS, et al: A comparison between bupivacaine instillation versus ilioinguinal/iliohypogastric nerve block for postoperative analgesia following inguinal herniorrhaphy in children. *Anesthesiology* 1990; 72(4):637–9.
2. Goldstein M: Surgical management of male infertility and other scrotal disorders. In *Campbell-Walsh Urology*, 9th edition. WB Saunders, Philadelphia: 2006.
3. Herr HW: Surgery of penile and urethral carcinoma. In *Campbell-Walsh Urology*, 9th edition. WB Saunders, Philadelphia: 2006.
4. Rozanski T, Bloom DA, Colodny A: Surgery of the scrotum and testis in childhood. In *Campbell-Walsh Urology*, 9th edition. WB Saunders, Philadelphia: 2006.

PENILE OPERATIONS

SURGICAL CONSIDERATIONS

Penectomy is the total or partial resection of the penis for squamous-cell carcinoma of the penile skin. If the tumor can be resected with a safe margin of at least 2 cm, partial penectomy is usually enough. A tourniquet is placed at the base of the penis, which is amputated at least 2 cm proximal to the tumor. The corpora cavernosa are sutured and the tourniquet is released, followed by inspection for bleeding. The edges of the urethra are sutured to the ventral skin and the lateral and dorsal skin edges are approximated over the ends of the corpora cavernosa. Often, an **inguinal lymph node biopsy** follows the penectomy.

Usual preop diagnosis: Squamous-cell carcinoma of the penile skin

Insertion of penile prosthesis is performed for impotence. The prosthesis is inserted into the corpora cavernosa (Fig. 9-18) through a penile or suprapubic incision. Penile prostheses are either malleable or inflatable. The latter have a reservoir in the retropubic space and a pump in the scrotum.

Usual preop diagnosis: Impotence

Hypospadias repair is performed primarily on children < 5 yr. (See Pediatric Urology, p. 1333.)

SUMMARY OF PROCEDURES

	Penectomy	Insertion of Penile Prosthesis
Position	Supine	⇐
Incision	Circumferential penile	Bilateral incisions at base of penis
Special instrumentation	None	⇐

SUMMARY OF PROCEDURES (cont'd)

	Penectomy	Insertion of Penile Prosthesis
Unique considerations	None	⇐
Antibiotics	None	Gentamicin 80 mg iv, slowly; ampicillin 2 g iv
Surgical time	2 h	⇐
Closing considerations	None	⇐
EBL	200 mL	⇐
Postop care	PACU → home	⇐
Mortality	< 1%	⇐
Morbidity	Penile hematoma: 5%	Malfunction: 10% Edema: 5% Infection: 2% Extrusion of the prosthesis: 1%
Pain score	5	5

PATIENT POPULATION CHARACTERISTICS

Age range	Adults	⇐
Incidence	< 1% of all males	1–2% of all males
Etiology	Poor hygiene	Organic impotence

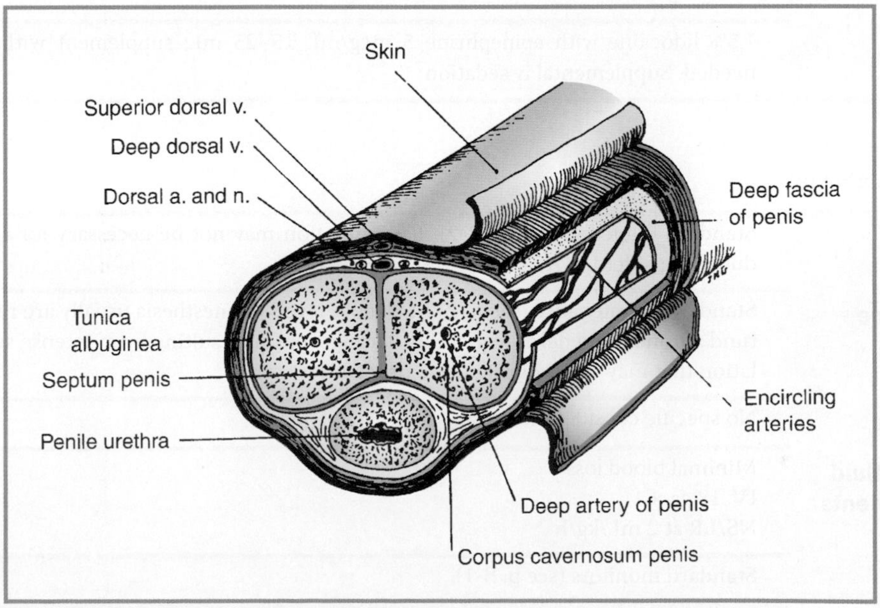

Figure 9-18. Anatomy of the penis. (Reproduced with permission from Hardy JD: *Textbook of Surgery*. JB Lippincott, 1988.)

ANESTHETIC CONSIDERATIONS

PREOPERATIVE

Patients presenting for insertion of a penile prosthesis are frequently elderly and often have preexisting medical problems, including CAD, CHF, PVD, cerebrovascular disease, COPD, and renal impairment. Preop evaluation should be directed toward the detection and treatment of these conditions prior to anesthesia.

Neurological	Patients presenting for insertion of a penile prosthesis often have Hx of diabetes or spinal cord injury. Note presence of neuropathy or Hx of autonomic hyperreflexia (AH) (see Anesthetic Considerations for Transurethral Procedures [except TURP], p. 861). Sx suggestive of AH include HA, flushing, nasal stuffiness, and HTN associated with voiding or noxious stimuli below the level of transection. It is important to document neurological deficits prior to regional anesthesia.
Hematologic	Coagulation defects may be present in patients with priapism. There is a high incidence of priapism in patients with sickle-cell anemia. **Tests:** Hct, if indicated from H&P.
Laboratory	Other tests as indicated from H&P.
Premedication	Sedation prn anxiety in adults (e.g., lorazepam 1–2 mg po 1–2 h prior to surgery; midazolam 1–2 mg iv in preop area).

INTRAOPERATIVE

Anesthetic technique: Spinal, caudal, or lumbar epidural and GA are acceptable, with choice dependent on length of procedure, patient age, coexisting disease, and patient preference. Sacral anesthesia (saddle block) is sufficient; lumbar epidural anesthesia may be less reliable than spinal or caudal at blocking sacral fibers.

Regional anesthesia:

Spinal	5% lidocaine 50 mg (controversial); 0.75% bupivacaine 10 mg in 7.5% dextrose; hyperbaric tetracaine 10 mg with epinephrine for longer procedures
Caudal	0.5% bupivacaine with epinephrine 5 mcg/mL 15–20 mL
Epidural	1.5% lidocaine with epinephrine 5 mcg/mL 15–25 mL; supplement with 5–10 mL as needed. Supplemental iv sedation

General anesthesia:

Induction	Standard induction (see p. B-2). ET intubation may not be necessary for shorter procedures; consider LMA.	
Maintenance	Standard maintenance (see p. B-2). Deeper levels of anesthesia usually are required to obtund autonomic reflexes (e.g., HTN, laryngospasm) resulting from intense surgical stimulation that may occur during these procedures.	
Emergence	No specific considerations	
Blood and fluid requirements	Minimal blood loss IV: 18 ga × 1 NS/LR at 2 mL/kg/h	
Monitoring	Standard monitors (see p. B-1).	
Complications	AH	See Anesthetic Considerations for Transurethral Procedures, p. 862.

POSTOPERATIVE

Complications	Urinary retention
Pain management	Morphine 0.05–0.1 mg/kg iv or fentanyl 25–50 mcg iv prn; ketorolac 30 mg im or iv

Suggested Readings

1. Herr HW: Surgery of penile and urethral carcinoma. In *Campbell-Walsh Urology*, 9th edition. WB Saunders, Philadelphia: 2006.
2. Lewis R: Penile prosthesis. In *Campbell-Walsh Urology*, 9th edition. WB Saunders, Philadelphia: 2006.
3. Lewis R: Surgery for erectile dysfunction. In *Campbell-Walsh Urology*, 9th edition. WB Saunders, Philadelphia: 2006.
4. Lynch DF, Schellhammer PF: Tumors of the penis. In *Campbell-Walsh Urology*, 9th edition. WB Saunders, Philadelphia: 2006.

SCROTAL OPERATIONS

SURGICAL CONSIDERATIONS

Description: Scrotal operations are minor, common urologic procedures, performed on an outpatient basis.

Simple orchiectomy is performed as an alternative to medical castration, using either estrogens or LH-RH agonists on men with metastatic prostate cancer for androgen ablation. It is always bilateral. A small scrotal incision is made and the testis delivered. The spermatic cord is cross-clamped, transected, and suture-ligated.

Usual preop diagnosis: Metastatic prostate cancer

Vasovasostomy is the reestablishment of the continuity of the vas deferens and restoration of fertility following a previously performed vasectomy. Through a small scrotal incision, the testis and spermatic cord are delivered. The site of previous vasectomy is identified and excised and the two ends of the vas deferens anastomosed. It is bilateral and requires the use of either the operating microscope or magnifying loupes.

Usual preop diagnosis: Infertility 2° vasectomy

Hydrocelectomy: The testis, with the surrounding hydrocele (Fig. 9-19), is delivered through a scrotal incision. The wall of the hydrocele is excised and the edges sutured around the epididymis to prevent recurrence.

Variant procedure or approach: Aspiration used as a temporizing approach since recurrence is almost 100%.

Usual preop diagnosis: Hydrocele

Spermatocelectomy: A spermatocele is a cyst of the epididymis, usually excised with the part of the epididymis from which it arises.

Variant procedure: Aspiration as a temporizing maneuver until the operation can be performed.

Usual preop diagnosis: Spermatocele or epididymal cyst

Insertion of testicular prosthesis: A small incision is made in the scrotal skin and a pouch is created by blunt dissection in dartos fascia. The prosthesis is placed in the pouch and fixed to the dartos fascia to prevent prosthesis migration.

Usual preop diagnosis: Absent testis, either congenital or following orchiectomy

Reduction of testicular torsion is an emergency operation which must be performed within 6 h of occurrence to prevent irreversible ischemic damage to the testis. Through a small scrotal incision, the testis is reduced and fixed to the dartos fascia to prevent retorsion.

Usual preop diagnosis: Acute testicular torsion

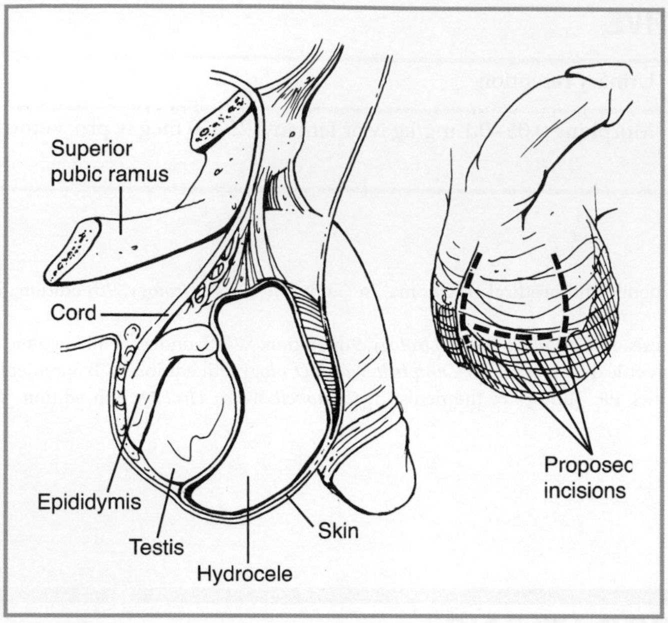

Figure 9-19. Scrotal hydrocele: scrotal incision.

SUMMARY OF PROCEDURES	
Position	Supine
Incision	Scrotal (Fig 9-19, inset)
Special instrumentation	Operating microscope: magnifying loupe for vasovasostomy
Antibiotics	None
Surgical time	1 h
EBL	Negligible
Postop care	PACU → home
Mortality	< 1%
Morbidity	Scrotal hematoma: 2% Wound infection: 2%
Pain score	4

PATIENT POPULATION CHARACTERISTICS	
Age range	All ages
Incidence	Common
Etiology	See preop diagnosis for each procedure, above.

ANESTHETIC CONSIDERATIONS

PREOPERATIVE

Patients presenting for scrotal operations typically fall into two groups: young, otherwise healthy patients and an older population who may present with metastatic prostate cancer accompanied by other medical conditions. The latter group is the focus of this preop evaluation.

Respiratory	Pulmonary disease may be present in elderly patients requiring orchiectomy. **Tests:** As indicated from H&P.
Cardiovascular	Cardiac disease may be present in elderly patients requiring orchiectomy. **Tests:** Consider ECG; others, if indicated from H&P.
Neurological	Document neurologic exam before regional anesthesia in patients with metastatic prostate carcinoma (spinal-cord or nerve-root compression may be present preop).
Musculoskeletal	✓ for presence of spinal metastases if orchiectomy is done for palliation of prostate carcinoma. Extensive lumbar metastases may preclude the use of spinal or epidural anesthesia (relative contraindication). **Tests:** L-spine films if Hx suggestive of spinal metastases.
Laboratory	Other tests as indicated from H&P.
Premedication	Sedation prn anxiety (e.g., lorazepam 1–2 mg po 1–2 h prior to surgery; midazolam 1–2 mg iv in preop area).

INTRAOPERATIVE

Anesthetic technique: Local anesthesia (with sedation) is acceptable for simpler operations (vasectomy, orchiectomy). Procedures that are longer or more complex may require spinal, epidural, or GA. A sensory level of T10 is required to block pain 2° testicular manipulation. Many of these procedures are done on an outpatient basis, and the anesthetic should be appropriately planned to facilitate early discharge.

Regional anesthesia:

Spinal	0.75% bupivacaine 10–12 mg. For shorter procedures(< 1 h), consider low-dose bupivacaine (0.75%, 7.5 mg) or mepivicaine (1.5%, 45 mg). Lidocaine may be used, but the incidence of transient neurologic symptoms is significant.
Epidural	1.5–2% lidocaine with epinephrine 5 mcg/mL, 15–20 mL; supplement with 5–10 mL as needed. Supplemental iv sedation with local or regional techniques (e.g., midazolam 1–2 mg, fentanyl 25–50 mcg iv prn anxiety or discomfort).

General anesthesia:

Induction	Standard induction (see p. B-2). Consider use of LMA.	
Maintenance	Standard maintenance (see p. B-2). Muscle relaxation usually not imperative. Deeper levels of anesthesia are usually required to obtund autonomic reflexes (e.g., HTN, taryngospasm) resulting from intense surgical stimulation that may occur during these procedures.	
Emergence	No specific considerations	
Blood and fluid requirements	Minimal blood loss IV:18 ga × 1 NS/LR @ 2 mL/kg/h	
Monitoring	Standard monitors (see p. B-1).	
Positioning	✓ and pad pressure points. ✓ eyes.	***NB:** peroneal nerve compression at lateral fibular head → foot drop.

POSTOPERATIVE

Complications	Peroneal nerve injury 2° lithotomy position	Peroneal nerve injury manifested by foot drop and loss of sensation on dorsum of foot. Seek neurology consultation.

Pain management	Ketorolac 30 mg im or iv in adults ± morphine 2–4 mg iv or fentanyl 25-50 mcg iv prn	Following orchiopexy, high incidence of postop pain, which may be reduced by ilioinguinal/iliohypogastric nerve blocks.

References

1. Hannallah RS, Broadman LM, Belman AB, et al: Comparison of caudal and ilioinguinal/iliohypogastric nerve blocks for control of post-orchiopexy pain in pediatric ambulatory surgery. *Anesthesiology* 1987; 66(6):832–4.
2. Rozanski T, Bloom DA, Colodny A: Surgery of the scrotum and testis in childhood. In *Campbell's Urology,* Vol 2, 7th edition. WB Saunders, Philadelphia: 1998, 2193–209.

PERINEAL OPERATIONS

SURGICAL CONSIDERATIONS

Urethroplasty: Urethral strictures that do not respond to transurethral dilation and incision are corrected with urethroplasty. A transverse or longitudinal perineal incision is made and carried down to the urethra, which is dissected free from surrounding tissues. The strictured area is excised and end-to-end anastomosis is performed over a catheter. Repair of a long urethral stricture may require placement of a patch from the scrotum, foreskin, or buccal mucosa.

Variant procedure: Transurethral incision and dilation, which is associated with a 30–50% recurrence rate.

Usual preop diagnosis: Urethral stricture, usually posttraumatic

Urethrectomy: Partial or total urethrectomy is done through a longitudinal perineal incision. The urethra is dissected free of surrounding tissues and followed proximally and distally from the membranous urethra to the external urethral meatus. In total urethrectomy, a tubularized skin graft is interposed between membranous urethra and perineal skin.

Usual preop diagnosis: Urethral carcinoma

Insertion of artificial urinary sphincter, performed for incontinence, consists of a perineal incision, through which a cuff is inserted around the bulbar urethra. A suprapubic incision is made to place the reservoir and pump, which inflates and deflates the cuff.

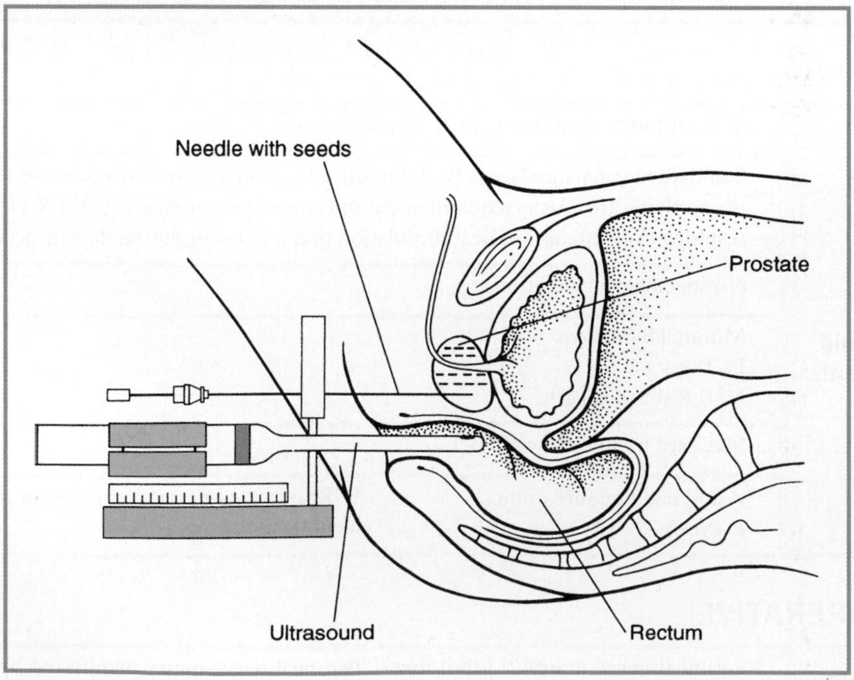

Figure 9-20. Transperineal brachytherapy of prostate gland.

Usual preop diagnosis: Urinary incontinence

Transperineal prostate seed implantation (brachytherapy): High doses of radiation can be delivered to the prostate by implanting radioactive seeds directly into the prostate gland. Using a transrectal ultrasound probe, radioactive seeds (iodine 125 or palladium 103) are implanted into the prostate (Fig. 9-20). The patient is placed in lithotomy position, and a rectal ultrasound probe, with a perineal grid attached, is introduced to image the prostate. Radioactive seeds are then placed transperineally using preloaded needles. Preop dosing calculations determine the number and location of the seeds. This procedure is done by a combined team of radiation oncologists and urologists. No special radiation precautions are necessary for the OR team.

Usual preop diagnosis: Prostate cancer

SUMMARY OF PROCEDURES

	Urethroplasty	Urethrectomy	Insertion of Sphincter	Brachytherapy
Position	Lithotomy	⇐	⇐	⇐
Incision	Perineal (Fig 9-6)	⇐	⇐ and scrotal (Fig. 9-19, inset)	None
Antibiotics	Gentamicin 80 mg im/iv	⇐	⇐	⇐
Surgical time	3 h	2 h	3 h	2 h
EBL	100 mL	300 mL	Minimal	⇐
Postop care	PACU → home	⇐	⇐	PACU, outpatient
Mortality	< 1%	⇐	⇐	⇐
Morbidity	Wound infection: 2%	⇐	⇐ Erosion of the urethra: 10% Extrusion of sphincter: 2%	Urinary retention
Pain score	3	3	4	3

PATIENT POPULATION CHARACTERISTICS

Age range	All ages	Adults	Older adults	50–80 yr
Incidence	< 1% of urologic procedures	⇐	2% of radical prostatectomy	10% of prostate cancer
Etiology	Traumatic strictures	Unknown	Radical prostatectomy (2%); incontinence	Aging

ANESTHETIC CONSIDERATIONS

PREOPERATIVE

This is a generally healthy patient population; preop considerations should be based on H&P.

Laboratory	Tests as indicated from H&P.
Premedication	Sedation prn anxiety in adults (e.g., lorazepam 1–2 mg po 1–2 h prior to surgery; midazolam 1–2 mg iv in preop area).

INTRAOPERATIVE

Anesthetic technique: Spinal or GA are acceptable, with choice dependent on length of procedure, position, patient age, coexisting disease, and patient preference. A sacral sensory level (saddle block) is usually sufficient. Lumbar epidural anesthesia may be less reliable at providing sacral anesthesia, and offers no advantages over the above techniques for shorter procedures, although caudal anesthesia may be an acceptable alternative.

Regional anesthesia:

Spinal	0.75% bupivacaine 10 mg in 7.5% dextrose: hyperbaric tetracaine 10 mg (with epinephrine [200 mcg] for longer procedures)
Caudal	0.5% bupivacaine with epinephrine 5 mcg/mL 15–20 mL. Supplemental iv sedation.

General anesthesia:

Induction	Standard induction (see p. B-2). Consider use of LMA.	
Maintenance	Standard maintenance (see p. B-2); muscle relaxation usually not required. Deeper levels of anesthesia are usually required to obtund autonomic reflexes (e.g., HTN, laryngospasm) resulting from intense surgical stimulation that may occur during these procedures.	
Emergence	No specific considerations	
Blood and fluid requirements	Minimal blood loss IV:18 ga × 1 NS/LR @ 2 mL/kg/h	
Monitoring	Standard monitors (see p. B-1)	
Positioning	✓ and pad pressure points. ✓ eyes.	Patients with arthritis or other musculoskeletal disorders may not tolerate the exaggerated lithotomy position, thus precluding the use of a regional technique. ***NB:** In lithotomy position, peroneal nerve compression at lateral fibular head → foot drop.
Complications	Anticipate ↓ BP on return from lithotomy position.	Rx: volume (200–500 mL NS/LR) or ephedrine (5 mg iv) may be necessary.

POSTOPERATIVE

Complications	Peroneal nerve injury 2° lithotomy position	Peroneal nerve injury manifested as foot drop with loss of sensation over dorsum of foot. Seek neurology consultation.
Pain management	Mild-to-moderate pain	Rx: morphine 0.05–0.1 mg/kg iv prn

VAGINAL OPERATIONS

SURGICAL CONSIDERATIONS

Description: Vaginal operations are performed by both urologists and gynecologists. They include the following:

Repair of vesicovaginal fistulas: The vaginal approach is usually recommended for small and distally located vesicovaginal fistulas; otherwise, a transabdominal repair is performed (see Open Bladder Operations, p. 883). An incision is made in the anterior vaginal wall around the fistula, which is excised. Bladder and vaginal walls are separated and closed with interposition of tissues or flaps to separate the incisions and prevent recurrence. A Foley catheter is left indwelling.

Variant approach: Transabdominal repair of vesicovaginal fistula (see Open Bladder Operations, p. 883).

Usual preop diagnosis: Vesicovaginal fistula

Operations to correct stress urinary incontinence: Many procedures have been designed to correct female urinary incontinence. They fall into two basic groups: (a) operations to correct hypermobility of the urethra, and (b) operations to correct nonfunctioning urethra. The operation most commonly used by urologists to correct hypermobility is the **Stamey procedure** (Fig. 9-21), or **vesical neck suspension.** The operation is performed through two small suprapubic incisions, one on each side of the midline, and an anterior vaginal incision. A nylon suture is placed in a loop from either side of the bladder neck and not around it. Cystoscopy is used to ensure proper placement and to prevent the suture from transversing the bladder. When the sutures are pulled up and tied over the anterior rectus sheath, they pull the bladder neck up to its original position behind the symphysis pubis and restore the acute posterior ureterovesical angle. A variant of this procedure is the **Raz bladder neck suspension,** where bolsters are not used.

Operations to correct a nonfunctioning urethra include **submucosal collagen injection** at the bladder neck or construction of a **sling.** Rectus fascia, fascia lata of the thigh or the vaginal wall can be used to construct a sling around the urethra. All these techniques involve a combined suprapubic and vaginal approach.

Sling operations are the most common procedures done for correction of stress incontinence. These procedures can be done vaginally or open via a suprapubic incision. A variety of materials, both natural and synthetic, have been used. Many modifications have been made with reference to the placement of anchorage of the sling; therefore, there are a large number of procedures with different names utilizing the same principle. Most slings are placed midurethra.

Variant approach: The **Marshall-Marchetti-Krantz operation,** which is performed retropubically, sutures the anterior portion of the urethra, bladder neck, and bladder to the pubic bone. Other modifications include laparoscopic suspensions and ligament surgery. Some patients have cystoceles and rectoceles, which can be repaired at the same time as the vaginal sling surgery.

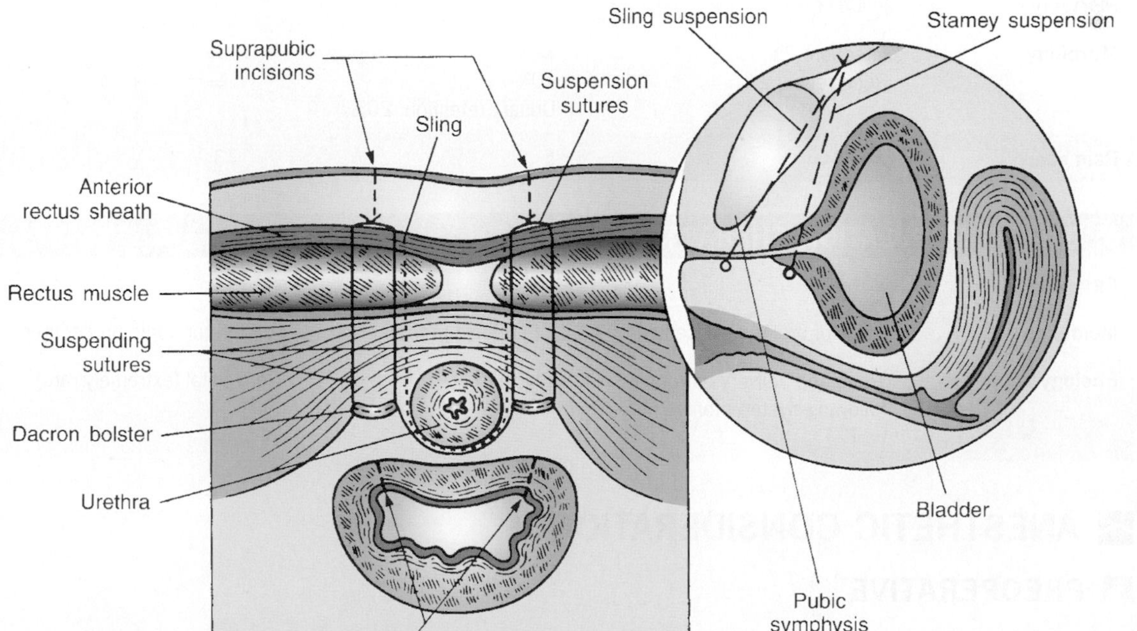

Figure 9-21. Stamey and sling procedures, sectional view; inset shows lateral view.

Usual preop diagnosis: Stress urinary incontinence

Excision of urethral diverticulum: Urethral diverticula are extremely rare and need excision only if they are the cause of recurrent UTIs. An incision is made in the anterior vaginal wall over the urethral diverticulum, which is dissected all around until it is attached only by its neck. It is excised and the neck closed. A Foley catheter is left indwelling, and the vaginal incision is closed.

Usual preop diagnosis: Recurrent UTI 2° infected urethral diverticulum

Repair of cystocele and rectocele: Some patients with urinary incontinence also present with prolapse of the bladder or rectum into the vagina. These can be repaired at the same time as incontinence surgery. A vaginal incision (anterior for cystocele, posterior for rectocele) is made and dissected laterally to free the bladder or rectum from the vagina. The defect is repaired and the redundant vaginal wall excised.

Usual preop diagnosis: Incontinence with pelvic prolapse, cystocele, or rectocele

SUMMARY OF PROCEDURES

	Repair of Vesicovaginal Fistula	Correction of Stress Incontinence	Excision of Urethral Diverticulum
Position	Lithotomy	⇐	⇐
Incision	Anterior vaginal	Anterior vaginal; suprapubic	Anterior vaginal
Special instrumentation	None	Cystoscope	None
Antibiotics	Gentamicin 80 mg iv, slowly	⇐	⇐
Surgical time	2 h	1 h	⇐
EBL	200 mL	500 mL	200 mL
Postop care	PACU → room	⇐	⇐
Mortality	< 1%	⇐	⇐
Morbidity	Infection: 2% Recurrence: 2%	⇐ 10% Urinary retention: 20%	⇐ ⇐
Pain score	3	5	3

PATIENT POPULATION CHARACTERISTICS

Age range	20–80 yr	⇐	⇐
Incidence	< 1% of urologic procedures	5% of urologic procedures	< 1% of urologic procedures
Etiology	Traumatic delivery; iatrogenic following hysterectomy (< 1%)	Childbirth	Congenital (extremely rare)

ANESTHETIC CONSIDERATIONS

PREOPERATIVE

This is a generally healthy patient population. Preop considerations should be based on H&P.

Laboratory	Tests as indicated from H&P.
Premedication	Standard premedication (see p. B-1).

INTRAOPERATIVE

Anesthetic technique: Spinal, continuous lumbar epidural, or GA are acceptable, with choice dependent on age, coexisting disease, and patient preference. A block level of T9-T10 is recommended for operations involving the bladder, whereas somewhat higher levels of anesthesia may be necessary if a suprapubic incision is made. Epidural anesthesia may be less reliable than spinal in providing sacral anesthesia.

Regional anesthesia:

Spinal	0.75% bupivacaine 10–12 mg (1.6 mL)
Epidural	2% lidocaine with epinephrine 5 mcg/mL, 15–20 mL. Supplemental iv sedation.

General anesthesia:

Induction	Standard induction (see p. B-2).	
Maintenance	Standard maintenance (see p. B-2). Muscle relaxation not imperative.	
Emergence	No specific considerations	
Blood and fluid requirements	Minimal blood loss IV: 18 ga × 1 NS/LR @ 2–4 mL/kg/h	
Monitoring	Standard monitors (see p. B-1).	
Positioning	✓ and pad pressure points. ✓ eyes.	***NB:** In lithotomy position, peroneal nerve compression at lateral fibular head → foot drop.
Complications	Anticipate ↓ BP when returning from lithotomy. Bladder perforation	Rx: volume (200–500 mL NS/LR) or ephedrine (5 mg iv) may be necessary. Bladder perforation may present as shoulder pain in the awake patient, but may go unnoticed in the patient under GA. Sx include unexplained HTN, tachycardia, ↓ BP (rare).

POSTOPERATIVE

Complications	Peroneal nerve injury 2° lithotomy position Bladder perforation (see above).	Peroneal nerve injury is manifested as foot drop with loss of sensation on dorsum of foot. Seek neurology consultation.
Pain management	Consider ketorolac 30 mg iv/im in adults; supplement with morphine 0.05–0.1 mg/kg iv prn.	

Suggested Readings

1. Leach GE, Trockman BA: Surgery for vesicovaginal and urethrovaginal fistula and urethral diverticulum. In *Campbell-Walsh Urology*, 9th edition. WB Saunders, Philadelphia: 2006.
2. Raz S, Stothers L, Chopra A: Vaginal reconstructive surgery for incontinence and prolapse. In *Campbell-Walsh Urology*, 9th edition. WB Saunders, Philadelphia: 2006.

SPECIAL CONSIDERATIONS FOR ROBOTIC-ASSISTED LAPAROSCOPIC PROCEDURES

ANESTHETIC CONSIDERATIONS

The anesthetic considerations for the majority of laparoscopic and robotic procedures on the urologic system are similar, and are thus summarized in this section rather than repeated for each individual procedure.

INTRAOPERATIVE

Anesthetic technique: In general, since laparoscopic surgery involves insufflation of the abdomen with CO_2, and may also require steep Trendelenburg position, GA with tracheal intubation and controlled ventilation is the technique of choice.

General anesthesia:

Induction	Standard induction (see p. B-1)	
Maintenance	Standard Maintenance (see p. B-2). Muscle relaxation advised.	
Emergence	Ensure airway patency (subcutaneous emphysema → airway compromise)	
Blood and fluid requirements	IV: 16–18 ga x 1 LR/NS @ 2–6 mL/kg/hr warm fluid, humidify gasses	Blood loss may be difficult to estimate. In general, less than for open procedures.
Monitoring	Standard monitors (see p. B-1) ± arterial line ± CVP	Consider invasive monitors for nephrectomy, prostatectomy
Positioning	✓ and pad pressure points.	Prolonged duration of robotic procedures in lithotomy position of special concern (peroneal nerve injury).
Complications	CO_2 insufflation	→ ↑ intra-abdominal pressure → ↓ venous return, ↓ BP; also ↑ airway pressure, ↑ $PCO_2/ETCO_2$. * **NB:** right mainstem intubation can occur because of shift of diaphragm cephalad.
	Retroperitoneal gas insufflation	→ subcutaneous emphysema (can track to head and neck → airway compromise), pneumothorax.
	VAE	Gas embolism via prostatic venous sinuses reported

POSTOPERATIVE

Complications	Peroneal nerve injury (foot drop) Upper airway obstruction	Other pressure point injuries may occur 2° subcutaneous emphysema tracking up to the head and neck
Pain management	Consider ketorolac 30 mg iv/im in adults	Pain less than for open procedures. Supplement with morphine 0.05–0.1 mg/kg iv prn, followed by PCA.
Tests	Hct	If excessive blood loss

Suggested Readings

1. Conacher ID, Soomro NA Rix D: Anaesthesia for laparoscopic urological surgery. *Br J Anaesth* 2004; 93(6): 859–64.
2. Nelson JB: Debate: open radical prostatectomy vs. laparoscopic vs. robotic. *Urol Oncol* 2007; 25(6): 490–3.
3. Zorn KC, Gofrit ON, Orvieto MA, et al: Da Vinci robot error and failure rates: single institution experience on a single three-arm robot unit of more than 700 consecutive robot-assisted laparoscopic radical prostatectomies. *J Endourol* 2007; 21(11):1341–4.

Urology

SECTION

10.0 ORTHOPEDIC SURGERY

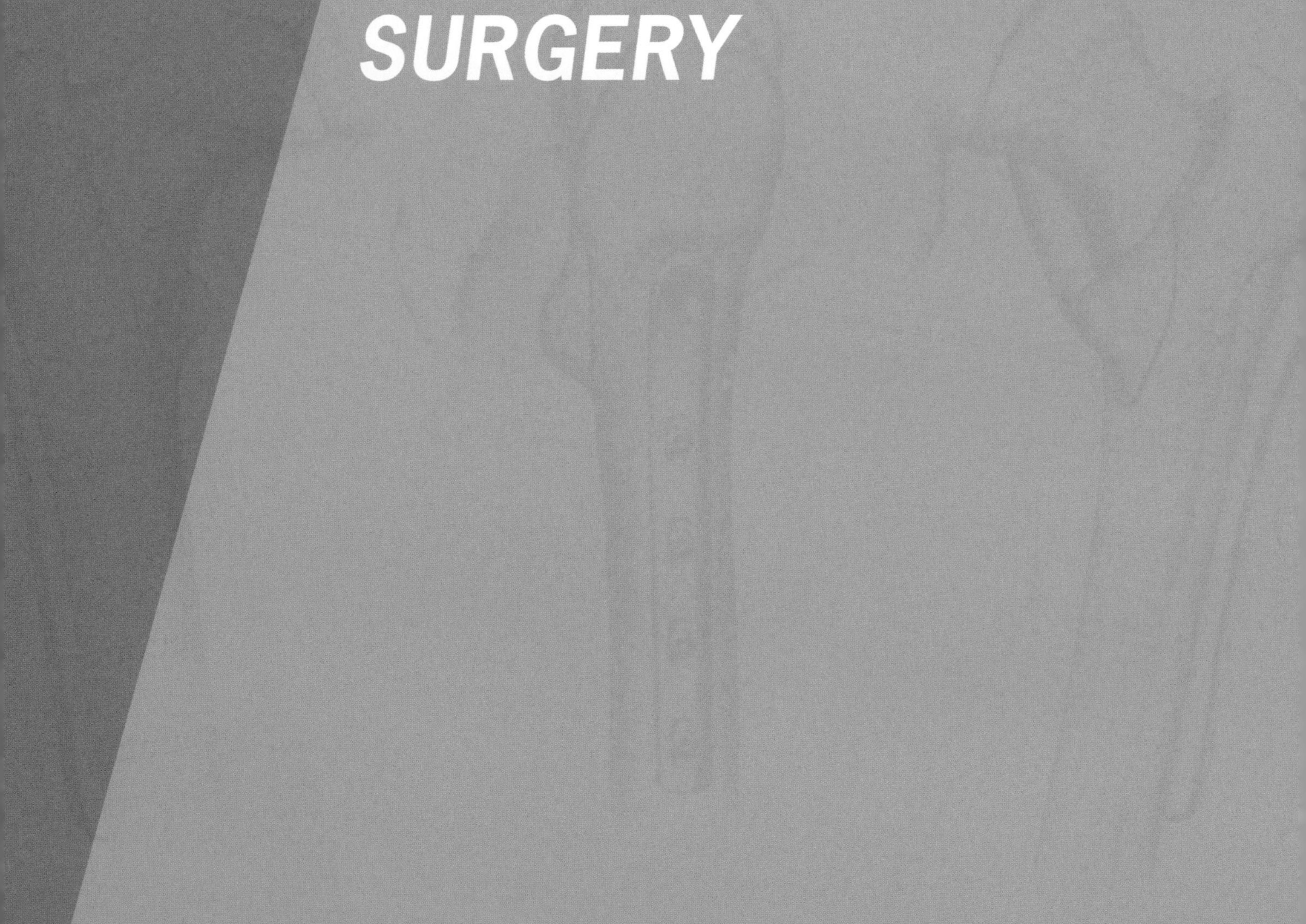

CHAPTER

10.1 Hand Surgery

SURGEONS

Vincent R. Hentz, MD

Kimberley Wirsing, MD

ANESTHESIOLOGIST

Lindsey Vokach-Brodsky, MB, ChB, FFARCS

DARRACH PROCEDURE

SURGICAL CONSIDERATIONS

Description: The **Darrach procedure** (Fig. 10.1-1) is a resection of the distal ulna. The distal 2 cm of the ulna is resected subperiosteally, and local soft tissues are used to stabilize and cover the remaining ulna. It is commonly performed in patients who have had a disruption of the distal radioulnar joint with subluxation of the ulna. It also is indicated for patients who have had a malunion of a distal radius fracture such that the radius has shortened relative to the ulna or is abnormally angulated, resulting in dorsal subluxation of the ulna and impingement of the ulnar head upon the carpus. This causes painful motion of the wrist and forearm and posttraumatic degenerative arthritis of the ulnar head, carpus, and sigmoid notch of the distal radius. Disorders of the distal radioulnar joint and degeneration of the ulnar head, which may lead to attrition rupture of the overlying extensor tendons, are common in rheumatoid arthritis. This dorsal prominence of the ulnar head is treated by **Darrach resection,** combined with a soft-tissue procedure to stabilize the remaining ulna. Osteoarthritic degeneration of the distal radioulnar joint, either 2° trauma (see above) or due to idiopathic osteoarthritis, responds well to this procedure.

Variant procedure or approaches: The Soavé-Kapandji procedure retains the articular portion of the distal ulna and fuses it to the sigmoid notch. The area of distal ulna that is resected is proximal to the joint; instability of the proximal stump may become problematic. Hemiresection with tendon interposition as well as distal ulnar arthroplasty are less common techniques for managing distal radio-ulnar arthritis.

Usual preop diagnosis: Arthritis or derangement of the distal radioulnar joint; rheumatoid arthritis; ulnar impingement syndrome; malunion of Colles' fracture or other fracture of the distal radius

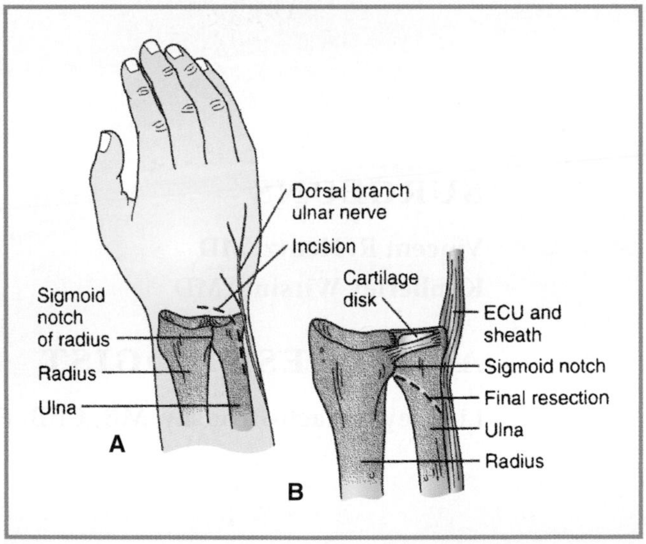

Figure 10.1-1. The Darrach procedure. **A:** Skin incision. Avoid dorsal cutaneous branch of the ulnar nerve. **B:** The distal ulna is resected at the radioulnar articulation just proximal to the sigmoid notch. (ECU = extensor carpi ulnaris) (Reproduced with permission from Chapman MW: *Chapman's Orthopaedic Surgery,* 3rd edition. Lippincott Williams & Wilkins: 2001.)

SUMMARY OF PROCEDURE	
Position	Supine, with arm extended on hand-surgery table
Incision	Dorsal-ulnar, over distal ulna
Special instrumentation	Pneumatic tourniquet

SUMMARY OF PROCEDURE (cont'd)	
Antibiotics	Cefazolin 1 g iv
Surgical time	1–2.5 h, depending on associated procedures
Tourniquet	150 mmHg above systolic; max time = 120 min
Closing considerations	Routine skin closure; postop splint placed at conclusion of procedure.
EBL	Minimal; performed under tourniquet control.
Postop care	PACU → home.
Mortality	None associated with procedure
Morbidity	Ulnar nerve injury: Rare Postop swelling (rarely requires specific treatment)
Pain score	5–7

PATIENT POPULATION CHARACTERISTICS	
Age range	Adult population
Male:Female	Slight predominance of females, due to incidence of malunion of Colles' fractures in women with senile osteoporosis as well as incidence of inflammatory arthropathies in women
Incidence	Not uncommon
Etiology	See Usual preop diagnosis, above.
Associated conditions	Rheumatoid arthritis

ANESTHETIC CONSIDERATIONS

See Anesthetic Considerations for Wrist Procedures, p. 914.

Suggested Reading

1. Nolan WB, Eaton RG: Darrach procedure for distal ulnar pathology derangements. *Clin Orthop* 1992;275:85–9.

DORSAL STABILIZATION AND EXTENSOR SYNOVECTOMY OF THE RHEUMATOID WRIST

SURGICAL CONSIDERATIONS

Description: This procedure is indicated for patients with rheumatoid arthritis and extensor tenosynovitis refractory to medical treatment, as well as extensor tendon ruptures and/or intercarpal synovitis. The procedure is performed under tourniquet control through a straight dorsal incision over the wrist. A **radical tenosynovectomy** of the extensor tendons in all six extensor compartments is carried out. Tendon ruptures or impending ruptures are repaired with tendon grafts or side-to-side anastomoses. Bone spurs are removed and a synovectomy of the distal radioulnar joint is carried out. A **modified Darrach procedure,** with resection or osteoplasty of the distal ulna, is usually performed. If there is evidence of synovitis within the wrist joint, a synovectomy is performed through a dorsal arthrotomy. A flap of the extensor retinaculum is transposed beneath the extensor tendons to reinforce the dorsal wrist ligaments and, thus, stabilize the wrist to prevent volar subluxation of the carpus. A posterior interosseous neurectomy is carried out at the same time. The remaining extensor retinaculum is divided into two transverse strips and one is used to stabilize the distal ulna. The second strip is placed dorsal to the extensor tendons so they will not bowstring during wrist extension.

Usual preop diagnosis: Rheumatoid arthritis with extensor tendon tenosynovitis; extensor tendon rupture; distal radioulnar joint synovitis and/or subluxation

SUMMARY OF PROCEDURE

Position	Supine, with arm extended on hand-surgery table
Incision	Dorsal wrist (Fig. 10.1-2)
Special instrumentation	Pneumatic tourniquet
Antibiotics	Cefazolin 1 g iv
Surgical time	2 h
Tourniquet	150 mmHg above systolic; max time = 120 min
Closing considerations	Postop splint
EBL	Minimal; tourniquet used until dressing in place.
Postop care	PACU → home.
Mortality	None associated with procedure
Morbidity	Extremity swelling (typically does not require treatment) Delayed healing 2° immunosuppression and steroid use Wound infection: Rare (unless patient is immunosuppressed)
Pain score	3–5

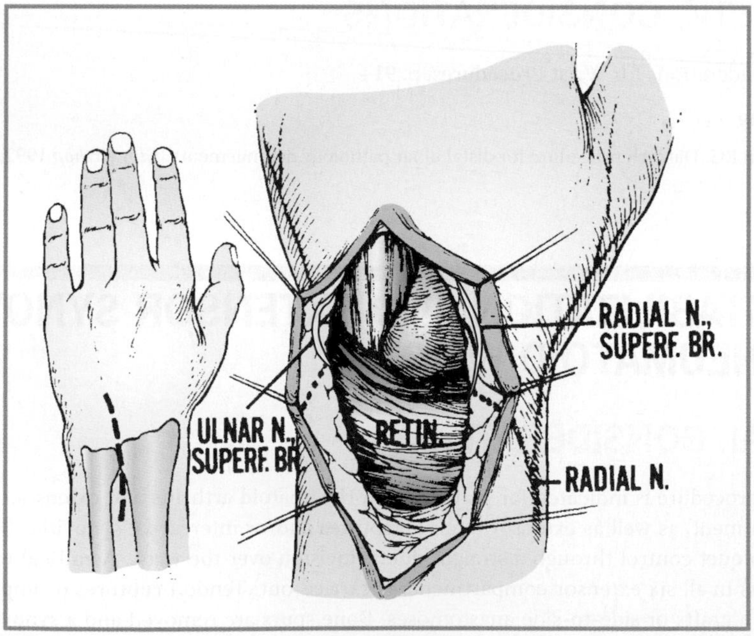

Figure 10.1-2. Incision and exposure for dorsal tenosynovectomy. Note superficial branches of radial and ulnar nerves protected in skin flaps. (Illustration by Elizabeth Roselius, 1988. Reproduced with permission from Green DP, RN Hotchkiss and WC Pederson, eds.: *Operative Hand Surgery,* 2nd edition. Churchill Livingstone: 1988.)

PATIENT POPULATION CHARACTERISTICS	
Age range	Procedure uncommon before 4th decade
Male:Female	As in all patients with rheumatoid arthritis, females more common.
Incidence	Not uncommon
Etiology	Connective tissue disorder; rheumatoid arthritis or variant
Associated conditions	All conditions associated with connective tissue disorders, including active rheumatoid arthritis, steroid dependency, immunosuppressive therapy, and/or skin fragility

ANESTHETIC CONSIDERATIONS

See Anesthetic Considerations for Wrist Procedures, p. 914.

Suggested Reading

1. Millender LH, Terrono AL: Synovectomy and tendon reconstruction. In *The Wrist.* Gelberman RH, ed. Raven Press, New York: 1994, 221–37.

METACARPOPHALANGEAL AND INTERPHALANGEAL JOINT ARTHROPLASTY AND ARTHRODESIS

SURGICAL CONSIDERATIONS

Description: **Joint replacement** in the hand is most commonly indicated in patients with rheumatoid arthritis with severe joint destruction → pain and dysfunction. Another option in these patients is arthrodesis or joint fusion, which involves removing the degenerative cartilaginous surfaces and using implanted metal to secure two opposing bone surfaces. Joint arthroplasty is rarely indicated in patients with osteoarthritis. The most common prostheses, made of silicone rubber and popularized by Swanson, differ from total joint replacement in the hip or knee in that they do not function as true joints, but rather as spacers in a **resection arthroplasty.** Most of the stability and motion of these joints depend on meticulous soft-tissue reconstructions involving tendon and ligament transfers, as well as intensive postop physical therapy. To obtain good results, patients must be well motivated and understand their disease process and what will be asked of them during the recovery period. The results for **metacarpophalangeal (MP) arthroplasty** are far better than those obtained in the proximal interphalangeal joints. **Proximal interphalangeal joint arthroplasty** is sometimes complicated by soft tissue deformities in rheumatoid arthritis such as swan-neck and boutonniere deformities. A swan-neck deformity consists of hyperextension of the PIP joint and flexion of the DIP joint. Conversely, a boutonniere deformity involves flexion at the PIP joint and hyperextension of the DIP joint. It is generally not indicated for the index finger due to the high stresses associated with pinch that may compromise the longevity or stability of an arthroplasty. **Distal interphalangeal (DIP) arthroplasty** is rarely performed, because these patients do well with fusions. The procedure for the MP joints is performed through a dorsal transverse incision under tourniquet control. The metacarpal heads are removed with an oscillating saw and the intramedullary canals reamed to accept the stems of the prostheses. After they have been placed with a no-touch technique, the capsule is closed and the supporting ligaments are reconstructed with centralization of extensor tendons. Technique for PIP joints is similar, although some surgeons will use a volar approach. A splint with support for each finger is placed at the conclusion of surgery. Reconstructive procedures of the wrist and fingers can be combined with arthroplasty.

Variant procedure or approaches: Some surgeons favor longitudinal incisions rather than a transverse incision for the approach to the MP joints. A volar approach to the PIP joint may be used.

Usual preop diagnosis: Rheumatoid arthritis or other connective-tissue disorder

SUMMARY OF PROCEDURE	
Position	Supine, with arm extended on hand-surgery table
Incision	Dorsal hand, transverse, or longitudinal
Special instrumentation	MP or PIP joint prostheses and associated instruments for preparing the medullary canal; power for bone cuts; K-wires, plates, or wire loop for fusion; pneumatic tourniquet
Antibiotics	Cefazolin 1 g iv
Surgical time	2.5 h
Tourniquet	150 mm above systolic; max time = 120 min
Closing considerations	Critical postop splinting
EBL	Minimal; tourniquet used throughout procedure.
Postop care	PACU → home.
Mortality	None associated with procedure
Morbidity	Swelling (may require early splitting of dressing) Wound infection: Rare (if it occurs, requires removal of prosthesis) Prosthesis infection: Rare
Pain score	3–6

PATIENT POPULATION CHARACTERISTICS	
Age range	>50 yr
Male:Female	As in rheumatoid arthritis, females predominate.
Incidence	Uncommon
Etiology	Rheumatoid arthritis or other connective-tissue disorder
Associated conditions	As in rheumatoid arthritis (e.g., skin fragility, steroid dependency, immunosuppression)

ANESTHETIC CONSIDERATIONS

See Anesthetic Considerations for Wrist Procedures, p. 914.

ARTHRODESIS OF THE WRIST

SURGICAL CONSIDERATIONS

Description: A variety of arthrodeses can be performed about the wrist. These include **radiopancarpal arthrodesis (total wrist fusion),** and radiolunate, radioscapholunate, and intercarpal arthrodeses (partial wrist fusions). Radiopancarpal arthrodesis is generally performed as a salvage procedure for wrist pathology that cannot be treated with a procedure that preserves wrist motion. These indications include: posttraumatic degenerative arthritis following fractures, dislocations and ligamentous injuries, idiopathic osteoarthritis, and/or rheumatoid arthritis. Predictable patterns of arthritis occur as a result of both scapholunate interosseous ligament injury (scapholunate advanced collapse) and scaphoid nonunion (scaphoid nonunion advanced collapse). As arthritic changes progress patients are no longer candidates for either reconstruction of the ligaments or fixation of the scaphoid. Another alternative to fusion is a proximal row carpectomy, which is a motion preserving procedure that may be used in patients without advanced capitolunate arthritis. In the nonrheumatoid patient, an effective procedure is an arthrodesis using an iliac crest bone graft fixed with plate and screws. More recent techniques with improved plate designs may not require iliac crest bone graft. As another option, local bone from the distal radius may be utilized. It has been shown that a position of fusion in 10–15° of dorsiflexion provides the greatest grip strength. In the rheumatoid patient, a technique using intramedullary fixation with a large-diameter Steinmann pin is preferred. Rheumatoid bone is osteoporotic, 2° disuse and chronic steroid administration and screw fixation is not ideal in this soft bone. Bone graft is obtained locally in these patients, usually from the resected ulnar head. **Radiolunate fusion** also is indicated in rheumatoid patients who have progressive ulnar translation of the carpus. The lunate acts to block this translation of the carpus. **Radioscapholunate fusion** is indicated in patients with radiocarpal arthritis. This procedure preserves about 50% of wrist motion that occurs at the midcarpal joint. Bone graft is necessary and is easily obtained from the distal radius through the same incision. There are a variety of **intercarpal arthrodeses,** including **triscaphe** (scaphotrapezial trapezoid), **scaphocapitate, lunotriquetral** and **four-corner** (capitate-hamate-triquetral-lunate). These procedures are indicated for the treatment of intercarpal arthritis, carpal instabilities due to intercarpal ligament tears and Kienböck's disease (aseptic necrosis of the lunate). The **Cloward cervical spine fusion instrumentation** is useful for obtaining a bicortical plug of bone from the iliac crest with minimal dissection. Local bone graft from the distal radius may be obtained using curettes or larger core needles.

Usual preop diagnosis: Posttraumatic arthritis; osteoarthritis or rheumatoid arthritis; Kienböck's disease; carpal instability

SUMMARY OF PROCEDURE

Position	Supine, with arm extended on hand-surgery table. The iliac crest may be prepped and elevated with a sandbag beneath the ipsilateral buttock.
Incision	Dorsal wrist, transverse or longitudinal
Special instrumentation	Pneumatic tourniquet; possibly power for preparation of opposing bone surfaces; K-wires, screws or special instrumentation for fusion
Unique considerations	Bone-graft donor site
Antibiotics	Cefazolin 1 g iv
Surgical time	2 h
Tourniquet	150 mmHg above systolic; max time = 120 min
Closing considerations	Immobilization with splints
EBL	Minimal; procedure is performed under tourniquet control. If iliac crest bone graft is used, there may be increased blood loss.
Postop care	PACU → home, sometimes admission for pain control and elevation
Mortality	None associated with procedure
Morbidity	Nonunion of fusion: ≤ 20%
Pain score	5–7, if no iliac graft; 6–9, if iliac graft used

PATIENT POPULATION CHARACTERISTICS

Age range	> 40 yr
Male:Female	Females predominate in rheumatoid arthritis; males in posttraumatic arthritis.
Incidence	Common
Etiology	Trauma (common); rheumatoid arthritis (common)
Associated conditions	Typical for rheumatoid arthritis (e.g., skin fragility, steroid dependency, immunosuppression)

ANESTHETIC CONSIDERATIONS

See Anesthetic Considerations for Wrist Procedures, p. 914.

Suggested Reading

1. Green DP, Pedereson WC, Hotchkiss RN, et al. eds: *Green's Operative Hand Surgery,* 5th edition. Churchill Livingstone, New York: 2005.

TOTAL WRIST REPLACEMENT

SURGICAL CONSIDERATIONS

Description: The major indication for this procedure is rheumatoid arthritis of the wrist. **Total wrist replacement (TWR)** is often recommended in patients with bilateral wrist disease. An arthrodesis will be carried out on the nondominant helping hand and a TWR on the dominant hand to preserve dexterity. Many surgeons prefer to avoid **bilateral wrist arthrodesis,** although some patients with bilateral fusions have been able to function relatively well. Currently available protheses are suitable only for low-demand patients, and are not indicated for high-demand patients with posttraumatic arthritis especially younger patients. These patients will do better with wrist arthrodesis. Silastic wrist prostheses are associated with a high failure rate and silicone synovitis, and their use has been abandoned by many surgeons. The most commonly used prostheses today are metal on ultra-high-molecular-weight polyethylene articulations that are fixed with methylmethacrylate cement or bone ingrowth into porous stems. The distal radius articular surface is resected to accept the implant, the proximal carpal row is resected and the distal carpus is prepared to accept the distal implant. All of these prostheses depend on intact, normally functioning wrist extensor tendons, especially the extensor carpi radialis brevis, for balance and function. Absence of this tendon is felt by many to be an absolute contraindication to this procedure. Because these tendons are so commonly affected by rheumatoid arthritis, the patient population for this procedure is limited. In addition to functioning tendons, meticulously accurate placement of the components in relation to the centers of rotation of the wrist is critical for success. If the centers of rotation of the prosthesis do not duplicate those of the normal wrist, early component loosening and failure is likely. Intraop radiographs are useful in verifying component position. These patients frequently have other upper extremity deformities that will require reconstruction. Because of the complexity of TWR, other reconstructive procedures are not carried out at the same time.

Usual preop diagnosis: Rheumatoid arthritis

SUMMARY OF PROCEDURE	
Position	Supine, with arm extended on hand-surgery table
Incision	Dorsal wrist
Special instrumentation	TWR instrumentation; power for bone cuts; pneumatic tourniquet
Antibiotics	Cefazolin 1 g iv
Surgical time	2 h
Tourniquet	150 mmHg above systolic; max time = 120 min
Closing considerations	Postop splint
EBL	Minimal; procedure performed under tourniquet control.
Postop care	PACU → home vs admission for pain control and elevation
Mortality	None associated with procedure

SUMMARY OF PROCEDURE (cont'd)	
Morbidity	Infection: Rare (but requires removal of prosthesis and methylmethacrylate cement, if used) Poor wound healing
Pain score	4–8

PATIENT POPULATION CHARACTERISTICS	
Age range	Rare before 4th decade; most in 6th and 7th decades
Male:Female	Females outnumber males, as in rheumatoid arthritis.
Incidence	Rare
Etiology	Rheumatoid arthritis
Associated conditions	Rheumatoid arthritis

ANESTHETIC CONSIDERATIONS

See Anesthetic Considerations for Wrist Procedures, p. 914.

Suggested Reading

1. Green DP, Hotchkiss, RN, Pederson, WC, et al, eds: *Operative Hand Surgery,* 5th edition. Churchill Livingstone, New York: 2005.

THUMB CARPOMETACARPAL JOINT FUSION/ ARTHROPLASTY/STABILIZATION

SURGICAL CONSIDERATIONS

Description: Patients with degenerative arthritis of the carpometacarpal (CMC) joint of the thumb present with subluxation, pain, and synovitis of the joint. A **synovectomy and ligament reconstruction** to restore stability will treat pain and may delay further degeneration. This procedure is performed through a curvilinear incision over the joint. A distally attached graft of the radial 1/2 of the flexor carpi radialis tendon is passed through a drill hole in the base of the metacarpal and woven into the joint capsule. In the later stages of degeneration, patients must be treated with either an arthroplasty or an arthrodesis. For more progressive arthritis a variety of **arthroplasty techniques** are available to the surgeon; most involve removal of degenerated articular surfaces, soft tissue interposition and often K-wire fixation to suspend the metacarpal is used. Cemented arthroplasty techniques were initially associated with a high loosening rate and fell out of favor. Newer designs and techniques do not have long-term follow-up yet. The status of the MCP joint of the thumb must be considered prior to CMC intervention. Hyperextension at the MCP joint will increase forces across any CMC procedure.

Variant procedure or approaches: Some surgeons choose to address CMC arthritis arthroscopically with joint debridement and sometimes material interposition.

Usual preop diagnosis: Osteoarthritis of CMC joint; basal joint arthritis; synovitis of CMC joint; CMC joint dislocation; trauma

SUMMARY OF PROCEDURE	
Position	Supine, with arm extended on hand-surgery table
Incision	Curvilinear over joint at base of thumb. If soft tissue interposition is used, additional incisions may be required.

SUMMARY OF PROCEDURE (cont'd)	
Special instrumentation	Pneumatic tourniquet; power if K-wire suspension is to be used
Antibiotics	Cefazolin 1 g iv
Surgical time	1.5–2 h
Tourniquet	150 mmHg above systolic; max time = 120 min
EBL	Minimal; procedures performed under tourniquet control.
Postop care	PACU → home
Mortality	None associated with procedure
Morbidity	Nonunion of arthrodesis: ≤ 20% Particulate synovitis (silicone rubber prostheses)
Pain score	8–9

PATIENT POPULATION CHARACTERISTICS	
Age range	Joint stabilization in 3rd–5th decades; arthroplasty and arthrodesis in 5th-8th decades
Male:Female	Basal joint instability and arthritis much more prevalent in women
Incidence	Common
Etiology	Trauma may play a role in producing instability. Intraarticular fracture of the base of the first metacarpal with a nonanatomic reduction → incongruence of the joint → post-traumatic arthritis. Rheumatoid arthritis → instability and degeneration of the joint. Congenital ligamentous laxity → unstable basal joints and arthritis in many patients.
Associated conditions	Rheumatoid arthritis; osteoarthritis; carpal tunnel syndrome (CTS)

ANESTHETIC CONSIDERATIONS FOR WRIST PROCEDURES

(Procedures covered: Darrach procedure; dorsal stabilization and extensor synovectomy of the rheumatoid wrist; metacarpophalangeal and interphalangeal joint arthroplasty; arthrodesis of the wrist; total wrist replacement; thumb carpometacarpal joint fusion/arthroscopy/stabilization)

PREOPERATIVE

Airway	Rheumatoid involvement of the C-spine, TMJ, and cricoarytenoid joint (CAJ) are common in this patient population. Erosion of cervical vertebrae → unstable C-spine (e.g., atlantoaxial subluxation) necessitates extreme care in head and neck manipulation. C-spine fusion (↓ neck ROM), TMJ arthritis (↓ mouth opening) and CAJ arthritis (laryngeal narrowing, hoarseness, DOE, stridor) portend difficult intubation and may necessitate awake fiber optic intubation (p. B-5). In the case of CAJ arthritis, use of a smaller ETT may be required.
Respiratory	Rheumatoid patients may exhibit Sx of pleural effusion (✓ CXR) or pulmonary fibrosis (dyspnea, diffuse rales, ↓ diffusing capacity, honeycomb appearance in CXR). **Tests:** Consider CXR, PFTs, ABGs in affected patients.
Cardiovascular	Rheumatoid patients may suffer from pericarditis, myocarditis, valvular disease, and cardiac conduction defects. Because of the physical limitations imposed by the disease process, it may prove difficult to evaluate these patients' cardiovascular status; hence, cardiology consultation, ECG, and ECHO may be useful in preparing for surgery. **Tests:** Consider ECG and ECHO, especially in patients with severe rheumatoid arthritis.

Neurological	Rheumatoid patients may have cervical or lumbar radiculopathies that should be documented carefully preop. In addition, peripheral neuropathy with consequent sensory/motor defects may be present. **Tests:** Consider C-spine radiographs to r/o occult subluxations in rheumatoid patients with neck pain or upper extremity radiculopathy.
Musculoskeletal	Bony deformities or muscle contractures may necessitate special attention to positioning.
Hematologic	Anemia, eosinophilia, and thrombocytosis may be present. Venous access may be difficult 2° vasculitis and ↑ skin fragility (steroid-induced). Virtually all of these patients will be on some type of anti-inflammatory medication that may result in anemia or Plt inhibition. Ideally, patients should discontinue NSAIDs at least 5 d preop; aspirin, 7 d preop.
Endocrine	Rheumatoid patients may be on oral corticosteroids and require supplemental periop steroids (e.g., 100 mg hydrocortisone q 8 h iv) to treat adrenal suppression, although the routine use of 'stress-dose steroids' has been questioned.
Laboratory	Hb/Hct serves as a minimum in otherwise healthy rheumatoid patients. Severe rheumatoid patients may require more extensive testing to screen for drug effects, etc. (e.g., serum electrolytes; glucose; kidney function tests; LFTs).
Premedication	Mild-to-moderate premedication (e.g., in adults, midazolam 1–2 mg iv, fentanyl 50–100 mcg iv, titrated to effect) is often desirable before placement of a regional block.

INTRAOPERATIVE

Anesthetic technique: Regional anesthesia, GA, or a combination of the two is commonly used. A brachial plexus block via the supraclavicular, axillary, or infraclavicular approach is excellent for this procedure; it is a means of avoiding tracheal intubation for GA if airway difficulty is anticipated. Furthermore, it decreases admission rate, speeds discharge from PACU in day surgery setting, and increases patient satisfaction. Intravenous regional anesthesia (Bier block) is most useful for short procedures (<1 h). If regional anesthesia is contraindicated, rheumatoid patients may require awake fiber optic intubation (see p. B-5).

Regional anesthesia: 1.5% mepivacaine, 30–40 mL for routine, superficial cases; 0.5% bupivacaine, or 0.5% ropivacaine, 30–40 mL for procedures >2.5 h or if extended analgesia is desired. Epinephrine (2.5–5mcg/mL) should be added whenever possible to decrease peak plasma concentrations of local anesthetics.

Infraclavicular block	The coracoid approach makes this a safe and effective regional technique. A single injection will provide anesthesia distal to the midhumerus. No additional injections are necessary, and the patient's arm does not need to be abducted for block placement. If intraop sedation is necessary, propofol (50–100 mcg/kg/min) by continuous infusion or intermittent bolus injection of opioid/benzodiazepine are good choices.
Axillary block	The medial aspect of the upper arm is innervated by the intercostobrachial nerve (T2) and requires a separate subcutaneous field block in the axilla, especially when a tourniquet is used. The lateral cutaneous nerve of the forearm, a sensory branch of the musculocutaneous nerve supplying sensation to the lateral forearm, is frequently missed by the axillary approach to the brachial plexus. Thus, a block of this nerve at the elbow or within the proximal coracobrachialis muscle is sometimes necessary. If intraop sedation is necessary, propofol (50–150 mcg/kg/min) by continuous infusion or intermittent bolus injection of opioid/benzodiazepine are good choices.
Bier block	The Bier block (intravenous regional anesthesia) is an excellent technique for short (<60 min), superficial wrist and hand surgeries. 40–50 mL of 0.5% lidocaine is commonly used. A very brief operative procedure may be an indication to reduce the dose of iv anesthetic agent by, for example, having the surgeon use a forearm tourniquet instead of an upper arm tourniquet. The OR staff should be alerted that iv regional anesthesia is being used, so that all are ready to proceed after the tourniquet is inflated (i.e., surgical prep ready to be performed; surgeons scrubbed, gowned, and gloved). Tourniquet pain and postop pain are reduced by adding ketorolac (20 mg) or clonidine (1 mcg/kg) to the lidocaine solution.

General anesthesia:

Induction	Standard induction (p. B-2) in patients with normal airways	
Maintenance	Standard maintenance (p. B-2)	
Emergence	Skin closure frequently is followed by application of a splint, and the patient should remain anesthetized during the splinting procedure. Cases with difficult airways require awake extubation.	
Blood and fluid requirements	Minimal blood loss IV: 18 ga × 1 NS/LR @ 1.5–3 mL/kg/h	IV placed in the contralateral upper extremity.
Monitoring	Standard monitors (p. B-1)	
Positioning	Special handling required. ✓ and pad pressure points. ✓ eyes. ✓ C-spine instability.	As with nearly all orthopedic cases, positioning is a subtle, yet crucial aspect of anesthetic management. Rheumatoid patients may have contractures that require special attention. Steroid-dependent patients require special handling because of fragile skin.
Infraclavicular block complications	Local anesthetic toxicity Inadequate block Intravascular injection Pneumothorax Persistent paresthesia	Less frequent occurrence, compared with axillary block. Pneumothorax is very rare with the lateral coracoid approach.
Axillary block complications	Local anesthetic toxicity Inadequate block Intravascular injection Persistent paresthesia Axillary hematoma Axillary artery thrombosis	Very minimal doses of local anesthetic can cause CNS toxicity if reverse flow occurs during an intraarterial injection. Axillary thrombosis is extremely rare.
Bier block complications	Local anesthetic toxicity Inadequate block Thrombophlebitis	Proper exsanguination and tourniquet function is critical. Tourniquet should remain inflated a minimum of 25 min. Systemic toxic reaction to the local anesthetic may occur as a result of tourniquet leak or inadvertent premature (<20 min) tourniquet release. Treatment is supportive. Sz are controlled with STP or midazolam, with appropriate airway protection. Even with a functioning tourniquet, it is possible to overcome tourniquet pressure by injecting too vigorously. Care must be taken when switching from proximal to distal tourniquet; never deflate proximal tourniquet until verifying that distal tourniquet is working.

POSTOPERATIVE

Pain management	PCA (p. C-3), in combination with regional block	Regional or combined regional-general anesthetic techniques are excellent for wrist procedures, especially with respect to postop pain management.
Tests	None routinely indicated.	

Suggested Readings

1. Gerancher JC: Upper extremity nerve blocks. *Anes Clin North Am* 2000; 18(2):1–16.
2. Green DP, Hotchkiss RN, Pederson WC, et al, eds: *Operative Hand Surgery,* 5th edition. Elsevier, New York: 2005.
3. Keenan MA, Stiles CM, Kaufman RL: Acquired laryngeal deviation associated with cervical spine disease in erosive polyarticular arthritis. *Anesthesiology* 1983; 58(5):441–9.
4. Marhofer P, Chan VW. Ultrasound-guided regional anesthesia: current concepts and future trends. *Anesth Analg* 2007; 104(5):1265–9.
5. Ramamurthy S, Anderson D: Anesthesia. In *Operative Hand Surgery,* 5th edition. Green DP, Hotchkiss RN, Pederson WC, et al, eds. Elsevier, New York: 2005, 25–54.
6. Salazar CH: Infraclavicular brachial plexus block. *Reg Anesth Pain Med* 1999; 24(5):411–6.
7. Sia, S: Axillary brachial plexus block using peripheral nerve stimulator: a comparison between double- and triple-injection techniques. *Reg Anesth Pain Med* 2001; 26(6):499–503.
8. Steinberg RB: The dose-response relationship of ketorolac as a component of intravenous regional anesthesia with lidocaine. *Anesth Analg* 1998; 86(4):791–3.
9. Vandam LD: Anesthesia for hand surgery. In *Flynn's Hand Surgery,* 4th edition. Jupiter JB, ed. Williams & Wilkins, Baltimore: 1991, 46–54.
10. White RH: Preoperative evaluation of patients with rheumatoid arthritis. *Semin Arthritis Rheum* 1985; 14(4):287–99.
11. Wilson JL: Infraclavicular brachial plexus block: parasagittal anatomy important to the coracoid technique. *Anesth Analg* 1998; 87(4):870–3.

EXCISION OF GANGLION OF THE WRIST

SURGICAL CONSIDERATIONS

Description: Ganglion cysts about the wrist most commonly occur dorsally, originating from the scapholunate joint. The second most common site is volar to the scaphotrapezial joint. To prevent recurrence, these synovial fluid-filled outpouchings of the joint capsule must be excised completely. This requires isolating the stalk of the cyst to its origin, and excising a small cuff of normal joint capsule with the cyst. The joint, therefore, must be entered for a complete excision. For patients with dorsal ganglia who have considerable preoperative pain a posterior interosseous neurectomy may be done at the same time as the excision. Older studies found that the recurrence rate was decreased by the use of GA, as opposed to local or regional anesthetics. This was due to the fact that a more complete excision was performed when the patient was under GA. Hand specialists today feel that regional anesthetics are quite acceptable for this procedure, as long as the surgeon performs a meticulous excision. Volar wrist ganglions commonly are near the radial artery, which is at risk during excision. A preop Allen test should be performed to ensure that, if the radial artery is interrupted, there will not be ischemia in the hand. Primary small dorsal ganglions may be approached arthroscopically.

Usual preop diagnosis: Ganglion cyst, primary or recurrent

SUMMARY OF PROCEDURE	
Position	Supine, with arm extended on hand-surgery table
Incision	Longitudinal or transverse directly over cyst
Special instrumentation	Pneumatic tourniquet
Antibiotics	Cefazolin 1 g iv
Surgical time	0.5–1.5 h
Tourniquet	150 mmHg above systolic; max time = 120 min
Closing considerations	Routine skin closure. Large recurrent cysts may require a repair of the wrist capsule. Splint applied in OR.
EBL	Minimal; performed under tourniquet control.

SUMMARY OF PROCEDURE (cont'd)	
Postop care	PACU → home
Mortality	None associated with procedure
Morbidity	Injury to radial artery: Rare (Because of the vascular interconnections between radial and ulnar arteries, loss of radial artery flow rarely → complications.)
Pain score	2–4

PATIENT POPULATION CHARACTERISTICS	
Age range	Adults
Male:Female	1:1
Incidence	Very common
Etiology	Unknown. Trauma has been associated with ~50% of ganglion cysts. Underlying carpal instabilities, such as scapholunate instability, have been implicated.
Associated conditions	Carpal instability; trauma (wrist sprains and strains)

ANESTHETIC CONSIDERATIONS

See Anesthetic Considerations following Repair of Flexor Tendon Laceration, p. 921.

PALMAR AND DIGITAL FASCIECTOMY

SURGICAL CONSIDERATIONS

Description: This procedure is indicated for the treatment of Dupuytren's contractures of the digits, which produces a neoplastic thickening of the palmar and digital fascia. These pathologic cords (whose active cell is the myofibroblast) contract and, through their connections with the skin, tendon sheath, and phalangeal bone, cause flexion contractures of the metacarpophalangeal, proximal interphalangeal, and distal interphalangeal joints. The disease is progressive, and the only treatment is surgical excision of the fascia. Research into nonsurgical options for treatment is ongoing, some surgeons perform needle aponeurectomy, which incises the diseased fascia, but does not remove it. In addition to the pathologic changes in the fascia of the hands, many patients also have thickening of the plantar fascia of the foot (Ledderhose disease) and the dorsal fascia of the penis (Peyronie's disease). Patients with severe contractures that have been neglected may require amputation. Because the pathologic fascia is so intimately connected to the skin, it is sometimes necessary to excise the skin and replace it with full-thickness skin grafts. The groin is an excellent donor site for these grafts.

Usual preop diagnosis: Dupuytren's contracture

SUMMARY OF PROCEDURE	
Position	Supine, with arm extended on hand-surgery table
Incision	Transverse or longitudinal palmar. Groin may be used as a full-thickness skin graft donor site.
Antibiotics	Cephazolin 1g iv
Surgical time	1–3 h

SUMMARY OF PROCEDURE (cont'd)	
Tourniquet	150 mmHg above systolic; max time = 120 min. Because of the need to deflate tourniquet so that hemostasis can be obtained, Bier block is not suitable.
Closing considerations	Must obtain meticulous hemostasis. Z-plasties and skin grafts used frequently.
EBL	Minimal; dissection done under tourniquet control. A small amount of blood loss occurs when tourniquet is released and hemostasis is obtained.
Postop care	PACU → home
Mortality	None associated with procedure
Morbidity	Hematoma (usually requires operative intervention) Skin necrosis (may require secondary skin grafting) Digital nerve and artery injury (Vascular injuries typically recognized immediately. An operating microscope may be needed, and the procedure will be prolonged.) Reflex-sympathetic dystrophy (so-called sympathetic "flare" reaction; requires prompt treatment, including stellate ganglion blockade)
Pain score	7–8

PATIENT POPULATION CHARACTERISTICS	
Age range	Typically, 40–60 yr
Male:Female	More common in males
Incidence	Common
Etiology	Definite heritance—associated with strong family Hx. Ethnic diathesis for northern Europeans with fair hair and skin, blue eyes. Almost never seen in Blacks. Experimental studies suggest that microhematomas 2° repetitive trauma may be important in the disease process.
Associated conditions	Cigarette smoking; alcoholism; antiseizure medications

ANESTHETIC CONSIDERATIONS

See Anesthetic Considerations following Repair of Flexor Tendon Laceration, p. 921.

REPAIR OF LACERATED TENDONS/NERVES

SURGICAL CONSIDERATIONS

Description: The prognosis and difficulty of a flexor tendon repair depends on the anatomic site of the laceration. There are five zones of injury in the upper extremity (Fig. 10.1-3). Zone I is distal to the flexor digitorum superficialis (FDS) tendon insertion and involves only the flexor digitorum profundus (FDP) tendon. Zone II extends from the entrance to the fibroosseous sheath at the metacarpal head to the FDS insertion. Lacerations usually involve both the FDS and FDP. These are the most difficult to repair and have the worst prognosis, as the tendons are apt to become scarred to each other and limit gliding. Zone III is the palm; Zone IV is at the level of the carpal canal; and Zone 5 is in the forearm. Lacerations in these areas are easier to repair and have good prognoses for restoration of tendon gliding and, thus, digit motion. Associated injuries to the neural structures are common. Digital nerve lacerations are seen in Zone II; median or ulnar nerve injuries, in Zone IV and proximal. Lacerations to the dorsal side of the hand involving the extensor tendons may be repaired in the emergency room as they often do not involve neurovascular

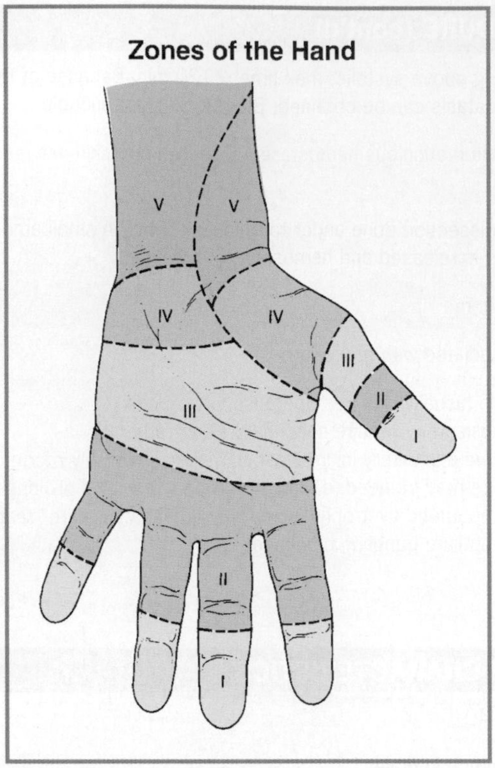

Figure 10.1-3. Zone classification of flexor tendon injuries. (Reproduced with permission from Scott-Conner CEH, Dawson DL: *Operative Anatomy,* 2nd edition. Lippincott Williams & Wilkins, 2003.)

structures, and the extensor digitorum communis tendon as well as the junctura tendinea may prevent retraction of the proximal tendon into the forearm. The exception to this is the thumb and radial dorsal hand where the extensor and abductor tendons may retract, and the dorsal sensory branch of the radial nerve is at risk.

In general, nerve injuries are repaired at the time of the tendon repair. Depending on the surgeon, an operating microscope or loupe magnification may be used. Tendons lacerated in the finger are often pulled back into the palm by muscular contraction. A palmar incision is required to retrieve the tendon, which must then be threaded carefully through the pulleys in the digit. Suture techniques for tendon repair create a juncture that is far weaker than an intact tendon. For this reason, the juncture must be protected from mechanical stress for a period of 8 wk or more. This is done by splinting the hand with the wrist and digits flexed so that the pull on the tendon by its muscle is limited. It is important that the patient emerges gently from anesthesia to limit the stress on the repair. The best results are obtained when repair is carried out within 7 d of the injury, although primary repair can be performed up to 3 wk. After 7 d, the muscle begins to undergo irreversible contracture. If the flexor tendon is advanced after this has occurred, a flexion contracture results. If a flexor tendon laceration is neglected, a palm-to-fingertip tendon graft, using a different flexor tendon, should be performed. If the tendon bed is suitable for gliding, the graft can be accomplished in one stage. If not, a Silastic tendon spacer (rubber rod) must be placed at the first stage; 6–8 wk later, a palm-to-fingertip graft is placed in the bed prepared with the Silastic rod. Tendon graft donor sites include the palmaris longus tendon and toe extensors.

A variant of the sharp flexor tendon laceration is the FDP avulsion from its insertion in Zone 1. This is the so-called "jersey finger"— initially named for the classic mechanism of someone grasping the jersey of a ball carrier. This injury occurs during forceful grasp, and most commonly affects the ring finger. The FDP tendon retracts to various predictable levels per the classification system of Leddy. Type I retracts in to the palm; this injury is most likely to disrupt the blood supply to the tendon via the vinculae. Type II retracts to the level of the PIP joint, and type III retracts to the level of the DIP joint. In general, these injuries should be explored and repaired within 7 days. Repair may require mini-suture anchors or a button/pull out suture through the nail/distal phalanx, because there is not sufficient tendon distally for a primary repair. If neglected, these patients should be treated with a **distal interphalangeal (DIP) arthrodesis.** A flexor tendon graft through an intact FDS tendon usually is not indicated, because tendon adhesions will commonly interfere with the function of the FDS, leading to decreased overall active motion of the digit. The most common complication is the development of tendon adhesions, which limit tendon gliding and digit motion. If these patients fail to improve within a 3- to 6-mo course of physical therapy, they require an operative tendolysis to lyse the adhesions.

Usual preop diagnosis: Flexor tendon laceration; FDP avulsion ("jersey finger"); digital nerve laceration; median nerve laceration

SUMMARY OF PROCEDURE

Position	Supine, with arm extended on hand-surgery table. The foot may be prepped for a graft.
Incision	Zig-zag (Brunner) within the digits, extensile approach hand or wrist
Special instrumentation	Pneumatic tourniquet, possibly operating microscope for nerve injuries
Antibiotics	Cefazolin 1 g iv
Surgical time	1–2 h; may be extended for nerve repair and treatment of associated injuries.
Closing considerations	Tendon and nerve repairs must be protected with splints before emergence from GA. Smooth extubation (see Emergence, below).
EBL	Minimal; procedure performed under tourniquet control.
Postop care	PACU → home
Mortality	None associated with procedure.
Morbidity	Tendon adhesions: 25% Rupture of tendon repair: <5% Infection: Rare
Pain score	2–4

PATIENT POPULATION CHARACTERISTICS

Age range	Adult population, rarely children.
Male:Female	Slight male predominance, due to occupational injuries
Incidence	Not uncommon
Etiology	Trauma

ANESTHETIC CONSIDERATIONS

(Procedures covered: excision of ganglion of the wrist; palmar and digital fasciectomy; repair of flexor tendon laceration)

PREOPERATIVE

The majority of patients presenting for these procedures are usually otherwise healthy. Many of them present for elective surgery as a result of progressive functional impairment and pain, and preop workup is routine.

Neurological	If regional anesthesia is contemplated, preexisting sensory or motor defects should be documented carefully.
Laboratory	Hb/Hct (healthy patients); otherwise, as indicated from H&P.
Premedication	Mild-to-moderate premedication (e.g., in adults, midazolam 1–2 mg iv, fentanyl 50–100 mcg iv, titrated to effect) is often desirable before placement of a regional block.

INTRAOPERATIVE

Anesthetic technique: Regional anesthesia (most common), GA, or a combination of the two may be used. Intravenous regional anesthesia (Bier block) is most useful for short procedures that last for < 1 h (see Anesthetic Considerations, p. 927). A brachial plexus block via the axillary or infraclavicular approach is excellent for this procedure. Because most of these procedures are done on an outpatient basis, brachial plexus block without GA is usually preferred to promote early "street-readiness."

Regional anesthesia: 1.5% mepivacaine 30–40 mL with alkalization for routine, superficial cases; 0.5% bupivacaine or 0.5% levobupivacaine/0.5% ropivacaine, if available, 30–40 mL for procedures > 2.5 h or if extended analgesia is desired. Epinephrine (2.5–5 mcg/mL) should be added whenever possible to decrease peak plasma concentrations of local anesthetics.

Ultrasound guided supraclavicular block	Using ultrasound guidance, the brachial plexus can be blocked at the supraclavicular level. Direct visualization of the plexus and surrounding structures reduces the risk of pneumothorax with this approach. This block provides adequate anesthesia for procedures distal to midhumerus.
Infraclavicular block	The coracoid approach makes this a safe and effective regional technique. A single injection will provide anesthesia distal to the midhumerus. No additional injections are necessary, and the patient's arm does not need to be abducted for block placement. If intraop sedation is necessary, propofol (50–100 mcg/kg/min) by continuous infusion or intermittent bolus injection of opioid/benzodiazepine are good choices.
Axillary block	The medial aspect of the upper arm is innervated by the intercostobrachial nerve (T2) and requires a separate subcutaneous field block in the axilla, especially when a tourniquet is used. The lateral cutaneous nerve of the forearm, a sensory branch of the musculocutaneous nerve supplying sensation to the lateral forearm, is frequently missed by the axillary approach to the brachial plexus. Thus, a block of this nerve at the elbow or within the proximal coracobrachialis muscle is sometimes necessary. If intraop sedation is necessary, propofol (50–100 mcg/kg/min) by continuous infusion or intermittent bolus injection of opioid/benzodiazepine are good choices.
Bier block	The Bier block (intravenous regional anesthesia) is an excellent technique for short (< 60 min), superficial wrist and hand surgeries. 40–50 mL of 0.5% lidocaine is commonly used. A very brief operative procedure may be an indication to reduce the dose of iv anesthetic agent by, for example, having the surgeon use a forearm tourniquet instead of an upper arm tourniquet. The OR staff should be alerted that iv regional anesthesia is being used, so that all are ready to proceed after the tourniquet is inflated (i.e., surgical prep ready to be performed; surgeons scrubbed, gowned, and gloved). Tourniquet pain and postop pain is reduced by adding ketorolac (20 mg) or clonidine (1 mcg/kg) to the lidocaine solution.

General anesthesia:

Induction	Standard induction (p. B-2)	
Maintenance	Standard maintenance (p. B-2)	
Emergence	Standard emergence (p. B-3). Skin closure is frequently followed by application of a splint; patient should remain anesthetized during splinting procedure.	
Blood and fluid requirements	Minimal blood loss IV: 18 ga × 1 NS/LR @ 1.5–3 mL/kg/h	An 18-ga iv catheter placed in the contralateral upper extremity should be adequate.
Monitoring	Standard monitors (p. B-1)	
Positioning	✓ and pad pressure points. ✓ eyes.	

Supraclavicular block complications	Inadequate block Intravascular injection Persistent parasthesia Local anesthetic toxicity Pnuemothorax	Ulnar nerve sparing
Infraclavicular block complications	Inadequate block Intravascular injection Pneumothorax Persistent paresthesia Local anesthetic toxicity	Less frequent occurrence, compared with axillary block. Pneumothorax is very rare with the lateral coracoid approach.
Axillary block complications	Local anesthetic toxicity Intravascular injection Inadequate block Persistent paresthesia Axillary hematoma Axillary artery thrombosis	Minimal doses of local anesthetic can cause CNS toxicity during an accidental intravascular injection. Sz should be treated with STP or midazolam titrated to effect, accompanied by airway control. If there is any question of a full stomach, intubation should be accomplished rapidly. Axillary thrombosis is very rare.
Bier block complications	Local anesthetic toxicity Inadequate block Thrombophlebitis	Proper exsanguination and tourniquet function is critical. Tourniquet should remain inflated a minimum of 25 min. Systemic toxic reaction to the local anesthetic may occur as a result of tourniquet leak or inadvertent premature (< 20 min) tourniquet release. Treatment is supportive. Sz are controlled with STP or midazolam, with appropriate airway protection. Even with a functioning tourniquet, it is possible to overcome tourniquet pressure by injecting too vigorously. Care must be taken when switching from proximal to distal tourniquet; never deflate proximal tourniquet until verifying that distal tourniquet is working.

POSTOPERATIVE

Pain management	Oral analgesics are usually sufficient.	The lingering analgesia of the brachial plexus block is often sufficient for pain relief in the recovery room; oral analgesic therapy can be instituted prior to discharging patient to home.
Tests	None routinely indicated.	

Suggested Readings

1. Brockway MS, Wildsmith JA: Axillary brachial plexus block: method of choice? *Br J Anaesth* 1990; 64(2):224–31.
2. Chan VW, Perlas A, Rawson R, et al: Ultrasound guided supraclavicular brachial plexus block. *Anesth Analg* 2003; 97(5):1514–7.
3. Gerancher JC: Upper extremity nerve blocks. *Anes Clin North Am* 2000; 18(2):1–16.
4. Goldberg ME, et al: A comparison of three methods of axillary approach to brachial plexus blockade for upper extremity surgery. *Anesthesiology* 1987; 66(6):814–16.
5. Green DP, Hotchkiss RN, Pederson WC, et al, eds: *Operative Hand Surgery,* 5th edition. Elsevier, New York: 2005.
6. Ramamurthy S, Anderson D: Anesthesia. In *Operative Hand Surgery,* 5th edition. Green DP, Hotchkiss RN, Pederson WC, et al, eds. Elsevier, New York: 2005, 25–54.
7. Sia S: Axillary brachial plexus block using peripheral nerve stimulator: a comparison between double- and triple-injection techniques. *Reg Anesth Pain Med* 2001; 26(6):499–503.
8. Salazar CH: Infraclavicular brachial plexus block. *Reg Anesth Pain Med* 1999; 24(5):411–6.
9. Steinberg RB: The dose-response relationship of ketorolac as a component of intravenous regional anesthesia with lidocaine. *Anesth Analg* 1998; 86(4):791–3.

10. Vandam LD: Anesthesia for Hand Surgery. In *Flynn's Hand Surgery,* 4th edition. Jupiter JB, ed. Williams & Wilkins, Baltimore: 1991, 46–54.
11. Wilson JL: Infraclavicular brachial plexus block: parasagittal anatomy important to the coracoid technique. *Anesth Analg* 1998; 87(4):870–3.

WRIST ARTHROSCOPY/REPAIR OF TRIANGULAR FIBROCARTILAGE COMPLEX TEARS

SURGICAL CONSIDERATIONS

Description: **Wrist arthroscopy** may be performed for either diagnostic or therapeutic indications. A smaller diameter version of the standard arthroscope is used for visualizing the wrist joint. All of the entry portals are on the dorsum of the wrist and course between the extensor compartments. Irrigation is used during the procedure and a cannula is routinely placed ulnar to the extensor carpi ulnaris tendon. Unlike the knee joint, where visualization is obtained by distention of the joint, in-the-wrist visualization is obtained by distraction. The digits are placed in finger traps and up to 10 lb of traction can be placed on the wrist. Specialized instrumentation is available to resect and débride intraarticular structures and to place sutures to repair torn ligaments. The **triangular fibrocartilage complex** is a source of ulnar-sided wrist pain. It is a term given to the soft tissues spanning the distal radio-ulnar joint. It is composed of the articular disk, radio-ulnar ligaments, ulnocarpal ligaments, extensor carpi ulnaris tendon sheath, and meniscus homologue. Advances in both imaging and arthroscopic techniques in the recent past have led to our ability to better treat patients with injuries to the triangular fibrocartilage complex (**TFCC**). The classification of these injuries credited to Palmer involves both traumatic and degenerative tears, which are associated with ulnar positive variance and ulnar impaction or impingement syndrome. If an open procedure, such as repair of an intercarpal ligament or an ulnar shortening procedure is contemplated following diagnostic arthroscopy, either GA or regional block is preferred.

Variant procedure or approaches: The standard approach is to suspend the forearm vertically in traction. The forearm also can be placed horizontally on the hand table in traction.

Usual preop diagnosis: Internal derangement of the wrist of unknown etiology; tears of the triangular fibrocartilage complex; intercarpal instability due to intercarpal ligament tears; scapholunate dissociation; luno-triquetral dissociation; fracture of distal radius; ulnar impingement syndrome.

SUMMARY OF PROCEDURE	
Position	Supine, with arm extended on hand-surgery table
Incision	Small incisions are made on the dorsum of the wrist for instrument insertion.
Special instrumentation	2.7-mm diameter arthroscope, 0 or 30° field of view; light source and video camera; television monitor; surgical power shaver; joint irrigation system; traction device for forearm; pneumatic tourniquet
Unique considerations	Patient is often awake and observes surgery on monitor.
Antibiotics	Cefazolin I g iv
Surgical time	30 min–2 h
Tourniquet	150 mmHg above SBP; max time = 120 min
Closing considerations	Arthroscopic portals are each closed with a single skin suture.
EBL	Minimal; procedure performed with tourniquet control.
Postop care	PACU → home

SUMMARY OF PROCEDURE (cont'd)

Mortality	None associated with procedure.
Morbidity	Infection: < 1% Swelling (2° to irrigation fluid): Common Nerve and artery damage: Uncommon
Pain score	1–3

PATIENT POPULATION CHARACTERISTICS

Age range	Adults
Male:Female	1:1
Incidence	Least common form of arthroscopy
Etiology	See Usual preop diagnosis, above.
Associated conditions	Antecedent trauma

ANESTHETIC CONSIDERATIONS

See Anesthetic Considerations following Carpal Tunnel Release, p. 927.

Suggested Reading

1. Green DP, Hotchkiss RN, Pederson WC, et al, eds: *Operative Hand Surgery,* 5th edition. Elsevier, New York: 2005.

CARPAL TUNNEL RELEASE

SURGICAL CONSIDERATIONS

Description: This is the most commonly performed procedure in hand surgery. It consists of the transection of the transverse carpal ligament through either an open-palmar or an endoscopic approach (Fig. 10.1-4). In patients

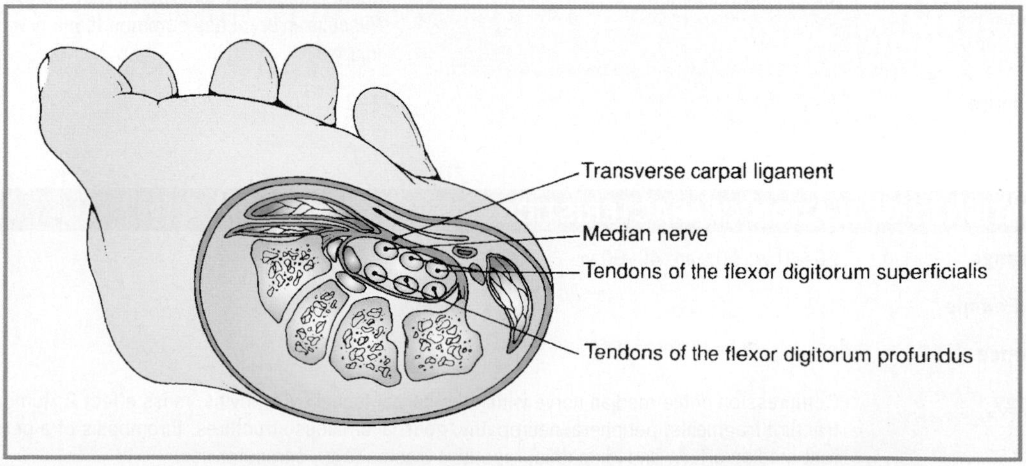

Figure 10.1-4. Exposure of the carpal tunnel. (Reproduced with permission from Scott-Conner CEH, Dawson DL: *Operative Anatomy,* 2nd edition. Lippincott Williams & Wilkins, 2003.)

with severe synovitis, as in rheumatoid arthritis, a synovectomy should be performed at the same time. If there is advanced thenar atrophy and weakness of thumb opposition, a tendon transfer may be done at that time. The most common transfer is the **Camitz opponensplasty,** in which the palmaris longus tendon is prolonged with palmar fascia and transferred to the thumb. Transfers of the extensor indicis proprius and superficial flexor tendons also can be performed. Surgeons differ in their approach to anesthesia for this procedure: some prefer local infiltration, whereas others prefer regional as there is less fluid edema.

Usual preop diagnosis: Carpal tunnel syndrome (CTS); median nerve compression at the wrist

SUMMARY OF PROCEDURES

	Open Carpal Tunnel Release	Endoscopic Carpal Tunnel Release
Position	Supine	⇐
Incision	Longitudinal incision in palm; may extend to forearm.	2 cm transverse at proximal flexion crease of wrist; some use a distal palmar incision also
Special instrumentation	Pneumatic tourniquet	Endoscopic carpal tunnel release system: endoscope, sheath and trocar, special cutting tools
Unique considerations	Although rare, damage to neurovascular structures	Danger of intraop injury to digital nerves, median nerve, tendons, superficial vascular arch
Antibiotics	Cefazolin 1 g iv	⇐
Surgical time	30–90 min	30 min
Tourniquet	150 mmHg above SBP; max time = 120 min	⇐
Closing considerations	Simple skin closure, some surgeons will splint	⇐
EBL	Minimal; performed under tourniquet control.	Minimal
Postop care	PACU → home	PACU-> home
Mortality	None associated with procedure	⇐
Morbidity	Overall complication rate: 4% Reflex sympathetic dystrophy (RSD): < 5% Hematoma: Rare Infection: Uncommon	⇐ Rare Complications of ulnar nerve palsy < 5% Tendon and nerve laceration: Rare (< 1%) Vascular injury: Less common than nerve injury
Pain score	1 –2	1–2

PATIENT POPULATION CHARACTERISTICS

Age range	20–80 yr; 50% are 40–60 yr
Male:Female	1:2
Incidence	Common
Etiology	Compression of the median nerve within the carpal tunnel by synovitis; mass effect 2° tumor or fracture fragments, peripheral neuropathy, gout, anomalous structures, thrombosis of a persistent median artery, and idiopathic; repetitive trauma (e.g., computer use)
Associated conditions	Rheumatoid arthritis; thyroid imbalance; diabetes; amyloidosis; multiple myeloma; alcoholism; hemophilia; pregnancy; menopause; gout; fractures of the distal radius; Kienböck's disease

ANESTHETIC CONSIDERATIONS

(Procedures covered: tendolysis of flexor or extensor tendon; wrist arthroscopy; carpal tunnel release)

PREOPERATIVE

In general, there are two patient populations involved: (a) healthy patients with Hx of wrist trauma, and (b) rheumatoid patients. (See Anesthetic Considerations for Wrist Procedures, p. 914, for discussion of preop concerns in the rheumatoid patient.)

Laboratory	Hb/Hct (healthy patients); otherwise, as indicated from H&P.
Premedication	Mild-to-moderate premedication (e.g., in adults, midazolam 1–2 mg iv, fentanyl 50–100 mcg iv, titrated to effect) is often desirable before placement of a regional block.

INTRAOPERATIVE

Anesthetic technique: Intravenous regional anesthesia is an excellent technique for procedures that are < 1 h. For longer procedures, an axillary or infraclavicular brachial plexus block is a good alternative. Both of these techniques are especially appropriate for outpatients.

Intravenous regional block	The Bier block (intravenous regional anesthesia) is an excellent technique for short (< 60 min), superficial wrist and hand surgeries. 40–50 mL of 0.5% lidocaine is commonly used. A very brief operative procedure may be an indication to reduce the dose of iv anesthetic agent by, for example, having the surgeon use a forearm tourniquet instead of an upper-arm tourniquet. The OR staff should be alerted that iv regional anesthesia is being used, so that all are ready to proceed after the tourniquet is inflated (i.e., surgical prep ready to be performed; surgeons scrubbed, gowned, and gloved). Tourniquet pain and postop pain are reduced by adding ketorolac (20 mg) or clonidine (1 mcg/kg) to the lidocaine solution.	
Blood and fluid requirements	Minimal blood loss IV: 18 ga × 1 NS/LR @ 1.5–2 mL/kg/h	An 18-ga iv catheter placed in the nonoperative upper extremity should be adequate.
Monitoring	Standard monitors (p. B-1)	
Positioning	✓ and pad pressure points. ✓ eyes.	
Intravenous regional block complications	Local anesthetic toxicity Inadequate block Thrombophlebitis	Proper exsanguination and tourniquet function are critical. A tourniquet should remain inflated a minimum of 25 min. Systemic toxic reaction to the local anesthetic may occur as a result of tourniquet leak or inadvertent premature (< 20 min) tourniquet release. Treatment is supportive. Sz are controlled with STP or midazolam, with appropriate airway protection. Even with a functioning tourniquet, it is possible to overcome tourniquet pressure by injecting too vigorously. Care must be taken when switching from proximal to distal tourniquet; never deflate proximal tourniquet until verifying that distal tourniquet is working.

POSTOPERATIVE

Pain management	Oral analgesics usually sufficient	Residual analgesia with iv regional anesthesia is minimal unless ketorolac or clonidine is used. Some iv opioid may be necessary until the patient is tolerating fluids in the recovery room.
Tests	None routinely indicated.	

Suggested Readings

1. Davies JA, Wilkey AD, Hall ID: Bupivacaine leak past inflated tourniquets during intravenous regional analgesia. *Anaesthesia* 1984; 39(10):996–9.
2. Gorgias NK: Clonidine versus ketamine to prevent tourniquet pain during intravenous regional anesthesia with lidocaine. *Reg Anesth Pain Med* 2001; 26(6):512–17.
3. Grice SC, Morell RC, Balestrieri FJ, et al: Intravenous regional anesthesia: evaluation and prevention of leakage under the tourniquet. *Anesthesiology* 1986; 65(3):316–20.
4. Ramamurthy S, Anderson D: Anesthesia. In *Operative Hand Surgery,* 5th edition. Green DP, Hotchkiss RN, Pederson WC, et al., eds. Elsevier, New York: 2005, 25–54.
5. Steinberg, RB: The dose-response relationship of ketorolac as a component of intravenous regional anesthesia with lidocaine. *Anesth Analg* 1998; 86(4):791–3.
6. Sukhani R, Garcia CJ, Munhall RJ, et al: Lidocaine disposition following intravenous regional anesthesia with different tourniquet deflation technics. *Anesth Analg* 1989; 68(5):633–7.
7. Vandam LD: Anesthesia for hand surgery. In *Flynn's Hand Surgery,* 4th edition. Jupiter JB, ed. Williams & Wilkins, Baltimore: 1991, 46–54.

FIXATION OF FRACTURES AND DISLOCATIONS OF THE WRIST AND HAND

SURGICAL CONSIDERATIONS

Description: Patients with fractures of the distal radius, distal ulna, carpus, metacarpals and phalanges that cannot be treated adequately with closed methods, require fixation. Difficult fractures may require a combination of techniques such as percutaneous pinning or external fixation in addition to **open reduction and internal fixation** (ORIF). The criteria for adequate treatment include anatomic reduction of the fracture fragments with focus on articular congruity and stable fixation for maintenance of this reduction. Cast/splint treatment or fixation of any kind is an effort to decrease motion at the fracture site and allow the body to produce a bony union with acceptable length, alignment and rotation. Patients with carpal/wrist fractures or dislocations may have signs of neurologic compromise, specifically the median nerve. Often a closed reduction will improve these symptoms, but if not urgent operative treatment is indicated. Most dislocations within the hand are reducible in the emergency room setting with adequate anesthesia; there are irreducible varieties that warrant immediate operative treatment. Vascular compromise of the hand associated with these injuries is rare, usually occurring in patients with severe crush or high-energy injuries. The devascularized hand is a surgical emergency, and revascularization must be carried out as soon as possible. High-energy injuries such as gunshot wounds may have significant soft-tissue components that must be treated. The possibility of a coexisting compartment syndrome should be considered; and a fasciotomy may be needed at the time of surgery. Open fractures are, by definition, contaminated and should be irrigated and débrided within 8 h of the injury. Surgical approaches depend on the nature and location of the fracture, but typically are longitudinal. Some fractures of the articular surface of the distal radius are amenable to percutaneous pin fixation using fluoroscopy and possibly arthroscopic assistance. Screw fixation of the scaphoid also can be accomplished via percutaneous methods using image guidance. This injury may be associated with a picture of perilunar instability. Damage to intercarpal ligaments may require open repair or reduction and percutaneous pinning. Intraoperative fluoroscopy often is utilized, as are standard portable radiographs to monitor and assess the quality of the reduction of the fracture.

Soft-tissue coverage of these injuries may be problematic, and **local flaps** or **free microvascular tissue transfers** may be indicated. Rarely are these procedures done with the initial operative debridement; an antibiotic bead pouch or wound vac may be used to temporize open wounds. Free transfers can come from the same limb (radial forearm flap, based on the radial artery; lateral upper arm flap, based on the posterior radial collateral artery) or a remote site (latissimus dorsi muscle, based on the thoracodorsal artery; or scapular skin flap, based on the circumflex scapular artery). Remote flaps require special patient positioning and draping. Microsurgical tissue transfers also may need special pharmacological considerations, such as the administration of heparin or dextran to prevent thrombosis of the anastomosis. These procedures also significantly increase operative time and equipment needs.

Usual preop diagnosis: Fractures of the distal radius (Colles', Barton's, Smith's are common eponyms); wrist dislocations (perilunate, lunate); fractures of the carpus, metacarpals, or phalanges; GSW; crush injuries; blast injuries

SUMMARY OF PROCEDURE	
Position	Supine, with arm extended on hand-surgery table.
Incision	Usually volar, longitudinal for distal radius; longitudinal either midaxial, midlateral or dorsal for phalanges; dorsal for metacarpals and carpal fractures; if symptoms of acute carpal tunnel syndrome, which warrants a volar incision
Special instrumentation	Fluoroscopy; internal and external fixation devices and power tools; pneumatic tourniquet,
Unique considerations	Associated injuries and soft-tissue problems in high-energy fractures
Antibiotics	Cephalosporin prophylaxis is indicated for the treatment of closed fractures. Open fractures may require the addition of an aminoglycoside or penicillin depending on the amount and type of contamination.
Surgical time	30 min–3 h.
Tourniquet	150 mmHg above SBP; max time = 120 min
Closing considerations	Some injuries require local flaps or free microsurgical tissue transfers for closure. Fasciotomy wounds may be left open. Splint applied at surgery.
EBL	Minimal for fracture treatment, as tourniquet control is used.
Postop care	PACU → home unless significant soft tissue injuries requiring additional procedures
Mortality	Usually 2° associated injuries
Morbidity	Loss of reduction, requiring repair Nonunion (requires additional surgical procedure) Infection
Pain score	3–9 (Great variation, probably depending on degree of median, ulnar, or dorsal radial sensory nerve involvement. Postop pain management is often problematic. Early use of stellate ganglion blocks may be beneficial in preventing the development of sympathetic mediated pain syndromes.)

PATIENT POPULATION CHARACTERISTICS	
Age range	All ages. More conservative approaches are used with elderly patients.
Male:Female	1:1
Incidence	Very common
Etiology	Trauma
Associated conditions	Traumatic injuries

ANESTHETIC CONSIDERATIONS

PREOPERATIVE

The majority of patients presenting for these procedures are relatively young and healthy. Most present for elective repair of a traumatic injury, and preop workup is routine. Replantation and some injuries, such as irreducible dislocations or open fracture, require immediate attention and necessitate emergency surgery and full-stomach considerations (see p. B-4).

Neurologic	If regional anesthesia is contemplated, pre-existing sensory or motor defects should be documented carefully preop.
Laboratory	Hb/Hct (healthy patients); otherwise, as indicated from H&P.
Premedication	Mild-to-moderate premedication (e.g., in adults, midazolam 1–2 mg iv, fentanyl 50–100 mcg iv, titrated to effect) is often desirable before placement of a regional block.

INTRAOPERATIVE

Anesthetic technique: GETA, regional anesthesia, or a combination is commonly used. A brachial plexus block is excellent for short (1–2 h) procedures on the wrist and hand. Ultrasound guided block may be performed with a supraclavicular or axillary approach. Using a nerve stimulator, infraclavicular or axillary approaches are usual. Regional anesthesia alone is a means of avoiding the risk of aspiration pneumonitis associated with GA in the patient with a full stomach whose operation must be done emergently (see Rapid-Sequence Induction of Anesthesia, p. B-4). A combination of regional and general anesthesia is appropriate for prolonged cases and those that require the use of bone grafts harvested from the iliac crest or a free-tissue transfer.

General anesthesia:

Induction	Standard induction (p. B-2)
Maintenance	Standard maintenance (p. B-2)
Emergence	Skin closure is frequently followed by application of a splint; patient should remain anesthetized during splinting procedure.

Regional anesthesia: 1.5% mepivacaine (40 mL) for routine superficial cases; 0.5% bupivacaine or 0.5% ropivacaine, 40 mL for procedures > 2.5 h or if extended analgesia is desired. Epinephrine (2.5–5 mcg/mL) should be added whenever possible to decrease peak plasma concentrations of local anesthetics.

Ultrasound guided supraclavicular block	Using ultrasound guidance the brachial plexus can be blocked at the supraclavicular level. Direct visualization of the plexus and surrounding structures reduces the risk if pneumothorax with this approach. This block provides adequate anesthesia for procedures distal to mid-humerus.	
Infraclavicular block	The coracoid approach makes this a safe and effective regional technique. A single injection will provide anesthesia distal to the mid-humerus. No additional injections are necessary, and the patient's arm does not need to be abducted for block placement. If intraop sedation is necessary, propofol (50–100 mcg/kg/min) by continuous infusion or intermittent bolus injection of opioid/benzodiazepine are good choices.	
Axillary block with nerve stimulator	The medial aspect of the upper arm is innervated by the intercostobrachial nerve (T2) and requires a separate subcutaneous field block in the axilla, especially when a tourniquet is used. The lateral cutaneous nerve of the forearm, a sensory branch of the musculocutaneous nerve supplying sensation to the lateral forearm, is frequently missed by the axillary approach to the brachial plexus. Thus, a block of this nerve at the elbow or within the proximal body of the coracobrachialis muscle is sometimes necessary. This block may also be performed under ultrasound guidance. Using this technique the musculocutaneous nerve is easily identified and blocked at the same time as the other nerves. If intraop sedation is needed, propofol (50 mcg/kg/min) by continuous infusion or intermittent bolus injection of opioid/benzodiazepine (e.g., midazolam 0.5–1.0 mg iv q 5 min and alfentanil 5–10 mcg/kg iv q min titrated to effect) are good choices.	
Blood and fluid requirements	Minimal-to-moderate blood loss IV: 18 ga × 1 NS/LR @ 1.5–3 mL/kg/h	An 18-ga iv catheter placed in the nonoperative upper extremity should be adequate.

Monitoring	Standard monitors (p. B-1)	
Positioning	✓ and pad pressure points. ✓ eyes.	
Infraclavicular block complications	Local anesthetic toxicity Inadequate block Intravascular injection Pneumothorax Persistent paresthesia	Pneumothorax is very rare with the lateral coracoid approach.
Axillary block complications	Inadequate block Intravascular injection Persistent paresthesia Axillary hematoma Axillary artery thrombosis	Minimal doses of local anesthetic can cause CNS toxicity during an accidental intravascular injection. Sz should be treated with propofol or midazolam titrated to effect, accompanied by airway control. If there is any question of a full stomach, then intubation should be accomplished rapidly. Axillary thrombosis is extremely rare.

POSTOPERATIVE

Pain management	Continuous nerve block can be considered in appropriate cases. PCA (p. C-3), in combination with regional block	Regional or combined regional-general anesthetic techniques are excellent for wrist procedures, especially with respect to postop pain management.
Tests	None routinely indicated.	

Suggested Readings

1. Brockway MS, Wildsmith JA: Axillary brachial plexus block: method of choice? *Br J Anaesth* 1990; 64(2):224–31.
2. Gerancher JC: Upper extremity nerve blocks. *Anes Clin North Am* 2000; 18(2):1–16.
3. Goldberg ME, et al: A comparison of three methods of axillary approach to brachial plexus blockade for upper extremity surgery. *Anesthesiology* 1987; 66(6):814–16.
4. Green DP: *Operative Hand Surgery*, 4th edition. Churchill Livingstone, New York: 1999.
5. Ramamurthy S, Anderson D: Anesthesia. In *Operative Hand Surgery*, 5th edition. Green DP, Hotchkiss RN, Pederson WC, et al, eds. Elsevier, New York: 2005, 25–54.
6. Salazar CH: Infraclavicular brachial plexus block. *Reg Anesth Pain Med* 1999; 24(5):411–6.
7. Sia, S: Axillary brachial plexus block using peripheral nerve stimulator: a comparison between double- and triple-injection techniques. *Reg Anesth Pain Med* 2001; 26(6):499–503.
8. Vandam LD: Anesthesia for hand surgery. In *Flynn's Hand Surgery*, 4th edition. Jupiter JB, ed. Williams & Wilkins, Baltimore: 1991, 46–54.
9. Wilson JL: Infraclavicular brachial plexus block: parasagittal anatomy important to the coracoid technique. *Anesth Analg* 1998; 87(4):870–3.

DIGIT AND HAND REPLANTATION

SURGICAL CONSIDERATIONS

Description: Patients with traumatic amputations of digits and the hand are candidates for emergency microsurgical replantation of these parts. In children, replantation is attempted for essentially all amputations. In the adult, replantation is carried out for amputations of the thumb, multiple digits, and amputations through the palm or proximal. In general, amputations of a single digit are not candidates for replantation, because of the minimal loss of function in relation to the long rehabilitation period and expected outcome. Certainly, a single digit amputated proximal to the insertion of the flexor digitorum superficialis (FDS) tendon (Zone II) (Fig. 10.1-3) should not be replanted. The condition of the amputated part plays an important role in the decision to proceed with replantation. A severely crushed, contaminated, or burned part cannot be expected to survive and function. In addition to the condition of the amputated part, the method of preservation and the time from initial injury play a role in deciding on whether or not replantation is attempted. The patients also may have associated traumatic injuries (i.e., intraabdominal bleeding with a positive peritoneal lavage, chest injuries), which will take preference over replantation. The patient's overall health status must be assessed and may play a role in deciding whether or not to proceed with replantation.

There are a variety of reasons that people suffer amputations. Some studies of these patients have shown an increased incidence of psychopathology, such as alcohol or substance abuse. More often than not these injuries occur in industrial accidents, or in a population of people using power tools at home. Rarely children will gain access to dangerous objects and self-inflicted injuries can occur. Because these procedures are emergent, patients often arrive at the hospital with full stomachs. Although regional anesthesia techniques provide peripheral vasodilation through their sympatholytic effect, surgeons prefer GA because of the unpredictable length of the procedures. While the patient is being readied for induction, the surgeon prepares the amputated part in the OR. At this time, the structures to be repaired are tagged, which saves a great deal of anesthetic time. When the patient is prepped and draped, the hand is irrigated and débrided, and the corresponding structures are tagged in similar manner. The amputated part is brought to the field and the actual replantation is performed. Once arterial blood flow is reestablished, the patient must be kept warm to prevent vasospasm. As with other microsurgical procedures, pharmacologic intervention is indicated to prevent thrombosis; iv heparin and dextran are normally administered. Skin grafts for soft-tissue coverage and vein grafts to replace segmental vascular defects are commonly used. Vein grafts can be obtained from the ipsilateral upper extremity or from the lower extremity, especially the dorsum of the foot. Either the lateral thigh or abdomen is an excellent donor site for split-thickness skin grafts. Rarely is an immediate microsurgical free-tissue transfer indicated for soft-tissue coverage.

Usual preop diagnosis: Traumatic amputation of the digits or hand

SUMMARY OF PROCEDURE	
Position	Supine, with arm extended on hand-surgery table
Incision	Incisions extend both proximal and distal to traumatic amputation to explore neurovascular structures as well as define the zone of injury. Lower extremity prepped and draped as donor site for vein grafts from dorsum of foot, split-thickness skin graft from the thigh.
Special instrumentation	Operating microscope; microsurgical instrumentation
Unique considerations	Emergency procedure
Antibiotics	Cefazolin 1 g iv
Surgical time	3–12 h
Tourniquet	150 mmHg above systolic; max time = 120 min
Closing considerations	Routine volar hand splint
EBL	< 500 mL
Postop care	ICU → requires monitoring in intensive nursing environment. Should be kept pain-free for extended period postop to minimize vessel spasm. Patients will benefit from postop sedation.
Mortality	Minimal for digit and hand. Mortality becomes an important issue when large amounts of muscle are part of the reattachment.
Morbidity	Loss of replanted part (vessel thrombosis): 10% Infection: Rare
Pain score	3–5

■ PATIENT POPULATION CHARACTERISTICS	
Age range	All ages, typically adults of working age
Male:Female	1:1
Incidence	Uncommon
Etiology	Trauma
Associated conditions	Substance abuse; alcoholism

ANESTHETIC CONSIDERATIONS

PREOPERATIVE

In general, there are two patient populations for hand replantation: (a) isolated hand injury patients (common), and (b) multiple trauma victims (rare).

Respiratory	As suggested by coexisting disease or acute trauma injuries. Evidence of occult chest injury, including pneumothorax and pulmonary contusion, should be sought. **Tests:** Consider CXR, ABGs in victims of significant trauma.
Cardiovascular	As suggested by coexisting disease or acute trauma injuries. ✓ for evidence of occult cardiac or mediastinal injuries, such as myocardial contusion or great vessel rupture. **Tests:** Consider CXR (with NG tube in place to assess mediastinal widening), and ECG in victims of significant trauma.
Neurological	As suggested by coexisting disease or acute trauma injuries. The possibility of closed head injury should be addressed in multiple-trauma victims. Verify integrity of C-spine. **Tests:** Consider head CT prior to beginning a long procedure under GA in a patient with evidence of head trauma; C-spine x-ray.
Gastrointestinal	All patients should be considered to have a full stomach and to be at risk for aspiration pneumonitis. In general, they should receive preop medication to reduce stomach volume and acidity (e.g., metoclopramide 10 mg iv and ranitidine 50 mg iv).
Hematologic	Multiple-trauma victims are likely to suffer from acute blood loss. Although blood loss from these procedures is generally modest, a preop T&C for several U PRBCs is wise for trauma patients. **Tests:** CBC
Metabolic	~50% of trauma victims are intoxicated. Anesthesia-related implications of ethanol intoxication include decreased anesthetic requirements, diuresis, vasodilation, and hypothermia.
Laboratory	As suggested by coexisting disease or acute trauma injuries. In general, most victims of significant trauma are best served by obtaining a wide variety of baseline lab studies to screen for unrecognized injury. These studies normally include: ABGs; UA; renal function tests; LFTs; serum amylase; tox screen.
Premedication	Full-stomach precautions: Na citrate 0.3 M 30 mL, metoclopramide 10-20 mg iv; H_2-blocker

INTRAOPERATIVE

Anesthetic technique: GETA, after rapid-sequence induction (see p. B-4). Because of the unpredictable length of these procedures and the possible need for bone and/or vessel grafts, regional anesthesia is not feasible as the primary technique. A concurrent, continuing brachial plexus block, however, will provide sympathetic blockade, as well as postop analgesia, and catheter placement should be considered before inducing GA. The hand injury repair may be done concurrently with other procedures in multiple-trauma victims.

Induction	Rapid-sequence induction (p. B-4) is mandatory in emergency cases, unless awake intubation is performed. C-spine fracture patients and those with facial injuries may require awake fiber optic intubation (p. B-5). Hemodynamically unstable, acute-trauma patients may be induced more safely with etomidate or ketamine.	
Maintenance	Standard maintenance (p. B-2) for stable patients. Hemodynamically unstable, acute-trauma victims undergoing emergency surgery may be better served by using a combination of medications designed to have minimal hemodynamic consequences (e.g., fentanyl for analgesia, vecuronium for muscle relaxation, and scopolamine or midazolam for amnesia). N_2O is best avoided in the trauma patient.	
Emergence	Difficult airway or full-stomach cases require awake extubation. Trauma victims who have undergone a prolonged procedure or who have significant associated cardiopulmonary injuries should remain intubated for postop mechanical ventilation.	
Blood and fluid requirements	Significant blood loss IV: 16 ga × 1 NS/LR @ 1.5–3 mL/kg/h + replacement of blood loss Fluid/blood warmers, heating blanket, warmed circuit humidifier	A 16-ga iv catheter in nonoperative upper extremity should be adequate in hemodynamically stable patients. Acute-trauma victims who are unstable require a minimum of two large-bore iv catheters or large-bore central lines.
Monitoring	Standard monitors (p. B-1)	Invasive hemodynamic monitoring and TEE should be considered in acute, multiple-trauma victims.
Positioning	✓ and pad pressure points. ✓ eyes.	
Complications	Hemodynamic instability	Previously unrecognized injuries (e.g., pneumothorax, cardiac tamponade, intracranial bleeding) should be considered as a cause of unexplained intraop hemodynamic instability in all acute-trauma victims.

POSTOPERATIVE

Complications	Sepsis ARDS
Pain management	PCA (p. C-3)
Tests	None routinely indicated.

Suggested Readings

1. Cullings HM, Hendee WR: Radiation risks in the orthopaedic operating room. *Contemp Orthop* 1984; 8:48–52.
2. Green DP, Hotchkiss RN, Pederson WC, et al, eds: *Operative Hand Surgery*, 5th edition. Elsevier, New York: 2005.
3. Johnstone RE: Acute trauma with multiple injuries. *Curr Opin Anesthesiol* 2000; 13(2): 175–9.
4. Morrison WA, McCombe D: Digital replantation. *Hand Clin* 2007; 23(1):1–12.
5. Nicholls BJ, Cullen BF: Anesthesia for trauma. *J Clin Anesth* 1988; 1(2):115–29.
6. Ramamurthy S, Anderson D: Anesthesia. In *Operative Hand Surgery*, 5th edition. Green DP, Hotchkiss RN, Pederson WC, et al, eds. Elsevier, New York: 2005, 25–54.
7. Soderstrom CA, Cowley RA: A national alcohol and trauma center survey. Missed opportunities, failures of responsibility. *Arch Surg* 1987; 122(9):1067–71.

CHAPTER

10.2 Shoulder/Arm Surgery

SURGEONS

Amy L. Ladd, MD
Andrew C. Karich, MD
Emilie V. Cheung, MD

ANESTHESIOLOGIST

Lindsey Vokach-Brodsky, MB, ChB, FFARCSI

ARTHROSCOPIC SHOULDER SURGERY

SURGICAL CONSIDERATIONS

Description: The role of arthroscopy in shoulder surgery has advanced tremendously in the past decade and is now routinely performed by most shoulder surgeons. Arthroscopic procedures include **subacromial decompression (SAD), distal clavicle resection (Mumford procedure), debridement** (for labral tear, infection, or synovitis), **rotator cuff (RC) repair, anterior capsule-labral repair** for recurrent dislocation (**Bankart repair**), **capsular plication** for multidirectional instability (MDI), **capsular release for frozen shoulder,** and **repair of SLAP lesions** (superior labral anterior-posterior tears).

Procedures done arthroscopically are less painful postoperatively than open procedures, because they produce less trauma to normal tissues. Rehabilitation is, therefore, facilitated. Interscalene block has been shown to provide good postop analgesia of shorter duration, but its clinical application with arthroscopic procedures is surgeon-dependent because the postoperative pain is usually moderate to mild. Some surgeons prefer only a general anesthesia for shoulder arthroscopy. The use of indwelling intra-articular pain catheters has fallen out of favor in the past few years due to multiple case reports of chondrolysis, a devastating complication characterized by end-stage arthrosis of the glenohumeral joint.

Arthroscopic shoulder surgery may be performed in the beach-chair or lateral decubitus position. Beachchair positioners are available with a trough for the head and a breakaway shoulder pad to provide important access to the posterior shoulder. The lateral decubitus position utilizes distal traction of 5–10 lbs, with the arm abducted 30–45°. Both are safe positions for the brachial plexus, because the shoulder is not excessively abducted. The "down" arm in the lateral position is placed in forward flexion, and an axillary roll is placed underneath the upper chest wall.

Initially, an 18-ga spinal needle is inserted into the glenohumeral joint, passing through the posterior deltoid and infraspinatus muscle and the posterior capsule of the joint (see shoulder anatomy, Fig. 10.2-1). Placement is verified by injecting saline to inflate the joint capsule. A stab incision is made using a No. 11 blade in the direction previously defined by the finder needle. Sharp, then blunt trocars are used to gain access to the joint and permit insertion of the arthroscopic device. Improper insertion of the instruments can injure the axillary or suprascapular nerves and the cartilage of the glenohumeral joint. Initial diagnostic arthroscopy is carried out through the posterior portal. Bupivacaine 0.5% with epinephrine 1:200,000 often is infiltrated into portals and the joint or subacromial space at the onset of surgery to help with hemostasis. An anterior portal is used for instrumentation within the glenohumeral joint. After joint arthroscopy, the scope is placed into the subacromial space, where a direct lateral portal is used for instrumentation. Accessory portals are established as needed, depending on the procedure performed. Joint debridement and anterior capsulolabral stabilization are usually performed through anterior portals. RC repair, subacromial bursectomy, acromioplasty, and distal clavicle resection are done within the subacromial space (deep to the deltoid and superficial to the RC). Epinephrine (1 mg/3 L) in the irrigation fluid and maintaining MAP < 80 mmHg help control bleeding, thus enhancing visualization during surgery.

Usual preop diagnosis: Rotator cuff tear; subacromial impingement; glenohumeral instability; AC arthritis; labral tear

SUMMARY OF PROCEDURE	
Position	Lateral decubitus or beachchair
Incision	Posterior arthroscopic portal, anterior instrumentation portal, lateral instrumentation portal for visualizing subacromial bursa; superior portal for semisitting position
Special instrumentation	Arthroscope; power burrs; arthroscopic shavers; suture-passing instruments; bone anchors; radiofrequency cautery
Unique considerations	Rigid eye patch over ipsilateral eye, to prevent corneal abrasion, suggested. Positioning of the head with appropriate support, removing upper section of operating table, if possible, for better access with semisitting position. ETT taped to opposite side of face. MAP ≤ 80.
Antibiotics	Cefazolin 1 g iv preop, particularly if bone work performed.
Surgical time	Positioning the patient is time-intensive; can add as much as 45 min. Reconstructive: 1–4 h Diagnostic: < 1–1.5 h

■ SUMMARY OF PROCEDURE (cont'd)	
EBL	Minimal: < 200 mL (less with use of epinephrine, electrocautery, and laser)
Postop care	Frequently outpatient; may be overnight if interscalene or supraclavicular block is given or reconstructive procedure performed. Intraarticular pain catheter commonly used.
Mortality	Rare
Morbidity	VAE possible Extravasation of fluid (NS or LR): > 50% Brachial plexus injury (lateral decubitus position): Rare Breakage of instruments: < 1% Infection: 0–3%
Pain score	4 (diagnostic); 5–7 (reconstruction)

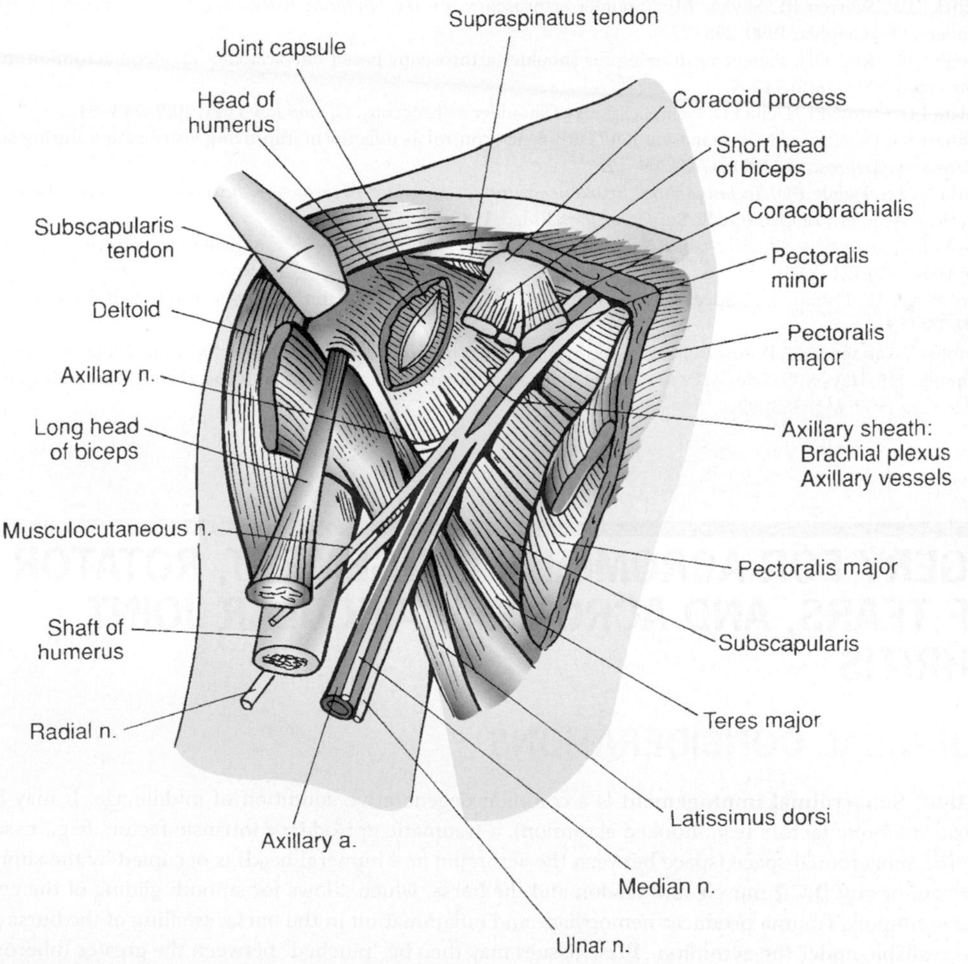

Figure 10.2-1. Anatomy of the shoulder joint, anterior. (Reproduced with permission from Hoppenfeld S, deBoer P, *Surgical Exposures in Orthopaedics: The Anatomic Approach*, 2nd edition. Lippincott Williams & Wilkins, 1994.)

PATIENT POPULATION CHARACTERISTICS	
Age range	15–40 yr (instability); 35–75 yr (rotator cuff and acromial pathology)
Male:Female	2:1–4:1
Incidence	Very common: > 50,000/yr
Etiology	Young patients: usually sports-related Older patients: cuff and acromial pathology; age-wear phenomenon Rotator cuff pathology and acromial impingement (frequently coexist)
Associated conditions	Cervical arthritis and radiculopathy with rotator cuff pathology

ANESTHETIC CONSIDERATIONS

See Anesthetic Considerations following Surgery for Shoulder Instability, p. 944.

Suggested Readings

1. Al-Kaisy A, McGuire G, Chan VW, et al: Analgesic effect of interscalene block using low-dose bupivacaine for outpatient arthroscopic shoulder surgery. *Reg Anesth Pain Med* 1998; 23(5):469–73.
2. Altchek DW, Carson EW: Arthroscopic acromioplasty. Current status. *Orthop Clin Am* 1997; 20(2):157–68.
3. Altchek DW, Warren RF, Skyhar MJ: Shoulder arthroscopy. In *The Shoulder.* Rockwood CA Jr, Matsen FA III, eds. WB Saunders, Philadelphia: 1990, 258–77.
4. Baechler MF, Kim DH: Patient positioning for shoulder arthroscopy based on variability in lateral acromion morphology. *Arthroscopy* 2002; 18(5):547–9.
5. Bigliani LU, Flatow EL, Deliz ED: Complications of shoulder arthroscopy. *Orthop Rev* 1991; 20(9):743–51.
6. Burkhart SS, Danaceau SM, Athanasiou KA: Turbulence control as a factor in improving visualization during subacromial arthroscopy. *Arthroscopy* 2001; 17(2):209–12.
7. Matthews LS, Fadale PD: *Technique and Instrumentation for Shoulder Arthroscopy: Instructional Course Lectures,* Vol 38. American Academy of Orthopedic Surgeons, Park Ridge: 1989.
8. Mileski RA, Snyder SJ: Superior labral lesions in the shoulder: pathoanatomy and surgical management. *J Am Acad Orthop Surg* 1998; 6(2):121–31.
9. Pearsall AW IV, Osbahr DC, Speer KP: An arthroscopic technique for treating patients with frozen shoulder. *Arthroscopy* 1999; 15(1):2–11.
10. Ruotolo C, Nottage WM, Flatow EL, et al: Controversial topics in shoulder arthroscopy. *Arthroscopy* 2002; 18(2 Supp 1):65–75.
11. Segmuller HE, Hays MG, Saies MD: Arthroscopic repair of glenolabral injuries with an absorbable fixation device. *J Shoulder Elbow Surg* 1997; 6(4):383–92.

SURGERY FOR ACROMIAL IMPINGEMENT, ROTATOR CUFF TEARS, AND ACROMIOCLAVICULAR JOINT ARTHRITIS

SURGICAL CONSIDERATIONS

Description: **Subacromial impingement** is a common degenerative condition of middle age. It may be related to extrinsic anatomic factors (e.g., hooked acromion), a traumatic episode, or intrinsic factors (e.g., tissue degeneration). The subacromial space (space between the acromion and humeral head) is occupied by the supraspinatus (superior rotator cuff [RC]) muscle and tendon and the bursa, which allows for smooth gliding of the cuff tendon under the acromion. Trauma produces hemorrhage and inflammation in the bursa; swelling of the bursa decreases the space available under the acromion. These tissues may then be "pinched" between the greater tuberosity of the humerus and the lateral aspect of the acromion (Fig. 10.2-2) with forward elevation or abduction of the arm. This further increases the inflammation, producing a vicious cycle.

Impingement of the anterolateral acromion on the insertion of the supraspinatus (along with poor vascularity of this part of the cuff) is a leading hypothesis for the etiology of degenerative **RC tears.**

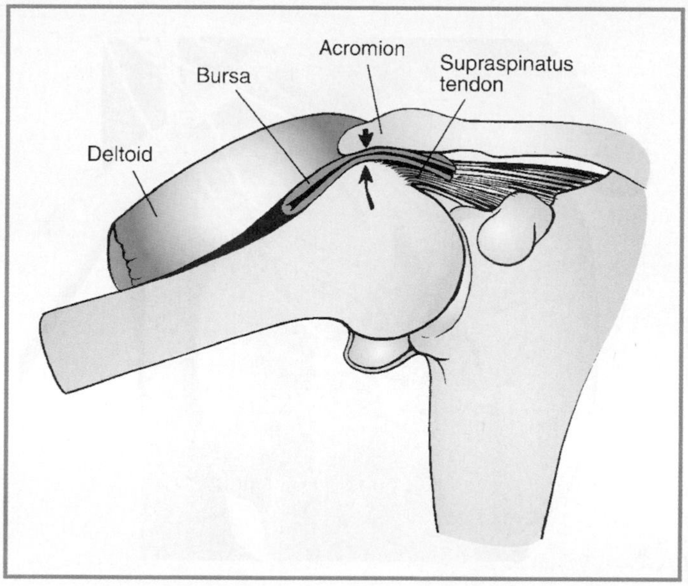

Figure 10.2-2. Abduction of the arm can impinge the subacromial bursa between the greater tuberosity and the undersurface of the acromion and coracoacromial ligament. (Reproduced with permission from Hoppenfeld S, deBoer P: *Surgical Exposures in Orthopaedics: The Anatomic Approach,* 2nd edition. Lippincott Williams & Wilkins, 1994.)

AC joint arthritis is a common radiographic finding in adults, but it is often asymptomatic. Distal clavicle excision is performed for clinically symptomatic AC joint arthritis.

Subacromial impingement: Surgical treatment of subacromial impingement is indicated when nonoperative treatment (e.g., cortisone injection, physical therapy) fails. Surgery involves shaving of the anterolateral aspect of the undersurface of the acromion (creating a flat surface, and providing more room in the subacromial space). This may be accomplished with open techniques in combination with open RC repair, but it is more commonly done arthroscopically. The bursa is usually inflamed and quite vascular. Bleeding may obscure arthroscopic visualization and is controlled with electrocautery, epinephrine in the irrigant, and by maintaining relative ↓ BP (MAP < 80 mmHg).

Rotator cuff tears: RC (Fig. 10.2-3) repair may be performed using the **direct lateral open approach, the mini-open (deltoid-splitting) approach** in conjunction with arthroscopy, or all arthroscopically. If a deltoid-splitting incision is used, care is taken not to extend the split more than 5 cm distal to the acromion because of possible injury to the axillary nerve, which innervates the deltoid 5 cm or more from the lateral aspect of the acromion. If the beach-chair position is used for open RC surgery or arthroscopy, the upper limb is draped free. The arm is manipulated, and traction is frequently applied. It is important that the head is secured (the head may be taped to the table or special beachchair positioner), the eyes are protected, and that the anesthesiologist frequently checks to see that the surgeon is not pulling the patient off the table (not always apparent from the surgeon's side of the drape). Traction on the brachial plexus is more likely in the lateral decubitus position 2° arm traction.

Open RC repair involves suturing the cuff insertion back to the greater tuberosity through drill holes or with suture anchors. Arthroscopic repair requires percutaneous anchor placement and arthroscopic suture-passing and knot-tying. Bleeding is minimal with the arthroscopic technique, but may approach 400 mL with an open procedure. Both require that the patient remain relaxed until all dressings are applied and he/she is fitted with an abduction sling. Patients typically are admitted for 24 h for pain control or if a drain is used.

AC joint disease: Surgery for **AC joint arthritis** is usually performed in conjunction with SAD and/or RC repair and may be done open or arthroscopically. It involves simple resection of the distal 5 mm of the clavicle through an incision directly over the joint or through an accessory anterior portal. Again, relative ↓ BP is required for the arthroscopic procedure.

Repair of AC joint dislocation ("shoulder separation") is uncommon. Most AC separations are treated non-operatively, because long-term functional results are the same or better than those treated surgically. Severe AC

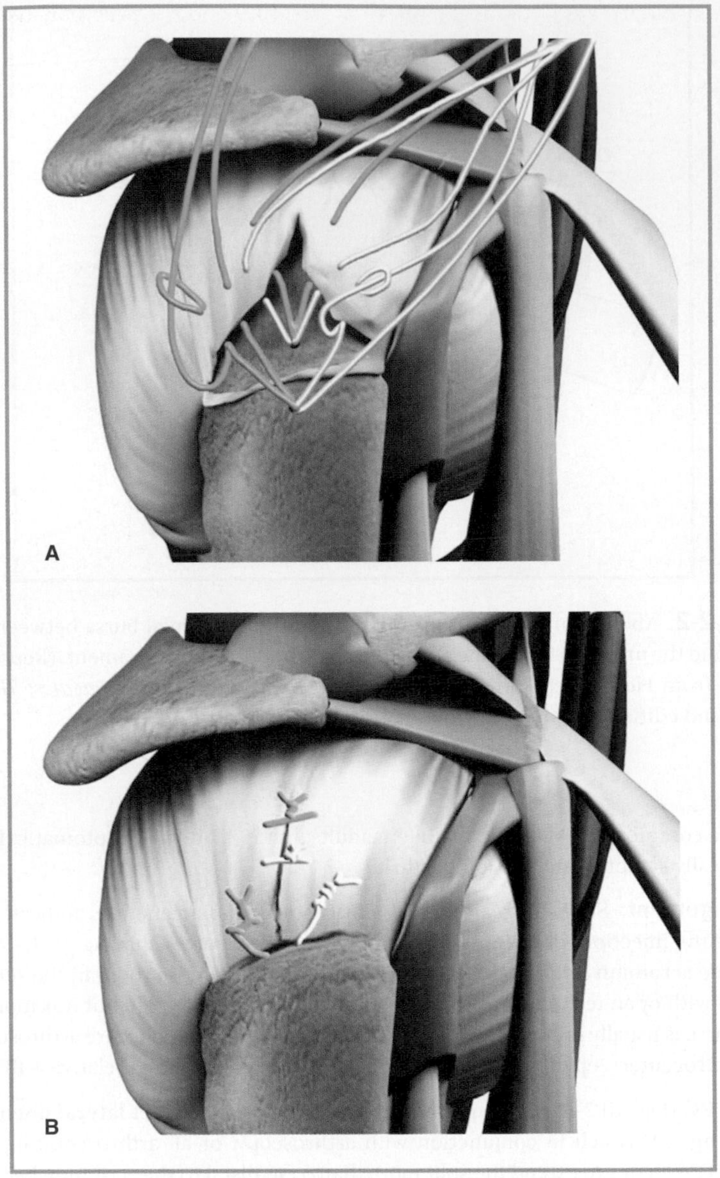

Figure 10.2-3. Lateral view of the right shoulder showing a rotator cuff repair. Reproduced with permission from Lafosse L, Brozska R, Toussaint B, et al. The outcome and structural integrity of arthroscopic rotator cuff repair with use of the double-row suture anchor technique. *J Bone Joint Surg,* 2007; 89:1533-41. **A:** Rotator cuff tear. **B:** Rotator cuff repair with suture anchors.

separations occasionally require surgery, when the dislocated clavicle is buttonholed posteriorly through the trapezius, the deltoid origin has been avulsed from the clavicle, or the clavicle is displaced inferiorly below the cricoid process. Repair is performed in the beachchair position with the incision carried out over the AC joint and distal third of the clavicle. The clavicle is reduced and held in place with a large screw into the base of the coracoid, a large suture wrapped around the coracoid, or with K-wires across the AC joint. The coracoclavicular ligament often is repaired or reconstructed with tendon graft, or the coracoacromial ligament is transferred from the edge of the acromion to the clavicle. Following reduction and fixation, the deltoid is reattached to the clavicle if it has been avulsed, and the patient is placed in an immobilizer after skin closure. The operation is technically challenging and the brachial plexus and subclavian vessels are at risk with screw placement and with inferior dislocations.

Usual preop diagnosis: RC tears (partial or complete); AC arthritis; impingement; bursitis; bicipital tendinitis; AC separation

SUMMARY OF PROCEDURE

Position	Beachchair; semisitting, ~40–70°; or lateral decubitus
Incision	Oblique, saber-type incision anteriorly over distal acromion; lateral or deltopectoral incision for wider exposure; deltoid-splitting incision for RC tears
Special instrumentation	Power equipment for bone work; self-retaining retractors for cuff repairs; suture anchors
Unique considerations	Rigid eye protection for ipsilateral eye and careful head positioning
Antibiotics	Cefazolin 1 g iv preop
Surgical time	1–3 h
Closing considerations	Muscle relaxation when mobilizing cuff and during closure. Arm in sling and swathe, or abduction pillow for large tears. Immobilizer should be positioned prior to awakening patient to minimize potential for rupture of repair.
EBL	200–400 mL
Postop care	Maintenance of position in sling and swathe; no active motion of shoulder girdle for 2 d–6 wk, depending on procedure.
Mortality	Rare
Morbidity	Infection: 1–5% Axillary nerve damage: < 2% Musculocutaneous nerve damage: < 2% Breakage of instruments: < 1% Brachial plexus damage (position-dependent) Suprascapular nerve at risk for RC mobilization
Pain score	5–8

PATIENT POPULATION CHARACTERISTICS

Age range	Rotator cuff tears > 40 yr (younger for athletes)
Male:Female	3:1
Incidence[3,4]	5–30% of general population affected by RC and acromial conditions, depending on age, thickness of tear, associated conditions
Etiology	Age-related; trauma (70% involved in light work)
Associated conditions	Bursitis; tendinitis; impingement; RC disease (especially in first-time glenohumeral dislocations > 40 yr); diabetes and renal failure; hypermobility

ANESTHETIC CONSIDERATIONS

See Anesthetic Considerations following Surgery for Shoulder Instability, p. 944.

Suggested Readings

1. Altchek DW, Carson EW: Arthroscopic acromioplasty. Current status. *Orthop Clin Am* 1997; 20(2):157–68.
2. Chelly JE, Greger J, Al-Samsam T, et al: Reduction of operating and recovery room times and overnight hospital stay with interscalene blocks as sole anesthetic technique for rotator cuff surgery. *Minerva Anestesiol* 2001; 67(9):613–19.
3. Cofield RH, Parvizi J, Hoffmeyer PJ, et al: Surgical repair of chronic rotator cuff tears. A prospective long-term study. *J Bone Joint Surg Am* 2001; 83A(1):71–7.
4. Flatow EL, Altchek DW, Gartsman GM, et al: The rotator cuff. Commentary. *Orthop Clin North Am* 1997; 28(2): 177–94.

5. Hata Y, Saitoh S, Murakami N, et al: A less invasive surgery for rotator cuff tear: mini-open repair. *J Shoulder Elbow Surg* 2001; 10(1):11–16.
6. Martin SD, Baumgarten TE, Andrews JR: Arthroscopic resection of the distal aspect of the clavicle with concomitant subacromial decompression. *J Bone Joint Surg Am* 2001; 83A:328–35.
7. Neer CS II: Impingement lesions. *Clin Orthop* 1983; 173:70–7.
8. Peterson CA II, Altchek DW: Arthroscopic treatment of rotator cuff disorders. *Clin Sports Med* 1996; 15(4):715–36.
9. Schlegel TF, Burks RT, Marcus RL, et al: A prospective evaluation of untreated acute grade III acromioclavicular separations. *Am J Sports Med* 2001; 29(6):699–703.
10. Tubiana R, McCullough CJ, Masquelet AC: *An Atlas of Surgical Exposures of the Upper Extremity.* JB Lippincott, Philadelphia: 1990.
11. Yamaguchi K, Ball CM, Galatz LM: Arthroscopic rotator cuff repair: transition from mini-open to all-arthroscopic. *Clin Orthop* 2001; 390:89–94.

SURGERY FOR SHOULDER INSTABILITY

SURGICAL CONSIDERATIONS

Description: **Shoulder instability** is classified as multidirectional (MDI)/atraumatic, or unidirectional/traumatic.

MDI is associated with generalized ligamentous laxity (e.g., Ehlers Danlos or Marfan syndromes, or idiopathic), and is treated primarily nonoperatively with physical therapy. Open or arthroscopic **capsular shift** is performed for recalcitrant cases. This involves "plication" of the capsule and/or labrum to decrease the capsular volume of the shoulder. Patients with MDI, known as "voluntary dislocators," frequently have psychiatric disorders and are very poor candidates for surgery.

Traumatic instability is usually anterior and is quite common in the young, active population. The shoulder is the most commonly dislocated joint. Recurrent dislocation in young, active patients is common (80–90%) and is associated with avulsion of the capsule/labrum from the anterior-inferior glenoid rim (Bankart lesion). The population undergoing a **Bankart repair** is almost invariably young and healthy. Older first-time dislocators (age >50 yr) more commonly sustain rotator cuff (RC) tears or fractures, which do not result in chronic instability, but may require operative reduction and RC repair or fracture fixation. Posterior traumatic dislocation is much less common and is associated with high-energy trauma, seizures, or electrocution.

Instability surgery is often preceded by exam under anesthesia and arthroscopic examination, either in the beachchair or lateral decubitus position. The essential feature of instability surgery, whether arthroscopic or open, is the reattachment of the anterior inferior capsulolabral complex back to the rim of the glenoid, thus re-establishing the normal "bumper" effect of the anterior-inferior labrum and decreasing the capsular volume of the shoulder. Nonanatomic procedures (reconstructive) are much less common, but are still performed occasionally. These include transfer of the coracoid process to the anterior glenoid rim (**Bristow or Latarjet procedure**).

The **open Bankart repair** is performed in the beachchair position using the deltopectoral approach, with the interval between the deltoid and pectoralis major. The subscapularis (anterior RC muscle) lies just anterior to the joint capsule (Fig. 10.2-4), and this is either detached from its insertion or split. The capsule may then be opened to visualize the joint and rim of the glenoid. The glenoid rim is decorticated, providing bleeding bone to promote healing, and the anterior capsule is reattached through drill holes in the glenoid or with suture anchors. The capsule often is imbricated (overlapping folds) if it is redundant.

The shoulder and deltoid are highly vascular; however, bleeding is usually slight, with careful surgical technique. Major nerves are close but out of the plane of the operative field. The **musculocutaneous nerve** may be stretched by excessive medial retraction of the coracobrachialis (especially if a coracoid osteotomy is used) and the **axillary nerve** may be injured if the surgeon strays too far inferiorly.

If a **subscapularis-releasing technique** is used, the muscle is reattached and must be protected postop. External rotation of the shoulder is prevented for several weeks while the repair heals, and the surgeon prefers that the patient remain anesthetized until a shoulder immobilizer is applied.

The **arthroscopic Bankart repair** is similar to the open procedure but is performed through two anterior portals with the scope coming in posteriorly. This procedure is less painful postop and allows for more rapid rehabilitation, because the subscapularis is not detached.

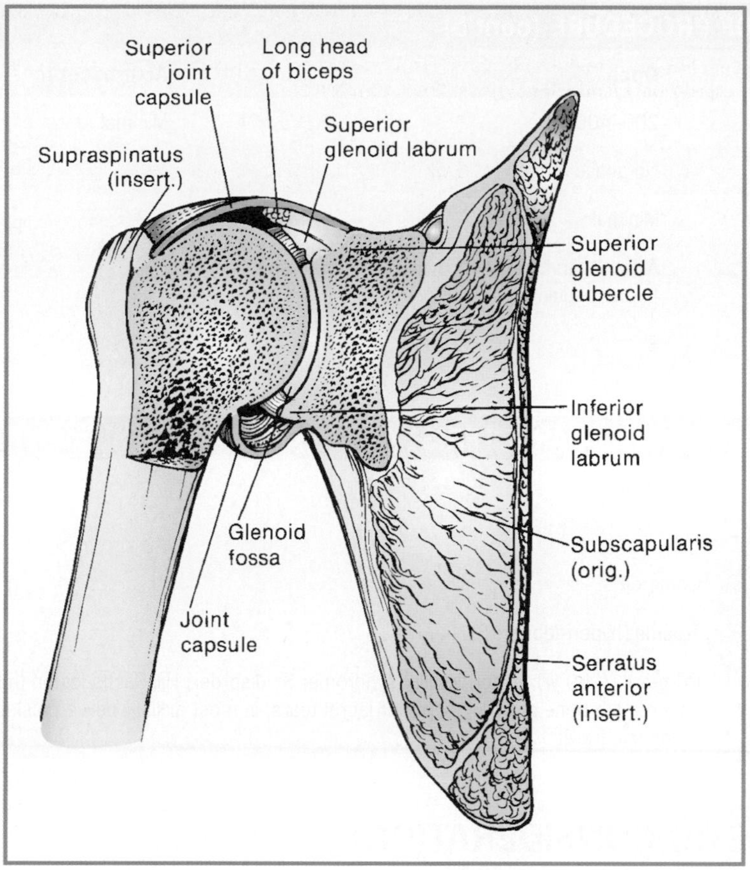

Figure 10.2-4. Cross section of the joint: The joint capsule is redundant inferiorly to allow abduction. The long head of the biceps tendon traverses the joint. The tendon is surrounded by synovium and, therefore, is anatomically intracapsular but extrasynovial. (Reproduced with permission from Hoppenfeld S, deBoer P: *Surgical Exposures in Orthopaedics: The Anatomic Approach,* 2nd edition. Lippincott Williams & Wilkins, 1994.)

Open surgery for posterior dislocation is similar to the open Bankart repair, but it is done in the lateral position and utilizes the interval between the infraspinatus and teres minor. The RC attachment is preserved, but the posterior deltoid is detached and must be protected postop.

Usual preop diagnosis: Recurrent traumatic anterior or posterior instability; MDI; fracture dislocation

SUMMARY OF PROCEDURES

	Open	Arthroscopic
Position	Beachchair for anterior; lateral decubitus for posterior	Lateral decubitus or beachchair
Incision	Deltopectoral (anterior); posterior approach (posterior)	Multiple small portals
Special instrumentation	Arthroscopic shaver; suture anchors; glenoid and humeral instrumentation	⇐ + arthroscopic instruments for suture passing and knot-tying
Antibiotics	Cefazolin 1 g iv preop if bone work performed.	⇐
Surgical time	2–4 h	⇐
Closing considerations	Continuous anesthesia until application of sling and swathe or abduction pillow	⇐

SUMMARY OF PROCEDURE (cont'd)		
	Open	**Arthroscopic**
EBL	200–400 mL	Minimal
Postop care	No active motion for 6 wk	⇐
Mortality	Minimal	⇐
Morbidity	Axillary nerve palsy: 15% (may be pre-existing) Suprascapular nerve injury	
Pain score	8	5

PATIENT POPULATION CHARACTERISTICS	
Age range	15–35 yr
Male:Female	2:1
Incidence	Common
Etiology	Trauma; hypermobility; Sz
Associated conditions	RC tears (> 50 yr); hypermobility syndrome; Sz disorder; Hill-Sachs lesion (humeral head defect) may require bone grafting; superior labral tears; in most axillary nerve palsies from the injury; iatrogenic (rare)

ANESTHETIC CONSIDERATIONS

(Procedures covered: shoulder arthroscopy; surgery for acromial impingement, RC tears, and AC disease; surgery for shoulder dislocations or instability)

PREOPERATIVE

Typically, three patient populations present for repair of RC tears or shoulder arthroscopy: (a) healthy post-trauma, (b) nonrheumatoid arthritic, and (c) rheumatoid arthritic. Individuals presenting for repair of shoulder dislocations also may include those with a joint hypermobility syndrome (e.g., Marfan or Ehlers-Danlos) or Sz disorder patients.

Respiratory	Arthritic patients may exhibit Sx of pleural effusion or pulmonary fibrosis. Hoarseness may indicate cricoarytenoid joint (CAJ) involvement → difficult intubation. (See Anesthetic Considerations for Wrist Procedures, p. 914.) Seizure disorder patients who suffer from recurrent shoulder dislocation as a result of frequent grand mal Sz also may suffer from occult aspiration pneumonia or pneumonitis. **Tests:** Consider CXR; PFTs; ABGs in debilitated rheumatoid patients
Cardiovascular	Arthritic patients may suffer from chronic pericardial effusions, valvular disease, and cardiac conduction defects. Patients presenting for shoulder stabilization because of joint hypermobility syndromes are likely to have valvular dysfunction and are vulnerable to aortic dissection 2° HTN. These patients may require antibiotic prophylaxis for bacterial endocarditis. **Tests:** Consider ECG, ECHO in patients with severe rheumatoid arthritis. Recent ECHO to assess valve function and aortic root size indicated in most patients with Marfan syndrome.
Neurological	Arthritic patients may have cervical or lumbar radiculopathies that should be documented carefully preop. For example, head flexion may cause cervical cord compression. Patients with severe Sz disorders can suffer from recurrent shoulder dislocations 2° frequent violent grand mal Sz. Such patients should be treated maximally for Sz disorder prior to elective surgery. Be aware that as many as 15% of shoulder dislocations can be accompanied by axillary nerve palsy, which should be documented carefully preop.

Neurological (cont'd)	**Tests:** Consider C-spine radiographs to r/o occult subluxations in arthritic patients with neck complaints or upper extremity radiculopathy. Verify therapeutic levels of antiepileptic medication in Sz disorder patients.
Musculoskeletal	Arthritic patients may have limited neck and jaw ROM and may require fiber optic intubation techniques. Bony deformities or muscle contractures may necessitate special attention to positioning. Patients with joint hypermobility syndromes presenting for shoulder surgery also may suffer other joint dislocations 2° positioning problems.
Hematologic	Virtually all patients will be on some type of anti-inflammatory medication that may result in anemia or Plt inhibition. Ideally, patients should D/C NSAIDs at least 5 d preop; aspirin, 7 d. In addition, selected patients with Ehlers-Danlos are known to have severe coagulation defects that may preclude the use of regional anesthesia. **Tests:** A coag profile is mandatory in Ehlers-Danlos patients.
Endocrine	Rheumatoid patients may be on oral corticosteroids and may require supplemental perioperative steroids (e.g., 100 mg hydrocortisone q 8 h iv) to treat adrenal suppression, although the routine use of "stress-dose steroids" has been questioned.
Laboratory	Hb/Hct (in healthy patients); other tests as indicated from H&P. Patients with Ehlers-Danlos syndrome should always have banked blood available for surgery, except for the most trivial of procedures.
Premedication	Mild-to-moderate premedication (e.g., in adults, midazolam 1–2 mg iv, fentanyl 50–100 mcg iv, titrated to effect) is often desirable before placement of a regional block.

INTRAOPERATIVE

Anesthetic technique: GETA or regional anesthesia (interscalene block), or a combination of the two techniques, can be used. A suprascapular block (when interscalene block is contraindicated) can be used for intraop → postop pain control in arthroscopic shoulder procedures. When logistically feasible, a combined technique is ideal. Unless contraindicated, a long-acting local anesthetic should be used in regional anesthesia for shoulder surgery to ameliorate postop pain.

General anesthesia:

Induction	Standard induction (see p. B-2). Arthritic patients may require awake fiber optic intubation (see p. B-5).
Maintenance	Standard maintenance (see p. B-2).
Emergence	Management of emergence and extubation should be routine, except in difficult airway cases which require awake extubation. Patients should remain anesthetized until the shoulder is immobilized.

Regional anesthesia:

Local anesthetics	2% lidocaine or 1.5% mepivacaine have similar onset times (10–15 min), and similar duration (4–6 h). If extended postop pain control is desired, 0.5% bupivacaine, or 0.5% ropivacaine (each with epinephrine 1:400,000) can be used. Onset is usually within 30 min, with duration up to 10–12 h. Ropivacaine may be preferred for peripheral nerve block due to its decreased cardiotoxicity.
Interscalene block	Anesthetics and doses (epinephrine [2.5–5 mcg/mL]) should be added to local anesthetic whenever possible to decrease peak plasma concentrations: • 2% lidocaine or 1.5% mepivacaine 30 mL for procedures ≤ 2.5 h. • 0.5% bupivacaine, levobupivacaine, or ropivacaine 30 mL for procedures lasting > 2.5 h. The skin on the top of the shoulder (C3-C4) and the medial aspect of the upper arm (T2) often require separate subcutaneous field blocks. Phrenic nerve block → hemidiaphragmatic paralysis is an inevitable consequence of the interscalene block, which may not be

Interscalene block (cont'd)	tolerated by patients with significant preexisting respiratory compromise. Major complications, such as total spinal or pneumothorax resulting from interscalene block, are extremely rare; therefore, this technique is suitable for use in outpatients. Interscalene block is contraindicated in patients with contralateral recurrent laryngeal nerve or phrenic nerve palsy (e.g., post CABG). If sedation is needed, midazolam (0.5–1.0 mcg boluses), alfentanil (0.125–0.25 mcg/kg/min by infusion) or propofol (50–100 mg/kg/min by infusion), given initially in subanesthetic doses and thereafter titrated to effect, are good choices.	
Blood and fluid requirements	Minimal-to-moderate blood loss IV: 18 ga × 1 NS/LR @ 1.5–3 mL/kg/h	IV catheter placed in contralateral upper extremity.
Monitoring	Standard monitors (see p. B-1). ± Precordial Doppler ± Arterial line	BP cuff should be placed on the arm for beach chair procedures. To help detect VAE, consider precordial Doppler monitoring when semisitting position used. Consider intraarterial BP monitoring for patients with hypermobility disorders because of risk for aortic dissection 2° HTN.
Positioning	✓ and pad pressure points. ✓eyes. ↑ VAE risk in semisitting position	Postural ↓ BP is the most common complication of the semisitting position. Changing to this position gradually can help prevent ↓ BP, as can the use of antiembolism stockings, plus fluid-loading the patient. Marfan and Ehlers-Danlos patients require very gentle positioning to prevent joint dislocations.
Interscalene block complications	Total spinal Accidental epidural injection Local anesthetic toxicity (Sz/dysrhythmias) Stellate ganglion block (Horner's syndrome) Laryngeal nerve block Phrenic nerve block Pneumothorax	Resuscitative equipment, including airway management tools, should be immediately available. When possible, nerve blocks should be performed in responsive and cooperative patients to minimize complications.
	Persistent paresthesia	May last ≤ 6 wk.
Other complications	↓ BP during surgical prep and positioning	↓ BP during long surgical preps normally can be avoided by using light inhalation anesthesia (e.g., isoflurane 0.3–0.5%) to ensure amnesia, with moderate muscle relaxation to prevent bucking on the ETT, and maintaining adequate hydration. Antiembolism stockings will help prevent venous pooling in lower limbs.
	Cardiac dysrhythmia VAE	Dysrhythmias may be 2° to irrigation fluids containing epinephrine.

POSTOPERATIVE

Pain management	PCA (see p. C-3) or regional block techniques.	Combined regional-general anesthetic techniques are excellent for shoulder procedures, especially with respect to postop pain management.
Tests	None indicated routinely.	

Suggested Readings

1. Bak H, Spring BJ, Henderson JP: Inferior capsular shift procedure in athletes with multidirectional instability based on isolated capsular and ligamentous redundancy. *Am J Sports Med* 2000; 28(4):466–71.

2. Borgeat A: Acute and nonacute complications associated with interscalene block and shoulder surgery. *Anesthesiology* 2001; 95(4):875–80.
3. Bottoni CR, Wilckens JH, DeBerardino TM, et al: A prospective, randomized evaluation of arthroscopic stabilization vs nonoperative treatment in patients with acute, traumatic, first-time shoulder dislocations. *Am J Sports Med* 2002; 30(4):576–80.
4. Dolan P, Sisko F, Riley E: Anesthetic considerations for Ehlers-Danlos syndrome. *Anesthesiology* 1980; 52(3):266–9.
5. Gerancher JC: Upper extremity nerve blocks. *Anes Clin N Am* 2000; 18(2):1–16.
6. Gill TJ, Micheli LJ, Gebhard F, et al: Bankart repair for anterior instability of the shoulder. Long-term outcome. *J Bone Joint Surg Am* 1997; 79(6):850–7.
7. Hoppenfeld S: *Surgical Exposures in Orthopaedics: The Anatomic Approach,* 2nd edition. Hoppenfeld S, deBoer P, eds. JB Lippincott, Philadelphia: 1994.
8. Keenan MA, Stiles CM, Kaufman RL: Acquired laryngeal deviation associated with cervical spine disease in erosive polyarticular arthritis. *Anesthesiology* 1983; 58(5):441–9.
9. Kim SH, Ha KI, Kim SH: Bankart repair in traumatic anterior shoulder instability: open vs arthroscopic technique. *Arthroscopy* 2002; 18(7):755–63.
10. Murphy DB: Upper extremity blocks for day surgery. *Tech in Reg Anes Pain Manag* 2000; 4(1):19–29.
11. Reginster JY, Damas P, Franchimont P: Anaesthetic risks in osteoarticular disorders. *Clin Rheum* 1985; 4:30–8.
12. Ritchie ED: Suprascapular nerve block for postoperative pain relief in arthroscopic shoulder surgery. *Anesth Analg* 1997; 84:1306–12.
13. Salathe M, Johr M: Unsuspected cervical fractures: a common problem in ankylosing spondylitis. *Anesthesiology* 1989; 70(5):869–70.
14. Sperber A, Hamberg P, Karlsson J, et al: Comparison of an arthroscopic and open procedure for posttraumatic instability of the shoulder: a prospective, randomized multicenter study. *J Shoulder Elbow Surg* 2001; 10(2):105–8.
15. Urmey WF, Talts KH, Sharrock NE: One hundred percent incidence of hemidiaphragmatic paresis associated with interscalene brachial plexus anesthesia as diagnosed by ultrasonography. *Anesth Analg* 1991; 72(4):498–503.
16. Verghese C: Anaesthesia in Marfan's syndrome. *Anaesthesia* 1984; 39(9):917–22.
17. Weiss KS, Savoie FH III: Recent advances in arthroscopic repair of traumatic anterior instability. *Clin Orthop* 2002; 400: 117–22.
18. Wells DG, Podolakin W: Anaesthesia and Marfan's syndrome: case report. *Can J Anaesth* 1987; 34(3+Pt 1):311–14.
19. White RH: Preoperative evaluation of patients with rheumatoid arthritis. *Semin Arthritis Rheum* 1985; 14(4):287–99.

GLENOHUMERAL SHOULDER ARTHROPLASTY

SURGICAL CONSIDERATIONS

Description: Shoulder replacement is performed for pain associated with end-stage arthritis. Primary osteoarthritis (wear-and-tear arthritis) is much less common in the shoulder than in the weight-bearing joints, such as the hip and knee. The most common causes of shoulder arthritis requiring **total shoulder arthroplasty (TSA)** are osteoarthritis, rheumatoid arthritis; avascular necrosis (AVN); posttraumatic arthritis, and rotator cuff tear arthropathy. Most patients are older than 65 years.

TSA involves replacement of the humeral head with a stemmed prosthesis and resurfacing the glenoid with a polyethylene component. Both components may be cemented or uncemented, depending on the surgeon's preference. **Hemiarthroplasty** involves only replacement of the humeral side. This is indicated when the humeral head is involved primarily and the glenoid is in good condition, as in severe proximal humerus fractures, AVN of the humeral head, and some chronic dislocators. Replacement of the glenoid is contraindicated in the presence of an unreconstructable massive RC tear because eccentric forces lead to rapid loosening of the glenoid component. Some revision cases require glenoid bone grafting, which increases the complexity and potential blood loss.

Shoulder arthroplasty utilizes the beachchair position and the deltopectoral incision (Fig. 10.2-5). The deltopectoral interval is developed. The subscapularis insertion is incised, and the muscle is reflected medially. The capsule is incised and the joint exposed. The humeral head is dislocated anteriorly, and the head is removed with an oscillating saw. Reamers and broaches are used to prepare the proximal humerus for the prosthesis. If the glenoid is to be resurfaced, it is done before implantation of the final humeral component. The labrum is excised and a motorized reamer is used to remove the cartilage of the glenoid. Glenoid drill holes are made to conform to the back of the prosthesis. The glenoid prosthesis is cemented into place, with the component held in position manually until the cement hardens (~15 min). Trial humeral components are placed, and the appropriate sizing of the head and stem are assessed. The final humeral component is inserted with or without cement. The joint is reduced, and the subscapularis is repaired. Skin closure is followed by placement of a sling or shoulder immobilizer. Postop management includes

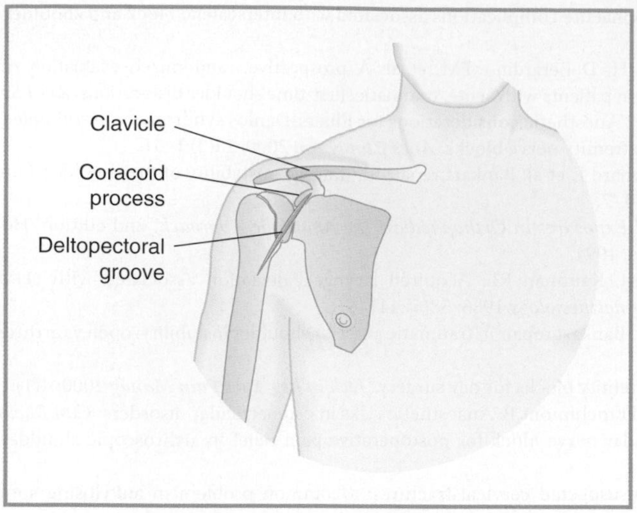

Figure 10.2-5. Incision in the deltopectoral groove. (Reproduced with permission from Hoppenfeld S, deBoer P: *Surgical Exposures in Orthopaedics: The Anatomic Approach,* 2nd edition. Lippincott Williams & Wilkins, 1994.)

early passive ROM, limiting active internal rotation, and passive external rotation until the subscapularis has healed. Additional limitations may be instituted in revision situations or if RC repair is performed.

Usual preop diagnosis: Rheumatoid arthritis; posttraumatic arthritis; AVN; RC arthropathy; 4–part proximal humerus fracture

SUMMARY OF PROCEDURE	
Position	Semisitting, beachchair
Incision	Deltopectoral incision (Fig. 10.2-5) or extended incision for complex revision
Special instrumentation	Glenoid and humeral instrumentation, in addition to usual shoulder instruments; mixing and introduction of cement
Unique considerations	Systemic illnesses of the patient; systemic complications of use of cement in the patient; precautions in pregnant staff working with methylmethacrylate; usage of laminar flow or UV lighting for total joint precautions, depending on the surgeon's preference and capabilities of the OR.
Antibiotics	Cefazolin 1 g iv preop, and 48 h postop
Surgical time	2–5 h
Closing considerations	Drain; sling and swathe
EBL	200–1,000 mL
Postop care	Immediate passive motion. No active internal rotation for 6 wk.
Mortality	< 1%
Morbidity	Blood loss Nerve injury: Rare ↓ BP 2° cement: Rare Infection
Pain score	8

Orthopedic Surgery

PATIENT POPULATION CHARACTERISTICS	
Age range	45–80 yr
Male:Female	1:1
Incidence	Uncommon
Etiology	Osteoarthritis; inflammatory arthritis; trauma; avascular necrosis; systemic disease
Associated conditions	Inflammatory disease; systemic disease; alcoholism; RC pathology; arthritis and radiculopathy; cervical arthritis

ANESTHETIC CONSIDERATIONS

PREOPERATIVE

Typically, three patient populations present for shoulder arthroplasty: (a) healthy post-trauma, (b) nonrheumatoid arthritic, and (c) rheumatoid arthritic.

Respiratory	Rheumatoid arthritic patients may exhibit Sx of pleural effusion or pulmonary fibrosis. Hoarseness may indicate cricoarytenoid joint (CAJ) involvement → difficult intubation. (See Anesthetic Considerations for Wrist Procedures, p. 914.) **Tests:** Consider CXR; PFTs; ABGs in debilitated rheumatoid patients.
Cardiovascular	Rheumatoid arthritic patients may suffer from chronic pericardial effusions, valvular disease, and cardiac conduction defects. **Tests:** Consider ECG and ECHO in patients with severe rheumatoid arthritis.
Neurological	Arthritic patients may have cervical or lumbar radiculopathies that should be documented carefully preop. For example, head flexion may cause cervical cord compression. **Tests:** C-spine radiographs to r/o occult subluxations in rheumatoid patients with neck complaints or upper extremity radiculopathy
Musculoskeletal	Arthritic patients may have limited neck and jaw ROM that may require special intubation techniques. Bony deformities or muscle contracture may necessitate special attention to positioning.
Hematologic	Virtually all nontrauma patients will be on some type of anti-inflammatory medication that may result in anemia or Plt inhibition. Ideally, patients should D/C NSAIDs at least 5 d preop.
Endocrine	Rheumatoid patients may be on oral corticosteroids and may require supplemental perioperative steroids (e.g., 100 mg hydrocortisone q 8 h iv) to treat adrenal suppression, although the routine use of "stress-dose steroids" has been questioned.
Laboratory	Hb/Hct (healthy patients); other tests as indicated from H&P.
Premedication	Mild-to-moderate premedication (e.g., in adults, midazolam 1–2 mg iv, fentanyl 50–100 mcg iv, titrated to effect) is often desirable before placement of a regional block.

INTRAOPERATIVE

Anesthetic technique: GETA or a combination of GETA and regional anesthesia can be used. An interscalene brachial plexus block in combination with GA is excellent for surgical procedures on the shoulder. Unless contraindicated, a long-acting local anesthetic should be used in regional anesthesia for shoulder surgery to ameliorate postop pain.

General anesthesia:

Induction	Standard induction (see p. B-2). Rheumatoid patients may require awake fiber optic intubation (see p. B-5).

Orthopedic Surgery

Maintenance	Standard maintenance (see p. B-2). Because of the typically long duration of these cases, the opioid selected as part of the balanced anesthetic technique may be given by continuous infusion (e.g., iv sufentanil [0.25–1.0 mcg/kg/h]). Some surgeons prefer muscle relaxation beyond that provided by volatile anesthetic. The surgeon may request reduction in BP: careful in sitting position to maintain cerebral circulation.
Emergence	Management of emergence and extubation should be routine except in difficult airway cases that require awake extubation. Emergence from anesthesia should be delayed until patient's shoulder is securely immobilized in the sling and swathe to prevent undesired movement of the newly placed prosthesis.

Regional anesthesia:

Local anesthetics	Significant discomfort may be associated with this procedure; therefore, extended postop pain control is desirable. When a single-shot technique is used, 0.5% bupivacaine, or 0.5% ropivacaine (each with epinephrine 1:400,000) can be used. Onset is usually within 30 min, with duration up to 10–12 h. Ropivacaine may be preferred for peripheral nerve block, due to its decreased cardiotoxicity. For continuous catheter techniques, a postop infusion of 6–8 mL/h of 0.2% of any of these agents is appropriate.	
Interscalene block	Typical anesthetics and doses. Note that epinephrine [2.5–5 mcg/mL] should be added to the local anesthetic whenever possible to decrease peak plasma concentrations: • 0.5% bupivacaine, or 0.5% ropivacaine, 30 mL. The skin on the top of the shoulder (C3-C4) and the medial aspect of the upper arm (T2) may require separate subcutaneous field blocks. Phrenic nerve block → hemidiaphragmatic paralysis is an inevitable consequence of the interscalene block, which may not be tolerated by patients with significant preexisting respiratory compromise. A continuous interscalene catheter may be placed for postop pain management. Major complications, such as total spinal or pneumothorax resulting from interscalene block, are extremely rare. Interscalene block is contraindicated in patients with contralateral recurrent laryngeal nerve or phrenic nerve palsy. If sedation is needed, midazolam (0.5–1.0 mg boluses), or propofol (25–100 mcg/kg/min by infusion), titrated to effect, are good choices.	
Blood and fluid requirements	Moderate-to-significant blood loss IV: 16 ga × 1 NS/LR @ 1.5–3.0 mL/kg/h	RBC recovery and reinfusion techniques (e.g., Cell Saver) are advisable because blood loss can be considerable. IV in nonoperative upper extremity.
Monitoring	Standard monitors (see p. B-1). Precordial Doppler	Consider invasive, hemodynamic monitoring in the debilitated or elderly patient. Since VAE is a possible complication of the semisitting position, consider using precordial Doppler for cases done in this position.
Positioning	✓and pad pressure points. ✓eyes. ↑ VAE risk	Postural ↓ BP is the most common complication of the semisitting position. Changing patient to this position gradually can help prevent ↓ BP, as can the use of antiembolism stockings and fluid-loading the patient. Care with neck positioning. Check head position intraoperatively as shoulder traction may lead to injury.
Interscalene block complications	Total spinal Epidural anesthesia Local anesthetic toxicity (Sz/dysrhythmias) Stellate ganglion block (Horner's syndrome) Laryngeal nerve block	Resuscitative equipment, including airway management tools, should be immediately available.

Interscalene block complications (cont'd)	Phrenic nerve block Pneumothorax Persistent paresthesia	 May last ≤ 6 wk.
Other complications	Potential for embolic event ↓ BP during prep and positioning	Because of the increased risk of VAE during shoulder arthroplasty, N_2O may be D/C'd during placement of humeral component. Use of methylmethacrylate cement has been associated with the sudden onset of ↓ BP and even cardiac arrest, presumably due to profound vasodilation ± associated VAE. ↓ BP during long surgical prep usually can be avoided by using light inhalation anesthesia (isoflurane 0.3–0.5%) to ensure amnesia, with moderate muscle relaxation to prevent bucking on ETT, and maintaining adequate hydration.

POSTOPERATIVE

Pain management	PCA (see p. C-3) or regional block/ catheter	Combined regional-general anesthetic techniques are excellent for shoulder procedures, especially for postop pain management.
Tests	None indicated routinely.	

Suggested Readings

1. Andersen KH: Air aspirated from the venous system during total hip replacement. *Anaesthesia* 1983; 38(12):1175–8.
2. Borgeat A: Acute and nonacute complications associated with interscalene block and shoulder surgery. *Anesthesiology* 2001; 95(4):875–80.
3. Cofield RH: Degenerative and arthritic problems of the glenohumeral joint. In *The Shoulder.* Rockwood CA Jr, Matsen FA III, eds. WB Saunders, Philadelphia: 1990, 678–749.
4. Cushner MA, Friedman RJ: Osteonecrosis of the humeral head. *J Am Acad Orthop Surg* 1997; 5(6):339–46.
5. Gartsman GM, Roddey TS, Hammerman SM: Shoulder arthroplasty with or without resurfacing of the glenoid in patients who have osteoarthritis. *J Bone Joint Surg Am* 2000; 82(l):26–34.
6. Goldberg BA, Smith K, Jackins S, et al: The magnitude and durability of functional improvement after total shoulder arthroplasty for degenerative joint disease. *J Shoulder Elbow Surg* 2001; 10(5):464–9.
7. Gray AT: Ultrasound-guided regional anesthesia: current state of the art. *Anesthesiology* 2006; 104:368–73.
8. Green A, Norris TR: Shoulder arthroplasty for advanced glenohumeral arthritis after anterior instability repair. *J Shoulder Elbow Surg* 2001; 10(6):539–45.
9. Keenan MA, Stiles CM, Kaufman RL: Acquired laryngeal deviation associated with cervical spine disease in erosive polyarticular arthritis. *Anesthesiology* 1983; 58(5):441–9.
10. Klein SM: Interscalene brachial plexus block with continuous catheter insertion system and a disposable infusion pump. *Anesth Analg* 2000; 91(6):1473–8.
11. Liu SS, Strodbeck WM, Richman JM, Wu CL: A comparison of regional versus general anesthesia for ambulatory anesthesia: A meta analysis of randomized controlled trials. *Anesth analg* 2005; 101:1634–42.
12. Murphy DB: Upper extremity blocks for day surgery. *Tech in Reg Anes Pain Manag* 2000; 4(1):19–29.
13. Newens AF, Volz RG: Severe hypotension during prosthetic hip surgery with acrylic bone cement. *Anesthesiology* 1972; 36(3):298–300.
14. Pohl A, Cullen DJ: Cerebral ischemia during shoulder surgery in the upright position: a case series. *J Clin Anesth* 2005; 17:463–9.
15. Reginster JY, Damas P, Franchimont P: Anaesthetic risks in osteoarticular disorders. *Clin Rheum* 1985; 4:30–8.
16. Salathe M, Johr M: Unsuspected cervical fractures: a common problem in ankylosing spondylitis. *Anesthesiology* 1989; 70(5):869–70.
17. Sanchez-Sotelo J, Cofield RH, Rowland CM: Shoulder hemiarthroplasty for glenohumeral arthritis associated with severe rotator cuff deficiency. *J Bone Joint Surg Am* 2001; 83–A(12):1814–22.
18. Shapiro J, Zuckerman JD: Glenohumeral arthroplasty: indications and preoperative considerations. *Instr Course Lect* 2002; 51:3–10.
19. White RH: Preoperative evaluation of patients with rheumatoid arthritis. *Semin Arthritis Rheum* 1985; 14(4):287–99.
20. Zuckerman JD, Scott AJ, Gallagher MA: Hemiarthroplasty for cuff tear arthropathy. *J Shoulder Elbow Surg* 2000; 9(3): 169–72.

SHOULDER GIRDLE PROCEDURES

SURGICAL CONSIDERATIONS

Description: Trauma about the shoulder girdle in young patients ranges from athletic injuries to life-threatening trauma. Some of these injuries include common athletic injuries, such as **acromioclavicular joint separations,** which rarely require surgery unless there are associated **acromial** or **clavicular fractures. Posterior sternoclavicular dislocations** may warrant surgical stabilization if the trachea is compressed. **Clavicle fractures,** frequently associated with **scapular fractures,** occasionally require open reduction.

Scapular fractures involving the glenoid also may require surgical stabilization. Extreme fractures involving the shoulder girdle (**scapulothoracic dissociations**) include scapular fracture, clavicle fracture, subclavian or axillary artery disruption, and brachial plexus injury. These may coexist with **proximal humerus fractures,** rib fractures, and pneumothorax. In the older, debilitated patient, the most common injury is proximal humeral fracture, which may be amenable to surgical stabilization or may be so comminuted as to warrant hemiarthroplasty.

A displaced proximal humerus fracture may require open reduction internal fixation with a plate and screws or hemiarthroplasty through a deltopectoral approach utilizing a beachchair position (see Surgery for Shoulder Instability, p. 942, and Glenohumeral Shoulder Arthroplasty, p. 947). A displaced clavicle fracture may require open reduction internal fixation with a plate and screws utilizing a beachchair or supine position. A scapular body fracture would be stabilized with a plate and screws via a posterior approach utilizing a prone or lateral position (see Surgery for Shoulder Instability, p. 942). As with other shoulder procedures, relaxation is necessary upon awakening the patient after the shoulder is placed into an immobilization device.

Usual preop diagnosis: Trauma about the shoulder girdle

SUMMARY OF PROCEDURES

	Anterior	Posterior
Position	Semisitting or prone	Lateral decubitus (scapula)
Incision	Anterior, superior, or oblique for acromioclavicular; supraclavicular for clavicle; deltopectoral for proximal humerus and glenoid	Posterior lateral border or medial border of scapula, spinous scapula, depending on location
Special instrumentation	Plates and screws; tension band wiring; proximal humerus replacement for comminuted fractures	⇐
Unique considerations	Multiple traumas warrant early stabilization; may require vascular repair and brachial plexus exploration.	⇐
Antibiotics	Cefazolin 1 g iv	⇐
Surgical time	2–10 h	⇐
Closing considerations	Fracture-dependent; most commonly requires application of sling and swathe.	⇐
EBL	200–1,200 mL or greater, depending on trauma	⇐
Postop care	May require ICU for multiple-trauma patients; otherwise, early mobilization with physical therapy	⇐
Mortality	Mortality dependent on associated conditions: Infection Neurologic injury Respiratory failure Massive blood loss Unrecognized pneumothorax Cardiac tamponade	⇐

SUMMARY OF PROCEDURE (cont'd)		
	Anterior	**Posterior**
Morbidity	Nerve injury (axillary, brachial plexus) Stiffness Poor healing	Axillary and suprascapular ⇐ ⇐
Pain score	6–10	6 (clavicle and AC joint) 8 (scapula and proximal humerus)

PATIENT POPULATION CHARACTERISTICS	
Age range	15–80 yr, depending on nature of trauma
Male:Female	5:1
Incidence	Common
Etiology	Trauma
Associated conditions	Axillary nerve palsy; musculocutaneous nerve palsy; brachial plexus injury; arterial disruption in high-energy trauma; brachial and great vessel injuries and posterior sternoclavicular dislocation pneumothorax

ANESTHETIC CONSIDERATIONS

See Anesthetic Considerations following Brachial Plexus Surgery, p. 955.

Suggested Readings

1. Butters KP: Fractures and dislocations of the scapula. In *Fractures in Adults,* Vol II, 4th edition. Rockwood CA Jr, Green DP, Bucholz RW, et al., eds. Lippincott-Raven, Philadelphia: 1996, 1163–92.
2. Collins DN, Harryman DT II: Arthroplasty for arthritis and rotator cuff deficiency. *Orthop Clin North Am* 1997; 20(2): 225–39.
3. Craig EV: Fractures of the clavicle. In *Fractures in Adults,* Vol II, 4th edition. Rockwood CA Jr, Green DP, Bucholz RW, et al., eds. Lippincott-Raven, Philadelphia: 1996, 1109–62.
4. Imatani RJ: Fractures of the scapula: a review of 53 fractures. *J Trauma* 1975; 15(6):473–8.
5. Neviaser RJ: Injuries to the clavicle and acromioclavicular joint. *Orthop Clin North Am* 1987; 18(3):433–8.
6. Richards RR, Sherman RM, Hudson AR, et al: Shoulder arthrodesis using a pelvic-reconstruction plate. A report of eleven cases. *J Bone Joint Surg* [Am] 1988; 70(3):416–21.
7. Rockwood CA Jr, Matsen FA III, eds: *The Shoulder.* WB Saunders, Philadelphia, 1990.
8. Rockwood CA Jr, Williams GR, Young CD: Injuries to the acromioclavicular joint. In *Fractures in Adults,* Vol II, 4th edition. Rockwood CA Jr, Green DP, Bucholz RW, et al., eds. Lippincott-Raven, Philadelphia: 1996, 1341–1414.
9. Rockwood CA Jr, Wirth MA: Injuries to the sternoclavicular joint. In *Fractures in Adults,* Vol II, 4th edition. Rockwood CA Jr, Green DP, Bucholz RW, et al., eds. Lippincott-Raven, Philadelphia: 1996, 1415–78.

BRACHIAL PLEXUS SURGERY

SURGICAL CONSIDERATIONS

Description: Brachial plexus injuries occur most commonly in two groups: traumatic birth injuries and high-energy trauma. Surgery ranges from exploration with neurolysis, to repairs, to cable nerve grafting. Typically, the latter requires grafting with the sural nerve, and nerve pedicle transfer, such as transfer of the spinal accessory nerve to denervated paralyzed muscle, combined with muscle transfers. C5-C6 is most commonly injured in obstetrical (Erb's) palsy. Injuries in adults are more commonly closed-traction. Similar to obstetrical palsy, they occur with an outstretched, abducted arm with the neck rotated in the opposite direction. The most severe form includes complete avulsion at the preganglionic level, presenting with a Horner's syndrome, winging of the scapula, and a flail arm.

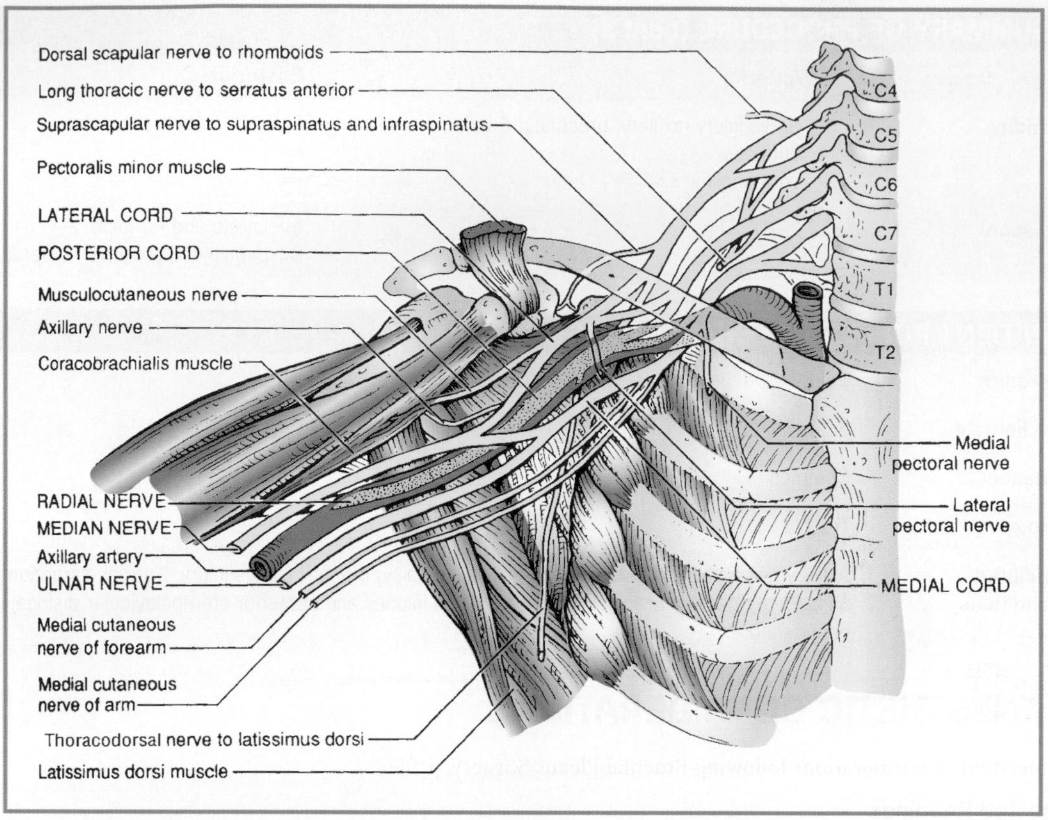

Figure 10.2-6. Brachial plexus: Its division into supraclavicular and infraclavicular portions is apparent. The proximal origin of the dorsal scapular nerve and the long thoracic nerve are demonstrated. The T1 spinal nerve arises below the head of the 1st rib. The relation of the cords of the plexus to the axillary artery at the level of the coracoid process (origin of the pectoralis minor and coracobrachialis muscles) is illustrated. The posterior cord and the radial nerve behind the axillary artery are stippled for clarity. (Reproduced with permission from Tindall GT, Cooper PR, Barrow DL: *The Practice of Neurosurgery,* Vol III. Williams & Wilkins, Baltimore, 1996.)

These are typically "supraclavicular" injuries, and have a poorer prognosis. Surgical exposure may proceed above the clavicle similar to an anterior neck dissection, or may require an extension below the clavicle. Occasionally, an osteotomy of the clavicle for extensive dissection is required. For axillary nerve dissection, a posterior approach also is used. Open injuries, such as gunshot or knife wounds, are typically "infraclavicular" and have a better prognosis. (See diagram of brachial plexus, Fig. 10.2-6.)

Usual preop diagnosis: Obstetrical palsy; adult trauma—most commonly motorcycle accident

SUMMARY OF PROCEDURE

Position	Lateral decubitus or semisitting
Incision	Supra- or infraclavicular, extensile to include deltopectoral incision. Clavicle osteotomy incision will provide for improved exposure. Supraclavicular incision used for supraclavicular brachial plexus.
Special instrumentation	Nerve stimulator
Unique considerations	Associated trauma
Antibiotics	Cefazolin 1 g iv preop

SUMMARY OF PROCEDURE (cont'd)	
Surgical time	4–10 h
Closing considerations	Other incisions if nerve grafts obtained.
EBL	400–2,000 mL
Mortality	Minimal
Morbidity	Bleeding Hematoma Pneumothorax Clavicular nonunion
Pain score	8

PATIENT POPULATION CHARACTERISTICS	
Age range	Infants and children: 3 mo–8 yr; adults: 20–40 yr
Male:Female	Adult: 5:1
Incidence	Infants: 0.3–8/1,000 births; adults: commonly associated with motorcycle accidents
Etiology	Obstetrical palsy; trauma
Associated conditions	None known

ANESTHETIC CONSIDERATIONS

(Procedures covered: shoulder girdle procedures; brachial plexus surgery)

PREOPERATIVE

With the exception of traumatic birth injuries, most of these patients are healthy males who have suffered major blunt or penetrating trauma. For the acute and subacute trauma victim, the major anesthesia-related concerns center on associated traumatic injuries. Many adult trauma victims with brachial plexus injuries will be operated on in the first few days after their injury. For infants (usually operated on at 6–12 mo), the major anesthesia-related concerns are those routinely associated with pediatric anesthesia (see Pediatric Orthopedic Surgery, p. 1354.). Approximately half of all trauma victims are intoxicated. The anesthesia-related implications of ethanol intoxication include: decreased anesthetic requirements, diuresis, vasodilation, and hypothermia.

Respiratory	As suggested by coexisting disease or acute trauma injuries. Look for evidence of occult chest injury, including pneumothorax (tachypnea, wheezing, ↓ BP, ↓ PaO_2, CXR changes) and pulmonary contusion (multiple rib fracture, ↓ PaO_2). **Tests:** Consider CXR and ABGs in victims of significant trauma; other tests as indicated from H&P.
Cardiovascular	As suggested by coexisting disease or acute trauma injuries. Look for evidence of occult cardiac or mediastinal injuries, such as myocardial contusion (e.g., ECG abnormalities typically consistent with ischemia) or great vessel rupture (e.g., widened mediastinum). **Tests:** Consider CXR (with NG tube in place to assess mediastinal widening) and ECG in victims of significant trauma; others as indicated from H&P.
Neurological	Victims of shoulder trauma are vulnerable to brachial plexus damage. Look for evidence of upper extremity nerve dysfunction and document any injuries preop. The possibility of closed-head injury also should be considered.

Neurological (cont.)	**Tests:** Head CT prior to beginning a procedure under GA in a patient with evidence of head trauma.
Musculoskeletal	As suggested by coexisting disease or acute trauma injuries. The amount of force necessary to produce a brachial plexus injury mandates a C-spine series to r/o C-spine fracture in all victims of brachial plexus trauma.
Laboratory	In general, most victims of significant trauma are best served by obtaining a wide variety of baseline lab studies to screen for unrecognized injury. These studies generally should include: Hct; CBC; ABGs; UA; renal function tests; LFTs; serum amylase.
Premedication	None

INTRAOPERATIVE

Anesthetic technique: GETA is preferred over regional techniques because of the unpredictable and prolonged length of these procedures and the need to evaluate brachial plexus function postop.

Induction	Rapid-sequence induction (see p. B-4) is mandatory in unscheduled cases, unless awake fiber optic intubation is performed (see Anesthetic Considerations for Thoracolumbar Neurosurgical Procedures, p. 122). C-spine fracture patients or those with facial injuries may require awake fiber optic intubation (see p. B-5) or other special airway techniques, as indicated from H&P. Hemodynamically unstable, acute-trauma patients can be induced more safely with etomidate (0.3–0.4 mg/kg iv) or ketamine (1–3 mg/kg iv).	
Maintenance	Balanced anesthesia with low-dose isoflurane (0.4–0.6%), iv sufentanil (0.25–1.0 mcg/kg/h), and N_2O in O_2 is suitable for stable patients. Hemodynamically unstable, acute-trauma victims undergoing emergency surgery are not likely to tolerate this regimen and are better served by using a combination of medications designed to have minimal hemodynamic consequences (e.g., fentanyl for analgesia, vecuronium for muscle relaxation, and scopolamine or midazolam for amnesia). N_2O is best avoided in the trauma patient. For brachial plexus surgery, some surgeons prefer minimal muscle relaxation after tracheal intubation so that a nerve stimulator can be used to help identify surgical anatomy.	
Emergence	Management of emergence and extubation should be routine except in difficult airway or full-stomach cases, which require that extubation be delayed until the patient's airway reflexes have returned and the patient is fully awake.	
Blood and fluid requirements	Significant blood loss IV: 14–16 ga × 1–2 NS/LR @ 1.5–3 mL/kg/h + replacement of blood loss @ 3 × volume Fluid warmer Airway humidifier	IV catheter placed in the nonoperative upper extremity is usually adequate in hemodynamically stable patients. Unstable, acute-trauma victims require a minimum of 2 large-bore iv catheters or large-bore central lines.
Monitoring	Standard monitors (see p. B-1). ± SSEP ± TEE	Invasive hemodynamic monitoring and TEE should be considered in acute, multiple-trauma victims. Some surgeons request SSEP to make continuous assessment of preop intact brachial plexus possible. When using SSEP monitoring, high doses of volatile anesthetic agents should be avoided because they adversely affect SSEP readings.
Positioning	✓and pad pressure points. ✓eyes. VAE risk	Postural ↓ BP is the most common complication of the semisitting position, particularly during the surgical prep period. SCD or antiembolism stockings may be beneficial. VAE is a potential complication of this position.

Orthopedic Surgery

Complications	Hemodynamic instability	Previously unrecognized injuries (e.g., pneumothorax, cardiac tamponade, intracranial bleeding) should be considered as a cause of unexplained intraop hemodynamic instability in all acute-trauma victims.
	Possible VAE	VAE risk is increased with patient in semisitting position.

POSTOPERATIVE

Complications	Sepsis ARDS	Many trauma victims survive the initial insult only to die later of sepsis or ARDS.
Pain management	PCA (see p. C-3).	
Tests	Based on concurrent injuries.	

Suggested Readings

1. Grundy BL: Intraoperative monitoring of sensory-evoked potentials. *Anesthesiology* 1983; 58(1):72–87.
2. Johnstone RE: Acute trauma with multiple injuries. *Curr Opin Anesthesiol* 2000; 13(2):175–9.
3. Leifert RD: Neurological problems. In *The Shoulder.* Rockwood CA Jr, Matsen FA III, eds. WB Saunders, Philadelphia: 1990, 750–8.
4. Nanakas AO: Injuries to the brachial plexus. In *The Pediatric Upper Extremity: Diagnosis and Treatment.* Bora FW Jr, ed. WB Saunders, Philadelphia: 1986, 247–58.
5. Thompson RW, Petrinec D, Toursarkissian B: I. Surgical treatment of thoracic outlet compression syndromes. II. Supraclavicular exploration and vascular reconstruction. *Ann Vasc Surg* 1997; 11(4):442–51.

ARM SURGERY

SURGICAL CONSIDERATIONS

Description: Surgical procedures on the arm are primarily for trauma or tumor surgery. Other procedures include extended approaches from the shoulder for significant trauma or tendon transfer. Exploration of peripheral nerves, most commonly of the radial nerve, are also included in this category, as are distal extensile approaches from the elbow for trauma or for lateral epicondylitis ("tennis elbow"). Depending on the lesion or fracture, the incision is developed through an internervous or intramuscular compartment. Procedures include **excisional biopsy** for soft tissue or bone tumors of the arm; **tumor excision,** which may be marginal, wide, or radical, depending on the tumor encountered; **tendon transfers,** such as pectoralis transfer to replace biceps function, used primarily for brachial plexus injuries; and **fractures and nonunion fractures of the humerus.** Positioning and location of incision is dependent on the level of the pathology. For example, for fractures involving the proximal half of the humerus, the standard **deltopectoral incision** may be extended distally along the interval between the biceps and triceps on the lateral aspect of the arm. This approach requires a beachchair (Figure 10.2-7) or, occasionally, supine position. Distal-third fractures are best approached posteriorly with the **triceps-splitting approach.** Distal fractures that extend into the elbow joint often require an olecranon osteotomy to visualize the fractured joint surface. Posterior approaches to the distal humerus are performed in either the lateral or prone position.

Usual preop diagnosis: Trauma; tumor

SUMMARY OF PROCEDURE	
Position	Supine; semisitting position for extended deltopectoral; lateral decubitus or prone for distal humerus fractures
Incision	Anterolateral approach; posterior approach in the lateral decubitus or prone position
Special istrumentation	Plate and screws; external fixators; intramedullary rods; occasionally, methylmethacrylate cement for tumor surgery; sterile tourniquet for distal humerus; I.I. for fracture surgery

SUMMARY OF PROCEDURE (cont'd)

Unique considerations	CT-guided sclerotherapy preop for vascular tumors; longitudinal incisions for biopsy and tumor excisions (not violating fascial planes)
Antibiotics	Cefazolin 1 g iv preop
Surgical time	45 min–6 h
Closing considerations	Drain frequently required.
EBL	Minimal—500+ mL, depending on pathology
Mortality	Varies with pathology
Morbidity	Bleeding Shoulder stiffness Nerve injury
Pain score	4–9

PATIENT POPULATION CHARACTERISTICS

Age range	Varies with procedure
Male:Female	Varies with procedure

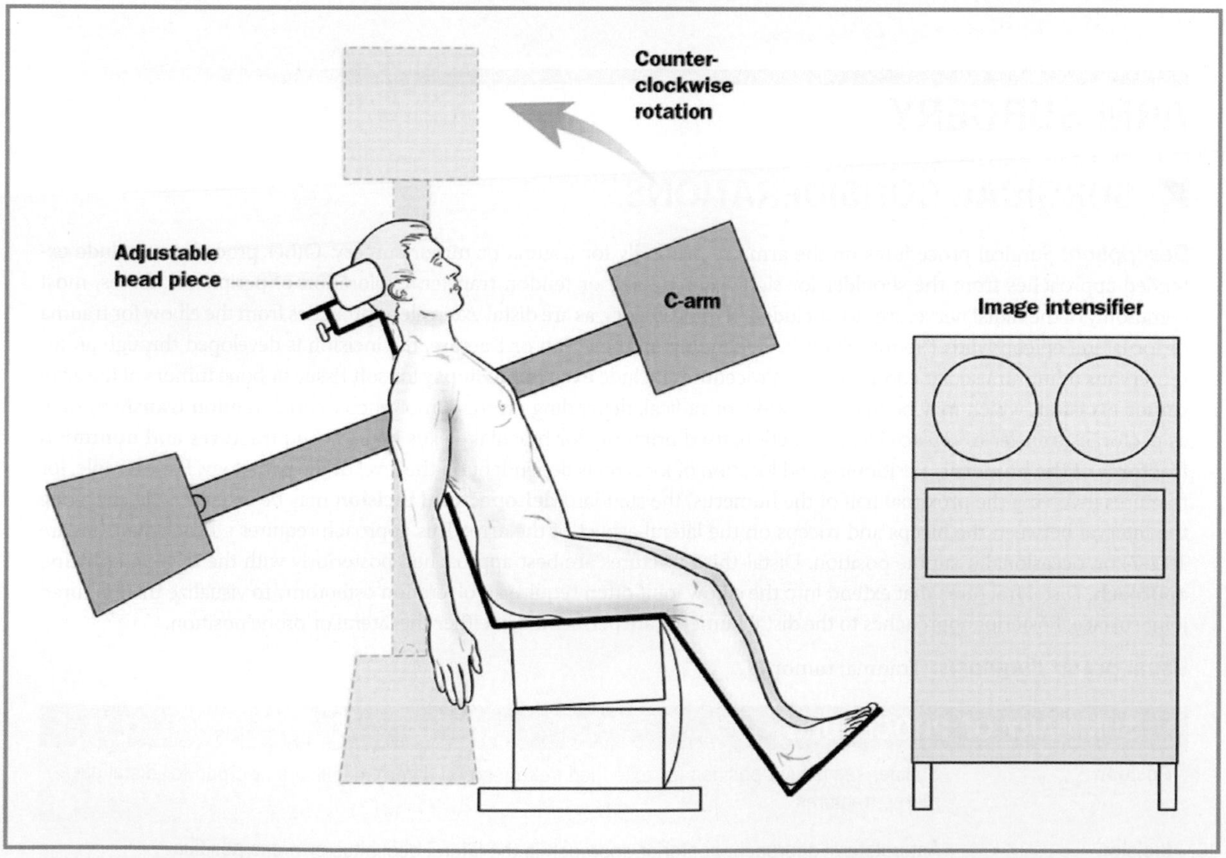

Figure 10.2-7. Beachchair positioning for shoulder surgery. Image intensification may be needed for intraoperative radiography (e.g., fracture surgery). (Reproduced by permission from Robinson CM, Page RS. Severely impacted proximal humerus fractures. *J Bone Joint Surg* 2004; 86:143-55.)

PATIENT POPULATION CHARACTERISTICS (cont'd)	
Incidence	Procedure-dependent
Etiology	Fractures; nerve entrapment (radial) following trauma; tumors
Associated conditions	Radial or ulnar nerve injury with humeral fractures

ANESTHETIC CONSIDERATIONS

PREOPERATIVE

Patients presenting for arm procedures are relatively young and otherwise healthy. Most of these patients present for elective repair of a traumatic injury. The preop workup is appropriate to patient's medical history. Some arm procedures, such as repair of a compound fracture, require immediate attention and necessitate emergency surgery and full-stomach considerations (p. B-4).

Laboratory	Hb/Hct (healthy patients); other tests as indicated from H&P.
Premedication	Mild-to-moderate premedication (e.g., in adults, midazolam 1–2 mg iv, fentanyl 50–100 mcg iv, titrated to effect) is often desirable before placement of a regional block.

INTRAOPERATIVE

Anesthetic technique: GA or regional anesthesia, or a combination of the two, can be used for surgical procedures on the arm. A brachial plexus block via the supraclavicular, infraclavicular or axillary approach is excellent for procedures on the distal arm. The interscalene approach to the brachial plexus is suitable for more proximal humerus procedures. Regional anesthesia alone is a means of avoiding the risk of aspiration pneumonitis associated with GA in the patient with a full stomach. Procedures longer than 3 h usually require general anesthesia in addition to regional. Regional anesthesia with sedation is usually well tolerated in shorter procedures.

General anesthesia:

Induction	Standard induction (see p. B-2) except in acute-trauma patients, where rapid-sequence induction is appropriate (see p. B-4).
Maintenance	Standard maintenance (see p. B-2).
Emergence	Management of emergence and extubation should be routine, except in difficult airway cases, which require awake extubation. Skin closure is frequently followed by application of a splint; patient should remain anesthetized during splinting procedure.

Regional anesthesia:

Local anesthetics	2% lidocaine or 1.5% mepivacaine have similar onset times (10–15 min), and similar duration (4–6 h). If extended postop pain control is desired, 0.5% bupivacaine, or ropivacaine (each with epinephrine 1:400,000) can be used. Onset is usually within 30 min, with duration up to 10–12 h. Ropivacaine may be preferred for peripheral nerve block due to its decreased cardiotoxicity.
Brachial plexus block	Supraclavicular, infraclavicular and axillary approaches are all suitable. Supraclavicular or infraclavicular blocks are better tolerated in fracture patients, because the arm need not be moved. Ultrasound guidance can improve speed and comfort during block placement. A peripheral nerve catheter may be placed to prolong pain relief in appropriate patients. • 2% lidocaine or 1.5% mepivacaine 30 mL for procedures lasting ≤ 2.5 h. • 0.5% bupivacaine, or ropivacaine 30 mL for procedures lasting > 2.5 h. If sedation is needed, midazolam (0.5–1.0 mg boluses), alfentanil (0.125–0.25 mcg/kg/min by infusion), or propofol (25–100 mcg/kg/min by infusion), titrated to effect, are good choices.

CHAPTER

10.3 Spine Surgery

SURGEON

Eugene J. Carragee, MD

ANESTHESIOLOGIST

C. Philip Larson, Jr., MD, CM

MINIMALLY INVASIVE POSTERIOR LUMBAR DISCECTOMY (MICRODISCECTOMY)

SURGICAL CONSIDERATIONS

Description: Since the mid-1990s, a number of techniques have been developed to allow the decompression of lumbar roots (removal of disc material) with as little trauma to the nerves and surrounding tissues as possible. In most instances, little or no bone is removed and, therefore, this is not technically a laminectomy or laminotomy. These minimally invasive procedures typically are carried out in healthy young or middle-aged adults with sciatica and are not done for more involved pathology, such as deformity, tumor, or infection. **Transpedicular fixation** and **short-segment fusions** may be attempted using modifications of these techniques.

Microdiscectomy approach: This can be done under GA, regional (epidural or spinal), or local anesthesia. The patient is placed in a prone or kneeling position and the posterior landmarks are palpated to identify the approximate level (e.g., L4/5); then the overlying skin is infiltrated with local anesthetic. A spinal needle is placed to the level of the lamina and an x-ray or fluoroscopic image is taken to confirm the level. A 1" incision is made over the proposed interspace and, using either traditional or specialized retractors, the soft tissue is displaced to expose the ligamentum flavum. With the use of an operating microscope, the ligamentum flavum is removed, the nerve retracted, and the extruded disc excised. For a single level, this should take between 30–90 min, depending on the size of the patient and whether there is any scarring or adhesions from previous surgery.

Variant approach: Percutaneous discectomy through a posterolateral approach is usually reserved for "contained discs"—protrusions into, but not through, the outer annulus of the disc. These are usually done under MAC with local anesthetic. The percutaneous instruments may be positioned using fluoroscopic guidance with or without a fiber optic light source and camera/monitor setup. The disc space is entered posterolaterally. The surgeon usually avoids anesthetizing the area around the nerve root so that the patient can alert the team if the root is struck by an instrument (quite painful). After the disc space is entered, fluoroscopic or camera images are used to guide the surgeon in the removal of herniated disc. The disc material can be removed with specialized grabbers or automatic power-driven shavers.

Usual preop diagnosis: Chronic back pain 2° herniated lumbar disc; lumbar radiculopathy

SUMMARY OF PROCEDURES

	Microdiscectomy	Percutaneous Discectomy
Position	Prone or kneeling, with bolster or frame support. The abdomen must hang free to decompress the epidural veins.	Prone or lateral decubitus
Incision	Posterior midline or slightly off midline, at the appropriate vertebral level	About 8–12 cm lateral to the midline at the appropriate vertebral level
Special instrumentation	Microscope; light source; specialized retraction and dissection instruments for working in a small, deep incision	Percutaneous instruments, including trocars, sounds, and arthroscopic-type grabbers and shavers; fluoroscopy; and, sometimes, camera/monitor and fiber optic light setup
Unique considerations	Often outpatient procedure. Need to make room for microscope at head of bed.	Patient must be alert enough to respond to pain if nerve roots are encountered.
Antibiotics	Cefazolin l g iv	⇐
Surgical time	0.5–1.5 h	1–2 h
Closing considerations	Minimal suturing	Usually no closure (Band-aids)
EBL	25–100 mL	Minimal
Postop care	PACU. Mobilization as soon as tolerated. Usually discharged within 24 h.	PACU → home. Mobilization as tolerated.

SUMMARY OF PROCEDURE (cont'd)

	Microdiscectomy	Percutaneous Discectomy
Mortality	Very rare	⇐
Morbidity	Nerve injury Dural laceration Infection	Failure to decompress the nerve adequately – ⇐
Pain score	4	2

PATIENT POPULATION CHARACTERISTICS

Age range	16–60 yr
Male:Female	3:2
Incidence	Common
Etiology	Degenerative; trauma (rare)

ANESTHETIC CONSIDERATIONS

PREOPERATIVE

Young and middle-aged adults are usually healthy; the elderly may have cardiovascular and/or pulmonary disease.

Musculoskeletal	Since these patients may have chronic back pain with radiculopathy, they may not be suitable candidates for regional anesthetic techniques. Postop exacerbation of symptoms may be incorrectly ascribed to the anesthetic technique. A careful motor and sensory evaluation of the lower extremities should be documented. Patients commonly taking centrally acting analgesics (e.g., Ultram); narcotics (e.g., Darvon, Darvocet, OxyContin, Percocet, Vicodin); NSAIDs (e.g., Feldene, Naprosyn, Relafen, Voltaren); or COX-2 inhibitors (Celebrex) often require higher doses of sedative-hypnotics and analgesics in the periop period.
Hematologic	Patients should stop taking aspirin or NSAIDs at least 2 wk before surgery. In addition, an INR or PT and PTT should be checked preop. **Tests:** Hct; Plt; INR
Laboratory	Other tests as indicated from H&P.
Premedication	Standard premedication (see p. B-1).

INTRAOPERATIVE

Anesthetic technique: Microdiscectomies are commonly done under GA; however, local or regional anesthetic techniques are suitable in selected patients. Care must be taken to avoid encroaching on the surgical site. Percutaneous discectomies typically require only MAC with sedation. These patients must be awake in order to alert the surgeon to inadvertent nerve root contact. In some centers, regional anesthesia (spinal or epidural) is the anesthetic of choice.

General Anesthesia:

Induction	Standard induction (see p. B-2). Consider using wire-reinforced ETT to prevent kinking, with patient in prone position.
Maintenance	Standard maintenance (see p. B-2). Usually 1–2 h operation. After exposure, further relaxant use is unnecessary.
Emergence	No special considerations
MAC	See p. B-3–B-4.

Regional anesthesia:

Spinal	Patient in sitting, lateral decubitus, or prone position for placement of subarachnoid block. Doses of local anesthetics should be adequate to provide a high lumbar level of sensory anesthesia (e.g., bupivacaine 6–10 mg with fentanyl 10 mcg).	
Epidural	Patient in sitting or lateral decubitus position for placement of epidural catheter. A test dose (e.g., 3 mL of 1.5% lidocaine with 1:200,000 epinephrine [5 mcg/mL]) is administered and the patient is observed for development of subarachnoid block or Sx of an intravascular injection. Titrate lidocaine 2% with epinephrine (3–5 mL at a time) until desired surgical level is obtained.	
Blood and fluid requirements	IV: 18–20 ga × 1 NS/LR @ 5 mL/kg/h	Blood not likely to be required.
Monitoring	Standard monitors (see p. B-1).	
Positioning	✓ and pad pressure points. ✓ eyes.	Prone position: Wilson frame or bolsters to support shoulders/hips and optimize ventilation. Knee-chest position: Andrews table. Place head in cushioned holder with cutout for eyes, nose, chin (e.g., Andrews Gentle-Rest pillow). Make certain nose and chin do not touch table. Pad elbows, knees, other pressure points.

POSTOPERATIVE

Complications	Urinary retention in the older patient Transient numbness/paresthesias, weakness	Rx: Consider catheterization. Due to nerve-root irritation from operation. Rx with analgesics and/or muscle relaxants (e.g., Flexeril, Robaxin, Soma).
Pain management	PCA (p. C-3) Ketorolac 30 mg iv Epidural analgesia (p. C-2)	PO analgesics may be suitable: acetaminophen and codeine (Tylenol #3 1– 2 tab q 4–6 h) or oxycodone and acetaminophen (Percocet 1 tab q 6 h)
Tests	As indicated by patient status	Patient usually discharged from hospital within 24–48 h.

Suggested Readings

1. Bookwalter J III, Busch M, Nicely D: Ambulatory surgery is safe and effective in radicular disc disease. *Spine* 1994; 19: 526–30.
2. Carragee E, Helms E, O'Sullivan G: Are post-operative activity restrictions necessary after posterior lumbar discectomy? A prospective study of outcomes in 50 consecutive cases. *Spine* 1996; 21:1893–7.
3. Javedan S, Sonntag VK: Lumbar disc herniation: microsurgical approach. *Neurosurgery* 2003; 52(l):160–4.
4. Maroon JC: Current concepts in minimally invasive discectomy. *Neurosurgery* 2002; 51(5 Suppl):137–45.
5. Rodriguez HE, Connolly MM, Dracopoulos H, et al: Anterior access to the lumbar spine: laparoscopic versus open. *Am Surg* 2002; 68(11):978–83.
6. Schick U, Dohnert J: Technique of microendoscopy in medial lumbar disc herniation. *Minim Invasive Neurosurg* 2002; 45(3):139–41.
7. Spengler DM: Lumbar disc herniation. In *Chapman's Orthopaedic Surgery,* 3rd edition. Chapman MW, ed. Lippincott Williams & Wilkins, Philadelphia: 2001, 3765–74.
8. Surgical treatment of lumbar disk disorders. *JAMA* 2006;296(20):2485–7.
9. Zahrawi F: Microlumbar discectomy: Is it safe as an outpatient procedure? *Spine* 1994; 19:1070–3.

ANTERIOR SPINAL RECONSTRUCTION AND FUSION—THORACIC AND THORACOLUMBAR SPINE

SURGICAL CONSIDERATIONS

Description: Traditionally, most spinal procedures have been approached posteriorly. The advent of surgical treatment for vertebral TB and postpolio spinal deformities during the 1960s saw the development of surgical approaches to the anterior spine. These procedures initially were reserved for patients with significant deformities, especially kyphosis. More recently, the treatment of traumatic, neoplastic, and degenerative conditions have been included in the anterior approach. Regardless of the condition under treatment, the approach is similar for a given level. There are several more or less distinct types of surgical exposures, depending on the level.

Cervicothoracic approach: Most cephalad and difficult is the approach to the upper thoracic spine (T1-T3). This generally includes a modified anterior cervical exposure with a caudal extension, including a resection of the clavicle, part of the manubrium, and sometimes the rib at the thoracic outlet. Dangers in this exposure are to the great vessels at the thoracic outlet, trachea (rare) and esophagus (more common), lung parenchyma, sympathetic ganglia, lymphatic duct (on the left), and brachial plexus. Once the spine is exposed and the discs and/or vertebrae are removed, the spinal cord is at risk. This procedure occasionally involves entering the thoracic cavity, in which case it is usually done intrapleurally—that is, through the parietal pleura. The lung needs to be collapsed at least partially. Spinal cord monitoring is usually performed; wake-up tests are not. Manipulation of the carotid artery and aortic arch may cause wide HR and BP fluctuations.

Transthoracic approach: Further down the spine, the levels from T5-T10 are more easily reached via a transthoracic approach Fig. 10.3-1. This involves a typical thoracotomy with the resection of a rib. The level of the rib resection is usually 1–2 levels above the highest vertebral level being approached. The great vessels and lung parenchyma are at risk, as is the thoracic duct (on the left). The patient is in the lateral decubitus position and the mediastinum and heart usually fall to the opposite side, out of harm's way. Risk to the spinal cord depends on the difficulty and extent of the vertebral disease and the reconstruction. Spinal cord monitoring usually is performed intraop. The need for

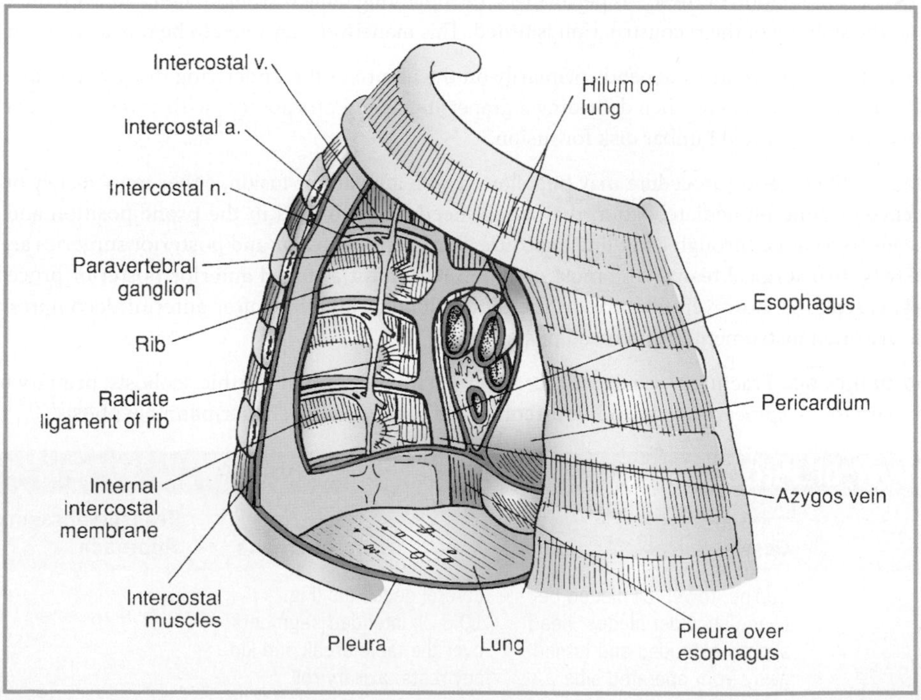

Figure 10.3-1. Surgical anatomy of the transthoracic approach. (Reproduced with permission from Hoppenfeld S, deBoer P: *Surgical Exposures in Orthopaedics.* JB Lippincott, Philadelphia: 1984.)

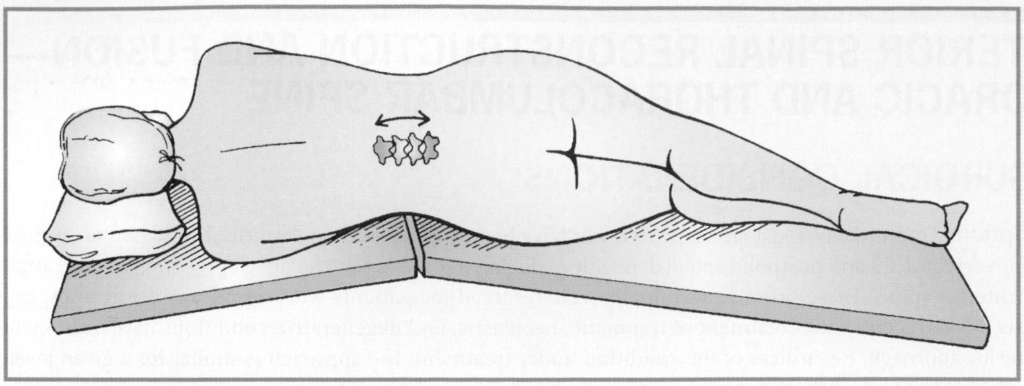

Figure 10.3-2. Patient position for transdiaphragmatic or retroperitoneal approach. (Reproduced with permission from Hoppenfeld S, deBoer P: *Surgical Exposures in Orthopaedics*. JB Lippincott, Philadelphia: 1984.)

the lung to be deflated varies with the extent of the exposure. In centers where this procedure is frequently performed and the surgeons are accustomed to the respiratory motion during operation, DLTs are not routinely used. Because there is no (intended) violation of the lung parenchyma, air leaks and parenchymal repairs are not common.

Transdiaphragmatic approach: When the exposure must transverse the diaphragm, a combined retroperitoneal and transthoracic approach is used. This requires the diaphragm to be sectioned circumferentially from the chest wall and spine. If only the very low segments of the thoracic spine (T10-T12) are exposed, the required deflation of the involved lung is minimal. The risks are the same as those encountered with the transthoracic or retroperitoneal approaches alone. Regardless of the level of exposure, the operating table may be used during the procedure to manipulate the spine for better exposure and to "lock in" implants, bone grafts, etc. Usually, the area of the spine to be exposed is centered above the "breaking" joint and kidney rests of the table (Fig. 10.3-2). After the initial exposure, the table is angled in the center with the head and legs pointing down and kidney rests elevated to "open up" the section of spine facing the surgeon. After removal of the disk, abscess, or tumor, a reconstruction—using bone graft, metal implants, bone cement, or a combination of these—is performed. The operating table is straightened and, with the spine in neutral alignment, the stability of the reconstruction is tested. This maneuver may need to be repeated several times.

The **morbidity** of these procedures depends primarily on the nature of the underlying disease. Obviously, bleeding and visceral injury are more likely when debriding a grapefruit-sized Potts abscess with several destroyed vertebrae than in removing a degenerated lumbar disk for fusion.

In some instances, the anterior procedure may be followed with a posterior fusion, either immediately or after 5–7 d of convalescence. If done immediately after, the patient needs to be placed in the prone position and the second procedure needs to be done through a midline exposure. Sometimes anterior and posterior surgeries are performed simultaneously by two surgical teams. The most common reason for a staged anterior/posterior procedure (in the United States) is scoliosis; however, fractures at the thoracolumbar junction, after anterior decompression and reconstruction, are often instrumented and fused posteriorly.

Usual preop diagnosis: Fractures (usually at thoracic lumbar junction); idiopathic scoliosis; primary neoplasm or metastatic disease to the spine; pyogenic or TB osteomyelitis of the spine; Scheuermann's kyphosis

SUMMARY OF PROCEDURES

	Cervicothoracic Approach	Transthoracic Approach	Transdiaphragmatic Approach
Position	Supine; towel roll placed between shoulder blades, head slightly extended and turned away from operated side	Lateral decubitus (Fig. 10.3-2); intended segments over the table break and kidney rests; axillary roll	⇐
Incision	Inverted "L" longitudinally along manubrium to sternal notch, then transversely above clavicle	Along a rib, two levels above the highest segment to be exposed	⇐

SUMMARY OF PROCEDURES (cont'd)

	Cervicothoracic Approach	Transthoracic Approach	Transdiaphragmatic Approach
Special instrumentation	Instrumentation rarely used. Strut grafts—using rib, fibula, clavicle or cement—may be used to replace excised vertebrae. ± DLT	For thoracolumbar scoliosis, a Zielke-type rod and screws may be used; more rigid instrumentation sometimes used in fractures. ± DLT	⇐ (More common to use instrumentation at the affected level than above.)
Unique considerations	Aortic arch and carotid manipulation may cause BP/HR changes. Postop respiratory distress well described.	During spinal reconstruction, manipulation of operating table may be essential to "lock in" graft or implant (see above).	⇐
Antibiotics	Cefazolin 1 g iv (+ gentamicin 80 mg iv, if indwelling bladder catheter)	⇐	⇐
Surgical time	2–6 h	⇐	⇐
Closing considerations	Patient usually transferred to bed prior to emergence; sudden jerking motions may dislodge graft or implant.	⇐	⇐
EBL	200–5000 mL. Blood loss is extremely variable; when bleeding occurs, it may be torrential from the aorta, vena cava, or iliac vessels and branches. In nontumor or infection cases, 200–400 mL is usual.	⇐	⇐
Postop care	Chest drain; NG suction usually needed; short period of ICU observation is usual.	⇐	⇐
Mortality	< 0.1%, except in cases of malignancy or sepsis	⇐	⇐
Morbidity	For elective degenerative cases: 5–10% overall	⇐	⇐
	DVT: 6%	⇐	⇐
	Neurological: 3%	⇐	⇐
	Infection: 1%	⇐	⇐
	Sexual dysfunction	⇐	⇐
	For sepsis or tumor: 50–80% (overall)	⇐	⇐
	Cardiorespiratory failure	⇐	⇐
	Sepsis	⇐	⇐
Pain score	7–8 (if patient sensate at level of surgery)	7–8 (if patient sensate at level of surgery)	7–8 (if patient sensate at level of surgery)

PATIENT POPULATION CHARACTERISTICS

Age range	12–30 yr (scoliosis surgery); > 40 (tumor and infection surgery); 15–35 yr (fractures)
Male:Female	1:1, except more scoliosis surgery in females (1:4) and more fractures in males
Incidence	20,000/yr
Etiology	Scoliosis: idiopathic (50%), neuromuscular (15%), congenital (5%); trauma (20%); infections, tumors (10%)
Associated conditions	Pulmonary HTN and impaired pulmonary function; neuromuscular scoliosis (poliomyelitis, CP, muscular dystrophy, Friedreich's ataxia); aspiration; cardiomyopathy

ANESTHETIC CONSIDERATIONS

See Anesthetic Considerations for Spinal Reconstruction and Fusion, p. 971.

Suggested Readings

1. Butler J, Schafer MF: Anterior approach to scoliosis. In *Chapman's Orthopaedic Surgery*, 3rd edition. Chapman MW, ed. Lippincott Williams & Wilkins, Philadelphia: 2001, 4011–30.
2. Hoppenfeld S, deBoer P: *Surgical Exposures in Orthopaedics: An Anatomic Approach*, 2nd edition. Lippincott Williams & Wilkins, Philadelphia: 1994, 215–302.
3. Jain AK: Treatment of tuberculosis of the spine with neurologic complications. *Clin Orthop* 2002; 398:75–84.
4. McLain RF, Benson DR: Operative treatment of thoracic and thoracolumbar fractures. In *Chapman's Orthopaedic Surgery*, 3rd edition. Chapman MW, ed. Lippincott Williams & Wilkins, Philadelphia: 2001, 3725–45.
5. McLain RF, Lieberman I: Surgical treatment of adult scoliosis. In *Chapman's Orthopaedic Surgery*, 3rd edition. Chapman MW, ed. Lippincott Williams & Wilkins, Philadelphia: 2001, 4101–14.
6. Taft E, Francis R: Evaluation and management of scoliosis. *J Pediatr Health Care* 2003; 17(1):42–4.
7. Tay BK, Deckey J, Hu SS: Spinal infections. *J Am Acad Orthop Surg* 2002; 10(3):188–97.

ANTERIOR SPINAL RECONSTRUCTION AND FUSION—LUMBOSACRAL SPINE

SURGICAL CONSIDERATIONS

Description: The same general considerations apply here as in thoracolumbar reconstruction segments. The thoracic cavity is not entered, nor is the diaphragm sectioned. Careful preop assessment is needed, as these patients may have a wide range of coexisting diseases. The same operative procedure is performed for removal of a degenerative disk in a healthy patient as is carried out to decompress the cauda equina in a debilitated patient with metastatic breast carcinoma.

Retroperitoneal approach: Below the diaphragm, exposure of the lumbar spine (L2-S1) can be performed through a retroperitoneal approach (Fig. 10.3-3). This often involves a flank incision, often with resection of the 11th or 12th rib. The patient lies in a decubitus or partial decubitus position. At risk here are the great vessels above and below the bifurcation of the aorta (L4-L5). The ureter crosses the operative field and must be identified and protected. The sympathetic chain may be damaged along the vertebrae, but the consequences of this are minimal. The presacral plexus further down may be injured and result in persistent retrograde ejaculation.

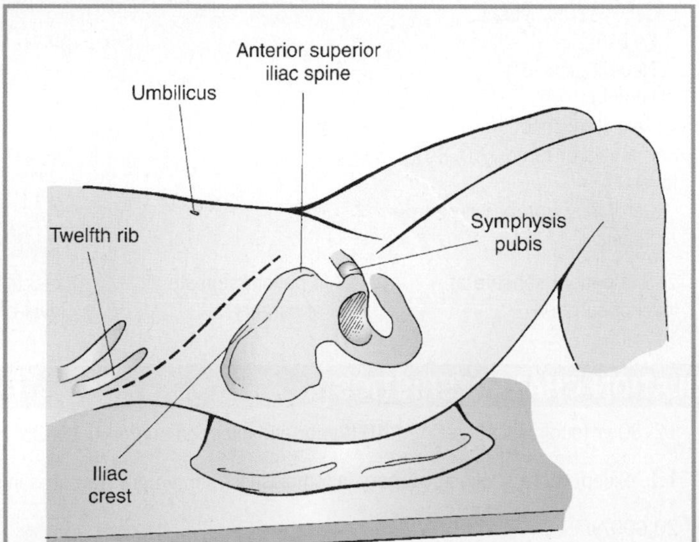

Figure 10.3-3. Retroperitoneal approach to lumbar spine. (Reproduced with permission from Hoppenfeld S, deBoer P: *Surgical Exposures in Orthopaedics*. JB Lippincott, Philadelphia: 1984.)

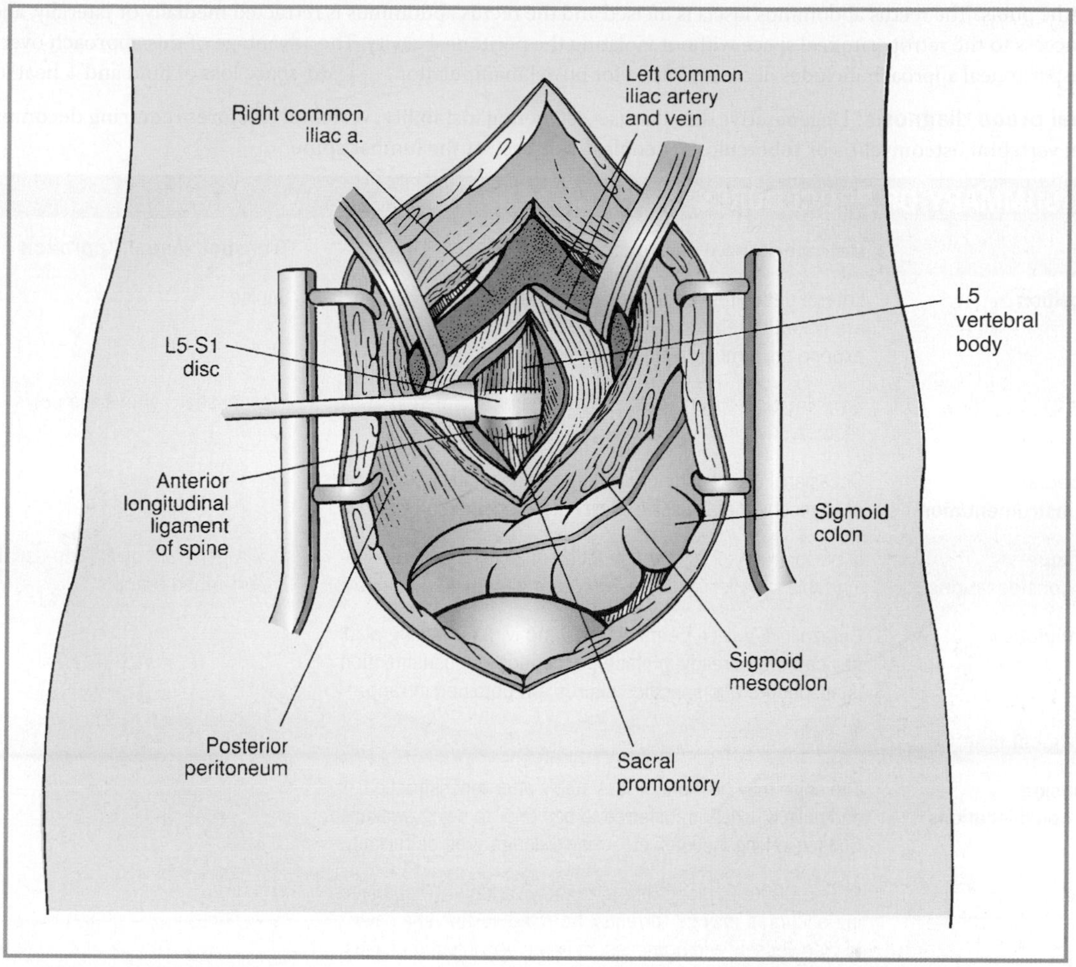

Figure 10.3-4. Transperitoneal approach to lumbosacral junction. (Reproduced with permission from Hoppenfeld S, deBoer P: *Surgical Exposures in Orthopaedics.* JB Lippincott, Philadelphia: 1984.)

A Pfannenstiel's incision may be used to approach L5/S1 or L4/5. Regardless of the level of exposure, the operating table is used during the procedure to manipulate the spine for better exposure and to "lock in" implants, bone grafts, etc. Usually the area of the spine to be exposed is centered above the 'breaking' joint and kidney rests of the table (Fig. 10.3-2). After initial exposure, the table is angled in the center with the head and legs pointing down and the kidney rests elevated to open up the section of spine facing the surgeon. After the removal of the disc, abscess, or tumor, a reconstruction—using bone graft, metal implants, bone cement, or a combination of these—is performed. The table is then straightened; with the spine in neutral alignment, the stability of the reconstruction is tested by this maneuver, which may need to be repeated several times.

In some instances, the anterior reconstruction and fusion is followed with a **posterior fusion,** either immediately or after 5–7 d of convalescence. If done immediately after, the patient needs to be positioned prone on the operating table, and the second procedure done through a midline exposure. Sometimes anterior and posterior surgeries can be performed simultaneously by two surgical teams. The most common reason for a staged anterior/posterior procedure (in the United States) was scoliosis. Recent trends in degenerative lumbar disk surgery indicate that anterior and posterior fusion has become more common with some evidence suggesting better results in fusion and pain relief.

Variant procedure or approaches: When the L5 vertebra and sacrum need to be exposed widely, a **transperitoneal approach** may be needed. This involves a laparotomy or Pfannenstiel's incision, displacement of the bowels out of the pelvis, and exposure of the lumbosacral junction (Fig. 10.3-4). The patient is supine for this procedure and the surgical risks are similar, as with other intraabdominal approaches.

In a recent modification to the retroperitoneal approach, the patient is placed in the supine position. In this **supine retroperitoneal approach,** an incision is made in either a longitudinal or transverse fashion between the umbilicus and the pubis. The rectus abdominus fascia is incised and the rectus abdominus is retracted medially or laterally, allowing access to the retroperitoneal space without violating the peritoneal cavity. The advantage of this approach over the transperitoneal approach includes decreased need for bowel manipulation, →↓ 3rd-space loss of fluid and ↓ heat loss.

Usual preop diagnosis: Degenerative disc disease; segmental instability; vertebral fractures requiring decompression; vertebral osteomyelitis or tuberculosis; neoplastic disease of the lumbar spine

SUMMARY OF PROCEDURES

	Retroperitoneal Approach (Lateral)	Transperitoneal Approach
Position	Lateral decubitus, affected side up. The up hip and knee are flexed to relax psoas muscle and allow its reflection to expose the lumbar vertebral bodies.	Supine
Incision	Flank incision curving anteriorly to the lateral margin of the rectus abdominus (Fig. 10.3-3)	Pfannenstiel's above the pubis
Special instrumentation	Occasional use of anterior instrumentation to stabilize fractures or to reconstruct the spine when entire vertebrae are removed	⇐
Unique considerations	In performing spinal reconstruction, manipulation of operating table is essential to "lock in" graft or implant (see above).	⇐+ A general bowel prep usually is performed preop.
Antibiotics	Cefazolin 1 g iv (+ gentamicin 80 mg iv, if indwelling bladder catheter already in place); exception is when infection is suspected and specific cultures are obtained intraop.	⇐
Surgical time	3–6 h	⇐
Closing considerations	The spine may be more or less stable after reconstruction, and patient usually transferred to bed prior to being awakened. Sudden jerking motions, etc., may dislodge graft or implant.	⇐
EBL	200–5,000 mL. Blood loss extremely variable. When bleeding occurs, it may be torrential from the aorta, vena cava, or iliac vessels and branches. In nontumor/infection cases, 200–400 mL is usual.	⇐
Postop care	Patients with degenerative conditions and elective surgeries normally recover in PACU and return to ward. Patients with infections, fractures, and tumors are usually observed in ICU for 24 h postop. Ileus for 24–72 h is usual; NG suction usually continues until bowel sounds and passing flatus are present. Generally, mobilization depends on final stability.	⇐
Mortality	Malignancy or sepsis: 1–2% Elective: < 0.1%	⇐ ⇐
Morbidity	In patients with malignancy, sepsis or fractures with cauda equina compression, overall serious complications: 25–50% Cardiopulmonary failure Neurologic deficit Pneumothorax Sepsis	⇐ ⇐ – – ⇐
Pain score	6	6

PATIENT POPULATION CHARACTERISTICS

Age range	Variable (infant–adult)
Male:Female	1:1, except more scoliosis surgery in females (1:4)
Incidence	Uncommon
Etiology	Infection (osteomyelitis, TB); trauma; congenital; neoplasia; idiopathic

ANESTHETIC CONSIDERATIONS FOR SPINAL RECONSTRUCTION AND FUSION

(Procedures covered: anterior reconstruction and fusion of thoracic, thoracolumbar, and lumbosacral spine)

PREOPERATIVE

Patients presenting for spinal reconstruction commonly have either idiopathic or acquired scoliosis, a complex deformity involving both lateral curvature and rotation of the spine, as well as an associated deformity of the rib cage. Types of scoliosis include: idiopathic, congenital, neuromuscular, myopathic, traumatic, tumor-related, and mesenchymal disorders. The majority of cases are idiopathic, with a male:female ratio of 1:4. Normally, the cervical spine and lumbar spine are lordotic, while the thoracic spine is kyphotic. Surgery is indicated when the curvature is severe (angulation beyond 40° in the thoracic or lumbar spine[7]) or progressing rapidly. The primary purpose of the operative correction of scoliosis is not to straighten the spine, but to prevent further curvature from developing. The instrumentation is intended to stabilize the spine until bony fusion of the spine has occurred. After the fusion is solid (6–12 mo), the instrumentation may be removed if it is broken, causes protrusions or lumps in the back, or the patient is having residual back pain. Nonscoliotic patients presenting for this surgery may have spinal instability as a result of trauma, metastatic carcinoma or infection (e.g., TB). These patients are usually healthy, apart from their underlying pathology. The patients with disseminated lung or breast cancer may need a careful workup with regard to respiratory, nutritional, and chemotherapeutic status. (See Anesthetic Considerations for Lobectomy, Pneumonectomy, p. 275, or Mastectomy, p. 652.)

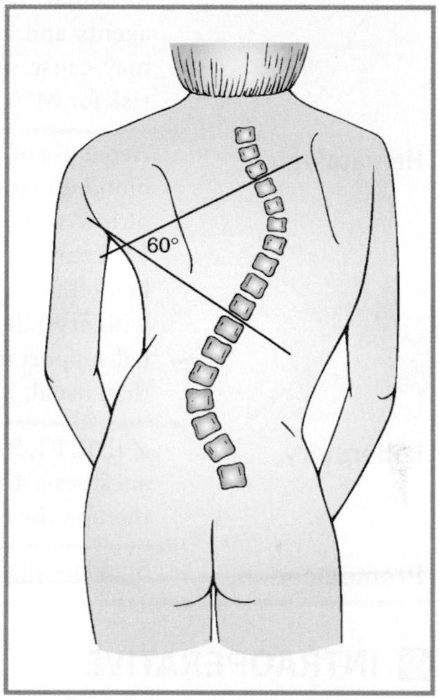

Figure 10.3-5. Cobb angle.

Respiratory

Respiratory impairment proportional to angle of lateral curvature (Cobb angle) (Fig. 10.3-5)

Cobb Angle:	30°–60°	60°– 90°	>90°
VC	↓ 25%	↓ 50%	↓ 70%
TLC	↓ 27%	↓ 37%	↓ 50%

Restrictive pattern: ↓ TLC + ↓ ↓ VC

- If VC >70% predicted, respiratory reserve is adequate.
- If VC < 40% predicted, postop ventilation usually is required.

Expect further significant (~40%) ↓ VC immediately postop, requiring 7–10 d to resolve.

↑ RR + ↓ TV →↑ dead space + ↓ alveolar ventilation → V/Q mismatch → hypoxemia.[12]

Patients with scoliosis of neuromuscular origin are more susceptible to aspiration and respiratory failure.

Tests: CXR; ABG; PFT; assess exercise tolerance by Hx.

Cardiovascular

↑ PVR (**NB:** independent of severity of scoliosis). High incidence of CHD and mitral valve prolapse.

Tests: ECG; ECHO—consult cardiologist if apical systolic murmur or other evidence of cardiovascular impairment is present.

Neurological

SSEPs (posterior cord) and MEPs (anterior cord) will be monitored in most patients who are undergoing spinal reconstruction. Some surgeons, however, may request that the patient be awakened intraop, after completion of the instrumentation, but before closure of the wound, to ensure that no motor deficits have developed as a result of the correction. Movement of the toes or feet bilaterally is sufficient to verify intact motor function. Inform the patient preop that this test will be performed, that it will only take a few minutes, that

Neurological (cont'd)	the patient will not be in severe pain while doing the test, and that full anesthesia will be reinstituted upon completion of the test. If focal neurological lesions exist preop as a result of disease (e.g., tuberculous spondylitis), their documentation is important to distinguish them from changes associated with correction.
Musculoskeletal	When the Cobb angle is > 25°, the degree of respiratory impairment will be significant, and the need for postop ventilatory support becomes more likely. Patients with muscular dystrophy may be more sensitive to myocardial depression from anesthetic agents and also may require postop ventilation 2° muscle weakness. Succinylcholine may cause severe rhabdomyolysis with hyperkalemia. These patients also may be at risk for MH.
Hematologic	Avoid use of Plt inhibitors 2 wk before surgery. Encourage autologous or directed-donor blood donations. Have at least 2 U PRBCs available at start of operation. Consider use of low-volume Cell Savers (e.g., Medtronic Autolog). Discuss use of controlled ↓ BP with surgeon. If anticipated blood loss is substantial, some institutions use isovolemic hemodilution by collecting 1–2 U blood at the start of anesthesia and replacing them with crystalloid or colloid solutions. Be aware that patients with previously placed spinal support (e.g., Milwaukee brace) for correction of scoliosis may have more blood loss than usual.
Laboratory	✓ INR, PT, PTT, and Plt count preop. ✓ Hct the morning of operation or after induction of anesthesia if autologous donations have been made since, with modest blood loss and fluid therapy, the Hct may rapidly ↓ to < 26%.
Premedication	Standard premedication (see p. B-1), if appropriate.

INTRAOPERATIVE

Anesthetic technique: GETA. For pediatric cases, preheat room to 78°F. For operations in the prone position, use a wire-reinforced tube to prevent kinking and airway obstruction. If a transthoracic approach is used, a DLT is necessary.

Induction	Standard induction (p. B-2). A DLT may facilitate surgical access in the patient undergoing an anterior correction. The smallest available DLT is size 28 Fr (OD = 8.9 mm), typically suitable for a child aged 12–14 yr.	
Maintenance	Standard maintenance (p. B-2). Monitoring of SSEP and MEP recordings are standard of care and performed in virtually all patients undergoing correction for scoliosis. For optimal monitoring a TIVA is preferred, thereby avoiding any inhalation anesthetics. The usual TIVA drugs are propofol 75–200 mcg/kg/min and remifentanil 0.02–0.5 mcg/kg/min. The larger doses are used at the start of anesthesia and surgery, and gradually lowered as a blood level of the agents is established. It is advisable to administer midazolam 3–5 mg at the start of anesthesia to minimize any possibility of recall in the early phase of anesthesia.	
Emergence	The patient's trachea usually is extubated at the conclusion of the operation, unless there is a question of lung function following a transthoracic approach and OLV. Some surgeons may place an epidural catheter before closure for postop pain management or perform intercostal injections for the transthoracic approach. Prior to emergence, scoliosis patients usually are fitted with a plaster mold to be used as a permanent brace that will be worn for several mo postop. Transfer from the operating table to bed must be smooth and gentle.	
Blood and fluid requirements	IV: 14–16 ga × 2 NS/LR @ 6–8 mL/kg/h not to exceed 40 mL/kg	Anticipate substantial blood loss with scoliosis surgery from extensive dissection of muscles from bony spine; less so with isolated thoracic fusion. It may vary from 25–100% of the patient's blood volume, although blood loss is usually less with the anterior approach (Dwyer's).

Blood and fluid requirements (cont'd)	Hetastarch 6% ≤ 20 mL/kg or albumin prn Warm all fluids. Humidify gases. T&C 2–4 U PRBCs. ± Cell Saver	Colloid is preferred since it will remain intravascular until metabolized. Low-volume units (e.g., Medtronic, AutoLog) are best.
Control of blood loss	Position to prevent venous engorgement. ↓ MAP to 60–70 mmHg. ± ↓ Hct to 25–28%.	Consider maintaining BP ≤ 20% below the lowest preop values to minimize blood loss during dissection. Generally maintain MAP > 60 mmHg in young, healthy patients, and > 85 mmHg in older patients, for spinal cord perfusion. Once dissection is complete, higher BP values acceptable. Maintain UO at 0.5–1 mL/kg/h during controlled hypotension.
Monitoring	Standard monitors (p. B-1) Arterial line CVP line Urinary catheter ± SSEP	CVP monitor helpful in selected, older patients to assess fluid Rx. Trends in CVP may be more reliable than measurement of UO to assess changes in volume status in patients in the prone and lateral positions.
Positioning	✓ and pad pressure points. ✓ eyes, neck.	**Prone:** Place head on cushioned head holder with cutout for eyes, nose, chin (e.g., Andrews Gentle-Rest pillow). Make certain that none of the face rests on bed. ✓ elbows, knees, feet. **Lateral:** Place head on donut in neutral position. Pad both arms in neutral position.
Wakeup test	30 min advance warning from surgeons is needed (sevoflurane). • Decrease inhalational agents. • Reverse muscle relaxants (and narcotics, if necessary). • Monitor train of four. • Request hand squeeze; if present, elicit bilateral foot movement. • Reinduce anesthesia with STP (2–3 mg/kg) or propofol (0.5–1 mg/kg). **Dangers:** Air embolus Dislodgement of spinal instrumentation Accidental extubation	The wake-up test assesses integrity of motor pathways in the ventral cord. Uncontrolled patient movement during wake-up test can result in accidental extubation or dislodgement of the spinal instrumentation. Unrestrained inspiratory efforts may provoke venous air embolism. The anesthesiologist must be prepared to rapidly reanesthetize the patient.
SSEP and MEPs	SSEP: Dorsal cord function only MEPs: Ventral cord function	SSEP and, more recently, MEP are being used routinely. The technician needs to know when there are substantive changes in doses of inhalation anesthetics or ventilation. Optimal EP recordings are obtained with TIVA anesthesia. One can discontinue TIVA at the start of closure and substitute sevoflurane until the operative procedure is concluded. Have fentanyl or meperidine ready for analgesia as the remifentanil effect wanes.
Complications	Spinal cord ischemia Massive blood loss Fat embolism	SSEP indications of spinal cord ischemia should be treated by restoring normal BP and by ↓ cord traction. Prompt transfusion may be necessary and blood should be available in the room (2–4 U PRBC).

POSTOPERATIVE

Complications	Pulmonary insufficiency Hypothermia Pneumothorax Dislodgement of internal fixation	Postop ventilation may be required in patients with severe respiratory impairment (see Preoperative Considerations, above). In addition, thoracotomy, surgical trauma to the diaphragm and fat embolism may further ↑ the risk of postop pulmonary insufficiency. Careful handling of patient in transfer is mandatory.
	Neurologic sequelae[27]	Neurologic sequelae probably remain the most feared complication, and it is important to document postop neurologic exam.
Pain management	PCA (p. C-3) Intrathecal morphine 0.1–0.25 mg by surgeon intraop, dependent on age of patient Thoracic/lumbar epidural opiates	Pain is a significant problem for postop scoliosis patients. Most need analgesia × 3–4 d. Preop consultation with patient (and parents) about different pain management techniques is important. See p. C-2.
Tests	CXR; ABG; Hct	✓ for pneumothorax and line placement.

Suggested Readings

1. Carragee EJ, Iezza A: Does acute placement of instrumentation in the treatment of vertebral osteomyelitis predispose to recurrent infection: long-term follow up in immune suppressed patients. *Spine* 2008; [in press].
2. Chapman MW: *Operative Orthopaedics,* 3rd edition. Lippincott Williams & Wilkins, Philadelphia: 1993, 4017–73.
3. Colovic V, Walker RW, Patel D, et al: Reduction of blood loss using aprotonin during spinal surgery in children for non-idiopathic scoliosis. *Paediatr Anaesth* 2002; 12(9):835.
4. Dwyer AF, Schafer MF: Anterior approach to scoliosis. Results of treatment in fifty-one cases. *J Bone Joint Surg* [Br] 1974; 56(2):218–24.
5. Fabregas N, Craen RA: Anaesthesia for minimally invasive neurosurgery. *Best Pract Res Clin Anaesthesiol* 2002; 16(1): 81–93.
6. Floman Y, Penny JN, Micheli LJ, et al: Combined anterior and posterior fusion in seventy-three spinally deformed patients: indications, results and complications. *Clin Orthop* 1982; 164:110–22.
7. Fritzell P, Flagg O, Wessberg P, et al: Chronic low back pain and fusion: a comparison of three surgical techniques: a prospective multicenter randomized study from the Swedish Lumbar Spine Study Group. *Spine* 2002; 27(11):1131–41.
8. Goldstein LA, Waugh TR: Classification and terminology of scoliosis. *Clin Orthop* 1973; 93:10–22.
9. Goodarzi M, Shier N, Ogden J: Epidural versus patient-controlled analgesia with morphine for postoperative pain after orthopedic procedures in children. *J Pediatr Orthop* 1993; 13:663–67.
10. Hagberg CA, Welch WC, Bowman-Howard ML: Anesthesia and surgery for spine and spinal cord procedures. In *Textbook of Neuroanesthesia with Neurosurgical and Neuroscience Perspectives.* Albin MS, ed. McGraw-Hill, New York: 1997, 1039–82.
11. Hoppenfeld S, deBoer P: *Surgical Exposures in Orthopaedics: the anatomic approach,* 2nd edition. Lippincott Williams & Wilkins, Philadelphia: 1994, 215–302.
12. Horlocker TT, Wedel DJ: Anesthesia for orthopaedic surgery. In *Clinical Anesthesia,* 4th edition. Barash PG, Cullen BF, Stoelting RK, eds. Lippincott Williams & Wilkins, Philadelphia: 2001, 1103–18.
13. Kafer ER: Respiratory and cardiovascular functions in scoliosis and the principles of anesthetic management. *Anesthesiology* 1980; 52(4):339–51.
14. Kostuik JP, Carl A, Ferron S: Anterior Zielke instrumentation for spinal deformity in adults. *J Bone Joint Surg* [Am] 1989; 71(6):898–906.
15. Larson CP: A rational approach to the prevention of blindness during posterior spine surgery. *Curr Rev Clin Anesth* 2008; [in press].
16. McMaster MJ: Anterior and posterior instrumentation and fusion of thoracolumbar scoliosis due to myelomeningocele. *J Bone Joint Surg* 1987; 69(1):20–5.
17. Morrissy RT: *Atlas of Pediatric Orthopaedic Surgery.* JB Lippincott, Philadelphia: 1992, 75–97.
18. O'Brien T, Akmakjian J, Ogin G, et al: Comparison of one-stage versus two-stage anterior/posterior spinal fusion for neuromuscular scoliosis. *J Pediatr Orthop* 1992; 12(5):610–15.
19. Perez-Cruet MJ, Fessler RG, Perin NI: Review: complications of minimally invasive spinal surgery. *Neurosurgery* 2002; 51(5 Suppl):26–36.
20. Phillips WA, Hensinger RN: Control of blood loss during scoliosis surgery. *Clin Orthop* 1988; 229:88–93.
21. Sinatra RS, Torres J, Bustos AM: Pain management after major orthopaedic surgery: current strategies and new concept. *J Am Acad Orthop Surg* 2002; 10(2):117–29.

22. Sloan TB, Heyer EJ: Anesthesia for intraoperative neurophysiologic monitoring of the spinal cord. *J Clin Neurophysiol* 2002; 19(5):430–43.
23. Slosar PJ: Indications and outcomes of reconstructive surgery in chronic pain of spinal origin. *Spine* 2002; 27(22):2555–63.
24. Smyth RJ, Chapman KR, Wright TA, et al: Pulmonary function in adolescents with mild idiopathic scoliosis. *Thorax* 1984; 39(12):901–4.
25. Smyth RJ, Chapman KR, Wright TA, et al: Ventilatory patterns during hypoxia, hypercapnia, and exercise in adolescents with mild scoliosis. *Pediatrics* 1986; 77(5):692–97.
26. Soriano SG, McCann ME, Laussen PC: Neuroanesthesia. Innovative techniques and monitoring. *Anesthesiol Clin North Am* 2002; 20(1):137–51.
27. Sudhir KG, Smith RM, Hall J, et al: Intraoperative awakening for early recognition of possible neurologic sequelae during Harrington-rod spinal fusion. *Anesth Analg* 1976; 55(4):526–8.
28. Tay BK, Deckey J, Hu SS: Spinal infections. *J Am Acad Orthop Surg* 2002; 10(3):188–97.

CHAPTER

10.4 Hip, Pelvis, Upper Leg Surgery

SURGEONS

James I. Huddleston, MD

Michael J. Bellino, MD

Stuart B. Goodman, MD, PhD, FRCSC, FACS

ANESTHESIOLOGISTS

Frederick G. Mihm, MD

Christoph Egger Halbeis, MD, MBA

OPEN REDUCTION AND INTERNAL FIXATION (ORIF) OF PELVIS OR ACETABULUM

SURGICAL CONSIDERATIONS

Description: Pelvic fractures present several challenging treatment problems. Surgical management is complex and often difficult in nature. Specialized training and equipment are required for a successful outcome. Major trauma mechanisms produce pelvic-ring injuries, and patients with pelvic-ring disruptions frequently have associated systemic injuries, which may be life-threatening (e.g., hemorrhagic shock). Pelvic stabilization and surgical control of hemorrhage may be performed acutely in the polytrauma patient who is hemodynamically unstable. This is in conjunction with an exploratory laparotomy performed by a trauma surgeon. The majority of patients with pelvic fractures who are treated operatively are taken to the OR on a delayed basis, after they have been stabilized. Pelvic fractures that do not heal are "nonunions," whereas those that heal in an unsatisfactory position are "malunions."

Anterior approaches to the pelvis include Pfannenstiel's and ilioinguinal incisions, which are utilized for reduction and fixation of dislocations and fracture/dislocations of the symphysis pubis, fractures of the pubic rami, and access to the anterior aspect of the sacroiliac (SI) joint. **Posterior approaches** to the pelvis involve either vertical or curved incisions along the iliac crest and are used for reduction and fixation of SI joint dislocations, fracture/dislocations of the SI joint, and fractures of the iliac wing and of the sacrum. These procedures are often lengthy and are staged, requiring changes in patient position. Reductions are facilitated by neuromuscular paralysis. The posterior approach requires a large operative field, which may prevent the use of an epidural catheter. In addition, postop anticoagulation for DVT prophylaxis is used uniformly, and may contraindicate the use of epidural catheters. The goal of pelvic reconstruction is to restore the anatomy and stability of the pelvis, which will decrease hemorrhage in the hemodynamically unstable patient, aid in mobilization of the multiply injured patient; and improve long-term function.

Usual preop diagnosis: Fractures of pelvis/acetabulum; nonunion/malunion of the pelvis/acetabulum

SUMMARY OF PROCEDURE	
Position	Supine (anterior); prone (posterior)
Incision	Pfannenstiel's, ilioinguinal (anterior); posterior, curving along iliac crest (posterior)
Special instrumentation	Radiolucent table; pelvic instruments and implants; Cell Saver; I.I.
Antibiotics	Cefazolin 1 g iv q 6–8 h × 24 h (vancomycin or clindamycin for 24 h if penicillin allergic)
Surgical time	1–6 h (anterior); 3–6 h (posterior)
Closing considerations	May require neuromuscular relaxation to aid reduction and closure; postop radiograph
EBL	≥ 1,000 mL
Postop care	Multiple-trauma patient → ICU; others → PACU
Mortality	10%+, dependent on extent of multiple trauma
Morbidity	Ileus: Common Neurologic injury: Common Genitourinary injuries: Not uncommon Failure of fixation: Rare Infection: Rare Malunion: Rare Nonunion: Rare
Pain score	9

PATIENT POPULATION CHARACTERISTICS	
Age range	Any age, but predominance of males < 30 yr
Male:Female	5:1
Incidence	1–2%
Etiology	Motorcycle and motor vehicle accidents (60–80%); falls (10–15%); crush injuries (5%); other (5%)
Associated conditions	Frequently associated with trauma to other organ systems, including head and neck, chest, abdomen, and extremities. These often will be addressed concurrently with pelvic or acetabular fracture.

ANESTHETIC CONSIDERATIONS

See Anesthetic Considerations for Procedures about the Pelvis and Hip (p. 989).

Suggested Readings

1. Burgess AR, Jones AL: Fractures of the pelvic ring. In *Fractures in Adults,* 4th edition. Rockwood CA Jr, Green DP, Bucholz RW, et al., eds. Lippincott-Raven, Philadelphia: 1996, 1575–1616.
2. Fishmann AJ, Greeno RA, Brooks LR, et al: Prevention of deep vein thrombosis and pulmonary embolism in acetabular and pelvic fracture surgery. *Clin Orthop* 1994; 305:133–7.
3. Guyton JL: Fractures of hip, acetabulum, and pelvis. In *Campbell's Operative Orthopaedics,* 10th edition. Canale ST, ed. Mosby-Year Book, St. Louis: 2003.
4. Jones A, Reinert C, Bucholz R: Complications of fractures of the pelvic ring and acetabulum. In *Complications in Orthopaedic Surgery,* 3rd edition. Epps CH Jr, ed. JB Lippincott, Philadelphia: 1994, 749–62.
5. Kane WJ: Complications of pelvic fractures and their treatment. In *Complications in Orthopaedic Surgery.* Epps CH Jr, ed. JB Lippincott, Philadelphia: 1986, 795–814.
6. LaVelle DG: Delayed union and nonunion of fractures. In *Campbell's Operative Orthopaedics,* 10th edition. Canale ST, ed. CV Mosby, St. Louis: 2003, 3125–67.
7. Leighton RK: Nonunions and malunions of the pelvis. In *Chapman's Orthopaedic Surgery,* Vol I, 3rd edition. Chapman MW, ed. Lippincott Williams & Wilkins, Philadelphia: 2001, 921–34.
8. Mears DC, Durbhakula SM: Fractures and dislocations of the pelvic ring. In *Chapman's Orthopaedic Surgery,* Vol I, 3rd edition. Chapman MW, ed. Lippincott Williams & Wilkins, Philadelphia: 2001, 531–86.
9. Mears DC, Rubash HE: *Pelvic and Acetabular Injuries.* Slack Inc., Thorofare NJ: 1986.
10. Prevezas N: Evolution of pelvic and acetabular surgery from ancient to modern times. *Injury* 2007; 38(4):397–409.
11. Rice PL Jr, Rudolph M:.Pelvic fractures. *Emerg Med Clin North Am* 2007; 25(3):795–802.
12. Tile M: Fractures of the acetabulum. In *Fractures in Adults,* 4th edition. Rockwood CA Jr, Green DP, Bucholz RW, et al., eds. Lippincott-Raven, Philadelphia 1996, 1617–58.
13. Tile M: *Fractures of the Pelvis and Acetabulum,* 2nd edition. Williams & Wilkins, Baltimore: 1995, 549–54.

CLOSED REDUCTION AND EXTERNAL FIXATION OF THE PELVIS

SURGICAL CONSIDERATIONS

Description: This procedure entails manipulating the pelvis to obtain an acceptable reduction by closed means under GA, and then applying an anterior external fixation device to maintain the reduction. The pins for the external fixator are inserted into the iliac crest either percutaneously or through small incisions. During this procedure, either radiographs or the I.I. is used to confirm that an acceptable reduction has been obtained. In some centers, this procedure is done in the emergency department as a life-saving procedure.

Usual preop diagnosis: Displaced fracture of the pelvis; unstable fracture of the pelvis

SUMMARY OF PROCEDURE	
Position	Supine
Incision	Percutaneously or through small incisions along the iliac crest.
Special instrumentation	External fixation; often performed on a radiolucent table using I.I.
Antibiotics	Cefazolin 1 g iv q 6–8 h × 24 h (vancomycin or clindamycin for 24 h if penicillin allergic); Combination antibiotics, if multiple severe, open fractures or other significant injuries are present.
Surgical time	1–1.5 h
EBL	Negligible from surgical procedure; however, anticipate large blood losses (4+ U) from the pelvic fracture alone.
Postop care	Multiple-trauma victim → ICU; others → PACU
Mortality	10% or more, depending on extent of multiple trauma; 50% in open fractures
Morbidity	Ileus: Virtually 100%; Sacroiliac (SI) pain: 15–30%+ Genitourinary problems, including bladder or urethral rupture: 13% Neurological deficit to lumbosacral plexus: 1–10% Malunion/severe deformity: 5% Leg-length discrepancy: 3–5% Impotence: 1–5% Residual instability: 1–3% Vascular complications: 1% Hypotension 2° to retroperitoneal hematoma: Common Respiratory distress: Common Gynecological and colorectal injuries: More common with open fractures/dislocations Delayed union, nonunion: Not uncommon Osteomyelitis: Rare Rupture of diaphragm: Rare
Pain score	7–10

Orthopedic Surgery

PATIENT POPULATION CHARACTERISTICS	
Age range	Any age, but predominance of males < 30 yr
Male:Female	5:1
Incidence	Common
Etiology	Motorcycle and motor vehicle accidents (60–80%); falls (10–15%); crush injuries (5%); other (5%)
Associated conditions	Frequently associated with trauma to other organ systems, including head and neck, chest, abdomen, and extremities. Patient sustaining a pelvic fracture also has a probability of having other injuries, including: musculoskeletal (85%); respiratory (60%); CNS (40%); GI (30%); urologic (12%); CVS (6%). These often will be addressed concurrently with the pelvic fracture.

ANESTHETIC CONSIDERATIONS

See Anesthetic Considerations for Procedures about the Pelvis and Hip (p. 989).

Suggested Readings

1. Bucholz RW, Brumback RJ: Fractures of the shaft of the femur. In *Fractures in Adults,* 4th edition. Rockwood CA Jr, Green DP, Bucholz RW, et al., eds. JB Lippincott, Philadelphia: 1996, 1827–1918.
2. Guyton JL: Fractures of hip, acetabulum, and pelvis. In *Campbell's Operative Orthopaedics,* Vol 3, 9th edition. Crenshaw AH, ed. Mosby-Year Book, St. Louis: 1998, 2042–80.

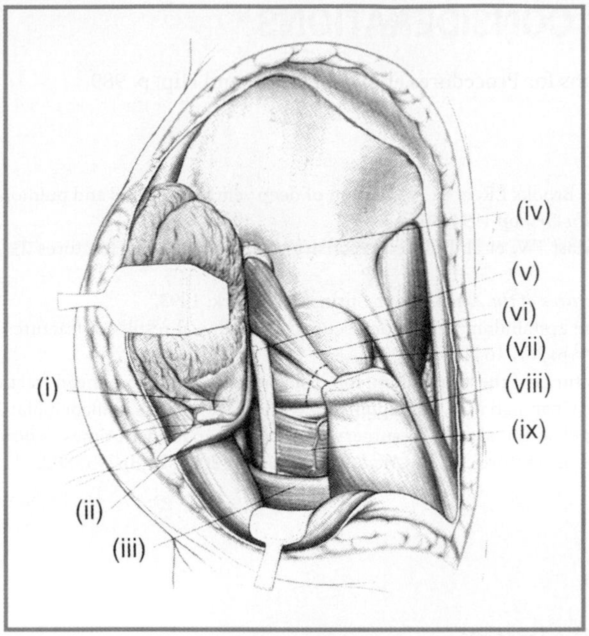

Figure 10.4-2. Extended iliofemoral approach: (i) Gluteus minimus tendon; (ii) gluteus medius tendon; (iii) gluteus maximus tendon; (iv) superior gluteal neurovascular bundle; (v) sciatic nerve; (vi) piriformis and conjoint tendons; (vii) hip joint capsule; (viii) greater trochanter; (ix) medial femoral circumflex artery overlying quadratus femoris. (Reproduced with permission from Sledge CB, ed: *The Hip*. Lippincott-Raven: 1998.)

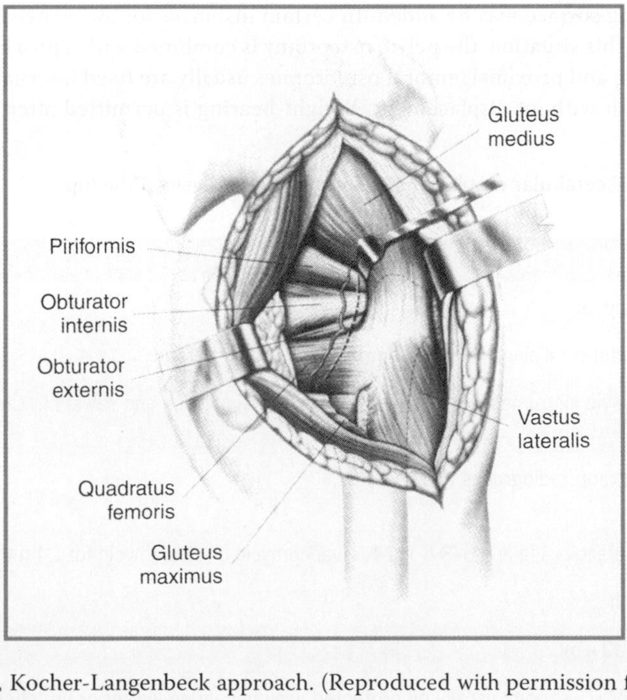

Figure 10.4-3. Kocher-Langenbeck approach. (Reproduced with permission from Sledge CB, ed: *The Hip*. Lippincott-Raven: 1998.)

ANESTHETIC CONSIDERATIONS

See Anesthetic Considerations for Procedures about the Pelvis and Hip, p. 989.

Suggested Readings

1. Fishmann AJ, Greeno RA, Brooks LR, et al: Prevention of deep vein thrombosis and pulmonary embolism in acetabular and pelvic fracture surgery. *Clin Orthop* 1994; 305:133–7.
2. Johnson EE, Matta JM, Mast JW, et al: Delayed reconstruction of acetabular fractures 21–120 days following injury. *Clin Orthop* 1994; 305:20–30.
3. Letournel E, Judet R: *Fractures of the Acetabulum*. Spring, New York: 1993.
4. Matta JM: Fractures of the acetabulum: reduction accuracy and clinical results of fractures operated within three weeks of injury. *J Bone Joint Surg* 1996; 78A:1632–45.
5. Olson SA, Matta JM: Fractures of the acetabulum, hip dislocations, and femoral head fractures. In *Chapman's Orthopaedic Surgery,* Vol I, 3rd edition. Chapman MW, ed. Lippincott Williams & Wilkins, Philadelphia: 2001, 587–616.
6. Prevezas N: Evolution of pelvic and acetabular surgery from ancient to modern times. *Injury* 2007; 38(4):397–409.
7. Rice PL Jr, Rudolph M: Pelvic fractures. *Emerg Med Clin North Am* 2007; 25(3):795–802.

OSTEOTOMY AND BONE GRAFT AUGMENTATION OF THE PELVIS

SURGICAL CONSIDERATIONS

Description: Acetabular insufficiency (acetabular dysplasia) is characterized by deficient anterior and lateral coverage of the acetabulum on the femoral head. This condition of the hip produces joint incongruity and instability, eventually leading to arthrosis and a dysfunctional hip joint. Treatment is aimed at reorienting the dysplastic acetabulum (Fig. 10.4-4). In children, bone grafting alone may be sufficient; in adults, however, pelvic osteotomy, to reorient or broaden the weight-bearing surface, is necessary. A supplemental bone graft to expand the weight-bearing surface may be added. In certain instances following pelvic osteotomy, incongruity of the hip may persist. In this situation, the pelvic osteotomy is combined with a proximal femoral osteotomy to restore congruence. Pelvic and proximal femoral osteotomies usually are fixed internally with screws and plates to allow early mobilization without displacement. Weight-bearing is permitted after healing of the osteotomy at ~8 wk.

Usual preop diagnosis: Acetabular dysplasia; developmental dysplasia of the hip

SUMMARY OF PROCEDURE	
Position	Supine
Incision	Anterior: ilioinguinal or iliofemoral and Smith-Peterson
Special instrumentation	Pelvic instruments and implants; special osteotomes and saws; I.I., Cell Saver
Unique considerations	Intraop radiographs and use of I.I.
Antibiotics	Cefazolin 1 g iv q 6–8 h × 24 h (vancomycin or clindamycin for 24 h if penicillin allergic)
Surgical time	3 h
EBL	500+ mL
Postop care	PACU → room; usually on protected, weight-bearing walker or crutches × 8 wk

SUMMARY OF PROCEDURE (cont'd)	
Mortality	Minimal
Morbidity	Ileus: 100% Leg-length discrepancy: Uniformly present after pelvic osteotomy Injury to lateral cutaneous nerve: Common (50%) Sciatic nerve: Uncommon (1%) Thromboembolism: 5–10% Wound infection: 1–5% Septic arthritis, osteomyelitis: 1–7% Delayed union, nonunion, malunion: 1–2% Genitourinary problems—urinary retention requiring catheterization: Common Hematoma: Common Hypotension 2° to retroperitoneal hematoma: Rare Vascular complications: Rare
Pain score	8

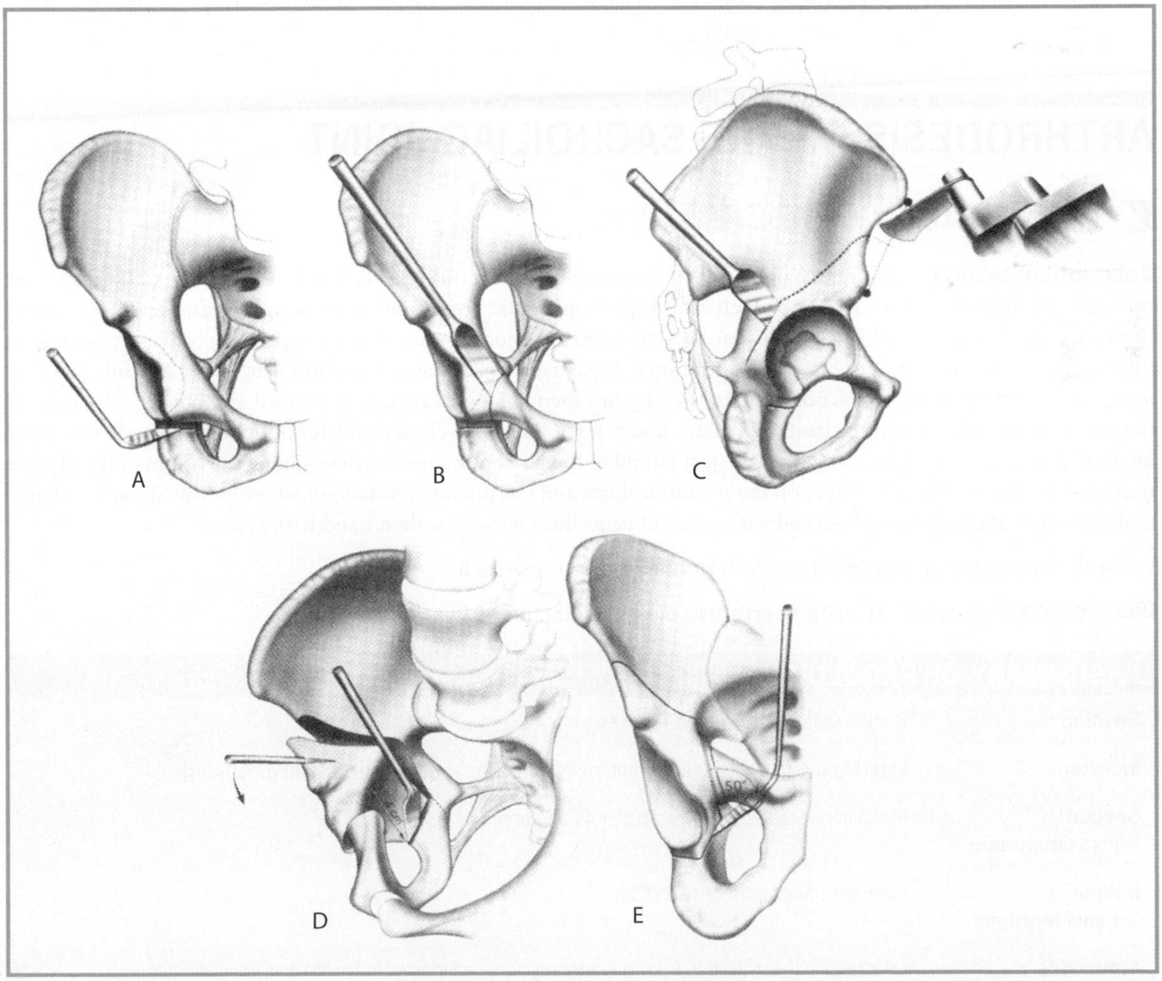

Figure 10.4-4. The Bernese periacetabular osteotomy. (Reproduced with permission from Ganz R, Klaue K, Vinh TS, et al: A new periacetabular osteotomy for the treatment of hip dysplasias: technique and preliminary results. *Clin Orthop* 1988; 232:26–36.)

PATIENT POPULATION CHARACTERISTICS	
Age range	20–50 yr
Male:Female	3–4 × higher incidence in females for congenital hip dysplasia; equal incidence for other causes
Etiology	Congenital hip dysplasia; neuromuscular disorders (cerebral palsy, meningomyelocele); pediatric trauma to acetabular growth plate
Associated conditions	Depends on Dx

ANESTHETIC CONSIDERATIONS

See Anesthetic Considerations for Procedures about the Pelvis and Hip (p. 989).

Suggested Readings

1. Chiari K: Iliac osteotomy in young adults. In *The Hip: Proceedings of the 7th Open Meeting of the Hip Society.* CV Mosby, St. Louis: 1979, 260–77.
2. Ganz R, Klaue, K, Vihn TS, et al: A new periacetabular osteotomy for the treatment of hip dysplasias. *Clin Orthop* 1988;232:26–36.
3. Hersch O, Casillas M, Ganz R: Indications for intertrochanteric osteotomy after periacetabular osteotomy for adult hip dysplasia. *Clin Orthop* 1998; 347:19–26.
4. Salter RB, Thompson GH: The role of innominate osteotomy in young adults. In *The Hip: Proceedings of the 7th Open Meeting of the Hip Society.* CV Mosby, St. Louis: 1979, 278–312.
5. Sutherland DH, Greenfield R: Double innominate osteotomy. *J Bone Joint Surg* 1977; 59(8):1082–91.

ARTHRODESIS OF THE SACROILIAC JOINT

SURGICAL CONSIDERATIONS

Description: In this procedure, a painful and/or unstable sacroiliac (SI) joint is fused, usually by excising the joint through an **anterior** or **posterior approach** and employing an iliac crest bone graft. Supplemental screw fixation of the joint is used. The incision follows the iliac crest from the anterior superior iliac spine past the convexity of the iliac tubercle; the aponeurosis of the external abdominal musculature is elevated from the iliac crest. The internal iliac fossa is exposed subperiosteally, posterior to the SI joint; then the joint cartilage is excised and packed with cancellous bone strips. The SI joint is fixed with plates and screws. Alternatively, a posterior approach to the SI Joint may be used. A straight vertical incision is made just lateral to the posterior superior iliac spine. The origin of the gluteus maximus is elevated from its origin off the posterior ilium and sacrum and reattached laterally. The SI joint is identified, débrided of cartilage, and packed with strips of cancellous bone. It is then fixed with screws.

Variant procedure or approaches: Anterior or posterior approach

Usual preop diagnosis: Arthritis or arthrosis of the SI joint; pelvic instability

SUMMARY OF PROCEDURE	
Position	Supine (anterior) or prone (posterior)
Incision	Lateral portion of ilioinguinal (anterior); posterior approach to SI joint (posterior)
Special instrumentation	Radiolucent table; pelvic instruments and implants; I.I.; Cell Saver
Unique considerations	Intraop radiographs or use of I.I.
Antibiotics	Cefazolin 1 g iv q 6–8 h × 24 h (vancomycin or clindamycin for 24 h if penicillin allergic)
Surgical time	2–3 h
EBL	250–500 mL

SUMMARY OF PROCEDURE (cont'd)	
Postop care	Usually on protected, weight-bearing walker or crutches × 6–8 wk; anticoagulation for DVT prophylaxis
Mortality	Extremely low
Morbidity	Ileus: Virtually always Osteomyelitis: < 1% Wound infection: < 1% Genitourinary problems; urinary retention requiring catheterization: Common Delayed union, nonunion, malunion, leg-length discrepancy: Not uncommon Neurological deficit; injury to lumbosacral plexus: Rare, unless present preop; L5 nerve root susceptible in anterior approaches Hypotension 2° to retroperitoneal hematoma: Rare Injury to bowel: Rare Vascular complications; injury to iliac arteries: Rare Thromboembolism
Pain score	7

PATIENT POPULATION CHARACTERISTICS	
Age range	20–50 yr
Male:Female	Increased incidence in males (trauma)
Incidence	Rare
Etiology	Trauma—postpelvic fracture dislocation; painful septic arthritis

ANESTHETIC CONSIDERATIONS

See Anesthetic Considerations for Procedures about the Pelvis and Hip (p. 989).

Suggested Readings

1. Christian CA, Donley BG: Arthrodesis of the ankle, knee and hip. In *Campbell's Operative Orthopaedics,* Vol 1, 9th edition. Crenshaw AH, ed. Mosby-Year Book, St. Louis: 1998, 145–88.
2. Guyton JL: Fractures of hip, acetabulum, and pelvis. In *Campbell's Operative Orthopaedics,* Vol 3, 9th edition. Crenshaw AH, ed. Mosby-Year Book, St. Louis: 1998, 2042–80.
3. Jones A, Reinert C, Bucholtz R: Complications of fractures of the pelvic ring and acetabulum. In *Complications in Orthopaedic Surgery,* 3rd edition. Epps CH Jr, ed. JB Lippincott, Philadelphia: 1994, 749–62.
4. Kane WJ: Complications of pelvic fractures and their treatment. In *Complications in Orthopaedic Surgery.* Epps CH Jr, ed. JB Lippincott, Philadelphia: 1986, 795–814.
5. LaVelle DG: Fractures of hip and pelvis. In *Campbell's Operative Orthopaedics,* 10th edition. Canale ST, ed. CV Mosby, St. Louis: 1998.
6. Prevezas N: Evolution of pelvic and acetabular surgery from ancient to modern times. *Injury* 2007; 38(4):397–409.
7. Rice PL Jr, Rudolph M: Pelvic fractures. *Emerg Med Clin North Am* 2007; 25(3):795–802.
8. Russell TA: Arthrodesis of the lower extremity and hip. In *Campbell's Operative Orthopaedics,* Vol 2, 9th edition. Crenshaw AH, ed. CV Mosby, St. Louis: 1998.

AMPUTATIONS ABOUT THE HIP AND PELVIS: DISARTICULATION OF THE HIP AND HINDQUARTER AMPUTATION

SURGICAL CONSIDERATIONS

Description: These surgical procedures accomplish an excision of the entire lower extremity. In a **hip disarticulation,** the amputation is performed through the hip joint. An anterior, racquet-shaped incision is made and all muscles crossing the hip joint are incised or detached. The femoral artery, vein, and nerve; obturator vessels; sciatic nerve; and deep vessels are isolated and ligated. The gluteal flap is brought anteriorly and sewn to the anterior portion of the incision. In a **hindquarter amputation,** excision of the lower extremity, hip joint and a portion of the pelvis is performed. Anterior and posterior incisions are used and the iliac wing is divided posteriorly and the symphysis pubis is disarticulated anteriorly. Either the common iliac or external iliac vessels are ligated, as are all nerves to the lower extremity. Usually the gluteal flap is drawn anteriorly for closure. These procedures are performed very rarely—for severe trauma, tumor, or infection—and are often life-saving surgeries. They often are performed in conjunction with a general surgeon, and standard bowel prep is done. The operations are long and tedious, with extensive blood loss, in patients who are usually systemically ill.

Usual preop diagnosis: Malignant tumor of femur, hip or pelvis; traumatic amputation to femur, hip, or pelvis; uncontrollable infection to leg, hip, or pelvis (e.g., clostridia)

SUMMARY OF PROCEDURES

	Hip Disarticulation	Hindquarter Amputation
Position	Supine	Lateral decubitus; stabilized by bean bag and/or kidney rests.
Incision	Anterior racquet type (rare)	Anterior and posterior
Unique considerations	Urinary catheter should be placed.	Urinary catheter; NG tube; scrotum strapped to opposite thigh; anus stitched closed/sealed.
Antibiotics	Cefazolin 1 g iv q 6–8 h × 24 h (vancomycin or clindamycin for 24 h if penicillin allergic)	⇐
Surgical time	3–4 h	4–5 h
EBL	1,000–2,000 mL (intraop blood salvage system recommended, except for tumors)	2,000–3,000 mL
Postop care	ICU	⇐
Mortality	Rare in patients undergoing elective amputation for trauma or localized tumor; higher for patients with debilitated trauma, chronic infection or extensive invasive malignant tumor; highest in clostridial infections: ~50%+	⇐
Morbidity	Anemia: Common Electrolyte abnormalities: Common Hematoma: Common Neurological injury to lumbosacral plexus or peripheral nerves: Common Paralytic ileus: Common Psychosocial problems: Common UTI: Common Flap necrosis: Not uncommon Incomplete excision with recurrence of tumor or infection: Not uncommon Injury to peritoneal or retroperitoneal contents, including bowel and bladder: Not uncommon Vascular injury—iliac, other vessels: Not uncommon	⇐ ⇐ ⇐ ⇐ ⇐ ⇐ ⇐ ⇐ ⇐ ⇐ ⇐
Pain Score	10	10

PATIENT POPULATION CHARACTERISTICS

Age range	Any age
Male:Female	Similar, except higher incidence in males for traumatic etiologies

PATIENT POPULATION CHARACTERISTICS (cont'd)	
Incidence	Uncommon
Etiology	Malignant tumor; trauma; infection—clostridial myonecrosis, chronic osteomyelitis, etc.

ANESTHETIC CONSIDERATIONS FOR PROCEDURES ABOUT THE PELVIS AND HIP

(Procedures covered: ORIF, pelvis, acetabulum; closed reduction, external fixation, pelvis; osteotomy and bone graft of pelvis; arthrodesis of SI joint; amputations about hip and pelvis: disarticulation of hip and hindquarter amputation)

PREOPERATIVE

Patients presenting for pelvic surgery generally fall into two categories: 1) Major trauma—pelvic fracture requires substantial force and seldom occurs alone. These patients require aggressive fluid resuscitation with large-bore iv's and invasive monitors (arterial line and CVP). If the patient can be made hemodynamically stable with volume resuscitation, a thorough evaluation for coexisting neurological, thoracic, or abdominal trauma should be undertaken before anesthesia. 2) Tumor resection and amputation of thigh, hip, and pelvis. Because of large intraop blood loss and 3rd-spacing of fluids, invasive hemodynamic monitoring is necessary. Although epidural anesthesia is seldom adequate for surgery, postop epidural analgesia is an effective means of controlling the tremendous pain caused by this type of surgery. Other patient populations covered in this section include otherwise healthy patients with congenital or acquired hip dysplasia presenting for augmentation procedures.

Respiratory	Trauma patients are at risk for hemothorax, pneumothorax, pulmonary contusion, fat embolism (preop and postop), and aspiration. A chest tube will be needed before surgery if either a hemothorax or pneumothorax is present. Pulmonary fat embolus occurs in 10–15% of patients with long-bone fractures, and can occur after isolated pelvic fractures. Sx include hypoxemia, tachycardia, tachypnea, respiratory alkalosis, mental status changes, conjunctival petechiae, fat bodies in the urine, and diffuse pulmonary infiltrates. Sx of pulmonary aspiration are similar to those of fat embolism. Preop therapy for either should include supplemental O_2 to correct hypoxemia (may necessitate mechanical ventilation) and meticulous fluid management to prevent worsening of pulmonary capillary leak. **Tests:** CXR, or others as indicated from H&P.
Cardiovascular	Blunt chest trauma can produce both cardiac contusion and aortic tear. Preop ECG and CPK isoenzymes will help evaluate the presence of myocardial injury. A wide mediastinal silhouette suggests aortic tear, which requires evaluation with TEE or angiography. **Tests:** Consider ECG; CPK isoenzymes; others as indicated from H&P.
Neurological	The possibility of coexistent neurologic trauma necessitates a thorough preop mental status review and peripheral sensory exam. A CT scan of the head is indicated for any patient with loss of consciousness prior to anesthesia.
Musculoskeletal	For trauma patients, C-spine films will evaluate the stability of the C-spine before neck manipulation during ET intubation. Thoracic and lumbar x-rays also should be evaluated for the presence of traumatic spinal deformity or instability that would require special stabilization in the anesthetized patient. **Tests:** C-spine x-rays or others as indicated from H&P.
Hematologic	Restore Hct to 25% prior to inducing anesthesia. Have available 1 blood volume (70 mL/kg) or 1 total erythrocyte mass (20 mL/kg) for intraop transfusion. Transfusions of more than 1 blood volume will require monitoring and possible replacement of Plts and coag factors. The incidence of DVT is very high in these patients, and prophylaxis with SCDs or low-dose sc heparin is indicated whenever feasible.
Renal	Renal injury commonly results from trauma to the collecting system, myoglobinuria from rhabdomyolysis and ischemic, acute, tubular necrosis from hypovolemia or aortic

Renal (cont'd)	dissection. Foley catheters should be placed only after urologic consultation for possible urethral tear. Suprapubic catheters are often necessary. Monitoring of UO is mandatory to detect intraop compromise of the collecting system, and to monitor adequacy of renal perfusion. **Tests:** Consider UA; BUN; Cr; others as indicated from H&P.	
Laboratory	Hct; electrolytes; other tests as indicated from H&P.	
Premedication	In hemodynamically stable patients, pain can be treated with morphine (1–2 mg iv q 10 min titrated to pain relief) prior to anesthesia.	

INTRAOPERATIVE

Anesthetic technique: GETA is indicated due to the duration and extent of the surgery, as well as the varied positions that are necessary to accomplish pelvic fixation. Regional anesthesia is generally inadequate for major pelvic surgery; however, in elective surgeries, serious consideration should be given to postop epidural analgesia.

Induction	A rapid-sequence induction (see p. B-4) is necessary for trauma patients to minimize aspiration risk. Elective cases can undergo a standard induction (see p. B-2).	
Maintenance	Standard maintenance (see p. B-2).	
Emergence	Extubate trauma patients when fully awake and protective airway reflexes have returned. Do not extubate patients with evolving pulmonary injuries (fat embolism, aspiration, or contusion). Monitoring in an ICU usually is indicated for trauma and cancer patients. Prolonged stays can be anticipated for patients with severe coexistent trauma.	
Blood and fluid requirements	Large blood loss IV: 14–16 ga × 2 NS/LR @ 8–12 mL/kg/h 2–4 U PRBC in OR Warm fluids. Humidify gases.	Expect large blood losses (from 0.5–2 or more blood volumes) with all but augmentation procedures. Cell-scavenging techniques are useful to reduce the requirement for blood. Care should be taken to ensure that cells have been adequately washed to minimize ↓ BP on reinfusion.
Control of blood loss	Deliberate hypotension Hemodilution	Patients with severe cardiovascular disease or carotid artery stenosis are not candidates for ↓ BP. Full replacement of any volume deficit is mandatory before inducing ↓ BP. Commonly used agents are isoflurane (1–3%) or esmolol (50–200 mcg/kg/min) ± SNP (0.25–3 mcg/kg/min). These agents are titrated to produce a 30% ↓ in preop MAP (but not < 60 mmHg).
Monitoring	Standard monitors (see p. B-1). Arterial line CVP line ± PA catheter ± TEE UO	Patients for shelf procedures may require only standard monitoring. Patients with myocardial dysfunction should have fluid and inotropic/pressor therapy, guided by continuous central venous saturation monitoring, a PA catheter and/or TEE.
Positioning	✓ and pad pressure points. ✓ eyes.	Meticulous padding of the chest, pelvis, and extremities is imperative to prevent nerve injury and ischemia of the extremities. ↓ BP → risk of neurovascular injury.

Complications	Hypothermia Damage to urinary collecting system Major blood loss Coagulopathy	Warming of hypothermic patient may unmask severe volume depletion that will increase fluid requirement to well above apparent losses.

POSTOPERATIVE

Complications	Nerve root damage Peripheral nerve damage	Preop or intraop damage to L4-S5 nerve roots and cauda equina, resulting in hemiplegia and bladder and bowel dysfunction. Neuropathy of the femoral, genitofemoral, and lateral femoral cutaneous nerves can result from pressure on the ilioinguinal ligament during surgery.
Pain management	IV morphine Spinal opiates	Morphine 1–2 mg iv q 10 min prn Epidural hydromorphone 50 mcg/mL infused at 100–250 mcg/hr, ± bupivacaine 0.125–0.25% at 4–8 mL/h, provides excellent analgesia.
Tests	Hct CXR Coag profile, as indicated.	

Suggested Readings

1. Fung DL: Anesthesia and pain management. In *Chapman's Orthopaedic Surgery,* 3rd edition, Vol I. Chapman MW, ed. Lippincott Williams & Wilkins, Philadelphia: 2001, 133–56.
2. Masursky D, Dexter F, McCartney CJ, et al: Predicting orthopedic surgeons' preferences for peripheral nerve blocks for their patients. *Anesth Analg* 2008; 106(2):561–7.
3. McCollough NC III: Complications of amputation surgery. In *Complications in Orthopaedic Surgery,* 3rd edition. Epps CH Jr, ed. JB Lippincott, Philadelphia: 1994.
4. Nutescu EA: Assessing, preventing, and treating venous thromboembolism: evidence-based approaches. *Am J Health Syst Pharm* 2007; 64(11 Suppl 7):S5–13.
5. Ranawat AS, Ranawat CS: Pain management and accelerated rehabilitation for total hip and total knee arthroplasty. *J Arthroplasty* 2007; 22(7 Suppl 3):12–5.
6. Rosencher N, Bonnet MP, Sessler DI: Selected new antithrombotic agents and neuraxial anaesthesia for major orthopaedic surgery: management strategies. *Anaesthesia* 2007; 62(11):1154–60.
7. Tooms RE: Amputations of lower extremity. In *Campbell's Operative Orthopaedics,* Vol 1, 9th edition. Crenshaw AH, ed. CV Mosby, St. Louis: 1998, 532–47.

ARTHROPLASTY OF THE HIP

SURGICAL CONSIDERATIONS

Description: **Total hip arthroplasty** is one of the most successful procedures in orthopedic surgery. In this procedure, the hip joint (Fig. 10.4-5) is approached through one of several standard incisions. The femoral head is dislocated from the acetabulum, and the arthritic femoral head and a portion of the neck are excised. The acetabulum is reamed to accept a cemented or cementless cup made of metal and plastic. The femoral stem and head are usually modular, allowing for numerous shapes, sizes, lengths, etc. The metallic femoral component may be cemented or cementless. A hybrid total hip combines a cemented femoral stem and a cementless acetabular cup. After relocation

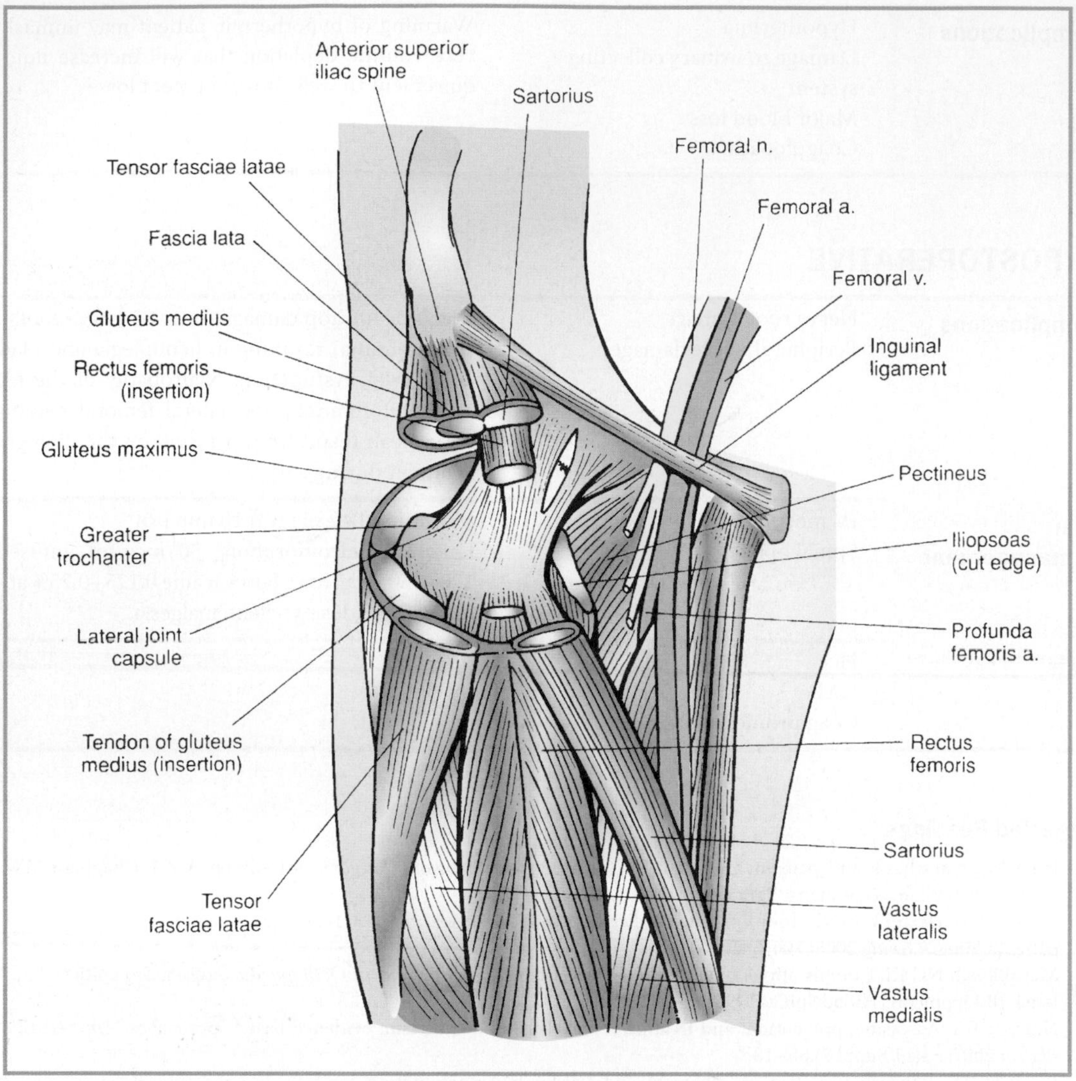

Figure 10.4-5. Surgical exposure of the hip joint. The hip joint may be exposed through a number of approaches. The relevant anatomical landmarks are shown here. (Reproduced with permission from Hoppenfeld S, deBoer P: *Surgical Exposures in Orthopaedics.* JB Lippincott, Philadelphia: 1984.)

of the new prosthetic hip joint and closure of the tissues, the patient may be given an abduction pillow to minimize the risk of dislocation. Mobilization takes place over the ensuing days.

Variant procedure or approaches: **Unipolar** (only the femoral side is replaced); **bipolar** (both the femoral side and the acetabular side are replaced; the acetabular cup is not fixed to the pelvis). **Revision procedures** are more arduous and time-consuming, as the "failed" or loose component(s) must be removed and the bone prepared to accept new cemented or cementless components. These procedures require more specialized equipment for extracting prostheses and cement, and rebuilding the femoral or acetabular bone stock (allografts, autografts, etc.). Often, special components are needed for implantation of a new prosthesis. In the **Girdlestone procedure (resection arthroplasty),** the components are removed, but not replaced. This procedure is usually performed for infection.

Usual preop diagnosis: Fracture of femoral neck; arthritis of hip; arthrosis of hip; loose (or malpositioned) hip prosthesis; chronic dislocation of hip arthroplasty; infected hip arthroplasty

SUMMARY OF PROCEDURES

	Unipolar, Bipolar, Total Hip Replacement	Revision, Total Hip Replacement	Girdlestone Resection Arthroplasty
Position	Supine (for anterior or anterolateral approaches); lateral decubitus position (for lateral or posterior approaches)	⇐	⇐
Incision	Anterolateral, lateral or posterolateral over hip joint	⇐	⇐
Special instrumentation	Appropriate prostheses and instrumentation	Special instruments for excising cement	⇐
Unique considerations	In lateral decubitus position, patient is usually stabilized by bean bag and/or kidney rests. SCDs used.	A trochanteric osteotomy may be performed.	⇐
Antibiotics	Cefazolin 1 g iv q 6–8 h × 24 h (vancomycin or clindamycin for 24 h if penicillin allergic)	⇐	⇐ after intraop cultures
Surgical time	2–3 h	3–6 h or more	3 h or more
EBL	250–750 mL (intraop blood retrieval system may be useful).	≥ 1,000 mL; intraop blood retrieval recommended.	⇐
Postop care	Patient's legs immobilized between abduction wedge; or operated leg suspended in a splint or placed in traction.	⇐	⇐
Mortality	1–2% (increasing with age)	⇐	⇐
Morbidity	DVT:	⇐	⇐
	• Without prophylaxis: ≥ 50%	⇐	⇐
	• With chemoprophylaxis and mechanical prophylaxis: 2–3%	⇐	⇐
	Heterotopic ossification: 3–50% (average, 13%; significant, 4–5%)	> 3–50%	⇐
	Intraop cementless fracture: 5–20%	⇐	⇐
	UTI: 7–14%	⇐	⇐
	Late aseptic loosening requiring revision: 5–10% (after 10 yr)	> 5–10%	⇐
	Wound infection: 1% • Primary psoriatic and diabetic patients: 5–10% • Primary OA: 1%	3–10%	⇐
	Hematoma (major): < 5%	⇐	5–10%
	Femoral/sciatic nerve injury: 0.7–3.5%	⇐	⇐
	PE: 1.8–3.4% (if no prophylaxis)	⇐	⇐
	Intraop cemented fracture: 1–3%	2–3%	1–3%
	Postopsubluxation/dislocation: 0.5–3%	⇐	–
	Vascular injury to iliac vessels: < 0.5%	> 0.5%	⇐
	Urinary retention requiring catheterization: Common	⇐	⇐
	GI bleed, MI, cholecystitis: Rare	⇐	–
			Neurological injury: 3–10%
Pain score	7	8	8

PATIENT POPULATION CHARACTERISTICS	
Age range	Hip fracture and cases of arthrosis of the hip joint: generally > 60 yr Arthritis of the hip (e.g., rheumatoid arthritis or juvenile rheumatoid arthritis, traumatic arthritis): all ages
Male:Female	Dependent on disease etiology
Incidence	Common: approximately 250,000/yr in United States
Etiology	Osteoarthritis; seropositive or seronegative arthritis; avascular necrosis; traumatic arthritis; congenital dislocation of the hip
Associated conditions	Dependent on primary conditions (e.g., rheumatoid arthritis patients may have numerous deformities, cardiorespiratory disease, etc.)

ANESTHETIC CONSIDERATIONS

See Anesthetic Considerations for Hip Procedures (p. 997).

Suggested Readings

1. Berry DJ: Primary total hip arthroplasty. In *Chapman's Orthopaedic Surgery,* 3rd edition, Vol III. Chapman MW, ed. Lippincott Williams & Wilkins, Philadelphia: 2001, 2769–94.
2. Bierbaum BE, Pomeroy DL, Berklacich FM: Late complications of total hip replacement. In *The Hip and its Disorders.* Steinberg ME, ed. WB Saunders, Philadelphia: 1991, 1061–96.
3. Harkey JW: Arthroplasty of hip. In *Campbell's Operative Orthopaedics,* Vol I, 9th edition. Crenshaw AH, ed. Mosby-Year Book, St. Louis: 1998, 473–520.
4. Malik A, Dorr LD: The science of minimally invasive total hip arthroplasty. *Clin Orthop Relat Res* 2007; 463:74–84.
5. Ranawat CS, Figgie MP: Early complications of total hip replacement. In *The Hip and its Disorders.* Steinberg ME, ed. WB Saunders, Philadelphia: 1991, 1042–60.
6. Shaw JA, Greer RB III: Complications of total hip replacement. In *Complications in Orthopaedic Surgery,* 3rd edition. Epps CH Jr, ed. JB Lippincott, Philadelphia: 1994, 1013–1106.

ARTHRODESIS OF THE HIP

SURGICAL CONSIDERATIONS

Description: In adults, this procedure is accomplished by fusing the femur to the acetabulum. Some form of internal fixation is usually employed; a spica cast is sometimes placed immediately postop or a few days later. The patient is usually not a good candidate for total hip arthroplasty (e.g., a young, healthy male with unilateral traumatic arthritis). The hip usually is fused in 30° of flexion, 10–30° of external rotation, and neutral-to-slight adduction. The surgical procedure may be performed through anterior, lateral, or posterior incisions with the lateral being most common. A **trochanteric osteotomy** facilitates exposure. After excising the cartilage surfaces, internal fixation, using screws ± a plate, is performed (Fig. 10.4-6).

Usual preop diagnosis: Arthritis or arthrosis of the hip; previous septic arthritis of the hip; recurrent subluxation or dislocation of the hip

SUMMARY OF PROCEDURE	
Position	Usually supine; occasionally lateral decubitus
Incision	Anterior or lateral thigh
Special instrumentation	Plates and screws or other internal fixation; reamers from surface replacement arthroplasty set also may be useful; intraop x-ray; fracture table

SUMMARY OF PROCEDURE (cont'd)

Unique considerations	Intraop radiographs or I.I. used with patient on fracture table
Antibiotics	Cefazolin 1 g iv q 6–8 h × 24 h (vancomycin or clindamycin for 24 h if penicillin allergic)
Surgical time	3–4 h
EBL	500–1,000 mL; Cell Saver recommended.
Postop care	Spica cast
Mortality	Extremely low
Morbidity	Limb shortening: Some shortening is always present Delayed union, nonunion, malunion: 10–15% Femoral shaft fracture: 5–10% Wound infection: < 1% Genitourinary problems: urinary retention requiring catheterization: Common Ileus: Common Late degenerative arthritis of other lower extremity joints or back: Common, many yr later Injury to iliac or femoral vessels: Rare Neurological deficit; injury to lateral cutaneous nerve, sciatic, or femoral nerves: Not uncommon Osteomyelitis: Rare Vascular complications: Rare Superior mesenteric artery syndrome causing duodenal obstruction: Extremely rare Thromboembolism: See Arthroplasty of the Hip, p. 993.
Pain score	9

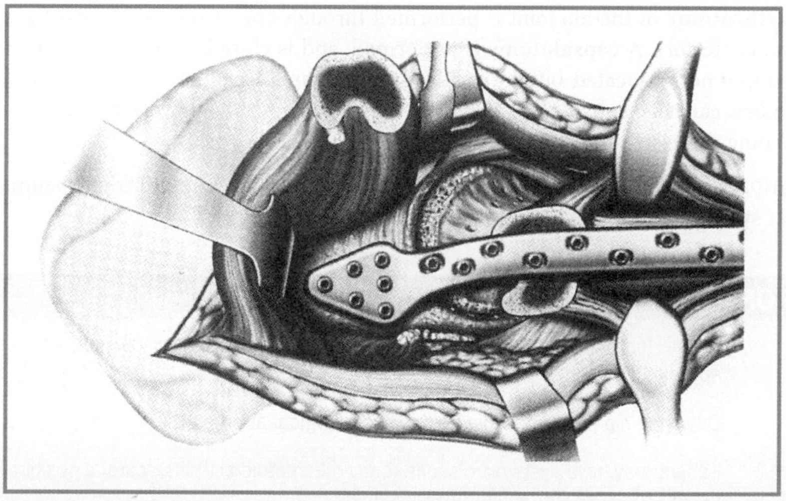

Figure 10.4-6. Application of cobra plate after it has molded to the shape of the acetabulum and femur, and initial fixation with one proximal + distal outrigger compression screws. (Reproduced with permission from Sledge CB, ed: *The Hip.* Lippincott-Raven: 1998.)

PATIENT POPULATION CHARACTERISTICS

Age range	18–50 yr
Male:Female	Usually males > females
Incidence	Rare

PATIENT POPULATION CHARACTERISTICS (cont'd)	
Etiology	Trauma, general; neuromuscular disorders (cerebral palsy, meningomyelocele); trauma to acetabular growth plate; congenital hip dysplasia
Associated conditions	Depends on etiology.

ANESTHETIC CONSIDERATIONS

See Anesthetic Considerations for Hip Procedures (p. 997).

Suggested Readings

1. Carnesale PG, Stewart MJ: Complications of arthrodesis surgery. In *Complications in Orthopaedic Surgery.* Epps CH Jr, ed. JB Lippincott, Philadelphia: 1986, 1289–1306.
2. Gill PS, Paprosky WG: Failed hip arthroplasty: revision and arthrodesis. In *Chapman's Orthopaedic Surgery,* 3rd edition, Vol III. Chapman MW, ed. Lippincott Williams & Wilkins, Philadelphia: 2001, 2795–2858.
3. Matta JM, Siebenrock KA, Gautier E, et al: Hip fusion through an anterior approach with the use of a ventral plate. *Clin Orthop* 1997; 337:129–39.
4. Russell TA: Arthrodesis of the lower extremity and hip. In *Campbell's Operative Orthopaedics,* Vol 2. Crenshaw AH, ed. CV Mosby, St. Louis: 1987, 1091–1130.

SYNOVECTOMY OF THE HIP

SURGICAL CONSIDERATIONS

Description: An **arthrotomy** of the hip joint is performed through one of several standard approaches (anterior, anterolateral, lateral, posterior). A **capsulotomy** is performed, and is closed with reabsorbable sutures later in the case. Generally, the hip is not dislocated, but the cartilage surfaces are inspected and documented. The synovium, as well as any loose bodies, cartilage flaps, and osteophytes, are excised. Although weight-bearing is usually protected, ROM and strengthening exercises are begun early.

Usual preop diagnosis: Chronic synovitis of hip; loose bodies in hip; juvenile and adult rheumatoid arthritis; pigmented villonodular synovitis; synovial chondromatosis

SUMMARY OF PROCEDURE	
Position	Supine for anterior or anterolateral surgical approaches; lateral decubitus for posterior approaches
Incision	Overlying hip joint, depending on specific surgical approach
Unique considerations	Patient may have systemic disease (e.g., rheumatoid arthritis); careful positioning of limbs is necessary to avoid fracture or skin slough.
Antibiotics	Cefazolin 1 g iv q 6–8 h × 24 h (vancomycin or clindamycin for 24 h if penicillin allergic)
Surgical time	2 h
EBL	< 500 mL
Mortality	Rare
Morbidity	Thromboembolism: 10–50% Neurovascular injury—femoral or sciatic nerve, or iliac vessels: < 3% Wound infection or dehiscence: < 3% Septic arthritis and osteomyelitis: < 1% (unless synovectomy is performed for infection). Avascular necrosis of femoral head: Rare (if hip is not dislocated).

SUMMARY OF PROCEDURE (cont'd)	
Morbidity (cont.)	Hematoma: Rare (if drainage tubes used). Inability to void, requiring urinary catheterization: Common
Pain score	7–8

PATIENT POPULATION CHARACTERISTICS	
Age range	< 60 yr
Male:Female	Dependent on disease etiology (e.g., preponderance of females in rheumatoid arthritis)
Incidence	Rare
Etiology	Septic arthritis (very common); rheumatoid arthritis, juvenile/adult (rare); pigmented villonodular synovitis (rare); trauma (rare)
Associated conditions	See Etiology, above.

ANESTHETIC CONSIDERATIONS FOR HIP PROCEDURES

(Procedures covered: hip arthroplasty, arthrodesis, synovectomy)

PREOPERATIVE

Osteoarthritis is the most common indication for hip arthroplasty. These patients are usually elderly and their anesthetic management is tailored to any concurrent disease. Rheumatoid and other inflammatory arthritides form another group of candidates for these procedures and the special anesthetic considerations for these patients are outlined below. Avascular necrosis of the hip is seen in patients with sickle-cell disease and in heart transplant patients.

Respiratory	Patients with rheumatoid arthritis frequently have associated pulmonary complications. SOB on performing activities of daily living or exercise (e.g., climbing a flight of stairs) warrants further evaluation with PFTs. Pulmonary effusions are common. Pulmonary fibrosis (rare) often manifests as cough and dyspnea. Rheumatoid arthritis involvement of the cricoarytenoid joints may produce glottic narrowing (requiring small ETT) and manifest as hoarseness. Arthritic involvement of the TMJ limits mouth opening and may necessitate special techniques (e.g., fiber optic or light wand) for ET intubation. **Tests:** As indicated from H&P.
Cardiovascular	The severity of the arthritis often limits exercise; thus, a dobutamine stress ECHO and/or dipyridamole/thallium imaging may be necessary for adequate cardiac evaluation in patients with poor exercise tolerance. HTN and cardiovascular disease are common in elderly patients (dysrhythmias/TIAs → fall → hip fracture). Rheumatoid arthritis is associated with pericardial effusion, cardiac valve fibrosis, cardiac conduction abnormalities and aortic regurgitation (AR). An ECG is indicated in all rheumatoid arthritis patients, and ECHO is indicated for patients with physical Sx suggestive of tamponade or cardiovascular disease. **Tests:** As indicated from H&P.
Neurological	In patients with rheumatoid arthritis, a thorough neurological exam preop often yields evidence of cervical nerve-root compression. Patients with arthritis involving the cervical spine should have lateral neck films preop to determine the stability of the atlanto-occipital joint. After the stability of the spine has been established, full ROM of the neck should be evaluated for evidence of further nerve-root compression or cerebral ischemia (suggesting vertebral artery compression). Evidence of cerebral ischemia mandates a neurovascular evaluation to plan intraop BP management. **Tests:** As indicated from H&P.

Musculoskeletal	Pain and ↓ joint mobility make positioning and regional anesthesia difficult in patients with arthritis.
Hematologic	Rheumatoid arthritis patients often have anemia. Also, anemia may be 2° NSAID gastritis. Patients with Hb > 12 g/dL are candidates for preop autologous blood donation. Hip fracture → potential large-volume blood loss at fracture site. DVT is common after hip surgery, and prophylaxis for its occurrence reduces mortality. Effective preventive measures include SCDs and sc heparin. NSAID-induced coagulopathy may preclude the use of regional anesthesia. **Tests:** As indicated from H&P.
Renal	Estimation of renal function may be useful to predict drug clearance and the need for invasive monitoring in this elderly population. **Tests:** As indicated from H&P.
Laboratory	Other tests as indicated from H&P.
Premedication	In the absence of limited pulmonary reserve or severe cardiac disease, a standard premedication (see p. B-2) is appropriate. Full-stomach precautions (p. B-5) may be necessary for patients in acute pain.

INTRAOPERATIVE

Anesthetic technique: GETA or regional anesthesia (may be difficult 2° pain on positioning).

General anesthesia:

Induction	The lateral position may mandate ET intubation for patients undergoing GA. A careful preop airway evaluation will determine the need for special airway techniques (e.g., fiber optic intubation or light wand). Aggravation of cricoarytenoid arthritis that is common in rheumatoid arthritis patients can be minimized if a small ETT (6–7 mm cuffed) is used. For otherwise healthy patients, standard induction (p. B-2) is appropriate.
Maintenance	Standard maintenance (p. B-2). Neuromuscular blockade facilitates the placement and testing of the prosthesis. In otherwise healthy patients, induced hypotension (e.g., ↓ 20%) →↓ blood loss.
Emergence	No special considerations

Regional anesthesia: Regional anesthesia offers the advantages of decreased periop DVT and pulmonary embolus, decreased intraop blood loss and a drier surgical field (which may improve conditions for cementing). However, induction of regional anesthesia, with its attendant positioning requirements, can be uncomfortable in patients with limited joint mobility. Rheumatoid arthritis patients, however, rarely have involvement of the lumbar spine, and regional anesthesia offers the advantages of decreased periop DVT, decreased intraop blood loss and no need for airway manipulation. Sedation or general anesthesia should be offered to supplement the regional technique. A typical dose for a subarachnoid block is 12.5–15 mg bupivacaine. 10–25 mcg of fentanyl and 100–200 mcg of morphine may be added for improved pain control up to 24 h postoperatively. Anesthesia to T10 is adequate. Full motor blockade is essential for placement of the prosthesis and assessment of the passive ROM. Lumbar epidural block (initial dose of 10–15 mL 2% lidocaine with epinephrine 1:200,000, administered over 10 min) has the advantage of slow onset, allowing time to treat the induced cardiovascular changes. Postop epidural opiates can provide excellent analgesia. Finally, a lumbar plexus block by the posterior approach (psoas compartment block) provides reliable postoperative analgesia, and hypotension and urinary retention are less common than with SAB or epidural analgesia. However, it is not sufficient for surgical anesthesia as the sole anesthetic. Continuous infusion is always initiated after the initial bolus of 15–20 mL of 0.125% bupivacaine or 0.2% ropivacaine.

Blood and fluid requirements	Major blood loss IV: 14–16 ga × 2 NS/LR @ 4–8 mL/kg/h	Cell scavenging helps reduce total transfusion requirement. Care should be taken to ensure that cells have been adequately washed to minimize ↓ BP on reinfusion.

Control of blood loss	Regional anesthesia Controlled hypotension	These techniques may be appropriate in selected patient populations.
Monitoring	Standard monitors (see p. B-1). ± CVP line ± Arterial line	Invasive monitoring is indicated in the presence of exercise-limiting cardiac or pulmonary disease.
Positioning	Axillary roll, bean bag ✓ and pad pressure points. ✓ eyes.	Meticulous padding of extremities and maintaining a neutral neck position are mandatory. A bean bag and axillary roll also are necessary to stabilize patient in the lateral position and to protect dependent arm from neurovascular compression injuries.
Complications	Methylmethacrylate: • ↓ BP 2° vasodilation • ↓ PaO_2 2° embolization • Cardiovascular collapse VAE Major blood loss DVT (femoral vein: 80%) Nerve damage Femur fracture	Microemboli of air, fat, bone fragments, and cement may occur during pressurized cementing which may lead to hypotension and hypoxia. Hypotension may be used to achieve a dry operating field, which improves cement penetration into the bone. However, significant hypovolemia must be avoided because this predisposes to a severe reaction to pressurized cementing. Systemic ↓ BP and pulmonary HTN may occur. Care should be taken to ensure that patient is adequately hydrated before and during the procedure, and pressors may be necessary to maintain BP (ephedrine 5–20 mg iv or epinephrine 10– 100 mcg iv and increasing the dose as necessary).

POSTOPERATIVE

Complications	Nerve damage DVT Continued blood loss	Sciatic nerve injury is evidenced by foot drop and an inability to flex the knee.
Pain management	Neuraxial regimens: • SAB	Intrathecal morphine 0.2–0.3 mg provides analgesia for up to 24 h after administration. May be administered along with bupivacaine for surgical anesthesia.
	• Epidural analgesia	Epidural bupivacaine 0.0125% 6–8 mL/h and hydromorphone 50 mcg/mL infused at 100–250 mcg/h provides good analgesia. Prior to removal of the epidural catheter a 0.2 mg bolus of hydromorphone may be given. Epidural catheters are typically removed on the morning of postoperative day 2. Low-molecular-weight heparin may be started 2 h after catheter removal.
	Continuous lumbar plexus (psoas compartment) block	Infusion with 0.2% ropivacaine or 0.125% bupivacaine maintained at 6–12 mL/h.
	Systemic regimens	Oral pain management with acetaminophen should be initiated immediately postoperatively (if not contraindicated). Patient-controlled analgesia (PCA) with IV morphine or hydromorphone may be initiated as alternative to neuraxial blocks or to supplement a continuous lumbar plexus (psoas compartment) block.

Tests	Hct CXR, if CVP was placed. Monitor UO

Suggested Readings

1. Dutkowsky JP: Miscellaneous nontraumatic disorders. In *Campbell's Operative Orthopaedics,* Vol 1, 9th edition. Crenshaw AH, ed. Mosby-Year Book, St. Louis: 1998, 787–856.
2. Fung DL: Anesthesia and pain management. In *Chapman's Orthopaedic Surgery,* 3rd edition, Vol I. Chapman MW, ed. Lippincott Williams & Wilkins, Philadelphia: 2001, 133–56.
3. Masursky D, Dexter F, McCartney CJ, et al: Predicting orthopedic surgeons' preferences for peripheral nerve blocks for their patients. *Anesth Analg* 2008; 106(2):561–7.
4. Ranawat AS, Ranawat CS: Pain management and accelerated rehabilitation for total hip and total knee arthroplasty. *J Arthroplasty* 2007; 22(7 Suppl 3):12–5.
5. Rosencher N, Bonnet MP, Sessler DI: Selected new antithrombotic agents and neuraxial anaesthesia for major orthopaedic surgery: management strategies. *Anaesthesia* 2007; 62(11):1154–60.

OPEN REDUCTION AND INTERNAL FIXATION (ORIF) OF PROXIMAL FEMORAL FRACTURES (FEMORAL NECK, INTERTROCHANTERIC, SUBTROCHANTERIC FRACTURES)

SURGICAL CONSIDERATIONS

Description: Fractures of the proximal femur are seen in two distinct populations: most commonly in elderly patients as the result of falls, and in younger patients following trauma. In elderly patients, the fracture occurs through osteoporotic bone in the femoral neck, intertrochanteric or subtrochanteric area (Fig. 10.4-9). Displaced femoral neck fractures are usually treated by **prosthetic replacement.** Nondisplaced or minimally displaced femoral neck fractures are usually treated by **closed reduction and percutaneous pinning** of the fracture. Intertrochanteric and subtrochanteric fractures, whether displaced or nondisplaced, are usually treated by **ORIF with a sliding hip screw and side plate, cephalomedullary nail, or blade plate** (Fig. 10.4-10). Prosthetic replacement is performed only rarely. Elderly patients frequently have numerous medical problems, which means that the fractures require prompt internal fixation/prosthetic replacement to facilitate early mobilization. In younger patients (16–40 yr), proximal femoral fractures are almost always treated by ORIF with screws, plates and screws, or intramedullary devices. These are normally much higher energy fractures, often associated with multiple traumas.

Variant procedure or approaches: Variants include: **percutaneous pinning** of nondisplaced femoral neck fracture; **ORIF of displaced femoral neck fracture** (also see Arthroplasty of the Hip, p. 991); **ORIF of intertrochanteric or subtrochanteric fracture.**

Usual preop diagnosis: Nondisplaced femoral neck fracture; displaced femoral neck fracture (those not requiring prosthetic replacement); intertrochanteric ± subtrochanteric fracture

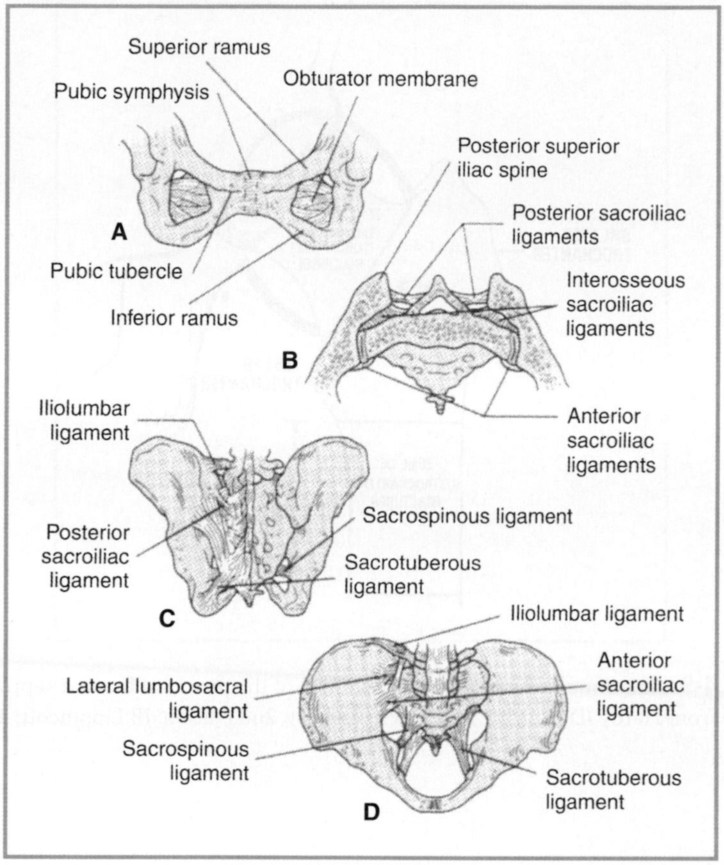

Figure 10.4-7. Schematic views of the pelvis with the principal ligamentous supports. **A:** Symphysis pubis fibrocartilage. **B:** Posterior SI ligaments. **C:** Posterior view. **D:** Anterior view. (Reproduced with permission from Chapman MW: *Chapman's Orthopaedic Surgery,* Vol 1, 3rd edition. Lippincott Williams & Wilkins, 2001.)

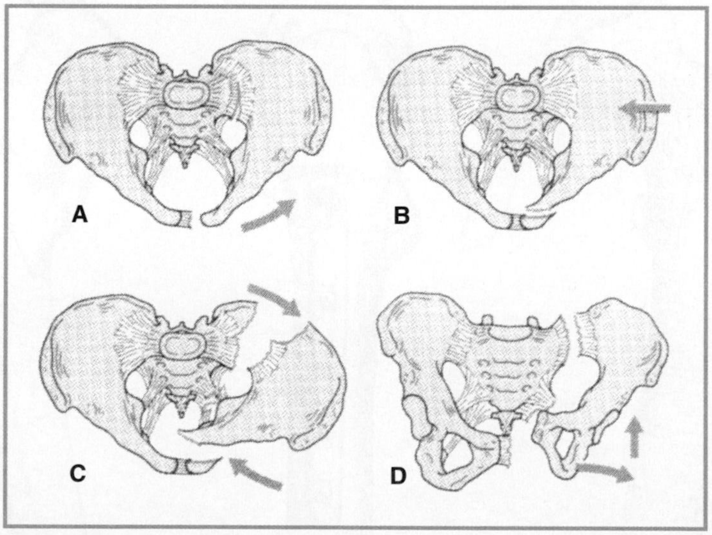

Figure 10.4-8. Schematic view of the principal pelvis injury patterns, as determined by the vector of the provocative blow. **A:** Anteroposterior compression or external rotation injury. **B:** Stable lateral compression or internal rotation injury. **C:** Unstable lateral compression or internal rotation injury. **D:** Unstable vertical shear disruption. (Reproduced with permission from Chapman MW: *Chapman's Orthopaedic Surgery,* Vol 1, 3rd edition. Lippincott Williams & Wilkins: 2001.)

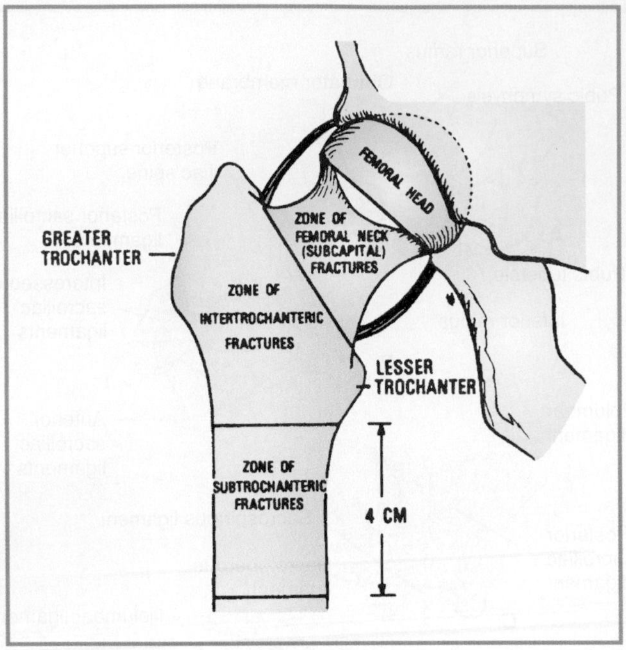

Figure 10.4-9. Anatomical classification of fractures of the proximal femur. (Reproduced with permission from Hardy JD: *Hardy's Textbook of Surgery,* 2nd edition. JB Lippincott: 1988.)

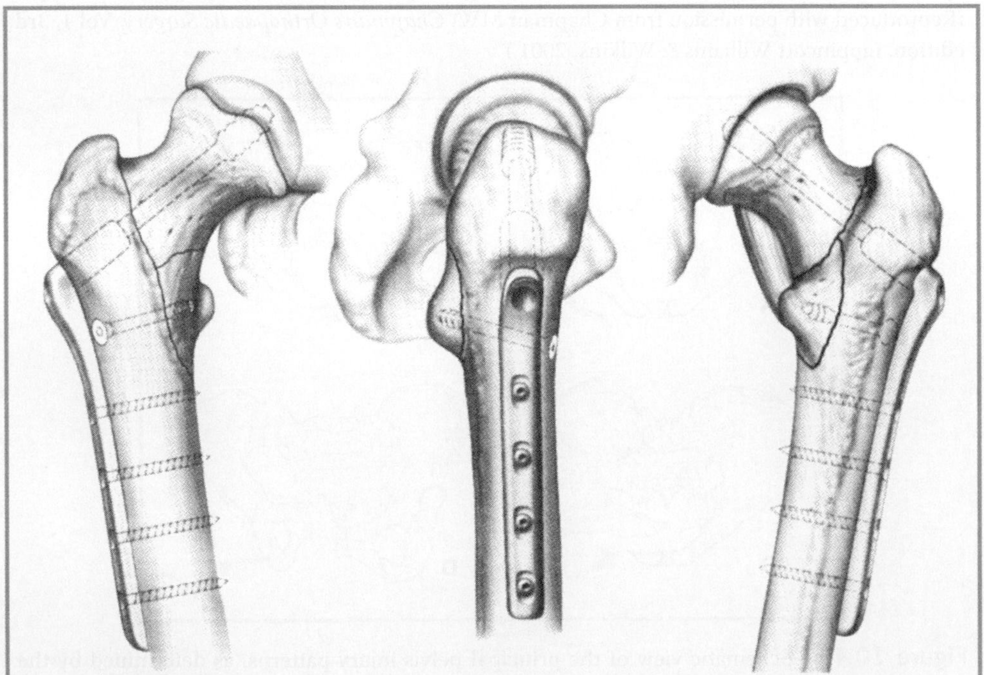

Figure 10.4-10. Intertrochanteric hip fracture treated with dynamic hip screw. (Reproduced with permission from Sledge CB, ed: *The Hip.* Lippincott-Raven: 1998.)

SUMMARY OF PROCEDURES

	Nondisplaced Femoral Neck Fracture	Displaced Femoral Neck Fracture	Intertrochanteric ± Subtrochanteric Fracture
Position	Supine, on fracture table	⇐	⇐
Incision	Proximal lateral thigh	⇐	⇐
Special instrumentation	Usually multiple percutaneous pins	Multiple screws or other devices	Screw-plate device or intramedullary device
Unique considerations	Fracture table and I.I. used. Percutaneous pinning may be accomplished with local anesthesia only.	⇐	⇐
Antibiotics	Cefazolin 1 g iv q 6–8 h × 24 h (vancomycin or clindamycin for 24 h if penicillin allergic)	⇐	⇐
Surgical time	1 h	1.5–2 h, including placing patient on fracture table and obtaining adequate reduction of fracture	1.5–3 h
EBL	< 100 mL	250–500 mL	500+ mL
Postop care	Generally PACU → room; if medically unstable, → ICU	⇐	⇐
Mortality	10–30% in first 12 mo postop in elderly; in younger patients, depends on other involved trauma.	⇐	⇐
Morbidity	Dysrhythmias: ~50%	⇐	⇐
	MI: ~50%	⇐	⇐
	Respiratory failure: ~50%	⇐	⇐
	Urinary retention requiring catheterization: ~50%	⇐	⇐
	UTI: ~50%	⇐	⇐
	Thromboembolism: 40%+	⇐	⇐
	Avascular necrosis and late segmental collapse: 10–20%	≥15–35%	1%
	Infection, deep: 2–17%	⇐	⇐
	Infection, superficial: 2–17%	⇐	⇐
	Septic arthritis: 2–17%	⇐	⇐
	Nonunion: 5–15%	20–30%	2%
	Malunion: < 10%	> 10%	10–20%
	Loss of reduction: < %5	> 10%	10%
	Hematoma	–	–
	Intraop comminution of the fracture	–	–
	Neurological injury: Rare	⇐	⇐
	Vascular injury: Rare	⇐	⇐
Pain score	5–6	7	8

PATIENT POPULATION CHARACTERISTICS

Age range	Usually > 60 yr (patients with an intertrochanteric fracture average 65–70 yr); occasionally, younger patients, 16–35 yr (as part of multiple-trauma situation)
Male:Female	Elderly 1:4–5
Incidence	Extremely common—about 5–100/100,000; femoral neck fractures are about twice as common as intertrochanteric fractures.

PATIENT POPULATION CHARACTERISTICS (cont'd)	
Etiology	Accidents and falls (may be 2° TIA, stroke, MI, dysrhythmia); pathological fracture; multiple trauma (younger patients); stress fracture
Associated conditions	Numerous serious medical conditions often present in elderly; senile dementia; multiple trauma often

ANESTHETIC CONSIDERATIONS

See Anesthetic Considerations for Lower-Extremity Procedures (p. 1059).

Suggested Readings

1. Chapman MW: Fractures of the hip and proximal femur. In *Chapman's Orthopaedic Surgery,* Vol I, 3rd edition. Chapman MW, ed. Lippincott Williams & Wilkins, Philadelphia: 2001, 617–70.
2. Guyton JL: Fractures of the hip, acetabulum, and pelvis. In *Campbell's Operative Orthopaedics,* Vol 3, 9th edition. Crenshaw AH, ed. CV Mosby, St. Louis: 1998, 2181–2280.
3. Kyle RF, Schmidt AH, Campbell SJ: Complications of the treatment of fractures and dislocations of the hip. In *Complications in Orthopaedic Surgery,* 3rd edition. Epps CH Jr, ed. JB Lippincott, Philadelphia: 1994, 443–86.
4. LaVelle DG: Delayed union and nonunion of fractures. In *Campbell's Operative Orthopaedics,* Vol 3, 9th edition. Crenshaw AH, ed. CV Mosby, St. Louis: 1998, 2579–2630.

OPEN REDUCTION AND INTERNAL FIXATION (ORIF) OF DISTAL FEMUR FRACTURES

SURGICAL CONSIDERATIONS

Description: ORIF of the distal femur fracture involves a longitudinal incision along the femoral shaft, obtaining reduction by direct visualization of the fracture fragments, and applying plates and screws along the femur for rigid internal fixation. An iliac crest bone graft may be necessary. Some intramedullary devices are also available for fixation of these fractures.

Usual preop diagnosis: Fracture of the distal femur; nonunion/malunion of the distal femur; degenerative arthritis of knee, with deformity

SUMMARY OF PROCEDURE	
Position	Supine. Patient usually arrives at OR in balanced traction if fracture is acute.
Incision	Anterior knee, lateral or medial thigh along the femoral shaft
Special instrumentation	Special plates, screws, rods, reduction clamps; radiolucent table; intraop blood salvage
Unique considerations	Usually requires intraop radiographs; tourniquet.
Antibiotics	Cefazolin 1 g iv q 6–8 h × 24 h (vancomycin or clindamycin for 24 h if penicillin allergic)
Surgical time	3 h (or more, depending on difficulty)
EBL	750 mL or more
Postop care	Multiple-trauma victim → ICU; others → PACU
Mortality	~3–4%, depending on the extent of multiple trauma
Morbidity	Nonunion: 4–33% Malunion: 4–31% Infection, osteomyelitis, septic arthritis; closed/open:

SUMMARY OF PROCEDURE (cont'd)	
	Grade I: 1–5% Grade II: 5–20% Grade III: > 20% Delayed union: 0–17% Vascular complications: 2–3% Neurological deficit to peripheral nerves, peroneal nerve: ~3% Compartment syndrome: Rare Hypotension: Rare Leg-length discrepancy: Rare Respiratory distress and fat embolism: Rare
Pain score	8

PATIENT POPULATION CHARACTERISTICS	
Age range	Any age; predominance of males < 40 yr (trauma); degenerative arthritis of knee < 60 yr. Special rare case is elderly patient with a supracondylar fracture above a total knee replacement.
Male:Female	5:1
Incidence	Common in trauma center patients; rare in cases of degenerative arthritis of knee (osteotomy) or elderly patient with a supracondylar fracture above a total knee replacement.
Etiology	Motorcycle and motor vehicle accidents; falls; industrial injury; degenerative arthritis of knee
Associated conditions	Frequently associated with trauma to other organ systems.

ANESTHETIC CONSIDERATIONS

See Anesthetic Considerations for Lower-Extremity Procedures. (p. 1059).

Suggested Readings

1. LaVelle DG: Delayed union and nonunion of fractures. In *Campbell's Operative Orthopaedics,* Vol 3, 9th edition. Crenshaw AH, ed. CV Mosby, St. Louis: 1998, 2579–2630.
2. Mize R, Johnson EE, Hohl M: Complications of fractures and dislocations of the knee. In *Complications in Orthopaedic* Surgery, 3rd edition. Epps CH Jr, ed. JB Lippincott, Philadelphia: 1994, 525–56.
3. Mize R: Supracondylar and articular fractures of the distal femur. In *Chapman's Orthopaedic Surgery,* 3rd edition, Vol I. Chapman MW, ed. Lippincott Williams & Wilkins, Philadelphia: 2001, 709–23.
4. Whittle AP: Fractures of lower extremity. In *Campbell's Operative Orthopaedics,* Vol 3, 9th edition. Crenshaw AH, ed. CV Mosby, St. Louis: 1998, 2042–2180.
5. Whittle AP: Malunited fractures. In *Campbell's Operative Orthopaedics,* 9th edition. Crenshaw AH, ed. Mosby, St. Louis: 1998, 2579–2630.
6. Wiss DA, Watson JT, Johnson EE: Fractures of the knee. In *Rockwood and Green's Fractures in Adults,* 4th edition. Rock-wood CA Jr, Green DP, Bucholz RW, Hickman JD, eds. Lippincott-Raven, Philadelphia: 1996, 1919–2000.

OPEN REDUCTION AND INTERNAL FIXATION (ORIF) OF THE FEMORAL SHAFT WITH PLATE

SURGICAL CONSIDERATIONS

Description: ORIF of the femoral shaft involves obtaining a reduction by open means, usually through a longitudinal lateral incision along the length of the femur, and applying plates and screws along the femur to maintain the reduction. An iliac crest bone graft may be necessary.

Usual preop diagnosis: Fracture of femur

SUMMARY OF PROCEDURE	
Position	Supine or lateral decubitus
Incision	Lateral thigh along length of femur ± iliac crest incision
Special instrumentation	Special plates, screws; reduction clamps; blood salvage device
Unique considerations	Fracture or radiolucent table; I.I. Patient usually arrives at OR in balanced traction.
Antibiotics	Cefazolin 1 g iv q 6–8 h × 24 h (vancomycin or clindamycin for 24 h if penicillin allergic)
Surgical time	3 h or more, depending on difficulty
EBL	750 mL; Cell Saver recommended.
Postop care	Multiple-trauma victims: ICU Others: PACU
Mortality	Dependent on extent of multiple trauma
Morbidity	Knee stiffness: 20–30% Delayed union, nonunion, malunion: 5–21% Leg-length discrepancy: 0–11% Failure of fixation: 5–10% Infection, osteomyelitis: < 5% Hypotension: Not uncommon Respiratory distress and fat embolism: Not uncommon, often subclinical Compartment syndrome: Rare Neurological deficit to peripheral nerves: Rare Vascular complications: Rare
Pain score	9

PATIENT POPULATION CHARACTERISTICS	
Age range	Any age, but predominance of males < 30 yr
Male:Female	5:1
Incidence	Unknown
Etiology	Motorcycle and motor vehicle accidents; falls; industrial injuries
Associated conditions	Frequently associated with trauma to other organ systems

Orthopedic Surgery

ANESTHETIC CONSIDERATIONS

See Anesthetic Considerations for Lower-Extremity Procedures (p. 1059).

Suggested Readings

1. Azer R, Rankin EA: Complications of femoral shaft fractures. In *Complications in Orthopaedic Surgery,* 3rd edition. Epps CH Jr, ed. JB Lippincott, Philadelphia: 1986, 487–524.
2. Bucholz RW, Brumback RJ: Fractures of the shaft of the femur. In *Rockwood and Green's Fractures in Adults,* 4th edition. Rockwood CA Jr, Green DP, Bucholz RW, et al., eds. JB Lippincott, Philadelphia: 1996, 1827–1918.
3. LaVelle DG: Delayed union and nonunion of fractures. In *Campbell's Operative Orthopaedics,* Vol 3, 9th edition. Crenshaw AH, ed. CV Mosby, St. Louis: 1998, 2579–2630.
4. Matta JM, Siebenrock KA, Gautier E, et al: Hip fusion through an anterior approach with the use of a ventral plate. *Clin Orthop* 1997; 337–129–39.
5. Whittle AP: Malunited fractures. In *Campbell's Operative Orthopaedics,* 9th edition. Crenshaw AH, ed. Mosby, St. Louis: 1998, 2579–2630.

INTRAMEDULLARY NAILING OF FEMORAL SHAFT

SURGICAL CONSIDERATIONS

Description: Intramedullary nailing of the femur is the standard procedure for fractures of the femoral shaft (Fig. 10.4.11). It is indicated for virtually any fracture, from the lesser trochanter to the distal femur, within 7 cm of the articular surface. The procedure also is used for the treatment of nonunions and malunions of the femoral shaft. Typically, the nail is placed in an anterograde fashion from proximal to distal. There are, however, indications in which the nail is inserted in a retrograde fashion from distal to proximal (e.g., bilateral femur fractures; ipsilateral femur and tibia fractures; distal femur fractures; and multiple-trauma, obese, and pregnant patients). Early fixation of femoral shaft fractures in severe polytrauma has several benefits. The advantages of early fixation of long bones include improved pain control, early mobilization, improved pulmonary function, and decreased morbidity and mortality.

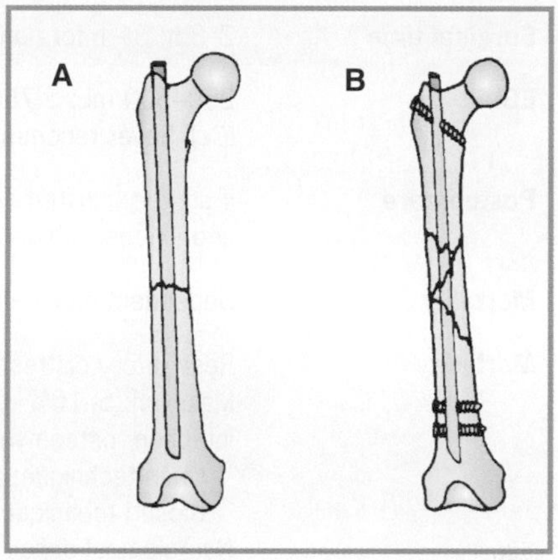

Figure 10.4-11. **A:** Simple and **(B)** locked intramedullary fixation of femoral shaft. (Reproduced with permission from Hardy JD: *Hardy's Textbook of Surgery,* 2nd edition. JB Lippincott, Philadelphia: 1988.)

Femoral nails are inserted after reaming the intramedullary canal, which allows a larger diameter implant and improves the mechanical properties of the bone implant interface. Reaming may produce systemic effects by embolic showering of medullary contents to the pulmonary vasculature, a phenomenon that has been documented by TEE. This situation may be exacerbated in the polytrauma patient with pulmonary injury, and may produce posttraumatic pulmonary failure. Patients with femur fractures may have associated injuries.

Patients may arrive from the ICU in skeletal traction or from the emergency department, especially in the case of an open fracture. Hemorrhage up to 1 L may be contained in the thigh following a femur fracture; therefore, patients may be hypovolemic at the start of the procedure. Since the procedure is essentially percutaneous, apparent blood loss may be underestimated because of the hemorrhaged blood contained in the thigh.

The patient is placed in the supine or lateral decubitus position on either a radiolucent table or a fracture table. Antegrade insertion of the nail requires a lateral incision several cm in length proximal to the greater trochanter. The hip abductors are split, and portal into the femoral canal is created in the piriformis fossa. The femoral canal is reamed over a guide wire. The intramedullary nail is then inserted into the intramedullary canal with gentle taps, using a hammer.

Retrograde insertion of the nail is performed through an incision several cm long over the anterior aspect of the knee. The knee joint is entered and the portal to the intramedullary canal is made in the nonweight-bearing portion of the intercondylar notch. The nail is inserted in the same fashion as the anterior nail. Cross-locking screws are commonly used, and they are inserted through the rod.

Variant procedure or approaches: The application of femoral nailing has been expanded to treat nonunions, malunions, posttraumatic deformities of the femur, and leg-length differences. Specialized additional equipment, such as an intramedullary saw or an external fixator, may be required for these procedures.

Usual preop diagnosis: Femur fracture; nonunion/malunion of the femur; leg-length discrepancy

SUMMARY OF PROCEDURE

Position	Supine or lateral decubitus
Incision	Proximal lateral thigh or anterior knee
Special instrumentation	Intramedullary nails; intramedullary saw for closed femoral shortening of femur; fracture or radiolucent table; I.I.

SUMMARY OF PROCEDURE (cont'd)	
Unique considerations	Patient may have multiple traumas with other associated injuries. Procedure is heavily dependent on I.I.
Antibiotics	Cefazolin 1 g iv q 6–8 h × 24 h (vancomycin or clindamycin for 24 h if penicillin allergic)
Surgical time	2–3 h; 3+ h for nonunion/malunion of femur or closed femoral shortening of femur
EBL	250–500 mL; ≥ 750 mL for nonunion/malunion of femur or closed femoral shortening of femur (Cell Saver recommended).
Postop care	If surgery performed acutely, patient is usually a multiple-trauma victim with numerous injuries and extensive blood loss; usually goes to ICU.
Mortality	Dependent on extent of trauma
Morbidity	Respiratory distress and fat embolism: 10% Malunion: 5–10% Infection, osteomyelitis: Open technique: 1–10% Closed technique: 0–1% Neurological deficit to peripheral nerves: 2% Vascular complications: ~2% (up to 15% have occult vascular abnormalities) Delayed union: 1% Nonunion: 1% Hypotension: Common in multiple-trauma situations Knee stiffness: Common Leg-length discrepancies: Not uncommon Compartment syndrome: Rare Failure of fixation: Rare
Pain score	6

PATIENT POPULATION CHARACTERISTICS	
Age range	Any age, but predominance of males < 30 yr
Male:Female	5:1
Incidence	Very common
Etiology	Motorcycle and motor vehicle accidents (60–80%); falls (5–10%); industrial injuries (5–10%); previous trauma (rare)
Associated conditions	Frequently associated with trauma to other organ systems.

Orthopedic Surgery

ANESTHETIC CONSIDERATIONS

See Anesthetic Considerations for Lower-Extremity Procedures (p. 1059).

Suggested Readings

1. Azer R, Rankin EA: Complications of femoral shaft fractures. In *Complications in Orthopaedic Surgery,* 3rd edition. Epps CH Jr, ed. JB Lippincott, Philadelphia: 1986, 487–524.
2. Bone LB, Johnson KD, Weigelt J: Early versus delayed stabilization of femoral fractures: a prospective randomized study. *J Bone Joint Surg* (Am) 1989; 71(3):336–40.
3. Bucholz RW, Brumback RJ: Fractures of the shaft of the femur. In *Rockwood and Green's Fractures in Adults,* 4th edition. Rockwood CA Jr, Green DP, Bucholz RW, et al., eds. Lippincott-Raven, Philadelphia: 1996, 1827–1918.
4. Chapman MW: Diaphyseal fractures of the femur. In *Chapman's Orthopaedic Surgery,* Vol I, 3rd edition. Chapman MW, ed. Lippincott Williams & Wilkins, Philadelphia: 2001, 671–708.
5. Chapman MW: Fractures of the hip and proximal femur. In *Chapman's Orthopaedic Surgery,* Vol I, 3rd edition. Chapman MW, ed. Lippincott Williams & Wilkins, Philadelphia: 2001, 617–70.

6. LaVelle DG: Delayed union and nonunion of fractures. In *Campbell's Operative Orthopaedics,* Vol 3, 9th edition. Crenshaw AH, ed. CV Mosby, St. Louis: 1998, 2579–2630.
7. Mize RD: Supracondylar and articular fractures of the distal femur. In *Chapman's Orthopaedic Surgery,* 3rd edition, Vol I. Chapman MW, ed. Lippincott Williams & Wilkins, Philadelphia: 2001, 709–23.
8. Pape HC, Regel G, Dwenger A: Influences of different methods of intramedullary femoral nailing on lung function in patients with multiple trauma. *J Trauma* 1993; 35(5):709–16.
9. Wenda K, Runkel M, Degeif J: Pathogenesis and clinical relevance of bone marrow embolism in medullary nailing—demonstrated by intraoperative echocardiography injury. *Injury* 1993; 24(Suppl 3):73–81.
10. Whittle AP: Malunited fractures. In *Campbell's Operative Orthopaedics,* 9th edition. Crenshaw AH, ed. Mosby, St. Louis: 1998, 2579–2630.

REPAIR OF NONUNION/MALUNION OF PROXIMAL THIRD OF FEMUR, PROXIMAL FEMORAL OSTEOTOMY FOR OSTEOARTHRITIS

SURGICAL CONSIDERATIONS

Description: Operations for nonunion/malunion of the proximal femur entail realigning the bones with a femoral osteotomy (as necessary); stabilizing the reduction with internal fixation (using a nail/plate-nail/rod device); and supplementing this with a bone graft. In young patients (< 50 yr) in whom early osteoarthritis of the hip spares some of the cartilage, the hip may be realigned with **proximal femoral osteotomy.** This entails cutting the bone at the level of the lesser trochanter, realigning the hip and stabilizing the osteotomy with internal fixation.

Variant procedure or approaches: Osteotomy of proximal 1/3 of femur for degenerative arthritis of hip

Usual preop diagnosis: Nonunion/malunion of proximal 1/3 of femur; early degenerative arthritis of hip

SUMMARY OF PROCEDURES

	Repair Nonunion/Malunion	Proximal Femoral Osteotomy
Position	Supine or lateral decubitus	⇐
Incision	Proximal lateral thigh	⇐
Special instrumentation	Plates, screws; reduction clamps; occasionally, an intramedullary device. Cell Saver recommended. Some surgeons use fracture or radiolucent table with I.I.	⇐
Antibiotics	Cefazolin 1 g iv q 6–8 h × 24 h (vancomycin or clindamycin for 24 h if penicillin allergic)	⇐
Surgical time	2 h for bone grafting alone; 3 h or more if difficult malunion	3 h
EBL	500–750 mL or more	500 mL +
Mortality	Rare: < 1%	⇐
Morbidity	Leg-length discrepancy: Common Technical complications/fixation failure: 1–5% Superficial, deep infection/osteomyelitis: 1% Malunion: Not uncommon Compartment syndrome: Rare Neurological deficit to peripheral nerves: Rare	– ⇐ ⇐ – ⇐ ⇐

SUMMARY OF PROCEDURE (cont'd)		
	Repair Nonunion/Malunion	**Proximal Femoral Osteotomy**
Morbidity (con't)	Vascular complications: Rare	⇐ Progressive pain/arthritis (by 5–10 yr): 40–50% Delayed union: 5–10% Nonunion: 1–5%
Pain score	8	8

PATIENT POPULATION CHARACTERISTICS		
Age range	Any age	⇐
Male:Female	1:1	⇐
Incidence	Rare	⇐
Etiology	Previous surgery (rare); previous trauma (rare)	Early degenerative arthritis of the hip (not uncommon)
Associated conditions	May accompany multiple traumas	⇐

ANESTHETIC CONSIDERATIONS

See Anesthetic Considerations for Lower-Extremity Procedures (p. 1059).

Suggested Readings

1. Barr RJ, Santore RF: Osteotomies about the hip. In *Chapman's Orthopaedic Surgery,* Vol 3, 3rd edition. Chapman MW, ed. Lippincott Williams & Wilkins, Philadelphia: 2001, 2723–68.
2. Kyle RF, Schmidt AH, Campbell SJ: Complications of the treatment of fractures and dislocations of the hip. In *Complications in Orthopaedic Surgery,* 3rd edition. Epps CH Jr, ed. JB Lippincott, Philadelphia: 1994, 443–86.
3. LaVelle DG: Delayed union and nonunion of fractures. In *Campbell's Operative Orthopaedics,* Vol 3, 9th edition. Crenshaw AH, ed. CV Mosby, St. Louis: 1998, 2579–2630.
4. Whittle AP: Malunited fractures. In *Campbell's Operative Orthopaedics,* Vol 3, 9th edition. Crenshaw AH, ed. CV Mosby, St. Louis: 1994, 2537–78.

CLOSED REDUCTION AND EXTERNAL FIXATION OF FEMUR

SURGICAL CONSIDERATIONS

Description: This procedure entails manipulating the femur to obtain an acceptable reduction by closed or limited-open means, then applying an external fixation device to maintain the reduction. The pins for the external fixator are inserted percutaneously or through small incisions. This method of treatment may be used for severe open fractures (e.g., grade III) with extensive bone and soft-tissue injury.

Usual preop diagnosis: Displaced, open fracture of the femur

SUMMARY OF PROCEDURE	
Position	Supine or lateral
Incision	Done percutaneously or through small incisions
Special instrumentation	External fixation device of surgeon's choice; radiolucent table with I.I.

SUMMARY OF PROCEDURE (cont'd)	
Unique considerations	Fracture is usually an open, extremely comminuted fracture in a multiple-trauma patient.
Antibiotics	Cefazolin 1 g iv q 6–8 h × 24 h (vancomycin or clindamycin for 24 h if penicillin allergic)
Surgical time	1 h
EBL	Operative blood loss usually 100–200 mL; however, blood loss may be extensive before surgery.
Postop care	Multiple-trauma victims → ICU; others → PACU
Mortality	Dependent on extent of trauma
Morbidity	Refracture: 2–12% Hypotension 2° blood loss and other injuries: Common Stiffness of knee: Common Delayed union, nonunion, malunion: More common in comminuted, open fractures Leg-length discrepancy: More common in severely comminuted fractures Osteomyelitis: More common in open fractures Respiratory distress: More common in multiple-trauma situations Amputation: Rare Compartment syndrome: Rare Neurological deficit to peripheral nerves: Rare Vascular complications: Rare
Pain score	9–10 (due to extensive open fracture)

PATIENT POPULATION CHARACTERISTICS	
Age range	Any age, but predominance of males < 30 yr
Male:Female	5:1
Incidence	Common
Etiology	Motorcycle and motor vehicle accidents; falls; industrial injury
Associated conditions	Frequently associated with trauma to other organ systems, including head and neck, chest, abdomen, and extremities; these will often be treated simultaneously with the femur fracture.

ANESTHETIC CONSIDERATIONS

See Anesthetic Considerations for Lower-Extremity Procedures (p. 1059).

Suggested Readings

1. Azer SN, Rankin EA: Complications of femoral shaft fractures. In *Complications in Orthopaedic Surgery,* 3rd edition. Epps CH Jr, ed. JB Lippincott, Philadelphia: 1986, 487–524.
2. Bucholz RW, Brumback RJ: Fractures of the shaft of the femur. In *Rockwood and Green's Fractures in Adults,* 4th edition. Rockwood CA Jr, Green DP, Bucholz RW, et al., eds. JB Lippincott, Philadelphia: 1996, 1827–1918.
3. Chapman MW: Diaphyseal fractures of the femur. In *Chapman's Orthopaedic Surgery,* Vol I, 3rd edition. Chapman MW, ed. Lippincott Williams & Wilkins, Philadelphia: 2001, 671–708.
4. LaVelle DG: Delayed union and nonunion of fractures. In *Campbell's Operative Orthopaedics,* Vol 3, 9th edition. Crenshaw AH, ed. CV Mosby, St. Louis: 1998, 2579–2630.
5. Whittle AP: Malunited fractures. In *Campbell's Operative Orthopaedics,* Vol 3, 9th edition. Crenshaw AH, ed. CV Mosby, St. Louis: 1994, 2537–78.

CHAPTER

10.5 Knee Surgery

SURGEONS

James I. Huddleston, MD
John J. Csongradi, MD
Stuart B. Goodman, MD, PhD, FRCSC, FACS

ANESTHESIOLOGISTS

Frederick G. Mihm, MD
Christoph Egger Halbeis, MD, MBA

ARTHROPLASTY OF THE KNEE

SURGICAL CONSIDERATIONS

Description: In this procedure, an arthrotomy of the knee joint is performed, and metallic and plastic components are used for replacement of the knee joint surfaces (**total knee replacement**). The femur, patella, and tibia are exposed; cartilage and minimal bone are excised with a saw. The new components may be cemented or uncemented. Alternatively, arthroplasty may be performed on only one compartment of the knee (i.e., medial/lateral **unicompartmental knee replacement**). In **revision procedures,** one or more components of the old joint are removed and new components are placed. In **resection or excision arthroplasty** of the knee, (usually for infection of the prosthesis), the components are removed, but not replaced.

Usual preop diagnosis: Arthritis of knee; arthrosis of knee; loose (or malpositioned) knee prosthesis; infected knee

SUMMARY OF PROCEDURES

	Knee Replacement	Revision	Resection/ Excision
Position	Supine	⇐	⇐
Incision	Anterior or anteromedial over patella	⇐	⇐
Special instrumentation	Appropriate prostheses and instrumentation	Special instruments for excising cement	⇐
Unique considerations	± Tourniquet; ± SCD	⇐	⇐
Antibiotics	Cefazolin 1 g iv q 6–8 h × 24 h (vancomycin or clindamycin for 24 h if penicillin allergic)	⇐	⇐
Surgical time	2 h	3–4 h or more	3 h
Closing considerations	In infected or complex revision cases (rare), a local or free flap is required.	⇐	⇐
EBL	300–500 mL	500–1,000 mL	⇐
Postop care	Bulky dressing or splint; continuous passive motion (CPM) may begin in the PACU or ward	⇐	Splint/cast
Mortality	Rare	⇐	⇐
Morbidity	DVT, without prophylaxis: 50–75%	⇐	⇐
	DVT, with prophylaxis (e.g., low-molecular-weight heparin, coumadin, SCD, antiembolism stockings): 2–3%	⇐	⇐
	Postop subluxation/dislocation of patella: 20%	> 30%	–
	Superficial wound necrosis: 10–15%	> 10–15%	≥ 10–15%
	Wound infection:	> 5–10%	Rare
	Primary rheumatoid or psoriatic arthritis, diabetes: 5–10%		
	Primary osteoarthritis (OA): 1%		
	PE: 1–7%	⇐	⇐
	Postop subluxation/dislocation of knee joint: 1–6%	≥ 1–6%	–
	Late aseptic loosening requiring revision after ~10 yr: 5%	–	–
	Peroneal nerve injury: 1–5%	> 1–5% (more common in difficult revisions)	1–5%
	Urinary retention requiring catheterization: Common	–	–

SUMMARY OF PROCEDURE (cont'd)

	Knee Replacement	Revision	Resection/ Excision
Morbidity (cont.)	Hematoma requiring reoperation: Rare	–	–
	Hypotension	–	–
	Knee stiffness	–	–
	Intraoperative fracture: Rare	⇐	⇐
	Wound dehiscence: Rare	–	–
	Fat embolism: Rare	–	–
	Vascular injury to popliteal vessels: Rare	–	–
Pain score	7	8	9

PATIENT POPULATION CHARACTERISTICS

Age range	Generally, > 60 yr. Arthritis of the knee (e.g., rheumatoid arthritis or juvenile rheumatoid arthritis); hemophilia, ≥ 18 yr
Male:Female	1:1
Incidence	Common (~400,000/yr in the United States)
Etiology	Arthrosis of the knee (degenerative joint disease [DJD] or OA); seropositive or seronegative arthritis; traumatic arthritis; hemophiliac arthropathy of the knee
Associated conditions	Dependent on primary condition (e.g. osteoarthritis)

ANESTHETIC CONSIDERATIONS

See Anesthetic Considerations for Knee Procedures (p. 1026).

Suggested Readings

1. Blaster RB, Matthews LS: Complications of prosthetic knee arthroplasty. In: *Complications in Orthopaedic Surgery,* 3rd edition. Epps CH Jr, ed. JB Lippincott, Philadelphia: 1994, 1057–86.
2. Burke DW, O'Flynn H: Primary total knee arthroplasty. In *Chapman's Orthopaedic Surgery,* 3rd edition. Chapman MW, ed. Lippincott Williams & Wilkins, Philadelphia: 2001, 2869–96.
3. Guyton JL: Arthroplasty of the ankle and knee. In: *Campbell's Operative Orthopaedics,* 9th edition. Crenshaw AH, ed. Mosby-Year Book, St. Louis: 1998, Vol 1, 232–94.
4. Insall JN: Total knee replacement. In: *Surgery of the Knee.* Insall JN, ed. Churchill Livingstone, New York: 1984, 587–695.
5. Kuper M, Rosenstein A: Infection control in total knee and total hip arthroplasties. *Am J Orthop* 2008; 37(1):E2–5.
6. NIH Consensus Statement on total knee replacement. *NIH Consens State Sci Statements.* 2003; 20(1):1–34.
7. Vince KG: Revision knee arthroplasty and arthrodesis of the knee. In *Chapman's Orthopaedic Surgery,* 3rd edition. Chapman MW, ed. Lippincott Williams & Wilkins, Philadelphia: 2001, 2897–2952.

ARTHRODESIS OF THE KNEE

SURGICAL CONSIDERATIONS

Description: In this procedure, the femur is fused to the tibia, obliterating the knee joint. Through a midline incision and anterior or median parapatellar arthrotomy, the cartilage surface and a small amount of bone are excised. The cut ends are opposed and aligned in 0–20° of flexion and 5–10% of valgus. The bones are stabilized with plates, screws, an intramedullary rod, or an external fixator.

Usual preop diagnosis: Arthritis or other arthrosis of the knee; previous septic arthritis of the knee; failed or infected knee arthroplasty

SUMMARY OF PROCEDURE	
Position	Usually supine
Incision	Anterior midline over knee
Special instrumentation	External fixator; internal fixation with plates and screws or intramedullary nail
Unique considerations	Intraop radiographs or I.I.; tourniquet
Antibiotics	Cefazolin 1 g iv q 6–8 h × 24 h (vancomycin or clindamycin for 24 h if penicillin allergic)
Surgical time	3 h (+ 1 h, if necessary, to excise total knee arthroplasty)
Closing considerations	Cast or splint while anesthetized
EBL	< 100 mL, if tourniquet and local fixation used. 500–1000 mL, if no tourniquet used, or if intramedullary procedures are used.
Mortality	Rare, but depends primarily on age and medical condition of patient.
Morbidity	Thromboembolism ≥ incidence following total knee replacement: DVT (without prophylaxis): 50–75% DVT (if prophylaxis used): 10–20% PE (if no prophylaxis; reduced if anticoagulation or SCDs used): 1–7% Failure of fusion (nonunion), malunion: 10% After failed knee replacement: 19–44% With Charcot joint: as high as 50% Pin tract infection: ≥ 1–10% Wound infection: 5% Deep infection and osteomyelitis Urinary retention requiring catheterization, UTI: Common Breakage or failure of internal or external fixation: Rare Fat embolism: Rare GI bleed, MI: Rare Hematoma: Rare Hypotension: Rare Intraop femoral or tibial fracture: Rare Neurological injury, usually popliteal nerve or peroneal nerve: Rare Superficial wound necrosis and wound dehiscence: Rare Vascular injury to popliteal vessels: Rare Amputation: Extremely rare (usually 2° acute arterial occlusion or uncontrollable local sepsis)
Pain score	9

PATIENT POPULATION CHARACTERISTICS	
Age range	Any age
Male:Female	1:1
Incidence	Rare
Etiology	Failed or infected total knee replacement (probably most common etiology); trauma to knee—unreconstructable, intraarticular fractures; total unstable knee or failed ligament repairs with severe DJD in a young patient

ANESTHETIC CONSIDERATIONS

See Anesthetic Considerations for Knee Procedures (p. 1026).

Suggested Readings

1. Blaster RB, Matthews LS: Complications of prosthetic knee arthroplasty. In: *Complications in Orthopaedic* Surgery, 3rd edition. Epps CH Jr, ed. JB Lippincott, Philadelphia: 1994, 1057–86.
2. Carnesale PG, Stewart MJ: Complications of arthrodesis surgery. In: *Complications in Orthopaedic Surgery,* 3rd edition. Epps CH Jr, ed. JB Lippincott, Philadelphia: 1994, 1279–1308.
3. Christian CA, Donley BG: Arthrodesis of the ankle, knee, hip. In: *Campbell's Operative Orthopaedics,* 9th edition. Canale ST, ed. Mosby-Year Book, St. Louis: 1998, Vol 1, 145–88.
4. Mize R, Johnson EE, Hohl M: Complications of fractures and dislocations of the knee. In: *Complications in Orthopaedic Surgery,* 3rd edition. Epps CH Jr, ed. JB Lippincott, Philadelphia: 1994, 525–56.
5. Vince KG: Revision knee arthroplasty and arthrodesis of the knee. In: *Chapman's Orthopaedic Surgery,* 3rd edition. Chapman MW, ed. Lippincott Williams & Wilkins, Philadelphia: 2001, 2897–2952.

OPEN REDUCTION AND INTERNAL FIXATION (ORIF) OF PATELLAR FRACTURES

SURGICAL CONSIDERATIONS

Description: In ORIF of patellar fractures, a short incision over the patella is used to perform a reduction by direct visualization of the fracture fragments of the patella. Since this is generally an intraarticular fracture, the fragments should be reduced precisely. The torn quadriceps retinaculum is also repaired. Part or all of the patella may be excised; pins, wires, and/or screws are normally used to fix the patellar fragments together internally. Thereafter, the knee is casted, or early motion of the knee is started.

Usual preop diagnosis: Fracture of patella; severe degenerative arthritis of patellofemoral joint

SUMMARY OF PROCEDURE	
Position	Supine
Incision	Anterior over patella
Special instrumentation	Wire, pins, screws as necessary
Unique considerations	Intraop radiographs may be obtained; tourniquet
Antibiotics	Cefazolin 1 g iv q 6–8 h × 24 h (vancomycin or clindamycin for 24 h if penicillin allergic)
Surgical time	1.5–2 h
Closing considerations	Splint or cast usually applied.
EBL	< 100 mL
Mortality	< 1%
Morbidity	Late degenerative arthritis of patellofemoral joint: ~50–60% DVT: ~5% Wound infection, septic arthritis, osteomyelitis: ~5% Delayed union, nonunion, malunion: ~2–5% Knee stiffness: Common Weakness: Common Avascular necrosis: Rare Complex regional pain syndrome: Rare Following patellectomy—quadriceps strength: ~75% of normal
Pain score	7

PATIENT POPULATION CHARACTERISTICS	
Age range	Any age; frequently seen in young, active, healthy adults.
Male:Female	1:1
Incidence	~1% of all skeletal injuries
Etiology	Trauma: falls (60%); motorcycle and motor vehicle accidents (25–35%); industrial injury (6%); degenerative arthritis of patellofemoral joint (rare)

ANESTHETIC CONSIDERATIONS

See Anesthetic Considerations for Knee Procedures (p. 1026).

Suggested Readings

1. Callaghan JJ, O'rourke MR, Saleh KJ. Why knees fail: lessons learned. *J Arthroplasty* 2004; 19(4 Suppl 1):31–4.
2. Mize R, Johnson EE, Hohl M: Complications of fractures and dislocations of the knee. In: *Complications in Orthopaedic Surgery,* 3rd edition. Epps CH Jr, ed. JB Lippincott, Philadelphia: 1994, 525–56.
3. Whittle AP: Fractures of lower extremity. In: *Campbell's Operative Orthopaedics,* Vol 3, 9th edition. Canale ST, ed. Mosby-Year Book, St. Louis: 1998, 2042–2180.
4. Whittle AP: Malunited fractures. In: *Campbell's Operative Orthopaedics,* Vol 3, 9th edition. Canale ST, ed. Mosby-Year Book, St. Louis: 1998, 2537–78.
5. Wiss DA, Watson JT, Johnson EE: Fractures of the knee. In: *Rockwood and Green's Fractures in Adults,* 5th edition. Rockwood CA Jr, Green DP, Bucholz RW, Heckman JD, eds. Lippincott-Raven, Philadelphia: 1996, 1919–71.

REPAIR OR RECONSTRUCTION OF KNEE LIGAMENTS

SURGICAL CONSIDERATIONS

Description: Collateral ligaments usually are repaired by direct suture or by stapling the torn ligaments to bone. Cruciate tears are generally repaired only if bone is avulsed at one end of the ligament, again with direct suture, staples, or screws. For collateral ligament repair, a longitudinal incision is made directly over the ligament medially or laterally. The ligament is exposed by deep dissection and elevation of skin flaps. The torn ligament is repaired by direct suture or by fixing it to bone with a screw or staple. Following closure, the knee is immobilized with a long leg splint or cast. Cruciate ligaments are repaired in similar fashion, except for the approaches: medial parapatellar (with anterior arthrotomy) for the anterior cruciate ligament (ACL) and posteromedial (with posterior arthrotomy) for the posterior cruciate ligament (PCL). Cruciate ligament reconstruction is performed for instability 2° intrasubstance tears of these ligaments. Homografts, such as a portion of the patellar tendon or semitendinosus tendon, normally are used, but allografts or synthetics also are available. (The ligaments of the knee are illustrated in Figs 10.5-1 and 10.5-2.)

Usual preop diagnosis: Trauma

SUMMARY OF PROCEDURES	Repair or Collateral Reconstruction	Repair or Cruciate Reconstruction
Position	Supine	⇐
Incision	Over collateral ligament	Anterior and lateral ACL or medial PCL
Special instrumentation	Staples	Drill guides, staples, screws
Unique considerations	Often arthroscopically assisted; tourniquet	⇐
Antibiotics	Cefazolin 1 g iv (vancomycin or clindamycin if penicillin allergic)	⇐
Surgical time	2 h	⇐

Orthopedic Surgery

SUMMARY OF PROCEDURES (cont'd)

	Repair or Collateral Reconstruction	Repair or Cruciate Reconstruction
Closing considerations	Splint or cast while anesthetized	⇐
EBL	100 mL	⇐
Postop care	PACU → room or home	⇐
Mortality	Minimal	⇐
Morbidity	Infection: < 1%	⇐
	Thrombophlebitis: < 5%	⇐
Pain score	4	7

PATIENT POPULATION CHARACTERISTICS

Age range	Young adult
Male:Female	2:1
Incidence	Common
Etiology	Trauma: 100%

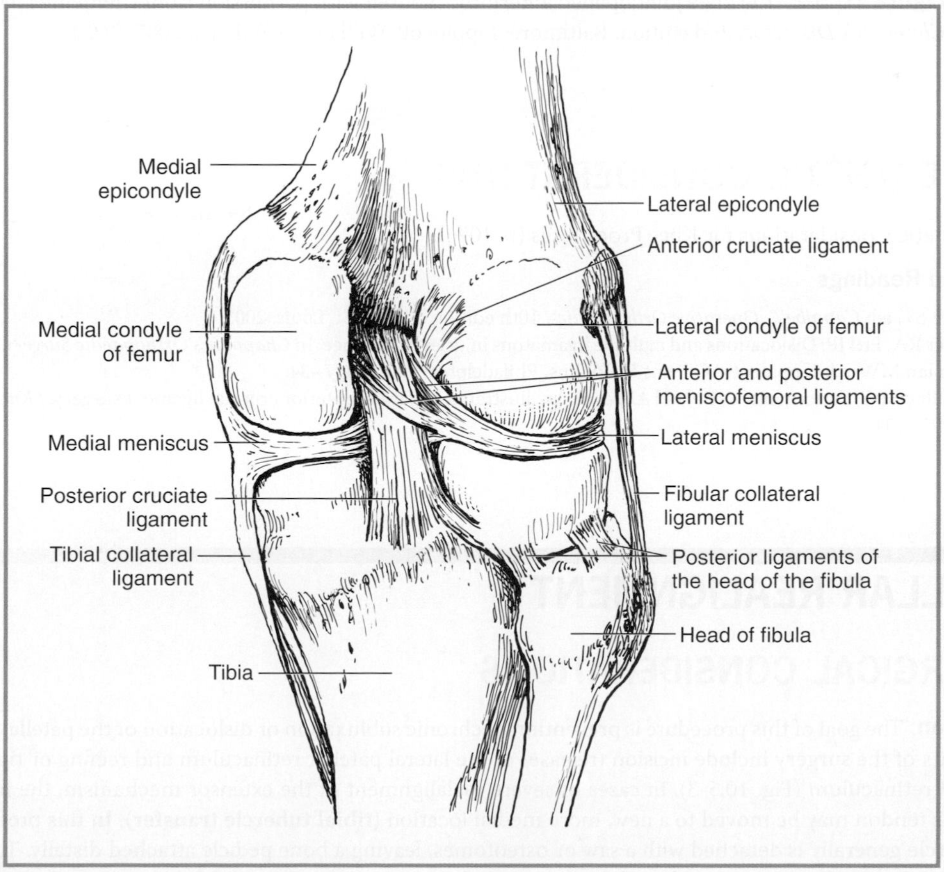

Figure 10.5-1. The cruciate ligaments (posterior view). (Reused with permission from Clemente CD. *Clemente's Dissector*, 2nd edition. Baltimore: Lippincott Williams & Wilkins, 2007: 270.)

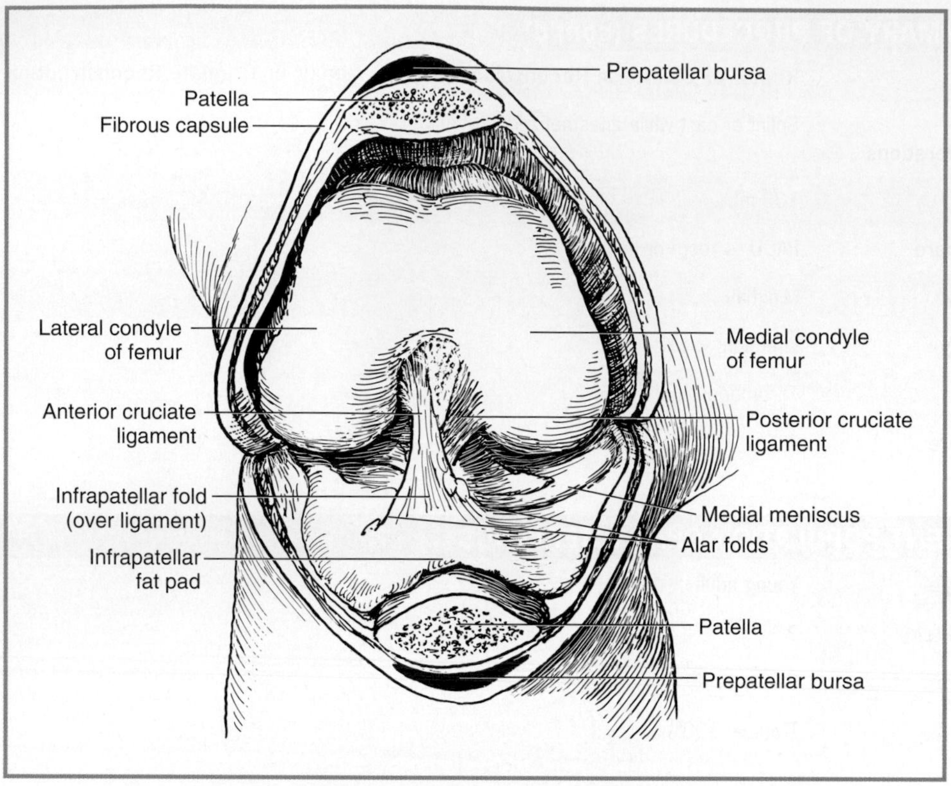

Figure 10.5-2. The knee joint opened anteriorly. (Reused with permission from Clemente CD. *Clemente's Dissector*, 2nd edition. Baltimore: Lippincott Williams & Wilkins, 2007: 269.)

ANESTHETIC CONSIDERATIONS

See Anesthetic Considerations for Knee Procedures (p. 1026).

Suggested Readings

1. Canale ST, ed: *Campbell's Operative Orthopaedics,* 10th edition. Mosby, St. Louis: 2003.
2. Marder RA, Ertl JP: Dislocations and multiple ligamatous injuries of the knee. In *Chapman's Orthopaedic Surgery,* 3rd edition. Chapman MW, ed. Lippincott Williams & Wilkins, Philadelphia: 2001, 2417–34.
3. McCulloch PC, Lattermann C, Boland AL, et al: An illustrated history of anterior cruciate ligament surgery. *J Knee Surg* 2007; 20(2):95–104.

PATELLAR REALIGNMENT

SURGICAL CONSIDERATIONS

Description: The goal of this procedure is prevention of chronic subluxation or dislocation of the patella. Soft tissue components of the surgery include incision (release) of the lateral patellar retinaculum and reefing or tightening of the medial retinaculum (Fig. 10.5-3). In cases of severe malalignment of the extensor mechanism, the insertion of the patellar tendon may be moved to a new, more medial location (**tibial tubercle transfer**). In this procedure, the tibial tubercle generally is detached with a saw or osteotomes, leaving a bone pedicle attached distally. The tubercle is then rotated medially on the pedicle and fixed in its new position with a screw. Many surgeons routinely perform an **anterior compartment fasciotomy** to prevent postop compartment syndrome.

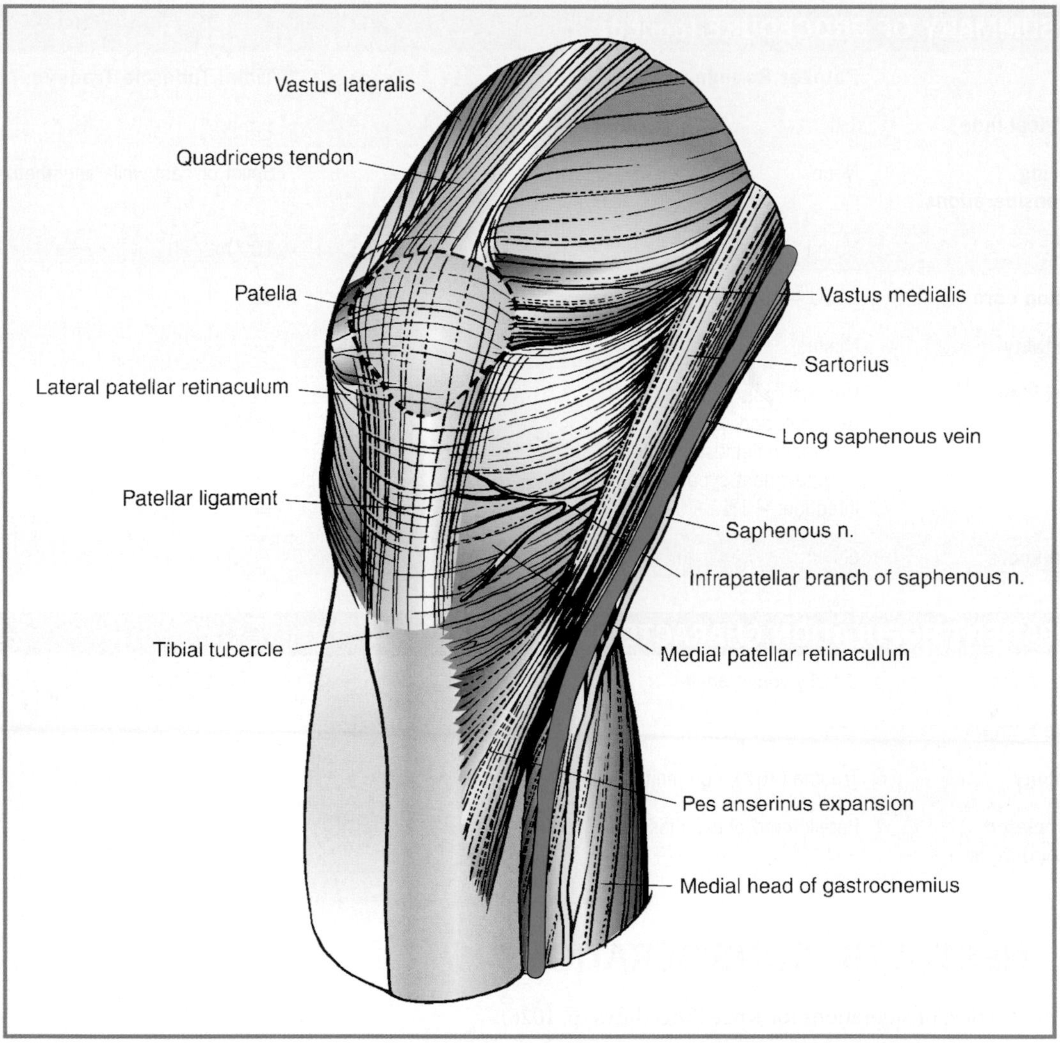

Figure 10.5-3. Outer layer of anteromedial aspect of the knee joint. Shows anatomy of the patellar retinaculum. (Reproduced with permission from Hoppenfeld S, deBoer P: *Surgical Exposures in Orthopaedics: The Anatomic Approach.* Lippincott Williams & Wilkins: 1994.)

Usual preop diagnosis: Chronic patellar subluxation or dislocation

SUMMARY OF PROCEDURES

	Patellar Realignment	Tibial Tubercle Transfer
Position	Supine	⇐
Incision	Anteromedial or anterolateral to knee	⇐
Special instrumentation	None	Screws or staples
Unique considerations	Tourniquet	⇐
Antibiotics	Cefazolin 1 g iv (vancomycin or clindamycin if penicillin allergic)	⇐

SUMMARY OF PROCEDURE (cont'd)

	Patellar Realignment	Tibial Tubercle Transfer
Surgical time	1 h	1.5 h
Closing considerations	None	Splint or cast while anesthetized
EBL	50 mL	100 mL
Postop care	PACU → room or home	⇐
Mortality	Minimal	⇐
Morbidity	Hemarthrosis: 100% Redislocation: 20% Thrombophlebitis: 10–20% Compartment syndrome: < 1% Infection: < 1%	5% 25% ⇐ ⇐ ⇐
Pain score	6	7

PATIENT POPULATION CHARACTERISTICS

Age range	Usually young adult
Male:Female	1:2
Etiology	Trauma (70%); congenital (30%)
Associated conditions	Patellofemoral dysphasia (60–70%)

ANESTHETIC CONSIDERATIONS

See Anesthetic Considerations for Knee Procedures (p. 1026).

Suggested Readings

1. Epps CH Jr, ed: *Complications in Orthopaedic Surgery,* 3rd edition. JB Lippincott, Philadelphia: 1994.
2. Griffin LY, Duralde XA: Adolescent sports injuries. In: *Chapman's Orthopaedic Surgery,* 3rd edition. Chapman MW, ed. Lippincott Williams & Wilkins, Philadelphia: 2001, 2493–2536.

ARTHROSCOPY OF THE KNEE

SURGICAL CONSIDERATIONS

Description: **Knee arthroscopy** is used to diagnose and treat intraarticular problems, most commonly torn meniscus, but the procedure is also used for ligament injuries (Fig 10.5-1, 10.5-2), osteochondral fractures, loose bodies, arthritis, and infections. In knee arthroscopy, multiple portals or entry points for the arthroscope and instruments generally are used. The most common portals are anteromedial and anterolateral adjacent to the patellar ligament. Other portals may be suprapatellar, parapatellar, and posterior. Portals are made by making a stab wound with a knife and then entering the joint with a combination of sharp and blunt trochars. A diagnostic inspection from one of the anterior portals is normally performed at the outset. A second portal is used with a nerve hook to manipulate intraarticular tissues. If resection or repair is performed, the appropriate instruments are inserted through one of the portals. Meniscus repair and cruciate reconstruction may require separate longitudinal incisions, which are usually posteromedial or posterolateral, for placement of sutures and/or drill holes.

Meniscectomy and/or **debridement** often are performed in conjunction with arthroscopy. **Cruciate ligament reconstruction** usually is performed with arthroscopic assistance. At the end of the procedure, the knee joint is copiously irrigated with NS or LR solution through one of the portals. Portals are closed with a single suture and Steri-Strips®; compression bandages are applied; and often a knee immobilizer is used.

Usual preop diagnosis: Torn meniscus; cruciate ligament tear; arthritis

SUMMARY OF PROCEDURES

	Arthroscopy	Meniscectomy/Debridement	Cruciate Reconstruction
Position	Supine	⇐	⇐
Incision	3–4.5 cm portals	⇐	⇐ + anterior midline and lateral
Special instrumentation	Arthroscopic video system; small biters and graspers	⇐ + shaver	⇐ + drill guides and drills; fixation screws
Unique considerations	Thigh holder; foot of table 90°; ± tourniquet	⇐	⇐
Antibiotics	Cefazolin 1 g iv (vancomycin or clindamycin if penicillin allergic)	⇐	⇐
Surgical time	0.5 h	1–2 h	2–3 h
Closing considerations	No splint; local anesthetic injected	⇐	⇐
EBL	Minimal	⇐	50 mL
Postop care	PACU → home	⇐	⇐ or overnight
Mortality	< 0.1%	⇐	⇐
Morbidity	Hemarthrosis: 5–20% Thrombophlebitis: < 2% Infection: 0.1% Stiffness: < 0.1%	5% ⇐ ⇐ < 4%	⇐ ⇐ ⇐ ⇐
Pain score	3	4	6

PATIENT POPULATION CHARACTERISTICS

Age range	10–70 yr (usually 20–40 yr)
Male:Female	2:1
Incidence	The most common arthroscopic procedure (85% of total)
Etiology	Trauma (~85%); arthritis (~10%); infection (~5%)
Associated conditions	Usually healthy; systemic arthritis (< 5%)

ANESTHETIC CONSIDERATIONS

See Anesthetic Considerations for Knee Procedures (p. 1026).

Suggested Readings

1. Coward DB: Principles of arthroscopy of the knee. In *Chapman's Orthopaedic Surgery*, 3rd edition. Chapman MW, ed. Lippincott Williams & Wilkins, Philadelphia: 2001, 2269–98.

2. McGinty JB, ed: *Operative Arthroscopy*. 3rd edition. Lippincott Williams & Wilkins, Philadelphia: 2002.
3. Silvis ML, Clinch CR, Tillett JS, et al: Clinical inquiries. What is the best way to evaluate an acute traumatic knee injury? *J Fam Pract* 2008; 57(2):116–8.

KNEE ARTHROTOMY

SURGICAL CONSIDERATIONS

Description: **Arthrotomy** of the knee is the opening of the joint for drainage, excision of intraarticular tissue (synovium, meniscus, loose bodies), ligament repair/reconstruction, or fracture fixation. The knee generally is opened with a parapatellar incision, either medial or lateral, and the joint capsule is incised just adjacent to the patella. After the intra-articular pathology is addressed, a tight capsular closure is performed, followed by subcutaneous tissue and skin closure.

Variant procedure or approaches: **Arthrotomy with debridement** may be used for infection or arthropathy which produces debris. In both cases, **synovectomy** may be necessary.

Usual preop diagnosis: Infection; trauma (fracture, sprain, torn meniscus); arthritis

SUMMARY OF PROCEDURES

	Arthrotomy	Arthrotomy with Debridement	Arthrotomy with Synovectomy
Position	Supine	⇐	⇐
Incision	Medial or lateral parapatellar	⇐	⇐
Special instrumentation	Tourniquet	⇐	⇐
Antibiotics	Cefazolin 1 g iv (vancomycin or clindamycin if penicillin allergic)	⇐	⇐
Surgical time	1 h	2 h	2 h
Closing considerations	Compressive dressing; may be splinted; suction drain	⇐	⇐
EBL	100 mL	⇐	⇐
Postop care	PACU → room	⇐	⇐
Mortality	Minimal	⇐	⇐
Morbidity	Hemarthrosis: 100% Degenerative arthritis: 5–20% Stiffness: 5% Thrombophlebitis: 5% Infection: 1 %	⇐ ⇐ ⇐ ⇐ 10%	⇐ ⇐ ⇐ ⇐ 20%
Pain score	7	7	8

PATIENT POPULATION CHARACTERISTICS

Age range	Infant–elderly (usually young adult)
Male:Female	1:1
Incidence	Common

Orthopedic Surgery

PATIENT POPULATION CHARACTERISTICS (cont'd)	
Etiology	Infection; trauma; arthritis
Associated conditions	Inflammatory arthritis (20%)

ANESTHETIC CONSIDERATIONS

See Anesthetic Considerations for Knee Procedures (p. 1026).

Suggested Reading

1. Epps CH Jr, ed: *Complications in Orthopaedic Surgery*, 3rd edition. JB Lippincott, Philadelphia: 1994.

REPAIR OF TENDONS—KNEE AND LEG

SURGICAL CONSIDERATIONS

Description: Acute ruptures of tendons in the lower limb are repaired by **direct suture** and sometimes reinforced with part of another tendon. At the knee, patellar tendon ruptures are most common; at the ankle, Achilles tendon ruptures are most common. A longitudinal incision generally is made directly over the tendon. The tendon sheath is opened and tendon ends reapproximated with a nonabsorbable tendon stitch. If necessary, the repair may be augmented by synthetic tape or fascia, or protected with a wire that takes tension off the repair. The tendon sheath is closed separately from the skin incision; and a cast or splint is applied. **Achilles tendon repair** and **posterior tibial tendon repair** require different positioning. For an Achilles tendon repair, the patient is placed prone, and a longitudinal incision is made just medial to the tendon, spanning the rupture. The tendon sheath is incised and carefully protected. Torn ends of the tendon are approximated with multiple tendon stitches and may be protected with a fascial flap developed from the gastrocnemius fascia. The tendon sheath is closed carefully, followed by skin wound closure. A splint or cast is applied with the foot in equinus (plantar flexion).

Usual preop diagnosis: Tendon rupture

SUMMARY OF PROCEDURES	Posterior Tendon Repair	Achilles Tendon Repair
Position	Supine	Prone
Incision	Over tendon	⇐
Special instrumentation	Wire or synthetic tape for augmentation	⇐
Unique considerations	Tourniquet	⇐
Antibiotics	Cefazolin 1 g iv (vancomycin or clindamycin if penicillin allergic)	⇐
Surgical time	1 h	⇐
Closing considerations	Splint or cast while anesthetized	⇐
EBL	Minimal	⇐
Postop care	PACU → room or home	⇐

SUMMARY OF PROCEDURES (cont'd)		
	Posterior Tendon Repair	**Achilles Tendon Repair**
Mortality	Minimal	⇐
Morbidity	Weakness: ~10% Wound slough: 5% Adhesions: < 1% Infection: < 1%	⇐ ⇐ ⇐ ⇐ Rerupture: 5–10%
Pain score	3	3

PATIENT POPULATION CHARACTERISTICS	
Age range	Any age
Male:Female	1:1
Incidence	Uncommon
Etiology	Trauma (90%); chronic tendinitis (10%)
Associated conditions	Obesity; diabetes mellitus (DM); inflammatory arthritis

ANESTHETIC CONSIDERATIONS FOR KNEE PROCEDURES

(Procedures covered: arthroplasty; arthrodesis; ORIF of patellar fractures; repair/reconstruction of ligaments; patellar realignment; arthroscopy; arthrotomy; tendon repair—knee and leg)

PREOPERATIVE

Trauma and osteoarthritis (OA) are the most common indications for these procedures. Trauma patients (e.g., those with sports injuries) are often young and healthy, whereas arthritic patients are often elderly, and anesthetic management must be tailored to any concurrent disease. Patients with rheumatoid and other inflammatory arthritides form another group of candidates for these procedures; the special anesthetic considerations for these patients are described in Anesthetic Considerations for Hip Procedures, p. 997. A final group of patients undergoing these procedures are hemophiliacs, who develop arthritis from recurrent bleeding into their joints. The hematologic management of these patients is discussed below.

Respiratory	These patients often have **rheumatoid arthritis** and associated pulmonary conditions. For example, pulmonary effusions are common. Limited respiratory reserve warrants further evaluation. Pulmonary fibrosis (rare) often manifests as a cough and dyspnea. Rheumatoid arthritis involving the cricoarytenoid joints may manifest as hoarseness, glottic narrowing, and difficult intubation. Arthritic involvement of the TMJ and cervical spine may further complicate airway management. **Tests:** As indicated from H&P.
Cardiovascular	The severity of the arthritis often limits exercise and makes assessment of cardiovascular status difficult. Dobutamine stress ECHO, and dipyridamole thallium imaging may be necessary for an adequate cardiac evaluation. Rheumatoid arthritis is associated with pericardial effusion, cardiac valve fibrosis, cardiac conduction abnormalities and aortic regurgitation (AR). **Tests:** ECG and others as indicated from H&P.
Neurological	In arthritic patients, a thorough preop neurological exam often yields evidence of cervical nerve root compression. After the stability of the neck has been established, the full range of neck motion should be evaluated for evidence of nerve compression or cerebral ischemia (suggesting vertebral artery compression). Consider preop lateral neck films to determine stability of atlantooccipital joint and evidence of vertebral spurs that may interfere with intubation. **Tests:** As indicated from H&P.

Musculoskeletal	Pain and ↓ joint mobility may make positioning and regional anesthesia difficult in this patient population.
Hematologic	**Hemophiliacs** require restoration of clotting factors preop. Administer 1 U of factor concentrate/kg body weight for each 2% increase necessary to achieve clotting factor activity of 40% normal. FFP contains l U/mL and cryoprecipitate 20 U/mL. Hemophilia B (Factor IX deficiency), but not hemophilia A (Factor VIII deficiency), can be treated with prothrombin complex concentrate; however, these products can activate clotting factors and → DIC. Approximately 10% of hemophiliacs develop antibodies to exogenous clotting factors, and the care of these patients should be guided by a hematologist. **Tests:** Hct; other tests as indicated from H&P.
Laboratory	Other tests as indicated from H&P.
Premedication	Standard premedication (see p. B-1). Preop patellar pain is treated effectively with a femoral nerve block at the inguinal ligament, using 10 mL of lidocaine 1.5% with epinephrine 1:200,000.

INTRAOPERATIVE

Anesthetic technique: For many of these patients, regional anesthesia may be the preferred technique, offering the advantages of ↓ blood loss, ↓ DVT, minimal respiratory impairment, and effective postop analgesia. Patients with rheumatoid arthritis rarely have involvement of the lumbar spine. Because rheumatoid arthritis frequently affects the C-spine, however, these patients may have limited range of neck motion, an unstable atlantooccipital joint, and cricoarytenoid and TMJ arthritis. Careful airway evaluation, therefore, is important to determine the appropriateness of special intubation techniques (e.g., fiber optic).

Regional anesthesia: A continuous peripheral nerve block (CPNB) provides similar effect on postop length of hospital stay and rehabilitation compared to an epidural pain management but has a lower incidence of side effects (urinary retention, hypotension, and dysesthesia). A combined femoral and sciatic nerve block provides superior pain control in the first 36 postoperative hours over a single, femoral nerve block. In addition to the nerve block, either a GA or a SAB is needed for the intraoperative phase since a CPNB does not reliably provide surgical anesthesia. Both nerves can be localized conventionally using a nerve stimulator or with ultrasound-guidance. A typical initial local anesthesia dose for each nerve is 20 mL of 0.5% bupivacaine or 0.75% ropivacaine.

An epidural block provides both intraop surgical anesthesia and postop pain control but it is contraindicated in patients receiving Coumadin postop. If the patient prefers not to receive a peripheral nerve or an epidural block, a subarachnoid block provides a useful alternative regional anesthesia technique, depending on the patient population (e.g., younger patients may be at ↑ risk of spinal headache following SAB). Anesthesia extending from S2 to T12 (T8, if tourniquet is used) is adequate for knee surgery. Full motor blockade is essential for fixation of the patella, or placement of the joint prosthesis and assessment of the passive ROM of the prosthesis. Typical drugs and doses include: subarachnoid—12.5–15 mg of 0.75% bupivacaine with morphine 0.2 mg; epidural—15–20 mL 2% lidocaine with epinephrine 1:200,000 in divided doses.

General anesthesia:

Induction	Standard induction (see p. B-2) is appropriate for patients with normal airways.	
Maintenance	Standard maintenance (see p. B-2). Neuromuscular relaxation facilitates the placement of the prosthesis. Hemophiliacs will require infusion of clotting factors. For hemophilia A and von Willebrand's disease, 1.5 U/kg/h; for hemophilia B, 0.75 U/kg/h.	
Emergence	The tourniquet is deflated around the time of emergence. In patients with moderate-to-severe lung disease, controlled ventilation should be continued until after the lactic acid that has accumulated in the leg has been metabolized (3–5 min), because these patients may be unable to increase ventilation to buffer this acid load.	
Blood and fluid requirements	IV: 14–16 ga × 1 NS/LR @ maintenance during the case, and 5–10 mL/kg bolus prior to tourniquet deflation	A tourniquet blocks intraop blood loss. When it is deflated, prepare for a 1–2 U blood loss over the ensuing h; more if the posterior tibial artery has been damaged in the dissection. Avoid under-resuscitation.

Control of blood loss	Tourniquet	Inflation pressure is typically 100 mmHg + systolic pressure. Maximum tourniquet time is 2 h, followed by a 30 min reperfusion interval, if further tourniquet time is necessary.
Monitoring	Standard monitors (see p. B-1). ± CVP line ± Arterial line	A CVP line is indicated if monitoring the CVP trend is expected to affect anesthetic care. Additional monitoring (CVO_2Sat, PA cath, TEE) may be indicated in special cases.
Positioning	✓ and pad pressure points. ✓ eyes.	In rheumatoid arthritic patients, meticulous padding of the extremities is mandatory.
Complications	Posterior tibial artery trauma Peroneal nerve palsy	A 20% ↓MAP is common on tourniquet deflation. Additional crystalloid (5–10 mL/kg) may be necessary to replace edema fluid and blood loss to the leg.

POSTOPERATIVE

Complications	Hemorrhage from the posterior tibial artery	✓ surgical drain output.
	Peroneal nerve palsy → foot drop	Examine patient for evidence of neurologic dysfunction and notify surgeons as necessary.
	Tourniquet-related nerve injury	
	Post-tourniquet syndrome (PTS)	PTS is a self-limiting condition in which the affected limb is edematous, pale, and weak.
Pain management	Neuraxial regimens: • Epidural anesthesia	Epidural bupivacaine 0.0125% infused at 6–8 mL/h with hydromorphone 50 mcg/mL infused at 100–250 mcg/h provides good analgesia. Prior to removal of the epidural catheter a 0.2 mg bolus of hydromorphone may be given. Epidural catheters are typically removed on the morning of postop day 2. Low-molecular-weight heparin may be started 2 h after catheter removal.
	• SAB	Intrathecal morphine 0.2–0.3 mg provides analgesia for up to 24 h. May be administered along with bupivacaine for surgical anesthesia.
	Peripheral regimens: • Single-shot peripheral nerve block (femoral or combined femoral/sciatic block)	These nerves may be blocked preop or postop as a pain rescue measure. A typical dose for each nerve is 20 mL of 0.5% bupivacaine or 0.75% ropivacaine.
	• CPNB	Continuous infusion of bupivacaine 0.125% through a standard infusion pump or a portable/disposable pump. Foley catheters are not required with peripheral nerve catheters.
	Systemic regimens:	Oral pain management with acetaminophen should be initiated immediately postoperatively (if not contraindicated). Patient-controlled analgesia (PCA) with IV morphine or hydromorphone may be initiated as alternative to neuraxial blocks or to supplement peripheral regimens.

Tests	Hct; other studies as indicated.	Patients with coagulopathies require replacement therapy for 6–10 d.

Suggested Readings

1. Choi PT, Bhandari M, Scott J, et al: Epidural analgesia for pain relief following hip or knee replacement. *Cochrane Database Syst Rev* 2003; 3:CD003071.
2. Epps CH Jr, ed: *Complications in Orthopaedic Surgery,* 3rd edition. JB Lippincott, Philadelphia: 1994.
3. Fowler SJ, Symons J, Sabato S, et al: Epidural analgesia compared with peripheral nerve blockade after major knee surgery: a systematic review and meta-analysis of randomized trials. *Br J Anaesth* 2008; 100(2):154–64.
4. Kuper M, Rosenstein A: Infection control in total knee and total hip arthroplasties. *Am J Orthop* 2008; 37(1):E2–5.
5. Rosenberg AG: Anesthesia and analgesia protocols for total knee arthroplasty. *Am J Orthop* 2006; 35(7 Suppl):23–6.
6. Scuderi GR: Preoperative planning and perioperative management for minimally invasive total knee arthroplasty. *Am J Orthop* 2006; 35(7 Suppl):4–6.

CHAPTER

10.6 Lower Leg, Ankle, Foot, and Other Lower-Extremity Procedures

SURGEON

John J. Csongradi, MD

ANESTHESIOLOGIST

Frederick G. Mihm, MD

OPEN REDUCTION AND INTERNAL FIXATION (ORIF) OF THE TIBIAL PLATEAU FRACTURE

SURGICAL CONSIDERATIONS

Description: **ORIF of the tibial plateau** or proximal tibia fracture involves making a longitudinal incision along the proximal leg, lateral to the knee, obtaining a reduction by direct visualization of the fracture fragments, and applying plates and screws along the tibia for rigid internal fixation. An iliac crest bone graft may be necessary. A **proximal tibial osteotomy** involves correcting malalignment (valgus and varus) of the lower extremity by excising a wedge of bone from the tibia and correcting the mechanical axis.

Usual preop diagnosis: Tibial plateau or proximal tibial fracture; nonunion/malunion of the tibial plateau or proximal tibia; degenerative arthritis of the knee, with varus or valgus deformity

SUMMARY OF PROCEDURES

	ORIF Tibial Plateau Fracture	Proximal Tibial Osteotomy
Position	Supine	⇐
Incision	Lateral to knee, usually; medial, rarely	Transverse or lateral incision
Special instrumentation	Special plates, screws; reduction clamps; radiolucent table	⇐
Unique considerations	Intraop radiographs or I.I.; tourniquet	⇐
Antibiotics	Cefazolin or cefamandole 1 g iv q 6–8 h × 48 h	⇐
Surgical time	~2.5–3 h; more, depending on difficulty	⇐
Closing considerations	Splint, cast while anesthetized	⇐
EBL	< 200 mL	⇐
Postop care	Multiple-trauma victim → ICU; others → PACU; ± CPM	PACU → ward
Mortality	Rare, except in severe multiple trauma	None
Morbidity	Compartment syndrome: 10–20% Wound infection: 7–15% DVT (symptomatic): 3–5% Delayed union, nonunion, malunion: < 5% Peripheral nerve damage: 3% Intraarticular fracture: 2% Hypotension (multiple trauma) Leg-length discrepancy Osteomyelitis, septic arthritis Respiratory distress and fat embolism Vascular complications	< 25% ~2% 2% ⇐ 0.2%
Pain score	7	7

PATIENT POPULATION CHARACTERISTICS

Age range	Any age; fracture most common in younger trauma patients and elderly Degenerative arthritis of knee, < 60 yr
Male:Female	1:1
Incidence	Common
Etiology	Trauma: falls, motorcycle and motor vehicle accidents, industrial injuries Degenerative: arthritis of knee

ANESTHETIC CONSIDERATIONS

See Anesthetic Considerations for Lower-Extremity Procedures, p. (1059).

Suggested Readings

1. Aglietti P, Chambat P: Fractures of the knee. In *Surgery of the Knee.* Insall JN, ed. Churchill Livingstone, New York: 1984, 395–490.
2. Egol KA, Koval KJ: Fractures of the tibial plateau. In *Chapman's Orthopaedic Surgery,* 3rd edition, Vol I. Chapman MW, ed. Lippincott Williams & Wilkins, Philadelphia: 2001, 737–54.
3. LaVelle DG: Delayed union and nonunion of fractures. In *Campbell's Operative Orthopaedics,* Vol 3. Canale ST, ed. CV Mosby, St. Louis: 1998, 2579–2630.
4. Mize R, Johnson EE, Hohl M: Complications of fractures and dislocations of the knee. In *Complications in Orthopaedic Surgery,* 3rd edition. Epps CH Jr, ed. JB Lippincott, Philadelphia: 1994, 525–56.
5. Whittle AP: Malunited fractures. In *Campbell's Operative Orthopaedics.* Canale ST, ed. Mosby, St. Louis: 1998, 2537–78.
6. Wiss DA, Watson JT, Johnson EE: Fractures of the knee. In *Rockwood and Green's Fractures in Adults,* 4th edition. Rockwood CA Jr, Green DP, Bucholz RW, et al., eds. Lippincott-Raven, Philadelphia: 1996.

INTRAMEDULLARY NAILING, TIBIA

SURGICAL CONSIDERATIONS

Description: In intramedullary nailing of the tibia, a metal nail is placed into the medullary canal of the tibia to stabilize (or prevent) a fracture. The affected leg generally is placed in traction, on a fracture table, via stirrup or calcaneal pin. Following the incision, an awl is used to make an entry hole in the proximal metaphysis of the tibia, through which a guide wire is introduced. The guide wire is placed across the aligned fracture, and the nail is introduced and driven over the guide wire. Before nail insertion, the medullary canal often is reamed to allow use of a larger nail. Most nails are interlocked both proximally and distally with screws that pass from the bone through holes in the nail.

Usual preop diagnosis: Fracture, nonunion or malunion of the tibia

SUMMARY OF PROCEDURE	
Position	Supine, on fracture table. Consider inducing anesthesia before moving patient.
Incision	Proximal longitudinal incision over the patellar tendon; stab wound for screws
Special instrumentation	Nails, screws, and insertion instruments; intramedullary reamers; I.I.
Antibiotics	Cefazolin 1 g iv preop
Surgical time	2 h
Closing considerations	No splint or cast
EBL	200 mL
Postop care	PACU → room
Mortality	Minimal
Morbidity	Compartment syndrome: < 5% Infection: < 2% Neuropraxia: < 1 %
Pain score	5

PATIENT POPULATION CHARACTERISTICS	
Age range	> 16 yr
Male:Female	5:1
Etiology	Trauma (95%); tumor (5%)
Associated conditions	Multiple trauma (50%); compartment syndrome (5%)

ANESTHETIC CONSIDERATIONS

See Anesthetic Considerations for Lower-Extremity Procedures, p. 1059.

Suggested Reading

1. Bucholz RW, Heckman JD, eds: *Rockwood and Green's Fractures in Adults,* 5th edition. Lippincott Williams & Wilkins, Philadelphia: 2001.

EXTERNAL FIXATION, TIBIA

SURGICAL CONSIDERATIONS

Description: Fractures of the tibia are fixed with percutaneous pins that are clamped to an external frame. Stainless steel pins are drilled into the proximal and distal fragments of the fracture through stab wounds in the skin and subcutaneous tissues. Usually 2–3 pins are placed on either side of the fracture. Pin clamps and an external frame are attached and the fracture aligned with the assistance of the I.I. or under direct vision. Following fracture alignment, the pin clamps and frames are tightened to hold fracture alignment. External fixation is often used with open fractures. **Small-pin fixators** (e.g., Ilizarov) are used for fracture fixation, leg lengthening, and treatment of bony defects. Wound irrigation and debridement often accompany application of the fixation frame.

Usual preop diagnosis: Tibial fracture; tibial nonunion or malunion; tibial shortening

SUMMARY OF PROCEDURE	
Position	Supine
Incision	Stab wounds. Small-pin fixator may require metaphyseal incision for osteotomy.
Special instrumentation	Pins; fixation frame; I.I.
Antibiotics	Cefazolin l g iv preop
Surgical time	0.5–1 h Small-pin fixator: 3–5 h
Closing considerations	May be open fracture (usually left open)
EBL	50 mL; small-pin fixator, 100 mL
Postop care	PACU → room
Mortality	Minimal
Morbidity	Infection: 15% Compartment syndrome: < 2% Neuropraxia: < 1%
Pain score	2–3

Orthopedic Surgery

PATIENT POPULATION CHARACTERISTICS	
Age range	All ages
Male:Female	5:1
Incidence	Common
Etiology	Trauma (95%); shortened limb (< 2%); ununited or malunited fracture (< 2%)
Associated conditions	Open fracture (95%); compartment syndrome (< 2%); congenital anomaly (< 1%)

ANESTHETIC CONSIDERATIONS

See Anesthetic Considerations for Lower-Extremity Procedures, p. 1059.

Suggested Reading

1. Bucholz RW, Heckman JD, eds: *Rockwood and Green's Fractures in Adults,* 5th edition. Lippincott Williams & Wilkins, Philadelphia: 2001.

OPEN REDUCTION AND INTERNAL FIXATION (ORIF) OF DISTAL TIBIA, ANKLE, AND FOOT FRACTURES

SURGICAL CONSIDERATIONS

Description: ORIF is nearly always required for displaced fractures involving the ankle or joints in the foot. A longitudinal incision is made over the fractured medial and/or lateral malleoli. Dissection is carried directly down to the bone and the fracture is identified and reduced under direct vision.

Open fractures may require **irrigation and debridement.** The fractures are realigned under direct vision and fixed and stabilized with pins, plates, and/or screws. An intraop radiograph is obtained to confirm reduction and placement of hardware. The incisions are closed and a splint or cast is applied.

Usual preop diagnosis: Fracture of the distal tibia, ankle, or foot

SUMMARY OF PROCEDURES

	ORIF Ankle	With Irrigation and Debridement
Position	Supine	⇐
Incision	Longitudinal over fracture site	⇐ + extension of existing wound
Special instrumentation	Pins, plates, and screws; tourniquet; x-ray or I.I.	⇐
Antibiotics	Cefazolin 1 g iv preop	⇐
Surgical time	2 h	2–3 h
Closing considerations	Splint or cast while anesthetized	Splint or cast; may leave wound open.
EBL	50 mL	100 mL
Postop care	PACU → room	⇐
Mortality	Minimal	⇐
Morbidity	Wound dehiscence: 10% Loss of reduction: 7% Infection: 3%	⇐ ⇐ 15%
Pain score	4	4

PATIENT POPULATION CHARACTERISTICS	
Age range	Infant–elderly (usually > 60 yr)
Male:Female	1:1
Incidence	~ 250,000 cases/yr in the United States
Etiology	Trauma: 100%
Associated conditions	Alcohol abuse; obesity; diabetes mellitus (DM)

ANESTHETIC CONSIDERATIONS

See Anesthetic Considerations for Lower-Extremity Procedures, p. 1059.

Suggested Readings

1. Bucholz RW, Heckman JD, eds: *Rockwood and Green's Fractures in Adults,* 5th edition. Lippincott Williams & Wilkins, Philadelphia: 2001.
2. Carragee EJ, Csongradi JJ, Bleck EE: Early complications in the operative treatment of ankle fractures. Influence of delay before operation. *J Bone Joint Surg* 1991; 73(l):79–82.
3. Epps CH Jr, ed: *Complications in Orthopaedic Surgery,* 3rd edition. JB Lippincott, Philadelphia: 1994.

REPAIR NONUNION/MALUNION, TIBIA

SURGICAL CONSIDERATIONS

Description: This procedure is used to treat a fracture that has not healed or was misaligned upon healing. The fracture is mobilized, usually grafted with autogenous or allograft bone, and realigned. With an anterior approach, a longitudinal incision is made anteromedial or anterolateral to the shaft of the tibia. Dissection is carried directly down to the bone and the nonunion identified. If the tibia is approached with a posterolateral incision, the patient is turned prone and a longitudinal incision is made just posterior to the fibula. Dissection is carried down posteriorly to the interosseous membrane, to the tibia, and the procedure becomes identical to the anterior approach. Tissue interposed between the bone ends may or may not be débrided. The cortex of the bone adjacent to the nonunion is roughened with an osteotome. Autogenous or allograft bone is placed adjacent to or in the nonunion site. In the case of a malunion, the bone may be osteotomized with a saw or osteotomes to allow realignment. If skeletal fixation is used, a plate may be attached to the bone through the same incision. Alternatively, an intramedullary nail may be placed through an incision anterior to the tibial tubercle. If an intramedullary device is used, the canal may be reamed with intramedullary reamers prior to placement of the nail. A third type of **skeletal fixation** is the external fixator that stabilizes the nonunion via percutaneous pins placed into the proximal and distal tibia, which are then spanned by a device with pin clamps at both ends. An intraop x-ray is often used to confirm fixation and placement of devices; alternatively, an I.I. may be used.

Variant procedure or approaches: Autogenous **bone grafting from the iliac crest** is commonly used to stimulate healing. An incision is made directly over the iliac crest and muscles are stripped from the crest and table of the ilium. Osteotomes and gouges are used to remove either the inner or outer table of the ilium and cancellous bone between the two tables. The wound is closed over a suction drain.

Usual preop diagnosis: Ununited or malunited fracture

SUMMARY OF PROCEDURES			
	Basic Repair	With Iliac Graft	With Skeletal Fixation
Position	Supine (prone with posterior lateral graft)	⇐	⇐

SUMMARY OF PROCEDURES (cont'd)	Basic Repair	With Iliac Graft	With Skeletal Fixation
Incision	Anteromedial or posterolateral to shaft of tibia	Anteromedial; parallel to iliac crest	
Special instrumentation	Tourniquet; x-ray or I.I.	⇐	Pins, plates, screws, rods, external fixator; tourniquet; x-ray or I.I.
Antibiotics	Cefazolin 1 g iv preop. (If infected nonunion anticipated, antibiotics are withheld until cultures are obtained.)	⇐	⇐
Surgical time	2 h	2.5 h	3 h
Closing considerations	Splint or cast applied while anesthetized.	⇐	No splint or cast
EBL	100 mL	200–300 mL	⇐
Postop care	PACU → room	⇐	⇐
Mortality	Minimal	⇐	⇐
Morbidity	Thrombophlebitis: 5% Compartment syndrome: 1% Infection: 1% Hematoma: < 1%	⇐ ⇐ ⇐ 5%	⇐ ⇐ ⇐ 1–3%
Pain score	5	8	5–8

PATIENT POPULATION CHARACTERISTICS	
Age range	10–80 yr (usually 20–40 yr)
Male:Female	5:1
Incidence	5–10% of tibia fractures; 50–75% of open fractures
Etiology	Trauma: 100%
Associated conditions	Poor nutrition (50%); infection (10%); metabolic disease (10%)

ANESTHETIC CONSIDERATIONS

See Anesthetic Considerations for Lower-Extremity Procedures, p. 1059.

Suggested Readings

1. Csongradi JJ, Maloney WI: Ununited lower limb fractures. *West J Med* 1989; 150(6):675–80.
2. Epps CH Jr, ed: *Complications in Orthopaedic Surgery,* 3rd edition. JB Lippincott, Philadelphia: 1994.
3. Goulet JA, Hak DJ: Nonunions and malunions of the tibia. In *Chapman's Orthopaedic Surgery,* 3rd edition, Vol I. Chapman MW, ed. Lippincott Williams & Wilkins, Philadelphia: 2001, 977–1000.

ARTHROSCOPY OF THE ANKLE

SURGICAL CONSIDERATIONS

Description: Ankle arthroscopy is usually a diagnostic procedure, although it may be used for debridement or removal of loose bodies. The ankle joint generally is inspected through anterolateral and anteromedial portals (entry

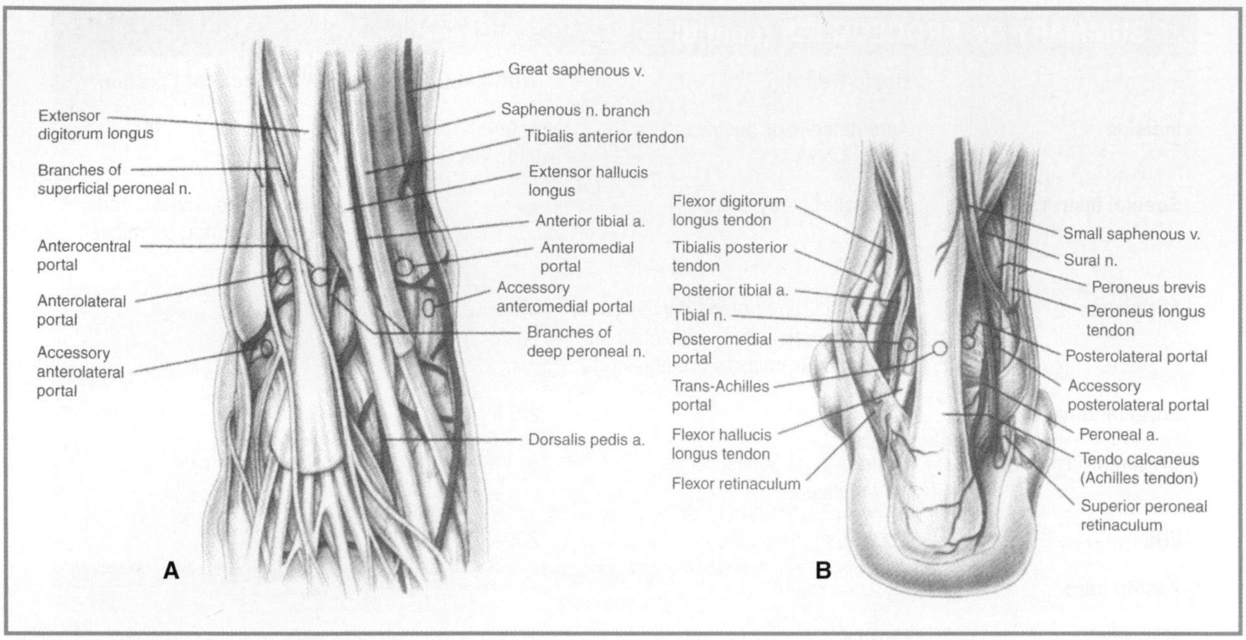

Figure 10.6-1. Portals for ankle arthroscopy. **A:** Anterior anatomy and portals. The anterolateral and anteromedial portals are used routinely. **B:** Posterior anatomy and portals. The posterolateral portal also is used routinely. (Reproduced with permission from Ferkel RD: *Arthroscopic Surgery: The Foot and Ankle.* Lippincott-Raven, 1996.)

wounds). Posterolateral and posteromedial portals also may be used. Each portal is made via a 5-mm stab wound in the skin (Fig. 10.6-1); then instrumentation is placed, using trochars. If the ankle joint is tight, a mechanical distractor (external fixator distraction apparatus spanning the ankle joint) may be used. The distractor is attached to the bones via percutaneous pins, as in the case of the application of an external fixator. The portals are closed with sterile tape or a single suture. **Debridement** may be used to reduce local or generalized articular damage.

Usual preop diagnosis: Trauma; infection; arthritis

SUMMARY OF PROCEDURES

	Arthroscopy	Arthroscopy + Debridement
Position	Supine	⇐
Incision	0.5 cm portals (incisions)	⇐
Special instrumentation	Arthroscopic video system; small biters and graspers	⇐ + shaver
Unique considerations	± Tourniquet. May use distractor with pins through tibia and calcaneus.	⇐
Antibiotics	Cefazolin 1 g iv preop (optional)	⇐
Surgical time	1 h	1–2 h
Closing considerations	No splint; incisions injected with local anesthetic.	⇐
EBL	Minimal	50 mL
Postop care	PACU → home	⇐
Mortality	< 0.01%	⇐
Morbidity	Hemarthrosis: 5% Thrombophlebitis < 2% Infection: < 1%	⇐ ⇐ ⇐
Pain score	2–3	3

PATIENT POPULATION CHARACTERISTICS	
Age range	12–70 yr (usually 20–40 yr)
Male:Female	1:1
Incidence	Uncommon
Etiology	Trauma (70%); arthritis (20%); infection (5%)
Associated conditions	Usually healthy; may have systemic arthritis.

ANESTHETIC CONSIDERATIONS

See Anesthetic Considerations for Lower-Extremity Procedures, p. 1059.

Suggested Readings

1. Ferkel RD, M[c]Grath SJ: Arthroscopy of the ankle. In *Chapman's Orthopaedic Surgery,* 3rd edition, Vol 3. Chapman MW, ed. Lippincott Williams & Wilkins, Philadelphia: 2001, 2441–66.
2. Lui TH: Arthroscopy and endoscopy of the foot and ankle: indications for new techniques. *Arthroscopy* 2007; 23(8):889–902.
3. McGinty JB, ed: *Operative Arthroscopy,* 3rd edition. Lippincott Williams & Wilkins, New York: 2002.

ANKLE ARTHROTOMY

SURGICAL CONSIDERATIONS

Description: Arthrotomy of the ankle is the opening of the joint for drainage, debridement, or fracture treatment. The joint usually is opened with an anterolateral midline or anteromedial longitudinal incision. Tendons and neurovascular structures are carefully retracted to expose the joint capsule, which is then opened in line with the skin incision. After intra-articular pathology is addressed, careful closure of the capsule is performed, taking care to obtain good hemostasis.

Usual preop diagnosis: Infection; trauma; arthritis

SUMMARY OF PROCEDURE	
Position	Supine
Incision	Anterior midline or anteromedial longitudinal
Special instrumentation	Tourniquet
Antibiotics	Cefazolin 1 g iv preop
Surgical time	1–2 h
Closing considerations	± Splint while anesthetized; may have suction drain.
EBL	Minimal
Postop care	PACU → room
Mortality	Minimal
Morbidity	Hemarthrosis: 20% Thrombophlebitis: 5% Infection: 1%
Pain score	5

PATIENT POPULATION CHARACTERISTICS	
Age range	Infant – elderly
Male:Female	1:1
Incidence	Rare
Etiology	Trauma (70%); arthritis (20%); infection (10%)
Associated conditions	Inflammatory arthritis; multiple trauma; immunosuppression

ANESTHETIC CONSIDERATIONS

See Anesthetic Considerations for Lower-Extremity Procedures, p. 1059.

Suggested Reading

1. Crenshaw AH, ed: *Campbell's Operative Orthopaedics,* 10th edition. Mosby, St. Louis: 2003.

ANKLE ARTHRODESIS

SURGICAL CONSIDERATIONS

Description: An **ankle fusion** may need to be performed for severe pain 2° arthritis of the ankle. In most cases, an anterior approach is made to the ankle joint. An alternative approach is through the medial malleolus. The ankle joint is exposed and the surfaces of the joint are débrided either with osteotomes or a burr. Cancellous bone is exposed on the distal tibia and talus, and the joint is clamped together either with a simple external fixation device with pins going through the distal tibia and talus, or with bone screws that go from the distal tibia into the talus. The wound is closed over a drain, and a splint may be applied.

Usual preop diagnosis: Arthritis of the ankle

SUMMARY OF PROCEDURE	
Position	Supine
Incision	Anterior midline over distal tibia
Special instrumentation	Tourniquet; external fixator or bone screws
Unique considerations	Intraop radiographs; tourniquet use
Antibiotics	Cefazolin 1 g iv preop
Surgical time	2 h
Closing considerations	May be splinted; suction drain.
EBL	100 mL
Postop care	PACU → room
Mortality	Minimal
Morbidity	Nonunion (late): 15% Thrombophlebitis: 10%

SUMMARY OF PROCEDURES (cont'd)	
Morbidity (con't)	Hematoma: 5% Wound dehiscence: 5% Infection: 1%
Pain score	8

PATIENT POPULATION CHARACTERISTICS	
Age range	All adult
Male:Female	1:1
Etiology	Degenerative arthritis; trauma; avascular necrosis of talus; septic arthritis
Associated conditions	Inflammatory arthritis; any disease requiring steroids

ANESTHETIC CONSIDERATIONS

See Anesthetic Considerations for Lower-Extremity Procedures, p. 1059.

Suggested Readings

1. Chapman MW, ed: *Operative Orthopaedics.* 3rd edition. Lippincott Williams & Wilkins, Philadelphia: 2000.
2. Crenshaw AH, ed: *Campbell's Operative Orthopaedics,* 10th edition. Mosby, St. Louis: 2003.

REPAIR/RECONSTRUCTION OF ANKLE LIGAMENTS

SURGICAL CONSIDERATIONS

Description: Lateral ankle ligaments may be repaired acutely, but generally are reconstructed at a later date, if necessary, with the peroneus brevis used in most reconstructions. An incision is made posterior to the distal fibula, curving around the lateral malleolus and ending in the anterolateral foot. The peroneus brevis tendon is identified and detached from its musculotendinous junction in the leg, and the peroneus brevis muscle is sutured to the peroneus longus tendon. A hole is drilled from anterior to posterior in the distal lateral malleolus; then the detached end of the peroneus brevis tendon is threaded through the hole. It is then attached to either the calcaneus or the talus, anterior to the lateral malleolus, with a staple or by suturing into a hole in the bone. The skin and subcutaneous tissues are closed and a splint or cast is applied.

Usual preop diagnosis: Lateral instability of the ankle

SUMMARY OF PROCEDURE	
Position	Supine or lateral decubitus
Incision	Posterolateral aspect of ankle
Special instrumentation	Bone staples; tourniquet
Antibiotics	Cefazolin, 1 g iv preop
Surgical time	2 h
Closing considerations	Splint or cast while still anesthetized.
EBL	Minimal
Postop care	PACU → room or home

SUMMARY OF PROCEDURES (cont'd)	
Mortality	Minimal
Morbidity	Infection: < 1% Rerupture: < 1% Wound dehiscence: < 0.1%
Pain score	5

PATIENT POPULATION CHARACTERISTICS	
Age range	Young adults
Male:Female	2:1
Etiology	Ankle sprain
Associated conditions	Alcohol abuse; obesity; diabetes mellitus (DM)

ANESTHETIC CONSIDERATIONS

See Anesthetic Considerations for Lower-Extremity Procedures, p. 1059.

Suggested Readings

1. Epps CH Jr, ed: *Complications in Orthopaedic Surgery,* 3rd edition. JB Lippincott, Philadelphia: 1994.
2. Marder RA: Ankle ligament injuries. In: *Chapman's Orthopaedic Surgery,* 3rd edition, Vol 3. Chapman MW, ed. Lippincott Williams & Wilkins, Philadelphia: 2001, 2473–84.

AMPUTATION THROUGH ANKLE (SYME)

SURGICAL CONSIDERATIONS

Description: Syme's amputation (Figs 10.6-2, 10.6-3) is ankle disarticulation with closure, using a posterior flap, including the heel pad. It is more functional than below-knee amputation, because patients can bear weight on the

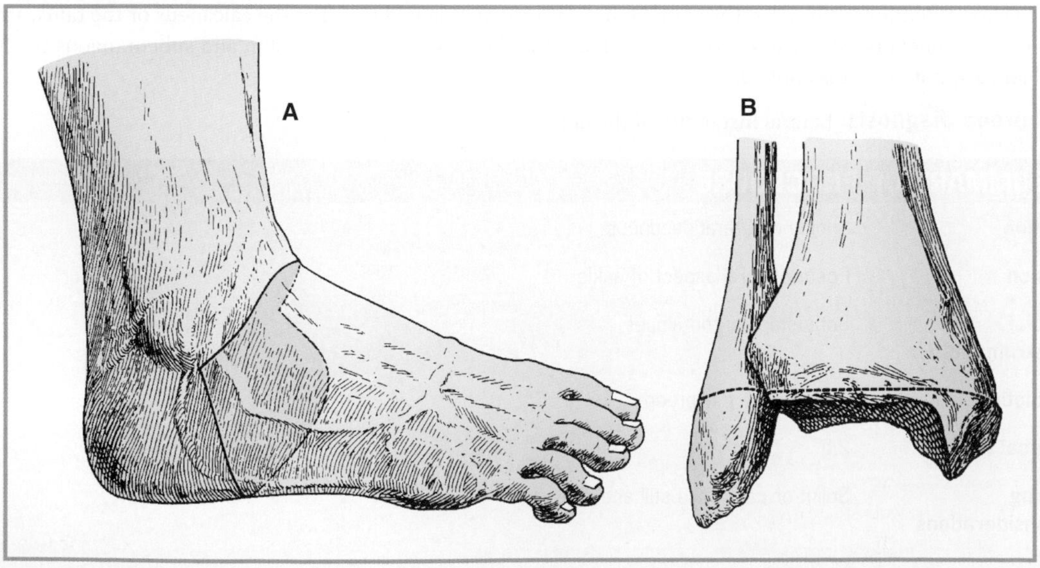

Figure 10.6-2. Syme's amputation. **A:** Skin incisions. **B:** Level of bone transection in adults. (Reproduced from Bohne WHO: *Atlas of Amputation Surgery.* Thieme Medical, 1987.)

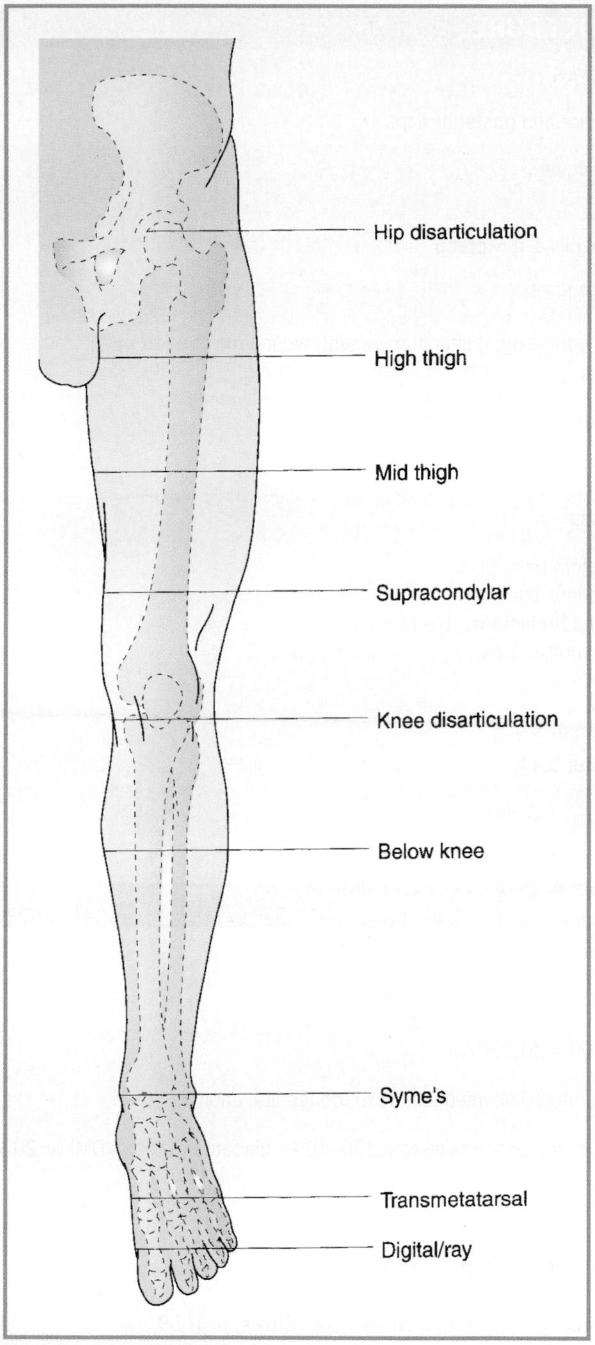

Figure 10.6-3. Common amputation levels for the lower extremity. (Reproduced with permission from Greenfield LJ, et al: *Surgery: Scientific Principles and Practices,* 3rd edition. Lippincott Williams & Wilkins, 2001.)

end of the stump; however, success is poor in patients with vascular disease or peripheral neuropathy. The posterior flap is dissected directly from the calcaneus, carefully preserving the tough heel pad and its blood supply. The heel pad is sutured directly to the distal tibia to prevent migration and to cover the bone end. The posterior flap is then sutured to the anterior flap with interrupted sutures and a compression dressing applied.

Usual preop diagnosis: Trauma; infection

SUMMARY OF PROCEDURE	
Position	Supine
Incision	Anterior and posterior flaps
Special instrumentation	Tourniquet
Antibiotics	Cefazolin 1 g iv preop
Surgical time	1.5–2 h
Closing considerations	Bulky dressing; if infection present, wound may be left open.
EBL	100 mL
Postop care	PACU → room
Mortality	Minimal
Morbidity	Phantom pain: 90% Infection: 10–15% Wound breakdown: 10–15% Pneumonia: 12% MI: 7% PE: 6% Hematoma: 5% Stroke: 5%
Pain score	5

PATIENT POPULATION CHARACTERISTICS	
Age range	Typically, > 60 yr
Male:Female	3:1
Incidence	20,000–30,000/yr
Etiology	Trauma (50%); infection (30%); congenital anomaly (5%)
Associated conditions	Peripheral vascular disease (30–40%); diabetes mellitus (DM) (< 20%)

ANESTHETIC CONSIDERATIONS

See Anesthetic Considerations for Lower-Extremity Procedures, p. 1059.

Suggested Readings

1. Bohne WHO, Ertl JP: Amputations of the lower extremity. In *Chapman's Orthopaedic Surgery,* 3rd edition, Vol 3. Chapman MW, ed. Lippincott Williams & Wilkins, Philadelphia: 2001, 3157.
2. Epps CH Jr, ed: *Complications in Orthopaedic Surgery,* 3rd edition. JB Lippincott, Philadelphia: 1994.

AMPUTATION, TRANSMETATARSAL

SURGICAL CONSIDERATIONS

Description: This amputation, usually for infection or ischemic necrosis of the toes, is performed at the mid-metatarsal level, leaving the patient able to walk without a prosthesis. A transverse dorsal incision is made at the transmetatarsal level, and a plantar incision is made beginning at the corners of the dorsal incision and extending distally to the metatarsal heads to create a long plantar flap. The plantar flap is reflected proximally to the midmetatarsal level and tapered distally. The metatarsals are sectioned with a saw, and nerves and tendons are sectioned proximal to the osteotomies. The plantar flap is then brought over the ends of the bones and sutured with interrupted sutures to the dorsal flap. A compression dressing is applied.

Variant procedure or approaches: Other partial-foot amputations, such as **midtarsal** and **ray amputation,** are much less common. They are managed in a fashion similar to that of the transmetatarsal amputation.

Usual preop diagnosis: Gangrene of the toes; infection

SUMMARY OF PROCEDURE	
Position	Supine
Incision	Dorsal and plantar flaps
Special instrumentation	Tourniquet
Antibiotics	Cefazolin 1 g iv preop
Surgical time	1–2 h
Closing considerations	Bulky dressing
EBL	50 mL
Postop care	PACU → room
Mortality	Minimal
Morbidity	Phantom pain: 90% Infection: 10–15% Wound breakdown: 10–15% Hematoma: 5%
Pain score	5

PATIENT POPULATION CHARACTERISTICS	
Age range	> 60 yr
Male:Female	3:1
Incidence	20,000–30,000 total amputations/yr
Etiology	Vascular disease (70%); infection (25%) trauma (< 5%); congenital anomalies (< 1%)
Associated conditions	Vascular disease (70%); diabetes mellitus (30%); pulmonary disease (30%)

ANESTHETIC CONSIDERATIONS

See Anesthetic Considerations for Lower-Extremity Procedures, p. 1059.

Suggested Readings

1. Bohne WHO, Ertl JP: Ampuations of the lower extremity. In *Chapman's Orthopaedic Surgery,* 3rd edition, Vol 3. Chapman MW, ed. Lippincott Williams & Wilkins, Philadelphia: 2001, 3152–5.
2. Canale ST, ed: *Campbell's Operative Orthopaedics,* 10th edition. Mosby, St. Louis: 2003.
3. Epps CH Jr, ed: *Complications in Orthopaedic Surgery,* 3rd edition. JB Lippincott, Philadelphia: 1994.

LENGTHENING OR TRANSFER OF TENDONS, ANKLE, AND FOOT

SURGICAL CONSIDERATIONS

Description: In cases of motor imbalance from neuromuscular disease or trauma, tendons are lengthened or transferred to a new insertion to partially restore balance or normalize joint motion. For **tendon lengthening,** a longitudinal incision generally is made directly over the tendon. Subcutaneous tissues and tendon sheath are incised to expose the tendon, which is transected with a Z-type incision. The tendon is placed in its lengthened position and the ends of the Z are closed with absorbable suture. If present, the tendon sheath is closed separately from the skin closure. In a **tendon transfer,** the tendon usually is cut close to its insertion and transferred to a new bony insertion, which often requires a separate incision. The tendon is attached to the bone either with a metal staple or by suturing it into a drill hole in the bone.

Variant procedure or approaches: Achilles tendon lengthening is used to bring the ankle out of equinus. A **posterior tibial tendon lengthening** and/or **posterior ankle capsulotomy** may accompany the procedure.

Usual preop diagnosis: Contracture of muscle

SUMMARY OF PROCEDURES

	Tendon Lengthening	Achilles Tendon Lengthening
Position	Supine	Prone
Incision	Over tendon; sometimes multiple incisions	Over tendon
Special instrumentation	Tourniquet	⇐
Antibiotics	If young, none; in elderly or infirm, cefazolin 1 g iv preop	⇐
Surgical time	2 h	1 h
Closing considerations	Splint or cast while anesthetized	⇐
EBL	10 mL	⇐
Postop care	PACU → room	PACU → room or home
Mortality	Minimal	⇐
Morbidity	Infection: < 1 %	⇐
Pain score	4	3

PATIENT POPULATION CHARACTERISTICS

Age range	Any age
Male:Female	1:1
Incidence	Rare
Etiology	Neuromuscular disease (80%); trauma (20%)
Associated conditions	Static encephalopathy/cerebral palsy (75%); other neuromuscular disease (25%)

ANESTHETIC CONSIDERATIONS

See Anesthetic Considerations for Lower-Extremity Procedures, p. 1059.

Orthopedic Surgery

Suggested Reading

1. Canale ST, ed: *Campbell's Operative Orthopaedics,* 10th edition. Mosby, St. Louis: 2003.

AMPUTATION ABOVE THE KNEE

SURGICAL CONSIDERATIONS

Description: In above-the-knee amputations, the distal part of the lower extremity is excised, starting just above the knee at the level of the distal third of the femur (Fig. 10.6–3). A stump is fashioned, and will require prosthetic fitting at a later time. The most commonly performed stumps incorporate anterior and posterior flaps of equal length. The underlying muscles (hamstrings and quadriceps) are either sewn to each other (**myoplasty**) or to bone (**myodesis**). In a **guillotine,** or **open amputation,** the stump is not fashioned (tissues are not closed) until later. This is a multistage procedure used for dirty, traumatic amputations, infection, or above-knee amputations with questionable survival, and usually is done as a life-saving measure. Internal fixation of part of the remaining femur may be indicated in traumatic amputations. The patient returns to the OR every 1–3 d for redebridement until closure of the clean stump can be performed.

Usual preop diagnosis: PVD or gangrene of lower extremity; trauma to lower extremity; open-femur fracture with traumatic amputation; tumor of lower extremity

SUMMARY OF PROCEDURE	
Position	Supine
Incision	Anterior and posterior on thigh
Special instrumentation	Amputation saw and rasp; drill for myodesis
Unique considerations	Patient often very ill from sepsis, chronic disease, or trauma
Antibiotics	Cefazolin or cefamandole 1 g iv q 6–8 h), ± gentamicin (80 mg iv q 8 h); adjust dosage for renal status, ± penicillin (1–2 million U iv q 4 h).
Surgical time	1–2 h
Closing considerations	Compressive dressing ± special stump sock
EBL	250 mL or more; higher for traumatic amputations
Postop care	Generally PACU → room (if medically unstable → ICU)
Mortality	Approximately 10–20%; higher in PVD (10–39%)
Morbidity	Phantom limb: 85–95% Phantom pain: 2–15% Wound infection ± deep infection: < 15% in PVD Respiratory failure or pneumonia: 10–15% MI: 7–10% Thromboembolism: 6–10% Cerebrovascular accident: 5–10% Contractures – flexion and abduction: Common Urinary retention requiring catheterization: Common Failure to heal ± wound dehiscence: Uncommon Hematoma: Rare Neuromas: Rare Reamputation: Rare UTI: Rare Contralateral amputation, especially in diabetics and those with PVD Postop depression
Pain score	7–10

PATIENT POPULATION CHARACTERISTICS

Age range	PVD, diabetic gangrene: 70–90% > 60 yr Multiple trauma with traumatic amputation, tumor of lower extremity: 18–35 yr
Male:Female	Overall, 3:1 Elderly, predominance of males Multiple trauma, 4–5:1 Tumor 1:1
Incidence	Common for PVD patients; rare for trauma or tumor
Etiology	PVD and diabetic gangrene (70–90%); multiple trauma (younger patients) (rare—usually with severe grade IIIC injuries with neurovascular severance); tumor (rare); uncontrollable infection (e.g., gas gangrene) (rare)
Associated conditions	Diabetes (70–80% of patients presenting for this procedure); numerous other serious medical conditions; multiple trauma in younger patients

ANESTHETIC CONSIDERATIONS

See Anesthetic Considerations for Above- and Below-Knee Amputation, p. 1050.

Suggested Readings

1. McCollough NC III, Epps CH Jr, Banks WJ Jr: Complications of amputation surgery. In *Complications in Orthopaedic Surgery,* 3rd edition. Epps CH Jr, ed. JB Lippincott, Philadelphia: 1994, 1279–1308.
2. Swiontkowski MF, Post PA: Surgical approaches to the lower extremity. In *Chapman's Orthopaedic Surgery,* 3rd edition, Vol I. Chapman MW, ed. Lippincott Williams & Wilkins, Philadelphia: 2001, 29–52.
3. Tooms RE: Amputations of lower extremity. In *Campbell's Operative Orthopaedics,* Vol 1, 9th edition. Canale ST, ed. Mosby-Year Book, St. Louis: 1998, 532–41.

AMPUTATION BELOW THE KNEE

SURGICAL CONSIDERATIONS

Description: Below-the-knee amputation is ablation of the lower limb, usually at the level of the midleg. A long, posterior flap normally is used to cover the stump. The condition of the soft tissues may dictate the level and/or type of flaps used. The procedure begins with an anterior transverse incision made over the midtibia. A long posterior flap, which is 2–3 times the diameter of the leg in length, is then made. The bone is exposed anteriorly and the anterolateral neurovascular structures and muscles are transected and ligated as appropriate (Fig. 10.6-4A). The bone is then transected with a bone saw, and the posterior structures are transected and ligated as appropriate. The amputated leg and foot are then removed from the table and the posterior flap is tapered and shaped for closure (Fig. 10.6-4B). Deep sutures are placed to secure the posterior muscles to the anterior tibia. The skin opening and subcutaneous tissues are closed with interrupted sutures. Finally, a drain is placed (sometimes), and either a compression dressing or an immediate postop cast is applied.

Variant procedure or approaches: Guillotine amputation may be used as the first of a two-stage procedure in infected or contaminated cases. With a guillotine amputation, the bone and soft tissues are transected very quickly in guillotine fashion at the midtibial level. Neurovascular structures are ligated as appropriate. These wounds are usually left open and a compression dressing applied.

Usual preop diagnosis: Dysvascular limb; infection; trauma

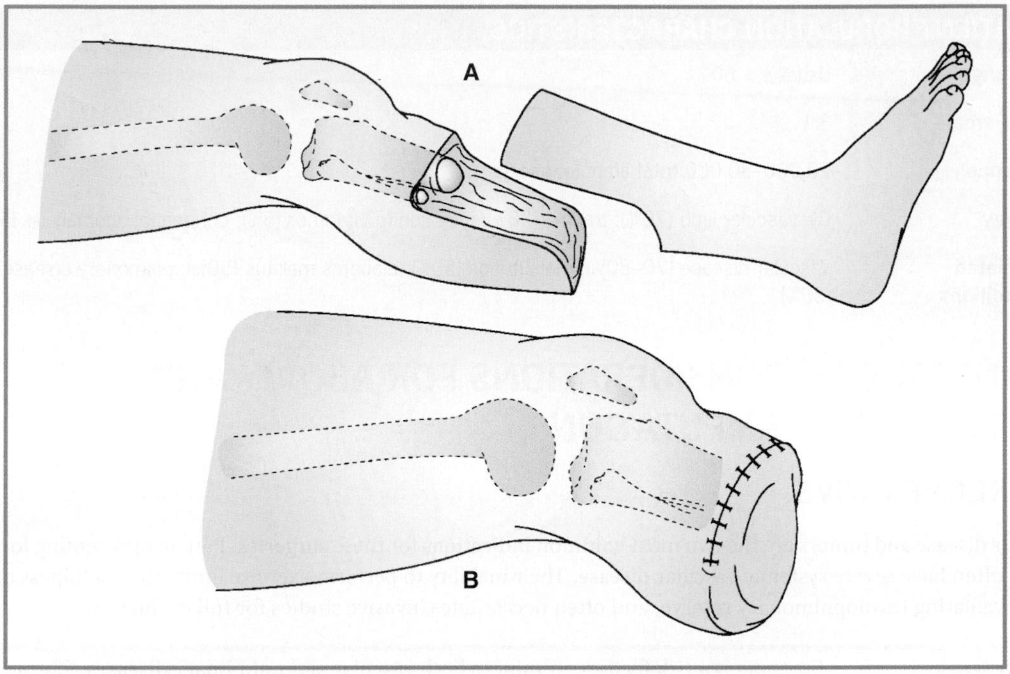

Figure 10.6-4. Below-knee amputation. **A:** The tibia is transected 1 cm proximal to the skin incision, and the fibula is transected an additional 1 cm proximal to the level of the tibial transection. The posterior calf muscles are incised along the plane of the skin incision. **B:** The posterior flap is rotated anteriorly and approximated. (Reproduced with permission from Greenfield LJ, et al, eds: *Surgery: Scientific Principles and Practice,* 3rd edition. Lippincott Williams & Wilkins, 2001.)

SUMMARY OF PROCEDURE

Position	Supine
Incision	Anterior and posterior flaps; for guillotine amputation, circumferential incision
Special instrumentation	Bone saw; tourniquet, if traumatic (tourniquet contraindicated if infected or avascular)
Antibiotics	Cefazolin 1 g iv preop
Surgical time	1.5 h; for guillotine amputation, 0.5 h
Closing considerations	May use cast; drain. Bulky dressing needed for guillotine amputation.
EBL	200 mL
Postop care	PACU → room
Mortality	10%
Morbidity	Phantom pain: 90% Infection: 10–15% Wound breakdown: 10–15% Pneumonia: 12% MI: 7% PE: 6% Hematoma: 5% Stroke: 5%
Pain score	5

PATIENT POPULATION CHARACTERISTICS	
Age range	Usually, > 60
Male:Female	3:1
Incidence	20,000–30,000 total amputations/yr
Etiology	Dysvascular limb (70%); trauma (20%); infection (5%); tumor (5%); congenital anomaly (< 1%)
Associated conditions	Vascular disease (70–80%); malnutrition (50%); diabetes mellitus (30%); pulmonary disease (30%)

ANESTHETIC CONSIDERATIONS FOR ABOVE- AND BELOW-KNEE AMPUTATION

PREOPERATIVE

Vascular disease and tumors are the two most common indications for these surgeries. Patients presenting for amputations often have severe systemic vascular disease. Their inability to perform exercise limits the usefulness of preop Hx in evaluating cardiopulmonary reserve, and often necessitates invasive studies for full evaluation.

Respiratory	Smoking is a risk factor common to both vascular and pulmonary diseases. Chronic bronchitis or COPD patients should have maximum medical therapy (e.g., inhaled bronchodilators, theophylline and steroids, when appropriate) prior to anesthesia. Regional anesthesia is an excellent choice for patients with severe pulmonary disease. **Tests:** As indicated from H&P.
Cardiovascular	Significant cardiovascular disease is present in ~30% of these patients. Particularly in diabetics, CAD is often silent. Dipyridamole thallium imaging of the heart can reveal the preop myocardium at risk of ischemia; however, therapy of stenotic coronary arteries usually can be undertaken only after the amputation. Medical management, to include β-blockers when tolerated, will reduce perioperative MIs. **Tests:** ECG; others as indicated from H&P.
Neurological	Peripheral and autonomic neuropathies may be present in the diabetic patient. Hence, these patients may be more susceptible to injury from malpositioning and are less able to tolerate the hemodynamic changes associated with regional anesthesia. Preexisting neurological deficits should be carefully documented. Autonomic neuropathy is diagnosed by any of the following: postural ↓ BP (in patient not bedridden); loss of sinus arrhythmia; resting ↑ HR; miosis–abnormal response to darkness.
Musculoskeletal	Rhabdomyolysis can occur in the presence of partial ischemia. (See Renal, below.)
Hematologic	Often a trial of heparin, warfarin, or thrombolytic therapy will have been undertaken before amputation. Coag studies, including PT, PTT, and bleeding time are, therefore, often necessary to determine the appropriateness of epidural or intrathecal anesthesia. Warfarin-induced elevation of the PT can be reversed preop with FFP 5–10 mL/kg body weight. This therapy may induce fluid overload in patients with poor cardiac reserve. For these patients, diuretics should be administered to maintain normovolemia. **Tests:** As indicated from H&P.
Renal	Limb ischemia can result in myoglobinemia from rhabdomyolysis. Evidence of progressive renal failure or rising CPK-MM fractions should be treated with hydration, forced alkaline diuresis and prompt amputation. **Tests:** Consider Cr; BUN; CPK enzymes; urine myoglobin.
Laboratory	Diabetic patients require preop control of blood glucose and periop glucose monitoring.
Premedication	Standard premedication (see p. B-1).

INTRAOPERATIVE

Anesthetic technique: Either regional or GA may be appropriate.

Regional anesthesia: Both SAB and epidural blocks are useful techniques. Subarachnoid anesthesia has the advantage of limited spread of the block above the level of surgery, while obtaining adequate blockade of the sacral roots that are resistant to low-dose epidural techniques. Epidural anesthesia allows for extending the duration of anesthesia and for the administration of postop epidural analgesia. Anesthesia from T12 (T8 with tourniquet) is adequate. Full motor blockade is not necessary. Typical drugs and doses include: subarachnoid—75 mg of 5% lidocaine in 5% dextrose (controversial) with morphine 0.2 mg; epidural—12–15 mL 2% lidocaine with epinephrine 1:200,000 in divided doses.

General anesthesia:

Induction	Standard induction (see p. B-2) is appropriate for patients with normal airways. Intubation is indicated for diabetic patients with gastroparesis. Beware of difficult airway in longstanding insulin-dependent diabetics.	
Maintenance	Standard maintenance (see p. B-2).	
Emergence	No special considerations	
Blood and fluid requirements	Moderate blood loss IV: 16 ga × 1 NS/LR @ 4–6 mL/kg/h	Expect 100–200 mL blood loss, mostly during cleaning of the wound made while developing a flap.
Control of blood loss	Tourniquet may be used.	Inflation pressure is typically 100 mmHg + systolic pressure. Maximum "safe" tourniquet time is 1.5–2 h, followed by a 5- to- (preferably) 15-min reperfusion interval, if further tourniquet is necessary.
Special considerations	Tourniquet deflation and limb reperfusion	Mild ↓ BP is common. In patients with moderate-to-severe lung disease, continue controlled ventilation until after the lactic acid accumulated in the ischemic leg is metabolized (3–5 min), because these patients may be unable to increase ventilation adequately to buffer this acid load.
Monitoring	Standard monitors (see p. B-1). ± CVP line ± Arterial line	Invasive monitoring is indicated in the presence of severe cardiac or pulmonary disease. Serial blood glucose determination should be made in the diabetic patient.
Positioning	✓ and pad pressure points. ✓ eyes.	Meticulous padding of the extremities is necessary to prevent ischemic skin ulceration in patients with vascular insufficiency.

POSTOPERATIVE

Complications	Hematoma Bleeding	✓ drains.
Pain management	Spinal opiates Epidural analgesia	Epidural hydromorphone 50 mcg/mL infused at 50–200 mcg/h provides excellent analgesia.
Tests	CXR if CVP was placed.	Other studies as indicated.

Suggested Readings

1. Bohne WHO, Ertl JP: Ampuations of the lower extremity. In *Chapman's Orthopaedic Surgery,* Vol 3, 3rd edition. Chapman MW, ed. Lippincott Williams & Wilkins, Philadelphia: 2001, 3149–74.

2. Fung DL: Anesthesia and pain management. In *Chapman's Orthopaedic Surgery,* Vol I, 3rd edition. Chapman MW, ed. Lippincott Williams & Wilkins, Philadelphia: 2001, 133–56.
3. McCollough NC III, Epps CH Jr, Banks WJ Jr: Complications of amputation surgery. In *Complications in Orthopaedic Surgery,* 3rd edition. Epps CH Jr, ed. JB Lippincott, Philadelphia: 1994, 1279–1308.
4. Sites BD, Brull R: Ultrasound guidance in peripheral regional anesthesia: philosophy, evidence-based medicine, and techniques. *Curr Opin Anaesthesiol* 2006; 19(6):630–9.
5. Tran D, Clemente A, Finlayson RJ: A review of approaches and techniques for lower extremity nerve blocks. *Can J Anaesth* 2007; 54(11):922–34.

FASCIOTOMY OF THE THIGH

SURGICAL CONSIDERATIONS

Description: Increased intracompartmental pressure in the thigh requires surgical release of tight skin and fascial structures (Fig. 10.6-5). This usually occurs after severe trauma to the thigh (e.g., crush injury, comminuted fracture, etc.), after prolonged vascular surgery (with ischemia to the thigh), or with infection. Compartment syndrome is a true emergency and must be treated within minutes of recognition. Failure to do so may result in loss of limb or death. Conventional devices may be used to measure intracompartmental pressure, which usually is abnormal if > 30–35 mmHg (normal = < 30 mmHg). **Fasciotomy of the thigh** involves incising the skin and fascia over the thigh and debriding any necrotic tissue. The wound is left open for later redebridement, delayed primary closure, or skin grafting. Thus, the fasciotomy begins a multistage procedure of incision and debridement with subsequent reconstruction.

Usual preop diagnosis: Compartment syndrome of thigh; crush injury to thigh; necrotizing fasciitis

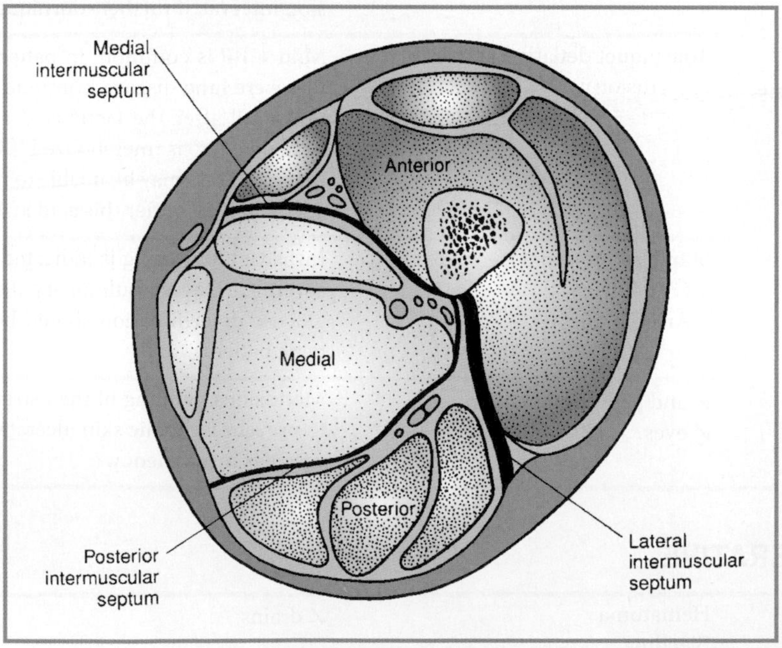

Figure 10.6-5. Cross-section of the thigh showing the 3 major compartments. (Reproduced with permission from Tarlow SD, Achterman C, Hayhurst J, Ovadin D: Acute compartment syndrome of the thigh. *J Bone Joint Surg* [Am] 1986; 68:1441.)

SUMMARY OF PROCEDURE	
Position	Supine or lateral decubitus
Incision	Lateral thigh

SUMMARY OF PROCEDURE (cont'd)	
Unique considerations	Patient may be very ill. If an ipsilateral femoral fracture is present with a compartment syndrome, the surgeon may want to perform ORIF, intramedullary nailing, or external fixation of the fracture.
Antibiotics	Cefazolin or cefamandole 1 g iv q 6 h
Surgical time	1.5–2 h for fasciotomy alone
Closing considerations	Wound left open and covered by sterile dressings.
EBL	250–500 mL
Postop care	If surgery is performed acutely, patient frequently will be a multiple-trauma victim with numerous injuries and extensive blood loss; usually goes to ICU.
Mortality	Dependent on extent of multiple trauma
Morbidity	Hypotension and fluid loss: Common Neurological deficit to peripheral nerves: Common, if decompression delayed Respiratory distress and fat embolism: Not uncommon, if concomitant femur fracture Vascular complications: Not uncommon Amputation: Rare, if decompression prompt Systemic sepsis: Rare Wound infection: Rare New compartment syndrome; insufficient fasciotomy: Rare
Pain score	7–8

PATIENT POPULATION CHARACTERISTICS	
Age range	Any age, but predominance of males < 30 yr
Male:Female	5:1
Incidence	Extremely rare
Etiology	Trauma—motorcycle and motor vehicle accidents, falls, industrial injury, crush injuries; post-surgery—local hematoma and swelling; thrombosis or disruption of blood supply to thigh (e.g., failed proximal vascular bypass surgery, aortic dissection, etc.); massive infection of thigh compartment (e.g., gas gangrene)
Associated conditions	Burns; drug and alcohol overdose; frequently associated with trauma to other organ systems

ANESTHETIC CONSIDERATIONS

See Anesthetic Considerations following Fasciotomy of the Leg, p. 1055.

Suggested Readings

1. Dutkowsky JP: Miscellaneous nontraumatic disorders. In *Campbell's Operative Orthopaedics,* Vol 1, 9th edition. Canale ST, ed. Mosby-Year Book, St. Louis: 1998, 787–856.
2. Meyer RS, Mubarak SJ: Compartment syndromes. In *Chapman's Orthopaedic Surgery,* 3rd edition. Chapman MW ed. Lippincott Williams & Wilkins, Philadelphia: 2001, 393–416.

FASCIOTOMY OF THE LEG

SURGICAL CONSIDERATIONS

Description: This procedure is the surgical decompression of fascial compartments for treatment or prevention of compartment syndrome. Patients are often very ill and unstable with other injuries or disease. Compartment

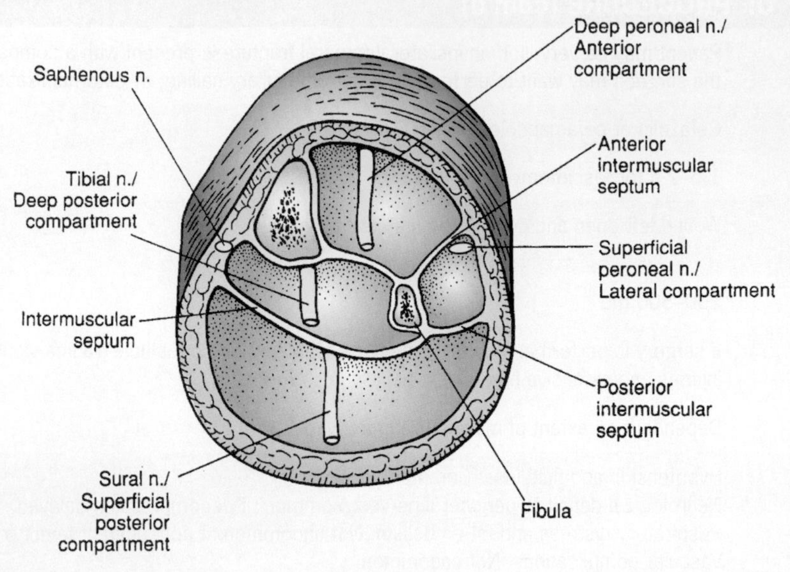

Figure 10.6-6. Cross-section of the left leg, middle lower third, showing the four compartments with associated peripheral nerves. (Reproduced with permission from Mubarak SJ, Owen CA: Double-incision fasciotomy of the leg for decompression in compartment syndromes. *J Bone Joint Surg* [Am] 1977; 59:184–7.)

syndrome is a true emergency and must be treated within minutes of recognition. Failure to do so may result in loss of limb or death. There are four compartments in the leg: anterior, lateral, deep posterior and superficial posterior (Fig. 10.6-6). Generally, all four compartments are released during the procedure. A **four-compartment fascial decompression** can be performed through two incisions—medial and lateral. A medial longitudinal incision is made just posterior to the tibia; through this incision, the superficial and deep posterior compartments are identified and the fascia incised in longitudinal fashion. A straight, lateral, longitudinal incision is made and the deep fascia overlying the anterior and lateral compartments is identified. The fascia of each compartment is then incised longitudinally. Skin incisions are rarely closed because of the swelling. A compression dressing is applied and splints may be used.

Usual preop diagnosis: Compartment syndrome; vascular trauma

SUMMARY OF PROCEDURE	
Position	Supine
Incision	Medial and lateral parallel to tibia
Unique considerations	Often associated with fracture; may require fixation.
Antibiotics	Cefazolin 1 g iv preop
Surgical time	30 min +
Closing considerations	Wounds left open; splint may be required.
EBL	100 mL
Postop care	PACU → room; vascular monitoring is carried out clinically via a pulse oximeter on toes.
Mortality	Minimal

SUMMARY OF PROCEDURE (cont'd)	
Morbidity	Myonecrosis: 50% Thrombophlebitis: 10–20% Infection: 10–15%
Pain score	3

PATIENT POPULATION CHARACTERISTICS	
Age range	All ages
Male:Female	1:1
Incidence	~5% of tibia fractures
Etiology	Trauma – blunt fracture, vascular (90%); drug overdose (10%); burns (< 5%); revascularization (< 5%)
Associated conditions	Multiple trauma (60%); vascular disease (15%)

ANESTHETIC CONSIDERATIONS FOR FASCIOTOMY OF THIGH AND LEG

PREOPERATIVE

Compartment syndromes and necrotizing fasciitis are the indications for these procedures (necrotizing fasciitis also may cause compartment syndrome). Patients with compartment syndrome often have no systemic disease, while patients with necrotizing fasciitis have a rapidly life-threatening infection that requires prompt surgical debridement and often is complicated by rhabdomyolysis and DIC.

Respiratory	Usually no special considerations, unless massive sepsis.
Cardiovascular	Sepsis is uniformly present in patients with necrotizing fasciitis. Management includes antibiotics and hemodynamic support with dopamine (5–15 mcg/kg/min) or epinephrine (0.02–0.25 mcg/kg/min), with therapy guided by invasive hemodynamic monitoring, which may include PA catheter.
Neurological	If fasciotomy is for compartment syndrome, there may be compromise of distal nerves and blood flow. Perform a thorough neurologic exam of the involved extremity to document preop deficits.
Hematologic	If infection is the indication for the fasciotomy, DIC is likely. Evaluate for pathologic bleeding. Administer factors necessary to correct coagulopathy during the procedure. **Tests:** CBC; PT; PTT; fibrinogen; fibrin split products; Plt count
Renal	Both necrotizing fasciitis and compartment syndrome often cause myoglobinuria and rhabdomyolysis. Myoglobinuria can be inferred from urine that is dipstick-positive for occult blood but microscopically free of RBCs in the absence of hemolysis (therefore, no free Hb in the urine).
Laboratory	Hct; serial K^+ levels if there is an active diuresis; other studies as indicated from H&P.
Premedication	Standard premedication (see p. B-1).

INTRAOPERATIVE

Anesthetic technique: Regional techniques are appropriate for compartment syndrome decompression, unless there is evidence of DIC or systemic infection. These surgeries are usually of short duration (< 1 h). Sepsis and hemodynamic instability usually mandate GETA for fasciotomy in patients with necrotizing fasciitis.

Regional anesthesia: Either subarachnoid or epidural blocks are useful in the absence of systemic infection or severe coagulopathy. Subarachnoid anesthesia has the advantage of adequate blockade of the sacral roots that are resistant to low-dose epidural techniques. Anesthesia from T10-S2 is adequate. Typical drugs and dosages include: subarachnoid—15 mg of 0.5% bupivacaine; epidural—12–15 mL 2% lidocaine with epinephrine 1:200,000 in divided doses.

General anesthesia:

Induction	Standard induction (see p. B-2).	
Maintenance	Standard maintenance (see p. B-2).	
Emergence	Consider postop ventilation for patients with impaired oxygenation or ongoing hemodynamic instability; otherwise, no special considerations.	
Blood and fluid requirements	IV: 16 ga × 1 (compartment syndrome) 14–16 ga × 2 (necrotizing fasciitis) NS/LR @ 4–6 mL/kg/h	To prevent renal damage, **insure adequate circulatory volume**; induce osmotic diuresis with mannitol 0.25 g/kg iv. Furosemide 10–100 mg also may be necessary to maintain diuresis. Replace UO with 0.5 NS + 50 mEq bicarbonate/L, or as guided by invasive monitoring.
Monitoring	Standard monitors (see p. B-1). UO ± Arterial line (± ABG) ± CVP or PA catheter	Fluid losses (3rd-spacing, bleeding) may be significant. Patients with necrotizing fasciitis require an arterial line and either a CVP or PA catheter to guide fluid and inotropic/pressor therapy.
Positioning	✓ and pad pressure points. ✓ eyes.	

POSTOPERATIVE

Complications	DIC Renal failure 2° rhabdomyolysis Hypo/hyperkalemia Sepsis syndrome, including ARDS	
Pain management	PCA or epidural analgesia	See p. C-3.
Tests	Hct Electrolytes UA (dipstick and microscopic)	For patients with sepsis: coag profile, including PT/PTT, fibrin split products, and Plt count

Suggested Readings

1. Bucholz RW, Heckman JD, eds: *Rockwood and Green's Fractures in Adults,* 5th edition. Lippincott Williams & Wilkins, Philadelphia: 2001.
2. Epps CH Jr, ed: *Complications in Orthopaedic Surgery,* 3rd edition. JB Lippincott, Philadelphia: 1994.
3. Meyer RS, Mubarak SJ: Compartment syndromes. In *Chapman's Orthopaedic Surgery,* 3rd edition. Chapman MW ed. Lippincott Williams & Wilkins, Philadelphia: 1993, 2001, 393–416.

BIOPSY, LEG AND FOOT

SURGICAL CONSIDERATIONS

Description: Biopsy is performed to excise tissues for pathologic evaluation, usually through a small, longitudinal wound. For **incisional biopsy,** a longitudinal incision is made over the mass. Overlying soft tissues are incised with minimal undermining. The area in question is incised and the biopsy removed, with care being taken to prevent spillage into the adjacent tissues. The pathologist often is asked to perform a frozen section to determine whether diagnostic tissue is present. The wound is closed with interrupted sutures and a compression dressing applied. A splint or cast may be used if a significant amount of bone has been removed. If the lesion is small, x-ray control or image intensification may be necessary for localization. **Needle biopsy** may be used for distinct osseous lesions to obtain small amounts of tissue for culture or histology. **Excisional biopsy** may be used for benign lesions like exostoses or lipomas.

Usual preop diagnosis: Tumor; infection

SUMMARY OF PROCEDURES

	Incisional Biopsy	Needle Biopsy	Excisional Biopsy
Position	Supine	⇐	⇐
Incision	Short longitudinal	Stab wound	Stab wound
Special instrumentation	Bone-cutting instruments; x-ray or I.I.	Trephine (e.g., Craig needle); x-ray or I.I.	X-ray or I.I.
Unique considerations	Tourniquet	⇐	⇐ (Bone graft may be necessary.)
Antibiotics	None (May be given postop.)	⇐	⇐
Surgical time	l h	0.5 h	0.5–2 h
Closing considerations	May be splinted.	Usually no splint	May be splinted.
EBL	50 mL	Minimal	100–200 mL
Postop care	PACU → room or home	⇐	PACU → room
Mortality	Minimal	⇐	⇐
Morbidity	Hematoma: 5% Tumor spread: < 5% Infection: < 1%	⇐ ⇐ ⇐	⇐ ⇐ ⇐
Pain score	3	2	3

PATIENT POPULATION CHARACTERISTICS

Age range	All ages
Male:Female	1:1
Incidence	Rare
Etiology	Tumor (75%); infection (25%)
Associated conditions	Metastatic disease; immune compromise

ANESTHETIC CONSIDERATIONS

See Anesthetic Considerations for Lower-Extremity Procedures, p. 1059.

Suggested Reading

1. Enneking WF: *Musculoskeletal Tumor Surgery.* Churchill Livingstone, New York: 1983.

BIOPSY OR DRAINAGE OF ABSCESS/ EXCISION OF TUMOR

SURGICAL CONSIDERATIONS

Description: This procedure involves obtaining a piece of tissue for histologic and/or bacteriologic Dx by closed, percutaneous means or by open biopsy. Subsequently, the area may be drained (abscess or infection) or an open excision of a tumor may follow (± internal fixation). For excision of tumors of the pelvis, acetabulum or femur, please consult the appropriate section describing fractures of the area. Each case must be individualized.

Variant procedure or approaches: Excision of infection or tumor of proximal or distal femur, femoral shaft, pelvis, or acetabulum.

Usual preop diagnosis: Femur: biopsy of mass; infection; osteomyelitis. Pelvis or acetabulum: biopsy of pelvis or acetabulum; drainage of abscess or infection of pelvis or acetabulum; osteomyelitis of pelvis or acetabulum; septic arthritis of acetabulum

SUMMARY OF PROCEDURE	
Position	Supine or lateral decubitus
Incision	Percutaneous, short or long; location depends on site of lesion.
Special instrumentation	Biopsy needles and instruments to take a core biopsy; bone cement may be used to plug biopsy site. Some surgeons use fracture table or radiolucent table with I.I.
Unique considerations	May require intraop frozen section and gram stain.
Antibiotics	After tissue has been obtained, cefazolin or cefamandole 1 g iv q 6 h × 48 h. A gram stain will help decide immediate antibiotic coverage, but cultures and sensitivities are ultimately necessary.
Surgical time	1 h for simple procedures; much longer (up to 12 h) for more extensive excisional procedures ± further reconstruction.
EBL	100–1,000 mL or more
Postop care	If procedure is extensive with much blood loss, or the patient is unstable or ill from chronic sepsis or invasive tumor, it is prudent to send patient to ICU.
Mortality	Dependent on extent of procedure. Biopsy or drainage of a small, localized abscess in soft tissue or bone is rarely life-threatening. Wide/radical excision of a malignant tumor in the pelvis or extremities is frequently life- and/or limb-threatening.
Morbidity	The following are dependent on site and procedure: Intraop fracture Nonunion Chronic osteomyelitis Compartment syndrome Residual instability of pelvis or hip joint Fracture of pelvis or acetabulum, nonunion Chronic osteomyelitis or septic arthritis Hypotension 2° to blood loss Respiratory distress Neurological injury to lumbosacral plexus, sciatic nerve, or other peripheral nerves Vascular injury to iliac or other vessels Injury to GI, genitourinary, or gynecological organs
Pain score	2–10

PATIENT POPULATION CHARACTERISTICS	
Age range	Any age; predominance of elderly patients with tumors
Male:Female	1:1
Incidence	Rare
Etiology	Benign and malignant tumors (common); infection (rare); previous surgery (rare); previous trauma (rare)
Associated conditions	Metastatic disease or other foci of infection

ANESTHETIC CONSIDERATIONS FOR LOWER-EXTREMITY PROCEDURES

(Procedures covered: ORIF of femur, tibia, ankle, and foot; intramedullary nailing of femur and tibia; closed reduction and external fixation of femur and tibia; distal tibia, ankle and foot procedures; repair nonunion/malunion of femur and tibia; ankle arthroscopy, arthrotomy, arthrodesis; repair/reconstruction, ankle ligaments; Syme's amputation; transmetatarsal amputation; tendon (ankle, foot) lengthening; biopsy of leg and foot; biopsy or drainage of abscess/excision of tumor)

PREOPERATIVE

Trauma victims comprise the largest group of patients for these procedures. Minimizing the time between fracture and surgery for open wounds significantly reduces the incidence of wound infection. Evaluations for other injury, adequacy of fluid resuscitation and preexisting conditions need to be undertaken promptly and used as a guide for anesthetic management. Patients with bone cancer form another subset of patients and often have concurrent medical conditions and have undergone chemotherapy or radiation therapy preop.

Respiratory	Pulmonary fat embolus occurs in 10–15% of patients following bone fracture. Sx include hypoxemia, ↑ HR, tachypnea, respiratory alkalosis, mental status changes, and conjunctival petechiae. Lab analysis may reveal fat in the urine. Preop therapy for this condition should include supplemental O_2 with mechanical ventilation, to correct hypoxemia, and meticulous fluid management to prevent worsening pulmonary capillary leak. **Tests:** Consider CXR; others as indicated from H&P.
Cardiovascular	Cardiac contusion or tamponade are possible if blunt chest trauma has occurred during the injury. A large volume of blood can be hidden around a long bone fracture site. ↑ HR, orthostasis, or ↓ BP indicate hypovolemia, and this should be corrected with crystalloid (10–40 mL/kg) or blood if Hct < 24%. In patients with a tibial or distal femur fracture, and who are presenting with hemodynamic instability and ongoing blood loss, consider applying a tourniquet to the thigh prior to induction. **Tests:** Consider ECG; CPK enzyme levels and ECHO will help evaluate the presence of cardiac injury.
Neurological	Perform a thorough neurological evaluation, including mental status and peripheral sensory exams. A CT scan of the head is indicated for any patient with prolonged loss of consciousness prior to anesthesia. Drug abuse is common in trauma patients and they should be asked specifically about any drug use. **Tests:** Patients with inappropriate behavior or a positive drug abuse Hx should undergo a urine and plasma drug screen.
Musculoskeletal	Consider cervical instability and obtain spine films if mechanism of injury included rapid deceleration or trauma to the head or neck. Myoglobinemia and ↑ K^+ may result from crush injury.

Orthopedic Surgery

Hematologic	Patients with cancer who have undergone chemotherapy and multiple transfusions often develop sensitivities to blood products and may require specialized blood products, such as leukocyte-poor PRBC or red cells negative for a particular antigen. The availability of these blood products should be confirmed before surgery. **Tests:** Hct and others as indicated from H&P.
Renal	**Tests:** UA
Laboratory	Other tests as indicated from H&P.
Premedication	Due to the risk of gastric aspiration, minimal or no premedication is given to trauma victims. For other patients, standard premedication (see p. B-1). Narcotic premedication (morphine 1–2 mg iv q 10 min titrated to effect) is appropriate for patients experiencing pain with movement.

INTRAOPERATIVE

Anesthetic technique: For trauma patients, regional anesthesia permits evaluation of mental status, provides intact airway reflexes, and ↓ blood loss. Combative patients and those requiring multiple concurrent surgical procedures or prolonged (> 2 h) procedures are often managed with GETA.

Regional anesthesia: Either subarachnoid or epidural blocks are useful techniques. Subarachnoid anesthesia has the advantage of adequate blockade of the sacral roots that are resistant to low-dose epidural techniques. Epidural anesthesia allows for the administration of postop epidural analgesia. Anesthesia from T12 (T8 with tourniquet) to S2 is adequate. Full motor blockade is desirable. Typical drugs and doses include: subarachnoid—15 mg of 0.5% bupivacaine with morphine 0.2 mg (omit if outpatient); epidural—12–15 mL 2% lidocaine with epinephrine 1:200,000 in divided doses (Na bicarbonate 0.1 mg/mL will speed onset of block).

General anesthesia:

Induction	Standard induction (see p. B-2) is appropriate for patients with normal airways. Trauma patients require a rapid-sequence induction (see p. B-5) and intubation with cricoid pressure to prevent gastric aspiration.	
Maintenance	Standard maintenance (see p. B-2). Trauma patients are often cold and require active warming if < 35°C (convection blanket and active humidifier). Warming the patient may unmask severe hypovolemia that should be corrected.	
Emergence	Trauma patients should have full return of protective airway reflexes and, given the possibility of fat embolus, evidence of adequate oxygenation on 50% O_2 prior to extubation.	
Blood and fluid requirements	IV: 14–16 ga × 2 NS/LR @ 4–8 mL/kg/h Warm fluids. Humidify gases.	Some fractures can involve large (30 mL/kg) blood losses that are hidden in the leg or thigh. Clinical signs of hypovolemia and serial Hct determination should guide fluid therapy.
Control of blood loss	Tourniquet	Inflation pressure is typically 100 mmHg + systolic pressure. Maximum "safe" tourniquet time is 1.5–2 h, followed by a 5– to- (preferably) 15-min reperfusion interval, if further tourniquet time is necessary.
Monitoring	Standard monitors (see p. B-1). ± Arterial line ± CVP line	Arterial/CVP lines indicated for patients with ↓BP not readily correctable with crystalloid infusion, massive blood loss (> 1 blood volume), or the need for postop ventilation.
Positioning	✓ and pad pressure points. ✓ eyes.	

Orthopedic Surgery

Special considerations	Release of tourniquet	A 20% ↓MAP is common on tourniquet deflation. Additional crystalloid (5–10 mL/kg) may be necessary to replace edema fluid and blood loss to the leg.
Complications	Fat embolism Myoglobinemia	

POSTOPERATIVE

Complications	Hypoxemia VTE (DVT)	May be 2° fat embolism. see VTE prophylaxis guidelines p. B-7
Pain management	Spinal opiates: Epidural anesthesia Spinal anesthesia	Epidural hydromorphone 50 mcg/mL infused at 100–250 mcg/h provides excellent analgesia. Intrathecal morphine 0.2–0.3 mg provides analgesia for up to 24 h after administration. (Monitor for delayed respiratory depression.)
Tests	Hct CXR, if CVP placed or oxygenation is impaired.	Other studies as indicated.

Suggested Readings

1. Fung DL: Anesthesia and pain management. In *Chapman's Orthopaedic Surgery,* 3rd edition, Vol I. Chapman MW, ed. Lippincott Williams & Wilkins, Philadelphia: 2001, 133–56.
2. Nutescu EA: Assessing, preventing, and treating venous thromboembolism: evidence-based approaches. *Am J Health Syst Pharm* 2007; 64(11 Suppl 7):S5–13.
3. Sites BD, Brull R: Ultrasound guidance in peripheral regional anesthesia: philosophy, evidence-based medicine, and techniques. *Curr Opin Anaesthesiol* 2006; 19(6):630–9.
4. Tran D, Clemente A, Finlayson RJ: A review of approaches and techniques for lower extremity nerve blocks. *Can J Anaesth* 2007; 54(11):922–34.
5. Warner WC Jr: General principles of infections. In *Campbell's Operative Orthopaedics,* Vol 1, 9th edition. Canale ST, ed. Mosby-Year Book, St. Louis: 1998, 563–77.
6. Williams BA, Matusic B, Kentor ML: Regional anesthesia procedures for ambulatory knee surgery: effects on in-hospital outcomes. *Int Anesthesiol Clin* 2005; 43(3):153–60.

SECTION

11.0 PLASTIC AND RECONSTRUCTIVE SURGERY

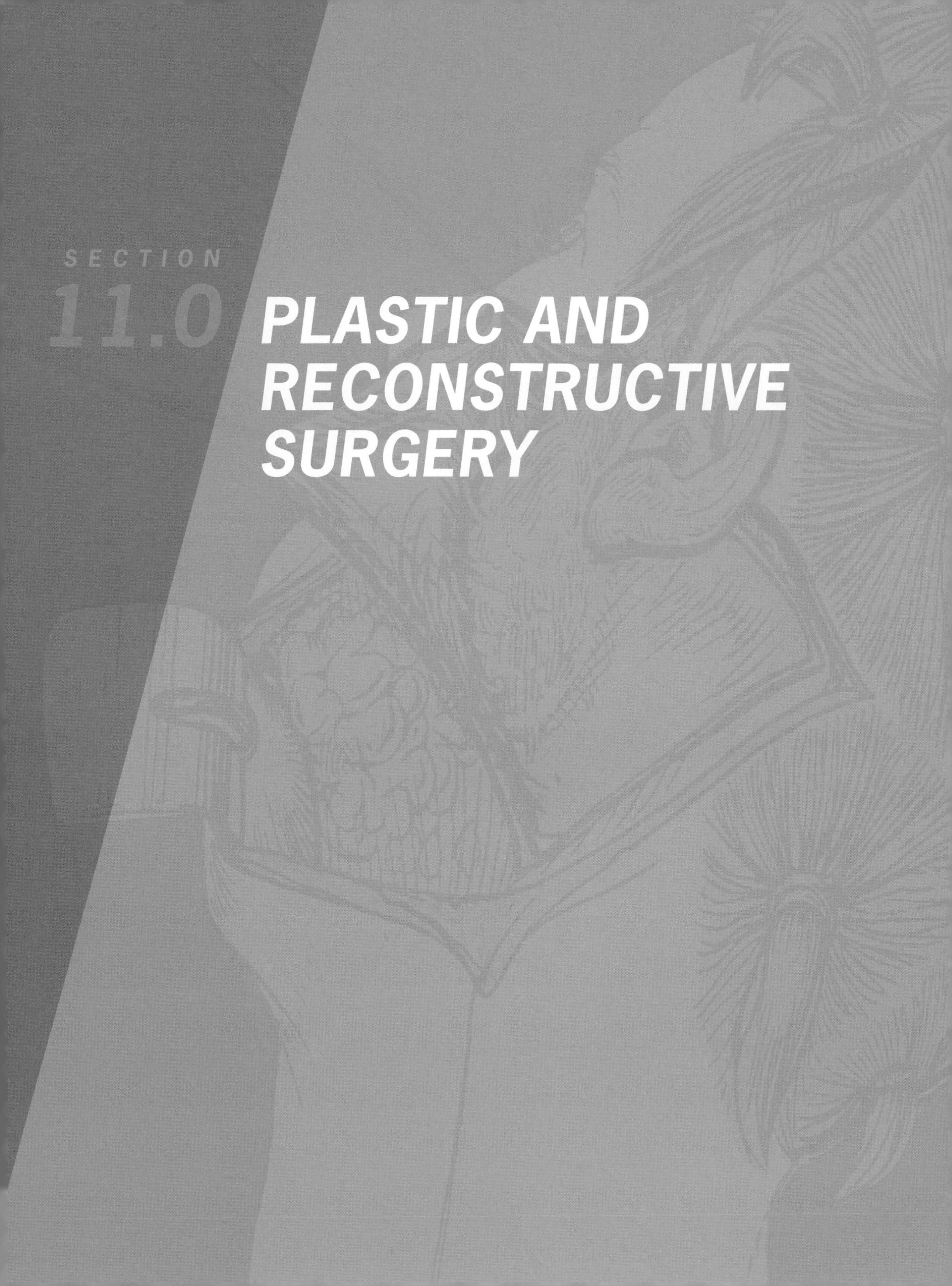

CHAPTER

11.1 Facial Cosmetic Surgery

SURGEONS

Angeline F. Lim, MD
Lonny L. Ross, MD, FRCSC
David M. Kahn, MD

ANESTHESIOLOGIST

Tara Cornaby, MD

INTRODUCTION TO COSMETIC FACIAL SURGERY

The presenting symptoms of the aging face are predictable, based on the effects of gravity, soft tissue atrophy, facial expression, ultraviolet radiation exposure, and connective tissue changes. Patients present with concerns about appearing tired, angry, or aged. They also may have functional difficulties, such as difficulty breathing or visual field obstruction due to drooping brows or eyelids. Other common complaints are wrinkles around the eyes and mouth, and a sagging or fatty chin and neck.

Cosmetic facial surgery aims to rejuvenate and restore the facial form by surgical manipulation of the hard and soft tissues. The techniques used involve any or all of the following: soft tissue release, resection, plication, and resuspension.

Facial aging takes place simultaneously in all areas of the face and neck; combined procedures are not uncommon. Generally in combined procedures, a browlift would precede a necklift, followed by a facelift. Blepharoplasty procedures can be performed at different times in the surgical scheme, because of their effect on eyelid tissue and brow posture. A rhinoplasty ideally is reserved for last, as it can cause bleeding and swelling that can obscure other facial surgical fields.

FACELIFT AND NECKLIFT

SURGICAL CONSIDERATIONS

FACELIFT (OR MELOPLASTY OR RHYTIDECTOMY)

Description: **Facelifts** and **midface lifts** are procedures to rejuvenate the face by surgical manipulation of the soft tissues between the inferior orbital rim and the inferior border of the mandible. The lips and nose are generally unaffected. Many types of "facelift" procedures have been developed to address the diverse challenges of facial aging and rejuvenation. Traditional facelift procedures took place in the subcutaneous plane, with some skin resection. Today, three planes of dissection are used (Fig. 11.1-1). **Subcutaneous dissection** continues to be popular, traversing the adipose tissue below the skin and many of the vessels supplying the skin. The **subSMAS** technique develops the plane between the superficial musculoaponeurotic system of the face (SMAS) and the parotid gland. Finally, **subperiosteal dissections** (midface lifts) have become popular, due to the decreased risk of postoperative hematomas. Combinations of these dissection planes also have been described. More recently, greater attention has been paid to minimal access techniques. Surgeries such as the minimal access cranial suspension lift, as well as adjunctive procedures such as the barbed suture lift, are being performed more frequently.

Local anesthetics with epinephrine are injected presurgically for the various procedures. A number of subcutaneous infiltration mixtures may be used, including one described by **Klein** that consists of NS 1,000 mL with 1.0 mL epinephrine (1:1000) and 50 mL of 1% lidocaine ± 12.5 mL of 8.5% sodium bicarbonate solution. It has been shown that with the use of this mixture, 5–7 times the traditionally accepted maximum dose of lidocaine with epinephrine can be injected safely into the subcutaneous space. Not only does this solution provide hemostasis and hydrodissection, but decreased operative time and excellent perioperative analgesia also have been attributed to its use.

Traditional incisions typically are made in the preauricular region with temporal and postauricular scalp extensions. The approaches for the subcutaneous and SMAS techniques resemble those used for bilateral facial palsy and parotid gland operations. The midface procedures may be carried out through intraoral, temporal, and/or lower-lid incisions and may be combined with other facelift procedures.

A typical facelift may begin with subcutaneous dissection of the facial skin flap (Fig. 11.1-2) on one side, with meticulous hemostasis accomplished with bipolar electrocautery. The SMAS layer can then be mobilized and resuspended. Some surgeons continue on the same side with skin resection and closure before beginning on the other side, while others temporarily pack the first side and perform an identical procedure on the opposite side. In the latter case, a second look for bleeding is made on each side after a waiting period.

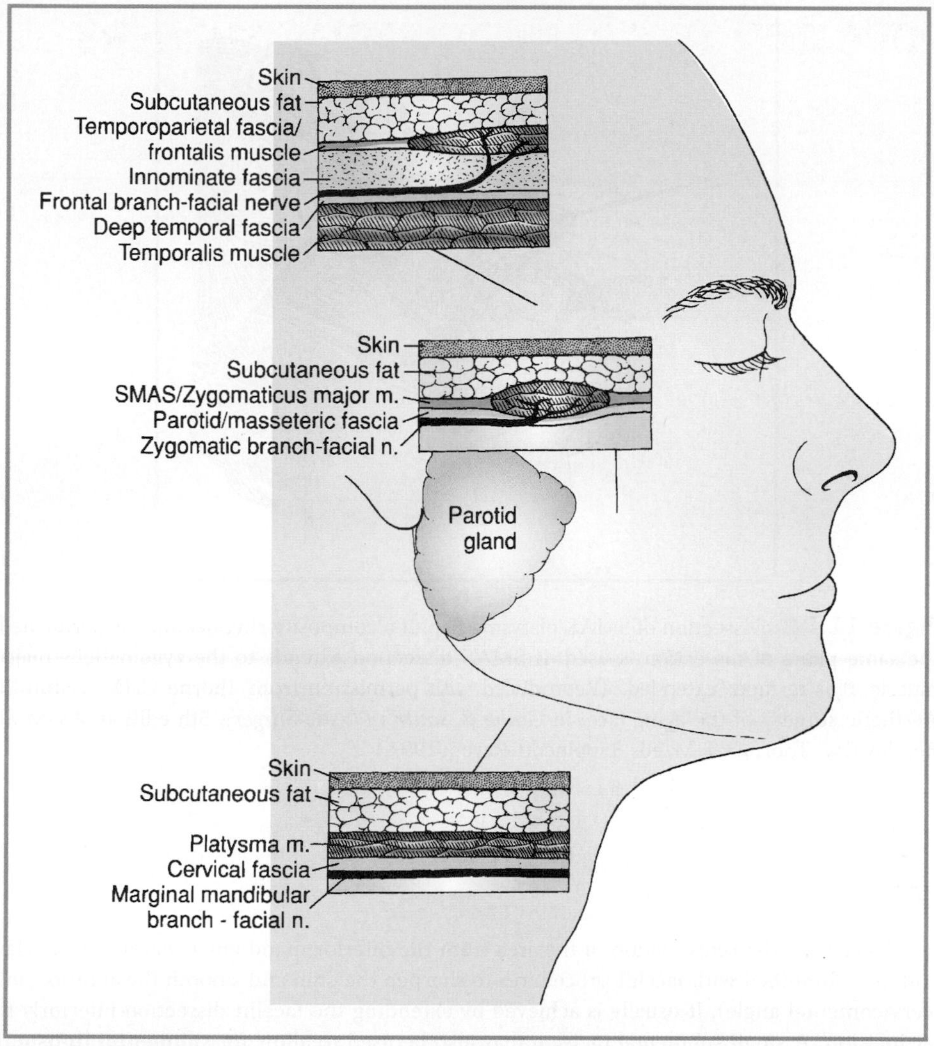

Figure 11.1-1. Anatomic layers of the face. Although the names vary, the arrangement persists, regardless of the area of the face. The facial nerve (CN VII) branches innervate their respective muscles of the SMAS layer via the deep surfaces. (Reproduced with permission from Thorne CHM, Aston SJ: Aesthetic surgery of the aging face. In *Grabb & Smith's Plastic Surgery,* 5th edition. Aston SJ, Beasley RW, Thorne CHM, eds. Lippincott-Raven: 1997.)

Hematoma is the most common complication of facelift surgery. Because hypertension is the most frequently encountered medical condition in the age group that typically presents for facelift, perioperative hypertension must be anticipated and treated pre-emptively to avoid development of hematoma. The risk is highest in male patients, perhaps due to increased perfusion of the bearded region, hormonal gender differences, or increased sebaceous gland density. Commonly used salicylates and other NSAIDS are contraindicated in the immediate preoperative period (i.e., within 10 days of surgery).

Smoking also has been shown to be detrimental to facelift results, especially with regard to skin flap survival. Ideally, patients should not smoke for two weeks before and after surgery.

One of the least desirable complications is injury to the facial nerve, which can produce a disastrous result following an elective cosmetic surgery. Many surgeons prefer that no paralytics be used during the procedure to allow for careful monitoring of facial nerve function.

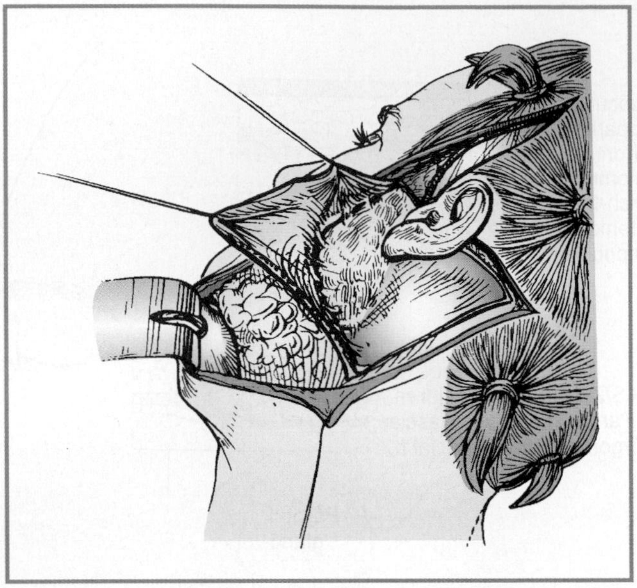

Figure 11.1-2. Dissection of SMAS/platysma flap. If a composite rhytidectomy is performed, the same plane of dissection is used. If SMAS dissection extends to the zygomaticus major muscle, it is termed "extended." (Reproduced with permission from Thorne CHM, Aston SJ: Aesthetic surgery of the aging face. In *Grabb & Smith's Plastic Surgery,* 5th edition. Aston SJ, Beasley RW, Thorne CHM, eds. Lippincott-Raven: 1997.)

NECKLIFT

Description: Necklift is the rejuvenation of the area from the inferior mandibular margin to the clavicles. This procedure often is combined with facelift procedures to sharpen the chin and smooth the anterior neck (i.e., improve the cervicomental angle). It usually is achieved by extending the facelift dissection inferiorly through the preauricular incision. A small submental incision may also be used to allow for **submental liposuction, lipectomy,** or **platysma muscle modifications** (plication, suspension, resection, or transection techniques).[8] Some platysmal suspension techniques require the facelift incisions to remain open with continuity in the subcutaneous plane laterally.

Variant procedures or approaches: **Laser resurfacing** (see p. 1080 and p. 1512), especially in the perioral and periorbital regions; **blepharoplasty** and **browlift** (see p. 1071) are common adjunct procedures.

Usual preop diagnosis: Facelift: facial rhytids (wrinkles/creases); solar or senile elastosis; jowling; deep nasolabial folds; tear troughs; nasojugal folds; malar bags. Necklift: "turkey gobbler" neck; platysmal bands; cervical laxity; cervical rhytids

SUMMARY OF PROCEDURES

	Facelift	Necklift	Midface lift
Position	Supine, reverse Trendelenburg	⇐	⇐
Incision	Preauricular, scalp	Extension of facelift incision + submental incision.	Intraoral ± subciliary or inferior lid
Special instrumentation	Infiltration equipment for super wet techniques; endoscopic equipment (more frequent with brow lifts)	⇐ ± liposuction instrumentation.	–

SUMMARY OF PROCEDURES (cont'd)

	Facelift	Necklift	Midface lift
Unique considerations	Oral intubation; ability to move ETT side-to-side. Watch for: oculocardiac reflex (OCR), retrobulbar hematoma with periorbital approaches.	⇐	⇐
	If laser is used:		
	• Special fire-retardant ETT and drapes	⇐	⇐
	• Laser eye protection for all in room		
	• Cannula-administered O_2 should be far away from laser (fire safety).		
	• Smoke evacuation system (See Facial Laser Resurfacing, p. 1080.)		
	Infiltration of large volumes of local with epinephrine in facelift and liposuction procedures.	⇐	–
Antibiotics + other meds	Cefazolin 1 g iv, (± methylprednisolone 125 mg iv). Antivirals periop if laser used (e.g., acyclovir 2,400 mg × 2 d preop and 14 d postop)	⇐	⇐
Surgical time	4–6 h	1–2 h	2–4 h
Closing considerations	Trendelenburg for final hemostasis ± drains	–	–
	Some surgeons prefer gentle ↑ in BP during hemostasis.	⇐	⇐
	Tissue thrombin agents may be used between the elevated flaps.	⇐	–
	Sensory nerve blocks by surgeon	⇐	⇐
	± Full head/face wrap before patient awakens	–	–
	Gentle, nonagitated awakening to prevent sudden ↑ BP.		
EBL	100–200 mL	⇐	⇐
Postop care	Monitor for hematoma: most common complaint is pain; therefore, r/o hematoma before increased analgesia or sedation.	⇐	⇐
	Lightly compressive dressing, ± drains: both removed at 24 h.	⇐	⇐
	2 wk no aspirin, moderate activity	⇐	⇐
Mortality	Rare	⇐	⇐
Morbidity	Early hematoma:	⇐	Very rare
	• Large expanding: 1–15% (return to OR)		
	• Small (> 30 mL): 10–15% (± aspiration in office)	⇐	
	Late hematoma (average = 9 d postop; 2° to exertion or aspirin use; from superficial temporal vessels)	⇐	–
	Infection: 0–0.33%	⇐	⇐
	Nerve injury:		
	• Motor (temporal/marginal mandibular branches)		Very rare
	• Temporary: 0.1–2.6%	⇐	
	• Permanent: 0–0.66%	⇐	
	• Motor (spinal accessory nerve): Rare	⇐	–
	Sensory injury:		
	• Great auricular nerve →↓ sensation in lower ½ of ear ± painful neuromas or paresthesias.		–
	• Lesser occipital nerve painful → neuroma.	⇐	–
	Alopecia: 0.4% (most temporary, along the incision)	⇐	–
	Skin slough: 14% (especially in retroauricular area) (12.5 × greater in smokers)		–
	Dehiscence: 0.1–0.35%	⇐	⇐
	Parotid cysts: Rare	⇐	–

SUMMARY OF PROCEDURES (cont'd)			
	Facelift	**Necklift**	**Midface lift**
	Poor cosmetic result: • Hyperpigmentation • Telangiectasia (pre-existing lesions may worsen) • Hypertrophic scarring • Keloids: Very rare • "Pixie" (pulled-down earlobe) deformity (technique-dependent) • Hairline shifts Ectropion (midface, approached via lid incisions only): Up to 3%	⇐	⇐
Pain score	3	3	3

PATIENT POPULATION CHARACTERISTICS	
Age range	> 35 yr
Male:Female	1:9 to 1:5 (increased from 1:17 in the 1970s.)
Incidence	104,055 facelift procedures in the United States (2006); sixth most common cosmetic plastic surgery procedure
Etiology	Facial rhytids 2° solar elastosis, senile elastosis, facial expression
Associated conditions	Cancers of the skin (basal cell carcinoma, squamous cell carcinoma and precursors, and melanoma), in solar elastosis cases, especially fair-skinned patients

ANESTHETIC CONSIDERATIONS

See Anesthetic Considerations following Browlift and Blepharoplasty, p. 1075.

Suggested Readings

1. Alster TS, Apfelberg DB, eds: *Cosmetic Laser Surgery: A Practitioner's Guide,* 2nd edition. Wiley-Liss, New York: 1999.
2. American Society of Plastic Surgeons web site: www.plasticsurgery.org.
3. Baker DC, Conley J: Avoiding facial nerve injuries in rhytidectomy. *Plast Reconstr Surg* 1979; 64(6):781–95.
4. Baker TJ, Gordon HL: Complications of rhytidectomy. *Plast Reconstr Surg* 1967; 40(1):31–9.
5. Brody GS: The tumescent technique for facelift. *Plast Reconstr Surg* 1994; 94:563.
6. Desnoyers Y, Custeau P, Berthiaume J: Anaesthesia for facial rhytidectomy. *Can Anaesth Soc J* 1979; 26(3): 222–4.
7. Dumanian GA, Bontempo FA, Johnson PC: Evaluation and treatment of the plastic surgical patient having a potential to bleed. *Plast Reconstr Surg* 1995; 96(1):211–18.
8. Feldman JJ: Corset platysmaplasty. *Plast Reconstr Surg* 1990; 85(3):333–43.
9. Goldwyn RM: Late bleeding after rhytidectomy from injury to the superficial temporal vessels. *Plast Reconstr Surg* 1991; 88(3):443–5.
10. Heinrichs HL, Kaidi AA: Subperiosteal face lift: A 200-case, 4-year review. *Plast Reconst Surg* 1998; 102(3):843–55.
11. Hester TR Jr, Codner MA, McCord CD, et al: Evolution of technique of the direct transblepharoplasty approach for the correction of lower lid and midfacial aging: maximizing results and minimizing complications in a 5-year experience. *Plast Reconstr Surg* 2000; 105(1):393–408.
12. Hochman M: Midface barbed suture lift. Facial Plast Surg Clin N Am 2007; (15):201–7.
13. Hoefflin SM: The extended supraplatysmal plane (ESP) face lift. *Plast Reconstr Surg* 1998; 101(2):494–503.
14. Kaye, BL: Complications of face-lift. Adv *Plast Reconstr Surg* 1990; 6:125–76.
15. Lemmon ML, Hamra ST: Skoog rhytidectomy: A five-year experience with 577 patients. *Plast Reconstr Surg* 1980; 65(3): 283–97.
16. Little JW: Three-dimensional rejuvenation of the midface: Volumetric resculpture by malar imbrication. *Plast Reconstr Surg* 2000; 105(1):267–85.
17. Mottura AA: The tumescent technique for face lifts? *Plast Reconstr Surg* 1995; 96(1):231.
18. Pitanguy I: Facial cosmetic surgery: A 30-year perspective. *Plast Reconstr Surg* 2000; 105(4):1517–27.
19. Rees TD, Lee YC, Coburn RJ: Expanding hematoma after rhytidectomy. *Plast Reconstr Surg* 1973; 51(2):149–53.
20. Schnur PL, Burkhardt BR, Tofield JJ: The second-look technique in face lifts: Does it work? *Plast Reconstr Surg* 1980; 65(3):298–301.

21. Schoen SA, Taylor CO, Owsley TG: Tumescent technique in cervicofacial rhytidectomy, *J Oral Maxillofac Surg* 1994; 52: 344–7.
22. Sullivan SA, Dailey RA: Endoscopic subperiosteal midface lift. *Opthal Plast Reconstr Surg* 2002; 18(5):319–30.
23. Tonnard P, Verpaele A, Monstrey S, et al: Minimal access cranial suspension lift: a modified S-lift. Plast Reconstr Surg 2002; 109(6):2074–86.

BROWLIFT AND BLEPHAROPLASTY

SURGICAL CONSIDERATIONS

BROWLIFT (OR FOREHEAD LIFT)

Description: Browlift is the resuspension of the brows and elimination of upper facial rhytids to restore the youthful appearance of the upper face. This procedure has a significant effect on the results of an upper blepharoplasty, with which it is frequently paired. Patients presenting for browlift usually have specific concerns about lateral brow hooding, forehead wrinkles, and glabellar creases that give them an angry appearance.

Like facelift procedures, browlifts have been performed in the subcutaneous plane, but the relatively avascular subgaleal and subperiosteal planes are more commonly used. The subgaleal and subperiosteal approaches have become more popular with the incorporation of **endoscopic techniques.** The incision may be a complete bicoronal or three to five small, interrupted access incisions along the hair line or within the hair-bearing scalp (Fig. 11.1-3). In the open technique, the bicoronal flap is dissected off the upper face (Fig. 11.1-4). The brows are elevated by **scalp resuspension ± resection**. Closure of the scalp helps maintain the resuspended position. The soft tissues may also be fixated directly to the cranium with screws or resorbable fixation devices and sutured to the temporal fascia to maintain

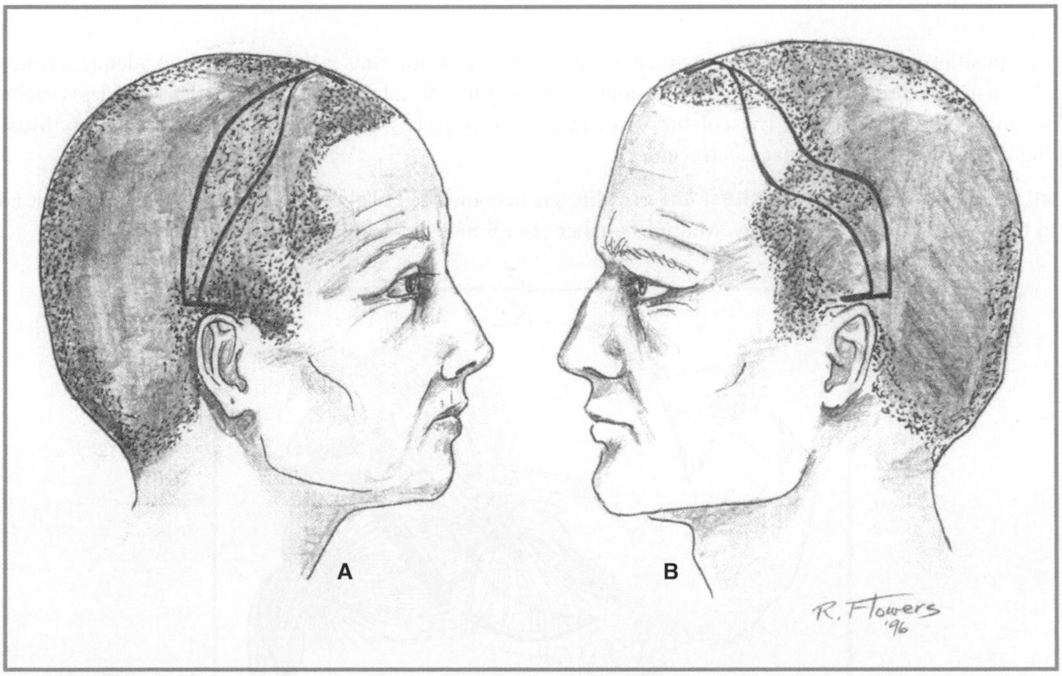

Figure 11.1-3. Incisions for forehead/brow lifting. Consistent blepharoplasty results demand appropriate frontal lifting technique. **A:** Standard coronal incision. **B:** Male and female balding incision. Note the posterior displacement of the ascending incision for maximum camouflage. Hair perimeter incisions are rarely necessary. The central brow corrects nicely from only parietotemporal scalp excisions (after appropriate supraperiosteal release). (Reproduced with permission from Flowers RS, DuVal C: Blepharoplasty and periorbital aesthetic surgery. In *Grabb & Smith's Plastic Surgery,* 5th edition. Aston SJ, Beasley RW, Thorne CHM, eds. Lippincott-Raven: 1997.)

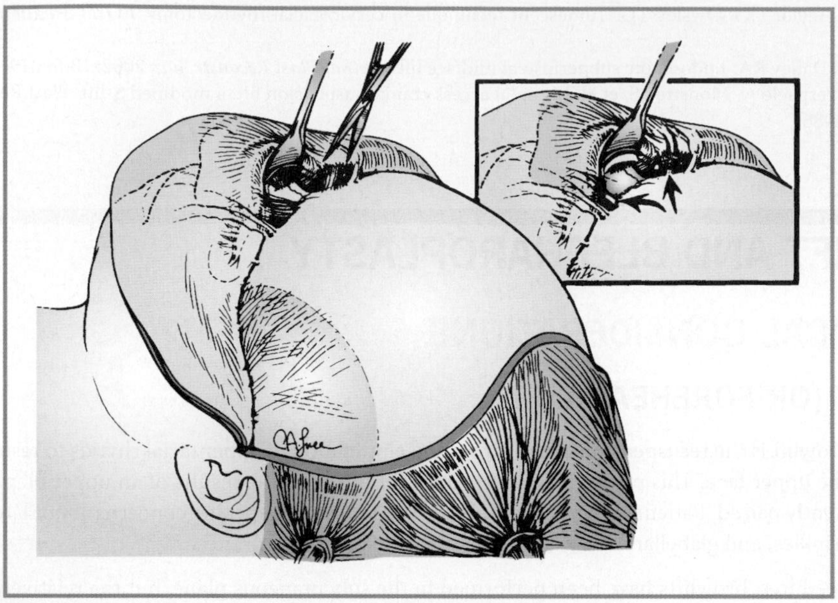

Figure 11.1-4. Exposure after subgaleal, supraperiosteal dissection of the forehead. The supraorbital nerves can be seen easily, but the supratrochlear nerves are more superficial and are hidden by the corrugator muscles. Scissors are used to tease through the corrugator muscles to locate the supratrochlear nerve branches. The muscle is then aggressively resected, preserving the sensory branches. (Reproduced with permission from Thorne CHM, Aston SJ: Aesthetic surgery of the aging face. In *Grabb & Smith's Plastic Surgery,* 5th edition. Aston SJ, Beasley RW, Thorne CHM, eds. Lippincott-Raven: 1997.)

their new positions. Release of the periosteum along the superior orbital rims is a prerequisite to adequate resuspension when using a subperiosteal approach. Elimination of the upper facial rhytids (i.e., glabellar wrinkles) is achieved by resection of the medial brow musculature (corrugator and procerus) from beneath the elevated flap. Muscular bleeding is controlled with bipolar electrocautery.

Variant procedures or approaches: The browlift has become the facial plastic surgery procedure most adaptable to the techniques of **endoscopy.** Multiple smaller (1–1.5 inch) incisions are used within the scalp for access,

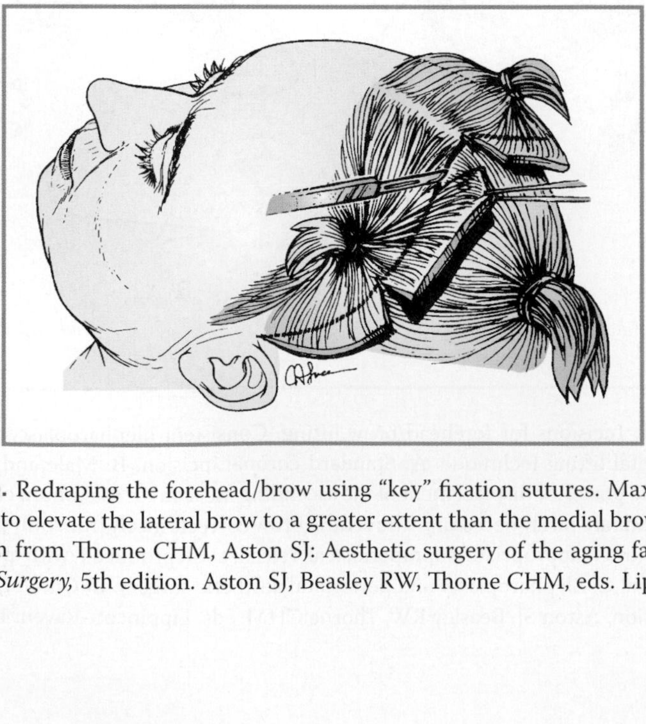

Figure 11.1-5. Redraping the forehead/brow using "key" fixation sutures. Maximal tension is placed laterally to elevate the lateral brow to a greater extent than the medial brow. (Reproduced with permission from Thorne CHM, Aston SJ: Aesthetic surgery of the aging face. In *Grabb & Smith's Plastic Surgery,* 5th edition. Aston SJ, Beasley RW, Thorne CHM, eds. Lippincott-Raven: 1997.)

SUMMARY OF PROCEDURES

	Browlift	Blepharoplasty
Position	Supine; table rotated 90 or 180°	⇐
Incision	Hairline, coronal; multiple scalp for endoscopic procedure	Upper: tarsal fold; lower: subciliary, transconjunctival
Special instrumentation	Fibrin glue, screws or resorbable fixation devices for suspension; endoscopic equipment	Bipolar electrocautery
Unique considerations	Local anesthetic with epinephrine	Retrobulbar hematoma; OCR; local anesthetic with epinephrine
Antibiotics	Cefazolin 1 g iv ± methylprednisolone 125 mg iv	⇐
Surgical time	1–2 h	⇐
Closing considerations	Place dressing before arousing patient. Gentle arousal from anesthesia (↑ in BP or emesis → risk of hematoma)	No dressing (ointment)
EBL	50 mL	Minimal
Postop care	PACU → room/home Lightly compressive dressing Head of bed elevated	⇐ Cool packs ⇐ Ophthalmic lubricant Vision checks
Mortality	Rare	⇐
Morbidity	Hematoma: Rare Alopecia: Rare (more common with bicoronal approach) Infection: < 1% Frontalis paralysis: Rare (usually transient) Poor cosmetic result Sensory nerve dysfunction Lagophthalmos	⇐ – ⇐ – ⇐ ⇐ ⇐ Blindness: Extremely rare Ectropion Entropion
Pain score	3	2–3

PATIENT POPULATION CHARACTERISTICS

Age range	Most ≥ 35 yr
Male:Female	Blepharoplasties: 1:4 Browlifts: 1:7.33
Incidence	Blepharoplasties: 233,200 (fourth most common cosmetic procedure in the United States, 2006) Browlifts: 55,525 (ninth most common cosmetic procedure in the United States, 2006)
Etiology	Facial rhytids secondary to solar elastosis, senile elastosis, facial expression, and increased muscle resting tone; Asian eyelids
Associated conditions	Cancers of the skin (basal cell carcinoma, squamous cell carcinoma and precursors, and melanoma) in solar elastosis cases, especially fair-skinned patients

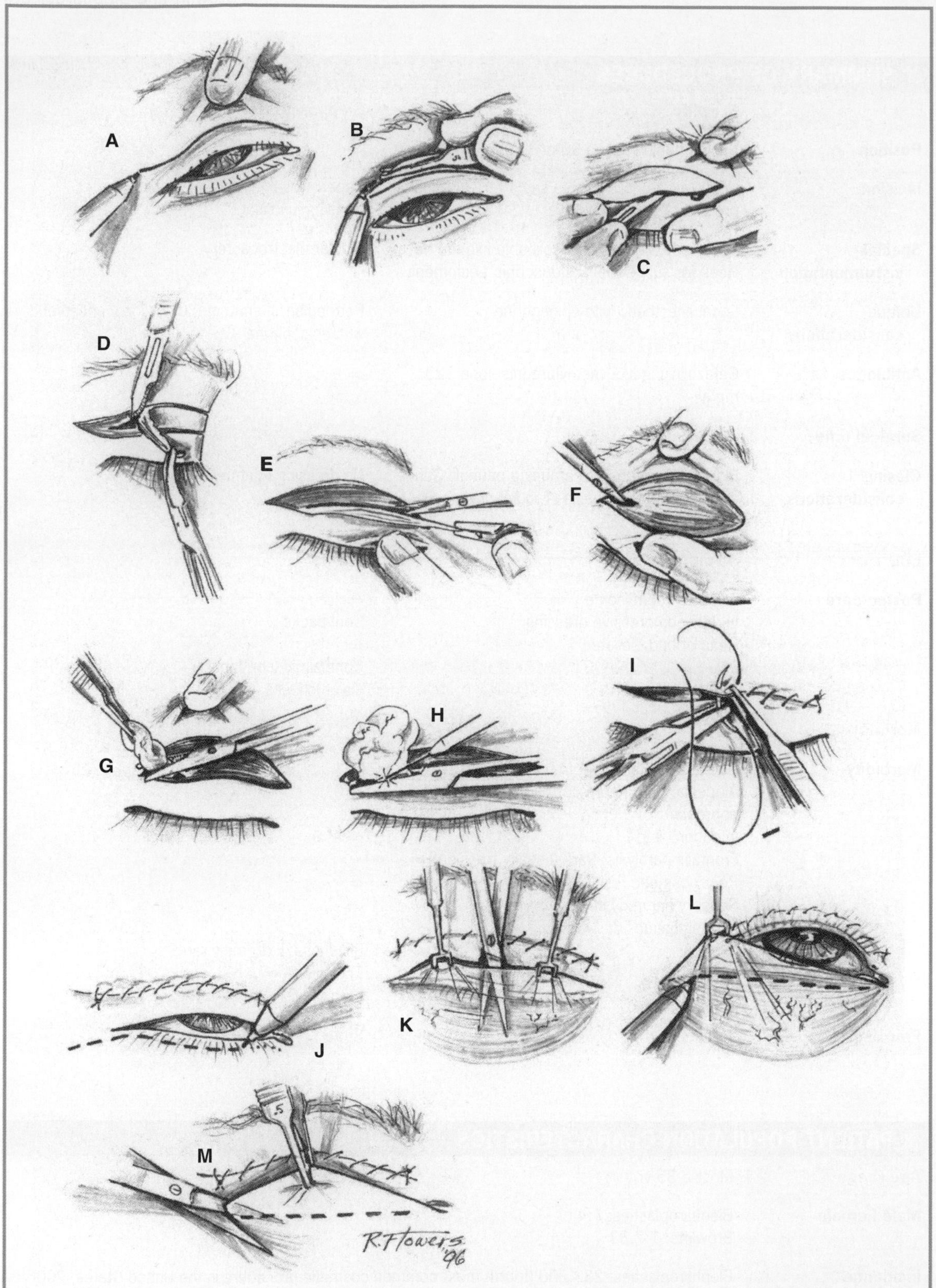

Figure 11.1-6. Traditional blepharoplasty technique. **A:** The caudal margin of the excision is marked and **(B)** the upper eyelid skin is pinched. Skin and muscle are excised **(C, D, E)**; excess or herniated fat is removed from medial and lateral compartments **(F, G, H)**; and the wound is closed **(I)**. On the lower lid, the traditional approach is flap elevation, consisting of skin or skin with attached muscle **(J, K)**. The skin is draped upward and outward so the surgeon can assess and remove excess skin **(L, M)**. (Reproduced with permission from Flowers RS, DuVal C: Blepharoplasty and periorbital aesthetic surgery. In *Grabb & Smith's Plastic Surgery*, 5th edition. Aston SJ, Beasley RW, Thorne CHM, eds. Lippincott-Raven: 1997.)

and small, elliptical excisions also may be used to achieve the desired effect. The muscle resection is accomplished endoscopically with very small biting forceps from beneath the flap.

Usual preop diagnosis: Brow ptosis; brow droop; upper facial rhytids (wrinkles or creases)

BLEPHAROPLASTY (OR LIDLIFT)

Description: Blepharoplasty (Fig. 11.1-6), or lidlift, is the surgical rejuvenation of the periorbital region to eliminate the tired and aged appearance of the eyes. Westernizing the Asian eyelid also has become quite commonplace. Presenting complaints include excess lid skin, prominent periorbital fat, and absence of upper lid folds. Blepharoplasty can involve resection of skin, muscle (orbicularis oculi), and fat. Many patients presenting for this procedure will require a simultaneous browlift to re-establish the baseline position of the brows, revealing the true amount of upper-lid redundancy. Eyelid ptosis repair also can be achieved in the same surgery.

Although a seemingly benign procedure, the manipulation of periorbital fat can have very serious consequences. Retrobulbar hematoma and blindness can occur postoperatively, and the oculocardiac reflex (OCR) can complicate the intraoperative course with bradycardia and hypotension. This generally resolves with elimination of the stimulus.

Blepharoplasty, as an isolated procedure, is often performed with local anesthetic and intravenous sedation so that patients can open and close their eyes during the surgery. This helps to achieve a good result and decreases the risk of lagophthalmos, which is especially important if a ptosis repair is also planned.

Variant Procedures or Approaches: CO_2 **laser blepharoplasty** techniques have proven effective, but must be done under the safety parameters of eye protection and fire and burn prevention (see p. 1080). With this technique, the fat and skin resections are achieved with a laser, replacing the use of a scalpel. Using the laser to gain some of the skin tightening associated with blepharoplasty has also been described.

Usual preop diagnosis: Blepharochalasis; periorbital fat; blepharoptosis; dermatochalasis; supratarsal fold absence; Asian eyelid

Suggested Readings

1. American Society of Plastic Surgeons web site: www.plasticsurgery.org.
2. Berkowitz RL, Jacobs DI, Gorman PJ: Brow fixation with the Endotine Forehead device in endoscopic brow lift. *Plast Reconstr Surg* 2005; 116(6):1761–7.
3. Flowers RS, Caputy GC, Flowers SS: The biomechanics of brow and frontalis function and its effect on blepharoplasty. *Clin Plast Surg* 1993; 20(2):255–68.
4. Flowers RS: The art of eyelid and orbital aesthetics: multiracial surgical considerations. *Clin Plast Surg* 1987; 14(4):703–21.
5. Matarasso A: The oculocardiac reflex in blepharoplasty surgery. *Plast Reconstr Surg* 1989; 83(2):243–50.
6. Mittelman H, Apfelberg DB: Carbon dioxide laser blepharoplasty—advantages and disadvantages. *Ann Plast Surg* 1990; 24(1):1–6.
7. Ortiz-Monasterio F, Barrera G, Olmedo A: The coronal incision in rhytidectomy—the brow lift. *Clin Plast Surg* 1978; 5(1):167–79.
8. Ramirez OM: Endoscopic techniques in facial rejuvenation: an overview. Part 1. *Aesth Plast Surg* 1994; 18:141–7.
9. Ramirez OM: Endoscopically assisted biplanar forehead lift. *Plast Reconstr Surg* 1995; 96(2):323–33.
10. Sacks SH, Lawson W, Edelstein D, et al: Surgical treatment of blindness secondary to intraorbital hemorrhage. *Arch Otolaryngol Head Neck Surg* 1988; 114:801–3.
11. Stasior OG, Ballitch HA II: Ptosis repair in aesthetic blepharoplasty. *Clin Plast Surg* 1993; 20(2):269–73.
12. Steinsapir KD, Shorr N, Hoenig J, et al: The endoscopic forehead lift. *Opthal Plast Reconstr Surg* 1998; 14(2):107–18.
13. Wolfe SA, Baird WL: The subcutaneous forehead lift. *Plast Reconstr Surg* 1989; 83(2):251–6.

ANESTHETIC CONSIDERATIONS

(Procedures covered: facelift, necklift; browlift, blepharoplasty)

PREOPERATIVE

Cosmetic facial surgery is elective and should be performed preferably on ASA I or II patients. Often, several cosmetic procedures (including facial laser resurfacing) are performed during the same surgical session. A preop discussion with the surgical team is important to help define the anesthetic plan. The above procedures are predominantly done under GA in the hospital, but can also be done under MAC with local anesthesia.

Airway	A careful inspection of the airway should be performed. Surgeon may request intraop manipulation of the oral ETT from side-to-side.
Cardiovascular	A thorough cardiovascular evaluation should be performed, because HTN is the most common medical condition in this patient population. Many procedures involve the use of significant amounts of local anesthetic with epinephrine, placing the patient at higher risk for HTN, dysrhythmias, and coronary artery spasm. Additionally, consider patient suitability for the use of controlled, mild controlled ↓ BP (particularly the facelift patient). **Tests:** ECG, if indicated from H&P.
Hematologic	✓ for recent aspirin/NSAID use. **Tests:** CBC, if indicated from H&P.
Laboratory	Others tests as indicated from H&P.
Premedication	Preop sedation with clonidine (adjunctive hypnotic and antihypertensive agent) or midazolam usually is appropriate. Preop steroids (dexamethasone 4–8 mg) also may be used to reduce postop pain and PONV, as well as swelling.

INTRAOPERATIVE

Anesthetic technique: Cases are predominantly done under GA, using an ETT or LMA, as appropriate. Several authors describe the use of a propofol/ketamine MAC or "dissociative anesthetic" in the office-based setting. There are varying descriptions of this technique, generally involving a propofol infusion with incremental ketamine boluses or infusion, resulting in elimination or significant reduction in the administration of iv opiates.

MAC with local anesthetic also is an option and may be advantageous for certain patients (e.g., with Hx of PONV) or for cases that benefit from a patient's intraop ability to follow commands (e.g., ptosis repair).

Induction	For those procedures done under GETA, a standard induction (see p. B-2) is appropriate. An oral RAE ETT may be used to minimize intrusion into the surgical field. For cases involving a laser, a shielded ETT manufactured for laser surgery should be used and the cuff filled with NS and methylene blue, rather than air. (Note: no cuffed ETT is 100% laser-proof; always use standard precautions.)
Maintenance	Standard maintenance (see p. B-2) with volatile anesthetic ± propofol infusion is appropriate in most cases. Muscle relaxation should be avoided in cases with facial nerve monitoring. Mild, controlled ↓ BP may be requested and used to facilitate hemostasis. HTN should be avoided and treated immediately if it occurs. Maintain anesthesia during application of head/face wrap.
Emergence	Antiemetic prophylaxis (e.g., ondansetron 4 mg iv) is recommended, as postop emesis greatly increases the likelihood of hematoma formation. Perform thorough oropharyngeal suctioning and ensure that all throat packing has been removed. A smooth emergence with no notable increase in BP is preferred.
Blood and fluid requirements	Blood loss generally minimal IV: 18 ga × 1 NS/LR @ 2–4 mL/kg/h
Monitoring	Standard monitors (see p. B-1)
Control of blood loss	Local infiltration with epinephrine Surgical hemostasis Mild degree of ↓ BP
Positioning	✓ and pad pressure points. Rotate OR table 90–180°. Scleral shields ± ophthalmic ointment

Plastic and Reconstructive Surgery

Complications	OCR Local anesthetic toxicity Retrobulbar hematoma	Remove inciting stimulus. Consider atropine 0.5 mcg and deepening anesthetic.

POSTOPERATIVE

Complications	PONV	Vigorous treatment of nausea is important.
Pain management	Local infiltration + iv/po narcotics, if needed	R/O expanding hematoma as cause of increasing pain.

Suggested Readings

1. Aasboe V, Raeder JC, Groegaard B: Betamethasone reduces postoperative pain and nausea after ambulatory surgery. *Anesth Analg* 1998; 87:319–23.
2. Friedberg BL: Propofol ketamine anesthesia for cosmetic surgery in the office suite. *Int Anesthesiol Clin* 2003; 41(2):39–50.
3. Richard MJ, Skues MA, Jarvis AP, et al: Total iv anesthesia with propofol and alfentanil: dose requirements for propranolol and the effect of premedication with clonidine. *Br J Anaesth* 1990; 65:157–63.
4. Yoho RA, Romaine JJ, O'Neil D: Review of the liposuction, abdominoplasty, and face-lift mortality and morbidity risk literature. *Dermatol Surg* 2005; 31:733–43; Erratum in: *Dermatol Surg* 2005; 31(9 Pt 1):1158.

RHINOPLASTY

SURGICAL CONSIDERATIONS

Description: **Rhinoplasty,** one of the greatest challenges of plastic surgery, is the surgical manipulation of the nasal form for aesthetic and/or functional improvement. In combination with nasal septal surgery, it is called **septorhinoplasty.** Common patient requests are for dorsal hump reduction and improved tip definition. Cosmetic surgery of the nose can be divided into four major types: **tip rhinoplasty, dorsal rhinoplasty, alarplasty,** and **septoplasty,** in addition to other ancillary procedures to enhance airway function.

Tip and **dorsal procedures** may be accomplished by either **reduction** or **augmentation.** Augmentation can be achieved with synthetic materials such as silicone, expanded fibrillated polytetrafluoroethylene polymer (Gore-Tex), porous polyethylene implants (Medpore), and hydroxyapatite. Cadaveric or autologous tissue (cartilage, bone, fascia, or dermis) also are utilized. Common donor sites for cartilage are the ear concha (via an anterior or posterior approach), the nasal septum (internal nasal approach), and the ribs. Bone harvest sites may include the outer table of cranium, the iliac crest, and the ribs. Dermal graft is commonly harvested from the groin and fascial graft harvest is often taken from the temporoparietal region. (Table 11.1-1 shows the range of open and closed rhinoplasty techniques.)

A throat pack is useful to prevent aspiration or ingestion of blood, as significant blood pooling can occur in the naso/oropharynx area, especially with nasal osteotomies used to narrow or straighten the nasal dorsum. Cases where such pooling is expected are safer under GA with a throat pack. Often rhinoplasties are done with local or regional (nasociliary and infraorbital blocks) anesthesia with sedation. Vasoconstrictor-soaked nasal packs (cocaine vs epinephrine vs oxymetazoline) are placed before the first incision.

The decision of open versus closed technique is based on patient requirements and surgeon preference. An **open approach** will utilize a transcolumellar incision to allow elevation of a nasal skin flap and degloving of the lower alar cartilages for direct and wide exposure of the nasal framework. **Closed approaches** use intercartilaginous, intracartilaginous, infracartilaginous, rim, hemitransfixion, and transfixion incisions (all hidden within the nose).

A typical **closed rhinoplasty** (Fig. 11.1-7) begins with dorsal work through intercartilaginous incisions. The dorsum may be reduced using a scalpel and/or rasps beneath the undermined dorsal skin and periosteum. The septum is addressed as necessary through a hemitransfixion incision (± cartilage harvest). Tip reduction by scalpel or scissor resection of the lower alar cartilage ± tip suture is next. Nasal osteotomies with an osteotome and mallet begin at the base of the nasal bones along the piriform aperture. Digital manipulation completes the fractures, and this is when most of the blood loss occurs. Dorsal and tip grafts are applied as necessary, with alar modifications made last. **Alar reduction** entails wedge resection of the lateral alar base and primary closure.

Table 11.1-1. Rhinoplasty Techniques

Open	Closed/Open	Closed
Incisions/skin flap elevation ↓ Tip analysis/cephalic crura excision ↓ Extramucosal tunnels ↓ Dorsal modification ↓ Caudal septum/anterior nasal spine ↓ Septoplasty/harvest ↓ Osteotomies ↓ Graft preparation ↓ Definitive dorsum/spreader grafts ↓ Tip: Columella strut/tip sutures ↓ Closure ↓ Alar base modification ↓ Dressing/postop management	Intercartilaginous/transfixion incisions ↓ Skin elevation/extramucosal tunnels ↓ Rasp bony hump/ excise cartilaginous hump ↓ Radix reduction ↓ Check profile line/septal angle ↓ Caudal septum/anterior nasal spine ↓ Infracartilaginous/ transcolumellar incisions ↓ Tip exposure and analysis ↓ Septal correction/harvest ↓ Osteotomies ↓ Definitive dorsum/spreader grafts ↓ Tip/columellar modification (excision/sutures/grafts) ↓ Closure ↓ Alar base modification ↓ Dressing	Transcartilaginous/ transfixion incision ↓ Skin elevation/extramucosal tunnels ↓ Rasp bony hump/ excise cartilage hump ↓ Radix reduction ↓ Check profile line/septal angle ↓ Caudal septum/anterior nasal spine ↓ Septoplasty/harvest ↓ Infracartilaginous incisions ↓ Alar cartilage delivery ↓ Excision/incision/sutures ↓ Osteotomies ↓ Grafts (spreader/dorsum/columella/tip) ↓ Closure ↓ Alar base modifications ↓ Dressing

Note: Only those steps appropriate for the individual case are performed.

Depending on the type of rhinoplasty performed, different dressings will be applied at the end of the procedure. When nasal bone osteotomies are used, the patient will require a dorsal nasal splint ± bilateral nasal packing. Nasal packing is generally removed at 24–72 hours postoperatively. When septal manipulation is needed, nasal packing or some sort of septal splint may be placed. The packs are generally removed within three days, but the splints can be maintained much longer and the nasal airways kept patent with vasoconstrictor nasal sprays.

Variant procedures or approaches: Placement of a **columellar strut (cartilage graft)** and **release of the tip depressor muscle** often are achieved via intraoral vestibular incisions (behind the upper lip).

Usual preop diagnosis: Posttraumatic nasal deformity (including disordered breathing, "saddle nose," crooked nose, septal deviation); developmental nasal deformities (bulbous tip, flat tip, drooping tip, broad dorsum, dorsal hump, alar widening, "Pinocchio nose"); congenital nasal malformation (cleft nasal deformities)

SUMMARY OF PROCEDURE

Position	Supine, table may be rotated 180°. If GA: oral ETT toward foot of bed, shoulder roll, neck extended, scleral lubricant, shields
Incision	External vs internal nasal incisions
Special instrumentation	Headlight
Unique considerations	Throat pack for expected nasopharyngeal bleeding. Intranasal vasoconstrictors.
Antibiotics	Cefazolin 1 g iv

SUMMARY OF PROCEDURE (cont'd)	
Surgical time	1–2.5 h
Closing considerations	Suction stomach via OG tube at the end of surgery. **Remove throat pack prior to extubation.** Internal and/or external nasal splints are placed for dressings.
EBL	Tip rhinoplasty: 20 mL Dorsum with osteotomies: 75–150 mL Septoplasty: + 50 mL
Postop care	PACU → room (most patients are home the same day). Ensure minimal PONV; elevate head of bed; no pressure on nose (e.g., O_2 mask).
Mortality	Rare
Morbidity	Infection: > 1% Adverse cosmetic result: Alar notching Alar collapse Dorsal irregularity Asymmetry Tip droop Adverse functional result (i.e., poor airway) Septal perforation
Pain Score	3 (4 with osteotomies)

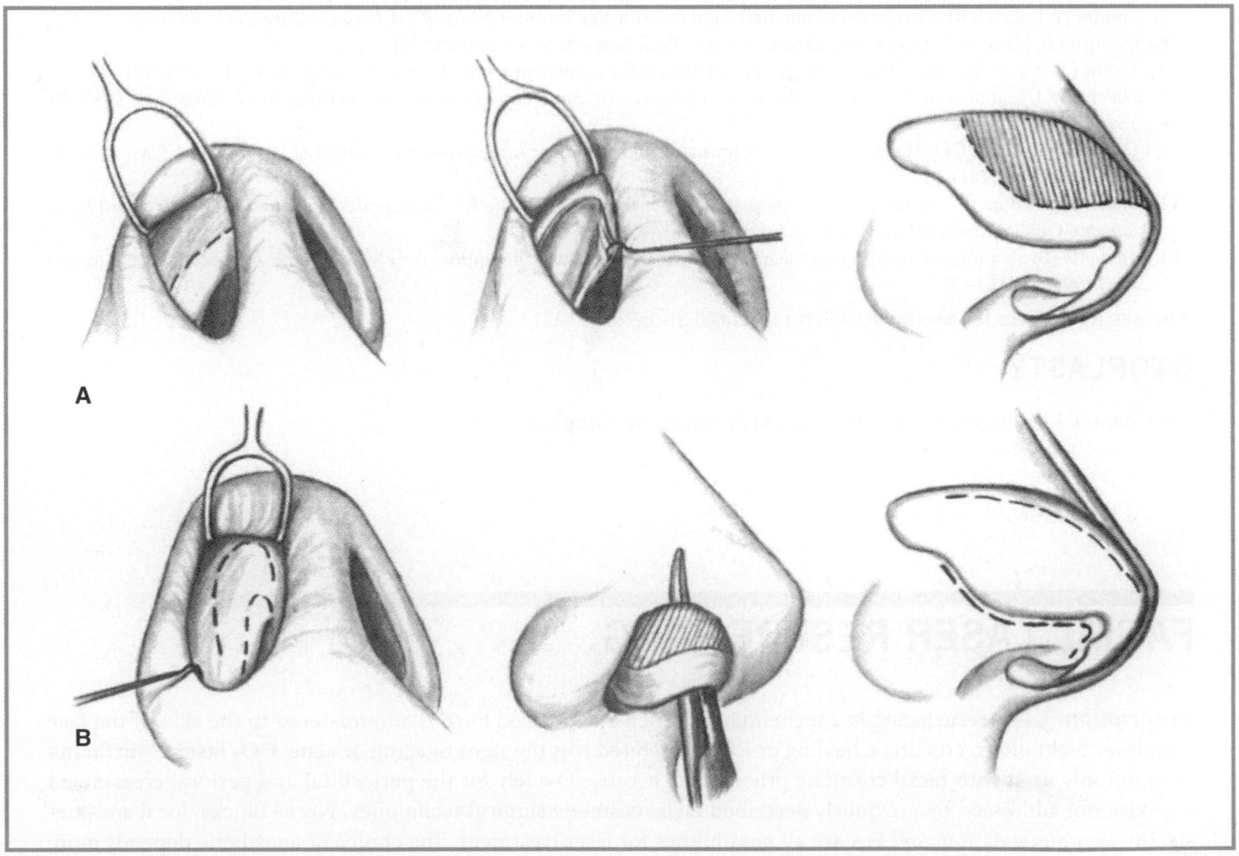

Figure 11.1-7. Closed rhinoplasty. **A:** Transcartilaginous approach using an intracartilaginous incision. **B:** Delivery approach, using a high intercartilaginous incision and a marginal incision to facilitate delivery of the lateral crura. (Reproduced with permission from Daniel RK: Rhinoplasty. In *Grabb & Smith's Plastic Surgery,* 5th edition. Aston SJ, Beasley RW, Thorne CHM, eds. Lippincott-Raven: 1997.)

PATIENT POPULATION CHARACTERISTICS	
Age Range	Most ≥ 15 yr
Male:Female[1]	1:1.7
Incidence[1]	307,258 (third most common cosmetic procedure in the United States, 2006)
Etiology	Developmental; acquired (post-traumatic); congenital (see Secondary Cleft Lip and Nasal Surgery, p. 1418).
Associated conditions	Breathing difficulties; psychosocial issues (body dysmorphic disorder)

ANESTHETIC CONSIDERATIONS

See Anesthetic Considerations for Nasal and Sinus Surgery, p. 245.

Suggested Readings

1. American Society of Plastic Surgeons web site: www.plasticsurgery.org, 444 East Algonquin Rd, Arlington Heights, IL 60005-4664.
2. Becker DG, McLaughlin RB, Loevner LA, et al: The lateral osteotomy in rhinoplasty: clinical and radiographic rationale for osteotome selection. *Plast Reconstr Surg* 2000; 105(5): 1806–19.
3. Byrd HS, Salomon J, Flood J: Correction of the crooked nose. *Plast Reconstr Surg* 1998; 102(6):2148–57.
4. Eppley BL: Alloplastic implantation. *Plast Reconstr Surg* 1999; 104(6):1761–83.
5. Gruber RP, Friedman GD: Suture algorithm for broad or bulbous nasal tip. *Plast Reconstr Surg* 2002; 110(7):1752–68.
6. Gruber RP: Lengthening the short nose. *Plast Reconstr Surg* 1993; 91(7):1252–8.
7. Gunter JP, Rohrich RJ: Correction of pinched nasal tip with alar spreader grafts. *Plast Reconstr Surg* 1992; 90(5):821–9.
8. Guyuron B: Nasal osteotomies and airway changes. *Plast Reconstr Surg* 1998; 102:856.
9. Molliex S, Navez M, Baylot D, et al: Regional anaesthesia for outpatient nasal surgery. *Br J Anaesthesia* 1996; 76:151–3.
10. Niechajev I, Haraldsson PO: Two methods of anesthesia for rhinoplasty in outpatient setting. *Aesth Plast Surg* 1996; 20: 159–63.
11. Owsley TG, Taylor CO: The use of Gore-Tex for nasal augmentation: A retrospective analysis of 106 patients. *Plast Reconstr Surg* 1994; 94(2):241–50.
12. Sheen JH: Adjunctive techniques in rhinoplasty: harvesting cranial bone for nasal grafts. In *Video Perspectives in Plastic Surgery.* Quality Medical Publishing, St. Louis: 1989, 1–32.
13. Tebbetts JB: Shaping and positioning the nasal tip without structural disruption: A new, systematic approach. *Plast Reconstr Surg* 1994; 94(l):61–77.

Also see References for Secondary Cleft Lip/Nasal Surgery, p. 1421.

OTOPLASTY

See Chapter 12.8 Surgery for Craniofacial Malformations, Otoplasty, p. 1423.

FACIAL LASER RESURFACING

Description: Laser resurfacing is a technique by which a controlled burn is administered to the skin of the face with laser technology, creating a healing process which reduces the signs of aging or acne. **CO_2 laser resurfacing** is commonly used with facial cosmetic procedures. It is used widely for the periorbital and perioral creases and wrinkles not addressed by previously described facial cosmetic surgical techniques. Nerve blocks, local anesthesia, intravenous sedation, and GA are all possibilities for laser treatment. The choice of anesthetic depends more on the specific surgical procedures to be performed first, as the laser procedure is usually adjunctive and added at the end. Facial laser resurfacing is done frequently in an office-based setting (see Chapter 14.0 Office-Based Procedures, p. 1512). Because laser resurfacing is usually an adjunct to another facial cosmetic procedure, the following discussion pertains primarily to the unique set of **safety issues** that must be addressed in the OR.

Ocular Hazards: These include direct and reflected injury to the eye. Everyone present, including the patient and all medical personnel, requires laser-specific (i.e., wavelength-specific) safety eyewear. Laser-specific scleral shields must be available for the patient in cases where the patient's eyewear would be in the operative field. Protective eyewear must be undamaged and have:

- Permanent labels with wavelength and optical density tolerance
- Side shields
- Damage threshold of > 10 sec
- No surface reflection
- Good fit
- Approval from the laser safety officer

Fire and reflectivity hazards: Many items used in the OR (e.g., drapes, sponges, plastic cannulas, etc.) are made of materials that can be fire hazards if not kept from interacting with the laser beam. Protection from fire and reflectivity is provided by:

- Having fire-retardant or moist draping
- Having water basin available
- Having a fire extinguisher readily available
- Avoiding all alcohol-containing prep solutions
- Avoiding use of plastic and rubber instruments (may melt or ignite)
- Using special fire-resistant ETTs or wet sponge protection for plastic ETTs to decrease the possibility of tube breach or ignition
- Avoiding open sources of O_2 (nasal cannulas, etc.)
- Avoiding metal or other reflective materials

Airborne contaminants: The laser destruction of cells releases carbon particles, microbials, DNA, and toxic fumes. Protection for the patient and medical personnel is provided by:

- Utilizing a smoke evacuation system 2 cm from created plume
- Wearing high-filtration masks. Note that these masks become less effective if moistened from perspiration during a long case; if the laser is to be used at the end of a case, changing masks before using the laser may be prudent.

ANESTHETIC CONSIDERATIONS

See Anesthetic Considerations following Browlift and Blepharoplasty, p. 1075, or Office-Based Laser Skin Resurfacing, p. 1513.

Suggested Readings

1. Alster TS, Apfelberg DB, eds: *Cosmetic Laser Surgery: A Practitioner's Guide,* 2nd edition. Wiley-Liss, New York: 1999.
2. Blakeley KR, Klein KW, White PF, et al: A total intravenous technique for outpatient facial laser resurfacing. *Anesth Analg* 1998; 87:827–9.

CHAPTER

11.2 Nonfacial Aesthetic Surgery

SURGEONS

Angeline F. Lim, MD
David M. Kahn, MD
George W. Commons, MD (*Liposuction*)

ANESTHESIOLOGISTS

Lindsey Vokach-Brodsky, MB, ChB, FFARCS
Bruce D. Halperin, MD (*Liposuction*)

AUGMENTATION MAMMOPLASTY

SURGICAL CONSIDERATIONS

Description: **Augmentation mammoplasty** is accomplished through the use of saline or silicone gel-filled breast implants. The surgery may be performed under GA or local anesthesia with sedation. The patient is positioned either with the arms abducted at 90° or with the hands on the abdomen. Local anesthetic (± epinephrine) is infiltrated into the skin at the incision site and under the glandular tissue. Implant insertion can be done through inframammary, periareolar, transaxillary, or transumbilical incisions. The implant is placed in a pocket that is created either beneath the mammary gland (subglandular), under the pectoralis muscle (submuscular), partially subglandular and partially submuscular (dual-plane), or beneath the pectoralis fascia (subfascial), depending on the surgeon's preference and the amount of tissue available. An endoscope may be used to assist with dissection of the pocket. When the implant is placed in the submuscular position, the pectoralis muscle is divided from its insertion along the inframammary fold and sometimes along the sternal insertion to allow the muscle to drape over the implant. Regardless of the location of the pocket, the surgical wound is carefully irrigated and inspected for hemostasis. Sizers, either predetermined volumes of silicone gel or adjustable saline- or air-filled temporary implants, may be used to help determine the appropriate final volume and placement. The patient may be placed in the seated position to assess the size, shape, and symmetry of the breasts. The sizers are then replaced with the permanent prostheses. If permanent saline implants are used, they are filled with saline until the desired volume is reached; gel-filled implants do not have alterable volumes. The wounds are closed, and dressings are applied (Fig. 11.2-1).

Augmentation mammoplasty usually is performed as an outpatient procedure, although some patients may want an overnight stay for pain management and antiemetics. PONV is not uncommon, and all efforts should be made to decrease its frequency.

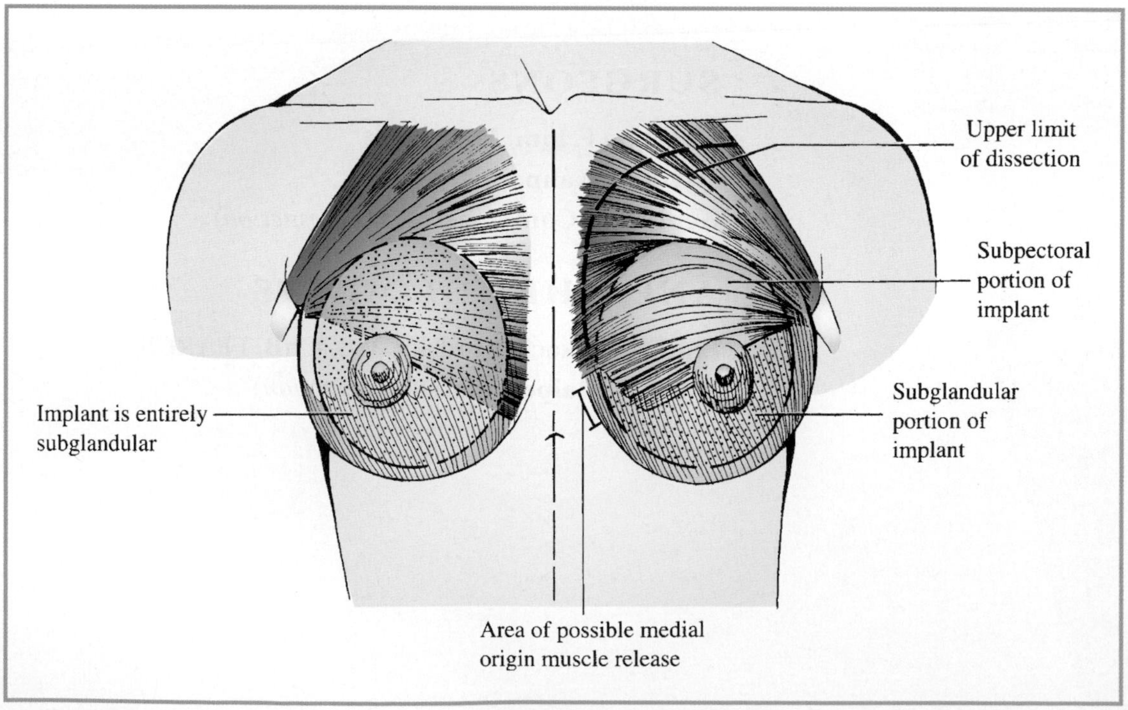

Figure 11.2-1. Breast augmentation. Implants may be placed in a subglandular or subpectoral position. (Reproduced with permission from Spear SL: *The Breast: Principles and Art.* Lippincott-Raven: 1998.)

Plastic and Reconstructive Surgery

Variant procedure or approaches: The endoscopic transumbilical approach is used much less frequently.

Preop Diagnosis: Hypomastia, breast ptosis

SUMMARY OF PROCEDURE	
Position	Supine
Incision	Inframammary; periareolar; transaxillary; or transumbilical
Antibiotics	Cefazolin 1 g iv
Unique considerations	May place patient in sitting position during procedure.
Surgical time	1 h
Closing considerations	May need patient in sitting position for application of dressings.
EBL	Minimal
Postop care	Outpatient procedure
Mortality	Rare
Morbidity	Prosthesis failure: 5% Capsular contracture: 5% Hematoma: 3% Infection: 2% Wound dehiscence: < 1% Cosmetic disappointments
Pain score	3–4

PATIENT POPULATION CHARACTERISTICS	
Age range	Typically 17–45 yr, but also may be done on the contralateral breast in a patient undergoing breast reconstruction.
Incidence	329,396 performed in the United States in 2006; the most common cosmetic surgical procedure
Etiology	Developmental; involution after breast feeding; age-related atrophy or ptosis
Associated conditions	Not common, but can be seen with Poland's syndrome.

ANESTHETIC CONSIDERATIONS

See Anesthetic Considerations following Mastopexy/Breast Lift, p. 1089.

Suggested Readings

1. Cooter RD, Rudkin GE, Gardiner SE: Day case breast augmentation under paravertebral blockade: a prospective study of 100 consecutive patients. *Aesthetic Plast Surg* 2007; 31(6):666–73.
2. Graf RM, Bernandes A, Rippel R, et al: Subfascial breast implant: a new procedure. *Plast Reconstr Surg* 2003; 111(2): 904–8.
3. McLaughlin JK, Lipworth L, Murphy DK, et al: The safety of silicone gel-filled breast implants: a review of the epidemiologic evidence. *Ann Plast Surg* 2007; 59(5):569–80.
4. See Suggested Readings Mastopexy/Breast Lift, p. 1090.
5. Tebbetts JB: Dual plane breast augmentation: optimizing implant-soft tissue relationships in a wide range of breast types. *Plast Reconstr Surg* 2001; 107(5):1255–72.

REDUCTION MAMMOPLASTY

SURGICAL CONSIDERATIONS

Description: Breast reduction surgery can be done as an outpatient procedure or with an overnight stay. One might choose to admit the patient overnight in a hospital setting to monitor for hematoma formation and evidence of decreased blood supply to the nipple-areola complex. For these patients, the pain from this procedure is relatively low; therefore, PONV tends to be the greater issue in the immediate postoperative period.

The traditional type of breast reduction performed in the U.S. is the **inferior pedicle technique** using a Wise pattern ("anchor-type" scar) for the skin excision (Fig. 11.2-2). Markings are made with the patient upright in the preoperative holding area. The areola is marked circumferentially with an areola sizer and incised. The remaining incision lines are scored with a scalpel. Next, the inferior pedicle, which contains the neurovascular supply to the nipple-areola complex, is deepithelialized. Excess skin and breast tissue are excised, preserving the pedicle of tissue that will compose the breast mound. The resected tissue from each breast, which can range from 200–1,000 g, is weighed as an adjunctive method of ensuring symmetry. Temporary skin closure with staples allows the patient to be placed in a sitting position so that the breasts can be evaluated for symmetry. When the surgeon is satisfied with the appearance of the breasts, they are closed with sutures. Drains may be placed, depending on surgeon preference (Fig. 11.2-2). After the skin has been closed, the location of the nipple and areola is marked and excised, and the nipple-areola complex is delivered and sutured into position. Soft, supportive dressings are placed.

A technique that has gained in popularity recently is the **vertical reduction mammoplasty**, which shares the fundamental principles of excision of excess breast tissue and preservation of blood flow to the nipple-areola complex, but differs in choice of skin incision and pedicle. Relatively more time is spent performing the tissue excision and pedicle shaping, but wound closure time is greatly decreased (resulting in a "lollipop-type" scar) compared with the traditional Wise-pattern technique.

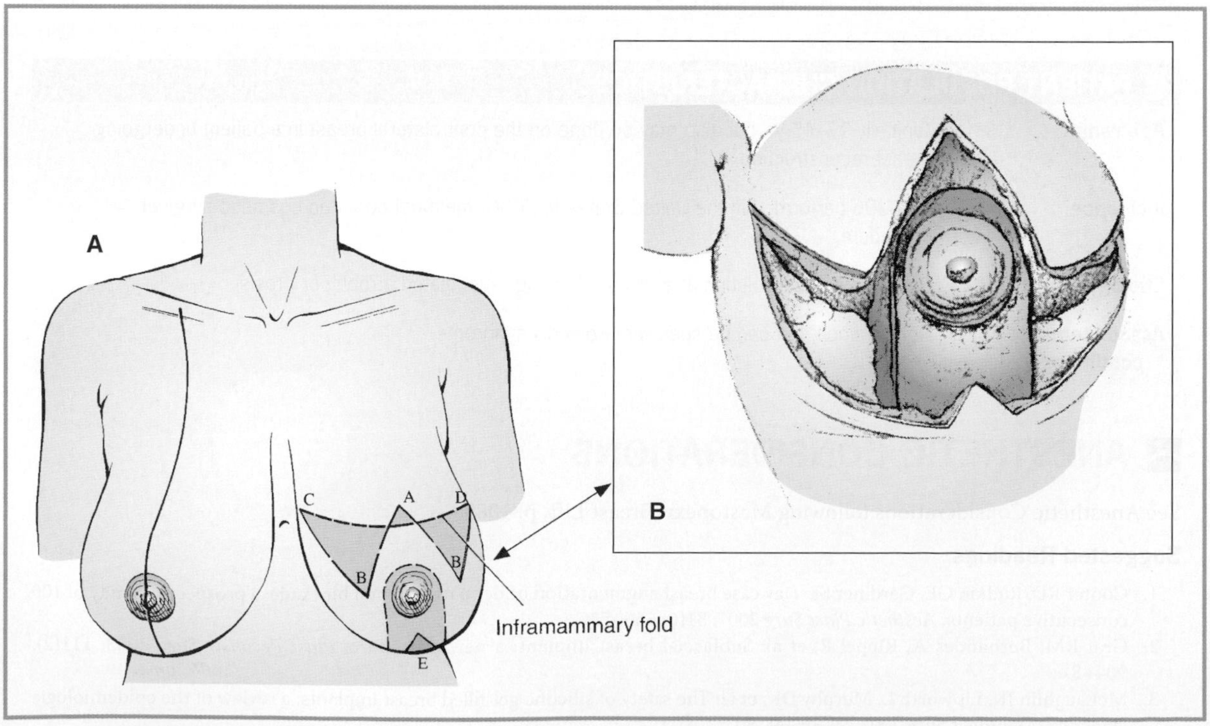

Figure 11.2-2. Reduction mammoplasty using an inferior pedicle technique. **A:** The skin and breast tissue on the medial and lateral sides of the pedicle are resected. **B:** The medial and lateral skin envelopes are sutured at the midline, leaving an inverted-T shaped scar. (Reproduced with permission from Spear SL: *The Breast: Principles and Art.* Lippincott-Raven: 1998.)

Variant procedure or approaches: Liposuction may be used in combination with this procedure. Reduction mammoplasty using liposuction alone has increased in popularity.

Preop diagnosis: Macromastia, gigantomastia, mammary hypertrophy

SUMMARY OF PROCEDURE	
Position	Supine, arm abducted 90°
Incision	Marked preop. Most have circumareolar incision with an inferior anchor-shaped extension (Fig. 11.2-2) or a short vertical component ("lollipop" scar).
Antibiotics	Cefazolin 1 g iv
Unique considerations	May place patient in sitting position during procedure to assess symmetry; Foley catheter; SCDs
Surgical time	2–5 h, depending on volume of reduction and technique
Closing considerations	May place patient in sitting position for application of dressings.
EBL	100–200 mL
Postop care	Outpatient or 24–h stay for pain/nausea management. Avoid the use of Toradol in the first 24 h because of the large, raw surface created between the skin flaps and breast tissue.
Mortality	Minimal
Morbidity	Dehiscence: 5% Infection: 1% Seroma/hematoma: < 1% (may require re-exploration) Skin flap necrosis Loss of nipple-areola complex (may require urgent reexploration) Loss of nipple-areola sensation Hypertrophic scarring Cosmetic disappointments
Pain score	3–4

PATIENT POPULATION CHARACTERISTICS	
Age range	25–65 yr
Incidence	104,455 performed in the United States in 2006[1]
Etiology	Developmental; child-bearing; obesity
Associated conditions	None common

ANESTHETIC CONSIDERATIONS

See Anesthetic Considerations following Mastopexy/Breast Lift, p. 1089.

Suggested Readings

1. Hall-Findlay, E: A simplified vertical reduction mammaplasty: shortening the learning curve. *Plast Reconstr Surg* 1999; 104(3):748–59.
2. Lejour M: Vertical mammaplasty and liposuction of the breast. *Plast Reconstr Surg* 1994; 94(1):100–14.
3. Lejour M: Vertical mammaplasty: early complications after 250 personal consecutive cases. *Plast Reconstr Surg* 1999; 104(3): 764–70.
4. Palmieri B, Benuzzi G, Costa A, et al: Breast reduction and subsequent cancer: a prophylactic perspective. *Breast* 2006; 15(4):476–81.
5. See Suggested Readings Mastopexy/Breast Lift, p. 1090.

MASTOPEXY/BREAST LIFT

SURGICAL CONSIDERATIONS

Description: Mastopexy procedures reduce the volume of the skin envelope to match the volume of the breast gland. Depending on the degree of ptosis ("droopy breasts") and the wishes of the patient, the ptosis may be treated by augmentation alone to increase the volume of the breast, by skin excision alone to reduce the skin envelope appropriately, or by a combination of a mastopexy and an augmentation.

The operation itself resembles a reduction mammoplasty, except that breast tissue is generally excised minimally or not at all, and an implant may be added (**mastopexy/augmentation**). The patient is marked before surgery in the upright position. After the induction of anesthesia, the arms are positioned either on the abdomen or abducted 90°. The procedure begins with the areola being marked circumferentially with an areola sizer, and then incised. Next, the skin flaps are elevated. The breast tissue is moved to a higher position on the chest wall, and the skin is redraped and tailor-tacked closed. The patient is placed in a sitting position to assess for symmetry and nipple location. The nipple-areola complex is then brought out into its new position, and dressings are applied.

Preop diagnosis: Breast ptosis

SUMMARY OF PROCEDURE	
Position	Supine
Incision	Circumareolar ± inferior vertical extension or complete anchor
Antibiotics	Cefazolin 1 g iv
Unique considerations	May place patient in sitting position during procedure.
Surgical time	2–4 h
Closing considerations	May place patient in sitting position for application of dressings.
EBL	> 100 mL
Postop care	Outpatient or 24-h stay
Mortality	Minimal
Morbidity	Wound healing: 5% Infection: 1% Seroma/hematoma: < 1% Hypertrophic scarring Cosmetic disappointments
Pain score	3–4

PATIENT POPULATION CHARACTERISTICS	
Age range	35–65 yr
Incidence	103,788 performed in the United States in 2006
Etiology	Age-related ptosis; involution after breastfeeding; weight loss
Associated conditions	None common

ANESTHETIC CONSIDERATIONS FOR MAMMOPLASTY/MASTOPEXY

PREOPERATIVE

Typically, three patient populations present for mammoplasty: (a) healthy individuals, for breast reduction/augmentation/lift or removal of an implant; (b) morbidly obese, for breast reduction; (c) breast cancer patients, for reconstruction after mastectomy. (For preop considerations in the morbidly obese patient, see Anesthetic Considerations for Abdominoplasty, p. 1094.) Breast cancer patients undergoing mastectomy with immediate reconstruction will not have had either chemotherapy or radiation. The following considerations are for breast cancer patients undergoing delayed reconstruction postchemotherapy.

Respiratory	Pulmonary fibrosis may complicate chemotherapy. Alkylating agents (e.g., cyclophosphamide and melphalan), used to treat breast cancer, have some pulmonary toxicity. Consider pulmonary fibrosis in a patient reporting dyspnea, nonproductive cough, and fever. **Tests:** Consider CXR; ABG, PFTs as indicated from H&P.
Cardiovascular	Cardiomyopathy and CHF may result from chemotherapy, especially doxorubicin (Adriamycin) > 550 mg/m^2. **Tests:** Consider ECG; ECHO, if indicated from H&P.
Neurologic	Note any previous damage to long thoracic nerves, as evidenced by winged scapula deformity.
Musculoskeletal	Avoid iv and BP cuff on mastectomy side.
Hematologic	Leukopenia, thrombocytopenia, and anemia from chemotherapy may be present. **Tests:** CBC; Plt count
Renal/Hepatic	Methotrexate can produce some renal and hepatic dysfunction. **Tests:** Cr; LFTs
Laboratory	Other tests as indicated from H&P, prior chemotherapy, obesity.
Premedication	Midazolam 1–2 mg iv immediately preop. Surgeon may want to mark the patient's skin preop, with patient standing. Delay premedication until this has been done.

INTRAOPERATIVE

Anesthetic technique: GETA

Induction	Standard induction (see p. B-2). ✓ with surgeons regarding use of a nerve stimulator during dissection (and the need to avoid muscle relaxants). Consider LTA to minimize coughing during position changes.	
Maintenance	Standard maintenance (see p. B-2). Surgeons may want patient sitting for part of the procedure. Pneumothorax should be considered with any change in lung inflation pressure, O_2 sat, or BP.	
Emergence	During some of the procedure and for application of dressing, patient may be moved to sitting position, with consequent coughing, bucking, etc. (Rx: deeper anesthesia, e.g., propofol 0.5 mg/kg or lidocaine 1 mg/kg.) Watch BP carefully and treat orthostatic hypotension if it occurs, usually with a fluid bolus if the patient is not fluid sensitive (Hx of CHF or renal failure).	
Blood and fluid requirements	IV 16–18 ga × 1 NS/LR @ 4–8 mL/kg/h	Minimal blood loss for simple reconstruction, augmentation, or reduction; larger blood losses anticipated for combined procedures (e.g., mastectomy with immediate reconstruction or flap reconstruction).

Monitoring	Standard monitors (p. B-1)	Arterial line in the morbidly obese
Positioning	Patient may need to be sitting for application of dressing.	Avoid HTN, bucking, and straining; these may cause or exacerbate bleeding at reconstruction site. Careful padding and unwrapping of arms to protect them during position change.

POSTOPERATIVE

Complications	Pneumothorax
Pain management	PCA (see p. C-3)

Suggested Readings

1. American Society of Plastic Surgeons web site: www.plasticsurgery.org
2. Arain MR, Buggy DJ. Anaesthesia for cancer patients. *Curr Opin Anaesthesiol* 2007; 20(3):247–53.
3. Baker, JL: Augmentation mammoplasty: general considerations. In *Surgery of the Breast: Principles and Art.* Spear SL, ed. Lippincott-Raven, Philadelphia: 1998, 845–54.
4. Elliott LF: Circumareolar mastopexy with augmentation. *Clin Plast Surg* 2002; 29(3): 337–47.
5. Hoffman, S: Inferior pedicle technique in breast reduction. In *Surgery of the Breast: Principles and Art.* Spear SL, ed. Lippincott-Raven, Philadelphia: 1998, 761–72.
6. Kuruba R, Koche LS, Murr MM. Preoperative assessment and perioperative care of patients undergoing bariatric surgery. *Med Clin North Am* 2007; 91(3):339–51.
7. Matarasso A. Suction mammoplasty: the use of suction lipectomy alone to reduce large breasts. *Clin Plast Surg* 2002; 29(3):433–43.
8. Vasconez HC, Holley DT: Use of the TRAM and latissimus dorsi flaps in autogenous breast reconstruction. *Clin Plast Surg* 1995; 22(1):153–66.
9. Warren AG, Morris DJ, Houlihan MJ, Slavin SA. Breast reconstruction in a changing breast cancer treatment paradigm. *Plast Reconstr Surg* 2008; 121(4):1116–26.

BRACHIOPLASTY

SURGICAL CONSIDERATIONS

Description: Brachioplasty is performed as outpatient surgery for patients who note "flabbiness" or a "bat-wing" appearance of their upper arms. Markings are done in the preoperative holding area with the patient upright, arms abducted and flexed. An incision is made starting along the chest wall or in the axilla, extending onto the upper arm and stopping before the elbow. Excess skin and soft tissue are excised, and the incision is closed, sometimes over a drain. Dressings are applied, often followed by a compression garment or ACE wraps.

Usual preop diagnosis: Upper arm laxity or redundancy, lipodystrophy.

SUMMARY OF PROCEDURE	
Position	Supine, arms abducted
Incision	From chest/axilla, extending along lower inner arm
Unique considerations	Both arms must be mobile and prepped circumferentially; SCDs
Antibiotics	Cefazolin 1 g iv

SUMMARY OF PROCEDURE (cont'd)	
Surgical time	1–2 h
EBL	Minimal
Postop care	Avoid ketorolac first 24–48 h
Mortality	Minimal
Morbidity	Seroma: 10% Hypertrophic scarring: 10% Dehiscence: 7.5% Infection: 5–7% Nerve injury: 5%
Pain score	3–4

PATIENT POPULATION CHARACTERISTICS	
Age range	20–65 yr
Male:Female	1:50
Incidence	14,886 performed in the United States in 2006
Etiology	Overweight; aging; massive weight loss
Associated conditions	Obesity

ANESTHETIC CONSIDERATIONS

PREOPERATIVE

Patients presenting for brachioplasty have often undergone gastric bypass surgery with massive weight loss. If morbidly obese an appropriate preoperative work up should be performed. IV access may be difficult. Consider need for IV access in lower limb or neck due to bilateral arm surgery. (See Anesthesia considerations in morbid obesity, p. 502.)

INTRAOPERATIVE

Anesthetic technique: GETA, routine monitors

Procedure may be combined with other plastic procedures, necessitating position changes.

Induction	Standard induction (see p. B-2) for healthy patients. Special considerations for the morbidly obese include prophylaxis for aspiration, followed by rapid-sequence induction in an appropriately positioned patient (see Fig. 7.2-6). If mandibular and cervical mobility are decreased by excessive soft tissue, plan awake fiber optic intubation (see p. B-5) with the patient sitting. Anticipate rapid O_2 desaturation during periods of hypoventilation, even with adequate preoxygenation.
Maintenance	Standard maintenance (see p. B-2). Calculate drug dosage on basis of lean body mass. In the obese, controlled ventilation with large TV and high inspired O_2 concentration is recommended. Positioning may be difficult and care must be taken to give adequate padding and support.
Emergence	Give antiemetics (ondansetron 4 mg) 20 min before conclusion of surgery.
Blood and fluid requirements	Minimal blood loss, 18 ga × 1 NS/LR @ 4–8 mL/h
Monitoring	Standard monitors

POSTOPERATIVE

Pain Management	PCA oral medications for outpatients
Tests	As indicated by patient condition

Suggested Readings

1. Hurwitz DJ, Holland SW: The L brachioplasty: an innovative approach to correct excess tissue of the upper arm, axilla, and lateral chest. *Plast Reconstr Surg* 2006; 117(2):403–11; discussion 412–3.
2. Knoetgen J 3rd, Moran SL: Long-term outcomes and complications associated with brachioplasty: a retrospective review and cadaveric study. *Plast Reconstr Surg* 2006; 117 (7): 2219–23.
3. Lockwood TE: Brachioplasty with superficial fascial system suspension. *Plast Reconstr Surg* 1995; 96(4):912–20.

ABDOMINOPLASTY

SURGICAL CONSIDERATIONS

Description: Patients who present for **abdominoplasty** have laxity in the abdominal wall musculature and excess skin and adipose tissue. This laxity may be associated with rectus muscle diastasis. **Liposuction** often is performed before abdominoplasty to remove additional adipose tissue and improve contour.

Incision lines are marked on the patient preoperatively in the upright position (Fig. 11.2-3). The umbilicus is circumscribed, with care taken to preserve its blood supply. An incision is made above the pubic hairline and extended

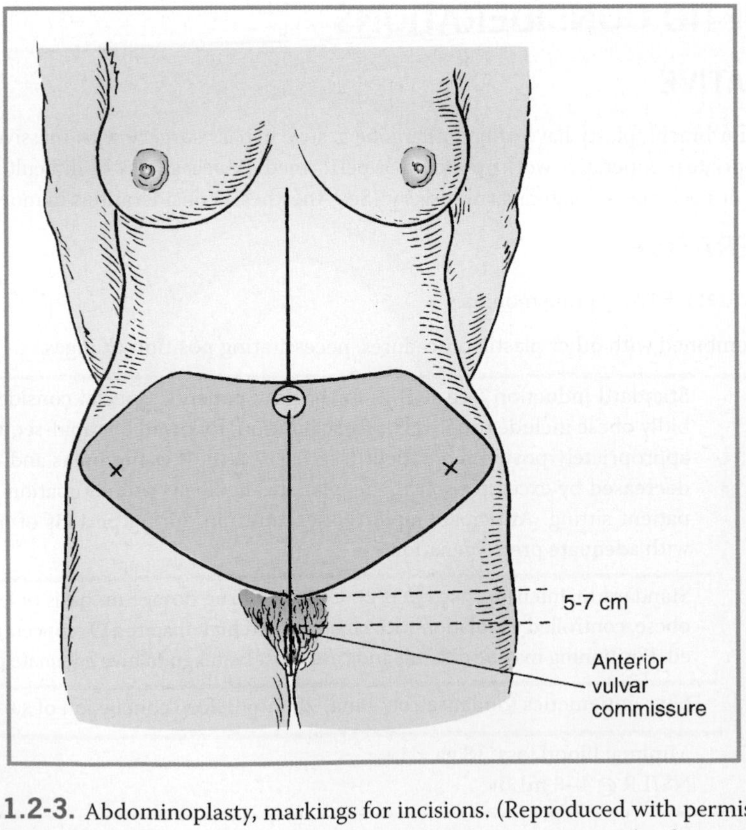

Figure 11.2-3. Abdominoplasty, markings for incisions. (Reproduced with permission from Aston SJ, Beasley RW, Thorne CHM: *Grabb & Smith's Plastic Surgery*, 5th edition. Lippincott-Raven: 1997.)

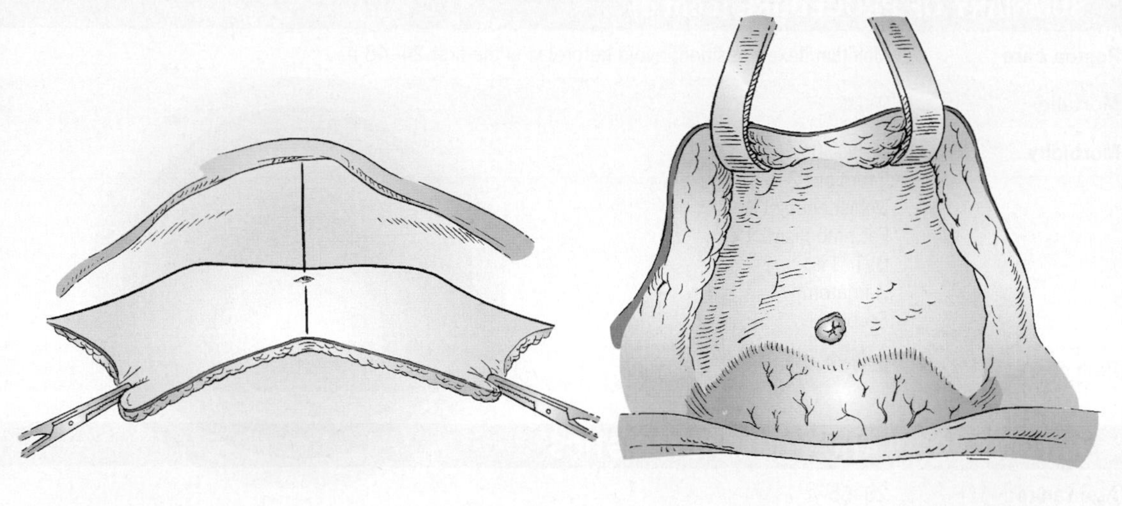

Figure 11.2-4. After the lower incision has been made and the abdominal flap has been elevated, the flap is pulled down to overlap the inferior incision, and the redundant soft tissue is excised in a tailor-tack fashion. (Reproduced with permission from Aston SJ, Beasley RW, Thorne CHM: *Grabb & Smith's Plastic Surgery*, 5th edition. Lippincott-Raven: 1997).

bilaterally to each anterior superior iliac spine. Electrocautery is used to raise a flap of skin, subcutaneous tissue, and fat at the level of the abdominal wall fascia. The dissection extends cephalad to the costal margin. The operating table is flexed to place the patient in the semi-Fowler position. The elevated flap is pulled down to overlap the inferior incision, and the redundant soft tissue is excised in a tailor-tack fashion (Fig. 11.2-4). The surgical area is inspected for hemostasis and irrigated. Sutures may be placed to plicate the abdominal wall musculature if there is laxity. Fibrin sealant may be sprayed to aid in hemostasis. The wound is closed over drains, and the umbilicus is brought out through a new incision. Dressings, which may include an abdominal binder, are applied. The patient is maintained in the semi-Fowler position during transfer from the operating table. The patient may elect to have the procedure as an outpatient or with an overnight stay in a monitored facility.

Variant procedure or approaches: Patients who require additional width reduction may have a fleur de lis abdominoplasty (vertical midline extension of incision and scar). Panniculectomy (simple resection of overhanging skin and soft tissue) can be performed alone without the fascial plication, particularly in the case of morbidly obese patients. Mini-abdominoplasty may be performed in those patients who require less extensive dissection.

Usual preop diagnosis: Abdominal wall laxity; rectus diastasis; lipodystrophy; redundant skin and soft tissue

SUMMARY OF PROCEDURE	
Position	Supine
Incision	Extended Pfannenstiel's; periumbilical; vertical midline extension if needed
Unique considerations	Foley catheter; SCDs
Antibiotics	Cefazolin 1 g iv
Surgical time	1.5–4 h
Closing considerations	Flex table to facilitate closure; patient must subsequently remain in semi-Fowler position.
EBL	~100 mL, not including blood contained in specimen.

SUMMARY OF PROCEDURE (cont'd)	
Postop care	Maintain flexed position; avoid ketorolac in the first 24–48 h.
Mortality	0–1%
Morbidity	Ileus: 10% Infection: 2–3% Dehiscence: 1% Fat embolism: 1% DVT: 1% Hematoma Seroma
Pain score	4–6

PATIENT POPULATION CHARACTERISTICS	
Age range	20–65 yr
Male:Female	1:25
Incidence	146,240 performed in the United States in 2006; fifth most common cosmetic surgical procedure.
Etiology	Overweight; laxity of skin after pregnancy; massive weight loss
Associated conditions	Obesity

ANESTHETIC CONSIDERATIONS

PREOPERATIVE

Typically, there are two patient populations for abdominoplasty: the generally healthy, and the morbidly obese. Some patients have Hx of amphetamine, cocaine, or thyroid hormone abuse, and ↑ incidence of hiatal hernia. The following considerations focus on the morbidly obese patient (body weight ≥ 2 × ideal weight. Ideal body weight can be estimated by subtracting 100 (male) or 105 (female) from height in cm).

Respiratory	In the morbidly obese patient, findings include: ↑ O_2 consumption, ↑CO_2 production, restrictive lung disease, ↓ FRC, ↓ ERV, ↓ VC,↓ IC, and ↓ PaO_2. These changes are exacerbated by the supine position. Younger patients may show alveolar hyperventilation in response to hypoxemia; older patients may not, and may retain CO_2. Patients may have obesity hypoventilation syndrome (Pickwickian syndrome) and sleep apnea; with intermittent airway obstruction, hypoxemia, and hypercarbia during sleep, which may → pulmonary HTN. Obese patients are at ↑ risk of pulmonary aspiration due to ↑ incidence of hiatal hernia, GERD, and ↑ gastric volumes (typically > 25 mL with pH < 2.5). See Premedication, below, for aspiration prophylaxis. **Tests:** Consider CXR, room-air ABG, and PFT (helpful, but generally do not predict postop complications, e.g., atelectasis, pneumonia).
Cardiovascular	↑ CO and ↑ blood volume → LVH. Chronic hypoxia and pulmonary compromise may produce right heart failure, ↓↓ exercise tolerance, ↑ risk of CAD, and pulmonary systemic HTN. Patients with LVH may have ↑ dysrhythmias. Some patients may have previously taken fenfluramine alone or in combination with phentermine for weight loss. Those patients should be evaluated for pulmonary HTN (e.g., dyspnea, central cyanosis, right axis deviation, and CXR changes) and valvular heart disease. **Tests:** ECG (↑HR, conduction abnormalities, LVH); CXR (cardiomegaly)

Metabolic	Increased incidence of diabetes, hypercholesterolemia, hypertriglyceridemia, liver abnormalities, ↓ plasma folate, B_{12}, ↑ incidence of cholelithiasis, nephrolithiasis. Determine whether electrolyte abnormalities are present in patient S/P ileojejunal bypass. **Tests:** As indicated from H&P.
Hematologic	Polycythemia suggests chronic hypoxemia (see Respiratory, above). **Tests:** Hb/Hct
Laboratory	Other tests as indicated from H&P.
Premedication	Sedative premedication is avoided in the morbidly obese due to their pulmonary compromise. Aspiration prophylaxis is essential: ranitidine 100 mg po or iv the evening before, and 60–90 min before surgery, plus nonparticulate antacid (Na citrate 0.3 M, 30 mL po) preinduction. Additionally, metoclopramide 10 mg iv may be given, although it has not been shown to be more effective in combination with an H_2-blocker than the H_2-blocker alone. For the healthy outpatient, midazolam 1–2 mg iv immediately preop may lessen anxiety.

INTRAOPERATIVE

Anesthetic technique: GETA. Morbidly obese patients may not tolerate the supine position for an extended period of time. Consider placement of thoracic epidural for postop pain control.

Induction	Standard induction (see p. B-2) for healthy patients. Special considerations for the morbidly obese include prophylaxis for aspiration (see above), followed by rapid-sequence induction in an appropriately positioned patient (see Fig. 7.2-6). If mandibular and cervical mobility are decreased by excessive soft tissue, plan awake fiber optic intubation (see p. B-5) with the patient sitting. Anticipate rapid O_2 desaturation during periods of hypoventilation, even with adequate preoxygenation.	
Maintenance	Standard maintenance (see p. B-2). Calculate drug dosage on basis of lean body mass. In the obese, increased plasma fluoride concentrations are found after anesthesia with halothane and enflurane; controlled ventilation with large TV and high inspired O_2 concentration is recommended. Because epinephrine infiltration generally is used to decrease blood loss, isoflurane is recommended as the least dysrhythmogenic of the inhalation agents in the presence of epinephrine. ***NB:** Midazolam has a prolonged half-life in obese patients, but awakening times from inhalational or narcotic-based anesthetics are comparable to those of nonobese patients.	
Emergence	Smooth emergence with minimal bucking, coughing, or retching to minimize tension on the suture line; give antiemetics (metoclopramide 10 mg and ondansetron 4 mg) 20 min before conclusion of surgery. Maintenance of flexed position will minimize tension on suture line. Small additional doses of narcotic (e.g., meperidine 10 mg) may be titrated to RR if patient is allowed to resume spontaneous respiration before the end of the case.	
Blood and fluid requirements	Moderate blood loss IV: 16–18 ga × 1 NS/LR @ 6–10 mL/kg/h	
Monitoring	Standard monitors (see p. B-1). ± Arterial line ± CVP line	Additional monitoring for the morbidly obese patient may include arterial and CVP lines.
Positioning	Flexed position Pillows under knees ✓ and pad pressure points. ✓ eyes.	Flexed position minimizes tension on suture line. Morbidly obese may require two OR tables side-by-side. Supine position may be poorly tolerated; monitor ventilation closely.
Complications	Fat emboli	More common during liposuction.

Plastic and Reconstructive Surgery

POSTOPERATIVE

Complications	Patients may have postop ileus of 1–2 d duration.	The morbidly obese should not be outpatients; they have an ↑ incidence of wound infection, DVT, PE, and postop pulmonary complications. Provide supplemental O_2 for the first 2 d postop. Keep patient in semisitting or flexed position to avoid undue stress on wound.
Pain management	Epidural narcotics or PCA may be used (p. C-3).	Monitor patient for postop respiratory depression.
Tests	Pulse oximetry	Maximum reduction of arterial saturation may occur on postop day 2–3.

Suggested Readings

1. Greminger RF: The mini-abdominoplasty. *Plast Reconstr Surg* 1987; 79(3):356–65.
2. Kuruba R, Koche LS, Murr MM: Preoperative assessment and perioperative care of patients undergoing bariatric surgery. *Med Clin North Am* 2007; 91(3):339–51.
3. Lockwood T: High-lateral-tension abdominoplasty with superficial fascial system suspension. *Plast Reconstr Surg* 1995; 96(3):603–15.
4. Matarasso A: Liposuction as an adjunct to a full abdominoplasty. *Plast Reconstr Surg* 1995; 95(5):829–36.
5. Ogunnaike BO, Jones SB, Jones DB, et al: Anesthetic considerations for bariatric surgery. *Anesth Analg*. 2002 Dec;95(6):1793–805.
6. Regatieri FL, Mosquera MS: Liposuction anesthesia techniques. *Clin Plast Surg* 2006; 33(1):27–37, vi.
7. Seung-Jun O, Taller SR: Refinements in abdominoplasty. *Clin Plast Surg* 2002; 29(1):95–109.
8. Vaughan RW, Wise L: Postoperative arterial blood gas measurements in obese patients: effects of position on gas exchange. *Ann Surg* 1975; 182(6):705–9.
9. Vistnes, LM: *Procedures in Plastic and Reconstructive Surgery: How They Do It*. Little, Brown, Boston: 1991.
10. Yoho RA, Romaine JJ, O'Neil D: Review of the liposuction, abdominoplasty, and face-lift mortality and morbidity risk literature. *Dermatol Surg* 2005; 31(7 Pt 1):733–43; Erratum in: *Dermatol Surg* 2005; 31(9 Pt 1):1158.

BODY LIFTS

SURGICAL CONSIDERATIONS

Description: With heightened awareness of the importance of nutrition and exercise as well as the advent of improved gastric bypass and restriction techniques, more patients with massive weight loss are presenting to plastic surgeons for treatment of the resultant skin excess and laxity. Patients frequently have multiple areas of concern, from the face (see **Facelifts**) to the breasts (see **Mastopexy**) to the abdomen and thighs. Often patients will require circumferential torso plasty (combining **Abdominoplasty** with a modified buttocks lift), and/or extensive lower body work (medial and lateral thigh lifts). All of these body lift procedures may be combined with **liposuction** for additional contouring.

The patient is marked in the standing position in the preoperative holding area. Depending on surgeon preference, the initial operative position may begin supine, lateral decubitus, or prone. Incisions are made, and the marked excess skin and soft tissues are elevated and excised. The patient's position is changed as needed to allow for access to all of the surgical areas. Drains are placed. During wound closure, care is taken to close in several layers, beginning with the strength layer of the superficial fascial system. Dressings are applied, and compression garments or ACE wraps may also be used. The patient may elect to have the procedure as an outpatient but frequently choose to stay overnight in a monitored facility.

Usual preop diagnosis: Thigh and buttock laxity; lipodystrophy; redundant skin and soft tissue

SUMMARY OF PROCEDURE	
Position	Multiple: supine, lateral decubitus, prone
Incision	Depending on the combination of procedures; may include circumferential waistline, transverse groin crease, possible medial thigh vertical extension
Unique considerations	Foley catheter; knee-high SCDs; appropriate pressure point padding
Antibiotics	Cefazolin 1 g iv
Surgical time	2–6 h
EBL	50–100 mL, not including blood contained in specimen
Postop care	Avoid ketorolac in the first 24–48 h; maintain semi-Fowler position for any procedures involving abdominoplasty
Mortality	Minimal
Morbidity	Seroma: 1–16% Dehiscence: 1–32% Skin necrosis: 1–10% Infection: 0.5–3.5% DVT/PE: 2–3%
Pain score	4–6

PATIENT POPULATION CHARACTERISTICS	
Age range	20–65 yr
Male:Female	1:4
Incidence	Thigh lift: 12,295 performed in the United States in 2006 Lower body lift: 10,323 performed in the United States in 2006
Etiology	Overweight; massive weight loss
Associated conditions	Obesity

ANESTHETIC CONSIDERATIONS

Patients may have had massive weight loss, or may be morbidly obese. (See anesthetic considerations for abdominoplasty, p. 1094). Body lift procedures may be combined with liposuction. (See anesthetic considerations, see p. 1099.)

Suggested Readings

1. Capella JF. Body lift. *Clin Plast Surg* 2008; 35(1):27–51.
2. Lockwood, TE: Fascial anchoring technique in medial thigh lifts. *Plast Reconstr Surg* 1988; 82(2):299–304.
3. Lockwood, TE: Lower body lift with superficial fascial system suspension. *Plast Reconstr Surg* 1993; 92(6):1112–22; discussion 1123–5.
4. Nemerofsky RB, Oliak DA, Capella JF: Body lift: an account of 200 consecutive cases in the massive weight loss patient. *Plast Reconstr Surg* 2006; 117(2):414–30.
5. Rohrich RJ, Gosman AA, Conrad MH, et al: Simplifying circumferential body contouring: the central body lift evolution. *Plast Reconstr Surg* 2006; 118(2): 525–35; discussion 536–8.
6. Strauch B, Herman C, Rohde C, et al: Mid-body contouring in the post-bariatric surgery patient. *Plast Reconstr Surg* 2006; 117(7):2200–11.

LIPOSUCTION

SURGICAL CONSIDERATIONS

Description: Liposuction remains the most commonly performed cosmetic surgical procedure in the United States. The surgical technique has changed since the introduction of the procedure in the late 1970s. For example, the preaspiration injection of epinephrine-containing wetting solution into the adipose tissue has expanded the use of the surgical procedure. Patients who desire a more dramatic cosmetic surgical result may now have larger volumes of fat removed safely, without losing large quantities of blood during surgery. All members of the surgical team must function in a coordinated fashion to avoid the many pitfalls associated with liposuction. Complications such as PE, fat emboli, fluid overload, toxicity from local anesthetics, and body-cavity perforation from both the wetting solution cannula and the suctioning cannula have been reported.

The current standards for performance of liposuction involve the use of an epinephrine-containing wetting solution injected into the subcutaneous tissue prior to aspiration. Most wetting solutions contain 1 L of LR, to which 1 mg of epinephrine and 200–500 mg of lidocaine are added. Epinephrine in the 1/1,000,000 concentration will provide excellent vasoconstriction in the adipose tissue before suctioning. The concentration of lidocaine depends on the primary anesthetic modality. For patients having GA or regional anesthesia, the lower concentration of local anesthetic will provide satisfactory postop analgesia. Higher concentrations of local anesthetic are needed for patients having liposuction under local anesthesia/MAC. Following administration of the wetting solution to the surgical region, 10–20 min is allowed for vasoconstriction to take place before suctioning. The large volume of local anesthetic and epinephrine-containing solution represents substantial risk to the patient (local anesthetic toxicity, HTN, cardiac arrhythmia, coronary insufficiency), along with the risk of perforation with the cannula.

Ultrasonic liposuction may be used to liquefy fat in the surgical region prior to or simultaneously with its removal. Power-assisted liposuction utilizes pressurized gases or an electrical motor to power the tip of the lipo cannula to improve the efficiency of the procedure. Complications reported during the use of the new technologies include seroma formation, increased blood loss, and increased risk of body cavity perforation.

Following completion of the surgery, incision sites are closed and sterile dressings are applied. Compressive garments may be worn by the patient for several d or wk, depending on the extent of the surgery. Discomfort in the surgical regions varies greatly from patient to patient, but may last from several d to several wk. Ultrasonic liposuction is now being used for the treatment of axillary osmidrosis (hyperhydrosis). Ultrasonic energy applied in the superficial planes of the skin of the axilla has successfully treated hyperhydrosis in a large number of patients. The procedure may be performed under local or general anesthesia.

Usual preop diagnosis: Obesity

SUMMARY OF PROCEDURE	
Position	According to body region (repositioning often required).
Incision	Incisions may be hidden in skin folds. The use of long injection and lipo cannulas will reduce the number of incisions.
Special instrumentation	Cannulas, aspirating machine; ultrasonic or power-assisted machinery
Antibiotics + other meds	Cefazolin 1 g. Dexamethasone 8 mg may be given during surgery.
Surgical time	2–7 h, depending on volume of resection and number of surgical sites
EBL	2–8% of total aspirate volume when using wetting solution before aspiration
Postop care	PACU for small-volume liposuction; hospitalization or postop monitoring for large-volume resection (> 5,000 mL)
Mortality	19.1/100,000

SUMMARY OF PROCEDURE (cont'd)	
Morbidity	Pulmonary emboli Fat emboli Fluid overload Local anesthetic toxicity Body cavity perforation Respiratory restriction from compressive garments has been noted in PACU.
Unique considerations	Wetting solution must be warmed before use to prevent hypothermia. Foley catheter monitoring is used for larger volume surgeries. TEDs, SCDs used on all cases.
Pain score	4–6

PATIENT POPULATION CHARACTERISTICS	
Age range	Teens–70 yr
Male:Female	< 1:9
Etiology	Quest for eternal youth

ANESTHETIC CONSIDERATIONS

PREOPERATIVE

Patients considering liposuction should be in ASA category I or II. The ideal candidate for surgery should be physically active and have maintained a stable weight Hx for 6 mo–1 yr. Preop consultation with the surgical team is necessary for finalizing the anesthetic plan. Current techniques use the injection of wetting solution to reduce blood loss and to deliver local anesthetics for postop analgesia. Most wetting solutions contain lidocaine 200–500 mg/L combined with epinephrine 1 mg/L (1/1,000,000). Typically, 1 mL of wetting solution will be used for each l mL of anticipated fat resection. Because of the demand for more dramatic results, larger fat resections (large-volume liposuction > 5,000 mL) are being performed. These large-volume procedures may require postop hospitalization for patient monitoring (fluid shifts, ↓ Hct, pulmonary edema). Large volumes of wetting solution often are used in these procedures and require limiting iv fluids during surgery. In contrast, small-volume liposuction often requires larger volumes of iv fluid administration because of the small volumes of wetting solution that would be available for postop hydration.

Respiratory	Postop discomfort following chest, upper back, and upper abdomen liposuction may interfere with respiration. Restrictive compression garments applied to the chest or upper abdomen also may restrict breathing. Patients with respiratory impairment may not be candidates for this procedure.
Cardiovascular	Patients with Hx of CHF or those with MVP may not be candidates for high-volume liposuction. Fluid management is based on volume status and the quantity of tumescent fluid injected during surgery. Tumescent solution injected into the subcutaneous tissue is absorbed over 48 h. Postop pulmonary edema has been reported 2° fluid overload in patients receiving larger volumes of tumescent injection. Some patients may have previously taken fenfluramine alone or in combination with phentermine for weight loss. Those patients should be evaluated for pulmonary HTN (e.g., dyspnea, central cyanosis, right axis deviation and CXR changes) and valvular heart disease. All weight control drugs should be D/C'd at least 2 wk before surgery.
Neurologic	Preop neurologic exam should be normal. Local anesthetic administration during tumescent injection may cause areas of numbness postop.
Hematologic	Vasoconstriction from epinephrine-containing wetting solutions greatly reduces blood loss to 2–8% of the total aspirate volume. Blood transfusion is rarely needed, even in larger volume resections. **Tests:** Hct

Laboratory	Other tests as indicated from H&P.
Premedication	Midazolam 1–2 mg or oral benzodiazepine (e.g., lorazepam 1 mg po 1–2 h preop)

INTRAOPERATIVE

Anesthetic technique: Local anesthesia may be suitable for smaller volume liposuction. Regional anesthesia (spinal, epidural) may be used when the surgical regions are appropriate for this type of anesthetic. Concerns have been raised because of vasodilation →↑ blood loss +↑ fat embolization with regional anesthesia. GA ensures patient comfort and allows liposuction to be done on all body regions. Airway and ventilation control also provides safety during the surgery. SCDs or foot/ankle compression devices are used for all patients to reduce the risk of PE.

Induction	Standard induction (see p. B-2). Steroids (dexamethasone 8 mg) may be used to reduce postop swelling and may be of benefit in the event of fat embolism.	
Maintenance	Standard maintenance (see p. B-2) with volatile anesthetics or propofol infusion. Neuromuscular blockade as appropriate. GA is maintained during application of compression garments.	
Emergence	Antiemetic prophylaxis with metoclopramide (10–20 mg) and ondansetron (4 mg) is appropriate. Careful monitoring of respiratory function is necessary when surgery has been performed on the chest, back or upper abdomen, since compression garments may limit respiration.	
Blood and fluid requirements	IV: 18 or 20 ga × 1 NS/LR	NS/LR volume determined by the needs of the case. Transfusion rarely needed, diuretics (e.g., furosemide 5–10 mg) may be needed for patients receiving large volumes of wetting solution. Larger intravenous fluid volumes are needed during smaller volume liposuction and restriction of IV fluid may be needed during large volume liposuction because of absorption of large volumes of wetting solution into the circulation.
Monitoring	Standard monitors (see p. B-1). ± Foley catheter	UO monitoring mandatory on all large-volume lipo cases. Careful temperature monitoring.
Positioning	✓ and pad pressure points. ✓ eyes. Repeat ✓s frequently.	Frequent intraop position checks are needed as patient position may change during surgery → potential for peripheral nerve injury. Documentation of avoidance of external ocular pressure Q 15 minutes while patients are in the prone position.
Complications	Local anesthetic toxicity Excess blood loss Volume overload Abdominal cavity perforation Peripheral nerve injury	Lidocaine 35–55 mg/kg has been shown to produce safe serum levels when used in a highly dilute solution (0.05–0.1%) with epinephrine for tumescent injection during liposuction. Peak plasma lidocaine level occurs 10–12 h after infusion. Peak epinephrine levels occur 5–6 h after infusion and leads to increases in cardiac index, heart rate.
	Hypothermia Fat embolism	Vigorous efforts needed to maintain body temperature (e.g., fluid warmer, Bair-Hugger).

POSTOPERATIVE

Complications	Hypoxemia	Consider fluid overload, fat embolism, pneumothorax or pulmonary edema in differential diagnosis (DDx).
	HTN	Consider fluid overload and epinephrine effect in DDx.
	Respiratory compromise	May be 2° compression garments and pain.
Pain management	PO analgesics IV opiates	Patients often will be comfortable 2° residual local anesthesia, which may persist for 8–24 h. Oral analgesics are usually satisfactory for postop pain control.
Tests	Hct Electrolytes	✓ Hct + Electrolytes following large-volume procedures.

Suggested Readings

1. Burk RW III, Guzman-Stein G, Vasconez LO: Lidocaine and epinephrine levels in tumescent technique liposuction. *Plast Reconstr Surg* 1996; 97:1379.
2. Commons GW, Chang CC, Vistnes D, Halperin BD: Role of liposuction in morbid obesity. In *Problems in General Surgery.* Lippincott Williams & Wilkins, Philadelphia: 2000.
3. Commons GW, Halperin BD, Chang CC. Large volume liposuction: a review of 631 consecutive cases over 12 years. *Plast Reconstr Surg* 2001; 108:1753.
4. Commons GW, Halperin BD: Considerations in large volume liposuction. *Sem Plast Surg* 2002; 16(2).
5. Do DV, Kelley LC. Tumescent anesthesia: evolution and current uses. Adv Dermatol. 2007;23:33–46.
6. Gilliland M, Commons GW, Halperin BD: Safety issues in ultrasonic assisted large volume lipoplasty. *Clin Plast Surg* 1999; 26(2)317–35.
7. Grazer FM, deJong RH: Fatal outcomes from liposuction: census survey of cosmetic surgeons. *Plast Reconstr Surg* 2000; 105(1):436–48.
8. Hunstad JP: Body contouring in the obese patient. *Clin Plast Surg* 1996; 23(4):647–70.
9. Kenkel JM et.al. Hemodynamic physiology and thermoregulation in Liposuction Plast Reconstr Surg 2004 Aug; 114 (2): 503–13.
10. Klein JA: Tumescent technique for regional anesthesia permits lidocaine doses of 35 mg/kg for liposuction. *J Dermatol Surg Oncol* 1990; 16:248–63.
11. Meister F: Possible association between tumescent technique and life-threatening pulmonary complications. *Clin Plast Surg* 1996; 23:642.
12. Ostad A, Kageymis N, Moy RL: Tumescent anesthesia with a lidocaine dose of 55 mg/kg is safe for liposuction. *Dermatol Surg* 1996; 22:921–7.
13. Pitman GH, Aker JS, Tripp ZD: Tumescent liposuction: a surgeon's perspective. *Clin Plast Surg* 1996; 23(4):633–41.
14. Rohrick RJ, Leedy JE, Swamy R, Brown SA, Coleman J, Fluid resuscitation in liposuction: a retrospective review of 89 consecutive patients *Plast Reconstr Surg* 2006 Feb; 117(2): 431–5.
15. Samdal F, Amland PF, Bugge JF: Blood loss during liposuction using the tumescent technique. *Aesthetic Plast Surg* 1994; 18(2):157–60.

CHAPTER

11.3 Craniofacial Surgery

SURGEONS

Stephen A. Schendel, MD, DDS, FACS
Joseph F. Looby, DO

ANESTHESIOLOGISTS

Tara Cornaby, MD
Richard A. Jaffe, MD, PhD

REPAIR OF FACIAL FRACTURES

SURGICAL CONSIDERATIONS

Description: Facial fractures are classified by location and the involved bones.

Upper and mid-face region: Frontal sinus fractures may involve the anterior wall alone, or also may involve the nasofrontal ducts and/or posterior wall. Nasofrontal duct disruption may require obliteration of the duct and sinus, which is done with an electric burr and loupe magnification to remove all mucosa before grafting the area with bone, fat, or pericranium. A posterior wall disruption is a fracture into the anterior cranial fossa that may require CSF leak repair ± cranialization of the sinus (complete removal of the posterior wall of the sinus). Each frontal bone forms a large component of the orbital roof and, as such, ocular injury or periorbital entrapment must be considered.

Fractures of the maxilla are classified as **LeFort I, II,** or **III,** depending on the level of the fracture (Fig. 11.3-2). **LeFort I** is a horizontal fracture, separating the teeth and lower maxillary components from the upper facial structures. **LeFort II** is a triangular fracture with a fracture line across the nose, below the infraorbital rims, and extending through the entire lower maxillary structures. **LeFort III** is essentially a disassociation of the cranium and face. In these cases, the maxilla is usually mobile or impacted posteriorly and occasionally closes off the posterior airway. Further mobility of the segments may be present with a sagittal split of the palate. Associated fractures in the maxillary region (Fig. 11.3-2) include fractures of the zygoma; orbital fractures (most commonly orbital floor), isolated nasal fractures; naso-orbital-ethmoid (NOE) fractures (usually with severe comminution of the upper face); and cranial base fractures with the potential for dural tears and CSF rhinorrhea. Added procedures which may be required to complete the repair of these fractures include **local flap closure** of a CSF leak and **primary bone grafting,** usually from cranium or distant sites, such as the ilium, to highly comminuted areas (e.g., NOE, orbital floors).

Lower face: **Fractures of the mandible** are classified by the type of fracture and location (Fig. 11.3-3), the most common being the subcondylar fracture. Fractures involving the mandibular body, such as a parasymphyseal fracture, may result in unstable mandibular segments. In cases of bilateral mandibular body fractures associated with symphyseal fractures, the mandible can be flail and fall posteriorly in the supine position, allowing the tongue to block off the airway. All of the fractures involving change in occlusion (LeFort maxillary and all mandibular fractures), require reestablishment of a normal occlusion by the application of arch bars and wires also called intermaxillary fixation (IMF). This may be combined with rigid fixation, most commonly internal plates. In some cases, rigid fixation will allow removal of the IMF at the end of the case; in others, IMF may be required for postop healing. Removal of the throat pack prior to final IMF is of paramount importance.

Trismus may be associated with any of the above injuries 2° direct injury to the muscles of mastication, but is more commonly associated with fractures of these muscular attachments (e.g., mandible, zygoma). Associated **dentoalveolar fractures** of the maxilla or mandible may require preop wiring in the ER. The intent is to hold steady those segments with tenuous stability and blood supply. Intubation techniques should avoid displacing these segments. Fractures not involving change in occlusion (e.g., orbital zygomatic, nasal fracture) can be orally intubated. Most fractures with a change in occlusion should be nasally intubated with RAE or 60° curved connector. Exceptions include edentulous segments allowing tube to pass versus edentulous patient with a splint fabricated for oral intubation. Another preop consideration is the amount of blood loss at the scene or in the ER. Facial and scalp vessels can bleed profusely (hypovolemia) and patients may arrive in the OR with both anterior and posterior nasal packs in place (difficult ventilation).

The **surgical approach** depends on the extent of fractures and associated lacerations. Periorbital incisions can be external, on or below the lower eyelid and over the brow, or internal, along the lower eyelid conjunctiva. Upper facial repair may include a bicoronal approach (Fig. 11.3-4) designed to peel the face off the upper facial skeleton via an ear-to-ear scalp incision. Rainey clips are used to minimize scalp bleeding. Of note, periorbital dissection to explore and repair NOE or orbital floor fractures involves some retraction on the globe. This may cause ↓HR and ↓BP via the oculocardiac reflex. The mandible can be approached through external, preauricular or inferior border, or intraoral incisions.

Variant procedure or approaches: **Endoscopic approaches** are being developed for multiple fracture sites. **Resorbable plates and screws,** especially for pediatric cases, can be applied through the same surgical approaches.

Usual preop diagnosis: Facial trauma

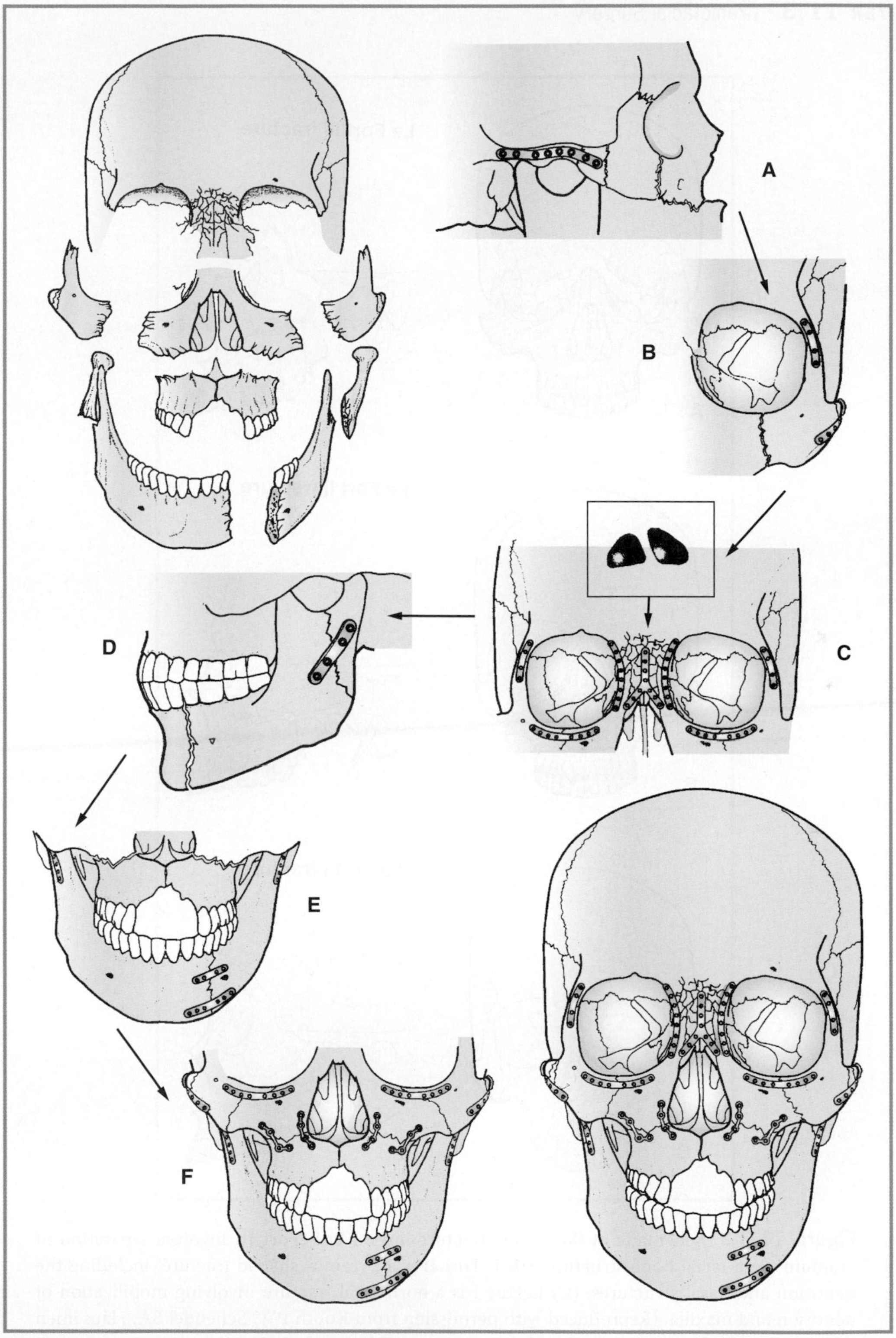

Figure 11.3-1. Panfacial fracture treatment protocol, based on reconstructing load-bearing structures of the facial skeleton. **(A)** Projection of the midface is created by reconstructing the zygomatic arches, starting from the stable part of the temporal bone. **(B)** The zygomas are fixed to the arches and to the frontal bone to create the final projection of the midface. **(C)** The width of the midface is reconstructed by repositioning the central midface (orbits and nose) to its correct position, in relation to the zygomas and frontal bone. Concomitantly, canthopexy is fixed and the frontal bone and sinus fractures are treated. (This procedure is independent of the occlusion.) **(D)** The posterior vertical height of the face is reconstructed by positioning and fixing the condylar fractures. **(E)** Intermaxillary fixation is applied and the mandible is reconstructed. **(F)** Finally, the LeFort I-level fractures are positioned to natural occlusion. (Reproduced with permission from Booth PW, Schendel SA, Hausamen J-E, eds: *Maxillofacial Surgery.* Churchill Livingstone, Edinburgh: 1999.)

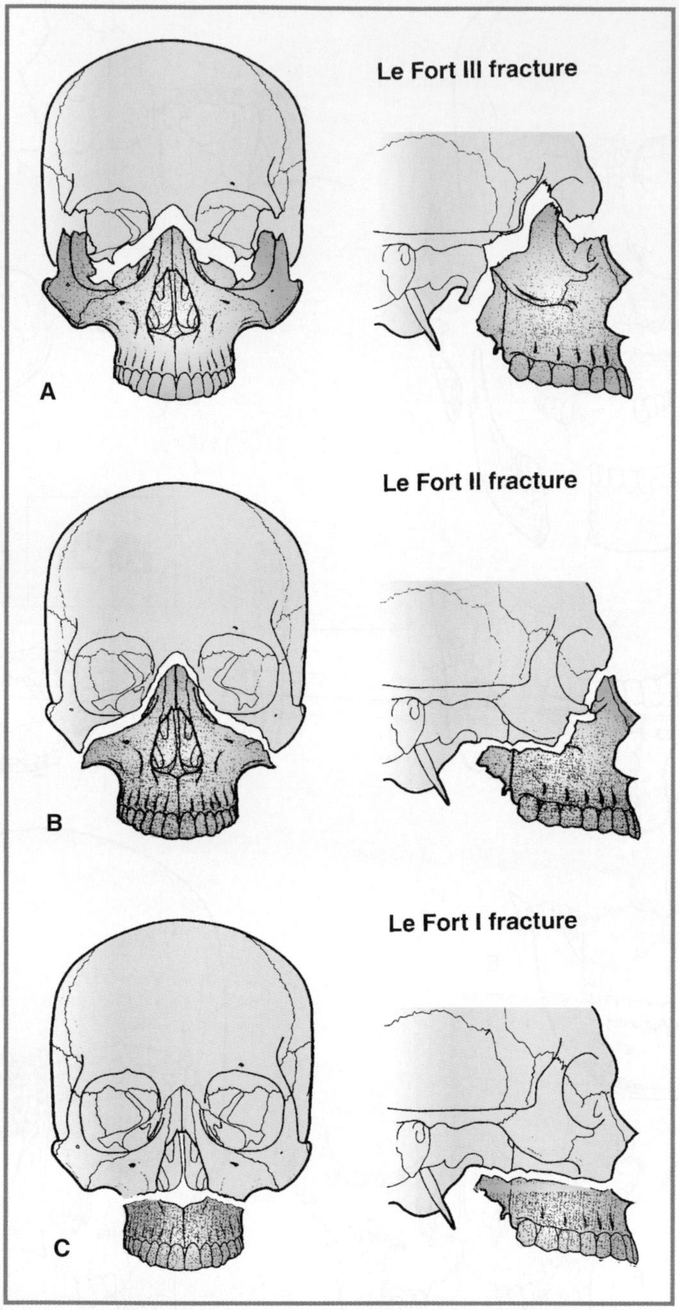

Figure 11.3-2. Schematic of the LeFort fracture lines. **(A)** LeFort III involves separation of cranium from facial bone structure. **(B)** LeFort II is a pyramid-shaped fracture, including the dentition and nasal structures. **(C)** LeFort I is a horizontal fracture involving mobilization of dentition and maxilla. (Reproduced with permission from Booth PW, Schendel SA, Hausamen J-E, eds: *Maxillofacial Surgery.* Churchill Livingstone, Edinburgh: 1999.)

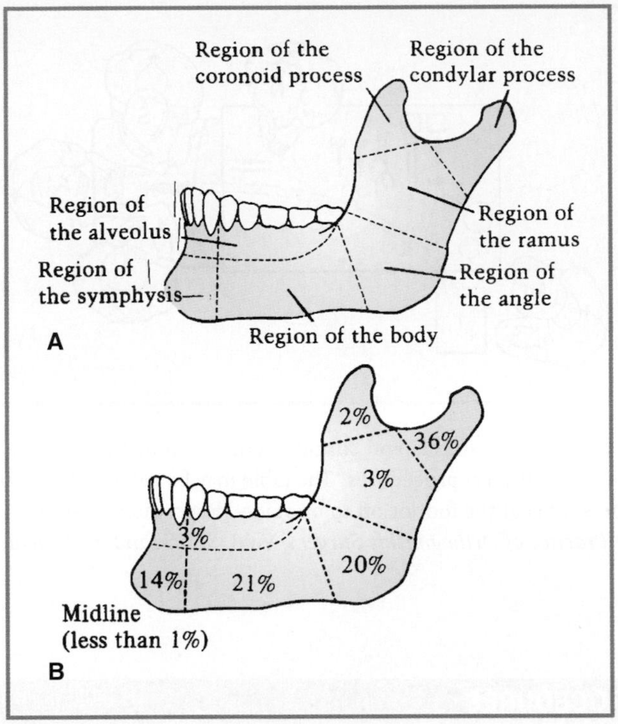

Figure 11.3-3. (**A**) Anatomic regions of the mandible and (**B**) frequency of fractures in those regions. (Reproduced with permission from Aston SJ, Beasley RW, Thorne CH, eds: *Grabb and Smith's Plastic Surgery,* 5th edition. Lippincott-Raven, Philadelphia: 1997.)

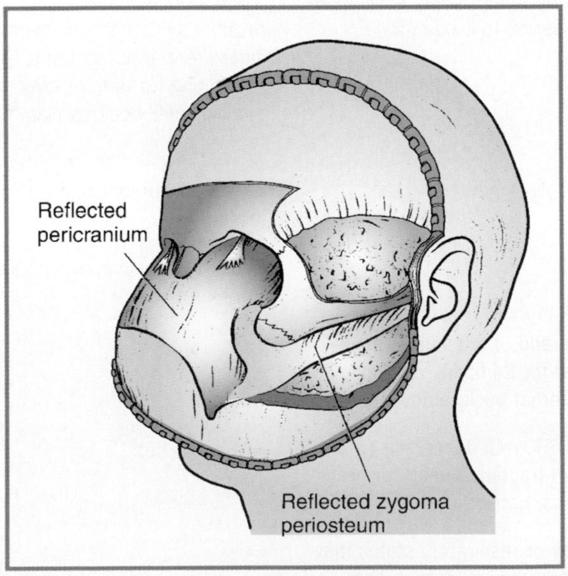

Figure 11.3-4. Bicoronal approach. (Reproduced with permission from Booth PW, Schendel SA, Hausamen J-E, eds: *Maxillofacial Surgery.* Churchill Livingstone, Edinburgh: 1999.)

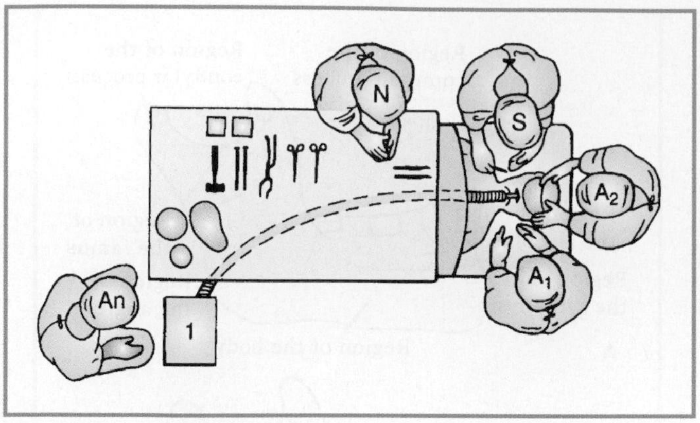

Figure 11.3-5. Standard anesthesia and surgical setup for a maxillofacial surgical procedure and certain craniofacial surgical procedures. The table may be rotated 90°–180° with anesthesia equipment and personnel at the foot or off to one side. (Reproduced with permission from Bell WH, ed: *Modern Practice of Orthognathic Surgery,* Vol I. WB Saunders, Philadelphia: 1990.)

SUMMARY OF PROCEDURES

	Mandibular	Maxillary Orbital/Zygomatic	Nasal
Position	Supine	⇐	⇐
Incision	Intraoral; lateral, submandibular	Intraoral, ± subciliary; possibly coronal	Closed reduction; possibly intranasal
Special instrumentation	Air power tools; plate fixation; headlight	⇐+ Periorbital malleable retractors; Rowe disimpaction forceps; acrylic dental split	⇐
Unique considerations	Nasal RAE (sutured to dentition or septum); throat pack; corticosteroids periop to ↓ edema.	Panfacial smash; airway swelling associated with head injury; burns or other system involvement. Consider preop tracheostomy. Close monitoring for and removal of stimulus until oculocardiac reflex recovery.	—
Antibiotics, etc.	Cefazolin 1 g iv	⇐ + Methylprednisolone 125 mg iv (adults)	⇐
Surgical time	1–3 h	1–6 h (bicoronal approach adds 1.5 h)	1 h
Closing considerations	NG at end of procedure, maintained for 24 h; IMF postop; **NB:** throat pack removal.	⇐	—
EBL	100–800 mL, depending on extent of fractures, need for graft harvest, patient age	⇐	⇐
Postop care	Airway or respiratory status may be compromised (preop and postop swelling/aspiration/associated injuries), requiring maintenance of intubation → ICU.	⇐	⇐

SUMMARY OF PROCEDURE (cont'd)

	Mandibular	Maxillary Orbital/Zygomatic	Nasal
Mortality	Minimal (↑ due to associated injuries and blood loss)	⇐	⇐
Morbidity	Trismus	⇐	–
	Poor occlusion	⇐	–
	Drooling	⇐	–
	Poor cosmetic result	⇐	⇐
	Chronic pain/sensation changes	⇐	⇐
	Loss of taste	Loss of smell	⇐
		Visual problems/epiphora	–
		Sinus problems	⇐
		Breathing difficulty	⇐
Pain score	4–8	4–8	4–8

PATIENT POPULATION CHARACTERISTICS

Age range	> 4 yr
Male:Female	1:1 (varies by age group)
Incidence	The most common are: nasal bones, zygoma and arch, mandible, and orbital floor (on the rise due to airbags in autos).
Etiology	**Adults:** Motor vehicle accidents (MVAs), mostly young males (43–67%); assaults (13–48.8%); sports-related (3.8%); falls (3.6%); gunshot wounds (3%) **Children:** Uncommon: only ~5% of all facial fractures occur in ages < 12 yr; falls (33%); MVA (28%); abuse (3%); dog bites (rare). 69% are periorbital or nasal.
Associated conditions	Airway compromise/closed head trauma (40%); extremity fractures (33%); thoracic injury (29%); open or radiographic brain injury (25%); intraabdominal (12%); globe injuries (11%); oral trauma (11%); pelvic fractures (10%); C-spine fractures (4–10%); T-L spine injuries (4%); shock; multisystem trauma; burns; massive soft-tissue loss. Mandibular fractures during MVAs are associated with a 65% incidence of life-threatening injuries and mortality of up to 8%; up to 1/3 of LeFort fractures will require intubation, most often due to upper respiratory tract blood and secretions.

ANESTHETIC CONSIDERATIONS

PREOPERATIVE

The forces required to produce facial fractures are considerable and frequently result in other associated trauma (e.g., closed head trauma; spine injuries; thoracic injury, including pneumothorax and myocardial contusion; intraabdominal bleeding). Soft-tissue injury to the tongue or larynx can make airway management difficult. When in doubt, a tracheostomy under local anesthesia or awake intubation should be considered. In mandible or maxillary fractures, nasal intubation is usually best, because the patient will be placed in intermaxillary fixation (IMF) (teeth brought together via wires or rubber bands) at the conclusion of the procedure. In malar or nasal bone fractures, the fixation may be precarious, making it undesirable to use mask ventilation at the termination of the procedure and necessitating awake extubation. Facial nerve monitoring may be required, contraindicating the use of muscle relaxants.

Frequently, the anesthesiologist's first encounter with these patients is in the ER, where prompt airway management decisions are essential—often before diagnostic imaging studies are complete. These patients should be treated with full-stomach precautions (see p. B-4) and may have already aspirated. Patients may be unable to open their mouths 2° pain or mechanical factors. The cause of limited mouth opening should be determined before induction of anesthesia. Several options exist. Often, the airway can be managed simply by inserting an oropharyngeal airway; failing this, an emergency intubation will be necessary. Blind nasal intubation should be avoided in patients with CSF rhinorrhea or other evidence of nasopharyngeal trauma, where the potential for creating false passages and additional trauma is significant. An awake oral intubation with topical anesthesia is often the safest approach. Emergency oral intubation may be complicated by an unstable C-spine and limited jaw opening, together with blood and debris in the oropharynx, making visualization difficult if not impossible. Often the only recourse is tracheostomy under local anesthesia. As with any trauma victim, attention is first directed toward maintaining the airway and restoration of fluid volume. The repair of the facial fracture may be carried out incidental to the primary trauma surgery or, more often, is deferred until the patient's condition is stabilized. This preop assessment will focus on the patient coming to the OR for semielective repair of a facial fracture.

Airway	**Semielective:** Usually, facial swelling and intraoral bleeding will have resolved, although mouth opening may be limited 2° pain or mechanical factors. Airway management requires knowledge of the fracture site(s). Patients with a maxillary fracture may benefit from an oral intubation to allow inspection of the nasopharynx before nasal intubation and definitive repair. The possibility of an awake fiber optic intubation (see p. B-5) should be discussed with the patient. Patients with an isolated orbital, zygomatic, or nasal fracture usually do not present airway management problems. The surgeon should be consulted regarding the preferred intubation route. **Trauma:** Airway and nasal obstruction following trauma can be extreme, as a result of soft-tissue swelling and accumulated blood and secretions. The extent of facial fractures, particularly in the midface, should be identified as they may preclude nasal intubation. Mandibular fractures may make access to the oropharynx difficult. Unstable dentoalveolar fractures may require preop wiring in the ER. In the case of massive trauma to the face, urgent tracheostomy should be considered. **Tests:** As indicated from H&P.
Respiratory	**Trauma:** Evaluate for associated trauma and respiratory insufficiency 2° aspiration. ✓ that chest tubes are functioning properly. **Tests:** CXR; others as indicated from H&P.
Cardiovascular	**Semielective:** Typically, several days will have elapsed since the initial trauma, and the patient should be hemodynamically stable. **Trauma:** Blunt chest trauma may be associated with myocardial contusion, pericardial effusion/tamponade, and aortic tear/dissection. **Tests:** ECG; others as indicated from H&P.
Neurological	**Semielective:** Document any neurological deficits and altered mental status. Meningitis may occur in patients with persistent CSF rhinorrhea or pneumocephalus. **Trauma:** Intracranial injury may be associated with facial fractures. Patients with head trauma may have ↑ ICP; therefore, appropriate methods (e.g., CO_2 ↓, fluid ↓, smooth induction/intubation) are used to prevent further ↑ ICP. Basilar skull fractures preclude passage of nasotracheal and NG tubes. In the presence of otorrhea or rhinorrhea, positive-pressure mask ventilation is inadvisable, due to the potential for causing pneumocephalus. **Tests:** Review skull and C-spine x-rays.
Musculoskeletal	**Semielective:** May be associated with other fractures and soft-tissue trauma that may affect patient positioning. **Trauma:** C-spine injuries are commonly associated with facial injuries. The C-spine should be cleared by clinical and x-ray exam before transport to OR. If C-spine cannot be cleared, intubation should be done with the head in a neutral position (splinted or with axial traction), using direct FOL (see p. B-5).
Hematologic	**Trauma:** Maxillary surgery may be associated with major blood loss and, for elective cases, autologous donation should be encouraged. **Tests:** Hct; others as indicated from H&P.
Laboratory	Other tests as indicated from H&P.
Premedication	Standard premedication (see p. B-1) is appropriate for nontrauma, neurologically intact patients with normal airways. **Trauma:** Trauma patients should be considered to have full stomachs, and sedative premedications are best avoided. Aspiration prophylaxis with 0.3 M Na citrate (30 mL po), ± metoclopramide 10 mg iv ± ranitidine 50 mg iv, should be considered.

INTRAOPERATIVE

Anesthetic technique: The majority of patients presenting for elective procedures are healthy and have normal airways. In the case of facial trauma, however, intubation of the trachea may be impossible. Hence, a tracheostomy under local anesthesia may be life-saving.

Induction	If there is any doubt regarding the ease of intubation, an awake FOL should be performed (see p. B-5). Nasal intubation is preferred for patients with mandibular and maxillary (Le-Fort) fractures involving a change in occlusion. Patients with orbital, zygomatic, or nasal fractures usually are intubated orally. In patients with normal airways, a standard induction (see p. B-2) is appropriate. Nasal or oral ETTs (RAE), or anode ETTs are commonly used to minimize intrusion into the surgical field.	
Maintenance	Standard maintenance (see p. B-2); muscle relaxation usually is required except with facial nerve monitoring. Controlled ↓ BP may be appropriate. Administration of an antiemetic (e.g., metoclopramide 10–20 mg iv and ondansetron 4 mg iv) is beneficial in patients who have their jaws wired or banded together.	
Emergence	Patients with difficult airways or with jaws wired together should be extubated when fully awake. Extubation over a tube-changer may be appropriate. A wire cutter (or scissors for elastic bands) should be at the bedside at all times. Ensure that all throat packing has been removed before extubation. Thorough oropharyngeal suctioning is essential. NG tube may be used postop, so consider placement prior to extubation. Some patients with multiple trauma or extensive soft-tissue swelling may require continued postop intubation and mechanical ventilation.	
Blood and fluid requirements	Moderate - large blood loss iv: 16–18 ga × 1–2 **Trauma:** NS/LR @ 6–8 mL/h **Other:** NS/LR @ 2–4 mL/h	Blood loss from facial fractures or orthognathic procedures can be extensive. T&C patient so blood is immediately available in OR.
Monitoring	Standard monitors (see p. B-1). ± Arterial line	Invasive monitoring may be required in patients with intracranial or other trauma, or for controlled ↓ BP. Muscle relaxants will interfere with facial nerve monitoring.
Control of blood loss	Surgical hemostasis	Surgical hemostasis should control most bleeding in these procedures.
	Topical vasoconstrictors	Topical vasoconstrictors, such as phenylephrine or cocaine, can be applied on the surgical field.
	Posterior oropharyngeal packing	Posterior oropharyngeal packing can keep blood from passing undetected into the upper GI tract.
	Controlled ↓ BP	Controlled ↓ BP often can be achieved simply by increasing volatile anesthetic levels.
Positioning	✓ and pad pressure points. ✓ eyes.	Some surgeons prefer that the OR table be rotated 90° or 180°. Be prepared with long hoses and appropriate connectors. Protect eyes with an ophthalmic ointment.
Complications	ETT damage	Nasal ETT may be wired inadvertently to the maxilla, making extubation difficult. In case of ETT damage, be prepared to reestablish the airway rapidly by re-intubation, usually over an intubating stylet or gum elastic bougie.
	Oculocardiac reflex	Notify surgeon (stop surgical stimulus). Consider atropine and increasing depth of anesthesia.

POSTOPERATIVE

Complications	Airway obstruction	Wire cutters (or scissors) should be available at bedside to facilitate emergent reintubation or other form of airway management. Consider retained throat pack.
	PONV	Multimodal treatment of nausea is important.
Pain management	Parenteral narcotics (see p. C-3) or PCA with antiemetics (see p. C-3).	Local anesthetic infiltrated at end of procedure.

Suggested Readings

1. Booth PW, Schendel SA, Hausamen J-E, eds: *Maxillofacial Surgery.* Churchill Livingstone, New York: 1999.
2. Carlin CB, et al: Facial fractures and related injuries. *J Craniomaxillofac Trauma* 1998; 4(2):44–8.
3. Fischer K, et al: Injuries associated with mandible fractures sustained in motor vehicle collisions. *Plast Reconstr Surg* 2001; 108(2):328–31.
4. Girotto JA: Long-term physical impairment and functional outcomes after complex facial fractures. *Plast Reconstr Surg* 2001; 108(2):312–27.
5. Greenberg AM, Prein J, eds: *Craniomaxillofacial Reconstructive and Corrective Bone Surgery.* Springer, New York: 2006.
6. Hoffmann JF: Naso-orbital-ethmoid complex fracture management. *Fac Plast Surg* 1998; 14(1):67–76.
7. Kellman RM, Marentette LJ: *Atlas of Craniomaxillofacial Fixation.* Raven Press, New York: 1995.
8. Kim KF, Doriot R, Morse MA, et al: Alternative to tracheostomy: submental intubation in craniomaxillofacial trauma. *J Craniofac Surg* 2005; 16(3):498–500.
9. Ng M, et al: Managing the emergency airway in LeFort fractures. *J Craniomaxillofac Trauma* 1998; 4(3):38–43.
10. Ng M, Saadat D, Sinha UK: Managing the emergency airway in Le Fort fractures. *J Craniomaxillofac Trauma* 1998; 4(4):38–43.
11. Pham AM, Strong EB. Endoscopic management of facial fractures. *Curr Opin Otolaryngol Head Neck Surg* 2006; 14(4):234–41.
12. Stanley RB Jr: Maxillofacial trama. In *Otolaryngology–Hand and Neck Surgery,* Vol I, 3rd edition. Cummings CW, Fredrickson JM, Harker LA, et al., eds. Mosby-Year Book, St. Louis: 1998, 453–85.
13. Strong EB, Sykes JM: Zygoma complex fractures. *Fac Plast Surg* 1998; 14(1):105–15.

LEFORT OSTEOTOMIES

SURGICAL CONSIDERATIONS

Description: LeFort osteotomies are used to correct maxillary deformities. The most common is the **LeFort I,** a transverse osteotomy, above the apices of the teeth, used to correct maxillary retrusion or maxillary vertical excess or deficiency. One of the goals in achieving improved function is to improve the occlusion, as classified by Angle (Fig. 11.3-6). One or both jaws may be moved to achieve normocclusion. An intraoral vestibular incision is used for this approach, followed by an osteotomy of the maxilla, with either a burr or a saw, and completed with osteotomes. The osteotomy extends through the maxillary sinus toward the ETT, within the piriform aperture. There is potential for nasal ETT damage with this maneuver. Of note, BP usually will increase at the start of the osteotomies, increasing bleeding if anesthesia/analgesia is inadequate. The maxilla is subsequently downfractured (Fig. 11.3-7) and mobilized with Rowe disimpaction forceps. This is when most of the bleeding occurs. Further interdental osteotomies creating multiple maxillary segments may be required. **LeFort II** or **LeFort III** maxillary osteotomies may be used to correct severe midfacial retrusion. In these cases, infraorbital incisions are used with either brow or coronal (Fig. 11.3-4) incisions. With maxillary advancements, iliac or cranial bone grafts are often necessary to close the bony gap created. Most of these patients have orthodontic appliances and will require

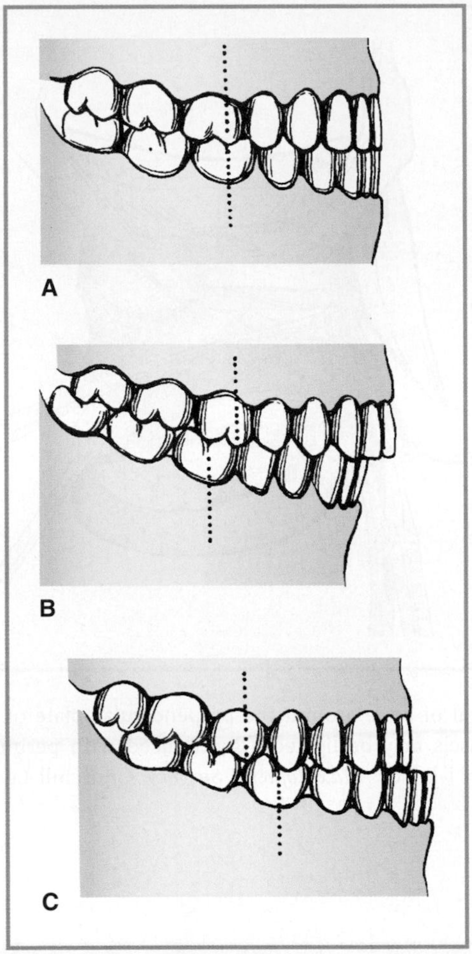

Figure 11.3-6. The Angle classification of occlusion. **(A)** Class I, normal occlusion. **(B)** Class II, retroocclusion or mandibular deficiency. **(C)** Class III, prognathic occlusion (maxillary deficiency or mandibular excess). The key relationships to be discerned are those of the first molar teeth, cuspids, and incisors. (Reproduced with permission from Aston SJ, Beasley RW, Thorne CH, eds: *Grabb and Smith's Plastic Surgery,* 5th edition. Lippincott-Raven, Philadelphia: 1997.)

intermaxillary fixation (IMF), with either wire or elastics at the end of the procedure, with or without a prefabricated splint. The maxilla is fixed rigidly in the new position with miniplates.

Variant procedure or approaches: Recently, **distraction osteogenesis** after LeFort osteotomy has been shown to be effective for correction of severe deformity that would be difficult to correct with single movements and internal fixation. This technique creates new bone as the osteotomized bones are slowly separated. No bone grafts are necessary. Distraction hardware is applied either internally or externally. External devices are stabilized via halo and compression bolts into the skull. IMF is not indicated, as the upper jaw must be free to be distracted in relation to the lower jaw. A second operation may be required for removal of distractor hardware. **Absorbable internal devices** also are available.

Usual preop diagnosis: Facial deformities; dentoskeletal dysplasia

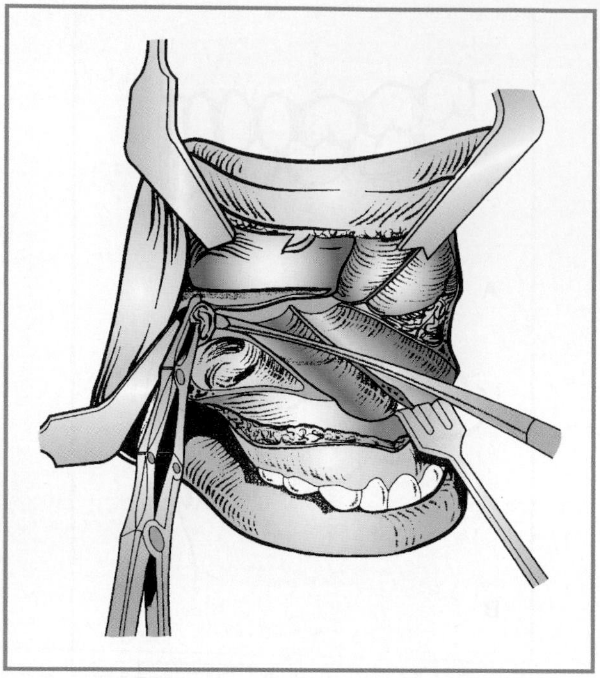

Figure 11.3-7. Removal of bone around the perpendicular plate of the palatine bone. The descending palatine vessels may be ligated. (Reproduced with permission from Booth PW, Schendel SA, Hausamen J-E, eds: *Maxillofacial Surgery.* Churchill Livingstone, Edinburgh: 1999.)

SUMMARY OF PROCEDURES

	LeFort I	LeFort II	LeFort III	Distractor
Position	Supine; table may be rotated 90° or 180°	⇐	⇐	⇐
Incision	Intraoral	Intraoral and facial ± coronal	⇐	⇐
Special instrumentation	Miniplates and screws; burr or saws	⇐	⇐	Distractors
Unique considerations	Jaw frequently closed (wires or elastic); nasal RAE or armored tube. ***NB: Keep SBP < 100 mmHg during osteotomy-closure.** With cranial bone graft harvest, the nasal ETT goes opposite to the donor side and is repositioned later.	⇐ ⇐	⇐ ⇐	No IMF ⇐
Antibiotics, etc.	Cefazolin 1 g iv; methylprednisolone 125 mg iv (adults)	⇐	⇐	⇐
Surgical time	3–6 h	⇐	⇐	⇐
Closing considerations	***NB: Throat pack removal.** NG at end of case × 24 h. NSAIDs contraindicated.	⇐	⇐	⇐
EBL	400–800 mL	⇐	⇐	⇐

SUMMARY OF PROCEDURE (cont'd)

	LeFort I	LeFort II	LeFort III	Distractor
Postop care	PACU → room	ICU × 1 d	⇐	⇐
Mortality	Rare	⇐	⇐	⇐
Morbidity	Relapse	⇐	⇐	⇐
	Infection	⇐	⇐	⇐
	Bone/tooth loss: Uncommon	⇐	⇐	⇐
	Severe intraop bleeding: Uncommon	⇐	⇐	⇐
	Blindness: Very rare	⇐	⇐	⇐
	Temporomandibular joint dysfunction	⇐	⇐	⇐
	Nasal obstruction	⇐	⇐	⇐
	Nasolacrimal obstruction	⇐	⇐	⇐
	Oronasal fistulas (multi-piece osteotomies, uncommon)	⇐	⇐	⇐
	Poor cosmetic result	⇐	⇐	⇐
	Sensory nerve dysfunction	⇐	⇐	⇐
				Distractor malfunction
Pain score	4	5	5	5

PATIENT POPULATION CHARACTERISTICS

Age range	15 yr–adulthood, usually < 30 yr
Male:Female	1:1
Incidence	Up to 5% of population
Etiology	Usually developmental in nature; also cleft lip and palate patients Rarely syndromic: Apert (1/100,000); Crouzon (1/25,000)
Associated conditions	Usually none with developmental cases; sleep apnea; or part of a recognized condition associated with congenital anomalies (e.g., cleft lip and palate, proptotic eyes, severe mitten-hand syndactylies)

ANESTHETIC CONSIDERATIONS

See Anesthetic Considerations following Mandibular Osteotomies/Genioplasty, p. 1119.

Suggested Readings

1. Ferraro JW, ed: *Fundamentals of Maxillofacial Surgery*. Springer, New York: 1997.
2. Frost DE: Orthognathic surgical techniques. In *Maxillofacial Surgery.* Booth PW, Schendel SA, Hausamen J-E, eds. Churchill Livingstone, Edinburgh: 1999, 1273–95.
3. Lo LJ, Hung KF, Chen YR: Blindness as a complication of LeFort I osteotomy for maxillary distraction. *Plast Reconstr Surg* 2002; 109(2):688–700.
4. Morris DE, Lo LJ, Margulis A: Pitfalls in orthognathic surgery: avoidance and management of complications. *Clin Plast Surg* 2007l; 34(3):e17–29.
5. Richardson D, Pospisil OA: Avoiding surgical complications in orthognathic surgery. In *Maxillofacial Surgery.* Booth PW, Schendel SA, Hausamen J-E, eds. Churchill Livingstone, Edinburgh: 1999, 1307–20.
6. Schendel SA, Mason ME: Adverse outcomes in orthognathic surgery and management of residual problems. *Clin Plast Surg* 1997; 24(3):489–505.
7. Scully JR, Matheson JD: Emergency airway management in the traumatized patient. In *Oral and Maxillofacial Trauma,* 2nd edition. Fonseca RJ, Walker RV, eds. WB Saunders, Philadelphia: 1997, 105–37.
8. Zellin G, Rasmusson L, Pålsson J, et al: Evaluation of hemorrhage depressors on blood loss during orthognathic surgery: a retrospective study. *J Oral Maxillofac Surg* 2004; 62(6):662–6.

MANDIBULAR OSTEOTOMIES/GENIOPLASTY

SURGICAL CONSIDERATIONS

Description: Mandibular deformities include either a retruded mandible or a prognathic mandible involving a malocclusion (Class II or III), and may occur in combination with a small chin (microgenia). Surgical correction of the basic mandibular deformity involves either advancing or retruding the mandible. The most common procedure for this is the **sagittal ramus split osteotomy (Obwegesser)** (Fig. 11.3-8). The mandible is split with the inferior alveolar nerve solely within the anterior segment, such that the tooth-bearing anterior segment can slide forward or backward to correct the original deformity. A variety of other techniques of mandibular osteotomies exist, often involving the ramus area of the mandible, and are performed via an intraoral approach.

In some very large deformities, an external incision (**Risdon** type) and bone graft placement may be necessary to complete the mandibular ramus reconstruction. Many patients will be treated for dentoskeletal deformities with a combination of LeFort movement and sagittal-split osteotomies of the mandible. When the mandible is set back, mandibular bone is resected and often can be used in combined procedures as bone graft for the LeFort osteotomy. This avoids cranial bone harvest and, therefore, avoids repositioning the ETT during the procedure for cranial bone access and avoids donor site morbidity. Occasionally, deformities may be corrected by mandibular body osteotomies.

Rigid fixation of mandibular osteotomies is often accomplished by the use of small miniplates and screws. Fixation also can be accomplished with elastic traction (rarely, wire fixation) between mandible and maxilla (IMF), placed either at the time of surgery, or several days following, and held in position for 1–2 wk. These procedures may be

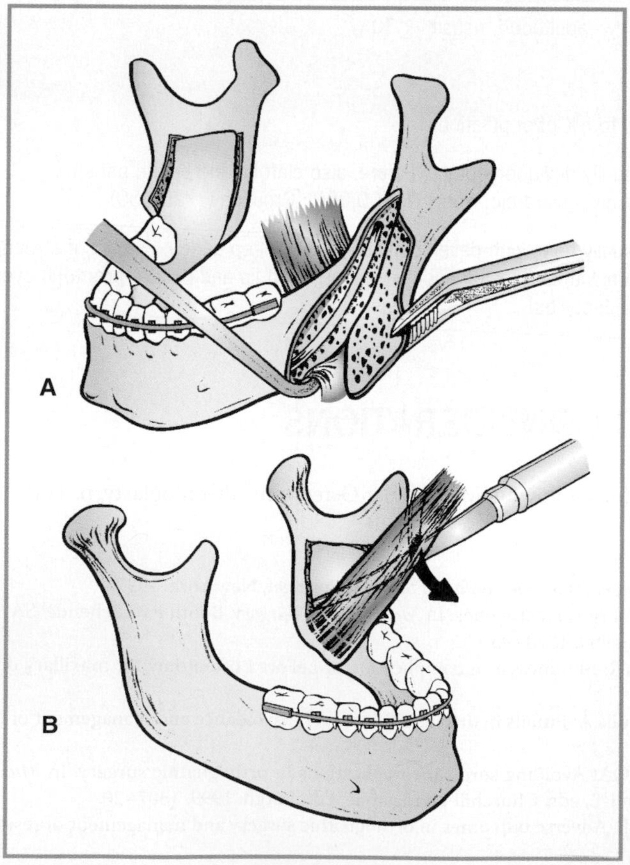

Figure 11.3-8. **(A, B)** "J" stripper used to remove muscle attachments from medial aspect of distal segment. Used through the osteotomy split. (Reproduced with permission from Booth PW, Schendel SA, Hausamen J-E, eds: *Maxillofacial Surgery.* Churchill Livingstone, Edinburgh: 1999.)

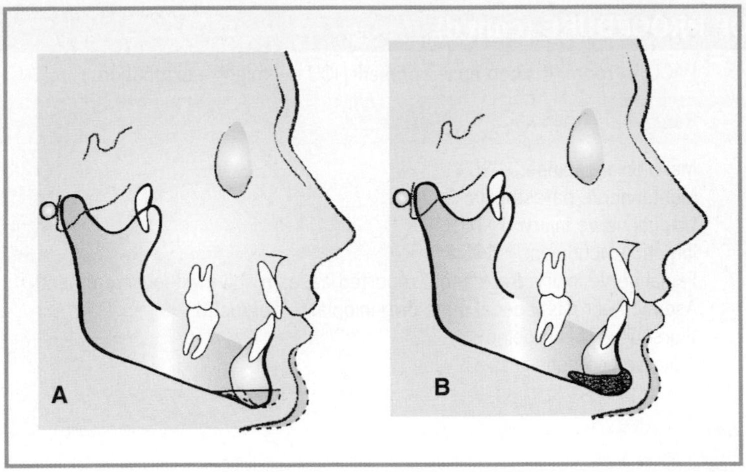

Figure 11.3-9. An osseous genioplasty **(A)** can be used to augment the chin, move it posteriorly, alter its vertical position or change the transverse position of the chin. Allopastic implants **(B)** can be used to augment the chin anteriorly. These are less effective for vertical augmentation. (Reproduced with permission from Booth PW, Schendel SA, Hausamen J-E, eds: *Maxillofacial Surgery.* Churchill Livingstone, Edinburgh: 1999.)

combined with a **genioplasty** to correct the chin deformity; or, genioplasty may be performed as an isolated procedure. The most common type is a horizontal osteotomy of the inferior mandible, with the chin segment repositioned with internal fixation (Fig. 11.3-9A). Augmentation of the chin also is accomplished with alloplastic onlay materials (Fig. 11.3-9B) placed via either the oral route or the extraoral route through a small submental incision. As an isolated procedure, genioplasty is performed most frequently with local anesthesia and sedation.

Variant procedure or approaches: **Distraction osteogenesis** is being used more frequently in treating certain acquired and congenital jaw deformities. This involves a partial mandibular osteotomy and placement of a distraction device (Fig. 11.3-10). Depending on the application, this may be an external or internal device. External devices are visible over the skin with percutaneous pins into the bone. Internal devices are placed beneath the oral soft tissues, with a single adjustment pin exposed.

Usual preop diagnosis: Mandibular deformity

SUMMARY OF PROCEDURE

Position	Supine; table may be rotated 90° or 180°. Nasal RAE tube toward head of bed (sutured through nasal septum), padded, and secured to forehead; shoulder roll; neck extended
Incision	Usually oral, but may be external in the submental or posterior mandibular area; preinjection with local anesthetic with epinephrine
Special instrumentation	Miniplates and screws; burrs/saws; osteotomes; distractor for distraction osteogenesis; throat pack
Unique considerations	Scleral lubricant and shields needed. Postop, patient may have IMF with inability to open the mouth. (IMF not used with distractor cases. ***NB: Remove throat pack** before extubation; thorough oro- and nasopharyngeal suction.
Antibiotics, etc.	Cefazolin 1 g iv; methylprednisolone 125 mg iv (adults)
Surgical time	Genioplasty: 0.5–1 h Mandibular osteotomy: 2–4 h
EBL	Genioplasty: 50 mL Mandibular osteotomy: 100–200 mL

SUMMARY OF PROCEDURE (cont'd)	
Postop care	PACU → room. If sleep apnea present, ICU overnight + extubation.
Mortality	Rare
Morbidity	Mandibular relapse: ≤ 30% Mental nerve paresthesia: 5–20% Lingual nerve injury: 1–16% Infection/nonunion: < 1% Facial nerve injury: Rare (most reported cases resolve without treatment) Aseptic necrosis (buccal plate or genioplasty fragment) Worsening TMJ problems Adverse cosmetic result
Pain score	4

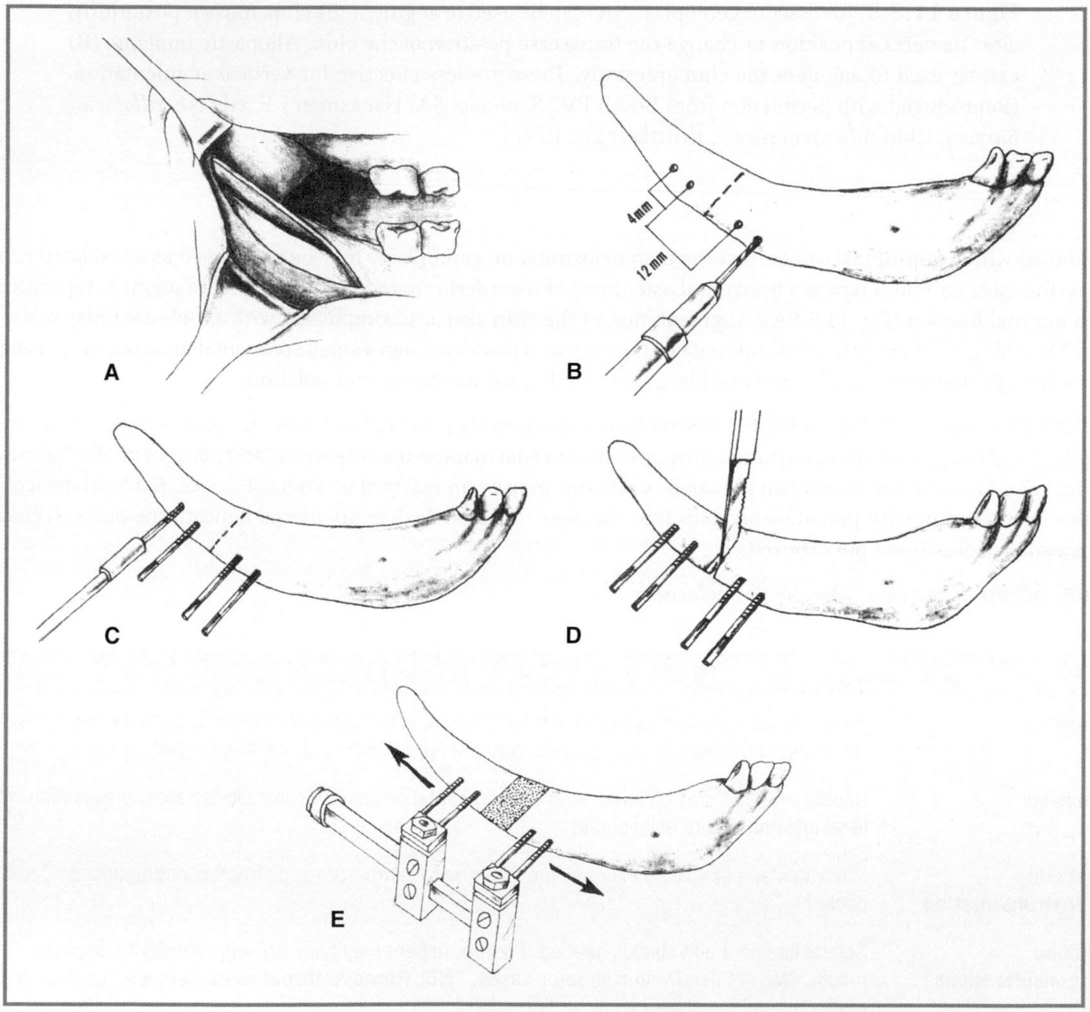

Figure 11.3-10. Mandibular distraction technique: **(A)** An intraoral incision is made along the oblique line of the mandibular remnant. **(B)** Sites of the pinholes and proposed osteotomy (interrupted line). **(C)** Pins have been inserted. **(D)** The osteotomy is performed. **(E)** Commencement of distraction with the appliance in position. The arrows designate the movement of the mandibular segments with formation of bony regenerate in the resulting gap. (Reproduced with permission from Aston SJ, Beasley RW, Thorne CH, eds: *Grabb and Smith's Plastic Surgery*, 5th edition. Lippincott-Raven, Philadelphia: 1997.)

PATIENT POPULATION CHARACTERISTICS	
Age range	Infant–adult
Male:Female	Unknown
Incidence	Unknown
Etiology	Developmental (90%); acquired (10%)
Associated conditions	Usually none with developmental cases; sleep apnea; congenitally small mandible may be associated with a large tongue and cleft palate (Pierre Robin syndrome), hemifacial microsomia (which may be associated with heart, vertebral, and other anomalies), Treacher Collins syndrome, or Nager's syndrome (many of the congenital cases may be tracheostomy- and gastrostomy-dependent, with associated TMJ ankylosis).

ANESTHETIC CONSIDERATIONS

(Procedures covered: LeFort osteotomies; mandibular osteotomies; genioplasty)

PREOPERATIVE

These surgeries are usually performed on patients with facial disproportion. In general, this patient population is young and healthy; however, many of them will present with challenging airway management problems. In addition, facial disproportion will often accompany congenital anomalies (e.g., Crouzon, Apert, Pierre Robin, and Treacher Collins syndromes). (For discussion of specific syndromes, see Anesthetic Considerations for Pediatric Orthopedic Surgery of the Pelvis and Lower Limbs, p. 1389).

Airway	As usual, a careful airway evaluation is essential since many of these patients have abnormal airway anatomy and may be difficult to mask ventilate or intubate. Visual inspection often reveals the reasons for the surgery and allows the anesthesiologist to determine the safest approach to intubation. When a difficult intubation is anticipated, the need for awake fiber optic intubation (see p. B-5) should be discussed with the patient.
Respiratory	Consider the anesthetic implications of associated congenital syndromes in this patient population. Obstructive sleep apnea (OSA, see p. 255) also may be associated with patients in need of mandibular surgery. **Tests:** As indicated from H&P.
Cardiovascular	As above, consider the implications of possible congenital syndromes. Assess whether patient is a suitable candidate for the use of controlled ↓ BP, particularly those undergoing maxillary procedures. **Tests:** As indicated from H&P.
Hematologic	Encourage autologous blood donation for maxillary procedures. **Tests:** Hct
Laboratory	Other tests as indicated from H&P.
Premedication	Standard premedication (see p. B-1) is usually appropriate.

INTRAOPERATIVE

Anesthetic technique: GETA

Induction	If there is any doubt regarding the ease of intubation or ability to mask ventilate, an awake FOL should be performed (see p. B-5). Nasal intubation is preferred for patients undergoing mandibular or maxillary osteotomies, as well as genioplasty. In patients with normal airways, a standard induction (see p. B-2) is appropriate. Nasal or oral ETTs (RAE), or anode ETTs, are commonly used to minimize intrusion into the surgical field.	
Maintenance	Standard maintenance (see p. B-2); muscle relaxation is usually required. Administration of an antiemetic (e.g., metoclopramide 10–20 mg iv and ondansetron 4 mg iv) is essential in patients who have their jaws wired or banded together.	
Emergence	Patients with difficult airways or with their jaws wired (or banded) together should be extubated when fully awake. Perform thorough oropharyngeal suctioning. If not placed previously, an NG tube should be placed before extubation. A wire cutter (or scissors for elastic bands) should be at the bedside at all times. Ensure that all throat packing has been removed before extubation.	
Blood and fluid requirements	Moderate - large blood loss iv: 16–18 ga × 1–2 NS/LR @ 5–8 mL/kg/h	Maxillary osteotomies may be associated with major blood loss (e.g., 1500–2000 mL). The majority of blood loss occurs when the maxilla is downfractured. Controlled ↓ BP (SBP < 90 mmHg) may be particularly useful during this part of the case, and blood should be readily available for this and all maxillary procedures.
Monitoring	Standard monitors (see p. B-1). ± Arterial line ± CVP line or 2nd iv	Direct arterial pressure measurements are useful for deliberate ↓ BP. Central venous access or a 2nd peripheral iv may be useful for vasodilator infusions.
Positioning	✓ and pad pressure points. ✓ eyes.	Eyes should be protected with an ophthalmic ointment and possible tarsorrhaphy by the surgeons. Some surgeons prefer to have the OR table rotated 90° or 180°. Be prepared with circuit-extension tubing.
Complications	ETT damage Hemorrhage	ETT may be cut during maxillary osteotomy, necessitating rapid reintubation.

POSTOPERATIVE

Complications	Airway obstruction PONV	Wire cutters (or scissors) should be available at bedside to facilitate emergent reinduction or other form of airway management. Consider retained throat pack. Multimodal treatment of nausea is important.
Pain management	Parenteral narcotics (see p. C-2) or PCA with antiemetics (see p. C-3).	

Suggested Readings

1. Blanco G, Melman E, Cuairn V et al: Fibreoptic nasal intubation in children with anticipated and unanticipated difficult intubation. *Paediatric Anaesthesia* 2001; 11(1):49–53.
2. Degoute CS: Controlled hypotension: a guide to drug choice. *Drugs* 2007;67(7):1053–76.
3. Denny A, Kalantarian B: Mandibular Distraction in Neonates: A Strategy to Avoid Tracheostomy. *Plast Reconstr Surg* 2002; 109(3): 896–904.

4. Frost DE: Orthognathic surgical techniques. In *Maxillofacial Surgery.* Booth PW, Schendel SA, Hausamen J-E, eds. Churchill Livingstone, Edinburgh: 1999, 1273–95.
5. Hunt JA, Hobar PC: Common craniofacial anomalies: the facial dysostoses. *Plast Reconstr Surg* 2002; 110(7):1714–28.
6. Morris DE, Lo LJ, Margulis A: Pitfalls in orthognathic surgery: avoidance and management of complications. *Clin Plast Surg* 2007; 34(3):e17–29.
7. Osses H, et al: Laryngeal mask for difficult intubation in children. *Paediatric Anaesthesia* 1999; 9(5):399–401.
8. Richardson D, Pospisil OA: Avoiding surgical complications in orthognathic surgery. In *Maxillofacial Surgery.* Booth PW, Schendel SA, Hausamen J-E, eds. Churchill Livingstone, Edinburgh: 1999, 1307–20.
9. Samchukov ML, Cope JB, Cherkashin AM, eds: *Craniofacial Distraction Osteogenesis,* Mosby-Year Book, St. Louis: 2001.
10. Schendel SA, Mason ME: Adverse outcomes in orthognathic surgery and management of residual problems. *Clin Plast Surg* 1997; 24(3):489–505.
11. Silva AC, O'Ryan F, Poor DB: Postoperative nausea and vomiting (PONV) after orthognathic surgery: a retrospective study and literature review. *J Oral Maxillofac Surg* 2006; 64(9):1385–97.

CHAPTER

11.4 Functional Restoration

SURGEONS

James Chang, MD
David M. Kahn, MD
Angeline Lim, MD

ANESTHESIOLOGIST

Tara Cornaby, MD

MICROSURGERY-FREE-FLAP RECONSTRUCTION

SURGICAL CONSIDERATIONS

Angeline Lim and James Chang

Description: Microsurgical reconstruction involves moving tissue from one site of the body to another (see Fig. 11.4-1, Table 11.4-1). This may be muscle, skin, bone, or any combination of these tissues. An artery and vein that supply the tissues are connected to an artery and vein at the new recipient site, thereby reestablishing blood flow and ensuring tissue survival. Once transplanted, the tissue is molded and shaped to replace the missing part. Vascular anastomoses are performed on vessels as small as 1.5 mm in diameter. Complex reconstructions may require 12 hours of GA with significant blood loss and fluid shifts. Patients with comorbid conditions may need additional medical tests before surgery to ensure that they are able to withstand this type of operation.

Peripheral, central, and arterial lines should be placed at the start of the case only after consultation with the reconstructive surgeon. For example, radial forearm flap may be injured by placement of a peripheral iv in the antecubital fossa or within the body of the flap. The neck is a common site for microvascular anastomoses in head and neck reconstruction. The placement of internal jugular lines should be discussed with the surgeon before surgery. The rectus muscle flap relies on the deep inferior epigastric vessels for its perfusion. Femoral arterial or venous line placement may injure these vessels and is, therefore, contraindicated. In bilateral breast reconstruction with free flaps, the iv lines should be placed in the lower extremities if possible. The reconstructive surgeon will try to operate in conjunction with the extirpative surgeon to minimize operating time. This often necessitates repositioning the patient as the case progresses.

Microsurgical reconstructions are often long operations, and large surface areas of the patient are exposed during the surgery. The patient's core temperature should be monitored closely with the use of a bladder or esophageal temperature probe. Body and fluid warmers should be used routinely to maintain the patient's body temperature. There is no

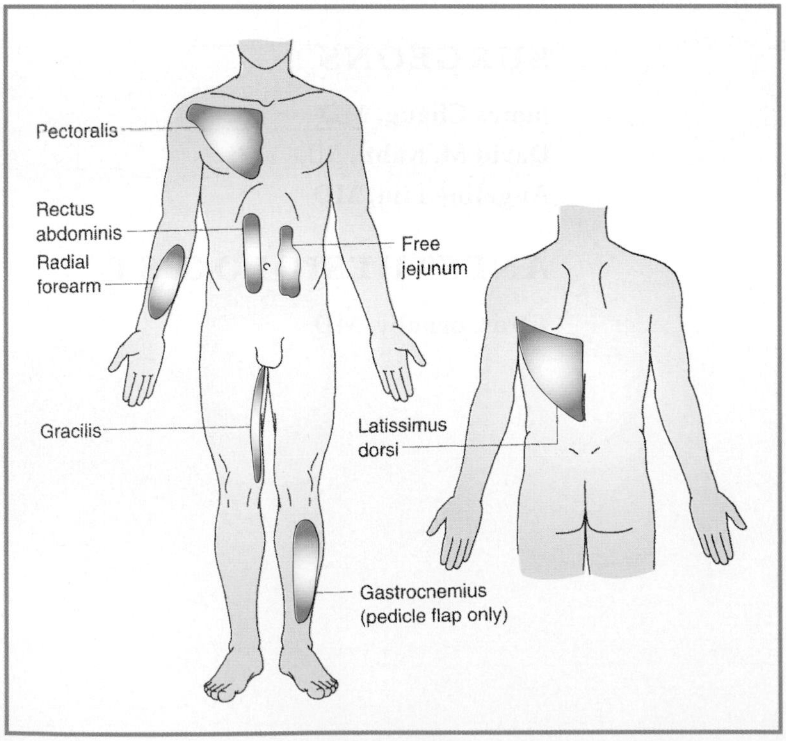

Figure 11.4-1. Locations of commonly used flaps. (Reproduced with permission from Greenfield, LJ, Mulholland MW, Oldham KT, et al, eds: *Surgery: Principles and Practice,* 2nd edition. Lippincott-Raven: 1997.)

Table 11.4-1. Types of Flaps

Reconstruction	Commonly Used Flaps	Location	Positioning
Head and neck	Fibula	Leg	Supine
	Radial forearm	Arm	Supine
	Scapula	Back	Lateral decubitus
	Iliac crest	Hip	Supine
	Anterolateral thigh	Thigh	Supine
	Gracilis	Thigh	Supine
Breast	TRAM	Abdomen	Supine
	Gluteal	Buttocks	Lateral decubitus
	Rubens/iliac crest	Hip	Supine
	Tensor fascia lata	Lateral thigh	Supine
	Latissimus dorsi	Back	Lateral decubitus
Lower extremity	Rectus abdominis	Abdomen	Supine
	Latissimus dorsi	Back	Lateral decubitus
	Serratus anterior	Back	Lateral decubitus
	Gracilis	Thigh	Supine

standard practice for anticoagulation in microsurgery. No randomized prospective clinical trial has definitively documented the efficacy of a particular type of anticoagulation in routine reconstructive microsurgery. Aspirin, dextran, and heparin are the most commonly used agents. Close communication between the surgeon and anesthesiologist is critical so that the desired agent is administered at the appropriate time.

The survival of the flap relies on the patency of the anastomosis. Thrombosis requires reexploration and may → complete loss of the tissue. Anastomotic patency is diminished by vasospasm or vascular constriction. The common causes of vasoconstriction include dehydration, hypothermia, pain, and administration of vasoconstrictors; therefore, during microsurgery, vasoconstrictors are contraindicated and should be given only when absolutely necessary, after consultation with the reconstructive surgeon. The patient must be adequately hydrated so that there is good perfusion to the transplanted tissue. Diuretics should be avoided. Postop pain control is important to prevent vasoconstriction on emergence from anesthesia. After surgery, patients are transferred to an area of the hospital where the free flap can be monitored. In many hospitals, this is an ICU.

Usual preop diagnosis: Trauma, cancer, chronic wounds, congenital anomalies, and burns are some of the common diagnoses that result in the need for microsurgical reconstruction.

SUMMARY OF PROCEDURE

Position	Requirements of the recipient site take precedence; optimal position for the donor site is then considered.
Incision	Each site will have specific incision.
Special instrumentation	Microscope; tourniquet for extremities
Unique considerations	Multiple surgical teams; avoid hypothermia; ± anticoagulation; if intraop nerve stimulation is planned, muscle relaxants should be avoided.
Antibiotics	Cefazolin (1 g iv) in uncomplicated cases; broader coverage in complicated circumstances
Surgical time	Simple flap: 4–6 h Complex cases: 8–12 h
Closing considerations	Splints and dressings should be secured before emergence.
EBL	Skin flap: 200 mL Muscle flap: 200–500 mL Bone flap: 500–1000 mL

SUMMARY OF PROCEDURE (cont'd)	
Postop care	ICU for flap perfusion monitoring
Mortality	< 2% (usually associated with coexisting disease)
Morbidity	Soft-tissue complications: 20–30% Vascular complications requiring reexploration: 5–10% Flap failure: 5%
Pain score	3–5

PATIENT POPULATION CHARACTERISTICS	
Age range	2–90 yr
Male:Female	1:1
Incidence	50–200/yr/major center
Etiology	Malignancy; trauma; chronic infection
Associated conditions	Complications of underlying disease (e.g., anemia)

ANESTHETIC CONSIDERATIONS

PREOPERATIVE

These surgeries are carried out on patients who have sustained major soft-tissue losses and require flap procedures to cover the defects. There are four typical patient populations presenting for this surgery: (a) those presenting for reconstruction following cancer surgery (e.g., radical neck dissection and mastectomy); (b) patients following trauma, usually with upper or lower-limb defects; (c) patients with congenital defects; and (d) previous burn victims. In general, these patients should present few problems for the anesthesiologist. In a patient with a congenital lesion, however, it is prudent to look for evidence of CHD, musculoskeletal deformities, and airway problems.

Respiratory	Exposure of the thorax to radiation may produce pathologic changes in the lungs and related structures, including pneumonitis (→ dyspnea, hypoxemia) that may progress to fibrosis (→↓ pulmonary compliance). Tracheal or bronchial fibrosis may → partial airway obstruction. Many burn patients have pulmonary pathology 2° smoke inhalation injury. The pathology usually include edema, inflammation, and loss of ciliary activity, but can vary depending on the length and amount of smoke exposure, as well as the composition of the material that burned. Patients with breast cancer may have been treated with chemotherapeutic agents (e.g., methotrexate, cyclophosphamide, bleomycin) that may cause pulmonary fibrosis, interstitial infiltrates, and pleural effusions. **Tests:** Consider CXR, PFT, and pulmonary consult.
Cardiovascular	Exposure of the heart to radiation may produce pathologic changes in the heart and related structures, including accelerated atherosclerotic changes, myocardial fibrosis, pericarditis, and valvular dysfunction. Patients with breast cancer may have been treated with doxorubicin (Adriamycin), which may produce cardiomyopathy (usually seen at total doses >550 mg/m^2) → CHF. XRT increases the incidence of clinically significant cardiomyopathy.
Hematologic	Myelosuppression may be present in patients with Hx of chemotherapy. **Tests:** CBC, with differential and Plt count
Laboratory	Other tests as indicated from H&P.
Premedication	Standard premedication (see p. B-1).

INTRAOPERATIVE

Anesthetic technique: GETA. Coordinate iv and/or invasive monitoring sites with the surgical team. Adjunctive regional anesthesia is an option for the appropriate patient who will not be anticoagulated. Some authors propose that the resultant vasodilation causes ↑ blood flow through the flap, but this has not been definitely shown in clinical trials.

Induction	Standard induction (see p. B-2) and intubation. Avoid succinylcholine in burn patients.	
Maintenance	Standard maintenance (see p. B-2). Muscle relaxation usually is required. The patient must be kept warm and well hydrated to minimize peripheral vasoconstriction, which might impair graft perfusion. Surgeon may request intraop anticoagulation, usually in the form of aspirin, dextran, or heparin.	
Emergence	Smooth emergence to avoid disrupting the surgical repair. Patients usually are transported to the ICU for continuous monitoring of flap perfusion.	
Blood and fluid requirements	Moderate blood loss IV: 16 ga × 1 NS/LR @ 4–5 mL/kg/h Warm fluids. Humidify gases.	Keep patient warm, and maintain a positive fluid balance. A Hct of 30–35% will provide adequate O_2 transport, while minimizing vi scosity. Dextran 40 usually is used to further ↓ viscosity, thereby ↑ flap blood flow.
Monitoring	Standard monitors (see p. B-1). UO ± Arterial line	An arterial line may be useful for prolonged procedures where regular ABGs and blood chemistries will be needed.
Positioning	✓ and pad pressure points. ✓ eyes.	These can be very lengthy surgeries, and careful monitoring of pressure points is essential.
Complications	Hypothermia	Maintain normal body temperature with warming blankets, fluid, and airway warmers.
	Decubitus ulcer	Pressure necrosis can occur in as little as 2 h. Carefully pad and repeatedly ✓ pressure points.
	Dextran reaction	Prophylactic use of very low molecular weight dextran (Promit) usually prevents allergic reactions to higher-molecular-weight dextran. Adult dose = 20 mL 1–15 min before dextran infusion.

POSTOPERATIVE

Complications	Arterial thrombosis Hematoma	May require reexploration. May require reexploration.
Pain management	Parenteral opiates (see p. C-2). PCA (see p. C-3).	Pain should be treated promptly to minimize reflex peripheral vasoconstriction and impaired graft perfusion.

Suggested Readings

1. Erni D, Banic A, Signer C, et al: Effects of epidural anaesthesia on microcirculatory blood flow in free flaps in patients under general anaesthesia. *Eur J Anaesthesiol* 1999; 16(10):692–8.
2. Evans BC, Evans GR: Microvascular surgery. *Plast Reconstr Surg* 2007; 119(2):18e–30e.
3. Hallock GG: The complete classification of flaps. *Microsurgery* 2004; 24(3):157–61.
4. Hynynen M, Eklund P, Rosenberg PH: Anaesthesia for patients undergoing prolonged reconstructive and microvascular plastic surgery. *Scand J Plast Surg* 1982; 16:201.
5. Khouris RK, Cooley BC, Kunselman AR, et al: A prospective study of microvascular free-flap surgery and outcome. *Plast Reconstr Surg* 1998; 102:711–21.

6. Lee RG, Baskin JZ: Improving outcomes of locoregional flaps: an emphasis on anatomy and basic science. *Curr Opin Otolaryngol Head Neck Surg* 2006; 14(4):260–4.
7. Lipa JE: Breast reconstruction with free flaps from the abdominal donor site: TRAM, DIEAP, and SIEA flaps. *Clin Plast Surg* 2007; 34(1):105–21.
8. Scott GR, Rothkopf DM, Walton RL: Efficacy of epidural anaesthesia in free flaps of the lower extremity. *Plast Reconstr Surg* 1993; 91:673.
9. Welch GW: Anesthesia for the patient with thermal injury. *Curr Rev Clin Anesth* 1992; 12:45.

MICROSURGERY-REPLANTATION

SURGICAL CONSIDERATIONS

Description: Patients who require replantation surgery are trauma victims and must be evaluated carefully preop, by both surgeons and anesthesiologists, to ensure that replantation is appropriate and that other injuries are not overlooked. In these cases, time is critical, as the amputated tissue is ischemic and may require immediate revascularization if it is to be salvaged. Coordination between the microsurgeon, anesthesiologist, and trauma team is important to minimize the time between injury and replantation.

As in any microsurgical procedure, it is critical to prevent vasoconstriction in these procedures. These patients may have experienced significant blood loss at the time of the trauma and require iv hydration and/or blood transfusion. The need for hemodynamic support often indicates another injury that may preclude transplantation. The patient may be hypothermic and require active rewarming. Vasoconstrictors and diuretics should be avoided unless absolutely necessary. During the replantation procedure, other tissues (e.g., skin, vein, bone) are required to aid in the reconstruction. These are routinely harvested from the leg, groin, or foot, which will be prepped into the surgical field.

The amputated stump is initially examined using loupe magnification. The arteries, veins, and nerves are dissected and tagged. The surgeon determines if the part is replantable. The amputated stump is prepared by dissecting the recipient arteries, veins, and nerves. The need for a vein graft may be determined at this time. The sequence of replantation varies; however, a general algorithm is:

Bone fixation → Extensor tendon repair → Flexor tendon repair → Nerve repair → Arterial and venous anastomoses → Skin closure

The replanted tissue must be monitored on an hourly basis to ensure continued viability. In many hospitals, this is performed in a microsurgical unit, while in others the ICU is used. Patients should be kept adequately hydrated, warm, and pain-free to prevent vasoconstriction and subsequent thrombosis. Vascular thrombosis requires immediate exploration and revision of the vascular anastomosis.

Specific variations of replantation procedures have unique features, as follows.

Replantation of fingers and hands: Generally, two surgeons work simultaneously. One surgeon at the back table explores the amputated parts, tagging significant nerves, vessels, and tendons. A second surgeon débrides the amputation sites and identifies the stumps of reparable structures. The surgeons then proceed with replantation. Generally, bone fixation and tendon repairs are performed first. Vessel and nerve repairs are performed next, using a microscope. The need for vein grafting and anticoagulation is determined intraop. Blood transfusions are rarely needed except when using anticoagulants.

Replantation of extremities: Replantation of arms or legs must be handled very efficiently since irreversible muscle damage occurs within 4 hours of ischemia. Generally, the sequence of surgery is similar to finger replantation, with the exception being that a temporary arterial circulation (using a dialysis shunt) is established as soon as possible to minimize ischemia time in an amputated part. Ongoing venous blood loss occurs while skeletal repairs are done, and transfusion is frequently required. Definitive vessel repairs (often requiring vein grafts) and nerve repairs are done under the microscope.

Scalp replantation: Scalp avulsions are caused by entanglement of hair in machinery. These amputations are frequently replantable, sparing the patient a grotesque and unstable deformity. Initial evaluation should include careful assessment of the C-spine, since the patient transiently hangs by the neck until the scalp separates. Initial blood loss can be significant and should be replaced preop. Replantation proceeds by identifying matching vessels at the margin of the defect and the avulsed scalp. The superficial temporal vessels are most commonly repaired, and use of vein grafts should be anticipated. Following the first artery repair, brisk bleeding generally occurs at the scalp margin until vein repairs are completed. This blood loss should be anticipated.

Usual preop diagnosis: Trauma

SUMMARY OF PROCEDURES

	Fingers/Hands	Extremities	Scalp
Position	Supine, injured arm extended	Supine	Supine or side (depending on vessel position)
Incision	Conventional hand exposure	Extension of injury; fasciotomies may be done.	Preauricular
Special instrumentation	Microscope; hand table; tourniquet	Microscope; tourniquet	Microscope; neurosurgical headrest
Unique considerations	Anticoagulation	⇐	RAE or anode tube; table, turned 180°
Antibiotics	Cefazolin 1g iv	⇐	⇐
Surgical time	1st finger: 3–4 h; 2 h/subsequent finger Hand: 4 h	4–8 h	4 h
Closing considerations	Splint applied before emergence.	Cast or splint applied before emergence.	Elevate head as much as possible.
EBL	100–200 mL	2–6 U	2–8 U
Postop care	ICU for monitoring	⇐	⇐
Mortality	None	Rare	None
Morbidity	Replant failure: 5–15%	Failure: 10–20%	Vascular occlusion → reexploration
Pain score	5–6	5–6	3–5

PATIENT POPULATION CHARACTERISTICS

Age range	Childhood-old age	⇐	Young adult
Male:Female	> 10:1	⇐	1:2
Incidence	250/yr/major center	Rare	⇐
Etiology	Trauma	⇐	⇐
Associated conditions	Other injuries	Other injuries, blood loss	C-spine injuries, blood loss

ANESTHETIC CONSIDERATIONS FOR REPLANTATION

PREOPERATIVE

In general, there are two patient populations for replantation procedures: (a) isolated limb and scalp injury patients (common), and (b) multiple trauma victims (rare). Most patients are otherwise healthy and the preop workup is routine.

Gastrointestinal	All of these patients should be considered to have full stomachs and, therefore, are at increased risk for aspiration pneumonitis. In general, they should receive preop medication to reduce stomach volume and acidity (e.g., metoclopramide 10 mg iv and ranitidine 50 mg iv) 30–60 min before induction, time permitting.
Metabolic	~50% of trauma victims are intoxicated. Anesthesia-related implications of acute ethanol intoxication include: ↓ anesthetic requirements, diuresis, vasodilation, and hypothermia.
Neurologic	Assess for possible head or C-spine injury, particularly in the trauma patient presenting with facial or scalp injuries.
Laboratory	As suggested by coexisting disease.
Premedication	Standard premedication (see p. B-1). Full-stomach precautions: Na citrate 0.3 M 30 mL immediately before induction of anesthesia.

INTRAOPERATIVE

Anesthetic technique: GETA, after rapid-sequence induction. These procedures are often lengthy, and regional anesthesia is usually not appropriate as the primary technique but may be considered as an adjunct.

Induction	Rapid-sequence induction (see p. B-4) is mandatory in emergency cases, unless awake intubation is performed. C-spine fracture patients or those with facial injuries may require awake fiber optic intubation (see p. B-5).	
Maintenance	Standard maintenance (see p. B-1) for stable patients.	
Emergence	Difficult airway or full-stomach cases require awake extubation.	
Blood and fluid requirements	Significant blood loss possible IV: 16 ga × 1–2 (extremity/scalp) IV: 18 ga × 1 (digit) NS/LR @ 1.5–3 mL/kg/h + 3 × blood loss Fluid/blood warmers, heating blanket, warmed circuit humidifier	A 16-ga iv catheter in a nonoperated upper extremity should be adequate in hemodynamically stable patients. Keep patient warm and hydrated to maximize perfusion to the replanted site. Avoid vasoconstrictors if possible.
Monitoring	Standard monitors (see p. B-1). ± Arterial line, CVP	Invasive hemodynamic monitoring should be considered in cases where large blood loss is anticipated.
Positioning	✓ and pad pressure points. ✓ eyes.	
Control of blood loss	Tourniquet may be used.	Inflation pressure is typically 100 mmHg greater than systolic pressure. Maximum 'safe' tourniquet time is 1.5–2 h, followed by a 5- (preferably) 15 min reperfusion interval, if further tourniquet time is necessary.
Special considerations	Tourniquet deflation and limb reperfusion	Mild ↓ BP is common. In patients with moderate-to-severe lung disease, continue controlled ventilation until after the lactic acid that has accumulated in the ischemic limb is metabolized (3–5 min), since these patients may be unable to increase ventilation adequately to buffer this acid load.
Complications	Hemodynamic instability	Previously unrecognized injuries (e.g., pneumothorax, cardiac tamponade, intracranial bleeding) should be considered as a cause of unexplained intraop hemodynamic instability in all acute-trauma victims.

POSTOPERATIVE

Complications	Reperfusion failure	May require immediate reexploration.
Pain management	PCA (see p. C-3)	
Tests	None routinely indicated.	Reimplant perfusion must be monitored.

Suggested Readings

1. Can DB, Kwon J: Anesthesia techniques and their indication for upper limb surgery. In *Surgery of the Hand and Upper Extremity*. Peimer CA, ed. McGraw-Hill, New York: 1996, 119–39.
2. Gayle L, Lineaweaver W, Buncke GM, et al: Lower extremity replantation. *Clin Plastic Surg* 1992; 18:437.
3. Goldner RD, Urbaniak JR: Replantation. In *Green's Operative Hand Surgery*. Green DP, Hotchkiss DP, Hotchkiss RN, et al., eds. Churchill Livingstone, San Francisco: 1999, 1139–58.
4. Ljungström KG: Dextran 40 therapy made safer by pretreatment with dextran 1. *Plast Reconstr Surg* 2007; 120(1):337–40.
5. Lloyd MS, Teo TC, Pickford MA, et al: Preoperative management of the amputated limb. *Emerg Med J* 2005; 22(7):478–80.
6. Morrison WA, McCombe D: Digital replantation. *Hand Clin* 2007; 23(1):1–12.
7. Sanders N, Anderson KR: Anesthesia for microsurgery. In *Microsurgery*. Buncke HJ, ed. LeaFebiger, Philadelphia: 1991, 729.
8. Strauch B, Greenstein B, Goldstein R, et al: Problems and complications encountered in replantation surgery. *Hand Clin* 1986; 2:389.
9. Yin JW, Matsuo JM, Hsieh CH, et al: Replantation of total avulsed scalp with microsurgery: experience of eight cases and literature review. *J Trauma* 2008; 64(3):796–802.

BREAST SURGERY—INTRODUCTION

David M. Kahn, Angeline Lim

Patients presenting for plastic surgery of the breast can be grouped into four basic categories along a continuum ranging from amastia/hypomastia to hypertrophy. Plastic surgery procedures are designed to create or make adjustments in the amounts of skin and glandular tissue or to make adjustments in their relationship to each other to create an aesthetic breast. The first type of patient is one who has acquired amastia after undergoing a mastectomy; it is this patient who is featured in this section on functional restoration. In this patient, the goal is to replace the missing tissue, both skin and glandular, with like tissue or an implant. The second type is a person presenting for augmentation mammoplasty (see p. 1084). In this situation, the breast is deficient of skin and glandular tissue. The third type is the patient who presents for a reduction mammoplasty (see p. 1086). In this situation, there is an excess of glandular tissue and skin. The fourth type is the patient who presents for a mastopexy or breast lift (see p. 1088). In this patient, there exists a discrepancy between the amount of glandular tissue present and the volume of the skin envelope, resulting in ptosis.

For all breast procedures, the patient's breasts are marked preop with the patient in either the sitting or standing position. This is a necessity, and its importance cannot be overstated. The appearance of the breasts in the supine position versus the upright position is significantly different due to the effects of gravity.

BREAST RECONSTRUCTION

SURGICAL CONSIDERATIONS

Description: The goal of breast reconstruction is to create an aesthetic breast that is symmetrical with the contralateral breast. Typically, this can be accomplished in three ways: expander/implant reconstruction; latissimus flap reconstruction, ± an implant; and TRAM flap reconstruction, performed using either a pedicled technique or a free-tissue transfer. Each type of reconstruction follows the principle of replacing glandular and cutaneous breast tissue. In patients undergoing mastectomy, reconstruction may be performed immediately after the mastectomy or it may be delayed and performed at a later date.

In **expander/implant reconstruction** (Fig 11.4-2), a tissue expander is placed underneath the pectoralis major muscle and a portion of the serratus anterior muscle, followed by skin closure. Thus, two layers exist above the implant—skin and muscle. The patient returns to the office for expansions, with saline being injected into the implant port. This is continued until the desired size is reached. Then, the patient returns to the OR for the exchange of the expander for a permanent implant that contains either saline or silicone gel as filler material. Except for the psychosocial aspects of patient management, much of the technique and perioperative concerns are similar to those for breast augmentation (see p. 1084).

Autologous breast reconstructions: Two types of flaps are used for these procedures—latissimus myocutaneous flap and transverse rectus abdominus muscle (TRAM) flap. The **latissimus dorsi myocutaneous flap** consists of the muscle with overlying skin that is rotated from the back to the anterior chest for the creation of a breast. The flap does not supply sufficient bulk to be used in breast reconstruction unless the contralateral breast is very small. Usually a breast implant is placed between the latissimus and pectoralis muscles, thus increasing the volume of the reconstruction. The patient is placed in the lateral decubitus position for the latissimus flap harvest. The incision is designed to surround the skin paddle. The ellipse of skin is incised, and the dissection then proceeds along the superficial surface of the latissimus muscle towards its lateral, superior, and inferior borders. Dissection is performed underneath the latissimus muscle to separate it from the deep tissues of the back. The muscle is released from its insertions on the posterior superior iliac crest, medial fascial attachments, and surrounding muscle attachments (i.e., serratus anterior, teres major). The flap is tunneled through the axilla, and the back wound is closed (Fig 11.4-3). The patient is then returned to the supine position. The muscle is disinserted from the humerus, if necessary, and brought out onto the anterior chest wall. At this point, the muscle is inset into the mastectomy defect. An implant or tissue expander may be placed under the muscle if necessary for size and symmetry. Often, the patient is placed in the seated or semi-Fowler position for closure. The incisions are closed over a drain and dressings are applied. The skin flap is monitored postop for signs of flap ischemia and congestion, which may necessitate a return to the OR.

The **TRAM flap** procedure replaces the breast with an ellipse of abdominal skin and subcutaneous tissue based on the rectus abdominus muscle (Fig 11.4-4). In selecting patients for a TRAM flap reconstruction, the patient must have adequate lower abdominal tissue to make a breast; however, obese patients, smokers, diabetics, and those with a Hx of prior abdominal surgery may have a higher incidence of complications and flap loss. The benefit of this procedure is that it creates a natural appearing breast from the patient's own tissue without an implant. As a bonus, the abdominal donor site is closed as though the patient had undergone abdominoplasty ('tummy tuck'). The myocutaneous perforators that arise from the superior epigastric and inferior epigastric arteries provide blood supply to

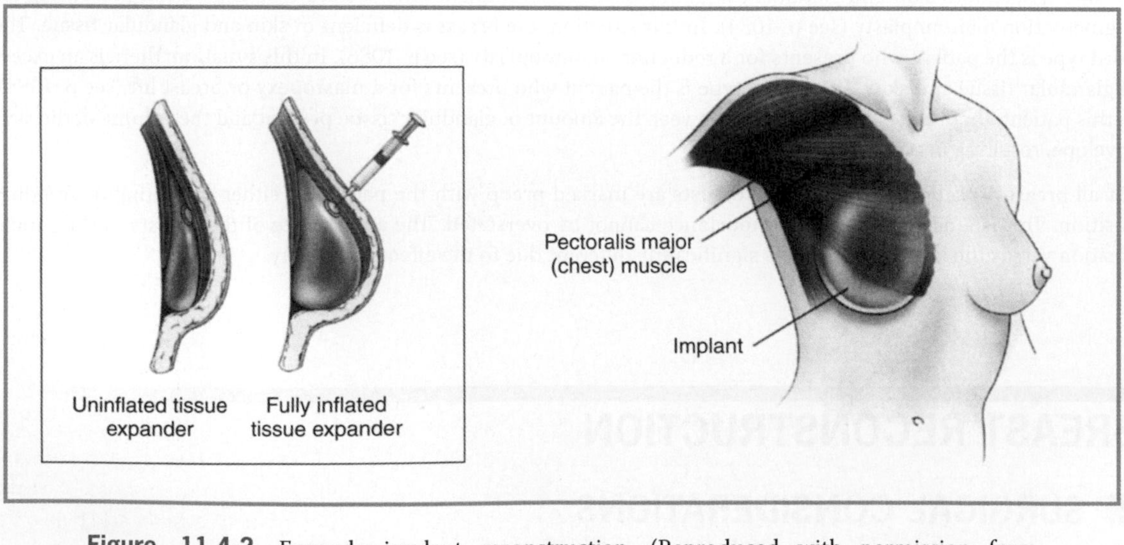

Figure 11.4-2. Expander-implant reconstruction. (Reproduced with permission from Greenfield LJ, et al, eds: *Surgery: Scientific Principles and Practices*, 3rd edition. Lippincott Williams & Wilkins, 2001.)

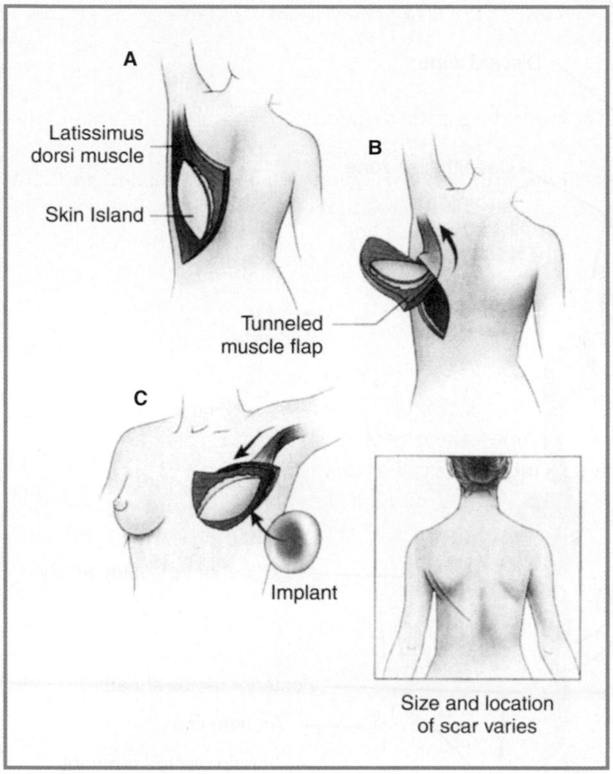

Figure 11.4-3. (A–C) Latissimus dorsi flap reconstruction. (Reproduced with permission from Greenfield LJ, et al, eds: *Surgery: Scientific Principles and Practices*, 3rd edition. Lippincott Williams & Wilkins, 2001.)

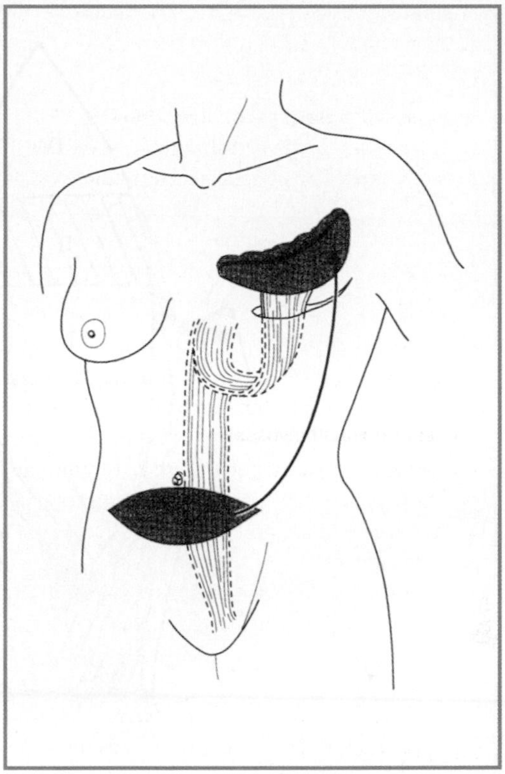

Figure 11.4-4. Breast reconstruction using free TRAM flap. (Reproduced with permission from Greenfield, LJ, et al, eds: *Surgery: Scientific Principles and Practice*, 2nd edition. Lippincott-Raven, 1997.)

the flap. This flap can be harvested in either a pedicled fashion, based on the superior epigastric artery, or as a free flap, based on the inferior epigastric artery. The inset of the flap and closure of the donor site are the same in both cases. The basic difference between the two methods of flap transfer is that, in the free TRAM procedure, the flap is removed from the abdomen, brought into the mastectomy wound, and the operating microscope is used to suture the vascular pedicle of the flap to the recipient vessels, either the thora-codorsal or internal mammary arteries. In the case of the pedicled TRAM flap, the flap is passed through a tunnel, created under the skin, maintaining the blood supply via the superior epigastric artery. The flap is brought out into the mastectomy wound where it is sutured into position.

Pedicled TRAM flap: The patient is marked preop in the upright position. The midline and inframammary folds are marked, as is the abdominal ellipse. The arms are placed at 90° abduction. The breasts and abdomen are prepped and draped. A general surgeon performs the mastectomy and, if possible, the TRAM flap harvest is started at the same time. Incising the skin along the superior marking of the abdominal ellipse begins the harvest of the flap. The upper abdominal skin and subcutaneous fat are elevated off the abdominal wall fascia up to the level of the costochondral cartilage, as in an abdominoplasty. The table is then flexed, and the upper skin and subcutaneous tissue is brought to overlap the TRAM flap to ensure that the location of the marked incision at the lower border of the flap will allow for abdominal closure. The patient is returned to the supine position. The skin and subcutaneous tissue of the flap are raised from a lateral to medial direction off the abdominal wall fascia until the lateral border of the rectus muscle is identified. Care is taken to preserve the myocutaneous perforators supplying the flap. The anterior rectus sheath is incised and the rectus muscle is elevated away from the posterior rectus sheath. The inferior epigastric vascular pedicle is identified and divided, preserving as much length as possible. The portion of the rectus muscle below the flap is transected so that the muscle, along with the overlying ellipse of skin and subcutaneous tissue can be rotated into the mastectomy site. A tunnel is created under the skin to connect the abdominal wound and mastectomy site. The flap is passed through this tunnel and rotated into position on the chest wall (Fig 11.4-5).

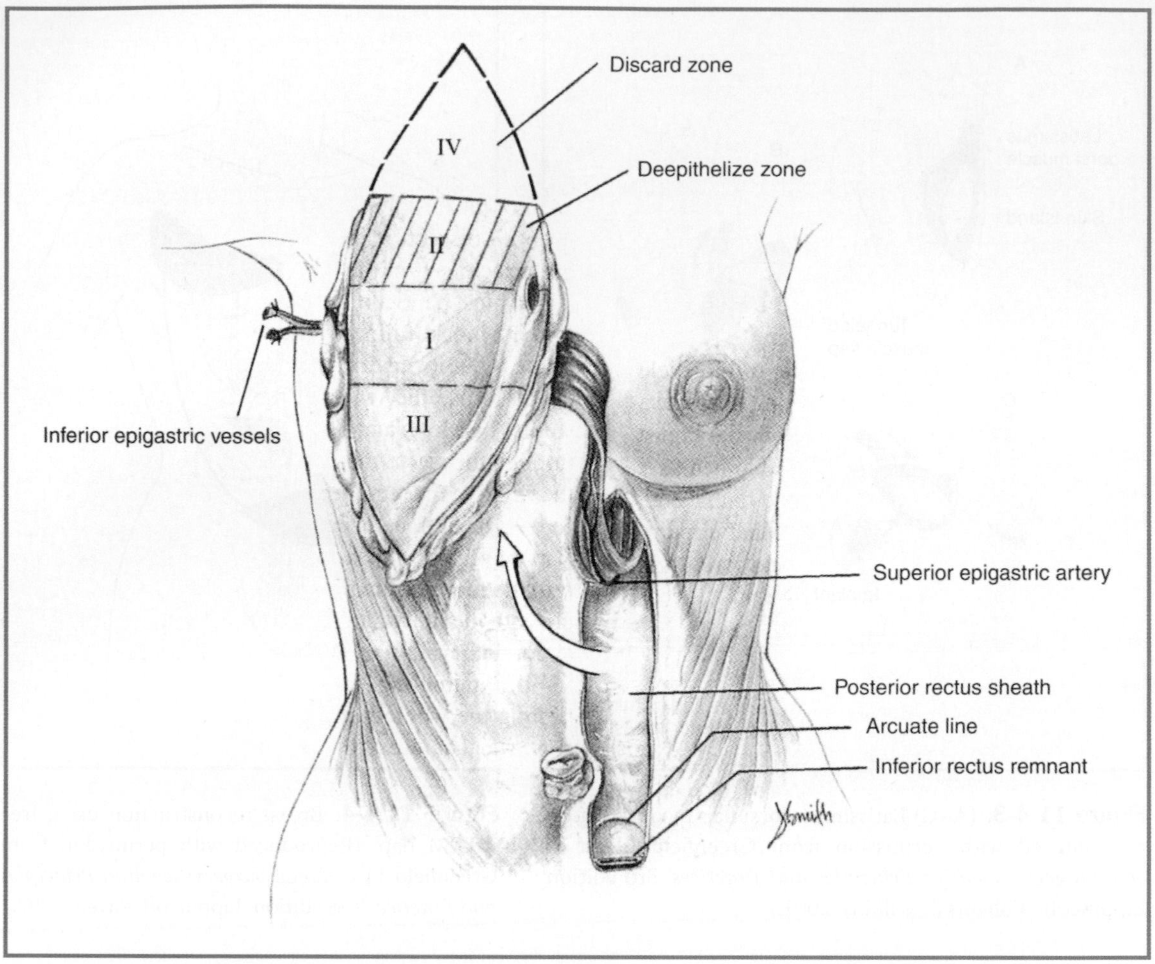

Figure 11.4-5. TRAM flap reconstruction of the breast. A contralateral pedicled TRAM flap has been elevated and will be tunneled under the skin to be inset at the mastectomy site. The zone of tissue furthest from the blood supply is discarded. A portion of the TRAM flap will be deepithelialized and placed under the mastectomy skin flaps. (Reproduced with permission from Spear SL: *Surgery of the Breast: Principles and Art.* Lippincott-Raven, 1998.)

In flap reconstructions, the harvested tissue receives its blood supply through a single artery and vein. It is important in these cases to maintain a stable BP that will allow for continued perfusion of the flap tissue. Vasopressors are to be avoided, as they will constrict the artery and thus restrict the inflow into the flap. It is preferred, if possible, to maintain a stable BP with volume replacement. Once the flap is in place at the mastectomy site, the table is again flexed as much as 45–60° for closure. Drains are placed within both the chest and abdominal wound beds. The flap is trimmed and sutured into position to create symmetry with the contralateral breast. The abdomen is closed in a fashion similar to an abdominoplasty. Many surgeons prefer that N_2O (which can distend the abdomen) be avoided during the abdominal closure. The surgeon will evaluate the flap to monitor for signs of ischemia and congestion. This is done both by clinical evaluation (color, temperature, and turgor) and by Doppler. If inflow or outflow is inadequate for flap survival, blood flow may be supplemented by performing a microvascular anastomosis between the inferior epigastric pedicle and the thoracodorsal vessels. In some cases, the surgeon may choose to convert the pedicled flap to a free flap.

Usual preop diagnosis: Carcinoma of the breast; radiation therapy; cardiovascular surgery; Poland syndrome

SUMMARY OF PROCEDURES

	Tissue Expander/Implant	Latissimus Dorsi Flap	TRAM Flap
Position	Supine	Lateral decubitus → supine	Supine
Incision	Breast	Posterior (supine); lateral (thorax)	Abdominal
Unique considerations	May have to place patient in sitting position during procedure; SCDs; Foley catheter if case > 3–4 h.	⇐	⇐ + Avoid use of N_2O.
Surgical time	1–2 h	4 h (+ mastectomy time)	6–8 h (free TRAM) 4 h (pedicled TRAM) (not including mastectomy time)
Closing considerations	Extensive dressing required	⇐	⇐ + Flex table for abdominal closure.
EBL	Minimal-100 mL	200–300 mL	200–400 mL
Postop care	PACU → room	⇐	⇐ (free TRAM flap → ICU)
Mortality	Rare	⇐	⇐
Morbidity	Capsular contraction: ± 30% Decreased sensation: 15% Hematoma: 2.2% Fat/skin necrosis: 1.7–1.9% Nipple areola necrosis: 1.4%	– ⇐ ⇐ ⇐ – Flap loss: Rare	– ⇐ ⇐ ⇐ – ⇐ Abdominal hernia: Infrequent
Pain score	5	5	5

PATIENT POPULATION CHARACTERISTICS

Age range	30–70 yr
Male:Female	Mostly female
Incidence	Breast reconstruction is performed in 9% of female population
Etiology	Cancer; trauma; idiopathic; radiation or postcardiovascular surgery
Associated conditions	Breast cancer; cardiovascular disease; S/P chemotherapy; pulmonary disease

ANESTHETIC CONSIDERATIONS

See Anesthetic Considerations for Breast and Chest-wall Reconstruction, p. 1137.

Suggested Readings

1. Abeloff MD, et al: Breast. In *Clinical Oncology*. Churchill Livingstone, New York: 1995.
2. American Society of Plastic Surgeons' Website: www.plasticsurgery.org.
3. Desidero DP, Kross RA, Bedford RF: Evaluation of the patient with oncologic disease. In *Principles and Practice of Anesthesiology*, 2nd edition. Longnecker DE, Tinker JH, Morgan GE Jr, eds. Mosby-Year Book, St. Louis: 1998, 379–96.
4. Spear SL, ed: Breast reconstruction. In *Surgery of the breast: Principles and art*. Lippincott-Raven, Philadelphia: 1998,335–672.
5. Spear SL: Primary implant reconstruction. In *Surgery of the Breast: Principles and Art*. Lippincott-Raven, Philadelphia:1998, 347–56.
6. Vasconez HC, Holley DT: Use of the TRAM and latissimus dorsi flaps in autogenous breast reconstruction. *Clin Plast Surg* 1995; 22(l):153–66.

CHEST-WALL RECONSTRUCTION

SURGICAL CONSIDERATIONS

Description: Chest-wall reconstruction is most commonly performed for infections, sternal dehiscence, tumor extirpation, and radiation injuries. Complications after median sternotomy make up a large number of these cases. The patients often have comorbidities and are at high risk for anesthetic and surgical complications. The goals of reconstruction are to provide a stable chest-wall for respiration, to eradicate infection, and to obtain a healed wound.

Sternal wound infections and dehiscences: Wound complications after median sternotomy include dehiscence of the sternum and mediastinitis. In these cases, radical debridement of all devitalized tissue is the cornerstone to a successful outcome. The initial debridement is, therefore, performed in conjunction with the cardiovascular surgeons. During this debridement, blood loss may be extensive, requiring transfusion. The resulting dead space around the heart and great vessels is obliterated, most commonly with **pectoralis major or rectus abdominis muscle (TRAM) flaps.** For patients who have failed the initial reconstruction or are not candidates for these flaps, a **latissimus dorsi muscle flap** may be used. In spite of radical excision of the sternum, the respiratory function of these patients remains adequate and no bony stabilization is required.

Tumor extirpation and radiation injury: Tumor resection or removal of osteoradionecrosis of the chest wall often involves the full-thickness removal of skin, muscle, and underlying rib cage. The rib cage may be reconstructed with prosthetic mesh or bone grafts. These structures are then covered with muscle flaps. The pectoralis major, rectus abdominis, and latissimus dorsi muscles are the muscle flaps most commonly used. After surgery, the patient's ventilatory capacity may be diminished by the rib resection, and this should be anticipated preop.

Usual preop diagnosis: Chest-wall infections; tumor; sternal dehiscence; radiation injuries

SUMMARY OF PROCEDURES

	Pectoralis Flap	Latissimus Flap	Rectus (TRAM) Flap
Position	Supine	Lateral decubitus → supine	Supine; table flexed
Incision	Chest	Posterolateral thorax	Abdominal
Antibiotics	Cefazolin 1 g	⇐	⇐
Surgical time	3 h	⇐	4–6 h
Closing considerations	✓ flap perfusion.	⇐	⇐
EBL	200–400 mL	⇐	300–500 mL
Postop care	PACU → room	⇐	⇐
Mortality	Rare	⇐	⇐
Morbidity	Thrombosis/flap failure Hematoma Fat/skin necrosis	⇐ ⇐ ⇐	⇐ ⇐ ⇐ Abdominal hernia: Infrequent
Pain score	4–5	4–5	4–5

PATIENT POPULATION CHARACTERISTICS

Age range	30–80 yr
Male:Female	1:1
Incidence	Uncommon

PATIENT POPULATION CHARACTERISTICS (cont'd)	
Etiology	Cancer; trauma; radiation; postcardiovascular surgery
Associated conditions	Breast cancer; cardiovascular disease; S/P chemotherapy; pulmonary disease; mediastinitis

ANESTHETIC CONSIDERATIONS FOR BREAST AND CHEST-WALL RECONSTRUCTION

PREOPERATIVE

These surgeries are performed most commonly for reconstruction following cancer surgery, such as radical neck dissection and mastectomy (see Anesthetic Considerations for the primary procedure), as well as complications after median sternotomy. The following considerations focus on patients undergoing reconstruction postchemotherapy.

Respiratory	Pulmonary fibrosis may complicate chemotherapy. Bleomycin (> 200 mg/m^2) carries the greatest risk of pulmonary toxicity (10%), but alkylating agents (e.g., cyclophosphamide and melphalan) may cause a degree of pulmonary toxicity as well. Avoid FiO_2 > 30% in bleomycin patients (to prevent progressive pulmonary fibrosis and edema). Patients presenting with complications from a prior sternotomy may have ↓ respiratory function/reserve and will require further work-up. **Tests:** CXR; ABG and PFTs as indicated from H&P.
Cardiovascular	Cardiomyopathy and CHF may result from chemotherapy, especially doxorubicin (Adriamycin) > 550 mg/m^2. Previous XRT increases risk of clinically significant cardiomyopathy. Patients with median sternotomy-related complications who have undergone prior cardiac surgery will require careful evaluation of their current cardiovascular status. **Tests:** ECG; ECHO, if indicated from H&P.
Neurological	Note any previous damage to long thoracic nerves, as evidenced by winged scapula deformity.
Musculoskeletal	It is traditional to avoid iv and BP cuff on mastectomy side.
Hematologic	Myelosuppression/toxicity from chemotherapuetic agents may be present. **Tests:** CBC; Plt count; coag profile; Hb/Hct
Renal/Hepatic	Methotrexate can produce renal and hepatic dysfunction. Elevated alkaline phosphatase may suggest metastatic bone invasion. **Tests:** Electrolytes; BUN; Cr; LFTs
Gastrointestinal	Tamoxifen, used in hormonal chemotherapy, can cause preop N/V and dehydration.
Laboratory	Other tests as indicated from H&P, prior chemotherapy.
Premedication	Midazolam 1–2 mg iv immediately preop, or Valium 5–10 mg po 1 h preop

INTRAOPERATIVE

Anesthetic technique: GETA

Induction	Standard induction (see p. B-2) and intubation. Avoid iv and NIBP monitoring on mastectomy side.
Maintenance	Standard maintenance (see p. B-2). Muscle relaxation is usually appropriate. These patients should be kept warm and well hydrated to minimize peripheral vasoconstriction, which might impair graft perfusion.
Emergence	During some of the procedure and for application of dressing, patient may be moved to sitting position, with consequent coughing, bucking, etc. (Rx: deeper anesthesia, e.g., propofol 0.5 mg/kg or lidocaine 1 mg/kg.) Watch BP carefully and treate orthostatic hypotension if it occurs, usually with a fluid bolus if the patient is not fluid-sensitive (e.g., Hx of CHF or renal failure).

Blood and fluid requirements	IV: 16 ga × 1 NS/LR @ 4–6 mL/kg/h Warm fluids. Humidify gases.	Extensive blood loss may occur with debridement of sternum in cases of infection or dehiscence. Keep patient warm and maintain a positive fluid balance. Hypothermia may impair flap perfusion.
Monitoring	Standard monitors (see p. B-1). UO	Use invasive monitoring in cardiovascular-challenged patients or in cases with significant expected blood loss, where regular ABGs and blood chemistries will be useful.
Positioning	✓ and pad pressure points. ✓ eyes.	
Complications	Pneumothorax Decubitus ulcer Dextran reaction	Pneumothorax should be considered with any ↑ lung inflation pressure, ↓ O_2 sat or ↓ BP. Pressure necrosis can occur in as little as 2 h. Carefully pad and repeatedly ✓ pressure points. Prophylactic use of very low molecular weight dextran (Promit) usually prevents allergic reactions to higher molecular weight dextrans. Adult dose = 20 mL (pediatric dose = 0.3 mL/kg) iv 1–2 min (maximum 15 min) before dextran infusion.

POSTOPERATIVE

Complications	Pneumothorax ↓ Flap perfusion	
Pain management	Parenteral opiates (see p. C-2). PCA (see p. C-3).	Pain should be treated promptly to minimize reflex peripheral vasoconstriction and impaired graft perfusion.

Suggested Readings

1. Buggy DJ, Kerin MJ: Paravertebral analgesia with levobupivacaine increases postoperative flap tissue oxygen tension after immediate latissimus dorsi breast reconstruction compared with intravenous opioid analgesia. *Anesthesiology* 2004; 100(2):375–80.
2. Hu E, Alderman AK: Breast reconstruction. *Surg Clin North Am* 2007; 87(2):453–67.
3. Roth DA: Thoracic and abdominal wall reconstruction. In *Grabb and Smith's Plastic Surgery,* 5th edition. Aston SJ, Beasley RW, Thorne CHM, eds. Lippincott-Raven, Philadelphia: 1997, 1023–30.
4. Skoracki RJ, Chang DW: Reconstruction of the chestwall and thorax. *J Surg Oncol* 2006; 94(6):455–65.

PRESSURE-SORE RECONSTRUCTION

SURGICAL CONSIDERATIONS

Description: Pressure sores occur when constant pressure is placed on an area of the body. They tend to occur in debilitated, bedridden, paralyzed, and wheelchair-bound patients. Multiple factors—including altered sensory perception, poor nutrition, incontinence, moisture, and shear forces—also may contribute to the formation of the pressure sores. The most common locations are the sacrum, ischium, and greater trochanter regions, as well as the heel and scalp.

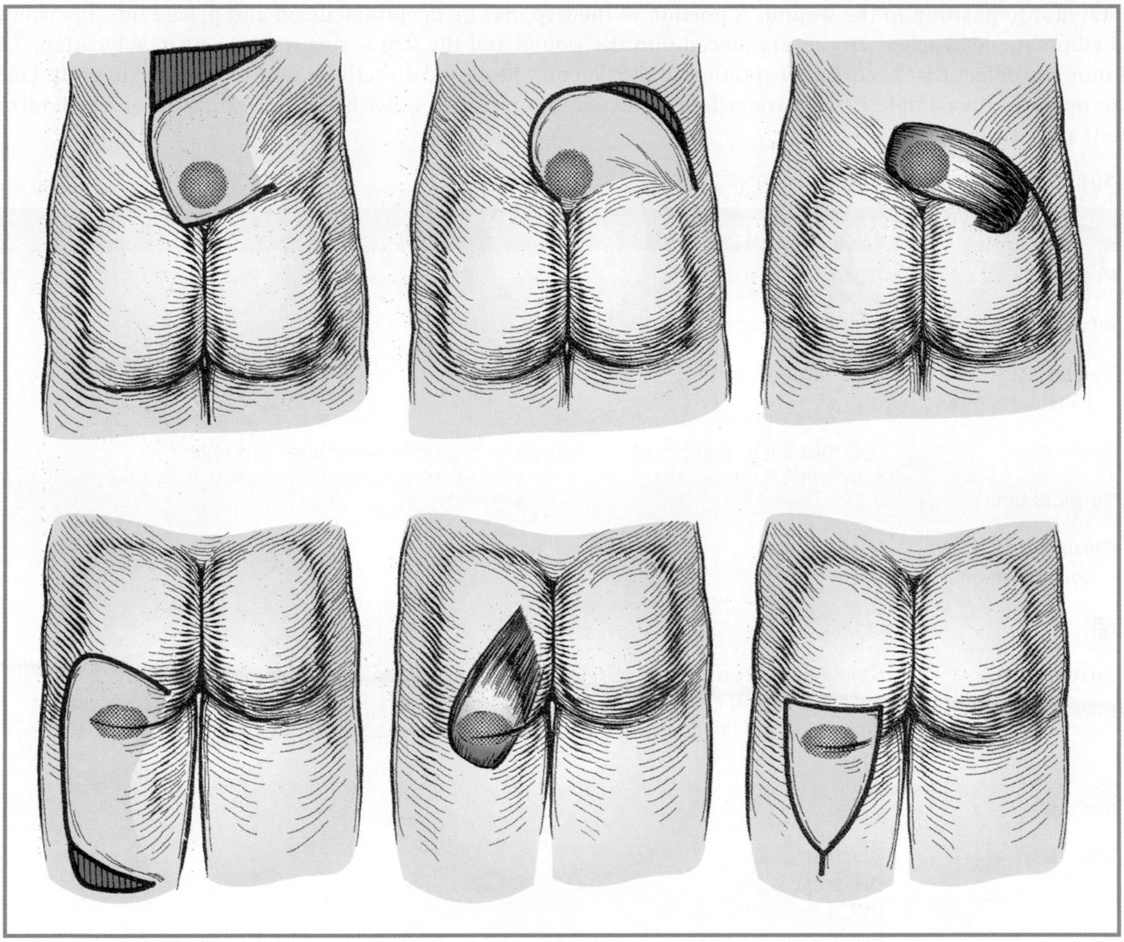

Figure 11.4-6. Commonly used flap designs for coverage of sacral and ischial pressure sores. (Reproduced with permission from Aston SJ, Beasley RW, Thorne CHM: *Grabb and Smith's Plastic Surgery,* 5th edition. Lippincott-Raven, 1997.)

The management of pressure sores is multidisciplinary and involves more than just debridement and wound closure. Patient compliance is the most important factor of wound management, as recurrence rates after closure are high. All components that contributed to the formation of the ulcer must be addressed before wound closure. This is best done in a team setting, with the goal of preventing further sores. In this effort, nutrition must be optimized; infection, muscle spasm, and contractures controlled; pressure relief measures instituted; and the psychological issues addressed. Once these are in place, wound reconstruction may begin.

Reconstruction is based on adequate debridement, elimination of dead space and pressure points, and closure of the wound with healthy, durable tissue. Multiple flap designs have been described for the coverage of pressure sores, depending on their location (Fig. 11.4-6). An important point in the design of a flap is the consideration for future reconstructions because of the high incidence of recurrent wounds. The choice of flap also needs to take into consideration the donor site morbidity. Skin-only flaps, fasciocutaneous flaps, and musculocutaneous flaps are commonly used.

The patient is placed in the prone position and may be jackknifed to facilitate exposure of the wound. Debridement of the wound is performed; and the bursa and underlying bony prominences may be removed. Hemostasis is obtained and the wound is irrigated with pulsed lavage. The flap to be used is designed over the vascular pedicle. The donor site for sacral, gluteal, and greater trochanteric wounds are typically the tissues of the buttocks and posterior thigh. The skin is incised and the flap is raised to include the appropriate layers of tissue, depending on whether a skin, fasciocutaneous, or musculocutaneous flap is to be used. The flap is then rotated into position in the wound. A portion of the flap may be deepithelialized and placed into the wound to eliminate dead space. Drains are placed into the wound and the flap is sutured into its new location. The donor site defect that occurs after rotation of the flap may be closed directly or may require a skin graft. Once the operation is complete, the patient is transferred to a pressure-relief bed (e.g., Clinitron or air-fluidized bed) and extubated.

Usual preop diagnosis: Pressure sores

SUMMARY OF PROCEDURE	
Position	Prone or lateral decubitus
Incision	Gluteal or posterior thigh
Unique considerations	Foley catheter; SCDs
Antibiotics	Cefazolin 1 g iv. Some surgeons may prefer broader polymicrobial coverage.
Surgical time	3 h
Closing considerations	None
EBL	200–300 mL
Postop care	Strict bed rest on a pressure-relief bed for up to 3 wk. Care must be taken to ensure that the patient is turned every 2 h so that excessive pressure is not transferred to a new location. Antibiotics and the control of urine and stool are important to prevent soiling of the suture lines.
Mortality	0–1%
Morbidity	Infection: 2–3% Dehiscence: 1% DVT: 1% Recurrence
Pain score	4–6 (depends on spinal cord status)

PATIENT POPULATION CHARACTERISTICS	
Age range	20–70 yr
Male:Female	Predominantly male
Etiology	Immobility; unrelieved pressure; altered sensation
Associated conditions	Paraplegia; debilitation; quadriplegia

ANESTHETIC CONSIDERATIONS

PREOPERATIVE

Typically, these surgeries are carried out on nonambulatory patients, with the spinal cord injury patient comprising a large subset. Anesthesia for plegic patients may well present several challenges, as discussed below.

Respiratory	Plegic patients may have intercostal muscle weakness → atelectasis and ↓ clearance of secretions → recurrent URIs and V/Q mismatching → hypoxemia. **Tests:** PFT; ABG; others as indicated from H&P.

Cardiovascular	Autonomic hyperreflexia (AH) may present as acute episodes of uninhibited hyperactivity in the patient with an injury level of T10-T7 or above. The main clinical signs are paroxysmal HTN and bradycardia, in response to stimulation below the lesion. Severe HTN can result in pulmonary edema, myocardial ischemia and cerebral hemorrhage. Identify triggering stimuli (e.g., bowel or bladder distension, cutaneous stimulation). T4 or higher lesions may →↓ BP on induction of GA or regional anesthesia, initiation of IPPV, or postural changes. **Tests:** ECG; others as indicated from H&P.
Neurological	✓ level of cord injury. AH in patient with spinal cord injury (see Cardiovascular, above) may manifest as headaches, sweating, facial flushing or syncope. Hyperreflexia below injury level.
Musculoskeletal	Immobility → skeletal muscle atrophy, osteoporosis, and decubitus ulcer formation.
Gastrointestinal	Spinal cord injury →↓ GI function → constipation/full stomach.
Renal	Chronic spinal cord injury → recurrent UTIs and calculi → renal failure. Foley catheter placement may → AH. **Tests:** UA; BUN; Cr; others as indicated from H&P.
Laboratory	Immobility →↑ Ca^{++}, → dysrhythmias and nausea. **Tests:** Others as indicated from H&P.
Premedication	Standard premedication (see p. B-1) is usually appropriate. Patients with limited respiratory reserve should receive minimal sedation. Nifedipine (10 mg sublingually 5 min or po 20 min before induction) may be used to blunt AH.

INTRAOPERATIVE

Anesthetic technique: GETA. If flap donor and recipient sites are confined to the lower half of the body, regional anesthesia may be considered for short procedures. Spinal or epidural anesthesia will minimize AH; however, anesthetic level may be difficult to assess and regional anesthesia may not be tolerated for prolonged surgery. Lighter levels of GA will not prevent AH.

Induction	Standard induction (see p. B-2) and intubation. Although the risk of ↑ K^+ 2° succinylcholine is reportedly decreased 6 mo after injury, NMRs are still preferred. AH may occur with Foley catheter placement.	
Maintenance	Standard maintenance (see p. B-2). Muscle relaxation is usually appropriate and may be necessary to reduce muscle spasticity. Avoid drugs that are primarily renally excreted in patients with CRI. Direct arterial vasodilators and alpha-adrenergic blocking agents should be readily available. Plegic patients are prone to hypothermia. These patients should be kept warm and well hydrated to minimize peripheral vasoconstriction, which might impair graft perfusion.	
Emergence	AH 2° distended bladder or rectum may occur on emergence from anesthesia.	
Blood and fluid requirements	IV: 16 ga × 1 NS/LR @ 4–6 mL/kg/h Warm fluids. Humidify gases.	Keep patient warm and maintain a positive fluid balance. Hypothermia may impair flap perfusion. Initial debridement of ulcer may be extensive and significant blood loss can occur. T&C as appropriate.
Monitoring	Standard monitors (see p. B-1). UO ± Arterial line	An arterial line may be useful in patients susceptible to AH and for prolonged procedures where regular ABGs and blood chemistries will be useful.
Positioning	✓ and pad pressure points. ✓ eyes.	Many of these patients may be osteoporotic, so great care should be used in moving and positioning.

Complications	Hypothermia	Patients with spinal cord injury often have impaired thermoregulation. Maintain normal body temperature with warming blankets, fluid, and airway warmers.
	AH	AH should be promptly controlled with SNP bolus (5–50 mcg) and infusion, while anesthesia is deepened. A continuous trimethaphan infusion (0.5–4 mg/min) is another option.
	Decubitus ulcer	Pressure necrosis can occur in as little as 2 h. Carefully pad and repeatedly ✓ pressure points.

POSTOPERATIVE

Complications	Respiratory Insufficiency	Quadriplegic Patients May Have ↓ Vc And ↓ Erv And Be Uniquely Susceptible To Residual Respiratory Depressant Effects.
	AH	AH may occur 2° distended bladder or rectum. Rx: phentolamine 1 mg Iv Q 1 min and/or SNP bolus/infusion; removal of stimulus.
Pain management	Parenteral opiates (see p. C-2). PCA (see p. C-3).	Pain should be treated promptly to minimize reflex peripheral vasoconstriction and impaired graft perfusion.

Suggested Readings

1. Bass MJ, Phillips LG: Pressure sores. *Curr Probl Surg* 2007; 44(2):101–43.
2. Bauer J, Phillips LG: MOC-PSSM CME article: pressure sores. *Plast Reconstr Surg* 2008; 121(1 Suppl):1–10.
3. Levi B, Rees R: Diagnosis and management of pressure ulcers. *Clin Plast Surg* 2007; 34(4):735–48.
4. Niazi ZB, Salzberg CA: Surgical management of pressure ulcers. *Ostomy Wound Manage* 1997; 43(3):44–52.

CHAPTER

11.5 Burn Surgery

SURGEON

Kenneth K. Yim, MD, FACS

ANESTHESIOLOGIST

Melissa T. Berhow, MD, PhD

FREE SKIN GRAFT FOR BURN WOUND (WITH TANGENTIAL EXCISION, EXCISION TO FASCIA, OR DEBRIDEMENT)

SURGICAL CONSIDERATIONS

Description: Until the mid-1970s, management of burn wounds involved daily debridement, hydrotherapy, and spontaneous eschar separation, with subsequent skin grafts applied to the granulated tissue. Operative management has become much more aggressive with the description of **tangential excision** by **Janzekovic.** There are two surgical approaches to burn wounds—tangential excision and fascial excision.

Tangential excision (TE) is the more frequently performed procedure. The concept of TE is extremely simple, but requires considerable experience and teamwork. Thin slices of burn eschar (burned, necrotic tissue), are shaved sequentially with manual or power dermatomes until a healthy wound bed is developed. Assessment of the wound bed is done with visualization of bleeding and/or the clinical appearance of the excised bed. Blood loss is generally diffuse and can be massive; therefore, communication between anesthesiologist and surgeon is essential. In large excision, PRBCs should be available in the OR before excision so that the anesthesiologist does not get behind in blood and fluid replacement.

Diffuse bleeding, especially dermal, is controlled by laparotomy pads soaked with warm 1:100,000 epinephrine solution. These pads are replaced every 3–5 min and, after ~10 min, are removed one at a time, with persistent bleeding points controlled by electrocautery. Although very high plasma epinephrine levels have been reported after major burn excision, systemic manifestations are very rare in acute burn patients (probably 2° chronic high-level endogenous catecholamine secretion).

TE in the extremities usually is accomplished with a pneumatic tourniquet to minimize blood loss. In some centers, subcutaneous injection of a diluted (1:1,000,000) epinephrine solution under the burn wound also is used to minimize blood loss; however, the resulting vasoconstriction makes the end-point of excision—i.e., bleeding—difficult to ascertain.

Fascial excision involves removing the burn eschar and all underlying fat en bloc to the level of muscle fascia, or beyond. Fascial excision can be performed more rapidly and with less blood loss than TE. Its disadvantages, however, are the marked cosmetic deformities and functional limitations that occur because of the loss of all soft tissue overlying the musculature. Because of its disadvantages, fascial excision is reserved for 4th-degree burns or for patients with very extensive, life-threatening, full-thickness (3rd-degree) burns.

In patients with serious burns (> 40% total body surface area [TBSA]), excision usually commences on postop day 2–5, after completion of fluid resuscitation, and is performed every 2–3 d, as the patient's condition permits. If eschar excision can be completed before secondary sepsis supervenes, management of the patient is easier and the complications and morbidity are lessened considerably.

The endpoints for surgical excision in large burns are: (a) operative time of 2–3 h; (b) core temperature of 35°C; or (c) blood loss of 10 U of PRBC. The violation of any of these parameters invites coagulopathy and increasing problems with hemostasis and VS stability. Adverse effects occurring after 3–4 h of operative time are usually the result of massive transfusion or hypothermia.

Due to loss of skin integrity and large exposed surfaces, these patients lose heat rapidly. Fluids, gases, and the OR should be warm, although there is no demonstrable benefit to warming the OR past the point of isothermic neutrality (~82°F [28°C]). Many surgeons, however, will maintain the room at ~ 100°F (38°C). All areas not in the operative field should be covered, and a warming blanket (Bair Hugger) is used frequently.

Coverage: After excision of wounds and attainment of hemostasis, wounds are covered, using either an autograft or temporary coverage with an allograft, xenograft, or synthetic/biologic dressing. An autograft is used for coverage when the wound bed is deemed suitable, a donor site is available, and the patient is stable. A split-thickness skin graft (STSG) often is used for coverage of a burn wound. Since a STSG is harvested at the dermal level, bleeding also is controlled with topical epinephrine-soaked laparotomy pads before application of dressings. Depending on the location of donor sites, many surgeons use subcutaneous infiltration of diluted (1:1,000,000) epinephrine in saline solution to smooth out irregularities (e.g., underlying ribs) or to create a flat surface (e.g., scalp) to physically improve the ease of taking skin grafts. A substantial volume of saline may be infiltrated, and this should be added into the total fluids administered to the patient.

Intraop position change may be necessary between the burn excision and the STSG harvest. For example, donor skin may be harvested from the back for application to the chest or abdomen.

The STSG is held temporarily in place with staples or sutures. Uncontrolled patient movement may dislodge the graft. To protect against this eventuality, grafts are secured with circumferential dressings and splints. This procedure may be time-consuming, and any uncontrolled patient movement should be avoided.

It has become apparent that early eschar excision is advantageous even if wounds are so extensive they cannot be covered with autografts. In this situation, temporary coverage of the excised wound is accomplished with the application of an allograft, porcine xenograft, or synthetic/biologic dressing. The wound is maintained in this way, with further debridement and biologic dressing changes as necessary, until autograft becomes available.

Usual preop diagnosis: Thermal, electrical, or chemical burn

SUMMARY OF PROCEDURES

	TE	Fascial Excision
Position	Supine, prone, or lateral	⇐
Incision	Anywhere eschar is to be excised.	⇐
Special instrumentation	Dermatomes, as determined by the surgeon—manual or powered.	–
Temperature considerations	Keep room T at ~82°F (28°C).	⇐
Unique considerations	Possible subcutaneous infiltration of diluted epinephrine-saline solution.	None
Antibiotics	Cefazolin (adult = 1g; child = 15 mg/kg) iv on induction of anesthesia	⇐
Surgical time	2–3 h	⇐
EBL	Massive; limit to 10 U PRBC transfusion	250–500 mL
Postop care	Generally, patients can be extubated at the end of these procedures, recovered in the PACU, and returned to the burn center. If patient remains intubated, generally he/she is transported directly to the burn center, where body T can be maintained more easily.	⇐
Mortality	18–40% (Mortality is a function of burn size, plus other associated conditions, especially inhalation injury [Figs 11.5-1, 11.5-2])	⇐
Morbidity	Massive blood loss Sepsis Infection 2° to catheters and lines	– ⇐ ⇐
Pain score	2–5 (Most patients are maintained on sustained-release methadone or iv morphine, for periop pain control.)	⇐

PATIENT POPULATION CHARACTERISTICS

Age range	All
Male:Female	More commonly male
Incidence	45,000 burn center admissions/yr
Etiology	Scald; flame burns; chemicals; electric burns
Associated conditions	Generally few, except in elderly patients

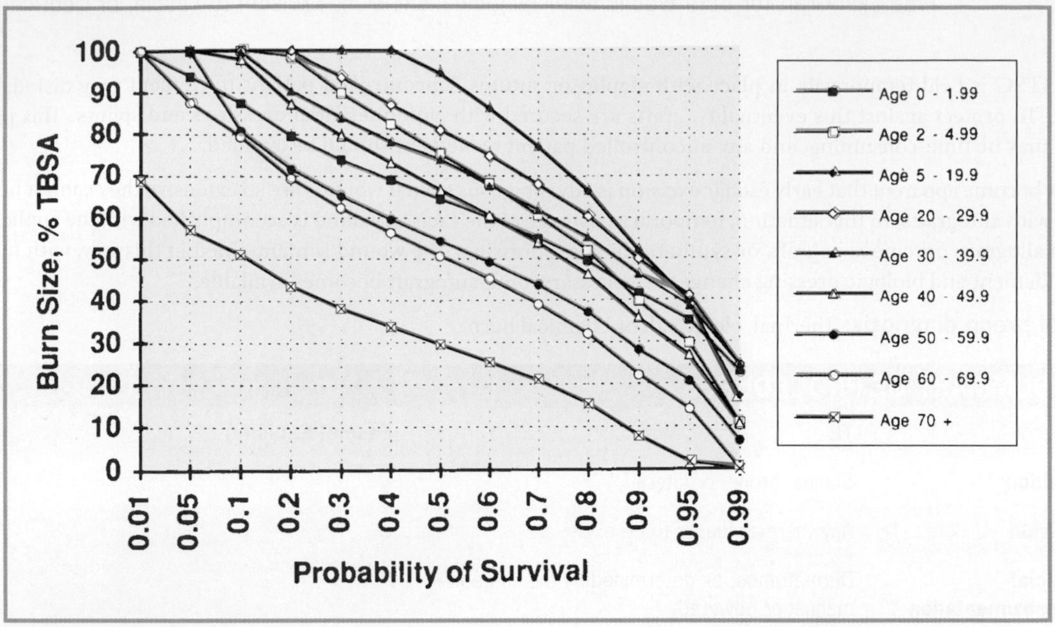

Figure 11.5-1. Probit Survival Curves for 6,417 patients by age groups. (Reproduced with permission from Saffle JR, Davis B, Williams P, et al: Recent outcomes in the treatment of burn injury in the United States: a report from the American Burn Association Patient Registry. *J Burn Care Rehab* 1995; 16:219–32.)

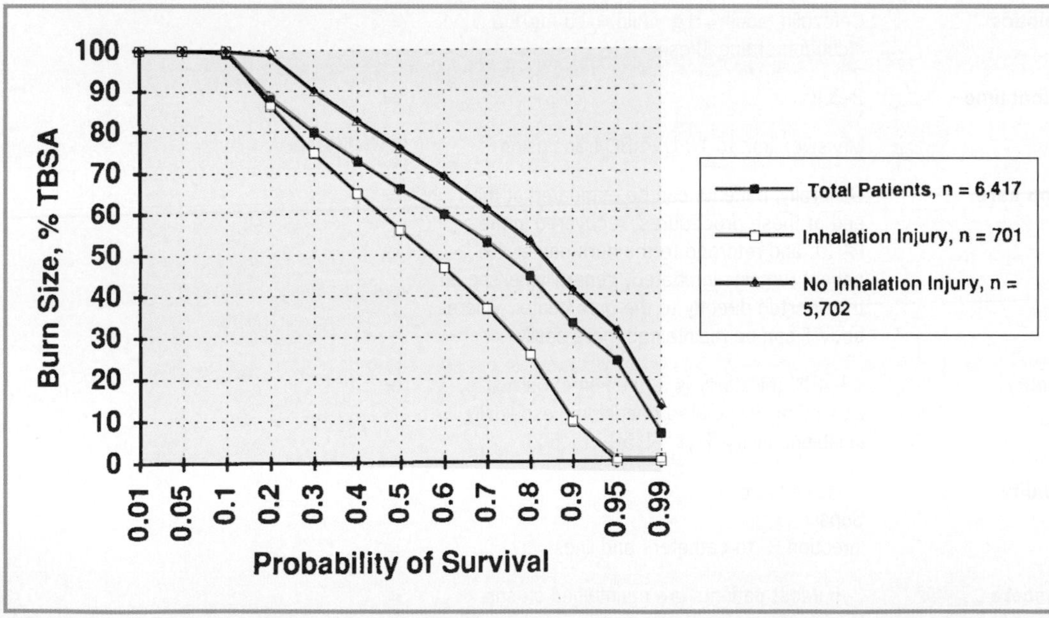

Figure 11.5-2. Probit Survival for patients with and without inhalation injury. (Reproduced with permission from Saffle JR, Davis B, Williams P, et al: Recent outcomes in the treatment of burn injury in the United States: a report from the American Burn Association Patient Registry. *J Burn Care Rehab* 1995; 16:219–32.)

Table 11.5-1. Burn wounds-Classified According to Depth of Burn

Degree	Burn Depth	Tissue Involved
1st degree	Superficial	Epidermis only
2nd degree	Partial thickness	Various thickness of dermis
3rd degree	Full thickness	Entire thickness of dermis
4th degree	To underlying tissue	Beyond dermis (e.g., subcutaneous fat, fascia, or muscle)

ANESTHETIC CONSIDERATIONS

PREOPERATIVE

Burn injuries may result in a broad spectrum of physiologic impairments. These vary, depending on the percent of TBSA burned, location of burns, age of the patient, time elapsed since initial injury, and interim treatment. Ideally, burn patients are fluid-resuscitated and stabilized before being brought to the OR. Typically, skin grafts to cover the burn area start on post-injury day 3. Blood loss and hypothermia are the predominant considerations during surgery on burn patients. Blood loss can be rapid and massive, as much as 8 U in 15 minutes, and can be difficult to estimate as it generally is not collected into the suction.

Respiratory	**Upper airway:** A patient with burns around the airway (e.g., singed nose hairs) should be intubated as early as possible. Direct inhalational/thermal injury and fluid resuscitation may make delayed intubation more difficult 2° upper airway edema. **Lower airway:** Physiologic derangements may include pulmonary edema and ARDS. Additionally, burn patients can be severely hypermetabolic (e.g., a patient with 40% TBSA burns may have twice the normal metabolic rate) with corresponding increased CO_2 production. These patients may have high PIPs and high minute-ventilation requirements. Pressure control ventilation and high levels of PEEP may be useful. Other possible effects of severe burns include: ↓ lung and chest-wall compliance, ↓FRC, ↑ A-a gradient, ↑ carboxyhemoglobinemia, and ↑ methemoglobinemia. **Tests:** ABG, depending on pulmonary status; CXR
Cardiovascular	The hypermetabolism associated with burns increases cardiac demand, and burn patients have greatly elevated circulating levels of catecholamines →↑↑HR + ↑ CO. **Tests:** As indicated from H&P.
Neurological	Evaluate for burn encephalopathy. Characterize baseline mental status before anesthesia to allow evaluation of recovery postop.
Musculoskeletal	Damaged muscle →↑ acetylcholine receptor density, resulting in ↓ sensitivity to nondepolarizing muscle relaxants and potentially fatal elevations of K^+ in response to succinylcholine. In burns > 5% TBSA, avoid succinylcholine after 24 h postburn and for at least 1 yr thereafter for burns > 10% TBSA (↑↑ K^+). Recovery of normal response to muscle relaxants does not occur until burns have healed completely.
Hematologic	Coagulopathies may result directly from the burn injury, as well as from rapid replacement of blood loss during operative procedures. **Tests:** Hb/Hct; electrolytes; coagulation profile
IV access	May be difficult; assess preop. Consider central line placement with a large-bore catheter, such as a Cordis.
Laboratory	Other tests as indicated from H&P.
Premedication	Patients are commonly placed on high-dose narcotics after the initial injury; additional narcotics are frequently required to provide adequate analgesia for transport and movement to the OR table.
Transport	For patients with severe ARDS, transportation from burn unit to OR may pose formidable challenges with regard to ventilation. Cardiopulmonary monitoring must be continued during transport; the ventilation system used in transport must be capable of delivering high minute-volumes, PEEP, and inspiratory pressures. These requirements may not be satisfied by standard bag-valve systems and may require a high-quality transport ventilator.

INTRAOPERATIVE

Anesthetic technique: GETA. Regional techniques are rarely feasible, given the multiple surgical sites for harvesting and grafting. LMAs are not recommended, given the potential for significant fluid resuscitation and subsequent airway edema, as well as the frequent repositioning of patient intraop.

Induction	If the patient is adequately volume-resuscitated, propofol (1.5–2.5 mL/kg iv) or thiopental (3–5 mg/kg) may be used. If the patient is intravascularly volume-depleted, etomidate (0.3 mg/kg) or ketamine (1–3 mg/kg) is recommended. Patients with extensive burns (> 30% TBSA) will develop a decreased sensitivity to nondepolarizing NMBs; therefore, 1.5 × the usual intubating dose of NMB is recommended: vecuronium (1.5 mg/kg), pancuronium (0.15 mg/kg), or rocuronium (1.5 mg/kg). If rapid-sequence induction is indicated, succinylcholine should not be used if the initial injury is > 24 h old. Under these circumstances, high-dose rocuronium (2 mg/kg) can be used. If the face is burned, awake FOI may be necessary and securing the ETT may be difficult. Alternatives to taping the ETT include suturing the tube to the teeth or using umbilical tape.	
Maintenance	Standard maintenance (see p. B-2). Physiologic derangements of the respiratory system (ARDS, pulmonary edema) and a hypermetabolic state may require minute-volumes > 30 L/min, and high inspiratory pressures and PEEP, for adequate ventilation. Depending on equipment availability, a Siemens or ICU ventilator (capable of PPV) may be necessary and possibly a ventilator capable of high frequency oscillatory ventilation. Intraop, surgeons may use epinephrine-soaked sponges to ↓ blood loss. Systemic absorption of epinephrine will cause tachycardia and increase the probability of dysrhythmias; therefore, it is best to avoid halothane or desflurane. Isoflurane and sevoflurane are acceptable.	
Emergence	Estimation of an adequate dose of narcotic to provide postop analgesia may be difficult since these patients are often receiving high doses of narcotics preop. Ketamine has been used with success in providing improved analgesia in the setting of escalating opioid doses. If large-volume resuscitation has occurred intraop, there is the possibility of clinically significant airway edema; use caution before extubating to ensure a patent airway.	
Blood and fluid requirements	Extensive blood loss IV: 14–16 ga × 2 or a Cordis NS/LR @ 8–10 mL/kg/h Keep UO @ 0.5–1 mL/kg/h. Blood: ~200 mL/1% BSA excised and grafted. Fluid warmer T&C 2–4 U PRBC (to keep ahead).	Blood must be in OR before induction. The major blood loss generally is associated with eschar excision, usually the first part of the procedure. For patients without contraindications to hemodilution (e.g., CAD, anemia), it is often better to delay PRBC transfusion until major blood loss is complete. IV hyperalimentation should be continued during surgery, or, replace with 10% dextrose infusion to avoid hypoglycemia. If sudden ↓ BP occurs during very rapid infusion of blood (>150 mL/min), consider using Ca^{++} to counteract the chelating effect of citrate. Avoid fluid overload, especially if patient has ARDS, is a small child, or is elderly. As the surgical site is superficial, there is not much 3rd-space loss.
Thermal considerations	Room = 80–82°F Warm all fluids. Humidify gases. Warming blanket Reflective head cover	Temperature must be monitored throughout the case. The surgeon may be notified if patient's core T is dropping.
Monitoring	Standard monitors (see p. B-1). ± CVP line PA catheter	ECG may require needle electrodes or alligator clip electrodes to skin graft if there is no skin availability to apply adhesive electrodes. The hemodynamically unstable patient should be monitored with a PA catheter.
Positioning	✓ and pad pressure points. ✓ eyes.	The burn patient may be uniquely susceptible to laryngeal or upper airway edema in the prone position; therefore, examination of the upper airway before extubation is recommended to avoid emergent reintubation.
Complications	Massive blood loss	

POSTOPERATIVE

Complications	Hypothermia Coagulopathy	May occur as the result of massive blood loss and replacement.
Transport	Continue cardiopulmonary monitoring. High minute-ventilation requirements ↑ PIP ↑ PEEP	Verify adequacy of transport ventilation system before departing OR.
Pain management	Oral methadone or sustained-release morphine sulfate IV fentanyl or morphine sulfate	Titrate analgesia to effect.
Tests	Hct, ABG, electrolytes, PT, PTT, Plt, if massive transfusion given.	

Suggested Readings

1. Barret JP: Burns reconstruction. *BMJ* 2004; 329:274–6.
2. Capan LM, Miller SM: Trauma and burns. In *Clinical Anesthesia,* 5th edition. Barash PG, Cullen BF, Stoelting RK, eds. Lippincott Williams & Wilkins, Philadelphia: 2006, 1279–97.
3. Edrich T, Friedrich A, Eltzschig HK: Ketamine for long-term sedation and analgesia of a burn patient. *Anest Analg* 2004; 99:893–5.
4. Gibran NS. Burns. In *Greenfield's Surgery: Scientific Principles and Practice.* Greenfield LJ, Mulholland, MW, Oldham KT, et al, eds. Lippincott Williams & Wilkins, Philadelphia: 2006, 239–69.
5. Heimbach DM: Early burn excision and grafting. *Surg Clin North Am* 1987; 67(1):93–107.
6. Janzekovic Z: A new concept in the early excision and immediate grafting of burns. *J Trauma* 1970; 10(2):1103–8.
7. Karaaslan P, Arsian G, Basaran O, et al: Anesthesia management in pediatric burn patients: experience of one center. *Burns* 2007; 33(1 Suppl 1):S50–1.
8. Moran KT, O'Reilly TJ, Furman W, et al: A new algorithm for calculation of blood loss in excisional burn surgery. *Am Surg* 1988; 54(4):207–8.

SECTION

12.0 PEDIATRIC SURGERY

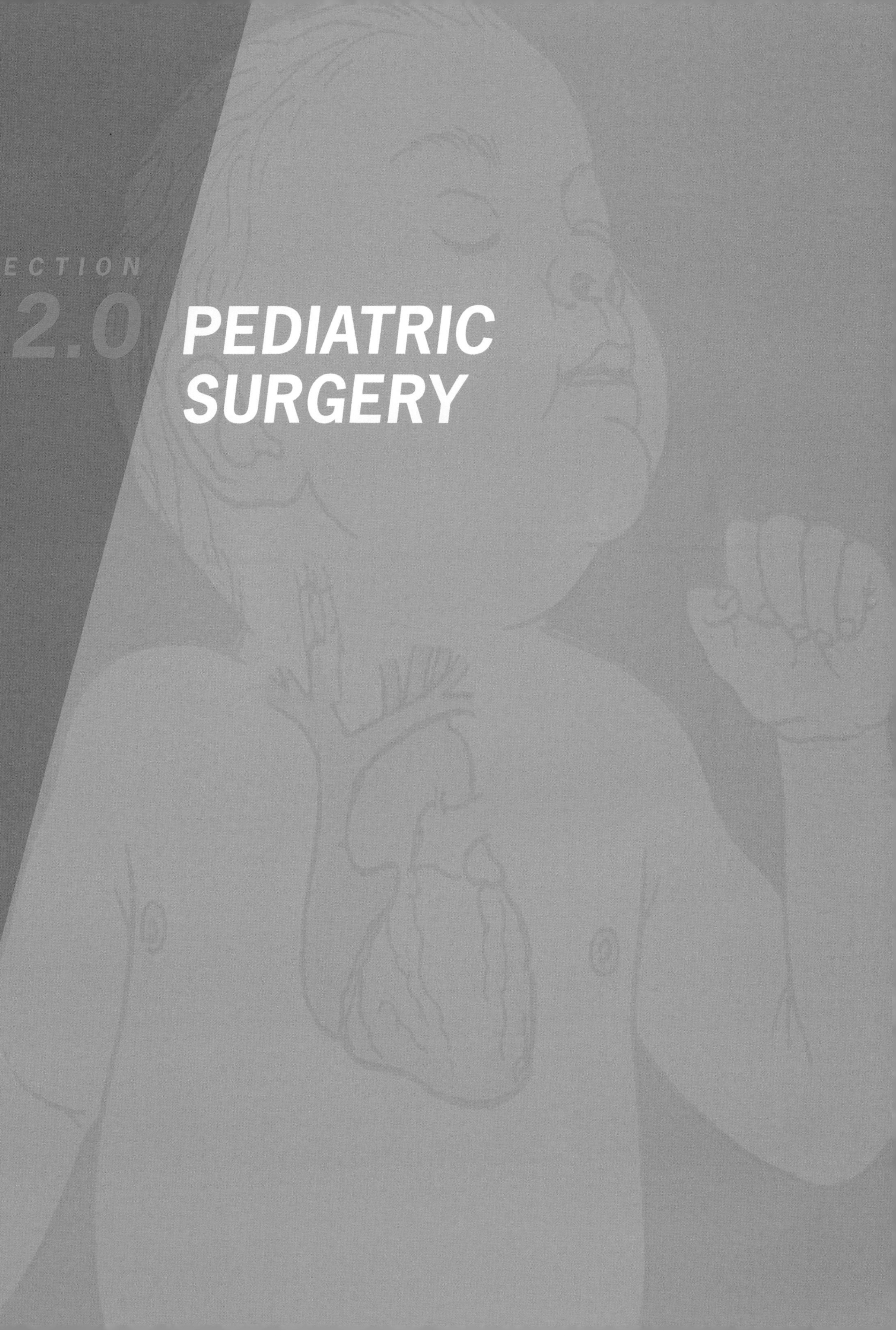

CHAPTER

12.1 Pediatric Neurosurgery

SURGEON

Michael Edwards, MD
Stephen L. Huhn, MD

ANESTHESIOLOGISTS

William W. Feaster, MD
Brian P. Struyk, MD

CRANIOFACIAL SURGERY

SURGICAL CONSIDERATIONS

Description: **Craniofacial surgery** is a broad term that refers to both cranial and/or facial reconstructive procedures for cranial dysostosis or craniofacial dysmorphism. Cranial dysostosis is the congenital maldevelopment of the cranial base and/or vault, 2° premature fusion of cranial sutures. More commonly referred to as **craniosynostosis,** the surgical correction of this disorder involves removal of the affected suture(s) and reconstruction of the cranial, orbital, or facial bones. The most common form of craniosynostosis—scaphocephaly—is caused by the fusion of the sagittal suture, which leads to a long and narrow calvarium. Other forms of craniosynostosis, in order of decreasing frequency, are coronal synostosis (brachycephaly), metopic synostosis (trigonocephaly), and lambdoidal synostosis. Deformational occipital plagiocephaly refers to flattening of the occiput 2° preferential sleep position and the resultant deformation of the skull. This condition is not a form of craniosynostosis and, despite the potential for significant flattening of the head, reconstructive surgery is not indicated. Crouzon and Apert syndromes are inherited craniofacial disorders associated with craniosynostosis and facial/orbital dysmorphism. The facial deformities common to Crouzon and Apert are shallow and misplaced orbits, exophthalmos, and midface hypoplasia. In each form of craniosynostosis, sporadic or predisposed, the abnormality is present at birth, but may not become recognizable until the rapid phase of brain growth, occurring in the 1st year of life, begins to accentuate the limitations on skull shape produced by the premature suture closure. In simple terms, the growth of the underlying brain drives the expansion of the skull, and closure of a suture produces reduced skull growth in the opposite direction.

Early recognition and correction of craniosynostosis results in the best cosmetic and neurologic outcome because, with release of the fused suture, the growing brain helps correct the abnormal cranial shape. Most procedures are scheduled during the 1st 6 mo of life; thus, the issue of blood volume and replacement becomes a critical factor for surgical and anesthetic consideration. The main principles of surgical treatment of craniosynostosis involve removal of the abnormal suture through a craniectomy or craniotomy, followed by reconstruction of the calvarium and/or orbit to overcome the cranial deformity and optimize the chance for normal cranial development. The surgery most often is done in conjunction with a pediatric neurosurgeon and a plastic surgeon. Patient positioning varies, depending on the approach to the craniectomy, and is generally prone for sagittal and lambdoidal synostosis, and supine for coronal and metopic synostosis. Another surgical principle important for synostosis surgery is to minimize intraop blood loss. The surgical team should make every effort to reduce blood loss during the procedure by infiltrating the scalp with 1:400,000 epinephrine, using point electrocautery, preserving the pericranium, and waxing the bone edges. The most common skin incision is a bicoronal opening that allows for access to the entire calvarium. The extent of the bone removal and reconstruction varies, depending on the type and number of sutures involved. Surgical correction of patients with Crouzon or Apert syndromes is often staged with correction of the cranial component, followed by a later procedure for the face, as described by Tessier and colleagues. Invariably, blood loss occurs from the scalp and bone, and the surgeon must remain mindful of the volume contained within the surgical field and readily communicate to the anesthesiologist when bleeding is felt to be either continuous or excessive. Injury to the underlying dural venous sinuses is rare, but the potential for catastrophic blood loss is great. Recent advances in endoscopy have lead to the development of minimally invasive techniques for craniosynostosis in some centers, and reports suggest that use of the endoscope reduces blood loss. Recombinant erythropoietin administered preop also has been studied in an attempt to reduce the need for intraop transfusion associated with repair of craniosynostosis. Subgaleal and epidural drains may be placed at the close of the procedure, and the patient is monitored closely in the PICU for postop bleeding that often requires additional transfusions in the 1st 24 h after surgery.

Usual preop diagnosis: Craniosynostosis (sagittal, coronal, metopic, lambdoidal); craniofacial dysmorphism; Apert syndrome; Crouzon syndrome

SUMMARY OF PROCEDURE	
Position	Supine or prone (less common); or table 180°
Incision	Bicoronal, biparietal, Meisterschnitt, midsagittal
Special instrumentation	Midas Rex craniotome; absorbable plates and screws, Colorado needle

SUMMARY OF PROCEDURE (cont'd)	
Unique considerations	↑ ICP and/or hydrocephalus may coexist. ↑ ICP is usually seen with multiple-suture synostosis; it also occurs in single-suture craniosynostosis, but is rare (< 5–10%). Hydrocephalus typically is seen in monogenic conditions (e.g., Apert, Crouzon). Most neurosurgeons shunt the hydrocephalus and treat the ↑ ICP prior to craniosynostosis surgery.
Antibiotics	Vancomycin (13–15 mg/kg) or ceftriaxone (25–50 mg/kg; avoid Ca^{++} containing solutions) for cranial surgery. Vancomycin or cloxacillin and cefotaxime (25–30 mg/kg) for craniofacial surgery involving nasal sinuses.
Closing considerations	Watch for ↑ blood loss from the scalp. To prevent excessive blood loss, reapproximate only one portion of the scalp at a time.
EBL	Highly variable; must be minimized. Amount depends on preoperative condition, on the number of sutures involved, age of the patient, and magnitude of the repair. Operative injury to the superior sagittal sinus may be catastrophic if hemostasis cannot be achieved or volume loss is excessive.
Postop care	PICU. Postop Hct/Hb levels required. Blood transfusion often necessary in infants (< 10 kg).
Mortality	< 1–2%
Morbidity	Meningitis CSF rhinorrhea ↑ ICP (2° skull reshaping) Venous thrombosis Neurological injury: Rare
Pain score	1–3

PATIENT POPULATION CHARACTERISTICS	
Age range	Newborn–young adult
Male:Female	1.2:1
Incidence	1/2000/yr
Etiology	Sporadic; heritable (monogenic and chromosomal syndromes); environmentally induced (amniotic bands, iatrogenic)
Associated conditions	Congenital defects (limbs, heart, brain, kidneys); hydrocephalus; encephalocele (sincipital/basal); fibrous dysplasia; craniometaphyseal dysplasia; holoprosencephaly

ANESTHETIC CONSIDERATIONS

PREOPERATIVE

Craniofacial surgery encompasses a wide variety of procedures, with the two most common being linear craniotomy for craniosynostosis (or premature closure of the cranial sutures) and reconstructive for congenital deformities of the forehead, orbit ridges, and nose. Craniosynostosis usually manifests itself in the 1st yr of life; surgery for other congenital deformities of the face and skull usually is performed from ages 1–8 yr.

Respiratory	As a result of midfacial deformities, some children may present difficult intubations. Their airways should be carefully evaluated preoperatively and preparations made for a difficult intubation.
Neurological	Presenting Sx in infants with craniosynostosis include: progressive head deformation, progressively increasing irritability, crying, failure to eat, and failure to grow in head circumference. These Sx may be due in part to ↑ ICP. On physical examination, one or more of the cranial sutures are fused. Infants with other types of craniofacial deformity usually have no Sx related to their abnormalities.

Laboratory	Tests as indicated from H&P. Preop Hct, Hgb, platelets, INR
Premedication	For children, midazolam 0.5 mg/kg po (see p. D-1) generally provides satisfactory preop sedation after ~30 min. For young children (< 5 yr) who refuse po meds, instillation of midazolam 0.3 mg/kg intranasally provides rapid amnesia, sedation, and easy separation from the parents.

INTRAOPERATIVE

Anesthetic technique: GETA using Pediatric circle. Forced air warmer. Warm room 75–80°F. Warm all fluids.

Induction	Standard pediatric induction (see p. D-1). Orotracheal tubes are preferred over nasotracheal tubes because the surgery may involve reflection of the scalp down over the eyes and nose, in which case a nasal tube would be in the way. Verify ETT placement (see p. D-2). Tape the tube firmly in place at one side of the mouth using benzoin adherent. When craniofacial surgery is performed, the surgeon usually places plastic corneal shields in the eyes or sutures the lids shut to protect the cornea from injury and may also suture the ETT in place.	
Maintenance	Standard maintenance (see p. D-2). Muscle relaxation is usually provided. Maintain a near-normal BP unless mild hypotension is requested to limit blood loss. Maintain normal temp by keeping the OR warm (78°F) and using warming lights and blankets as needed. Ventilation is controlled to $PetCO_2$ = 35–40 mmHg with a mechanical ventilator from the start of anesthesia until the surgical wound is closed.	
Emergence	No specific considerations. The ETT is removed at the conclusion of the anesthetic. Patient usually goes to the PICU for observation.	
Blood and fluid requirements	Large blood loss iv: 18–20 ga × 1–2 NS/LR @ 4 mL/kg/h 5% albumin Fluid warmer	Administer crystalloid via a continuous infusion pump or Volutrol. Blood is often necessary. It is advisable to begin transfusion early in course of surgery, to avoid getting behind. In smaller children, it is better to administer warmed blood by syringe, in 10 mL increments. Serial Hct determinations are useful. Blood salvage techniques may be used when large blood loss is anticipated.
Monitoring	Standard monitors (see p. D-1). ± Foley catheter ± Doppler ± Arterial line ± CVP line	If operation is anticipated to last several hours, a Foley catheter should be inserted. If patient is semi-sitting, a Doppler ultrasound probe may be placed on the chest to monitor for air embolism. Invasive monitoring is often appropriate. ↑ K^+ and ↓ Ca^{++} are most common following transfusions with blood or FFP.
Positioning	OR table usually rotated 180°. ✓ and pad pressure points. ✓ eyes.	Ensure access to airway by placing a Mayo stand over the chest area.
Complications	Major blood loss VAE	Treatment of venous air embolism–Notify surgeon who will locate entry point and flood with saline, D/C N_20, attempt to aspirate air from CVP, lower head of bed, compress jugular veins to decrease the rate of air entry, CPR as needed. PEEP is not recommended and may be deleterious. VAE more likely if dural sinus entered.

POSTOPERATIVE CONSIDERATIONS

Complications	Bleeding Extubation Hypovolemia	Major complications from these operations are uncommon.
Pain management	Parenteral opioids (see p. E-1). Avoid oversedation.	Fentanyl 1–2 mcg/kg q 60 min or morphine 0.05–0.1 mg/kg q 2 h.
Tests	Hct/Hb Coagulation parameters	Hct/Hb levels are necessary to determine adequacy of blood replacement.

Suggested Readings

1. Dahmani S, et al: Perioperative blood salvage during surgical correction of craniosynostosis in infants. *Br J Anesth* 2000; 85(4):550–5.
2. Fearon JA, Weinthal J: The use of recombinant erythropoietin in the reduction of blood transfusion rated in craniosynostosis repair in infants and children. *Plast Reconstr Surg* 2002; 109(7):2190–6.
3. Fearon JA: Reducing allogenic blood transfusions during pediatric cranial vault surgical procedures: a prospective analysis of blood recycling. *Plast Reconstr Surg* 2004; 113(4):1126–30.
4. Hoffman HJ, Hendrick EB: Early neurosurgical repair in craniofacial dysmorphism. *J Neurosurg* 1979; 51(6):796–803.
5. Hoffman HJ: Congenital malformations of the spine and skull. In *Practice of Surgery.* Goldsmith HS, ed. Harper & Row, New York; 1980.
6. Jimenez DF, Barone CM, Cartwright CC, et al: Early management of craniosynostosis using endoscopic-assisted strip craniectomies and cranial orthotic molding therapy. *Pediatrics* 2002; 110:97–104.
7. Karl HW, Keifer AT, Rosenberger JL et al: Comparison of the safety and efficacy of intranasal midazolam or sufentanil for preinduction of anesthesia in pediatric patients. *Anesthesiology* 1992: 76(2):209–15.
8. Shillito J Jr, Matson DD: Craniosynostoses: a review of 519 surgical patients. *Pediatrics* 1968; 41(4):829–53.
9. Tessier P, Guiot G, Rougerie J, Delbet JP, et al: Cranio-naso-orbito-facial osteotomies. Hypertelorism. *Ann Chir Plast* 1967; 12(2):103–18.
10. Tessier P: Relationship of craniostenoses to craniofacial dysostoses and to faciostenoses: a study with therapeutic implications. *Plast Reconstr Surg* 1971; 48(3):224–37.
11. Tessier P: Total facial osteotomy. Crouzon's syndrome, Apert's syndrome: oxycephaly, scaphocephaly, turricephaly. *Ann Chir Plast* 1967; 12(4):273–86.

CLOSURE OF MYELOMENINGOCELE

SURGICAL CONSIDERATIONS

Description: Myelomeningocele is a neural tube defect characterized by failure of the spinal cord to fuse posteriorly during primary neurulation. This results in an open neural placode joined to the incomplete epithelial defect, usually located in the thoracolumbar spine, and rarely in the cervical spine. Associated CNS conditions are hydrocephalus and Chiari II hindbrain malformation, both of which usually contribute more to long-term morbidity than the spinal cord defect itself. The presence of the myelomeningocele may be detected before birth by high-resolution ultrasound and/or elevated maternal serum alpha fetoprotein, as well as fetal MRI scans. The incidence of neural tube defects is declining in the United States due to maternal dietary folate supplementation and prenatal Dx and selective termination.

The fundamental goals of surgery are preservation of neural tissue, reconstitution of a normal intrathecal environment, and complete skin closure to prevent a spinal fluid leak. Despite a very thin parchment of dystrophic epithelium attached to the placode, most myelomeningoceles leak spinal fluid from the time of birth. Because of the risk of ventriculitis associated with the exposed subarachnoid space, closure of the myelomeningocele is recommended within 72 h after birth. Infants with neural tube defects have a higher incidence of other congenital anomalies, including hydronephrosis, malrotation of the gut, VSD or ASD, and craniofacial disorders. The neonate should be screened for these potential abnormalities before undergoing surgery and, in general, this can be accomplished within 24 h after birth. During the procedure, the child is in the prone position. The defect is dissected so that the various anatomic layers can be separated. The edges of the placode (spinal cord) are mobilized from the adjacent epithelium and often imbricated to form a closed tube. The laterally displaced dura is dissected from the fascia and closed over the spinal cord, thus reconstituting the elements of the spine, except for the lamina defect that is not reconstructed. An attempt is made to mobilize the lumbosacral fascia as a separate layer and the subcutaneous and skin layers comprise the final layer. In cases of large defects, local skin or myocutaneous flaps may be necessary to cover the spinal defect adequately. Progressive hydrocephalus usually presents within days to weeks after closure of the myelomeningocele, but ~15% of patients will present at birth with significant hydrocephalus that requires early insertion of a VP shunt. Finally, in rare circumstances, prominent vertebral angulation, or kyphosis, at the defect could necessitate vertebrectomies to re-establish normal spinal alignment, usually at an older age.

Variant procedure or approaches: The efficacy of **intrauterine myelomeningocele repair** is currently being explored through a randomized multicenter trial, and the results may alter future approaches in favor of intrauterine closure if the incidence of hydrocephalus is reduced in these patients.

Usual preop diagnosis: Myelomeningocele; meningocele; myelodysplasia; spina bifida

SUMMARY OF PROCEDURE

Position	Prone
Incision	Surrounding the defect, preserving skin that can be utilized in the closure. Use of plain lidocaine (0.25%) local anesthetic decreases blood loss.
Special instrumentation	Loupes or operating microscope (optional)
Unique considerations	Concomitant hydrocephalus, lower brain stem dysfunction. Need for blood replacement rare in straightforward cases. Latex precautions should be used in all cases. (p. G-1)
Antibiotics	Ceftriaxone (50 mg/kg iv), or if Ca^{++} containing solutions are required use vancomycin (13–15 mg/kg iv, slowly),
Surgical time	1.5–3 h
Closing considerations	Skin closure may be complex and require rotation of flaps or aid of plastic surgeon.
EBL	Negligible–25 mL (in most cases)
Postop care	Neonatal nursery. Postop, child often nursed on stomach or side. Head size and head ultrasound are used to monitor for development of hydrocephalus, which may require shunting at a later date.
Mortality	Approaching zero
Morbidity	Meningitis/ventriculitis Hind brain dysfunction Wound infection CSF leak Apnea, vocal cord paralysis
Pain score	3–5

PATIENT POPULATION CHARACTERISTICS

Age range	Newborn (diagnosed at birth)
Male:Female	~1:1
Incidence	1/1000 live births
Etiology	Congenital

PATIENT POPULATION CHARACTERISTICS (cont'd)

Associated conditions	Hydrocephalus; lower extremity weakness; bowel and/or bladder dysfunction (neurogenic bladder) and/or hydronephrosis; scoliosis; Chiari II malformations; congenital cardiac anomalies **NB: Latex allergy is increased in this population. Latex precautions should be used beginning with the 1st operation. See Appendix G.

ANESTHETIC CONSIDERATIONS

PREOPERATIVE

Myelomeningoceles are congenital abnormalities of the spinal cord that result in a saccular protrusion near the base of the spine. The sac, containing neural elements and CSF, can vary in size from very small to a volume that occupies the whole lower spinal region. The Dx may be suspected from maternal alpha-fetoprotein screening, fetal ultrasound, or prenatal MRI and is confirmed at birth. It is generally believed that immediate removal of the sac and covering of the defect with skin is desirable to preserve neurological function and avoid infections. These newborns, therefore, usually are brought to surgery within 24–48 h after birth.

Cardiovascular	May have associated congenital anomalies. **Test:** ECHO
Neurological	Although difficult to assess at this age, newborns may have motor and/or sensory deficits in the lower extremities, neurogenic bladder, and lower cranial nerve dysfunction. Most have an Arnold-Chiari malformation, which requires a ventriculoperitoneal shunt within days of the spine repair.
Renal	May have associated congenital anomalies. **Tests:** Renal ultrasound
Laboratory	Routine preop studies
Premedication	None necessary
Other	**NB**: Latex Precautions for all patients (beginning from birth). See p. G-1.

INTRAOPERATIVE

Anesthetic technique: GETA using Pediatric circle; forced air warmer; Warm room to 75–80°F.

Induction	Before induction, the patient is placed in the supine position, and the back defect is protected by a sterile donut or rolls to prevent pressure on or rupture of defect. Patients usually will come to the OR with an iv in place, allowing for a standard iv induction. (See p. D-1). If not, a standard inhalational induction followed by establishment of iv access is indicated. See p. D-1. Sevoflurane is preferred because of its low blood-gas partition coefficient and absence of airway irritability, which allows a smooth, rapid induction. Oral ETT intubation usually follows muscle relaxation with rocuronium (0.6–1 mg/kg) or vecuronium (0.1 mg/kg). Atropine (0.05–0.1 mg) may be administered before intubation to reduce secretions and to prevent reflex bradycardia. Verify ETT placement and tape tube securely in place at one side of the mouth with benzoin adherent to facilitate prone positioning.
Maintenance	Sevoflurane 2–3% or desflurane 7% or less, with N_2O or air/O_2 mixture to maintain arterial O_2 sat at 95–97%. Depending on duration of operation, additional doses of rocuronium (0.3 mg/kg) or vecuronium (0.1 mg/kg) may be needed. Maintain a near-normal BP. Maintain normal temp by keeping OR warm (78°F) and using warming lights and blankets as needed. Ventilation is controlled to maintain $PetCO_2$ = 35–40 mmHg with a mechanical ventilator or manually, from the start of anesthesia until surgical wound is closed.
Emergence	These patients almost always remain intubated for the 1st 24 h. The newborn is nursed in the prone or lateral positions for the 1st few days postop.

Blood and fluid requirements	iv: 22–24 ga × 1 D10 @ 2–4 mL/kg/h (newborn) D10 ¼ NS @ 4 mL/kg/h (> 24 h) Warm fluids.	Administer crystalloid, usually D10 ¼ NS, via a continuous infusion pump, etc. Blood is rarely, if ever, necessary.
Monitoring	Standard monitors (see p. D-1).	
Positioning	✓ and pad pressure points. ✓ eyes.	Prone with shoulders and hips on bolsters to elevate abdomen off operating table. Head turned to the side, which results in the ETT being furthest from the bed. ✓ tube placement by listening for bilateral breath sounds after repositioning.

POSTOPERATIVE

Complications	CSF leak Wound healing complications Infection Hydrocephalus Renal Failure
Pain management	Parenteral opioids (see p. E-3).

Suggested Readings

1. Cochrane D, Irwin B, Chambers K: Clinical outcomes that fetal surgery for myelomeningocele needs to achieve. *Eur J Pediatr Surg* 2001; 22(Suppl 1):S18–20.
2. Cohen AR, Robinson S: Early management of myelomeningocele. In *Pediatric Neurosurgery: Surgery of the Developing Nervous System,* 4th edition. McLone DG, ed. WB Saunders, Philadelphia: 2001, 241–60.
3. Cragen J, Roberts H, Edmonds L, et al: Surveillance for anencephaly and spina bifida and the impact of prenatal diagnosis-Unites States, 1985–1994. *Morbid Mortal Wkly Rep* 1995; 44(S–4): 1–13.
4. Reigel DH: Myelomeningocele repair. In *Pediatric Neurosurgery: Surgery of the Developing Nervous System,* 4th edition. McLone DG, ed. WB Saunders, Philadelphia: 2001, 261–5.
5. Tulipan N, Sutton LN, Bruner JP et al: The effect of intrauterine myelomeningocele repair on the incidence of shunt-dependent hydrocephalus. *Pediatr Neurosurg* 2003; 38(l):27–33.

SURGICAL CORRECTION OF SPINAL DYSRAPHISM

SURGICAL CONSIDERATIONS

Description: **Occult spinal dysraphism** covers a spectrum of spinal anomalies generally related to defects in secondary neurulation, in contrast to a myelomeningocele, which occurs as a result of defective primary neurulation. These forms of congenital spinal defects are covered by intact skin and share the common pathophysiology of spinal cord tethering. Occult spinal dysraphism includes tight filum terminale, intramedullary lipoma, lipomyelomeningocele, split cord malformations (diastematomyelia), dermal sinus tracts, meningocele manque, neuroenteric cyst, and myelocystocele. Each of these lesions can result in a tethering, or stretching, of the spinal cord as the vertebral axis elongates during normal growth. The fixed spinal cord is stretched by the growing spine, resulting in neurological dysfunction, most likely as a result of reduced spinal cord blood flow. Excision of the lesion and release of the tethering elements is recommended to prevent either the onset or worsening of cord dysfunction.

The surgical principles for correction of occult spinal dysraphism involve excision of the intradural lesion and release of the tissue element that is tethering the spinal cord, while preserving the normal neural structures. In cases of tight filum terminale, this is easily accomplished with little threat to the spinal cord or nerve root function, whereas excision of lipomyelomeningoceles may be extremely challenging procedures. Any tethering lesion needs to be carefully separated from the spinal cord and adjacent nerve roots without disrupting neurological function. Intraop neurophysiological monitoring may be a useful adjunct to monitor cord and nerve root function during the dissection and release of the tethering lesion. Following the intradural procedure, closure of the dura and myofascial layers are critical in prevention of postop spinal fluid leaks; and dural grafts may be necessary in some cases.

Usual preop diagnosis: Tethered spinal cord; fat filum terminale; lipomyelomeningocele; lipoma of the filum; diastematomyelia; spinal dysraphism; dermal sinus tract; caudal agenesis

SUMMARY OF PROCEDURE

Position	Prone
Incision	Posterior midline centered over abnormality
Special instrumentation	Operating microscope; laser
Unique considerations	Blood replacement with loss of significant amount of blood in the infant (rare). Minimal latex exposure
Antibiotics	Ceftriaxone (50 mg/kg iv; do not use with Ca^{++} containing solutions); or vancomycin (13–15 mg/kg iv slowly)
Surgical time	1.5–5 h (longer for diastematomyelia and lipomyelomeningocele)
Closing considerations	Surgeon often wants to test integrity of dural closure with Valsalva maneuver: sustained (10–20 sec) inspiratory pressure at 20–40 cmH_2O.
EBL	5–100 mL
Postop care	Patient often kept flat postop to protect dural closure.
Mortality	Approaching zero
Morbidity	Infection Neurological deficit Aseptic meningitis CSF leak Urinary dysfunction; Check preop renal function, renal U/S
Pain score	3–5
Other	Latex precautions See p. G-1.

PATIENT POPULATION CHARACTERISTICS

Age range	Newborn-adults
Male:Female	~1:1
Incidence	Uncommon
Etiology	Congenital
Associated conditions	Ankle/foot deformity (talipes); neurologic impairment; neurogenic bowel/bladder; scoliosis; vertebral abnormalities; VACTERL/VATER association (vertebral, anal, cardiac, tracheoesophageal, renal, and limb anomalies); cutaneous anomaly over spine; syringomyelia; caudal agenesis; urinary anomalies; check abdominal ultrasound, renal function prior to OR

ANESTHETIC CONSIDERATIONS

PREOPERATIVE

A variety of spinal abnormalities fall under the category of spinal dysraphism, the most common being a tethered cord or a lipoma of the spinal cord. In the case of the tethered cord, there may be a Hx of myelomeningocele repair at birth. Most patients range from 3–16 yr. of age.

Neurological	Presenting Sx in older children are usually pain in the lower back radiating into the legs and/or progressively worsening motor or sensory deficits in the anal region or involving the lower extremities (document carefully).
Musculoskeletal	Lower extremity foot deformity as well as sensory or motor deficits may be present and should be carefully documented.
Renal	Renal function may be impaired in patients with Hx of recurrent UTIs. **Tests:** UA; BUN; Cr; others as indicated from H&P.
Laboratory	Other tests as indicated from H&P.
Premedication	For children, midazolam 0.5 mg/kg po (see p. D-1) generally provides satisfactory preop sedation after ~30 min. For young children (< 5 yr) who refuse po meds, instillation of midazolam 0.3 mg/kg intranasally provides rapid amnesia, sedation, and easy separation from parents.
Latex allergy	Latex precautions should be used in all patients even at 1st operation. Meningomyelocele patients may have developed a latex allergy (see p. G-1).

INTRAOPERATIVE

Anesthetic technique: GETA

Induction	Standard induction (see p. D-1) with sevoflurane, N_2O, and O_2. This is followed by establishment of iv access, then ETT intubation with the use of a muscle relaxant (e.g., rocuronium 1 mg/kg or vecuronium 0.15 mg/kg). Sevoflurane is preferred because of its rapid, smooth induction. Tape the tube firmly in place at one side of the mouth, using benzoin adherent to facilitate prone positioning. Latex precautions.	
Maintenance	Standard maintenance (see p. D-2). Upon completion of placement of the dural graft, and before closure of the wound, the surgeon will want to check the integrity of the graft to eliminate any CSF leaks. The surgeon will ask that positive pressure be applied to the airway to at least 20 cmH_2O for 10–20 sec. If graft leaks are detected, they will be repaired and the test repeated.	
Emergence	The ETT is removed at the conclusion of the anesthetic. The patient may be nursed flat in the prone or lateral position for the 1st few days postop to lessen the chance of a CSF leak developing.	
Blood and fluid requirements	iv: 18–20 ga × 1 NS/LR @ 4–6 mL/kg/h	In children, administer fluids via a volumetric infusion set. Blood is rarely necessary.
Monitoring	Standard monitors (see p. D-1). ± Foley catheter ± UO	If the operation is anticipated to last several hours, or in the case of neurogenic bladder, a Foley catheter should be inserted.
Positioning	✓ and pad pressure points. ✓ eyes.	Prone with the shoulders and hips on bolsters to elevate the abdomen off the operating table. Head turned to the side, resulting in the ETT being furthest from bed. ✓ tube placement by listening for bilateral breath sounds after repositioning.

Complications	Severe bradycardia Latex allergy	Manipulation of the spinal cord may produce ↓↓ HR reflexly. See p. G-1 for latex allergy considerations.

POSTOPERATIVE

Complications	Possible neurological deficits Infection CSF leak Urinary retention Incontinence	Major complications from this operation are uncommon, but include new neurological deficits from irritation of the spinal cord during surgery, localized infection, and CSF leak from the wound site.
Pain management	Parental opioids or PCA (see p. E-3–E-4).	

Suggested Readings

1. Oakes WJ: Management of spinal cord lipomas and lipomyelomeningoceles. In *Neurosurgery Update II.* Wilkins RH, Rengachary S, eds. McGraw-Hill, New York: 1991, 345–52.
2. von Koch CS, Quinones-Hinojosa A, Gulati M et al: Clinical outcome in children undergoing tethered cord release utilizing intraoperative neurophysiological monitoring. *Pediatr Neurosurg* 2002; 37(2):81–6.
3. Warf BC: Pathophysiology of tethered cord syndrome. In *Pediatric Neurosurgery: Surgery of the Developing Nervous System,* 4th edition. McLone DG, ed. WB Saunders, Philadelphia: 2001, 282–8.
4. Yamada S, Iacono RP: Tethered Cord Syndrome. In *Disorders of the Pediatric Spine.* Pang D, ed. Raven Press, New York: 1995, 159–74.

CRANIOTOMY FOR VEIN OF GALEN MALFORMATION

SURGICAL CONSIDERATIONS

Description: A vein of Galen malformation is a large, AV fistula between arteries, mainly of the posterior cerebral circulation, and a massively enlarged vein of Galen (deep venous drainage of the brain). Patients can present with high-output CHF (infants), progressive macrocephaly from hydrocephalus (infants, children, adults), or, rarely, IC hemorrhage in adult patients. Most cases present at birth or during the infant years, and immediate care is often directed toward stabilizing cardiac function related to CHF. Patients undergoing surgery with high output CHF carry the highest risk of periop mortality. Many patients will have some degree of accompanying hydrocephalus, but decisions regarding the placement of ventricular shunts are best postponed until the malformation has been treated, as hydrocephalus may improve with reduction in intracranial venous pressure. High output CHF is addressed by treating the fistula. Embolization via the arterial or venous system minimizes resistance or reduces flow in the fistula, improving cardiac function.

Treatment is directed at staged occlusion of the arterial feeders to the AV fistula and eventually thrombosis of the fistula itself from the venous side. Open microsurgical techniques, endovascular methods, or a combination of both may be used to reduce flow through the malformation. With reduction in the aneurysmal flow, CO will decrease, SVR will improve, and mixed venous PO_2 will decrease. Because of the high mortality associated with treatment by surgery alone and the advances in endovascular techniques, vein of Galen malformations currently are managed without direct primary surgical approaches. Surgery, as an option, is more likely to occur in the setting of staged or attempted embolizations. Subtemporal, midline occipital, or bilateral occipital craniotomies can be used to isolate and occlude arterial feeders to the malformation. Stereotactic radiosurgery has been used successfully as an adjunct to embolization for surgery.

Variant procedure or approaches: Alternative approaches may access the torcular (confluence) of venous sinuses through a burr hole to allow direct retrograde placement of thrombogenic coils in the AV fistula.

Usual preop diagnosis: Vein of Galen aneurysm; IC hemorrhage; hydrocephalus; progressive neurologic deficits; current management focuses on embolization in the cath lab prior to surgical repair.

SUMMARY OF PROCEDURE

Position	Lateral decubitus, Concorde (modified prone), or semisitting; for burr hole, lateral
Incision	Temporal or occipital; for burr hole, occipital
Special instrumentation	Operating microscope, microscopic instruments; intraop angiography; for burr hole, endovascular catheters and equipment; intraop SSEP monitoring
Unique considerations	Careful attention to blood loss in infants Central venous access and A-line mandatory
Antibiotics	Vancomycin (1 g iv slowly q 12 h for adults; 10–15 mg/kg iv slowly q 6 h for children); cefotaxime (1 g iv q 6 h for adults; 40 mg/kg iv q 6 h for children)
Surgical time	3–5 h
Closing considerations	Meticulous hemostasis; avoid ↓ BP or HTN (MAP 80–90 adults; 70–80, children).
EBL	< 250 mL
Postop care	Monitor for ↑ ICP (use of extraventricular drain) as a result of venous HTN 2° rapid occlusion of AV fistula. ICU × 1–3 d.
Mortality	Approaches 100% if high output CHF not resolved
Morbidity	Deep venous infarct: 5–10% Hydrocephalus Stroke Subdural hygroma Infection: Rare
Pain score	3–4

PATIENT POPULATION CHARACTERISTICS

Age range	Birth–3 yr (typically)
Male:Female	1:1
Incidence	Rare
Etiology	Congenital
Associated conditions	Other intracranial vascular malformations; high-output CHF

ANESTHETIC CONSIDERATIONS

PREOPERATIVE

Vein of Galen vascular malformations are rare congenital abnormalities representing < 1% of all malformations. They are usually diagnosed in infants because of high output CHF and may cause an abnormal increase in head size due to the aneurysmal dilation and obstruction of the dural sinus. The abnormal vasculature constitutes a high-flow shunt, much like an AVM. If left untreated, the morbidity and mortality are high; however, treatment with radiologic embolization is superior to surgical excision and also is associated with lower morbidity and mortality rates.

Cardiovascular	Because these lesions constitute high-flow shunts through the brain, the infants are prone to develop high output CHF, which is fatal in more than 40% of patients. Newborns present with h/o CHF.
Neurological	Infants usually present with an abnormal head size, Sz disorder, or bizarre neurological signs, such as high-pitched crying, posturing, failure to eat or thrive, etc.
Laboratory	CT; MRI; cerebral angiography. The infant may need sedation and anesthetic management to obtain adequate diagnostic studies. Check renal function.
Premedication	For children, midazolam 0.5 mg/kg po (see p. D-1) generally provides satisfactory preop sedation after ~30 min. For young children (< 5 yr) who refuse po meds, instillation of midazolam 0.3 mg/kg intranasally provides rapid amnesia, sedation, and easy separation from the parents.

INTRAOPERATIVE

Anesthetic technique: GETA, with the goals being the same as those for IC vascular malformations.

Induction	Whenever possible, an iv induction is preferred. STP 2–3 mg/kg or propofol 1–2 mg/kg, fentanyl 2–3 mcg/kg, and rocuronium 0.6–1 mg/kg or vecuronium 0.1 mg/kg are satisfactory induction agents.	
Maintenance	Isoflurane ≤ 1%, sevoflurane 2–3% or desflurane ≤ 7%, with N_2O or air 60–70% to keep O_2 sat = 95–98%. Depending on duration of operation, additional doses or NMBs may be administered as needed to maintain a single-twitch response to nerve stimulation. Maintain a near-normal BP. Ventilation is controlled to maintain $PetCO_2$ = 35–40 mmHg with a mechanical ventilator or manually, from the start of anesthesia until surgical wound is closed. Mild hypothermia (32–35°C) may be requested by the surgeon. Normovolemia should be maintained.	
Emergence	Plan to leave ETT in place for at least 24 h postop; infant should receive controlled ventilation and sedation during that interval.	
Blood and fluid requirements	IV: 20–22 ga × 1–2 Central venous access = subclavian (no IJ, as may compromise cerebral circulation)	Replace blood as it is lost (cc for cc). Limit crystalloid fluid therapy to no more than 10 mL/kg above UO.
Control of brain volume	Same as for AVMs (see p. 21).	
Monitoring	Same as for AVMs (see p. 21).	
Control of BP	Goal = normal range for age Neonate: 55–70/40 (HR = 180) 1 yr: 70–100/60 (HR = 140)	BP should be kept in the normal range for the infant with close monitoring from an arterial catheter. If HR becomes excessive, esmolol infusion is useful.
Positioning	Same as for AVMs.	
Complications	Coagulopathy	If large volumes of blood are needed, a coagulopathy may ensue. Monitoring of coagulation status during surgery is mandatory.
	Hypothermia	After the aneurysm is surgically corrected, hypothermia needs to be continued for 24–72 h.

POSTOPERATIVE

Complications	Neurological deficits IC hemorrhage Heart failure
Pain management	Fentanyl 0.5–1 mcg/kg. MSO_4 0.05–0.1 mg /kg.
Tests	Same as for AVMs (see p. 22). Patients will need a CT or MRI under anesthesia postop in the AM

Suggested Readings

1. Herman JM, Hamilton MG, Spetzler RF: Vein of Galen malformations: surgical indications and techniques. In *Neurovascular Surgery,* Carter LP, Spetzler RF, eds. McGraw-Hill, New York: 1994, 1041–8.
2. Horowitz MB, Jungreis CA, Quisling RG, et al: Vein of Galen aneurysms: a review and current perspective. *AJNR Am J Neuroradiol* 1994; 15(8):1486–96.
3. Lasjaunias P, Rodesch G, Pruvost P et al: Treatment of vein of Galen aneurysmal malformation. *J Neurosurg* 1989; 70(5): 746–50.
4. McIntyre LA, Furgeson DA, Hebert PC, et al. Prolonged therapeutic hypothermia after traumatic brain injury in adults. *JAMA* 2003; 289:2992–9.
5. Moriarity JL, Steinberg GK: Surgical obliteration for vein of Galen malformation: a case report. *Surg Neurol* 1995; 44:365–70.
6. Shann F: Hypothermia for traumatic brain injury: how soon, how cold, and how long? *Lancet* 2003; 362:1950–1951.

VENTRICULOSCOPY AND THIRD VENTRICULOSTOMY

SURGICAL CONSIDERATIONS

Description: Ventriculoscopy is the technique of intraop visualization of the lateral, 3rd, and, occasionally, 4th ventricles using fiber optic endoscopes inserted through standard cranial burr holes. The ventriculoscope permits direct inspection and limited navigation within the ventricle for both diagnostic and therapeutic purposes, and often is most commonly applied in the setting of hydrocephalus. In addition to CT scans, preop MRI exam of the brain is obtained to better depict the anatomy of the ventricular system, which is distorted frequently by congenital lesions. The enlarged ventricles produced by the hydrocephalus contribute to the safety and feasibility of most endoscopic approaches, enabling a variety of procedures. The endoscope can be used to fenestrate multicompartmental periventricular or arachnoid cysts, position ventricular catheters during shunt insertion, biopsy or, in some cases, resect intraventricular tumors. Neuroendoscopy generally does not help in the initial cannulation of the ventricle (a common misconception).

Endoscopic ventriculoscopy may be performed through either frontal or parietal-occipital approaches, with the patient typically supine with the neck slightly flexed. Standard small incisions similar to shunt insertions are used. A twist drill or burr hole is created and the ventricle cannulated by insertion of the shunt catheter or an introducer with a peel-away sheath (for larger endoscopes). Endoscopes vary in size from 1.1 mm, for use inside a standard shunt catheter, to larger endoscopes (12–14 Fr), equipped with working channels, for more complex intraventricular procedures. After the ventricle is "tapped" through conventional methods, the endoscope can be inserted and the ventricular anatomy identified. After the intraventricular anatomic landmarks—such as the choroid plexus—are recognized, the scope can be navigated to the site of interest. Smaller endoscopes are used to position the catheter in the optimal ventricular location during shunt placement or revision. Larger endoscopes equipped with channels for instrumentation are used for biopsy, tumor resection, cyst aspiration, or fenestration procedures. Most scope systems have a separate channel for fluid irrigation if minor bleeding or debris obscure visibility.

Intraop complications associated with neuroendoscopic procedures include: minor or major intraventricular hemorrhage; air entrapment (pneumocephalus); injury to paraventricular structures (basal ganglia, hypothalamus, brain

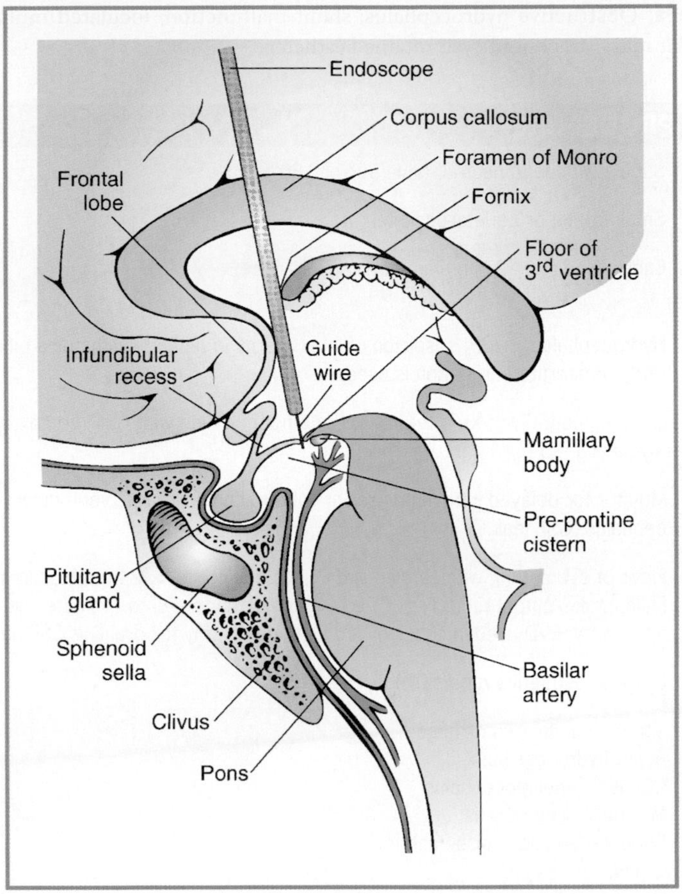

Figure 12.1-1. Endoscopic 3rd ventriculostomy. The figure depicts fenestration of the floor of the 3rd ventricle by a blunt probe inserted through the endoscope.

stem); cardiorespiratory depression; and delayed arousal from anesthesia. Intraventricular hemorrhage is caused by direct or indirect injury to ependymal and extraependymal blood vessels. Fortunately, most bleeding encountered is minor, but may be sufficient to interfere with visualization and illumination of the ventricle. Cardiorespiratory depression and cardiac arrhythmia are due, at least in part, to phenomena attributed to ↑ ICP from excessive irrigation without equal extracranial egress, rate of fluid instillation, and/or nonisothermic irrigant irritating the hypothalamic nuclei adjacent to the 3rd ventricle.

Third ventriculostomy is one of the more common endoscopic procedures and refers to fenestration of the floor of the 3rd ventricle to create a communication between the 3rd ventricle and the basilar cistern (Fig. 12.1-1). The technique is most commonly applied to patients with obstructive, or noncommunicating, hydrocephalus, although broader indications are being explored. This form of hydrocephalus results from impaired CSF flow through the Sylvian aqueduct or 4th ventricle outlets. For patients with noncommunicating hydrocephalus, successful 3rd ventriculostomy allows CSF communication between the 3rd ventricle and the interpeduncular subarachnoid space, thereby alleviating the hydrocephalus and avoiding shunt placement. The fenestration is conducted first by direct visualization of the floor of the 3rd ventricle and then by perforation of the ependymal and arachnoid tissue between the mammillary bodies and the infundibular recess. The perforation can be dilated by inflation of a balloon catheter passed through the fenestration. Because of the proximity to the brain stem—in addition to the complications encountered with ventriculoscopy—3rd ventriculostomy carries the additional risk of mesencephalic injury, hypothalamic dysregulation, cranial nerve injury, and hemorrhage from the basilar artery and adjacent perforating vessels. Minor bleeding can be controlled easily by steady irrigation. In the event of excessive bleeding, conversion to an open craniotomy is unlikely to improve control of the hemorrhage. Patients also may be prepped for shunt insertion in the event the ventriculostomy is aborted because of unfavorable 3rd ventricular anatomy. A temporary extraventricular drain (EVD) may be left in place following some procedures to control CSF drainage postop and/or to allow assessment of ICP.

Usual preop diagnosis: Obstructive hydrocephalus; shunt malfunction; loculated multicompartmental hydrocephalus; intraventricular mass; arachnoid cyst; retained catheter

SUMMARY OF PROCEDURE

Position	Supine with head neutral; table 90° or 180°
Incision	Small frontal or parietal-occipital
Special instrumentation	Endoscope (1.1–6 mm diameter); video system
Unique considerations	Hydrocephalus, ↑ ICP; suspicion of latex allergy in patients with spina bifida (see p. G-1). Body temperature irrigation is used.
Antibiotics	Ceftriaxone (50 mg/kg q 24 h iv × 2; do not combine with Ca^{++} containing solutions); or vancomycin (13–15 mg/kg iv)
Closing considerations	Monitor for delayed intraventricular or subdural hemorrhage, ventricular collapse, acute hydrocephalus, CSF leak.
Postop care	Floor or ICU setting with cardiac and O_2 sat monitoring × 24 h. Measurement of serum sodium. Fluid intake/output recording. CT to r/o hemorrhage and to evaluate ventricular volume may be necessary. EVD used in cases of 3rd ventriculostomy for draining CSF and testing ICP.
Mortality	0–7% (most series report 0%)
Morbidity	Intraventricular hemorrhage Acute hydrocephalus CSF leak/pneumocephalus Meningitis/ventriculitis Subdural effusions or hematoma Cranial nerve palsy Hemiparesis Diabetes insipidus SIADH Temperature dysregulation
Pain score	2–4

PATIENT POPULATION CHARACTERISTICS

Age range	Newborn–adult
Male:Female	1:1
Incidence	3/1000 live births (congenital only)
Etiology	Congenital and acquired
Associated conditions	Hydrocephalus; spinal dysraphism; Chiari malformation; posthemorrhagic hydrocephalus; arachnoid cyst

ANESTHETIC CONSIDERATIONS

PREOPERATIVE

Ventricular shunts are inserted to ameliorate hydrocephalus or cyst formations, which are either congenital or acquired.

Cardiovascular	↑ ICP →↑ BP & ↓↓ HR (Cushing's response) **Tests:** As indicated from H&P.

Neurological	The most common presenting Sx is HA. If hydrocephalus is severe, Sx of ↑ ICP (>15 mmHg) (e.g., N/V, drowsiness, papilledema, Sz, and focal neurological defects) develop.	
Laboratory	Tests as indicated by H&P, CT, and/or MRI.	
Premedication	Usually not required; should be avoided in patients with ↑ ICP.	

INTRAOPERATIVE

Anesthetic technique: GETA with pediatric circle; forced air warmer.

Induction	If ↑ ICP, iv induction with STP (3–6 mg/kg) or propofol (1.5–3.5 mg/kg) is preferred, because of their ability to decrease cerebral blood volume and, hence, ICP. ETT intubation is accomplished with the use of a nondepolarizing NMB (e.g., vecuronium [0.1 mg/kg] or rocuronium [0.7–1 mg/kg]).	
Maintenance	Isoflurane <1% or sevoflurane < 2% inspired with N_2O/O_2 mixture to maintain O_2 sat ~99%. Depending on duration of operation, additional doses of vecuronium (0.1 mg/kg) or rocuronium (0.2 mg/kg) may be needed. Maintain normal T in children by keeping OR warm (78°F) and using warming lights as needed. Ventilation is controlled mechanically (ventilator) or manually from the start of anesthesia until the surgical wound is closed. TV and frequency are adjusted so that $PetCO_2$ = 35–40 mmHg. Hyperventilation and hypocarbia are undesirable because they make cannulation of the ventricle(s) more difficult for the surgeon. Maintain normotension.	
Emergence	ETT is removed at the conclusion of the anesthetic. Prophylactic antiemetic (eg. ondansetron 0.1 mg/kg, max = 4 mg) should be given 30 min before extubation.	
Blood and fluid requirements	iv: 18–20 ga × 1 (22 ga for children) NS/LR @ 4–6 mL/kg/h	Administer crystalloid (via measured volume system in a child). Blood is rarely, if ever, necessary.
Management of ICP	Low normal $PaO_2 \geq 100$ Minimize fluids Isoflurane < 1% or Sevoflurane < 2% Hyperventilate to $PaCO_2$ = 25–30 mmHg ($PetCO_2$ = 20–25 mmHg)	Patients with malfunctioning VP shunts may be on the steep portion of the intracranial compliance curve such that any increase in intracranial volume may ↑↑ ICP. Transient increases in ICP are tolerated, provided that they are promptly terminated. Sustained increases in ICP > 25–30 mmHg are associated with severe neurological injury and poor outcome.
Monitoring	Standard monitors (see p. D-1).	
Positioning	Table turned 180° ✓ and pad pressure points. ✓ eyes.	Supine with a bolster under the shoulder on the operative side. The head, chest, and abdomen are prepped, so all anesthesia equipment and lines must be at the sides of the patient.
Complications	Infection Valve malfunction	Major complications from this operation are uncommon, but include infection at the valve site or in the tubing, and malfunction of the valve, either draining too little or too much CSF.

POSTOPERATIVE

Pain management	Children < 2 yr: Tylenol suppositories (up to 40 mg/kg intraop, then 10–15 mg/kg q 4 h). Fentanyl 0.5–1 mcg/kg MSO_4 0.05–0.1 mg/kg	New shunts are painful as a result of subcutaneous tunneling.

Suggested Readings

1. Drake JM: Ventriculostomy for treatment of hydrocephalus. *Neurosurg Clin North Am* 1993; 4(4):657–66.
2. Grant JA, McLone DG: Third ventriculostomy: a review. *Surg Neurol* 1997; 47:210–12.
3. Grotenhuis JA: *Manual of Endoscopic Procedures in Neurosurgery.* Uitgeverij Machaon, Nijmegen: 1995.
4. Handler MH, Abbott R, Lee M: A near-fatal complication of endoscopic third ventriculostomy: case report. *Neurosurg* 1994; 35(3): 525–8.
5. Jones RFC, Kwok BCT, Stening WA, et al: The current status of endoscopic third ventriculostomy in the management of non-communicating hydrocephalus. *Minim Invasive Neurosurg* 1994; 37:28–36.
6. Jones RFC, Kwok BCT, Stening WA, et al: Third ventriculostomy for hydrocephalus associated with spinal dysraphism: indications and contraindications. *Eur J Pediatr Surg* 1996; 6(Suppl 1):5–6.
7. Kirolous RW, Javadpour M, May P, et al: Endoscopic treatment of suprasellar and third ventricle-related arachnoid cysts. *Childs Nsrv Syst* 2001; 17(12)713–8.
8. Walker ML, Petronio J, Carey CM: Ventriculoscopy. In *Pediatric Neurosurgery: Surgery of the Developing Nervous System.* Cheek WR, Marlin AE, McLone DG, et al., eds. WB Saunders, Philadelphia: 1994, 572–81.

PEDIATRIC BRAIN ARTERIOVENOUS MALFORMATIONS (AVM)

SURGICAL CONSIDERATIONS

Description: An arteriovenous malformation is the most common cause of non-traumatic intracranial hemorrhage in childhood. It consists of direct connections between arteries and veins without an interposed capillary network and leads to a tangle of malformed vessels and channels (the nidus), carrying blood at arterial pressure. They may occur in any location of the brain, brain stem, or spinal cord; however, cerebral malformations are the most common. The arterial vessels deliver blood to the veins at systolic blood pressure, and that may cause bleeding. The lack of an interposed capillary network prevents local oxygen delivery leading to focal ischemia (steal) and seizures. This steal may result in a progressive neurologic deficit. In addition, venous congestion with arterial pressure blood may produce neurologic symptoms due to venous congestion and reduced perfusion to surrounding brain. AVMs can vary in size from lesions having only one feeding vessel to very complex lesions with multiple feeders and draining veins encompassing an entire hemisphere. It is estimated that 80–90% involve the cerebral hemisphere. Most are conical in shape with the apex near the ventricle. Small AVMs are more likely to exhibit spontaneous hemorrhage, resulting in headache, neurologic deficit, coma, and rarely death. Aneurysms within the nidus of the AVM (nidal aneurysm) or involving the feeding arteries are the most likely source of bleeding. The risk of hemorrhage is reported to be 2% per year. It is reported that after a hemorrhage the risk may be as high as 6% during the subsequent year. AVMs residing in the brainstem or cerebellum are more likely to result in permanent neurologic deficit or death if hemorrhage develops compared to those in the hemispheres. Recurrent headache or new onset seizure may herald the symptomatic AVM. However, the sudden onset of headache often followed by neurologic deficit should lead to an imaging study (CT or MRI) to demonstrate the lesion. If no lesion is identified, a lumbar puncture to confirm the presence of subarachnoid blood is indicated. Although CT angiography (CTA) or magnetic resonance angiography (MRA) is very sensitive in the diagnosis of AVM, four-vessel cerebral angiography is still the gold standard to confirm the presence and define the anatomy of these lesions. If the initial angiogram following a hemorrhage is nondiagnostic, the study should be repeated in 1–3 months, after resolution of hematoma and local compression of the vessels in the nidus. The ideal treatment of AVMs is complete surgical excision which removes the risk of hemorrhage, decreases or eliminates seizures and may alleviate or resolve neurologic symptoms of "cerebral steal" or venous congestion. A treatment decision for AVMs depends on size, location, and complexity, presence of associated aneurysms, as well as patient age, neurologic status, surgical expertise, and requires consideration of family and patient preference. The surgeon's decision to treat or observe a child with an AVM is complex with the ultimate goal of preservation of neurologic function. Some lesions situated in eloquent or deep regions of the brain are best observed or considered for interventional and/or stereotactic radiosurgery rather than craniotomy and resection. Angiography and embolization is most often performed under general anesthesia in the radiology suite. However, operating rooms have been constructed that can be used for complex angiographic procedures, open neurosurgical operations, magnetic-resonance imaging and image guided surgery. During angiography and embolization, physiologic monitoring (sensory and motor evoked potentials) is usually carried out. Careful blood pressure control is mandatory, and mild hypothermia (33° C) may be desirable. The duration of anesthesia is usually measured in hours, and post embolization the children are cared for in the PICU. Frequently, multiple episodes of embolization over weeks or even months are required for large or complex AVMs before the lesion is amenable to surgery or radiosurgery. However, embolization as the sole treatment for AVMs is not recommended; rather it should be used as an adjunct to surgery or to decrease size in order to successfully treat with radiosurgery. Surgery is most often performed under GA. In older teenagers with lesions in eloquent cortex, especially those involving speech, awake craniotomy and direct brain mapping may be used. Obtaining adequate brain relaxation may be difficult using awake techniques. For most children GA is recommended. The use of image guidance helps in localization of the lesion allowing for more precise placement of the craniotomy flap and better localization of subcortical lesions. Intubation should be completed without the patient straining or becoming hypertensive so as to decrease the risk of hemorrhage. Mild hyperventilation is begun to decrease and maintain the $PaCO_2$ to 30–35 mmHg. A lumbar subarachnoid drain may be used to allow for brain relaxation and access to deep lesions. At least two peripheral intravenous lines, an arterial line, pulse oximeter, Foley catheter, and a CVP line are placed. The use of mild (33° C) or moderate hypothermia requiring central cooling (e.g. Innercool-type device) may be undertaken. Minimal isotonic fluids should be administered and the serum Na^+ is kept in the 140–150 mEq range. If needed, hypertonic (3%) saline is administered. Mannitol and/or Lasix may be given to aid in brain relaxation if a lumbar drain is not placed. The use of dexamethasone (1-2 mg/kg/d; max 16 mg/d) is controversial, but is used more often than not. Anticonvulsants are not routinely administered unless there is a history of seizures. Routine prophylactic antibiotics (eg. Ceftriaxone) are given 30–60 min before the skin incision. If intraop angiography is to be used, the catheter sheath is placed in the femoral artery and covered beneath a sterile dressing. The patient is carefully positioned on the table and a radiolucent headholder is applied to the skull. Evoked potential monitoring electrodes are placed and baseline potentials are established (special anesthetic techniques are required and motor paralytic agents are minimized or avoided). Image guidance is established and the patient is draped and padded to avoid pressure points, allow access to the femoral arterial sheath, and allow a clear line of sight to the image-guidance system. The skin incision is infiltrated with 1/4–1/2% bupivacaine with 1/200,000 or 1/400,000 epinephrine to minimize skin bleeding. After the elevation of the bone flap, either CSF drainage via the lumbar drain or hypertonic agents are used to allow for minimal brain retraction and/or manipulation during the approach and resection of the AVM. If planned temporary occlusion of a major feeding vessel is required, barbiturates may be administered. Surgery may be prolonged and intraop angiography performed on multiple occasions during the procedure. MAP is maintained at the preop resting levels or within a set range determined by the surgical team using SNP and other vasoactive agents. In order to prevent perfusion pressure breakthrough and cerebral swelling, hypertension is avoided. If the procedure is prolonged, the AVM very complex, or a subtotal or planned staged removal is the surgical outcome, then the patient should remain intubated and ventilated postoperatively. Strict control of MAP is mandatory, and the range is based on the patient's age, AVM complexity, location, use of and degree of hypothermia, and preop blood pressure. Intraop MRI scans are being studied at many institutions. MRI requires very careful planning to allow the patient's head to be moved or rotated into the MRI donut during the operative procedure. MRI eliminates the ability to perform evoked potential monitoring. The use of this advanced technology, albeit attractive, produces a complex and hostile operating room environment and increases the anesthesia workload. Its benefit for AVM surgery is as yet to be determined.

Summary of Procedures: See Chapter 1, Craniotomy for intracranial aneurysms, p. 5.

Anesthetic Considerations: See Chapter 1, Craniotomy for intracranial aneurysms, p. 6.

Suggested Readings

1. Brain Trauma Foundation, American Association of Neurological Surgeons, Congress of Neurological Surgeons: Guidelines for the management of severe traumatic brain injury. Prophylactic hypothermia. *J Neurotrauma* 2007; 24(Suppl1):S21–5.
2. Hamilton MG, Spetzler RF: The prospective application of a grading system for arteriovenous malformations. *Neurosurgery* 1994; 34(1):2–6.
3. Lawton MT, Hamilton MG, Spetzler RF: Multimodality treatment of deep arteriovenous malformations: thalamus, basal ganglia, and brain stem. *Neurosurgery* 1995;37:29.
4. McIntyre LA, Furgeson DA, Hebert PC, et al: Prolonged therapeutic hypothermia after traumatic brain injury in adults. *JAMA* 2003; 289:2992–9.
5. Robin PH. Arteriovenous malformations. In *Principles and Practice of Pediatric Neurosurgery*. Albright AL, Pollack IF, Adelson PD, eds. New York, Thieme: 2008, 983–1003.
6. Smyth MD, Sneed PK, Ciricillo SF, et al. Stereotactic radiosurgery for pediatric intracranial arteriovenous malformations: the University of California at San Francisco experience. *J Neurosurg* 2002; 97(1):48–55.

anesthesia is usually measured in hours, and post embolization the children are cared for in the PICU. Frequently multiple episodes of embolization over weeks or even months are required for large or complex AVMs before the lesion is amenable to surgery or radiosurgery. However, embolization as the sole treatment for AVMs is not recommended; rather it should be used as an adjunct to surgery or to decrease size in order to more easily treat with radiosurgery. Surgery is most often performed under GA. In older teenagers with lesions in eloquent cortex, especially those involving speech, awake craniotomy and direct brain mapping may be used. Obtaining adequate brain relaxation may be difficult using awake techniques. For most children GA is recommended. The use of image guidance helps in localization of the lesion allowing for more precise placement of the craniotomy flap and better localization of subcortical lesions. Intubation should be completed without the patient straining or becoming hypertensive so as to decrease the risk of hemorrhage. Mild hyperventilation is begun to decrease and maintain the $PaCO_2$ to 30–35 mm Hg. A lumbar subarachnoid drain may be used to allow for brain relaxation and access to deep lesions. At least two peripheral intravenous lines, an arterial line, pulse oximeter, Foley catheter, and a CVP line are placed. The use of mild (35°C) or moderate hypothermia requires a central cooling (e.g., [illegible] type device) may be undertaken. [illegible] should be administered and the serum Na is kept in the 140–150 range. If needed, hypertonic (3%) saline [illegible] administered. Mannitol and/or Lasix may be given to aid in brain relaxation if a lumbar drain is not placed. The use of dexamethasone (1–2 mg/kg, max 10 mg/d) is controversial, but is used more often than not. Anticonvulsants are routinely administered unless there is a history of seizures. Routine prophylactic antibiotics (e.g., Cefazolin) are given 30–60 min before the skin incision. If intraop angiography is to be used, the catheter sheath is placed in the femoral artery and covered with a sterile dressing. The patient is carefully positioned on the table and a radiolucent head holder is applied to the skull. Evoked potential monitoring electrodes are placed and baseline potentials are established. If special anesthetic techniques are required and motor paralytic agents are minimized or avoided. Image guidance is established and the patient is [illegible] and padded to avoid pressure points. Easy access to the femoral artery [illegible] and allow a clear unobstructed view for the image guidance system. The skin incision is infiltrated with [illegible] or 1:200,000 epinephrine to minimize skin bleeding. After the elevation of the bone flap, the lumbar drain may be opened or hyperosmolar agents are used to allow for minimal brain retraction and/or [illegible] during the approach and resection of the AVM. If planned temporary occlusion of a major feeding vessel [illegible] may be administered. Surgery may be performed and intraop angiography performed to [illegible] during the procedure. MAP is maintained at the preop resting levels or within a set range determined [illegible] SSEP and other vasoactive agents. To reduce normal perfusion pressure breakthrough [illegible] hypotension is avoided. If the procedure is prolonged, the AVM very complex, or a subtotal [illegible] is the surgical outcome, then the patient should remain intubated and ventilated postoperatively [illegible] is mandatory, and the ranges is based on the patient's age, AVM complexity, location, use [illegible] hypothermia, and preop blood pressure. Intraop MRI scans are being studied at many institutions [illegible] careful planning to allow the patient's head to be moved or rotated into the MRI bore during the [illegible] the ability to perform evoked potential monitoring. The use of this advanced [illegible] requires a complex and more expensive room environment and increases the [illegible] surgery is yet to be determined.

[illegible] Craniotomy for supratentorial [illegible], p. [illegible]
[illegible] Chapter 1, Craniotomy for infratentorial [illegible], p. 6

[illegible] American Association of Neurological Surgeons, Congress of Neurological Surgeons. Guidelines [illegible] brain injury [illegible] 2003 [illegible] S21–[illegible]
[illegible] The [illegible] of a [illegible] malformations [illegible]
[illegible] multimodality treatment of deep arteriovenous malformations [illegible]
[illegible] et al. Prolonged [illegible] hypothermia [illegible]
[illegible] In [illegible] 2008; [illegible]
[illegible] radiosurgery for pediatric intracranial arteriovenous malformations [illegible] 2002; 97 [illegible]

CHAPTER

12.2 Pediatric Ophthalmic Surgery

SURGEON

D. M. Alcorn, MD

ANESTHESIOLOGISTS

Brian P. Struyk, MD

Alice A. Edler, MD

STRABISMUS SURGERY

SURGICAL CONSIDERATIONS

Description: Surgical correction of strabismus is a common procedure in ophthalmic practice, as strabismus occurs in 3–5% of the general population. Strabismus surgery is the most common pediatric eye surgery performed. The goal of this procedure is to correct the ocular misalignment caused by this condition. This can be achieved by several methods: (a) **weakening the muscles** (either by recession, marginal myotomy, or inserting a spacer), (b) **strengthening the muscles,** by shortening their length (resection), moving the muscle's insertion toward the limbus (advancement), or tightening the muscle's fibers (plication or tuck), or (c) by **transposing the muscles.** Surgery can be performed on any of the four recti muscles (medial rectus, lateral rectus, superior rectus, and/or lateral rectus muscle) or the two oblique muscles (superior oblique and inferior oblique).

Often, **forced duction testing (FDT)** is performed during surgery to determine if there is evidence of limited ductions. This helps to differentiate a paretic muscle vs a restriction that may limit motility. The eyes should be immobile during FDT as well as during surgery. If succinylcholine has been used, at least 20 min should pass before performing duction testing, since succinylcholine causes contraction of extraocular muscles. Alternatively, a different muscle relaxant may be used.

Eye position under GA is well documented: the eyes will become more divergent and this tendency is increased in misaligned eyes; therefore, exotropic eyes appear more outwardly deviated and esotropic (inward deviation) eyes actually appear straighter (less esotropic). Hence, it is important that the surgeon have solid measurements preoperatively.

The surgery usually is performed through one of two possible approaches. The **limbal incision** is made at the junction of the cornea and the conjunctiva, with radial relaxing incisions in the quadrants on either side of the muscle. The other is a **fornix** or **cul-de-sac incision,** which is made ~4–8 mm from the limbus in the quadrant adjacent to the muscle on which to operate. This approach is subposterior to tenon's capsule. Comfort and cosmesis immediately postop are superior with the fornix incision.

Variant procedure or approaches: In very cooperative older children, an **adjustable suture** technique may be used. Unlike fixed sutures, the adjustable suture technique allows modification of the position of the muscle. An adjustable suture involves temporarily positioning the muscle, but not finally tying it down until the patient is awake and has been remeasured. After the patient is free of the effects of anesthesia, measurements are retaken, and the muscle is placed in its optimum position, to properly align the eyes, and then securely tied down. This adjustment may be performed the same day of surgery or the following day. **Adjustable strabismus surgery** ideally reduces the frequency of reoperations by eliminating undesirable early postop undercorrections or overcorrections and increases the rate of surgical success.

Although GA is most commonly used, strabismus surgery may be done using a **retrobulbar, peribulbar, subtenon,** or **subconjunctival block**, or even **topical anesthesia**. Both topical and peribulbar anesthesia have the advantage of providing good akinesia and anesthesia but without the risks associated with a retrobulbar injection (e.g., hemorrhage, optic nerve damage, ocular perforation). When using topical anesthesia, this may be augmented by the use of minimal sedation and/or antianxiety medications.

Usual preop diagnosis: Strabismus

SUMMARY OF PROCEDURE	
Position	Supine
Incision	Limbal or fornix
Antibiotics	Topical and/or subconjunctival antibiotics at completion of case
Unique considerations	Ask surgeons if they want neuromuscular blockade. If using succinylcholine, would need to wait 20 min before doing FDT. Keep patient under stable anesthesia, so the eyes are immobile and not drifting. Postop vomiting is common after strabismus surgery, with an incidence of 40–88%. Topical tetracaine may aide in diminishing postop pain.
Surgical time	Dependent upon type of surgery and number of muscles; usually 20–90 min.

SUMMARY OF PROCEDURE (cont'd)	
EBL	Minimal
Mortality	Rare
Morbidity	Failure to achieve desired alignment Infection Hemorrhage Anterior segment ischemia
Postop care	PACU with discharge home within a few hours. Typically no eye patches.
Pain Score	2–4

PATIENT POPULATION CHARACTERISTICS	
Age range	Children (most common)
Male:Female	1:1
Incidence	~5% of population
Etiology	Generally idiopathic; muscle palsies may be associated with trauma, inflammation, tumors, and/or ischemia; restrictive strabismus may occur with thyroid disease (Graves disease), fibrosis syndromes, or 2° to a scleral buckle or mass.
Associated conditions	↑ incidence in premature infants, small-for-gestational-age infants, those with a positive family Hx of strabismus, craniosynostosis syndromes, or associated CNS disease

ANESTHETIC CONSIDERATIONS

PREOPERATIVE

In children, strabismus is the most frequent ophthalmic condition requiring surgical repair. Although most patients with this condition are otherwise healthy, there is an increased incidence of strabismus in children with cerebral palsy and other neurological disorders. Although many adult eye surgeries can be performed under regional anesthesia (retrobulbar or peribulbar block), in children GA is almost always required to ensure good surgical conditions. The anesthesiologist should be aware of the potential problems associated with strabismus surgery, including: increased risk of malignant hyperthermia (MH), occurrence of the oculocardiac reflex (OCR), and increased incidence of PONV. Because individuals at risk for MH often have musculoskeletal abnormalities, such as strabismus or ptosis, it is important to obtain a thorough family Hx of anesthetic problems. Avoid the use of succinylcholine since it can induce a tonic contracture of the extraocular muscles, which can interfere with the FDT (see above). The surgeon performs FDT by grasping the eye at the limbus, slightly proptosing the eye, and moving it into each field of gaze in order to determine if the strabismus is a result of paretic or restrictive extraocular muscles. This helps in formulating the surgical plan.

Anesthetic technique: GETA, LMA

Induction	Following standard pediatric induction (see p. D-1), a vagolytic dose of atropine (0.02 mg/kg) or glycopyrrolate (0.01 mg/kg) may be given to attenuate oculocardiac and oculorespiratory reflexes. The use of sevoflurane as an inhalation agent, however, significantly decreases the occurrence of these two vagally mediated responses. FDT may be performed by the surgeon at this time, before the use of muscle relaxants. Subsequently, NMB (e.g., rocuronium 0.6 mg/kg) can be used to assist ET intubation.
Maintenance	Techniques can include either inhalation agents or TIVA. The use of N_2O may ↑ risk for PONV, despite use of prophylactic antiemetics. If a propofol drip is used, suggested dose ranges are 150–175 mcg/kg/min. Postop analgesia should include fentanyl (1–2 mcg/kg) and acetaminophen (30–40 mg/kg prn × 1). Preferred antiemetic medications include ondansetron (0.1 mg/kg up to 4 mg), metoclopramide (0.1 mg/kg up to 10 mg), or dexamethasone (0.15 mg/kg up to 5 mg); consider "super" hydration with 30 cc/kg of LR solution. Combination therapy with drugs from different antiemetic drug classes is most effective.

Emergence	In specific cases, the surgeon may request "deep extubation.' This can be accomplished with a high concentration of inhalational anesthetic (e.g., 2% sevoflurane). The ETT is removed, and an oral airway is placed. The patient is then gradually allowed to awaken, taking care to monitor for the development of laryngospasm.	
Blood and fluid requirements	iv: 20–22 ga NS/LR to replace calculated deficit and maintain requirements.	
Monitoring	Standard monitors (see p. B-1). Temperature	
Positioning	Supine or supine with shoulder roll.	
Complications	Oculocardiac reflex (OCR)/ oculorespiratory reflex (ORR)	Traction on extraocular muscles can result in vagally mediated slowing of HR (> 20% of baseline), ± junctional, ventricular, or supraventricular arrhythmias. Additionally, depressed spontaneous ventilation may occur. Both of these complications are significantly decreased with use of sevoflurane or desflurane anesthesia. OCR/ORR tends to fatigue with repeated manipulation. Treatment includes release of tension on extraocular muscles and administration of vagolytic agents (atropine or glycopyrrolate).
	Malignant hyperthermia (MH)	Consider MH if the following are noted: unexplained tachycardia; ↑ $ETCO_2$; muscular rigidity, masseter spasm; ↑ temperature (a late sign). To evaluate, obtain ABGs, CK, and myoglobin. MH produces ↓ PaO_2, ↑ $PaCO_2$, ↑ K^+, and acidosis. If MH is suspected, discontinue volatile agents immediately. Stop surgery as soon as possible, hyperventilate patient with 100% O_2 at > 10 L/min. Give dantrolene 2.5 mg/kg iv ASAP. Treat acidosis with bicarbonate (1–2 mEq/kg), and treat hyperkalemia (insulin 0.1 U/kg + 1 ml/kg D50, CaCl 10 mg/kg or Ca gluconate 10–50 mg/kg). Cool the patient and hydrate to maintain urine output. Further doses of Dantrolene may be necessary (up to 30 mg/kg).
	Accidental extubation	Surgical repositioning or removal of surgical drapes may result in accidental extubation. ETT should be firmly secured and anesthesiologist should be attentive to changes in positioning or removal of drapes.

POSTOPERATIVE

Complications	PONV MH	See above for rescue doses of antiemetics. See above.
Pain management	Continue po acetaminophen (10–12 mg/kg q 4 h) + antiemetics as needed.	Occasional need of opioid analgesics.

Suggested Readings

1. Alexander JP: Reflex disturbances of cardiac rhythm during ophthalmic surgery. *Brit J Ophthal* 1975; 59(9):518–23.
2. Alison CE, Delange JJ, Koole FD et al: A comparison of the incidence of the oculocardiac and oculorespiratory reflexes during sevoflurane and halothane anesthesia for strabismus surgery in children. *Anesth Analg* 2000; 90(2):306–10.
3. Anninger W, Forbes B, Quinn G et al. The effect of topical tetracaine eye drops on emergence behavior and pain relief after strabismus surgery. *J AAPOS* 2007; 11(3):273–6.

4. Braun U, Feise J, Muhlendyck H: Is there a cholinergic and adrenergic phase of the oculocardiac reflex during strabismus surgery? *Acta Anaesthesiol Scand* 1993; 37(4):390–5.
5. Eberhart LH, Morin AM, Guber D et al. Applicability of risk scores for post operative nausea and vomiting in adults to paediatric patients. *Br J Anaesth* 2004; 93(3):386–92.
6. France NK, France TD, Woodburn JD, et al: Succinylcholine alteration of the forced duction test. *Ophthalmol* 1980; 87(2): 1282–7.
7. Goodarzi M, Matar MM, Shafa M et al. A prospective randomized blinded study of the effect of intravenous fluid therapy on postoperative nausea and vomiting in children undergoing strabismus surgery. *Pediatric Anesthesia* 2006 Jan; 16(1):49–53.
8. Hill R, Lubarsky DA, Phillips-Bute B et al. Cost effectiveness of prophylactic antiemetic therapy with ondansetron, droperidol or placebo. *Anesthesiology* 2000; 92(4):958–67.
9. Hopkins PM: Malignant hyperthermia: advances in clinical management and diagnosis. *Br J Anaesth* 2000; 85(1):118–28.
10. http://medical.mhaus.org/PubData/PDFs/treatmentposter.pdf
11. Keaney A, Diviney D, Hartes et al. Postoperative behavioral changes following anesthesia with sevo-flurane. *Paediatr Anaesth* 2004; 14(10):866–70.
12. Kovac AL: Management of postoperative nausea and vomiting in children. *Paediatr Drugs* 2007; 9(1):47–69.
13. Malmgren W, Akeson J. Similar excitation after sevo-flurane anesthesia in young children given rectal morphine or midazolam as premedication. *Acta Anesthesiol Scand* 2004; 48:1277–82.
14. Oh AY, Yun MJ, Kim HJ et al. Comparison of Desflurane with Sevoflurane for the incidence of occulocardiac reflex in children undergoing strabismus surgery. *Br J Anaesth* 2007 Aug; 99(2):262–5.
15. Tramer M, Moore A, McQuay H: Prevention of vomiting after paediatric strabismus surgery: a systematic review using the numbers-needed-to-treat method. *Br J Anaesth* 1995; 75(5):556–61.
16. Watcha M, Simeon R, White PF, et al: Effect of propofol on the incidence of postoperative vomiting after strabismus surgery in pediatric outpatients. *Anesthesiology* 1991; 75(2):204–9.

CHAPTER

12.3 Pediatric Otolaryngology

SURGEONS

Anna H. Messner, MD
Kay W. Chang, MD

ANESTHESIOLOGISTS

Michael Chen, MD
Cathy R. Lammers, MD
Gregory B. Hammer, MD

MYRINGOTOMY AND TYMPANOSTOMY TUBE PLACEMENT

SURGICAL CONSIDERATIONS

Description: Tympanostomy (PE or pressure equalizing) tubes are placed in the patient with chronic serous otitis media (fluid in the middle ear for > 3 mo) or recurrent acute otitis media (6 or more episodes of otitis media over the prior yr). Occasionally, PE tubes are placed in a child with meningitis of otitic origin or with acute otitis media that is unresponsive to antibiotics. The patient is supine and the OR table in the 0° position. The microscope is positioned over the bed and the head turned to expose the ear. An ear speculum is inserted into the ear canal, cerumen is removed, and an incision is made in the tympanic membrane. Fluid is sometimes suctioned from the middle ear; then, a tympanostomy tube is inserted into the ear, straddling the tympanic membrane. Antibiotic ear drops frequently are inserted into the external auditory canal. Sometimes lidocaine and/or oxymetazoline drops are also inserted into the ear canal. The surgeon moves to the other side of the table, the microscope is repositioned, the head is turned, and the procedure is repeated on the other ear.

Usual preop diagnosis: Chronic serous otitis media (CSOM); recurrent acute otitis media (RAOM)

SUMMARY OF PROCEDURE	
Position	Supine; head to anesthesia
Incision	Tympanic membrane
Special instrumentation	Operating microscope
Antibiotics	No parenteral antibiotics (except for SBE prophylaxis); topical antibiotic ear drops
Surgical time	5–10 min. Patients with stenotic ear canals (e.g., Down syndrome) can take longer.
EBL	None
Postop care	PACU → home
Mortality	Rare
Morbidity	Bleeding from ear Purulent drainage from ear (otorrhea)
Pain score	1–3

PATIENT POPULATION CHARACTERISTICS	
Age range	3 mo+ (most common, 1–3 yr)
Male:Female	1:1
Incidence	Very common
Etiology	Chronic middle ear infections
Associated conditions	Cleft palate

ANESTHETIC CONSIDERATIONS

PREOPERATIVE

The majority of children presenting for PE tubes are < 3 yr and generally in good health. Many of these children, however, have recurrent URI, which contributes to edema of the eustachian tubes, predisposing to episodes of acute otitis media. Intervals between URI may be brief, and scheduling surgery during these interludes is often impractical.

Children with mild URI generally can be anesthetized safely for PE tube placement, because tracheal intubation is generally not performed. Surgery should be delayed for patients with acute, febrile illnesses, and in those with Sx referable to the lower airways (e.g., productive cough, wheezing). Surgery need not be delayed if fever is 2° acute otitis media.

Respiratory	Surgery in patients with URI Sx referable to the extrathoracic airway alone is generally not delayed. These Sx include nasal congestion and/or discharge and mild conjunctivitis. Fever accompanied by productive cough and wheezing are Sx of lower respiratory tract involvement and should prompt rescheduling of the procedure 2–3 wk after these Sx have abated. In borderline cases (e.g., those with rales auscultated on chest exam but no other lower tract Sx), O_2 sat may be measured by pulse oximetry. Procedures in patients with $SpO_2 <$ 95% should be deferred.
Laboratory	None
Premedication	Some practitioners advocate withholding premedication, as the duration of action of the premed may outlast the surgery. In general, however, we administer oral midazolam to patients > 9 mo (see p. D-1) and have not found a significant related delay in discharge from PACU. Parental presence in the OR may obviate the need for premedication in selected cases.

INTRAOPERATIVE

Anesthetic technique: GA via face mask

Induction	A standard inhalation induction with sevoflurane and $O_2 \pm N_2O$ is performed with routine monitoring. An oral airway commonly is inserted, as soft tissue obstruction may occur when the head is turned fully to the side during surgery. CPAP 5–8 cmH_2O also may be useful in maintaining airway patency. Following induction, a one-time dose of rectal acetaminophen (30–40 mg/kg) may be given for postop analgesia. (↓ rectal dose if po acetaminophen is given at home or as premedication.)	
Maintenance	Marked agitation ("emergence delirium") has been noted following emergence from sevoflurane and other inhaled agents. A variety of strategies have been used to minimize this phenomenon, including nasal or IM fentanyl (1–2 mcg/kg) or ketamine. Since an iv catheter is not placed routinely, iv drugs are not usually given.	
Emergence	For bilateral procedures, the potent inhaled anesthetic is D/C'd before or during the 2nd myringotomy to facilitate prompt emergence. N_2O is continued until the completion of surgery. As the patient is awakening, gentle oropharyngeal suctioning is performed.	
Blood and fluid requirements	None	
Monitoring	Standard monitors (see p. D-1).	
Positioning	✓ and pad pressure points. ✓ eyes.	
Complications	Laryngospasm	Secretions → laryngospasm 2° irritation of the vocal cords, especially in children with URI. Rx: 100% O_2 and CPAP or manual ventilation with PEEP ≤ 20–25 cm H_2O. Rarely, succinylcholine (2–4 mg/kg im) may be needed if a significant decrease in SpO_2 occurs and ventilation is not possible. Atropine (0.01–0.02 mg/kg) should be given in the same syringe to mitigate the bradycardia associated with succinylcholine. Oropharyngeal suctioning and manual ventilation usually result in resolution of the laryngospasm. Rarely, tracheal intubation may be indicated for recurrent laryngospasm.

POSTOPERATIVE

Complications	Laryngospasm	Laryngospasm may occur, and should be treated as described above.
Pain management	Acetaminophen 10–15 mg/kg po Ibuprofen 10 mg/kg Hydrocodone 0.15 mg/kg po	Consider previously administered po and/or pr dosing.

Suggested Readings

1. Haupert MS, Pascual C, Mohan A et al: Parental satisfaction with anesthesia without intravenous access for myringotomy. *Arch Otolaryngol Head Neck Surg* 2004; 130(9):1025–8.
2. Hoffmann KK, Thompson GK, Burke BL, et al: Anesthetic complications of tympanostomy tube placement in children. *Arch Otolaryngol Head Neck Surg* 2002; 128(9):1040–3.
3. Pappas AL, Fluder EM, Creech S et al: Postoperative analgesia in children undergoing myringotomy and placement equalization tubes in ambulatory surgery. *Anesth Analg* 2003; 96(6):1621–4.
4. Tait AR, Knight PR: The effects of general anesthesia on upper respiratory tract infections in children. *Anesthesiology* 1987; 67:930–5.
5. Tobias JD, Lowe S, Hersey S, et al. Analgesia after bilateral myringotomy and placement of pressure equalization tubes in children: acetaminophen vs acetaminophen with codeine. *Anesth Analg* 1995; 81:496–500.

TONSILLECTOMY AND ADENOIDECTOMY

SURGICAL CONSIDERATIONS

Description: The dissection is carried out with the patient supine, shoulders slightly elevated by a shoulder roll (typically, a rolled towel). A mouth gag is inserted, and a small suction catheter is passed through the nose and brought out the mouth to elevate the soft palate and expose the nasopharynx. The adenoids are viewed with a mirror and/or palpated. A curette, adenotome, microdebrider or suction electrocautery is used to remove the adenoids; then, typically, the nasopharynx is packed. There are two major types of tonsillectomy: total tonsillectomy and subtotal (partial) tonsillectomy. The traditional total tonsillectomy is performed by grasping the tonsil with Allis forceps and pulling it medially. A vertical incision is made in the anterior tonsillar pillar with a sickle knife, scissors, or electrocautery instruments; then, the tonsil is dissected from the surrounding tissue and removed. A snare may be used to amputate the inferior pole of the tonsil before removal. Hemostasis is obtained through use of packs and suction electrocautery. After hemostasis has been obtained in the tonsillar fossae, the pack is removed from the nasopharynx, and hemostasis is achieved in the nasopharynx using suction electrocautery. Tonsils can also be completely removed using radiofrequency (Coblation), bipolar scissors, bipolar forceps or laser. The same approach and set-up is used for a subtotal tonsillectomy which can be performed using radiofrequency or a microdebrider. The literature on incisional local anesthetic injection is mixed with some studies reporting benefit and some showing no benefit. Therefore, injection is not generally recommended.

Usual preop diagnosis: Obstructive sleep apnea (OSA); chronic tonsillitis and/or adenoiditis; tonsillar and adenoid hypertrophy; asymmetric enlargement of tonsils (to r/o cancer)

SUMMARY OF PROCEDURE	
Position	Supine, shoulder roll, head extended; table turned 90°; surgeon at head of table
Incision	Intraoral mucosal
Special instrumentation	Mouth gag (McIvor, Crowe-Davis, Dingman)

SUMMARY OF PROCEDURE (cont'd)	
Unique considerations	Observe for compression of ETT or accidental extubation when mouth gag is manipulated. Patients with Down syndrome may need to be evaluated preop for possible atlantoaxial subluxation, as the neck is typically extended. Steroids (e.g., dexamethasone 0.5 mg/kg) used routinely by some practitioners.
Antibiotics	Not used routinely.
Surgical time	30 min
EBL	10–200 mL. Monitor closely.
Postop care	Lateral position; suction in midline only. Most commonly, PACU → home. Overnight stay, if < 2 yr or other comorbidities.
Mortality	Rare
Morbidity	Bleeding: 2–3% Aspiration: Rare Tooth damage: Rare
Pain score	Adenoidectomy, 3–5; tonsillectomy, 6–9

PATIENT POPULATION CHARACTERISTICS	
Age range	1 yr+ (most common, 2–8 yr)
Male:Female	1:1
Incidence	300,000 cases/yr in the United States
Etiology	OSA; chronic infection; peritonsillar abscess; snoring. (R/O lymphoma, carcinoma, lymphoproliferative disease.)
Associated conditions	Down syndrome

ANESTHETIC CONSIDERATIONS

PREOPERATIVE

While most children presenting for tonsillectomy and/or adenoidectomy are healthy, a variety of medical problems may coexist. Severe adenoidal hyperplasia may cause nasopharyngeal obstruction, obligate mouth breathing, failure to thrive 2° poor feeding, and disturbances of speech and sleep. Chronic nasal obstruction may result in narrowing of the upper airway and dental and facial changes (so-called 'adenoidal facies'). Tonsillar hyperplasia may cause airway obstruction, OSA, CO_2 retention, cor pulmonale, and failure to thrive. Most of these changes are reversible with removal of the adenoids and tonsils. Children presenting f or adenoidectomy/tonsillectomy also frequently have URI (see Anesthetic Considerations for Myringotomy and Tympanostomy Tube Placement p. 1181).

Respiratory	See discussion under Anesthetic Considerations for Myringotomy and Tympanostomy Tube Placement (see p. 1181).
Dental	Examination of the airway should include inspection of the teeth. Parents should be advised that loose teeth may be dislodged during placement of the mouth gag or laryngoscopy.
Cardiovascular	In children with severe OSA, CXR and EKG should be done to evaluate the presence of cor pulmonale. If significant RVH and/or cardiomegaly are present, consider ECHO and consultation by pediatric cardiologist.
Hematologic	A careful Hx is taken for Sx of easy bruising or bleeding. If present, a CBC with Plt count, as well as PT, INR, PTT, and bleeding time are performed. In patients with a negative Hx, we order no preop lab tests.

Premedication	Children with severe OSA (airway obstruction) who are very anxious may receive a reduced dose of oral midazolam (see p. D-1) in a well-monitored environment (e.g., with an experienced RN or member of the anesthesia team present). SpO_2 should be monitored following administration of premedication.

INTRAOPERATIVE

Anesthetic technique: GETA

Induction	Standard inhalation induction (see p. D-1); airway obstruction during induction is common in these patients, and usually is alleviated with placement of an oral airway and administration of CPAP: 10–20 cm H_2O. An iv catheter should be placed as soon as possible to facilitate administration of muscle relaxant if needed with glycopyrrolate (4–6 mcg/kg) to reduce oral secretions. Some practitioners prefer not to paralyze these patients due to the brevity of the procedure; propofol may be given before laryngoscopy. For patients with severe OSA, consider iv induction to facilitate prompt placement of the ETT. An oral RAE ETT is used and taped securely in the midline position to facilitate placement of the mouth gag. A cuffed ETT may be desirable because, in combination with a throat pack, it minimizes the risk of entry of blood and oral secretions into the trachea during surgery. Care should be exercised in ensuring that the inferior part of the oral RAE tube is long enough for the cuff to pass beyond the vocal cords. A short tube may easily dislodge with changes in head position, or the cuff may cause vocal cord trauma. Bilateral breath sounds and chest excursion should be confirmed after placement of the mouth gag, which may cause kinking and obstruction of the ETT. Acetaminophen (30–40 mg/kg) may be given pr after induction. (↓ dose if po acetaminophen given with premedications.)	
Maintenance	Standard maintenance (see p. D-2). An intermediate-acting NMR (e.g., rocuronium 0.6–1.0 mg/kg or vecuronium 0.1 mg/kg) may given to facilitate tracheal intubation. Opioids (e.g., fentanyl 2–3 mcg/kg, morphine sulfate 0.1–0.15 mg/kg) are given for postop analgesia. The use of propofol, ± remifentanil, instead of anesthetic vapor, may ↓ the incidence of PONV, which is common following tonsillectomy/adenoidectomy. Administration of ondansetron (0.1 mg/kg, up to 4 mg) is controversial due to some evidence that it can mask postop bleeding, with retained blood in the stomach. Dexamethasone 0.25–1.0 mg/kg may be given to reduce airway edema and PONV.	
Emergence	Blood and secretions should be suctioned from the oropharynx and stomach following the completion of surgery. The patient should be fully awake before tracheal extubation, which may be performed supine or in the lateral position with the head down. Verify removal of throat packs. Alternatively, extubating under deep anesthesia decreases coughing, but requires vigilance to avoid airway obstruction and aspiration at emergence and during transport to PACU.	
Blood and fluid requirements	IV: 22 or 20 ga × 1 NS/LR @ 5–10 mL/h	Blood loss is typically ~4 mL/kg and may accumulate in the stomach → N/V (unless prevented by antiemetics).
Monitoring	Standard monitors (see p. D-1).	
Positioning	✓ and pad pressure points. ✓ eyes.	
Complications	Airway obstruction ETT dislodgement/kinking	 Usually caused by insertion/manipulation of mouth gag.

POSTOPERATIVE

Complications	Airway obstruction	Retention of throat pack → airway obstruction. Remove with Magill forceps. Recurrent airway obstruction may require application of positive pressure via face mask (CPAP vs manual ventilation with PEEP) ± placement of an oral airway. Severe postop airway obstruction is more common in patients < 2 yr. In these patients, admission to PICU may be necessary. CPAP via face mask or nasal mask may be helpful. On rare occasions, tracheal intubation and mechanical ventilation are required until swelling of the airway resolves.
	Hemorrhage	Bleeding may occur in the immediate postop period or several d later. Patients present with anemia and hypovolemia, as well as airway compromise and a full stomach 2° swallowed blood. IV fluids, including blood, should be given before induction. Rapid-sequence intubation (see p. B-4) should be performed with cricoid pressure in preparation for surgical treatment.
Pain management	Morphine 0.025–0.05 mg/kg	May be given incrementally in PACU. Subsequently, acetaminophen with or without hydrocodone 0.15 mg/kg is given. Local anesthetic injection by the surgeon into the tonsillar and adenoidal beds ↓ postop opioid requirements.

Suggested Readings

1. Colclasure JB, Grahamm SS: Complications of outpatient tonsillectomy and adenoidectomy: a review of 3,340 cases. *Ear Nose Throat J* 1990; 69:155–60.
2. Francis A, Eltaki K, Bash T, et al: The safety of preoperative sedation in children with sleep-disordered breathing. *Int J Pediatr Otorhinolaryngol.* 2006; 70(9):1517–21.
3. Linden BE, Gross CW, Long TE, et al: Morbidity in pediatric tonsillectomy. *Laryngoscope* 1990; 100:120–4.
4. Mather SJ, Peurtrell JM: Postoperative morphine requirements, nausea and vomiting following anaesthesia for tonsillectomy. Comparison of intravenous morphine and non-opioid analgesic techniques. *Paediatr Anaesth* 1995; 5:185–8.
5. Park AH, Pappas AL, Fluder E, et al: Effect of perioperative administration of ropivacaine with epinephrine on postoperative pediatric adenotonsillectomy recovery. *Arch Otolaryngol Head Neck Surg* 2004; 130(4):459–64.
6. Smith SL, Pereira KD: Tonsillectomy in children: indications, diagnosis and complications. *ORL J Otorhinolaryngol Relat Spec.* 2007; 69(6):336–9.

BRONCHOSCOPY/ESOPHAGOSCOPY

SURGICAL CONSIDERATIONS

Description: Flexible bronchoscopy is performed when the dynamics of the larynx and trachea need to be visualized. The child is supine on the OR table, which is turned 90–180°. With the child sedated or under GA, but breathing spontaneously, the bronchoscope is passed through the nose into the pharynx by way of an adapter attached to a standard anesthesia mask. Alternatively, the bronchoscope can be passed through an LMA if visualization of the pharynx is not required. The larynx is viewed with the patient breathing spontaneously so that vocal cord movement can be observed; then the anesthesia is deepened and the bronchoscope passed into the trachea. The trachea and bronchi are viewed and, when indicated, bronchoalveolar lavage or bronchial biopsy can be performed.

Rigid bronchoscopy is preferred when direct ventilation of the trachea is required and/or when foreign bodies (FBs) need to be removed. It also can be used for Dx of airway lesions. Direct laryngoscopy is performed and topical anesthetic is applied to the larynx and trachea. The rigid bronchoscope is passed through the vocal cords into the trachea. The anesthesia tubing is connected to the bronchoscope and the patient is ventilated through the scope. If a FB is present, the telescope within the bronchoscope will be removed and optical forceps inserted through the bronchoscope to remove the FB. During the time when the telescope is being changed, a leak will be present in the ventilation system.

Usual preop diagnosis: Airway obstruction; stridor; bronchial FB; pneumonia (requiring bronchoalveolar lavage); tracheal or bronchial lesion

Flexible or rigid esophagoscopy can be performed for diagnostic or therapeutic (removal of FB) purposes. Flexible esophagoscopy can be performed under sedation; however, GETA is preferred for rigid esophagoscopy. The esophagoscope is inserted through the mouth into the esophagus, and the entire length of the esophagus is viewed. If a FB is to be removed with the rigid esophagoscope, the telescope and forceps are passed through the lumen of the esophagoscope. If a FB (especially food stuff) is to be removed with the flexible esophagoscope, the scope may need to be passed several times.

Esophageal dilation may be performed in one of several ways. Balloon dilation can be performed with the flexible esophagoscope. Alternatively, a guide wire can be passed through the esophagoscope, then Savary/Gilliard dilators, in successively larger sizes, are passed over the wire. Another option is to remove the esophagoscope after the stenosis has been visualized; then, Maloney or Hurst dilators are passed blindly through the mouth and into the esophagus. Care must be taken to avoid accidental extubation of the patient while the dilators are being inserted and removed.

Usual preop diagnosis: GERD; esophageal FB; esophageal stricture

SUMMARY OF PROCEDURES

	Bronchoscopy	Esophagoscopy
Position	Patient supine; table turned 90°	⇐
Unique considerations	Ventilate through rigid bronchoscope. Ventilate via mask with adapter for flexible bronchoscope or via LMA. Dexamethasone (0.5 mg/kg) may be indicated, if glottic or subglottic edema is present.	Observe for accidental extubation. ETT taped to left side of mouth.
Antibiotics	None	⇐
Surgical time	10 min–1.5 h	15 min–1 h
EBL	None	< 10 mL
Postop care	Watch for airway compromise; PACU.	PACU
Mortality	Rare	⇐
Morbidity	Laryngospasm Laryngeal edema Dental trauma	Esophageal perforation Bleeding ⇐
Pain score	3–4	3–4

PATIENT POPULATION CHARACTERISTICS

Age range	Newborn+
Male:Female	1:1
Incidence	Common
Associated conditions	Bronchoscopy requiring bronchial alveolar lavage (BAL): immunocompromised patient Esophageal stricture: tracheoesophageal fistula (TEF) Esophageal FB: esophageal stricture

ANESTHETIC CONSIDERATIONS

See Anesthetic Considerations following Laryngoscopy, Supraglottoplasty, Excision of Laryngeal Lesions, p. 1188.

LARYNGOSCOPY, SUPRAGLOTTOPLASTY, EXCISION OF LARYNGEAL LESIONS

SURGICAL CONSIDERATIONS

Description: **Flexible laryngoscopy** typically is performed in the clinic setting, but may be performed in the OR in an unstable or uncooperative child. The patient should be breathing spontaneously, and will be in a sitting (with support) or supine position. Topical anesthesia and vasoconstrictors are applied to the nose; then the scope is passed through the nose into the pharynx, and the larynx is viewed. Vocal cord function is best assessed with the child only mildly sedated.

Diagnostic direct laryngoscopy is performed with the child in a supine position, table turned 90°, with a small shoulder roll in place. The laryngoscope is introduced and, with a lifting motion, a thorough exam of the oropharynx, hypopharynx, and larynx is performed. If more than a brief exam is to take place, the vocal cords are anesthetized with topical lidocaine to help prevent laryngospasm. A telescope (often connected via camera to a video monitor), or bronchoscope, may be passed through the vocal cords to observe the trachea and major bronchi.

Microlaryngoscopy with removal/ablation of laryngeal lesions—most commonly papillomas, nodules, or polyps—is accomplished by suspending the laryngoscope from the Mayo stand or OR table, using a suspension apparatus. The patient continues to breathe spontaneously or is paralyzed and jet-ventilated. Papillomas may be removed with a cup forceps, microdebrider, or laser. When the laser is used, the patient's eyes and face are covered with a damp cloth. OR personnel must wear protective glasses. A microscope with the laser attached is positioned so that the laser beam passes through the laryngoscope onto the vocal folds. Alternatively, the laser may be held by the surgeon and passed through an optical fiber.

Young infants with severe laryngomalacia may undergo a **supraglottoplasty** for relief of airway obstruction. The laryngoscope is suspended and the laser or microlaryngeal instruments are used to remove redundant aryepiglottic fold tissue.

Usual preop diagnosis: Diagnostic laryngoscopy: hoarseness; airway obstruction; stridor. Operative laryngoscopy: laryngeal papillomas; laryngeal nodules; laryngeal web; laryngeal polyps; subglottic hemangioma or cysts; severe laryngomalacia

SUMMARY OF PROCEDURE	
Position	Supine; table turned 90°; shoulder roll
Special instrumentation	± Jet ventilation; laryngoscope suspension apparatus; video equipment; operating microscope
Unique considerations	Potential laser precautions; patient usually not intubated; dexamethasone 0.5–1.0 mg/kg to prevent laryngeal edema; laryngeal topical lidocaine 0.4 mg/kg.
Antibiotics	None
Surgical time	15–90 min
EBL	< 5 mL
Postop care	Observe for airway obstruction in PACU.

SUMMARY OF PROCEDURE (cont'd)	
Mortality	Rare
Morbidity	Laryngospasm Laryngeal edema Dental trauma
Pain score	3–5

PATIENT POPULATION CHARACTERISTICS	
Age range	Newborn +
Male:Female	1:1
Incidence	Occasional
Etiology	Papillomas: Most commonly, viral infection contracted from mother during vaginal delivery Nodules, polyps: Vocal abuse, gastropharyngeal reflux Subglottic hemangioma: Unknown Subglottic cyst: Prior intubation Laryngeal cysts, webs: Congenital malformation Laryngomalacia: Unknown
Associated conditions	Chronic hoarseness, stridor; GERD; FTT

ANESTHETIC CONSIDERATIONS

(Procedures covered: bronchoscopy; esophagoscopy; laryngoscopy; supraglottoplasty; excision of laryngeal lesions)

PREOPERATIVE

Direct laryngoscopy (DL) is performed most commonly for patients with stridor. In infants, stridor is most often 2° laryngomalacia, with vocal cord paralysis and obstructive airway lesions being less common. Patients with severe laryngomalacia and those with post-transplant lymphoproliferative disease involving the epiglottis may undergo supraglottoplasty. Older children may present with stridor 2° laryngeal masses or papillomatosis, for which laser excision may be performed. A careful H&P is contributory to Dx, after which flexible laryngoscopy in the ENT clinic can be confirmatory.

Laryngoscopy and **rigid bronchoscopy** also are performed for the removal of airway foreign bodies (FBs). A Hx of choking and/or coughing while eating is usually elicited. Children may present with agitation, wheezing, and cyanosis. This condition constitutes a true surgical emergency and the patient should be taken to the OR as soon as possible.

Airway/ Respiratory	Stridor usually is worsened with crying or agitation, and often is less severe during sleep.
Dental	Any loose teeth may be dislodged.
Laboratory	No routine tests indicated. In stable patients with suspected FB aspiration, CXR may be obtained.
Premedication	Because stridor often is decreased during quiet breathing and sleep, premedication with oral midazolam is usually beneficial in patients > 9 mo. Children with FB aspiration generally should not be given po medications. They may benefit from small doses of iv midazolam. EMLA or ELA-max® cream may be applied 45 or 20 min (respectively) in advance to iv sites for topical anesthesia.

INTRAOPERATIVE

Anesthetic technique: GA. Primary and backup plans for airway management during the procedure should be discussed in detail with the ENT surgeon in advance of anesthetic induction.

Induction	Mask induction is followed by placement of an iv catheter, if not already in place. In cases where vocal cord function must be evaluated, spontaneous breathing is maintained under sevoflurane in 100% O_2. Alternatively, propofol (2–3 mg/kg) ± ketamine (1–2 mg/kg) may be used for induction followed by a continuous infusion (see below).	
Maintenance	Before removal of the face mask for DL, a deep level of anesthesia is achieved. During DL, blow-by O_2 is administered. For patients in whom vocal cord function must be assessed a gradual reduction of inhalational anesthesia or an iv anesthetic infusion should →↑ vocal cord excursion. Supraglottoplasty and laser excision of laryngeal lesions may be performed with intermittent mask anesthesia. Propofol ± remifentanil or ketamine may be used, thereby avoiding contamination of the OR with inhaled anesthetics while providing continuous anesthesia. In general, the trachea is not intubated, as even a small ETT will interfere with the surgical procedure. For patients who are paralyzed or hypoventilating, jet ventilation may be maintained using a Sanders jet ventilator (see Fig 3-4, p. 199). Intermittent jets of 100% O_2 are delivered with a high-pressure (40–55 psi) gas source through a tube incorporated into the laryngoscope blade. As the jet is pointed toward the glottic opening, gas is entrained by the Venturi effect. Manual jet ventilation is performed while chest excursion is observed to ensure that excessive inflating pressures and volumes are avoided. During jet ventilation, anesthesia is maintained with iv agents. Propofol is infused with remifentanil or ketamine. (Remifentanil 0.1 mg may be added to each 10 mL of propofol in a single syringe; e.g., for a propofol infusion of 100 mcg/kg/min, remifentanil 0.1 mcg/kg/min is delivered. Ketamine 1–3 mg/mL of propofol may be added as an alternative to remifentanil). **NB:** fire hazard during laser surgery is minimal in the absence of a combustible material (e.g., plastic) in the field. An FiO_2 of 1.0 may, therefore, be used safely, unless a plastic ETT is in place. For selected laser procedures involving the tissues around the glottis, a metal or metal-wrapped ETT may be used. When a plastic ETT is in place, the lowest possible FiO_2 is used (O_2/air mixture) to maintain an acceptable SpO_2. During rigid bronchoscopy, ventilation is performed through a side port of the bronchoscope. Assisted, spontaneous ventilation under deep inhalational anesthesia may be maintained. Alternatively, iv anesthesia with or without muscle relaxation may be preferred, as described above. For FB cases, maintenance of spontaneous ventilation generally is preferred to avoid distal displacement of the FB. Gentle, assisted ventilation may be required, however, to ensure adequate oxygenation and ventilation.	
Emergence	A conventional ETT sometimes is placed after removal of the laryngoscope or bronchoscope, as laryngospasm following these procedures is common. Tracheal extubation is performed with the patient fully awake and following complete reversal of neuromuscular blockade, if applicable.	
Blood and fluid requirements	IV: 22 ga × 1 NS/LR @ 3–5 mL/kg/h	Blood loss is minimal.
Monitoring	Standard monitors (see p. D-1).	
Positioning	Table rotated 90° ✓ and pad pressure points. ✓ eyes.	Shoulder roll/neck extension for surgery Eyes covered with wet sponges or goggles when laser in use.
Complications	Hypoventilation Hypoxemia Airway injury Pneumothorax	Adjust Sanders jet; mask ventilation prn. 2° jet ventilation, DL/bronchoscope

Complications (cont'd)	Laryngospasm Eye injury Airway fire	Rx: 100% O_2, CPAP vs manual ventilation/PEEP Remove ETT; irrigate with NS; resume ventilation with 100% O_2 when fire extinguished.

POSTOPERATIVE

Complications	Dental trauma Bleeding Eye trauma Pneumothorax	
Pain management	Acetaminophen (10–15 mg/kg) po q 6 h ± Hydrocodone 0.15 mg/kg or codeine 1 mg/kg q 4 h	
Tests	CXR	If respiratory distress or ↓ SpO_2 present.

Suggested Readings

1. Farrell PT: Rigid bronchoscopy for foreign body removal: anaesthesia and ventilation. *Paediatr Anaesth* 2004; 14(1):84–9.
2. Jaggar SI, Haxby E: Sedation, anaesthesia and monitoring for bronchoscopy. *Paediatr Respir Rev* 2002; 3(4):321–7.
3. Naguib ML, Streetman DS, Clifton S, et al: Use of laryngeal mask airway in flexible bronchoscopy in infants and children. *Pediatr Pulmonol* 2005; 39(1):56–63.
4. Nicklaus PJ, Kelley PE: Management of deep neck infection. Review. *Pediatr Clin North Am* 1996; 43(6):1277–96.
5. Shott SR: Down syndrome: analysis of airway size and a guide for appropriate intubation. *Laryngoscope* 2000; 110(4):585–92.
6. Thompson DM: Abnormal sensorimotor integrative function of the larynx in congenital laryngomalacia: a new theory of etiology. *Laryngoscope* 2007; 117(6 Pt 2 Suppl 114):1–33.
7. Weeks DG: Laboratory and clinical description of the use of jet-Venturi ventilator during laser microsurgery of the glottis and subglottis. *Anesth Rev* 1985; 12:32–6.
8. Yellon RF: Prevention and management of complications of airway surgery in children. *Paediatr Anaesth* 2004; 14(1):107–11.
9. Zalzal GH: Stridor and airway compromise. *Pediatr Clin North Am* 1989; 36:1389–1402.

REMOVAL OF BRANCHIAL CLEFT CYST OR THYROGLOSSAL DUCT CYST

SURGICAL CONSIDERATIONS

Description: Branchial cleft cysts and tracts typically present in the lateral neck; thyroglossal duct cysts, in the midline. Removal consists of making an incision in the neck around the opening of the tract (if present), or over the palpable cyst, and following the tract superiorly to its origin. A **Sistrunk procedure** is performed in the case of a thyroglossal duct cyst, and involves the removal of the middle section of the hyoid bone.

Usual preop diagnosis: Branchial cleft cyst; thyroglossal duct cyst

SUMMARY OF PROCEDURE	
Position	Supine; head 180° from anesthesia; oral intubation
Incision	Horizontal neck
Antibiotics	Clindamycin 12 mg/kg or cefazolin 25 mg/kg

SUMMARY OF PROCEDURE (cont'd)	
Surgical time	45–90 min
EBL	10–50 mL
Postop care	Routine
Mortality	Rare
Morbidity	Bleeding/neck hematoma Infection Recurrence of cyst Damage to CN XI, XII
Pain score	4–6

PATIENT POPULATION CHARACTERISTICS	
Age range	Newborn–adult
Male:Female	1:1
Etiology	Congenital
Associated conditions	Branchio-oto-renal (BOR) syndrome

ANESTHETIC CONSIDERATIONS

See Anesthetic Considerations following Incision/Drainage of Deep Neck Abscess (p. 1192).

INCISION/DRAINAGE OF DEEP NECK ABSCESS

SURGICAL CONSIDERATIONS

Description: Children with deep neck abscesses (retropharyngeal, parapharyngeal, peritonsillar) are at risk for acute airway obstruction; therefore, the abscesses are drained on an emergent basis. Retropharyngeal and peritonsillar abscesses typically are drained through an intraoral approach; parapharyngeal abscesses, through an external neck approach. In each case, the child must be intubated orally and placed in the supine position. The anesthesiologist or otolaryngologist who is intubating the child must be prepared for abnormal pharyngeal anatomy 2° the abscess. Care must be taken that the abscess is not ruptured in the intubation process. In most cases, the child can be extubated immediately after the abscess is drained; however, in a small number of cases, the child may need to remain intubated until the pharyngeal edema subsides.

Usual preop diagnosis: Retropharyngeal, parapharyngeal, or peritonsillar abscess

SUMMARY OF PROCEDURE	
Position	Supine; table turned 90–180°; oral intubation
Incision	Intraoral (retropharyngeal or peritonsillar abscess); lateral neck (parapharyngeal abscess)
Unique considerations	Acute airway obstruction can occur with induction. Care must be taken to avoid rupture of abscess on intubation; ± dexamethasone 0.5 mg/kg.
Antibiotics	Clindamycin 10 mg/kg

Pediatric Surgery

SUMMARY OF PROCEDURE (cont'd)	
Surgical time	30–90 min
EBL	< 30 mL
Postop care	May remain intubated postop.
Mortality	Rare
Morbidity	Aspiration (if abscess ruptures spontaneously) Airway obstruction 2° aspiration or edema Bleeding
Pain score	5

PATIENT POPULATION CHARACTERISTICS	
Age range	Most common, 6 mo–3 yr; can occur at any age.
Male:Female	1:1
Incidence	Uncommon
Etiology	URI

ANESTHETIC CONSIDERATIONS

(Procedures covered: excision of branchial cleft and thyroglossal duct cyst; incision/drainage of neck abscess)

PREOPERATIVE

These patients generally are otherwise healthy children. A cystic hygroma (cystic lymphangioma), as with other neck masses, may cause airway obstruction and difficult intubation.

Respiratory	The size and extent of the neck mass should be defined carefully in an effort to detect the potential for airway compromise and to avoid soft-tissue trauma during intubation, with consequent acute airway obstruction. Inspiratory stridor suggests supraglottic obstruction, while expiratory stridor is associated with subglottic/intrathoracic obstruction. These patients should have had prior CT/MRI imaging; scans and anesthesia records for these studies should be reviewed. **Tests:** CXR; CT/MRI
Cardiovascular	Cervical masses may be adherent to and/or cause compression of the great vessels. **Tests:** CT/MRI
Hematologic	T&C for cystic hygroma, or if a cervical mass involves great vessels or extends into the mediastinum. **Tests:** Hct
Laboratory	Other tests as indicated from H&P.
Premedication	If > 9–12 mo and asymptomatic, midazolam (0.5–0.75 mg po) 30 min prior to arrival in OR. Avoid all premedication in patients with significant potential for airway compromise.

INTRAOPERATIVE

Anesthetic technique: GETA

Induction	Standard pediatric induction (see p. D-1) in patients without airway compromise. When airway obstruction is present, iv should be secured prior to mask induction, which may be done with sevoflurane in 100% O_2. As the plane of anesthesia deepens, gently assist ventilation. Give atropine (0.01–0.02 mg/kg iv) prior to laryngoscopy. If partial airway obstruction exists, maintain spontaneous ventilation with CPAP and perform laryngoscopy at ~3 MAC of volatile agent. FOB should be available. Have full range of ETT sizes available, since airway narrowing may be present. Once airway is secured, proceed with neuromuscular blockade (e.g., rocuronium 0.6–1.0 mg/kg or vecuronium 0.1 mg/kg).	
Maintenance	Standard pediatric maintenance (see p. D-2). Surgeon may infiltrate incision with local anesthetic. Limit lidocaine to 5 mg/kg when used without epinephrine, or 7 mg/kg when used with epinephrine, and bupivacaine to 2.5 mg/kg.	
Emergence	Reverse neuromuscular blockade with neostigmine (0.07 mg/kg iv) and atropine (0.02 mg/kg iv). Extubate when fully awake.	
Blood and fluid requirements	Minimal blood loss usually IV: 20–22 ga × 1 Great vessel involvement: IV: 20 ga × 1–2 NS/LR @ 3 mL/kg/h	Minimal 3rd-space losses. Each mL blood loss can be replaced with 3 mL NS/LR. When great vessels involved, place at least 1 iv in lower extremity. Blood loss can be quite sudden; have blood available in OR.
Monitoring	Standard monitors (see p. D-1). ± Arterial line, 22 ga	An arterial line is used when there is risk of large blood loss or periop airway compromise.
Positioning	✓ and pad pressure points. ✓ eyes.	
Complications	ETT dislodged/loss of airway Laryngospasm Bronchospasm Hemorrhage	ETT must be secured carefully. Liberal use of benzoin adherent. Avoid tension on ETT by circuit hoses. Hold ETT during surgeon's intraoral examination to prevent accidental extubation.

POSTOPERATIVE

Complications	Subglottic edema Upper airway obstruction from Edema related to tumor resection Recurrent laryngeal nerve injury	Dexamethasone (0.5–1 mg/kg iv) and nebulized racemic epinephrine (1.25%) with mist O_2 to treat subglottic edema.
Pain management	Morphine (0.025–0.1 mg/kg iv q 2–4 h) Acetaminophen (10–15 mg/kg po/pr q 6 h)	The majority of these procedures are performed on outpatient basis (except cystic hygroma).

Suggested Readings

1. Gregory GA, ed: *Pediatric Anesthesia,* 4th edition. Churchill Livingstone, New York: 2002.
2. Motoyama EK, Davis PC, eds: *Smith's Anesthesia for Infants and Children,* 5th edition. CV Mosby, St. Louis: 1990.
3. Tapper D: Head and neck-sinuses and masses. In *Pediatric Surgery.* Ashcraft KW, Holder TM, eds. WB Saunders, Philadelphia: 1993, 923–34.

LARYNGOTRACHEAL RECONSTRUCTION, CRICOTRACHEAL RESECTION, LARYNGOTRACHEOPLASTY

SURGICAL CONSIDERATIONS

Description: A **laryngotracheal reconstruction** (LTR, laryngotracheoplasty) or **cricotracheal resection** (CTR) is performed in the patient with moderate-to-severe subglottic stenosis. Typically, the procedure starts with a diagnostic bronchoscopy. In most of these patients, a tracheotomy will already be present. During the procedure, the tracheotomy tube may be switched for an anode tube, which is sutured or taped to the chest. A horizontal neck incision is made over the cricoid cartilage. The strap muscles are separated in the midline, and the laryngeal cartilage and trachea are exposed. In a LTR a vertical incision (laryngofissure) is made through the inferior portion of the thyroid cartilage, through the cricoid cartilage, and down to the tracheotomy site. Either before or after the airway is exposed, costal cartilage, auricular cartilage, or thyroid cartilage will be harvested for use as a graft. The cartilage graft is then sutured into the anterior airway, keeping the laryngofissure incision open. Sometimes, a posterior cartilage graft is necessary in a severely stenotic airway, and this is placed after making an incision through the posterior cricoid. The initial exposure for a CTR is the same as a LTR but instead of placing a cartilage graft(s), the anterior portion of the cricoid cartilage and stenotic portion of the trachea are removed and the trachea pulled superiorly and sutured to the thyroid and remaining cricoid cartilages.

In a single-stage procedure, the ETT is removed intraop before the anterior cartilaginous incisions are closed, and replaced with an oral or nasal ET tube. This ETT is kept in place for 2–7 d as a stent around which the airway heals. In a two-stage procedure, the tracheotomy tube is kept in place. In this circumstance, there may be a stent superior to the tracheotomy tube, or a T-shaped tracheotomy tube may be used.

A **cricoid split** is most commonly performed in the NICU baby who fails extubation due to subglottic stenosis. Diagnostic bronchoscopy is performed; then the baby is reintubated or the bronchoscope is left in the airway and the procedure is performed over the bronchoscope. A laryngofissure is performed but no cartilage graft placed. Typically, an ETT 1/2 size larger than the previously placed ETT is inserted.

Usual preop diagnosis: Subglottic stenosis, subglottic hemangioma

SUMMARY OF PROCEDURE	
Position	Supine, shoulder roll
Incision	Horizontal neck
Unique considerations	After the cut is made into the airway, a leak may be present, depending on position of the cuff (if present).
Antibiotics	Clindamycin 10 mg/kg
Surgical time	Laryngotracheal reconstruction (LTR, laryngotracheoplasty), Cricotracheal reconstruction 1.5–4 hours Cricoid split: 45 min
EBL	5–30 mL
Mortality	Rare
Morbidity	Pneumothorax Bleeding Infection Stent or ETT dislodgement Residual/recurrent subglottic stenosis
Pain score	4–6; 6–8 if costal cartilage harvested.

PATIENT POPULATION CHARACTERISTICS	
Age range	Newborn–adult
Male:Female	1:1
Incidence	Rare
Etiology	ETT intubation; congenital
Associated conditions	Prematurity with prolonged NICU course

ANESTHETIC CONSIDERATIONS

PREOPERATIVE

These procedures are performed in patients with subglottic stenosis with a lesion that is either congenital or acquired. Congenital subglottic stenosis varies with regard to the length of trachea involved and the degree of stenosis. Segmental stenosis may occur in the region of the cricoid cartilage, midtrachea, or just above the carina. Sx are severe retractions, especially with agitation or intercurrent URI, dyspnea, and stridor. If the stenotic segment is short and severe, excision with primary anastomosis may be performed. If the involved segment is long, tracheoplasty is usually performed.

Acquired subglottic stenosis occurs as a complication of prolonged tracheal intubation and mechanical ventilation, most commonly in premature neonates with severe lung disease (infant respiratory distress syndrome [IRDS]). The stenotic lesion usually is limited to the level of the cricoid cartilage, and is treated with the cricoid split procedure. In addition to tracheal stenosis, tracheomalacia may be present.

Respiratory	Patients may be intubated and mechanically ventilated in the PICU. A variable degree of lung disease may be present; some patients may be on minimal ventilatory support, while others may require relatively high F_iO_2 and/or inflating pressures. Some patients will have an indwelling tracheostomy tube that bypasses the stenotic lesion, and may be cared for at home. **Tests:** As indicated from H&P.
Cardiovascular	Although not common, cor pulmonale with RVH may be present 2° chronic lung disease.
Hematologic	Anemia is common, especially in infants with chronic lung disease. **Tests:** Hct
Premedication	Infants in PICU usually are receiving a regimen of sedative and analgesia drugs. These should be continued until the patient is transported to the OR, with supplemental doses given preop as needed. Tolerance may be present, and drug doses should be titrated to achieve an adequate level of sedation.

INTRAOPERATIVE

Anesthetic technique: GETA

Induction	In intubated or trached patients with iv access, an iv induction is performed; otherwise, a mask induction is done with inhalation agents. Care should be taken to preserve upper airway patency, as even mild obstruction tends to exacerbate tracheal collapse. Following induction, tracheal intubation is performed with an ETT smaller than normal for age. In patients with severe stenosis, an ETT as small as 2.5 mm may be required. A cuffed tube is recommended and the surgeon should be careful not to damage the cuff during the procedure. If prolonged sedation and mechanical ventilation are planned postop, central venous access should be considered.

Maintenance	Plans for postop mechanical ventilation are discussed with the surgeon. In those patients for whom mechanical ventilation is planned for > 24 h, high-dose opioid anesthesia is appropriate (e.g., fentanyl 20–50 mcg/kg), as well as a long-acting muscle relaxant (pancuronium). A mixture of air and O_2 is used to minimize the risk of airway fire.	
Emergence	The majority of patients are transported to the PICU with indwelling ETT and residual sedation, narcosis, and neuromuscular blockade. These patients should be transported with iv sedation (propofol, benzodiazepine, or dexmedetomidine). Emergent reintubation poses a higher risk in these patients should an accidental extubation occur.	
Blood and fluid requirements	IV: 24 or 22 ga × 1 NS/LR @ maintenance	Blood loss < 30 mL
Monitoring	Standard monitors (see p. D-1).	
Positioning	✓ and pad pressure points. ✓ eyes.	
Complications	Tracheal edema Injury to neck structures: Trachea Vascular structures Recurrent laryngeal nerve injury	Rx: dexamethasone (0.5–1 mg/kg)

POSTOPERATIVE

Complications	Tracheal disruption (leak)	Presents with subcutaneous emphysema of the neck, face and chest wall.
	Recurrent laryngeal nerve injury	May cause vocal cord dysfunction.
Sedation/ analgesia	Heavy sedation	To minimize head and neck movement and tracheal wound disruption while ETT is in place.

Suggested Readings

1. Allen TH, Stevens IM: Prolonged endotracheal intubation in infants and children. *Br J Anaesth* 1985; 37:566–73.
2. Cotton RT: Pediatric laryngotracheal stenosis. *J Pediatr Surg* 1984; 19:699.
3. Vinograd I, Klim B, Efrati Y: Airway obstruction in neonates and children: surgical treatment. *J Cardiovasc Surg* 1994; 35: 7–12.

Pediatric Surgery

CHOANAL ATRESIA REPAIR

SURGICAL CONSIDERATIONS

Description: Infants born with bilateral choanal atresia typically have severe airway distress shortly following birth, because neonates are obligate nose breathers. The distress resolves after the child is intubated or a McGovern nipple (large nipple with cross-cuts in the end) or oral airway is positioned in the oral cavity. These infants undergo primary repair of the atresia within the first few days of life. Children with unilateral choanal atresia usually do not have severe respiratory distress and, thus, surgery is often postponed until a later age.

Intranasal repair involves opening up the atretic area with choanal dilators, urethral sounds, a microdebrider or drill. Endoscopic sinus instruments are used to view the choanae and remove the posterior nasal septum. Sometimes an intranasal stent is placed. If a transpalatal repair is performed, a Dingman mouth gag is placed in the mouth, a palatal flap is raised and the posterior portion of the hard palate and posterior septum is removed. A stent is positioned in the nose. The infant should be able to breathe spontaneously through the nose at completion of either procedure.

Usual preop diagnosis: Bilateral or unilateral choanal atresia

SUMMARY OF PROCEDURE	
Position	Supine; rotate bed 90–180°
Incision	Intranasal or intraoral
Special instrumentation	Choanal dilators; Dingman mouth gag
Antibiotics	Clindamycin 10 mg/kg
Surgical time	30 min–2 h
EBL	< 10 mL
Postop care	Observation in PICU for respiratory distress
Mortality	Rare
Morbidity	Bleeding Pressure necrosis to nasal ala from stent Infection Airway obstruction if stents become malpositioned
Pain score	3–6

PATIENT POPULATION CHARACTERISTICS	
Age range	Newborn–young child
Male:Female	1:1
Incidence	Rare
Etiology	Congenital
Associated conditions	Coloboma, heart disease, atresia choanae, retarded growth, genital anomalies, and ear deformities (CHARGE) association (see Anesthetic Considerations, below).

ANESTHETIC CONSIDERATIONS

PREOPERATIVE

Because many neonates are nasal breathers, choanal atresia may present with cyanosis at rest, resolving with crying or placement of an oral airway. Unilateral atresia is usually asymptomatic; bilateral lesions usually → respiratory distress in the neonatal period, but occasionally are asymptomatic. Although choanal atresia is most commonly an isolated anomaly, it may present as part of the CHARGE association.

Respiratory	Classic findings include cyanosis at rest, resolving with crying.
Cardiovascular	When part of the CHARGE association, cardiac defects include tetralogy of Fallot, ASD, VSD, PDA, AV canal, or right-side aortic arch.
Neurologic	When part of the CHARGE association, a variety of CNS abnormalities may be present. Hypoxia 2° airway obstruction may cause CNS impairment and Sz.
Premedication	Repair of choanal atresia usually is performed in infancy, and premedication is not indicated.

INTRAOPERATIVE

Anesthetic technique: GETA

Induction	Standard pediatric induction (see p. D-1). Airway obstruction may develop during induction of anesthesia. Early placement of an oral airway is recommended to relieve airway obstruction. An oral RAE ETT is preferred, especially if a transpalatal repair is planned using a Dingman mouth retractor.	
Maintenance	Inhalational or iv anesthesia is maintained during the procedure. During the first mo of life, opioids (other than remifentanil) should be avoided generally because of the risk of postop respiratory depression. For infants undergoing repair after the first mo of life, small doses of fentanyl (1–2 mcg/kg) or morphine sulfate (0.05–0.1 mg/kg) may be given. Muscle relaxation does not need to be maintained following tracheal intubation.	
Emergence	Nasal stents placed following the repair must be secure and free of secretions prior to tracheal extubation. Patients must be fully awake and capable of maintaining patency of their oropharynx in the event of postop swelling and transient obstruction of the nasopharynx.	
Blood and fluid requirements	IV: 24 or 22 ga × 1 NS/LR @ maintenance	Blood loss is usually < 10 mL; may be greater in older infants.
Monitoring	Standard monitors (see p. D-1) .	
Positioning	✓ and pad pressure points. ✓ eyes.	
Complications	Airway obstruction Bleeding	2° obstruction or displacement of nasal stents into oral pharynx especially in older infants

POSTOPERATIVE

Complications	See Intraop Complications, above.	
Pain management	Acetaminophen po/pr	Small doses of opioid may be given iv immediately post-op, with special attention to avoid respiratory depression/ obstruction.

Suggested Readings

1. Harris J, Robert E, Kfallfen B: Epidemiology of choanal atresia with special reference to the CHARGE association. *Pediatrics* 1997; 99:363–7.
2. Menasse-Palmer L, Bogdanow A, Marion RW: Choanal atresia. *Pediatr Rev* 1995; 16:475–6.
3. Prescott CA: Nasal obstruction in infancy. *Arch Dis Child* 1995; 72:287–9.

PEDIATRIC TRACHEOSTOMY

SURGICAL CONSIDERATIONS

Description: A **tracheostomy** is performed in the infant or child with upper airway obstruction (subglottic stenosis, laryngeal web, etc.) or in the child in whom prolonged mechanical ventilation is anticipated. In most cases, the child will already be intubated and the procedure will be performed over the ETT. In selected infants, the tracheostomy can be performed with a rigid bronchoscope in the airway through which the patient is being ventilated. A midline horizontal neck incision is made just inferior to the cricoid cartilage. The dissection is carried out in the midline until the trachea is reached. In children, the tracheal incision is vertical. Stay sutures may be placed in the right and left sides of the trachea on either side of the incision to facilitate replacement of the tracheotomy tube should it become displaced. Alternatively, a **starplasty** can be performed where the tracheal incision is made in the shape of a "+", the skin incision an "x", and the skin is sutured to the trachea. A large air leak will be present as soon as the tracheal incision is made. As the ETT or bronchoscope is being removed, a tracheostomy tube is inserted in the neck. The ventilation tubing is moved and connected to the tracheotomy tube which is secured with neck sutures and/or ties around the neck. The starplasty has the advantage that in case the tracheotomy tube is dislodged accidentally, it can be fairly easily re-inserted, even on the first postoperative day, providing an additional safety factor over the conventional approach.

Usual preop diagnosis: Ventilator dependence; subglottic stenosis

SUMMARY OF PROCEDURE	
Position	Supine; head to anesthesia; shoulder roll; neck extended
Incision	Horizontal neck
Special instrumentation	Tracheostomy hook
Unique considerations	Patient is draped to allow easy access to ETT. When trachea is opened, a large air leak may be present.
Antibiotics	Clindamycin 10 mg/kg or cefazolin 25 mg/kg
Surgical time	30 min–1 h
EBL	< 10 mL
Postop care	Close observation in PICU. CXR immediately following procedure to r/o pneumothorax.
Mortality	Intraoperative: rare. Postop 1–3%, usually 2° tracheostomy tube plugging or dislodgement.
Morbidity	Pneumothorax Subcutaneous emphysema Bleeding Infection Plugging Skin abrasion around trach edges or trach ties in patient with short, chubby neck
Pain score	3–5

PATIENT POPULATION CHARACTERISTICS	
Age range	Newborn–adult
Male:Female	1:1
Incidence	Uncommon
Etiology	Anatomical airway obstruction; ventilatory dependence; high, spinal-cord, or head injury
Associated conditions	Prematurity; trauma

ANESTHETIC CONSIDERATIONS

See Anesthetic Considerations following Tracheostomy in Chapter 3.0 Otolaryngology (p. 187).

horizontal neck incision is made just inferior to the cricoid cartilage. The dissection is carried out in the midline until the trachea is reached. In children the tracheal incision is vertical. Stay sutures may be placed in the right and left sides of the trachea on either side of the incision to facilitate replacement of the tracheostomy tube should it become displaced. Alternatively, a starplasty can be performed where the tracheal incision is made in the shape of a "+", the skin incision an "X," and the skin is sutured to the trachea. A large air leak will be present as soon as the tracheal incision is made. As the ETT or bronchoscope is being removed, a tracheostomy tube is inserted in the neck. The ventilation tubing is moved and connected to the tracheostomy tube which is secured with neck sutures and/or ties around the neck. The starplasty has the advantage that in case the tracheostomy tube is dislodged accidentally it can be fairly easily re-inserted, even on the first postoperative day, providing an additional safety factor over the conventional approach.

Usual preop diagnosis: Ventilator dependence; subglottic stenosis

Position	Supine, arms to anesthesia, shoulder roll, neck extended
Incision	Horizontal neck
Special instrumentation	Tracheostomy tools
Unique considerations	Patient is draped to allow easy access to ETT. When trachea is opened, ... present.
Antibiotics	[illegible]
Surgical time	30 min–1 h
EBL	< 10 mL
Postop care	Close observation ... CXR immediately following procedure to r/o pneumothorax.
Mortality	[illegible]
Morbidity	Pneumothorax Subcutaneous emphysema Bleeding Infection Plugging
	Skin ulceration around tracheostomy ... with short, chubby neck

Comorbidities

Upper airway obstruction, ventilatory dependence, ... spinal cord or head injury, ... trauma

ANESTHETIC CONSIDERATIONS

See Anesthetic Considerations following Tracheostomy in Chapter 5.0 Otolaryngology (p. ...).

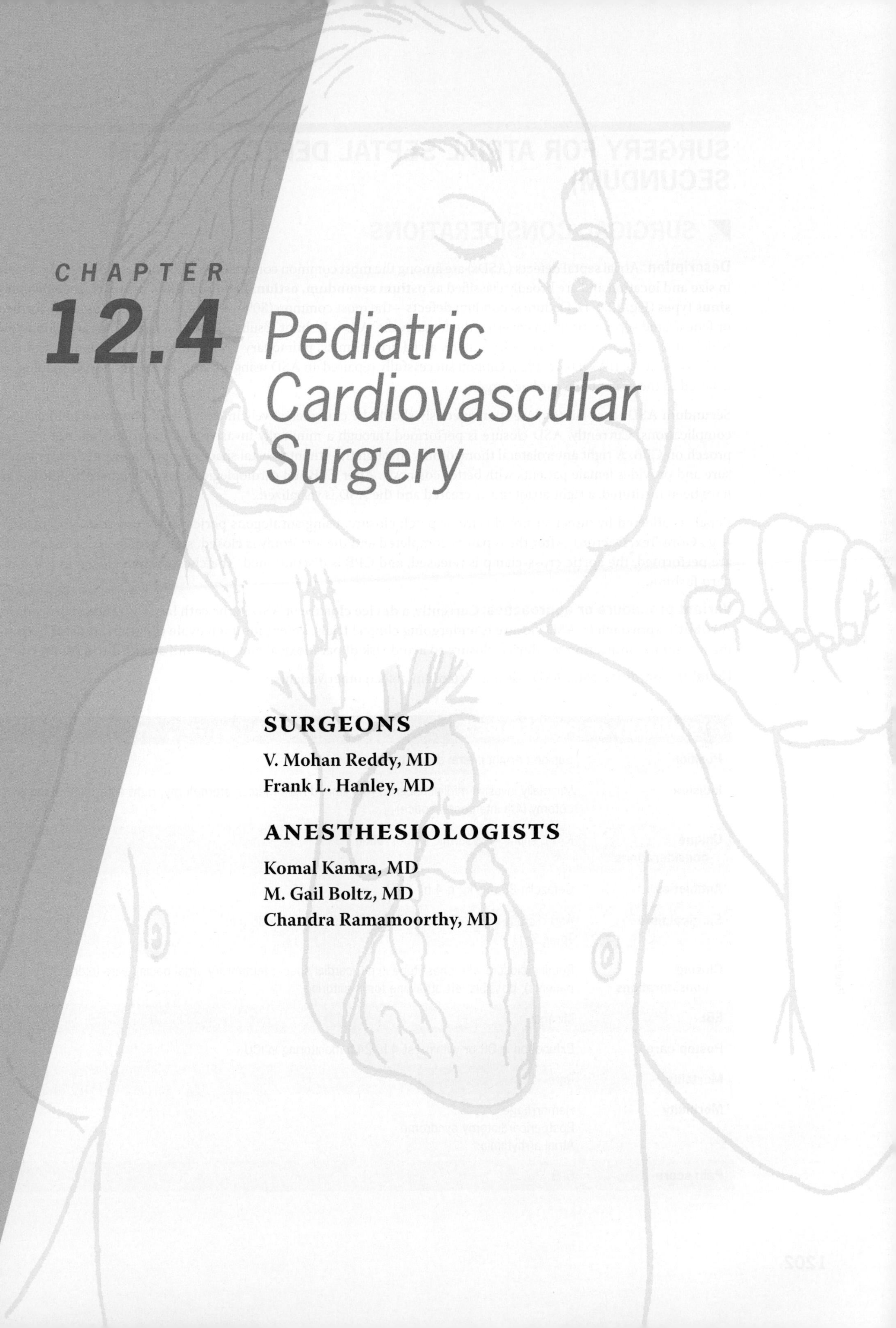

CHAPTER

12.4 Pediatric Cardiovascular Surgery

SURGEONS

V. Mohan Reddy, MD

Frank L. Hanley, MD

ANESTHESIOLOGISTS

Komal Kamra, MD

M. Gail Boltz, MD

Chandra Ramamoorthy, MD

SURGERY FOR ATRIAL SEPTAL DEFECT (OSTIUM SECUNDUM)

SURGICAL CONSIDERATIONS

Description: Atrial septal defects (ASDs) are among the most common congenital cardiac defects. ASDs vary widely in size and location and are broadly classified as **ostium secundum, ostium primum, sinus venosus,** and **coronary sinus** types (Fig. 12.4-1). Ostium secundum defects—the most common (80%)—result from an incompletely formed or fenestrated septum primum covering the fossa ovalis. A L→ R shunt results in augmented pulmonary blood flow which, if left uncorrected, may → RV failure, atrial arrhythmias, pulmonary HTN, and rarely, pulmonary vascular occlusive disease (PVOD). In 1953, Gibbon successfully repaired an ASD using a pump-oxygenator and, in doing so, ushered in the era of open cardiac surgery.

Secundum ASDs that fail to close spontaneously should be closed electively in early childhood to avoid long-term complications. Currently, ASD closure is performed through a minimally invasive midline partial sternotomy approach on CPB. A right anterolateral thoracotomy through the 4th intercostal space also provides satisfactory exposure and provides female patients with better cosmesis. After CPB and cardioplegic arrest or ventricular fibrillation have been instituted, a right atriotomy is created and the ASD is visualized.

Repair is affected by direct suture closure or patch closure, using autologous pericardium or prosthetic material (e.g., Gore-Tex, Dacron). After the repair is completed and the atriotomy is closed, standard de-airing maneuvers are performed, the aortic cross-clamp is released, and CPB is discontinued. The chest is then closed in the standard fashion.

Variant procedure or approaches: Currently, a **device closure** of ASD in the cath lab is a standard procedure. A **robotic approach** to ASD closure is undergoing clinical trials. Patent foramen ovale (PFO) in adults is becoming a common indication for device closure to avoid risk of paradoxical embolism and stroke during surgery.

Usual preop diagnosis: ASD; ostium secundum defect; other variants

SUMMARY OF PROCEDURE	
Position	Supine or right lateral decubitus (thoracotomy)
Incision	Minimally invasive midline incision with limited right median sternotomy; right anterolateral thoracotomy (4th intercostal space)
Unique considerations	R→ L shunt → systemic embolization
Antibiotics	Cefazolin 25 mg/kg q 4 h
Surgical time	Aortic cross-clamp or ventricular fibrillation time: 10–30 min Total: 2 h
Closing considerations	Routine closure with chest tube in pericardial space; temporary atrial pacing wire (older patients); possible left atrial line for monitoring
EBL	Minimal
Postop care	Extubation in OR or within 1st 4 h; 24-h monitoring in ICU
Mortality	Rare
Morbidity	Hemorrhage Postpericardiotomy syndrome Atrial arrhythmias
Pain score	6–8

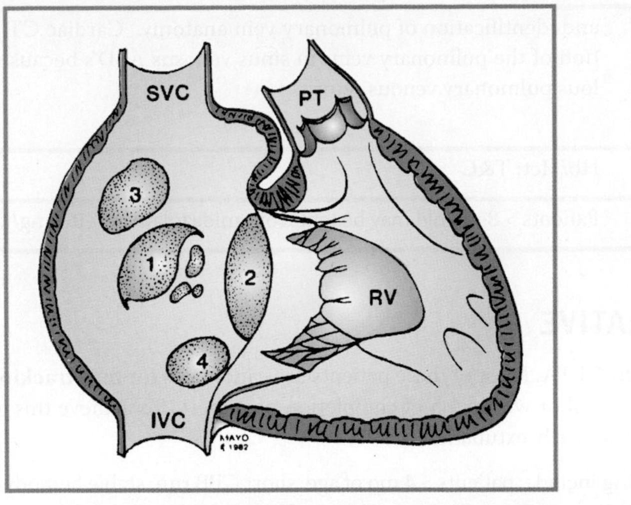

Figure 12.4-1. Location of ASDs, numbered in decreasing order of frequency: 1 = secundum; 2 = primum; 3 = sinus venosus; 4 = coronary sinus type. IVC = inferior vena cava; PT = pulmonary trunk; RV = right ventricle; SVC = superior vena cava. (Reproduced with permission from the Mayo Foundation for Education and Research.)

PATIENT POPULATION CHARACTERISTICS

Age range	Neonate–adults
Male:Female	1:2
Incidence	10–15% of congenital heart defects
Etiology	Unknown; sometimes associated with syndromes such as Holt-Oram.
Associated conditions	ASD may coexist with nearly any of the other recognized congenital cardiac anomalies, but is more commonly associated with pulmonary stenosis (10%), partial anomalous pulmonary venous return (7%), VSD (5%), PDA (3%), and mitral stenosis (2%). ASDs are also part of other malformations, including tricuspid atresia, total anomalous pulmonary venous connection (TAPVC), and mitral atresia.

ANESTHETIC CONSIDERATIONS

PREOPERATIVE

Pathophysiology	Although the secundum ASD is the most common, periop management varies little among all types of ASDs (including ostium primum, sinus venosus, and coronary sinus types). One principle guideline in all L→R shunts is the estimation of shunt flow: Q_p:Q_s. This is determined by the amount of pulmonary blood flow (Q_p), size of the defect, and the PVR and SVR. Patients are generally asymptomatic until the Q_p:Q_s ratio exceeds 3.0. As the shunt flow increases, Sx of pulmonary overcirculation may develop (e.g., failure to thrive, tachypnea at rest, and feeding difficulties). L→R shunt →↑ pulmonary blood flow (Q_p) →↑ PA pressures →↑ PVR → RV overload → RV failure. The larger the area of the defect, the greater the shunt.
Cardiovascular and Respiratory	Most infants with ASDs are asymptomatic. The ASDs are detected on cardiac auscultation (fixed splitting of S2). Young children may have h/o frequent URIs. Cyanosis is rare and indicates shunt reversal and development of pulmonary HTN. Surgical closure is advocated as these patients are at risk for paradoxical embolism, stroke, and bacterial endocarditis. Unlike ventricular septal defects (VSDs), ASDs rarely close spontaneously. Endovascular closure in the cath lab may be suitable for some patients, obviating the need for CPB. **Tests:** EKG: normal or RVH. CXR: cardiomegaly and ↑ pulmonary vascular markings. ECHO. TEE: essential for locating and estimating size of defect, other valvular abnormalities,

Cardiovascular and Respiratory (cont'd)	and identification of pulmonary vein anatomy. Cardiac CT may be indicated for delineation of the pulmonary veins in sinus venosus ASD's because of the association of anomalous pulmonary venous return.
Laboratory	Hb/Hct; T&C
Premedication	Patients > 8 mo old may benefit from midazolam 0.5–0.7 mg/kg po 20 min before induction.

INTRAOPERATIVE

Anesthetic technique: GETA. Most of these patients are candidates for **fast-tracking**—the practice of extubation of cardiac patients in the OR or within 4 h of completion of surgery. To achieve this goal, the anesthetic technique must be adjusted to permit early extubation.

Criteria for fast-tracking include: patients > 4 mo of age, short CPB run, stable hemodynamic profile, minimal inotropic support, normal acid-base status, and adequate surgical hemostasis. Patients who are pacemaker-dependent are not suitable candidates for fast-tracking. Generally, patients selected for fast-tracking have undergone repair of a secundum ASD, VSD (no evidence of postop pulmonary HTN), bidirectional Glenn and Fontan procedures, or a RV → PA conduit change. For patients with a single ventricle, resumption of spontaneous ventilation decreases intrathoracic pressure and improves the transthoracic (PA-LA) pressure gradient. This increases venous return and improves CO.

Induction	Following inhalation induction using sevoflurane (O_2/N_2O), an iv is placed and intubation facilitated with rocuronium (1 mg/kg). After ET intubation, an arterial line is placed for close BP monitoring. **Fast-track:** Intravenous techniques are used for fast-tracking patients who are not candidates for regional anesthesia (e.g., parent preference, spine abnormality, age). Inhalation induction (sevoflurane ± N_2O) is followed by placement of a PIV and arterial line. Fentanyl (2–5 mcg/kg) and a muscle relaxant (e.g., rocuronium 1 mg/kg) are administered and the airway is secured. Then, either an infusion of remifentanil (0.1–0.4 mcg/kg) is started or single bolus iv methadone (0.2 mg/kg; max dose 20 mg) is administered. Propofol may also be used after separation from CPB and in transport to the ICU, where it is weaned and discontinued prior to extubation. **Non fast-track:** For patients who are not candidates for fast-tracking, the standard anesthetic is fentanyl 20–40 mcg/kg in divided doses with supplemental isoflurane before and during CPB. Additional midazolam (0.1–0.3 mg/kg) may be administered to prevent recall and awareness. Smaller children generally tolerate an inhalation induction with sevoflurane in 50% N_2O + O_2. After induction, iv access is established and rocuronium (1 mg/kg), followed by volatile anesthetic and supplemental iv fentanyl. An iv induction should be used in patients with significant pulmonary HTN and/or RV failure. IV induction is accomplished with etomidate 0.1–0.3 mg/kg or ketamine 0.5–1 mg/kg, followed by a muscle relaxant (e.g., vecuronium 0.1 mg/kg).
Maintenance	In the maintenance of anesthesia, isoflurane may be used with iv techniques before, during, and after CPB. In patients in whom immediate postop extubation is planned, anesthesia is maintained using a volatile agent in air + O_2, N_2O is turned off after induction to avoid expansion of any intraop VAE. In patients with pulmonary HTN, RV failure and/or other medical conditions requiring postop mechanical ventilation, a high-dose narcotic technique may be appropriate (e.g., fentanyl 50–150 mcg/kg ± inhalation agent).
Emergence	If the choice is made to extubate the patient receiving remifentanil in the OR, isoflurane is terminated during skin closure, muscle relaxant is reversed, and the remifentanil is turned off when the dressing is applied. When the patient meets standard extubation criteria (e.g., –25 cmH_2O NIF, spontaneous ventilation, adequate sat), remove the ETT and document spontaneous ventilation. If the patient is not extubated in the OR, transport the patient to the ICU sedated with remifentanil (0.1–0.4 mcg/kg/min) or low-dose

Emergence (cont'd)	propofol (25–75 mcg/kg/min), and extubate in the ICU. If the patient received methadone, standard criteria for extubation are used. Vasodilators are usually not required for BP control. O_2, bag, mask, airway equipment, and emergency drugs should be available during transport.	
Blood and fluid requirements	IV: appropriate for patient's size × 1–2 LR @ TKO Blood warmer ✓ for air bubbles. T&C 1 U PRBC.	**NB:** It is critical to avoid iv bubbles in all patients with intracardiac shunts. Meticulous attention must be paid to clearing the iv tubing and stopcocks of any bubbles to avoid paradoxical air embolism and possible stroke. Have blood available in the OR. Blood transfusion may be required in patients < 10 kg.
Monitoring	Standard monitors (see p. D-1). Cerebral oximetry T (two sites) Arterial line CVP line Urinary catheter ACT monitoring TEE	ABG, electrolytes, and Hct should be checked as needed during the procedure. Place at least two O_2 probes to ensure readings during critical times. Avoid dorsalis pedis and posterior tibial arterial lines (inaccurate 2° spasm post-CPB). Femoral arterial line may be used. Double lumen CVP in IJ preferable. TEE monitoring is used to assess anatomy and repair. On CPB, if the aorta is not cross-clamped, monitor for intra-cardiac air.
Positioning	✓ and pad pressure points. ✓ eyes.	
Pre-CPB	Heparinization (200–400 U/kg) ✓ ACT > 480 sec. ✓ NMB. ✓ UO.	Heparin is added to the prime (1–3 U/mL). Confirm that antibiotics have been given 30–60 min before skin incision and repeat q 4–6 h per protocol.
CPB	Hypothermia ✓ adequate flow and pressure during CPB. Ventilation stopped ✓ face for venous congestion. ✓ ABG and ACT. ✓ UO. Blood should be available.	The patient is not actively cooled for secundum ASD closure. Temperature is allowed to drift to 33–34°C. Secundum ASD may be repaired using ventricular fibrillation instead of cardioplegia with aortic cross- clamping.
Transition off CPB	Rewarming Vasoactive infusions started at 32°C. Flush lines. Zero transducers. Suction ETT. Resume ventilation.	Surgeon will de-air heart, and this maneuver is monitored with TEE. Dopamine 3–5 mcg/kg/min. Observe inflation of both lungs.
Post-CPB	Reversal of heparin with protamine ✓ UO. ± Modified ultrafiltration (MUF)	1 mg of protamine will reverse 100 U of residual heparin (4 mg/kg may be needed in neonates). MUF uses the CPB machine to remove excess water and inflammatory mediators. It has been shown to transiently ↓ postop edema and improve cardiopulmonary function. This technique is not routinely performed at Stanford.
Complications	Air embolism (VAE) Supraventricular dysrhythmias Heart block Ventricular dysfunction	Potential for paradoxical embolization Likely 2° atriotomy

POSTOPERATIVE

Complications	Bleeding
Tests	ABG Electrolytes; Hct CXR

Suggested Readings

1. Allen HD, Driscoll DJ, Shaddy RE et al. *Moss and Adams' Heart Disease in Infants, Children, and Adolescents*, 7th edition. Lippincott Williams & Wilkins, Philadelphia: 2007.
2. Bent ST: Anesthesia for left-to-right shunt lesions. In: *Anesthesia for Congenital Heart Disease*, 1st edition. Andropoulos S, Andropoulos R, eds. Blackwell Futura, CITY: 2005, 297–317.
3. Castaneda AR, Jonas RA, Mayer JE Jr, et al: Atrial septal defect. In: *Cardiac Surgery of the Neonate and Infant*. EDITORS. WB Saunders, Philadelphia: 1994, 143–55.
4. Emmanouilides GC, Allen HD, Riemenschneider TA, et al: Atrial septal defects. In: *Clinical Synopsis of Moss and Adams' Heart Disease in Infants, Children, and Adolescents*. Williams & Wilkins, Baltimore: 1998, 243–52.
5. Kopf GS, Laks H: Atrial septal defects and cor triatriatum. In: *Glenn's Thoracic and Cardiovascular Surgery*, 6th edition. Baue AE, ed. Appleton & Lange, Stamford: 1996: 1115–25.
6. Mainwaring RD, Lamberti JJ: Atrial septal defects. In *Mastery of Cardiothoracic Surgery*. Kaiser LR, Kron IL, Spray TL, eds. Lippincott-Raven, Philadelphia: 1998, 677–86.
7. Reitz BA, Yuh DD, eds: *Congenital Cardiac Surgery*. McGraw-Hill, New York: 2002.
8. Torracca L, Ismeno G, Alfieri O: Totally endoscopic computer-enhanced atrial septal defect closure in six patients. *Ann Thorac Surg* 2001; 72(4):1354–7.
9. Wilson NJ, Smith J, Prommete B, et al: Transcatheter closure of secundum atrial septal defects with the amplatzer septal occluder in adults and children-follow-up closure rates, degree of mitral regurgitation and evolution of arrhythmias. *Heart Lung Circ* 2008; 17(4)318–24.

SURGERY FOR ATRIOVENTRICULAR CANAL DEFECT

SURGICAL CONSIDERATIONS

Description: Atrioventricular (A-V) canal defects comprise a spectrum of congenital cardiac anomalies stemming from the embryonic maldevelopment of endocardial cushions. This leads to the absence of septal tissue immediately above and below the level of the A-V valves and defects in the A-V valves in continuity with these septal defects. **Partial A-V canal defects** (or **ostium primum atrial septal defects**) involve the atrial septum and mitral valve, whereas **complete A-V canal defects** involve the atrial and ventricular septa and have a common atrioventricular valve. Intermediate or transitional A-V canal have varying degree of pathology between the above two common patterns. Pathophysiologically, these defects result in L → R shunting at the atrial and/or ventricular levels, leading to pulmonary HTN and CHF. A-V valvular insufficiency is also frequently observed with these defects, contributing to the early development of CHF.

Palliative repair of A-V canal defects consists of **pulmonary artery banding** (Fig. 12.4-2) to reduce excessive pulmonary blood flow. Palliation is rare and is reserved for very small infants with complicating conditions, such as RSV and other pneumonias. **Total correction** is now performed routinely, even in neonates. Repair consists of the closure of atrial and ventricular septal defects (VSDs) with closure of the cleft in the anterior leaflet of the mitral valve, and repair of associated defects, such as a patent ductus arteriosus (PDA) or secundum atrial septal defect (ASD). The septal defects may be repaired with either a **"two-patch technique,"** consisting of a Dacron or pericardial patch on the ventricular septum and pericardial patch on the atrial septum, or a single patch (pericardium) covering both ASDs and VSDs. A modified single patch technique where the A-V valve is plastered down to the ventricular septum is currently used by some surgeons.

Partial A-V canal defects: Exposure is obtained through a standard median sternotomy. CPB is instituted with aortic cross-clamping and cardioplegic arrest. Through a right atriotomy, the mitral valve cleft is sutured. A pericardial

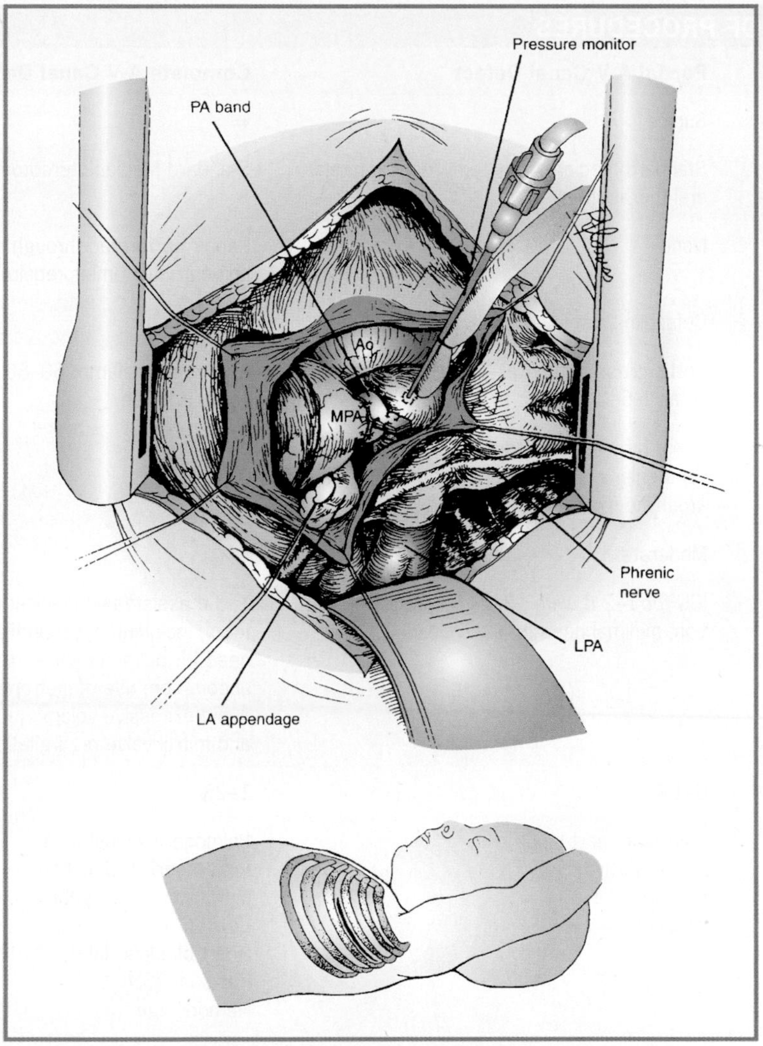

Figure 12.4-2. Placement of pulmonary artery band. PA = pulmonary artery; Ao = aorta; MPA = main pulmonary artery; LPA = left pulmonary artery; LA = left atrial. (Reproduced with permission from Kaiser LR, Kron IL, Spray TL, eds: *Mastery of Cardiothoracic Surgery*. Lippincott-Raven, Philadelphia: 1998.)

patch is placed across the top of the ventricular septum, around the coronary sinus orifice, and along the free edge of the superior portion of the ASD. The atriotomy is closed and the aorta unclamped after de-airing. The patient is rewarmed and weaned from bypass.

Complete A-V canal defects: Following median sternotomy, CPB is instituted with aortic cross-clamping and cardioplegic arrest. In the **single-patch technique,** one patch is used to close both the ASD and VSD components. The anterior and posterior bridging leaflets often are divided and resuspended to the patch, thereby creating two separate valves. The cleft in the left AV valve is usually closed. If AV valve regurgitation is present, repair is undertaken. In the two-patch technique, two separate patches are used to close the ASD and VSD, and the common AV valve is sandwiched in between the two patches. Repair of AV valve is the same in either technique. Closure of the right atrium, de-airing, aortic unclamping, rewarming, and resuscitation of the heart are commenced, and CPB is discontinued. Closure proceeds in the standard fashion. In ~5% of patients with complete A-V canal defects, tetralogy of Fallot (TOF) or left ventricular outflow tract obstruction (LVOTO) has to be addressed surgically.

Usual preop diagnosis: A-V canal defects (complete, intermediate, or partial); endocardial cushion defects

SUMMARY OF PROCEDURES

	Partial A-V Canal Defect	Complete A-V Canal Defect
Position	Supine	⇐
Incision	Standard median sternotomy/right anterolateral thoracotomy	Standard median sternotomy
Unique considerations	None	Repair performed through a right atriotomy; no ventriculotomies required.
Antibiotics	Cefazolin 25 mg/kg q 4 h	⇐
Surgical time	Aortic cross-clamp: 30–40 min Total: 1.5–2 h	Aortic cross-clamp: 60–80 min Total: 2.5–3 h
Closing considerations	Chest tube in pericardial space; temporary ventricular pacing wire; possibly right or left atrial line for monitoring	⇐
EBL	Moderate	⇐
Postop care	ICU for 1–2 d, with 12–24 h assisted ventilation; minimal need for inotropes.	1–3 d assisted ventilation; pulmonary HTN protocol, including hyperventilation and sedation; need for pulmonary vasodilators (e.g., NO) is uncommon; use of inotropes for adequate CO. Avoid excessive volume to prevent distension and mitral valve regurgitation.
Mortality	0–1%	1–2%
Morbidity	Transient heart block Atrial dysrhythmias Hemorrhage Infection	Pulmonary vasospasm Right heart dysfunction Mitral valve regurgitation Low CO Heart block/atrial dysrhythmias Residual VSD Hemorrhage
Pain score	6–10	6–8

PATIENT POPULATION CHARACTERISTICS

Age range	1–20 yr (usually 2–3 yr)	2–6 mo (occasionally older; rarely, adults)
Male:Female	1:1	⇐
Incidence	0.5–1% of congenital heart defects	⇐
Etiology	Down syndrome: Rare, in patients with partial A-V canal defect	Commonly associated with Down syndrome (75% in patients with complete A-V canal defect)
Associated conditions	Left A-V valve insufficiency	Pulmonary HTN, left A-V valve insufficiency, minor associated cardiac anomalies (e.g., PDA or ASD); major associated anomalies (e.g., TOF, LVOTO)

ANESTHETIC CONSIDERATIONS

PREOPERATIVE

Pathophysiology	A-V canal defects may be either partial or complete. The partial A-V canal has no interventricular communication and has an ostium primum ASD. There is often a cleft in the anterior leaflet of the mitral valve → MR. The complete A-V canal has communication at both the arterial and ventricular levels with a single A-V valve that is regurgitant. Like all L → R shunt lesions, the degree of shunt depends on relative resistances in the systemic and pulmonary circuits. Patients with large L → R shunts are at risk of developing pulmonary HTN, requiring early surgical correction.
Respiratory	Look for pulmonary congestion or any infectious process. Pulmonary HTN can be present in patients with partial or complete A-V canal defects. **Tests:** CXR: enlarged heart + increased pulmonary markings
Cardiovascular	Complete A-V canal → CHF and biventricular failure. **Tests:** ECG: RAE, RVE; ECHO diagnostic; rarely cardiac cath may be indicated to assess PVR.
Down syndrome	A-V canal defects account for 40% of cardiac defects in the Down syndrome patient. These patients are at risk of atlantoaxial instability (20%); therefore, avoid excessive flexion-extension of the head and neck. Additional airway considerations (subglottic stenosis, large tongue, hypotonia) make these patients unsuitable for fast-tracking and early extubation.
Laboratory	See ASD, p. 1204.
Premedication	Midazolam 0.5–0.75 mg/kg po.

INTRAOPERATIVE

Anesthetic technique: GETA

Induction	Typically, mask sevoflurane in air and O_2. If the iv is in place, ketamine 1–2 mg/kg or fentanyl 10 mcg/kg and rocuronium 1 mg/kg. Verify ETT position (see p. D-2). In children with Down syndrome, anticipate difficult airway and atlantoaxial instability. Avoid excessive neck flexion. In this population, The non-Down partial AV canal defects may be candidates for early or immediate extubation if the intracardiac defects are small and surgery uncomplicated.	
Maintenance	Air-oxygen with volatile anesthetic and narcotics is the standard. In patients requiring postop mechanical ventilation, fentanyl 50–100 mcg/kg total, rocuronium prn, and midazolam (0.1–0.2 mg/kg) ± volatile agent (FiO_2 = 1) is used.	
Emergence	Patients undergoing repair of complete A-V canal defects are seldom suitable for fast-tracking. On conclusion of procedure, the patient is taken to PICU, intubated, ventilated, sedated, and monitored. Transport to ICU.	
Blood and fluid requirements	IV: 22–24 ga × 2 LR @ TKO Blood products	See Table 12.4-2, p. 1226.
Monitoring	See ASD, p. 1205. TEE	TEE is used to assess left A-V valve regurgitation, valvular function, residual shunt, and ventricular function.
CPB	Management of CPB is discussed in Intraoperative Considerations for TOF, p. 1205.	In the immediate post-CPB period, TEE exam is valuable for evaluation of ventricular function and residual mitral valve regurgitation.

Complications	Air embolism	Avoid air embolism in A-V canal patients (shunt reversal → paradoxical embolization).
	A-V block, ventricular dysfunction	A-V block may be temporary 2° edema and/or cardioplegic arrest. Permanent injury can occur to the conduction system at the A-V node or bundle of His with repair of the VSD. Temporary atrial and ventricular pacing wires are placed.
	Persistent bleeding	
	Pulmonary HTN	See treatment for pulmonary HTN (see p. 430).

POSTOPERATIVE

Complications	Residual VSD/ASD AV valve regurgitation	
Tests	TEE	Analysis of post repair function is best done by TEE.

Suggested Readings

1. Allen HD, Driscoll DJ, Shaddy RE, et al., eds. *Moss and Adams' Heart Disease in Infants, Children, and Adolescents,* 7th edition. Lippincott Williams & Wilkins, Philadelphia: 2007.
2. Bent ST: Anesthesia for left-to-right shunt lesions. In *Anesthesia for Congenital Heart Disease,* 1st edition. Andropoulos S, Andropoulos R, eds. Blackwell Futura, 2005, 297–317.
3. Castaneda AR, Jonas RA, Mayer JE Jr, et al: Atrioventricular canal defect. In *Cardiac Surgery of the Neonate and Infant.* WB Saunders, Philadelphia: 1994, 167–86.
4. Kouchoukos NT, Blackstone EH, Doty DB, et al: Atrial septal defect. In *Kirklin, Barrett, Boyes Cardiac Surgery.* Churchill Livingstone, Philadelphia: 2003, 800–49.
5. Reitz BA, Yuh DD, eds: *Congenital Cardiac Surgery.* McGraw-Hill, New York: 2002.
6. Vick WG, Titus JL: Defects of the atrial septum including the atrioventricular canal. In *The Science and Practice of Pediatric Cardiology.* Garson A, Bricker JT, McNamara DG, eds. Lea & Febiger, Philadelphia: 1990.

SURGERY FOR VENTRICULAR SEPTAL DEFECT

SURGICAL CONSIDERATIONS

Description: Ventricular septal defect (VSD) is the most common congenital cardiac anomaly. VSDs can occur anywhere in the interventricular septum (Fig. 12.4-3). One of the most common locations is the perimembranous (conoventricular) in the region of membranous septum near the tricuspid and aortic valves. Supracristal (subarterial) defects are common in the Pacific Rim population. Muscular defects occur in the inlet, trabecular, or outlet muscular septum. A-V canal defects are present under the septal leaflet of the tricuspid valve. Physiologically, these defects result in L→ R shunting in proportion to the defect size. Untreated, this defect can → RV volume overload and CHF in infancy and irreversible pulmonary HTN later in life. As PVR rises, shunt reversal to a R→ L shunt can occur, producing hypoxemia and cyanosis; this is known as Eisenmenger's syndrome and occurs in ~10% of untreated, nonrestrictive VSDs (rare). Moderate-to-large VSDs that remain open > 6 mo of age should be closed. Severe, intractable CHF in infants refractory to medical therapy (e.g., diuretics, digoxin), or ↑ PVR in infants > 6 mo are indications for earlier VSD repair.

Lillehei, et al performed the first successful VSD repairs using normothermic cross-circulation in 1955. Kirklin subsequently described successful VSD closure using extra-corporeal circulation in 1957. VSD repair is performed now through a median sternotomy on CPB with bicaval cannulation. Deep hypothermia (18°C) with circulatory arrest is used in neonates < 1800 g to facilitate repair. After CPB and cardioplegic arrest have been instituted, a right atriotomy is created and the VSD is visualized by retracting the tricuspid valve leaflets. The VSD is then closed with a

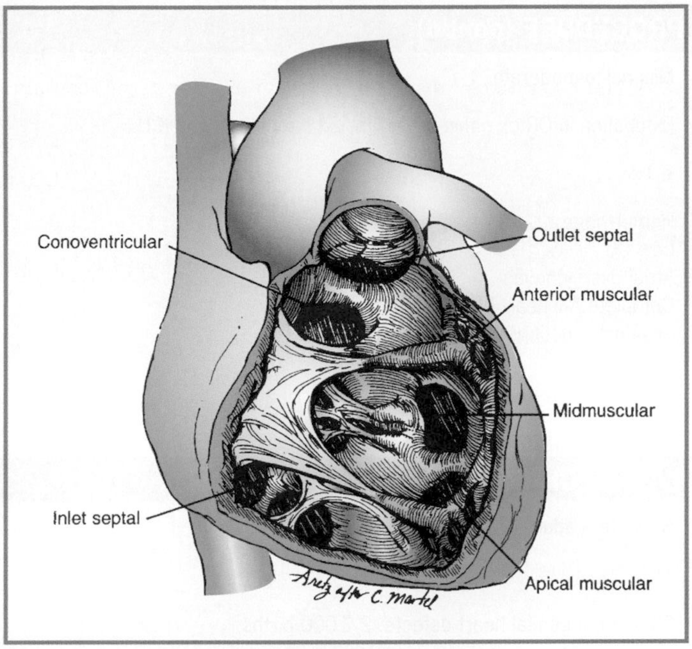

Figure 12.4-3. The right ventricular free wall has been resected to show the VSDs: conoventricular = perimembranous; conal septal = outlet septal (subpulmonary); inlet septal = A-V canal type. Muscular (trabecular) defects may be midmuscular, anterior, or apical. The penetrating bundle is closely related to the inferior margin of the conoventricular defect and diverges away from this margin into the trabecular septomarginalis beneath the muscle of Lancisi. (Reproduced with permission from Kaiser LR, Kron IL, Spray TL, eds: *Mastery of Cardiothoracic Surgery*. Lippincott-Raven, Philadelphia: 1998.)

patch (e.g., pericardium, Gore-Tex, Dacron), with care being taken not to place sutures through the nearby conduction fiber bundles or the aortic valve. After the repair is completed and the atriotomy is closed, standard deairing maneuvers are performed, the aortic cross-clamp is released, and CPB is discontinued. The chest is then closed in the standard fashion.

Variant procedure or approaches: Supracristal defects may be more easily exposed through a pulmonary arteriotomy, while some inferiorly located muscular VSDs may be better accessed through a right ventriculotomy. Multiple VSDs or "Swiss cheese" ventricular septum can be a challenging surgical problem. Many can be closed with the approaches described above. Some may require a combined surgical and device closure. Palliative pulmonary artery banding may be required in Swiss cheese muscular VSD, with the hope that many of the VSDs may close spontaneously. At a 2nd stage, the remaining VSDs are closed and the PA band is removed. Currently, device closure of muscular VSDs is experimental in the USA but is being used often in other countries.

Usual preop diagnosis: VSD

SUMMARY OF PROCEDURE

Position	Supine
Incision	Standard median sternotomy
Antibiotics	Cefazolin 25 mg/kg q 4 h
Surgical time	Aortic cross-clamp: 15–45 min Total: 2–3 h
Closing considerations	Routine closure with chest tube in the pericardial space; temporary ventricular pacing wire; possibly right/left atrial and/or pulmonary arterial lines for monitoring

SUMMARY OF PROCEDURE (cont'd)	
EBL	Minimal-to-moderate
Postop care	Extubation in OR or within several h; 24 h monitoring in ICU.
Mortality	≤ 1%
Morbidity	Hemorrhage Low CO Atrial dysrhythmias Complete A-V heart block Residual shunting; tricuspid regurgitation
Pain score	6–8

PATIENT POPULATION CHARACTERISTICS	
Age range	Neonate – adult
Male:Female	1:1
Incidence	20% of congenital heart defects; 2/1000 births
Associated conditions	PDA (6%); coarctation of the aorta (5%); congenital AS (2%); congenital mitral valve disease (2%); also part of other malformations, including TOF, TGA, DORV, tricuspid atresia; truncus arteriosus; others

ANESTHETIC CONSIDERATIONS

PREOPERATIVE

Pathophysiology	VSDs are classified by their location and degree of shunt flow. Large VSDs offer little resistance to flow and are nonrestrictive (RV = LV pressure). Small VSDs (restrictive) may close spontaneously in early childhood. Patients with large VSDs present with CHF and other signs of pulmonary over-circulation (Q_p:Q_s > 3.0). Cyanosis indicates pulmonary HTN and shunt reversal (Eisenmenger's syndrome).
Cardiovascular and respiratory	Infants may present with feeding difficulty and failure to thrive (FTT). Children with small VSDs may be asymptomatic, while children with larger VSDs may have ↓ exercise tolerance, fatigue, frequent URIs and Sx of CHF. A holosystolic murmur can be heard best at the left lower sternal border. Cyanosis is absent unless there is R → L shunting (suggesting pulmonary HTN). **Tests:** Obtain EKG, CXR, ECHO. If pulmonary HTN is suspected, cardiac catheterization is performed for measurement of PA pressures. If PA pressures are elevated, O_2 and NO responsiveness is tested. VSDs may be closed surgically or by a device in the cath lab if pulmonary HTN is not present.
Laboratory	Hct; electrolytes (children on diuretic Rx); others as indicated from H&P.
Premedication	See ASD (see p. 1204).

INTRAOPERATIVE

Anesthetic technique: The anesthetic management of a patient with VSD (without pulmonary HTN and CHF) is similar to the patient with ASD. These patients may be candidates for fast-tracking and early extubation. Refer to fast-tracking in ASD section (see p. 1204). For patients with unrestrictive VSDs, avoid factors that ↓ PVR and ↑ shunt flow. This will compromise DBP and coronary perfusion. For patients who are not candidates for fast-tracking, the standard anesthetic is fentanyl 20–40 mcg/kg in divided doses with supplemental isoflurane before and during CPB. Additional midazolam (0.1–0.3 mg/kg) may be administered to prevent recall and awareness.

Blood and fluid requirements	IV: appropriate for patient size × 1–2 LR @ TKO Blood warmer T&C	Minimize administration of iv fluids. Both ventricles are volume-overloaded in large VSDs.
Monitoring	Standard monitors (see p. D-1). Arterial line Surgical LA line Urinary catheter ACT monitoring TEE	A transthoracic LA line may be placed by the surgeon if there is concern about postop mitral valve and LV dysfunction. In the immediate post-CPB period, TEE exam is valuable for evaluation of residual VSD and ventricular function.
Pre-CPB	See ASD (see p. 1205).	
CPB	See ASD (see p. 1205).	Most VSDs are closed under mild/moderate hypothermic CPB (28–32°C).
Transition off CPB	See ASD (see p. 1205).	
Post-CPB	Maintenance of adequate filling pressure (LA = 5–10 mmHg) Temporary pacemaker wires TEE Pulmonary HTN	Placed in patients with conduction disturbances; pacemaker wires are placed routinely, but may not be connected to a pacemaker. ✓ for residual shunt and ventricular and valvular function.

POSTOPERATIVE

Complications	Persistent bleeding Heart block Ventricular dysfunction/failure	May occur particularly after perimembranous VSD closure Especially in patients with ventriculotomy Dx: TEE
Tests	ABGs Electrolytes; Hct; coags prn CXR	

Suggested Readings

1. Bent ST: Anesthesia for left-to-right shunt lesions. In *Anesthesia for Congenital Heart Disease*, 1st edition. Andropoulos S, Andropoulos R, eds. Blackwell Futura, 2005, 297–317.
2. Castaneda AR, Jonas RA, Mayer JE Jr, et al: Ventricular septal defect. In *Cardiac Surgery of the Neonate and Infant.* WB Saunders, Philadelphia: 1994, 187–201.
3. Emmanouilides GC, Allen HD, Riemenschneider TA, et al: Ventricular septal defects. In *Clinical Synopsis of Moss and Adams' Heart Disease in Infants, Children, and Adolescents.* Williams & Wilkins, Baltimore: 1998, 264–85.
4. Knott-Craig CJ: Ventricular septal defects. In *Mastery of Cardiothoracic Surgery.* Kaiser LR, Kron IL, Spray TL, eds. Lippincott-Raven, Philadelphia: 1998, 687–96.
5. Kouchoukos NT, Blackstone EH, Doty DB, et al. Ventricular septal defect. In *Kirklin, Barrett, Boyes Cardiac Surgery.* Churchill Livingstone, Philadelphia: 2003, 850–910.

SURGERY FOR PATENT DUCTUS ARTERIOSUS

SURGICAL CONSIDERATIONS

Description: Patent ductus arteriosus (PDA) usually is located between the proximal descending thoracic aorta and the main PA. Pathophysiologically, this results in L → R shunting and augmented pulmonary blood flow, which, if left untreated, may lead to pulmonary HTN and CHF. A relatively common congenital heart anomaly, comprising 12–15% of CHDs, PDA was first successfully ligated by Gross in 1938. Early administration of indomethacin may promote ductal closure in many premature infants, obviating surgical intervention; however, this mode of therapy generally is contraindicated in the setting of renal insufficiency or intracranial bleeding.

Surgical ductal closure is indicated for significant L → R shunting. The ductus usually can be exposed via a small, left, posterolateral thoracotomy in the 4th intercostal space or via the thoracoscopic approach. The ductus is identified and dissected with special care taken to avoid injury to the phrenic and left recurrent laryngeal nerves (Fig. 12.4-4). The ductus is interrupted with a surgical clip in neonates; in older children, the ductus is double- or triple-ligated or divided between vascular clamps, and the ends are oversewn. A small thoracostomy tube is placed, and the thoracotomy is closed. The thoracostomy tube is removed in the OR immediately after the chest is closed or a few hours later.

Variant procedure or approaches: **Percutaneous coil embolization** and **thoracoscopic clip ligation** are standard alternative approaches. A **robotic approach** is experimental.

Usual preop diagnosis: PDA

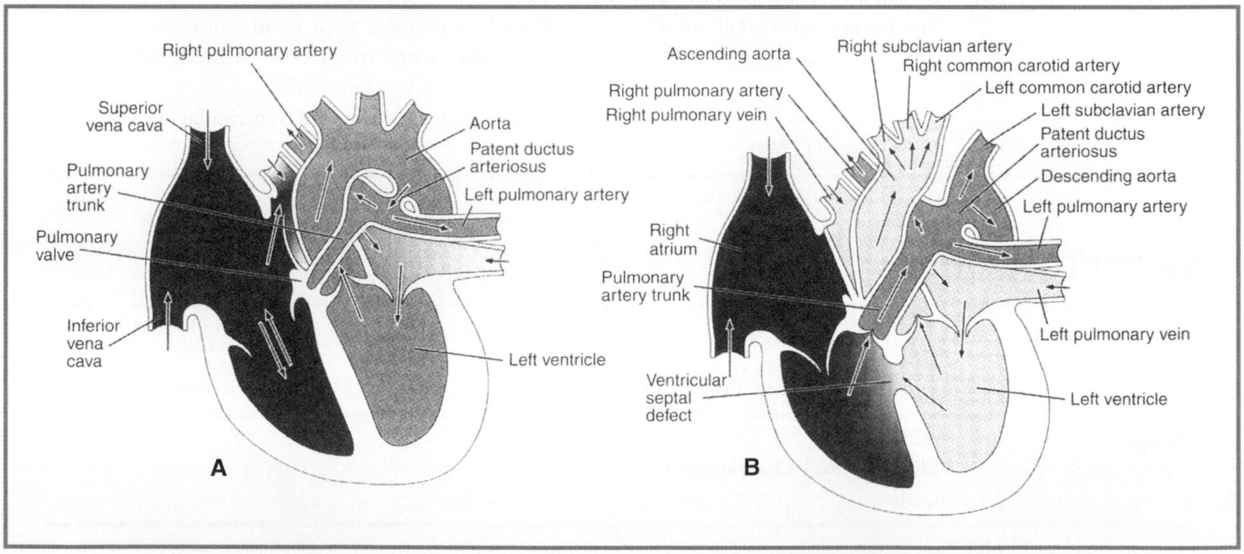

Figure 12.4-4. PDA. **(A)** Ductal dependency for pulmonary blood flow in pulmonary valvular atresia. The ductus arteriosus must be open for blood to enter the pulmonary arteries; as the ductus arteriosus closes, pulmonary blood flow is lost, and the patient becomes cyanotic. **(B)** Dependence on the ductus arteriosus for perfusion of the distal aorta is shown in a patient with interrupted aortic arch. Left ventricular blood (oxygenated) is able to cross the VSD and enter the PA, where it mixes with right ventricular blood. The flow is then distributed to the branch PAs and across the ductus arteriosus to the descending aorta. (Reproduced with permission from Ungerleider RM, Plunkett MD, Gaynor JW: Congenital heart disease. In *Surgery of Infants and Children*. Oldham KT, Colombani PM, Foglia RP, eds. Lippincott-Raven, Philadelphia: 1997).

SUMMARY OF PROCEDURE	
Position	Right lateral decubitus
Incision	Small left posterolateral thoracotomy; 3rd or 4th intercostal space
Antibiotics	Cefazolin 25 mg q 4 h
Surgical time	30–60 min
Closing considerations	Routine closure ± left thoracostomy tube
EBL	Minimal
Postop care	24 h observation in ICU; extubation in the OR or within several h
Mortality	Rare
Morbidity	Hemorrhage Recurrent laryngeal nerve injury Chylothorax
Pain score	6–8

PATIENT POPULATION CHARACTERISTICS	
Age range	1 mo–adulthood
Male:Female	1:2
Incidence	12–15% of congenital heart defects
Etiology	Failure of complete ductal closure

ANESTHETIC CONSIDERATIONS

PREOPERATIVE

Closure of PDA in the preterm infant is done at the bedside in the NICU. These patients are intubated, mechanically ventilated, hemodynamically unstable, and may require inotropic support. The premature infant requiring surgical closure of PDA typically presents because indomethacin Rx has failed or is contraindicated. They often have primary pulmonary disease and multisystem organ problems. In these infants, the symptoms of large L → R shunt and pulmonary overcirculation → cardiac and respiratory failure and ventilator dependence. The ductal runoff causes ↓ DBP and compromises coronary blood flow and other organ perfusion. Older patients may be eligible for endovascular closure in the cath lab, leaving a small percentage for open surgical closure in the OR. Surgical closure may be performed with video-assisted thoracoscopy (VAT) or via thoracotomy. The following discussion for anesthetic management covers open thoracotomy only. In older asymptomatic patients, risk of bacterial endocarditis necessitates closure.

Cardiovascular	Clinical presentation depends on the size of the ductus. An infant with a large ductus can present in CHF with tachypnea, tachycardia, diaphoresis, failure to thrive (FTT), and hepatosplenomegaly. A continuous systolic murmur heard best at the left upper sternal border and widened pulse pressure with bounding pulses may be present. **Tests:** CXR: Normal or cardiomegaly with ↑ PA size and ↑ pulmonary vascular markings. EKG: Normal or LVH/RVH. ECHO diagnostic: documents patency, evaluates left-sided cardiac chamber sizes and aortic arch anatomy, and estimates size of shunt.
Laboratory	Hct; others as indicated from H&P.
Premedication	Not indicated in premature infants. Midazolam 0.5–0.7 mg/kg po 20 min prior to induction for children > 9 mo having routine PDA closure.

Pediatric Surgery

INTRAOPERATIVE

Anesthetic technique: Most children presenting for elective closure of PDA via thoracotomy are candidates for thoracic epidural analgesia, while for those undergoing thoracoscopic closure, an epidural is not required. In patients > 25 kg, placement of a DLT for selective ventilation of the right lung will improve surgical access. In general these patients are candidates for early extubation in the OR (see fast-track in ASD, p. 1204).

Induction	At the bedside of the preterm infant, anesthesia can be provided with ketamine (1–2 mg/kg) and muscle relaxant (e.g., rocuronium 1 mg/kg iv). Small doses of fentanyl (2–5 mcg/kg) may be given for supplemental analgesia. During lateral decubitus positioning, careful attention to the airway and close monitoring of BP is necessary. Children presenting in the OR for elective operation tolerate an inhalation induction with sevoflurane in 50% N_2O + O_2. Once the patient is anesthetized, iv access is established, followed by oral intubation, with administration of a muscle relaxant (e.g., rocuronium 1 mg/kg).	
Maintenance	In patients for whom immediate postop extubation is planned, anesthesia is maintained with isoflurane in air + O_2.	
Emergence	Patients are extubated awake. Post-thoracotomy, an effective regional anesthetic is helpful for fast-tracking.	
Epidural	Thoracic level T8-10 preferred. For neonates < 10 kg a caudal catneter can be advanced to thoracic levels. Initial bolus of bupivacaine (0.25%, 0.3 mL/kg) with hydromorphone (5–10 mcg/kg) ± clonidine (0.5–1 mcg/kg). Infuse bupivacaine (1/8%) at 0.3–0.5 mL/h during surgery. Check coagulation parameters prior to placing epidural. If < 10 kg, caudal approach can be used.	
Blood and fluid requirements	IV: 22–24 × 1–2 Continue iv dextrose. Blood warmer T&C ✓ for air bubbles.	Blood loss may become significant if the ductus is torn during ligation. Have blood available for rapid transfusion. Clear air bubbles from iv tubing and stopcocks (potential bidirectional shunt → paradoxical embolism).
Monitoring	Standard monitors (see p. D-1). ± Arterial line ± CVP line	In preterm infants monitoring of the preductal BP (right arm) and a postductal saturation monitor (usually lower extremity) are required because of possible inadvertent ligation of the descending aorta. Place BP cuff on preductal (right arm) and pulse oximeter on the foot to monitor flow in the ascending and descending aorta. Inadvertent aortic occlusion →↓ LE pulses/pressure/perfusion. Inadvertent PA occlusion →↓ SpO_2 + ↓ $ETCO_2$. Bradycardia may occur during manipulation of the ductus. The DBP will ↑ postligation.
Positioning	✓ and pad pressure points. ✓ eyes.	
Complications	Occlusion of aorta or PA Torn ductus → hemorrhage Residual PDA Lung trauma ± pneumothorax	

POSTOPERATIVE

Complications	Recurrent laryngeal nerve injury Vagus nerve injury	
Tests	Hct CXR	Other tests as indicated.

Suggested Readings

1. Bent ST: Anesthesia for left-to-right shunt lesions. In *Anesthesia for Congenital Heart Disease,* 1st edition. Andropoulos S, Andropoulos R, eds. Blackwell Futura, 2005, 297–317.
2. Burke RP: Patent ductus arteriosus. In *Mastery of Cardiothoracic Surgery.* Kaiser LR, Kron IL, Spray TL, eds. Lippincott-Raven, Philadelphia: 1998, 657–62.
3. Castaneda AR, Jonas RA, Mayer JE Jr, et al: Patent ductus arteriosus. In *Cardiac Surgery of the Neonate and Infant.* WB Saunders, Philadelphia: 1994, 203–13.
4. Emmanouilides GC, Allen HD, Riemenschneider TA, et al: Patent ductus arteriosus. In *Clinical Synopsis of Moss and Adams' Heart Disease in Infants, Children, and Adolescents.* Williams & Wilkins, Baltimore: 1998, 286–308.
5. Haas G: Patent ductus arteriosus and aortopulmonary window. In *Glenn's Thoracic and Cardiovascular Surgery,* 6th edition. Baue AE, ed. Appleton & Lange, Stamford: 1996, 1137–61.

SURGERY FOR COARCTATION OF THE AORTA

SURGICAL CONSIDERATIONS

Description: Coarctation of the aorta is a congenital narrowing of the upper descending aorta, typically located at the juxtaductal region (Fig. 12.4-5). Coexisting intracardiac defects are not uncommon. Surgical repair of aortic coarctation, first performed by **Crafoord** in 1944, consisted of resection of the narrowed aortic segment, followed by an **end-to-end repair.** The same year, **Blalock** and **Park** proposed an alternative technique in which the left subclavian artery was divided distally and sutured into the descending thoracic aorta, creating a bypass. Subsequently, the use of an onlay prosthetic graft to widen the area of coarctation and the use of a **subclavian artery flap** were described by **Waldhausen. Prosthetic interposition tube graft repairs** have been described in patients with diffuse aortic hypoplasia. Patients with an associated intracardiac L → R shunt (e.g., VSD) may require concomitant pulmonary artery banding following repair of the coarctation.

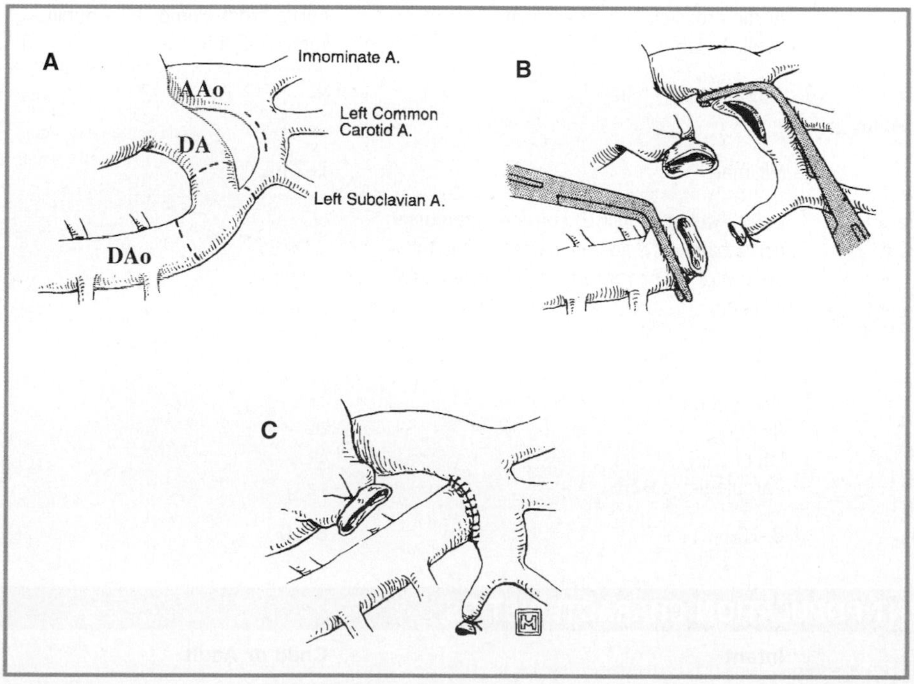

Figure 12.4-5. Redrawn with permission from Younoszai AK, Reddy VM, Hanley FL, et al: Intermediate term follow-up of the end-to-side aortic anastomosis for coarctation of the aorta. *Ann Thorac Surg* 2002; 74(5):1631–4.

In infants, a left posterolateral thoracotomy approach is used. The lung is retracted anteriorly and the pleura are incised vertically over the aorta, along the left subclavian artery and the descending aorta. The aortic arch, all the arch branches, and the descending aorta are thoroughly mobilized. The PDA/ligamentum arteriosus is ligated and divided. Vascular clamps are placed across the aortic arch and the descending aorta. The aortic arch clamp also partially occludes the distal ascending aorta. The aortic isthmus is ligated. The coarctated segment and all ductal tissue from the descending aorta are excised. An aortotomy is made in the aortic arch (may extend on to the distal ascending aorta) and the descending aorta is anastomosed to the aortic arch. Rarely if a subclavian flap angioplasty is performed, the distal left subclavian artery is ligated and opened longitudinally down into the aorta, across the coarctation and into the descending aorta. The subclavian flap is then turned down and anastomosed to the descending aorta across the coarctated segment. Patch aortoplasty is performed by creating a longitudinal aortotomy above and below the coarctation and suturing a generously sized patch onto the defect. Following repair, the aortic cross-clamps are released, and hemostasis is secured. A pleural drainage tube is placed and the pleura are sutured over the aorta, followed by standard closure.

Variant procedure or approaches: In adults and older children (teens), **balloon dilatation with stent placement** is an acceptable alternative.

Usual preop diagnosis: Coarctation of the aorta

SUMMARY OF PROCEDURES

	Infant	Child or Adult
Position	Right lateral decubitus	⇐
Incision	Posterolateral left thoracotomy, 3rd-4th interspace	⇐
Unique considerations	Right upper limb arterial line. Avoid iv or arterial lines in left arm. Mild hypothermia and surface cooling (35°C).	Collateral circulation is adequate if distal aortic MAP > 50 mmHg. In rare cases of inadequate collateral circulation, left atrial-to-descending-aorta or femoral bypass should be considered. Mild hypothermia of 35° may be useful.
Antibiotics	Cefazolin 25 mg/kg q 4 h	⇐
Surgical time	Aortic cross-clamp: 12–20 min Total: 1–1.5 h	Aortic cross-clamp: 10–15 min Total: 2–2.5 h
Closing considerations	Thoracostomy tube	⇐
EBL	Minimal	1–2 mL/kg
Postop care	Early extubation in ICU; consider intercostal nerve block or epidural analgesia; careful control of MAP may require SNP or esmolol infusion.	⇐
Mortality	< 1%	⇐
Morbidity	Chylothorax Bleeding Infection Paraplegia: < 0.5%	⇐ ⇐ ⇐ ⇐
Pain score	8–10	8–10

PATIENT POPULATION CHARACTERISTICS

	Infant	Child or Adult
Age range	1 wk–1 yr	1 yr–adult
Male:Female	2:1; 1:1 for coarctations with associated defects	⇐

PATIENT POPULATION CHARACTERISTICS (cont'd)	Infant	Child or Adult
Incidence	5–8% of congenital heart defects	5% of congenital heart defects
Etiology	Unknown. Ductal sling may be the single most contributory factor.	⇐
Associated conditions	PDA (50%); VSD (36%); congenital mitral stenosis (7%); single ventricle (7%); TGA/VSD (7%)	Usually an isolated defect. When repaired at a later age, bicuspid aortic valve.

ANESTHETIC CONSIDERATIONS

PREOPERATIVE

Pathophysiology	Coarctation is a narrowing of the aortic arch, most commonly occurring at the junction of the ductus arteriosus. The clinical presentation of the neonate or infant with coarctation depends on: (a) location and degree of obstruction, (b) rate at which high-grade stenosis develops, (c) patency of the ductus, (d) PVR, and (e) associated cardiac anomalies. Neonates with critical stenosis will demonstrate ductal-dependent aortic flow. With the ductus open and ↑ PVR, the neonate may be asymptomatic. R→L ductal flow, enhanced by ↑ PVR, may → palpable lower extremity pulses, obscuring the Dx. As the ductus closes (after 4–10 d), lower torso hypoperfusion will become significant (acidemia, gut ischemia, cold lower extremities). Neonates may present in shock and require prompt resuscitation and surgery. Patients with mild-to-moderate stenosis and no associated abnormalities will be asymptomatic with upper extremity HTN and diminished lower extremity pulses.
Respiratory	**Tests:** CXR (cardiomegaly, characteristic aorta, PE)
Cardiovascular	**Neonates:** Neonates present with "critical" coarctation and are ductal-dependent. If the ductus is closing, PGE_1 may reopen the duct—or at least relax juxtaductal tissue—and improve perfusion. PGE_1 treatment may allow time for ECHO assessment of associated lesions. **Infants:** Present with upper extremity hypertension and murmur. Imaging studies such as MRI or CT scan may be needed to confirm diagnosis if gradient is not well detected by echo. **Older children:** Often present with HTN, HA, and diminished or absent femoral pulses. The indication for operation is similar to that of infants. Systemic HTN and LVH may not resolve following repair. **Tests:** ECHO; ECG; ABG; CXR—rib notching 2° collateral vessels. (This is a late finding.) Recently cardiac MRI or CT angio of the chest are used to diagnose coarctations and other associated anomalies.
Renal	**Tests:** BUN; Cr; electrolytes
CNS	PGE_1 is associated with apnea in the newborn. Generally, the neonate is intubated once the prostaglandin infusion is started.
Laboratory	Hct; T&C
Premedication	Not appropriate in severely ill infants. Otherwise, midazolam 0.5–0.7 mg/kg po (maximum of 20 mg). For children > 25 kg, lorazepam 1–2 mg po 2 h before surgery.

INTRAOPERATIVE

Anesthetic technique: GETA. For the neonate, fast-tracking is not appropriate.

Induction	In neonates, an iv induction with fentanyl 2–5 mcg/kg and rocuronium is appropriate. Avoid ↓ SVR and myocardial depression, while maintaining a normal HR. Inhalation induction (sevoflurane and O_2) is well tolerated in the older patients. In most infants and children, single-lumen ETT is sufficient. In children selective ventilation of the right lung with a DLT will facilitate surgery.	
Maintenance	A narcotic technique (10–20 mcg/kg fentanyl ± volatile agent) is appropriate for critically ill neonates. Consider mild hypothermia (34–35°C) for CNS protection. The operation usually is via a left thoracotomy. The aortic arch, isthmus, and descending aorta are mobilized. 100 U/kg of heparin may be given. The ductus arteriosus is ligated, then the aortic arch and descending aorta are occluded. The anesthesiologist should observe the arterial line trace closely during proximal occlusion and immediately inform the surgeon of any damping. Upper and lower extremity cuff pressures are measured. When early postop extubation is planned, see fast-tracking (see p. 1204).	
Emergence	Infants and children undergoing elective operation can usually be extubated in the OR. In young infants, systolic pressure consistently > 120 mmHg should be treated and an esmolol and or SNP infusion may have to be started in the OR. In neonates or infants with compromised cardiac function, extubation should be delayed until their clinical status has improved. Dopamine or milrinone may be required. A chest tube is left in place to monitor blood loss or the appearance of a chylous effusion.	
Blood and fluid requirements	IV: appropriate for patient size × 1–2 LR @ TKO (D5 LR in neonates) Blood warmer T&C 1–2 U.	As a rule, infants and children undergoing coarctation repair will not require transfusion. Infrequently, however, sudden and substantial blood loss can occur, necessitating rapid transfusion. Adequate iv access and immediate availability of blood is essential in this operation.
Monitoring	Standard monitors (see p. D-1).	
	RUE arterial line ± CVP	BP must be monitored above and below the level of coarctation. A right radial arterial line allows BP monitoring during occlusion of the aortic arch. If a percutaneous radial arterial line cannot be placed, a surgical cutdown should be performed or a right axillary arterial line should be placed.
	BP cuffs × 2 (UE + LE)	Both upper and lower extremity cuff pressures should be monitored.
	Temperature	Monitor rectal temperature and maintain it below 35°C
	NIRS	Both cerebral and somatic ✓ ABG, glucose, Hct at intervals.
Control of BP	Anesthetic depth	In neonates and infants, GA is usually sufficient to control BP during aortic cross-clamp; however, SNP may be necessary to control BP in some patients.
Aortic cross-clamping	± Heparin 100 U/kg Ductus arteriosus ligated Aorta cross-clamped × 2 ✓ arterial line for damping. Ischemia time = 10–20 min Maintain distal perfusion. Lactic acidosis →↓ SVR + ↓BP.	Aortic cross-clamping presents an acute afterload to the LV. In preparation for release of cross-clamp, decrease or eliminate volatile anesthetic. Have blood and other volume available. $NaHCO_3$ is frequently required (1–2 mEq/kg). ✓ ABG and treat accordingly.

Complications	Spinal cord ischemia HTN Bleeding Hypothermia Residual coarctation	

POSTOPERATIVE

Complications	Paraplegia HTN Bleeding GI bleed Abdominal pain and ileus Recurrent laryngeal nerve injury Chylous effusion Residual or recurrent coarctation	Incidence = 0.14–0.4%. The cause is likely 2° spinal cord ischemia. Occurs infrequently. Attributable to mesenteric arteritis. Neonates are at risk for GI reperfusion injury following repair. These patients are kept npo for 12–24 h.
Tests	CXR Hct ABGs	

Suggested Readings

1. Allen HD, Clark EB, Gutgesell HP, et al, eds. *Moss and Adams' Heart Disease in Infants, Children, and Adolescents*, 6th edition. Lippincott Williams & Wilkins, Philadelphia: 2001.
2. Castaneda AR, Jonas RA, Mayer JE Jr, et al: Aortic coarctation. In *Cardiac Surgery of the Neonate and Infant*. WB Saunders, Philadelphia: 1994, 333–52.
3. DeSilva A, Stratman G: Anesthesia for left-sided obstructive lesions. In *Anesthesia for Congenital Heart Disease*, 1st edition. Andropoulos S, Andropoulos R, eds. Blackwell Futura, 2005, 322–3.
4. Emmanouilides GC, Allen HD, Riemenschneider TA, et al: Left ventricular and pulmonary outflow abnormalities. In *Clinical Synopsis of Moss and Adams' Heart Disease in Infants, Children, and Adolescents*. Williams & Wilkins, Philadelphia: 1998, 464–500.
5. Kouchoukos NT, Blackstone EG, Doty DB, et al. Coarctation of the aorta and interrupted aortic arch. In *Kirklin, Barrett, Boyes Cardiac Surgery*. Churchill Livingstone, Philadelphia: 2003, 1315–76.
6. Reitz BA, Yuh DD, eds: *Congenital Cardiac Surgery*. McGraw-Hill, New York: 2002.
7. Ungerleider RM: Coarctation of the aorta. In *Mastery of Cardiothoracic Surgery*. Kaiser LR, Kron IL, Spray TL, eds. Lippincott-Raven, Philadelphia: 1998, 704–15.

SURGERY FOR TETRALOGY OF FALLOT

SURGICAL CONSIDERATIONS

Description: In **tetralogy of Fallot (TOF),** the RV infundibulum is maldeveloped, resulting in RV outflow tract obstruction (RVOTO), a large malalignment (overriding aorta) VSD, RVH (see Fig. 12.4-6) and, occasionally, an ASD (**pentalogy of Fallot**). TOF is the most common cyanotic congenital cardiac defect. Pathophysiologically, RVOTO leads to significant R → L shunting across a nonrestrictive VSD, which, in turn, leads to inadequate pulmonary blood flow and varying degrees of cyanosis. The variation in presentation depends primarily on the severity and type of RVOTO.

Patients with TOF were first treated palliatively beginning in 1944, with the introduction of the **Blalock-Taussig** (B-T) **systemic-to-pulmonary artery shunt.** This procedure augments pulmonary blood flow and, hence, systemic oxygenation. Currently, however, most cases of TOF are treated routinely with early complete correction between 3–12 mo of age. Neonatal repair is performed in infants who are severely cyanotic (SaO_2 < 80%), have ductal-dependent pulmonary blood flow, or have cyanotic spells. Initial palliation with the B-T procedure is now reserved

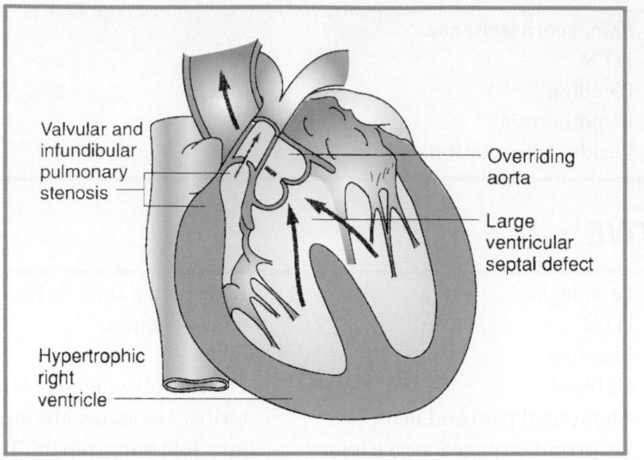

Figure 12.4-6. Anatomic features of tetralogy of Fallot. The primary morphologic abnormality, anterior and superior displacement of the infundibular septum, results in malalignment VSD, overriding the aortic valve and obstructing RV outflow. RV hypertrophy is a secondary occurrence. (Reproduced with permission from Greenfield LJ, Mulholland MW, Oldham KT, et al, eds: *Surgery: Scientific Principles and Practice,* 2nd edition. Lippincott-Raven Publishers, Philadelphia: 1997.)

for patients with severe pulmonary arterial hypoplasia and (by some surgeons) for an anomalous left anterior descending coronary artery originating from the right coronary artery.

Surgical correction is performed through a standard median sternotomy on standard CPB with moderate hypothermia. During cooling, the modified B-T shunt, if present, is ligated and divided, followed by aortic cross-clamping, cardioplegic arrest, and topical cooling. The pulmonary valve and RVOT are accessed through a longitudinal pulmonary arteriotomy and the tricuspid valve (via a right atriotomy), respectively. RVOTO is treated as necessary by infundibular muscle resection, pulmonary valvotomy or valvectomy, and patch augmentation of the main PA or its branches. Autologous pericardium, Gore-Tex, or other type of synthetic/biologic material may be used for patch widening the RVOT at any level, from the RV to the PAs. The primary goal in relieving the RVOTO is to save the pulmonary valve, avoid a trans-cannular patch, and minimize pulmonary valve insufficiency. The VSD, accessed through the tricuspid valve, is closed with a patch (pericardial/Dacron) in the standard fashion with care being taken to avoid injury to the bundle of His.

Variant procedure or approaches: In patients with severe hypoplasia or atresia of the RVOT, or in patients with an anomalous origin of the LAD coronary artery from the right coronary artery, a **Rastelli procedure** is performed. This operation consists of patch closure of the VSD and reconstruction of the RVOT in which a conduit, in the form of a cryopreserved homograft or valved prosthesis, is placed between the RV and the PA.

Usual preop diagnosis: TOF; cyanotic CHD; severe cyanotic spells; failure to thrive (FTT)

SUMMARY OF PROCEDURES

	Neonate Repair	Infant and Adult Repair With Standard CPB
Position	Supine	⇐
Incision	Standard median sternotomy	⇐
Unique considerations	R → L shunt → systemic embolization	⇐
Antibiotics	Cefazolin 25 mg/kg q 4 h	⇐
Surgical time	Aortic cross-clamp: 30–60 min CPB: 90–120 min Total: 3–4 h	30–50 min 75–100 min 3–4 h

SUMMARY OF PROCEDURE (cont'd)

	Neonate Repair	Infant and Adult Repair With Standard CPB
Closing considerations	Chest tube in pericardial (and possibly pleural) space, if opened; temporary ventricular pacing wires; routine right- and left-atrial lines for monitoring.	⇐
EBL	Moderate	⇐
Postop care	ICU × 2–3 d. 1–3 d assisted ventilation; inotropes for RV dysfunction	ICU for 1–2 d
Mortality	~2%	⇐
Morbidity	Junctional tachycardia Atrial dysrhythmias Hemorrhage Infection Low CO Stroke Heart block Residual VSD Transient, right-side CHF	⇐ ⇐ ⇐ ⇐ ⇐ ⇐ ⇐ ⇐ ⇐
Pain score	8–10	8–10

PATIENT POPULATION CHARACTERISTICS

Age range	Neonate-adult (usually < 6 mo)
Male:Female	3:2
Incidence	10% of congenital cardiac defects
Etiology	22g microdeletion is seen in some patients, who also may have DiGeorge syndrome; higher than expected prevalence of older maternal age at time of conception of affected children.
Associated conditions	A-V canal; PDA; previous systemic-to-pulmonary arterial shunt; anomalous left coronary artery from pulmonary artery (ALCAPA); metabolic acidosis (profound hypoxia); right-sided aortic arch

ANESTHETIC CONSIDERATIONS

PREOPERATIVE

Pathophysiology	The clinical presentation of TOF is dependent on the wide anatomic variation of this tetrad. The critical factor is the degree of RVOTO, which determines the amount of R → L shunting across the VSD. This obstruction is dynamic and can be related to RV infundibular spasm, and variations in pH, $PaCO_2$ and PaO_2. The onset of hypercyanotic episodes in an infant < 3 mo of age is the indication for complete surgical repair.
"TET" spells	Hypercyanotic episodes, or "TET" spells: These constitute medical and surgical emergencies; however, they are seen less frequently due to early surgical intervention. TET spells may present in early infancy and are related to infundibular spasm resulting in ↑ R→ L shunting. If untreated, these episodes can progress to unconsciousness, Sz, and death. For management of TET spells, see Table 12.4-1, p. 1224
Respiratory	Infectious/asthmatic pulmonary processes will complicate preop and postop cardiopulmonary function. Optimize pulmonary function preop. **Tests:** CXR: ↓ pulmonary vascular markings and characteristic heart shape.

Pediatric Surgery

Table 12.4-1. Treatment for TET Spells

Treatment Modalities	Effect
1. Knee-chest position	↑ SVR.
2. Abdominal compression	Simulates squatting. ↑ SVR.
3. Volume administration	↑ preload, opens RVOT.
4. O_2	Pulmonary vasodilator
5. Anesthesia and sedation	Negative inotropy → reduced RVOT spasm.
6. Alpha-agonist (phenylephrine)	↑ SVR. Dose: 10 mcg/kg bolus and repeat.
7. Beta-blockers (esmolol)	Negative inotropy. Dose: 50 mcg/kg bolus.

Cardiovascular	CHF is not the usual presentation for an unrepaired Tet. An understanding of the patient's anatomic defects and their pathophysiology (e.g., is their RVOTO fixed or dynamic?) is essential for formulating the anesthetic plan. Avoid prolonged fasting to prevent profound decreases in preload on induction. **Tests:** ABG; ECG: ✓ for RVH, right axis deviation (RAD) ± complete or incomplete RBBB. CXR: ✓ heart size, "coeur en sabot" (elevation of apex 2° RVH, RAE). Cardiac cath and ECHO: Locate site of pulmonary outflow obstruction, VSD, bronchopulmonary collaterals, PDA, abnormal patency of previous surgical shunts (e.g., B-T shunt). Define aortic arch anatomy, abnormal coronary or subclavian arteries, tricuspid regurgitation/aortic insufficiency (TR/AI), ventricular function.
Hematologic	Polycythemia (typical with chronic O_2 sat < 90%) →↑blood viscosity → thromboembolic events. Polycythemia →↓Plt + coagulopathy. Extreme polycythemia (> 70) may require isovolemic hemodilution intraop. **Tests:** CBC; Plt; bleeding time; coag profile
Laboratory	Electrolytes if on diuretics; otherwise, tests as indicated from H&P.
Premedication	As required to ↓ anxiety, avoid TET spells and facilitate separation from parents. Midazolam 0.5–0.75 mg/kg po 20 min before induction in a monitored setting.

INTRAOPERATIVE

Anesthetic technique: GETA. Patients with TOF, pulmonary atresia, and MAPCAS (major aortopulmonary collaterals) requiring unifocalization, present a challenge for surgical and anesthetic management. Special periop requirements include: placement of cuffed ETTs is necessary. OLV also may be required to facilitate surgical exposure. Bronchial bleeding 2° extensive surgical dissection requires frequent ETT suctioning. A significant portion of the procedure is done off-CPB, and hemodynamic instability with ST segment changes may occur during surgical dissection. Closely monitor blood loss and replace mL/mL with PRBCs. Avoid air bubbles in iv tubing/stopcocks. In older patients presenting for conduit change or revisions, massive blood loss should be anticipated.

Induction	Typically mask induction with sevoflurane, O_2 ± air. If iv in place, ketamine (1–2 mg/kg) and/or fentanyl (10 mcg/kg) with rocuronium (1 mg/kg) ± volatile agent. Avoid ↓↓SVR. Verify ETT position (see p. D-2).
Maintenance	For patients not undergoing unifocalization, anesthesia is maintained with isoflurane or sevoflurane. TET spells can occur 2° surgical manipulation. Hypercyanotic episodes can occur during surgical dissection for cannulation before CPB. The surgeon can provide direct aortic compression or urgently proceed to CPB. Refer to Table 12.4-1 for other treatment. For patients who are undergoing unifocalization, hypoxic pulmonary vasoconstriction is blunted by the use of volatile anesthetic agents, causing a further decrease in arterial saturation. As a result, we prefer to use total intravenous anesthesia with propofol/ketamine/midazolam infusion. Antifibrinolytics, such as Amicar, are routinely given to redo-patients to reduce blood loss.

Emergence	Patients are transported to ICU monitored, intubated, and ventilated.	
Blood and fluid requirements	IV: 22–24 ga × 2 LR @ TKO T&C PRBC	Blood in OR before incision. For all repeat sternotomy patients, have blood available for immediate administration. Have massive transfusion system set up for older pateints.
Monitoring	Standard monitors Urinary catheter Arterial line (usually radial) CVP line TEE: Transthoracic LA land PA line: have transducers available.	Double-lumen CVP placed in IJ or femoral vein. During MAPCAS dissection and RVOT change with beating heart close monitoring of TEE for function and air.
Pre-CPB	Heparinization (4 mg/kg) ACT > 400 sec MAP ~70 mmHg ✓ muscle relaxation. ✓ pupils. ✓ UO.	In the pre-CPB period, crystalloid and/or 5% albumin is administered as needed to compensate for bleeding and 3rd-space losses.
CPB	Ventilation stopped. Hypothermia: ~28°C to 32°C Hct 30 typical during CPB ✓ adequate flow/pressure. ✓ anesthetic/NMB levels. ✓ pupils. ✓ face for venous congestion. ✓ ABG, electrolytes, UO, Hct, and ACT q 30 min.	Furosemide (0.5–1 mg/kg) for ↓ UO and hemoconcentration.
Transition off CPB	Rewarming Vasoactive infusions started at 32°C. Flush lines. TEE Zero transducers. Suction ETT. Resume ventilation. Observe lung inflation. Supplement NMB and deepen anesthesia. Rewarm to 36°C. ✓ bilateral breath sounds. ✓ ABGs, electrolytes, Hct (~40). ✓ ACT (> 400). ✓ ECG: pacing may be necessary.	Surgeons de-air heart, which can be monitored by TEE. A measurement of the RV and LV pressure ratio helps to judge adequacy of repair of the RVOTO. TEE also is used to evaluate the anatomy, the repair, and pressures. Infants are at risk for development of junctional ectopic tachycardia (JET). Avoid excessive warming > 37°C. Have amiodarone (5–10 mg/kg load) available.
Post-CPB	Inotropic support (dopamine, milrinone, epinephrine, and CaCl) Rx pulmonary HTN (↓PVR): $FiO_2 = 1$ $PaCO_2$ ~35 Early use of inhaled nitric oxide (40 ppm) AV sequential pacemaker (heart block not uncommon). Transthoracic PA or LA line placed to monitor hemodynamics. Reverse anticoagulation.	↓ RV compliance is expected. RV afterload reduction is essential, initially through ventilatory efforts: clear unobstructed ventilation; do not allow wheezing (albuterol pm); use gentle hyperventilation on 100% O_2. Inotropic support of RV also typically is used—dopamine/initially and epinephrine reserved for severe RV dysfunction. Milrinone 0.5 mcg/kg/min and $CaCl_2$10–20 mg/kg/h are routine in infants.

Table 12.4-2. Blood Product Utilization[8]

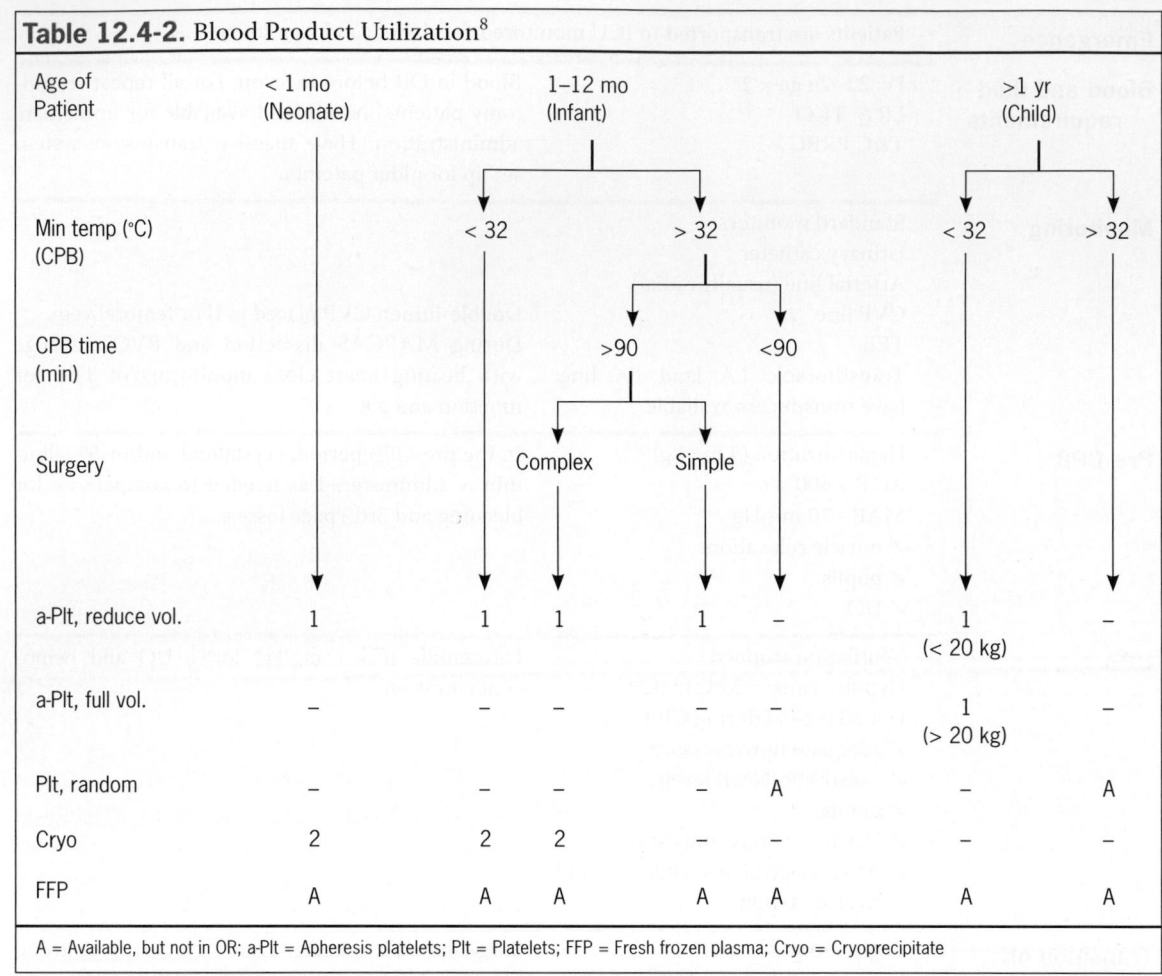

Age of Patient	< 1 mo (Neonate)	1–12 mo (Infant)				>1 yr (Child)	
Min temp (°C) (CPB)		< 32	> 32	> 32	> 32	< 32	> 32
CPB time (min)			>90	>90	<90		
Surgery			Complex	Simple			
a-Plt, reduce vol.	1	1	1	1	–	1 (< 20 kg)	–
a-Plt, full vol.	–	–	–	–	–	1 (> 20 kg)	–
Plt, random	–	–	–	–	A	–	A
Cryo	2	2	2	–	–	–	–
FFP	A	A	A	A	A	A	A

A = Available, but not in OR; a-Plt = Apheresis platelets; Plt = Platelets; FFP = Fresh frozen plasma; Cryo = Cryoprecipitate

Post-CPB (cont'd)	Rx coagulopathy	See Table 12.4-2 for blood product utilization. MUF uses the CPB machine to remove excess H_2O and inflammatory mediators (↓ edema and improved cardiopulmonary function).
Positioning	✓ and pad pressure points. ✓ eyes.	
Complications	See Postoperative Complications, below.	

POSTOPERATIVE

Complications	Persistent bleeding Persistent RVOTO Dysrhythmias (JET)	For neonatal repairs, a PFO is left surgically open to allow RV decompression via a R → L intraatrial shunt. This often will result in a ↓ systemic O_2 sat. TEE will confirm the existence of intra-atrial shunting.
Tests	ABGs + electrolytes Coag profile CXR: ✓ line, ETT placement.	

Suggested Readings

1. Allen HD, Clark EB, Gutgesell HP, et al., eds: *Moss and Adams' Heart Disease in Infants, Children, and Adolescents,* 6th edition. Lippincott Williams & Wilkins, Philadelphia: 2001.
2. Castaneda AR, Jonas RA, Mayer JE Jr, et al: Tetralogy of fallot. In *Cardiac Surgery of the Neonate and Infant.* WB Saunders, Philadelphia: 1994, 215–34.
3. Emmanouilides GC, Allen HD, Riemenschneider TA, et al: Tetralogy of fallot. In *Clinical Synopsis of Moss and Adams' Heart Disease in Infants, Children, and Adolescents.* Williams & Wilkins, Philadelphia: 1998, 409–33.
4. Karl TR: Tetralogy of fallot. In *Glenn's Thoracic and Cardiovascular Surgery,* 6th edition. Baue AE, ed. Appleton & Lange, Stamford: 1996, 1211–19.
5. Kouchoukos NT, Blackstone EG, Doty DB, et al. Ventricular Septal Defect with pulmonary stenosis or atresia. In *Kirklin, Barrett, Boyes Cardiac Surgery.* Churchill Livingstone, Philadelphia: 2003, 946–1075.
6. Perryman RA, Jaquiss DB: Tetralogy of fallot. In *Mastery of Cardiothoracic Surgery.* Kaiser LR, Kron IL, Spray TL, eds. Lippincott-Raven, Philadelphia: 1998, 831–8.
7. Reitz BA, Yuh DD, eds: *Congenital Cardiac Surgery.* McGraw-Hill, New York: 2002.
8. Schmitz ML, Ullah S: Anesthesia for right sided obstructive lesions eds In *Anesthesia for Congenital Heart Disease,* 1st edition. Andropoulos S, Andropoulos R, eds. Blackwell Futura, 2005, 332–8.
9. Williams GD, Bratton SL, Riley EC, et al: Association between age and blood loss in children undergoing open-heart surgery. *Ann Thorac Surg* 1998; 66:870–6.

SURGERY FOR TOTAL ANOMALOUS PULMONARY VENOUS CONNECTION

SURGICAL CONSIDERATIONS

Description: Total anomalous pulmonary venous connection (TAPVC) is a rare congenital cardiac malformation in which the entire pulmonary venous return empties either directly into the systemic venous channels via anomalous veins or the right atrium (Fig. 12.4-7). An interatrial R → L shunt, in the form of a PFO or an ASD, is required to maintain systemic output and, hence, survival in the postnatal period. The objective of surgical correction is to redirect the entire pulmonary venous return to the left atrium.

TAPVC was first successfully repaired in 1956 by Lewis and Varco at the University of Minnesota by joining the pulmonary venous sinus to the left atrium and closure of the ASD. Although mortality for this lesion was initially quite high, particularly in infants with obstruction of the pulmonary veins, improvements in intraop and postop management have permitted successful correction in most neonates and infants. There are four TAPVC drainage patterns as defined by Darling, et al. These include **supracardiac** (45%), **cardiac** (25%), **infracardiac** (25%), and **mixed** patterns (5%) of venous drainage. The anomalous drainage in supracardiac TAPVC is usually by a left vertical vein into the innominate vein. In cardiac TAPVC, drainage is usually into the coronary sinus and occasionally into the right atrium. In infracardiac TAPVC, drainage is usually into the portal vein. The mixed type consists of combinations of the other three varieties of TAPVC.

When pulmonary venous drainage is obstructed, patients present with cyanosis severe pulmonary edema, pulmonary HTN, and ↓ CO. Symptomatic TAPVC is repaired at any age. TAPVC with obstruction is a true surgical emergency. Critically ill neonates with obstructed pulmonary venous return must undergo emergent correction after initial stabilization (i.e., intubation/ventilation, diuretics). Occasionally, preop ECMO may be required.

In most cases, the right and left pulmonary veins drain into a common pulmonary venous sinus, allowing for its anastomosis to the left atrium for a definitive repair. Through a standard median sternotomy, the aortic and venous cannulae are placed and CPB with cooling is initiated. The aorta is cross-clamped, immediately followed by cardioplegic arrest. The cardiac apex is lifted up, and the pulmonary veins are identified through the posterior pericardium. The left atrium is then opened transversely with extension onto the left atrial appendage, followed by the direct anastomosis of the pulmonary venous confluence to the left atrium. Finally, via a right atriotomy, the ASD or PFO is closed. The heart is de-aired, aortic cross-clamp is released, and the patient is rewarmed and separated from bypass. Successful outcomes are dependent on early and immediate correction of TAPVC with obstruction, before lung damage ensues. Other important factors include repair without residual obstruction and postop control of pulmonary HTN.

Variant procedure or approaches: Alternatively, repair of TAPVC may be accomplished through a right atriotomy and across the atrial septum, constructing the anastomosis between the pulmonary venous confluence and left atrium from within the left atrium or through a transverse sinus approach.

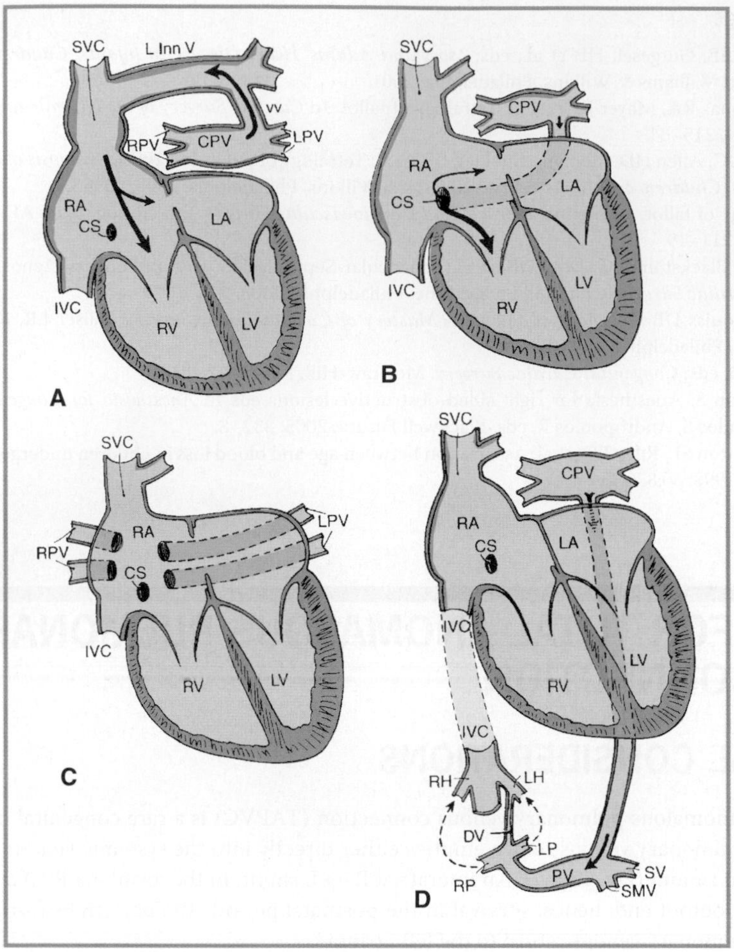

Figure 12.4-7. Common forms of TAPVC: **(A)** TAPVC to the left innominate vein (L inn V) by way of a vertical vein (VV). **(B)** TAPVC to coronary sinus (CS). The pulmonary veins join to form a confluence designated as the common pulmonary vein (CPV), which connects to the coronary sinus. **(C)** TAPVC to right atrium (RA) The left and right pulmonary veins (LPV and RPV) usually enter the RA separately. **(D)** TAPVC to the portal vein (PV). The PVs form a confluence, from which an anomalous channel arises. (Reproduced with permission from Emmanouilides GC, Allen HD, Riemenschneider TA, et al: *Clinical Synopsis of Moss and Adams' Heart Disease in Infants, Children, and Adolescents.* Williams & Wilkins, Philadelphia: 1998.)

Usual preop diagnosis: TAPVC; total anomalous venous return; total anomalous pulmonary venous drainage—all of these ± obstruction and either supracardiac, cardiac, or mixed types

SUMMARY OF PROCEDURE

Position	Supine
Incision	Standard median sternotomy
Unique considerations	Patients often require urgent or emergency surgery. Obligatory R → L shunting → risk of systemic embolization. Myocardial preservation using blood or crystalloid cardioplegia, in addition to topical myocardial hypothermia, is used.
Antibiotics	Cefazolin 25 mg/kg q 4 h
Surgical time	Aortic cross-clamp: 30–60 min Circulatory arrest: occasionally, 30–45 min Total: 2–3 h

SUMMARY OF PROCEDURE (cont'd)	
Closing considerations	A fine polyvinyl catheter inserted through the free wall of the right ventricle and advanced into the pulmonary trunk will allow monitoring for pulmonary HTN. A chest tube is inserted into the pericardial space; temporary ventricular pacing wires are placed. Left atrial lines normally needed.
EBL	Moderate
Postop care	2–6 d of assisted ventilation, sedation and hyperventilation; pulmonary vasodilators, including isoproterenol, PGE1, SNP; inotropes as needed for right heart dysfunction. Sometimes, if pulmonary injury is severe or pulmonary HTN is uncontrollable, ECMO may be indicated.
Mortality	2–10%, depending on presence of preop pulmonary venous obstruction and metabolic acidosis.
Morbidity	Pulmonary vasospasm: 25–40% Low CO: 10% Hemorrhage: 2–3%
Pain score	8–10

PATIENT POPULATION CHARACTERISTICS	
Age range	1 d–20 yr (usually < 1 mo)
Male:Female	4:1 in infracardiac type; equal distribution in other types
Incidence	0.5–2% of congenital heart defects
Etiology	Failure of fusion of the pulmonary vein evagination (from posterior left atrium) with the pulmonary venous plexus surrounding the lung buds.
Associated conditions	PDA present in nearly all infants within the first few wk of life and in about 15% of cases overall. VSD occasionally occurs (may be associated with TOF, DORV, interrupted aortic arch, and other lesions).

ANESTHETIC CONSIDERATIONS

PREOPERATIVE

Pathophysiology	In the supradiaphragmatic connection, all the pulmonary venous return drains into the right atrium via a vertical vein. When this vein or confluence is stenotic or obstructed, severe pulmonary HTN, cyanosis, pulmonary edema, and shock ensue. This is a true surgical emergency, requiring immediate intervention. An ASD or PFO is essential for survival.
Respiratory	In patients with obstructed TAPVR, expect severe pulmonary edema and pulmonary HTN. **Tests:** ✓ CXR: ↑ heart size, ↑ pulmonary vascularity, "figure-of-8," or "snowman" cardiac silhouette.
Cardiovascular	ECHO findings: large RV and small LA. Cardiac interventricular cath for balloon or blade septostomy in patients with restrictive ASD may be necessary to improve R → L shunting. **Tests:**✓ ECG for right axis deviation (RAD), RAE and RVH.
Laboratory	ABG and Hct; other tests as indicated from H&P.
Premedication	Generally not indicated and not necessary in severely ill infants.
Transport of critically ill newborn	All critically ill neonates are intubated, ventilated, and often are on PGE_1 and/or dopamine infusions for hemodynamic stability. To facilitate transport of these patients, notify the nurse in advance, and request all drips transferred to OR syringe pumps. Maintain a dextrose-containing infusion during and after transport to ensure normoglycemia. Verify that the transport monitor has ECG, SaO_2 and invasive pressure transducers. Resuscitation medications and airway equipment must accompany the patient.

INTRAOPERATIVE

Anesthetic technique: GETA. Profound hypothermic CPB (16–18°C) with low flow may be required. Patients who weigh < 3.0 kg and the ICU ventilator are used in the OR, because this allows for maximum flexibility in ventilator support.

Induction	Infants are often severely ill and come to the OR intubated and ventilated, with invasive lines and inotropic support. Verify ETT placement. Patients are subject to rapid cardiovascular decompensation. Rocuronium (1 mg/kg) is given, as is fentanyl (1–3 mcg/kg) as tolerated. Volatile agents are rarely tolerated in obstructed TAPVC.	
Maintenance	Fentanyl (20–50 mcg/kg) in divided doses on CPB. Rocuronium prn, midazolam 0.1–0.2 mg/kg. FiO_2 = 1.0. Ventilation maneuvers to ↓ PVR. (See Post-CPB, p. 1225.)	
Emergence	Transport to ICU intubated and ventilated. If NO used in OR, must have delivery system ready for transport to ICU. There may be continued requirement for inotropic support.	
Blood and fluid requirements	IV: 22–24 ga × 2, taped securely LR @ TKO Continue iv dextrose in neonates. 5% albumin PRBC Blood warmer	Avoid air bubbles with R → L shunt—can cause systemic embolization of air. ✓ blood glucose. Avoid hyperglycemia, especially during profound hypothermic CPB. See Table 12.4-2 for blood product utilization.
Monitoring	Standard monitors (see p. D-1). Transthoracic LA, PA, RA lines	Severely ill infants usually present with invasive monitoring and ETT. ✓ correct placement of UAC and UVC preop.
Complications	Bleeding	
	Refractory pulmonary HTN	Pulmonary HTN may be difficult to control. Ventilation maneuvers (e.g., ↓ $PaCO_2$; 100% O_2), vasodilators, and deep anesthesia to ↓ PVR. NO is started for refractory pulmonary HTN; if NO (40 ppm) is unsuccessful, ECMO may be instituted. In these instances sternum is not closed.
	Biventricular failure	Inotropic support (dopamine, milrinone, epinephrine, calcium chloride)
	Overdose of NO → methHb	✓ metHb while on NO therapy.

POSTOPERATIVE

Complications	See above.	
Tests	ABG	Only if on NO
	Hct; electrolytes; coags	
	Methemoglobin	
	CXR	

Suggested Readings

1. Allen HD, Clark EB, Gutgesell HP, et al, eds. *Moss and Adams' Heart Disease in Infants, Children, and Adolescents,* 6th edition. Lippincott Williams & Wilkins, Philadelphia: 2001.
2. Bent ST: Anesthesia for left-to-right shunt lesions. In *Anesthesia for Congenital Heart Disease,* 1st edition. Andropoulos S, Andropoulos R, eds. Blackwell Futura, 2005, 297–317.
3. Castaneda AR, Jonas RA, Mayer JE Jr, et al: Total anomalous pulmonary venous connection. In *Cardiac Surgery of the Neonate and Infant.* WB Saunders, Philadelphia: 1994, 157–66.
4. Cope JT, Kron IL: Anomalies of pulmonary venous return and cor triatriatum. In *Mastery of Cardiothoracic Surgery.* Kaiser LR, Kron IL, Spray TL, eds. Lippincott-Raven, Philadelphia: 1998, 867–79.
5. Emmanouilides GC, Allen HD, Riemenschneider TA, et al: Venous abnormalities. In *Clinical Synopsis of Moss and Adams' Heart Disease in Infants, Children, and Adolescents.* Williams & Wilkins, Philadelphia: 1998, 349–68.

6. Kouchoukos NT, Blackstone EG, Doty DB, et al. Total Ventricular Septal Defect with pulmonary stenosis or atresia. In *Kirklin, Barrett, Boyes Cardiac Surgery*. Churchill Livingstone, Philadelphia: 2003, 946–1075.
7. Reitz BA, Yuh DD, eds: *Congenital Cardiac Surgery*. McGraw-Hill, New York: 2002.

SURGERY FOR COMPLETE TRANSPOSITION OF THE GREAT ARTERIES

SURGICAL CONSIDERATIONS

Description: Complete **transposition of the great arteries (TGA)** is a congenital cardiac defect in which the aorta arises from the RV and the PA arises from the LV (Fig. 12.4-8). TGA is associated with an intact ventricular septum (TGA/IVS) or a ventricular septal defect (TGA/VSD). Pathophysiologically, this discordant ventriculoarterial configuration results in systemic and pulmonary circulations placed in a parallel (normally in series) configuration. Thus, a L → R shunt in the form of an atrial septal defect (ASD), VSD, or patent ductus arteriosus (PDA) is required to permit oxygenated blood to enter the "right-sided" systemic circulation. The earliest surgical treatment for TGA was described by **Blalock** and **Hanlon** in 1950 with a procedure in which an **atrial septectomy** was performed, improving the mixing of pulmonary and systemic blood at the atrial level. In the 1950s, a variety of partial physiologic corrections were developed in which the pulmonary veins or the vena cava were transposed to the alternate atria. Palliative treatment was advanced by **Rashkind's** description of a **balloon atrial septostomy** in 1966. More complete physiologic correction was obtained by **atrial switch** operations, described by **Senning** in 1959 and **Mustard** in 1963, in which systemic and pulmonary venous return were baffled to the appropriate ventricles. Postop complications with the atrial switch operations, however, led to the development of the more "anatomic" **arterial switch** operations described by **Jatene, Yacoub,** and others beginning in the 1970s. By 1987, the arterial switch operation in neonates was widely accepted as the standard approach to TGA.

Total correction is now performed routinely in the first 2 wk of life. The heart is exposed through a standard median sternotomy and CPB is instituted. The aortic cross-clamp is applied, followed by cardioplegic arrest and induced hypothermia. The ascending aorta is transected just above the sinotubular junction at and the pulmonary trunk is transected just proximal to its bifurcation. Two buttons from the "neopulmonary artery" (former aortic root) containing the origins of the left and right coronary arteries are transposed and anastomosed to the "neoaorta" (former main pulmonary trunk). The distal aortic segment is swung beneath the PA bifurcation **(Lecompte maneuver)**. Pericardial patches are used to repair the defects resulting from excision of the coronary artery buttons, and any associated ASDs and/or VSDs are repaired. The distal aortic segment is anastomosed to the neoaorta and the distal bifurcated pulmonary artery segment is anastomosed to the neopulmonary artery. If hypothermia has been induced, a brief period of circulatory arrest facilitates repair of the ASD and/or VSD, if present. The aortic cross-clamp is removed and rewarming is begun during the neopulmonary arterial anastomosis. CPB is then discontinued and closure is routine.

Variant procedure or approaches: In children with TGA and VSD, additional cardiac anomalies are common. These include pulmonary stenosis, pulmonary atresia, straddling atrioventricular valves, hypoplasia of ventricular chambers, and coarctation or interruption of aorta. Dynamic or structural subpulmonic obstruction is also more common in TGA and VSD than in TGA/IVS.

Rastelli procedure: The VSD is baffled to the aorta with construction of a RV→PA valved conduit and is the procedure of choice for patients with TGA/VSD and pulmonary atresia or significant valvular pulmonary stenosis. Often the VSD may have to be enlarged to prevent LVOT obstruction. Alternatively in some cases an aortic root translocation may be required.

Coronary arteries in TGA: Abnormalities in the origin and course of coronary arteries are common in TGA and, in the past, influenced the success of surgery. A simple rule that accounts for virtually all variations is that the coronaries arise from the sinuses of Valsalva, which face the pulmonary artery, and follow the shortest route to their ultimate destination. Only a small number pose a problem in switching the great arteries.

Usual preop diagnosis: Complete TGA; transposition of the great vessels; transposition ± VSD; ASD; PDA

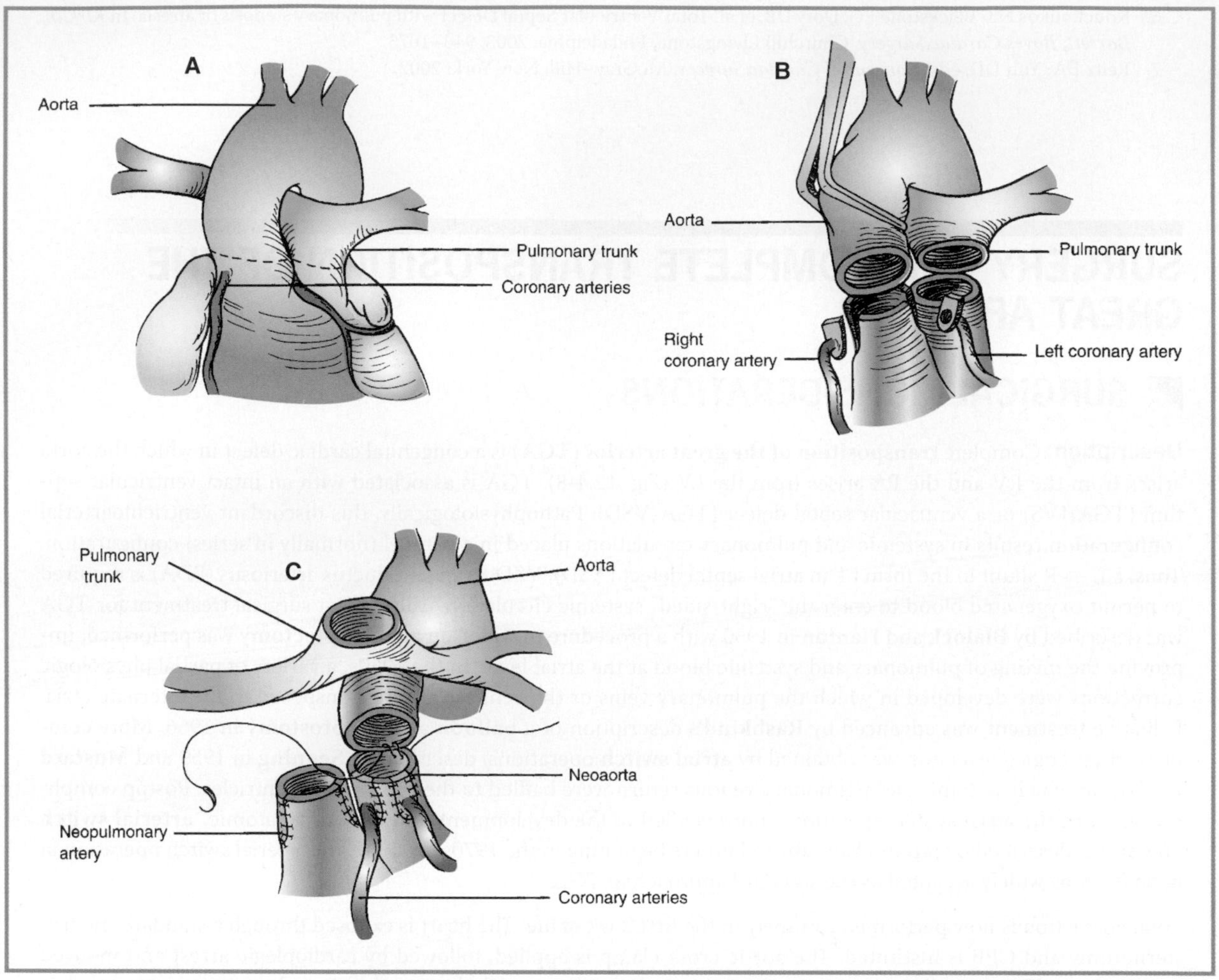

Figure 12.4-8. TGA: **(A)** Typical anatomy of transposition of the great vessels, with the aorta anterior and slightly to the right of the pulmonary artery. The coronary arteries can be seen arising from the aorta. **(B)** Repair is best accomplished by an arterial switch procedure in infancy. The great vessels are transsected, and the coronary arteries are removed from the aorta and placed into the proximal pulmonary artery (neoaorta). **(C)** The distal aorta is brought behind the pulmonary artery bifurcation (Lecompte maneuver), and the neoaorta anastomosis is completed. (Reproduced with permission from Ungerleider RM, Plunkett MD, Gaynor JW: Congenital heart disease. In *Surgery of Infants and Children*. Oldham KT, Colombani PM, Foglia RP, eds. Lippincott-Raven, Philadelphia: 1997.)

SUMMARY OF PROCEDURE	
Position	Supine
Incision	Standard median sternotomy
Unique considerations	Operation to be performed before LV pressure falls substantially 2° ↓PVR.
Antibiotics	Cefazolin 25 mg/kg q 4 h
Surgical time	Aortic cross-clamp: 45–90 min No circulatory arrest Total: 3 h

SUMMARY OF PROCEDURE (cont'd)	
Closing considerations	Routine closure with chest tube in the pericardial space; temporary ventricular pacing wire; possible right or left atrial line for monitoring.
EBL	Moderate
Postop care	1–5 d of assisted ventilation; pulmonary HTN protocol consisting of hyperventilation and sedation and use of pulmonary vasodilators; inotropes for adequate CO.
Mortality	1–3%
Morbidity	Hemorrhage Atrial dysrhythmias ↓CO Coronary artery kinking and myocardial ischemia Pulmonary HTN
Pain score	8–10

PATIENT POPULATION CHARACTERISTICS	
Age range	1–21 d; ≤ 3–6 mo in TGA/VSD
Male:Female	2:1; for TGA/IVS, 3.3:1
Incidence	7–8% of congenital heart defects
Etiology	Usually no associated syndromes or other noncardiac abnormalities
Associated conditions	ASD; VSD; PDA; LVOTO; pulmonary atresia; coarctation of the aorta

ANESTHETIC CONSIDERATIONS

PREOPERATIVE

Pathophysiology	In TGA, the pulmonary and systemic circulations flow in parallel, unlike the normal series circulation. Deoxygenated blood returns to the right heart and is pumped to the aorta and systemic circulation without passing through the lungs for gas exchange. The oxygenated blood returns via the pulmonary veins and recirculates through the LV back into the lungs. Survival depends on mixing of pulmonary and systemic blood at some level (ASD, VSD, PDA). In the absence of a septal defect, a balloon atrial septostomy (Rashkind) may be required before surgery to promote mixing.
Respiratory	Some patients are maintained preop on PGE_1, to maintain ductal patency. PGE_1 can cause apnea; therefore, mechanical ventilation may be required. **Tests:** CXR: ✓ enlarged heart and pulmonary edema.
Cardiovascular	Patients with VSD have ↑ pulmonary blood flow, ↑ intercirculatory mixing → CHF. Marked cyanosis is seen in patients with TGA and intact ventricular septum, O_2 sat depends on degree of mixing (Q_P/Q_S ratio). **Tests:** EKG: right axis deviation (RAD) and RVH. ECHO. Cardiac cath defines anatomy, coronary arteries, septal defects, PFO, PDA, bronchopulmonary collaterals, LVOT, pulmonic valve function and pressures, including PVR and LV:RV ratio. Balloon atrial septostomy (Rashkind-Miller) is required to improve mixing in some patients.
Laboratory	Hct; coags; other tests as indicated from H&P.

Premedication	Generally not necessary in children < 9 mo.
Transport of critically ill newborn	All critically ill neonates are intubated, ventilated, and often are on PGE_1 and/or dopamine for hemodynamic stability. To facilitate transport of these patients, notify the nurse in advance and request all drips transferred to OR syringe pumps. An air-O_2 blender should be available so the inspired O_2 concentration can be adjusted as needed. Verify that the transport monitor has EKG, SaO_2 and invasive pressure transducers. Resuscitation medications and airway equipment must accompany the patient. Patients can be transported on room air with gentle manual ventilation, taking care to avoid hyperventilation. Avoid oversedation and use of muscle relaxants before transport.

INTRAOPERATIVE

Anesthetic technique: GETA

Induction	Neonates with TGA and intact ventricular septum are placed on PGE_1 to maintain ductal patency and promote mixing of pulmonary and systemic blood. Anesthetic management is based on maintaining a balance between systemic and pulmonary blood flows. Excessive pulmonary blood flow →↓ systemic perfusion. IV induction with ketamine, fentanyl (e.g., 2–15 mcg/kg incrementally) and muscle relaxant (e.g., rocuronium 1 mg/kg) is the technique of choice. Inotropic infusion and PRBC transfusion may be required to support BP.	
Maintenance	For patients with inadequate intercirculatory mixing and ↓ pulmonary blood flow, treatment should include ventilation maneuvers to ↓ PVR (see TOF, Post-CPB, p. 1225) and improve mixing. Deep GA helps to blunt reactive pulmonary HTN. Avoid ↓ HR →↓ CO in infants with limited myocardial reserve.	
Emergence	Control aortic BP and treat any coagulopathy. Monitor LA pressures closely. ✓ for myocardial ischemia, which can be 2° coronary air emboli or at the implantation site of the coronaries. Transport to ICU intubated and ventilated.	
Blood and fluid requirements	IV: 22–24 ga × 1–2 taped securely LR @ TKO	Avoid air bubbles in patients with R → L and L → R shunts.
	Continue iv dextrose in neonates. 5% albumin	See Table 12.4-2 for blood products utilization. Administer blood and products slowly, with close monitoring of LAP. Overtransfusion can cause systemic HTN, LA dilation, or pulmonary edema, producing additional suture line bleeding or mitral regurgitation.
Monitoring	Standard monitors (see p. D-1).	Severely ill infants often present with invasive monitoring and mechanical ventilation. Correct placement of UAC and UVC should be checked preop. Also verify position of ETT.
	Transthoracic monitoring lines (RA, LA, or PA)	Placed routinely on rewarming, before weaning from CPB. These are for monitoring and administration of inotropes and other medications. The LV can be deconditioned may be dysfunctional and require inotropic support (dopamine, milrinone, epinephrine, and CaCl infusion). During weaning from CPB, it is critical to monitor LAP, as a reflection of left-sided filling, simultaneously with RA pressure monitoring.
	TEE	Abnormalities in coronary perfusion may manifest as changes in EKG rhythm and should be closely followed. TEE is useful both as a monitor of function and volume status. ECMO may be needed for severe ventricular dysfunction.

CPB	Management of CPB is discussed in Intraoperative Considerations for TOF, (p. 1225).	Low flow or moderate hypothermic CPB. Cool with pH stat management (T corrected ABG). Warm on reperfusion with alpha stat management.
Complications	Bleeding LV dysfunction and failure Myocardial ischemia Residual structural defects Dysrhythmias Pulmonary HTN	In patients with TGA and IVS, the LV may be inadequate to support the systemic circulation. The LV becomes deconditioned after the PVR drops in early infancy. The LV is then unable to function as the systemic ventricle. Inotropic support (dopamine and epinephrine) and afterload reduction (SNP or amrinone) may be necessary to separate from CPB. ECMO may be required for severe ventricular dysfunction.

POSTOPERATIVE

Complications	Hypothermia Bleeding Dysrhythmias Myocardial ischemia LV failure	Ischemia 2° coronary artery stenosis, stretching, spasm, or compression. Spasm can be treated with NTG and ↑ aortic pressure. If the now-anterior PA dilates (↓ PaO_2, ↑$PaCO_2$, ↓T, ↓ pH, excessive or too little PIP, or RV failure), the coronary arteries may be compressed. Measures to ↓ PA pressure are often essential.
Tests	ABGs; electrolytes; coag profile CXR TEE	✓ line, chest tube placement; ✓ for pneumothorax.

Suggested Readings

1. Castaneda AR, Jonas RA, Mayer JE Jr, et al: D-transposition of the great arteries. In *Cardiac Surgery of the Neonate and Infant*. WB Saunders, Philadelphia: 1994, 409–38.
2. Castaneda AR, Mayer JE: Neonatal repair of transposition of the great arteries. In *Fetal and Neonatal Cardiology*. Long WA, ed. WB Saunders, Philadelphia: 1990.
3. du Plessis AJ, Jonas RA, Wypij D, et al: Perioperative effects of alpha-stat versus pH-stat strategies for deep hypothermic cardiopulmonary bypass in infants. *J Thorac Cardiovasc Surg* 1997; 114:991–1001.
4. Emmanouilides GC, Allen HD, Riemenschneider TA, et al: Great artery anomalies. In *Clinical Synopsis of Moss and Adams' Heart Disease in Infants, Children, and Adolescents*. Williams & Wilkins, Philadelphia: 1998, 501–14.
5. Kouchoukos NT, Blackstone EH, Doty DB, et al: Complete transposition of the great arteries. In *Kirklin, Barrett, Boyes Cardiac Surgery*. Churchill Livingstone, Philadelphia: 2003, 1438–1508.
6. Quaegebeur JM, Auteri JS: Transposition of the great arteries. In *Glenn's Thoracic and Cardiovascular Surgery*, 6th edition. Baue AE, ed. Appleton & Lange, Stamford: 1996, 1393–1407.
7. Spray TL: Transposition of the great arteries. In *Mastery of Cardiothoracic Surgery*. Kaiser LR, Kron IL, Spray TL, eds. Lippincott-Raven, Philadelphia: 1998, 785–99.

SURGERY FOR TRUNCUS ARTERIOSUS

SURGICAL CONSIDERATIONS

Description: Truncus arteriosus is a rare cardiac anomaly in which there is a common aortopulmonary trunk originating from the base of the heart by way of a single, semilunar valve (truncal valve). This single great artery gives rise to the pulmonary, systemic, and coronary circulations. A nonrestrictive VSD is almost always found immediately below the truncal valve. An anatomic classification scheme proposed by **Collett** and **Edwards** in 1949 describes four types of truncus. In **type I** truncus (60%), a single arterial trunk gives rise to the aorta and main PA (Fig. 12.4-9A). In **type II** truncus (20%), the right and left PAs arise separately from the posterolateral aspect of the truncus. **Type III**

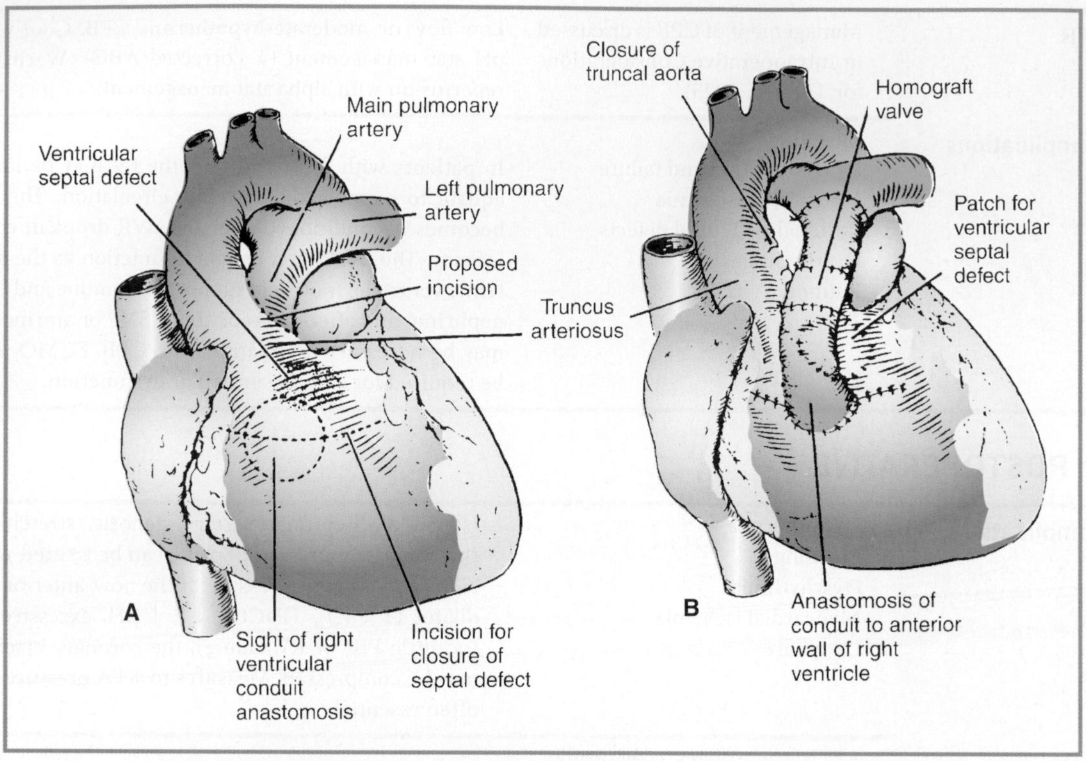

Figure 12.4-9. Truncus arteriosus. (**A**) Cohen-Edwards (Type I). (**B**) Surgical correction involves the separation of the main PA from the truncus, VSD patch closure and insertion of a conduit between the RV and the distal main PA. (Reproduced with permission from Way LW: *Current Surgical Diagnosis and Treatment,* 10th edition. Lange Medical Publications, City: 1973.)

truncus (10%) designates cases in which the two PAs also originate from the posterior truncus, but with widely separated orifices. In **type IV** truncus (10%), the PA branches are absent with pulmonary blood flow derived from aortopulmonary collaterals. Pathophysiologically, there is significant L→R shunting at the truncal and ventricular levels, leading to unrestricted pulmonary blood flow, CHF, and pulmonary HTN. Patients become symptomatic in infancy 2° CHF when the PVR ↓ and CO ↑. Untreated, 90% of infants die within 6 mo.

The first total repairs of this congenital anomaly were reported in the early 1960s and included the insertion of **nonvalved artificial conduits** and **aortic allograft and valve conduits.** In the early and mid-1970s, repair was performed at younger ages, with abandonment of palliative banding of the PA branches. Currently, early primary repair is carried out during the first few weeks of life.

Through a median sternotomy, the truncus and PA branches are dissected and cannulation for CPB is performed. The PAs are snared to block pulmonary flow during perfusion. Hypothermia is induced and the aorta is cross-clamped. The PAs are separated from the main truncus, the resultant aortic defect is repaired with a patch, and a valved homograft (12–14 mm) is prepared. An end-to-end anastomosis of the distal homograft to the PA opening is performed, the VSD is closed through a right ventriculotomy, and the proximal end of the homograft is then anastomosed to the right ventriculotomy (Fig. 12.4-9B). The heart is de-aired, the aorta is unclamped, rewarming and resuscitation are performed, and CPB is discontinued.

There are several **special considerations** associated with this repair that warrant mention. The truncal valve may exhibit insufficiency, necessitating valve repair or replacement using a cryopreserved aortic or pulmonary homograft. In older infants, the PVR may be elevated and pulmonary hypertensive crises should be anticipated. In some patients, an associated interruption of the aortic arch has to be addressed and increases the complexity of the procedure. Coronary artery abnormalities are common in patients with truncus arteriosus and may contribute to their mortality.

Usual preop diagnosis: Truncus arteriosus (types I, II, III, IV)

SUMMARY OF PROCEDURE

Position	Supine
Incision	Standard median sternotomy
Antibiotics	Cefazolin 25 mg/kg q 4 h
Surgical time	Aortic cross-clamp: 30–90 min Total: 2.5–3 h
Closing considerations	Routine closure with chest tube in the pericardial space; temporary ventricular pacing wire; possible right or left atrial line for monitoring
EBL	Moderate
Postop care	1–5 d of assisted ventilation; pulmonary HTN protocol consisting of hyperventilation and sedation and use of pulmonary vasodilators. Inotropes for adequate CO.
Mortality	< 3%
Morbidity	Hemorrhage Atrial dysrhythmias Pulmonary vasospasm Truncal valve insufficiency ↓CO
Pain score	8–10

PATIENT POPULATION CHARACTERISTICS

Age range	3 wk–6 mo
Male:Female	1:1
Incidence	1.7–4.6% of congenital heart defects
Etiology	No known etiology
Associated conditions	Coexisting interrupted aortic arch or coarctation with PDA (10–20%); right aortic arch (16%); mitral valve anomalies (10%); moderate-size or large ASD (10%); DiGeorge syndrome

ANESTHETIC CONSIDERATIONS

PREOPERATIVE

Pathophysiology	A single, common aortopulmonary artery—the truncus—overlies the two ventricles and VSD. Depending on the configuration, the truncus gives rise to coronary and pulmonary arteries and ascending aorta. Complete mixing of systemic and pulmonary circulations occurs at the VSD and truncal valve, resulting initially in cyanosis. After birth, as PVR decreases, significant L → R shunting occurs at the level of the VSD. This causes pulmonary blood flow and CHF. If present, truncal valve insufficiency causes ventricular dilatation and low diastolic coronary perfusion, → myocardial ischemia. If untreated, 80% die of CHF in the 1st yr. Early total correction is indicated.
Airway	The facial anomalies (e.g., micrognathia) in DiGeorge syndrome may make intubation difficult.
Respiratory	Typically, these infants present with the respiratory Sx of CHF (dyspnea, tachypnea, hypoxemia). **Tests:** CXR: ↑ pulmonary markings and wide mediastinum.

Pediatric Surgery

Cardiovascular	Frequently, neonates are intubated and ventilated for hemodynamic support. Arterial saturation > 85% indicates excessive pulmonary blood flow. This may be controlled by the use of hypoxic gas mixtures (17–19% FiO_2), inspired CO_2 (3–5%), and PEEP. **Tests:** EKG. ECHO: Usually diagnostic. Identifies the origin of the PA from the common trunk and the presence (subtype A) or absence (subtype B) of a VSD. Evaluates truncal valve competency.	
Endocrine	In DiGeorge syndrome, thymic hypoplasia occurs with hypoparathyroidism and symptomatic hypocalcemia. **Tests:** ✓ Ca^{++} levels; parathyroid hormone	
Premedication	Not indicated.	
Transport to OR	See Transport of the Critically Ill Newborn (see p. 1229).	

INTRAOPERATIVE

Anesthetic technique: GETA

Induction	The goal for induction is maintenance of hemodynamic stability. If not intubated prior to induction, do not preoxygenate or hyperventilate. IV induction with ketamine (1–2mg/kg), fentanyl (2–4 mcg/kg) and muscle relaxant (e.g., rocuronium 1 mg/kg) is preferred. After ETT is secured, avoid hyperventilation and maintain arterial saturation 75–85%. Keep DBP > 20 mmHg to maintain coronary perfusion. Treat ↓ BP on induction with additional inotropes, transfusion of blood, or occlusion of a PA by the surgeon as soon as the chest is opened.	
Maintenance	Fentanyl (20–50 mcg/kg). Rocuronium as needed ± midazolam 0.2 mg/kg ± volatile agent. FiO_2 = 0.21. Avoid hyperventilation (↓ PVR →↑ shunt + CHF). PEEP may be useful to maintain PVR. The surgeon may leave a PFO to serve as a "pop-off" to preserve systemic perfusion when ↑ PVR and RV dysfunction occur. A transthoracic left atrial line is frequently placed for monitoring. In some cases, the sternum may be left open due to chest-wall and mediastinal edema and the presence of the anterior RV-PA conduit (Rastelli conduit).	
Emergence	Transport to ICU intubated and ventilated. Maintain narcotic and muscle relaxant infusions (e.g., fentanyl and vecuronium) for initial postop period (2–3 d) to minimize pulmonary hypertensive crises.	
Blood and fluid requirements	See Tetralogy of Fallot (TOF).	Continue dextrose infusion in neonates. See Table 12.4-2, p. 1226 for blood product utilization.
Infusions	Inotropic support	These patients require inotropic support (dopamine, milrinone, epinephrine, and CaCl infusion).
Monitoring	Standard monitors + LA, RA, PA lines TEE	 Transthoracic lines TEE is helpful to assess function, truncal valve competency, RV function, and the direction of atrial shunt.
Positioning	See TOF (p. 1225).	
CPB	See TOF (p. 1225).	
Complications	Pulmonary HTN Truncal valve insufficiency Coronary artery insufficiency Residual lesion	

POSTOPERATIVE

Complications (cont'd)	Bleeding	
	Pulmonary hypertensive crisis	Frequent in patients > 1 mo old. Rx: NO, sedation, PGE_1, hyperventilation.
	A-V block	Generally temporary, injury to conduction system unlikely because it is remote from VSD closure. Occasionally, a pacemaker may be required.
	Ventricular dysfunction	May require inotropic support.
	Residual lesions	Residual VSD, severe truncal valve incompetence or obstruction, obstruction of coronary flow, LVOTO.

Suggested Readings

1. Allen HD, Clark EB, Gutgesell HP, et al, eds. *Moss and Adams' Heart Disease in Infants, Children, and Adolescents,* 6th edition. Lippincott Williams & Wilkins, Philadelphia: 2001.
2. Castaneda AR, Jonas RA, Mayer JE Jr, et al: Truncus arteriosus. In *Cardiac Surgery of the Neonate and Infant.* WB Saunders, Philadelphia: 1994, 281–93.
3. Emmanouilides GC, Allen HD, Riemenschneider TA, et al: Truncus arteriosus. In *Clinical Synopsis of Moss and Adams' Heart Disease in Infants, Children, and Adolescents.* EDITORS. Williams & Wilkins, Philadelphia: 1998, 434–41.
4. Kouchoukos NT, Blackstone EH, Doty DB, et al. Truncus arteriosus. In *Kirklin, Barrett, Boyes Cardiac Surgery.* Churchill Livingstone, Philadelphia: 2003, 1200–22.
5. Ramamoorthy C, Tabbutt S, Kurth CD, et al: Effects of inspired hypoxic and hypercapnic gas mixtures on cerebral oxygen saturation in neonates with univentricular heart defects. *Anesthesiology* 2002; 96:283–8.
6. Reitz BA, Yuh DD, eds: *Congenital Cardiac Surgery.* McGraw-Hill, New York: 2002.
7. Spray TL: Truncus arteriosus. In *Mastery of Cardiothoracic Surgery.* Kaiser LR, Kron IL, Spray TL, eds. Lippincott-Raven, Philadelphia: 1998, 759–70.
8. Tabbutt S, Ramamoorthy C, Montenegro LM, et al: Impact of inspired gas mixtures on preoperative infants with hypoplastic left heart syndrome during controlled ventilation. *Circulation* 2001; 104(Supp I):I159–64.

SURGERY FOR TRICUSPID ATRESIA

SURGICAL CONSIDERATIONS

Description: In tricuspid atresia, there is a developmental failure of the tricuspid valve, isolating the RA from the RV. There are three types of tricuspid atresia, based on the relationship of the great vessels to the ventricles, otherwise known as **ventriculoarterial concordance.** Type I, the most common (60–80%), consists of normal ventriculoarterial concordance. Type II (15–25%) consists of *d*-transposition, and Type III (3%) consists of *l*-transposition. In most cases of tricuspid atresia, the RV is hypoplastic, an ASD is present, and pulmonary blood flow is restricted 2° pulmonary stenosis or atresia. Together, these malformations lead to R → L shunting and varying degrees of cyanosis. Those patients with unobstructed pulmonary blood flow develop pulmonary overcirculation and CHF. Consequently, the initial palliative surgical management of this defect depends on the magnitude of pulmonary blood flow; the initial procedure may be either a modified **Blalock-Taussig systemic-to-PA shunt** or a **PA band.** The subsequent definitive surgical management consists of a bidirectional **Glenn shunt** and a modified **Fontan procedure.** Patients undergo these operations sequentially or, in rare cases, directly to the definitive Fontan operation.

The systemic-to-PA shunt, developed by **Blalock** and **Taussig** in 1944, was the first palliative treatment for this condition. Later, other shunts were introduced by **Potts** (descending aorta-to-left PA) and **Waterston** (ascending aorta-to-right PA). In 1958, Glenn described a shunt from the SVC to the right PA applied specifically to patients with tricuspid atresia. A modification of this shunt to a **bidirectional cavopulmonary anastomosis** was performed clinically by **Azzollina** in 1974 and has since gained widespread acceptance. In 1971, Fontan proposed a surgical repair for tricuspid atresia based on separation of the right and left circulations. Subsequent modifications to Fontan's original operation were designed to bypass the RV and direct systemic venous return to the pulmonary circulation. The most recent modifications divert vena caval blood directly to the PA—now referred to as a **total cavopulmonary**

connection (modified Fontan). In 1988, **Laks** suggested leaving a small ASD between the right and left circulations, creating a R → L shunt for the purposes of augmenting systemic CO while still maintaining adequate oxygenation.

Modified Blalock-Taussig (B-T) shunt: In neonates with tricuspid atresia or other single ventricle variants with low pulmonary blood flow, a modified B-T shunt is the procedure of choice. The preferred approach is through a mid-sternotomy. The right PA and the right innominate and subclavian arteries are mobilized. The patient is heparinized and clamps are applied on the right PA and the innominate/subclavian arteries. Arteriotomies are performed and a Gore-Tex tube graft is interposed and anastomosed to the right PA and the subclavian/innominate arteries. The size of shunt (3–4 mm) is dictated by patient size and arterial anatomy. Alternatively, the procedure can be performed via right thoracotomy or through a left thoracotomy if the morphology dictates a left-sided shunt. A midline approach can be used for any variation of the shunt and also gives the option of using CPB in case of patient instability.

Pulmonary artery banding: In patients with tricuspid atresia or other variants of single ventricle and increased pulmonary blood flow, PA banding is performed to protect the pulmonary vascular bed, prevent pulmonary HTN, and prevent CHF. A midline sternotomy is the preferred approach. The main PA is exposed and a 2–3 mm wide strip of Silastic band is placed around the main PA and tightened to adjust the pulmonary blood flow. The goal is a SaO_2 of ~80–85%.

Bidirectional Glenn shunt: A standard median sternotomy approach is used. If concomitant intracardiac repairs are not anticipated, the bidirectional Glenn shunt may be performed without CPB by placing a temporary shunt between the high SVC and the RA. If the patient has a preexisting Blalock-Taussig shunt on the right, it is divided after instituting CPB. A shunt on the left side may be left open, while the bidirectional Glenn shunt is created on the right. The SVC is divided and the cardiac end is oversewn. The remaining caval end is anastomosed end-to-side to the superior aspect of the right PA (Fig. 12.4-10A).

Fontan procedure: The heart is accessed via a standard median sternotomy. Previously placed systemic-to-PA shunts are dissected and occluded prior to bypass. Bicaval cannulation and CPB with hypothermia are used. The IVC is transected at its PA junction and a Gore-Tex tube graft is interposed end-to-end between the IVC and the inferior surface of the right PA. This operation, in conjunction with the previously performed bidirectional Glenn shunt, establishes a total cavopulmonary connection (Fig. 12.4-1B). After completing the anastomosis, the aortic cross-clamp is removed, the heart is rewarmed and the patient is weaned from CPB. Fenestration of the Fontan

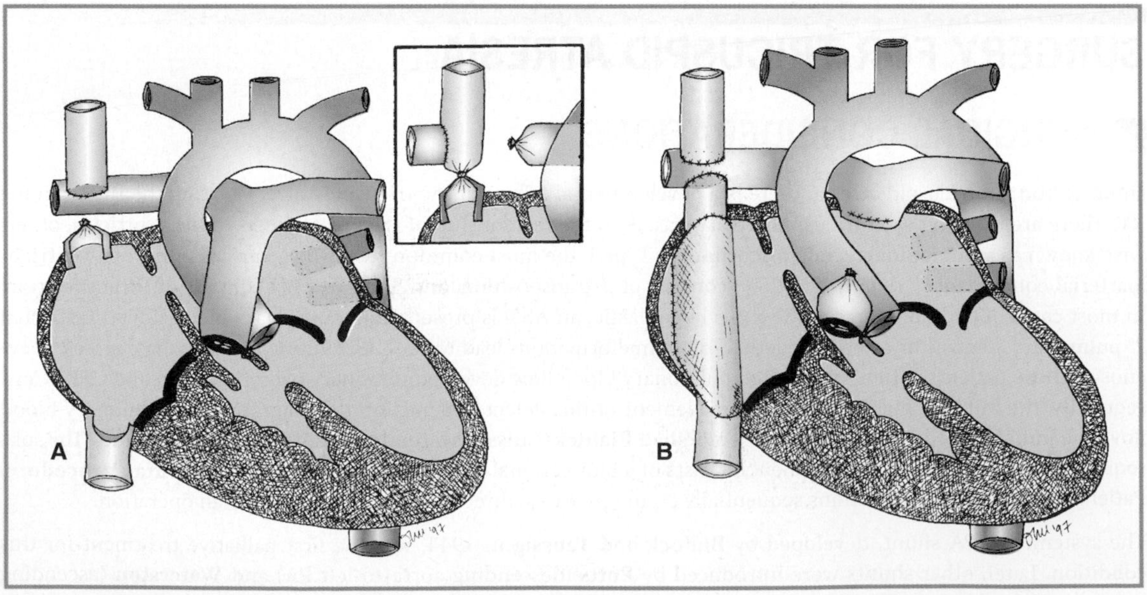

Figure 12.4-10. Surgery for tricuspid atresia. **(A)** Bidirectional Glenn shunt. Inset shows classic unidirectional Glenn shunt. **(B)** Lateral tunnel Fontan operation. (Reproduced with permission from Emmanouilides GC, Allen HD, Riemenschneider TA, et al: *Clinical Synopsis of Moss and Adams' Heart Disease in Infants, Children, and Adolescents.* Williams & Wilkins, Philadelphia: 1998.)

circuit may be desirable in high-risk patients, but is generally not required in patients with tricuspid atresia and good ventricular function. Our current standard is to perform the Fontan procedure without using cardiopulmonary bypass.

Variant procedure or approaches: **A RA→RV connection** can be performed in patients with tricuspid atresia without pulmonary obstruction and an adequately functioning RV. This is accomplished with a direct anastomosis or a valved/nonvalved conduit (e.g., aortic homograft, Dacron graft).

Usual preop diagnosis: Tricuspid atresia after B-T shunt or PA banding; univentricular heart or single ventricle after shunt or band; cyanotic congenital heart disease

SUMMARY OF PROCEDURES

	Bidirectional Glenn Shunt	Cavopulmonary Fontan Procedure
Position	Supine	⇐
Incision	Standard median sternotomy	⇐
Unique considerations	Particulate or gaseous emboli from iv lines can become systemic emboli.	Areas of PA stenosis need to be repaired concomitantly; subaortic obstruction needs to be considered if there is a restrictive VSD and the great vessels are transposed.
Antibiotics	Cefazolin 25 mg/kg q 4 h	⇐
Surgical time	If a simple anastomosis is constructed, the aorta is not cross-clamped. Total: 1.5–2 h	⇐ Total: 3–4 h
Closing considerations	Chest tube in the pericardial space; temporary ventricular pacing wire; possible atrial monitoring line to assess ventricular filling pressure	Chest tube in the pericardial space; possible pleural tubes; temporary ventricular and atrial pacing wires; possible atrial line to correlate with CVP to determine the transpulmonary gradient
EBL	Moderate	⇐
Postop care	Cardiac ICU; early extubation to minimize positive intrathoracic pressure	ICU or early extubation; inotropes for ventricular function, including low-dose dopamine, milrinone for afterload reduction. Maintain sinus rhythm, A-V pacing, if required.
Mortality	< 2%	2–4%
Morbidity	Bleeding Infection Atrial dysrhythmias ↑SVC pressure Upper extremity edema (SVC syndrome) ↓CO Cyanosis 2° ↓pulmonary blood flow Pulmonary arteriovenous fistula	Pleural effusions – ⇐ – – ⇐ – Protein-losing enteropathy (late)
Pain score	8–10	8–10

PATIENT POPULATION CHARACTERISTICS

Age range	4 mo–1 yr	2–5 yr
Male:Female	1:1	⇐
Incidence	1–3% of congenital heart defects	⇐

PATIENT POPULATION CHARACTERISTICS (cont'd)	
Etiology	Unknown ⇐
Associated conditions	TGA; AV valve insufficiency requiring repair or replacement; residual PA obstruction from previous procedures; dextrocardia; asplenia or polysplenia syndromes

ANESTHETIC CONSIDERATIONS

PREOPERATIVE

Pathophysiology	This is characterized by absence of the tricuspid valve and a hypoplastic RV with no communication between RA and RV. Survival in the neonatal period depends on presence of an interatrial communication. The degree of cyanosis reflects the size of the VSD and magnitude of RVOTO. Thirty percent of patients have CHF from pulmonary overcirculation 2° a large VSD and unobstructed RVOT and may require PA banding. Tricuspid atresia requires staged palliation, beginning with the establishment of adequate pulmonary blood flow. Patients undergo a balloon septostomy or a systemic-pulmonary artery shunt (B-T shunt) in the newborn period to augment pulmonary blood flow. Subsequently, at 3–4 mo of age, they undergo cardiac catheterization, and a palliative bidirectional Glenn shunt (SVC→PA) is performed and the B-T shunt is ligated. The Glenn shunt reduces the volume load of the systemic ventricle. The final palliative procedure—the Fontan operation—is done between 1.5–3 yr of age, where the IVC is connected to the PA via an extracardiac conduit. The pulmonary and systemic circulations are now in series.
Respiratory	Identify any infectious or asthma-related problems. Optimizing pulmonary function is imperative as the pulmonary blood flow will be supplied passively from the systemic venous return. **Tests:** CXR; O_2 sat
Cardiovascular	**Tests:** EKG, ECHO, cath
Laboratory	Hct; others as indicated by H&P.
Premedication	Midazolam 0.5–0.75 mg/kg po 20 min before induction in children > 9 mo old

INTRAOPERATIVE/POSTOPERATIVE

For intraop and postop considerations for tricuspid atresia, see Anesthetic Considerations for Surgery for HLHS (see p. 1248).

Suggested Readings

1. Emmanouilides GC, Allen HD, Riemenschneider TA, et al: Tricuspid valve abnormalities. In *Clinical Synopsis of Moss and Adams' Heart Disease in Infants, Children, and Adolescents.* Williams & Wilkins, Philadelphia: 1998, 369–84.
2. Kouchoukos NT, Blackstone EH, Doty DB, et al: Tricuspid atresia and management of single ventricle physiology. in *Kirklin, Barrett, Boyes Cardiac Surgery.* Churchill Livingstone, Philadelphia: 2003, 1113–76.
3. Mayer JE Jr: Tricuspid atresia single ventricle and the Fontan operation. In *Mastery of Cardiothoracic Surgery.* Kaiser LR, Kron IL, Spray TL, eds. Lippincott-Raven, Philadelphia: 1998, 848–57.

SURGERY FOR DOUBLE-OUTLET RIGHT VENTRICLE

SURGICAL CONSIDERATIONS

Description: In double-outlet right ventricle (DORV), at least 50% of both of the great arteries arise from the RV. By necessity, there is a VSD that is usually large, but may in some cases be restrictive or, rarely, multiple and muscular.

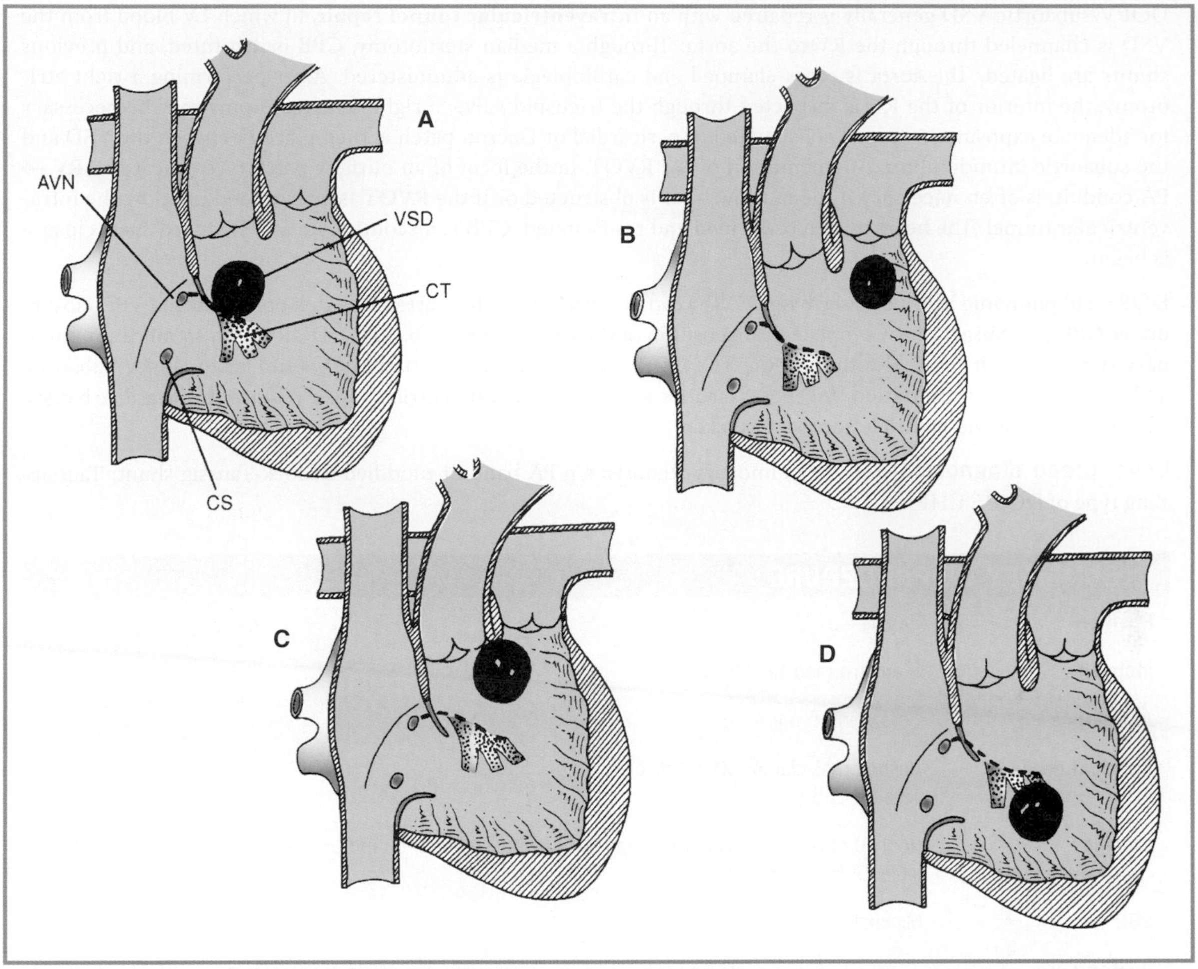

Figure 12.4-11. Types of double-outlet right ventricle classified by the relationship of the VSD to the great arteries. The location of the atrioventricular node and conduction tissue is depicted. **(A)** Subaortic VSD. **(B)** Subpulmonary VSD. **(C)** Doubly committed VSD. **(D)** Noncommitted VSD. AVN = atrioventricular node; CS = coronary sinus; CT = conduction tissue. (Reproduced with permission from Kaiser LR, Kron IL, Spray TL, eds: *Mastery of Cardiothoracic Surgery.* Lippincott-Raven, Philadelphia: 1998.)

The VSD may be located primarily below the aorta (**DORV/subaortic VSD**) (Fig. 12.4-11A), below the pulmonary valve (**DORV/subpulmonic VSD,** or **Taussig-Bing DORV**) (Fig. 12.4-11B), below both great vessels (doubly committed, Fig. 12.4-11C), or remote from both great vessels (noncommitted, Fig. 12.4-11D). In DORV/subaortic VSD, oxygenated LV blood is directed to the aorta and deoxygenated systemic venous return from the RV is directed to the PA, resulting in minimal-to-no cyanosis. L → R shunting across the VSD, however, leads to pulmonary overcirculation, pulmonary HTN, and CHF. In DORV/subpulmonic VSD, oxygenated LV blood is directed to the PA and deoxygenated systemic venous return from the RV is directed to the aorta → pulmonary overcirculation and significant cyanosis. If early PA banding or primary correction is not performed in patients with pulmonary overcirculation, PVOD may result at an early age. In patients with some degree of pulmonary stenosis (usually infundibular), R → L shunting and cyanosis results; the natural history resembles that of patients with tetralogy of Fallot.

The first repairs of DORV were described by **Kirklin** in 1957. The Taussig-Bing DORV was first corrected in 1967. In recent years, management has been simplified for this variant by combining the **arterial switch operation** with an **intraventricular baffle to the pulmonary valve.** From a surgical standpoint, the anatomic variations and past attempts at correction may lead to unique intraop challenges. For example, if a previous Blalock-Taussig shunt has been performed, it needs to be controlled prior to initiating CPB. A previous pulmonary band may require removal and PA reconstruction.

DORV/subaortic VSD generally is repaired with an **intraventricular tunnel repair,** in which LV blood from the VSD is channeled through the RV to the aorta. Through a median sternotomy, CPB is instituted, and previous shunts are ligated. The aorta is cross-clamped and cardioplegia is administered. After performing a right atriotomy, the interior of the RV is inspected through the tricuspid valve; a right ventriculotomy may be necessary for adequate exposure. A tunnel constructed of pericardial or Dacron patch is then placed between the VSD and the subaortic infundibulum. Augmentation of the RVOT, in the form of an outflow patch or extracardiac RV → PA conduit, is often necessary if the outflow tract is obstructed or if the RVOT is encroached upon by the intraventricular tunnel. The heart is then rewarmed and resuscitated, CPB is discontinued, and standard chest closure is begun.

DORV/subpulmonic VSD (Taussig-Bing DORV) can be corrected with an arterial switch operation and VSD closure under CPB (see Surgery for Complete Transposition of the Great Arteries, p. 1231). DORV with significant pulmonary stenosis repair resembles that for the TO. DORV with doubly committed VSD is similar to DORV/subaortic VSD. DORV with uncommitted VSD poses a surgical challenge. A two-ventricle repair requires intracardiac baffles. Alternatively, a single-ventricle approach is taken.

Usual preop diagnosis: DORV ± pulmonary stenosis; s/p PA band or modified Blalock-Taussig shunt; Taussig-Bing type of DORV; CHF

SUMMARY OF PROCEDURE

Position	Supine
Incision	Standard median sternotomy
Antibiotics	Cefazolin 25 mg/kg q 4 h
Surgical time	Aortic cross-clamp: 30–80 min Total: 2–3.5 h
Closing considerations	Routine closure with chest tube in the pericardial space; temporary ventricular pacing wire; possible LA line for monitoring
EBL	Minimal
Postop care	ICU for 1–4 d of controlled ventilation; possible pulmonary HTN protocol in cases of unrestricted pulmonary blood flow (see description of management for A-V canal defect, p. 1206).
Mortality	~2%
Morbidity	Hemorrhage ↓CO Atrial dysrhythmias RV dysrhythmias Intraventricular tunnel obstruction Baffle leakage; residual RVOTO Heart block
Pain score	8–10

PATIENT POPULATION CHARACTERISTICS

Age range	3–24 mo
Male:Female	1:1
Incidence	1–3% of congenital heart defects
Etiology	No specific correlations or associated conditions
Associated conditions	Pulmonary stenosis; complete A-V canal defect; coarctation of the aorta; interruption of the aortic arch; straddling tricuspid valve

ANESTHETIC CONSIDERATIONS

PREOPERATIVE

Pathophysiology	Both great vessels arise from the RV and there is a single, large VSD, whose location may vary (subaortic, subpulmonic). The pathophysiology varies according to the VSD location and other concomitant cardiac anomalies, such as aortic stenosis (AS) or pulmonary stenosis (PS). Those with subaortic VSD present with minimal or no cyanosis, but may have pulmonary overcirculation and CHF. In infants with PS in addition to subaortic VSD, the physiology is similar to TOF. In DORV with subpulmonic VSD, deoxygenated venous return from RV is directed to the aorta, leading to cyanosis. The oxygenated LV output is directed through the VSD into the PA, leading to pulmonary overcirculation. This physiology resembles TGA. The surgical approach may consist of VSD closure, or TOF or TGA repair.

Anesthetic management: Is dictated by specific surgical repair. See sections on VSD, TOF, and TGA, for Anesthetic Considerations (p. 1212, 1223, 1233).

Suggested Readings

1. Emmanouilides GC, Allen HD, Riemenschneider TA, et al: Great artery anomalies. In *Clinical Synopsis of Moss and Adams' Heart Disease in Infants, Children, and Adolescents.* Williams & Wilkins, Philadelphia: 1998, 501–14.
2. Kanter KR: Double-outlet ventricles. In *Mastery of Cardiothoracic Surgery.* Kaiser LR, Kron IL, Spray TL, eds. Lippincott-Raven, Philadelphia: 1998, 771–84.
3. Kouchoukos NT, Blackstone EH, Doty DB et al. Double outlet right ventricle. In *Kirklin, Barrett, Boyes Cardiac Surgery.* Churchill Livingstone, Philadelphia: 2003, 1509–40.

SURGERY FOR HYPOPLASTIC LEFT HEART SYNDROME

SURGICAL CONSIDERATIONS

Description: Hypoplastic left heart syndrome (HLHS) represents a spectrum of left-sided cardiac malformations centered around a markedly hypoplastic LV, and an atretic or hypoplastic aortic valve and ascending aorta; the mitral valve is also usually hypoplastic or atretic (Fig. 12.4-12). Consequently, the RV supports both the pulmonary and systemic circulations. The pulmonary venous return (PVR) enters the RA via an ASD, and the admixture of systemic and pulmonary venous return is delivered into the RV and main PA. Systemic flow is delivered into the aorta by way of a typically large PDA. Cyanosis, CHF, and systemic hypoperfusion result as PVR decreases and pulmonary blood flow increases at the expense of systemic blood flow.

Until the mid-to-late 1980s, patients born with this anomaly usually died within the first 2 wk of life, with survival beyond 6 wk being very rare. A palliative surgical treatment was reported by Norwood in 1983. This treatment of HLHS comprises staged operations, with the first stage designated as the **Norwood operation.** The procedure is directed toward establishing effective CO from the RV to the systemic circulation and to support the pulmonary circulation with a systemic-to-pulmonary arterial shunt. An adequate atrial septal communication is essential.

Stage I (Norwood): A midline sternotomy approach is used. The innominate artery (alternatively, the main PA or ascending aorta, if it is of adequate size) and RA appendage are cannulated and CPB with cooling is instituted. The arch vessels and proximal descending thoracic aorta are dissected. Deep hypothermia with low-flow CPB technique is used. During arch reconstruction, cerebral blood flow is maintained, although many surgeons prefer total circulatory arrest. The ductus arteriosus is then divided and the pulmonary end is oversewn. Next, the main PA is divided and the distal PA is oversewn. An aortotomy is created, extending from the interior aspect of the aortic arch through the lateral aspect of the ascending aorta to the level of the transected pulmonary trunk. The entire aortic arch complex is then augmented, creating a "neoaorta" from the proximal portion of the transected main PA, which is anastomosed to the ascending aorta and arch. A cryopreserved homograft patch is used to facilitate the repair. The RA is

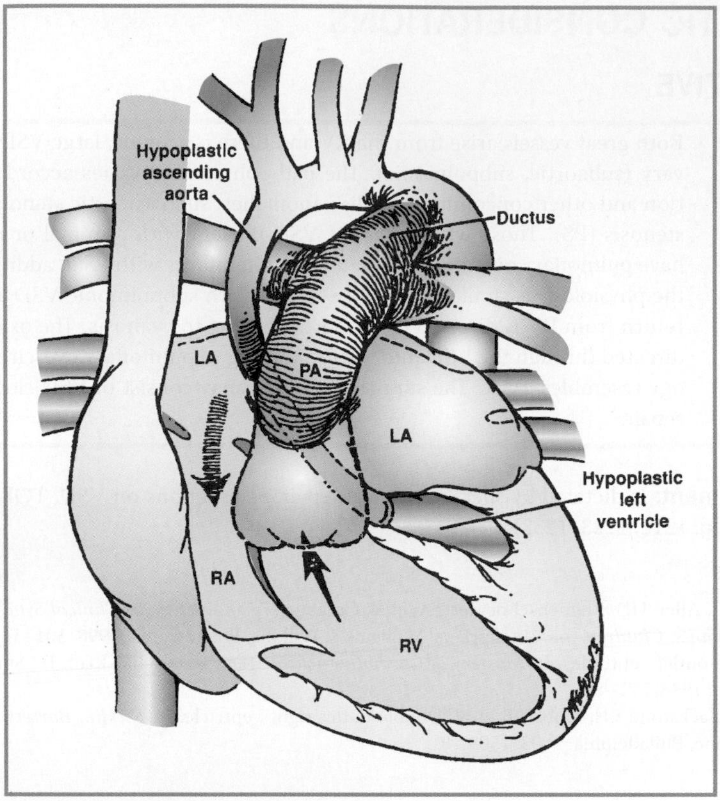

Figure 12.4-12. The anatomic features of hypoplastic left heart syndrome. The right atrium (RA), right ventricle (RV), and main pulmonary artery (PA) are larger than in neonates with normal circulation. LA = left atrium. (Reproduced with permission from Kaiser LR, Kron IL, Spray TL, eds: *Mastery of Cardiothoracic Surgery*. Lippincott-Raven, Philadelphia: 1998.)

opened and the atrial septum is excised to maximize the size of the interatrial communication. The heart is de-aired and rewarming is started with full CPB. If circulatory arrest was used, the cannulae are reinserted, and rewarming begins. Finally, a B-T systemic-to-PA shunt is created to provide pulmonary blood flow. The patient is weaned from CPB, a pericardial drainage tube is placed, and the chest is closed in standard fashion.

Currently, a modification of the Norwood procedure strongly advocated by Japanese surgeons is being adopted by many surgeons worldwide, including us. This involves abandoning the modified B-T shunt in favor of RV-PA shunt ± valve. This modification eliminates the diastolic run-off and preserves coronary blood flow. The major advantage is a stable early postop course. The long-term implications of right ventriculotomy in a systemic RV are not known at the present time.

Stage II (bidirectional Glenn procedure): As the PVR normally falls in the weeks after the first-stage operation, excessive pulmonary blood flow from the B-T shunt may → RV volume overload and CHF. The 2nd-stage procedure for HLHS is intended to reduce the volume load on the single ventricle, while maintaining adequate pulmonary blood flow. This operation consists of a bidirectional cavopulmonary (Glenn) shunt (see Surgery for Tricuspid Atresia, p. 1239), and usually is performed in children 4–6 mo old.

Stage III (Fontan procedure): The 3rd and final stages of the Norwood procedure usually are performed about 6–12 mo after the 2nd stage and consist of the completion of the Fontan procedure (see Surgery for Tricuspid Atresia, p. 1239). It is designed to divide the systemic venous return from the pulmonary venous return by establishing continuity from the IVC to the confluence of the PA and SVC.

Variant procedure or approaches: Successful cardiac transplantation for this condition was performed by **Bailey** in 1985. Cardiac transplantation is associated with a lower operative mortality; however, a significant number of neonates on the waiting lists do not receive donor hearts. Moreover, cardiac transplantation is associated with lifelong immunosuppression and its associated risks.

Usual preop diagnosis: HLHS; mitral and aortic atresia

SUMMARY OF PROCEDURE	
Position	Supine
Incision	Standard median sternotomy
Unique considerations	Hypothermia (< 18° C) ± circulatory arrest; manipulation of PVR and SVR, both preop and postop, is extremely important, with the FiO_2 and ventilation being crucial in regulating pulmonary blood flow. For very high pulmonary blood flows and O_2 sats > 85%, consider the addition of N_2 to lower the FiO_2 to < 20%; use of afterload reduction to manipulate SVR and ↓ ventricular work.
Antibiotics	Cefazolin 25 mg/kg q 4 h
Surgical time	Aortic cross-clamp: 30–60 min Circulatory arrest (if used): 30–45 min Total: 2.5–3.5 h
Closing considerations	Sternum often left open, with chest tube in the pericardial space, with closure delayed until POD 2–4; temporary ventricular pacing wire; possible left atrial line for monitoring
EBL	Minimal-to-moderate
Postop care	2–7 h of controlled ventilation; moderate need for inotropic drugs; balancing PVR and SVR to optimize pulmonary blood flow and systemic CO.
Mortality	10–20%
Morbidity	Hemorrhage Infection ↓CO RV dysfunction Inadequate/excessive pulmonary blood flow Tricuspid regurgitation
Pain score	8–10

PATIENT POPULATION CHARACTERISTICS	
Age range	5–30 d
Male:Female	2:1
Incidence	3–5% of congenital heart defects
Etiology	Often associated with genetic disorders, but no single associated defect
Associated conditions	CNS defects (29%); microencephaly (25–27%); VSD (5%); TGA

ANESTHETIC CONSIDERATIONS

PREOPERATIVE

Pathophysiology

HLHS is characterized by a hypoplastic or atretic aortic and mitral valves associated with hypoplasia of the LV, ascending aorta, and aortic arch. Pulmonary venous return enters the LA and then passes into the RA via an ASD or the PFO. Rarely, pulmonary venous return is via TAPVC to the RA. The systemic circulation is supplied entirely through the ductus arteriosus. Perfusion of the ascending aorta, coronary arteries, and transverse arch is retrograde via the ductus. Maintenance of adequate systemic perfusion relies on ductal patency and is achieved with continuous administration of PGE_1. Maintaining ↑ PVR by ↓ FiO_2 to 0.17–0.20, or by adding CO_2 to breathing gas mixture, may be necessary. As the ductus closes, the systemic perfusion is compromised, → ischemia, acidosis, and eventually death. Survival is dependent on maintaining ductal patency, and adequacy of mixing at the atrial level and a balance between PVR and SVR to ensure adequate pulmonary and systemic perfusion.

Cardiovascular	**Tests:** EKG; RAE/RVH; ECHO: assessment of tricuspid or common AV valve regurgitation. Severe TR is a contraindication for 1st stage repair.	
Neurological	Preop head ultrasound to r/o intracranial pathology (e.g., hemorrhage). Periop neurological monitoring, including cerebral oximeter can be useful, either both hemispheres or left cerebral hemisphere and flank (somatic oxygenation)	
Laboratory	BUN; Cr; Hb/Hct; Plt count	
Premedication	Not indicated.	
Transport to OR	See Transport of the Critically Ill Newborn (p. 1229).	

INTRAOPERATIVE

Anesthetic technique: GETA

Induction	On arrival in the OR, monitors are applied and ventilation should be adjusted to maintain arterial O_2 sat = 75–85%. Avoid hyperventilation (→↑pulmonary blood flow). Arterial sat > 85% will cause systemic hypoperfusion. See Truncus Arteriosus, p. 1238.	
Maintenance	Fentanyl (20–40 mcg/kg) with muscle relaxant (Rocuronium 1 mg/kg) in divided doses on CPB. Volatile anesthetics on CPB. Midazolam (0.1–0.2 mg/kg) as tolerated.	
Emergence	Transport to ICU intubated, ventilated, and monitored.	
Blood and fluid requirements	See Tetralogy of Fallot (TOF) (p. 1224). See Table 12.4-2, p. 1226, for blood product utilization.	Blood loss can be due largely to dilutional coagulopathy and multiple suture lines.
Infusions	See Truncus Arteriosus.	
Monitoring	See Truncus Arteriosus (p. 1238).	
CPB	See TGA (p. 1235).	
Transition off CPB and Post-CPB	See TOF (p. 1225).	After Stage I (Norwood) surgical repair, the blood flow continues to be supplied in a parallel fashion from the single ventricle. At Stanford, a small homograft conduit is placed from the RV to PA (Kashimoto modification) instead of the traditional modified B-T shunt. This prevents the diastolic run-off of the B-T shunt and improves coronary perfusion. Optimal PaO_2 30–50 mmHg with MAP 40–50 mmHg.

POSTOPERATIVE

Complications	Bleeding Pulmonary overcirculation Myocardial dysfunction and failure Aortic arch obstruction Pulmonary HTN CNS injury

Suggested Readings

1. Allen HD, Clark EB, Gutgesell HP, et al eds. *Moss and Adams' Heart Disease in Infants, Children, and Adolescents*, 6th edition. Lippincott Williams & Wilkins, Philadelphia: 2001.
2. Emmanouilides GC, Allen HD, Riemenschneider TA, et al: Left ventricular outflow abnormalities. In *Clinical Synopsis of Moss and Adams' Heart Disease in Infants, Children, and Adolescents*. Williams & Wilkins, Philadelphia: 1998, 501–14.

3. Jacobs ML, Norwood WI: Hyperplastic left heart syndrome. In *Pediatric Cardiac Surgery: Current Issues.* Jacobs ML, Norwood WI, eds. Butterworth-Heinemann, Stoneham: 1992, 182–92.
4. Jacobs ML, Norwood WI: Hypoplastic left heart syndrome. In *Glenn's Thoracic and Cardiovascular Surgery*, 6th edition. Baue AE, ed. Appleton & Lange, Stamford: 1996, 1271–81.
5. Jacobs ML: Hypoplastic left heart syndrome. In *Mastery of Cardiothoracic Surgery*. Kaiser LR, Kron IL, Spray TL, eds. Lippincott-Raven, Philadelphia: 1998, 858–66.
6. Kirkham FJ: Recognition and prevention of neurological complications in pediatric cardiac surgery. *Pediatr Cardiol* 1998; 19:331–45.
7. Kouchoukos NT, Blackstone EH, Doty DB, et al: Aortic atresia and other forms of hypoplastic left heart physiology. In *Kirklin, Barrett, Boyes Cardiac Surgery*. Churchill Livingstone, Philadelphia: 2003, 1377–1400.
8. Nicolson SC, Steven JM, Jobes DR: Hypoplastic left heart syndrome. In *Pediatric Cardiac Anesthesia,* 3rd edition. Lake CL, ed. Appleton & Lange, Stamford: 1998, 337–52.
9. Ramamoorthy C, Tabbutt S, Kurth CD, et al: Effects of inspired hypoxic and hypercapnic gas mixtures on cerebral oxygen saturation in neonates with univentricular heart defects. *Anesthesiology* 2002; 96:283–8.
10. Reitz BA, Yuh DD, eds: *Congenital Cardiac Surgery*. McGraw-Hill, New York: 2002.
11. Sano S, Ishino K, Kado H, et al. Outcome of right ventricle to pulmonary artery shunt in first stage palliation of hypoplastic left heart syndrome–a multi-institutional study. *Ann Thorac Surg* 2004; 78(6):1951–7.
12. Tabbutt S, Ramamoorthy C, Montenegro LM, et al: Impact of inspired gas mixtures on preoperative infants with hypoplastic left heart syndrome during controlled ventilation. *Circulation* 2001; 104(Supp I):I159–64.

3. Jacobs ML, Norwood WI. Hypoplastic left heart syndrome. In: Pediatric Cardiac Surgery: Current Issues. Jacobs ML, Norwood WI, eds. Butterworth-Heinemann: Stoneham 1992; 182–92.
4. Jacobs ML, Norwood WI. Hypoplastic left heart syndrome. In: Glenn's Thoracic and Cardiovascular Surgery, 6th edition. Baue AE, ed. Appleton & Lange: Stamford 1996; 1271–81.
5. Jacobs ML. Hypoplastic left heart syndrome. In: Mastery of Cardiothoracic Surgery. Kaiser LR, Kron IL, Spray TL, eds. Lippincott-Raven: Philadelphia 1998; 858–66.
6. Jonas RA. Recognition and prevention of neurological complications in pediatric cardiac surgery. Pediatr Cardiol 1998; [illegible].
7. Kouchoukos NT, Blackstone EH, Doty DB, et al. Aortic atresia and other forms of hypoplastic left heart physiology. In: Kirklin/Barratt-Boyes Cardiac Surgery. Churchill Livingstone: Philadelphia 2003; 1377–1400.
8. Nicolson SC, Steven JM, Jobes DR. Hypoplastic left heart syndrome. In: Pediatric Cardiac Anesthesia, 3rd edition. Lake CL, ed. Appleton & Lange: Stamford 1998; [illegible].
9. Ramamoorthy C, Tabbutt S, Kurth CD, et al. Effects of inspired hypoxia and hypercapnia on oxygenation in neonates with univentricular heart defects. Anesthesiology 2002; [illegible].
10. [illegible] Yuh DD, eds. Congenital Cardiac Surgery. McGraw-Hill: New York [illegible].
11. Sano S, Ishino K, Kado H, et al. Outcome of right ventricle-to-pulmonary artery shunt in first-stage palliation of hypoplastic left heart syndrome: a multi-institutional study. Ann Thorac Surg 2004; [illegible].
12. Tabbutt S, Ramamoorthy C, Montenegro LM, et al. Impact of inspired gas mixtures on preoperative infants with hypoplastic left heart syndrome during controlled ventilation. Circulation 2001; 104(Suppl I):[illegible].

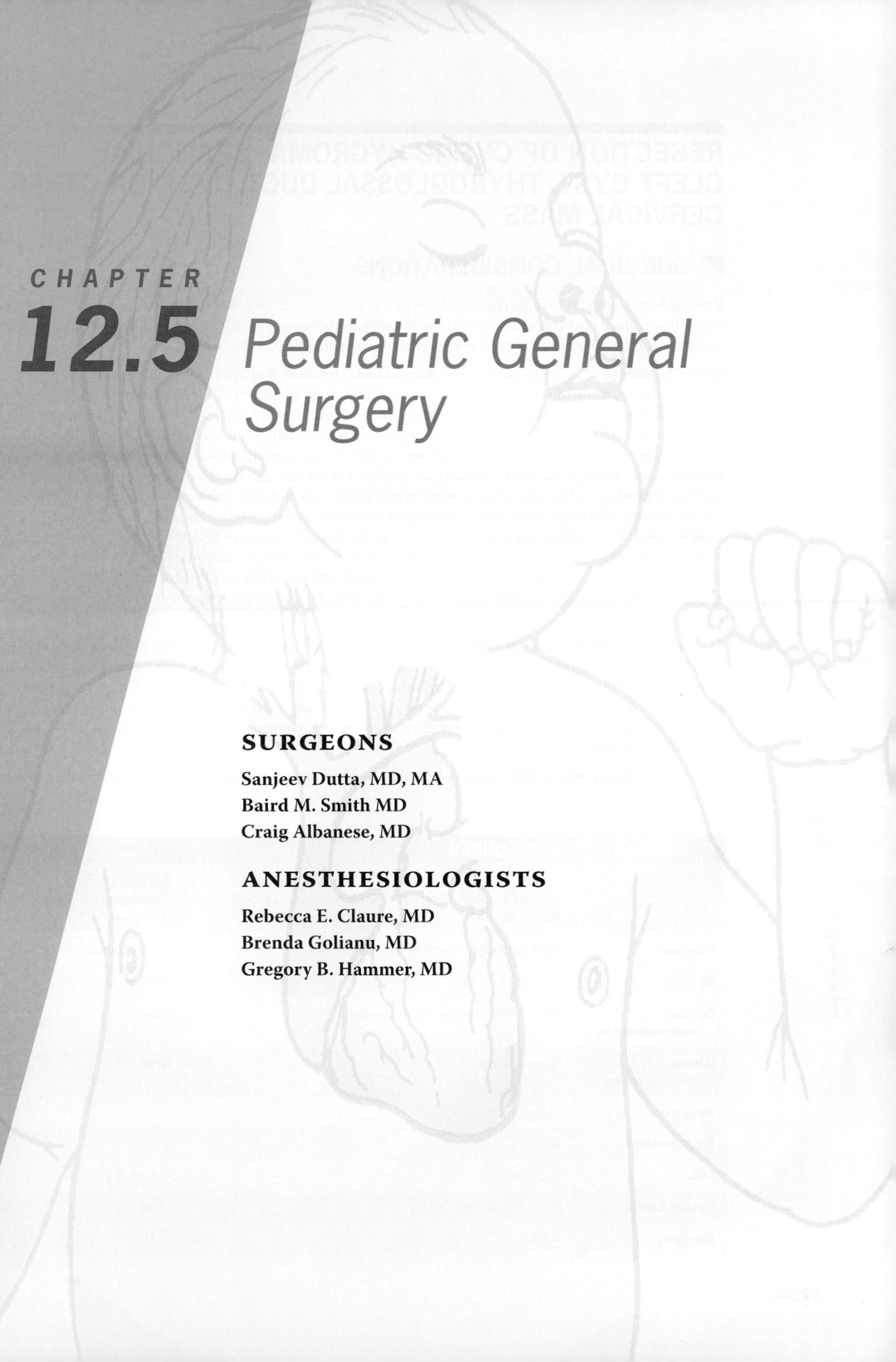

CHAPTER

12.5 Pediatric General Surgery

SURGEONS

Sanjeev Dutta, MD, MA
Baird M. Smith MD
Craig Albanese, MD

ANESTHESIOLOGISTS

Rebecca E. Claure, MD
Brenda Golianu, MD
Gregory B. Hammer, MD

RESECTION OF CYSTIC HYGROMA, BRANCHIAL CLEFT CYST, THYROGLOSSAL DUCT CYST, OR OTHER CERVICAL MASS

SURGICAL CONSIDERATIONS

Description: Common lesions requiring dissection in the neck and floor of the mouth include branchial cleft remnants; thyroglossal duct remnants; vascular malformations (hemangiomas); lymphatic malformations (cystic hygromas); and infected or enlarged lymph nodes refractory to antibiotic therapy.

Surgical approach: Ideally, an acutely inflamed node (*typically Staphylococcus aureus*) usually is incised and drained; a chronically infected node (e.g., cat-scratch disease, atypical TB) or an enlarged node (lymphoma) is excised. Remnants of the first and second (rarely third) branchial clefts are lateral masses found and excised from (respectively), the parotid region anterior to the ear, sometimes extending to the external auditory canal, or the anterior border of the sternocleidomastoid muscle, sometimes extending through the carotid bifurcation to the tonsillar fossa. Thyroglossal duct remnants are midline lesions that involve the central portion of the hyoid bone and may extend up to the base of the tongue. When acutely infected and resistant to a course of antibiotics, they can be drained; when quiescent, thyroglossal duct remnants are excised. Occasionally, it is advantageous for the anesthesiologist to digitally depress the tongue near the foramen cecum to help the surgeon know when the dissection approaches this structure. Vascular and lymphatic malformations may overlap; they tend to be lateral and are sometimes extensive. Significant blood loss may result and resection may involve tedious dissection of neurovascular structures, including the carotid sheath, brachial plexus, sympathetic chain, phrenic nerve, and cranial nerves V, VII, X, XI, and XII.

Transaxillary subcutaneous **endoscopic surgery** allows an alternate approach to resecting these lesions. This approach involves using tiny incisions placed in the ipsilateral axilla through which endoscopic ports are placed and tunneling under the skin to the neck, aided by carbon dioxide insufflation, to resect benign lesions using laparoscopic tools. This is a very new approach and not widely practiced; however, it appears to be safe and effective for a wide variety of lesions, including thyroid and parathyroid lesions. It completely avoids a neck incision, which can be cosmetically unappealing.

Usual preop diagnosis: Cystic hygroma; branchial cleft cyst/fistula; thyroglossal duct cyst; atypical mycobacterial adenitis

SUMMARY OF PROCEDURES

	Lateral Lesions (Branchial Cleft Remnant Lymph Node, Vascular + Lymphatic Malformations)	Midline Lesions (Thyroglossal Duct Remnants)
Position	Neck extended, turned to contralateral side	Neck extended
Incision	Oblique	Transverse
Special instrumentation	Facial nerve monitor; nerve stimulator	None
Unique considerations	Nerve testing	None
Antibiotics	Cefazolin 25 mg/kg iv	⇐
Surgical time	1–6 h	1 h
EBL	5–20 mL/kg	< 5 mL/kg
Postop care	PICU; airway monitoring	None
Mortality	< 2%	< 1%

SUMMARY OF PROCEDURE (cont'd)

	Lateral Lesions (Branchial Cleft Remnant Lymph Node, Vascular + Lymphatic Malformations)	Midline Lesions (Thyroglossal Duct Remnants)
Morbidity	Airway compromise Fluid accumulation Infection	⇐ ⇐ ⇐
Pain score	3–4	3–4

PATIENT POPULATION CHARACTERISTICS

Age range	Newborn–school age
Male:Female	1:1
Incidence	Common
Etiology	Developmental anomaly; mycobacteria
Associated conditions	Hygroma-mediastinal airway involvement; branchial cleft

ANESTHETIC CONSIDERATIONS

PREOPERATIVE

These patients generally are otherwise healthy children. Cervical masses, including cystic hygroma (cystic lymphangioma), may cause airway obstruction and difficult intubation.

Respiratory	The size and extent of the cervical mass should be defined carefully in an effort to detect the potential for airway compromise and to avoid soft-tissue trauma during intubation. Inspiratory stridor suggests supraglottic obstruction, while expiratory stridor is associated with subglottic/intrathoracic obstruction. These patients should have had prior CT/MRI imaging, and all records for these studies, including anesthesia records, should be reviewed. **Tests:** CXR ± CT/MRI scans
Cardiovascular	Cervical masses may be adherent to and/or cause compression of the great vessels. **Tests:** CT/MRI scans
Hematologic	T&C for cystic hygroma, or if a cervical mass involves great vessels or extends into the mediastinum. **Tests:** Hct
Laboratory	Other tests as indicated from H&P.
Premedication	If patient > 7–9 mo, and asymptomatic, consider midazolam (0.5–0.75 mg/kg po) 30 min. prior to arrival in OR. Use premedication cautiously in patients with potential airway compromise.

INTRAOPERATIVE

Anesthetic technique: GETA with pediatric circuit; OR temperature 75–80°; forced air warmer on OR table; use air/O_2 mixture for ventilation; maintain SpO_2 between 92–94% to minimize retinopathy in premature infants at risk.

Induction	Standard pediatric induction (see p. D-1) in patients without airway compromise. IV access should be secured before induction when airway compromise is present or suspected. Mask induction with sevoflurane in 100% O_2. As plane of anesthesia deepens, gently assist

Induction (cont'd)	ventilation. (Keep PIP < 20 cmH_2O). Prior to laryngoscopy, consider atropine (0.02 mg/kg, minimum dose 0.1 mg), if < 1 month, to prevent vagal response. If partial airway obstruction exists, maintain spontaneous ventilation and perform laryngoscopy under deep anesthesia (e.g., ~3 MAC of volatile agent). FOB should be available. Have full range of ETT sizes available, since airway narrowing may be present. Once airway is secured, proceed with NMB (e.g., rocuronium 0.6 mg/kg iv, or vecuronium 0.1 mg/kg iv), unless monitoring facial nerve function.	
Maintenance	Standard pediatric maintenance (see p. D-2). Surgeon may infiltrate incision with local anesthetic. Limit bupivacaine to 2.5 mg/kg (maximum: 10 mL of 0.25 % bupivacaine).	
Emergence	Reverse neuromuscular blockade with neostigmine (0.07 mg/kg) and glycopyrrolate (0.01 mg/kg). Confirm air leak around ETT and extubate when fully awake.	
Blood and fluid requirements	Minimal blood loss usual IV: 20–22 ga × 1; 2nd iv if great vessel involvement NS/LR @ 3 mL/kg/h	Minimal 3rd-space losses. Each mL blood loss can be replaced with 3 mL NS/LR. When great vessels are involved, place at least one iv in lower extremity. Blood loss can be quite sudden; have blood available in OR.
Monitoring	Standard monitors (see p. D-1) ± Arterial line, 22 ga	An arterial line is used when there is risk of large blood loss or to assist management of ventilation
Positioning	✓ and pad pressure points. ✓ eyes.	
Complications	ETT dislodged/loss of airway Laryngospasm Bronchospasm Hemorrhage	ETT must be carefully secured. Liberal use of benzoin. Avoid tension on ETT by circuit hoses. Hold ETT during surgeon's intraoral examination.

POSTOPERATIVE

Complications	Subglottic edema Upper-airway obstruction from edema related to tumor resection Recurrent laryngeal nerve injury	Dexamethasone (0.5–1 mg/kg) and nebulized racemic epinephrine (2.25%) with mist O_2.
Pain management	Morphine (0.05–0.1 mg/kg q2 h), hydromorphone (0.01 mg/kg–0.015 mg/kg q 1 h), acetaminophen (10–15 mg/kg po/ pr q 6 h)	
Tests	As indicated.	

Suggested Readings

1. Foley DS, Fallat ME: Thyroglossal duct and other congenital midline cervical anomalies. *Semin Pediatr Surg* 2006; 15(2):70–5.
2. Gregory GA, ed: *Pediatric Anesthesia,* 4th ed. Churchill Livingstone, New York: 2002, 664–6.
3. Gross, E, Sichel JY: Congenital neck lesions. *Surg Clin North Am* 2006; 86(2):383–92.

ESOPHAGUS-FOREIGN BODY REMOVAL AND DILATION

SURGICAL CONSIDERATIONS

Description: Flexible, diagnostic **esophagogastroduodenoscopy—a** common procedure in pediatrics—usually is performed under GA or heavy sedation in an endoscopy suite or special procedure area. **Rigid esophagoscopy**

usually is performed for therapeutic indications such as removal of a foreign body (FB), dilation of an esophageal stricture, or injection of varices. The procedure is similar for each diagnosis and generally is performed with ET intubation. FB removal is normally a very short procedure, while dilation and variceal injection can be prolonged and may require multiple insertions/removals of the endoscope. Compression of the trachea distal to the ETT by the rigid esophagoscope is a common occurrence. **Radial balloon dilation,** which involves less shear stress than repeatedly passing a bougie catheter, is becoming a popular method of dilation. This is done under endoscopic and fluoroscopic guidance, and is accompanied by a very low rate of complications.

Usual preop diagnosis: Esophageal FB; stricture; esophageal varices

SUMMARY OF PROCEDURE

Position	Supine, head to the side for rigid esophagoscopy
Special instrumentation	Rigid esophagoscopes; forceps; dilators
Unique considerations	Esophagoscope may obstruct airway; dilation may perforate esophagus.
Surgical time	5 min–2 h
Closing considerations	Abrupt ending
EBL	< 5 mL/kg
Postop care	Airway support
Mortality	< 5%
Morbidity	Esophageal perforation: 2–5%
Pain score	2–3

PATIENT POPULATION CHARACTERISTICS

Age range	Newborn–school age
Male:Female	1:1
Incidence	1/1000
Etiology	Varices – portal HTN; FB – possible stricture
Associated conditions	Esophageal atresia – stricture; portal HTN – varices

ANESTHETIC CONSIDERATIONS

PREOPERATIVE

Esophagoscopy for FB removal is usually performed in healthy infants and toddlers, although it can occur in any age group. All of these patients should be treated with full-stomach precautions (see p. B-4). Esophageal dilation is usually performed in three distinct patient populations: (a) those with prior tracheoesophageal fistula (TEF) repair; (b) those with prior ingestion of a caustic substance; and (c) those with skin and connective tissue diseases (e.g., epidermolysis bullosa [EB]).

Respiratory	Patients with TEF may have residual BPD or chronic lung disease, or subglottic stenosis due to prolonged intubation. Check anesthesia records for ETT size used. Those with prior caustic ingestion may have Hx of pulmonary aspiration, with resultant chemical pneumonitis and/or fibrosis. Patients with EB may have limited mouth opening and require special care regarding placing and securing of ETT. **Tests:** CXR, if clinically indicated.

Cardiovascular	There may be persistent congenital cardiac anomalies in the TEF patient. **Tests:** EKG, ECHO as indicated. Cardiology consultation, as needed.
Laboratory	No routine lab analyses are required if patient has no underlying chronic illnesses.
Premedication	For esophageal dilation, patient preference is extremely important since some patients have undergone this procedure several times. For FB removal, iv access is usually recommended before induction, though a mask induction may be selected by the anesthesiologist as well.

INTRAOPERATIVE

Anesthetic technique: GETA, using a pediatric circuit. Room temperature should be maintained at 75–80°F. Forced air warmer may be used.

Induction	If the patient is presenting for dilation alone and has no evidence to suggest reflux or retained food in the esophagus, a standard inhalation or iv induction may be performed. Rapid-sequence induction is usually appropriate for FB removal. Atropine (0.02 mg/kg if < 1 mo, minimum 0.1 mg) may be administered to attenuate bradycardia from intubation. Preoxygenate for 2–3 min. Apply cricoid pressure. Propofol (2–3 mg/kg) or STP (3–5mg/kg), followed by rocuronium (1 mg/kg) or succinylcholine (1–2 mg/kg). Intubate trachea with age-appropriate ETT. If succinylcholine was used, consider additional neuromuscular blockade.	
Maintenance	Maintain anesthesia with volatile agent/N_2O/O_2 or propofol (100–250 mcg/kg/min) + remifentanil (0.05–0.2 n mcg/kg/min). Supplement inhalation anesthetic with small doses of fentanyl (e.g., 1–2 mcg/kg) or morphine (0.05–0.1 mcg/kg). Maintain neuromuscular blockade or deep plane of anesthesia. Movement must be avoided with rigid esophagoscopy.	
Emergence	Extubate when fully awake. Neostigmine (0.07 mg/kg) and glycopyrrolate (0.01 mg/kg) to reverse neuromuscular blockade. Do not attempt reversal of neuromuscular blockade until first twitch of train-of-four has returned.	
Blood and fluid requirements	IV: 20–22 ga × 1 NS/LR @ 4–6 mL/kg/h	
Monitoring	Standard monitors (see p. D-1) Peripheral nerve stimulator	
Positioning	✓ and pad pressure points. ✓ eyes. ✓ radial pulse of dependent arm.	Axillary roll as needed; avoid brachial plexus compression.
Complications	Esophageal perforation Aspiration Accidental extubation Stridor 2° subglottic edema	Esophageal perforation, more common with rigid esophagoscopy, may lead to pneumothorax (R > L)

POSTOPERATIVE

Complications	Residual neuromuscular blockade Pneumothorax, esophageal perforation	
Pain management	Minimal postop pain	If patient reports marked substernal discomfort, suspect esophageal perforation.
Tests	None	

Pediatric Surgery

Suggested Readings

1. Lan LC, Wong KK, Lin SC, et al: Endoscopic balloon dilatation of esophageal strictures in infants and children: 17 years' experience and a literature review. *J Pediatr Surg* 2003; 38(12):1712–5.
2. Li, ZS, Sun ZX, Zou DW, et al: Endoscopic management of foreign bodies in the upper-GI tract: experience with 1088 cases in China. *Gastrointest Endosc* 2006; 64(4):485–92.
3. Motoyama EK, Davis PJ, eds: *Smith's Anesthesia for Infants and* Children, 7th edition. Mosby-Elsevier, Philadelphia: 2006:818.
4. Rodgers BM, McGahren ED III: Esophagus. In *Surgery of Infants and Children.* Oldham KT, Colombani PM, Foglia RP, eds. Lippincott-Raven, Philadelphia: 1997, 1005–20.

REPAIR OF TRACHEOESOPHAGEAL FISTULA AND ESOPHAGEAL ATRESIA

SURGICAL CONSIDERATIONS

Description: The majority of infants with tracheoesophageal fistulae (TEF) have an associated esophageal atresia (EA), as shown in Fig. 12.5-1 (Type C). The Dx is made presumptively when a NG tube cannot be advanced past 8–13 cm and gas is present in the stomach. The complications of aspiration (gastric contents come up the fistula into the trachea) and GI distention compromising respiration (from passage of air down the fistula into the intestines) are

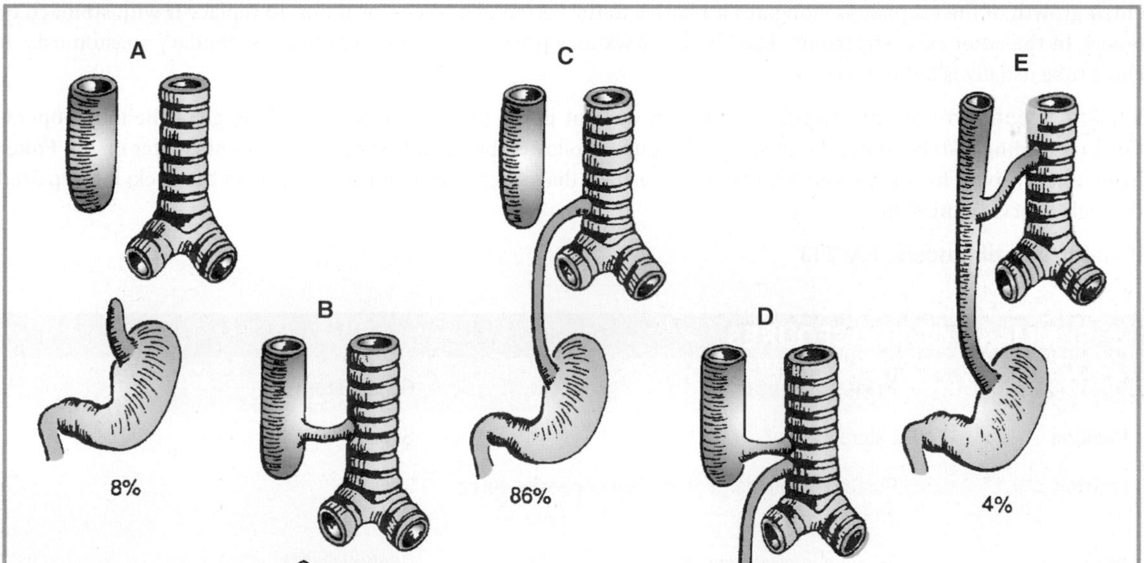

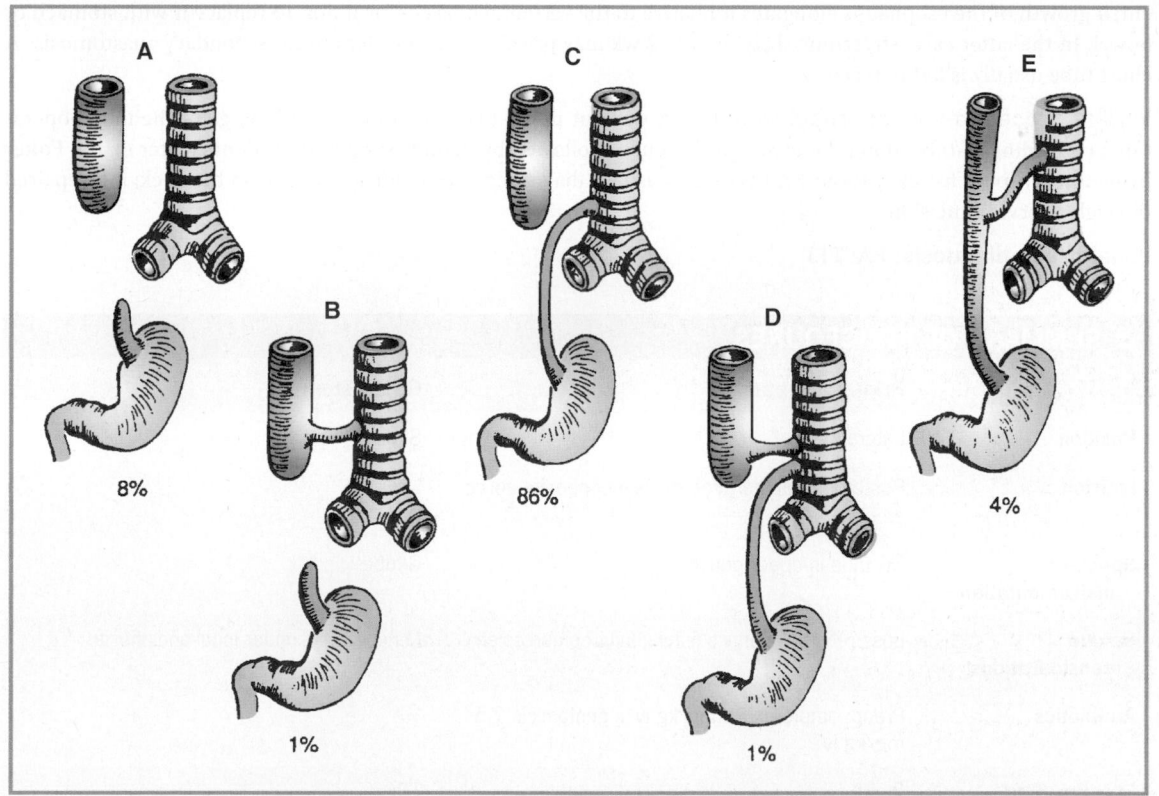

Figure 12.5-1. Types of esophageal atresia: **(A)** pure esophageal atresia; **(B)** proximal fistula; **(C)** esophageal atresia, distal fistula; **(D)** proximal and distal fistula; **(E)** pure tracheoesophageal fistula. (Redrawn from Ravitch MM, et al, eds: *Pediatric Surgery*, Vol 1, 3rd edition. Year Book Medical Publishers, Chicago: 1979.)

diminished by repair within a few days of birth. Primary repair without gastrostomy is routine. The absence of stomach and bowel gas suggests a pure EA without fistula (Type A). A staged procedure—initial gastrostomy with deferred thoracotomy—may be used in babies < 1 kg, those with pure EA, or with more critical associated anomalies.

Surgical approach: The operation is performed in left-lateral decubitus position through a 4th **interspace right** thoracotomy. Preop EKG is advised to look for cardiac anomalies and confirm a normal left-sided aortic arch. In the case of a right-sided arch (10%), most surgeons approach the fistula through a **left thoracotomy.** Debate continues as to whether the best approach is retropleural or transpleural. The former is slower, but it may diminish the chances of empyema when the esophageal anastomosis leaks transiently.

Another approach is **thoracoscopy.** There is now extensive experience with this approach, and it is proven to be a safe and effective method of repair in children, even those with complex congenital heart disease. It is performed using three or four trocars in the modified (prone) left-lateral decubitus position, causing the lung to drop forward as 5 mmHg capnothorax is achieved. Dividing the azygous vein is necessary to find the subjacent fistula, branching off the posterior aspect of the trachea (Type C). The right bronchus, aorta, and (rarely) left bronchus may be mistaken for this structure. Division of the fistula may dramatically improve ventilation; until this moment it is sometimes necessary to operate in short 3- to 5-min. bursts, relaxing lung and mediastinal retraction for 1–2 min. when saturations descend to critical levels. Afterwards, the proximal fistula is located (when the anesthesiologist pushes downward on the indwelling [Replogle] tube) and then is dissected upwards into the root of the neck to achieve sufficient length for anastomosis. After the posterior wall of the anastomosis is complete, some surgeons will ask for the NG tube to be replaced by a small (5 or 6 Fr) feeding tube, which is advanced into the stomach, separating the anterior from posterior esophageal wall during closure and permitting enteric feeds during the customary 1 week before an esophagram is performed. This tube must be fixed in place, because it has a tendency to become dislodged. Because neck hyperextension, as would occur during direct laryngoscopy, places significant tension on the anastomosis, post-operative reintubation is to be avoided. When the length of native esophagus is too short, even after lengthening maneuvers, both ends can be tied to the prevertebral fascia or attached to monofilament sutures and brought tangentially out of the back skin (Foker). In the former case, one reoperates months later, after differential growth of the esophagus elongates it relative to the vertebral bodies—or if not, to replace it with stomach or bowel. In the latter case, stretching daily over 1–2 wk may provide sufficient length for secondary anastomosis. A chest tube usually is left in place.

Variant procedures or approaches: Pure EA without fistula (Type A) indicates a long gap—the initial operation is a feeding G-tube along the lesser gastric curve, followed by definitive operation months later or the **Foker procedure.** A pure fistula without EA (Type E) is usually diagnosed later in life and occurs in the neck; it is repaired through a cervical incision.

Usual preop diagnosis: EA; TEF

SUMMARY OF PROCEDURES

	Primary Repair	Gastrostomy
Position	Lateral	Supine
Incision	Posterolateral thoracotomy (side opposite aortic arch)	LUQ
Special instrumentation	NG tube in upper pouch	G-tube
Unique considerations	Loss of ventilation via fistula; lung compression	May be done under local anesthesia.
Antibiotics	Preop: ampicillin 25 mg/kg iv + gentamicin 2.5 mg/kg iv	⇐
Surgical time	2–4 h	1 h
Closing considerations	Extubation favored	Local anesthetic; wound infiltration
EBL	10 mL/kg	5 mL/kg

SUMMARY OF PROCEDURE (cont'd)

	Primary Repair	Gastrostomy
Postop care	NICU; humidified mist; avoid CPAP and neck hyperextension	⇐
Mortality	1–20%, depending on associated anomalies	5%
Morbidity	Stricture: 20–40% Leak: 10–20% Aspiration Atelectasis Stridor	– – ⇐ – –
Pain score	7–8	3–4

PATIENT POPULATION CHARACTERISTICS

Age range	Days–weeks
Male:Female	1:1
Incidence	1 in 4,000 births
Etiology	Unknown
Associated conditions	Vertebral, anal, TEF, renal (or radial) anomalies (VATER association); vertebral, anal, cardiac, TEF, renal, limb anomalies (VACTERL association); trisomy 13, 18; hydrocephalus

ANESTHETIC CONSIDERATIONS

PREOPERATIVE

EA and TEF usually are detected in the first day of life, although TEF without atresia may be difficult to diagnose until the patient experiences recurrent pneumonia, cyanosis associated with feeding, or abdominal distention. The fistula is usually at the distal trachea near the carina. Because of the risk of pulmonary aspiration, gastrostomy may be performed within hours of detection. Associated conditions frequently associated with TEF include prematurity (30–40%) and congenital anomalies such as cardiac (20–35%), VATER and VACTERL associations (see above). Routine neonatal preop evaluation includes: serum electrolytes, glucose and hematocrit. Patient should be well-hydrated and should have adequate urine output.

Respiratory	The upper esophageal pouch should be suctioned to minimize aspiration. These patients frequently have respiratory insufficiency 2° prematurity (RDS), or aspiration pneumonitis, and may be intubated and on mechanical ventilation. **Tests:** CXR, ABG
Cardiovascular	Associated cardiac abnormalities include: VSD, PDA, tetralogy of Fallot, ASD, and coarctation of the aorta. At risk for pulmonary HTN with R → L shunt. **Tests:** EKG, ECHO, catheterization as indicated.
Gastrointestinal	Associated GI anomalies may occur (e.g., imperforate anus, midgut malrotation, duodenal atresia, pyloric stenosis).
Musculoskeletal	Musculoskeletal anomalies are usually of little anesthetic significance, except for possible C-spine involvement.
Hematologic	For the first 2–3 mo of life, the O_2-carrying capacity of blood is increased because of the presence of fetal Hb with its ↓ sensitivity to 2,3-DPG. A shift to the right of the O_2 sat curve results in ↑ O_2 –Hb affinity. As a result, tissue oxygenation may be reduced, especially with anemia (Hb < 12 g/dL @ < 2–3 mo). Although TEF repair is not usually associated with significant blood loss, a T&C is indicated. **Tests:** Hct; T&C; others as indicated from H&P.

Laboratory	Serum electrolytes, ABG, blood glucose, to determine metabolic state.
Premedication	Usually none

INTRAOPERATIVE

Anesthetic technique: Combined GETA/epidural, using a pediatric circuit. Warm room to 75–80°F and use forced air warmer. If the child is otherwise healthy and extubation is planned within 48 hours, consider placing a caudal or lumbar epidural catheter (see p. D-4) after airway is secured and the child is anesthetized. Patients with large fistulas may need awake gastrostomy or a Fogarty catheter placed via the gastrostomy, using FOB, to occlude the distal end of the fistula. Alternatively, the Fogarty catheter can be used to occlude the proximal end of the fistula via the trachea.

Induction	Atropine (0.02 mg/kg iv in children < 1 mo, minimum 0.1 mg) is given before induction to ablate vagal response to laryngoscopy. IV induction with care during ventilation to minimize PIP and potential inflation of stomach. Advance ETT to right mainstem and withdraw until bilateral breath sounds are present. Rotate ETT so the bevel faces posteriorly (to prevent intubation of the fistula). Have flexible pediatric bronchoscope available to verify placement of ETT and site of TEF. Keep air leak around ETT to a minimum (leak at 18–35 cm H_2O) to minimize alterations in ventilation 2° changes in chest and pulmonary compliance.	
Maintenance	Avoid high FiO_2 if possible in premature neonates at risk for retinopathy. Use air/O_2 mixture for ventilation to maintain O_2 sat between 95–100%. Use low PIPs to avoid gastric distention by gases passing through fistula. Careful adjustment of ventilation will be necessary during surgical retraction of lung or during insufflation if procedure is done thoracoscopically. Manual ventilation can be helpful in assessing pulmonary compliance. If the patient is not tolerating manipulation by the surgeon, brief breaks may be necessary to restore ventilation and oxygenation. Air/O_2/opioid (e.g., fentanyl 5–10 mcg/kg/h) propofol or low-dose volatile technique is preferred because of better hemodynamic stability. Muscle relaxation (rocuronium 0.6mg/kg iv, vecuronium 0.1 mg/kg) is usually necessary. If epidural is used, GA drug requirements will be reduced. Frequent tracheal suctioning may be needed.	
Emergence	Extubation in OR is preferable, but not always possible. Supplement O_2 as necessary to keep SpO_2 = 95–100% (PaO_2 = 60–80 mmHg). Cardiac or pulmonary complications, or any question regarding adequacy of ventilation mandate continued intubation and ventilation. Reintubation may compromise the new anastomosis.	
Blood and fluid requirements	Blood loss usually minimal IV: 22–24 ga × 2 NS/LR (maintenance) @: 4 mL/kg/h – 0–10 kg 5% albumin	Continue dextrose-containing solution from NICU. Replace 3rd-space losses (6–8 mL/kg/h) with NS/LR. Replace blood loss with 5% albumin mL for mL blood loss; maintain Hct > 35%.
Monitoring	Standard monitors (see p. D-1). Left axillary precordial stethoscope Arterial line (24 ga)	ABG, Hct, and glucose q 60 min
Positioning	✓ and pad pressure points. ✓ eyes. Axillary roll Arms should be positioned to be visible and easily available to anesthesiologist.	The patient is turned to the left-lateral decubitus position for a right thoracotomy. Monitor breath sounds in dependent lung. Consider using bronchoscope to recheck tube position.
Complications	Hypothermia Metabolic acidosis Hypo- or hyperventilation Aspiration Pneumothorax Atelectasis Mucus plug	ETT placement may interfere with TEF closure. Migration of ETT above fistula may lead to leak through gastrostomy and difficult ventilating. Typically in ETT or large bronchi

POSTOPERATIVE

Complications	Apnea Pneumothorax Hypoventilation Tracheal leak Inadequate NMB reversal Recurrent laryngeal nerve injury Pneumonia	Maintenance of normothermia lessens incidence of apnea, hypoventilation, and metabolic acidosis. Spontaneous hip flexion is the most reliable indication of adequate neuromuscular function.
Pain management	Acetaminophen: 10–20 mg/kg pr q 4 h prn Fentanyl 0.5–1.0 mcg/kg iv q 60 min prn Dilaudid 0.01– 0.015 mg/kg iv Morphine 0.05 mg/kg–0.1 mg/kg iv Epidural analgesia (see E-5)	
Tests	ABG; Hct	

Suggested Readings

1. Andropoulus DB, Row RW, Betts JM: Anesthetic and surgical airway management during tracheoesophageal fistula repair. *Paediatr Anesth* 1998; 8:313–19.
2. Beasley SW: Esophageal atresia and tracheoesophageal fistula. In *Surgery of Infants and Children*. Oldham KT, Colombani PM, Foglia RP, eds. Lippincott-Raven, Philadelphia: 1997, 1021–34.
3. Chittmittrapap S, Spitz L, Kiely EM, et al: Anastomotic leakage following surgery for esophageal atresia. *J Pediatr Surg* 1992; 27(1):29–32.
4. Goh DW, Brereton RJ: Success and failure with neonatal tracheo-oesophageal anomalies. *Br J Surg* 1991; 78(7):834–7.
5. Gregory GA, ed: *Pediatric Anesthesia*, 4th ed. Churchill Livingstone, New York, 2002:440–3.
6. Holcomb GW 3rd, Rothenberg SS, Bax KM, et al: Thoracoscopic repair of esophageal atresia and tracheoesophageal fistula: a multi-institutional analysis. *Ann Surg* 2005; 242(3):422–8.
7. Holzki J: Bronchoscopic findings and treatment in congenital tracheo-oesophageal fistula. *Paediatric Anaesthesia* 1992; 2:297–303.
8. Krosnar S, Baxter A: Thoracoscopic repair of esophageal atresia with tracheoesophageal fistula: anesthetic and intensive care management of a series of eight neonates. *Pediatric Anesthesia* 2005; 15:541–6.
9. Liu LM, Pang LM: Neonatal surgical emergencies in anesthesiology. *Clin North Am* 2001; 19(2):272–6.
10. Motoyama EK, Davis PJ, eds: *Smith's Anesthesia for Infants and Children*, 7th edition. Mosby-Elsevier, Philadelphia 2006:550–2.
11. Rice-Townsend S, Ramamoorthy C, Dutta S: Thoracoscopic repair of a type D esophageal atresia in a newborn with complex congenital heart disease. *J Pediatr Surg* 2007; 42(9):1616–9.

MEDIASTINAL MASS—BIOPSY OR RESECTION

SURGICAL CONSIDERATIONS

Description: **Mass lesions** in the mediastinum are classified as anterior, middle, and posterior, based on their relationship to the heart, which occupies the middle mediastinum. **Anterior tumors** include lymphomas, thyroid tumors, teratomas, and thymomas. Large lymphomas and, less commonly, teratomas or metastatic germ cell tumors may cause **anterior mediastinal mass syndrome** and/or **SVC compression.** Patients will use accessory muscles, refuse to lie flat, may have a suffused face with venous distention, and are at great risk for distal airway obstruction during induction. As often as possible, operations are performed quickly with the patient awake and semirecumbent. Steroids are very effective in shrinking lymphomas, causing massive cell death such that tumor histology may demonstrate only necrosis after 36 hours. Preop preparation includes a rigid bronchoscope, plans to advance the ETT into a mainstem bronchus, and consideration of the need to rapidly roll the patient prone. These masses often are approached through a **3rd-rib anterior mediastinotomy (Chamberlain procedure)** or thoracoscopically. For patients with compromised airway, light sedation and core-needle biopsy under image guidance (e.g., ultrasound or CT scan) is preferable. **Middle mediastinal tumors** include esophageal duplications, bronchogenic cysts, lymphangiomas and variants, pericardial cysts, and lymph nodes. They are typically approached through a 5th-intercostal space posterolateral thoracotomy or thoracoscopically. **Posterior mediastinal lesions** are usually neurogenic tumors; less commonly, neuroenteric cysts. The former may communicate with the spinal cord through the intervertebral foramina, giving them the appearance of central narrowing ("dumbbell tumor"). They usually arise from the sympathetic ganglia and, when high in the chest, excision may cause Horner's syndrome. They are approached thoracoscopically or via posterolateral thoracotomy.

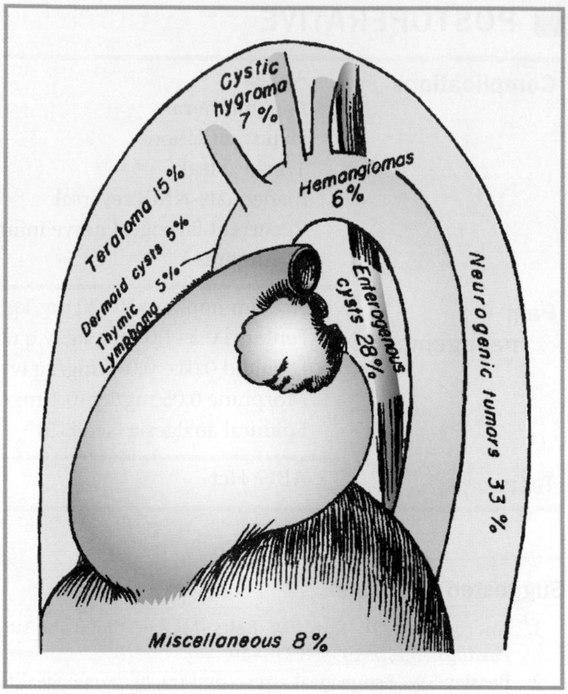

Figure 12.5-2. Distribution of mediastinal cysts and tumor. (Reprinted with permission from Ravitch MM, et al: *Pediatric Surgery*. Year Book Medical Publishers, Chicago: 1986.)

Surgical approach: The potential for blood loss and airway compromise must always be anticipated when operating on chest lesions adjacent to the great vessels and tracheobronchial tree. When SVC or anterior mediastinal mass syndromes are suspected, they may be confirmed clinically and should be discussed among surgeon, anesthesiologist, and oncologist. **Thoracoscopy** is the gold standard for biopsy. In the absence of an adequate workspace, a mini-thoracotomy may be necessary, but adequate biopsy for diagnostic purposes can typically be achieved with core needle biopsy.

Variant Procedure: In the past, it was a dictum that at least 1 cm^2 of tumor was needed for architecture to diagnose and classify lymphomas. In the age of histochemistry and chromosomal studies, this is less true. Sometimes the Dx can be made on bone marrow aspirate, pleural effusion aspirate, or a Tru-Cut needle biopsy. These alternatives should be considered when large anterior mediastinal masses are encountered.

Usual preop diagnosis: Neuroblastoma; teratoma; duplication cyst of foregut; mediastinal mass (lymphoma)

SUMMARY OF PROCEDURES

	Lateral Thoracotomy	Median Sternotomy
Position	Lateral	Supine or semirecumbent
Incision	Posterolateral	Median, parasternal
Special instrumentation	None	Bronchoscope; ± CPB
Unique considerations	Airway or cardiovascular collapse after induction in anterior mediastinal masses	⇐
Antibiotics	Preop: ampicillin 25 mg/kg iv + gentamicin 2.5 mg/kg iv; intraop: cephalosporin irrigation (1 g/500 mL NS)	⇐
Surgical time	2–4 h	1–4 h
Closing considerations	Lung inflation; intercostal block; epidural catheter	⇐
EBL	10–30 mL/kg	10–50 mL/kg
Postop care	Aggressive respiratory therapy; analgesia	⇐

SUMMARY OF PROCEDURE (cont'd)

	Lateral Thoracotomy	Median Sternotomy
Mortality	< 5%, except symptomatic anterior masses	⇐
Morbidity	Atelectasis/respiratory Cardiovascular collapse with anterior masses	⇐ ⇐
Pain score	7–8	6–7

PATIENT POPULATION CHARACTERISTICS

Age range	Newborn—teens
Male:Female	1:1
Incidence	1/5000
Etiology	Unknown
Associated conditions	Cervical or axillary cystic hygroma; hemangioma; SVC syndrome

ANESTHETIC CONSIDERATIONS

PREOPERATIVE

The clinical presentation of a mediastinal mass is often nonspecific in an otherwise healthy child. Often, a routine CXR (for some incidental Sx) will show the presence of an anterior mediastinal mass. These patients may suffer acute cardiorespiratory compromise on induction of anesthesia. A careful preop workup is essential to ensure that GA is absolutely necessary before proceeding. This includes a non-diagnostic bone marrow aspirate/biopsy and drainage of pleural fluid, and consideration of peripheral lymph node biopsy.

Respiratory	Respiratory Sx (e.g., dyspnea, cough, stridor, wheezing) are extremely important in guiding additional studies. Note that, when mild airway compromise is present in the awake patient, this can indicate that total obstruction may occur when the patient is anesthetized or after muscle relaxation. The ability to lie supine without respiratory compromise should be determined, but does not guarantee adequate air exchange after receiving sedation or anesthesia. Tracheal and bronchial compression from the tumor may be positional. Preop radiation therapy may ↓ tumor mass and relieve airway obstruction. **Tests:** CXR; chest CT/MRI; echocardiogram; supine-sitting flow/volume loops can be useful for evaluating location and extent of airway obstruction in patients who are cooperative > 5 years; Oxygen saturation or ABG is indicated if symptomatic.
Cardiovascular	Sx of a mediastinal mass may include SVC syndrome (e.g., venous engorgement of head and neck, edema of upper body). Other Sx and signs may include syncope and headaches (↑ ICP) made worse in the supine position, JVD, papilledema. Cardiac insufficiency may occur due to tumor compression. **NB:** In severely symptomatic patients or large mediastinal masses, consider necessity for cardiopulmonary fem-fem bypass standby. **Tests:** ECHO; EKG if symptomatic
Musculoskeletal	If thymoma present, ✓ for Sx of myasthenia gravis. **Tests:** Presence of acetylcholine-receptor antibodies
Laboratory	Electrolytes; CBC; T&C for 2–4 U, depending on body weight and tumor size; other tests as indicated from H&P.
Premedication	If patient > 7–9 mo consider premedication with midazolam (0.5 mg/kg). Use premedication cautiously in patients with large masses, or those that are symptomatic.

INTRAOPERATIVE

Anesthetic technique: GETA using pediatric circle. OR temperature 75–80°; forced air warmer.

Induction	An iv is mandatory. Placement of an arterial catheter may be indicated in patients with large masses or in symptomatic patients. If SVC syndrome is present, it is important to have iv access in the lower extremity. Glycopyrrolate (0.01 mg/kg iv) is given to dry secretions and prevent bradycardia 2° deep inhalation induction and laryngoscopy. An awake FOB and intubation in the sitting position may be necessary. Alternatively, a mask induction with sevoflurane/O_2 in the semi-Fowler's (reclining) position may be appropriate. Intubation should be performed with preservation of spontaneous ventilation. Have small styletted ETTs available, in the event of tracheal compression. FOB is useful to confirm ETT placement and to evaluate trachea/bronchi. Use muscle relaxants with caution, because the change from spontaneous to positive pressure ventilation may not be tolerated and may lead to obstruction. **NB:** Surgeon must be present (with rigid bronchoscope immediately available) in the event of acute airway obstruction on induction. If obstruction is unabated, options include median sternotomy and femoral-femoral bypass. **NB:** A simple positional change (e.g., supine to lateral, prone or sitting) may relieve cardiorespiratory collapse.	
Maintenance	Spontaneous ventilation/assisted ventilation with volatile agent and 100% O_2 may be appropriate. Supplemental epidural analgesia may be administered if a major resection is planned as opposed to a small incision for biopsy (see p. D-2). Have surgeon infiltrate wound with bupivacaine 0.25% to reduce volatile anesthetic and opiate requirements.	
Emergence	Confirm air leak around ETT (with cuff deflated). Have all emergency airway equipment available and surgeon present. Patient should be fully awake before extubation.	
Blood and fluid requirements	Usually minimal blood loss IV: 18–24 ga × 2, depending on age NS/LR @ 10–20 mL/kg iv	If mediastinoscopy is performed, sudden blood loss from torn great vessel may occur. Volume-loading with NS/LR before induction may be appropriate to minimize cardiovascular effects of deep inhalational induction.
Monitoring	Standard monitors (see p. D-1) Arterial line	Esophageal or precordial stethoscope is earliest monitor of airway obstruction. If obstruction worsens acutely, be prepared to change to lateral-decubitus or prone position, which may help alleviate tracheal, bronchial compression and cardiovascular collapse.
Positioning	✓ and pad pressure points. ✓ eyes.	
Complications	Cardio/Respiratory failure Loss of airway Hypotension	These cases require great attention to detail. All efforts must be made to maintain spontaneous ventilation. Preparations must be made for resuscitation.

POSTOPERATIVE

Complications	Respiratory failure Pneumothorax	Anesthesiologist must be readily available in the PACU to manage acute airway problems.
Pain management	Ketorolac 0.5 mg/kg(up to 30 mg) iv q 6 h × 24 h Epidural analgesia PCA (see p. E-3–E-4)	Cervical biopsy/mediastinoscopy have minimal postop pain and can be effectively treated with NSAID and local anesthetic infiltration. Use opiates cautiously.
Tests	Hct, ABG, CXR, as clinically indicated.	

Suggested Readings

1. Ferrari LR, Bedford RF: General anesthesia prior to treatment of anterior mediastinal masses in pediatric cancer patients. *Anesthesiology* 1990; 72(6):991–5.
2. Golianu B, Hammer GB: Pediatric thoracic anesthesia. *Curr Opin Anaesth* 2005; 18(1):5–11.
3. Gregory GA, ed: *Pediatric Anesthesia*, 4th ed. Churchill Livingstone, New York: 2002, 445–7.
4. Hammer GB: Anesthetic management for the child with a mediastinal mass. *Pediatric Anaesth* 2004; 14:95–7.
5. Narang S, Harte BH, Body SC: Anesthesia for patients with a mediastinal mass. *Anesth Clin North Am* 2001; 19(3):559–79.
6. Neuman GB, Weingarten AE, Abramowitz RM, et al: The anesthetic management of the patient with an anterior mediastinal mass. *Anesthesiology* 1984; 60(2):144–7.
7. Rodgers BM, McGahren ED III: Mediastinum and pleura. In *Surgery of Infants and Children.* Oldham KT, Colombani PM, Foglia RP, eds. Lippincott-Raven, Philadelphia: 1997, 915–34.
8. Tsao K, St Peter SD, Sharp SW, et al: Current application of thoracoscopy in children. *J Laparoendosc Adv Surg Tech A* 2008; 18(1):131–5.
9. Vas L, Naregal F, Nail V: Anaesthetic management of an infant with mediastinal mass. *Pediatr Anaesth* 1999; 9(5):439–43.
10. Watcha MF, et al: Comparison of ketorolac and morphine as adjuvants during pediatric surgery. *Anesthesiology* 1991; 76(3): 368–72.

NEONATAL LUNG RESECTION

SURGICAL CONSIDERATIONS

Description: Neonatal lung resection is performed for a few disorders relatively unique to children, including congenital cystic adenomatoid malformations (CCAM); sequestrations (intralobar 75%, extralobar 25%); congenital lobar overdistention (CLO, formerly called "emphysema"); and congenital pulmonary cysts (Fig. 12.5-3). Many lesions are asymptomatic; they are diagnosed by antenatal ultrasound or later when a CXR is performed for other reasons. CCAMs may compromise respiration and are at low risk for subsequent malignant degeneration. Sequestrations represent little danger, but they are frequently fed by a large artery of near-aortic caliber (often from below the diaphragm)

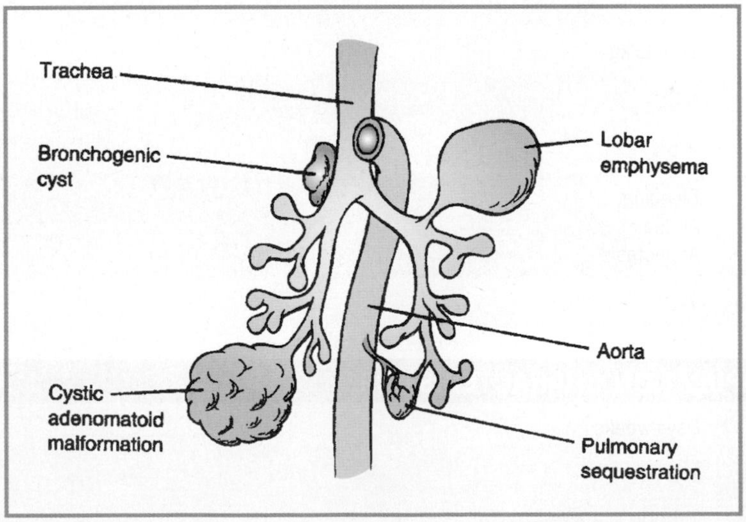

Figure 12.5-3. Classic developmental abnormalities of the tracheobronchial tree. (Reproduced with permission from Oldham KT, Colombani PM, Foglia RP: *Surgery of Infants and Children.* Lippincott-Raven, 1997. After Haller JA Jr, Golladay ES, Pickard LR, et al: Surgical management of lung bud anomalies: lobar emphysema, bronchogenic cyst, cystic adenomatoid malformation, and intralobar pulmonary sequestration. *Ann Thorac Surg* 1979; 28:34.)

with independent venous drainage back into the vena cava, causing significant L → R shunting. CLO resection is performed when the volume of ineffective, dilated lung compresses adjacent functioning lobes, compromising their function. (This condition is worsened by artificial ventilation with high pressure.) The key therapy is surgical—opening the hemithorax enables an oversized lobe to herniate through the incision, decompressing the healthy lung beneath. Most resections are performed on a ventilated lung because it is difficult to selectively intubate small airways.

Surgical approach: Patients undergoing lateral thoracotomy through the 4th, 5th, or 6th intercostal space benefit from preop placement of an epidural catheter. In some institutions, thoracoscopic resection may be performed. Significant blood loss is possible (infrequent). Often ventilation improves when the aberrant lung segment is removed. A large CCAM, intralobar sequestration, or CLO usually requires formal **lobectomy.** Smaller CCAMs, pulmonary cysts, and extralobar sequestrations are treated with lesser resections. A chest tube usually is left in place at the end of the case.

Variant procedures or approaches: Thoracoscopic lobectomy is increasingly practiced, and at our institution is the preferred method of lung resection. It can be performed safely and effectively, and avoids the morbidity and poor cosmesis of a thoracotomy. Upper-lobe resections can be technically more challenging, but are still possible with thoracoscopy. Insufflation of the hemithorax with 7 Hg carbon dioxide can aid in lung collapse.

Usual preop diagnosis: CCAM; sequestration; CLO; pulmonary cysts; congenital diaphragmatic hernia; pneumothorax

SUMMARY OF PROCEDURE

Position	Lateral decubitus
Incision	Lateral thoracotomy
Special instrumentation	Pediatric rib retractor
Unique considerations	Rapid thoracotomy improves ventilation in CLO. Aggressive high-pressure ventilation should be avoided.
Antibiotics	Cefazolin 25 mg/kg
Surgical time	2 h
Closing considerations	Extubation preferable and aided by epidural catheter.
EBL	10 mL/kg
Postop care	NICU
Mortality	< 5%
Morbidity	Bleeding Air leak Atelectasis
Pain score	7–8

PATIENT POPULATION CHARACTERISTICS

Age range	Days-weeks
Male:Female	1:1
Incidence	1/5000 live births
Etiology	Bronchopulmonary foregut maldifferentiation
Associated conditions	**Extralobar sequestration:** may occur below the diaphragm. **Sequestrations:** may be associated with high-output heart failure and diaphragmatic hernia. **CCAM:** may cause hydrops fetalis and fetal death. Intermediate forms of sequestration and CCAM exist.

ANESTHETIC CONSIDERATIONS

PREOPERATIVE

In general, children have significantly decreased respiratory reserve compared with adults because:

1. FRC is closer to RV in children, thereby making airway closure more likely.
2. O_2 consumption is higher (6–8 mL/kg/min vs 3 mL/kg/min).
3. In adults, the decubitus position increases blood flow to the ventilated, dependent lung, while decreasing perfusion to the operated nondependent lung. In children, the nondependent lung may actually receive greater perfusion than the dependent lung, which may be due to a more compliant chest wall in infants and young children.

Premedication	In children > 7–9 mo, consider midazolam 0.5–0.7 mg/kg po or 1–2 mg iv. If airway obstruction or severe pulmonary disease is present, use premedication judiciously.

INTRAOPERATIVE

Anesthetic technique: Combined epidural/GETA, using a pediatric circle forced-air warmer; OR warmed to 75–80°F; use warming pad on OR table, and warm iv fluids.

Induction	Either inhalation or iv induction may be performed. (For OLV, see below.) The trachea is intubated. An arterial line is indicated for children having a thoracotomy and for VATS in patients with significant lung disease. A CVP is generally not required if iv access is adequate.	
One-lung ventilation (OLV) in pediatric patients	OLV is used to allow deflation of the operative lung, which is especially useful during VATS. Alternatively, the surgeon may insufflate CO_2 to compress the operative lung. OLV also isolates the lungs to help prevent contamination of the nonoperative lung with blood or purulent fluid from the operative lung. The **three techniques for OLV** in infants and children include: Use of a **single-lumen tube:** a single-lumen tube is advanced into the mainstem bronchus of the nonoperative lung. FOB may be placed through ETT to confirm placement. Disadvantages: may obstruct upper lobe bronchus; cannot suction operative lung; may not have complete collapse of operative lung. Use of a **balloon-tipped catheter or bronchial blocker:** For placing blocker OUTSIDE the ETT: Operative lung intubated with ETT, guide wire passed through ETT, BB advanced over guide wire; second smaller ETT placed in trachea, alongside the BB. BB also can be advanced under direct visualization with FOB guidance via ETT. For placing blocker THROUGH ETT, multiport adapters allow oxygenation while positioning. Disadvantages: requires small ETT, FOB, or fluoroscopy. Use of a **double-lumen tube (DLT):** Can be placed for older children (see table below for approximate sizes). (See Lobectomy, Pneumonectomy, for details.)	
Maintenance	Standard maintenance (see p. D-2). Muscle relaxation is appropriate. Inhalation agent or TIVA (see p. B-2) may be used; 100% O_2 or O_2/air mixture; N_2O is avoided. Fentanyl 2–5 mcg/kg or other iv opioid should be given when epidural is not in place.	
Emergence	In most cases, the patient can be extubated at the end of surgery. An OG tube should be placed before, and suctioned prior to extubation. Ensure ability to oxygenate and ventilate adequately before extubation.	
Blood and fluid requirements	IV: 18–22 ga × 2 NS/LR @ maintenance	Potential for moderate blood loss. Transfuse to maintain Hct > 23. If > 2 mo of age, dextrose-containing solutions are not required.

Table 12.5-1. Tube Selection for OLV in Children

Age (yr)	ETT (Inner Diameter)	Fogarty Catheter	Arndt Blocker	Univent Tube	DLT (Fr)
0.5–1	3.5–4.0	3	n/a		
1–2	4.0–4.5	4	n/a		
2–4	4.5–5.0	4	5		
4–6	5.0–5.5	5	5		
6–8	5.5–6	6	5	3.5	
8–10	6.0 cuffed	6	5	3.5	26
10–12	6.5 cuffed	6	7	4.5	26–28
12–14	6.5–7.0 cuffed	6	7	4.5	32
14–16	7.0 cuffed	7	7	6.0	35
16–18	7.0–8.0 cuffed	7	7 or 9	7.0	35

Monitoring	Standard monitors (see p. D-1). ± Arterial line (22 ga) ± CVP Foley catheter ± TEE	For thoracotomy, ABG, Hct, and glucose should be evaluated as clinically indicated; UO monitored and kept at 1 mL/kg/h. CVP may be useful to evaluate fluid status if large fluid shifts or blood loss is anticipated, or if significant cardiac or respiratory compromise is present.
Positioning	✓ and pad pressure points. ✓ eyes.	
Complications	Hypoxia	DDX: Movement of ETT or BB, compromising OLV; bronchospasm; obstruction of ETT by kinking or secretions; pre-existing disease.
	Hypercarbia	Permissible during OLV (40–50 mmHg) to minimize barotrauma.
	↓ BP	Blood loss; hypovolemia; ↓ venous return 2° ↑ intrathoracic pressure

POSTOPERATIVE

Complications	Atelectasis Hypoventilation	Encourage deep breathing, hyperventilation.
	Hypoxia	Supplemental O_2
	Pneumothorax	Check breath sounds, chest wall motion, CXR. May require chest tube.
Pain management	Thoracic epidural	Lumbar (or caudal if < 8 kg and < 1 yr) epidural catheter may be placed and threaded up to thoracic levels.(NB- 1st dilate space with NS prior to threading catheter; ultrasound guidance may also be used to guide placement)
	Ketorolac 0.5 mg/kg iv q 6 h × 48–72 h	max 30mg/dose, if needed to enhance analgesia
Tests	Hct ABG CXR	

Suggested Readings

1. Dinesh K: Single lung ventilation in pediatric anesthesia. *Anesth Clin North Am* 2005; 23:693–708.
2. Gregory GA, ed: *Pediatric Anesthesia*, 4th edition. Churchill Livingstone, New York: 2002, 428–34.
3. Hammer GB, Harrison TK, Vricella LA, et al: Single lung ventilation in children using a new paediatric bronchial blocker. *Pediatr Anesth* 2002; 12:69–72.
4. Hammer GB: Single lung ventilation in infants and children. *Pediatr Anesth* 2004; 14:98–102.
5. Rothenberg SS, Albanese CT: Experience with 144 consecutive pediatric thoracoscopic lobectomies. *J Laparoendosc Adv Surg Tech A* 2007; 17(3):339–41.

DRAINAGE OF EMPYEMA

SURGICAL CONSIDERATIONS

Description: Most empyemas occur in otherwise healthy children when a necrotizing pneumonia causes a parapneumonic effusion that becomes infected. The infected fluid (empyema) has the tendency to become solid over days to weeks. It compresses the diseased lung and responds poorly to antibiotics because it is remote from the circulatory system. Three phases of empyema are recognized, and the key variable determining outcome is fibrin. The early or **exudative phase** occurs when the effusion becomes purulent—liquid pus without fibrin is successfully treated with a chest tube if it is recognized early (uncommon). The second phase, **fibrinopurulent,** occurs over the next days as thick strands of infected fibrin replace exudative fluid. It is the most common phase and is most expeditiously treated by **thoracoscopic ± open empyemectomy.** The last phase, **organized,** occurs when all exudate has been replaced by thick, infected fibrin, compressing the lung and adhering to both visceral and parietal pleura. Fortunately, this stage is rare in children; tedious **thoracoscopic decortication** may be successful, but often **thoracotomy** is required and the procedure is bloody. Some previously common organisms (e.g., *Haemophilius influenzae*) are decreasing with the advent of pediatric vaccines; *Streptococcus pneumonia, Staphylococcus aureus,* and *Streptococcus pyogenes* remain common pathogens, joined more recently by gram-negative rods. Significant bleeding is not uncommon and bronchopleural fistulae, if not already present, may occur when dead lung adheres to débrided overlying fibrin.

Surgical approach: Ipsilateral long-term venous access (peripherally inserted central or subclavian catheter) is placed before or during surgery. In larger children, a BB may protect the healthy lung from pus, which may extrude from the infected side into the trachea during operation. A **two- or three-port thoracoscopic technique** is most common, aided by hermetic trochars used with 5 mmHg intrathoracic pressure (unless a bronchopleural fistula exists). The first port is placed into a pre-existing chest tube site or the largest known pocket of pus/fibrin observed on preop imaging. Gradually, this space is enlarged until the remaining ports can be inserted under direct vision. As fibrin and pus are removed, trapped lung is liberated and the procedure continues somewhat tediously until the entire lung is free and most fibrin is removed. One or two large-bore chest tubes are placed at the end of the procedure.

Alternate approach is placement of one or more pigtail chest tubes and flushing the chest cavity with a fibrinolytic agent (e.g., tissue plasminogen activator). There is debate whether this approach may result in longer hospital stays, and thoracoscopy remains the gold standard.

SUMMARY OF PROCEDURES

	Thoracoscopic	Thoracotomy
Position	Contralateral decubitus	⇐
Incision	Three ports	5th interspace
Special instrumentation	Suction irrigator; chest tube	Rib retractor; suction; chest tube
Unique considerations	5 mmHg capnothorax	—

SUMMARY OF PROCEDURE (cont'd)		
	Thoracoscopic	**Thoracotomy**
Antibiotics	Cefuroxime (25 mg/kg) and clindamycin (10 mg/kg)	⇐
Surgical time	1.5 h	2 h
Closing considerations	Local anesthetic	± Epidural catheter
EBL	10–20 mL/kg	⇐
Postop care	May be septic for 24 h Extubation ideal	⇐ ⇐
Mortality	< 5%	< 10% when used for advanced disease
Morbidity	Air leak Bleeding Sepsis Atelectasis Pneumatocele	⇐ ⇐ ⇐ ⇐ ⇐
Pain Score	3–4	7–8

PATIENT POPULATION CHARACTERISTICS	
Age range	1–17 yr
Male: Female	1:1
Incidence	1/150 pneumonias
Etiology	Bacteria infect pleural effusion.
Associated conditions	Chronic granulomatous disease (uncommon)

ANESTHETIC CONSIDERATIONS

See Anesthetic Considerations for Pediatric Thoracic Surgery, p. 1267.

Suggested Readings

1. Choudry DK. Single lung ventilation in pediatric anesthesia. *Anesth Clin North Am.* 2005;23:693–708.
2. Fuller MK, Helmrath MA. Thoracic empyema, application of video-assisted thoracic surgery and its current management. *Curr Opin Pediatr.* 2007 Jun;19(3):328–32.
3. Golianu B, Hammer GB. Pediatric thoracic anesthesia. *Curr Opin in Anesth.* 2005;18(1):5–11.

REPAIR OF PECTUS EXCAVATUM/CARINATUM

SURGICAL CONSIDERATIONS

Description: Pectus excavatum ("funnel chest") is a sternochondral deformity more common in boys and of greater frequency than pectus carinatum ("pigeon chest"). Both may be associated with scoliosis, spontaneous pneumothorax, and Marfan syndrome—for which children of appropriate body habitus should be screened. It is difficult to confirm significant cardiorespiratory compromise in other than very severe excavatum lesions;

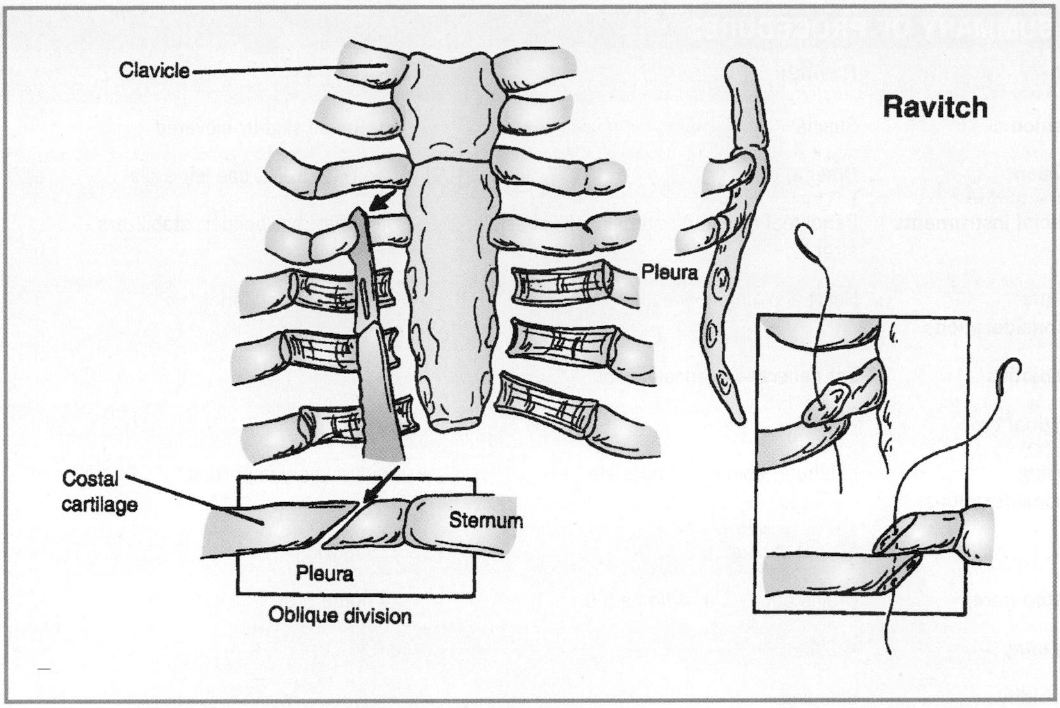

Figure 12.5-4. Ravitch approach: The costal cartilage immediately above the most cephalad abnormal costal cartilage is divided obliquely from medial to lateral, as shown. This is often at the level of the second costal cartilage, at the manubrial-sternal junction. The divided normal costal cartilages are allowed to overlap, the medial portion being anterior and the lateral being posterior. Suture fixation of the transected cartilage provides immobilization, ensuring sternal support at this level (inset). (Reproduced with permission from Oldham KT, Colombani PM, Foglia RP: *Surgery of Infants and Children.* Lippincott-Raven, 1997.)

transient pains are common and psychosocial distress is often the impetus for repair. The timing of repair is variable; some surgeons preferring to operate on younger children (5–6 yr) because of the ease and decreased bleeding, whereas others prefer doing surgery during adolescence to prevent possible recurrence during puberty.

Surgical approach: The classic **Ravitch** approach involves an omega-shaped chest incision in the supine position. The pectus muscles are detached from the sternum and 3–5 pairs of costochondral cartilages are resected, leaving the perichondrium for subsequent cartilage regeneration (Fig. 12.5-4). A transverse osteotomy of the upper sternum corrects its appearance. In some excavatum patients, a metal bar or "strut" may be placed beneath the sternum but on top of the ribs. If used, the strut is removed 2 yr later in a short operation through a small lateral incision. Hemovac drains are placed beneath the skin to trap bleeding from cut bony surfaces; chest tube(s) are placed if the pleura or pericardium is violated. Significant blood loss from cut surfaces of bones and cartilage occurs in older patients.

A newer approach (**Nuss Procedure**), is now widely practiced. This involves placement of a curvilinear stainless steel bar (pectus bar) via lateral axillary incisions through the ribspace under thoracoscopic guidance beneath the sternum at the point of maximal sternal depression. The bar travels through both hemithoraces anterior to the heart and lungs; when "flipped" 180° it exerts powerful forces backwards on the ribs and forward on the sternum. Sometimes fixation devices must be added to the ribs to keep the bar from "flipping back" into original position. A chest tube is not always necessary; however, very significant pain results, optimally treated with an epidural catheter. The rapid change of chest-wall shape also has caused thoracic outlet syndrome.

Usual preop diagnosis: Pectus excavatum; carinatum

Pediatric Surgery

SUMMARY OF PROCEDURES

	Ravitch	Nuss
Position	Supine	⇐, R side slightly elevated
Incision	Omega, chest	Two right axilla, one left axilla
Special instruments	Periosteal elevators; sternal saw; possible strut	Steel bar; bar bender; stabilizers
Unique considerations	Heart and lungs beneath	Cosmetically superior
Antibiotics	1st generation cephalosporin	⇐
Surgical time	~3 h	≤1 h
Closing considerations	Extubate; epidural, if possible	Epidural very important
EBL	10–20 mL/kg	< 5 mL/kg
Postop care	Drains out 1–3 d → home 5 d	→ home 5 d
Mortality	< 2%	⇐
Morbidity	Bleeding Recurrence Pneumothorax Cardiac injury	⇐ Bar "flips" Thoracic outlet syndrome ⇐
Pain score	5–6	8–9

PATIENT POPULATION CHARACTERISTICS

Age range	5 yr–adolescent
Male:Female	5–9:1
Incidence	Uncertain
Etiology	Relationship with reactive airway disease
Associated conditions	Marfan syndrome (5%); mitral valve prolapse (5%)

ANESTHETIC CONSIDERATIONS

PREOPERATIVE

Pectus excavatum (a condition in which there is concave depression of the lower sternum) may be associated with CHD and restrictive lung disease. If the deformity is present without cardiac or pulmonary disease, the patient is asymptomatic and the procedure is cosmetic. Surgery usually occurs between 12–15 yr of age. **Pectus carinatum** (a convex lower sternum) usually is repaired for cosmetic reasons only and usually during the teenage years. Cardiac abnormalities (VSD, PDA, mitral valve anomalies) may be associated with the pectus disorder.

Respiratory	Restrictive lung disease 2° chest-wall deformity may be present. If a longstanding condition, patient may have chronic hypoxemia, with resultant pulmonary HTN and polycythemia. If patient has exercise limitations, there is a need to differentiate between cardiac and pulmonary components. **Tests:** CXR: AP, lateral; PFTs; ABG, if symptomatic

Cardiovascular	In both conditions, CHD should be investigated if present. Pulmonary HTN may be 2° pulmonary overcirculation (e.g., VSD), or chronic hypoxemia. **Tests:** ECG; ECHO	
Laboratory	Hct; T&C; electrolytes	
Premedication	If patient is an asymptomatic child, midazolam (0.75 mg/kg po or 1–2 mg iv).	

INTRAOPERATIVE

Anesthetic technique: GETA, using a pediatric circle; forced air warmer; maintain OR temperature 75–80°.

Induction	IV or mask induction. With restrictive lung disease, there is ↓ FRC, which will shorten the time to alveolar equilibration for the volatile anesthetics. Hypercarbia will aggravate pulmonary HTN; institute early manual hyperventilation. Tracheal intubation, facilitated by neuromuscular blockade (rocuronium 1 mg/kg, vecuronium 0.1 mg/kg). Use appropriately sized ETT (see p. D-2). With uncuffed ETT, keep air leak to minimum (>20 cmH_2O) to avoid alterations in alveolar ventilation with changes in chest and pulmonary compliance.	
Maintenance	Standard maintenance with inhalational anesthetic, TIVA or combination. Insertion of thoracic lumbar epidural catheter will provide for supplemental anesthesia and treatment of postop pain and is highly recommended. Use morphine/hydromorphone-bupivacaine mixture (see p. D-2). If no epidural is placed, bolus with long acting iv opioid (morphine 0.1 mg/kg, hydromorphone 15 mcg/kg) for postoperative pain control.	
Emergence	Plan for extubation in OR. Ensure adequate reversal of neuromuscular blockade with neostigmine (0.07 mg/kg iv) and glycopyrrolate (0.014 mg/kg iv).	
Blood and fluid requirements	Usually minimal blood and 3rd-space losses IV: 18 or 20 ga × 1 NS/LR @ 3–5 kg/h	With chronic hypoxemia or right-side heart disease, maintain Hct > 30. If otherwise healthy, maintain Hct > 22.
Monitoring	Standard monitors (see p. D-1)	Arterial line if pulmonary HTN present.
Positioning	✓ and pad pressure points. ✓ eyes.	Elbow padding to avoid ulnar nerve compression. Careful positioning to avoid nerve compression.
Complications	Pneumothorax Atelectasis Subglottic edema	

POSTOPERATIVE

Complications	Respiratory insufficiency Pneumothorax	2° splinting, preexisting restrictive pulmonary disease, nerve injury related to positioning
Pain management	Epidural (thoracic) or PCA	Standard epidural infusion (see p. E-5). Ketorolac (0.5 mg/kg (p. E-3–E-4) iv q 6 h × 24–72 h), if needed, in addition to the above measures

Suggested Readings

1. Arn PH, Scherer LR, Haller JA Jr, et al: Outcome of pectus excavatum in patients with Marfan syndrome and in the general population. *J Pediatr* 1989; 115(6):954–8.
2. Chidambaram B, Mehta AV: Currarino-Silverman syndrome (pectus carinatum type 2 deformity) and mitral valve disease. *Chest* 1992; 102(3):780–2.
3. Davis JT, Weinstein S: Repair of the pectus deformity: results of the Ravitch approach in the current era. *Ann Thorac Surg* 2004; 78(2):421–6.

4. Derveaux L, Ivanoff I, Rochette F, et al: Mechanism of pulmonary function changes after surgical correction for funnel chest. *Eur Respir J* 1988; 1(9):823–5.
5. Golianu B, Hammer G: Pediatric thoracic anesthesia. *Curr Opin Anesth* 2005; 18(1):5–11.
6. Goretsky ML, Kelly RE, Croituru D, et al: Chest wall anomalies: pectus excavatum and pectus carinatum. *Adolesc Med Clin* 2004; 15(3):455–71.
7. Gregory GA, ed: *Pediatric Anesthesia,* 4th edition. Churchill Livingstone, New York: 2002:447–9.
8. Kandel J, Haller JA: Chest wall and breast. In *Surgery of Infants and Children*. Oldham KT, Colombani PM, Foglia RP, eds. Lippincott-Raven, Philadelphia: 1997, 871–82.
9. Motoyama EK, Davis PJ, eds: *Smith's Anesthesia for Infants and Children,* 7th edition. Mosby-Year Book, St. Louis, 2006: 700–1.

ESOPHAGEAL REPLACEMENT, COLON INTERPOSITION, GASTRIC TUBE PLACEMENT

SURGICAL CONSIDERATIONS

Description: Esophageal replacement in children usually is performed for caustic stricture or esophageal atresia (EA) refractory to other therapy. Caustic esophageal strictures—usually in toddlers following lye ingestion—are becoming less common; esophageal replacement is indicated after failed attempts at balloon dilation (BD). Patients with EA may have a primary replacement for known long-gap atresia (Type A), or will have a secondary replacement after failed attempts at anastomosis (all types). There is no good long-term esophageal replacement; a segment of colon, stomach, or (rarely) jejunum is the best surrogate.

Surgical approach: Depending on anatomy and surgeon preference, the **distal dissection** occurs in the abdomen and/or chest; the **proximal anastomosis** occurs in the chest or neck. Position changes with redraping may be required, depending on the selection of incisions. The esophageal substitute usually is brought through the bed of the esophagus with small risks to the pulmonary vessels, recurrent laryngeal nerves, and brachiocephalic vein. The **retrosternal approach** may be safer but is less optimal in children because of long-term problems with obstruction and emptying.

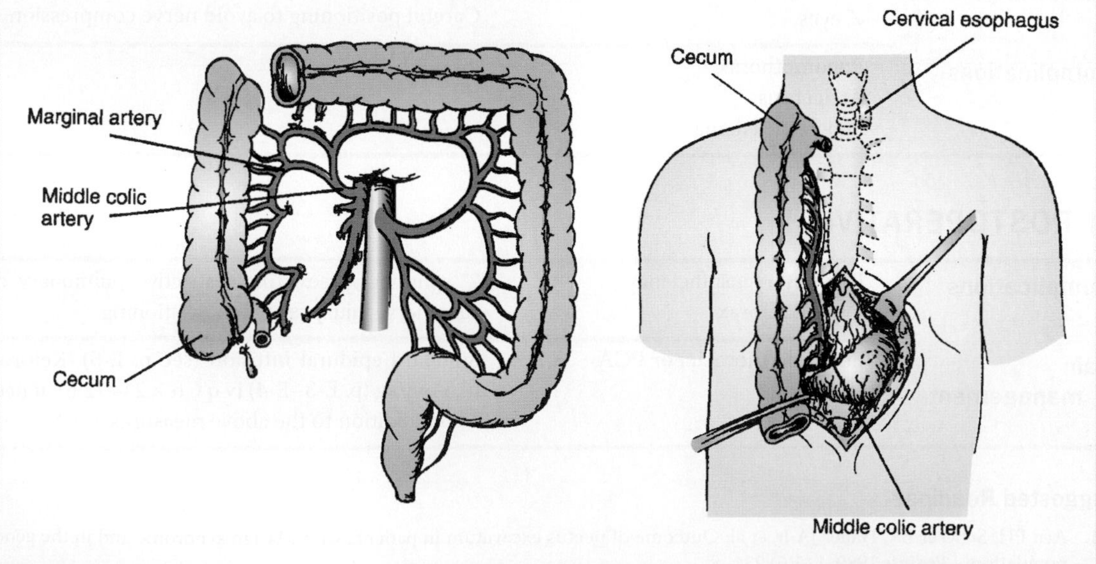

Figure 12.5-5. Esophageal replacement using a right colon interposition in a retrosternal position. (Reproduced with permission from Oldham KT, Colombani PM, Foglia RP: *Surgery of Infants and Children*. Lippincott-Raven, 1997.)

Variant procedures or approaches: Colon is the most frequent substitute, with the transverse colon attached to either the R colon (isoperistaltic) or L colon (reverse peristaltic) being used. When the stomach is used, it may be pulled up entirely from the abdomen through the chest with **gastroesophageal anastomosis** in the neck **(Orringer)**; alternatively, a **gastric tube** of greater (common) or lesser curve maybe constructed for cervical or thoracic anastomosis. Small bowel is used only when other substitutes are inappropriate—because an additional microvascular anastomosis is needed for graft survival.

Usual preop diagnosis: EA; caustic stricture

SUMMARY OF PROCEDURE	
Position	Supine, tilted; or supine, ± lateral
Incision	Abdominal and cervical ± thoracotomy
Special instrumentation	Bougie (upper esophagus)
Antibiotics	Preop: ampicillin 25 mg/kg iv + gentamicin 2.5 mg/kg iv
Surgical time	3–5 h (4–6 h with position change)
EBL	20–40 mL/kg
Postop care	PICU
Mortality	< 5%
Morbidity	Respiratory failure Anastomotic leak Sepsis Stricture
Pain score	7–8

PATIENT POPULATION CHARACTERISTICS	
Age range	1–5 yr
Male:Female	2:1
Incidence	~200/yr in the United States
Etiology	Caustic ingestion; EA
Associated conditions	Caustic stricture; imperforate anus; VACTERL association

ANESTHETIC CONSIDERATIONS

PREOPERATIVE

These patients usually are children presenting with a Hx of caustic substance ingestion and subsequent development of esophageal stricture. They frequently have undergone multiple esophageal dilations under GA. Previous anesthesia records should be obtained. Preop, these patients are admitted for bowel prep and, consequently, may be hypovolemic.

Gastrointestinal	Varying degrees of esophageal reflux may be present. Preop H_2-blocker administration may be appropriate (e.g., ranitidine 1.0 mg/kg iv). If a gastrostomy is present, it should be vented. **Tests:** Electrolytes

Pediatric Surgery

Hematologic	Anemia due to poor nutrition **Tests:** CBC; T&C	
Laboratory	Other tests as indicated from H&P.	
Premedication	IV may already be in place and midazolam (1–2 mg iv) can be administered in holding area. Alternatively, midazolam usually can be given (0.5–0.75 mg/kg po) 30 min. before surgery.	

INTRAOPERATIVE

Anesthetic technique: GETA, using a pediatric circle. Forced-air warmer; heating pad on OR table. Warm room to 75–80°F. An epidural catheter (for intraop and postop pain management) may be placed once child is anesthetized and airway is secured.

Induction	IV induction preferred. If reflux concerns present, preoxygenate for 2–3 min and perform rapid-sequence induction and intubation with cricoid pressure (see p. B-4). Use appropriately sized ETT (see p. D-2). Continue neuromuscular blockade with vecuronium (0.1 mg/kg) or rocuronium (0.6 mg/kg).	
Maintenance	Use air/O_2/isoflurane. Avoid N_2O to minimize increase in size of possible pneumothorax during mediastinal dissection, use appropriate use of NMB with train-of-four monitoring, and dose epidural catheter as needed (see. p. D-3).	
Emergence	Possible extubation in OR vs postop intubation.	
Blood and fluid requirements	Blood loss moderate IV: 22 ga × 2 NS/LR @ –10 mL/kg/h	Replace 3rd-space losses with NS/LR (~10 mL/kg/h). Replace blood loss mL for mL with albumin 5%. Transfuse to maintain Hct > 22.
Monitoring	Standard monitors (see p. D-1) CVP: 4 Fr DL or 5Fr TL ± Arterial line (22 ga) Foley catheter	CVP line used for postop TPN (maintain 1 lumen for that purpose). Marked arterial waveform variation with ventilation is a sensitive indicator of hypovolemia. ABG/Hct prn.
Positioning	Shoulder roll ✓ and pad pressure points. ✓ eyes.	Beware of tracheal extubation with head extension. If necessary, reconfirm ETT position with laryngoscopy.
Complications	Hypoventilation Hypothermia Pneumothorax Dysrhythmias Aspiration	Suprasternal dissection involves traction on trachea and recurrent laryngeal nerve. Mediastinal pull-through may damage great vessels and → pneumothorax, manipulation-induced dysrhythmias, impaired chest-wall compliance.

POSTOPERATIVE

Complications	Subglottic edema Hypoventilation Pneumothorax Recurrent laryngeal nerve injury Mediastinitis	Inadequately treated pain → hypoventilation.
Pain management	Epidural analgesia (see p. E-5). Acetaminophen (10–20 mg/kg pr q 4 h prn) Ketorolac (0.5 mg/kg iv up to 15 mg q 6 h × 24–72 h)	
Tests	CXR Hct	

Suggested Readings

1. Anderson KD: Esophageal substitution. In *Pediatric Surgery.* Holder TM, Ashcraft KW, eds. WB Saunders, Philadelphia: 1980, 284–91.
2. Cywes S, Millar AJW, Rode H, et al: Corrosive strictures of the oesophagus in children. *Pediatr Surg Int* 1993; 8:8–13.
3. Schecter NL, Berde CB, Yaster M, eds: *Pain in Infants, Children, and Adolescents,* 2nd edition. Lippincott, Williams & Wilkins, Philadelphia: 2003, 363–96.

REPAIR OF CONGENITAL DIAPHRAGMATIC HERNIA

SURGICAL CONSIDERATIONS

Description: Congenital diaphragmatic hernia (CDH; Bochdalek Hernia) remains a potentially lethal anomaly due to pulmonary HTN, pulmonary hypoplasia, and associated cardiac dysfunction. In utero Dx allows for delivery at (ideally) or transport to a tertiary center with sophisticated ventilatory support techniques. Early NG tube placement is important to minimize distention of the intrathoracic viscera. Surgery transiently worsens pulmonary HTN and may cause "persistent fetal circulation," in which the fetal circulation reopens to shunt blood around the lungs, causing further hypoxemia, hypercarbia, and acidosis—all stimuli for further pulmonary HTN. Thus, in the sickest newborns, surgery is delayed until after cardiorespiratory stabilization, with an arsenal of supportive measures, including: low-pressure, high-frequency ventilation; passive hypercapnia; oscillating or jet ventilation; NO; and even ECMO, which is becoming less common with the success of the former methods. When ECMO (with anticoagulation) is used, diaphragm repair may be performed: **early during ECMO** (less swelling, more bleeding); **late during ECMO** (more swelling, ability to "come off" if bleeding); or **after ECMO** (less bleeding, less swelling, little recourse if surgery worsens ventilation). (For a description of ECMO, see p. 1503.) When the intestines are reduced from the chest, there is sometimes insufficient room in the abdomen, in which case, an abdominal silo is placed transiently.

Surgical approach: Left-side lesions (Fig. 12.5-6) are 7x more frequent than right; repair is traditionally performed through a subcostal incision, but increasingly a laparoscopic or thoracoscopic approach is being utilized. In children with significant hypercarbia and/or pulmonary hypertension, insufflation with carbon dioxide may not be tolerated, precluding this approach. However infants are surprisingly resilient to intrathoracic insufflation and respiratory acidosis can be effectively managed with hyperventilation.

Small defects cause few ventilation problems and are closed primarily. Larger defects are associated with more challenging ventilation and require prosthetic mesh augmentation, either with synthetic or biologic mesh. Recurrent defects may be approached through the abdomen or chest and sometimes require transfer of muscle flaps (interior oblique). Unless ECMO is used, a chest tube is not necessary.

Variant procedure: **In utero therapies** for CDH, including tracheal occlusion, have not been shown to improve survival. Although the defect commonly originates in the posterolateral diaphragm (Bochdalek), less common retrosternal defects (Morgagni) present later in life without the same degree of cardiorespiratory compromise.

Usual preop diagnosis: Diaphragmatic hernia; Bochdalek's hernia (posterolateral diaphragm)

SUMMARY OF PROCEDURE	
Position	Supine (lateral for thoracic approach)
Incision	Subcostal (posterolateral for thoracic approach)
Special instrumentation	Pre- and postductal arterial monitors
Unique considerations	Reactive pulmonary vasculature
Antibiotics	Preop: ampicillin 25 mg/kg iv + gentamicin 2.5 mg/kg iv

SUMMARY OF PROCEDURE (cont'd)

Surgical time	1–2 h
Closing considerations	Assess for changes in ventilation (e.g., PIP, pre- and postductal ABG).
EBL	5–10 mL/kg
Postop care	Paralysis maintained; hyperventilation; fentanyl infusion @ 2–5 mcg/kg/min
Mortality	15–50% without ECMO 25–30% with ECMO
Morbidity	Pulmonary HTN Respiratory failure Sepsis Intestinal obstruction/dysfunction
Pain score	6–7 (7–8 for thoracic approach)

PATIENT POPULATION CHARACTERISTICS

Age range	Newborn–wk or mo
Male:Female	1–2:1
Incidence	1 in 4000
Etiology	Unknown
Associated conditions	Malrotation (40–100%); congenital heart disease (23%- VSD, ASD, PDA, TOF); renal anomalies (rare); esophageal atresia (rare); CNS abnormalities (e.g., myelomeningocele, hydrocephalus) (rare)

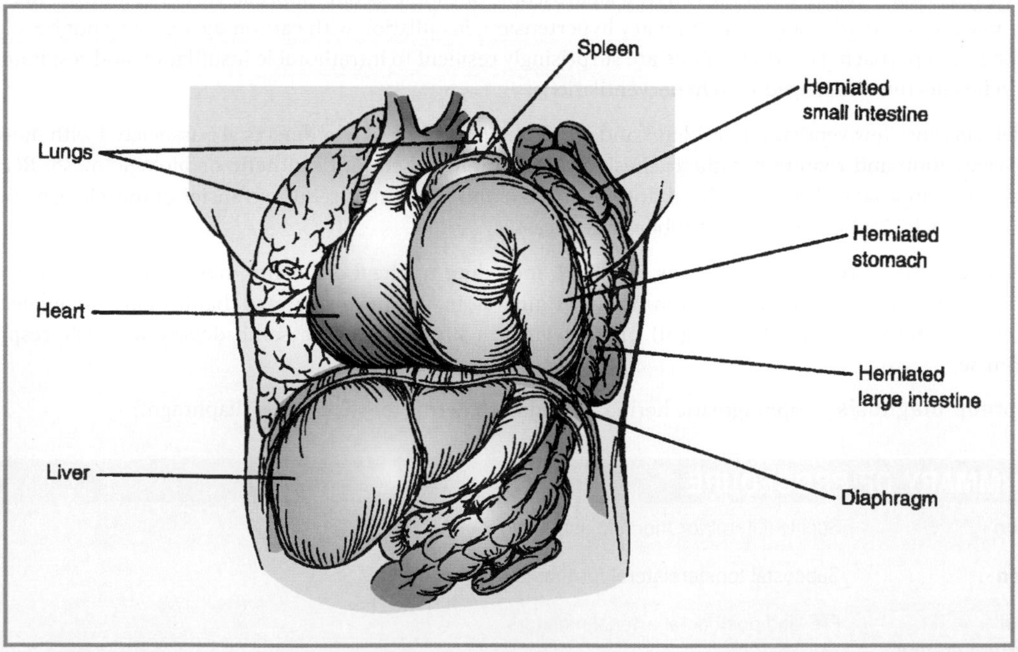

Figure 12.5-6. Left-sided congenital diaphragmatic hernia demonstrating translocation of the abdominal viscera into the left hemothorax and displacement of the mediastinum to the contralateral side. (Reproduced with permission from Oldham KT, Colombani PM, Foglia RP: *Surgery of Infants and Children.* Lippincott-Raven, Philadelphia: 1997.)

ANESTHETIC CONSIDERATIONS

PREOPERATIVE

These infants present with varying degrees of respiratory distress. Surgery is performed after the child has been stabilized medically. The majority are already mechanically ventilated, sedated, and paralyzed in the NICU prior to anesthesia consultation. The anesthesiologist needs to be aware of the distinction between early and late diaphragmatic hernias. Late events (occurring near or even after delivery) are associated with mature, well developed lungs and minimal problems with ventilation. These babies often can be extubated in the early postop period, facilitated by epidural analgesia. Some infants may be on ECMO (see p. 1505).

Respiratory	The lung on affected side is variably hypoplastic and the lung on the contralateral side is compressed and also may be hypoplastic. Pulmonary hypoplasia is most severe in patients with early herniation, and may be minimal in cases of late (even postnatal) herniation. The prognosis is correlated with magnitude of pulmonary hypoplasia and pulmonary muscular abnormalities present on the contralateral side. There is ↓ compliance, → risk for hypoventilation. ↑ PIP →↑ risk for pneumothorax. Persistent pulmonary HTN and progressive hypoxemia may be present. **Tests:** CXR; ABG
Cardiovascular	R → L shunting may occur at level of PDA or preductally (e.g., PFO). The degree of R → L shunting may be dramatically increased by ↑ pulmonary vasoconstriction (2° ↓ PO_2, ↑ PCO_2, ↑ pH, ↑ sympathetic tone) → severe systemic hypoxemia. ↓ CO 2° persistent pulmonary HTN and hypoxemia will lead to metabolic acidosis. **Tests:** CXR; ABG; preoperative echocardiogram needed
Neurological	Myelomeningocele and/or hydrocephalus may be present. Repeated bouts of hypoxemia predispose to intraventricular hemorrhage (IVH) in preterm infant. These areas of hemorrhage have loss of cerebral autoregulation and BP increases are directly transmitted to the microvasculature, with ↑ risk of recurrent hemorrhage and edema. **Tests:** Head ultrasound
Hematologic	Hct should be maintained at 35%. HbF has ↑ affinity for O_2 and ↓ sensitivity to 2,3-DPG. This will aggravate cellular hypoxia in the patient with compromised circulatory status. Confirm that vitamin K was administered at birth. **Tests:** CBC; T&C; PT; PTT
Metabolic	Dextrose supplementation needed due to negligible glycogen stores in neonate. In patients with CHF, diuretic administration leads to ↓ K^+. **Tests:** Electrolytes; glucose; BUN; Cr
Gastrointestinal	Constant NG/OG suction. Gastric distention will worsen ventilation.
Laboratory	Other tests as indicated from H&P.
Premedication	None

INTRAOPERATIVE

Anesthetic technique: GETA, using a pediatric circle. Forced air warmer. Warm room to 75–80°. Use pressure-limited ventilation (PIP < 30 cmH_2O). Continue NO if administered preop. Maintain body temperature as close to 37°C as possible. Warm room to 75–80°F. Consider use of NICU ventilator, particularly if high RR (> 30/min) is required.

Induction	Transported from NICU to OR by anesthesia team. If infant is already intubated, confirm paralysis prior to transport to lessen the risk of patient movement and inadvertent extubation. Transport with full monitoring (ECG, pulse oximetry, arterial pressure tracing). Have airway equipment available (Miller 1 laryngoscope blade, ET 3.0–3.5 with stylets, neonatal mask). Resuscitation drugs (e.g., epinephrine 1 and 10 mcg/mL) should be drawn up.

Induction (cont'd)	Syringe with NS/LR flush. Prior to any further anesthetic administration, reestablish all monitoring in OR. For nonintubated patients, rapid-sequence induction (p. B-4) is appropriate. Atropine (0.02 mg/kg iv) given prior to induction to counteract bradycardia. If necessary to mask ventilate, avoid high inflation pressures, as this may further dilate the bowel. Place an OG tube prior to induction. Avoid N_2O and maintain PIPs as low as possible. For patients with late herniations and healthy lungs, consider caudal epidural catheter advanced to thoracic space instead of iv opioids, and early extubation (OR or NICU); (see p. D-4). If surgery is performed on ECMO, give high-dose iv opioids (may be given in ECMO circuit) and muscle relaxant.	
Maintenance	Opiate-based anesthetic (fentanyl 10–25 mcg/kg iv total), if no epidural in place, with isoflurane supplementation. Ventilate with air/O_2 to maintain O_2 saturation 95–100%, as measured by preductal ABGs/pulse oximetry. Avoid hypoxia, acidosis, hypothermia, which will ↑ pulmonary vasoconstriction. Keep CO_2 normal or slightly ↑ (permissive hypercapnia). Continue neuromuscular blockade with pancuronium, rocuronium, or vecuronium. May need to momentarily pause surgery to restore adequate oxygenation and ventilation.	
Emergence	Transport back to NICU with full monitoring, airway equipment, and drugs.	
Blood and fluid requirements	Blood loss minimal IV: 22–24 ga × 2 NS/LR @ 4 mL/kg/h maintenance	These infants are fluid-restricted in NICU. Continue dextrose-containing solution from NICU. If umbilical venous line not present, dopamine may be infused via peripheral iv with dextrose solution serving as the carrier fluid. In emergency, NS/LR, albumin 5%, PRBCs (Hct < 50%) may be given via umbilical artery line.
Monitoring	Standard monitors (see p. D-1) Right-side precordial stethoscope Arterial line (umbilical or radial – 24 ga); if possible, right hand (preductal) ± Umbilical vein line Preductal and postductal pulse oximetry	Contralateral pneumothorax is detected using a right axillary precordial stethoscope. ABG, Hct, glucose q 30–60 min. Changes in pre- and postductal pulse oximetry provide early warning of R→L shunt/pulmonary HTN. (L hand postductal SaO_2 will drop with R→L shunt.
Positioning	✓ and pad pressure points. ✓ eyes.	
Complications	Pneumothorax Hypoventilation Hypothermia Metabolic acidosis R → L shunting CHF	With acute deterioration in O_2 sat, pneumothorax on unaffected side is likely. Do not attempt to expand lungs vigorously. Hypoplasia, not atelectasis, is the primary problem. Keep PIP <30 cmH_2O, if possible.

POSTOPERATIVE

Complications	Same as Intraoperative Complications, above.	Severely affected neonates will usually have been stabilized on high-frequency jet ventilation or ECMO. The goal is to schedule semi-elective surgery when the neonate is medically stable. In case of acute deterioration in the OR, discuss with NICU criteria for initiation of HFJV or ECMO for infants whose oxygenation continues to worsen.

Complications (cont'd)		High-frequency jet ventilation may be an option prior to ECMO. Post-operatively, these neonates go through a "honeymoon period" of up to 24 h, after which they may develop ↑ pulmonary HTN and deteriorate clinically.
Pain management	Fentanyl (0.5–2.0 mcg/kg/h iv) Epidural analgesia	Tachyphylaxis can develop in 24–48 h.
Tests	CXR ABG Hct Glucose Electrolytes	

Suggested Readings

1. Arca MJ, Barnhart DC, Lelli JL Jr, et al: Early experience with minimally invasive repair of congenital diaphragmatic hernias: results and lessons learned. *J Pediatr Surg* 2003; 38(11):1563–8.
2. Azarow K, Messineo A, Pearl R, et al: Congenital diaphragmatic hernia: a tale of two cities: the Toronto experience. *J Pediatr Surg* 1997; 32:395–400.
3. Bikhazi GB, Davis PJ: Anesthesia for neonates and premature infants. In *Smith's Anesthesia for Infants and Children,* 6th edition. Motoyama EK, Davis PJ, eds. Mosby-Year Book, St. Louis: 2006, 545–50.
4. Cook DR, Marcy JH, eds: *Neonatal Anesthesia,* 1st edition. Appleton Davies, Pasadena: 1988.
5. Falconer AR, Brown RA, Helms P, et al: Pulmonary sequelae in survivors of congenital diaphragmatic hernia. *Thorax* 1990; 45(2):126–9.
6. Goldsmith JP, Karokin EH, eds: *Assisted Ventilation of the Neonate,* 2nd edition. WB Saunders, Philadelphia: 1988.
7. Gregory GA, ed: *Pediatric Anesthesia,* 4th edition. Churchill Livingstone, New York: 2002, 434–40.
8. Holcomb GW 3rd, Ostlie DJ, Miller KA: Laparoscopic patch repair of diaphragmatic hernias with surgisis. *J Pediatr Surg* 2005; 40(8):E1–5.
9. Liu LM, Pang LM: Neonatal surgical emergencies in anesthesiology. *Clin North Am* 2001; 19(2):268–72.
10. Stehling L, ed: *Common Problems in Pediatric Anesthesia,* 2nd edition. Mosby-Year Book, St. Louis: 1992, 7–11.
11. Wilson JM, Lund DP, Lillehei CW, et al: Congenital diaphragmatic hernia: a tale of two cities: the Boston experience. *J Pediatr Surg* 1997; 32:401–5.
12. Wilson JM, Lund DP, Lillehei CW, et al: Congenital diaphragmatic hernia: predictors of severity in the ECMO era. *J Pediatr Surg* 1991; 26(9):1028–33.
13. Yang EY, Allmendinger N, Johnson SM, et al: Neonatal thoracoscopic repair of congenital diaphragmatic hernia: selection criteria for successful outcome. *J Pediatr Surg* 2005; 40(9):1369–75.

PYLOROMYOTOMY FOR PYLORIC STENOSIS

SURGICAL CONSIDERATIONS

Description: Pyloric stenosis due to idiopathic hypertrophy of the muscular layers of the antrum and pylorus occurs in infants from 1 to 3 months of age, causing projectile vomiting with subsequent dehydration and metabolic alkalosis. Surgical division of the hypertrophied fibers—**pyloromyotomy**—is the treatment of choice. Preop hydration and electrolyte replacement are becoming less frequently needed, as early Dx by ultrasound becomes more common. Aspiration (of food or barium contrast) is avoided by NG suction.

Surgical approach: The operation is performed through either a RUQ, periumbilical, or three laparoscopic incisions. The RUQ incision is now less utilized, while laparoscopic approach in experienced hands can be performed very quickly and effectively. With the open approach, the serosa and hypertrophic muscle of the pylorus are divided with a scalpel handle or Benson spreader. With the laparoscopic approach, a special bladed instrument and blunt retraction are used to perform the myotomy. The anesthesiologist is typically asked to instill 40–60 cc of saline by orogastric tube into the stomach so that leaks can be detected. Careful inspection for a mucosal tear will avoid a

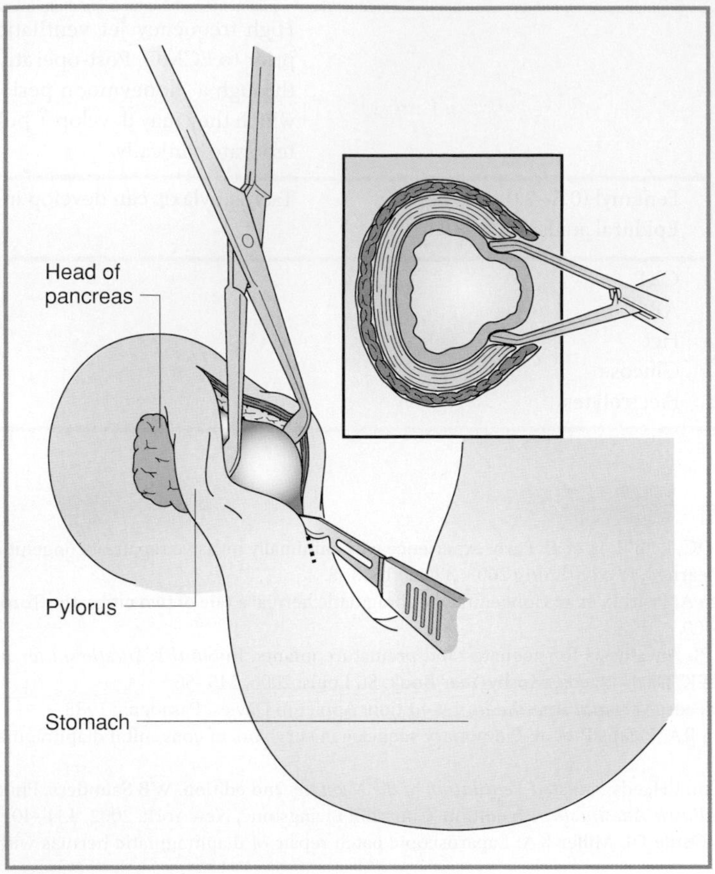

Figure 12.5-7. Ramstedt pyloromyotomy for infantile hypertrophic pyloric stenosis. The cross-sectional view shows herniation of the submucosa into the myotomy site, indicative of an adequate myotomy. (Reproduced with permission from Sato TT, Oldham KT: Pediatric abdomen. In *Surgery: Scientific Principles and Practice,* 3rd edition. Greenfield LJ, Mulholland MW, Oldham KT, et al., eds. Lippincott Williams & Wilkins, Philadelphia: 2001.)

subsequent leak, the most common serious complication. Mucosal injury is treated by a simple repair or by closing the entire myotomy and creating a new one at an alternate site.

Usual preop diagnosis: Pyloric stenosis; gastroenteritis; GERD

SUMMARY OF PROCEDURE	
Position	Supine
Incision	Transverse; RUQ; periumbilical, or three laparoscopic ports
Special instrumentation	Benson pyloric spreader; arthrotome (laparoscopy)
Intraop antibiotics	Cefazolin 25 mg/kg iv
Surgical time	0.5–1 h
EBL	< 5 mL/kg
Postop care	Cardiac/apnea monitoring
Mortality	0.3%

SUMMARY OF PROCEDURE (cont'd)	
Morbidity	Duodenal perforation Incomplete myotomy with recurrent vomiting Dehiscence Hernia
Pain score	4–5

PATIENT POPULATION CHARACTERISTICS	
Age range	1–12 wk
Male:Female	4:1
Incidence	3/1000 births
Etiology	Unknown
Associated conditions	Has occurred following repair of other congenital anomalies, such as esophageal atresia, omphalocele.

ANESTHETIC CONSIDERATIONS

PREOPERATIVE

Patients with pyloric stenosis are usually term infants that present in the first month of life with mild-to-moderate dehydration 2° intractable vomiting. While in past these infants usually presented with moderate to severe dehydration, diagnosis by ultrasound has led to earlier intervention, thereby minimizing the degree of electrolyte imbalance. Correction of volume deficit and metabolic abnormalities is the first line of treatment. Surgery should proceed only after patients are medically stabilized, adequate urine output is assured, and metabolic alkalosis is corrected. These procedures are usually done with laparoscopy.

Cardiovascular	Mild-to-moderate dehydration (50–100 mL/kg) is common and this deficit should be replaced with NS over ~12 h. **Tests:** Urinary Cl > 20 mEq/L or plasma Cl > 100 mEq/L, when fluid volume restored.
Metabolic	Protracted vomiting → dehydration with hypochloremic hypokalemic metabolic alkalosis. Up to 30% of infants may be hyperkalemic. ↓ K^+ should be treated once alkalemia is resolved and UO is confirmed. **Tests:** ABGs; electrolytes; Ca^{++}; glucose
Gastrointestinal	Full-stomach precautions (see p. B-4). Prior to induction, it is necessary to pass an OG tube several times to adequately decompress the stomach.
Laboratory	Hct; other tests as indicated from H&P.
Premedication	None

INTRAOPERATIVE

Anesthetic technique: GETA, using a pediatric circle. Forced-air warmer. Warm OR to 75–80° F. Use air/O_2 mixture to maintain O_2 sat @ 95–100%. Maintain body temperature close to 37°C.

Induction	An iv catheter should be in place prior to induction for preop fluid management. Decompress stomach with NG or OG tube. Atropine (0.02 mg/kg iv, 0.1 mg minimum) commonly

Induction (cont'd)	given before stomach decompression. Preoxygenate 2–3 min. Rapid-sequence induction with cricoid pressure should be performed, using propofol (2–3 mg/kg) or STP (4 mg/kg iv) and succinylcholine (1–2 mg/kg iv) or rocuronium (1 mg/kg). Use awake laryngoscopy if difficulty with intubation is anticipated. Intubate trachea with a appropriately sized uncuffed tube, usually 3.5 mm. Air leak should be between 20–30 cm H_2O pressure. If succinylcholine is used, further NMB with rocuronium (0.6 mg/kg) or vecuronium (0.1 mg/kg) will be necessary. If a laparoscopic technique is used, confirm adequate ventilation bilaterally after insufflation of the abdomen.	
Maintenance	Volatile agent (isoflurane) and air/O_2 or N_2O/O_2. Avoid opioids to lessen risk of postop apnea due to tendency to hypoventilate due to previous metabolic alkalosis. Maintain muscle relaxation. Surgeon should infiltrate wound site with bupivacaine 0.25% (with epinephrine 1:200,000)—not to exceed 2.5 mg/kg (1 mL/kg), for postop pain relief. Rectal acetaminophen 30 mg/kg can be administered.	
Emergence	Reverse NMB with appropriate agent (see p. D-3). Prior to extubation, suction stomach contents via NG/OG tube. Extubate when fully awake.	
Blood and fluid requirements	Minimal blood loss IV: 22 ga × 1 NS/LR @ (maintenance)	Minimal 3rd-space loss
Monitoring	Standard monitors (see p. D-1)	
Positioning	✓ and pad pressure points. ✓ eyes.	
Complications	Aspiration	

POSTOPERATIVE

Complications	Apnea Hypoglycemia (rare)	Pulse oximetry/apnea monitor × 24 h. Differential diagnoses of apnea include hypoglycemia and hypothermia. Rx for hypoglycemia: dextrose 0.5 g/kg iv
Pain management	Acetaminophen (10–15 mg/kg po, 20 mg/kg pr q 6 h prn)	For child with severe dehydration and electrolyte abnormalities, ICU admission may be necessary.
Tests	None routinely indicated.	

Suggested Readings

1. Andropoulos DB, Heard MB, Johnson KL, et al: Postanesthetic apnea in full-term infants after pyloromyotomy. *Anesthesiology* 1994; 80(1):216–9.
2. Goh DW, Hall SK, Gornall P, et al: Plasma chloride and alkalemia in pyloric stenosis. *Br J Surg* 1990; 77(8):922–3.
3. Gregory GA, ed: *Pediatric Anesthesia*, 4th edition. Churchill Livingstone, New York: 2002, 579–80.
4. Liu LM, Pang LM: Neonatal surgical emergencies in anesthesiology. *Clin North Am* 2001; 19(2):265–8.
5. Maher M, Hehir DJ, Horgan A, et al: Infantile hypertrophic pyloric stenosis: long-term audit from a general surgical unit. *Ir J Med Sci* 1996; 165(2):115–7.
6. Oldham KT: Introduction to neonatal intestinal obstruction. In *Surgery of Infants and Children.* Oldham KT, Colombani PM, Foglia RP, eds. Lippincott-Raven, Philadelphia: 1997, 1181–2.
7. Schwartz D, Connelly NR, Manikantan P, et al: Hyperkalemia and pyloric stenosis. *Anesth Analgesia* 2003; 97:355–7.
8. Scorpio RJ, Tan HL, Hutson JM: Pyloromyotomy: comparison between laparoscopic and open surgical techniques. *J Laparoendosc Surg* 1995; 5(2):81–4.
9. Vegunta RK, Woodland JH, Rawlings AL, et al: Practice makes perfect: progressive improvement of laparoscopic pyloromyotomy results, with experience. *J Laparoendosc Adv Surg Tech A* 2008; 18(1):152–6.

ABDOMINAL TUMOR: RESECTION OF NEUROBLASTOMA, WILMS' TUMOR, HEPATOBLASTOMA

SURGICAL CONSIDERATIONS

Description: Pediatric abdominal tumors occur most commonly in children 1–4 yr old, may be massive, and usually arise from the sympathetic chain (including adrenal gland), kidney, or liver. Neuroblastoma and Wilms' tumors are the most common; hepatic tumors (including hemangiomas) are less common but challenging. Because they originate in sympathetic tissue, many neuroblastomas produce catecholamines; however, these rarely have hemodynamic consequences.

Surgical Approach: At first operation, a central line is placed and very large neuroblastomas and hepatoblastomas are biopsied; definitive resection follows neoadjuvant therapy. Small neuroblastomas, small hepatoblastomas, and even large Wilms' tumors (without vascular extension or bilateral involvement) may be excised primarily. The principles of operation for these tumors are similar, beginning with a generous incision (transverse, midline, or thoracoabdominal), depending on tumor location and surgeon preference. The incision may be extended into the chest if control of the suprahepatic vena cava is necessary. Epidural anesthesia is ideal. Mobilization of the tumor from adjacent structures may precede vascular control when the latter is difficult to obtain early, as is often the case. Tumors encasing vessels may be divided to preserve end-organ blood supply. Neuroblastomas tend to invade local structures. Wilms' tumors and hepatoblastomas tend to push aside adjacent structures. Wilms' tumors are bilateral in 10–15% of cases and are prone to vascular extension into the renal vein, IVC, and (rarely) right atrium. Major hepatic resections are sometimes required for hemangiomas that cause CHF or thrombocytopenia (Kasabach-Merritt syndrome).

Laparoscopic assistance is limited generally to biopsy of these lesions for tissue diagnosis. Some hepatoblastomas may be amenable to laparoscopic liver resection. Small, localized neuroblastomas, and posterior mediastinal neural crest lesions are quite amenable to laparoscopic or thoracoscopic resection.

Usual preop diagnosis: Neuroblastoma; Wilms' tumor; hepatoblastoma

SUMMARY OF PROCEDURES

	Neuroblastoma	Wilms' Tumor	Hepatic Resections
Position	Supine, 15° lift	⇐	⇐
Incision	Transverse, possible thoracic extension (Fig. 12.5-8)	⇐	⇐
Special instrumentation	None	Bypass instruments	CUSA; laser; argon beam coagulator
Unique considerations	Rarely, hormonally active; may wrap blood vessels	Atrial tumor; ivC may be obstructed →↓ ↓ CO.	Possible CHF; Plt trapping
Antibiotics	Cefotaxime 25 mg/kg	⇐	⇐
Surgical time	3–6 h	⇐	⇐
Closing considerations	None	⇐	Hypoglycemia
EBL	20–50 mL/kg	⇐	20–100 mL/kg
Postop care	PICU	± PICU	PICU
Mortality	< 5%	⇐	⇐
Morbidity	Intestinal obstruction: 10% Postop respiratory atelectasis	⇐ ⇐	– ⇐ Hypoglycemia: 10% Bile leak: 5–10%
Pain score	7–8	7–8	7–8

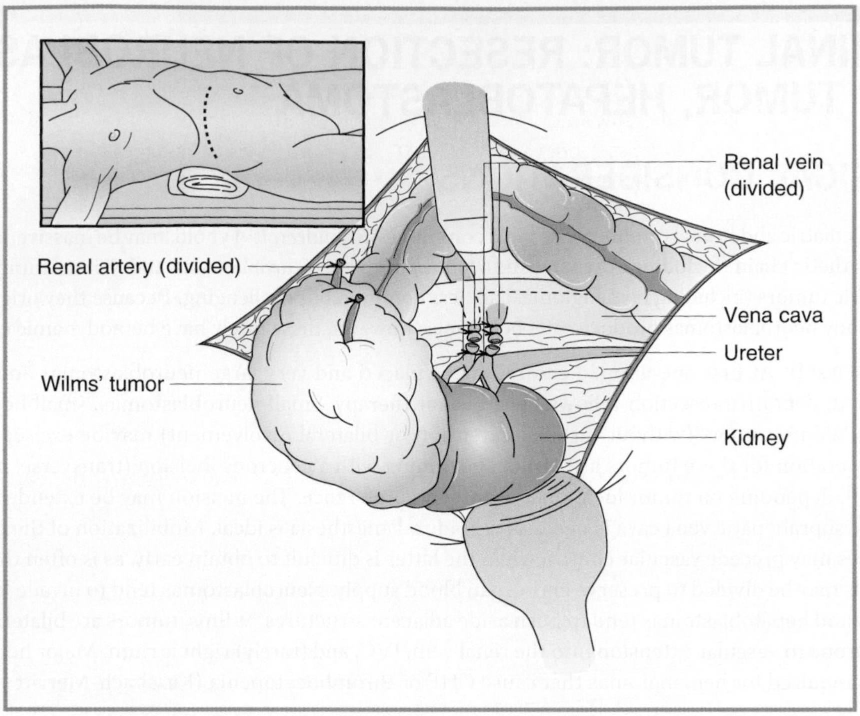

Figure 12.5-8. Operative approach to resection of a right renal Wilms' tumor. Insert shows transverse incision. (Reproduced with permission from Laquaglia MP: Childhood tumors. In *Surgery: Scientific Principles and Practice,* 3rd edition. Greenfield LJ, Mulholland MW, Oldham KT, et al, eds. Lippincott Williams & Wilkins, Philadelphia: 2001.)

PATIENT POPULATION CHARACTERISTICS

	Neuroblastoma	Wilms' Tumor	Hepatic Resections
Age range	Few months—school age	⇐	⇐
Male:Female	1:1	⇐	⇐
Incidence	1/10,000	< 1/10,000	⇐
Etiology	Unknown	⇐	⇐
Associated conditions	Beckwith-Wiedemann syndrome; aniridia; hemihypertrophy; HTN (rare)	None	⇐

ANESTHETIC CONSIDERATIONS

PREOPERATIVE

Neuroblastoma, Wilms' tumor (nephroblastoma), and hepatoblastoma commonly present as abdominal masses in infants and children < 4 yr old. Abdominal pain, fever, and ↑ BP (2° ↑ catecholamines or renal ischemia) are often associated findings. These patients may have received chemotherapy or XRT preop, and the timing of surgery may be based on multiple factors.

Respiratory	There may be respiratory compromise (as a result of a large abdominal mass pushing up on the diaphragm), which may worsen in the supine position. Wilms' tumor commonly metastasizes to the lungs. **Tests:** CXR, if indicated from H&P.

Cardiovascular	↑ BP is associated with both Wilms' tumor and neuroblastoma, and volume status should be assessed carefully. Tumor bulk may impede venous return by occluding the IVC. Wilms' tumor may extend through the IVC into the right atrium. These patients may have received chemotherapy, for example adriamycin or doxorubicin, which is associated with cardiac toxicity. (Most commonly at doses > 200 mg/m^2). Cardiology consultation may be appropriate. **Tests:** Echocardiogram
Renal	Wilms' tumor may present with hematuria and other GU anomalies such as horseshoe kidney, duplication of urinary tract, aplastic or hypoplastic kidneys. Renal function is usually normal unless both kidneys are affected. **Tests:** BUN; Cr
Endocrine	Neuroblastomas are associated with ↑ catecholamine production. Preop adrenergic blockade (as would be required for a pheochromocytoma) is usually not necessary. **Tests:** Urine VMA and HVA
Gastrointestinal	Persistent, watery diarrhea (→ hypovolemia, ↓ K^+) is associated with neuroblastoma 2° VIP secretion. Intestinal compression from tumor may ↑ risk of gastric aspiration. A surgical bowel prep may cause additional fluid and electrolyte disturbances. **Tests:** Electrolytes
Hematologic	Severe anemia and thrombocytopenia may be present. Blood should be available because of possible massive intraop blood loss. **Tests:** CBC; T&C. ✓ availability of parental/directed donor blood, if requested. ✓ PT, PTT.
Laboratory	Other tests as indicated from H&P.
Premedication	In patients at risk for gastric aspiration, prophylaxis with ranitidine (0.8 mg/kg iv) should be considered. Patients >12 mo may benefit from midazolam (0.5–0.75 mg/kg po) 30 min. before surgery.

INTRAOPERATIVE

Anesthetic technique: Combined epidural/GETA, using a pediatric circle; forced air warmer; warm OR to 75°–80F; warm all iv fluids.

Induction	IV catheter insertion before induction may be preferable. An upper extremity or EJ site is preferred due to potential for obstruction of IVC during surgery. A modified rapid-sequence induction is recommended in those patients with a large intraabdominal mass compressing the GI tract. Otherwise, standard pediatric induction (see p. D-1) is appropriate. Children < 6–9 mo may benefit from a preinduction dose of atropine (0.2 mg/kg iv) to ablate vagal response to laryngoscopy.	
Maintenance	Standard maintenance (see p. D-2). Muscle relaxation is appropriate. HTN associated with tumor manipulation can be treated with SNP (0.5–2.0 mcg/kg/min) or esmolol (50–150 mcg/kg/min). Labetalol boluses (0.1 mg/kg iv) may also be used with caution, taking into account potential for blood loss and hypotension.	
Emergence	In most instances, patient can be extubated at the end of surgery. Suction NG tube and confirm air leak around ETT before extubation. If there is no air leak, consider laryngeal edema and need for continued intubation.	
Blood and fluid requirements	Potential for large blood loss/ moderate 3rd-space loss IV: 18–20 ga × 1–2 NS/LR @ maintenance	Tumor resection may be associated with massive blood loss, especially with IVC or renal vein involvement. Avoid placement of iv catheter in lower extremities. 5% albumin may be useful to replace 3rd- space losses (8–10 mL/kg/h). Transfuse to maintain Hct > 23. If > 2 mo of age, dextrose-containing solutions are not required.

Monitoring	Standard monitors (see p. D-1) Arterial line: 22 ga CVP line: 4 Fr (subclavian or IJ) confirm position by CXR	ABG, Hct, blood glucose should be measured hourly. CVP measurement may be useful to evaluate fluid status. Monitor UO and keep at 1 mL/kg/h.
Positioning	✓ and pad pressure points. ✓ eyes.	
Complications	Hypotension HTN PE Hypothermia Hypoventilation	↓ BP 2° blood loss or IVC obstruction or PE ↑ BP 2° tumor or adrenal manipulation 2° tumor embolization usually from IVC →↓ BP. 45% of patients had hypotension after tumor excision, suggesting that catecholamines are present; Rx may require volume loading/pressor support Abdominal retractors and packing will interfere with ventilation.

POSTOPERATIVE

Complications	Atelectasis Hypoventilation	
Pain management	Epidural or iv opiates Ketorolac 0.5 mg/kg iv q 6 × 2 d	See p. E-5 for dosing schedule.
Tests	Hct ABG CXR	

Suggested Readings

1. Charlton GA, Sedgwick J, Sutton DN: Anaesthetic management of renin-secreting nephroblastoma. *Br J Anaesth* 1992; 69(2):206–9.
2. Creagh-Barry P, Sumner E: Neuroblastoma and anaesthesia. *Paed Anaesth* 1992;2:147–52.
3. Gregory GA, ed: *Pediatric Anesthesia,* 4th edition. Churchill Livingstone, New York: 2002: 611–12.
4. Hammer GH: Pediatric thoracic anesthesia. *Anesth Analgesia* 2001; 92:1449–1964.
5. Kain ZN, Shamberger RS, Holzman RS: Anesthetic management of children with neuroblastoma. *J Clin Anesth* 1993; 5(6): 486–91.
6. Lacreuse I, Valla JS, de Lagausie P, et al: Thoracoscopic resection of neurogenic tumors in children. *J Pediatr Surg* 2007; 42(10):1725–8.
7. Leclair MD, de Lagausie P, Becmeur F, et al: Laparoscopic resection of abdominal neuroblastoma. *Ann Surg Onco.* 2008; 15(1):117–24.
8. Mayhew JF: Intraoperative hyperthermia in a child with neuroblastoma. *Ped Anesthesia* 2006; 16:890–91.
9. Motoyama EK, Davis PJ, eds: *Smith's Anesthesia for Infants and Children,* 7th edition. CV Mosby-Year Book, St. Louis: 2006: 691–93.
10. Nagabuchi E, Ziegler MM: Neuroblastoma. In *Surgery of Infants and Children.* Oldham KT, Colombani PM, Foglia RP, eds. Lippincott-Raven, Philadelphia: 1997, 593–614.
11. Ritchey ML, Andrassy RJ, Kelalis PP: Pediatric urologic oncology. In *Adult and Pediatric Urology,* Vol 3, 3rd edition. Gillenwater JY, Grayhack JT, Howards SS, et al, eds. Mosby-Year Book, St. Louis: 1996, 2675–93.
12. Shochat SJ: Renal tumors. *Surgery of Infants and Children.* Oldham KT, Colombani PM, Foglia RP, eds. Lippincott-Raven, Philadelphia: 1997, 581–92.
13. Tagge EP, Tagge DU: Hepatoblastoma and hepatocellular carcinoma. *Surgery of Infants and Children.* Oldham KT, Colombani PM, Foglia RP, eds. Lippincott-Raven, Philadelphia: 1997, 633–44.

LAPAROTOMY FOR INTESTINAL PERFORATION, NECROTIZING ENTEROCOLITIS

SURGICAL CONSIDERATIONS

Description: Necrotizing enterocolitis (NEC) is an ischemic/inflammatory condition of the entire GI tract, most commonly affecting the terminal ileum, occurring in stressed, premature infants, often after feeding with formula. It may resolve with conservative management (npo, antibiotics, NG suction) or progress to necrosis and perforation, treated by resection and stoma formation or drainage procedure, according to patient weight and surgeon preference. Isolated ileal perforation—occurring without precedent pneumatosis intestinalis—may be a different disease entity; it is sometimes treated by primary repair. Infants with NEC may be septic, thrombocytopenic, and coagulopathic, with organ dysfunction related to prematurity, and have marginal ventilation. Despite expeditious surgery, several blood volumes may be lost and hypothermia may develop. Unstable infants may have surgery performed in the NICU.

Surgical approach: If not already present, central venous access is established at the time of surgery. A transverse laparotomy incision enables inspection of all intestines; dead bowel is resected, a proximal stoma is created in the healthy bowel, and a distal mucous fistula is created to protect potentially viable bowel. Less commonly, a **Hartmann's pouch** is created (distal intestine remains inside without stoma). When proximal bowel is of intermediate viability, a second-look operation is wise.

Variant procedures or approaches: The role of **drainage procedures** is undetermined; some who advocate their use in < 1 kg neonates are less enthusiastic about larger children. The procedure involves placement of a RLQ Penrose drain into the abdominal cavity as a bedside procedure. It is quick, relatively easy, and attended by little bleeding or hypothermia. Between 60–80% of drained children subsequently will require laparotomy.

Usual preop diagnosis: Perforated NEC

SUMMARY OF PROCEDURES

	Resection	Drainage
Position	Supine	⇐
Incision	Transverse	RLQ
Special instrumentation	None	Penrose drains
Unique considerations	Temperature support	⇐
Antibiotics	Ampicillin 50 mg/kg + gentamicin 2.5 mg/kg + clindamycin 10 mg/kg iv preop	⇐
Surgical time	1–2.5 h	0.5 h
EBL	10–100 mL/kg	1–2 mL/kg
Postop care	NICU	⇐
Mortality	20–25%	16–20%
Morbidity	Respiratory failure Sepsis Stricture Intracranial hemorrhage	⇐
Pain score	6–7	3–4

PATIENT POPULATION CHARACTERISTICS

Age range	Newborn–weeks
Male:Female	> 1:1
Incidence	5–8% NICU admissions
Etiology	Multifactorial, including intestinal ischemia; bacterial colonization; perinatal stress; immaturity; hypoxia; hyperosmolar feeding; splanchnic ischemia
Associated conditions	Prematurity (80–90%); respiratory distress; PDA

ANESTHETIC CONSIDERATIONS

PREOPERATIVE

Most (80–90%) of these patients are premature infants (< 36 wk gestational age) presenting with sepsis. Respiratory Distress Syndrome (RDS) is often present 2° prematurity of the lungs, and pulmonary insufficiency is likely present. In addition to sepsis, significant 3rd-space losses contribute to hypovolemia and metabolic acidosis. If the patient is extremely unstable, consider surgical intervention at the bedside in the NICU.

Respiratory	Premature infants are at risk for RDS. These infants are usually on mechanical ventilation with ↑ FiO_2 prior to surgery. They also are at ↑ risk for pneumonia, pneumothorax, and pulmonary edema. ✓ ventilator settings and recent ABG in preparation for OR mechanical ventilation. **Tests:** CXR; ABG
Cardiovascular	Likely hemodynamic instability 2° to sepsis and/or under-resuscitation. Inotropes. (e.g., dopamine 5–10 mcg/kg/min) may be required to maintain adequate CO. Associated cardiac anomalies (e.g., VSD, PDA) can lead to CHF, further complicating fluid management. Pulmonary overcirculation and intrinsic pulmonary disease contribute to pulmonary HTN. **Tests:** CXR; ABG; ECHO
Neurological	Intraventricular hemorrhage (IVH) may be 2° to prematurity or birth asphyxia. These hemorrhagic regions have impaired autoregulation, and wide variations in BP (20–30 mmHg) can aggravate ischemia/hemorrhage. In addition, these patients may have a seizure disorder. **Tests:** Head ultrasound, if indicated from H&P.
Renal	Presence of PDA and previous Rx with NSAID can lead to impaired renal perfusion and clearance. Aggravating factors are aminoglycoside antibiotics, sepsis, and CHF. **Tests:** BUN; Cr
Metabolic	Metabolic acidosis 2° to sepsis and/or CHF will further worsen myocardial function. Neonate has minimal glycogen stores and impaired ability to mobilize calcium. **Tests:** ABG; Ca^{++}; glucose; electrolytes
Hematologic	DIC, and associated thrombocytopenia, anemia may be present. **Tests:** CBC, PT, PTT, fibrinogen, T-antigen; availability of irradiated, washed RBCs and instrumentation (plasma can contain antibody against T-antigen that causes hemolysis).
Laboratory	Others as indicated from H&P
Premedication	None

INTRAOPERATIVE

Anesthetic technique: GETA, using a pediatric circle. Warm OR to 75°–80°F. Forced-air warmer and warming pad on OR table. Use air/O_2 mixture for ventilation and maintain SpO_2 between 92–94% (PaO_2 < 70 mmHg) to minimize risk of retinopathy. Avoid high concentrations of O_2. Consider use of NICU ventilator if patient requires ↑ RR or ↑ PIPs. Epidural catheter insertion is not recommended in the presence of sepsis.

Induction	These patients usually are intubated. If not, intubate with full-stomach precautions (see p. B-4).Suction stomach. Give atropine 0.02 mg/kg iv (0.1 mg minimum dose) before laryngoscopy. Preoxygenate for 1 min. Miller 0/1 blade with O_2 side port, if available. Apply cricoid pressure until airway secured. ETT should have leak at 18–35 cm H_2O pressure.	
Maintenance	Opioid technique (fentanyl 10–30 mcg/kg iv total)—avoid myocardial depression from volatile agents. Avoid N_2O (↑ bowel size). Muscle relaxation required.	
Emergence	Postop ventilation generally required. Transport to NICU with full monitoring (pulse oximetry, ECG, arterial line). Have laryngoscope and appropriately sized mask and ETT available. Extra volume (albumin 5% in 20 mL syringes) may be needed during transport.	
Blood and fluid requirements	Anticipate moderate-to-large blood and fluid losses. IV: 22–24 ga × 2 (or 1 + CVP)	Neonates are usually fluid-restricted in NICU to lessen incidence of PDA. 3rd- space losses are usually significant. Rx: ↑ BP with volume before increasing dopamine. Maintain solution Hct > 35%. Albumin 5% (10 mL/kg iv) boluses as needed. Crystalloid/colloid > 100 mL/kg total not uncommon. Hct, glucose, Ca^{++}, ABG, Plt count, PT/PTT, electrolytes q 30–60 min. I-stat if available.
	Continue dextrose-containing solution from NICU to avoid hypoglycemia. Warm fluids.	Because of the potentially large blood loss/kg, ensure that blood replacement is available in the room, and that additional factor replacement is available on call.
Monitoring	Standard monitors (see p. D-1) A-line pref. preductal (RUE) ± CVP line 3 Fr	CUP line is not as important as arterial line for intraop care, but may be useful for administering inotropic drugs.
Positioning	✓ eyes ✓ pad pressure points	
Complications	Hypothermia Metabolic acidosis Hypovolemia	Aggressive volume replacement and maintaining normothermia will prevent or ameliorate metabolic acidosis. Bicarbonate replacement = base deficit × wt (kg) × 0.3.
	Hyperkalemia 2° blood products(rare)	Minimized by requesting that newest blood available be sent up. If blood is irradiated, it may need to be washed prior to transfusion. (check w/ blood bank for policy).
	Pneumothorax	↓ O_2 sats, ↑ PIPs. ✓ for mucus plugging or mainstem intubation.
	Hypocalcemia	Frequent blood sampling is necessary. Rx: $CaCl_2$ (10 mg/kg iv) in dilute solution via CUP line or Ca gluconate (30 mg/kg iv) via peripheral line.
	Hypoglycemia	Continue 10% dextrose infusion from NICU.

POSTOPERATIVE

Complications	Hypovolemia due to blood loss, and 3rd-spacing Metabolic acidosis and/or sepsis Pulmonary edema Retinopathy of prematurity (ROP)

Pain management	Morphine (0.05–0.10 mg/kg iv) q 1–2 h prn or via continuous infusion for initial 24–48 h
Tests	CBC Electrolytes, Ca++, Glucose ABG CXR, if central line placed.

Suggested Readings

1. Ade-Ajayi N, Kiely E, Drake D, et al: Resection and primary anastomosis in necrotizing enterocolitis. *J R Soc Med* 1996; 89(7):385–8.
2. Diaz JH, ed: *Perinatal Anesthesia and Critical Care.* WB Saunders, Philadelphia: 1991.
3. Ein SH, Shandling B, Wesson D, et al: A 13-year experience with peritoneal drainage under local anesthesia for necrotizing enterocolitis perforation. *J Pediatr Surg* 1990; 25(10):1034–7.
4. Gregory GA, ed: *Pediatric Anesthesia*, 4th edition. Churchill Livingstone, New York: 2002, 363–4.
5. Grosfeld JL, Molinari F, Chaet M, et al: Gastrointestinal perforation and peritonitis in infants and children: experience with 179 cases over ten years. *Surgery* 1996; 120(4):650–5.
6. Kosloske AN: Necrotizing enterocolitis. In *Surgery of Infants and Children.* Oldham KT, Colombani PM, Foglia RP, eds. Lippincott-Raven, Philadelphia: 1997, 1201–14.
7. Liu LM, Pang LM: Neonatal surgical emergencies in anesthesiology. *Clin North Am* 2001; 19(2):277–9.
8. Luzzatto C, Previtera C, Boscolo R, et al: Necrotizing enterocolitis: late surgical results after enterostomy without resection. *Eur J Pediatr Surg* 1996; 6(2):92–4.
9. Motoyama EK, Davis PJ, eds: *Smith's Anesthesia for Infants and Children*, 7th edition. Mosby-Elsevier, Philadelphia: 2006, 552–5.

REPAIR OF BILIARY ATRESIA AND CHOLEDOCHAL CYSTS

SURGICAL CONSIDERATIONS

Description: "Biliary atresia" is a misnomer, because the pathology seems to be an ascending progressive fibrosis of the biliary tree ultimately manifested by intrahepatic bridging fibrosis and cirrhosis. The obstruction develops postnatally, typically in an otherwise healthy 4- to 6-wk-old girl, though it may be confused with neonatal hepatitis or with the cholestasis seen in sick neonates fed intravenously. Preop studies often are not diagnostic, and there is some time pressure because of dismal surgical outcomes when a definitive operation is performed after 8–10 wk of age. **Todani** classified choledochal cysts into five types. The first type is the most common: a fusiform ballooning of the extrahepatic bile ducts often involving the gallbladder. Cysts are prone to bile stasis, obstruction, and malignant conversion in adulthood. Some are detected when they become symptomatic; an increasing number are detected on antenatal ultrasound.

Surgical approach: Following preop administration of vitamin K, operation for biliary atresia begins through a transverse RUQ incision (or laparoscopically) for liver biopsy and operative cholangiography. Ascent of contrast into the liver and descent into the duodenum excludes biliary atresia and will terminate the operation. Failure to establish patency of the biliary tree is indication to extend the incision to excise the gallbladder and extrahepatic biliary tree. In doing so, the portal vein and hepatic artery are skeletonized up to the base of the liver (called the portal or hepatic "plate.") (Fig. 12.5-9) This region is excised (attended by some bleeding) in the hope that bile will drain from the liver above into a Roux-en-Y loop of jejunum, which is sewn to the undersurface of the liver (**portoenterostomy** or **Kasai procedure**). There is currently little support for early liver transplantation. **Choledochal cyst resection** involves a smaller incision, possible cholangiogram, and dissection similar to the Kasai procedure, but only to a level above the cyst (frequently, the bifurcation of the hepatic ducts). Liver biopsy is not always required and cirrhosis is uncommon. Bleeding may result when an inflamed cyst is adherent to the portal vein or hepatic artery. The distal end of the cyst

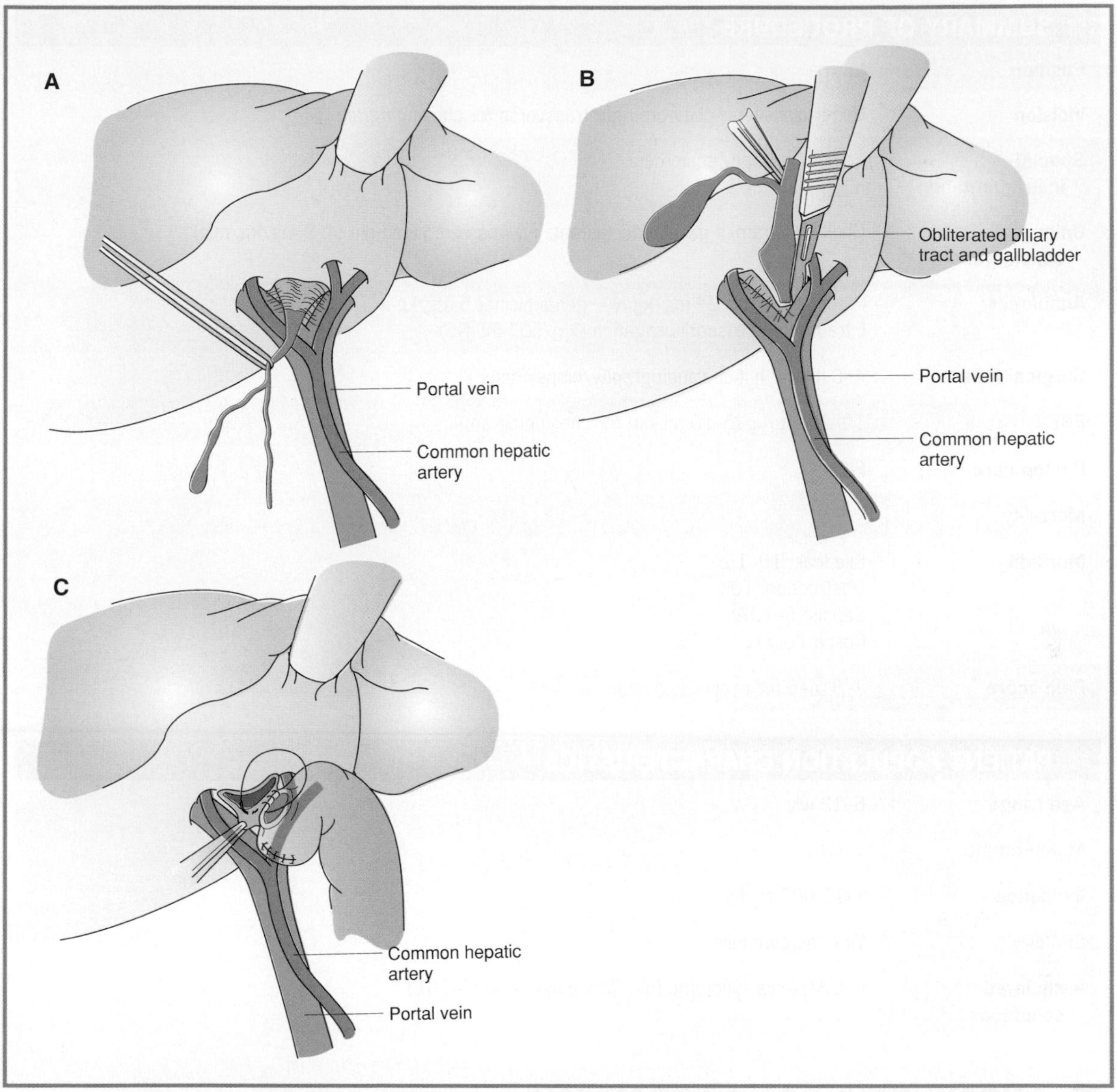

Figure 12.5-9. The essential features of the portoenterostomy for biliary atresia include appropriate mobilization **(A)** and transection **(B)** of the fibrous biliary tract remnant. **(C)** Creation of a Roux-en-Y jejunal conduit with biliary enteric anastomosis completes the procedure. (Reproduced with permission from Sato TT, Oldham KT: Pediatric abdomen. In *Surgery: Scientific Principles and Practice,* 3rd edition. Greenfield LJ, Mulholland MW, Oldham KT, et al, eds. Lippincott Williams & Wilkins, Philadelphia: 2001.)

is ligated, the body of it excised, and the proximal bile duct (usually the common hepatic duct) sewn to a Roux-en-Y limb of jejunum.

Both operations can be performed using laparoscopy, with or without robotic assistance. Dissection is carried out laparoscopically, an Roux limb is created outside the abdomen by bringing the intestine out of an umbilical wound then replacing it back into the belly, and the final reconstruction is performed laparoscopically.

Usual preop diagnosis: Biliary atresia; choledochal cyst; obstructive jaundice

SUMMARY OF PROCEDURE	
Position	Supine
Incision	Upper transverse-chevron; right transverse for cholangiogram
Special instrumentation	Cholangiography equipment
Unique considerations	Cholangiogram, if gallbladder patent; ↑ glucose requirement (4–8 mg/kg/min)
Antibiotics	Preop: ampicillin 25 mg/kg iv + gentamicin 2.5 mg/kg iv Intraop: cephalosporin irrigation (1 g/500 mL NS)
Surgical time	4–6 h (1–2 h if cholangiography/biopsy only)
EBL	10–20 mL/kg (5–10 mL/kg for cholangiogram)
Postop care	PICU
Mortality	< 5%
Morbidity	Bile leak: 10–15% Obstruction: 10% Sepsis: 5–10% Respiratory failure: 5%
Pain score	7–8 (4–5 for cholangiogram)

PATIENT POPULATION CHARACTERISTICS	
Age range	6–12 wk
Male:Female	> 1:1
Incidence	1/15,000 births
Etiology	Viral; autoimmune
Associated conditions	NB: Asplenia syndrome (5–10%); polysplenia (5–10%)

ANESTHETIC CONSIDERATIONS

PREOPERATIVE

Biliary atresia is a postnatal inflammatory disorder of the hepatobiliary tree resulting in fibrosis, cirrhosis, and obstructive jaundice. The Kasai procedure is indicated if the diagnosis of biliary atresia is made in the first 3–4 mo of life. If the Kasai procedure is unsuccessful, the patient may require a liver transplant.

Gastrointestinal	Hepatic function preserved initially (i.e., normal albumin synthesis). Cholestatic jaundice usually present. There may be impaired elimination of drugs, particularly NMBs. Glucose homeostasis is usually normal.
Hematologic	Anemia 2° chronic disease. Impaired vitamin K absorption 2° lack of bile salts. Elevated PT will variably correct with vitamin K administration (phytonadione 1 mg im/iv given during the week before surgery). Have FFP available if PT not corrected after vitamin K. **Tests:** PT; PTT; CBC; T&C
Laboratory	Electrolytes: BUN, Cr, LFTs, albumin, bilirubin, direct and indirect, glucose, others as indicated from H&P. Confirm availability of blood products (PRBCs, FFP).
Premedication	None

INTRAOPERATIVE

Anesthetic technique: GETA/epidural, using a pediatric circle. Warm OR to 75°–80°F; use forced-air warmer, warming pad on OR table. (Remember: majority of heat loss is radiant).

Induction	Mask induction is appropriate if no iv in place. NMB (e.g., rocuronium 0.6–1 mg/kg) to facilitate tracheal intubation, using appropriately sized ETT (usually 3.5–4.0 uncuffed ETT) (with leak at 18–35 cmH_2O). If coagulation factors are normal, consider epidural or caudal catheter, and advance to thoracic position.	
Maintenance	Isoflurane/air/O_2; no N_2O, to avoid bowel distention. Continue muscle relaxant to facilitate abdominal closure.	
Emergence	Patient usually extubated in OR and transported to PACU or, in the case of prolonged surgery and/or significant blood loss, to PICU with O_2 and monitors in place.	
Blood and fluid requirements	Moderate blood loss IV: 22 ga × 1–2 NS/LR @ 10 mL/kg/h Albumin 5%	Potential for large 3rd-space losses. Plan 10 mL/kg/h of NS/LR for replacement, and be prepared for sudden blood loss. Use albumin 5%, or NS/LR to replace blood loss; transfuse to maintain Hct > 22%. If dextrose infusion required, give 4–6 mg/kg/min.
Monitoring	Standard monitors (see p. D-1) Urinary catheter NG tube Arterial line (22–24 ga) ± CVP line	Hct, blood glucose, ±ABG q 1–2 h and prn. Maintain UO @ 1 mL/kg/h. The presence of ↑↑ BP variations with respiration is a useful indicator of hypovolemia. CVP may be indicated for intravascular volume monitoring.
Positioning	✓ padding – heels, elbows, occiput. ✓ eyes.	
Complications	Hypothermia Hypovolemia Hypoventilation Metabolic acidosis	In upper abdominal surgery, the retractors and abdominal packing may limit diaphragmatic excursion, thus requiring higher PIP to adequately ventilate the patient. ETT leak (PIP) > 20 cmH_2O to ensure adequate ventilation. ETT position may also change with packing, resulting in R mainstem intubation, requiring repositioning.

POSTOPERATIVE

Complications	Hypovolemia Transfusion-associated disease Atelectasis Cholangitis	3rd-space losses continue in the immediate postop period. Postop mechanical ventilation with TV 10– 12 mL/kg and PEEP 3–5 cmH_2O to minimize atelectasis.
Pain management	Fentanyl (1–2 mcg/kg/iv q 1 h prn) MSO_4 (0.05–0.1 mg/kg iv q 2–4 h prn)	Epidural analgesia if catheter in place (see p. E-5). Bupivicaine dose should be limited to 0.25–0.3 mg/kg 2° decreased hepatic clearance and serum protein binding capacity.
Tests	Hct ABG	

Suggested Readings

1. Dutta S, Woo RK, Albanese CT: Minimal access portoenterostomy: advantages and disadvantages of standard laparoscopic and robotic techniques. *J Laparoendosc Adv Surg Tech A* 2007; 17(2):258–64.
2. Engelskirchen R, Holschneider AM, Gharib M, et al: Biliary atresia—a 25-year survey. *Eur J Pediatr Surg* 1991; 1(3): 154–60.
3. Flake AW: Disorders of the gallbladder and biliary tract. In *Surgery of Infants and Children.* Oldham KT, Colombani PM, Foglia RP, eds. Lippincott-Raven, Philadelphia: 1997, 1405–14.

4. Green DW, Howard ER, Davenport M: Anesthesia, perioperative management and outcome of correction of extrahepatic biliary atresia in the infant: a review of 50 cases in the King's College Hospital Series. *Pediatr Anesth* 2000; 10(6):581–9.
5. Karrer FM, Hall RJ, Stewart BA, et al: Congenital biliary tract disease. *Surg Clin North Am* 1990; 70(6):1403–18.
6. Karrer FM, Lilly JP: Biliary atresia. In *Surgery of Infants and Children.* Oldham KT, Colombani PM, Foglia RP, eds. Lippincott-Raven, Philadelphia: 1997, 1395–1404.
7. Kasai M, Suzuki H, Ohashi E, et al: Technique and results of operative management of biliary atresia. *World J Surg* 1978; 2(5):571–9.
8. Katz J, Steward DJ, eds: *Anesthesia and Uncommon Pediatric Diseases,* 2nd edition. WB Saunders, Philadelphia: 1993.
9. Le D, Woo RK, Sylvester KG, et al: Laparoscopic resection of type 1 choledochal cysts in pediatric patients. *Surg Endosc* 2006; 20(2):249–51.
10. Meunier JF, Goujard E, Dubousset AM, et al: Pharmakokinetics of bupivacaine after continuous epidural infusion in infants with and without biliary atresia. *Anesthesiology* 2001; 95(1):87–95.
11. Woo RK, Le D, Albanese CT, et al: Robot-assisted laparoscopic resection of a type I choledochal cyst in a child. *J Laparoendosc Adv Surg Tech A* 2006; 16(2):179–83.

REPAIR OF ABDOMINAL WALL DEFECTS: OMPHALOCELE/GASTROSCHISIS

SURGICAL CONSIDERATIONS

Description: **Omphalocele** is a herniation of bowel and sometimes viscera into an enlarged umbilical cord that may be categorized as small (< 2 cm, sometimes called a 'hernia of the cord'); medium (2–5 cm defect); or giant (≥ 6 cm and containing liver). The larger the defect, the more difficult the repair for lack of skin and muscle; primary repair is virtually never possible for giant defects. Omphaloceles are associated with genetic defects (trisomy 21) and may be part of other syndromes (e.g., OEIS, pentalogy of Cantrell, which includes cardiac defects). The surprisingly tough membrane of the umbilical cord protects the intestines from exposure to amniotic fluid. **Gastroschisis** is not associated with chromosomal anomalies or syndromes. It involves a 1–2 cm defect to the right of the umbilicus, through which bowel, and sometimes stomach or gonads, extrude and are exposed to the sclerosing effects of amniotic fluid, causing variable degrees of "peel" (bowel-wall thickening).

Surgical approach: Central venous catheter placement precedes or accompanies the initial operation. Enlargement of the defect is sometimes necessary to permit visceral reduction, provided there is sufficient abdominal domain. If not, reduction will cause bowel ischemia and respiratory embarrassment. Some surgeons will use a maximal transduced bladder or stomach pressure (20 mmHg) or maximal PIP (35 mmHg) as an indicator that primary repair is dangerous. In this case, a prosthetic abdominal wall of Silastic is created (or purchased) and applied to the edges of the defect, creating a tubular prominence called a 'silo'. In the NICU the silo is gradually reduced in size over 3–10 d, whereupon the abdomen is closed primarily (Fig. 12.5-10). Small and medium size omphaloceles are treated similarly. Return of intestinal function will take 3–7 d for omphaloceles and 1–4 wk for gastroschisis.

Variant procedures or approaches: Sutureless approaches to both gastroschisis and omphalocoele are emerging, and can be effective means of closing these defects with outstanding cosmetic results. For giant omphalocoele, sclerosing solutions (silver sulfasalazine, tincture of mercurochrome) can be applied to cause epithelialization. Many months later, the resulting unsightly bulge may be excised and closure of the abdominal defect attempted without undue respiratory or bowel compromise. Alternatively compression wraps applied around the abdomen work to reduce bowel content over a period of months. The remaining fascial defect decreases in size until it resembles an umbilical hernia, which may close spontaneously or require later minor surgical closure. With gastroschisis, sutured closure of the fascial defect is unnecessary. In cases where the bowel can be primarily reduced, the remnant umbilical cord is used as a biological dressing over the defect, and a large plastic dressing is applied (e.g., Tegaderm). The defect closes spontaneously over the ensuing weeks, and re-epithelialization occurs, as bowel function returns. For irreducible bowel, a silo is applied and sequential reduction is performed. After the bowel is reduced completely, a plastic dressing with absorbant nonstick gauze is applied and spontaneous closure

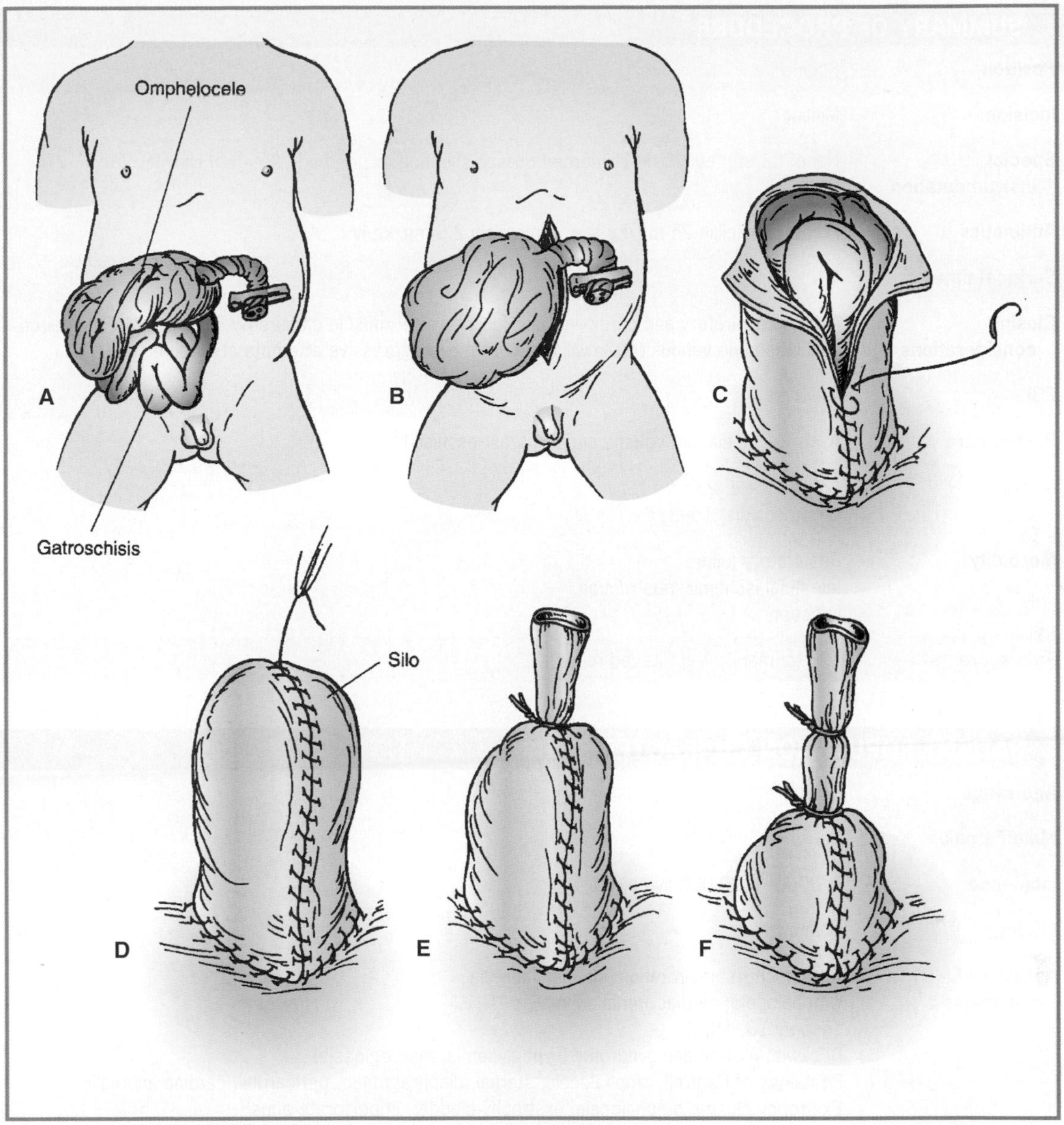

Figure 12.5-10. Management of gastroschisis and omphalocele (both shown together): **(A)** Gastroschisis defect. **(B)** Extension of opening with midline incision (optional). **(C)** Use of silo if primary closure is not possible. **(D)** Finished silo. **(E, F)** Staged ligation of silo with reduction of silo contents into abdominal cavity proper. (Reproduced with permission from Oldham KT, Colombani PM, Foglia RP: *Surgery of Infants and Children.* Lippincott-Raven, Philadelphia: 1997.)

ensues. Cosmetic results are typically superior to suture closure, and there is never a concern for high ventilatory pressures.

Variant procedures or approaches: Giant omphaloceles are sometimes treated without initial attempts at definitive surgery. Instead, the amniotic membrane retaining the intestinal contents is treated with daily applications of a **sclerosing solution** (silver sulfasalazine, tincture of mercurochrome). This causes the membrane to thicken and eventually epithelialize. Many months later, the resulting unsightly bulge may be excised and closure of the abdominal defect attempted without undue respiratory or bowel compromise.

Usual preop diagnosis: Omphalocele; gastroschisis; pentalogy of Cantrell; exstrophy cloaca

SUMMARY OF PROCEDURE

Position	Supine
Incision	Midline
Special instrumentation	None; for staged repair, reinforced Silastic sheeting or pre-made (Bentec) silo
Antibiotics	Preop: ampicillin 25 mg/kg iv + gentamicin 2.5 mg/kg iv
Surgical time	2 h
Closing considerations	Assess respiratory and cardiovascular function after muscle closure by PIP, ABG, MAP. Impaired ventilation and venous return will result from overaggressive attempts at closure.
EBL	5–10 mL/kg
Postop care	Assisted ventilation; volume support (gastroschisis)
Mortality	Omphalocele: 28% Gastroschisis: 15–23%
Morbidity	Respiratory failure Intestinal ischemia/obstruction Infection
Pain score	5–6 (primary); 4–5 (staged repair)

PATIENT POPULATION CHARACTERISTICS

Age range	Newborn
Male:Female	1:1
Incidence	1/3000–1/10,000 live births
Etiology	Unknown
Associated conditions	Gastroschisis: malrotation, intestinal atresia Omphalocele: cardiac, renal anomalies Trisomy 13, 18, 21 Beckwith-Wiedemann syndrome (hypoglycemia, macroglossia) Pentalogy of Cantrell: omphalocele, sternal, diaphragmatic, pericardial, cardiac anomalies Exstrophy cloaca: omphalocele, exstrophy bladder, imperforate anus

ANESTHETIC CONSIDERATIONS

PREOPERATIVE

Newborns with omphalocele/gastroschisis present for urgent surgery. The large exposed surface area of abdominal contents allows substantial evaporative heat and fluid losses. Omphalocele is associated with other congenital anomalies (e.g., VSD, Beckwith-Wiedemann syndrome [infantile gigantism, macroglossia, hypoglycemia]). The majority of these patients should be medically stabilized in the nursery before coming to the OR.

Respiratory	If premature (< 36 wk gestational age), infant is at ↑ risk for RDS and respiratory insufficiency. **Tests:** CXR; ABG
Cardiovascular	With omphalocele, there is a 20% incidence of cardiac anomalies (VSD, PDA). Check for murmur. **Tests:** ECHO for omphalocele, or if murmur is found.

Gastrointestinal	Intestinal atresia may be present. Hypovolemia from evaporative loss and under-resuscitation likely; check for evidence of dehydration, urine output, ABG. Full stomach precautions (see p. B-4).
Endocrine	Beckwith-Wiedemann associated with hypoglycemia (term infant glucose should be > 36 mg/dL). **Tests:** Glucose; electrolytes
Laboratory	CBC; T&C; PT; PTT; UA; ABG

INTRAOPERATIVE

Anesthetic technique: GETA, using a pediatric circle; warm OR to 75°–80°F; forced-air warmer, warming pad on OR table. (Remember majority of heat loss is radiant.)

Induction	Atropine (0.02 mg/kg iv; minimum dose, 0.1 mg) is given before induction in patients < 9 mo to ablate vagal response to laryngoscopy. Pass an OG tube to decompress stomach. Assure adequate intravascular volume status (capillary refill < 2 sec; warm, pink extremities). Preoxygenate with 100% O_2 for 2–3 min. prior to rapid-sequence intubation. Propofol (2–3 mg/kg) or STP (4 mg/kg) and rocuronium (1 mg/kg) or succinylcholine (1–2 mg/kg) iv administered to facilitate tracheal intubation. Use appropriately sized ETT to keep air leak at 18–35 cmH_2O. Lower pressure air leak may make ventilation difficult if primary closure of abdomen is accompanied by significant rise in intraabdominal pressure. For small defects, place an epidural catheter inserted via the caudal or lumbar route after intubation. If positioning for the epidural catheter insertion is difficult, do not proceed; use IV Fentanyl or morphine for pain management. An epidural catheter may be placed at the end of the case for postop analgesia.	
Maintenance	Avoid high FiO_2. Use air/O_2 mixture for ventilation to maintain O_2 sat 95–100% and PaO_2 < 100. If no epidural is placed, then use a primarily narcotic-based technique with fentanyl (10–25 mcg/kg iv total), low-dose isoflurane as needed. Note initial PIP prior to abdominal closure. Maintain neuromuscular blockade to facilitate abdominal closure. If an epidural catheter is available, dose with local anesthetic and opiate (see p. D-5) to supplement inhalation iv agent.	
Emergence	Remain intubated postop unless defect is very small. Transport to NICU on 100% O_2.	
Blood and fluid requirements	Marked 3rd-space fluid loss Minimal-moderate blood loss IV: 22–24 ga × 1–2, upper extremities NS/LR @ 4 mL/kg/h	Continue dextrose-containing solution from NICU. Replace 3rd-space losses (10– 15+ mL/kg/h). Replace blood loss with albumin 5% and/or blood mL for mL. Maintain Hct > 30%. Lower extremities usually edematous due to abdominal venous and lymphatic compression.
Monitoring	Standard monitors (see p. D-1) Arterial line (24-ga radial) ± CVP – 3 Fr if large repair planned Urinary catheter ± intragastric catheter	ABG pre- and postabdominal closure. Hct, glucose, electrolytes q 60 min. CVP; reserve 1 lumen for postop TPN. Respiratory variation on arterial waveform is sensitive indicator of hypovolemia.
Positioning	✓ and pad pressure points. ✓ eyes.	Arms positioned to have ready access to arterial line.
Complications	Hypothermia Hypovolemia Respiratory insufficiency/hypoventilation Atelectasis Volume overload/pulmonary edema	Some institutions monitor intraabdominal pressure during closure. If intragastric pressure is > 20 mmHg and CVP increases by 4 mmHg with initial primary closure, it should be converted to a staged repair. Raised abdominal pressure will cause an acute restrictive ventilatory defect and promote abdominal visceral ischemia.

POSTOPERATIVE

Complications	Respiratory failure Bowel ischemia/necrosis Renal failure Peritonitis Sepsis/metabolic acidosis Pneumothorax RDS Hypothermia	1. Respiratory insufficiency due to raised abdominal pressure; may require release of repair and converting to a staged repair. 2. Abdominal 3rd spacing will persist in immediate postop period → ↓ intraabdominal pressure → bowel ischemia + ↓ renal perfusion. Persistent metabolic and/or respiratory acidosis mandates staged repair.
Pain management	Continuous epidural or iv infusion (see p. E-5)	
Tests	ABG Hct Glucose Electrolytes, Ca^{++}	UO maintained at > 0.5 mL/kg/h

Suggested Readings

1. Gregory GA, ed: *Pediatric Anesthesia,* 4th edition. Churchill Livingstone, New York. 2002:574–7.
2. Lee SL, Beyer TD, Kim SS, et al: Initial nonoperative management and delayed closure for treatment of giant omphaloceles. *J Pediatr Surg* 2006; 41(11):1846–9.
3. Liu LM, Pang LM: Neonatal surgical emergencies in anesthesiology. *Clin North Am* 2001; 19(2):276–7.
4. Motoyama EK, Davis PJ, eds: *Smith's Anesthesia for Infants and Children,* 7th edition. Mosby-Elsevier, Philadelphia: 2006, 542–5.
5. Novotny DA, Klein RL, Boeckman CR: Gastroschisis: an 18-year review. *J Pediatr Surg* 1993; 28(5):650–2.
6. Sandler A, Lawrence J, Meehan J, et al: A "plastic" sutureless abdominal wall closure in gastroschisis. *J Pediatr Surg* 2004; 39(5):738–41.
7. Sauter ER, Falterman KW, Arensman RM: Is primary repair of gastroschisis and omphalocele always the best operation? *Am Surg* 1991; 57(3):142–4.
8. Schier F, Schier C, Stute MP, et al: 193 cases of gastroschisis and omphalocele–postoperative results. *Zentralbl Chir* 1988; 113(4):225–34.
9. Tracy TF Jr: Abdominal wall defects. In *Surgery of Infants and Children.* Oldham KT, Colombani PM, Foglia RP, eds. Lippincott-Raven, Philadelphia: 1997, 1083–94.
10. Tsakayannis DE, Zurakowski D, Lillehei CW: Respiratory insufficiency at birth: a predictor of mortality for infants with omphalocele. *J Pediatr Surg* 1996; 31(8):1088–90.
11. Yaster M, Buck JR, Dudgeon DL, et al: Hemodynamic effects of primary closure of omphalocele/gastroschisis in human newborns. *Anesthesiology* 1988; 69:84–8.

PULL-THROUGH FOR HIRSCHSPRUNG'S DISEASE

SURGICAL CONSIDERATIONS

Description: Congenital aganglionosis, called **Hirschprung's disease** (HD), begins at the dentate line of the anus and extends proximally for a variable distance. It produces functional obstruction because the involved bowel is tonically contracted. The "transition zone" to ganglionic bowel occurs in the distal colon in 80% of cases; in 10%, it occurs in the small bowel. Sx range from mild-to-severe constipation, sometimes complicated by toxic enterocolitis. When severe, it may be life-threatening and mandates a rapid **loop colostomy**. Three classical operations (**Swenson, Soave, Duhamel**) and a newer perineal one-stage pull-through (**POOP**) were developed to remove or bypass the affected bowel (Fig. 12.5-11). Today, classic three-stage operations are being reduced to one or two stages, often assisted by laparoscopy.

Surgical Approach: Initial diagnosis is with contrast enema, followed by a transanal rectal biopsy to demonstrate absence of ganglion cells. Standard surgical approach in a neonatally diagnosed Hirschsprung's disease is now a **one-stage neonatal repair,** using a Soave or Swenson procedure, which avoids a colostomy and may be performed via a

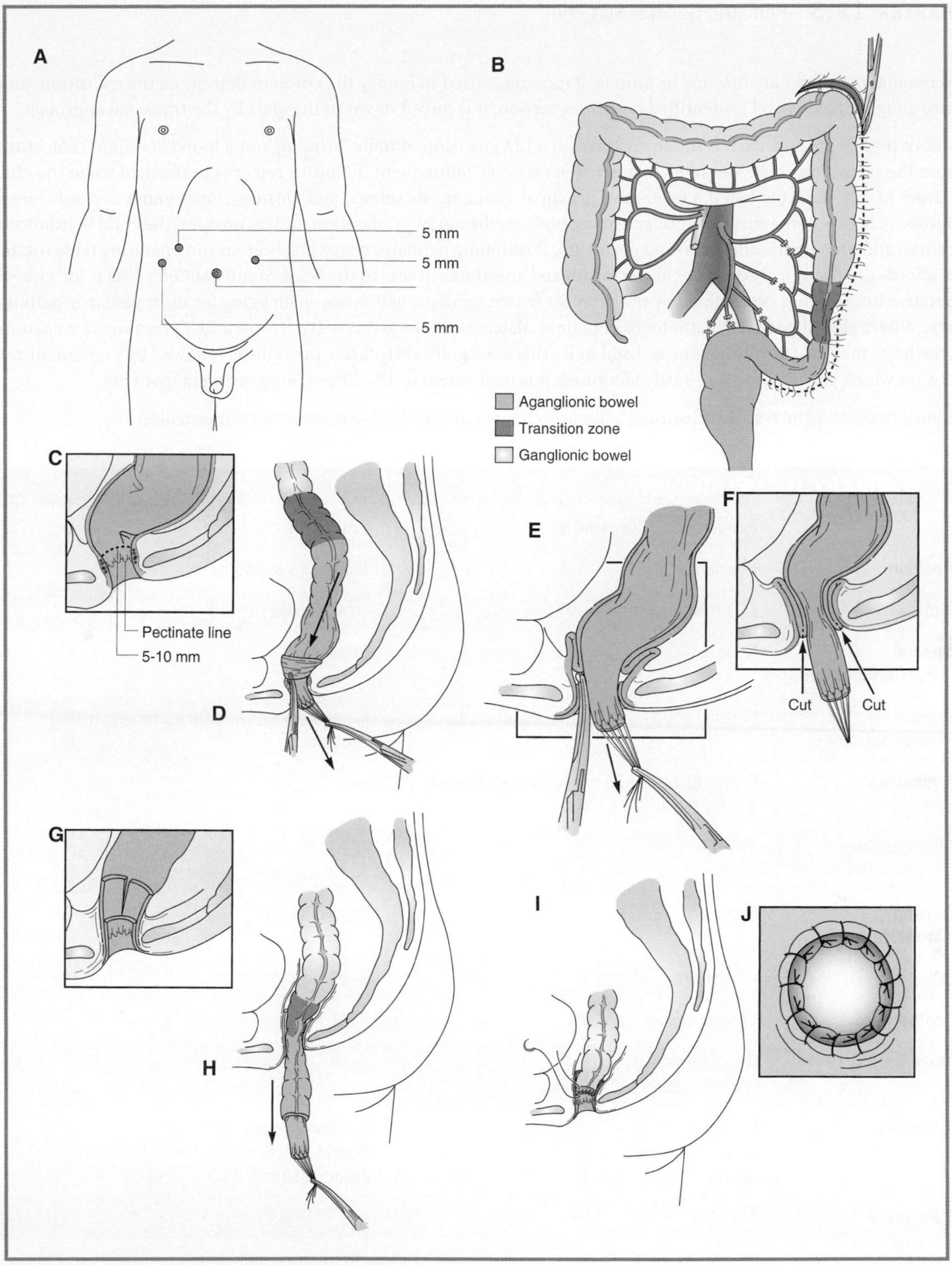

Figure 12.5-11. Laparoscopically assisted pull-through for Hirschsprung's disease. **(A)** Sites for operative trocar placement. **(B)** Division of colon and rectal mesentery with mobilization of proximal colon. **(C)** Circumferential incision in rectal mucosa 5–10 mm cephalad to the pectinate line. **(D)** Mucosal traction sutures to facilitate further dissection from rectal muscular cuff. **(E)** Transanal submucosal dissection is continued cephalad to meet the caudal extent of the transperitoneal rectal dissection. **(F)** Circumferential incisions of rectal muscular cuff. **(G)** Rectal muscular cuff is split posteriorly to accommodate the pull-through segment (segment is not shown here). **(H)** Rectum and sigmoid colon are pulled through the rectal muscular cuff to the anastomotic sites. **(I)** Colon is transected at appropriate site with confirmation of ganglion cells by frozen section. **(J)** Transanal, end-to-end single layer colorectal anastomosis. (Reproduced with permission from Sato TT, Oldham KT: Pediatric abdomen. In *Surgery: Scientific Principles and Practice,* 3rd edition. Greenfield LJ, Mulholland MW, Oldham KT, et al, eds. Lippincott Williams & Wilkins, Philadelphia: 2001.)

circumanal incision. Laparoscopy or umbilical incision is used to biopsy the colon to determine the transition zone. Once ganglionated bowel is identified on frozen section, it is pulled down to the anus by the transanal approach.

A more traditional approach is to biopsy through a LLQ incision initially, bringing out a loop ("leveling") colostomy above the transition zone, identified using frozen sections. Subsequent definitive repair is performed when the child is larger in one stage (or two if a protective proximal stoma needs subsequent closure). Positioning depends on the approach chosen; some surgeons prefer a lower body antibacterial preparation, others position the child in lithotomy position and prepare the abdomen and perineum. Positioning neonates transversely across an operating table rotated 90° affords good surgical access to the perineum and anesthesia access to the head. Significant bleeding is infrequent; operative time often is determined by the delay for frozen sections, which are challenging for most pediatric pathologists. Where skilled pediatric pathologists are unavailable, some surgeons will perform a RUQ transverse colostomy in the hope that the transition zone is distal to it. This is a significantly faster procedure, followed by permanent sections on which ganglia are more easily identified; it is inadequate in 10–20% of 'long-segment' patients.

Usual preop diagnosis: Hirschsprung's disease; congenital aganglionosis; congenital megacolon

SUMMARY OF PROCEDURES

	Preliminary Colostomy	Pull-through
Position	Supine	Supine → lithotomy
Incision	LLQ transverse	Low transverse
Special instrumentation	None	Staplers
Unique considerations	Frozen section to confirm ganglion cells	No monitors or iv lower extremity; frozen sections
Antibiotics	Preop: ampicillin 25 mg/kg iv + gentamicin 2.5 mg/kg iv	⇐
Surgical time	1–1.5 h	1–2 h (POOP) 3–4 h (Duhamel, Swenson, Soave)
Closing considerations	None	Reprep/drape
EBL	< 5 mL/kg	5–10 mL/kg
Postop care	Cardiac/apnea monitor	PICU
Mortality	With enterocolitis: 10% Without enterocolitis: 0–2%	< 5%
Morbidity	Prolapse Stricture Hernia	Anastomotic leak: 5% Wound infection: 4% Pelvic abscess: 3%
Pain score	4	6–7

PATIENT POPULATION CHARACTERISTICS

Age range	Newborn–18 mo (normally)	1 yr
Male:Female	4:1	⇐
Incidence	1/5000	⇐
Etiology	Unknown	⇐
Associated conditions	Trisomy 21 (5%); GU anomalies (< 5%); neurofibromatoses	⇐

ANESTHETIC CONSIDERATIONS

PREOPERATIVE

Children with Hirschsprung's disease (congenital aganglionosis) may have had prior colostomies and may present for colorectal reanastomosis. They may be mildly malnourished, but otherwise healthy.

GI	Diarrhea may be present with associated malabsorption state. **Tests:** Electrolytes
Laboratory	Hct; T&C
Premedication	For infants > 7–9 mo, consider midazolam 0.5–0.75 mg/kg po administered 30 min. before induction.

INTRAOPERATIVE

Anesthetic technique: Combined epidural/GETA, using a pediatric circle; warm OR to 75–80°F; forced-air warmer.

Induction	Mask induction is preferable, unless iv is already in place. Keep air leak around ETT to 18–35 cmH_2O. For more involved procedure, consider placement of epidural catheter.	
Maintenance	Low-dose volatile agent and air/O_2 with muscle relaxation for majority of cases. During last 30 min, N_2O can be substituted for air. Epidural anesthesia will provide the majority of analgesia, but not the degree of muscle relaxation that will be necessary. Supplemental muscle relaxants (e.g., pancuronium or vecuronium 0.1 mg/kg), therefore, are required.	
Emergence	The goal is to extubate at end of case. Reverse neuromuscular blockade with neostigmine (0.07 mg/kg iv) and atropine (0.02 mg/kg) or glycopyrrolate (0.01 mg/kg).	
Blood and fluid requirements	Mild blood loss IV: 20–22 ga × 1–2 in upper extremities NS/LR @ maintenance	These cases are usually not associated with large blood losses. Plan 10 mL/kg/h of crystalloid for replacement. Use 5% albumin for rapid volume expansion; transfuse to maintain Hct > 23%. As a result of bowel prep, patient may require 10–20 mL/kg iv of NS/LR to offset volume deficit.
Monitoring	Standard monitors (See p. D-1) Urinary catheter ± Arterial line (22 ga)	ABG, Hct, blood glucose prn. Maintain UO @ 1 mL/kg/h. Arterial line helpful for monitoring BP, lab draws, and presence of respiratory variations as indicator of volume status.
Positioning	✓ padding, particularly over lateral fibular head (common peroneal nerve). ✓ eyes.	
Complications	Hypothermia Hypovolemia	Majority of heat loss is radiant (skin), but potential for large volume shifts mandates warming fluids.

POSTOPERATIVE

Complications	Hypothermia Hypovolemia	
Pain management	Continuous epidural	Bupivacaine +/- hydromorphone, clonidine will provide analgesia for 8–16 h (see p. E-4).
Tests	Hct if sig. blood loss	

Suggested Readings

1. Georgeson KE, Robertson DJ: Laparoscopic-assisted approaches for the definitive surgery for Hirschsprung's disease. *Semin Pediatr Surg* 2004; 13(4):256–62.
2. Puri P: Hirschsprung disease. In *Surgery of Infants and Children.* Oldham KT, Colombani PM, Foglia RP, eds. Lippincott-Raven, Philadelphia: 1997, 1277–1300.
3. Raffensperger JG, ed: *Swenson's Pediatric Surgery,* 5th edition. Appleton & Lange, Norwalk: 1990, 555–78.
4. Swenson O, Sherman JO, Fisher JH, et al: The treatment and postoperative complications of congenital megacolon: a 25-year followup. *Ann Surg* 1975; 182(3):266–73.

PULL-THROUGH FOR IMPERFORATE ANUS, CLOACA

SURGICAL CONSIDERATIONS

Description: **Imperforate anus anomalies** are classified as **high** or **low,** depending on whether the distal rectum ends above or below the levator muscle. Usually the rectum terminates as a "fistula" entering the perineum or pelvic structures anterior to the external anal sphincter. Rarely the rectum ends blindly, often associated with Trisomy 21. If the fistula terminates on the perineum, it is called a "perineal fistula" or "anterior anus." In girls, it often terminates inside the fourchette but outside the hymen, called a "vestibular" fistula. Fistulas to the vagina or uterus are rare; when they occur, they may be in conjunction with urethral anomalies. This combined structure—including rectum, vagina, and urethra—is called a 'cloaca.' In boys, the fistula often ends in the urethra, occasionally the prostate, and rarely the bladder neck.

Surgical approach: At birth, associated conditions (e.g., VACTERL syndrome) are excluded while one waits 24 hours for the appearance of meconium through a sometimes-hard-to-see perineal fistula. The operation is then performed according to the estimated site of the fistula. Low lesions are dilated or repaired; high lesions are treated with a divided RLQ colostomy. Definitive repair of high lesions occurs after months following contrast studies. This operation—called a **perineal sagittal anorectoplasty (PSARP)** or **Pena procedure**—is performed in the prone jackknife position. If the fistula is high, it occasionally will be necessary to turn the patient over for abdominal mobilization of the sigmoid colon.

Laparoscopic approaches are quickly replacing the PSARP, especially for high lesions. High lesions are also amenable to early **laparoscopic mobilization and pull-through.** This can be done with low fistulas as well, but dissection of the common wall between the urethra and fistula must be performed with care.

Usual preop diagnosis: Imperforate anus

SUMMARY OF PROCEDURES

	Low Lesions	High Lesions
Position	Supine, lithotomy	Prone, possible turn to spine or lithotomy
Incision	Midline perineal	Midline sacral, transverse abdominal
Special instrumentation	Muscle stimulator	⇐ + Urethral sound; vaginal pack
Unique considerations	None	Pressure points; prone position
Antibiotics	Preop: ampicillin 25 mg/kg iv + gentamicin 2.5 mg/kg iv	⇐
Surgical time	1–1.5 h	3–6 h
EBL	< 5 mL/kg	5–20 mL/kg

SUMMARY OF PROCEDURE (cont'd)		
	Low Lesions	**High Lesions**
Postop care	Apnea monitor if neonate	PICU
Mortality	20%, due to associated anomalies	≤ 40%, due to associated anomalies
Morbidity	Anal stenosis: 5–10% Mucosal prolapse: 5%	⇐ Intestinal obstruction: 5–10% Neurogenic bladder: < 5% Urethral stricture: 1–3%
Pain score	3–4	5–6

PATIENT POPULATION CHARACTERISTICS		
Age range	Newborn–6 mo	12–18 mo
Male:Female	1.5:1	⇐
Incidence	1/5000	⇐
Etiology	Unknown	⇐
Associated conditions	CHD (common); esophageal atresia (15%); GU anomalies; sacral/spinal cord anomalies; VATER association	⇐

ANESTHETIC CONSIDERATIONS

PREOPERATIVE

Definitive repair is performed via the sacral and/or perineal route at ~12 mo. Children with rectal or anal agenesis without fistula will have had colostomies in newborn period. Other anomalies (e.g., VATER association, VSDs, vertebral anomalies, anal agenesis, tracheoesophageal fistula [TEF]), esophageal atresia (EA), and/or renal or radial bone abnormalities may be present.

Respiratory	If VATER association present, ✓ cervical spine film and neck ROM. Avoid extreme head flexion. If prior TEF repair, concerns as previously noted in Anesthetic Considerations for Repair of Tracheoesophageal Fistula/Esophageal Atresia, p. 1259. **Tests:** CXR; cervical spine film
Cardiovascular	Patients with VATER association have a 20% incidence of CHD (e.g., VSD). Obtain cardiology consultation prior to surgery. **Tests:** ECHO
Gastrointestinal	Colostomy may be present; thus, anesthesia records may be available for review.
Renal	Renal abnormalities may be present. **Tests:** BUN; Cr; electrolytes
Musculoskeletal	Radial bone deformities may be present. There is no evidence to suggest that VATER patients are at ↑ risk for malignant hyperthermia (MH).
Laboratory	Hct; T&C (✓ parental/directed donor blood availability.)
Premedication	If > 7–9 mo, consider midazolam (0.5–0.75 mg/kg po) 30 min. prior to arrival in OR.

INTRAOPERATIVE

Anesthetic technique: Combined epidural/GETA, using a pediatric circle or Bain circuit with humidified and warmed gases. Warm OR to 75°–80°F; heating pad on OR table.

Induction	Awake intubation if airway management problems anticipated; otherwise, standard pediatric induction (see p. D-1). Secure iv access and administer muscle relaxant (e.g., vecuronium or pancuronium [0.1 mg/kg]) to facilitate ET intubation. Maintain air leak at > 15–35 cmH_2O. Lumbar epidural catheter inserted after induction.	
Maintenance	Volatile agent/air/O_2 with epidural analgesia (2 mL 0.25% bupivacaine or Chirocaine @ start, 1 mL/h maintenance), or morphine (0.1 mg/kg iv) or fentanyl (2–5 mcg/kg iv). Maintain neuromuscular blockade as surgically indicated.	
Emergence	Usually extubated at end of case. Reverse neuromuscular blockade with neostigmine (0.07 mg/kg iv) and atropine (0.02 mg/kg iv). Ability to flex hips is a sign of adequate reversal.	
Blood and fluid requirements	Moderate blood/3rd-space losses IV: 20–22 ga × 2 NS/LR@ maintenance	Place iv's in upper extremities, since positioning of legs may impede venous flow. Maintain Hct > 22. This age group does not require dextrose infusions. 3rd- space losses ~5 mL/kg/h.
Monitoring	Standard monitors (see p. D-1) Urinary catheter ± 24 ga radial arterial line	Maintain UO @ 0.5–1 mL/kg/h. Marked arterial wave-form variation with ventilation is a sensitive indicator of hypovolemia. ABG/Hct/glucose prn.
Positioning	✓ and pad pressure points. ✓ eyes.	Patient may be turned during procedure.
Complications	Metabolic acidosis Hypovolemia →↓ BP Hypothermia	Mild metabolic acidosis may occur with significant bleeding, or when 3rd-space losses are replaced with bicarbonate-deficient fluids (NS, albumin 5%, PRBCs).

POSTOPERATIVE

Complications	Subglottic edema Respiratory depression 2° to opiates	
Pain management	Continuous epidural analgesia. Fentanyl (1–2 mg/kg iv q 1 h prn), Morphine (0.05–0.1 mg/kg iv q 1–4 h) Dilaudid (0.002 mg/kg iv q 1 h)	See p. E-4. Aggressive pain management warranted.
Tests	Hct ABG Electrolytes	

Suggested Readings

1. DeVries PA, Pena A: Posterior sagittal anorectoplasty. *J Pediatr Surg* 1982; 17(5):638–45.
2. Motoyama EK, Davis PJ, eds: *Smith's Anesthesia for Infants and children*, 7th edition. Mosby-Elsevier, Philadelphia: 2006, 556–7.
3. Paidas C, Pena A: Rectum and anus. In *Surgery of Infants and Children*. Oldham KT, Colombani PM, Foglia RP, eds. Lippincott-Raven, Philadelphia: 1997, 1323–64.
4. Schecter NL, Berde CB,Yaster M, eds: *Pain in Infants, Children, and Adolescents*. Lippincott Williams & Wilkins, Philadelphia: 2002.
5. Smith EI, Tunell WP, Williams GR: A clinical evaluation of the surgical treatment of anorectal malformations (imperforate anus). *Ann Surg* 1978; 187(6):583–92.
6. Sydorak RM, Albanese CT. Laparoscopic repair of high imperforate anus. *Semin Pediatr Surg* 2002; 11(4):217–25.

REPAIR OF INGUINAL & UMBILICAL HERNIAS, HYDROCELE

SURGICAL CONSIDERATIONS

Description: Inguinal hernia repair (**herniorrhaphy**) and its variant, **hydrocele repair,** are the most frequently performed operations in pediatric surgery. Most pediatric hernias are indirect; they occur when the processus vaginalis (a small pouch of peritoneum dragged down to the scrotum during gonadal descent) fails to obliterate. Infants, particularly the premature, are more likely than toddlers to develop bilateral and incarcerated hernias. Hydroceles are identical to hernias in origin but have a smaller neck and derive their name because this neck is so small that only intraperitoneal fluid, not bowel, can pass through it. Hydroceles tend to close spontaneously (~80%) during the first 2 years of life; those that fail to resolve are repaired at ~2 years. Hydroceles are termed 'communicating' when they empty/fill with postural change. Umbilical hernias have a tendency to close over the first 5 years of life (~95%), and are repaired when large (> 2 cm) or persistent. Complications of hernia/hydrocele repair include damage to the vas deferens or testicular vessels, metachronous contras-lateral hernias (~10%) if just one side is repaired initially, and a very low incidence of infertility when bilateral repairs are undertaken. Bleeding, if any, is minor, recurrence uncommon (≤ 1%) and bowel resection is rarely necessary even when a hernia is incarcerated. Overnight admission for apnea monitoring is suggested in premature children (≤ 48–60 wk corrected age). **Hydrocele repair** complications are similar to those of herniorrhaphy. **Umbilical hernia repairs** have very few complications. Acetaminophen pr at the beginning of the procedure aids postop pain management.

Surgical approach: Inguinal hernias and hydroceles are repaired through a lower-lateral abdominal skin crease incision (more recently, laparoscopically), permitting separation of the sac from spermatic cord structures, followed by high ligation ± distal fenestration (in hydroceles). Umbilical hernia repair is performed through a transverse incision in the infraumbilical skin fold, through which the sac is resected from the undersurface of the skin and healthy fascial edges closed.

Usual preop diagnosis: Inguinal hernia; umbilical hernia; hydrocele

SUMMARY OF PROCEDURES

	Inguinal	Umbilical
Position	Supine	⇐
Incision	Inguinal, bilateral	Infraumbilical
Unique considerations	Prematurity	Abdominal compression if hernia large
Antibiotics	None	⇐
Surgical time	40 min	⇐
Closing considerations	Nerve block, caudal	Umbilical block
EBL	5 mL/kg	⇐
Postop care	Apnea monitor; hospitalization for premature infants	None
Mortality	< 1%	⇐
Morbidity	Apnea Recurrence	None
Pain score	3–5	3–5

PATIENT POPULATION CHARACTERISTICS		
Age range	Premature–adolescent	> 2 yr
Male:Female	5:1	N/A
Incidence	1–2%	1%
Etiology	Patent processus vaginalis	Persistent umbilical defect
Associated conditions	Gonadal dysgenesis (Rare)	None

ANESTHETIC CONSIDERATIONS

PREOPERATIVE

Hernia repair is most commonly performed in otherwise healthy infants in the first 2 years of life, often on an outpatient basis. It is also performed on premature infants (< 36 wk gestational age at birth) and other neonates requiring intensive care. Premature infants are particularly prone to inguinal hernias. Postop apnea can occur in infants ≤ 50–60 wk postconceptual age, particularly if the infant was premature, has neurologic disease, anemia, or required intensive care in the early neonatal period. Infants ≤ 50 wk post-conception usually require overnight admission Br monitoring (post-op apnea and ↓ HR).

Respiratory	Bronchopulmonary dysplasia (BPD), tracheomalacia, and subglottic stenosis are consequences of prolonged mechanical ventilation and immature lungs at birth. ✓ prior NICU Hx. ↓ FRC and ↑ PVR make infants with this disease more susceptible to hypoxia. They may require supplemental nasal O_2 on a chronic basis. **Tests:** CXR
Cardiovascular	Prior PDA ligation is possible. These patients may be on diuretic therapy for intrinsic lung disease (e.g., BPD) with resultant decreased intravascular volume. **Tests:** CXR; electrolytes
Neurological	Premature infants may be prone to seizure disorders. Premature infants have immature respiratory centers and may exhibit paradoxical apneic/bradycardic episodes in response to hypoxemia. **Tests:** Anticonvulsant levels
Hematologic	Anemia is common at ~3 mo of age (physiologic nadir) and increases risk of postop apnea.
Tests	Hct; PT; PTT; Plt, as indicated from H&P.
Laboratory	Other tests as indicated from H&P.
Premedication	If appropriate (e.g. infants > 8 mo), midazolam (0.5–0.75 mg/kg po) 30 min. prior to arrival in OR.

INTRAOPERATIVE

Anesthetic technique: Typically, GETA or LMA (± caudal or ilioinguinal/iliohypogastric block), using a pediatric circle. An alternative in ex-preterm infants at high risk for postop apnea is spinal anesthesia without GA (see p. E-4), though this is practice more rarely. Warm OR to 75°–80° F and use a forced-air warmer

Induction	Mask induction in children with sevoflurane/N_2O/O_2. Secure iv. If appropriate, position child for placement of caudal anesthetic: bupivacaine 0.25% ± epinephrine 1:200,000 @ 1 mL/kg. If child otherwise healthy and >18 mo old, can proceed with LMA; otherwise, tracheal intubation is preferred. If premature, consider atropine. Intubation may be facilitated with rocuronium (1 mg/kg) or vecuronium (0.1 mg/kg).

Maintenance	Standard pediatric inhalational anesthetic (see p. D-2) is appropriate. With caudal anesthetic or nerve block, decrease amount of volatile anesthetic and avoid or reduce opiates. If LMA and spontaneous ventilation is used, deepen anesthetic to 2 MAC of inhalational agents at incision to minimize risk of laryngospasm. Caudal bupivacaine onset time ~15 min.	
Emergence	Reverse neuromuscular blockade with neostigmine (0.07 mg/kg iv) and atropine (0.02 mg/kg iv). Extubate only when fully awake.	
Blood and fluid requirements	Negligible blood loss IV: 22–24 ga × 1 NS/LR @ maintenance	Infants receiving diuretics will require 10–20 mL/kg iv of NS/LR to avoid ↓ BP 2° volatile anesthetics. In children < 1 mo old, use dextrose-containing iv solution (e.g., D10W for maintenance, LR for replacement fluids)
Monitoring	Standard monitors (see p. D-1)	Premature infants may become hypoglycemic. ✓ blood glucose during surgery.
Positioning	✓ and pad pressure points. ✓ eyes.	
Complications	Laryngospasm Bronchospasm Local anesthetic toxicity Hypothermia Hypoglycemia	Rx bronchospasm: albuterol inhaler, mist, mask, deepen anesthesia

POSTOPERATIVE

Complications	Apnea/bradycardia Subglottic edema	Can ↓ incidence of apnea/bradycardia by administering caffeine (10 mg/kg iv) intraop or in NICU/PACU.
Pain management	Field block Acetaminophen (10–20 mg/kg po q 4–6 h prn)	If no caudal used, a field block (bupivacaine 0.25% 2–3 mL) at end of surgery reduces pain in the immediate postop period. It is usually performed by the surgeon.
Tests/monitoring	Apnea monitor and pulse oximeter for 12–18 h for: all patients < 44 wks, born before 37 wks with current age <52 wks; and premature infants <60 wks	Caffeine is no substitute for monitoring and attentive parents/nurses.

Suggested Readings

1. Beckerman RC, Brouillette RT, Hunt CE, eds: *Respiratory Control Disorders in Infants and Children.* Williams &Wilkins, Baltimore: 1991, 161–77.
2. Cote CJ, Zaslavsky A, Downes JJ, et al: Postoperative apnea in former preterm infants after inguinal herniorrhaphy. A combined analysis. *Anesthesiology* 1995; 82(4):809–22.
3. Hanallah RS, Welborn LG, McGill WA: Postanesthetic apnea in full-term infants. *Anesthesiology* 1994; 81(1):264–5.
4. Rescorla FJ: Hernias and umbilicus. *In Surgery of Infants and Children*. Oldham KT, Colombani PM, Foglia RP, eds. Lippincott-Raven, Philadelphia: 1997, 1069–82.
5. Stehling L, ed: *Common Problems in Pediatric Anesthesia,* 2nd edition. Mosby-Year Book, St. Louis: 1992, 69–85.
6. Walther-Larsen S, Rasmussen LS: The former preterm infant and risk of post-operative apnoea: recommendations for management. *Acta Anaesthesiol Scand* 2006; 50(7):888–93.
7. Welborn LG, Greenspun JC: Anesthesia and apnea. Perioperative considerations in the former preterm infant. *Pediatr Clin North Am* 1994; 41(1):181–98.

SURGERY FOR THE UNDESCENDED TESTICLE

SURGICAL CONSIDERATIONS

Description: Also called "cryptorchidism," this occurs when a testicle fails to follow the usual pattern of descent. Testicles begin fetal life just inferior to the kidney and, through differential growth, migrate to the base of the ipsilateral hemiscrotum, attached there by the gubernaculum. Problems occur when testicular descent does not occur, occurs partially, or occurs incorrectly. Testicles that are found in the abdomen, inguinal canal, perineum, thigh, suprapubic fat, or contralateral scrotum may be associated with subsequent problems, including infertility and malignant degeneration. Transposition and fixation of the testicles into their normal location (**orchidopexy**), does not eliminate these problems; rather, it places the testicle in a position where it can be more easily evaluated and may mitigate the progressive infertility thought to occur when testicles remain outside the scrotum. Because testicular descent is a dynamic process, cryptorchidism is not addressed until 18–24 mo of life, because a significant portion of initially cryptorchid testes will descend into the scrotum during this time.

Surgical approach: The operation begins in a similar fashion to a hernia repair, as 95% of cryptorchid testes have an associated hernia sac. One exception is if the testicle is thought to be **intraabdominal.** In this circumstance, many surgeons will begin with a laparoscopic abdominal examination, using the vas deferens and testicular vessels to locate the testis. If it is high in the abdomen, it may be brought immediately to the perineum (difficult if the testicular vessels are short), or a two-step **Fowler-Stevens** approach is undertaken. In this approach, the gubernacular vessels supplying the inferior pole of the testis are encouraged to hypertrophy by division of the spermatic vessels, and the testicle is left in the abdomen near the internal ring. At a second operation ~6 months later, the testicle is brought down, much as in the primary operation following hernia repair. This involves creation of a passage down to the base of the ipsilateral hemiscrotum, through which the testicle is advanced as far as the vas deferens permits. The tough outer layer of the testicle—the tunica albuginea—is then attached to the scrotum in a subcutaneous pocket outside the dartos fascia to discourage migration back up to a high location. There is scant blood loss; however, there is a small risk to testicular viability. Small, high, abnormal testes with short vessels and vas associated with poor gubernacular vessels are deemed better removed than left in a high location where malignant degeneration might go undetected. A caudal block may be preferable to injection of local anesthesia at multiple sites.

Usual preop diagnosis: Undescended testicle; cryptorchidism

SUMMARY OF PROCEDURES

	Orchidopexy	First of Two-stage Repair
Position	Supine	⇐
Incision	Lower groin crease	Laparoscopic or open
Special instrumentation	–	One to three ports if laparoscopic
Unique considerations	Length of vas and vessels	Length of vas deferens
Antibiotics	None	⇐
Surgical time	1–1.5 h	30 min
EBL	< 5 mL/kg	⇐
Postop care	Home	⇐
Mortality	< 1%	⇐
Morbidity	Bleeding Orchiectomy	⇐
Pain score	4–5	2–3

PATIENT POPULATION CHARACTERISTICS	
Age range	18–24 mo
Incidence	1/2000 births
Etiology	Unknown
Associated conditions	Prematurity; gastroschisis; intersex anomaly; Turner's syndrome (potential for airway, cardiac, and renal problems)

ANESTHETIC CONSIDERATIONS

See Anesthetic Considerations for Pediatric Urology, Inguinoscrotal Procedures, p. 1339.

Suggested Readings

1. Kogan SJ, Gill B: Cryptorchidism and pediatric hydrocele/hernia. In: *Glenn's Urologic Surgery,* 5th edition. Graham SD Jr. Glenn JF, eds. Lippincott Williams & Wilkins, Philadelphia: 1998; 833–42.
2. Rozanski TA, Bloom DA: Male genital tract. In: *Surgery of Infants and Children: Scientific Principles and Practice.* Oldham KT, Colombani PM, Foglia RP, eds. Lippincott-Raven, Philadelphia: 1997, 1550–2.
3. Thorup J, Haugen S, Kollin C, et al: Surgical treatment of undescended testes. *Acta Paediatr* 2007; 96(5):631–7.

RESECTION OF SACROCOCCYGEAL TERATOMA

SURGICAL CONSIDERATIONS

Description: Occasionally during gestation, a group of cells composing all three germ layers segregates and begins autonomous development as a teratoma. When this occurs just anterior to the coccyx, the tumor may remain small and local, or grow up into the abdomen or down into the peritoneum, attaining sizes as large as the child itself. Although a few centers attempt fetal surgery for very large lesions, in most hospitals the child is delivered by the appropriate route (cesarian delivery for large external lesions) and the mass is addressed in the neonatal period or whenever it is diagnosed thereafter. Most (though not all) sacrococcygeal teratomas (SCTs) are initially benign; however, they may soon transform into malignancy beginning at 2 months of age.

Surgical approach: Small teratomas are approached prone from the rectum; larger ones, with high blood flow, may first have an intraabdominal procedure to ligate feeding vessels and mobilize the tumor. Once prone, a V-shaped incision is created down to the posterior aspect of the anteriorly displaced anus. Surgical principles of dissection include avoiding entry into the rectum (a colostomy is rarely necessary); meticulous hemostasis, including ligation of the median sacral artery; and removal of the coccyx, from which the tumor arises and may recur. At the end of the procedure, the levator muscles are brought together and the anus is suspended from the presacral fascia. Bleeding can be massive, and adjacent structures (bowel, bladder, and presacral nerve plexus) are distorted and prone to injury.

Usual preop diagnosis: Sacrococcygeal teratoma.

Differential diagnosis: May appear similar to meningomyelocele.

SUMMARY OF PROCEDURE	
Position	Prone, sometimes preceded by supine
Incision	Perineal chevron, sometimes preceded by transverse abdominal
Special instrumentation	Hegar dilators
Unique considerations	Intraabdominal blood supply

SUMMARY OF PROCEDURE (cont'd)	
Antibiotics	Ampicillin 25 mg/kg and gentamicin 2.5 mg/kg
Surgical time	2–5 h
Closing considerations	Extubation depends on duration and blood loss
EBL	20–80 mL/kg
Postop care	NICU, prone
Mortality	Fetal, due to hydrops and high flow state; < 10% neonatal
Morbidity	Bleeding Colostomy Pelvic nerve damage → bowel and bladder dysfunction Recurrence and/or malignant degeneration

PATIENT POPULATION CHARACTERISTICS	
Age range	1–2 mo
Male:Female	1:1
Incidence	1/15,000 births
Etiology	Unknown
Associated conditions	Constipation; heart failure; Currarino's triad; malignant degeneration

ANESTHETIC CONSIDERATIONS

PREOPERATIVE

Sacrococcygeal teratoma is a rare tumor of infancy. Sometimes diagnosed prenatally, it also can present as late as 18–24 mo. Patients may present with urinary obstruction by the tumor mass; lower extremity pain, numbness, or weakness; or bowel obstruction. ~10% may have a sacral anomaly or myelomeningocele.

Respiratory	There may be respiratory compromise as a result of a large abdominal mass pushing up on the abdominal contents and the diaphragm. **Tests:** CXR, if indicated from H&P.
Cardiovascular	Sacrococcygeal teratoma may be associated with high-output cardiac failure due to AV fistulae within the tumor. Consultation with a cardiologist may be appropriate. **Tests:** ECG; ECHO may be necessary.
Renal	Postrenal obstruction may compromise renal function. **Tests:** BUN; Cr
Gastrointestinal	Intestinal compression by the tumor may cause ↑ risk of gastric aspiration. **Tests:** Electrolytes
Hematologic	This tumor may be associated with coagulopathy. **Tests:** PT; PTT; INR
Laboratory	Other tests as indicated from H&P.
Premedication	In patients at risk for gastric aspiration, prophylaxis with metoclopramide (0.1 mg/kg iv) and ranitidine (0.8 mg/kg iv) should be considered. Patients > 10 mo may benefit from midazolam (0.5–0.75 mg/kg) po 30 min. before surgery. If iv is present, iv midazolam 0.05–0.1 mg/kg may be used (e.g., for 10 kg child, 0.5–1 mg midazolam).

INTRAOPERATIVE

Anesthetic technique: GETA, using a pediatric circle; warm OR to 75–80°F; warm all iv fluids. Due to risk of coagulopathy and the possibility of spine malformations, epidural catheter usually is not considered.

Induction	Usually an inhalation induction. If an iv is present, then an iv induction is performed. A modified rapid-sequence induction is recommended in those patients with a large intraabdominal mass compressing the GI tract. Otherwise, standard pediatric induction (see p. D-1) is appropriate. An uncuffed tube normally is used. The appropriate size for the ETT is one that will allow a small leak around the tube when positive pressure is applied (18–35 cmH_2O).	
Maintenance	Standard maintenance (see p. D-3). Muscle relaxation is appropriate.	
Emergence	Depending on blood loss and fluid requirements, the patient may need to remain intubated at the end of the procedure. If extubation is elected, suction NG and confirm air leak around ETT before extubation. If there is no air leak, consider laryngeal edema and the need for continued intubation.	
Blood and fluid requirements	Potential for massive blood loss. IV: Two large-bore iv catheters (e.g., 22–18 ga)	Tumor resection may be associated with massive blood loss, due to large pelvic venous bed, AV fistula, coagulopathy. Close monitoring of Hct is necessary, along with correction of acidosis and Ca^{++} replacement.
Monitoring	Standard monitor (see p. D-1) Central line Arterial line (22 ga)	

POSTOPERATIVE

Complications	Bleeding Coagulopathy Hypoventilation Laryngeal edema	PICU usually required. Maintain normothermia; correct metabolic acidosis. Postop ventilation requirement due to hypoventilation, laryngeal edema.
Pain management	Fentanyl 1 mcg/kg/h iv Morphine 0.1 mg/kg/h	Approximate doses; titration required.
Tests	ABG Hct PT/PTT	

Suggested Readings

1. Cowles RA, Stolar CJ, Kandel JJ, et al: Preoperative angiography with embolization and radiofrequency ablation as novel adjuncts to safe surgical resection of a large, vascular sacrococcygeal teratoma. *Pediatr Surg Int* 2006; 22(6):554–6.
2. Robinson S, Laussen PC, Brown TCK, et al: Anaesthesia for sacrococcygeal teratoma–a case report and a review of 32 cases. *Anaesth Intens Care* 1992; 20:354–86.
3. Sasaoka N, Kitamura S, Kninouchi K, et al: Perinatal and perianesthetic management of the sacrococcygeal teratoma in a neonate. *Masui* 1998; 47(12):1482–5.

ANESTHESIA FOR MINIMALLY INVASIVE SURGERY IN PEDIATRIC PATIENTS

Gregory B. Hammer

In recent years there has been a significant increase in the practice of minimally invasive surgery in pediatric patients. Specific considerations for these surgeries (as in adult patients) include the effects of pneumoperitoneum on respiratory and cardiac function. ↑ abdominal pressure →↓ diaphragmatic excursion, ↑ atelectasis, and V/Q mismatch. ↑ CO_2 levels can be difficult to control with mechanical ventilation; thus, manual ventilation may be necessary. There is risk of pneumothorax and pneumomediastinum. Use of Trendelenburg position further decreases FRC and lung compliance, and increases the work of breathing. Cephalad movement of the carina may cause endobronchial intubation. Venous return may be impaired, causing ↓ CO. These effects are most pronounced in children < 6 months old. These children also may be at risk for reversal of L → R shunts through a patent foramen ovale (PFO) or ductus arteriosus.

Minimally invasive procedures that are frequently performed in pediatrics include: appendectomy, pyloric stenosis, hernia repair, Nissen fundoplication, cholecystectomy, splenectomy, laparoscopically assisted bowel resection, thoracoscopy (VATS), and congenital diaphragmatic hernia repair. The general principles for anesthesia for minimally invasive surgery in pediatric patients are as follows:

PREOPERATIVE

1. Be vigilant about respiratory and cardiac function. Note baseline lung function (SaO_2, CXR, ABG); ✓ for any cardiac defects (e.g., L → R shunt, ↓ CO).
2. ✓ PT/PTT if epidural is considered (usually not placed for laparoscopy or thoracoscopy, but it should be considered at the end of the procedure if the decision is made to do open surgery).
3. Blood should be available for major cases including VATS for empeyema. Although there usually is little blood loss with minimally invasive surgery, the potential for large-vessel disruption exists.

Premedication	In patients at risk for aspiration, prophylaxis with ranitidine (0.8 mg/kg iv) should be considered. Patients > 7–9 mo may benefit from midazolam (0.5–0.75 mg/kg po) 30 min before surgery.

INTRAOPERATIVE

Anesthetic technique: GETA, using a pediatric circle; forced-air warmer; warm OR to 70–75°F; warm iv fluids.

Induction	Inhalation induction using sevoflurane, N_2O, followed by iv placement. If patient is at risk for aspiration, rapid-sequence induction is appropriate. For ET intubation in children < 6–8 yr of age, an uncuffed tube is preferred, with the goal being to attain a seal allowing for a leak of 18–35 cmH_2O. A cuffed tube (usually a half size smaller than the appropriate uncuffed tube) also may be used for children > 2 yr old. If OLV is required, see Anesthetic Considerations for Pediatric Thoracic Surgery p. 1267, for placement. Note distance of end of ETT from carina. As abdominal girth is increased during CO_2 insufflation, it is common for the tube to advance to an endobronchial position.	
Maintenance	Standard maintenance (see p. D-3). Muscle relaxation is appropriate. An OG tube is placed to empty the stomach of any residual premedication and excess air introduced during PPV. Continued communication between anesthesiologist and surgeon is essential. Pay attention to changes in positioning (e.g., Trendelenburg), intraabdominal pressure (n1= 15 cmH_2O), airway pressures, BP.	
Emergence	In most cases, the patient can be extubated at the end of surgery.	
Blood and fluid requirements	IV: 22–20 ga catheter × 1 Maintenance fluids	Potential for 3rd-space and blood loss, especially with VATS surgery for empyema.
Monitoring	Standard monitors (see p. D-1) ± Arterial line Urinary catheter	Consider arterial line if patient has significant cardiac or respiratory compromise.
Positioning	✓ and pad pressure points. ✓ eyes.	

Complications	↑ CO_2 (40–50 mmHg) (common) ↑ PIP (common) Endobronchial intubation (common) Difficult ventilating (common) Hypovolemia Pneumothorax Pneumomediastinum (rare) Inadvertent cannulation of vessel (rare)	 2° Trendelenburg position, ↑ abdominal girth. In thoracoscopy, if SLV is used, may need to raise lung and ventilate transiently. → ↓ CO. Rx: crystalloid or albumin 10–20 mL/kg. CO_2 embolus (rare)

POSTOPERATIVE

Complications	Respiratory function impairment Bleeding Residual subcutaneous CO_2 Pneumothorax	Respiratory function may still be significantly impaired in the postop period and should be monitored closely.
Pain management	Ketorolac 0.5 mg/kg iv q 6 h MSO_4 0.05–0.1 mg/kg	If significant intraoperative bleeding, avoid ketorolac for 24 h post-op

Suggested Readings

1. Bissonnette B, Dalens BJ: *Pediatric Anesthesia.* McGraw-Hill, New York: 2002.
2. Cote CJ, Todres ID, Ryan JF, et al: *A Practice of Anesthesia for Infants and Children.* WB Saunders, New York: 2001.
3. Gregory GA: *Pediatric Anesthesia,* 4th edition. Churchill Livingstone, New York: 2002.
4. Pennant JH: Anesthesia for laparoscopy in the pediatric patient. *Anesth Clin North Am* 2001; 19(1):69–88.
5. Wedgewood J, Doyle E: Anesthesia and laparoscopic surgery in children. *Pediatric Anesthesia.* 2001; 11:391–9.

EX UTERO INTRAPARTUM TREATMENT (EXIT) PROCEDURE

SURGICAL CONSIDERATIONS

Description: The EXIT (Ex Utero Intrapartum Treatment) strategy was developed as a means of establishing an airway after iatrogenic occlusion of the fetal trachea to promote lung growth for fetuses with severe congenital diaphragmatic hernia (CDH). The EXIT strategy can be viewed as a "half" delivery in which a **hysterotomy** is performed, only the head and shoulders are "delivered", and uterine relaxation is maintained by high concentrations of an inhalational anesthetic and intravenous tocolytics, ensuring the maintenance of uteroplacental blood flow and gas exchange. Using this strategy, operations as long as 3 hours on uteroplacental "bypass" have been performed without significant maternal bleeding and uterine contraction. It provides time to perform procedures such as direct laryngoscopy, bronchoscopy, tracheotomy, arterial and venous access, administration of surfactant, resection of neck or lung masses, and cannulation for ECMO (extracorporeal membrane oxygenation) support, thereby converting a potential emergent crisis into a controlled situation.

Surgical Technique: A successful EXIT procedure is a carefully orchestrated event in which all members of the OR team have specific roles and responsibilities. The scrubbed personnel consist of two pediatric/fetal surgeons, a maternal-fetal medicine specialist/obstetrician, a pediatric anesthesiologist, a neonatologist, and a nurse. Unlike the EXIT procedure, a conventional Cesarean delivery makes no attempt to prevent bleeding from the hysterotomy since hemostasis is achieved by return of uterine tone following the relatively rapid delivery of the fetus. Because of the significant hemorrhage from a conventional hysterotomy, the EXIT procedure is carried out using a **hemostatic**

uterine stapling device (US Surgical CS 57, US Surgical/Tyco, Norwalk, CT). First, a low transverse skin crease incision is used. The decision to use a Mallard versus Pfannenstiel fascial incision is determined by uterine size (e.g. presence/absence polyhydramnios) and placental position. If the operation is performed in the late 3rd trimester and the placenta is posterior or fundic, the lower uterine segment can be opened and the uterus left in situ. An anterior or previa placenta often necessitates moving the uterus out of the abdomen/pelvis. The hysterotomy in this situation is not in the lower uterine segment. Intraop ultrasonography is critical to map placental position. If polyhydramnios is present, amnioreduction is performed to avoid underestimation of the proximity of the placental edge to the hysterotomy. Two applications of the uterine stapler are usually necessary for an adequate opening. Bleeding often occurs where the staple lines fail to intersect and is easily controlled with suture ligation. Only the necessary fetal parts are delivered in order to maintain uterine volume and avoid vigorous contractions and placental separation. A **sterile pulse oximeter** is attached to the palm of the fetal hand. It is covered with foil and Tegaderm tape to prevent aberrant readings due to the operating room lights. The long oximeter cord is passed across the field to the anesthesiologist. The fetal eyes are covered with a warm wet laparotomy pad. The fetus is continuously bathed in warm saline. Care is taken not to manipulate or unnecessarily expose the umbilical cord in order to avoid spasm of the vessels. Sterile instruments that need to be available include a laryngoscope with at least two different sized blades and extra bulbs (batteries are not sterilized and are inserted separately), two sizes of a rigid bronchoscope, a light cord, various endotracheal (some with surfactant adapters) and tracheostomy tubes, endotracheal tube stylettes, a hand bag device with a manometer and sterile tubing that is passed off the field to an oxygen source, a sterile neonatal stethoscope, and a sterile syringe filled with surfactant (if necessary). IV access is obtained if possible. Alternatively, a mixture of fentanyl, and a NMB agent such as pancuronium can be administered im (deltoid) to the fetus immediately after the hysterotomy. After the airway is obtained and secured, the umbilical cord is clamped and divided and the child taken to the resuscitation table by the neonatologist. The placenta is delivered and the uterus closed in the standard fashion. Oxytocin is administered immediately prior to clamping the umbilical cord to enhance uterine tone.

Indications: Clinical situations in which the fetal airway or cardiovascular well-being is significantly threatened by conventional Cesarean or vaginal delivery are candidates for the EXIT strategy. Some examples are:

- Intrinsic laryngotracheal anomalies resulting in congenital high airway obstruction syndrome (CHAOS): laryngeal web/atresia/cyst/stenosis, tracheal stenosis/atresia
- Extrinsic airway compression: cervical teratoma/lymphangioma (may or may not result in CHAOS)
- Epignathus
- Severe hydrops from a cystic adenomatoid malformation of the lung after 32 weeks gestation
- EXIT to ECMO for severe CDH with congenital heart disease
- Delivery of thoracoomphalopagus twins
- Delivery of twins discordant for a potentially obstructing neck lesion

SUMMARY OF PROCEDURES	
Position	L uterine displacement
Incision	Low transverse
Special Instructions	Fetal monitoring
Unique Considerations	Need to maintain uterine relaxation
Child	Fetal hypoxia, bradycardia
Antibiotics	Cefazolin 1 gm iv
Surgical Time	2 h
Closing Considerations	Extubation
Post-operative care	Variable–moderate
Mortality	Rare
Morbidity	Risk of hemorrhage

STERILE EQUIPMENT (ON SURGICAL FIELD)	
ETT	2.5, 3.0, 3.5 uncuffed, and available stylets
Laryngoscopes and blades	Miller 0,1 Wis-Hipple 1,1.5
LMA	1, 1.5
Suction catheters	6 Fr, 8 Fr
Other	Mask, capnograph tubing, oral airways, umbilical tape, steri strips, stethoscope

NON-STERILE EQUIPMENT READILY AVAILABLE	
Fiberoptic bronchoscope	appropriate for neonatal airway
Ambu-bag	
Additional oxygen source	

Maternal Risks and Outcomes: The most serious and immediate maternal risk during the EXIT procedure is **intraop hemorrhage**. This may result from **uterine atony**, and can be minimized by decreasing the concentration of the inhalational anesthetic and administering oxytocin before umbilical cord ligation. This, in combination with the hemostatic uterine stapling device, has kept the average maternal blood loss well within the accepted range for traditional Cesarean delivery. In addition, **placental injury** may occur during hysterotomy, resulting in hemorrhage. This has occurred in the setting of polyhydramnios, in which the edge of the placenta was compressed, obscuring it from view by the ultrasonographer. It is advisable to perform intraop amnioreduction in cases with severe polyhydramnios with a potentially nearby placenta before performing an EXIT procedure to allow better placental visualization. In one study, the short-term maternal outcomes after 34 EXIT procedures were compared to those from 52 non-laboring patients who underwent non-emergent primary cesarean delivery of singleton fetuses. The rates of chorioamnionitis and endometritis, and the postop hematocrit and hospital stays were similar between groups. The incidence of **wound infection** was increased in those undergoing EXIT procedure (15%) compared to controls (2%).

Lower uterine segment transverse hysterotomy is preferred for the EXIT procedure as it allows the possibility of future vaginal delivery. However, a low anterior placenta or an extremely large neck mass may make this incision impossible. In such cases, a classical hysterotomy is necessary which would preclude future vaginal deliveries because of the risk of uterine rupture during labor. Thus, all pregnant women should be counseled that Cesarean delivery may be required for all future pregnancies and that there is an increased risk of abnormal placentation with subsequent pregnancies.

ANESTHESIA CONSIDERATIONS

The features which distinguish the EXIT procedure from a conventional Cesarean delivery are, in large part, due to the anesthetic management. Of paramount importance is the uterine relaxation achieved with an inhalational agent, most commonly isoflurane. Isoflurane has been administered in concentrations up to 2.5% to completely anesthetize the fetus in order to allow fetal laryngoscopy, bronchoscopy, tracheostomy or tumor resection. Preservation of uteroplacental gas exchange with high concentrations of maternal isoflurane is well tolerated by the fetus for EXIT procedures lasting up to 180 min. Careful attention to the maintenance of maternal systemic blood pressure, often with the use of phenylephrine and ephedrine, is essential in order to safely use the high concentration of isoflurane required for uterine relaxation. Intraop fluid administration is kept to an absolute minimum 2° the postop predisposition to maternal pulmonary edema while on tocolytic agents. Occasionally, additional uterine relaxation is required, even when the end-tidal isoflurane concentration is ≥ 2.5%. This suggests that extensive manipulation of the uterus, (e.g., forward displacement of the uterus to perform a posterior hysterotomy because of an anterior placenta), may stimulate the uterus to contract, even if high concentrations of isoflurane are used. For this situation, the intraop use of nitroglycerine provides excellent temporary uterine relaxation and is well-tolerated. Pulmonary edema does not occur as a result of intraop intermittent dosing of nitroglycerine when it is used as an adjunct for uterine relaxation.

PREOPERATIVE

Conduct a rigorous preop evaluation of the mother, including CV history; evaluate all fetal anomalies in question. The most common indication for an EXIT procedure is the presence of a prenatally diagnosed neck mass which is anticipated to result in severe airway obstruction following birth; severe micrognathia, mandibular hypoplasia may also require this approach.

Full Stomach Precautions	Pretreatment with Bicitra 30 mL po, ranitidine 50 mg iv
Positioning	Left uterine displacement

INTRAOPERATIVE

Anesthetic technique: GETA, rapid-sequence induction. Primary goal is to maintain complete uterine relaxation, to support materal-fetal gas exchange, and assure fetal oxygenation. Uterine blood flow is not auto-regulated, but directly related to MAP.

Maintain blood pressure with phenylephrine as necessary. Maintain fluid resuscitation to moderate due to propensity of pulmonary edema while on tocolytic agents. High concentration of isoflurane or sevoflurane to maintain uterine relaxation. Nitroglycerin can also be used to facilitate relaxation. Intrauterine infusion with normal saline may be necessary to preserve uterine volume and prevent separation of placenta.

Induction	Rapid sequence induction, with propofol, or STP, and succinylcholine. (see p. B-4)	
Maintenance	Volatile agent at high concentration to maintain uterine relaxation	
Special considerations	Coordination necessary between maternal anesthesia team, surgical team and pediatric anesthesia regarding cord clamping and delivery. Cord is clamped, volatile agent immediately discontinued, N_20 continued, fentanyl and midazolam given; oxytocin bolus and continuous infusion of oxytocin titrated to uterine response. Once hemostasis is achieved, and uterine tone is restored, anesthetic agents are restarted.	
Care of fetus/ neonate	Infant: delivery of fetal head and upper extremity. Commence fetal monitoring with fetal scalp electrode, O_2 Sat monitoring (normal SaO_2 – 65–75%). If possible, place iv catheter. Alternatively, additional anesthetic can be administered IM via deltoid muscle (fentanyl 2–3 mcg/kg, pancuronium 0.1 mg/kg.). After the airway is secured, the cord is clamped and delivery completed. Once airway secure, O_2 sat should increase to >90%. If unable to secure, consider surgical intervention. Secure ETT with umbilical tape, steri-strips. Secure iv access if not obtained previously. Hemodynamic management may include resuscitation with iv fluids, transfusion. Transfer to NICU unless further immediate surgical intervention needed.	
Emergence	Usually extubated	
Blood and fluid requirements	Moderate blood loss IV: 16–18 ga × 1–2	Blood products available in room due to potential for hemorrhage; Cautious crystalloid administration due to potential for pulmonary edema related to the use of tocolytics.
Monitoring	Standard monitors A-line	CVP to guide fluid resuscitation
Positioning	L-uterine displacement	
Complications	Maternal hemorrhage Uterine atony	

POSTOPERATIVE

Complications (maternal)	Hemorrhage	✓ H/H regularly (e.g., 30 min. for the 1st h); transfuse as necessary
	Pulmonary edema	2° overly aggressive resuscitation, prolonged use of NTG
Complications (neonate)	Hypovolemia	2° fetal hemorrhage via umbilical cord
	Respiratory compromise	2° aspiration, over-resuscitation-ventilatory support as necessary
Tests	CXR to verify ETT position	
Pain Management	Maternal	Patient-controlled analgesia
	Neonate	Fentanyl 1–2 mcg/kg iv q 1° prn; MSO_4 (0.05–0.1 mg/kg iv q 2–4°)

Suggested Readings

1. Bouchard S, Johnson MP, Flake AW, et al: The EXIT procedure: experience and outcome in 31 cases. *J Pediatric Surgery* 2002; 37(3):418–26.
2. Crombleholme TM, Albanese CT: The fetus with airway obstruction. In: *The Unborn Patient. The Art and Science of Fetal Therapy*. Harrison MR, Evans MI, Adzick NS, et al, eds. WB Saunders, Philadelphia: 2001, 357–71.
3. Hedrick HL: Ex utero intrapartum therapy. *Semin Pediatr Surg* 2003; 12:190–5.
4. Hirose S, Sydorak RM, Tsao K, et al: Spectrum of intrapartum management strategies for giant fetal cervical teratoma. *J Pediatr Surg* 2003; 38:446–50.
5. Mychalishka GB, Bealor JF, Graf JL, et al: Operating on placental support: the ex utero intrapartum treatment (EXIT) procedure. *J Pediatr Surg* 1997; 32:227–30.
6. Myers LB: *Anesthesia for Ex Utero Intrapartum Treatment (EXIT Procedure)*. BC Decker Inc, Hamilton: 2005.
7. Noah MM, Norton ME, Sandberg P, et al: Short-term maternal outcomes that are associated with the EXIT procedure, as compared with cesarean delivery. *Am J Obstet Gynecol* 2002; 186:773–3.
8. Otteson TD, Jackam DJ, Mandell DL: The ex utero intrapartum treatment (EXIT) procedure. *Arch Otolaryng. Head and Neck Surg* 2006; 132:686–9.

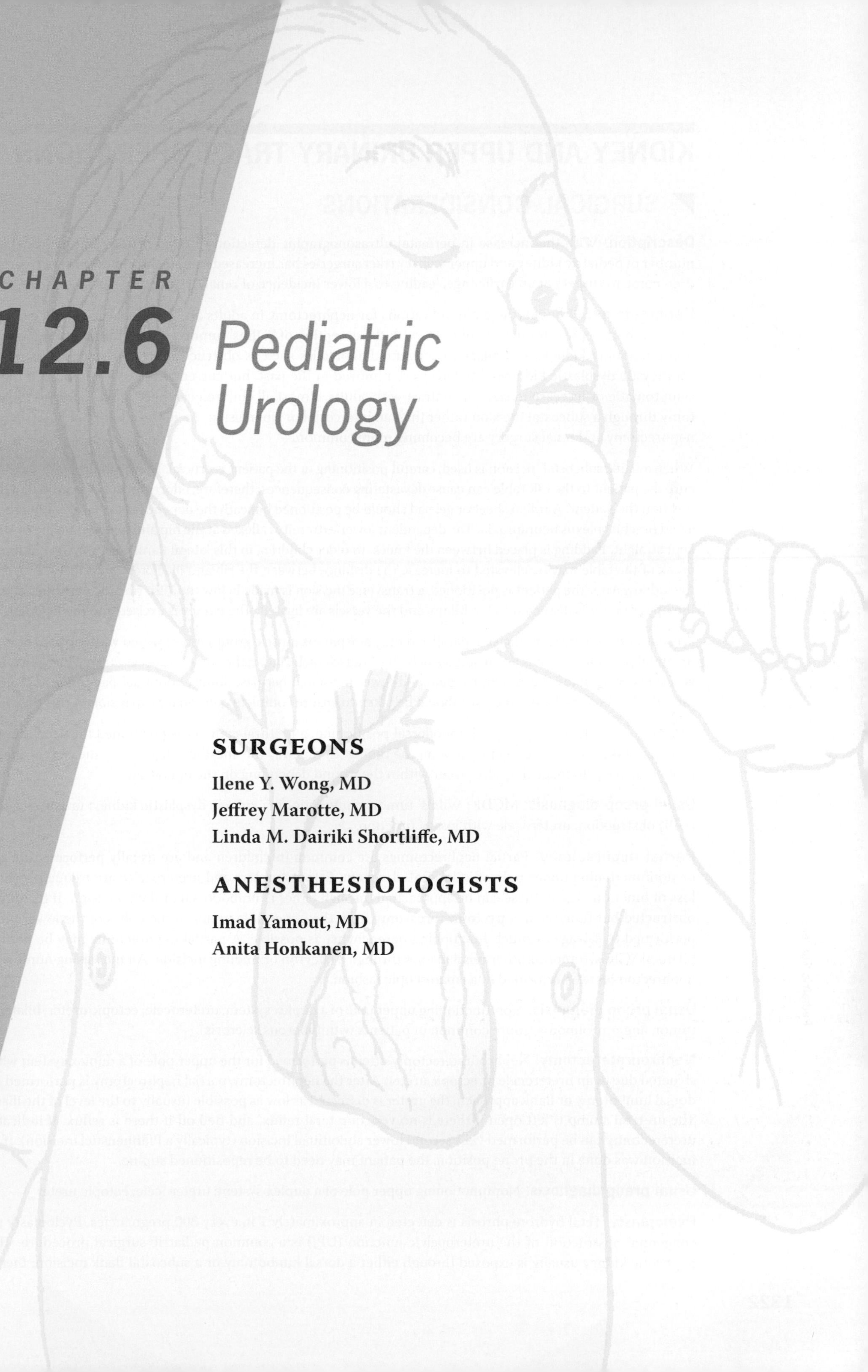

CHAPTER

12.6 Pediatric Urology

SURGEONS

Ilene Y. Wong, MD
Jeffrey Marotte, MD
Linda M. Dairiki Shortliffe, MD

ANESTHESIOLOGISTS

Imad Yamout, MD
Anita Honkanen, MD

KIDNEY AND UPPER URINARY TRACT OPERATIONS

SURGICAL CONSIDERATIONS

Description: With the increase in perinatal ultrasonographic detection of renal masses and hydronephrosis, the number of pediatric kidney and upper urinary tract surgeries has increased significantly in the past two decades. Children come to surgery at an earlier age, leading to a lower incidence of renal dysfunction.

Nephrectomy: Although the main indications for nephrectomy in adults are renal-cell carcinoma or benign renal tumors, most nephrectomies in children (with the exception of Wilms' tumors) are performed to remove poorly or nonfunctioning kidneys secondary to congenital anomalies such as obstruction or end-stage reflux nephropathy. Multicystic dysplastic kidneys (MCDK) were removed in the past, but currently are only removed if they become symptomatic or increase in size. In contrast with adults, almost all children can have good exposure for a nephrectomy through a subcostal incision rather than an intercostal or rib incision. As in the adult population, laparoscopic nephrectomy and renal surgery are becoming more common.

When a flank/subcostal incision is used, careful positioning of the patient is crucial. Failure to properly stabilize and secure the patient to the OR table can cause devastating consequences; therefore, efforts must be coordinated to properly position the patient. A rolled sheet or gel pad should be positioned beneath the dependent axilla, elevating the thorax to avoid brachial plexus neurapraxia. The dependent lower extremity is flexed at the hip and knee, while the overlying leg is kept straight. Padding is placed between the knees. In older children, in this lateral flank position, the kidney rest at the break of the table may be elevated to increase the distance between the rib and iliac crest, thus increasing exposure of the kidney. After the patient is positioned, a transverse incision is made below the 12th rib. The peritoneum is reflected, the upper ureter is dissected to the hilum, and the vessels are ligated. The kidney is excised and the wound is closed.

The lumbodorsal incision (incision parallel to the paraspinous muscle group) is performed with the patient in the prone or lateral position. This has an advantage of being a muscle-splitting, rather than a muscle-cutting incision and, as such, is associated with less postoperative pain and fewer incisional hernias. Some abdominal padding usually is added to raise the lumbodorsal area, and care should be taken to ensure complete pulmonary expansion in this position.

Most often in either the flank or lumbodorsal positioning, a urethral catheter is positioned for dependent drainage with care taken to avoid body pressure on the tubing. In this way the anesthesiologist may measure urinary output, though urinary drainage may also occur within the wound depending on the operation.

Usual preop diagnosis: MCDK; Wilms' tumor; nonfunctioning kidney; dysplastic kidney; ureteropelvic junction (UPJ) obstruction; ureterocele with loss of function.

Partial nephrectomy: Partial nephrectomies are common in children and are usually performed for a partially or nonfunctioning upper pole of a duplicated system. Ectopic ureters and ureteroceles are frequently the cause of loss of function. Again, these can be approached through either a lumbodorsal or flank incision. If the upper pole is obstructed but functional, a **pyeloureterostomy** from the upper pole ureter to the pelvis of the lower pole may be performed to salvage as much functioning parenchyma as possible. A partial nephrectomy may be performed for bilateral Wilms' tumor or other renal masses through a chevron or midline incision. An increasing number of partial nephrectomies are performed in a laparoscopic fashion.

Usual preop diagnosis: Nonfunctioning upper pole of a duplex system; ureterocele; ectopic ureter; bilateral Wilms' tumor, angiomyolipoma (more common in patients with tuberous sclerosis).

Nephroureterectomy: Nephroureterectomy often is performed for the upper pole of a duplex system which is obstructed due to an ureterocele or ectopic ureter. After the nephrectomy/partial nephrectomy is performed through a dorsal lumbotomy or flank approach, the ureter is dissected as low as possible (usually to the level of the iliac vessels). The ureteral stump is left open if there is no vesicoureteral reflux, and tied off if there is reflux. If indicated, distal ureterectomy can be performed via a second lower abdominal incision (typically a Pfannenstiel incision). If the initial incision was done in the prone position, the patient may need to be repositioned supine.

Usual preop diagnosis: Nonfunctioning upper pole of a duplex system; ureterocele; ectopic ureter

Pyeloplasty: Fetal hydronephrosis is detected in approximately 1 in every 300 pregnancies. Pyeloplasty to correct congenital obstruction of the ureteropelvic junction (UPJ) is a common pediatric surgical procedure. The hydronephrotic kidney usually is exposed through either a dorsal lumbotomy or a subcostal flank incision; therefore, the

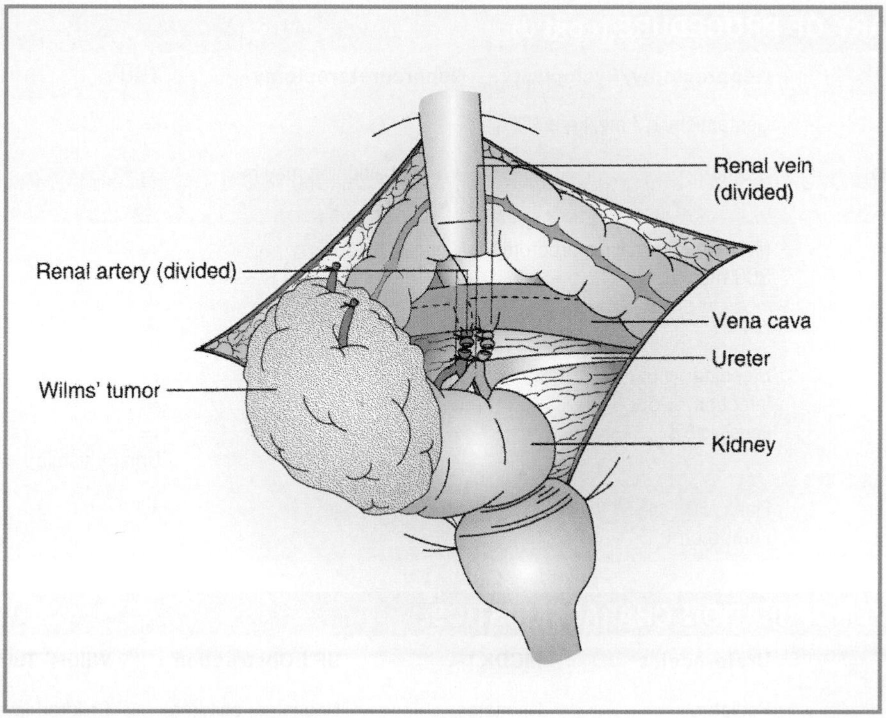

Figure 12.6-1. Anatomy for nephrectomy. (Reproduced with permission from Greenfield LJ, Mulholland MW, Oldham KT, et al: *Surgery: Scientific Principles and Practice*, 3rd edition. Lippincott Williams & Wilkins, Philadelphia: 2001.)

patient may be in a prone or modified lateral decubitus position (See details related to subcostal or lumbodorsal incision above). In most instances, the operation is performed entirely retroperitoneally with exposure of the upper ureter and renal pelvis. The abnormal UPJ usually is excised, followed by an end-to-end anastomosis (**dismembered pyeloplasty** or **Anderson-Hynes pyeloplasty**). If the renal pelvis is large and intrarenal and dependent drainage is not possible via a conventional pyeloplasty, an **ureterocalicostomy** may be performed by removing an area of thin renal parenchyma and anastomosing the ureter to a lower pole calyx. At the conclusion of the procedure, a perirenal Penrose drain typically is placed near the anastomosis, and, depending on surgeon preference, a ureteral stent or nephrostomy tube may be used. A urethral catheter may or may not be left after the procedure. Recently, more of these procedures have been performed robotically or laparoscopically.

Usual preop diagnosis: Fetal hydronephrosis 2° UPJ obstruction; hydronephrosis with a decrease in kidney function and/or flank pain

Transureteroureterostomy (TUU): This procedure, in which a ureter is anastomosed to the contralateral ureter, is used when there is problematic drainage of the distal ureter into the bladder. It is sometimes required to salvage a failed reimplantation or to transform a conduit-type diversion to an orthotopic neobladder or augmented native bladder. This technique can also be used to provide drainage in ureteral trauma. A midline or Pfannenstiel's, incision is used, and the peritoneum is entered. The ureters are dissected and the affected ureter is retroperitonealized and brought to the contralateral side anterior to the great vessels. It is anastomosed to the contralateral ureter end-to-side with absorbable suture. If required, the recipient ureter is then reimplanted into the neobladder or augmented bladder.

Usual preop diagnosis: Failed ureteral reimplant; undiversion; distal ureteral trauma

SUMMARY OF PROCEDURES

	Nephrectomy/Pyeloplasty	Nephroureterectomy	TUU
Position	Flank/prone	Supine/flank	Supine
Incision	Dorsal lumbotomy; subcostal; flank; midline	Subcostal flank 2nd incision: Pfannenstiel	Midline or Pfannenstiel

SUMMARY OF PROCEDURE (cont'd)

	Nephrectomy/Pyeloplasty	Nephroureterectomy	TUU
Antibiotics	Gentamicin 1.7 mg/kg iv	⇐	⇐
Surgical time	2.5 h	3 h (repositioning may be required)	⇐
EBL	Minimal; if partial nephrectomy, 300 mL	Minimal	⇐
Mortality	< 1%	⇐	⇐
Morbidity	Bleeding: < 5% Infection: < 5% Ileus: < 5%	⇐ ⇐ ⇐	⇐ ⇐ ⇐ Urinary fistula : < 5%
Pain score	Flank: 10 Lumbotomy: 5	10	10

PATIENT POPULATION CHARACTERISTICS

	Ureteroceles	MCDK*	UPJ Obstruction	Wilms' Tumor
Age range	Pediatric	Neonates	Neonates, children	Children (average, 4 yr)
Male:Female	1:4	⇐	M > F	M < F in the United States
Incidence	1:2000	⇐	1:500 birth	1:100,00
Etiology	Congenital	⇐	⇐	Genetic: WT1 gene
Associated conditions	UPJ; VUR; duplicated collecting system	⇐	VUR**; renal insufficiency	Hemihypertrophy, aniridia, HTN, Beckwith-Weidemann syndrome

*MCDK = multicystic dysplastic kidney
**VUR = vesicoureteral reflux

Suggested Readings

1. Kelalis PP, Maizels M, Das S, et al: Kidney reconstruction. In *Atlas of Pediatric Urologic Surgery.* Hinman F Jr, ed. WB Saunders, Philadelphia: 1994, 112–17, 123–43.
2. Marshall FF, Massad C, Hensle TW, et al: Kidney excision. In *Atlas of Pediatric Urologic Surgery.* Hinman F Jr, ed. WB Saunders, Philadelphia: 1994, 155–88.
3. Richey ML: Pediatric urologic oncology. In *Adult and Pediatric Urology,* Vol 3, 4th edition. Gillenwater JY, Grayhack JT, Howards SS, et al, eds. Mosby-Year Book, St. Louis: 2002, 2623–46.
4. Ritchy ML: Pediatric urologic oncology. In *Campbell's Urology,* 8th edition. Walsh PC, Retik AB, Vaughn ED, et al, eds. WB Saunders, Philadelphia: 2002, 2649–94.
5. Shaffer BS: Pearls and perils of patient positioning. *AUA Update Series* 1995;14:178–83.

ANESTHETIC CONSIDERATIONS

PREOPERATIVE

In infants and children, most upper urinary tract surgical procedures are performed to preserve or restore renal function. Patients may present with renal function that varies from minimally abnormal, requiring little or no modification of anesthetic plan, to end-stage renal disease (ESRD) with its associated abnormalities, including hypoproteinemia, chronic anemia, and serum electrolyte disturbances. A careful preop workup is required to determine the presence or absence of abnormal physiologic factors that will affect anesthesia management. For most cases, the workup will have been performed by the patient's physicians before surgery and will provide the rationale for the surgical procedure. Such nonspecific findings as anorexia, headache, nausea, excessive tiredness, alterations in urine output, and the presence of edema will alert the clinician to the likelihood of renal failure.

Renal abnormalities often are present as one component of a congenital malformation syndrome (e.g., polycystic kidneys, cerebrohepatorenal syndrome). In formulating the anesthetic plan, drugs eliminated by the kidney (e.g., pancuronium, meperidine, etc.) should be avoided.

Respiratory	An evaluation of pulmonary function, including auscultation of the lungs, may indicate the presence of pulmonary edema (uremic lung) or a pleural effusion. **Tests:** ABG; CXR; pulse oximetry
Cardiovascular	HTN is commonly seen in these patients, who may be taking antihypertensive medications and diuretics. In severe cases, CHF or pulmonary edema may be present, necessitating the use of cardioactive drugs and diuretics to optimize the patient's clinical condition before surgery. **Tests:** ABG; CXR; digitalis level; electrolytes
Renal	In cases requiring unilateral urinary tract surgery, the opposite kidney is usually normal. In the presence of renal insufficiency, a detailed evaluation of renal function is essential. Chronic metabolic acidosis may be present 2° poor kidney function, electrolyte abnormalities (↑ K+, ↓ Ca^{++}, ↑ or ↓ Na), hypovolemia, hypervolemia, and/or poor tissue perfusion. Children with ESRD will have been dialyzed before surgery. Preop K^+ < 6 mEq/L is usually safe. These patients may have an AV fistula, which must be protected during surgery (padded, no BP cuff). More commonly, a double-lumen central venous catheter will have been placed for hemodialysis (e.g., Permacath, etc). **Tests:** UA; UO; serum electrolytes; BUN; Cr; total protein; A/G ratio; ABG
Gastrointestinal	Renal failure is associated with increased incidence of delayed gastric emptying and gastroesophageal reflux. Modified rapid sequence induction should be considered.
Hematologic	Anemia, bone marrow depression, and coagulopathies are common in patients with poor renal function, particularly platelet dysfunction. An Hct of 15–18 kg/dL is not uncommon. **Tests:** Hb/Hct, PT/PTT; Plt count
Medications	Patients with ESRD will be taking many medications, which may influence the anesthetic plan. For example, chronic steroid therapy → Cushing facies, glycosuria; therefore, ✓ blood sugar and ✓ airway. Patients taking digitalis or diuretics →↓ K^+ → arrhythmias. Aminoglycosides → prolongation of neuromuscular blockade. If possible, avoid renal toxic drugs in patients with renal insufficiency (e.g., NSAIDs, aminoglycosides, etc.).
Premedication	Standard pre-op medication if renal function is normal (see p. D-1). Patients with ESRD may have increased sensitivity to sedatives; doses should be titrated carefully to effect.

INTRAOPERATIVE

Anesthetic technique: GETA ± epidural. (Platelet dysfunction should be assumed in ESRD and the risk/benefit of epidural placement carefully weighed). Warm OR to 70–75°F; use warming pad on OR table and forced-air warming.

Induction	Mask induction is preferable, unless iv is already in place. If an indwelling Permacath is to be accessed, heparin should be aspirated from the lumen before use. Routine use of dialysis catheters is discouraged due to need for strict sterile technique in handling of the catheter to avoid line infection. Succinylcholine should not be used in renal failure patients due to risk of K^+ release in borderline hyperkalemic patients. In the presence of renal insufficiency, antibiotics (e.g., aminoglycosides) may interfere with the metabolism of muscle relaxants and prolong their effect, and may further compromise renal function. Tracheal intubation, facilitated by a NMR (e.g., cisatracurium 0.2–0.3 mg/kg) is appropriate in patients with renal insufficiency. In appropriate patients (normal coags and no platelet dysfunction), epidural anesthesia with bupivacaine (see p. E-6) may reduce anesthetic requirements and provide postop analgesia (**NB:** local anesthetic clearance may be impaired in ESRD). Maintain muscle relaxation with cisatracurium in patients with renal insufficiency; otherwise, intermediate long-acting relaxants are appropriate (e.g., rocuronium, vecuronium, etc.).

Maintenance	Standard pediatric maintenance (see p. D-3). Moderate hyperventilation may be beneficial (→↓ K^+ + ↑ pH).	
Emergence	Reverse neuromuscular blockade with neostigmine and atropine or glycopyrrolate (see p. D-3).	
Blood and fluid requirements	IV × 1 in upper extremities NS @ (maintenance): 4 mL/kg/h (1–10 kg) + 2 mL/kg/h (11–20 kg) + 1 mL/kg/h (> 20 kg)	Usually minimal blood loss; however, renal surgery may be associated with ↑ blood loss. Transfuse with whole blood or PRBCs as needed to maintain an adequate Hct, based on physiologic response (usually 25–30%). If K+ is high and patient has ESRD use freshest PRBC or washed PRBC to minimize the K+ load. Minimal iv flush should be administered in the presence of oliguric renal insufficiency. Fluids in excess can lead to pulmonary edema especially in an aneuric patient. Avoid K+ containing crystalloid infusions.
Monitoring	Standard monitors (see p. D-1). ± Arterial line	Place arterial line in patients with significant renal failure; ✓ serum electrolytes and ABG frequently.
Positioning	✓ and pad pressure points. ✓ eyes.	✓ eyes frequently if prone or flank positions are used.
Complications	Peripheral nerve injury Eye trauma Hemorrhage Dysrhythmia	

POSTOPERATIVE

Complications	Hypovolemia Anemia Hypothermia Electrolyte abnormalities Coagulopathy Metabolic/respiratory acidosis	
Pain management	Acetaminophen (see p. E-4). Narcotics by epidural catheter (see p. E-6) or PCA (see p. E-4)	In renal failure, reduce analgesic doses by 50% to minimize cumulative effects. Note: morphine-6-glucuronide is renally excreted and accumulates in patients with renal failure. It leads to increased analgesia. Morphine-3-glucuronide is antanalgesic, and likewise increases in patients with ESRD. It is therefore preferred to use Dilaudid iv for treatment of postop pain in ESRD patients.
Tests	As indicated.	

Suggested Readings

1. Berry F: Anesthesia for genitourinary surgery. In *Pediatric Anesthesia,* 3rd edition. Gregory GA, ed. Churchill Livingstone, New York: 1994.
2. Davis PJ, Hall S. Deshpande JK, et al: Anesthesia for general, urologic and plastic surgery. In *Smith's Anesthesia for Infants and Children,* 6th edition. Motoyama EK, Davis PS, eds. Mosby-Year Book, St. Louis: 1996.

TRANSURETHRAL PROCEDURES

SURGICAL CONSIDERATIONS

Description: Transurethral procedures are not as common in children as they are in adults; however, the instrumentation, general principles, and considerations are similar. The most common pediatric endoscopic procedures are: **cystoscopy** and **vaginoscopy**, primarily as diagnostic procedures; **removal of foreign bodies** (FBs) including indwelling ureteral stents; **transurethral incision of urethral stricture**, for congenital lesions or complications of urethral surgery; **transurethral incision of posterior urethral valves** (PUV); **transurethral incision of ureterocele**; **subureteric injection for vesicoureteral reflux**; and **endoscopic injection for urinary incontinence**.

The positioning and techniques are identical to those in the adult. Careful attention to positioning is required when the pediatric patient is placed in the lithotomy position. The patient can remain supine if a flexible cystoscope is used. The most frequent neurological complication from lithotomy position may be injury to the common peroneal nerve → foot drop and sensory deficit. After the patient is positioned, a lubricated cystoscope or resectoscope (7–18 Fr) is introduced through the urethra. In infants, posterior urethral valves may be resected using a small cutting electrode or a laser, while a resectoscope is used in older children. With the advent of prenatal ultrasonography, posterior urethral valves (hydronephrosis and azotemia) often are resected in the neonatal period.

Often, transurethral procedures for urinary stone disease (**ureteral stent placement, cystolithalopaxy, ureteroscopy**) require fluoroscopy, which may bring with it both equipment considerations (fluoro-compatible moving tables) and positioning requirements to allow C-arm placement.

Foreign bodies or stones are removed using forceps, after crushing or pulverization with a laser, if necessary. Eye protection should be worn by all operating room staff if a laser is used. Occasionally, ureteral stents are placed/removed (after renal transplants, for instance) and an intraoperative retrograde pyelogram is performed to evaluate the upper tract collection system. During cystoscopy, localization of the ureteral orifices may be difficult 2° inflammation, prior bladder surgery, or congenital ectopia. The anesthesiologist may be asked to administer IV indigo carmine (this has potential effects of ↑ BP and may appear to ↓ O_2 sat), which will filter through the kidneys and produce blue urine to assist with locating the ureteral orifices.

Because most endoscopic procedures are short and the prostate and large resections are not involved, fluid absorption toxicity is rare, as opposed to that seen during "TURP syndrome." The operative team, however, must still be aware of the metabolic consequences of fluid reabsorption, as this can also occur through catastrophic ureteral or bladder perforation during endoscopic procedures in addition to the routine water reabsorption through venous channels.

By surgeon choice, lidocaine gel may be injected transurethrally at the completion of the transurethral procedure to avoid postoperative urethral irritation. Postoperatively some surgeons administer phenazopyridine (Pyridium) via nasogastric tube to decrease catheter irritation.

Usual preop diagnosis: Intravesical foreign body; bladder calculus; bladder outlet obstruction; urethral stricture; ureterocele; hematuria; urethral/vaginal mass; posterior urethral valves, urogenital sinus

SUMMARY OF PROCEDURE	
Position	Lithotomy
Incision	None
Special instrumentation	Cystoscope, resectoscope, catheters, stents, video camera unit, laser (optional)
Unique considerations	Use of cautery, fluoroscopy, PUV (prematurity or azotemia). Children with an obstructing ureterocele and pyelonephrosis may be at risk for urosepsis and should have close hemodynamic monitoring
Antibiotics	If infected urine preop, gentamicin 1.7 mg/kg iv
Surgical time	Cystoscopy: 10 min Transurethral procedure: 1 h

SUMMARY OF PROCEDURE (cont'd)	
EBL	Minimal
Postop care	PACU; basic catheter management, with oral Pyridium in the PACU for bladder analgesia
Mortality	< 1%
Morbidity	Bleeding Urethral stricture Infection Overdistention in augmented bladder
Pain score	2

PATIENT POPULATION CHARACTERISTICS	
Age range	0–18 yr
Male:Female	Posterior urethral valves, strictures: male only Ureterocele 1:6 Vesicoureteral reflux 1:4
Incidence	1/1,000–1/5,000
Etiology	Posterior urethral valves; vesicoureteral reflux; intravesical FB; bladder calculus; bladder outlet obstruction; urethral stricture; ureterocele
Associated conditions	Spina bifida; paraplegia/quadriplegia; repeat cystoscopies; strictures; bladder stones; latex allergy

ANESTHETIC CONSIDERATIONS

See Anesthetic Considerations for Transurethral Procedures, Open Bladder Procedures, Penile Surgery, Genital Procedures, p. 1336.

Suggested Readings

1. Strand WR, Bloom DA: Pediatric endourology. In *Adult and Pediatric Urology,* Vol 3, 4th edition. Gillenwater JY, Grayhack JT, Howards SS, et al., eds. Mosby-Year Book, St. Louis: 2002, 2719–28.
2. Warner MA: Lower extremity neuropathies associated with lithotomy positions. *Anesthesiology* 2000; 93:938–42.

OPEN BLADDER OPERATIONS

SURGICAL CONSIDERATIONS

Description: Open bladder operations commonly performed on children include **ureteral reimplantation** for correction of vesicoureteral reflux, obstructive megaureters, or ureterocele; **vesicostomy (Blocksom);** and **bladder neck operations.**

Ureteral reimplantation: Vesicoureteral reflux (VUR) is one of the most common abnormalities of the urinary tract in children and is present in about 25–50% of those who have UTI. Although VUR resolves spontaneously in many children, there are a number of indications for correction of VUR. These include: (a) high-grade VUR, (b) progressive VUR and renal scarring, (c) failure to resolve within several years, (d) other bladder surgery, (e) breakthrough UTIs, and (f) poor medical compliance.

Ureteral reimplantations can be performed using different approaches to the bladder (e.g., extravesical, intravesical, or a combined approach); however, these different approaches require a similar exposure and abdominal incision. In general, these are extraperitoneal rather than intraperitoneal operations. Initially, cystoscopy may be performed to

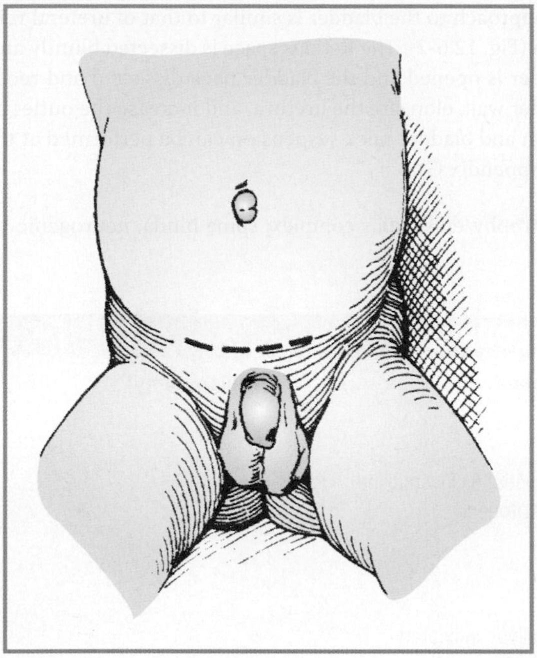

Figure 12.6-2. A Pfannensteil's incision in Langer's lines is a low transverse incision that provides good access to the bladder and other pelvic organs and good cosmesis. (Reproduced with permission from Hinman F: *Atlas of Pediatric Urologic Surgery*, 2nd edition. WB Saunders, Philadelphia: 1994.)

plan a potentially complex reimplantation (e.g., duplex systems, ectopia, or periureteral diverticula). A lower abdominal suprapubic (Pfannensteil) incision (Fig. 12.6-2) is usually made, the fascia is opened and the bladder exposed. Sufficient muscle relaxation is required to enable the surgeon to place a self-retaining retractor to expose the bladder. The anesthesiologist also may be asked to limit N_2O to decrease the amount of peritoneal contents bulging toward the bladder surgical field. The bladder is then opened (intravesical approach) and the ureter(s) is (are) reimplanted, or the bladder is mobilized to expose the posterolateral ureter, which is then reimplanted (extravesical approach). When required, ureteral stents are brought to the abdominal skin through the bladder wall. A Penrose drain is typically left in place, which is either brought through the incision or through a separate skin puncture.

Obstructive megaureters and ureteroceles are other conditions that may require ureteral reimplantation. The abdominal exposure and indications do not differ significantly from ureteral reimplantation for VUR; however, tailoring of the ureter by reducing its caliber and excising redundant tissue or plicating it may be necessary. A procedure on the bladder neck also may be required if an ureterocele extends distally through the bladder outlet. Regional anesthesia techniques—specifically caudal or epidural analgesia—have gained popularity for these procedures. They have been shown to decrease postoperative pain medication requirements. Although the majority of patients void 6–9 hours after surgery, there may be ↑ risk of urinary retention after a caudal block has been administered. The surgeon's preference on whether an indwelling urethral or ureteral catheters will be left at the conclusion of the procedure should be known and discussed before consideration to giving a caudal block is entertained.

Usual preop diagnosis: VUR; obstructive megaureter; ureterocele

Vesicostomy: Infants and very young children may require bladder drainage until definitive bladder or urethral surgery. A vesicostomy may be performed, allowing the urine to flow continuously from a small, lower abdominal vesicocutaneous fistula. A 2-cm transverse incision is made halfway between the umbilicus and the pubis, and the bladder is dissected extraperitoneally to expose the dome. The bladder is opened at the dome (urachus) and is anastomosed to abdominal skin with absorbable sutures, creating a small fistula.

Usual preop diagnosis: Posterior or anterior urethral valves; severe VUR; neurovesical dysfunction; prune-belly syndrome

Bladder neck operations: These procedures usually are required in patients with severe anomalies, such as exstrophy, or severe incontinence due to an incompetent bladder neck. These are more complex procedures, with dissection often difficult. The approach to the bladder is similar to that of ureteral reimplantation, using a lower abdominal (Pfannenstiel) incision (Fig. 12.6-2). The Retzius space is dissected bluntly and the anterior bladder wall and pubic bone exposed. The bladder is opened and the bladder neck dissected and reconstructed. Various techniques to tubularize the anterior bladder wall, elongate the urethra, and increase the outlet resistance have been described. Bilateral ureteral reimplantation and bladder neck suspension can be performed at the same time. One special consideration is latex allergy (see Appendix G).

Usual preop diagnosis: Exstrophy/epispadias complex; spina bifida; neurogenic bladder; incontinence; bladder-neck reconstruction

SUMMARY OF PROCEDURES

	Reimplantation	Vesicostomy	Bladder Neck
Position	Supine	⇐	⇐
Incision	Pfannenstiel or low midline extraperitoneal	⇐	⇐
Unique considerations	None	⇐	Latex allergy (see p. G-1)
Antibiotics	None unless indicated	⇐	Gentamicin 1.7 mg/kg iv, slowly
Surgical time	1.5 h	45 min	2 h
EBL	Minimal	→	200 mL
Postop care	PACU; ± urethral catheter ± stents. Anticholenergics for bladder spasms; belladonna and opioid suppositories, if given, must be monitored because of the potential of oversedation and respiratory depression. Older children may benefit from epidural anesthesia.	PACU	Urethral catheter 4–7 d; PACU → ward
Mortality	< 1%	⇐	⇐
Morbidity	Infection: < 3% Bleeding: < 3% Urinary retention: Unilateral: < 5% Bilateral: 8–10% Ureteral obstruction Persistent reflux	⇐ ⇐ – 	⇐ < 5% Urinary retention ⇐
Pain score	7	4	7

PATIENT POPULATION CHARACTERISTICS

Age range	1 mo–teenage	⇐	⇐
Male:Female	1:4	1:1	⇐
Incidence	1%	⇐	⇐
Etiology	Unknown	Congenital	⇐
Associated conditions	UTI; renal failure	⇐	⇐

ANESTHETIC CONSIDERATIONS

See Anesthetic Considerations for Transurethral Procedures, Open Bladder Procedures, Penile Surgery, Genital Procedures, p. 1336.

Suggested Readings

1. Canning DA, Koo HP, Duckett JW: Anomalies of the bladder and cloaca. In *Adult and Pediatric Urology*, Vol 3, 3rd edition. Gillenwater JY, Grayhack JT, Howards SS, et al, eds. Mosby-Year Book, St. Louis: 1996, 2445–88.
2. Dixon Walker R: Vesicoureteral reflux and urinary tract infection in children. In *Adult and Pediatric Urology*, Vol 3, 3rd edition. Gillenwater JY, Grayhack JT, Howards SS, et al, eds. Mosby-Year Book, St. Louis: 1996, 2459–95.
3. King LR: Vesicoureteral reflux, megaureter, and ureteral reimplantation. In *Campbell's Urology*, Vol 2, 6th edition. Walsh PC, Retik AB, Stamey TA, et al, eds. WB Saunders, Philadelphia: 1992, 1689–1742.
4. Smith GHH, Duckett JW: Urethral lesions in infants and children. In *Adult and Pediatric Urology*, Vol 3, 3rd edition. Gillenwater JY, Grayhack JT, Howards SS, et al, eds. Mosby-Year Book, St. Louis: 1996, 2411–43.
5. Wilton NT: Postoperative pain management for pediatric urologic surgery. *Urologic Clin North Am* 1995; 22(1):189–201.

BLADDER AUGMENTATION

SURGICAL CONSIDERATIONS

Description: A variety of pathologies may be associated with neurogenic bladder, including spina bifida, cerebral palsy and spinal cord injury. Failure of bladder storage and/or compliance may cause urinary incontinence or high voiding pressures leading to upper tract deterioration. In such cases, and in cases where infectious or fibrotic processes have caused a reduction in bladder capacity, the patient may be a candidate for **bladder augmentation** with native intestine, colon, stomach or ureter (in the case of significantly dilated upper tracts). A **continent catheterizable stoma** may be performed at the same time due to the frequent need for catheterization subsequent to the procedure. Patients with limited mobility who require urethral catheterization can also opt for the placement of a continent catheterizable stoma using appendix or ileum. This may be done as a separate procedure with or without augmentation. These patients have often had many operations and the operative team needs to consider possible latex sensitivity (see Appendix G).

In some cases for treatment of urinary incontinence, bladder augmentation and stoma formation is combined with closure of the bladder neck or insertion of an **artificial urethral sphincter.**

Patients with neurogenic bowel may become dehydrated more easily during bowel preparation prior to surgery. Although traditionally mechanical bowel preparation for 1–2 days prior to surgery is recommended, growing evidence in the general surgery literature suggests that bowel preparation does not reduce wound infections and anastomotic leaks and may actually increase ileus rates. Anesthesiologists should be aware of the length and extent of preop bowel preparation in case the patient has became dehydrated or suffered electrolyte imbalance due to this process. Special consideration should be made for patients who have ventriculoperitoneal (VP) shunts; typically care is made to sequester the shunt in sterile feation, keeping it away from any spillage from bowel segments.

Bladder Augmentation: Bladder augmentation is usually performed on children with a small capacity bladder, resulting from congenital abnormalities or fibrosis with resulting poor compliance. Cystoscopy may or may not be performed in association. The patient is usually in supine position and the operation may be performed through a lower midline or Pfannenstiel incision. The bowel and bladder are mobilized, with wide intraperitoneal exposure so that consideration to insensible loss may be large in small children. The relevant bowel segment is harvested, and the remaining native bowel is reanastomosed across the defect in the standard stapled or hand-sewn fashion. The "patch" of bowel segment is then sewn on to the bladder using running absorbable suture to minimize risk of subsequent nidus for bladder calculi. At the end of the procedure, a suprapubic tube is placed to decompress the bladder and allow irrigation of mucus produced by the bowel segments. Postoperatively, nasogastric decompression is maintained until return of bowel function, and perioperative antibiotics are usually continued for a minimum of 3 days.

Usual preop diagnosis: Spinal cord injury, spina bifida, cerebral palsy; urinary incontinence; bladder tuberculosis, schistosomiasis, interstitial cystitis.

Continent catheterizable stoma (Mitrofanoff appendicovesicostomy or Monti tube): In the case of a child who needs lifetime catheterization, a continent catheterizable abdominal stoma is often preferred due to its greater ease of catheterization, particularly for children with motor impairment. Use of the appendix as a flap-valve conduit between the bladder and the abdominal wall was first described by Mitrofanoff in 1980. Operative setup is similar to that of a bladder augmentation. After amputation of the appendix, its base is brought through the abdominal wall to form a stoma at the umbilicus. The tip of the appendix is amputated to create a tube, and a small submucosal trough is made in the posterolateral bladder and an indwelling catheter is placed in the channel to maintain patency immediately postoperatively. Other continent stomas that can be catheterized may be constructed from short segments of bowel.

Usual preop diagnosis: Spina bifida, spinal cord injury or cerebral palsy with neurogenic bladder; urinary retention or urinary incontinence, limited mobility.

SUMMARY OF PROCEDURES

	Bladder Augmentation	Continent Catheterizable Stoma
Position	Supine	⇐
Incision	Lower midline incision	⇐
Special instrumentation	Catheter in bladder/suprapubic tube, NG tube	Catheter in bladder/suprapubic tube, NG tube, catheter in stoma
Unique considerations	Spina bifida pts may have latex allergy	Pts with chronic catheterization may have infected urine; treat with preop antibacterial irrigation and culture specific antibiotics
Antibiotics	Broad spectrum antibiotics (e.g., 3rd generation cephalosporin)	⇐
Surgical time	3.5 h	4.5 h (with augmentation) or 1.5 h (without augmentation)
EBL	100 cc	⇐
Postop care	PACU – > ward	⇐
Mortality	<1%	⇐
Morbidity	Electrolyte abnormalities, growth retardation (>50%) Bladder calculi (10–50%) Rupture of augmented bladder (5–10%) Small bowel obstruction (3%) Bladder cancer (1%)	Stomal stenosis (30–40%)

ANESTHETIC CONSIDERATIONS

See Anesthetic Considerations for Transurethral Procedures, Open Bladder Procedures, Penile Surgery, Genital Procedures (p. 1336).

Suggested Readings

1. Adams MC, Joseph DB: Urinary tract reconstruction in children. In *Campbell-Walsh Urology*, Vol 4, 9th edition. Wein A, Kavoussi L, Novick AC, et al, eds. WB Saunders, Philadelphia: 2007.
2. Camey M, Thuroff J, Reddy P, et al: Principles of bladder substitution. In *Atlas of Urologic Surgery*, 2nd edition. Hinman F Jr ed. WB Saunders, Philadelphia: 1992, 768–82.
3. Gilbert SM, Hensle TW: Metabolic consequences and long-term complications of enterocystoplasty in children: a review. *J Urol* 2005; 173(4):1080–6.

PENILE SURGERY

SURGICAL CONSIDERATIONS

Description: Pediatric penile operations usually correct congenital urethral abnormalities or involve circumcision. The most common surgical operation performed in the United States, **circumcision,** consists of the excision of the preputial skin to expose the glans. It can be performed for either religious, ethnic, social, or medical reasons (e.g., phimosis or recurrent balanitis).

Circumcision: Freehand circumcision involves excising preputial skin using two incisions to remove a sleeve of penile skin to fully expose the glans. At times, various clamps (Gomco, Mogen, etc.) can be used to circumcise in the newborn period. Most circumcisions performed in the operating room on older children or those with penile skin anomalies will be free-hand excisions of the foreskin. Newer considerations regarding analgesia even in the neonate recommend a penile block for this procedure. In older children being circumcised, both caudal and penile block can offer similar duration of anesthesia (4–8 h) but school-age children may, however, be bothered more by leg numbness and inability to void from the caudal block, and this should be taken into consideration.

Usual preop diagnosis: Phimosis, balanitis, family preference for circumcision

Hypospadias is the abnormal opening of the urethral meatus resulting from incomplete development of the urethra. The defect can be located anywhere from the corona of the glans to the perineum. Accordingly, surgical correction can require limited reconstruction as in the **meatal advancement granuloplasty (MAGPI)** procedure or extensive dissection and reconstruction requiring 3–4 hours of surgery. While most pediatric urologists perform one-stage reconstruction for the majority of hypospadias, some more extensive cases and surgeon choice may plan for a two-staged repair. Postoperative urethral instrumentation should be avoided because catheterization of the newly formed urethra could cause disruption of the repair. An artificial erection is obtained by infusion of normal saline into the corpora to judge need for and adequacy of repair. Significant fluid may be used and absorbed during artificial erection in the small child.

The surgeon may choose not to use a urethral catheter in distal hypospadias repairs and some midshaft repairs. In such cases, caudal anesthesia should be avoided due to risk of urinary retention and risks of surgical complications relating to need for postoperative catheterization. A **penile nerve block** may be helpful in such cases with care given to avoiding a penile hematoma or disrupting penile anatomy or blood flow to the dorsal penis. In all cases, postoperative urethral instrumentation should be avoided because catheterization of the newly formed urethra could cause disruption of the repair. Catheters, when placed, are usually secured by stitching to the glans penis. Often at the conclusion of the surgery the surgeon may require an additional 3–5 minutes of anesthesia to properly apply dressings to protect the hypospadias repair.

In reoperative cases for repair of fistulae or other complications, bladder or buccal mucosa may be needed to create a new urethra. Use of buccal mucosa is popular but may require access to the patient's mouth and inner buccal area.

Usual preop diagnosis: Hypospadias ± chordee; fistula repair; epispadias repair; penile torsion; concealed penis

SUMMARY OF PROCEDURES

	Circumcision	Hypospadias
Position	Supine	⇐
Incision	Circumferential penile	⇐ + ventral penis
Special instrumentation	None	Optical magnification
Unique considerations	1% lidocaine with 1:100,000 epinephrine for better hemostasis.	Tourniquet; injectable NS for artificial erection; 1% lidocaine. If a catheter is placed, liberal IV fluids may be given.
Antibiotics	None	⇐
Surgical time	30 min	1.5–4 h

SUMMARY OF PROCEDURE (cont'd)

	Circumcision	Hypospadias
EBL	Minimal	< 50 mL
Postop care	Outpatient	Outpatient or ward ± urethral catheter
Mortality	< 1%	⇐
Morbidity	Infection: 2% Hematoma: 2%	⇐ ⇐ Urethrocutaneous fistula (5–20%), urethral stricture, urethral diverticulum.
Pain score	2	5

PATIENT POPULATION CHARACTERISTICS

Age range	Neonates-children	> 4 mo
Incidence	61%	1:300
Etiology	Acquired	Congenital
Associated conditions	Infection	Cryptorchidism; inguinal hernia; bifid scrotum

ANESTHETIC CONSIDERATIONS

See Anesthetic Considerations for Transurethral Procedures, Open Bladder Procedures, Penile Surgery, Genital Procedures (p. 1336)

Suggested Readings

1. Elder JS: Hypospadias. In *Campbell's Urology*, Vol 3, 8th edition. Walsh PC, Retik AB, Vaughn ED, et al, eds. WB Saunders, Philadelphia: 2002, 2334–6.
2. Snodgrass W, Baskin LS: Abnormalities of the genitalia in boys and their surgical management. In *Adult and Pediatric Urology*, Vol III, 4th edition. Gillenwater JY, Grayhack JT, Howards SS, et al, eds. Mosby-Year Book, St. Louis: 2002, 2509–32.
3. Wilton NT: Postoperative pain management for pediatric urologic surgery. *Urologic Clin North Am* 1995,22(1):189–201.
4. Weksler N, Atias I, Klein M, et al: Is penile block better than caudal epidural block for post-circumcision analgesia? *J Anesth* 2005; 19(1):36–39.

GENITAL PROCEDURES (CLITOROPLASTY, VAGINOPLASTY, URETHROPLASTY)

SURGICAL CONSIDERATIONS

Description: Masses of the introitus include urethral prolapse, prolapsed ectopic ureterocele, and rhabdomyosarcoma. Genitoplasty usually is performed in female patients with abnormal genitalia, e.g., ambiguous genitalia resulting from abnormal steroidogenesis (congenital adrenal hyperplasia [CAH], danazol exposure) and urogenital sinus or cloacal anomalies.

Urethral prolapse repair: With the patient in a lithotomy position, a simple circumferential incision is made at the junction between the prolapsed mucosa and the urethral meatus. The prolapsed tissue is excised, and anastomosis is performed with absorbable suture. Introital rhabdomyosarcoma often requires open or transurethral biopsy of the mass, and is usually treated with chemotherapy.

Vaginoplasty/clitoroplasty: These procedures are performed in patients with ambiguous genitalia, and are usually associated with hormonal imbalance (CAH). The initial procedure usually requires reduction of the enlarged clitoris and reconstruction of the labioscrotal folds. With the patient in a lithotomy position, skin incisions are made to allow partial resection of the corporal bodies and glans with nerve sparing. Periclitoral skin flaps are used to reconstruct the clitoris and labial folds. Vaginoplasty is performed through a perineal approach by creating an urethrovaginal septum. The vagina usually can be pulled into its normal position between the urethra and rectum, and anastomosed to perineal skin flaps using absorbable sutures. Vaginoplasty can be performed with clitoroplasty in an infant. If performed later in life (puberty), a vaginoplasty with complex flaps and bowel interposition is necessary. Many of these patients are on long-term corticosteroid replacement therapy and, therefore, preop stress-dosing of steroids may be indicated; if a long, complicated intraabdominal procedure is anticipated, an abdominoperineal approach is required. A loop of sigmoid colon or ileum is isolated, along with its mesentery, and is brought through the perineal incision. It is then anastomosed proximally to the vagina and distally to skin flaps. Also, these procedures may be used for **gender reassignment** if masculinization of the ambiguous genitalia in a genotypic male is not possible.

Usual preop diagnosis: Ambiguous genitalia; CAH; cloacal exstrophy; urogenital sinus persistence; danazol exposure

SUMMARY OF PROCEDURE

Position	Lithotomy
Incision	Perineal
Special instrumentation	Loupes
Unique considerations	Steroid replacement may be necessary (CAH)
Antibiotics	Gentamicin 1.7 mg/kg iv (children)
Surgical time	2–4 h
EBL	10–15 mL
Postop care	± Urethral catheter
Mortality	< 1%
Morbidity	Infection: < 5% Bleeding: < 5% Flap necrosis: < 5%
Pain score	6

PATIENT POPULATION CHARACTERISTICS

Age range	Clitoroplasty: 3–6 mo; vaginoplasty: puberty
Incidence	1:30,000 births (ambiguous genitalia)
Etiology	Congenital
Associated conditions	Hypothalamic-pituitary axis suppression; adrenal hyperplasia; steroid replacement therapy

Suggested Readings

1. Hussman D: Intersex. In *Adult and Pediatric Urology*, Vol 3, 4th edition. Gillenwater JY, Grayhack JT, Howards SS, et al, eds. Mosby-Year Book, St. Louis: 2002, 2533–64.
2. Rink R, Kaefer M: Surgical management of intersexuality, cloacal malformations, and other genitalia in girls. In *Campbell's Urology*, Vol 4, 8th edition. Walsh PC, Retik AB, Vaughn ED, et al., eds. WB Saunders, Philadelphia: 2002, 2428–68.

ANESTHETIC CONSIDERATIONS FOR TRANSURETHRAL PROCEDURES, OPEN BLADDER PROCEDURES, PENILE SURGERY, GENITAL PROCEDURES

PREOPERATIVE

Typically, infants and children presenting for these procedures are otherwise healthy, with some notable exceptions. **Vesicoureteral reflux** may be associated with renal dysplasia and HTN. The **prune-belly (Eagle-Barrett) syndrome** includes dystrophic abdominal musculature, requiring an evaluation of pulmonary function. **Bladder and cloacal exstrophy** may be accompanied by a spinal cord abnormality (e.g., tethered cord, spina bifida).Congenital cardiac anomalies may be present, and an evaluation should be performed prior to surgery.

Pediatric urology patients with lower urinary tract dysfunction and underlying neurologic disorders (e.g., myelomeningocele), and exstrophy are at risk for developing latex allergy as a result of repeated urethral catheterizations or surgical procedures. (See p. G-1)

Circumcision and hypospadias repair are most commonly performed in the first two years of life in otherwise healthy children.

Respiratory	Prune-belly syndrome: pulmonary function may be decreased. ✓ for Hx of respiratory compromise. Post-op ventilatory support may be necessary. ✓ adequate reversal of NMB and force of cough. **Tests:** CXR; others as indicated from H&P.
Renal	Renal anomalies may be present as part of a congenital malformation complex. **Tests:** As indicated from H&P.
Endocrine	Surgery for genital disorders usually are performed to reshape anatomic abnormalities 2° congenital endocrine disorders. Ambiguous genitalia are associated with congenital adrenal abnormalities. They are usually detected in the first month of life and may lead to severe salt-losing crises with ↑ Na^+ and ↓ K^+. The electrolyte status of these patients must be evaluated in the preop period. Treatment consists of steroid replacement. **Tests:** Electrolytes; blood sugar
Premedication	If > 7–9 months of age, consider midazolam premedication (0.5–0.75 mg/kg) po, or 1–2 mg iv (see p. D-1).

INTRAOPERATIVE

Anesthetic technique: GA (ETT or LMA) using a pediatric circle. A combined technique with epidural or caudal anesthesia is often used. For small children, warm OR to 70–75°F. Use warming pad on OR table.

Induction	For patients < 5–10 yr, standard mask induction with sevoflurane/N_2O/O_2. Older patients may agree to standard iv induction, facilitated by the use of topical local anesthetic cream or patch (see p. D-1). For open-bladder and complex genital procedures, an indwelling epidural catheter for intraop and postop pain relief is recommended.	
Maintenance	Standard pediatric maintenance (see p. D-2). With epidural anesthesia, volatile and/or iv anesthetic requirements are reduced.	
Emergence	Typically, no special considerations. Carefully evaluate patient for adequate ventilation prior to extubation in those with prune-belly syndrome.	
Blood and fluid requirements	Minimal blood loss IV: 22 or 24 ga × 1 NS/LR @ (maintenance): 4 mL/kg/h (1–10 kg) + 2 mL/kg/h (11–20 kg)	Complex cases may be associated with significant blood loss, and require transform with whole blood or PRBC.

Monitoring	Standard monitors (see p. D-1). ± Arterial line	Place arterial line for measurement of arterial gases. ✓ Hct and blood glucose if significant blood loss or long case is anticipated, in patients with concurrent renal dysfunction.
Positioning	✓ and pad pressure points. ✓ eyes.	
Complications	Nerve damage	In lower extremities, ✓ if padding is insufficient with lithotomy position.

POSTOPERATIVE

Complications	Prune belly: hypoventilation Adrenogenital syndrome: adrenal insufficiency	Assisted ventilation may be required.
Pain management	Acetaminophen Epidural (p. E-6) or PCA (p. E-4) analgesia IV opiates	See p. E-4. Ditropan or ketorolac will ↓ bladder spasm. Ketorolac → renal insufficiency. Do not use if renal function is abnormal.

Suggested Readings

1. Berry F: Anesthesia for genitourinary surgery. In *Pediatric Anesthesia,* 3rd edition. Churchill Livingstone, New York: 1994.
2. Davis PJ, Hall S, Deshpande JK, Spear RM: Anesthesia for general, urologic and plastic surgery. In *Smith's Anesthesia for Infants and Children,* 6th edition. Motoyama EK, Davis PJ, eds. Mosby-Year Book, St. Louis: 1990.
3. Sheldon CA, Snyder HM III: Principles of urinary tract reconstruction. In *Adult and Pediatric Urology,* Vol 1, 3rd edition. Gillenwater JY, Grayhack JT, Howards SS, et al, eds. Mosby-Year Book, St. Louis: 1996, 249–50, 2394–5.

INGUINOSCROTAL PROCEDURES

SURGICAL CONSIDERATIONS

Description: Undescended testis (cryptorchidism), hydrocele, and inguinal hernia are common in pediatric urology, and surgery is usually performed on an outpatient basis. Testicular torsion is one of the few true pediatric urologic emergencies because testicular infarction will occur within hours of the torsion. Testicular tumors in children, accounting for 1–2% of all pediatric solid tumors, are more frequently benign than those in adults, and represent the main indication for **radical or simple orchiectomy.**

Orchiopexy: Orchiopexy for a palpable undescended testis is performed through a small inguinal incision. A nonpalpable testis may warrant diagnostic laparoscopy as the initial procedure; otherwise, the external oblique fascia is opened, exposing the inguinal canal. An initially nonpalpable testis may become palpable with anesthetic relaxation. The testis is localized and the cord is dissected to gain adequate length for scrotal fixation, without torsion or tension, to prevent postop ischemia and atrophy. If the testicle is high and adequate inguinal mobilization is not possible, dissection into the retroperitoneum may be required. The scrotal pouch is created by skin incision two-thirds the way down to the scrotum and blunt dissection between the skin and dartos muscle. The testis is fixed with suture material.

Both ilioinguinal nerve block and caudal analgesia appear to be equally effective in management of postorchiopexy pain, but parents should be counseled on the small risk of postoperative urinary retention. When inguinal block is contemplated prior to incision, this should be discussed with the surgeon. At times, inguinal infiltration distorts the anatomy and may perforate the hernia sac, thus turning a relatively simple operation into a more complex one.

Alternatively, the block may be performed at the end of the procedure or the wound irrigated with 0.25% bupivacaine, which provides excellent postoperative analgesia and facilitates early discharge from the surgical recovery unit. (Also see Surgery for the Undescended Testicle, p. 1310.)

Usual preop diagnosis: Cryptorchidism; nonpalpable testis

Testicular torsion is a pediatric urologic emergency. There is no definitive diagnostic imaging study, although Doppler and isotope scans of the testis can be useful. At times, symptoms of testicular torsion may be indistinguishable from epididymitis or torsion of the testicular appendages (embryonic remnants). The testis is delivered through a scrotal incision, examined, detorsed, and assessed for viability. If the testis is nonviable, a **simple scrotal orchiectomy** is performed. If the testicle is viable, it is fixed in a **scrotal dartos pouch.** The contralateral testis is fixed in a similar fashion. A torsion of a testicular appendage usually is treated medically with pain control and anti-inflammatory agents. If this condition is discovered at surgical exploration, the diseased tissue is excised, the testis is simply reinserted in the scrotum, and the wound is closed. It should be noted that neonatal (antenatal) or perinatal torsion may be performed in the newborn period. It the diagnosis is unclear this operation may be performed at times through an inguinal incision.

Usual preop diagnosis: Testicular torsion; torsion of the testicular appendage

Hydrocelectomy–inguinal hernia repair: This procedure is performed through an inguinal incision and dissection of the inguinal canal. The patent processus vaginalis is carefully dissected from the cord structures; the peritoneal sac is ligated at the level of the internal inguinal ring; and the wound is closed after evacuation of the hydrocele liquid. (Also see Repair of Inguinal and Umbilical Hernias, Hydrocele, p. 1307.)

Usual preop diagnosis: Hydrocele; inguinal hernia

Radical orchiectomy: While simple orchiectomy is performed through a scrotal incision, radical orchiectomy (used when testicular cancer is suspected) is performed through an inguinal incision. The external oblique fascia is opened, and the spermatic cord is isolated and clamped at the level of the internal ring. The testis is delivered through the incision and examined. If the testis is felt to contain malignancy, the cord is ligated and divided at the level of the internal inguinal ring. If there is uncertainty in the Dx, a biopsy can be performed.

Usual preop diagnosis: Testicular mass

SUMMARY OF PROCEDURES

	Hydrocelectomy, Hernia Repair	Orchiopexy, Orchiectomy
Position	Supine	⇐
Incision	Inguinal/scrotal	⇐ + Can be extended to reach retroperitoneum ± laparoscopic exploration.
Antibiotics	None	⇐
Surgical time	1 h	⇐
EBL	Minimal	⇐
Postop care	PACU → home	⇐
Mortality	< 1%	⇐
Morbidity	Infection: 1–2% Recurrence: 1%	Testicular atrophy: 7%
Pain score	5	5

PATIENT POPULATION CHARACTERISTICS

Age range	1 yrs–puberty	Cryptorchidism: 1–2 yr Torsion: 0–18 yr
Incidence	1–4%	Cryptorchidism: 3% Torsion: 1:4000
Etiology	Congenital	⇐

ANESTHETIC CONSIDERATIONS

PREOPERATIVE

Orchiopexy, orchiectomy, hydrocelectomy, and hernia repair are performed most commonly in otherwise healthy children.

Renal	With phimosis, there may be Hx of UTIs. Possible pyelonephritis. Hematuria requires GU workup. **Tests:** UA; renal function (BUN, Cr), as clinically indicated.
Laboratory	Hct; others as indicated from H&P.
Premedication	If > 7 to 9 months of age, consider midazolam (0.5–0.75 mg/kg po) before induction. If > 10 yr old: standard premedication (see p. D-1).

INTRAOPERATIVE

Anesthetic technique: GETA or LMA/mask anesthetic, using a pediatric circle with humidified and warmed gases. A combined technique with caudal anesthesia often is used for nonendoscopic procedures. For small children, warm OR to 70–75°F. Use warming pad and/or forced air warming on OR table.

Induction	In younger patients, mask induction is customary before iv placement. If the surgical procedure will be > 30 min, tracheal intubation or LMA is preferred. Intermediate-acting NMR (e.g., vecuronium 0.1 mg/kg iv or rocuronium 0.6 mg/kg iv) is administered to facilitate tracheal intubation. If appropriate, caudal anesthesia can be obtained using bupivacaine or levobupivacaine 0.125 or 0.25% with epinephrine 1: 200,000; 1 mL/kg up to 10 mL total. Test dose of 1 mL should be given after a negative aspiration through the catheter or needle. A positive test dose, in contrast to adults epidural test dose, could be indicated by an increase in HR, a decrease in HR, a decrease in BP, or ST-T wave changes. The caudal local anesthetic dose should be fractionated with frequent aspirations. The addition of clonidine (1–2 mg/kg) to the caudal block intensifies and prolongs the analgesia, with minimal sedation. Acetaminophen 30–40 mg/kg PR may be given following intubation.	
Maintenance	Standard pediatric maintenance (see p. D-3). If no regional block is performed, at least 2 MAC anesthesia is required prior to skin incision to prevent laryngospasm in nonintubated patients. Caudal anesthesia can be used to provide the majority of analgesia in nonendoscopic procedures.	
Emergence	If neuromuscular blockade is used, reverse with neostigmine (0.07 mg/kg iv) and atropine (0.02 mg/kg iv) or glycopyrrolate (0.01 mg/kg). Extubate when patient is fully awake or deep.	
Blood and fluid requirements	Negligible blood loss IV: 20–22 ga × 1 NS/LR @ maintenance	Pediatric maintenance: 4 mL/kg/h (0–10 kg) + 2 mL/kg/h (11–20 kg) + 1 mL/kg/h (>20 kg)
Monitoring	Standard monitors (see p. D-1)	
Positioning	✓ and pad pressure points. ✓ eyes.	Ocular compression/corneal abrasion may occur with oversized mask.
Complications	Laryngospasm	Rx: 100% O_2, jaw thrust, positive pressure. If iv is present, first deepen the level of anesthesia with propofol. If necessary, administer succinylcholine (1–2 mg/kg iv) in addition to atropine (0.02 mg/kg iv). If no iv, can give succinylcholine 3 mg/kg im, atropine 0.02 mg/kg im.

Complications (cont'd)	Intravascular local anesthetic administration	Epinephrine in caudal anesthetic (to detect intravascular administration) does not significantly prolong analgesia.

POSTOPERATIVE

Complications	Bleeding	
Pain management	Caudal or regional block Acetaminophen (10–20 mg po, and 10 mg q6h pr; 30–40 mg pr on 1st dose, followed by 20 mg q 6 h prn)	Optimal analgesia and presence of parents in PACU will minimize child's agitation/movement/crying.

Suggested Readings

1. Berry FA: Anesthesia for genitourinary surgery. In *Pediatric Anesthesia,* 3rd edition, Gregory GA, ed. Churchill Livingstone, New York: 1994, 571–606.
2. Motoyama EK, Davis PS, eds: *Smith's Anesthesia for Infants and Children,* 6th edition. Mosby-Year-Book, St. Louis: 1996.
3. Rozanski TA, Bloom DA: Male genital tract. In *Surgery of Infants and Children.* Oldham KT, Colombani PM, Foglia RP, eds. Lippincott-Raven Publishers, Philadelphia: 1997, 1543–58.
4. Schneck FX, Bellinger MF: *Campbell's Urology,* Vol 4, 8th edition. Walsh PC, Retik AB, Vaughn ED, et al, eds. WB Saunders, Philadelphia: 2002.
5. Tobias JD: Caudal epidural block: a review of test dosing and recognition of systemic injection in children. *Anesth Analg* 200;93(5):1156–61.
6. Wilton NT: Postoperative pain management for pediatric urologic surgery. *Urologic Clin North Am* 1995; 22(1):189–201.

LAPAROSCOPIC PROCEDURES

SURGICAL CONSIDERATIONS

Description: Laparoscopy has become a useful technique for many pediatric urologists. It is used widely to locate the impalpable testis via **diagnostic laparoscopy**, with subsequent **laparoscopic orchidopexy** as needed, and has gained popularity for many procedures. Among them are **laparoscopic nephrectomy, partial nephrectomy, nephroureterectomy, adrenalectomy, pyeloplasty,** and **varicocelectomy.** More recently, robotic laparoscopic procedures are becoming increasingly prevalent, with **robotic pyeloplasty** and **ureteral reimplantation** being among the most common. Advantages to the use of the robot include improved 3D visualization and instrument control; however, approximately 20–45 minutes of robot set-up time should be calculated into the time under anesthesia.

As in adults, pneumoperitoneum is created by insufflating CO_2 (to a pressure of 14–16 mmHg) either through the Veress needle technique or after trocar insertion in the peritoneal cavity through a small, 1-cm periumbilical incision under direct vision **(Hasson technique)**. Other trocars (2, 5, or 10 mm) are then inserted, as necessary, under direct laparoscopic vision, avoiding abdominal wall vessels and internal organs.

Impalpable testis: If diagnostic laparoscopy reveals blind ending vessels, confirming the absence of a testis, the procedure is terminated and no inguinal incision is made. An inguinal testis remnant usually indicates either antenatal testicular ischemia or torsion. If the vessels are seen to enter the inguinal ring, the laparoscopy is ended and inguinal exploration is performed. If the testis is located intraabdominally, it is evaluated for size and location to determine whether to proceed to **orchiectomy** or a one- to two-stage (**Fowler Stevens**) **laparoscopic orchiopexy.** Laparoscopic ligation of the vessels may be done with placement of the testis into a scrotal pouch (**darto pouch**) in one stage, if adequate cord length permits. In other situations, **laparoscopic or open dissection** in the retroperitoneum may be performed. A 2nd-stage Fowler Stevens is performed after ligation of the gonadal vessels to allow adequate collateral vascular development before the intraabdominal testis is brought into the scrotum. Laparoscopic orchiectomy or **gonadectomy** also may be performed in intersex situations for a dysgenetic (streak), nonviable gonad, or for a gonad in which inadequate cord length exists.

Usual preop diagnosis: Nonpalpable testis; cryptorchidism

Varicocele ligation: Through a transperitoneal approach identical to that of the approach for diagnostic laparoscopy, the spermatic veins are isolated from the abdominal wall and are ligated with metallic clips to reduce the varicocele. The primary complications from this procedure are hydrocele and varicocele recurrence.

Usual preop diagnosis: Varicocele

Heminephrectomy, nephroureterectomy, and pyeloplasty: With the patient in the lateral-decubitus position, the initial trocar is inserted extraperitoneally on the anterior axillary line just below the 12th rib. The prone position has also been described for a retroperitoneal approach. Gas dissection is used to open the retroperitoneal space, and kidney dissection is performed. In a nephrectomy, the hilar vessels are ligated with metallic clips. The kidney is then retrieved through the 10-mm port by morcellating it or the incision can be dilated or elongated. Laparoscopic pyeloplasty is carried out using the same principles as open pyeloplasty, namely dismembering the ureter from the renal pelvis, spatulation of the ureter, and careful reassembly of the ureteropelvic unit.

Usual preop diagnosis: UPJ obstruction; infected or nonfunctioning kidney; HTN; multicystic or dysplastic kidney; protein-losing nephropathy in ESRD

Robotic vesicoureteral reimplantation: After initial cystoscopy to determine that there is adequate size for a robotic procedure, the patient is placed in a supine position with legs splayed. A urinary catheter is placed. At that time a Hassan port is placed through a midline incision one third of the way from the umbilicus to the pubis. The bladder is cleared and a balloon trocar is placed through a cystotomy into the bladder, followed by two robotic working ports. Adequate leg padding and solid securing of the patient to the bed are necessary. The robot is then docked, coming in from the direction of the patient's feet and the patient is dropped into the Trendelenburg position, which provides improved exposure of the pelvic organs, allowing bowel to drop away. At this point either extravesical or intravesical repair may be attempted. Primary complications following robotic reimplant include bladder leak, transient obstruction and persistent reflux.

Usual preop diagnosis: Vesicoureteral reflux

SUMMARY OF PROCEDURES

	Undescended Testis / Varicocele	Robotic Reimplant	Renal Surgery
Position	Supine; 15° Trendelenburg	Supine, legs splayed, Trendelenburg	Lateral decubitus
Incision	5–10-mm umbilical port + one or two additional ports	12-mm umbilical port and 5–8-mm working ports × 2	Four ports usually necessary
Special instrumentation	Bladder catheterization, NG tube	Cystoscopy, Bladder catheterization	⇐
Unique considerations	Secure child firmly to avoid movement with table tilting. Intraabdominal pressure = 14–16 mmHg. Lower pressure may be needed if pulmonary mechanics are compromised. Urethral catheter commonly placed.		⇐
Antibiotics	None	As necessary per preop urine culture	⇐
Surgical time	30 min to 1 h	3–5 h	2.5 h (nephrectomy) to 4 h (pyeloplasty)
EBL	Minimal	⇐	⇐
Postop care	PACU → home	PACU → ward	PACU → ward
Mortality	< 1%	⇐	⇐

SUMMARY OF PROCEDURE (cont'd)

	Undescended Testis / Varicocele	Robotic Reimplant	Renal Surgery
Morbidity	Overall: 0.6–5%	⇐	⇐
	Trocar misplacement: bowel perforation	⇐	⇐
	Vascular/organ thermal injury from electrocautery	⇐	⇐
	CO_2 embolus	⇐	Bleeding < 5%
	Grounding pad thermal injury	bladder leak	
	Trocar site bleeding, trocar hernia	transient obstruction	
	Varicocele only: Recurrent varicocele (1–11%), hydrocele (1–5%)	recurrent reflux	
Pain score	2	4	4

PATIENT POPULATION CHARACTERISTICS

Age range	10 mo–18 yr
Male:Female	Male (cryptorchidism)
Incidence	3% of newborn boys
Etiology	Congenital
Associated conditions	Renal insufficiency

ANESTHETIC CONSIDERATIONS

During mask induction care should be taken to avoid excessive positive pressure with consequent insufflation of the stomach. An OGT should be placed immediately after induction and intubation to remove air from the stomach, decreasing the risk of gastric puncture with placement of trochars, and improving surgical view during procedure. Creation of a pneumoperitoneum as part of a laparoscopic procedure impairs ventilation and can restrict venous return. The use of Trendelenburg and lithotomy positions can further worsen the respiratory changes that occur. Anesthetic considerations for pediatric patients undergoing laparoscopic procedures are further considered in 12.5 (Anesthesia for Minimally—Invasive Surgery in Pediatric Patients, p 1313). Severely limited patient access in robotic assisted surgery makes it difficult to respond to the patient. A practice trial maneuvering the cumbersome robotic equipment should be performed to ensure rapid access to the patient in case of emergency. Care should be taken not to move operating room table after robotic arm/instruments are placed in order to avoid patient injury.

Suggested Readings

1. Farber GJ, Bloom DA: Pediatric endourology. In *Adult and Pediatric Urology,* Vol 3, 3rd edition. Gillenwater JY, Grayhack JT, Howards, SS, et al, eds. Mosby-Year Book, St. Louis: 1996, 2739–47.
2. Mariano ER, Furukawa L, Woo RK, et al: Anesthetic concerns for robot-assisted laparoscopy in an infant. *Anesth Analg* 2004;99(6):1665–7.
3. McDougall EM, Gill IS, Clayman RV: Laparoscopic urology. In *Adult and Pediatric Urology,* Vol 1, 3rd edition. Gillenwater JY, Grayhack JT, Howards, SS, et al, eds. Mosby-Year Book, St. Louis: 1996, 829–912.
4. Peters CA: Robotically assisted surgery in pediatric urology. *Urol Clin N Am* 2007;31(4):743–752.
5. Sweeney DD, Smaldone MC, Docimio SG: Minimally invasive surgery for urologic disease in children. *Nat Clin Prac Urol* 2007;4(1):26–38.

CHAPTER

12.7 Pediatric Orthopedic Surgery

SURGEONS

James G. Gamble, MD, PhD
Lawrence A. Rinsky, MD
James Chang, MD
Amy L. Ladd, MD

ANESTHESIOLOGISTS

Komal Kamra, MD
Alice A. Edler, MD
R. J. Ramamurthi MD FRCA

PERCUTANEOUS PINNING OF DISPLACED SUPRACONDYLAR HUMERUS FRACTURE

SURGICAL CONSIDERATIONS

Description: Supracondylar fractures of the humerus are the most common elbow fractures in children, and the most common pediatric fractures requiring reduction under GA. They have a justifiable reputation for complications because of the risk to the brachial artery, and a high incidence of median or radial nerve palsies. The most serious potential complication is a compartment syndrome of the forearm, resulting in the need for emergency reduction and fasciotomy.

The vast majority of these injuries result from falling on an outstretched arm with the elbow extended elbow—a extremely common childhood event. Type 1 supracondylar fractures are minimally displaced and usually stable. They can be managed with a splint alone. Most supracondylar fractures are either Type 2 or Type 3 completely displaced fractures and require general anesthesia for **closed reduction and percutaneous pinning.**

Flexion type supracondylar fractures are more likely to require open reduction than extension type injuries.

Documentation of the neurovascular examination is mandatory immediately before anesthesia and upon awakening. If the neurovascular status is normal, and if the patient has eaten recently, it may be safe to wait 6–8 hours with continued monitoring of the neurovascular status. Reduction is obtained by a combination of traction and manipulation. Complete muscular relaxation is essential during the reduction maneuver. Usually two small, smooth, Kirschner wires are inserted under fluoroscopic control. Many surgeons prefer to use the intensifier screen as a platform; thus requiring the patient to be at the edge of the OR table. Occasionally, the fracture cannot be reduced closed, and an open reduction is necessary. In that case, the arm is reprepped and a small, lateral incision is made to openly visualize and reduce the fracture. The same type of smooth pin fixation is then used. Prolonged skeletal traction, although used

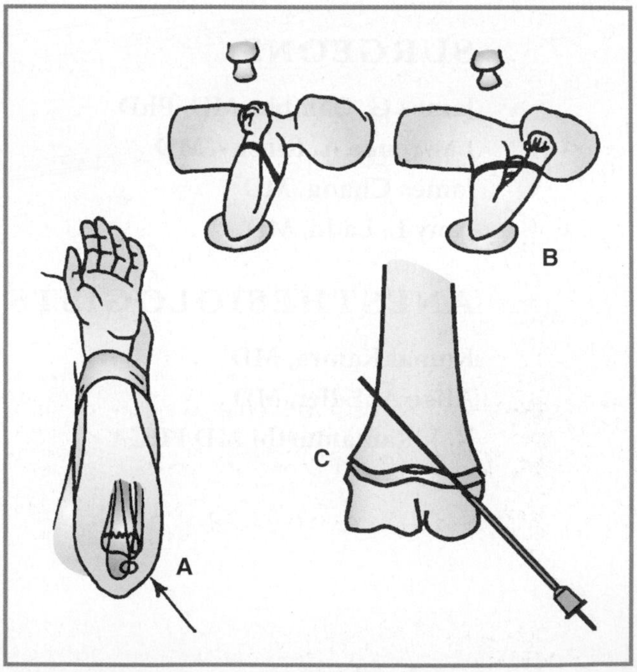

Figure 12.7-1. Percutaneous pinning of supracondylar humerus fracture. (**A**) The fracture is manually reduced and held with elbow flexed. (**B**) Fracture reduction is assessed with I.I. (**C**) The fracture is stabilized with percutaneous K-wires. (Reproduced with permission from Chapman MW: *Chapman's Orthopaedic Surgery,* 3rd edition. Lippincott Williams & Wilkins, Philadelphia: 2001.)

in the past, is rarely used and the standard of care is reduction and percutaneous pinning. Following the pinning, either a splint or well padded cast is applied before the patient is awakened.

Usual preop diagnosis: Supracondylar fracture of the elbow

SUMMARY OF PROCEDURES

	Percutaneous Pinning	Open Reduction
Position	Usually supine, occasionally prone or lateral	⇐
Incision	None	1" lateral
Special instrumentation	Power drill, image intensifier or FluoroScan	⇐
Unique considerations	Full-stomach; impending compartment syndrome	⇐
Antibiotics	Usually none	Cefazolin 25 mg/kg
Surgical time	30–60 min	30–90 min
Closing considerations	Cast or splint	⇐
EBL	Minimal	⇐
Postop care	PACU → room; close neurovascular monitoring	⇐
Mortality	Rare	⇐
Morbidity	Late angular deformity, especially cubitus varus: 10% Nerve palsy (typically radial nerve) from the fracture itself: 7% Compartment syndrome (Volkmann's contracture): < 0.5% (some degree of vascular spasm or loss of radial pulse much more common) Stiffness, myositis ossificans Ipsilateral fracture	⇐ ⇐ ⇐ ⇐ ⇐
Pain score	3–5	3–6

PATIENT POPULATION CHARACTERISTICS

Age range	3–10 years with peak age range of 5–8 yr.
Male:Female	1.6:1
Incidence	Frequent
Etiology	Trauma, usually a fall
Associated conditions	Usually normal, healthy child

ANESTHETIC CONSIDERATIONS

See Anesthetic Considerations for Upper Extremity Procedures, see p. 1353.

Suggested Readings

1. Bell C, Kain Z: Acute pediatric pain management. In *The Pediatric Anesthesia Handbook*. Mosby, St. Louis: 1997.
2. Dormans JP, Squillante R, Sharf H: Acute neurovascular complications with supracondylar humerus fractures in children. *J Hand Surg*; 1995;20(1):1–4.

3. Garbuz DS, Leitch K, Wright JG: The treatment of supracondylar fractures in children with an absent radial pulse. *J Pediatr Orthop* 1996;16(5):594–6.
4. Gordon JE, Patton CM, Luhmann SJ, et al: Fracture stability after pinning of displaced supracondylar distal humerus fractures in children. *J Pediatr Orthop* 2001;21(3):313–18.
5. Kasser JR, Beaty JH: Supracondylar fractures of the distal humerus. In *Fractures in Children.* Beaty JH, Kasser JR, eds. Lippincott-Raven, Philadelphia: 2001, 577–624.
6. Mehan ST, May CD, Kocher MS: Operative management of displaced flexion supracondylar humerus fractures in children. *J Pediatr Orthop* 2007;27:551–6.
7. Mehlman CT, Strub WM, Roy DR, et al: The effect of surgical timing on the perioperative complications of treatment of supracondylar humeral fractures in children. *J Bone Joint Surg Am* 2001;83A(3):323–7.
8. Otsuka NY, Kasser JR: Supracondylar fractures of the humerous in children. *J Am Acad Orthop Surg* 1997;5(l):19–26.
9. Pullerits J, Holzman R: Pediatric neuraxial blockade. *J Clin Anesth* 1993;5(4):342–54.
10. Salem MR, Klowden AS: Anesthesia for orthopaedic surgery. In *Pediatric Anesthesia,* 3rd edition. Gregory G, ed. Churchill Livingstone, New York: 1994, 607–56.
11. Shaw BA, Kasser JR, Emans JB, et al: Management of vascular injuries in displaced supracondylar humerus fractures without arteriography. *J Orthop Trauma* 1990;4(l):25–9.

CLOSED OR OPEN REDUCTION OF DISPLACED LATERAL CONDYLE HUMERUS FRACTURE

SURGICAL CONSIDERATIONS

Description: Lateral condylar fractures of the distal humerus are second only to supracondylar fractures in frequency. Initial radiographs of lateral condyle fractures can look deceptively normal; however, since these fractures cross the physis (growth plate) and enter the articular surface, they require anatomic reduction to restore joint surface congruity and to avoid a premature physeal arrest. In addition, the elbow may be unstable and dislocate if the fracture extends into the trochlea of the humerus. Accurate and stable reduction minimizes the risk of nonunion, a well-known complication resulting from unsuspected rotation of the fracture fragment and by traction forces of the extensor muscles attaching to this condyle. Unlike supracondylar fractures, neurovascular complications are rare with lateral condyle fractures.

Although minimally displaced fractures can be treated with a cast, 60% of lateral condyle fractures are displaced and require manipulation and pinning. Casting without manipulation, and thus requiring no anesthesia, is indicated for stable fractures that are displaced less than 2 mm. **Closed reduction and percutaneous pinning** under fluoroscopic control requires general anesthesia, and is indicated for stable fractures with 2–4 mm displacement. **Open reduction and pinning** is necessary for fractures that are unstable, rotated, or displaced more than 4 mm. Muscular relaxation is advantageous when performing either a closed or open reduction of the fracture. A sterile tourniquet is used for cases requiring open reduction.

Usual preoperative diagnosis: Displaced lateral condyle humerus fracture

SUMMARY OF PROCEDURES

	Closed Reduction/Pinning	Open Reduction/Pinning
Position	Supine	⇐
Incision	None	1–2" lateral
Instrumentation	Power drill, fluoroscopy	⇐
Unique considerations	None	⇐
Antibiotics	Usually none	Cefazolin 25 mg/kg
Surgical time	30–60 min	45–90 min

SUMMARY OF PROCEDURE (cont'd)		
	Closed Reduction/Pinning	**Open Reduction/Pinning**
Closing considerations	Cast or splint	⇐
EBL	Negligible	⇐
Postoperative care	PACU → room	⇐
Mortality	Rare	⇐
Morbidity	Delayed or nonunion Cubitus valgus (more common) or varus Lateral condylar overgrowth Physeal arrest Osteonecrosis of lateral trochlea Ulnar nerve palsy	⇐ ⇐ ⇐ ⇐ ⇐ ⇐ Avascular necrosis of trochlea
Pain score	3–5	3–6

PATIENT POPULATION CHARACTERISTICS	
Age range	5–10 yr; average = 6 yr
Incidence	15% of all elbow fractures; more common in summer
Etiology	Trauma
Associated conditions	Usually normal, healthy child

ANESTHETIC CONSIDERATIONS

See Anesthetic Considerations for Upper Extremity Procedures, see p 1353.

Suggested Readings

1. Foster DE, Sullivan JA, Gross RH: Lateral humeral condylar fractures in children. *J Pediatr Orthop* 1985; 5(1):16–22.
2. Launay F, Leet AI, Jacopin S, et al: Lateral humeral condyle fractures in children: a comparison of two approaches to treatment. *J Pediatr Orthop* 2004; 24:385–91.
3. Mintzer CM, Waters PM, Brown DJ, et al: Percutaneous pinning in the treatment of displaced lateral condyle fractures. *J Pediatr Orthop* 1994; 14(4):462–5.
4. Thomas DP, Howard AW, Cole WG, et al: Three weeks of Kirschner wire fixation for displaced lateral condylar fractures of the humerus in children. *J Pediatr Orthop* 2001; 21(5):565–9.

ASPIRATION AND INJECTION OF UNICAMERAL BONE CYST

SURGICAL CONSIDERATIONS

Description: Unicameral bone cysts (UBC) are benign lesions typically located in the metaphyseal regions of long bones, most commonly in the proximal humerus of a growing child. The cyst is rarely a source of pain until presentation (typically after a fracture). The benign radiographic appearance allows clinicians to follow most lesions without the need for surgical biopsy. Surgical care is indicated when the UBC is of sufficient size and location to cause mechanical weakening of the bone and predispose to a pathologic fracture. The goals of surgical care are to confirm the diagnosis of UBC and to reestablish the mechanical integrity of the bone. Diagnosis of a UBC is made by percutaneous aspiration of the lesion, using a standard 16–18-gauge spinal needle under general anesthesia. Fluoroscopic guidance facilitates needle placement. The presence of clear, straw-colored fluid confirms diagnosis of UBC. An alternative diagnosis, such as aneurismal bone cyst, is more likely if frank blood is aspirated. If the lesion contains no fluid, it may be a nonossifying fibroma.

Open biopsy may be necessary if the diagnosis is unclear. However, most cases can be treated adequately with percutaneous aspiration and injection of a radiopaque dye to verify that the entire cavity is contiguous. If the cystic cavity is loculated by bony trabecula, a **curette** or **percutaneous Kirschner** wire is used to convert the lesion into a unicompartmental space so the subsequent injection will easily access the entire lesion. Scraping the inner cyst walls also helps to disrupt the cyst lining and is thought to improve the chance of filling in the cavity. The final surgical step is to introduce a second 'venting' needle into the cyst to allow lavage with sterile saline, followed by injection of the cavity with a substance to promote new bone formation. Historically, methylprednisolone has been used, but more recent evidence suggests a higher success rate when autologous bone marrow is injected. **Injectable allograft bone** preparations also can supplement the bone marrow injection. Care must be taken to avoid aspirating from the first needle after the second has been placed, to avoid intraosseous air embolism.

Usual preoperative diagnosis: Unicameral bone cyst

SUMMARY OF PROCEDURES

	Percutaneous	Open
Position	Supine	⇐
Incision	None	Length of cyst
Instrumentation	Spinal needles, Kershner wires, I.I.	Curettes
Unique considerations	Risk of air embolus	Additional time for intraop pathology evaluation
Antibiotics	Usually none	Cefazolin 25 mg/kg
Surgical time	30–60 min	60–90 min
Closing considerations	None	Cast or splint
EBL	Minimal	⇐
Postop care	PACU → home	PACU → room/home
Mortality	Rare	⇐
Morbidity	Infection Iatrogenic fracture Growth arrest: rare	⇐ ⇐ ⇐
Pain score	0–2	3–6

PATIENT POPULATION CHARACTERISTICS

Age range	5–15 yr; not found in adults
Male:Female	1:3
Incidence	20% of benign bone lesions; most common location is the proximal humerus (67%), followed by the proximal femur (15%)
Etiology	Unknown. Venous obstruction → fluid transudate containing high levels of interleukin-1 and interleukin-6, which stimulate osteoclasts
Associated conditions	Usually normal, healthy child. Initial presentation typically follows a pathologic fracture.

ANESTHETIC CONSIDERATIONS

See Anesthetic Considerations for Upper Extremity Procedures, see p. 1353.

Suggested Readings

1. Alvarez RG, Arnold JM.: Arthroscopic assistance in minimally invasive curettage and bone grafting of a calcaneal unicameral bone cyst. *Foot Ankle Int* 2007;28:1198–99.
2. Bensahel H, Jehanno P, Desgrippes Y, et al: Solitary bone cyst: controversies and treatment. *J Pediatr Orthop* 1998;7(4): 257–61.
3. Killian JT, Wilkenson L, White S, et al: Treatment of unicameral bone cyst with demineralized bone matrix. *J Pediatr Orthop* 1998;18(5):621–4.
4. Rougraff BT, Kling TJ: Treatment of active unicameral bone cysts with percutaneous injection of demineralized bone matrix and autogenous bone marrow. *J Bone Joint Surg* 2002;84A(6):921–9.
5. Yandow SM, Lundeen GA, Scott SM, et al: Autogenic bone marrow injections as a treatment for simple bone cyst. *J Pediatr Orthop* 1998;18(5):616–20.

RELEASE FOR TORTICOLLIS

SURGICAL CONSIDERATIONS

Description: **Congenital muscular torticollis** is a painless tilting of the head due to contracture of the sternocleidomastoid muscle. The head tilts toward the involved side and rotates toward the opposite side (a "cocked-robin" posture such that the chin points to the opposite side). It is associated with breech and difficult deliveries, as well as other musculoskeletal disorders, such as metatarsus adductus, hip dysplasia, and talipes equinovarus. Multiple theories regarding the etiology of congenital muscular torticollis have been proposed, including fibrosis of the sternocleidomastoid muscle following a peripartum intramuscular bleed, fibrosis resulting from a compartment syndrome of the sternocleidomastoid muscle, intrauterine crowding, and a primary myopathy of the sternocleidomastoid muscle. Eighty percent of cases of torticollis are a result of this congenital contracture of the sternocleidomastoid muscle. Less common etiologies—such as congenital cervical spine malformations (e.g., Klippel-Feil syndrome), neurologic disorders, a cranial or cervical neoplasm, inflammatory conditions (e.g., Grisel's syndrome), or an ocular dysfunction—should also be excluded. Congenital muscular torticollis is seen more frequently on the right side. A persistent torticollis will lead to skull and facial deformities (plagiocephaly). If the child sleeps prone, he will usually lie with the affected side down, resulting in flattening of the face on that side. If the child sleeps supine, flattening of the contralateral skull occurs. This plagiocephaly will become permanent if the torticollis persists and is left untreated.

Initial treatment includes physical therapy for stretching exercises. For children less than 1 year of age, a program of sternocleidomastoid muscle stretching is recommended, with 90% of cases being resolved with this treatment. After 2 years of age, nonoperative treatment is not likely to be effective. Children with persistent torticollis and an unacceptable amount of facial asymmetry preferably are treated surgically before the age of 3 years; however, some improvement in facial asymmetry has been shown even in children surgically treated up to 8 years of age.

Surgical options include a **unipolar release,** a **bipolar release, middle-third transection,** or a **complete resection.** Unipolar release involves division of the distal insertion of the sternocleidomastoid muscle and usually is performed for a mild deformity. Bipolar release entails division of both the sternocleidomastoid origin and insertion, and usually is done for more marked involvement. **Z-plasty** of the clavicular head or transfer of the clavicular head to the sternal head may be done to maintain a more normal cosmetic contour of the neck. Potential surgical complications include injury to the spinal accessory nerve, jugular veins, carotid vessels, and the facial nerve. Postop, patients may perform simple stretching exercises, but they often require bracing to maintain a corrected alignment.

Usual preoperative diagnosis: Congenital muscular torticollis

SUMMARY OF PROCEDURES		
	Unipolar	**Bipolar**
Position	Supine	⇐
Incision	Transverse, 1.5 cm superior to sternum and clavicle over muscle insertion	⇐ + 1 cm distal to mastoid process behind ear at muscle origin
Unique considerations	Plagiocephaly	⇐
Antibiotics	Cefazolin 25 mg/kg	⇐
Surgical time	30 min	45 min
EBL	Minimal	⇐
Postoperative care	PACU → room/home	⇐
Mortality	Rare	⇐
Morbidity	Hypertrophic scar Loss of normal muscle contour	⇐ ⇐ Spinal accessory nerve injury
Pain score	3–5	3–5

PATIENT POPULATION CHARACTERISTICS	
Age range	Onset at birth, surgery after age 1 yr
Male:Female	1:1
Incidence	1/500
Etiology	Fibrosis of sternocleidomastoid; possible intrauterine or perinatal muscle compartment syndrome
Associated conditions	Usually normal, healthy child; hip dysplasia in 20%

ANESTHETIC CONSIDERATIONS

See Anesthetic Considerations for Upper Extremity Procedures, see p. 1353.

Suggested Readings

1. Ballock RT, Song KM: The prevalence of nonmuscular causes of torticollis in children. *J Pediatr Orthop* 1996; 16(4):500–4.
2. Davids JR, Wenger DR, Mubarak SJ: Congenital muscular torticollis: sequela of intrauterine or perinatal compartment syndrome. *J Pediatr Orthop* 1993;13(2):141–7.
3. Ferkel RD, Westin GW, Dawson EG, et al: Muscular torticollis: a modified surgical approach. *J Bone Joint Surg* 1983;65A: 894–900.
4. Von Heideken J, Green DW, Burke SW, et al: The relationship between developmental dysplasia of the hip and congenital muscular torticollis. *J Pediatr Orthop* 2006;26:805–8.
5. Wirth CJ, Hagena FW, Wuelker N, et al: Biterminal tenotomy for the treatment of congenital muscular torticollis. Long-term results. *J Bone Joint Surg Am* 1992;74(3):427–34.

POLLICIZATION OF A FINGER

SURGICAL CONSIDERATIONS

Description: This procedure is indicated in the infant with congenital absence or hypoplasia of the thumb. A normal finger—usually the index finger—with its tendon, nerve, and vascular supply is shortened and rotated into the position of the thumb (Fig. 12.7-2). Tendon transfers are performed to substitute for the absent or hypoplastic thenar muscles. These patients may have many other associated congenital anomalies, which should be ruled out prior to surgery.

Variant procedure or approaches: There are several different surgical techniques, which share the basic transposition and rotation of the finger to the thumb position.

Usual preop diagnosis: Aplastic thumb; hypoplastic thumb; radial club hand; radial longitudinal deficiency

SUMMARY OF PROCEDURE

Position	Supine, with arm extended on hand-surgery table
Incision	Multiple incisions on the hand
Special instrumentation	Pneumatic tourniquet; magnification loupes
Antibiotics	Cefazolin 25 mg/kg (children)
Surgical time	3–4 h
Tourniquet	100 mmHg above systolic; max time = 120 min
Closing considerations	Complex skin flaps are necessary. A plaster splint is placed while the patient is still anesthetized.
EBL	Minimal; performed under tourniquet control.
Postop care	PACU → overnight admission for observation or perfusion to the transposed finger
Mortality	Minimal
Morbidity	Ischemia (loss of digit): Rare Skin flap necrosis: Moderately common
Pain score	1–2

PATIENT POPULATION CHARACTERISTICS

Age range	1–2 yr is ideal time for surgery. Procedure should be done before patient begins school.
Male:Female	1:1
Incidence	Overall, about 1/20,000 live births require a variant of this procedure.
Etiology	Unknown; also associated with thalidomide ingestion.
Associated conditions	Associated congenital anomalies of the upper extremity, esophagus, spine, and lower extremities Absence of radius (radial club hand), common Various forms of syndactylies, common Abnormalities of the hematopoietic system (Fanconi's syndrome), cardiovascular system (ASDs in Holt-Oram syndrome), spine, and GI system, along with hypothyroidism, are frequently associated.

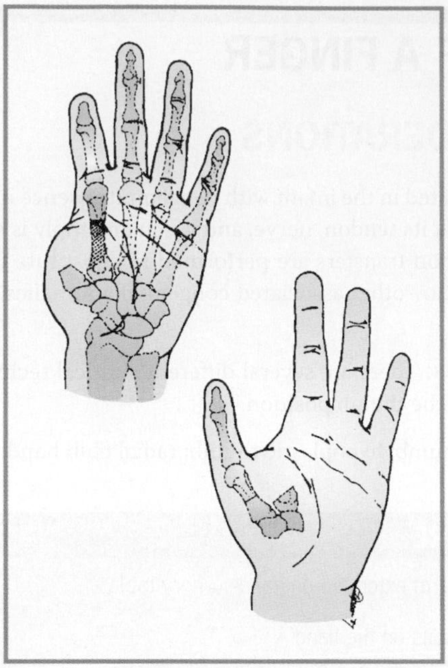

Figure 12.7-2. Pollicization of a finger. (Reproduced with permission from Chapman MW: *Chapman's Orthopaedic Surgery,* 3rd edition. Lippincott Williams & Wilkins, Philadelphia: 2001.)

ANESTHETIC CONSIDERATIONS

See Anesthetic Considerations for Upper Extremity Procedures, see p. 1353.

Suggested Reading

1. Light TR: Amputations of the hand. In *Chapman's Orthopaedic Surgery,* Vol 2, 3rd edition. Chapman MW, ed. Lippincott Williams & Wilkins, Philadelphia: 2001, 1454–5.

SYNDACTYLY REPAIR

SURGICAL CONSIDERATIONS

Description: Syndactyly refers to congenital failure of separation of two or more fingers. It is complete if it extends to the ends of the fingers; incomplete syndactyly extends short of the finger ends. A **simple syndactyly repair** joins fingers by only skin and fibrous tissues. A **complex syndactyly repair** signifies fusion of adjacent phalanges or interposition of accessory phalanges, with frequent abnormalities of the neurovascular structures. Surgical separation is performed in the first few years of life for functional, as well as aesthetic reasons. The technique involves creation of a dorsal, proximally based skin flap to recreate the web. A zigzag dorsal and palmar incision is then created, separating from the distal end in a proximal direction. The digital nerve and arteries are dissected proximally as far as possible. Primary closure is almost never possible, and supplemental full-thickness skin graft harvested from the groin is used to complete the closure. Usually only one site is done at a time per hand; and, never should both sides of a digit be released, because of risk to the vascular supply. It is not always possible to save all the bony elements. Patients with conditions such as Apert syndrome must undergo careful evaluation of the airway.

Usual preop diagnosis: Syndactyly of fingers; bifid finger, thumb/finger

SUMMARY OF PROCEDURE	
Position	Supine
Incision	Zigzag between digits; skin graft donor site from groin
Special instrumentation	Magnification loupes always necessary. Tourniquet is mandatory.
Unique considerations	Groin skin also must be taken for graft closure.
Antibiotics	Usually none
Surgical time	2–4 h
Closing considerations	Above-the-elbow cast or splint to keep incision away from mouth and other hand of the infant or child
EBL	20 mL
Postop care	PACU → home, if simple syndactyly
Mortality	None associated with procedure.
Morbidity	Partial slough of flaps or skin graft requiring revision Scarring and some stiffness of fingers Angulatory deformities late, occasionally depending on degree of involvement of the skeleton and joint
Pain score	1–3

PATIENT POPULATION CHARACTERISTICS	
Age range	6 mo–5 yr
Male:Female	2:1
Incidence	1/2,000 births (the most common significant congenital hand anomaly)
Etiology	Family Hx (10–40%); failure of differentiation in the 6th–8th wk of intrauterine life
Associated conditions	Polydactyly, accessory phalanges; Apert syndrome; Poland syndrome

ANESTHETIC CONSIDERATIONS

See Anesthetic Considerations for Upper Extremity Procedures, see p 1353.

Suggested Readings

1. Bauer TB, Tondra JM, Trusler HM: Technical modification in repair of syndactylism. *Plast Reconstr Surg* 1956;17:385–92.
2. Chang J, Danton TK, Ladd AL, et al: Reconstruction of the hand in Apert's syndrome: a simplified approach. *Plast Reconstr Surg* 2002;109(2):465–70.
3. Ezaki M, Kay SP, et al: In *Green's Operative Hand Surgery.* Green DP, Hotchkiss RN, Pederson WC, eds. Churchill Livingstone, Philadelphia: 1993, 325.

ANESTHETIC CONSIDERATIONS FOR UPPER EXTREMITY PROCEDURES

(Procedures covered: percutaneous pinning; displaced supracondylar humerus fracture; closed/open reduction; displaced lateral condylar humerus fracture; aspiration/injection unicameral/bone cyst; torticollis release; pollicization of finger; syndactyly release)

PREOPERATIVE

The majority of children presenting for repair of upper extremity fractures are otherwise healthy. Most of these patients present for repair of a traumatic injury; thus, the preop workup is routine. Some arm procedures, such as repair of a compound fracture, require immediate attention and necessitate emergency surgery and full-stomach considerations (see p. B-4).

Laboratory	Tests as indicated from H&P.
Premedication	Standard premedication (see p. D-1).

INTRAOPERATIVE

Anesthetic technique: GETA or LMA, since small children rarely tolerate regional anesthesia alone. In the older patient, regional anesthesia may be appropriate, and can reduce the risk of aspiration pneumonitis associated with GA in the patient with a full stomach. A combined technique offers the advantages of reduced anesthetic requirements and postop pain relief; however, regional anesthesia is relatively contraindicated in patients with neurovascular damage.

General anesthesia:

Induction	Standard induction (see p. D-1) except in acute-trauma patients, where rapid-sequence induction is appropriate (see p. B-5).
Maintenance	Standard maintenance (see p. D-3).
Emergence	Management of emergence and extubation should be routine, except in difficult airway cases, which require awake extubation. Skin closure is frequently followed by application of a splint; patient should remain anesthetized during splinting procedure.

Regional anesthesia:

Ultrasound guidance: Ultrasound-guided nerve block techniques are increasingly used in the pediatric anesthesia. The use of ultrasonography increases the ability to position the needle as close to the nerve as possible avoiding inadvertent trauma to the adjacent structures. Direct visualization also helps in optimizing the volume and distribution of the local anesthetic thus improving the safety and efficacy of the block.

Anesthetics and doses	See Table 12.7-1.
Interscalene block	Phrenic nerve block → hemidiaphragm paralysis is an inevitable consequence of the interscalene block. Major complications (e.g., total spinal or pneumothorax) resulting from interscalene block are very rare; therefore, this technique is suitable for outpatients. Interscalene block is contraindicated in patients with contralateral recurrent laryngeal nerve or phrenic nerve palsy.
Infraclavicular block	The infraclavicular approach to brachial plexus block has the advantage of blocking the axillary and musculocutaneous nerves. The coracoid approach is shown to be safer than the classical approach. Use of ultrasonography increases the efficacy and safety of this block.
Axillary block	The medial aspect of the upper arm is innervated by the intercostobrachial nerve (T2) and requires a separate subcutaneous field block in the axilla, especially when a tourniquet is used. The lateral cutaneous nerve of the forearm, a sensory branch of the musculocutaneous nerve supplying sensation to the lateral forearm, is frequently missed by the axillary approach to the brachial plexus. Thus, a block of this nerve at the elbow is sometimes necessary. The dose volume of local anesthetic required varies with the height and weight of the child. As a rule, the child's body surface area can be used as an approximate proportion of the usual adult volume (e.g., a 1.7 M^2 adult will require 40 mL of local anesthetic; a 1 M^2 patient requires 20–25 mL). Care must be taken to avoid local anesthetic overdose (see Table 12.7-1).

Table 12.7-1. Maximum Recommended Doses of Ansthetics for Regional Anesthesia

Drug	mg/kg (*with epinephrine)	Duration (min)
Lidocaine	5 (*7)	45–180
Bupivicaine	2.5 (*3)	180–600
Ropivacaine	3	180–600
Tetracaine	1.5	180–600
2-Chloroprocaine	8 (*10)	30–60
Procaine	8 (*10)	60–90

Supplemental sedation	Supplemental sedation may be accomplished with use of propofol by continuous infusion (50–150 mcg/kg/min).	
Blood and fluid requirements	Minimal blood loss IV: 20 ga × 1 NS/LR @ 1.5–3 mL/kg/h	IV catheter should be placed in the contralateral upper extremity.
Monitoring	Standard monitors (see p. D-1).	
Positioning	✓ and pad pressure points. ✓ eyes.	
Interscalene block complications	Total spinal Epidural anesthesia IV injection (Sz/dysrhythmias) Stellate ganglion block (Horner's syndrome) Laryngeal nerve block Phrenic nerve block Pneumothorax	Resuscitative equipment, including airway management tools, should be immediately available.
Infraclavicular block complications	Hematoma Pneumothorax Inadvertent intravascular injection	The coracoid approach has reduced risk of complications.
Axillary block complications	Inadequate block Intravascular injection Peripheral nerve damage Axillary hematoma Axillary artery thrombosis Pneumothorax	Very minimal doses of local anesthetic can cause CNS toxicity if reverse flow occurs during an intraarterial injection. Axillary thrombosis and pneumothorax are extremely rare.

POSTOPERATIVE

Pain management	PCA (see p. E-4). Regional block	Combined regional-GA provides excellent postop pain management.
Tests	None routinely indicated.	

Suggested Readings

1. Marhofer P, Greher M, Kapral S: Ultrasound guidance in regional anaesthesia. *Br J Anaesth.* 2005;94(1):7–17.
2. Marhofer P, Sitzwohl C, Greher M, et al: Ultrasound guidance for infraclavicular brachial plexus anesthesia in children. *Anaesthesia* 2004;59:642–6.

POSTERIOR SPINAL INSTRUMENTATION AND FUSION

SURGICAL CONSIDERATIONS

Description: **Posterior spinal instrumentation** refers to implanted metal rods affixed to the spine to correct and internally splint the deformed spine. Originally designed for scoliosis, posterior spinal instrumentation is commonly performed simultaneously with **spinal fusion** for a variety of diagnoses, including fracture, tumor, degenerative changes, and developmental spinal deformity. Although posterior spinal instrumentation with the ratcheted **Harrington rod** gained widespread usage in the 1970s, it is no longer used by spinal surgeons. The current standard is a hook-rod system, such as the **Cotrel-Duboussett** (C-D), the **Texas Scottish Rite Hospital** (TSRH), the **Miami Modular Orthopaedic Spinal System** (MOSS) and the **Universal Spine System** (USS). Regardless of the surgeon's choice of instrumentation, the spine is approached by an extensive midline posterior incision, in which a subperiosteal exposure (typically T2-5 down to L1-4) is used to elevate all the paraspinous muscles as far laterally as the tips of the transverse processes. Typically, 4–8 hooks are affixed to the posterior spinal elements (lamina, pedicles, or transverse processes) on both the concave and convex sides of the spine (Figure 12.7-3). These points of spinal fixation are then joined to two contoured rods. By compressing along the convex surfaces and distracting along the concave surfaces, some degree of rotational correction is possible. Some spine surgeons advise the patient to wear a brace for the initial months following surgery; however, body casts are no longer necessary.

Sublaminar wire loops (Fig. 12.7-4) are commonly used instead of the hook-rod method of spinal instrumentation when treating neuromuscular spinal deformity (e.g., cerebral palsy, muscular dystrophy, myelomeningocele, or spinal muscular atrophy). This alternative construct provides more points of fixation to the spine and eliminates the need for postop bracing. When a large degree of pelvic obliquity is a component of the patient's deformity, the instrumentation often is extended into the iliac wings (Fig. 12-7.5).

Somatosensory evoked potentials (SSEP) and **motor evoked potentials** (MEP) are used routinely in centers where spinal deformity correction surgery is common. Close coordination among the surgeon, spinal cord monitoring personnel, and anesthesiologist is necessary to properly recognize adverse intraop spinal events and to minimize the occurrence of false-positive findings. Many spine surgeons also request that an intraop wake-up test be performed to further verify spinal cord function.

Usual preop diagnosis: Scoliosis (usually idiopathic or neuromuscular); kyphosis (increased round back); reconstruction for tumor, trauma, or other.

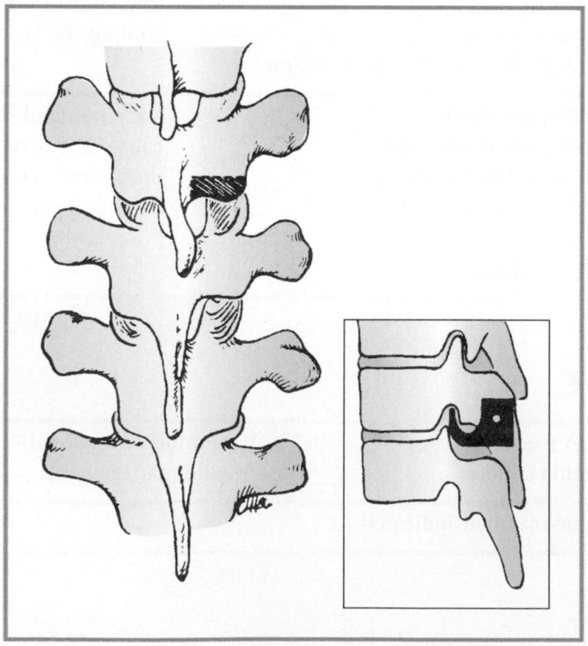

Figure 12.7-3. Placement of a standard pedicle hook, in a hood-rod device. (Reproduced with permission from Chapman MW, ed: *Operative Orthopaedics,* 3rd edition. Lippincott Williams & Wilkins, Philadelphia: 2001.)

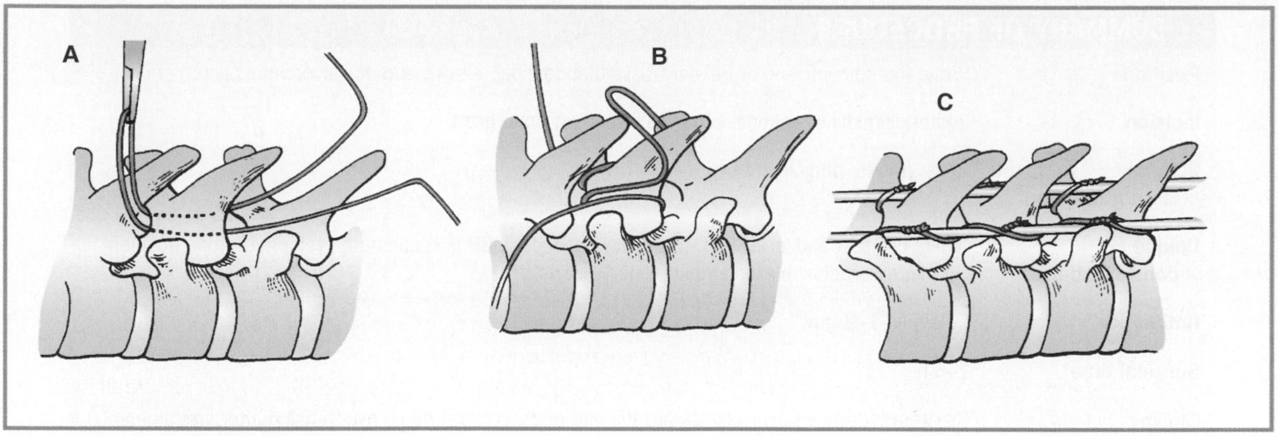

Figure 12.7-4. An example of passing and attaching sublaminar wires. (Reproduced with permission from Chapman MW, ed: *Operative Orthopaedics,* 3rd edition. Lippincott Williams & Wilkins, Philadelphia: 2001.)

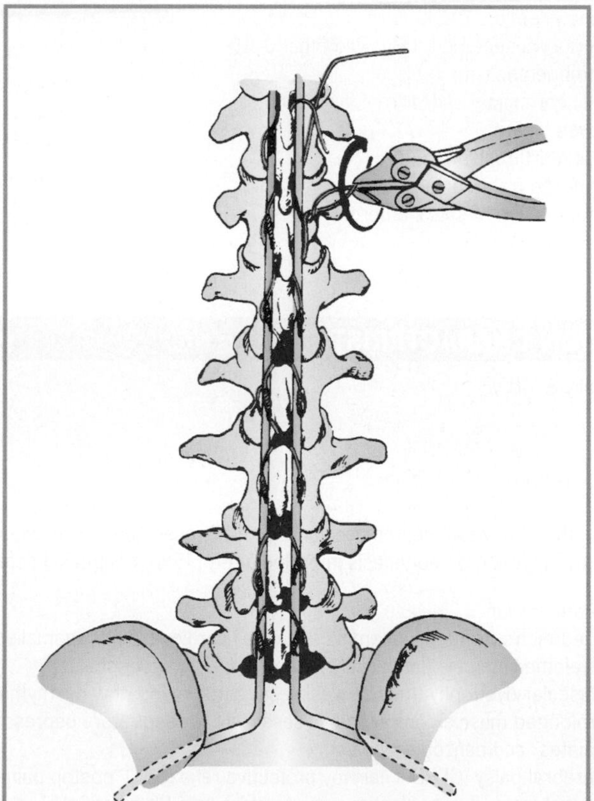

Figure 12.7-5. Positioning rods in pelvis; sublaminar wires being tightened. (Reproduced with permission from Chapman MW, ed: *Operative Orthopaedics,* 3rd edition. Lippincott Williams & Wilkins, Philadelphia: 2001.)

SUMMARY OF PROCEDURE

Position	Prone (on spinal frame or bolsters); avoid abdominal, elbow, and ocular compression.
Incision	Posterior midline; optional separate iliac crest bone graft
Special instrumentation	Rods, hooks, pedicle screws, wires
Unique considerations	"Wake up" test and/or SSEPs; frequently, induced ↓ BP is requested; prolonged prone positioning places brachial plexus and ulnar nerve at risk.
Antibiotics	Cefazolin 1–2 g iv
Surgical time	2–6 h
Closing considerations	Greatest blood loss typically toward the end of procedure. Avoid hypotension after instrumentation is implanted.
EBL	1,200–3,000 mL
Postop care	ICU: 1–2 d
Mortality	0–0.5%
Morbidity	Acute ileus: Very common Genitourinary infection: 5–7% Hematoma, massive bleeding: 1–5% Pneumothorax, pneumonia, atelectasis: 1–5% Hook dislodgement requiring reoperation: 0–2% Wound infection: 0–2% Superior mesenteric artery syndrome: 0–1% Thromboembolism: < 1% Spinal cord injury and/or root injury: 0.6% Delayed: Pseudarthrosis: 0–5% Late rod fracture: 0–5% Progression of spinal deformity: 0–2%
Pain score	7–9

PATIENT POPULATION CHARACTERISTICS

Age range	Usually 8–40 yr
Male:Female	1:5
Incidence	1–2/10,000
Etiology	Idiopathic (50–75%); neuromuscular (20–30%); associated with syndromes such as osteochondral dystrophies, osteogenesis imperfecta, etc. (5%); congenital scoliosis (2–5%)
Associated conditions	*Neuromuscular:* Friedreich's ataxia (myocarditis and other cardiovascular anomalies; sudden death) Myelomeningocele (latex allergy, chronic UTI, hydrocephalus) Muscular dystrophy (muscle weakness, cardiomyopathy, dysrhythmias, succinylcholine → prolonged muscle contraction, ↑ sensitivity to respiratory depressant effect of barbiturates, opiates, and benzodiazepines) Cerebral palsy (GERD,↓ ;airway protective reflexes, ↑ postop pulmonary complications, malnourishment, Sz, medication may interfere with Plt function) Higher incidence of MH *Connective tissue disease:* Ehlers-Danlos and Marfan syndromes (avoid ↑ BP → aortic dissection; ↑ risk of pneumothorax). Osteogenesis imperfecta (position and intubate with great care). Congenital osteochondral dystrophies

ANESTHETIC CONSIDERATIONS

See Anesthetic Considerations for Spinal Reconstruction and Fusion, (see p. 971).

Suggested Readings

1. Auerbach JD, Lonner BS, Antonacci MD, et al: Perioperative outcomes and complications related to teaching residents and fellows in scoliosis surgery. *Spine* 2008;33(10):1113–8.
2. Bridwell KHL: Spinal instrumentation in the management of adolescent scoliosis. *Clin Orthop* 1997;335:64–72.
3. Borgeat A, Blumenthal S: Postoperative pain management following scoliosis surgery. *Curr Opin Anaesthesiol* 2008;21(3): 313–6.
4. Dubousset J, Cotrel Y: Application technique of Cotrel-Dubousset instrumentation for scoliosis deformities. *Clin Orthop* 1991;264:103–10.
5. Heller KD, Wirtz DC, Siebert CH, et al: Spinal stabilization in Duchenne muscular dystrophy: principles of treatment and record of 31 operative treated cases. *J Pediatr Orthop* 2001;10(1):18–24.
6. Thomson JD, Banta JV: Scoliosis in cerebral palsy: an overview and recent results. *J Pediatr Orthop* 2001;10(1):6–9.
7. Torre-Healy A, Samdani AF: Newer technologies for the treatment of scoliosis in the growing spine. *Neurosurg Clin N Am* 2007;18(4):697–705.

ANTERIOR SPINAL FUSION FOR SCOLIOSIS

SURGICAL CONSIDERATIONS

Description: **Anterior spinal fusion** is performed through a transthoracic and/or retroperitoneal approach to the vertebral bodies, in which the intervertebral discs are removed and a bone graft is placed between the vertebral bodies. The disc removal ("release") loosens the spine and allows greater deformity correction than posterior-only procedures. Often, no instrumentation is used anteriorly when the anterior fusion is performed as a first stage to a "front-and-back" fusion. (In such cases, posterior spinal instrumentation is subsequently implanted to correct the spinal deformity.) Anterior spinal instrumentation is performed when a posterior spinal fusion is not needed (e.g., idiopathic thoracolumbar or lumbar scoliosis).

When **instrumentation of the anterior spine** is performed, the surgical approach is through a flank incision, then through a rib bed on the convex side of the curve (usually the 10th rib). The retroperitoneal plane is entered and developed by blunt dissection behind the transversus abdominis muscle. The pleural cavity is entered, and the diaphragm usually must be divided circumferentially near its costal origin and around posteriorly to the spine. The prevertebral areolar plane is then entered and the segmental vessels to each vertebral body are clipped or cauterized in the midline. The psoas muscle is elevated off the lateral aspects of the vertebral bodies. Each disc in the fusion area (usually 3–5 discs) is excised back to the posterior longitudinal ligament. Next, vertebral screws (e.g., **Texas Scottish Rite Hospital** [TSRH], **Miami Modular Orthopaedic Spine System** [MOSS], **Universal Spine System** [USS] instrumentation) are inserted transversely across the appropriate bodies and joined at their heads by a rod (Figs 12.7-6 and 12.7-7). Bone graft (typically from the rib harvested during the surgical approach) is placed within each discectomy level. A chest tube is placed before closure of the thoracic cavity.

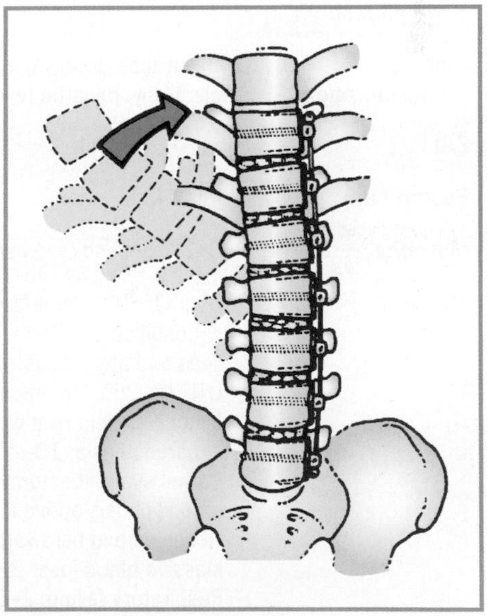

Figure 12.7-6. Dwyer instrumentation used to make spinal correction. (Reproduced with permission from Crenshaw AH, ed: *Campbell's Operative Orthopaedics,* 8th edition. Mosby-Year Book, St. Louis: 1992.)

Usual preop diagnosis: Idiopathic or neuromuscular scoliosis

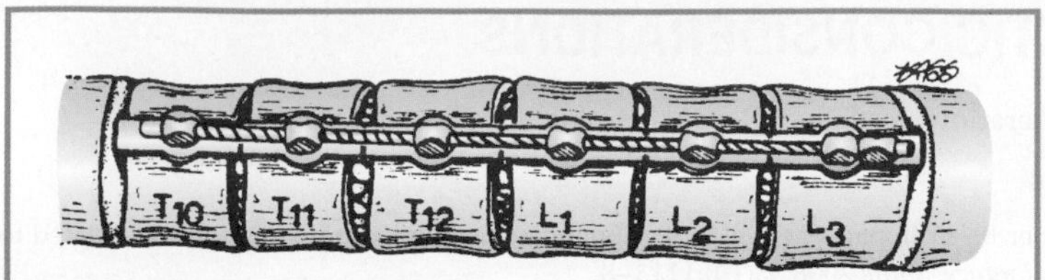

Figure 12.7-7. Instrumentation from T10-L3 (Zielke). (Reproduced with permission from Chapman MW,ed: *Operative Orthopaedics,* 3rd edition. Lippincott Williams & Wilkins, Philadelphia: 2001.)

SUMMARY OF PROCEDURES

	Fusion with Instrumentation	Release (No Instrumentation)
Position	Full lateral decubitus (Fig. 12.7-8)	⇐
Incision	Flank: over rib at top vertebra in the curve (usually T9-T11)	⇐
Special instrumentation	Screws, staples, rods	None
Unique considerations	Flex OR table at thoracolumbar junction until disc removal and deformity correction. Procedure often followed by posterior spinal fusion. Proximity of great vessels → potential for major bleeding. Patients with neuromuscular scoliosis often have poor generalized nutrition. SSEP/MEP often used to monitor spinal cord function.	⇐ Uninstrumented release is always followed by posterior spinal fusion with instrumentation.
Antibiotics	Cefazolin 25 mg/kg iv	⇐
Surgical time	3–4 h	2–3 h
Closing considerations	Chest tube always used; hypotension, if used electively, must be reversed before closure.	⇐
EBL	500–2,000 mL	250–2,000 mL
Postop care	ICU 1–2 d	⇐
Mortality	0–2%, depending on underlying conditions	⇐
Morbidity	Overall: 30%, depending on underlying condition	20%
	Ileus and atelectasis: ~50%	⇐
	UTI: 10–25% (common in spina bifida)	⇐
	Minor transient root weakness, or paraesthesia: 10–20%	1–5%
	Partial sympathectomy: Common	⇐
	Late kyphosis above instrumentation: 5–10%	–
	Nonunion and hardware failure: 5%	–
	Massive blood loss: 2–5%	⇐
	Respiratory failure: 1–2%	⇐
	Pneumonia: 1%	⇐
	Paraplegia (acute anterior spinal artery syndrome): <1%	⇐
	Thromboembolism: Rare (<5% in children)	⇐
Pain score	5–8	4–7

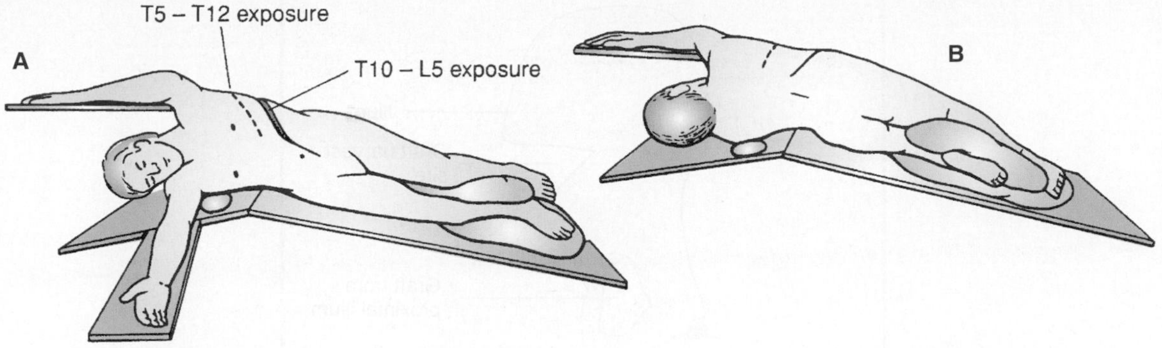

Figure 12.7-8. Lateral decubitus position (diagrammatic) for anterior spinal procedures: (**A**) anterior view; (**B**) posterior view. Roll is placed under axilla to minimize axillary artery compression. Skin incision for exposure of T5–T12 is shown with the dotted line. (Reproduced with permission from Chapman MW, ed: *Operative Orthopaedics,* 3rd edition. Lippincott Williams & Wilkins, Philadelphia: 2001.)

PATIENT POPULATION CHARACTERISTICS	
Age range	5–35 yr
Male:Female	Idiopathic: 1:10 Neuromuscular: 1:1
Incidence	< 1/10,000
Etiology	Idiopathic scoliosis; neuromuscular disease (especially cerebral palsy, spina bifida, polio, myopathies, muscular dystrophies); other genetic bone dysplasias; Marfan syndrome
Associated conditions	See Associated Conditions for Posterior Spinal Instrumentation and Fusion, p. 1356.

ANESTHETIC CONSIDERATIONS

See Anesthetic Considerations for Spinal Reconstruction and Fusion, (see p. 971).

Suggested Readings

1. Betz RR, Harms J, Clement DH III, et al: Comparison of anterior and posterior instrumentation for correction of adolescent thoracic idiopathic scoliosis. *Spine* 1999;24(3):225–39.
2. Betz RR, Shufflebarger H: Anterior versus posterior instrumentation for the correction of thoracic idiopathic scoliosis. *Spine* 2001;26(9):1095–1100.
3. Hammmerberg KW, Rodts MF, DeWald RL: Zielke instrumentation. *Orthopedics* 1988;11(10):1365–71.
4. Kaneda K, Shono Y, Satoh S, et al: New anterior instrumentation for the management of thoracolumbar and lumbar scoliosis. Application of the Kaneda two-rod system. *Spine* 1996;21(10):1250–61.

PELVIC OSTEOTOMY

SURGICAL CONSIDERATIONS

Description: Pelvic osteotomy is used to improve hip instability in cases of developmental hip dysplasia. The purpose of the procedure is to improve the coverage of the femoral head and stimulate appropriate growth of the shallow

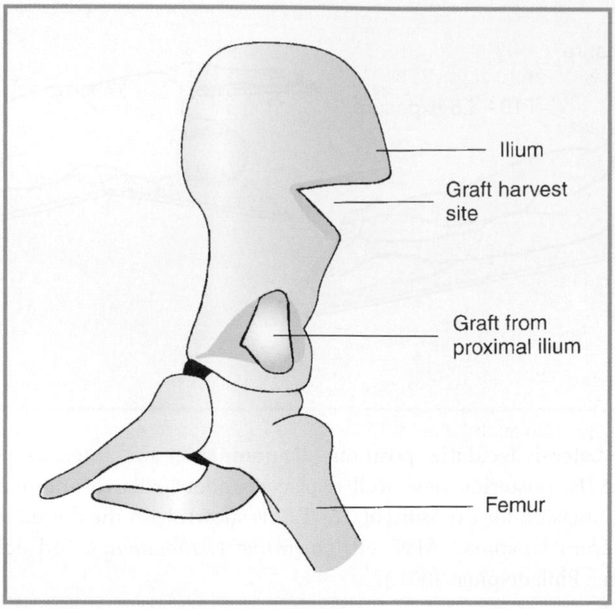

Figure 12.7-9. Pemberton osteotomy: A triangular graft is cut from the proximal ilium, and the graft is carefully wedged into the osteotomy site. (Reproduced with permission from Chapman MW: *Chapman's Orthopaedic Surgery,* 3rd edition. Lippincott Williams & Wilkins, Philadelphia: 2001.)

acetabulum. It is frequently performed in conjunction with open reduction, and occasionally with femoral osteotomy. The surgical approach is made along the iliac crest, exposing the external (gluteal) surface of the iliac bone, and sometimes the internal (iliac) surface as well. The pelvis is osteotomized closely above the acetabulum, and sometimes through the pubis and ischium, depending on the direction of rotation and reorientation desired. Pelvic osteotomies either reorient an intact acetabular hyaline cartilage surface or are designed as salvage procedures to enlarge the acetabulum by fibrocartilage metaplasia (see Acetabular Augmentation and Chiari, p. 1364). **Salter's innominate osteotomy** is the classic reorientation osteotomy, in which a complete cut of the supraacetabular iliac bone allows rotation through the symphysis pubis. **Pemberton's operation** is a slightly more difficult incomplete iliac osteotomy, rotating on the triradius cartilage (Fig. 12.7-9), which is at the center of the acetabulum in young children. The **Steel, "Dial"** or **Eppright osteotomies** are the most difficult reorientation procedures. In each, the acetabulum is freed totally from any bony contact with the remainder of the pelvis and rotated into better position.

Usual preop diagnosis: Acetabular dysplasia due to congenital or developmental hip dislocation

SUMMARY OF PROCEDURES

	Salter	Pemberton	Steel, Dial
Position	Supine or slightly lateral	⇐	⇐
Incision	Oblique or longitudinal anterior hip	⇐	⇐
Special instrumentation	Steinmann pins	Special curved, custom osteotomes	Steinmann pins
Unique considerations	Frequently follows previous unsuccessful open-hip surgery.	⇐	⇐+ additional ischial incision
Antibiotics	Usually, cefazolin 25 mg/kg iv	⇐	⇐
Surgical time	1.5–2 h	2–3 h	2–4 h

SUMMARY OF PROCEDURES (cont'd)	Salter	Pemberton	Steel, Dial
Closing considerations	Hip spica	⇐	⇐
EBL	100–300 mL	⇐	200–600 mL
Postop care	PACU → room; care as needed for spica cast	⇐	⇐
Mortality	Minimal	⇐	⇐
Morbidity	Avascular necrosis of the hip: 5–6%	–	–
	Persistent hip subluxation: 5%	⇐	⇐
	Infection: 1%	⇐	⇐
	Sciatic or perineal palsy: <0.1%	⇐	⇐
	Excess bleeding from superior gluteal artery: Rare	⇐	Occasional
	Ileus: Rare	⇐	Occasional
Pain score	2–5	2–5	3–6

PATIENT POPULATION CHARACTERISTICS			
Age range	18 mo–6 yr, if dislocated 18 mo–10 yr, if only subluxated	18 mo–7 yr	12 yr
Male:Female	1:2	⇐	⇐
Incidence	1/10,000	1/10,000	1/10,000
Etiology	Congenital and/or developmental hip dysplasia: 98% Perthes disease: 1%	⇐	⇐
Associated conditions	Torticollis: < 1%	⇐	⇐
	Other joint contractures in cases of neuromuscular dislocation: <1%	⇐	⇐

ANESTHETIC CONSIDERATIONS

See Anesthetic Considerations for Pediatric Orthopedic Surgery of the Pelvis and Lower Extremities, see p. 1389.

Suggested Readings

1. Ganz R, Klaue K, Vinh TS, et al: A new periacetabular osteotomy for the treatment of hip dysplasias. *Clin Orthop Rel Res* 1998;232:26–36.
2. Millis MB, Kaelin AJ, Schluntz K, et al: Spherical acetabular osteotomy for the treatment of acetabular dysplasia in adolescents and young adults. *J Pediatr Orthop* 1994;3:47–53.
3. Pogliacomi F, De Filippo M, Costantino C, et al: 2006: the value of pelvic and femoral osteotomies in hip surgery. *Acta Biomed* 2007;78(1):60–70.
4. Pemberton PA: Pericapsular osteotomy of the ilium for the treatment of congenitally dislocated hips. *Clin Orthop* 1974;98: 41–54.
5. Salter RB, Duboi JP: The first fifteen years' personal experience with innominate osteotomy in the treatment of congenital dislocation and subluxation of the hip. *Clin Orthop* 1974;98:72–103.
6. Sanchez-Sotelo J, Trousdale RT, Berry DJ, et al: Surgical treatment of developmental dysplasia of the hip in adults: I. Nonarthroplasty options. *J Am Acad Orthop Surg* 2002;10(5):321–33.

7. Staheli LT: Surgical management of acetabular dysplasia. *Clin Orthop* 1991;264:111–21.
8. Steel HH: Triple osteotomy of the innominate bone. *J Bone Joint Surg* 1973;55(2):343–50.
9. Tonnis D, Arning A, Block M, et al: Triple pelvic osteotomy. *J Pediatr Orthop* 1994;3:54–67.
10. Vitale MG, Skaggs DL: Developmental dysplasia of the hip from six months to four years of age. *J Am Acad Orthop Surg* 2001;9(6):401–11.
11. Waters P, Kurica K, Hall J, et al: Salter innominate osteotomies in congenital dislocation of the hip. *J Pediatr Orthop* 1988; 8(6):650–5.

ACETABULAR AUGMENTATION (SHELF) & CHIARI OSTEOTOMY

SURGICAL CONSIDERATIONS

Description: Acetabular augmentation is a "salvage" procedure used to deepen the hip socket when a realignment osteotomy of the pelvis and/or femur would not adequately cover the femoral head. This is accomplished by securing strips of cortical cancellous bone graft onto the proximal surface of the hip capsule. The surgical approach is anterior to the hip, elevating the gluteal muscles subperiosteally from the outer surface of the ilium. The reflected head of the rectus femoris tendon is elevated, and a domed-shaped slot is created just above the capsular attachment to the ilium. Abundant cortical cancellous strips of bone graft are then harvested from the upper two thirds of the outer wall of the ilium. These bone grafts have a natural curve and lie on the convexity of the hip capsule. No internal fixation, other than suture repair, is used to hold the bone graft in place. This creates a large bony augmentation (shelf) over the uncovered femoral capsule.

Variant procedure or approaches: The bone graft may be taken as a large, sculpted, solitary, cortical cancellous strut or wedge, or more commonly, as curved "shavings" anchored in a dome-shaped slot just above the hip capsule. In the **Chiari procedure,** a complete dome-shaped osteotomy allows lateral displacement of the ilium just above the proximal hip capsule (Fig. 12.7-10). The line of the osteotomy corresponds more or less with the slot of the shelf procedure. In either case, the result is abundant bony coverage over the hip capsule, which undergoes metaplasia into fibrocartilage.

Usual preop diagnosis: Acetabular dysplasia (shallow socket) due to congenital hip dislocation or developmental neurologic subluxation

Pediatric Surgery

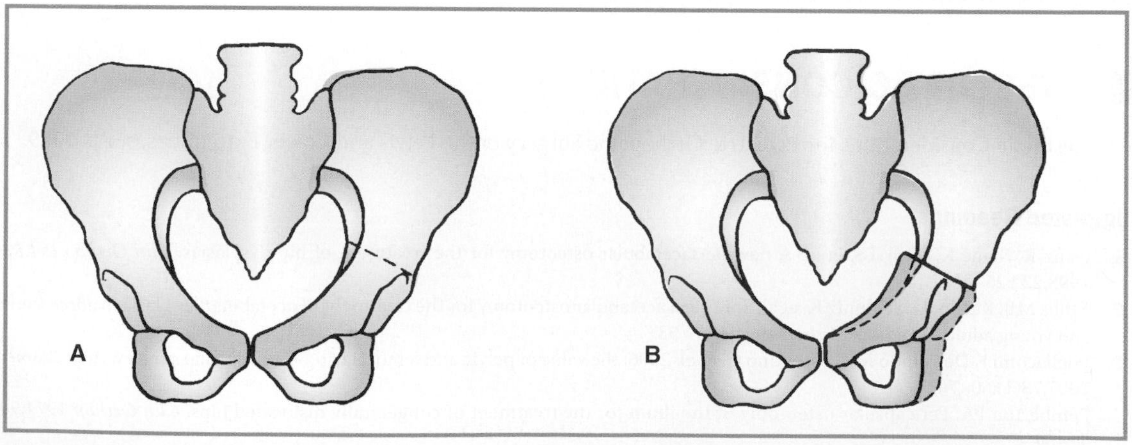

Figure 12.7-10. Chiari osteotomy: (**A**) Line of osteotomy. (**B**) Completed osteotomy. (Reproduced with permission from Crenshaw AH, ed: *Campbell's Operative Orthopaedics*, 8th edition. Mosby-Year Book, St. Louis: 1992.)

SUMMARY OF PROCEDURES

	Acetabular Augmentation	Chiari Osteotomy
Position	Supine or slightly tilted up (reverse Trendelenburg)	⇐or lateral decubitus
Incision	Oblique or longitudinal; anterior hip region	⇐
Special instrumentation	Usually no internal fixation; I.I. or intraop x-ray	Two large screws or pins; I.I. or intraop x-ray
Antibiotics	Cefazolin 25 mg/kg iv	⇐
Surgical time	1.5–3 h	⇐
Closing considerations	Unilateral or 1.5 spica cast mandatory	Spica cast (optional)
EBL	100–500 mL	200–800 mL
Postop care	PACU → room. Care as necessary for cast.	⇐
Mortality	Minimal	⇐
Morbidity	Lateral femoral cutaneous nerve dysfunction: 30–50% Infection: 1%	Sciatic or peroneal palsy: 2% Possible need for later C-section: Rare
Pain score	4–6	4–6

PATIENT POPULATION CHARACTERISTICS

Age range	6–35 yr
Male:Female	1:1.5
Incidence	< 1/10,000 in general population; in neuromuscular population (e.g., cerebral palsy, poliomyelitis residuals): 5–10%
Etiology	Neuromuscular hip subluxation with shallow acetabulum; residual shallow acetabulum (poor coverage from congenitally dislocated hip)
Associated conditions	Cerebral palsy; polio; spina bifida; myopathy; congenital atrophies; Charcot-Marie Tooth disease

ANESTHETIC CONSIDERATIONS

See Anesthetic Considerations for Pediatric Orthopedic Surgery of the Pelvis and Lower Extremities, see p. 1389.

Suggested Readings

1. Betz RR, Kumar Si, Palmer CT, et al: Chiari pelvic osteotomy in children and young adults. *J Bone Joint Surg* 1988;70(2): 182–91.
2. Chiari K: Medial displacement osteotomy of the pelvis. *Clin Orthop* 1974;98:55–69.
3. Fong HC, Lu W, Li YH, et al: Chiari osteotomy and shelf augmentation in the treatment of hip dysplasia. *J Pediatr Orthop* 2000;20(6):740–4.
4. Morrissy RT: *Atlas of Pediatric Orthopaedic Surgery.* JB Lippincott, Philadelphia: 1992.
5. Piontek T, Szulc A, Gowacki M, et al: Distant outcomes of the Chiari osteotomy 30 years follow up evaluation. *Ortop Traumatol Rehabil* 2006;8(1):16–23.
6. Staheli LT, Chew DE: Slotted acetabular augmentation in childhood and adolescence. *J Pediatr Orthop* 1992;12(5): 569–80.

7. Summers BN, Turner A, Wynn-Jones CH: The shelf operation in the management of late presentation of congenital hip dysplasia. *J Bone Joint Surg* 1988;70(1):63–8.
8. White RE Jr, Sherman FC: The hip shelf procedure. A long-term evaluation. *J Bone Joint Surg* 1980;62(6):928–32.
9. Zuckerman JD, Staheli LT, McLaughlin JF: Acetabular augmentation for progressive hip subluxation in cerebral palsy. *J Pediatr Orthop* 1984;4(4):436–42.

OBER FASCIOTOMY, YOUNT-OBER RELEASE

SURGICAL CONSIDERATIONS

Description: **Ober's fasciotomy** is performed to release flexion, abduction, and external rotation contracture at the hip. This contracture usually occurs as a result of profound flaccid paralysis → prolonged positioning in a so-called "frog" position of 90° flexion, abduction, and lateral rotation at the hips. This results in tightening of the iliotibial (IT) band (the greatly thickened lateral aspect of the fascia lata) and related structures. The operation is performed through an anterolateral incision just distal to the iliac crest. All of the fascial investments of the tensor, sartorius, and, at times, the rectus femoris and gluteus medias and minimus are divided, while preserving any normal-appearing muscle fibers. The limb is stretched into progressively more adduction and extension, until a neutral position can be obtained. The **Yount procedure** is added when the knee also is contracted in a flexed mode due to tightness of the IT band. The Yount procedure consists of further resection of a segment of the IT band and a lateral intermuscular septum through a separate distal mid-lateral longitudinal incision just above the knee. An oblique segment of the IT band and septum are removed and not repaired.

Usual preop diagnosis: Flaccid paralysis and "frog"-type contracture due to poliomyelitis, myelomeningocele, or myopathy

SUMMARY OF PROCEDURES

	Ober Fasciotomy	Yount-Ober Release
Position	Supine; both legs must be prepped and draped to well above the iliac crest area for intraop stretching.	⇐
Incision	Oblique iliac crest	Mid-lateral longitudinal above knee joint, ~10 cm
Unique considerations	Patients with sensory and motor loss have a tendency to get pressure sores.	⇐
Antibiotics	Usually none	⇐
Surgical time	1 h/side	30 min/side
Closing considerations	Bilateral above-knee casts	⇐
EBL	< 150 mL	< 50 mL
Postop care	PACU → room; extensive physical therapy program of stretching exercises. Myopathic patients at risk for postop respiratory compromise.	⇐
Mortality	Minimal	⇐
Morbidity	Hematoma: ~1% Fracture of atrophied bone postop: < 1% Infection < 1% Pressure sores from positioning or casts: < 1%	⇐ ⇐ ⇐ ⇐
Pain score	3–4	3–4

PATIENT POPULATION CHARACTERISTICS	
Age range	2–15 yr
Male:Female	1:1
Incidence	Extremely rare in children born in the United States; however, polio is seen commonly in south-east Asian and Latin-American immigrants.
Etiology	Polio; myelomeningocele; myopathy or dystrophy
Associated conditions	Other contractures; incontinence; pressure sores in myelomeningocele

ANESTHETIC CONSIDERATIONS

See Anesthetic Considerations for Pediatric Orthopedic Surgery of the Pelvis and Lower Extremities, see p. 1389.

Suggested Readings

1. Beaty JH: Paralytic disorders. In *Campbell's Operative Orthopaedics,* 8th edition. Crenshaw AH, ed. Mosby-Year Book, St. Louis: 1992, 2412–16.
2. Irwin CE: The iliotibial band, its role in producing deformity in poliomyelitis. *J Bone Joint Surg* 1949;31:141–52.
3. Ober FR: The role of the iliotibial band and fascia lata as a factor in the causation of low-back disabilities and sciatica. *J Bone Joint Surg* 1936;18:105–19.
4. Yount CC: The role of the tensor fasciae femoris in certain deformities of the lower extremities. *J Bone Joint Surg* 1926;8:171–82.

HIP, OPEN REDUCTION & FEMORAL SHORTENING

SURGICAL CONSIDERATIONS

Description: **Open reduction of the hip** replaces a dislocated femoral head into the anatomic acetabulum, at times after an unsuccessful attempt to reduce the hip by closed means. A developmental dislocation presents with a more normal acetabulum and occurs around birth or later. A teratologic congenital dislocation of the hip occurs early in utero, and, as a result, has a high–riding dislocation with a poorly developed acetabulum, presenting much more difficulty in obtaining and maintaining reduction. The most common surgical approach is through an extended anterior incision. The hip capsule is exposed circumferentially, after division and tagging of the origins of the rectus, femoris, and sartorius muscles, and retraction of the tensor and gluteal muscles. The iliopsoas tendon is either lengthened or divided. The capsule is opened in an oblique fashion, the ligamentum teres is excised, and any obstacle to reduction is removed. The femoral head is replaced in the socket, and the capsule is repaired in a "vest-over-pants" imbrication, with the hip reduced under direct visualization (Fig. 12.7-11). A medial approach through the adductor region can be used in very young children (<18 mo), but does not allow a capsular repair. If femoral shortening is necessary, the surgical excision is either extended anterolaterally, or a separate lateral incision is made longitudinally over the proximal femur.

Variant procedure or approaches: Most children < 2 years old can simply have the hip repositioned—closed or open—and subsequently have normal hip development. In older children, especially with a high dislocation, a segment of the femur is removed subtrochanterically to allow reduction without pressure (thus allowing "descent" of the femoral head). If the acetabulum is very shallow, a pelvic osteotomy may be added.

Usual preop diagnosis: Developmental dislocation of hip; teratologic congenital dislocation of hip

SUMMARY OF PROCEDURES		
	Open Reduction	**Open Reduction + Femoral Shortening**
Position	Supine	⇐
Incision	Oblique ("bikini") along the iliac crest or medial longitudinal over joint	⇐ + anterolateral thigh over joint

SUMMARY OF PROCEDURES (cont'd)

	Open Reduction	Open Reduction + Femoral Shortening
Special instrumentation	None	Plates and screws
Unique considerations	Preliminary arthrogram and, often, attempted closed reduction. I.I. is used.	⇐
Antibiotics	Usually cefazolin 25 mg/kg iv	⇐
Surgical time	1.5–3 h	2–4 h
Closing considerations	Hip spica cast applied on child's spica frame. **NB:** Do not wake patient until last radiograph is taken, in case cast has to be reapplied.	⇐
EBL	< 100 mL	100–400 mL
Postop care	PACU → room; care as necessary for spica cast	⇐
Mortality	Minimal	⇐
Morbidity	Avascular necrosis of femoral head Stiffness and late arthritis Limb-length discrepancy Marked scrotal or labial swelling: temporary Redislocation Infection	⇐ ⇐ ⇐ ⇐ ⇐ ⇐
Pain score	2–4	3–5

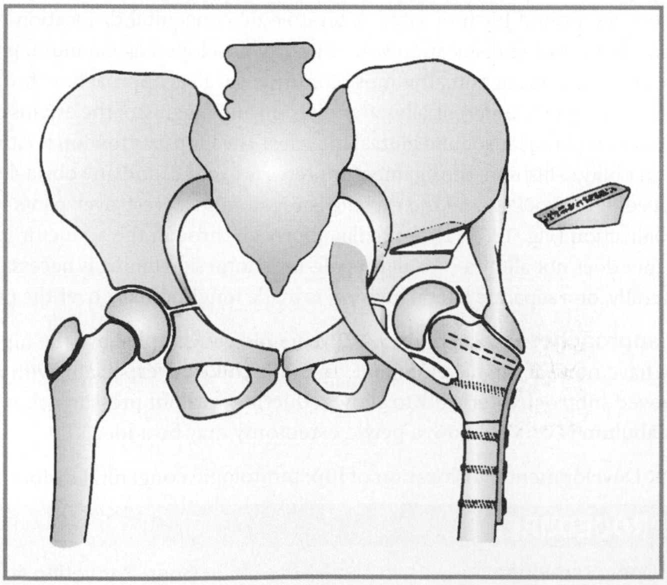

Figure 12.7-11. Open reduction with femoral shortening. (Reproduced with permission from Crenshaw AH, ed: *Campbell's Operative Orthopaedics,* 8th edition Mosby-Year Book, St. Louis: 1992.)

PATIENT POPULATION CHARACTERISTICS	
Age range	Closed reduction: 3 mo–3 yr Open reduction: 6 mo–10 yr Open reduction femoral shortening: 2–14 yr
Male:Female	1:5 (approximate)
Incidence	1:10,000
Etiology	Genetic background; breech presentation; first-born girl
Associated conditions	Arthrogryposis; Larsen's disease; myelomeningocele; chromosomal anomalies; congenital torticollis; cerebral palsy

ANESTHETIC CONSIDERATIONS

See Anesthetic Considerations for Pediatric Orthopedic Surgery of the Pelvis and Lower Extremities, see p. 1389.

Suggested Readings

1. Coleman SS: *Congenital Dysplasia and Dislocation of the Hip.* Mosby-Year Book, St. Louis: 1978.
2. Ferguson AB: Primary open reduction of congenital dislocation of the hip using a median adductor approach. *J Bone Joint Surg* 1973;55:671–89.
3. Galpin RD, Roach JW, Wenger DR, et al: One-stage treatment of congenital dislocation of the hip in older children, including femoral shortening. *J Bone Joint Surg* 1989;71(5):734–41.
4. Hogan KA, Blake M, Gross RH: Subtrochanteric valgus osteotomy for chronically dislocated, painful spastic hips. Surgical technique. *J Bone Joint Surg* 2007;89(Suppl 2):226–31.
5. Moseley CF: Developmental hip dysplasia and dislocation: management of the older child. *Instr Course Lect* 2001;50: 547–53.
6. Morrissy RT: *Atlas of Pediatric Orthopaedic Surgery.* JB Lippincott, Philadelphia: 1992:137–54.
7. Rab GT: Surgery for developmental dysplasia of the hip. In *Chapman's Orthopaedic Surgery,* 3rd edition. Chapman MW, ed. Lippincott Williams & Wilkins, Philadelphia: 2001:4241–58.
8. Schoenecker PL, Strecker WB: Congenital dislocation of the hip in children. Comparison of the effects of femoral shortening and of skeletal traction in treatment. *J Bone Joint Surg* 1984;66(1):21–7.
9. Wenger, DR, Lee CS, Kolman B: Derotational femoral shortening for developmental dislocation of the hip: special indications and results in the child younger than 2 years. *J Pediatr Orthop* 1995;15(6):768–79.

ADDUCTOR RELEASE OR TRANSFER, PSOAS RELEASE

SURGICAL CONSIDERATIONS

Description: The adductor tendons and often the iliopsoas tendon are released in spastic and other neurologic conditions (especially cerebral palsy). The goal is to allow greater abduction by decreasing the strength of the adductors and flexors. The releases are also performed for other causes of hip contracture due to developmental hip dislocation, juvenile arthritis, etc. The procedure is performed with the patient supine, using a medial groin incision in which the tendons (usually the adductor longus, brevis, and gracilis) are isolated and divided by electrocautery. In the classic procedure, popularized by **Banks** and **Green,** the anterior branch of the obturator nerve is divided on the surface of the adductor brevis to affect more permanent adductor weakness. This procedure is now less popular, because the denervated muscles can undergo denervation fibrosis resulting in recurrent contracture. The iliopsoas tendon may be released at its insertion on the lesser trochanter, in the base of the adductor incision; or, just the tendinous portion of the combined iliopsoas may be released at the pelvic rim, which produces a more modest degree of the flexor lengthening. Some surgeons transfer the adductor longus and gracilis muscles proximally and laterally, suturing them to the ischium to convert the adductors to hip extensors by changing their mechanics.

Usual preop diagnosis: Adduction and flexion contracture of the hip with subluxation due to cerebral palsy, acquired encephalopathy, or progressive neurologic disorder.

SUMMARY OF PROCEDURES

	Adductor Release	Adductor Transfer	Psoas Release
Position	Supine	Supine or lithotomy	⇐
Incision	Medial proximal groin, longitudinal or transverse	Transverse medial groin	Anterior groin
Unique considerations	Frequently bilateral; often poor hygiene, especially if severe contracture; proximity to perineum	⇐	⇐
Antibiotics	± cefazolin 25 mg/kg iv	⇐	⇐
Surgical time	1 h	1.5 h	1 hr
Closing considerations	Bilateral leg casts or double spica cast	⇐	⇐
EBL	< 100 mL	⇐	⇐
Postop care	PACU → room; care as necessary for spica cast	⇐	⇐
Mortality	Minimal	⇐	⇐
Morbidity	Hematoma, drainage Infection: < 1% Recurrence of adduction deformity	⇐ ⇐	⇐ ⇐
Pain score	2–4	2–4	2–4

PATIENT POPULATION CHARACTERISTICS

Age range	2–20 yr
Male:Female	1:1
Incidence	0 in general population; 30% of cerebral palsy patients (0.6–5.9/1,000)
Etiology	Cerebral palsy (90%); slowly progressive degenerative neurologic conditions (8–10%); head injury and drowning (1–2%)
Associated conditions	Multiple other contractures; GERD; poor general nutrition; mental retardation

Pediatric Surgery

ANESTHETIC CONSIDERATIONS

See Anesthetic Considerations for Pediatric Orthopedic Surgery of the Pelvis and Lower Extremities, see p. 1389.

Suggested Readings

1. Banks HH, Green WT: Adductor myotomy and obturator neurectomy for the correction of adduction contracture of the hip in cerebral palsy. *J Bone Joint Surg* 1960;42:111–26.
2. Bleck EE: The hip in cerebral palsy. *Orthop Clin North Am* 1980;11(1):79–104.
3. Kalen V, Bleck EE: Prevention of spastic paralytic dislocation of the hip. *Dev Med Child Neurol* 1985;27(l):17–24.
4. Miller F, Cardoso Dias R, Dabney KW, et al: Soft-tissue release for spastic hip subluxation in cerebral palsy. *J Pediatr Orthop* 1997;17(5):571–84.

5. Presedo A, Oh CW, Dabney KW, et al: Soft-tissue releases to treat spastic hip subluxation in children with cerebral palsy. *J Bone Joint Surg* 2005;87:832–41.
6. Reimers J, Poulsen S: Adductor transfer versus tenotomy for stability of the hip in spastic cerebral palsy. *J Pediatr Orthop* 1984;4(1):52–4.
7. Rinsky LA: Surgery for cerebral palsy. In *Chapman's Orthopaedic Surgery,* 3rd edition. Chapman MW, ed. Lippincott Williams & Wilkins, Philadelphia: 2001, 4485–504.
8. Root L, Spero CR: Hip adductor transfer compared with adductor tenotomy in cerebral palsy. *J Bone Joint Surg* 1981;63(5): 767–72.

PINNING OF SLIPPED CAPITAL FEMORAL EPIPHYSIS (SCFE)

SURGICAL CONSIDERATIONS

Description: Slipped capital femoral epiphysis is a mechanical failure of the proximal femoral growth plate. During the rapid growth period, the shearing stress of the body weight on the proximal femoral growth plate may cause the femoral head (capital epiphysis) to gradually move relative to the femoral neck through the physis or growth cartilage. The displacement occurs over weeks-to-months, with the head appearing to move posteriorly and inferiorly on the neck. Percutaneous **in situ pinning** (no reduction) is the most common treatment. The goal is to prevent further slipping and subsequent arthritis by causing closure of the growth plate. The procedure must be performed under radiographic control (usually I.I.), using a variety of threaded pins or screws which are passed through the neck into the femoral head. Currently, the favored technique uses one cannulated screw, which is passed percutaneously over a guide wire from the anterolateral aspect of the proximal femur.

Variant procedure or approaches: Although most slips are chronic, occasionally following mild trauma, an acute slip will supervene. Following severe trauma, a previously normal hip with an open physis (growth plate) may suffer an acute displacement. In such acute slips, some degree of reduction may be possible, and two pins are usually necessary. Because pin-related complications are common, some surgeons prefer to close the growth plate by open drilling and curettement, with bone grafting across the cartilaginous plates. This is performed through an anterior incision, opening the hip capsule widely from an oblique groin incision. No pins are used, but an iliac bone graft is placed across the physis. A body spica cast is frequently needed. After the physis is closed, if there is severe residual deformity, a corrective osteotomy is performed in the trochanteric region (see Proximal Femoral Osteotomy, Southwick procedure, p. 1375).

Usual preop diagnosis: Acute or chronic SCFE

SUMMARY OF PROCEDURES

	Pinning of SCFE	Variant Open Epiphysiodesis
Position	Supine	⇐
Incision	Short, proximal thigh or stab incision	Anterolateral groin
Special instrumentation	Guide wires; cannulated screws; I.I.; fracture table	I.I. (recommended)
Unique considerations	Frequently bilateral (≤ 20%); often obese	⇐
Antibiotics	Cefazolin 1 g iv	⇐
Surgical time	0.5–2 h	1–3 h

SUMMARY OF PROCEDURES (cont'd)		
	Pinning of SCFE	**Variant Open Epiphysiodesis**
Closing considerations	None	Frequently needs spica cast
EBL	Negligible	200–500 mL
Postop care	PACU → room	Body spica cast, occasionally
Mortality	Minimal	⇐
Morbidity	Unsuspected pin penetration: ≤ 37% Avascular necrosis: ≤ 33% (in acute slip cases) Chondrolysis, hip stiffness: 1–28% Fracture after pin removal : <1% Infection: < 1%	⇐ ⇐ ⇐ ⇐
Pain score	2–3	2–3

PATIENT POPULATION CHARACTERISTICS	
Age range	10–16 yr
Male:Female	2–3:1
Incidence	1–3/100,000 (higher in African Americans)
Etiology	Excessive loading of the growth plate (obesity or increased angle of inclination of the physis) Insufficient tensile strength of collagen and proteoglycans around the femoral neck Increased thickness of the physis as from excessive growth hormone, hypogonadism, hypothyroidism, hyperparathyroidism, renal osteodystrophy, almost any other significant endocrinopathy Radiation therapy
Associated conditions	Obesity; endocrinopathies; renal osteodystrophy

ANESTHETIC CONSIDERATIONS

See Anesthetic Considerations for Pediatric Orthopedic Surgery of the Pelvis and Lower Extremities, see p. 1389.

Suggested Readings

1. Aadalen RJ, Weiner DS, Hoyt W, et al: Acute slipped capital femoral epiphysis. *J Bone Joint Surg*; 1974;56(7):1473–87.
2. Aronsson DD, Loder RT, Breur GJ, et al: Slipped capital femoral epiphysis: current concepts. *J Am Acad Orthop Surg* 2006;14:666–79.
3. Asnis SE: The guided screw system in slipped capital femoral epiphysis. *Contemp Orthop* 1985;11:27–31.
4. Dobbs MB, Weinstein SL: Natural history and long-term outcomes of slipped capital femoral epiphysis. *Instr Course Lect* 2001;50:571–5.
5. Lee FY, Chapman CB: In situ pinning of hip for stable slipped capital femoral epiphysis on a radiolucent operating table. *J Pediatr Orthop* 2003;23(1):27–9.
6. Lehman WB, Menche D, Grant A, et al: The problem of evaluating *in situ* pinning of slipped capital femoral epiphysis: an experimental model and a review of 63 consecutive cases. *J Pediatr Orthop* 1984;4(3):297–303.
7. Loder RT: Unstable slipped capital femoral epiphysis. *J Pediatr Orthop* 2001;21(5):694–9.
8. Loder RT, Aronsson DD, Dobbs MB, et al: Slipped capital femoral epiphysis. *Inst Course Lect* 2001;50:555–70.
9. Morrissy RT: *Atlas of Pediatric Orthopaedic Surgery.* JB Lippincott, Philadelphia: 1992, 212–44.
10. O'Brien ET, Fahey JJ: Remodeling of the femoral neck after *in situ* pinning for slipped capital femoral epiphysis. *J Bone Joint Surg*: 1977;59(1):62–8.

FLEXIBLE INTRAMEDULLARY NAILING OF LONG-BONE FRACTURES

SURGICAL CONSIDERATIONS

Description: The purpose of flexible nailing of long bones is to obtain stability with minimal surgical risk. This method is applicable to both lower- and upper-extremity fractures. Casting is unnecessary in many cases because of the balanced dynamic forces exerted by the elastic memory of the implanted precontoured nails. This is particularly appealing when treating femur fractures that otherwise would require spica casting and prolonged immobility. This technique results in a high rate of fracture union, promoted by the implant load-sharing characteristics with a modulus of elasticity that is close to bone, thereby avoiding stress shielding. The flexible nailing technique for treatment of femur fractures in children also avoids the risk of avascular necrosis of the femoral head because of a more distal entry point on the bone, compared to standard rigid intramedullary nails that enter the medullary canal at the base of the femoral neck, where the primary vascular supply to the femoral head is located.

The child is placed supine on a radiolucent operating table, although some surgeons prefer to use a fracture table when treating femur fractures with this method. The surgeon performs a closed reduction of the fracture with fluoroscopy assistance, proceeding to an open incision and reduction only if an acceptable fracture reduction cannot be achieved with closed techniques. After the fracture is aligned, a small incision for each nail is made on the extremity proximal to the physis at the knee. A drill is used to create an entry point in the cortex of the bone, and each nail is contoured before insertion through this entry point. No intramedullary reaming is performed before nail insertion. The rare need for cast application is judged by intraop imaging for rotational and angular stability.

Usual preop diagnosis: Fracture

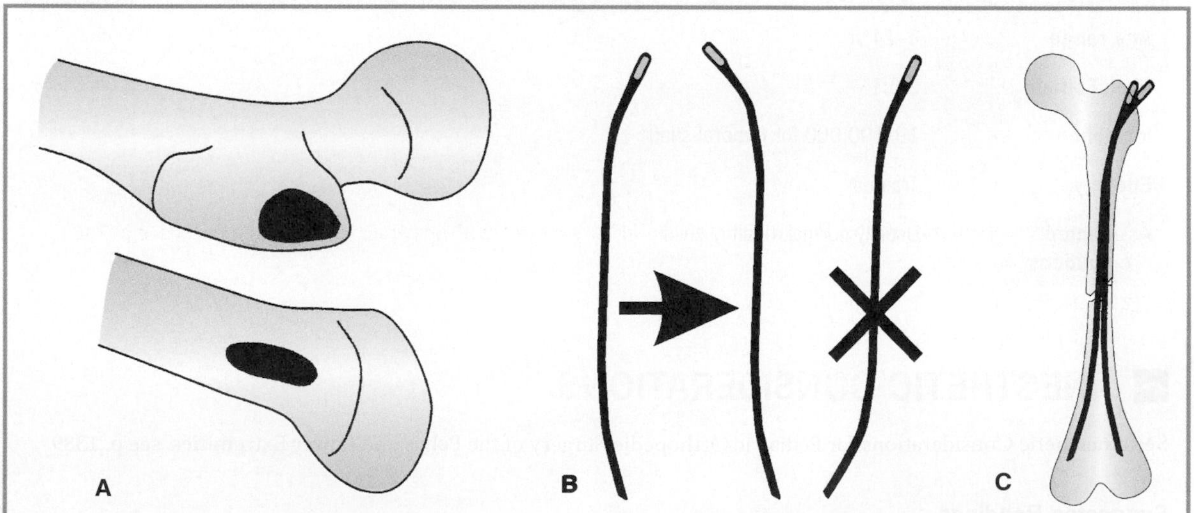

Figure 12.7-12. Intramedullary nailing. (**A**) Nail entry site through greater trochanter (antegrade) or distal metaphysic (retrograde). (**B**) Nails are contoured before insertion. (**C**) Fracture stabilized with two antegrade nails. (Reproduced with permission from Chapman MW: *Chapman's Orthopaedic Surgery,* 3rd edition. Lippincott Williams & Wilkins, Philadelphia: 2001.)

SUMMARY OF PROCEDURES

	Closed Reduction	Open Reduction
Position	Supine; may be performed on fracture table if femoral.	⇐
Incision	2–3 cm at entry site for each nail	Incision at fracture site and 2–3 cm at entry site for each nail
Instrumentation	Intramedullary nails, power drill, I.I.	⇐
Unique considerations	Blood loss from fracture; muscle relaxation may be necessary to obtain reduction.	⇐
Antibiotics	Cefazolin 25 mg/kg	⇐
Surgical time	45–60 min	60–90 min
Closing considerations	May supplement with cast.	⇐
EBL	Minimal	50–200 mL
Postoperative care	PACU → room	⇐
Mortality	Rare, except in multitrauma	⇐
Morbidity	Nonunion, malunion Shortening Infection Painful instrumentation	⇐ ⇐ ⇐ ⇐
Pain score	4–7	4–7

PATIENT POPULATION CHARACTERISTICS

Age range	6–14 yr
Male:Female	2.6:1
Incidence	19/100,000 for femoral shaft
Etiology	Trauma
Associated conditions	Usually normal, healthy child

Pediatric Surgery

ANESTHETIC CONSIDERATIONS

See Anesthetic Considerations for Pediatric Orthopedic Surgery of the Pelvis and Lower Extremities, see p. 1389.

Suggested Readings

1. Hedlund R, Lindgren U: The incidence of femoral shaft fractures in children and adolescents. *J Pediatr Orthop* 1986;6(1):47–50.
2. Hinton RY, Lincoln A, Crockett MM, et al: Fractures of the femoral shaft in children. Incidence, mechanisms, and sociodemographic risk factors. *J Bone Joint Surg* 1999;81(4):500–9.
3. Mazda K, Khairouni A, Pennecot GF, et al: Closed flexible intramedullary nailing of femoral shaft fractures in children. *J Pediatr Orthop* 1997;6(3):198–202.
4. Rathjen KE, Riccio AI, De La Garza D: Stainless steel flexible intramedullary fixation of unstable femoral shaft fractures in children. *J Pediatr Orthop* 2007;27:432–41.
5. Vrsansky P, Bourdelat D, Al Faour: Flexible stable intramedullary pinning technique in the treatment of pediatric fractures. *J Pediatr Orthop* 2000;20(1):23–7.

PROXIMAL FEMORAL OSTEOTOMY

SURGICAL CONSIDERATIONS

Description: Femoral osteotomy is performed in the inter- or subtrochanteric area to redirect the femoral head more superiorly (valgus) or inferiorly (varus) and/or for rotational correction of excessive medial/femoral torsion (anteversion). A plate and screws are commonly used, but an **external fixator** and/or spica cast may be placed instead. The usual surgical approach is direct lateral over the proximal shaft of the femur, beginning at the greater trochanter. The deep fascia is split and the underlying vastus muscle is elevated subperiosteally to expose the femoral shaft. Normally, a power saw is used to make the osteotomy; and, depending on the correction desired, there are a variety of internal fixation devices which can be used.

Variant procedure or approaches: Different named plates (e.g., AO blade, Coventry screw, Richards screw, Wagner, etc.) may be used to affix the proximal to the distal femoral segments. A 1–4-cm segment of femur may be removed in cases of superior hip dislocation to allow soft-tissue relaxation and descent of the femoral head into the socket. Most proximal femoral osteotomies are performed in the subtrochanteric area, but some are performed in the intertrochanteric or base of the neck (**Kramer compensating**). The **Southwick osteotomy** is a more complicated example of a subtrochanteric osteotomy, which corrects for three directions (varus, lateral rotation, and extension).

Usual preop diagnosis: Developmental hip subluxation; excessive hip anteversion; residual deformity from Perthes disease; coxa vara; slipped capital femoral epiphysis (SCFE); residual deformity

SUMMARY OF PROCEDURES

	Varus Derotation Osteotomy + Plate and Screws	External Fixator	Southwick or Kramer
Position	Supine	⇐	⇐
Incision	Lateral thigh or, occasionally, long anterior thigh	⇐	⇐
Special instrumentation	Plate and screws; power drill and saw; I.I.	External fixator; multiple pins; I.I.	Plate and screws; power drill and saw; I.I.
Unique considerations	Fracture or radiolucent table	⇐	⇐
Antibiotics	± Cefazolin 25 mg/kg iv	⇐	⇐
Surgical time	1.5–2.5 h		2–4 h
Closing considerations	Spica cast, frequently	± Spica cast	Spica cast, occasionally
EBL	250–750 mL	⇐	500–1,000 mL
Postop care	PACU → room. Spica cast; Nonweight-bearing ~6 wk; no full weight-bearing, 3 mo.	⇐	⇐
Mortality	Minimal	⇐	⇐
Morbidity	Persistent hip dysplasia: 5–20% (depending on etiology)	⇐	⇐
	Excess blood loss from a perforating branch of the profunda femoris: < 1%	⇐	⇐
	Infection: < 1%	⇐	⇐
	Loss of fixation, instrument failure: < 1%	⇐	⇐
	Nonunion: < 1%	⇐	⇐
	Persistent hip stiffness: < 1%	⇐	⇐
	Avascular necrosis: Rare	⇐	⇐
Pain score	6–8	6–8	6–8

PATIENT POPULATION CHARACTERISTICS	
Age range	2–21 yr
Male:Female	1:1
Incidence	Depending on Dx
Etiology	Coxa varum, coxa valgum due to muscle imbalance; hip dislocation; excessive medial femoral torsion (anteversion); osteochondrodystrophies (dwarfing syndromes); Perthes disease; SCFE
Associated conditions	Cerebral palsy; myelomeningocele, neuromyopathies; congenital hip dislocation; occasionally, hypothyroidism as a cause of SCFE

ANESTHETIC CONSIDERATIONS

See Anesthetic Considerations for Pediatric Orthopedic Surgery of the Pelvis and Lower Extremities, see p. 1389.

Suggested Readings

1. Beauchesne R, Miller F, Moseley C: Proximal femoral osteotomy using the AO fixed-angle blade plate. *J Pediatr Orthop* 1992;12(6):735–40.
2. Hau R, Dickens DR, Nattrass GR, et al: Which implant for proximal femoral osteotomy in children? A comparison of the AO (ASIF) 90 degree fixed-angle blade plate and the Richards intermediate hip screw. *J Pediatr Orthop* 2000;20(3):336–43.
3. Kramer WG, Craig WA, Noel S: Compensating osteotomy at the base of the femoral neck for slipped capital femoral epiphysis. *J Bone Joint Surg* 1976;58(6):796–800.
4. Morrissy RT: *Atlas of Pediatric Orthopaedic Surgery.* JB Lippincott, Philadelphia: 1992, 264–304.
5. Raney EM, Grogan DP, Hurley ME, et al: The role of proximal femoral valgus osteotomy in Legg-Calve-Perthes disease. *Orthopedics* 2002;25(5):513–17.
6. Southwick WO: Osteotomy through the lesser trochanter for slipped capital femoral epiphysis. *J Bone Joint Surg* 1967;49(5):807–35.

EPIPHYSIODESIS

SURGICAL CONSIDERATIONS

Description: Epiphysiodesis is performed in skeletally immature adolescents to eliminate or retard growth of the longer limb in cases of leg-length discrepancy (anisomelia). The timing of the procedure is critical, based on the child's bone age and discrepancy, which are plotted on a graph or computer program. The procedure is most commonly performed through small incisions (1") about the knee, centered on the growth plate (physis) of the distal femur or proximal tibia. The original **Phemister technique** (Fig. 12.7-13) is an approach in which a ¾"–1¼" square or rectangular block of bone is removed using a box chisel centered on the physis, visualized directly. The bone block is rotated 90° or 180° and reinserted, causing a bony bridge across the physis. **Blount** subsequently used stout, reinforced staples to bracket the physis and "lock it." This provides a theoretical advantage of reversibility (i.e., if staples are removed, growth may resume if the procedure was performed at too early an age). More recently, a **percutaneous technique** of simply drilling directly across the cartilaginous physeal growth plate, causing a bony bridge, has been used. This is accomplished through small stab incisions, under fluoroscopic control.

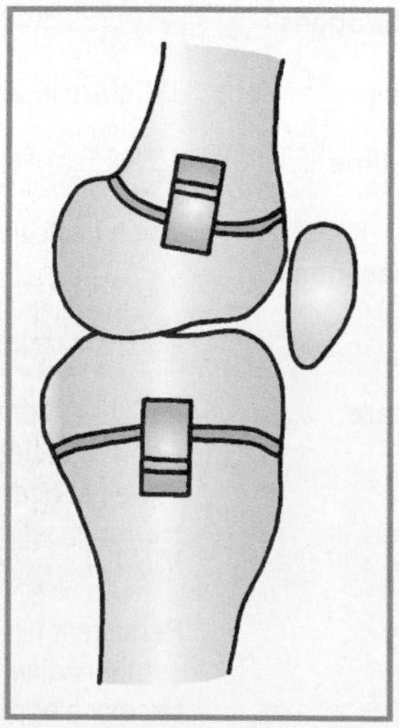

Figure 12.7-13. Phemister method of epiphysiodesis (block of bone reversed, then reinserted to form osseous bar). (Reproduced with permission from Chapman MW: *Chapman's Orthopaedic Surgery,* 3rd edition. Lippincott Williams & Wilkins, Philadelphia: 2001.)

Usual preop diagnosis: Limb-length discrepancies of 2–5 cm in adolescents (willing to accept a slight diminution in adult stature)

SUMMARY OF PROCEDURES

	Open Epiphysiodesis	Percutaneous Epiphysiodesis	Epiphyseal Stapling
Position	Supine, with tourniquet	Supine	Supine, with tourniquet
Incision	3–4 cm longitudinal incision, medial and laterally centered incisions over distal femoral and/or proximal tibial epiphysis	1 cm, same area as open epiphysiodesis	4–5 cm, same area as open epiphysiodesis
Special instrumentation	Box chisel	Drill point and sleeve	Heavy, reinforced staples
Unique considerations	Tourniquet used	I.I. control mandatory; tourniquet (optional)	⇐
Antibiotics	± Cefazolin 25 mg/kg iv	⇐	⇐
Surgical time	1 h	⇐	⇐
Closing considerations	Cylinder cast or knee immobilizer	⇐	⇐
EBL	< 50 mL	⇐	⇐
Postop care	PACU → room; crutches for comfort	⇐	⇐
Mortality	Minimal	⇐	⇐
Morbidity	Under- or overcorrection with regard to length: 5–10%	⇐	⇐
	Wound problems: < 5%	⇐	⇐
	Asymmetric growth arrest → valgus or varus deformity: 2–5%	⇐	⇐
	Anterior or lateral compartment syndrome: 1 %	–	–
	Fracture: 1 %	–	–
	Peroneal palsy: < 1 %	–	–
Pain score	3–5	2–3	3–5

PATIENT POPULATION CHARACTERISTICS

Age range	9–14 yr (adolescents, usually healthy with limb-length discrepancy 2–6 cm)
Male:Female	1:1
Incidence	< 1/1,000
Etiology	Idiopathic hemihypertrophy; neurologic (e.g., polio, hemiplegia); congenital deformities of the lower extremities (e.g., congenitally short femur, fibular hemimelia); osteomyelitis; development of tumorous conditions (e.g., enchondromatosis); traumatic growth plate injuries occurring near puberty; epiphyseal problems related to hip (slipped epiphysis, sequelae of Perthes disease); Klippel-Trenaunay-Weber syndrome
Associated conditions	Other contractures in neurologic conditions (e.g., polio); neurofibromatosis, AV fistulae; Wilms' tumor (rare)

ANESTHETIC CONSIDERATIONS

See Anesthetic Considerations for Pediatric Orthopedic Surgery of the Pelvis and Lower Extremities, see p. 1389.

Suggested Readings

1. Blair VP III, Walker SJ, Sheridan JJ, et al: Epiphysiodesis: a problem of timing. *J Pediatr Orthop* 1982;2(3):281–4.
2. Blount WP, Clarke GR: Control of bone growth by epiphyseal stapling. *J Bone Joint Surg* 1949;31:464–78.
3. Bowen JR, Torres RR, Forlin E: Partial epiphysiodesis to address genu varum or genu valgum. *J Pediatr Orthop* 1992;12(3):359–64.
4. Johnston CE II, Beuche MJ, Williamson B, et al: Epiphysiodesis for management of lower limb deformities. *Instr Course Lect* 1992;41:437–44.
5. Kemnitz S, Moens P, Fabry G: Percutaneous epiphysiodesis for leg length discrepancy. *J Pediatr Orthop* 2003;12(1):69–71.
6. Liotta FJ, Ambrose TA II, Eilert RE: Fluoroscopic technique vs Phemister technique for epiphysiodesis. *J Pediatr Orthop* 1992;12(2):248–51.
7. Moseley CF: A straight line graft for leg length discrepancies. *Clin Orthop* 1978;136:33–40.
8. Phemister DB: Operative arrestment of longitudinal growth of bones in the treatment of deformities. *J Bone Joint Surg* 1933;15:1–15.
9. Scott AC, Urquhart BA, Cain TE: Percutaneous vs modified Phemister epiphysiodesis of the lower extremity. *Orthopedics* 1996;19(10):857–61.
10. Waseem M, Fischer J, Paton RW. Partial percutaneous epiphyseodesis in patients with congenital abnormalities of the growth plates. *J Pediart Orthop B* 2004;13:39–42.

SOFIELD PROCEDURE

SURGICAL CONSIDERATIONS

Description: The **Sofield procedure,** or "**fragmentation rodding,**" is most commonly performed for deformity of the long bone, and to prevent recurrent fracture, usually a result of osteogenesis imperfecta. The procedure involves exposure of at least one end and a varying amount of the bony shaft. If the deformity is severe, the entire shaft is exposed via a longitudinal incision, usually laterally. The bone is divided (osteotomized) into the minimum number of segments that will allow a straight intramedullary rod to traverse the segments (usually 2–4 osteotomies). The construct is justly referred to as a "shish kebab." It is needed less frequently in the upper extremities.

Variant procedure or approaches: Because a growing bone will elongate beyond the end of a simple intramedullary rod after 1–2 years, the resulting unsupported portion of the bone will be liable to fracture or new deformity. To obviate this problem, **Bailey** and **Dubow** developed an **elongating rod system**, consisting of an outer tubular rod sleeve (the female portion) and an inner obturator portion (male). Both ends of the telescoping rod are anchored in the ends of the bones. The system elongates much like a car radio antenna and decreases the need for frequent revisions. The surgical technique is, however, identical to any fragmentation rodding, except that both ends of the bone must be exposed.

Usual preop diagnosis: Osteogenesis imperfecta; fibrous dysplasia (occasionally); rickets; congenital pseudarthrosis of the tibia

SUMMARY OF PROCEDURE	
Position	Supine
Incision	Lateral for femur; anterolateral for tibia
Special instrumentation	± fluoroscopy (I.I.) table
Unique considerations	Tendency to hyperthermia; other bones may fracture in more severe cases, even as a result of a BP cuff. If dentinogenesis imperfecta is present, extreme care should be taken during intubation to prevent tooth trauma. In these patients, neck motion is often limited.
Antibiotics	Cefazolin 25 mg/kg iv

SUMMARY OF PROCEDURE (cont'd)	
Surgical time	1–1.5 h/tibia; 1.5–2.5 h/femur (often done sequentially on the same day)
Closing considerations	Double spica cast if femur is rodded.
EBL	Depending on patient age and size, as well as use of a tourniquet for the femur, 50–250 mL; for the tibia, 50–100 mL
Postop care	PACU → room; avoid trauma to teeth, mouth, or other bones in PACU.
Mortality	< 1% (usually related to severe restrictive lung disease, in the most severely involved cases)
Morbidity	Intraop hyperthermia: common Intraop fracture of other bones or teeth Late rod migration: common Late refracture: common Nonunion: rare Exuberant callus simulating osteosarcoma: rare Infection: < 1% of rodding Radial nerve palsy (in cases of humerus or radius rodding)
Pain score	2–3 (It is surprising how little discomfort these children have, especially the 2nd or 3rd time a bone is rodded.)

PATIENT POPULATION CHARACTERISTICS	
Age range	2–25 yr
Male:Female	1:1
Incidence	1/20,000 (osteogenesis imperfecta); other etiologies much less common
Etiology	Congenital (hereditary deficit in collagen synthesis), most commonly as autosomal dominant or spontaneous mutation: All cases
Associated conditions	Dentinogenesis imperfecta; diminished vital capacity due to associated kyphoscoliosis ↓ hearing due to otosclerosis and impingement of the 8th cranial nerve; pelvic distortion causing chronic constipation; basilar impression and other C-spine abnormalities causing brain stem compression or even hydrocephalus (rare)

ANESTHETIC CONSIDERATIONS

See Anesthetic Considerations for Pediatric Orthopedic Surgery of the Pelvis and Lower Extremities, see p. 1389.

Suggested Readings

1. Bailey RW, Dubow HE: Evolution of the concept of an extensible nail accommodating to normal longitudinal bone growth: clinical considerations and implications. *Clin Orthop* 1981;159:157–70.
2. Gamble JG, Strudwick WJ, Rinsky LA, et al: Complications of intramedullary rods in osteogenesis imperfecta: Bailey-Dubow rods versus non-elongating rods. *J Pediatr Orthop* 1988;8(6):645–9.
3. Marafioti RL, Westin GW: Elongating intramedullary rods in the treatment of osteogenesis imperfecta. *J Bone Joint Surg* 1977;59(4):467–72.
4. Peluso A, Cerullo M: Malignant hyperthermia susceptibility in patients with osteogenesis imperfecta. *Paediatr Anaesth* 1995;5(6):398–9.
5. Pozo JL, Crockard HA, Ransford AO: Basilar impression in osteogenesis imperfecta. A report of three cases in one family. *J Bone Joint Surg* 1984;66(2):233–8.
6. Rodriquez RP, Bailey RW: Internal fixation of the femur in patients with osteogenesis imperfecta. *Clin Orthop* 1988;159: 126–33.
7. Sofield HA, Millar EA: Fragmentation, realignment and intramedullary rod fixation of deformities of the long bones in children. A ten-year appraisal. *J Bone Joint Surg* 1959;41:1371–91.

8. Stockley I, Bell MJ, Sharrad WJ: The role of expanding intramedullary rods in osteogenesis imperfecta. *J Bone Joint Surg* 1989;71(3):422–7.
9. Wilkinson JM, Scott BW, Clarke AM, et al: Surgical stabilization of the lower limb in osteogenesis imperfecta using the Sheffield Telescopic Intramedullary Rod System. *J Bone Joint Surg* 1998;80(6):999–1004.

LIMB LENGTHENING

SURGICAL CONSIDERATIONS

Description: Limb lengthening usually is performed in the lower extremity for congenital or acquired leg-length discrepancies of at least 5 cm. Lesser discrepancies are dealt with by bone shortening or epiphysiodesis of the long side. The basic principles include: (a) application of an adjustable, external fixator; (b) "low-energy," transverse bone cut (osteotomy without use of a power saw) through a small, longitudinal incision over the involved bone; (c) preservation of the periosteal sleeve; (d) gradual lengthening, usually 1 mm/day in fractional adjustments; and (e) when the desired limb length is obtained, either use bone graft and plate acutely or leave until the bone gap fills in and stabilizes (average 38 d/cm gained).

Limb lengthening dates back to the early 1900s, but it fell into disfavor because of the high rate of major complications. **Wagner** improved the technique by introducing a simplified, unilateral, large-pin fixator, but performed the osteotomy in the midshaft and began lengthening immediately (Fig. 12.7-14). This technique usually requires a bone graft and later plating as a second operation to obtain healing. **DeBastiani** uses a similar large-pin fixator (**Orthofix**), but performs the osteotomy more toward the end of the bone (metaphysis) and waits a week before beginning the lengthening. Spontaneous healing is usual. **Ilizarov** introduced a more complex, but more adaptable, small-pin transfixation system with a circular fixator. In a similar fashion, the Ilizarov method stretches the healing callus (callotasis). Typically, 4–10 cm/bone are gained with any of the above techniques.

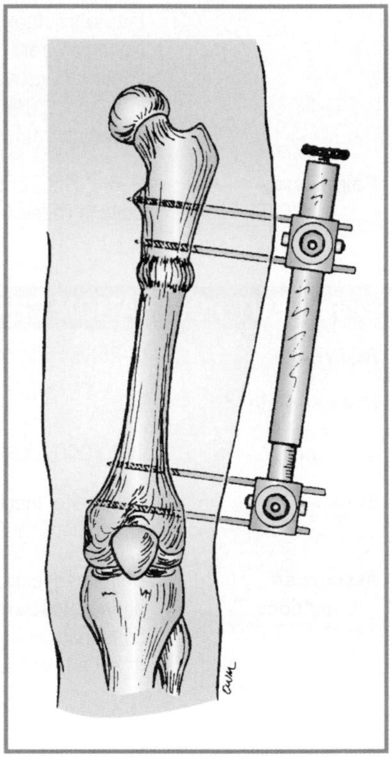

Figure 12.7-14. Wagner apparatus for leg lengthening. (Reproduced with permission from Chapman MW, ed: *Operative Orthopaedics,* 2nd edition. JB Lippincott, Philadelphia: 1993.)

Usual preop diagnosis: Congenital or acquired anisomelia (limb-length discrepancy) due to overgrowth or growth retardation > 5 cm.

Pediatric Surgery

SUMMARY OF PROCEDURES

	Wagner	Orthofix	Ilizarov
Position	Supine	⇐	⇐
Incision	Longitudinal midshaft	Longitudinal proximal shaft (metaphyseal)	⇐
Special instrumentation	I.I.; Wagner device (Fig.12.7-13); large bone pins	I.I.; Orthofix device; large bone pins	Ilizarov frame ("Erector set"); multiple 1.5–1.8 mm small-diameter wires

SUMMARY OF PROCEDURES (cont'd)

	Wagner	Orthofix	Ilizarov
Unique considerations	Acute lengthening may cause ↑ BP.	–	Frame should be prepped prior to surgery because of "fiddle factor."
Antibiotics	Cefazolin 25 mg/kg iv	⇐	⇐
Surgical time	1–2 h	⇐	2–4 h
EBL	< 100 mL	⇐	⇐
Postop care	PACU → room; early initiation of physical therapy and/or CPM machine	⇐	⇐
Mortality	Minimal	⇐	⇐
Morbidity	While the device remains in place, at least one of the following complications is usual; frequently, several occur before healing is complete:	⇐	⇐
	• Joint stiffness or localized pin infection: Very common (50% temporary)	⇐	⇐
	• Edema, swelling, pressure sores: Common	⇐	⇐
	• Joint subluxation: Common	⇐	⇐
	• Psychological decompensation due to pain: Common	⇐	⇐
	• Premature consolidation: Common	⇐	⇐
	• Skin necrosis: Common	⇐	⇐
	• Wound infection: Common	⇐	⇐
	• Localized osteomyelitis: Common	⇐	⇐
	• Axial deviation of the bone: Common	⇐	⇐
	• Delayed union, nonunion, late fracture: Common	⇐	⇐
	• Pin penetration of a vessel or nerve: Rare	⇐	⇐
	• Compartment syndrome: Rare	⇐	⇐
	Sudeck's atrophy: Rare	⇐	⇐
Pain score	7–8	7–8	7–8

PATIENT POPULATION CHARACTERISTICS

Age range	10–30 yr
Male:Female	1:1
Incidence	Dependent on underlying Dx (common in polio)
Etiology	Congenital deficiencies of the lower extremities (e.g., proximal focal femoral deficiency, congenitally short femur, fibular hemimelia, etc.); osteomyelitis, traumatic growth plate injury, fracture; asymmetric neurologic conditions (e.g., polio or cerebral palsy); congenital hemihypertrophy
Associated conditions	Hip and knee contractures; in cases of polio, other deformities, and weaknesses; AVM; congenital or developmental hip dislocation

ANESTHETIC CONSIDERATIONS

See Anesthetic Considerations for Pediatric Orthopedic Surgery of the Pelvis and Lower Extremities, p. 1389.

Suggested Readings

1. Abbott LC: The operative lengthening of the tibia and fibula. *J Bone Joint Surg* 1927;9:128–52.
2. Aronson J: Limb-lengthening, skeletal reconstruction, and bone transport with the Ilizarov method. *J Bone Joint Surg* 1997;79(8):1243–58.
3. DeBastiani G, Aldegheai R, Renzi-Briviol, et al: Limb lengthening by callus distraction (callotasis). *J Pediatr Orthop* 1987;7(2):129–34.
4. Friend L, Widmann RF: Advances in management of limb length discrepancy and lower limb deformity. *Curr Opin Pediatr* 2008;20(1):46–51.
5. Murray JH, Fitch RD: Distraction histiogenesis: principles and indications. *J Am Acad Orthop Surg* 1996;4(6):317–27.
6. Noonan KJ, Leyes M, Forriol F, et al: Distraction osteogenesis of the lower extremity with use of monolateral external fixation. A study of two hundred and sixty-one femora and tibiae. *J Bone Joint Surg* 1998;80(6):793–806.
7. Wagner H: Operative lengthening of the femur. *Clin Orthop* 1978;136:125–42.

PATELLAR REALIGNMENT

SURGICAL CONSIDERATIONS

Description: Patellar realignment encompasses over 100 procedures designed to prevent lateral subluxation and dislocation of the patella. These disorders include a spectrum of malalignments of the patella, ranging from simple excess lateral tilt, recurrent partial subluxation, and recurrent episodic dislocation, to irreducible chronic dislocation. As such, the surgical procedures also encompass a spectrum of complexities, depending on the degree of instability. Nowadays, an arthroscopic inspection often is performed first. The basic principles of the repair include both proximal and distal realignment. **Proximal realignment** includes: (a) lateral release, which is the division of the contracted lateral patellar retinacular joint capsule and other tight lateral tissue—the first step in all surgical repair; (b) medial tightening, including reefing and/or advancement of the medial capsule and vastus medialis muscle insertion; and (c) distal realignment, consisting of redirection of the patellar tendon more medially (and sometimes more anteriorly).

Variant procedure or approaches: **Arthroscopic or open lateral release** is the simplest and first-step procedure. It may be sufficient when there is only subluxation and not true dislocation; and it has the advantage of being an outpatient procedure. For frank dislocation, an open "proximal realignment" also includes the medial tautening. If this is not sufficient to hold the patella centralized and if the patient has open epiphyses (< 16 yr), the lateral half of the patellar tendon may be released (distal realignment) and reattached medially (**Roux-Goldthwait**) or the patella may be held medially by tenodesing the semitendinosus tendon to it. In skeletally mature patients, the bony insertion of the patellar tendon is osteotomized and transferred medially (**Trillat**) or anteriomedially (**Macquet**).The **Hauser procedure** of distal and medial transfer of the tibial tubercle has had a very poor long-term outcome and is seldom performed.

Usual preop diagnosis: Lateral patellar subluxation; recurrent dislocation; congenital or chronic lateral patellar dislocation

Pediatric Surgery

SUMMARY OF PROCEDURES

	Proximal Realignment	Trillat	Macquet
Position	Supine, with tourniquet	⇐	⇐
Incision	Anterior transverse or longitudinal or oblique, about the knee, or arthroscopic	Anterior longitudinal	Transverse or oblique
Special instrumentation	None	Single bone screw	⇐

SUMMARY OF PROCEDURES (cont'd)

	Proximal Realignment	Trillat	Macquet
Unique considerations	Tourniquet	⇐	May use iliac or bank bone graft.
Antibiotics	Optional, cefazolin 25 mg/kg iv	Usually, cefazolin 25 mg/kg iv	⇐
Surgical time	1.5 h	1–2 h	⇐
Closing considerations	Cylinder cast	⇐	Skin closure may be difficult, depending on elevation of tibial tubercle.
Postop care	PACU → home, if arthroscopic	PACU → room	⇐
EBL	< 100 mL	⇐	⇐
Mortality	Minimal	⇐	⇐
Morbidity	Recurrence: 5–10%	⇐	⇐
	Late stiffness or ↑ knee pain: 5%	⇐	⇐
	Superficial wound dehiscence or infection: ≤ 5%	<5%	≤ 5%
	Anterior compartment syndrome of the leg (Hauser procedure): 1–5%	⇐	⇐
	Deep infection: 1–2%	⇐	⇐
	Peroneal palsy: < 1%	⇐	⇐
Pain score	4–6	4–6	4–6

PATIENT POPULATION CHARACTERISTICS

Age range	2–20 yr (most commonly, 13–20 yr)
Male:Female	1:3
Incidence	Subluxation: Very common Recurrent dislocation: Rare Congenital dislocation: Very rare
Etiology	Generalized ligamentous laxity; familial tendency; congenital hypoplasia at a lateral femoral condyle; abnormal attachment or contracture of the IT band; medial femoral torsion or genu valgum; trauma
Associated conditions	Diffuse hyperlaxity syndromes (Ehlers-Danlos, Marfan, etc.); nail patella syndrome (hypoplastic nails and dislocated radial heads, as well as hypoplastic patellae)

ANESTHETIC CONSIDERATIONS

See Anesthetic Considerations for Pediatric Orthopedic Surgery of the Pelvis and Lower Extremities, see p. 1389.

Suggested Readings

1. Baker RH, Carroll N, Dewar FP, et al: The semitendinosus tenodesis for recurrent dislocation of the patella. *J Bone Joint Surg* 1972;54(l):103–9.
2. Chrisman OD, Snook GA, Wilson TC: A long-term prospective study of the Hauser and Roux-Goldthwait procedures for recurrent patellar dislocation. *Clin Orthop* 1979;144:27–30.
3. Cox JS: Evaluation of the Roux-Elmslie-Trillat procedure for knee extensor realignment. *Am J Sports Med* 1982;10(5):303–10.

4. Fondren FB, Goldner JL, Bassett FH III: Recurrent dislocation of the patella treated by the modified Roux-Goldthwait procedure. A prospective study of forty-seven knees. *J Bone Joint Surg* 1985;67(7):993–1005.
5. Hughston J, Walsh WM: Proximal and distal reconstruction of the extensor mechanism for patellar subluxation. *Clin Orthop* 1979;144:36–42.
6. Maquet P: Mechanics and osteoarthritis of the patellofemoral joint. *Clin Orthop* 1979;144:70–3.
7. Morrissy RT: *Atlas of Pediatric Orthopaedic Surgery.* JB Lippincott, Philadelphia: 1992, 425–38.
8. Mulford JS, Wakeley CJ, Eldridge JD: Assessment and management of chronic patellofemoral instability. *J Bone Joint Surg Br* 2007;89(6):709–16.
9. Tachdjian MO: *Pediatric Orthopaedics.* WB Saunders, Philadelphia: 1990, 1551–95.
10. Trillat A, DeJour H, Louette A: Diagnostic et traitement des subluxations récidiventes de la rotule. *Rev Chir Orthop* 1964;50:813–24.
11. Wall JJ: Compartment syndrome as a complication of the Hauser procedure. *J Bone Joint Surg* 1979;61(2):185–91.

TENDON TRANSFER, LENGTHENING (POSTERIOR TIBIAL)

SURGICAL CONSIDERATIONS

Description: Extremity tendons may be lengthened (for contracture) or transferred to change the muscle force vector and compensate for paralysis or paresis of other muscle groups. Originally used for the treatment of poliomyelitis sequelae, these lengthenings and transfers are now used for a variety of deformities 2° more common neuromuscular disorders, such as cerebral palsy, muscular dystrophies, Charcot-Marie-Tooth disease, traumatic nerve palsies, etc. Basic principles are that the muscles to be transferred should be at least grade 4/5 strength, and that the loss of normal function should be well compensated. The posterior tibial muscle (PTM) is a representative example, but many extremity muscles have one or more described lengthenings or transfers. Such procedures frequently are combined with other transfers or fusions.

For moderate spastic ankle varus, the simplest procedure, **PTM lengthening,** is accomplished by an intramuscular myotendinous "slide." This refers to simply cutting the tendinous fibers well within the distal muscle belly and leaving a small gap in the tendon, while the surrounding muscle fibers remain intact. An alternative for spastic varus is the **split posterior tibial transfer** of the PTM. Four short, 2–3-cm incisions are used to expose and dissect half of the posterior tibia tendon at its insertion on the navicular. Then half of the tendon is passed proximally up its sheath to a second incision just posterior to the distal tibial shaft medially. The freed half tendon is passed laterally to the peroneal tendon sheath just distal to the lateral malleolus, where, through a final incision, the tendon is anastomosed to the peroneus brevis.

For complete flaccid foot drop (e.g., peroneal nerve palsy), the entire posterior tibial tendon is transferred. First, it is detached at its medial insertion, delivered proximally at the distal tibia posteriorly, passed **anteriorly** through a window in the interosseous membrane, and then subcutaneously passed to the mid-dorsal surface of the foot, where it is fixed into the middle cuneiform by a pull-out stitch.

Usual preop diagnosis: Flaccid or spastic developmental deformity, such as varus or valgus foot neuromuscular disease

SUMMARY OF PROCEDURES

	Lengthening	Split Transfer	Anterior Transfer
Position	Supine	⇐	⇐
Incision	Longitudinal posteromedial calf	Medial foot; posteromedial calf; lateral ankle; lateral foot	Medial foot; posteromedial calf; anterior ankle; dorsal foot
Special instrumentation	None	Tendon passer	Pull-out suture; buttons
Unique considerations	Underlying neurologic disease. Usually added to other procedures (e.g., Achilles tendon lengthenings).	⇐	⇐

SUMMARY OF PROCEDURES (cont'd)

	Lengthening	Split Transfer	Anterior Transfer
Antibiotics	Usually none	⇐	⇐
Surgical time	30 min	1 h	⇐
Closing considerations	Below-knee cast	⇐	⇐
EBL	< 20 mL	< 50 mL	⇐
Postop care	PACU or room	⇐	⇐
Mortality	Rare	⇐	⇐
Morbidity	Over- or undercorrection Hematoma Drainage: < 1%	⇐ ⇐ ⇐	⇐ ⇐ ⇐
Pain score	1–3	3–4	3–4

PATIENT POPULATION CHARACTERISTICS

Age range	3–30 yr
Male:Female	1:1
Incidence	Dependent on Dx
Etiology	Poliomyelitis; cerebral palsy, spina bifida; traumatic peroneal nerve injury; neuropathies, myopathies (e.g., Charcot-Marie-Tooth disease)
Associated conditions	Multiple other contractures

ANESTHETIC CONSIDERATIONS

See Anesthetic Considerations for Pediatric Orthopedic Surgery of the Pelvis and Lower Extremities, see p. 1389.

Suggested Readings

1. Barnes MJ, Herring JA: Combined split anterior tibial-tendon transfer and intramuscular lengthening of the posterior tibial tendon. Results in patients who have a varus deformity of the foot due to spastic cerebral palsy. *J Bone Joint Surg* 1991;73(5):734–8.
2. Green NE, Griffin PP, Shiavi R: Split posterior tibial-tendon transfers in spastic cerebral palsy. *J Bone Joint Surg* 1983;65(6):748–54.
3. Greene WB: Cerebral palsy. Evaluation and management of equinus and equinovarus deformities. *Foot Ankle Clin* 2000;5(2):265–80.
4. Hoffer MD, Barakat G, Koffman M: 10-year follow-up of split anterior tibial tendon transfer in cerebral palsied patients with spastic equinovarus deformity. *J Pediatr Orthop* 1985;5(4):432–4.
5. Miller G, Hsu JD, Hoffer MM, et al: Posterior tibial tendon transfer: a review of the literature and analysis of 74 procedures. *J Pediatr Orthop* 1982;2(4):363–70.
6. Morrissy RT: *Atlas of Pediatric Orthopaedic Surgery.* JB Lippincott, Philadelphia: 1992, 645–68.
7. Richards BM: Interosseous transfer of tibialis posterior for common peroneal nerve palsy. *J Bone Joint Surg* 1989;71(5):834–7.
8. Rinsky LA: Surgery for cerebral palsy. In *Chapman's Orthopaedic Surgery,* 3rd edition. Chapman MW, ed. Lippincott Williams & Wilkins, Philadelphia: 2001, 4485–504.
9. Woo R: Spasticity: Orthopedic perspective. *J Child Neurol* 2001;16(1):47–53.

TRIPLE ARTHRODESIS AND GRICE PROCEDURE (EXTRA-ARTICULAR SUBTALAR ARTHRODESIS)

SURGICAL CONSIDERATIONS

Description: **Triple arthrodesis** is used to realign the hind foot of skeletally mature patients with significant fixed or flexible deformities of multiple etiologies. The technique involves denuding the cartilaginous surfaces of the talonavicular, talocalcaneal (subtalar), and calcaneocuboid joints and fusing them. The approach is always through an oblique lateral sinus tarsi incision and often an additional short medial incision over the talonavicular joint. For supple (passively correctable) deformities, the fusion is performed easily in situ. Fixed deformities are more difficult; but, basically, any deformity (valgus, varus, planus, cavus, etc.) can be corrected by resecting appropriate wedges of bone. Fixation is usually internal with pins, screws, or staples, in addition to an external cast.

Variant procedure or approaches: Because the triple arthrodesis removes growth cartilage, it is unsuitable in growing children (< 12–14 yr). **Grice** developed an **extraarticular subtalar fusion** which can be performed as early as age 3. It is basically a block of autologous bone graft placed between the talus and the calcaneus to stabilize a valgus heel. Tibial, fibular or, preferably, iliac autologous graft is used through the same lateral sinus tarsi incision as for a triple arthrodesis.

Usual preop diagnosis: Varus or cavovarus foot deformities; severe valgus or equinovalgus

SUMMARY OF PROCEDURES

	Triple Arthrodesis	Grice Procedure
Position	Supine, slightly tilted up on the operative side	⇐
Incision	2" oblique over the sinus tarsi; optional medial incision	⇐
Special instrumentation	Pins, screws, or rods	Pin or screw
Unique considerations	Intraop x-ray to confirm pin position	Iliac or tibial autologous graft
Antibiotics	Usually, cefazolin 25 mg/kg iv up to 1 gm	Cefazolin 25 mg/kg iv up to 1 gm
Surgical time	1–2 h	1.5 h
Closing considerations	Above-the-knee cast	⇐
EBL	< 100 mL	< 50 mL
Postop care	PACU → room	⇐
Mortality	Rare	⇐
Morbidity	Superficial skin slough Superficial infection Nonunion of at least one arthrodesis site (usually talonavicular) Aseptic necrosis of the talus: Rare	⇐ ⇐ ⇐ ⇐
Pain score	6–8	4–5

PATIENT POPULATION CHARACTERISTICS

Age range	> 12 yr (triple arthrodesis); 3–10 yr (Grice)
Male:Female	1:1
Incidence	< 1% (depends on diagnosis and severity of deformity)

PATIENT POPULATION CHARACTERISTICS (cont'd)	
Etiology	Neuromuscular imbalance (most cases); congenital malformations (e.g., coalitions, severe pes planus); incompletely treated or overcorrected clubfoot; postfracture of calcaneus or talus
Associated conditions	Poliomyelitis; cerebral palsy (↑ GERD, ↓ airway protective reflexes, ↑ postop pulmonary complications); myelomeningocele; Charcot-Marie-Tooth disease (↑ sensitivity to muscle relaxants); congenital tarsal coalition

ANESTHETIC CONSIDERATIONS

See Anesthetic Considerations for Pediatric Orthopedic Surgery of the Pelvis and Lower Extremities, see p. 1389.

Suggested Readings

1. Dennyson WG, Fulford GE: Subtalar arthrodesis by cancellous grafts and metallic internal fixation. *J Bone Joint Surg* 1976;58(4):507–10.
2. Duncan JW, Lovell WW: Hoke triple arthrodesis. *J Bone Joint Surg* 1978;60(6):795–8.
3. Grice DS: An extra-articular arthrodesis of the subastragalar joint for correction of paralytic flat feet in children. *J Bone Joint Surg* 1952;34:927–40.
4. Mann RA, Mann JA: Arthrodesis of the foot and ankle. In *Chapman's Orthopaedic Surgery,* 3rd edition. Chapman MW, ed. Lippincott Williams & Wilkins, Philadelphia: 2001, 3057–72.
5. Morrissy RT: *Atlas of Pediatric Orthopaedic Surgery.* JB Lippincott, Philadelphia: 1992, 589–99.

SURGICAL CORRECTION OF CLUBFOOT

SURGICAL CONSIDERATIONS

Description: **Turco** popularized the one-stage surgical correction of resistant (uncorrected by casting) clubfoot (talipes equinovarus) in 1971. The orthopedic literature, however, is replete with reports of varying techniques for surgical correction of clubfoot. The three components of the deformity are: (a) hindfoot equinus (back of the heel is up); (b) varus (rolled inwardly); and (c) forefoot adductus (medial deviation). Beyond this, however, there exists considerable disagreement as to the pathologic anatomy, ideal skin incision, position, and which structures to release. Most surgeons vary the degree of release in proportion to the degree of deformity, often performing release of the same deep structures through totally different skin incisions. The most important structures released include: the entire posterior capsule of the ankle and subtalar joint; capsule of the subtalar, talonavicular, and calcaneal cuboid joints; tendo-Achilles, posterior tibial tendon, and usually the toe flexors; and origin of the abductor, halluces, and the plantar fascia. The navicular is repositioned on the talus and usually held with a small pin.

Variant procedure or approaches: **Turco's procedure** is essentially a posteromedial procedure only and is performed through one incision on the medial aspect of the foot. **Crawford** described a much more extensile approach through an incision (**Cincinnati**) that runs from anteromedial, around the back of the tendo-Achilles, and then anterolateral to the calcaneal cuboid joint. This approach is also used by **McKay**, **Simons** and others for a more complete release. If there is severe equinus deformity, however, the incision is difficult to close posteriorly when the foot is brought up. **Carroll** accomplishes much the same correction using a separate medial and posterolateral incision.

Usual preop diagnosis: Resistant idiopathic clubfoot; secondary clubfoot due to paralysis

SUMMARY OF PROCEDURES			
	Turco	**Cincinnati/McKay/Simons**	**Carroll**
Position	Supine	Prone or supine	Supine
Incision	Straight medial foot	Transverse from the navicular bone medially posteriorly across the heel cord, then laterally to the cuboid	Medial zigzag and posterolateral longitudinal

Pediatric Surgery

SUMMARY OF PROCEDURES (cont'd)

	Turco	Cincinnati/McKay/Simons	Carroll
Special instrumentation	Usually loupe magnification; small K wires to hold reduction	⇐	⇐
Unique considerations	Tourniquet mandatory and often bilateral	⇐	⇐
Antibiotics	Cefazolin 25 mg/kg iv	⇐	⇐
Surgical time	1–2 h/foot	⇐	⇐
Closing considerations	Well padded, loose-fitting, above-the-knee cast × 10–14 d	⇐	⇐
EBL	< 30 mL	⇐	⇐
Postop care	PACU → room	⇐	⇐
Mortality	Rare	⇐	⇐
Morbidity	Mild, persistent deformity: very common Hematoma: 2% Superficial infection: 1–2% Avascular necrosis Overcorrection valgus, planus Pressure changes of the navicula Wound dehiscence or necrosis Transection of posterior tibial nerve or artery branch: Rare (except in patients who have had multiple operations)	⇐	⇐
Pain score	2–5	2–5	2–5

PATIENT POPULATION CHARACTERISTICS

Age range	3 mo–6 yr
Male:Female	2:1 (idiopathic type)
Incidence	1.2/10,000 live births (idiopathic type)
Etiology	Genetic, or hereditary effects; neuromuscular defects of the calf muscles; primary defect of formation of the talus and/or other tarsal bones; shortened ligaments and muscles
Associated conditions	Arthrogryposis (difficult intubation; ±VSD, other CHD); Larsen's syndrome (difficult intubation, ± ↑ICP); Freeman-Sheldon syndrome (difficult intubation); osteochondral dystrophies (e.g., diastrophic dwarfism); spinal dysraphism; tethered spinal cord; congenital constricting bands; poliomyelitis

ANESTHETIC CONSIDERATIONS

See Anesthetic Considerations for Pediatric Orthopedic Surgery of the Pelvis and Lower Extremities, see p 1389.

Suggested Readings

1. Beat JH: Congenital anomalies of the lower extremity. In *Campbell's Operative Orthopaedics,* 8th edition. Crenshaw AH, ed. Mosby-Year Book, St. Louis: 1992, 2075–91.

2. Carroll NC: Congenital clubfoot: pathoanatomy and treatment. *AAOS Instr Course Lect* 1987;36:117–21.
3. Crawford AH, Marxen JL, Osterfeld DL: The Cincinnati incision: a comprehensive approach for surgical procedures of the foot and ankle in childhood. *J Bone Joint Surg* 1982;64(9):1355–8.
4. Cummings RJ, Davidson RS, Armstrong PF, et al: Congenital clubfoot. *J Bone Joint Surg* 2002;84A(2)290–308.
5. Lichtblau S: A medial and lateral release operation for clubfoot. *J Bone Joint Surg* 1973;55(7):1377–84.
6. McKay DW: New concept of and approach to club foot treatment: section II–correction of the club foot. *J Pediatr Orthop* 1983;3(1):10–21.
7. Morrissy RT: *Atlas of Pediatric Orthopaedic Surgery.* JB Lippincott, Philadelphia: 1992, 523–8.
8. Simons GW: Complete subtalar release in clubfeet: part I–a preliminary report. *J Bone Joint Surg* 1985;67(7):1044–55.
9. Simons GW: Complete subtalar release in clubfeet: part II–comparison with less extensive procedures. *J Bone Joint Surg* 1985;67(7):1056–65.
10. Turco VJ: Resistant congenital club foot-one-stage posteromedial release with internal fixation. A follow-up report of a fifteen-year experience. *J Bone Joint Surg* 1979;61(6A):805–14.
11. Turco VJ: Surgical correction of the resistant club foot. One-stage posteromedial release with internal fixation: a preliminary report. *J Bone Joint Surg* 1971;53(3):477–97.

ANESTHETIC CONSIDERATIONS FOR PEDIATRIC ORTHOPEDIC SURGERY OF THE PELVIS AND LOWER EXTREMITIES

(Procedures covered: pelvic osteotomy; acetabular augmentation & Chiari osteotomy; Ober fasciotomy; Yount Ober release; hip, open reduction; adductor release and/or transfer; psoas release; pinning of SCFE; femoral osteotomy; epiphysiodesis; Sofield procedure; limb lengthening; tendon transfer or lengthening; triple arthrodesis, Grice procedure; correction of clubfoot)

PREOPERATIVE

Children undergoing orthopedic procedures of the lower extremities typically fall into two groups: (a) post-trauma but otherwise healthy, and (b) those with a variety of chronic medical problems, including cerebral palsy, congenital hip dislocation, limb deformities, osteogenesis imperfecta, juvenile rheumatoid arthritis, epidermolysis bullosa, and various myopathies and muscular dystrophies. The anesthesiologist should review the anesthetic implications of these various syndromes or diseases (see Table 12.7-2). Many of these patients will have cardiac, respiratory, endocrine, and metabolic derangements, as well as airway abnormalities that may affect anesthetic management. In addition, the surgical procedures may run the gamut from a simple syndactyly repair of the toes with little blood loss to pelvic osteotomies (in small children) with blood loss approaching the patients blood volume. Many patients with slipped capital femoral epiphysis (SCFE) are obese and require anesthetic techniques that minimize the risk of aspiration.

Respiratory	Patient's preop activity level is a good indication for baseline respiratory function. Careful assessment is necessary as associated anomalies may affect airway or lungs. Chronic otitis 2° eustachian tube dysfunction is common. Postpone surgery (~2–3 wk) if Sx of acute URI (e.g., runny nose, fever, sore throat, cough) are present. **Tests:** As indicated from H&P (although PFTs are not currently recommended as a routine part of the preanesthetic evaluation of the scoliosis patient).
Cardiovascular	Some pediatric patients with congenital musculoskeletal anomalies presenting for orthopedic procedures have coexisting cardiovascular anomalies. Preop review of patient's H&P is essential. Patients should not be accepted for orthopedic surgery and anesthesia until they are in the best possible physical and emotional condition. For children with CHD or who require cardiac medication, it is advisable to consult with a pediatric cardiologist before surgery. ***NB:** The consequences of VAE may be disastrous (e.g., cerebral or myocardial embolization) in patients with R→ L shunt lesions. All iv lines, injection ports, and syringes should be air-free. **Tests:** EKG; Hct; baseline SaO_2 ; CXR, as necessary

Pediatric Surgery

Table 12.7-2. Preop Anesthesia Considerations for Pediatric Orthopedic Diseases

General Considerations	Pediatric orthopedic patients may present with a spectrum of congenital and acquired problems. Congenital malformations and deformations include clubfoot, developmental dislocation of hip, and congenital limb deficiencies. Acquired conditions include trauma, infections, and growth disturbance. A variety of patients with neuromuscular disorders present for orthopedic procedures and present special challenges to the anesthesiologist (e.g., cerebral palsy, spina bifida, muscular dystrophy). Other syndromes and chronic conditions with orthopedic manifestations include osteogenesis imperfecta, juvenile rheumatoid arthritis, and epidermolysis bullosa. The anesthesiologist should review and understand the anesthetic implications of these various syndromes.
Specific Disease	**Anesthetic Considerations**
Achondroplasia	± Unstable spine: preop neuro and ortho exams are critical. Careful positioning necessary; prevent compression of cervicomedullary junction by placing a bolster under shoulders. Difficult iv access. ± GERD 2° obesity. Anticipate difficult mask fit and intubation. Possible choanal stenosis/narrow nasopharynx; may preclude nasal airway/nasal intubation and placement of NG tube. Smaller ETTs are needed. ± Restrictive lung disease and chronic respiratory infections common.
Apert syndrome	C-spine fusion and small nasopharynx. Hypoplastic maxilla, prominent mandible/cleft palate. Difficult laryngoscopy and ET intubation. ± Tracheal stenosis/abnormal tracheal cartilage. Possible choanal stenosis/atresia; may preclude nasal airway, nasal ETT, and NG tube placement. Difficult vascular access. ±Craniosynostosis → ↑ ICP. ± CHD.
Arthrogryposis	Poor cervical mobility; TMJ ankylosis; possibility of difficult intubation. IV access and positioning difficult 2° flexion or contracture deformity. 10% incidence of CHD.
Cerebral palsy	Communication difficulties. Scoliosis → restrictive lung disease. ± GERD. ↑ sensitivity to succinylcholine. ↑ resistance to NMRs. MAC decreased. Contractures → restricted access for examination and positioning. ± Latex allergy. Difficult iv access.
Juvenile rheumatoid arthritis	Poor cervical mobility; TMJ ankylosis; possibility of difficult intubation. ± Restrictive pulmonary disease. ± Restrictive pericarditis and tamponade.
Klippel-Feil syndrome	Limited C-Spine mobility → difficult intubation. Impaired renal drug excretion.
Marfan syndrome	Atlantoaxial instability: Evaluate C-spine before laryngoscopy. Care in positioning needed. May require larger than normal doses of spinal epidural anesthesia 2° height. Aortic dilatation → aortic insufficiency ± aortic dissection/aneurysm. Avoid ↑ BP. Anticipate difficult intubation 2° narrow palate. Lung cysts → pneumothorax.
Muscular dystrophy	Possible cardiomyopathy: Avoid cardiac depressant drugs. ↑ sensitivity to muscle relaxants. MH susceptibility. ↓ gastric emptying and weak laryngeal reflexes. Avoid succinylcholine. May have MVR and cardiac conduction abnormalities. May require postop ventilation.
Myopathies	Avoid all muscle relaxants and respiratory depressants. Postop ventilation may be necessary.
Osteogenesis imperfecta	Bones fracture easily (e.g., with BP cuff): Use extreme care in positioning and intubation. Hypermetabolic fever may occur during anesthesia. Plt dysfunction: Difficult airway. Use atropine with caution as it may exacerbate pyrexia. CHD may require antibiotic prophylaxis. ± Difficult airway. ± Restrictive lung disease. Deafness may make communication difficult.
Septic arthritis	Infection/systemic toxicity slows gastric emptying; requires rapid-sequence intubation (Appendix B-4). Dehydration 2° ↑ T and ↓ fluid intake → hypovolemia/hemodynamic instability. Rx: adequate fluid resuscitation with balanced salt solution.

Neurological

For patients with cerebral palsy presenting for orthopedic surgery, preop understanding of their intellectual functional capacity is necessary. Information about patient's behavioral or intellectual abilities is usually best obtained from parents or guardian. If patient is on seizure-control medication, it is recommended that the medication be continued until surgery. All patients who require Ober fasciotomy or Yount release will have profound weakness of lower extremities, if not of the entire body. Must be careful in choice of muscle relaxant (generally avoid depolarizing agents). Many patients with muscular dystrophy

Neurological (cont'd)	present for repeated orthopedic procedures. Patients with congenital muscular dystrophy (especially Duchenne's or Becker's) can have significant associated cardiac dysfunction. A pediatric cardiologist should be involved in the preanesthetic evaluation of their LV function, size, LV ejection fraction, shortening fraction, and ECHO exam. It is important to note that asymptomatic carriers of these X-linked muscular dystrophies can have associated ECHO and EKG abnormalities.
Hematologic	Complications of blood loss remain a major anesthetic consideration in pelvic osteotomies, especially in small children or those who have ↑ bleeding 2° osteogenic bone or bleeding disorders. There is no hard-and-fast rule for an acceptable amount of blood loss before transfusion therapy begins; each case must be individualized. Patients who need ↑ O_2-carrying capacity (e.g., congenital heart disease, sickle cell anemia (SSA), evidence of V/Q mismatch from preexisting pulmonary disease) will require transfusion at lower levels of blood loss than otherwise healthy children. Blood transfusion therapy must be considered after the loss of 15–20% of the patient's total blood volume. Predonation is limited by age, size, and level of cooperation with blood-collecting techniques. Hemodilution is not used frequently in pediatrics. Cell salvaging can introduce both intracellular and surgical debris back into circulation.
Laboratory	Tests as indicated from H&P.
Premedication	Premedication for separation anxiety (e.g., midazolam) and facilitating induction. Care must be taken if premedication is used in patients with respiratory or cardiac dysfunction. Dosage must be individualized (see p. E-4). Children with valvular disease, prosthetic valves, and/or most forms of CHD, as well as postcardiac-correction patients, should receive antibiotics for bacterial endocarditis prophylaxis preop.

INTRAOPERATIVE

Anesthetic technique: As indicated in the preop considerations, these patient populations cover a vast spectrum, from fit and healthy children to those suffering from a variety of clinical syndromes with airway and cardiorespiratory problems. Thus, anesthesia needs to be tailored to the individual patient. Some older children may benefit from regional anesthesia with sedation. Some may do well with a combined regional/GA technique, whereas still others with difficult airways may require awake FOB (see p. B-5). The following sections address some of these concerns.

Induction	**Otherwise healthy:** Standard pediatric (< 12 yr) (see p. D-1) or adult induction (see p. B-2). **Difficult airway:** A mask induction and FOL during spontaneous respiration should be considered. Alternatives include use of LMA/intubating LMA, FOL or light wand stylet, retrograde wire intubation, and tracheostomy. **Muscle abnormalities:** These patients may be very sensitive to muscle relaxants, have gastric hypomotility, and may be predisposed to MH. Induction should be accomplished by nontriggering agents (e.g., propofol 1–2 mg/kg and rocuronium 0.5–1 mg/kg) if necessary for intubation. Succinylcholine usually is contraindicated in these patients. Dantrolene must be available, but it need not be administered prophylactically. A study of MH patients showed that 32 out of 89 had preexisting musculoskeletal abnormalities. **Cardiorespiratory compromise**: Inhalational induction, when administered cautiously, may be used safely in this group of patients. Intramuscular (e.g., ketamine 4–8 mg/kg im) inductions are usually safe and effective in neonates and infants with severe cardiac disease.
Maintenance	**Otherwise healthy:** Standard pediatric maintenance (see p. D-3). **Muscle abnormalities:** Maintenance of anesthesia with a nontriggering agent (e.g., N_2O, opiates) and short-acting NMRs is prudent. A peripheral nerve stimulator should be used to monitor muscle relaxation, as the effects of muscle relaxants may be unexpectedly prolonged. **Cardiorespiratory compromise**: The maintenance of anesthesia in this group most commonly is accomplished by use of inhalational agents, additional narcotics, or other iv agents, depending on patient tolerance and postop plans for ventilatory management.

Emergence	**Otherwise healthy:** If a muscle relaxant is used, reverse with neostigmine (0.07 mg/kg) and glycopyrrolate (0.01 mg/kg iv) or edrophonium (0.5 mg/kg) and atropine (0.015 mg/kg iv). Make sure patient is awake and able to protect airway. A vital capacity of >15 mL/kg is considered an adequate sign of recovery of respiratory reserve. **Muscle abnormalities:** Anticipate postop respiratory impairment. Suction airway carefully. The response to neostigmine is unpredictable and may precipitate myotonia. Continued postop mechanical ventilation may be required. **Cardiorespiratory compromise:** Tourniquet release may cause significant. ↓ CO and ↓ BP, requiring temporary inotropic support. Otherwise, emergence as in normal patients.

Regional anesthesia: Used in patients undergoing lower extremity surgery.

Caudal epidural	In young children, the epidural space can be reached easily by the caudal epidural approach, with less risk of dural puncture than with thoracic or lumbar epidural approaches. There is minimal risk of cord injury at the level of the sacrococcygeal ligament. The dural sac, however, can extend to the level of the third or fourth sacral vertebra in the newborn; therefore, care must be taken to avoid an inadvertent intrathecal injection. Bupivacaine or leuobupivacaine provide reliable, long-lasting anesthesia and postop analgesia when given via the caudal epidural route. Bupivacaine 0.25% with epinephrine 1:200,000 (1 mL/kg) provides 3–6 h of analgesia for all procedures below the umbilicus. In infants (< 2.5 kg), a more dilute solution is used (0.125% or 0.175%) and the volume can be increased to remain below the toxic dose range (2.5 mg/kg). Intraop anesthesia with bupivacaine 0.25% with epinephrine 1:200,000 is given as a bolus with volumes determined by level desired (0.05 mL/kg/segment, not to exceed l mL/kg). Preservative-free clonidine (1–2 mcg/kg) as an additive to bupivacaine caudal anesthesia has been shown to increase the efficacy and duration of the analgesia.	
Continuous epidural infusion	Use bupivacaine 0.1–0.125% at rate of 0.1 mL/kg/h in patients < 5 yr; thereafter, patients may require 0.05–0.15 mL/kg/h.	
Peripheral nerve blocks	Use of ultrasonography helps to improve the efficacy and safety of these blocks.Femoral, obturator and lateral cutaneous nerve of thigh can be blocked by doing a lumbar plexus block at the level of the L4 vertebra or by doing a 3-in-1 block at the groin. Sciatic nerve can be blocked in the posterior thigh at the apex of the popliteal fossa. If used in combination, these blocks can provide excellent post-oerative analgesia for most of the lower limb procedures with minimal side effects. Catheters can be left in place for providing continuous post-operative analgesia. With the availability of safer and less expensive programmable pumps, most of the blocks can be done even for outpatient procedures and the children can be sent home on these pumps.	
Blood and fluid requirements	IV: 22 ga or greater × 1–2 NS/LR 4 mL/kg/h: 0–10 kg + 2 mL/kg/h: 11–20 kg + 1 mL/kg/h: >20 kg (e.g., 25 kg = 65 mL/h) Warm fluids for long cases.	There may be rapid fluid shifts in pediatric patients undergoing orthopedic procedures. Close monitoring and adequate fluid replacement will ensure hemodynamic stability. In hip or pelvis surgery, blood loss may be substantial, and adequate iv access is important as blood transfusion may be required.
Control of blood loss	Tourniquet: 120-min limit	Use of pneumatic tourniquets has become common practice in peripheral orthopedic procedures. They reduce intraop blood loss; however, they cause pain and, upon removal, and release products of anaerobic metabolism.

Monitoring	Standard monitors (see p. D-1). ± Arterial line ± CVP line Temperature	Most pediatric patients presenting for extremity surgery do not require invasive monitoring. An arterial or CVP line may be helpful, depending on patient's medical condition, length of surgery, and anticipated blood loss.
Positioning	✓ and pad pressure points. ✓ eyes.	Patients with osteogenesis imperfecta or osteoporosis are at risk for fractures and joint dislocations and require special care in positioning.
Complications	MH	Early Sx of MH include: Tachycardia, tachypnea, unstable BP, dysrhythmias, cyanotic mottling of skin, rapid rise in T (1°/15 min), discolored urine, metabolic acidosis, respiratory acidosis, hyperkalemia, myoglobinuria. Rx: stop surgery and anesthesia immediately; hyperventilate with 100% O_2; administer dantrolene sodium iv (starting dose = 1–2 mg/kg q 5–10 min; maximum cumulative dose = 10 mg/kg) by rapid infusion. Procainamide (15 mg/kg) over 15 min may be required for dysrhythmias. Initiate cooling, correct acidosis and hyperkalemia. Maintain UO of at least 2 mL/kg/hr. Monitor patient in ICU until danger of subsequent episodes is over (24 h).

POSTOPERATIVE

Complications	MH Respiratory insufficiency	For MH considerations, see above.
Pain management	PCA Parenteral opiates Spinal/epidural opiates	(see p. E-4).

Suggested Readings

1. American Heart Association: Prevention of bacterial endocarditis. AHA Committee on Rheumatic Fever; Endocarditis and Kawasaki Disease of the Council on Cardiovascular Disease in the Young. *JAMA* 1990;264(22):2919–22.
2. Baum VC, O'Flaherty JE: *Anesthesia for Genetic, Metabolic, and Dysmorphic Syndromes of Childhood.* Lippincott Williams & Wilkins, Philadelphia: 1999.
3. Bell C, Kain Z: Acute pediatric pain management. In *The Pediatric Anesthesia Handbook.* Mosby, St. Louis: 1997.
4. Bernstein R. Rosenberg AD: *Manual of Orthopedic Anesthesia and Related Pain Syndromes.* Churchill Livingstone, New York: 1993.
5. Britt BA, Kalow W: Malignant hyperthermia: a statistical review. *Can Anaesth Soc J* 1970;17(4):293–315.
6. Brownell AK, Paasuke RT, Elash A, et al: Malignant hyperthermia in Duchenne muscular dystrophy. *Anesthesiology* 1983;58(2):180–2.
7. Brustowicz RM, Moncorge C, Koka BV, et al: Metabolic responses to tourniquet release in children. *Anesthesiology* 1987; 67(5):792–4.
8. Ceviz N, Alehan F, Alehan D, et al: Assessment of left ventricular systolic and diastolic functions in children with merosin-positive congenital muscular dystrophy. *Int J Cardiol* 2003;87(2–3):129–33.
9. Glassman SD, Rose SM, Dimar JR, et al: The effect of postoperative nonsteroidal anti-inflammatory drug administration on spinal fusion. *Spine* 1998;23(7):834–8.
10. Grain L, Cortina-Borja M, Forfar C, et al: Cardiac abnormalities and skeletal muscle weakness in carriers of Duchenne and Becker muscular dystrophies and controls. *Neuromuscul Disord* 2001;11(2):186–91.
11. Howell TK, Patel D: Plasma paracetamol concentrations after different doses of rectal paracetamol in older children. A comparison of 1 g vs. 40 mg × kg(-1). *Anaesthesia* 2003;58(1):69–73.
12. Lemos J, Helay W: Blood transfusion on orthopedic operations. *J Bone Joint Surg* 1996;78:1260–70.

13. Loder RT, Aronson DD, Greenfield ML: The epidemiology of bilateral slipped capital femoral epiphysis. A study of children in Michigan. *J Bone Joint Surg* [Am] 1993;75(8):1141–7.
14. Melacini P, Fanin M, Danieli GA, et al: Cardiac involvement in Becker muscular dystrophy. *J Am Coll Cardiol* 1993;22(7): 1927–34.
15. Pullerits J, Holzman R: Pediatric neuraxial blockade. *J Clin Anesth* 1993;5(4):342–54.
16. Salem MR, Klowden AJ: Anesthesia for orthopedic surgery. In *Pediatric Anesthesia,* 4th edition. Gregory GA, ed. Churchill Livingstone, New York: 2001, 617–62.
17. Shimada Y, Yoshiya I, Tanaka K, et al: Crying vital capacity and maximal inspiratory pressure as clinical indicators of readiness for weaning of infants less than a year of age. *Anesthesiology* 1979;51(5):456–9.
18. Tait AR, Knight PR: The effects of general anesthesia on upper respiratory tract infections in children. *Anesthesiology* 1987;67(6):930–5.
19. Takasaki M, Dohi S, KawabataY, et al: Dosage of lidocaine for caudal anesthesia in infants and children. *Anesthesiology* 1977;47(6):527–9.
20. Tetzloff JE, ed: *Clinical Orthopedic Anesthesia.* Butterworth-Henemann, Boston: 1995.
21. Wedel DJ: *Orthopaedic Anesthesia.* Churchill Livingstone, New York: 1993.
22. Wongprasartsuk P, Stevens J: Cerebral palsy and anesthesia. *Ped Anesth* 2002; 12:296–303.

SURGERY FOR EPIDERMOLYSIS BULLOSA

SURGICAL CONSIDERATIONS

Description: Epidermolysis bullosa (EB) is a disabling inherited condition affecting the skin and submucosa. Recessive dystrophic EB is the most common type requiring surgical treatment. Children develop lesions associated with minimal trauma, which most commonly result in contractures of the hands and feet, mouth, and esophagus. Special care is required in handling patients with EB, because minor trauma from iv or EKG lead placement can cause severe blistering. Hand surgery typically involves opening up the contracted fingers by removing the cocoon of epidermis. The defects are grafted with full-thickness skin grafts, typically taken from the abdomen. Following sedation or anesthesia, the affected extremity is gently sponged with dilute chlorhexidine solution. A tourniquet is not applied since it is typically not required. A wrist block is administered by the surgeon. The cocoon of scar tissue is removed, the fingers manipulated to expose the defects, and a full-thickness skin graft is harvested. Generous Bactroban ointment and nonadhesive dressings are placed on the hand and a well-padded cast is applied at the end of the procedure. Adhesive tape is avoided throughout the procedure.

Usual preop diagnosis: EB

SUMMARY OF PROCEDURE	
Position	Supine
Incision	As necessary to relieve skin contractures on the hands
Antibiotics	Cefazolin 20–40 mg/kg iv up to 1 gm.
Surgical time	1–2 h. Positioning, iv placement and sedation/anesthesia are time-consuming, often longer than the procedure itself.
EBL	< 100 mL
Postop care	PACU → home. Return in 2 wk for intraop removal of cast, dressing change, and first splint application. Splinting and special gloves are the mainstay of postop treatment.
Mortality	None associated with procedure
Morbidity	Trauma from positioning and monitoring → new blisters
Pain score	7–9 (similar to 2nd-degree burns)

PATIENT POPULATION CHARACTERISTICS	
Age range	1–20 yr; older patients with precancerous or cancerous hand lesions
Male:Female	2–3:1
Incidence	Extremely rare
Etiology	Inherited
Associated conditions	Malnutrition; esophageal strictures; generalized skin contractures; malignant transformation of skin lesions

ANESTHETIC CONSIDERATIONS

PREOPERATIVE

EB is a heterogenous group of rare hereditary disorders characterized by blister formation in the skin in response to minor trauma, friction, or pressure. The most minor form of EB is EB simplex, in which the blisters heal without scarring. The junctional form often is diagnosed at birth, with blisters caused by the physical trauma of delivery. These patients develop severe scarring and have a short life expectancy. Patients with the recessive dystrophic form may have strictures of the oropharynx, larynx, and esophagus. Patients may be on long-term corticosteroid treatment. Periop hydrocortisone treatment may be required to compensate for adrenal suppression.

Airway	A careful airway evaluation is essential, since these patients may have a difficult airway 2° mucous membrane and skin involvement in the area of the oropharynx, face, and neck. Patients with EB also may have limited mouth opening and neck movement as the result of scarring and contractures. Poor dentition: ✓ for loose teeth.
Skin	Because of the fragility of skin and mucous membranes in patients with EB, the anesthetic plan should be designed to prevent even the slightest trauma to skin and mucous membranes.
Gastrointestinal	The most common sites of involvement are the oropharynx, esophagus, and anus. Dysphagia, esophageal stricture and constipation are common, and are the major causes of morbidity, nutritional deficiencies, and growth retardation. Esophageal dilatation, insertion of NG feeding tubes, gastrostomy, and colonic interposition have been performed in patients with EB. Esophageal stricture increases the risk of regurgitation and aspiration, and precautions to avoid aspiration should be taken.
Musculoskeletal	Skin lesions can be painful, and some patients will be on chronic opiate medication for pain management.
Hematologic	Chronic blood loss from denuded skin can → anemia and hypoalbuminemia. **Tests:** CBC
Laboratory	Other tests as indicated from H&P.
Premedication	Adequate premedication is essential to minimize movement during induction. An orally administered combination of midazolam (0.6 mg/kg) and ketamine (3.5 mg/kg) facilitates the atraumatic placement of iv lines in the OR. Glycopyrrolate 0.01 mg/kg can be given as antisialagogue. EMLA cream can be applied without adhesive dressing.

INTRAOPERATIVE

Patients are placed on sheepskin to cushion pressure points. The following should be available: Albolene liquefying cleanser, Surg-O-Flex (flexible tubular bandage), Vaseline gauze, Zeroform, Kerlix, Webril, cotton umbilical tape, and Coban wrap. No adhesive tape is used. Adhesive portions of EKG leads and electrocautery dispersion plates are removed; the leads and plates are secured to the patient, using Webril or Surg-O-Flex. BP cuff must be applied over multiple layers of cotton padding. Carefully trim the adhesive off the pulse oximetry probe, wrap around the palm or finger, and wrap Coban around the probe. Alternatively, use adult clip-on probe. Anesthesia masks, ETTs, temperature probes, and all attached monitoring equipment are lubricated with Albolene. Venipuncture can be difficult, and the iv lines are secured with Vaseline gauze and Coban.

Anesthetic technique: GETA is the preferred method of anesthesia when upper airway manipulation is required or airway protection is compromised. Anticipate difficult airway. Planned FOL is safer than DL. Use smaller ETT to avoid formation of laryngeal bullae. ETT and laryngoscope blade, if used, should be well lubricated. Smaller than normal LMA has been used, with the shaft and cuff lubricated. Secure tube with umbilical tape. James, et al, reported 309 anesthetics performed on 73 patients with recessive dystrophic EB without the occurrence of laryngeal bullae, postop stridor, or "airway embarrassment." The safety of GETA, however, is not well documented in junctional EB patients, where columnar epithelium can be involved. Avoid succinylcholine 2° risk of ↑ K^+ 2° muscle atrophy. NMRs prolong duration of action 2° ↓ muscle mass and changes in volume of distribution 2° hypoalbuminemia, which results from ill health and poor nutritional status.

IV anesthesia: Ketamine has been utilized for patients with EB undergoing surgical procedures. For iv anesthesia, use a loading dose of midazolam 0.1–0.2 mg/kg with ketamine 0.25–0.5 mg/kg, followed by a continuous infusion of ketamine (1 mg/kg/h) and midazolam (0.1 mg/kg/h). Glycopyrrolate can be used as an antisialagogue in these patients. Alternatively, propofol (50–100 mg/kg/h) with remifentanil (0.05–0.1 mg/kg/h) infusions may be used. Titrate both medications according to patient's response to the surgical stimulation.

Local anesthesia: At our institution, local anesthetic infiltration has not been associated with any serious sequelae; however, Kubota, et al, have recommended against the use of local anesthetic infiltration.

Regional anesthesia: In some patients with EB, regional anesthesia techniques allow maintenance of airway patency, involve minimal epidermal/dermal damage, and can offer prolonged postop pain relief. Brachial plexus anesthesia, epidural anesthesia, and spinal anesthesia have been used successfully in patients with EB.

Emergence	Adequate postop analgesia and parental presence in the PACU may help prevent excessive struggling and skin trauma during emergence and recovery. Plastic O_2 delivery masks should be avoided as they have sharp edges. Avoid rectal route for pain management, as it may cause perianal trauma and blistering. Acetaminophen, ketorolac, and opiates can be used for postop analgesia. PONV should be avoided by using combination antiemetic therapy. Pruritus, a common side effect of opiates, should be treated promptly.

Suggested Readings

1. Lin YC, Golianu B: Anesthesia and pain management for pediatric patients with dystrophic epidermolysis bullosa. *J Clin Anesth* 2006;18(4):268–71.
2. Borgeat A, Blumenthal S: Postoperative pain management following scoliosis surgery. *Curr Opin Anaesthesiol* 2008;21(3):313–6.
3. Broster T, Placek R, Eggers G: Epidermolysis bullosa: anesthetic management for cesarean section. *Anesth Analg* 1987;66:341–3.
4. Campiglio GL, Pajardi G, Rafanelli G: A new protocol for the treatment of hand deformities and recessive dystrophic epidermolysis bullosa (13 cases). *Ann Chir Main Memb Super* 1997;16(2):91–100, discussion 101.
5. Ergun G, Lin A, Dannenberg A, et al: Gastrointestinal manifestations of epidermolysis bullosa: a study of 101 patients. *Medicine* 1992;71(3):121–7.
6. Farber N, Troshynski T, Turco G: Spinal anesthesia in an infant with epidermolysis bullosa. *Anesthesiology* 1995;83:1364–7.
7. Herod J, Denyer J, Goldman A, et al: Epidermolysis bullosa in children: pathophysiology, anaesthesia and pain management. *Paediatr Anesth* 2002;12:388–97.
8. Iohom G, Lyons B: Anaesthesia for children with epidermolysis bullosa: a review of 20 years' experience. *EU J Anesthesiology* 2000;18:745–54.
9. Fine JD, Johnson LB, Weiner M, et al: Tracheolaryngeal complications of inherited epidermolysis bullosa: cumulative experience of the national epidermolysis bullosa registry. *Laryngoscope* 2007;117(9):1652–60.
10. Kelly R, Koff H, Rothaus K, et al: Brachial plexus anesthesia in eight patients with recessive dystrophic epidermolysis bullosa. *Anesth Analg* 1987;66:1318–20.
11. Kubota Y, Norton M, Goldenberg S, et al: Anesthetic management of patients with epidermolysis bullosa undergoing surgery. *Anesth Analg* 1961;40(2):244–50.
12. Ladd AL, Kibele A, Gibbons S: Surgical treatment and postoperative splinting of recessive dystrophic epidermolysis bullosa. *J Hand Surg* [Am] 1996;21(5):888–97.
13. Patch MR, Woodey RD: Spinal anaesthesia in a patient with epidermolysis bullosa dystrophica. *Anaesth Inten Care* 2000;28:446–8.
14. Spielman F, Mann E: Subarachnoid and epidural anaesthesia for patients with epidermolysis bullosa. *Can Anaesth Soc J* 1984;31(5)549–51.
15. Yee C, Gunter J, Manley C: Caudal epidural anesthesia in an infant with epidermolysis bullosa. *Anesthesiology* 1989;70:149–51.
16. Yonker-Sell A, Connolly L: Twelve-hour anaesthesia in a patient with epidermolysis bullosa. *Can J Anaesth* 1995;42(8):735–9.

CHAPTER

12.8 Surgery for Craniofacial Malformations

SURGEONS

Stephen A. Schendel, MD, DDS, FACS
Lawrence M. Shuer, MD (*Craniosynostosis*)
Joseph F. Looby, DO

ANESTHESIOLOGISTS

Louise Furukawa, MD
Gregory B. Hammer, MD

SURGICAL CORRECTION OF CRANIOSYNOSTOSIS

SURGICAL CONSIDERATIONS

Description: Premature fusion of cranial sutures, or **craniosynostosis,** causes various well-recognized patterns of cranial vault and facial deformities. Rarely, these are related to conditions such as Crouzon, Apert, Saethre-Chotzen, and Pfeiffer syndromes. Single or multiple sutures can be involved, the most common being the sagittal suture. This condition is called **scaphocephaly,** in which the cranial vault is bitemporally narrow, with AP elongation. **Anterior or posterior plagiocephaly** involves a single coronal suture or lambdoid suture and is characterized by flattening of the forehead on the affected side. **Oxycephaly** ('tower-head deformity') involves bilateral coronal sutures, with a flat, high forehead, whereas **brachycephaly** also involves the cranial base sutures, and results in bitemporal bulging, midfacial hypoplasia, an anterior open bite, and hypertelorism. These patients may have severe sleep apnea and can pose a challenge for airway management. **Trigonocephaly** (triangular head shape) (Fig. 12.8-1), with a keel-shaped forehead and hypoteloric tendency, involves the metopic suture.

Surgical correction of these craniofacial anomalies requires a combined plastic surgery and neurosurgery team approach involving the release or resection of the affected suture and simultaneous correction of the asymmetric skull by **bone-flap repositioning or advancement.** Frontal/orbital abnormalities are addressed with **bifrontal craniotomy** and **floating forehead advancement,** along with advancement of the supraorbital bar **(fronto-orbital advancement)** (Fig. 12.8-2). For example, in plagiocephaly, because of the unilateral coronal synostosis, the frontal bone is retruded and the superior orbital rim is elevated and retruded on this side. Craniectomy is performed, the forehead is removed, the involved coronal suture is resected, and the supraorbital bar is cut above the orbit and down to the lateral orbital wall across the midline. The bar is bent, advanced on the involved side—sometimes up to 1.5 cm—and fixed in this position. Additional bone strips are taken from the posterior cranium and split for use as graft material; the other bone pieces are replaced and fixed with wires, suture, or restorable plates.

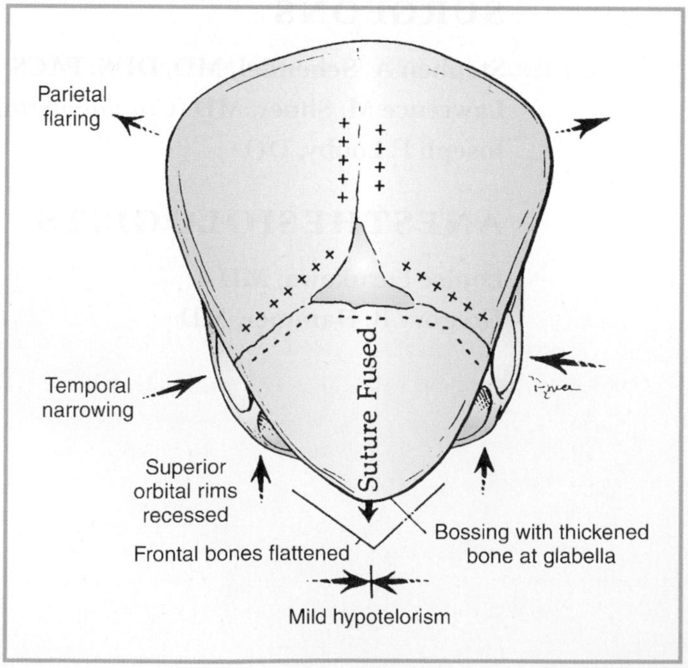

Figure 12.8-1. Skull shape abnormalities in metopic synostosis: Regions of reduced bone deposition (---). Regions of compensatory increased bone deposition (+++). (From Belfrey ME, Pershing JA, et al: Surgical Treatment of Metopic Synostosis. In *Neurosurgical Clinics of North America.* Pershing JA, Jane JA, eds. WB Saunders, Philadelphia: 1991, used with permission.)

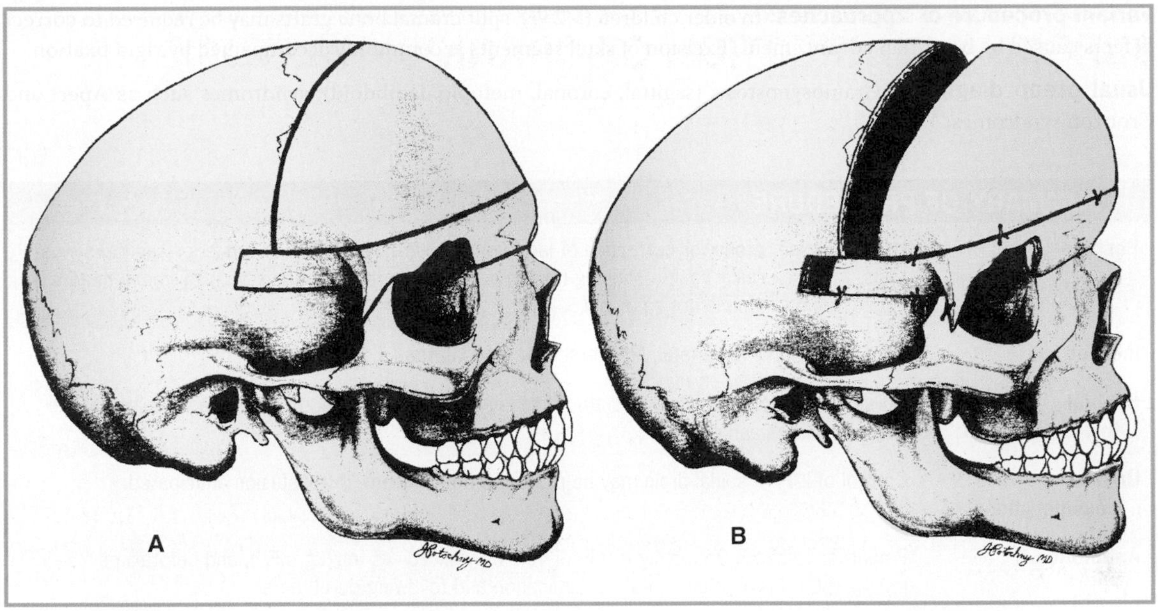

Figure 12.8-2. Fronto-orbital advancement. **(A)** Lines of osteotomy for forehead and supraorbital bar advancement. **(B)** Fronto-orbital advancement in a tongue-in-groove manner and fixation with wires. (Reproduced with permission from Aston SJ, Beasley RW, Thorne CH, eds: *Grabb and Smith's Plastic Surgery,* 5th edition. Lippincott-Raven, Philadelphia: 1997.)

Patient positioning, type of headrest, and incision all vary, depending on location of the suture abnormality. If the deformity is mostly posterior (e.g., a sagittal or plagiocephaly case), a prone approach with biparietal or midsagittal incision can be used. Resection of the involved suture and **barrel staving** of the cranium, with grafting for reshaping, works well. Reconstruction as above usually is accomplished at ~3–6 months of age. Brain mass doubles in size the first 6 months and triples by 3 years of age, when ~80% of the brain growth is completed (the driving force for cranial vault growth).

All procedures are extradural. Dural tears, if they occur, are repaired to prevent CSF leak and CNS infection.

In the syndromic cases, the cranial synostosis deformity is treated similarly to the procedure described, usually before the age of 12 months, with a view to midfacial advancement of the primary dentition at maturity either by **LeFort III or monobloc advancement.** (See p. 1116 LeFort Osteotomies, and p. 1403 Major Secondary Craniofacial Surgical Procedures.)

Postsurgical orthopedic distraction devices like the **Delaire mask** also can be used to encourage midfacial growth. The syndromic cases may require repeat craniotomy and reshaping at a young age if signs of ↑ ICP appear. Other synostotic cases also should be monitored for ↑ ICP and the need for urgent secondary craniotomy. Marchac and Renier detected ↑ ICP in 13% of single-suture synostosis and 42% of multisuture synostosis. ↑ ICP may increase the risk of dural breach during craniotomy 2° cranial bone resorption and thinning.

Blood loss can be significant at first incision through the vessel-rich scalp. Rainey clips are applied immediately to minimize blood loss. In anticipation of major blood loss, transfusion should be started with the first incision. Severe life-threatening blood loss can occur if the sagittal sinus is breached, and neurosurgical repair must be accomplished quickly. Elevation of the bone flaps usually causes diffuse bleeding, which is stopped easily with irrigated bipolar cautery and thrombin-soaked sponges. It is useful to have the patient in the reverse Trendelenburg position from the start. Diffuse bleeding at the cut bone edges and over the bone surfaces can be further controlled with bone wax. Focal bleeding from around the orbit and in the temporal fossa region subperiosteally also can be controlled with bone wax. A LeFort/monobloc component to the surgery increases blood loss, especially during the initial mobilization of the facial segment. Local anesthetic with epinephrine injected, and/or on sponge packs for pressure, will control the diffuse mucosal bleeding. BP control is also paramount. Electrocautery and Ligaclips to larger vessels (e.g., descending palatine pedicles) may be necessary.

Variant procedure or approaches: In older children (> 2 yr), split cranial bone grafts may be required to correct defects caused by bone-flap advancement. Excision of skull segments is commonly accompanied by rigid fixation.

Usual preop diagnosis: Craniosynostosis (sagittal, coronal, metopic, lambdoid); syndromes such as Apert and Crouzon syndromes; ↑ ICP

SUMMARY OF PROCEDURE

Position	Usually supine; prone for correction of lambdoidal suture synostosis or posterior sagittal synostosis. If entire cranial vault reshaping (multiple sutures), special padded occipital-cheek headrest, because pin fixation is not safe until > 2 yr.
Incision	Usually bicoronal, biparietal, Meisterschnitt, midsagittal
Special instrumentation	Horseshoe headrest, usually pediatric; occasionally, Gardiner tongs; Midas Rex craniotome; resorbable plates and screws
Unique considerations	Control of ICP — spinal drain may be placed. Blood in room, if transfusion anticipated.
Antibiotics	Pediatric: cefazolin 25 mg/kg q 8 h, or vancomycin 10–15 mg/kg q 6 h, and cefotaxime 25–50 mg/kg q 6 h for oropharyngeal contamination and following dural tears
Surgical time	2–6 h
Closing considerations	Blood loss with Rainey clip removal. Full head-wrap dressing causes head/neck movement → bucking.
EBL	200–800 mL; may be formidable.
Postop care	ICU: 1–2 d (further transfusion often necessary in 1st 2 h to replace drain losses)
Mortality	0.6–1.6%
Morbidity	Major complications: 14.3% Bone infection: 3–7% Meningitis CSF leak: 4.5% ↑ ICP Air embolus: < 1% Blindness: < 1% Massive bleeding: < 1% Venous thrombosis Neurologic injury: Rare
Pain score	4

PATIENT POPULATION CHARACTERISTICS

Age range	2–24 mo (primary correction)
Male:Female	1:1
Incidence	Non syndromic: 1/10,000 births (most sporadic; few familial patterns) Crouzon syndrome: 1/25,000 Apert syndrome: 1/100,000
Etiology	Idiopathic; however, some are associated with specific genetic conditions (e.g., Crouzon and Apert syndromes). Other cases may be 2° ↓ brain growth.
Associated conditions	Hydrocephalus; ↑ ICP; mental retardation; airway problems; ocular abnormalities; exotropia (29% Crouzon or Apert syndromes); lagophthalmus; exorbitism

ANESTHETIC CONSIDERATIONS

PREOPERATIVE

Patients may have craniofacial anomalies—particularly Apert and Crouzon syndromes—which are associated with midface hypoplasia, obstructive sleep apnea and in some cases difficult intubation. Hence, detailed preop airway evaluation is necessary. Children with single-suture craniosynostosis are usually healthy. Surgery is often performed between 3–6 months of age, preferably when the infant weighs > 5 kg.

Respiratory	Patients with long-standing upper-airway obstruction due to choanal atresia, mandibular and maxillary hypoplasia, or other causes, may have chronic hypoventilation and hypoxia and may experience episodes of apnea. If the patient has Sx of acute URI, delay elective surgery at least 2 wk. The presence of fever, cough, and abnormal chest auscultation necessitates radiographic evaluation and pediatric consultation. **Tests:** As indicated from H&P.
Airway	Be aware of other congenital anomalies affecting the patient's airway, such as Apert, Klippel-Feil, Goldenhar, Pierre-Robin, Treacher-Collins, or Crouzon syndromes. Review any previous anesthetic records for patient to gain insights into appropriate airway management (e.g., FOI may be necessary). Consider elective tracheostomy under local anesthesia in patients with severe airway abnormalities.
Cardiovascular	Consider the coexistence of congenital cardiopulmonary anomalies, particularly in patients with Apert syndrome (autosomal dominant trait, craniosynostosis, syndactyly of hands and feet). Preop evaluation of a patient with a known or suspected heart defect should include thorough H&P, ECG, Hct, baseline O_2 sat, and CXR. For children with Sx of cardiac dysfunction or those requiring cardiac medication, it is advisable to consult with a pediatric cardiologist to optimize the patient's condition prior to surgery. **Tests:** Preop EKG indicated for patients with CHD; others as indicated from H&P.
Neurological	If only the sagittal suture is involved, ICP is usually normal. If more than one suture is involved, brain growth will be impaired, the patient will be developmentally delayed, and intracranial HTN may be present.
Hematologic	Surgery in early infancy (< 9 mo) is common; thus, allowable blood loss is small; blood transfusion usually is required. **Tests:** Hct; PT; PTT; T&C blood.
Laboratory	Other tests as indicated from H&P.
Premedication	Patients >9–10 mo old may benefit from premedication with midazolam (0.5–0.75 mg/kg po). Antibiotic prophylaxis for CHD (e.g., ampicillin 25 mg/kg + gentamicin 2.5 mg/kg iv) may be warranted (see AHA guidelines).

INTRAOPERATIVE

Anesthetic technique: GETA. Anticipate possible difficult airway. Heat OR to 78–80°. Forced air warmer. Heat all fluids to body temperature.

Induction	Surgery for craniectomies is extradural. Either mask induction with N_2O and inhalational agent or iv induction is suitable for the infant with a normal airway. If ICP is suspected to be elevated, consider mild hyperventilation after loss of consciousness. For a difficult airway, intubation may be facilitated by using an FOI while patient is awake or anesthetized and spontaneously ventilating. In rare situations, tracheostomy, under sedation and local anesthesia, may be necessary. Consider suturing ETT to prevent accidental extubation. In prone cases, unsutured endotracheal tubes can slip through tape due to pooling of oral or nasal secretions.

Pediatric Surgery

Maintenance	Maintenance anesthesia with inhalational agent or balanced (iv) anesthesia and long-acting muscle relaxant, should be adequate. Surgery may be prolonged. Control of ICP may be necessary (see below). A remifentanil infusion 100–300 ng/kg/min provides profound intraop analgesia and rapid awakening.	
Emergence	Prompt awakening to allow neurological evaluation is an important goal. Excessive facial edema, particularly in patients with preoperative sleep apnea may require the patient to remain intubated postoperatively.	
Blood and fluid requirements	Anticipate large blood loss. IV× 2 (as large as possible LR @: 4 mL/kg/h – 0–10 kg + 2 mL/kg/h – 11–20 kg + 1 mL/kg/h – > 20 kg (e.g., 25 kg = 65 mL/h) Warm all fluids. Humidify gases.	Have 1–2 U PRBC or whole blood available in the room. Use LR for replacing deficit, maintenance, and 3rd-space fluid loss. Replace blood loss with colloid and PRBC mL for mL. Significant blood loss begins with scalp incision; allowable blood loss is small, so that it is important to begin transfusion early before hypovolemia occurs. EBV for an infant in this age group is 75 mL/kg. A good rule is to infuse a volume of blood equal to 10% of EBV prior to incision in the healthy infant after discussion with the attending surgeon regarding expected blood loss. Avoid NS (acidosis, ↑ bleeding) in children < 5 yr. Beware of ↑ K^+ and ↓ Ca^{++} associated with massive transfusion.
Control of ICP	Hyperventilation Osmotic diuretic Loop diuretic	In some cases, it may be desirable to ↓ ICP. This can be accomplished by ↑ ventilation ($PaCO_2$ = 25–30 mmHg), diuretics (furosemide 1 mg/kg iv).
Monitoring	Standard monitors (Appendix D-1). ± Arterial line ± CVP line ± Precordial Doppler ± Urinary catheter	Arterial cannulation for BP, monitoring of ABG, Hct, electrolytes, etc. ↑ K^+ and ↓ Ca^{++} are most common following transfusion with whole blood or FFP. VAE has been reported during craniectomies in infants; hence, a precordial Doppler and CVP line will be helpful. CVP may be particularly helpful in the infant with marginal cardiovascular status for volume assessment and drug administration. Close attention to $ETCO_2$ and, if available, ETN_2 monitoring is useful. If VAE is suspected the surgical field should be flooded and the head lowered immediately. CVP may be particularly helpful in the infant with marginal cardiovascular status for volume assessment and drug administration and if peripheral iv access is limited. Precordial or esophageal stethoscope is useful in cases where the patient is turned 180° or in cases of marginal pulmonary function.
Positioning	✓ and pad pressure points. ✓ eyes.	Positioning depends on surgical approach; most are performed with patient prone; however, use of the head-up position is not uncommon.
Complications	Oculocardiac reflex (OCR) → ↓↓ HR and ↓↓ BP	Notify surgeons and Rx with atropine 0.02 mg/kg iv.
	VAE	Be prepared to make prompt Dx of VAE (↓ $ETCO_2$, change in Doppler sounds, ↑ ETN_2 ↓ O_2 sat, ↓ BP, ↑ HR) and Rx: notify surgeons, flood wound, ± head down, aspirate CVP, ± vasopressors.

POSTOPERATIVE

Complications	Hypovolemia with ↓ BP Hypothermia Airway Complications	Inadequate volume replacement may result in ↓ BP and acidosis. ✓ Hct to establish need for further fluid or blood therapy. Excessive facial edema, history of a marginal airway preoperatively, or severe obstructive sleep apnea with sensitivity to opioids may necessitate maintenance of a secure airway postoperatively
Pain management	Parenteral opioids (see p. E-4).	
Tests	Followup Hct postop	Transfuse to keep Hct ≥ 30%.

Suggested Readings

1. Chiaretti A, Pietrini B: Safety & efficacy of remifentanil infusion in craniosynostosis repair in infants. *Ped Neurosurg* 2002;36(1):55–6.
2. Davies DW, Munro IR: The anesthetic management and intraoperative care of patients undergoing major facial osteotomies. *Plast Reconstr Surg* 1975;55(1):50–5.
3. Harris MM, Yemen TA, Davidson A, et al: Venous embolism during craniectomy in supine infants. *Anesthesiology* 1987;67(5):816–19.
4. Huang M, Mouradian WE, Cohen SR, et al: The differential diagnosis of abnormal head shapes: separating craniosynostosis from positional deformities and normal variants. *Cleft Palate Craniofacial J* 1998;35(3):204–11.
5. Koh JL, Gries H: Perioperative management of pediatric patients with craniosynostosis. *Anesthesiol Clin* 2007;25(3):465–81.
6. Marchac D, Renier D, Jones BM: Experience with the "Floating Forehead." Br *J Plast Surg* 1988;41(1):1–15.
7. Muhling J: Surgical treatment of craniosynostosis. In *Maxillofacial Surgery*. Booth PW, Schendel SA, Hausamen J-E, eds. Churchill Livingstone, Edinburgh: 1999, 877–88.
8. Palmisano BW, Rusy LM: Anesthesia for plastic surgery. In *Pediatric Anesthesia,* 4th edition, Gregory GA, ed. Churchill Livingstone, New York: 2002, 707–45.
9. Posnick JC: Surgical management of Crouzon, Apert and related syndromes. In *Maxillofacial Surgery*. Booth PW, Schendel SA, Hausamen J-E, eds. Churchill Livingstone, Edinburgh: 1999, 863–75.
10. Tessier P: Relationship of craniostenoses to craniofacial dysostoses and to faciostenoses: a study with therapeutic implications. *Plast Reconstruct Surg* 1971;48(3):224–37.

MAJOR SECONDARY CRANIOFACIAL SURGICAL PROCEDURES

SURGICAL CONSIDERATIONS

Description: These procedures usually are performed on children ≥ 5 years. There are two basic approaches. The first involves advancement of the upper face and frontal bone, frequently described as a **monobloc** (Fig. 12.8-3) or **frontofacial advancement.** The second variation, called **facial bipartition** or **periorbital osteotomy,** is for correction of telorbitism (widely spaced eyes), usually accomplished by a combined extra- and intracranial approach, using both plastic and neurosurgery teams.

Variant procedure or approaches: Many different variations of the above-named procedures can be performed; however, from an anesthetic standpoint, they are not significantly different. The use of **cranial bone grafts** and **rigid fixation** have shortened these somewhat lengthy procedures. Other bone grafts, however, from ribs and iliac crest, are occasionally required. These procedures frequently last ≥ 6 hours and blood loss can be very heavy. Reconstruction of the forehead and orbital area following a tumor excision, for example, uses a similar approach, but requires additional bone grafts.

Usual preop diagnosis: Craniofacial malformations; craniofacial deformities; telorbitism or hypertelorism; craniofacial dysostosis

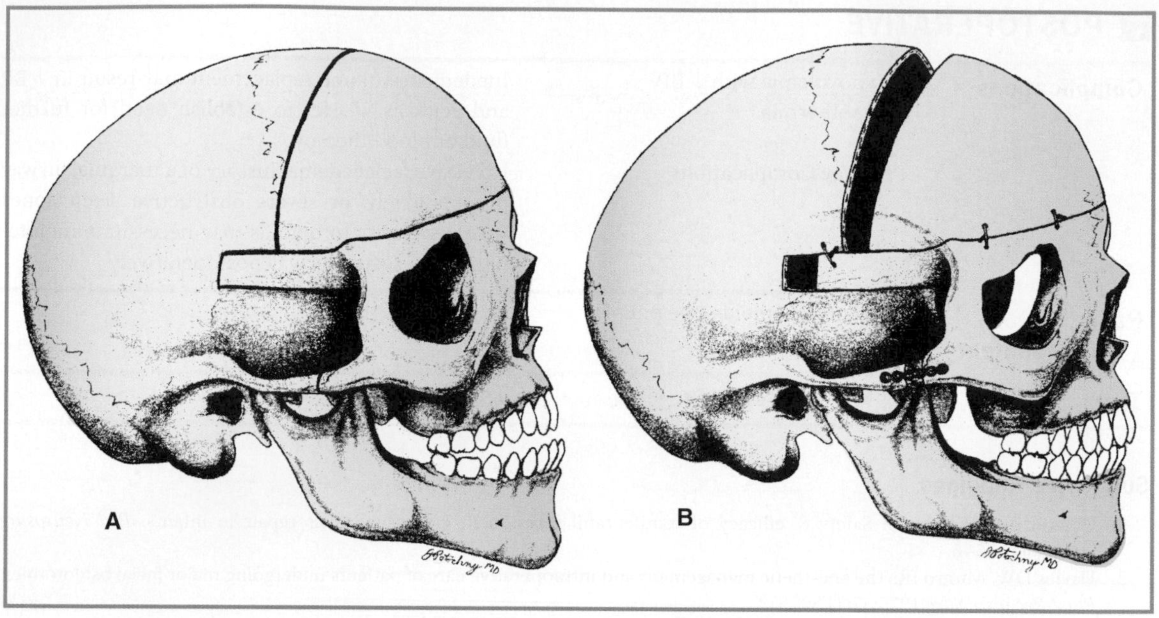

Figure 12.8-3. Monobloc advancement. **(A)** Lines of osteotomy for monobloc osteotomy. **(B)** Advancement of midface, orbits, and frontal bone, and stabilization with bone grafts and miniplates. (Reproduced with permission from Aston SJ, Beasley RW, Thorne CH, eds: *Grabb and Smith's Plastic Surgery,* 5th edition. Lippincott-Raven, Philadelphia: 1997.)

SUMMARY OF PROCEDURES

	Monobloc/Frontofacial Advancement	Facial Bipartition, Periorbital Osteotomies
Position	Supine	⇐
Incision	Bicoronal, oral	Bicoronal, infraorbital
Special instrumentation	Horseshoe headrest, usually pediatric; disimpaction forceps; Midas Rex craniotome; resorbable plates and screws; mini/micro titanium plates and screws; ± distraction device to supplant bone grafting and rigid fixation.	⇐
Unique considerations	Control of ICP: spinal drain may be placed, hyperventilation. Blood in room for anticipated transfusion.	⇐
Antibiotics	Cefazolin 25 mg/kg q 8 h or vancomycin 10–15 mg/kg q 6 h, and cefotaxime 25–50 mg/kg q 6 h for oropharyngeal contamination and following dural tears	⇐
Surgical time	4–10 h	⇐
Closing considerations	Blood loss with Rainey clip removal for suturing. Full head-wrap dressing → head/neck movement with awakening.	⇐
EBL	400–800 mL; may be formidable	⇐
Postop care	ICU: 1–2 d; Monitor Hct.	⇐
Mortality	0.6–1.6%	⇐

SUMMARY OF PROCEDURES (cont'd)		
	Monobloc/Frontofacial Advancement	Facial Bipartition, Periorbital Osteotomies
Morbidity	Major complications: 14.3%	⇐
	Bone infection: 3–7%	⇐
	Meningitis	⇐
	Infection rates higher if:	⇐
	Adults rather than children (10 ×)	⇐
	Longer OR times and longer hospital stay	⇐
	Tracheostomy	⇐
	Foreign body (plates/screws/other alloplast)	⇐
	Anterior fossa entered	⇐
	Large dead space (e.g., in adult nongrowing brain)	⇐
	CSF leak: 4.5%	⇐
	↑ ICP	⇐
	Air embolus: < 1%	⇐
	Blindness: < 1%	⇐
	Massive bleeding: < 1%	⇐
	Venous thrombosis	⇐
	Neurological injury: Rare	⇐
Pain score	6	6

PATIENT POPULATION CHARACTERISTICS	
Age range	3–20 yr
Male:Female	1:1
Incidence	Crouzon syndrome: 1/25,000 Apert syndrome: 1/100,000
Etiology	Congenital (80%); occasionally trauma or tumor (20%)
Associated conditions	Depends greatly on the syndrome or disease entity. See Craniosynostosis, p. 1398.

ANESTHETIC CONSIDERATIONS

PREOPERATIVE

Craniofacial syndromes often are associated with maxillofacial deformities, mandibular abnormalities and challenging airway management.

Respiratory	Patients with long-standing upper airway obstruction due to choanal atresia, mandibular and maxillary hypoplasia, etc., may have chronic hypoventilation and hypoxia, and may have apnea episodes. If Sx of acute URI, delay elective surgery at least 2 wk. The presence of fever, cough, and abnormal chest auscultation necessitates radiographic evaluation and pediatric consultation. **Tests:** As indicated from H&P.
Airway	Be aware of other congenital anomalies affecting the airway, such as Apert, Goldenhar, Klippel-Feil, Pierre Robin, Treacher Collins, or Crouzon syndromes. Review any previous anesthetic records for insights into airway management (e.g., need for FOI). Consider elective tracheostomy under local anesthesia in patients with severe airway abnormalities.

Cardiovascular	Frequency of CHD is increased in patients with craniofacial abnormalities. Preop evaluation of patient with known or suspected heart defect should include H&P, ECG, Hct, baseline O_2 sat, and CXR. For children with Sx of cardiac dysfunction or those requiring cardiac medication, it is advisable to consult with a pediatric cardiologist to optimize patient's condition prior to surgery. **Tests:** Preop ECG indicated for patients with CHD; others as indicated from H&P.
Neurological	Neurologic deficits, if any, should be documented preop.
Laboratory	Hb/Hct; therapeutic drug levels for patients taking anticonvulsants.
Premedication	Premedication is helpful for patients > 1 yr – oral midazolam 0.5–0.75 mg/kg or oral ketamine 6 mg/kg about 30–60 min before induction.

INTRAOPERATIVE

Anesthetic technique: GETA, with special consideration given to associated CHD, pulmonary, and airway problems.

Induction	In an otherwise healthy patient, inhalational induction with subsequent placement of iv lines is appropriate. Muscle relaxants facilitate intubation but should be used only when adequate mask ventilation can be assured. An oral RAE ETT is useful for this procedure and should be secured carefully in place (often by suturing). Intubation in a patient with airway abnormalities may be facilitated by using an FOI with patient awake or lightly anesthetized and spontaneously ventilating. In rare situations, tracheostomy, under sedation and local anesthesia, may be necessary.	
Maintenance	Standard pediatric maintenance (see p. D-2). Consider use of remifentanil infusion (100–300 ng/ kg/min) for supplemental analgesia and to facilitate rapid awakening.	
Emergence	Extubate trachea when patient is awake and protective airway reflexes have returned. Patients with reactive airway disease may require deep extubation.	
Blood and fluid requirements	Anticipate large blood loss. IV: 18 ga × 1–2 NS/LR @: 4 mL/kg/h – 0–10 kg + 2 mL/kg/h – 11–20 kg + 1 mL/kg/h –> 20 kg (e.g., 25 kg = 65 mL/h) Warm fluids. Humidify gases.	The goal of intraop fluid therapy is to replace preop deficits, intraop fluid, electrolyte, and blood losses, while providing maintenance fluids. Half of the calculated deficit (hours fasting × hourly maintenance fluid requirement) generally is replaced during the 1st h of anesthesia and the balance over the next 1–2 h. Surgical manipulation of tissue will cause 3rd-space fluid loss proportional to the degree of surgical trauma and tissue exposure. It may range from 0–10 mL/kg/h.
Control of blood loss	Deliberate ↓ BP	Deliberate ↓ BP can be accomplished by use of SNP, esmolol, or potent inhalational agents titrated to effect (MAP 50–60 mmHg).
Monitoring	Standard monitors (see p. D-1). Arterial line ± CVP line	Arterial line is essential for monitoring BP during deliberate ↓ BP and for ABGs and blood chemistries.
Control of ICP	Hyperventilation Mannitol Loop diuretics CSF drainage (> 1 yr)	For some procedures, it is essential to reduce intracranial volume to facilitate surgical access. If prolonged brain retraction is required, postop cerebral edema may ensue.

Positioning	✓ and pad pressure points. ✓ eyes.	Positioning head above the heart facilitates venous drainage, but also increases the incidence of VAE. Do not hyperextend or hyperflex the head and neck. Flexion of the neck will move the ETT downward (mainstem intubation); extension will move the ETT upward (cuff leak).
Complications	Displacement of ETT	Suture ETT to alveolar ridge.
	Oculocardiac reflex (OCR)→ ↓↓ HR ↓ BP	Notify surgeon. Rx: atropine 0.02 mg/kg.
	VAE Major blood loss	VAE should be suspected if sudden ↑ ETN_2, ↓ $ETCO_2$, ↓ O_2 sat, ↓ BP, ↑ HR. Notify surgeon, flood surgical field with NS, support patient hemodynamically and D/C N_2O.

POSTOPERATIVE

Complications	↑ ADH secretion Diabetes insipidus (see Appendix D-1).	SIADH or DI may follow brain manipulation and may require pharmacologic intervention for Rx.
	Cerebral edema	Cerebral edema may →↑ ICP (headache, N/V, ↓ mental status, etc.)
	Pneumothorax Bleeding	Pneumothorax (Sx = ↑ respirations, wheezing, ↓ BP, ↓ CO, ↓ O_2 sat) may occur 2° rib resection for bone graft. ✓ CXR.
Pain management	PCA (see p. E-4).	
Tests	Hct	

Suggested Readings

1. Christianson L: Anesthesia for major craniofacial operations. *Int Anesthesiol Clin* 1985;23(4):117–30.
2. David DJ, Cooter RD: Craniofacial infection in 10 years of transcranial surgery. *Plast Reconstruct Surg J* 1987;80(2):213–23.
3. MacLennan FM, Robertson GS: Ketamine for induction and intubation in Treacher Collins syndrome. *Anesthesia* 1981;36(2):196–8.
4. Nargozian C: The airway in patients with craniofacial abnormalities. *Paediatr Anaesth* 2004;14(1):53–9.
5. Posnick JC: Surgical management of Crouzon, Apert and related syndromes. In *Maxillofacial Surgery*. Booth PW, Schendel SA, Hausamen J-E, eds. Churchill Livingstone, Edinburgh: 1999, 863–75.
6. Rasch DK, Browder F, Barr M, et al: Anaesthesia for Treacher Collins and Pierre Robin syndromes: a report of three cases. *Can Anaesth Soc J* 1986;33(3P+l):364–70.
7. Williams JK, Longaker MT: Surgical complications of craniofacial surgery. In *Maxillofacial Surgery*. Booth PW, Schendel SA, Hausamen J-E, eds. Churchill Livingstone, Edinburgh: 1999, 905–16.
8. Wolfe SA, Morrison G, Page LK, et al: The Monobloc Frontofacial Advancement: do the pluses outweigh the minuses? *Plast Reconstr Surg* 1993;91(6):977–87.

CLEFT LIP REPAIR—UNILATERAL/BILATERAL

SURGICAL CONSIDERATIONS

Description: Cleft lip may be either unilateral or bilateral, associated frequently with clefts of the alveolus and palate. Surgical repair involves the design and execution of geometric flaps on the medial and lateral

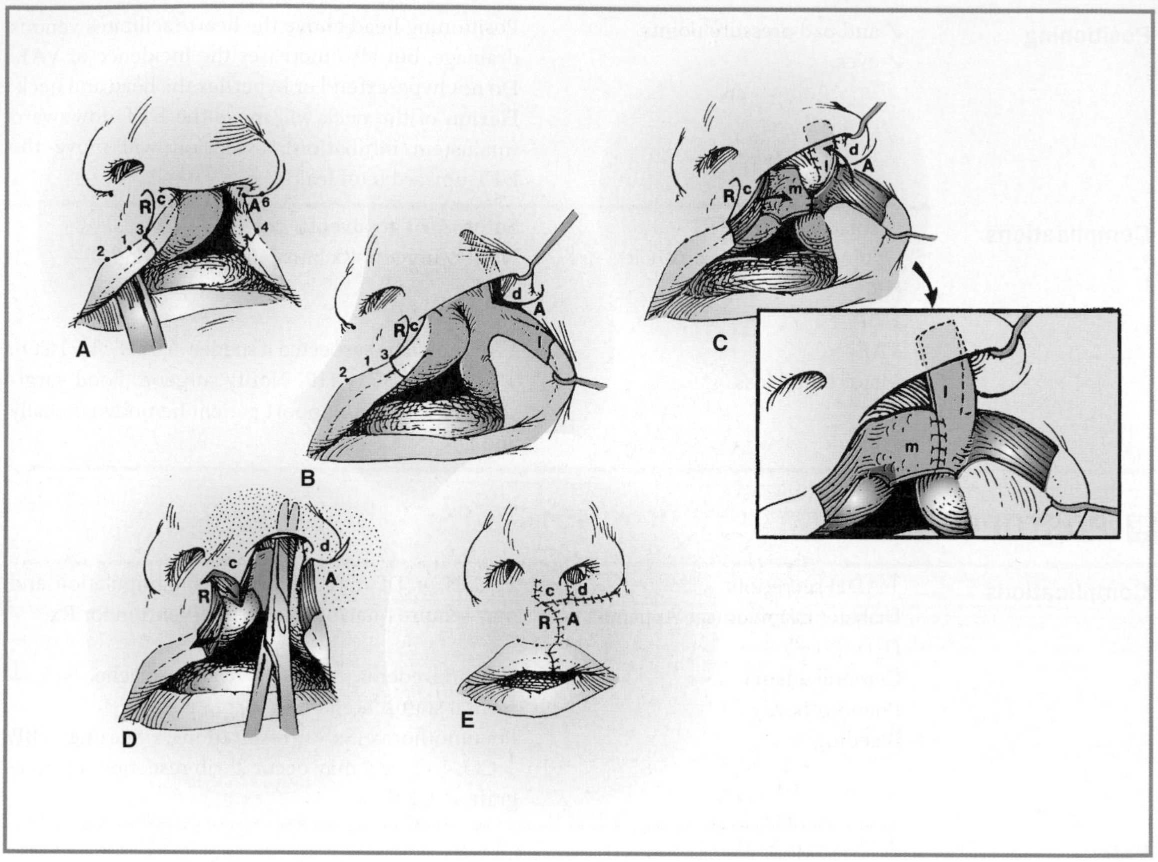

Figure 12.8-4. Step-by-step unilateral complete cleft rotation advancement: m = medial mucosal flap; l = lateral mucosal flap. (Reproduced with permission from Aston SJ, Beasley RW, Thorne CH, eds: *Grabb and Smith's Plastic Surgery,* 5th edition. Lippincott-Raven, Philadelphia: 1997.)

sides of the cleft and primary repair of the cleft nasal deformity. The most common unilateral technique is the **rotation advancement flap of Millard** (Fig. 12.8-4). Multiple bilateral lip repairs have been described, some repairing both sides simultaneously and some one side at a time (Fig. 12.8-5). Technique depends on the amount of prolabial and lateral element tissue available. Recently, **primary nasal repair** has been coupled with these bilateral procedures. These nasal repairs involve extensive mobilization of the alar cartilages and transfer of tissue up into the cleft nasal vestibule and floor, with nasal stents often placed. All of these factors can decrease or occlude nasal airway breathing. Although only a minority of neonates has been found to be true nasal obligatory breathers, this should be kept in mind for those postop patients with respiratory distress.

Variant procedure or approaches: Other approaches commonly performed are those of the **Davies-** or **Tennison** -type (Z-plasty) lip repairs (Fig. 12.8-6). In large clefts, a lip adhesion may be performed as an initial stage several months before the actual definitive correction of the cleft lip. This procedure basically involves creating a wound on either side and suturing the muscles, mucosa, and skin together. The procedure itself is very short (~45 min). **Presurgical orthopedic devices** may be placed and manipulated, instead of a lip adhesion, to bring a wide, bony cleft into better opposition for a tension-free complete repair. These are custom-fitted and may be fixed with pins to the palate. They are removed in the OR at time of repair.

Usual preop diagnosis: Cleft lip/palate

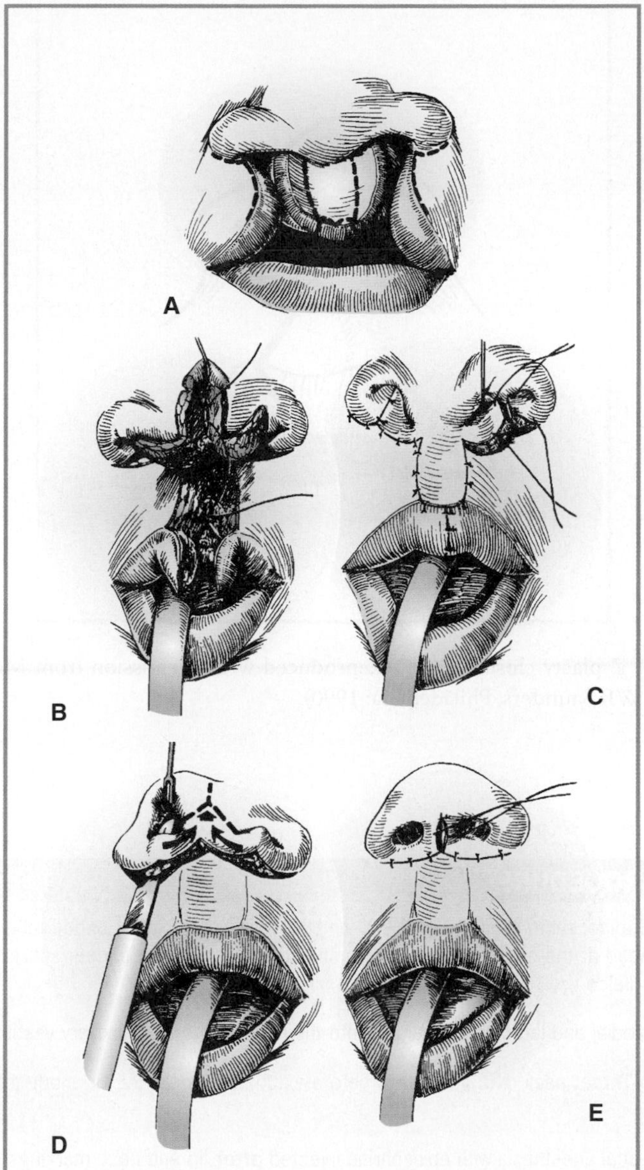

Figure 12.8-5. Banked fork-flap procedure. In the first stage **(A-C)**, bilateral straight line repairs are done after the prolabium is divided vertically into three forks. The central limb is used to construct the center of the lip. The lateral forks are 'banked' at the alar bases for later use in constructing a columella. At the second stage **(D-E)**, bipedicle flaps from the nasal floor, which include the banked forks, are used in combination with a membranous septum incision to elongate the columella and increase tip projection. (Reproduced with permission from Aston SJ, Beasley RW, Thorne CH, eds: *Grabh and Smith's Plastic Surgery,* 5th edition. Lippincott-Raven, Philadelphia: 1997. After Millard DR Jr: Closure of bilateral cleft lip and elongation of columella by two operations at infancy. *Plast Reconstr Surg* 1971;47:324–31.)

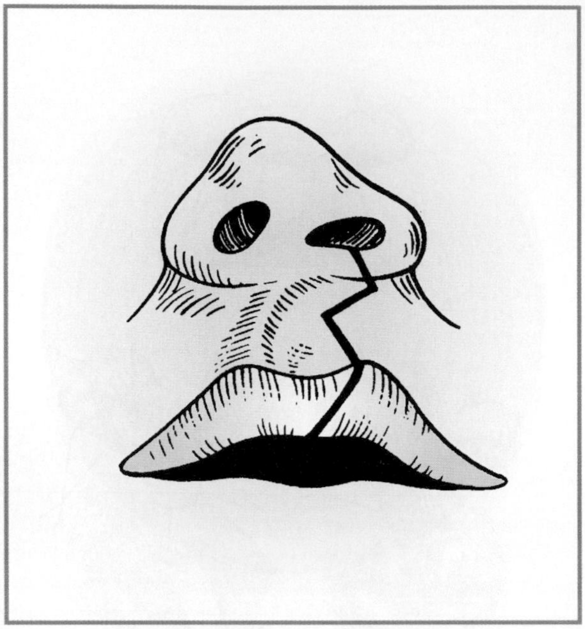

Figure 12.8-6. Z-plasty closure of lip. (Reproduced with permission from McCarthy JG, ed: *Plastic Surgery*. WB Saunders, Philadelphia: 1990).

SUMMARY OF PROCEDURE	
Position	Supine; table rotated either 90° or 180°, with oral RAE or anode tube toward chin; patient's head at the edge of head of bed; shoulder roll; neck extended; entire face exposed; scleral shields
Incision	Medial and lateral cleft margins into the nose and in the maxillary vestibule on the cleft side
Special instrumentation	* Throat pack (**NB:** ✓ removal before extubation); oral RAE or anode tube.
Unique considerations	Local anesthesia with epinephrine injected **after** lip and nose markings complete. Pediatric patients should wake up in an unagitated state, because undue crying may place excessive tension on the repair. Immediate elbow restraints for children × 2 wk.
Antibiotics	Cefazolin 25 mg/kg iv
Surgical time	1.5 h (bilateral usually ½ h longer) Lip adhesion: 45 min
Closing considerations	Nasal stent; swelling and ointment may occlude nasal airway; smooth emergence important.
EBL	5–10 mL (higher with palatoplasty)
Postop care	Elbow restraints × 2 wk; PACU → room overnight → home POD 1.
Mortality	Minimal
Morbidity	Infection Wound breakdown Hypertrophic scars
Pain score	4

PATIENT POPULATION CHARACTERISTICS	
Age range	1 wk–6 mo
Male:Female	2:1—cleft lip and palate. Isolated cleft palate more common in females.
Incidence	1/750 for Caucasians; more common in Asians; less in African Americans. Left cleft more common than right; both more common than bilateral, in the ratio of 6:3:1.
Etiology	Multifactorial, including both genetic and environmental aspects
Associated conditions	Associated anomalies are seen in ~29% of cleft lip cases, and may include major chromosomal deletions and/or duplications, along with possible severe mental retardation and CHD.

ANESTHETIC CONSIDERATIONS

See Anesthetic Considerations for Lip and Nose Surgery, (p. 1421).

Suggested Readings

1. Arosarena OA: Cleft lip and palate. *Otolaryngol Clin North Am* 2007;40(1):27–60.
2. Grayson BH, Cutting CB: Presurgical nasoalveolar orthopedic molding in primary correction of the nose, lip, and alveolus of infants born with unilateral and bilateral clefts. *Cleft Palate Craniofac J* 2001;38(3):193–8.
3. Gundlach KKH: Etiology, prevalence, growth and trends in cleft lip, alveolus and palate. In *Maxillofacial Surgery*. Booth PW, Schendel SA, Hausamen J-E, eds. Churchill Livingstone, Edinburgh: 1999, 991–1003.
4. Mommaerts Y: The traditional 'Millard' approach to lip and palate repair. In *Maxillofacial Surgery*. Booth PW, Schendel SA, Hausamen J-E, eds. Churchill Livingstone, Edinburgh: 1999, 1029–45.
5. Mulliken JB: Primary repair of bilateral cleft lip and nasal deformity. *Plast Reconstr Surg* 2001;108(1):181–94.
6. Schendel SA: Unilateral cleft lip repair–state of the art. *Cleft Palate-Craniofac J* 2000;37(4):335–41.
7. Sullivan WG: Respiratory distress following cleft lip repair: the role of obligatory nasal breathing in the infant. *Ann Plast Surg* 1988;20(6):590–2.
8. Winters JC, Hurwitz DJ: Presurgical orthopedics in the surgical management of unilateral cleft lip and palate. *Plast Reconstruct Surg J* 1995;95(4):755–64.

PALATOPLASTY

SURGICAL CONSIDERATIONS

Description: Cleft palate can be seen as either an isolated condition or in conjunction with clefting of the lip. The mildest form of cleft palate is the submucous, or occult cleft, in which there is no visible cleft but, rather, a nonunion of the soft-palate muscles. This is followed by the incomplete soft-palate cleft and, finally, the complete cleft, which includes soft and hard palates and may extend through the alveolar portion of the maxilla. Repair involves mobilizing the lateral soft tissue and moving it toward the midline to close the cleft and elongate the palate, if necessary. The most important goal of cleft-palate repair is the attainment of normal speech. Children with unrepaired or inadequately repaired clefts develop nasal-sounding speech patterns termed *rhinolalia*. Cleft-palate repair, therefore, usually is done when the child is 9–18 months old, before consequential speech development. In addition to closing the cleft itself, an important goal of palate repair is normal anatomic approximation of the levator palati muscles, which are responsible for oronasal valving in speech and swallowing. The cleft palate is closed by elevating the mucoperiosteum from the underlying bones and approximating it in the midline (**von Langenbeck technique**) (Fig. 12.8-7) or using a V-Y type of retrodisplacement and closure (**Wardill-Kilner technique**). In either method, the levator muscles are specifically dissected and the levator sling is reconstructed. A layered closure usually is accomplished, including repositioning of the uvular muscles.

There are several different approaches to the muscle reconstruction in the soft palate, generally termed **intravelarveloplasties.** Z-plasty of the soft palate, also called a **Furlow procedure,** (Fig. 12.8-8) has been used to lengthen the palate and reorient the palatal muscles across the cleft. The other procedures basically involve direct closure of the muscles and a push-back to lengthen the palate.

Usual preop diagnosis: Cleft palate

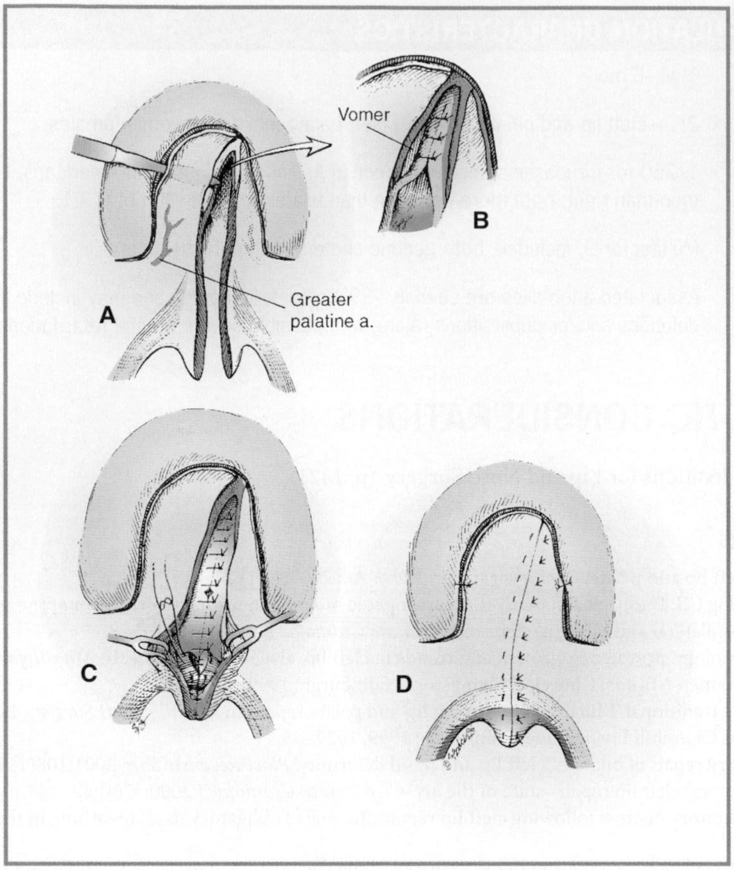

Figure 12.8-7. Palatoplasty technique. **(A)** Cleft palate closure after healing of gingivoperiosteoplasty at 11–12 mo of age. Bilateral, unipedicled mucoperiosteal flaps, based on the greater palatine arteries, are elevated. **(B)** Anteriorly, the nasal floor is repaired by suturing the vomerine mucosa to the nasal mucosa on the cleft side. **(C)** The levator muscles are dissected free from the oral and nasal mucosa and released from the posterior edge of the hard palate. The levator muscles are approximated to each other in the midline. **(D)** The oral mucosa is reapproximated in the midline with interrupted horizontal mattress sutures. (Reproduced with permission from Aston SJ, Beasley RW, Thorne CH, eds: *Grabb and Smith's Plastic Surgery,* 5th edition. Lippincott-Raven, Philadelphia: 1997.)

SUMMARY OF PROCEDURE

Position	Supine; table rotated 90°–180° with oral RAE tube extending down the midline of the lower jaw and taped to the chin.
Incision	Edges of the cleft palate and, possibly, the alveolar and pterygomandibular raphe areas.
Special instrumentation	Dingman mouth gag (when setting the gag, communication between surgeon and anesthetist allows ETT compression to be noted early); usually, a headlight; oropharyngeal pack
Unique considerations	The gag may be released intermittently to allow reperfusion of the tongue; each manipulation may affect the ETT. Minimal-to-moderate amount of blood in the oropharynx at end of procedure—should be carefully suctioned. Also, there may be some respiratory difficulties on emergence. Traction with a tongue suture often proves helpful in restoring patient's airway (maintained 24 h). Usually, oral or nasopharyngeal airways should not be placed in children.
Antibiotics	Cefazolin 25 mg/kg q 5–6 h (up to 1 g) × 5 d

SUMMARY OF PROCEDURE (cont'd)

Surgical time	1–1.5 h
Closing considerations	Child should not wake up crying and hypertensive. Tongue suture may be placed prior to extubation. **NB:** Dingman gag will stick to the ETT; therefore, holding the tube with a forceps deep in the oropharynx and careful removal of the gag avoids accidental extubation.
EBL	50 mL
Postop care	Elbow restraints; PACU → room; → home next day. OG tube placed, suctioned, and removed.
Mortality	Rare
Morbidity	Recurrent bleeding (requiring early return to OR): Rare Hematoma under palate Dehiscence of palate
Pain score	4

PATIENT POPULATION CHARACTERISTICS

Age range	6–18 mo
Male:Female	1:3 (isolated cleft palate)
Incidence	1/1,000
Etiology	Failure of fusion of the palatal shelves from anterior to posterior. (Can be due to a persistent high-tongue position in utero, increased facial width, reduced facial mesenchyme and/or drugs such as steroids, anticonvulsants, and benzodiazepines, or infection.)
Associated conditions	Multiple associated conditions. Most common is the Pierre Robin syndrome, in which cleft palate is found in association with glossoptosis and a micrognathic retruded mandible. These children frequently have airway obstruction and, even at an older age, may have sleep apnea. Other associations include Klippel-Feil syndrome, Treacher Collins syndrome, CHD, chronic URI, chronic otitis media, subglottic stenosis.

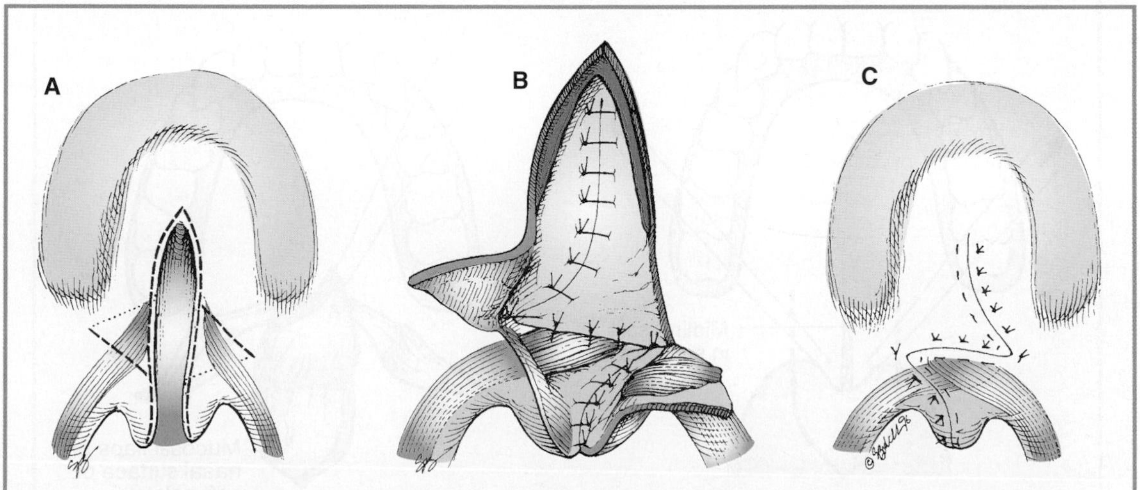

Figure 12.8-8. Double opposing Z-plasty closure of an isolated cleft palate. **(A)** Design of the incisions. **(B)** Muscle included in the posteriorly based flap. **(C)** Final result with recreation of the levator sling. (Reproduced with permission from Aston SJ, Beasley RW, Thorne CH, eds: *Grabb and Smith's Plastic Surgery,* 5th edition. Lippincott-Raven, Philadelphia: 1997.)

ANESTHETIC CONSIDERATIONS

See Anesthetic Considerations for Lip and Nose Surgery, p. 1421.

Suggested Readings

1. Arosarena OA: Cleft lip and palate. *Otolaryngol Clin North Am* 2007;40(1):27–60.
2. Gundlach KKH: Etiology, prevalence, growth and trends in cleft lip, alveolus and palate. In *Maxillofacial Surgery*. Booth PW, Schendel SA, Hausamen J-E, eds. Churchill Livingstone, Edinburgh: 1999, 991–1003.
3. Kirschner RE, Wang P, Jawad AF, et al: Cleft-palate repair by modified Furlow double-opposing Z-Plasty: *The Children's Hospital of Philadelphia Experience, Plastic and Reconstructive Surgery* 1999;104(7):1998–2014.
4. Mommaerts Y: The traditional 'Millard' approach to lip and palate repair. In *Maxillofacial Surgery*. Booth PW, Schendel SA, Hausamen, J-E, eds. Churchill Livingstone, Edinburgh: 1999, 1029–45.

PHARYNGOPLASTY

SURGICAL CONSIDERATIONS

Description: Following the initial repair of palatal clefts, some children or young adults demonstrate continued hypernasal speech patterns, a condition called "velopharyngeal incompetence." This can be 2° a short soft palate, a large nasopharynx, or a soft palate that has inadequate movement either 2° scarring or due to neurogenic problems. The typical repair would be a superiorly based **pharyngeal flap** (Fig. 12.8-9) to the soft palate.

Variant procedure or approaches: The **Jackson modification of the Orticochea flap** uses the posterior tonsillar pillars, which consist of the palatopharyngeus muscle and overlying mucosa, to create a competent oronasal

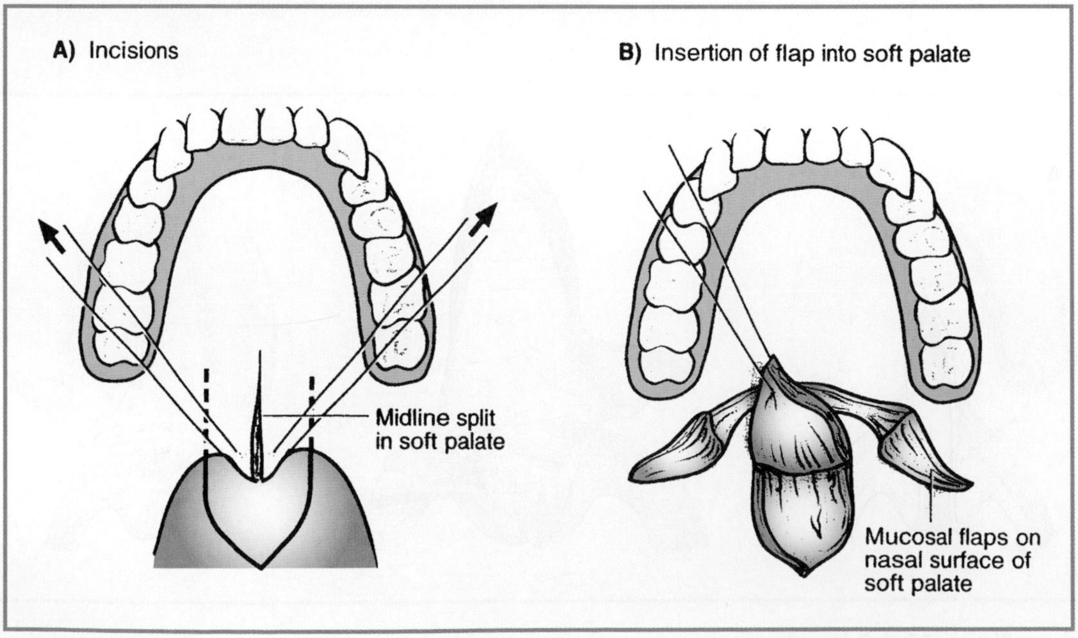

Figure 12.8-9. Pharyngeal flap, superiorly based. (Reproduced with permission from Booth PW, Schendel SA, Hausamen J-E, eds: *Maxillofacial Surgery*. Churchill Livingstone, Edinburgh: 1999.)

Pediatric Surgery

sphincter (Fig. 12.8-10). The flaps are based superiorly and repositioned horizontally to meet above and behind the soft palate. Although they act to augment the posterior pharyngeal wall, they also are intended to maintain their innervation and, therefore, augment sphincter activity. A posterior pharyngeal wall implant also may be placed.

Usual preop diagnosis: Velopharyngeal incompetence

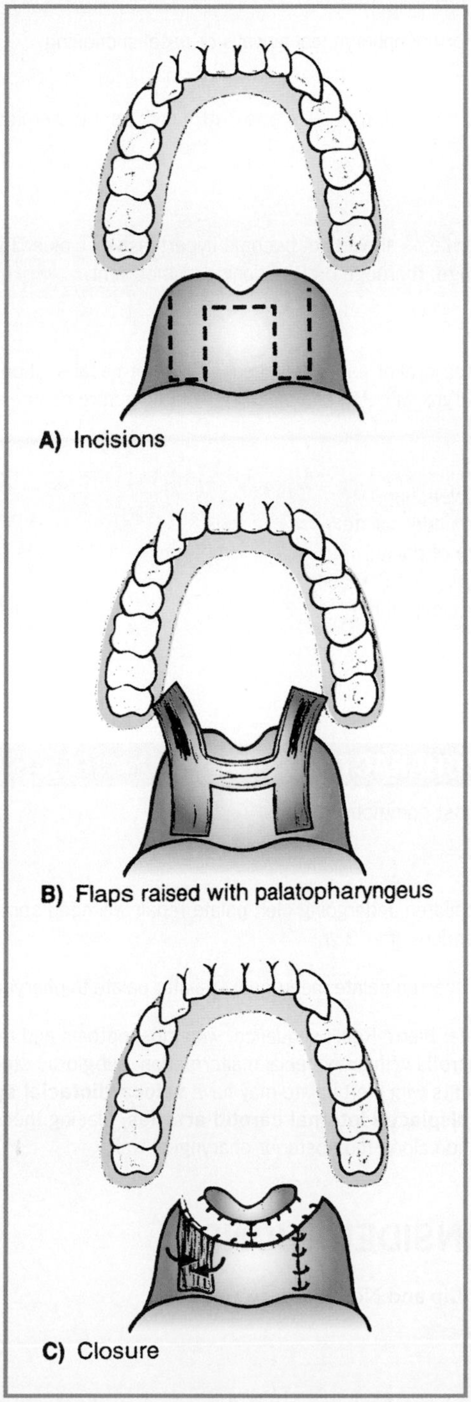

Figure 12.8-10. Sphincter pharyngoplasty. (Reproduced with permission from Booth PW, Schendel SA, Hausamen J-E, eds: *Maxillofacial Surgery*. Churchill Livingstone, Edinburgh: 1999.)

SUMMARY OF PROCEDURE	
Position	Supine, table rotated 90° or 180°; oral RAE tube extending down the midline chin and taped in position.
Incision	Involves incisions in soft and hard palates and in the posterior pharyngeal wall.
Special Instrumentation	Dingman mouth gag (caution with removal and manipulation re ETT); headlight
Unique considerations	Avoid oral or nasopharyngeal airways or nasal suctioning.
Antibiotics+ other meds	Cefazolin 25 mg/kg q 6–8 h (up to 1 g) × 3 d; periop steroids, depending on preop airway.
Surgical time	1–1.5 h
Closing considerations	Pediatric patients should not become hypertensive (↑ bleeding).There will be some nasopharyngeal drainage; thorough oral suctioning is important.
EBL	50–100 mL
Postop care	Avoid postop oral or nasopharyngeal airways or nasal suctioning. Be aware of possible occlusion of nasopharynx with flap and bleeding. Tongue suture can be placed for 24 h.
Mortality	Rare
Morbidity	Recurrent bleeding Hematoma under palate Dehiscence of palate Nasopharyngeal obstruction Secondary sleep apnea
Pain score	4

PATIENT POPULATION CHARACTERISTICS	
Age range	3–11 yr most common
Male:Female	1:1
Incidence	~15% of children undergoing cleft palate repair will need some type of secondary palatal lengthening procedure after 3 yr.
Etiology	Short and scarred palate; neurogenic palate; palate-to-pharyngeal ratio that is too small.
Associated conditions	Sleep apnea; Pierre Robin sequence, with gloscoptosis and micrognathia. Treacher Collins syndrome; microtia with craniofacial malformation; subglottic stenosis; CHD. Of special interest: some patients with cleft palate may have **velocardiofacial syndrome.** These children may have **medially displaced internal carotid arteries,** placing these major arteries in harm's way during dissection along the posterior pharyngeal wall.

ANESTHETIC CONSIDERATIONS

See Anesthetic Considerations for Lip and Nose Surgery, (p 1421).

Suggested Readings

1. Boorman JG, Bharathwaj S: Secondary palatal surgery and pharyngoplasty. In *Maxillofacial Surgery*. Booth PW, Schendel SA, Hausamen J-E, eds. Churchill Livingstone, Edinburgh: 1999, 1083–99.
2. Jackson IT: Sphincter pharyngoplasty. *Clin Plastic Surg* 1985;12(4):711–17.

3. Markus AF, Precious DS: Secondary surgery for cleft lip and palate. In *Maxillofacial Surgery*. Booth PW, Schendel SA, Hausamen J-E, eds. Churchill Livingstone, Edinburgh: 1999, 1057–72.
4. Sloan GM: Posterior pharyngeal flap and sphincter pharyngoplasty: the state of the art. *Cleft Palate Craniofac J* 2000; 37(2):112–22.

Also see Suggested Readings for Cleft Lip, (p 1421).

ALVEOLAR CLEFT REPAIR WITH BONE GRAFT

SURGICAL CONSIDERATIONS

Description: Alveolar cleft occurs as both bony and soft-tissue defects in the alveolar portion of the maxilla in the position of the lateral incisor tooth; thus, an oral/nasal fistula exists with this deformity. The size of the cleft is variable; it may be unilateral or bilateral and is associated with cleft lip and palate. The alveolar segments are often collapsed such that orthodontic expansion is required before bone graft and repair. These devices are maintained to stabilize the graft in situ for a 3-month healing period. The surgical procedure involves raising mucosal-gingival-periosteal flaps, advancing them, and performing a layered closure, starting with the nasal floor and working toward the oral cavity. A bone graft is placed in between these two layers to consolidate the upper arch. Cancellous bone usually is taken from the iliac crest or corticocancellous bone from the outer table of the skull.

Most commonly, the bone is harvested from the ilium. This can be accomplished via limited access and a trephine or via an open technique, depending on the amount of bone required. This portion of the procedure, especially by open technique, can add 50–100 mL of blood loss. Most nasal and lip revision surgery should be put off until the alveolus is reconstructed, since this is the base on which the lip and nose sit.

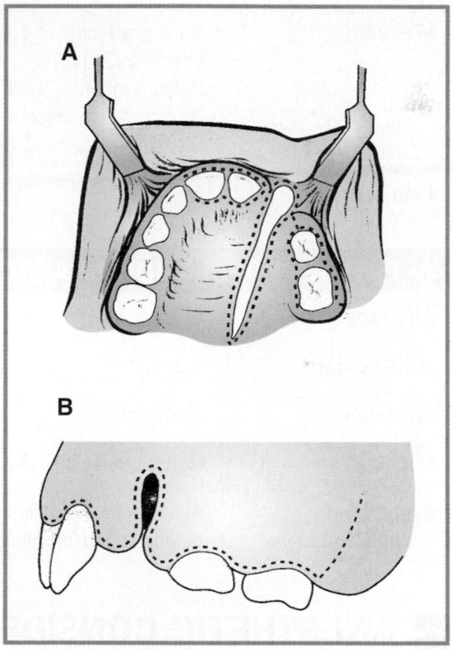

Figure 12.8-11. Gingivoalveoloplasty (GAP). Gingival and mucosal incisions are shown on the palate **(A)** and vestibular **(B)** surfaces, extending along the cleft borders. (Reproduced with permission from Booth PW, Schendel SA, Hausamen J-E, eds: *Maxillofacial Surgery*. Churchill Livingstone, Edinburgh: 1999.)

Variant procedure or approaches: In young children, the alveolar cleft procedure may be performed without the use of bone grafts at the time of lip or hard palate closure (**gingivoalveoloplasty,** Fig. 12.8-11) with the hope that preop alignment of the clefted alveolus and periosteal creation of new bone will fill the bony defect and allow subsequent normal tooth eruption. This is not always complete, and some of these children will need later bone grafting at age 7–8 years, before eruption of the permanent canine teeth.

Usual preop diagnosis: Congenital alveolar cleft

SUMMARY OF PROCEDURE

Position	Supine; table rotated 90°–180° ± roll under hip (bone harvest)
Incision	Oral, with the addition of iliac crest incision or scalp incision, either parasagittal or coronal
Special instrumentation	Throat pack; Dingman mouth gag; headlight. Two instrument setups used, to prevent cross-contamination from oral to iliac surgical sites.

SUMMARY OF PROCEDURE (cont'd)	
Unique considerations	Important to ensure that the hip iliac crest bone graft site is on the opposite side from the anesthesiologist if the table is rotated only 90°. Midline oral RAE tube to chin. Care when manipulating Dingman, as it sticks to ETT.
Antibiotics	Cefazolin 25 mg/kg (up to 1 g) iv preop
Surgical time	1.5–2.5 h
Closing considerations	***NB:** Ensure that throat pack has been removed. Pediatric patients should not wake up in agitated state. Noncleft-side oral mouth gag and gentle oral suctioning permissible; avoid nasal suctioning, especially from the cleft side.
EBL	100–200 ml
Postop care	PACU → ward; walking POD 1 or 2 post-iliac graft.
Mortality	Rare
Morbidity	Bone graft loss: 2–10% Infection: 2–10% Refistulization: 2–10% Prolonged hip discomfort (bone graft donor site) Bleeding—oral or at bone donor site
Pain score	6

PATIENT POPULATION CHARACTERISTICS	
Age range	8–12 yr
Male:Female	2:1
Incidence	Unknown
Etiology	Multifactorial, including both genetic and environmental aspects
Associated conditions	Associated anomalies are seen in ~29% of cleft lip cases; and may include major chromosomal deletions and/or duplications, with the possibility of severe developmental delay, CHD.

ANESTHETIC CONSIDERATIONS

See Anesthetic Considerations for Lip and Nose Surgery, (p. 1421).

Suggested Readings

1. Brusati R, Mannucci N: Primary repair of the lip and palate using the Delaire philosophy. In *Maxillofacial Surgery*. Booth PW, Schendel SA, Hausamen J-E, eds. Churchill Livingstone, Edinburgh: 1999, 1005–28.
2. Posnick JC: *Craniofacial and Maxillofacial Surgery in Children and Young Adults.* WB Saunders, Philadelphia: 2000, 785–980.
3. Stassen LFA: Alveolar bone grafting–how I do it. In *Maxillofacial Surgery*. Booth PW, Schendel SA, Hausamen J-E, eds. Churchill Livingstone, Edinburgh: 1999, 1047–55.
4. Wolfe SA, Kawamoto HK: Taking the iliac bone graft: a new technique. *J Bone Joint Surg* 1978;60-A(3):411.

Also see Suggested Readings for Cleft Lip. p. 1421.

SECONDARY CLEFT LIP/NASAL SURGERY

SURGICAL CONSIDERATIONS

Description: Secondary deformities of the nose and lip develop, following the initial repair of either bilateral or unilateral cleft lip deformities. These subsequent deformities depend on the extent of the initial congenital anomaly,

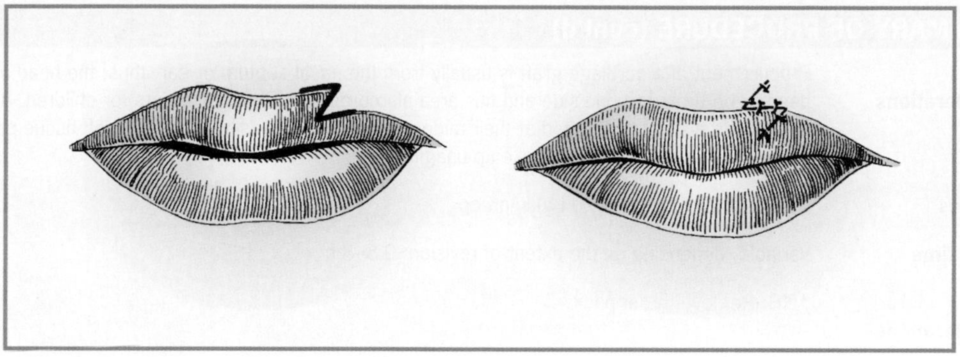

Figure 12.8-12. Z-plasty to correct notching of the vermillion border. (Reproduced with permission from Aston SJ, Beasley RW, Thorne CH, eds: *Grabb and Smith's Plastic Surgery,* 5th edition. Lippincott-Raven, Philadelphia: 1997. Originally from Millard DR Jr: *Cleft Craft: The Evolution of Its Surgery*. Little & Brown, 1976.)

the quality of the surgical repair, and resulting oral/facial function. Revision can vary from a minimal scar revision (Fig. 12.8-12), to a complete opening and reconstruction of the lip and nose, with or without ancillary procedures such as **septorhinoplasty ± cartilage grafting, forked flaps** (Fig. 12.8-13), **fascial lip augmentation, or Abbe-Estlander flap** (lip-switch flap) (Fig. 12.8-14).

Occasionally, the individual born with a cleft lip and palate is severely deficient in tissue of the upper lip. This occurs most frequently in the bilateral condition. Correction involves switching tissue from the midline of the lower lip to the central portion of the upper lip, maintaining a pedicle of soft tissue between the lips, which usually contains the labial artery on one side. This pedicle normally is cut between 7–11 days. The redundant tissue in the mid portion of the upper lip is transferred to the columellar portion of the nose at the same time, which elongates this section (Fig. 12.8-14). To avoid disruption of the flap, the older child should be cautioned to avoid wide mouth opening in the postop period.

Usual preop diagnosis: Secondary cleft deformity

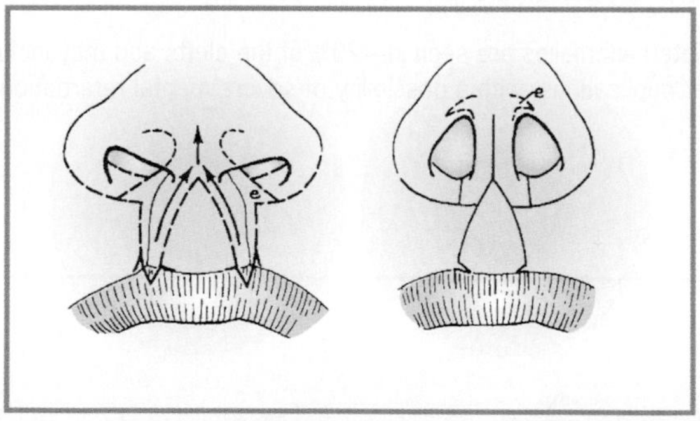

Figure 12.8-13. Short columella associated with the bilateral cleft nose, elongated by forked flaps. (Reproduced with permission from Aston SJ, Beasley RW, Thorne CH, eds: *Grabb and Smith's Plastic Surgery,* 5th edition. Lippincott-Raven, Philadelphia: 1997.)

SUMMARY OF PROCEDURE

Position	Supine, table rotated 90°–180°; oral RAE; nasal RAE tube when working on lips only (especially if lips are held closed by a flap pedicle, making extubation more difficult).
Incision	Variable, in lip or nasal areas. (See Figs 12.8-12, 12.8-13, 12.8-14.)
Special instrumentation	Throat pack; possibly rhinoplasty instruments; oral RAE tube; head light; loupe magnification.

SUMMARY OF PROCEDURE (cont'd)

Unique considerations	Procurement of a cartilage graft is usually from the nasal septum or ear; thus, the head may need to be turned to one side and this area also prepped. Elbow restraints for children. A switch flap leaves the lips connected at their midportion by a thin, easily damaged, soft-tissue pedicle; therefore, the patient should wake up unagitated.
Antibiotics	Cefazolin 25 mg/kg (up to l g) iv preop
Surgical time	Variable, depending on the extent of revision: 0.5–3 h
Closing considerations	***NB:** Remove throat pack.
EBL	Minimal–75 mL
Postop care	May be obligatory mouth breathing post-rhinoplasty, or lips may be held mostly closed by the pedicle and swelling of a lip-switch flap; consider oral-pharyngeal airway; avoid wide mouth opening. PACU → room; elbow restraints in young children.
Mortality	Rare
Morbidity	Infection Wound breakdown Flap necrosis: < 1% (with lip switch) Bleeding
Pain score	3–5 (depending on extent of procedure)

PATIENT POPULATION CHARACTERISTICS

Age range	2–50 yr
Male:Female	1:1
Incidence	20–60% of patients with primary clefts
Etiology	Unsatisfactory outcome of previous lip/nose surgery
Associated conditions	Associated anomalies are seen in ~29% of the clefts and may include major chromosomal deletions or duplications, with a possibility of severe mental retardation.

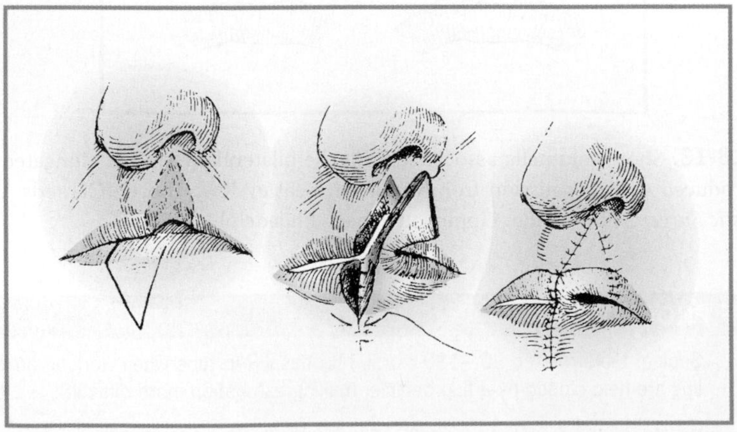

Figure 12.8-14. Abbe-Estlander flap. Note lips sutured together. (Reproduced with permission from Converse JM, ed: *Reconstructive Plastic Surgery,* Vol 3, 2nd edition. WB Saunders, Philadelphia: 1977.)

ANESTHETIC CONSIDERATIONS

See Anesthetic Considerations for Lip and Nose Surgery, p. 1421.

Suggested Readings

1. Palmisano BW: Anesthesia for plastic surgery. In: *Pediatric Anesthesia,* 3rd edition. Gregory GA, ed. Churchill Livingstone, New York: 1994, 699–741.
2. Sadove AM, Eppley BL: Correction of secondary cleft lip and nasal deformities. *Clin Plastic Surg* 1993;20(4):793–801.
3. Talmant JC: Cleft rhinoplasty. In *Maxillofacial Surgery.* Booth PW, Schendel SA, Hausamen J-E, eds. Churchill Livingstone, Edinburgh: 1999, 1133–71.

ANESTHETIC CONSIDERATIONS FOR LIP AND NOSE SURGERY

(Procedures covered: cleft lip repair; palatoplasty; pharyngoplasty; alveolar cleft repair with bone graft; secondary cleft lip/nasal surgery)

PREOPERATIVE

The anesthesiologist should be aware of the parents' feelings about their child with a congenital malformation. The whole family needs to be treated with sensitivity and compassion. Cleft lip closure may be carried out as early as the first week of life in the healthy neonate; however, many surgeons and anesthesiologists find the 'rule of ten' helpful: the child should have an Hb >10 g, be 10 wk old, and weigh 10 lbs. The hard palate usually is closed between the ages of 1–5 yr; however, the soft palate should be closed prior to speech development (12–15 mo). **Palatoplasty** and **pharyngoplasty** usually are carried out from 1–15 years. Patients with these midline facial defects are most likely to have other associated anomalies, including CHD, subglottic stenosis, and Pierre-Robin or Treacher-Collins syndromes. In patients with severe OSA, post-op edema may impair ventilation. The possibility of remaining instubated post-op should be discussed with the surgical team and the family.

Respiratory	Careful assessment is necessary as associated anomalies may affect airway or lungs. Chronic otitis 2° eustachian tube dysfunction is common. Treat with antibiotics before surgery. Postpone surgery (~2 wk) if Sx of acute URI present (e.g., runny nose, fever, sore throat, cough). Chronic aspiration may be associated with cleft lip/palate. **Tests:** as indicated from H&P.
Airway	Be aware of other congenital anomalies affecting the airway, such as Apert, Goldenhar, Klippel-Feil, Pierre Robin, or Treacher Collins syndromes. Review any previous anesthetic records for insights into airway management. Consider fiber optic intubation (FOI) in patients with suspected difficult airway. Also consider elective tracheostomy under local anesthesia in patients with severe airway abnormalities. Patients with severe subglottic stenosis may require preop tracheostomy. Patients with difficult airways or severe obstructive sleep apnea undergoing palatal surgery should be evaluated for ICU monitoring postoperatively.
Cardiovascular	CHD is frequently associated with cleft palate. Preop evaluation of a patient with a known or suspected heart defect should include thorough H&P, EKG, Hct, baseline O_2 sat, and CXR. For children with Sx of cardiac dysfunction or those requiring cardiac medication, it is advisable to consult with a pediatric cardiologist to optimize the patient's condition prior to surgery. **Tests:** Preop ECG indicated for patients with CHD; others as indicated from H&P.
Nutritional	Infants with cleft lip/palate may have problems with oral feeding. Assess nutritional status from physical exam and by comparison to expected growth for age. **NB:** NPO after midnight for solids. Patients should continue to have clear liquids up until 2 h preop.
Neurological	Delayed development of speech is common in the older child with cleft palate. Some of these children may be hearing impaired. Preop preparation and discussion is important to minimize the impact of these communication problems.

Psychological	Many patients with orofacial congenital malformations require multiple procedures; emotional support and psychological assessment of these patients are essential. Preoperative visits and consultation with play-therapists can be helpful, particularly if the child with a difficult airway will need a preoperative IV.
Hematologic	High incidence of iron deficiency anemia; T&C for 1 U PRBC (cleft palate). **Tests:** Hct
Laboratory	Other tests as indicated from H&P.
Premedication	< 9 mo old rarely needs premedication; > 9 mo old, may benefit form midazolam (0.5–0.75 mg/kg po); alternatively ketamine (5 mg/kg po) ~30 min preop may be used.

INTRAOPERATIVE

Anesthetic technique: GETA; warm room to 75–80°F; forced air warmer.

Induction	Typically, an inhalational induction (sevoflurane ± N_2O/O_2) while patient is breathing spontaneously. Airway obstruction is best treated with an oral airway. Anticipate difficult laryngoscopy if large, prepalatal cleft present. Intubate with oral RAE tube and secure in midline of lower lip. In patients with difficult airways, preoperative IV and FOI is the technique of choice. IV glycopyrrolate and nebulized local anesthetics may facilitate FOI. Avoid muscle relaxants for difficult intubations until ETT is placed. For children with difficult airways and a small posterior pharynx, consider preop dexamethasone 0.5 mg/kg IV to decrease palatal edema. After induction, consider morphine 0.1 mg/kg, ketamine 0.1 mg/kg for analgesia.	
Maintenance	Standard pediatric maintenance (see p. D-3) ± muscle relaxant. Airway is shared with the surgeons. The Dingman mouth gag is used for surgical exposure and may inadvertently compress the ETT or cause an endobronchial intubation. Monitor PIP before and after placement of Dingman. Flexion of the neck also may cause endobronchial intubation. Extension of the neck may cause complete or partial extubation. Adequacy of ventilation should be checked after every position change. Bilateral breath sounds should be equal after final positioning. In cases with the table turned 180°, a precordial stethoscope placed over the left chest can help elucidate endobronchial tube migration. ETT should be sutured to the alveolar ridge. In palatoplasty, the palate is infiltrated with epinephrine (in lidocaine usually) →↓ blood loss + ↑ dysrhythmias (halothane > sevoflurane). ↑ $PaCO_2$ →↑ dysrhythmias.	
Emergence	*Pharyngeal (throat) packs are usually placed to prevent aspiration of blood. **NB:** Packs must be removed before extubating the trachea. Consider laryngoscopy to inspect airway and remove blood and clots before extubation. A tongue stitch is useful postop following cleft palate surgery. It may be used to pull the tongue forward to relieve postop respiratory obstruction. Extubation in the lateral (tonsillar) position is useful in promoting drainage of blood and secretions.	
Blood and fluid requirements	IV: 18–20 ga × 1 NS/LR @: 4 mL/kg/h – 0–10 kg + 2 mL/kg/h –11–20 kg + 1 mL/kg/h – > 20 kg (e.g., 25 kg = 65 mL/h)	Blood loss replaced by 3:1 crystalloid or 1:1 colloid (e.g., 5% albumin or 6% hetastarch). Rarely, a blood transfusion may be indicated for hemorrhage.
Monitoring	Standard monitors (see p. D-1)	
Positioning	✓ and pad pressure points. ✓ eyes.	

Pediatric Surgery

Complications	Obstructed ETT→ ↑ PIP Mucous plugging Hemorrhage	✓ ETT to see that it is not partially or completely obstructed by mouth gag. ✓ bilateral breath sounds.

POSTOPERATIVE

Complications	Retained throat pack Airway edema → croup Hemorrhage Obstructive sleep apnea	✓ for retained throat pack if there are Sx of airway obstruction in immediate postop period. Rx of postintubation croup consists of cool, humidified, 100% O_2 mask, or nebulization 2.25% racemic epinephrine (0.5 ml in 3 mL NS). Racemic epinephrine is given for its vasoconstrictor, rather than its bronchodilator, effect. If posterior pharyngeal edema is present, consider dexamethasone 0.5 mg/kg iv.
Pain management	Acetaminophen (10–15 mg/kg po or 20–30 mg/kg pr) q6H Fentanyl 1 mcg/kg iv; Morphine 0.05–0.1 mg/kg iv q 2–3 h prn	Avoid oversedation in patients with Abbe-Estlander repair 2° airway obstruction. Aim for child to be mildly sedated (decreases bleeding), but not obstructing; intraop morphine, ketamine helpful to ensure smooth awakening.
Tests	Hct, if indicated.	Others as indicated.

OTOPLASTY

SURGICAL CONSIDERATIONS

Description: There are a number of congenital ear malformations. The two most frequently encountered in the OR are **prominent ear** and **microtia.** Both conditions can be unilateral or bilateral.

Prominent ears are usually an isolated finding. The ear is examined in thirds to determine where the prominence lies, and the surgery is tailored to correct the specific excesses. The antihelical fold is usually flattened and requires reshaping. The prominence of the ear, as measured by its projection from the mastoid process, is decreased accordingly. This usually involves an elliptical skin incision in the posterior ear area, dissection over the mastoid, and one, or a combination of three techniques—mattress sutures, cartilage scoring, and/or resection.

Variant procedure or approaches: All procedures are similar, with minor differences in suturing and amount of resected tissue. In addition to the posterior incisions, an anterior incision can be used in some approaches.

Microtia is within the congenital anomaly spectrum of hemifacial microsomia, and the associated facial malformation may include a small asymmetric jaw, creating a difficult intubation. Reconstruction is most often accomplished with autologous rib graft as a multistaged procedure. This donor site comes with the attendant risks of pneumothorax and hemothorax (Fig. 12.8-15). Stage one is the creation of a cartilaginous framework, with placement into a cutaneous pocket symmetric with the normal ear, if present (Fig. 12.8-16). Stage one is accomplished once the rib cartilage has grown to sufficient size—usually, ~6–7 years of age. Stage two requires transposition of the lobule 3 months after stage one. Stage three is the elevation with skin graft of the framework from the head posteriorly. Stage four is the creation of a tragus and conchal excavation.

Variant procedure or approaches: Recently, **porous polyethylene implants** have been used to avoid donor-site morbidity, and **temporoparietal fascial flaps** provide coverage to avoid alloplastic extrusion.

Usual preop diagnosis: Ear malformation; prominent ears; microtia; anotia

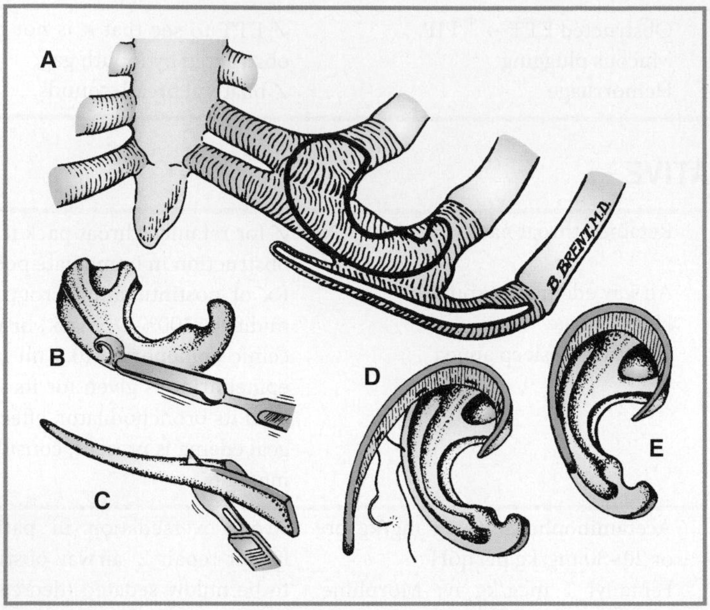

Figure 12.8-15. Fabricating an ear framework from costal cartilage. **(A)** Donor site: the contralateral thorax. The helical rim is obtained from a 'floating' rib cartilage, the main pattern from the synchondrosis of two cartilages. **(B)** Sculpting the main block. **(C)** Thinning the 'floating' rib cartilage to produce a delicate helical rim. **(D)** Affixing the rim to the main framework block. **(E)** Completed framework. (Reproduced with permission from Aston SJ, Beasley RW, Thorne CH, eds: *Grabb and Smith's Plastic Surgery,* 5th edition. Lippincott-Raven, Philadelphia: 1997.)

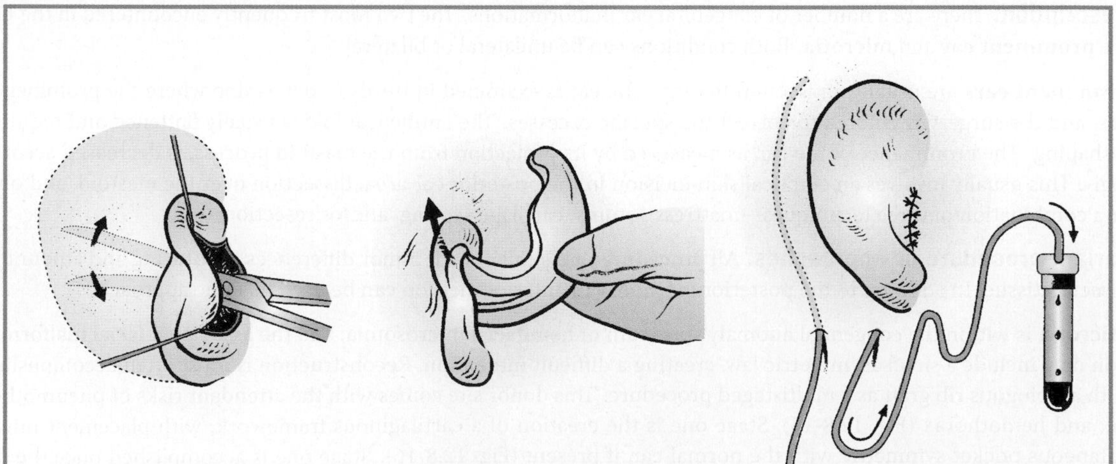

Figure 12.8-16. The cutaneous "pocket." The vestigial native cartilage is excised; then a skin pocket is created. To provide tension-free accommodation of the framework, the dissection is carried out well beyond the proposed auricular position. Using two silicone catheters, the skin is coapted to the framework by means of vacuum tube suction. (Reproduced with permission from Booth PW, Schendel SA, Hausamen J-E, eds: *Maxillofacial Surgery*. Churchill Livingstone, Edinburgh: 1999.)

SUMMARY OF PROCEDURE	
Position	Supine; table rotated either 90° or 180°; oral intubation
Incision	Posterior ear; occasionally anterior ear; microtia, stage-dependent; and chest wall
Unique considerations	Head turned from side-to-side during operation.
Antibiotics	Cefazolin 25 mg/kg (up to 1 g) iv preop
Surgical time	2–4 h (depends on unilateral vs bilateral); 1st stage microtia much longer
Closing considerations	Ear dressing requires 5–10 min at end of procedure. Delicate vacuum test-tube drainage system in 1st stage microtia repair fixed to head dressing.
EBL	10–100 mL
Postop care	PACU → room
Mortality	Rare
Morbidity	**Protruding ears:** Hematoma formation: < 1% Infection: < 1 % Asymmetrical ear reduction: < 1% Suture extrusion < 1% **Microtia:** Pneumothorax or hemothorax Hematoma, infection, and skin loss: 1.6% (total) Overgrowth: 41%
Pain score	4

PATIENT POPULATION CHARACTERISTICS	
Age range	6+ yr
Male:Female	2:1
Incidence	Unknown
Etiology	**Microtia:** 9.2% bilateral; 32% left vs 58% right; 4.9% recurrence within immediate family **Protrusion:** Also seen among family members. Most are bilateral.
Associated conditions	**Protruding ears:** none known **Microtia:** Brachial arch deformities: bone/soft tissue deficit, 36.5%; facial nerve weakness, 15.2%; cleft lip ± palate, 4.3%; macrostomia, 2.5%; urogenital defects, 4%; cardiovascular malformations, 2.5%; other, 1.6%

ANESTHETIC CONSIDERATIONS

See Anesthetic Considerations for Ear Surgery, Chapter 3.0 Otolaryngology, p 229.

Suggested Readings

1. Brent B: Ear reconstruction. In *Maxillofacial Surgery*. Booth PW, Schendel SA, Hausamen J-E, eds. Churchill Livingstone, Edinburgh: 1999, 1419–28.
2. Brent B: Technical advances in ear reconstruction with autogenous rib cartilage grafts: personal experience with 1200 cases. *Plastic Reconstruct Surg J* 1999;104(2):319–38.

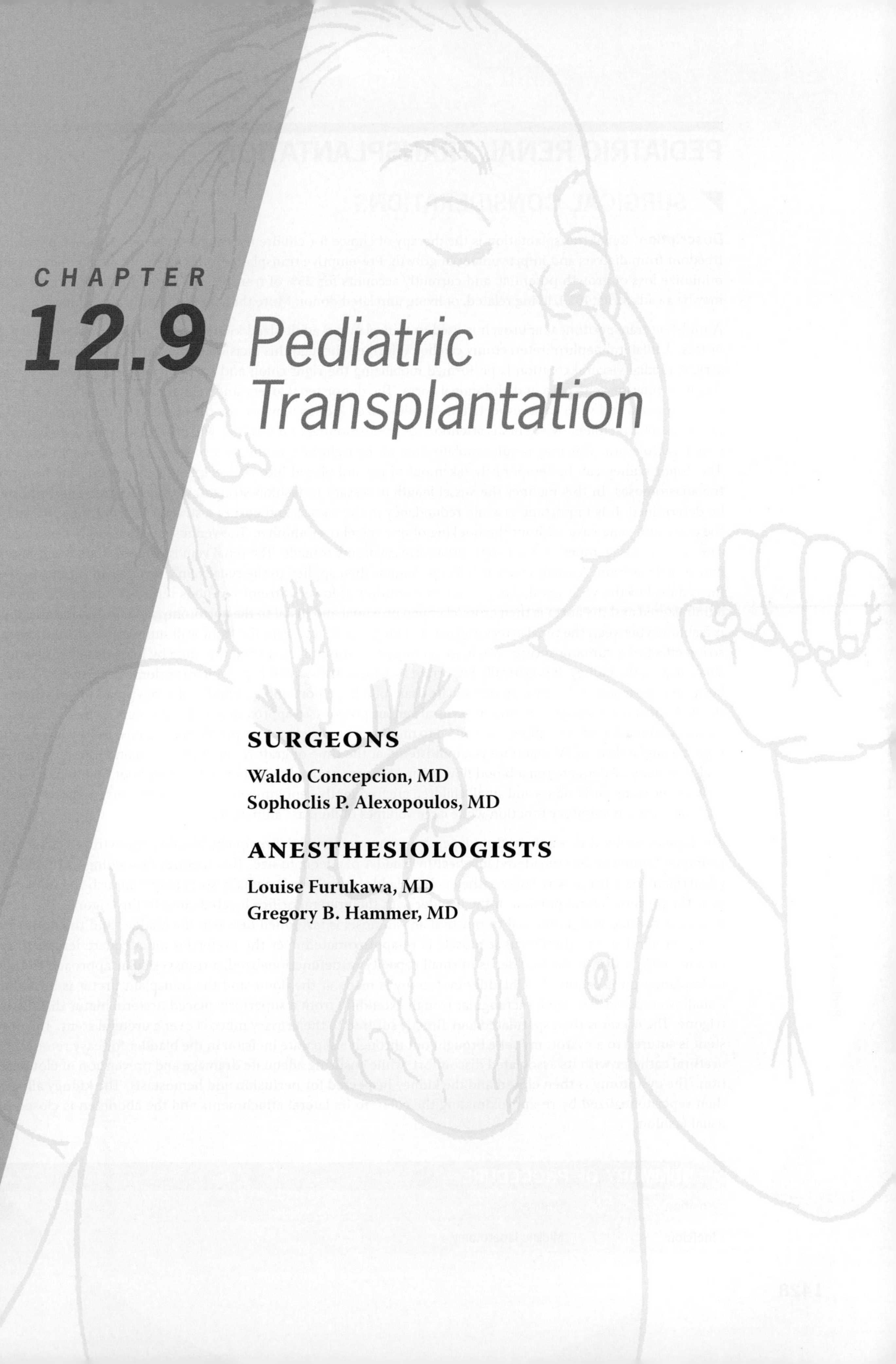

CHAPTER

12.9 Pediatric Transplantation

SURGEONS

Waldo Concepcion, MD
Sophoclis P. Alexopoulos, MD

ANESTHESIOLOGISTS

Louise Furukawa, MD
Gregory B. Hammer, MD

PEDIATRIC RENAL TRANSPLANTATION

SURGICAL CONSIDERATIONS

Description: Renal transplantation is the therapy of choice for children with end-stage renal disease providing for freedom from dialysis and improvement in growth. Pre-emptive transplantation is recommended when possible to minimize loss of growth potential, and currently accounts for 25% of transplants. The source of the renal allograft may be a cadaveric (40%), living related, or living unrelated donor. More than 90% of donors are adults.

A mid-line transperitoneal approach is used to transplant an adult-sized kidney (ASK) into a child weighing 20 kg or less. A bilateral nephroureterectomy can be performed through this incision at the same time should it be necessary. A medial visceral rotation is performed mobilizing the right colon and small bowel mesentery to expose the recipient inferior vena cava and abdominal aorta. The donor renal artery and vein are anastomosed directly to the recipient aorta and vena cava respectively. An adult-sized kidney may occupy the majority of the right upper quadrant in a small recipient. Meticulous attention to the positioning of the kidney will prevent kinking or twisting of the donor vasculature. This may require mobilization of the right lobe of the liver or even hepatectomy in some cases. The donor kidney can be temporarily taken out of ice and placed into the recipient to determine the best site for the anastomoses. In this manner the vessel length necessary to fashion straight, yet tension-free anastomoses can be determined. It is important to avoid redundancy in the vessels and ensure a straight lie from the renal hilum to the aorta and vena cava without the hooking of one vessel over another. The venous anastomosis is fashioned first. The vena cava is clamped, and an appropriate size cavotomy is made. The renal vein is sutured to the vena cava in an end-to-side fashion. A small vascular bulldog clamp is then applied to the renal vein above the anastomosis to allow for removal of the vena caval clamp and reconstitution of lower extremity venous return to the heart. Heparin is administered and the aorta is then cross-clamped proximal and distal to the aortotomy. An end-to-side anastomosis is fashioned between the renal artery and aorta, taking care to interrupt the front wall sutures and prevent the purse-string effect of a running suture. Warm ischemia can be minimized during this time by intermittently placing iced slush around the kidney. It is critically important to achieve substantial hypervolemia prior to reperfusion of the ASK because reperfusion will cause an immediate drain of a large portion of a child's relatively small blood volume into the ASK. This necessitates bringing the central venous pressure to approximately 18–20 cm H_2O before reperfusion with a combination of crystalloid and colloid to minimize tissue edema. As prophylaxis against ischemia-reperfusion injury, a single dose of IV mannitol is administered at the time of graft re-vascularization and low-dose dopamine is also initiated. Adequate renal blood flow to an ASK cannot be obtained in children without maintenance of a hypervolemic state, and infants and small children are frequently kept intubated for 24 to 48 hours postop to maintain control of their respiratory function while large volumes of fluid are administered.

The type of ureteral re-implantation depends on the quality of the recipient bladder. An extravesicular ureteral re-implantation can be considered in a healthy bladder of adequate size. This requires distending the bladder with GU irrigant via a three-way Foley catheter. The bladder is reflected medially so as to accomplish the implantation near the postero-lateral portion of the bladder with the ureteral orifice located close to the trigone. The detrusor muscle is divided and a mucosal to mucosal anastomosis is fashioned between the bladder and the donor ureter over a ureteral stent. The detrusor muscle is re-approximated over the ureter for an adequate length to create an anti-reflux valve. If the bladder is of small capacity or defunctionalized, a transvesicular approach to ureteral re-implantation is required. A bladder cystotomy is made at the dome and the transplant ureter is brought into a shallow, mucosa-denuded, rectangular trough extending from a superiorly placed ureteral hiatus distally to the trigone. The ureter is then spatulated and directly sutured to the urinary mucosa over a ureteral stent. The ureteral stent is sutured to a cystotomy tube brought out through a separate incision in the bladder for easy removal of the urethral catheter with its associated discomfort, while ensuring adequate drainage and prevention of clot obstruction. The cystotomy is then closed and the kidney inspected for perfusion and hemostasis. The kidney allograft is then reperitonealized by re-approximating the colon to its lateral attachments and the abdomen is closed in the usual fashion.

SUMMARY OF PROCEDURE	
Position	Supine
Incision	Midline laparotomy

SUMMARY OF PROCEDURE (cont'd)	
Special instrumentation	Self-retaining retractor Vascular instruments Foley catheter (three-way)
Unique considerations	Recipient hypervolemia (CVP 18–20 mm H_2O) Mannitol Dopamine Immunosuppression Potassium free I.V. fluids
Antibiotics	Cephalosporin
Surgical Time	3–5 h
EBL	Minimal
Postop Care	Maintain hypervolemia (CVP > 10 mm Hg) Maintain adequate SBP > 120 mm Hg with dopamine Maintain high UO with a combination of I.V. fluids + Lasix. Goal 150–200 cc/h ICU postop Transplant ultrasound postop
Mortality	< 2%
Morbidity	Primary nonfunction: 2.6% Vascular thrombosis: 10.3% Renal artery stenosis: 0.7% Other technical: 1.3% Bleeding: 2% Wound infection: 5%
Pain Score	7

ANESTHETIC CONSIDERATIONS FOR KIDNEY TRANSPLANTATION IN INFANTS AND CHILDREN

PREOPERATIVE

Patients presenting for renal transplantation tend to fall into two groups: (a) children in the infant/toddler age group who suffer from congenital syndromes (congenital nephrotic syndrome, severe polycystic kidney disease, obstructive uropathies, FSGS) or (b) the older child who may have a variety of conditions including severe autoimmune nephropathies. These children are often the recipient of a living related transplant and as such, the surgery proceeds as a somewhat elective procedure. Most patients have been on a well-established regimen of peritoneal or hemodialysis.

Airway	Some renal conditions may have associated syndromes and dysmorphia. A thorough airway examination as well as perusal of old anesthetic records should reveal any potential airway problems.
Respiratory	Patients with autoimmune diseases (e.g. lupus) may have pulmonary involvement. Any patient presenting with signs and symptoms of URI should be allowed adequate time for resolution of heightened airway reactivity. Children born with large polycystic kidneys may have pulmonary hypoplasia. **Tests:** Pulmonary Function Tests
Cardiovascular	Relatively long-standing hypertension and LVH can be seen in this patient population and may require bilateral nephrectomies prior to or during the transplantation. Adequate control of hypertension should be achieved during the preoperative admission period. **Tests:** EKG, echocardiogram

Gastrointestinal/ Hepatic	Patients with polycystic kidney disease may also have hepatic dysfunction and require future liver transplantation. Patients with congenital nephrotic syndrome tend to be hypoalbuminemic and may be on continuous albumin infusions. **Tests:** Albumin, LFTs, PT, PTT if applicable
Renal	Most patients are well-maintained on hemodialysis or peritoneal dialysis. Other common electrolyte abnormalities are metabolic acidosis, hypocalcemia, and hypermagnesemia. Be aware of current weight relative to dry weight as some patients may present with dehydration in the postdialysis period. **Tests:** Serum electrolytes, BUN and Creatinine
Hematologic	Anemia and platelet dysfunction are commonly seen. **Tests:** CBC, Platelet count
Premedication	Most children will require a premedication to allay separation anxiety. Oral midazolam 0.5–0.75 mg/kg or IV midazolam 0.1 mg/kg (maximum 2 mg) is usually sufficient.

INTRAOPERATIVE

Anesthetic technique: GETA. Epidural anesthesia may be a possibility; however, hypotension must be avoided. There are also risks of epidural hematoma due to dysfunctional platelets.

Induction	An inhalational induction with standard monitors will work well in patients without prior IV access. Patients in the infant/toddler age group may have significant venous access problems, and the hemodialysis catheter (if present) may be used provided that sufficient heparinized blood has been aspirated from the dead-space of the catheter lumen. Use of muscle relaxation once IV access has been established is necessary for adequate surgical visualization and mobilization.	
Maintenance	Standard balanced anesthetic maintenance. Titration of a long-acting narcotic is recommended although high doses of meperidine should be avoided due to accumulation of normeperidine. Adequate muscle relaxation is especially important in the patient under 20 kg to facilitate surgical exposure. Any coughing or straining can result in vascular injury. Significant hypothermia can be seen when the iced organ is placed in the peritoneum. Tachycardia is frequently seen following reperfusion of the ASK due to this large volume and low-resistance circuit. Urine output should be closely monitored post-reperfusion.	
Emergence	Most smaller children will remain intubated in anticipation of large fluid shifts due to volume loading. Older children can be extubated in the OR. All patients are sent to the ICU for monitoring of hemodynamics and urine output.	
Management of reperfusion	**Blood and fluids:** Maintenance IV fluids without K Volume loading Albumin loading	Preop fluid status is variable. Albumin boluses (10cc/kg) may be needed. Since crystalloid may → visceral edema and complicate surgery. Volume loading for a CVP of 15–20 (or titrated to kidney turgor post-perfusion) with albumin, is usually requested by the surgeon in anticipation of reperfusion.
	Blood may be required Warm all fluids	PRBC transfusion may be needed if CUP or BP response to albumen is insufficient.
	Promoting diuresis	Doses of mannitol (0.5 g/kg) and furosemide (1 mg/kg) are also given prior to reperfusion.
	Pressor support	Dopamine 3–5 mcg/kg/min is started.
Monitoring	Standard Monitors (see p. D-1) Arterial line CVP (2–3 lumen)	Adequate blood pressure to perfuse the ASK is crucial as is sufficient preload (CVP 10–15) prior to reperfusion.

Monitoring (cont'd)	Hct/electrolytes	Goal Hct after reperfusion is about 25. (higher Hct can lead to occlusion of the renal artery). Electrolytes must be closely followed especially in the setting of blood transfusion or large volume albumin infusion. Hyperkalemia and hypocalcemia must be corrected.
	Urine Output	Goal UOP after reperfusion is about 5–10 mL/kg/h. Urine output must be continually monitored after ureteral implantation.
	PIP	Follow ventilation pressures as patients can go into pulmonary edema from the large volume challenge.
	Temperature control	Hypothermia must be avoided in all children. Placement of the iced donor kidney can drop the temperature by as much as 1.5°C.
Complications	Ventilatory difficulties Electrolyte abnormalities Hypotension/inadequate renal perfusion Low urine output	

POSTOPERATIVE

Complications	Electrolyte abnormalities Ventilatory difficulties Inadequate pain control in the face of hypotension Hemorrhage Clot retention given small catheter size	
Pain Management	Fentanyl 1 mcg/kg iv Small doses of ketamine (eg 1–5 mg iv) can be used for analgesia if patient is intubated	Care must be taken in the administration of iv opioids to prevent hypotension.

Suggested Readings

1. Coupe N, O'Brien M, Gibson P, et al: Anesthesia for pediatric renal transplantation with and without epidural analgesia–a review of 7 years experience. *Paediatr Anaesth* 2005;15(3):220–8.
2. Fine RN, Ho M, Tejani A: The contribution of renal transplantation to final adult height: a report of the North American Renal Transplant Cooperative Study (NAPRTCS). *Pediatr Nephrol* 2001;16:951–6.
3. Giessing M, Muller D, Winkelmann B, et al: Kidney transplantation in children and adolescents. *Transplant Proc* 2007;39(7):2197–201.
4. Hammer G, Chuljian P, Al-Uzri A, et al: Intraoperative management of small children undergoing kidney transplantation. *Am J Anesthesiol* 1997;24:37–9.
5. Salvatierra O, Alfrey E, Tanney DC, et al: Superior outcomes in pediatric renal transplantation. *Arch Surgery* 1997;132:842–9.
6. Salvatierra O Jr, Millan M, Concepcion M: Pediatric renal transplantation with considerations for successful outcomes. *Semin Pediatr Surg* 2006;15(3):208–17.
7. Salvatierra O, Tanney D, Mak R, et al: Pediatric renal transplantation and its challenges. *Transplant Rev* 1997;11:51–69.
8. Shapiro R: Living donor kidney transplantation in pediatric recipients. *Pediatr Transplant* 2006;10(7):844–50.
9. Smith JM, Fine RN, McDonald RA: Current state of pediatric renal transplantation. *Front Biosci* 2008;13:197–203.
10. Smith JM, Stablein DM, Munoz R, et al: Contributions of the transplant registry: the 2006 annual report of the North American Pediatric Trials and Collaborative Studies (NAPRTCS). *Pediatr Transpl* 2007;11(4):366–73.
11. Uejima T: Anesthetic management of the pediatric patient undergoing solid organ transplantation. *Anesthesiol Clin North America* 2004;22(4):809–26.

PEDIATRIC LIVER TRANSPLANTATION

SURGICAL CONSIDERATIONS

Description: Liver transplantation was first pioneered in the 1960s as a life-saving experimental procedure for children with end-stage liver disease (ESLD). Since then, it has developed into the accepted treatment modality for pediatric patients with ESLD or fulminant hepatic failure. The indications for liver transplantation in children are broad and range from cholestatic cirrhosis secondary to biliary atresia to inborn errors of metabolism that, if untreated, result in devastating neurological injury.

The current liver allocation system prioritizes pediatric recipients based on a calculated numerical value known as the Pediatric End-Stage Liver Disease (PELD) score. The PELD score was validated as a model for predicting the 3-month wait-list mortality. Although exemption points can be petitioned for on a case-by-case basis, a patient's degree of illness generally correlates with his PELD. Absolute contraindications for liver transplantation include irreversible encephalopathy, uncontrollable infection, and untreatable extrahepatic malignancy. A general contraindication is poor quality of life postoperatively.

The main constraint to pediatric liver transplantation compounding the pre-existing organ shortage involves the donor-to-recipient size ratio. The minimum acceptable graft-to-body weight ratio to provide adequate postop liver function is 1%. However, the suitability of a donor is more often determined by the maximum amount of donor liver that a recipient can accommodate in his abdominal cavity. This results in the utilization of several different types of grafts in pediatric liver transplantation.

Type of Graft	Artery	Portal Vein	Venous Outflow	Biliary Reconstrution
Cadaveric Full Size	Celiac Trunk	Main PV	Full VC	Main HD
Cadaveric Reduced Size	Celiac Trunk	Main PV	Full VC	Main HD
Cadaveric Left Lobe	Common HA	Left PV	Left HV	Left HD
Cadaveric Left Lateral Segment	Common HA	Left PV	Left HV	Left HD
Live Donor Left Lateral Segment	Left HA	Left PV	Left HV	Left HD

Although the type of graft used determines certain technical aspects of the hepatectomy and implantation, the general sequence of events consists of:

Recipient hepatectomy
Anhepatic phase (during which portal venous inflow and hepatic venous outflow are reconstituted)
Allograft reperfusion
Reconstitution of hepatic arterial inflow
Biliary reconstruction

A bilateral subcostal incision is used with a midline subxiphoid extension as needed. The abdomen is explored and adhesions are lysed taking care to suture-ligate varices in patients with portal hypertension. This portion of the procedure may be tedious and bloody in patients with prior liver surgery. The falciform ligament is divided down to the suprahepatic vena cava. The left coronary ligament is divided and the left lateral segment is mobilized from the diaphragm. The lesser omentum is divided and the lesser sac entered. The peritoneum of the hepatoduodenal ligament is divided and a hilar dissection is performed. The connective and vascular tissue of the hepatoduodenal ligament is carefully divided taking care to suture-ligate any varices en masse until the common bile duct is identified. This portion of the procedure may result in significant blood loss in patients with severe portal hypertension. The common bile duct is then suture-ligated, and divided high in the hilum of the liver. The hepatic artery is similarly identified, suture ligated, and divided. The portal vein is then completely skeletonized. The right lobe of the liver is then mobilized. The infra and suprahepatic vena cava are encircled taking care not to injure the right adrenal vein, right renal vein, or inferior phrenic veins. High central-venous pressures during this portion of the procedure can exacerbate portal hypertension and make variceal bleeding difficult to control. However, the patient must have adequate circulatory volume to support the interruption of subdiaphragmatic venous return to the heart without developing vasopressor refractory hypotension. The portal inflow is then occluded with a vascular clamp followed by occlusion of the infrahepatic and suprahepatic vena cava. The recipient liver and retrohepatic vena cava are excised, and donor liver implantation begins. In the piggyback technique the liver is completely mobilized from the retrohepatic vena cava by individually ligating the short hepatic veins draining directly from the liver to the cava. The liver is excised with preservation of the retrohepatic vena cava and venous return can be restored prior to implantation by moving the vascular clamp to the junction of the vena cava with the hepatic veins.

The goal of the surgical team during the anhepatic phase is to minimize the duration of caval disruption with its associated intestinal edema and variceal congestion. The hepatic vein outflow is first reconstructed by fashioning the suprahepatic caval anastomosis. In the **piggyback technique,** there is no infrahepatic caval anastomosis and an end-to-end portal vein anastomosis is fashioned next. The liver is flushed with albumin prior to reperfusion to minimize the risk of cardiac arrest 2° ↑ K^+ and ↓ pH. Venous outflow is then re-established by removing the suprahepatic caval or hepatic venous clamp prior to opening the portal venous anastomosis. In a standard procedure the infrahepatic caval clamp is also removed. Reperfusion is the portion of the procedure associated with significant hemodynamic lability, as large volume shifts may occur → pulmonary HTN and RV failure. Alternatively, the release of systemic inflammatory mediators may result in vasodilatation and significant ↓ BP. The anesthesia team needs to be ready to pharmacologically intervene. Hemostasis is achieved prior to arterial reconstruction. Patients who receive cut down or split livers performed ex-vivo may have significant bleeding from the cut surface of the liver.

The donor hepatic artery is typically anastomosed in an end-to-end fashion to the recipient common hepatic artery. In situations of large size discrepancy or poor recipient hepatic artery quality, an anastomosis may be fashioned directly to the supraceliac aorta. This requires aortic cross-clamping with its associated risk of ischemia/reperfusion injury and renal failure. The surgical team should notice the immediate production of bile and resolution of coagulopathy with clot formation in patients with a well functioning graft. The biliary reconstruction can then be performed in an end-to-end fashion if possible but frequently requires a Roux-en-Y reconstruction. If a Roux-en-Y is performed the bowel is divided distal to the ligament of Treitz and the distal limb is brought up to the bile duct. Intestinal continuity is restored with an end-to-side enteroenterostomy and a hepaticojejunostomy is fashioned to the Roux limb. Abdominal drains are typically left along the cut surface in split or cut down livers due to the increased incidence of bile leaks.

The pediatric patient is then taken to the intensive care unit. In patients with end-to-end arterial anastomosis, the patient should be maintained in hypervolemic state to ensure adequate hepatic perfusion in the immediate postop period.

SUMMARY OF PROCEDURE

Position	Supine with arms tucked
Incision	Bilateral subcostal with midline subxiphoid extension as needed
Special instrumentation	Thompson liver retractor; Vascular instruments; Argon beam coagulator; Arterial and central venous access (above and below diaphragm); Foley catheter
Unique considerations	Hypothermia requiring covering extremities with plastic to minimize convective heat loss, active rewarming Encephalopathy requiring ICP monitoring Hypoxemia secondary to hepatopulmonary syndrome Hyperkalemic cardiac arrest on reperfusion Air embolism on reperfusion RV failure on reperfusion Pressor refractory hypotension with vena caval disruption DIC/fibrinolysis on reperfusion Severe acidosis Renal failure requiring intraoperative CVVH Coagulopathy and hemorrhage requiring massive transfusion Hypoglycemia
Antibiotics	Zosyn (piperacillin + tazobactam) 80 mg of piperacillin component/kg/8h.
Surgical Time	4–6 h
EBL	300–1,500 mL (1–5 U)

SUMMARY OF PROCEDURE (cont'd)	
Postop Care	Maintain infusion hypervolemia in end-to-end arterial reconstructions. Heparin infusion, Dextran infusion, and aspirin for end-to-end arterial reconstructions ICU postop Monitor closely for signs of bleeding. Monitor closely for acidosis or worsening coagulopathy suggestive of graft dysfunction - Transplant ultrasound postop.
Mortality	2–5%
Morbidity	Primary nonfunction: <5% Portal vein thrombosis: 2–5% early, 10% late Hepatic artery thrombosis: 5–10% Bile leak: 10–20% Bleeding: 10% Wound infection: 5% Reoperation: 18%
Pain Score	10

PATIENT POPULATION CHARACTERISTICS	
Age range	0–18 yr
Male:Female	1:1
Incidence	500–600 transplants annually
Etiology	Biliary atresia 35–40%; TPN related 15%; Metabolic diseases 10%; Acute hepatic necrosis 10–15%; Hepatoblastoma 3%; Autoimmune 3%; Congenital hepatic fibrosis 2–3%

ANESTHETIC CONSIDERATIONS

PREOPERATIVE

Indications for liver transplant (LT) in children include (a) progressive subacute or chronic primary liver disease, such as biliary atresia, (b) metabolic disease of the liver, (c) fulminant hepatic failure, (d) hepatic tumors, and (e) retransplantation for hepatic graft failure. The most common disorder for which LT is performed in children is **biliary atresia,** accounting for more than 50% of patients. It is the most common cause of chronic cholestasis in infants and children. For the majority of these patients, a Kasai portoenterostomy is performed in early infancy. Even in those infants in whom bile flow is achieved, however, progressive liver failure commonly ensues, resulting in cirrhosis, portal HTN, and malnutrition. Complications include coagulopathy, esophageal varices, hypersplenism with splenomegaly and thrombocytopenia, ascites, and growth failure. Recurrent cholangitis following the Kasai procedure may lead to progressive hepatic injury and repeated hospitalizations for IV antibiotic therapy. Children with metabolic liver disease represent the second largest group of patients presenting for LT. Of these, **alpha-1-antitrypsin deficiency** is most prevalent, followed by tyrosinemia and Wilson's disease. LT may also be indicated in patients with metabolic liver disorders presenting solely with extrahepatic manifestations. Oxalosis, or primary hyperoxaluria, is a metabolic liver disease presenting with renal failure due to deposition of oxalate in the renal tubules. These children generally have normal hepatic synthetic function and do not have portal hypertension. Metabolic liver diseases including protein C, protein S, and anti-thrombin III deficiency may present with portal vein thrombosis, portal hypertension, and hypoxemia due to intrapulmonary shunting, and may be treated with LT. Unlike the patients with biliary atresia or alpha-1-antitrypsin deficiency, these children may have normal synthetic liver function and appear relatively healthy.

Respiratory	Previous prolonged intubation may have caused subglottic stenosis. Ascites, pleural effusions, and hepatosplenomegaly cause a reduction in lung volumes in children with liver failure. Intrapulmonary R $\rightarrow$ L shunting through abnormally dilated pulmonary arterioles and impaired hypoxic pulmonary vasoconstriction may cause severe hypoxemia.

Respiratory (cont'd)	Pulmonary edema may result from hypoalbuminemia and I.V. fluid administration, impairing oxygenation as well as ventilation. Supplemental oxygen and, in advanced cases, mechanical ventilation may be required preop. **Tests:** CXR, ABG in hepatopulmonary syndrome
Circulatory	Chronic liver failure may be accompanied by a hyperdynamic circulatory state with ↓ SVR + ↑ CO. On the other hand, cardiomyopathy and/or pulmonary HTN may be present and CO may actually be diminished. These changes appear to be less common in children than adults. **Tests:** Echocardiogram
Neurologic	Hepatic encephalopathy is a life-threatening complication of ESLD. Causes include accumulation of toxins such as ammonia, GABA agonists, and other neuroactive substances. Cerebral metabolism and the blood-brain barrier may also be abnormal in advanced liver disease. The clinical manifestations of hepatic encephalopathy range from mild somnolence to coma. **Tests:** Head CT to rule out bleed. Rarely, ICP monitoring may be indicated, especially in cases of fulminant hepatic failure.
Hematologic	In addition to the coagulation problems secondary to poor hepatic synthetic function, patients with ESLD may have anemia and thrombocytopenia. Anemia may arise from malnutrition and bleeding. Thrombocytopenia may be a result of splenic sequestration. Both conditions are worsened by dilutional effects from increased plasma volume. **Tests:** CBC, PT/INR/PTT, fibrinogen
Hepatic	Decreased concentrations of the vitamin K-dependent clotting factors II, VII, IX and X may lead to severe bleeding. Deficiency of clotting factors may be caused by hepatic synthetic dysfunction as well as malabsorption of vitamin K 2° ↓ bile salts in the gastrointestinal tract or antibiotic therapy. Hypoalbuminemia contributes to low serum oncotic pressure which predisposes to intravascular hypovolemia, interstitial edema, ascites, and pleural effusions. ESLD results in diminished hepatic drug clearance reduced hepatic blood flow and hepatic extraction ratio. **Tests:** LFTs, albumin, bilirubin, PT/INR/PTT, fibrinogen, NH_3
GI	Gastrointestinal variceal hemorrhage in patients with portal hypertension is common. Aspiration of blood during an acute bleed can lead to pulmonary decompensation. Previous need for a Blakemore tube should be noted and one should be available for intraoperative use. Large protuberant abdomens usually warrant rapid sequence or modified rapid sequence induction with rocuronium. Most patients are already on proton pump inhibitors and some will be on an octreotide drip. Octreotide (a somatostatin mimic) is incompatible with most TPN solutions and usually requires a separate IV for infusion.
Renal	Most children with relative long-term hepatic insufficiency coming to transplant have chronically been on diuretic therapy for management of their ascites This can result in severe alteration of electrolytes. Hepatorenal syndrome requiring hemodialysis or CVVH is not uncommon in fulminant hepatic failure. Preop discussion MUST occur with the nephrology team as to the feasibility of intraop CVVH or an intraop dialysis run. For small children with limited vascular access, the dialysis catheter may be needed for fluid resuscitation purposes. Communicate with the blood bank to request both washed units of blood (which take about 1 h to prepare) or freshest units of RBCs. Correction of metabolic acidosis while on dialysis is also preferred. **Tests:** Serum electrolytes, BUN, Cr
Metabolic	Many children with liver failure have severely impaired glycogen metabolism. Preop dextrose infusion (TPN) must be continued intraop. Either the TPN solution or a D25 mixture run at equivalent grams of dextrose per h can be used. Preop consultation with the geneticist is invaluable in the management of complex metabolic disorders. **Tests:** Serum glucose

Premedication	IV midazolam is usually required to facilitate separation from parents. Ketamine 0.5–1 mg/kg iv is also effective in those children with paradoxical reactions to benzodiazepines.
Preop Prep	Preparation of the room including iv fluids and medications may take 1 h. Underbody forced air warmers are used since the infant is prepped from sternum to pubis. The following drips are routinely prepared: dextrose containing carrier, epinephrine, dopamine, and calcium chloride. Rocuronium and fentanyl drips may be used. The following resuscitation drugs must be readily available at a variety of concentrations; epinephrine, phenylephrine, ephedrine, and atropine. Drugs to treat hyperkalemia should be unit dosed and drawn up, including sodium bicarbonate 1 mEq/kg, calcium chloride 10–20 mg/kg, dextrose with insulin (0.5 g/kg dextrose and 0.2 U/kg insulin). A variety of ET tubes should be ready. Extreme changes in chest wall and pulmonary compliance can occur during the surgery resulting from large volumes of fluids given and changes in chest wall compliance from surgical retraction and placement of a sometimes large organ in the abdomen. A cuffed tube may be invaluable in providing the ability to alter ETT leak to allow for sufficient ventilation at different stages of the operation. Other equipment includes TEE, ultrasound to aid in vascular access, and rapid infusion systems (for larger children and teens).

INTRAOPERATIVE

Anesthetic technique: GETA with postop ventilation.

Induction	A modified rapid-sequence induction with rocuronium (0.6 mg/kg) follows placement of standard monitors (see D-1). Provide continuous glucose infusion throughout.
Maintenance	Standard maintenance (see D-3) with volatile agent, muscle relaxation, and fentanyl 10–50 mcg/kg. During periods of instability when vapor concentrations may be low, IV ketamine 1 mg/kg can be used. Nitrous oxide is avoided to prevent bowel distention. PEEP is useful to prevent atelectasis exacerbated by surgical retraction of the diaphragm. Antibiotics are dosed per surgical protocol. ABGs are drawn frequently depending on the degree of blood loss. Establishment of vascular access can be very difficult and may take 1–2 h. Use of ultrasonic guidance can be helpful especially in the profoundly coagulopathic patient. Care should be taken to keep the patient warm during this period of vascular access. Major vascular access should be restricted to the SVC distribution since the IVC will be clamped. In cases of "piggy-back" transplantation, the caval clamp time is usually reduced and if vascular access is severely limited, IVC distribution veins may be used. This should be discussed with the surgical team.
Preanhepatic phase	This phase of surgery begins with surgical incision and concludes when the hepatic/portal vessels are clamped. Opening of the abdomen and drainage of ascites will often improve ventilation. Blood loss during mobilization of the liver may be copious in the presence of portal HTN or adhesions from previous surgeries. "Maintenance fluids" may include FFP and blood. Use of platelets and cryoprecipitate should be discussed with the surgical team as a hypercoagulable state is undesirable when the graft hepatic artery and/or portal vein are small. Hypercoagulability should also be avoided if venovenous bypass is planned. (not commonly used in children <30–40 kg). Large variations in blood pressure and cardiac filling pressures are common during this phase of surgery due to the manipulation and rotation of the liver. Intermittent kinking of the vena cava can occur. The anesthesiologist must be constantly aware of the progress of surgery and communicate any protracted periods of hypotension due to surgical manipulation. Transfusion of blood/products may result in hyperkalemia, hypocalcemia and hypothermia. All products need to be warmed. A calcium chloride infusion (10 mg/kg/h) can be used to maintain the serum ionized calcium >1.0, and helps avoid BP associated with bolus administration of calcium. Hyperkalemia is treated with furosemide (1 mg/kg), correcting acidosis and infusing dextrose and insulin as required. Goals of this stage in preparation for the anhepatic phase include: (a) serum potassium < 4, (b) correction of metabolic acidosis,

Preanhepatic phase (cont'd)	(c) ionized calcium > 1.0–1.2, (d) adequate urine output (0.5 – 1 mL/kg/h), (e) adequate blood pressure at the lowest CVP possible, (f) hematocrit in the 30 range, and (g) euthermia. Mild hyperthermia may help mitigate the hypothermia created by the iced donor liver during the anhepatic phase. Frequent arterial blood-gas sampling is necessary. Hourly sampling is a minimum, and extreme blood loss may necessitate sampling every 15 min. Blood loss and third space losses are considerable in this phase of surgery. Edema of internal organs and eventually the transplanted liver is undesirable. Closure of the small abdominal cavity with an edematous liver can cause pressure necrosis as well as abdominal compartment syndrome.
Anhepatic phase	The anhepatic phase begins with clamping of the hepatic vessels and ends with reperfusion of the donor liver. Problems during this phase include fibrinolysis, acidosis, and hypothermia. Communication must exist between surgical and anesthetic teams regarding the amount of bleeding present and which products should be used to treat it. Respiratory alkalosis may be desirable to compensate for existing or projected metabolic acidosis. Correct any metabolic acidosis with bicarbonate. Placement of the iced donor liver usually decreases the core temperature by 1.5°C. This coupled with pre-existing hypothermia can increase coagulopathic bleeding. The anhepatic phase can be as short as 15 min or longer than 1 h depending on surgical difficulty. In the case of short anhepatic times, the metabolic goals should have been achieved in the preanhepatic phase. Anticipation and preparation for reperfusion should be ongoing. A split liver transplant usually entails more bleeding upon reperfusion, so the appropriate blood products must be present in the room. Anticipation and preparation for reperfusion should be ongoing. Reperfusion takes place after the portal vein and bicaval anastomoses are complete. In the piggy back liver transplant, anhepatic time is reduced since only the hepatic vein(s) and portal vein require anastomosis. Prior to tying the anastomotic suture, the liver is flushed to remove any air from the vessels. A 10-min warning to unclamp is usually given to the anesthesia team. Last minute electrolyte corrections can be made. The patient is then placed on 100% O_2, low dose epinephrine infusion may be started (0.03–0.05 mcg/kg/min), and inhalational agent should be decreased or turned off. IV midazolam or ketamine may be given to ensure amnesia.
Postperfusion phase	This phase begins with slow unclamping of the portal vein and vena cavae with reperfusion of the donor liver. Unclamping may be associated with hemodynamic instability and even cardiac arrest. Hypotension, tachycardia, dysrhythmias, hypothermia, severe acidosis, coagulopathy and air- or thromboembolism can occur. During the unclamping the anesthesiologist must simultaneously watch the uniform reperfusion of the liver as well as the blood pressure and ECG waveform. Increased T waves or widening of the QRS complex should be assumed to represent hyperkalemia. IV fluids in the form of RBCs or albumin should be ready in the event of anastomotic bleeding or bleeding from the cut edge of a split liver graft. A small amount of epinephrine (1–2 mcg) as well as a bolus of calcium chloride (10 mg/kg) may help maintain hemodynamic stability during unclamping. When giving IV fluids watch the liver for swelling. The hepatic artery anastomosis is then completed, prior to which the surgeon may request that a dose of heparin (10 U/kg) be given. Once the graft is well-perfused and bleeding is controlled, methylprednisolone (15 mg/kg) is given. Care should be taken at this point to avoid hyperglycemia as it can lead to osmotic diuresis and hemoconcentration. Volatile agent can be restarted and the FiO_2 can be reduced. Blood gas tensions and coagulation parameters should be checked. Care should be taken to maintain the hematocrit between 25 and 30, because relative polycythemia may lead to hepatic artery thrombosis. The biliary system will be constructed either with a duct-to-duct reconstruction, or, in cases of the small child or the patient with biliary atresia, with a roux-en-Y choledochojejunostomy. Patients with previous Kasai procedures will have an existing roux limb and biliary reconstruction takes places quickly. Construction of a new roux limb may take 1–2 h. During this time, it is important to keep up with third space losses and avoid hemoconcentration while avoiding congestion of the liver. Vasopressors may be required.

Emergence	The patient is taken to the ICU intubated and usually paralyzed to facilitate ventilation. Extubation is deferred to the ICU team.	
Blood and fluid requirements	Massive blood loss expected. IV × 2 as large as tolerated based on age. Arterial line in radial and femoral 2–3 lumen CVP line.	IV access restricted to SVC destribution. Avoid hand veins for large volume fluid administration, because infiltration is difficult to detect. Two arterial lines may be necessary since extreme vasoconstriction may dampen peripheral arterial line; femoral line interrupted if aortic clamping occurs. Avoid IV solutions containing lactate. Normosol preferred over NS due to lower sodium content. Administer blood based on hemodynamics and ABG since EBL is difficult to measure.
	Warm all fluids	**Fluids to have available:** Normosol, or normal saline, PRBC, FFP, Cryo and platelets; 5% albumin
	UO 0.5–1 mL/kg/h	Rapid infusion system if child is large
Monitoring	Standard Monitors ETN_2 Arterial line × 2	Five-lead EKG. Bladder temp if child is large enough. Carefully insert nasopharyngeal temp probe.
	I-STAT CVP	I-STAT (bedside arterial blood gas sampling) system is useful.
	TEE	Take care during insertion of TEE due to varices. May be difficult to use, because continuous orogastric decompression is needed.
Coagulation management	PT PTT plt count fibrinogen FSP	Pre-existing coagulopathy is very common. Coagulopathy may necessitate administration of products during line placement. Discuss use of cryo and platelets with surgical team prior to administration. Postreperfusion, treat clinical bleeding not lab values.
Positioning	Pad and protect lines Pad pressure points ✓ Retraction devices	Wrap all stopcocks near patient. Use gel headrest to protect occiput. Check for pressure points due to surgical retraction devices.
Temperature	Warming blanket Control fluid warmers Wrap patient	Underbody forced air warming. Hotline, Ranger, or rapid infusion system. The patient is wrapped with Webril and saran wrap for warmth and to keep patient dry.
Complications	Coagulopathy Hemorrhage Air embolism Cardiac arrest Metabolic acidosis IV infiltration	

POSTOPERATIVE

Monitoring	Serial LFTs PT, PTT Lactate Glucose Bilirubin	Initial LFTs are quite high depending on level of preservation injury. Bile production and normal glucose level are good signs.

Complications	Bleeding Hepatic artery thrombosis Portal vein thrombosis Biliary leak Primary graft nonfunction Rejection Infection Intracranial bleed Electrolyte abnormalities Alkalosis Renal Failure	Most care is deferred to the ICU team. Postop vascular ultrasounds are followed. Hepatic artery thrombosis is ominous and patients are often relisted for transplant if this complication occurs. Hypertensive swings in the coagulopathic patient can lead to intracranial hemorrhage.

Suggested Readings

1. Alonso EM, Besedovsky A, Emerick K, et al: General criteria for pediatric transplantation. In *Transplantation of the Liver,* 2nd Edition. Busuttil RW, Klintmalm GB, eds. WB Saunders, Philadelphia: 2005, 287–302.
2. De Goyet JV, Rogiers X, Ott JB: Split-liver transplantation for the pediatric and adult recipient. In *Transplantation of the Liver,* 2nd Edition. Busuttil RW, Klintmalm GB, eds. WB Saunders, Philadelphia: 2005, 689–28.
3. Esquivel CO: Current status and outcome of pediatric liver transplantation. *Clin Liever Dis* 1997;1(2):397–415.
4. Esquivel CO, Nakazato P, Cox K, et al: The impact of liver reductions in pediatric liver transplantation. *Arch Surg* 1991; 126:1278–86.
5. Farmer DG, Venick RS, McDiarmid SV, et al: Predictors of outcomes after pediatric liver transplantation: an analysis of more than 800 cases performed at a single institution. *J Am Coll Surg* 2007;204:904–14.
6. Hammer GB, Krane EJ: Anesthetic considerations for liver transplantation in children. *Pediatr Anesth* 2001;1:3–18.
7. Kerkar N, Emre S: Issues unique to pediatric liver transplantation. *Clin Liver Dis* 2007;11(2):323–35.
8. Vanatta JM, Esquivel CO: Status of liver transplantation in infants <5 kg. *Pediatr Transpl* 2007;11(1):5–9.

SECTION 13.0

OUT-OF-OPERATING ROOM PROCEDURES

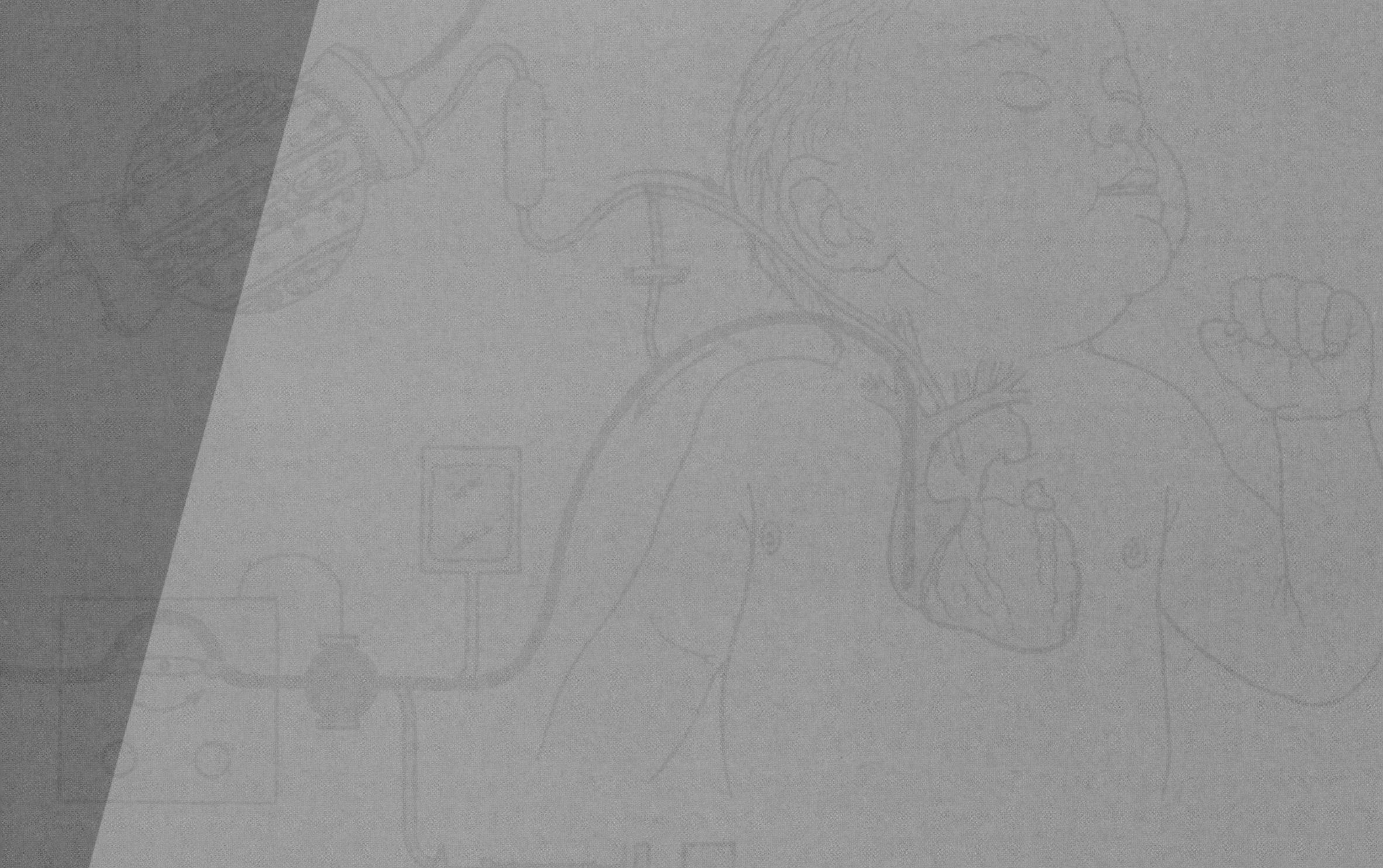

CHAPTER

13.1 Out-of-Operating Room Procedures—Adult

SURGEONS

Charles DeBattista, MD (*Electroconvulsive therapy*)
Joan K. Frisoli, MD, PhD (*TIPS*)
Stephen T. Kee, MD (*Tracheobronchial stenting, RF ablation*)
L. Bing Liem, DO (*DC cardioversion, ICD*)
Michael P. Marks, MD (*Interventional neuroradiology*)
Erik J. Sirulnick, MD (*DC cardioversion, ICD*)
Daniel Y. Sze, MD, PhD (*Image-guided procedures*)

ANESTHESIOLOGISTS

John Brock-Utne, MD, PhD
Jens Lohser, MD, MSc, FRCPC
Richard A. Jaffe, MD, PhD
Leland H. Hanowell, MD

ANESTHESIA FOR OUT-OF-OPERATING ROOM PROCEDURES

GENERAL COMMENTS

Advances in the fields of radiology, cardiology, and neurology have led to an increase in the number of anesthesia procedures performed away from the OR. In line with these changes, the ASA has provided guidelines for the safe delivery of anesthesia at locations remote from the OR environment.

Anesthetic considerations for out-of-OR locations (modified from ASA Guidelines[1]) include:

- Primary and backup O_2 sources (e.g., piped O_2 + 1 full E cylinder)
- Adequate and reliable suction
- Adequate and reliable scavenging system (for inhalational anesthesia)
- Self-inflating hand resuscitator bag with ability to deliver at least 90% O_2
- Adequate anesthetic drug supplies and equipment
- Adequate monitoring equipment to allow adherence to the "Standards of Basic Anesthetic Monitoring"[2]
- Sufficient electrical outlets connected to an emergency power supply
- Wet locations (e.g., cysto, arthroscopy, labor, and delivery) should be equipped with either an isolated electrical source or circuits with ground-fault interrupters.
- Adequate illumination for patient observation and monitoring equipment (flashlight backup)
- Sufficient space for expeditious access to patient, machine, and support equipment
- Emergency cart with defibrillator immediately available
- Immediate access to skilled anesthesia support personnel

Suggested Readings

1. American Society of Anesthesiologists: *Guidelines for Non-Operating Room Locations*. American Society of Anesthesiologists, Park Ridge: 1997.
2. American Society of Anesthesiologists: *Standards for Basic Anesthesia Monitoring*. American Society of Anesthesiologists, Park Ridge: 1998.
3. Melloni C: Anesthesia and sedation outside the operating room: how to prevent risk and maintain good quality. *Curr Opin Anaesthesiol* 2007; 20(6):513–9.
4. Pino RM: The nature of anesthesia and procedural sedation outside the operating room. *Curr Opin Anaesthesiol* 2007; 20(4): 347–51.

ELECTROCONVULSIVE THERAPY (ECT)

PROCEDURAL CONSIDERATIONS

Description: Electroconvulsive therapy (ECT) is the transcutaneous application of small electrical stimuli to the brain to produce generalized seizures for the treatment of selected psychiatric disorders, such as severe depression. There are several important aspects of ECT that are of relevance to the anesthesiologist. The first is the uncontrolled motor activity associated with generalized seizures. Prior to introduction of GA, the most common injuries associated with ECT were compression fractures of the vertebral bodies and broken limbs from violent tonic clonic motor activity. Even with complete paralysis, the masseter muscles are directly stimulated to contract during seizure induction. As a result, the most common injury currently associated with ECT is broken teeth.

A second consequence of ECT induction is that the electrical stimulus can cause contraction of cranial musculature and a brief dilation of meningeal blood vessels, resulting in postictal headaches in up to 40% of patients. Patients < 50 yr and those with a Hx of migraine headaches appear most at risk for post ECT headaches that may occasionally require aggressive pain management. Finally, ECT may be a significant hemodynamic stressor. Initially, central parasympathetic centers are activated, resulting in bradydysrhythmias in ~30% of patients. Brief sinus pauses are not uncommon. The initial parasympathetic effects are followed by sympathetically mediated increases in HR and

BP up to 20–30% above baseline. Mean arterial blood pressure has been known to double in some instances. These cardiovascular responses can persist for minutes to an hour or more after the procedure is completed.

The optimal position for ECT is supine. Occasionally, the head is kept slightly raised to help maintain an adequate airway and decrease anxiety. Patients typically come to ECT quite anxious about the procedure. ECT is generally performed in a PACU, or specialized ECT suite. In many centers, outpatients make up the majority of patients seen for ECT. The electrical stimulus is applied through plastic adhesive leads prepared with a contact gel. These leads are usually applied to the forehead in a bitemporal or right unilateral placement. Monitoring typically includes a two-lead electroencephalogram (EEG) and frequently an electromyogram (EMG) to measure motor activity. A BP cuff is inflated to act as a tourniquet and prevent neuromuscular blockade in the distal limb. Thus, an arm or leg can be used to measure motor duration of the seizure. A special ECT device is used to generate the appropriate electrical stimulus. Seizures are typically 30–90 sec in duration, and the entire procedure—from the induction of anesthesia to patient awakening—is generally < 15 min. The recovery period averages 45–90 min and allows for monitoring of vital signs, as well as the opportunity for the postictal confusion to clear. Patients can wake up mildly confused-to-frankly delirious and require close nursing supervision. Postictal agitation is also quite common and may require an intervention. Treatments are typically performed every other day, and the average number of treatments is 6–12 in the acute management of major depression. However, ECT treatments currently tend to be tapered rather than stopped abruptly. Thus, the frequency of treatments may go from 3/week for acute treatment, to 1/week, 2/month, and finally 1/month. Maintenance ECT with a frequency ranging from every few weeks to every few months is commonly prescribed for those patients who respond to ECT but fail to benefit from pharmacotherapy.

The most common morbidities associated with ECT include headaches and myalgias. Postictal confusion is the rule and some anterograde and retrograde memory loss occurs in most patients who have completed an acute course of ECT. Memory loss is typically confined to the period immediately before, during, and immediately after an acute series of ECT. There tends to be a cumulative memory loss with subsequent ECT treatments within a given series. In most patients, memory deficits largely subside in the first 1–3 months following an acute series of treatments. In rare instances, autobiographical memory loss has been reported for months or years after an ECT series has been completed. Long-term memory loss appears to be more common with bilateral lead placement. In addition, ECT-related mortality is estimated at approximately 4/10,000. Cardiac events account for 67% of all ECT-related deaths, with malignant arrhythmias and MIs accounting for most fatalities. Pulmonary events (obstruction, pulmonary edema, or emboli) account for most additional mortality. Cerebrovascular infarctions or hemorrhages have rarely been reported with ECT.

Usual preop diagnosis: Depression; mania; catatonia; refractory psychosis

SUMMARY OF PROCEDURE

Position	Supine
Incision	None
Special instrumentation	Seizure generator & electrodes; EEG/EMG monitors
Unique considerations	Requires muscle relaxation to prevent injury. 50–80 mg of succinylcholine is usually sufficient. Using larger dose of succinylcholine can lead to patient waking up while paralyzed. Non-disposable bite blocks are required to prevent dental injury. Apply tourniquet (BP cuff) to one arm before administration of muscle relaxant. A slow heart rate preop may require atropine. A high BP preop may require aggressive hypotensive Rx with beta blockers, phentolamine, hydralazine etc. If the seizure duration is not > 25 sec, then another seizure may be ordered. Give more induction agents needed. Because one arm is not paralyzed, asking the patient to squeeze your fingers will tell you that she/he is awake.
Antibiotics	None
Procedure time	Setup: 5–10 min Treatment: < 10 min (seizure duration 25–280 sec)
Postop care	PACU → room or home
Mortality	4/10,000
Morbidity	HA/myalgias/nausea: Common Confusion/memory loss: Common. Be aware that postoperative hypoxia can present with confusion.

SUMMARY OF PROCEDURES (cont'd)

Morbidity (cont'd)	Cardiac dysrhythmias: 10–40% (brief asystole common). Keep a close eye on the EKG. MI: Rare Pulmonary edema from excessive IV fluids: not uncommon. Pulmonary aspiration and/or negative pressure pulmonary edema: Rare CVA: Rare
Pain score	2–3 (HA)

PATIENT POPULATION CHARACTERISTICS

Age range	≥ 18 yr. ECT is rarely performed in adolescent and preadolescents; however, patients in their 90s are sometimes candidates for ECT. There is a preponderance of geriatric patients on many ECT services.
Male:Female	1:2
Incidence	The lifetime prevalence of major depression (the primary indication for ECT) is ~17%; 26% of women and 12% of men are affected. < 1% of patients with major depression undergo ECT; and approximately 400,000 ECT procedures are performed in North America annually.
Associated conditions	Substance abuse (30% of all depressed patients meet criteria for alcohol or drug abuse); panic attacks (30% of depressed patients); psychotic symptoms (14% of patients); HTN and sinus tachycardia; dehydration; self-inflicted trauma. Pregnancy.

ANESTHETIC CONSIDERATIONS

PREOPERATIVE

Patients presenting for ECT usually have failed to respond to antidepressants; however, most will continue to take psychotherapeutic agents. Many of the older patients will be taking other medications for coexisting medical conditions. Drug interactions are an important consideration for the anesthesiologist (see Drug Interactions, p. F-1). The most commonly used medications are listed in Table 13.1-1.

Anesthesia for ECT may seem to be a benign procedure; however, these cases—which seldom take > 20 minutes—can prove very challenging, especially in the geriatric population. ECT can place significant stress on the cardiovascular system; therefore, particular care should be taken to evaluate and optimize the patient's

Table 13.1-1. Commonly Used Medications in the Treatment of Depression

Tricyclic	MAOI	SSRI	SNRI and other Antidepressants
amitriptyline (Elavil, others) amoxapine (Asendin) desipramine (Norpramin) doxepin (Sinequan) imipramine (Tofranil) maprotiline (Ludiomil) nortriptyline (Pamelor) Protriptyline (Vivactil) trimipramine (Surmontil)	isocarboxazid (Marplan) phenelzine (Nardil) tranylcypromine (Parnate) transdermal selegiline (Emsam) **Lithium** (Often used as an adjunctive agent/mood stabilizer in depression)	fluoxetine (Prozac) paroxetine (Paxil) sertraline (Zoloft) fluvoxamine (Luvox) citalopram (Celexa) escitavopram (Lexapro)	venlafaxine (Effexor) duloxetine (Cymbalta nefazodone (Serzone) mirtazapine (Remeron) bupropion (Wellbutrin) trazodone (Desyrel) **Atypical Antipsychotics** (Used Adjunctively) olanzapine (Zyprexa) quetiapine (Seroquel) aripiprazole (Abilify) risperidone (Risperdal) ziprasidone (Geodon)

MAOI = monoamine oxidase inhibitor
SSRI = selective serotonin reuptake inhibitor
SNRI = selective norepinephrine/serotonin reuptake inhibitor

pretreatment cardiovascular status. ECT usually takes place in remote locations, so the anesthesiologist must ensure that the location is properly equipped and complies with ASA Guidelines for Out-of-OR Procedures (see p. 1444) and Standards for Basic Anesthesia Monitory.

Respiratory	These patients will require airway management and PPV. Hence, preop assessment of the airway must focus on the ease of mask ventilation and the potential need for ET intubation (e.g., airway compromise or severe GERD).
Cardiovascular	A recent MI (< 3 mo) is a contraindication to ECT. Relative contraindications include aortic aneurysm, angina, CHF, and thrombophlebitis. The presence of dysrhythmias, a pacemaker, or ICD is not a contraindication for ECT. For the patient with a pacemaker, a means (e.g., a magnet) should be available to convert the pacemaker to an asynchronous mode. **Tests:** As indicated from H&P.
Gastrointestinal	Patient should be npo. Patients with Sx of GERD should be pretreated with Na citrate (30 mL po), ranitidine (50 mg iv) and metoclopramide (10 mg iv). ET intubation should be considered for all patients at risk for aspiration.
Neurological	ECT is relatively contraindicated in the presence of ↑ ICP, and recent CVA (< 3 mo), intracranial mass lesions or recent intracranial surgery (< 3 mo).
Endocrine	Presence of a pheochromocytoma (Sx of which may be confused with a psychiatric disorder) is a contraindication to ECT. < 1% of hypertensive patients will have a pheochromocytoma.
Genetic	✓ for family Hx of pseudocholinesterase deficiency. Mivacurium (0.15 mg/kg) is a suitable alternative to succinylcholine. **Tests:** Dibucaine number (normal ≥ 80) and serum cholinesterase level, if indicated from H&P.
Hepatic	Hepatotoxicity has been associated with use of MAOI. **Tests:** Consider LFTs for patients on chronic MAOI therapy.
Orthopaedic	In patients susceptible to bone fracture (e.g., severe osteoporosis, osteoporosis imperfecta), an increased succinylcholine dosage (1.5 mg/kg) is given to ensure profound muscle relaxation. Patients with severe rheumatoid arthritis may have unstable C-spine, and extreme care should be taken during positioning of head and neck.
Ophthalmologic	Retinal detachment is a relative contraindication to ECT. Succinylcholine should be avoided in patients with glaucoma treated with cholinesterase-inhibitors (e.g., echothiophate). Mivacurium (0.15 mg/kg) is a suitable alternative.
Pregnancy	Pregnancy is not a contraindication for ECT (even in the third trimester). After the 4th mo, the need for full-stomach precautions requires rapid-sequence induction and ET intubation (see p. B-4). Left uterine displacement should be maintained during treatment. Monitor fetal heartbeat.
Psychiatric Drugs	Patients receiving tricyclic antidepressants (TCAs) may have an exaggerated pressor response to direct-acting sympathomimetic drugs, with the potential for tachycardia, dysrhythmias, and hyperthermia. The response to indirect-acting sympathomimetic drugs (e.g., ephedrine) may be attenuated in these patients. TCAs also will increase the effects of anticholinergic drugs (e.g., glycopyrrolate, atropine). Patients receiving MAOIs will exhibit exaggerated responses to indirect-acting sympathomimetic drugs (e.g., ephedrine). Additionally, in these patients succinylcholine metabolism is inhibited (↑ NMB), and meperidine is contraindicated (↑↑ BP, ↑ Sz, ↑↑ T). It is probably unnecessary to discontinue TCAs or MAOIs prior to ECT, as long as these interactions can be avoided. Lithium should be discontinued for at least 3 d prior to ECT to avoid delayed recovery and subsequent posttreatment agitation and confusion. Lithium also is associated with ↑ NMB (succinylcholine and pancuronium). SSRIs have been associated with prolonged ECT-induced seizure duration, and adverse behavioral/neurological effects following haloperidol administration (use droperidol and metoclopramide with caution). No adverse interactions have been reported between anesthetic agents and SSRIs or SNRIs.

Laboratory	Tests as indicated from H&P.
Premedication	Although usually not required, some patients may benefit from an antisialagogue (glycopyrrolate 0.2 mg iv). Patients with Hx of postop N/V will benefit from a prophylactic antiemetic (e.g., ondansetron 4 mg iv). Patients with postseizure muscle pain and headache may benefit from ketorolac (30 mg iv). Some patients will require 500-1,000 mg caffeine iv to decrease seizure threshold. The caffeine effect should be manifest in 5 min. Verapamil (not adenosine, which is blocked by caffeine) should be available to control supraventricular tachycardia (0.07–0.25 mg/kg over 2 min). Esmolol and diltiazem are alternative drugs for control of HR.

INTRAOPERATIVE

Anesthetic technique: A review of previous anesthetic records is very helpful in formulating the anesthetic plan and in anticipating physiological changes unique to each patient. Usually brief iv anesthesia (mask oxygenation and ventilation) with profound muscle relaxation is required to prevent patient injury during seizures. Prior to induction, a tourniquet (BP cuff) is applied to the non-iv arm and inflated to a pressure above systolic. This prevents neuromuscular blockade distal to the cuff and permits direct monitoring of seizure activity. Preop BP control (e.g., labetalol 5–20 mg, diltiazem 10–20 mg iv, or esmolol 0.5–1 mg/kg iv in increments) is often necessary.

Induction	Preoxygenation should be attempted in all patients. In some patients who are intolerant of a mask, a less intrusive blow-by technique may be tried. Anesthesia is induced with either STP (1.5–3 mg/kg), sodium methohexital (0.5–1 mg/kg), or etomidate (0.1–0.2 mg/kg). An induction close of etomidate will block stress-induced cortisol production for up to 24 h. Propofol (1–1.5 mg/kg) may be used, but may shorten seizure duration. TCAs and MAOIs can increase sleep time. After tourniquet inflation, succinylcholine (1 mg/kg) is injected to induce paralysis. Hyperventilation is carried out to enhance seizure activity. A bite block is placed and then the patient is ready for ECT. In barbiturate-tolerant patients, remifentanil (1–3 mcg/kg) has been used as a means of reducing the barbiturate dose, thereby permitting adequate seizure duration. Patients receiving remifentanil need minimal postseizure BP control.	
Maintenance	Given the brevity of this procedure, maintenance of anesthesia is rarely a concern; however, occasionally a second or third treatment may be necessary if the seizures are of inadequate duration (< 25 sec) and quality. In this case, a subsequent dose (10–30 mg) of succinylcholine may be needed. Assisted ventilation is necessary until spontaneous ventilation resumes. Of major concern during the seizure period is the hypertensive response. Some patients may need to be treated prior to induction of anesthesia with either labetalol (5–20 mg iv) or esmolol (10 mg q 1 min) to control HR/BP. SNP (5–50 mcg/bolus iv) is useful to control BP in refractory cases.	
Emergence	Patients should be awake within 5–10 min postseizure and often are disoriented. Small doses of midazolam (e.g., 0.25–0.5 mg iv) may help to control agitation. ASA guidelines for postanesthesia care should be followed (see p. 1444).	
Blood and fluid requirements	No blood loss IV: 20 ga × 1 NS/LR @ TKO	
Monitoring	Standard monitors (see p. B-1) Tourniquet EEG EMG	Seizure activity is usually monitored by a psychiatrist observing the tourniqueted limb and by measuring EMG and EEG activity. (These monitors are usually an integral part of the ECT seizure generator.)
Positioning	Supine	

Complications	Dysrhythmias	Brief periods of asystole and profound bradycardia are not uncommon (usually related to parasympathetic overactivity). Treatment is rarely necessary.
	Tachydysrhythmias	Responds well to esmolol (10–15 mg iv) or lidocaine (1 mg/kg iv), although treatment is usually unnecessary.
	↑ BP	↑ BP readily responds to esmolol (10–30 mg), or labetalol (5–20 mg). In refractory cases, 10–50 mcg of SNP may be necessary.
	Dental damage Pulmonary edema Aspiration	Use of bite block is essential. Dental damage is not prevented by muscle relaxation (direct electrical stimulation of facial and jaw muscles).

POSTOPERATIVE

Complications	HA, myalgias	Rx: ketorolac 30 mg iv
	N/V	Rx: ondansetron 4 mg iv
	Disorientation	Rx: midazolam 0.25–0.5 mg iv
	Memory impairment	
	MI/ischemia	
	Dysrhythmias	
	Pulmonary edema/aspiration	
	↑ BP	Prolonged ↑ BP is unusual and may suggest the need for further workup.

Suggested Readings

1. Cohran M, DeBattista C, Schmiesing C, et al: Negative pressure pulmonary edema. A potential hazard in patients undergoing ECT. *J ECT* 1999; 15:168–70.
2. DeBattista C, Cohran M, Barry JJ, et al: Fetal heart decelertation during ECT induced seizures: is it important? *Acta Anaesth Scand* 2003;47:101–3.
3. Ding Z, White PF: Anesthesia for electroconvulsive therapy. *Anesth Analg* 2002;94:1351–64.
4. Saito S: Anesthesia management for electroconvulsive therapy: hemodynamic and respiratory management. *J Anesth* 2005;19(2):142–9.
5. Smith D, Angst M, Brock-Utne JG, et al: Seizure duration with remifentanil/methohexital vs. methohexital in middle aged patients undergoing ECT. *Acta Anaesth Scand* 2003;47:1064–6.
6. Wagner KJ, Mollenberg O, Rentrop M, et al: Guide to anesthetic selection for electroconvulsive therapy. *CNS Drugs* 2005; 19(9):745–58.

INTERVENTIONAL NEURORADIOLOGY

PROCEDURAL CONSIDERATIONS

The indications for endovascular therapy for the brain and spine have continued to grow with the technical strides made in both devices and imaging during the past decade. Endovascular therapy is now widely used in the treatment of intracranial aneurysms, arteriovenous malformations (AVMs), arteriovenous fistulas (AVFs), and tumors. It also is extensively used in revascularization of the cerebral circulation in the setting of acute stroke or for the treatment of stenoses with angioplasty and/or stent. Many of these procedures can be performed with the patient awake; however, GA or deep sedation often is used to minimize patient movement during procedures that require careful catheter and device control for safe operation. These procedures can be divided into three broad categories: (a) embolization, (b) aneurysm therapy, and (c) cerebral revascularization.

EMBOLIZATION

This therapy may be used for a variety of lesions, including AVMs in the brain; dural AVFs; Vein of Galen malformations; vascular neoplasms, such as meningiomas, hemangiomas, glomus tumors, and juvenile nasal angiofibromas; and for treatment of epistaxis.

AVM embolization usually is performed as an adjunct to radiosurgery or microsurgery, although in selected cases, embolization may be the definitive treatment. Brain AVMs are generally parenchymal lesions with multiple feeding pial arteries and draining veins. The goal of embolization is to reduce the size and shunt burden presented by the AVM before either radiosurgery or microsurgical resection. Liquid embolic agents are preferred, with n-butyl cyanoacrylate (NBCA) and ethylene vinyl alcohol copolymer (EVOH) being the two materials currently used for the procedure. Embolization often is preceded by neurophysiologic testing, which may include the superselective injection of amobarbital into the portion of the intracranial circulation being considered for embolization. Some centers perform the procedure with the patient awake to allow for more thorough clinical testing prior to embolization, while others prefer the patient to have general anesthesia to minimize patient motion.

Dural arteriovenous fistulas involve the dural sinuses, most commonly in the area of the cavernous, transverse, and sigmoid sinuses. Because of their location, these malformations usually are supplied from meningeal vessels. A cavernous sinus fistula also may develop as a direct large-hole fistula between the internal carotid artery and the cavernous sinus. Patients may have a variety of symptoms depending upon the location, size and drainage pattern of the dural fistula. The embolization process for these dural-based lesions differs somewhat from the technique used for pial-based brain AVMs. Arterial embolization may be used, but venous embolization is often used to definitively occlude the fistula. Embolization of meningeal arteries may be preceded by clinical testing for cranial nerve deficits. This usually is accomplished with the superselective injection of lidocaine before embolization and it often preferred to have the patient awake for this procedure. If arterial embolization is utilized, a liquid embolic (NBCA or EVOH) is often utilized; however a particulate embolic may also be used. Particle embolization is often done with polyvinyl alcohol particles (PVA). The venous embolization is usually done with platinum coil occlusion.

Vein of Galen malformations are congenital lesions that may present in infants or children. Presenting symptoms include CHF, hydrocephalus, and neurodevelopmental delay. These lesions often require a staged approach, and present a special challenge in the neonate or infant. In general, arterial embolization is performed as the initial endovascular approach, and a liquid embolic agent is used. In some cases, this may be augmented by a venous approach, with embolization using platinum coils.

Tumor embolization usually is performed as an adjunct to the surgical resection of highly vascular tumors (e.g., meningiomas, hemangiomas, hemangioblastomas, glomus tumors, and juvenile nasal angiofibromas). Generally, arterial embolization of meningeal supply vessels is done before surgery, using PVA or trisacryl gelatin microspheres. Physiologic testing with super-selective injection of lidocaine often precedes embolization. When there is tumor encasement of a major artery the patient may also undergo balloon test occlusion followed by permanent occlusion to reduce the risk of intraoperative bleeding.

ANEURYSM THERAPY

Endovascular therapy is the treatment of choice for many intracranial aneurysms, and it consists of either direct intra-aneurysmal obliteration with detachable platinum coils or occlusion of the parent artery to produce thrombosis of the aneurysm. A randomized, controlled trial has shown better clinical outcome for patients treated with aneurysm coiling than surgical clipping in the setting of subarachnoid hemorrhage. Narrow-necked aneurysms may be treated using a microcatheter to introduce coils directly into the aneurysm. Wide-necked aneurysms are more difficult to treat using this technique. Balloon remodeling often is used for treatment of wide-necked aneurysms. This technique involves placing a balloon over the ostium of the aneurysm. The balloon is intermittently inflated with each coil insertion to prevent coil prolapse into the parent vessel. Fenestrated stents have also become available to treat wide-necked aneurysms. These are introduced into the parent artery over the ostium of the aneurysm, which is then coiled through the fenestrations. Parent artery occlusion is still used for some giant or fusiform aneurysms. It generally is done in a two-step process. Test occlusion is initially performed with a balloon-tipped catheter and the patient is evaluated using clinical testing and neurophysiological monitoring. The testing may be done with controlled hypotension to improve the test sensitivity. If the patient tolerates test occlusion, a permanent occlusion is usually done using detachable balloons and/or coils.

CEREBRAL REVASCULARIZATION

Acute stroke thrombolysis or thrombectomy is performed up to 8 h after the onset of symptoms in the middle and anterior cerebral artery circulations (carotid territory) and at some centers up to 24 h after the onset of symptoms in the vertebrobasilar territory. The FDA has recently approved a device for mechanical embolectomy in the setting of stroke. In addition, many endovascular therapists employ intra-arterial thrombolytics either alone or combined with a mechanical thrombectomy device. Other devices including baskets, ultrasound, suction thrombectomy catheters, and intracranial stents have been proposed or are in development.

Angioplasty and stent placement for symptomatic atherosclerotic stenosis in the cerebrovascular circulation is becoming more widely performed in lieu of medical or direct surgical therapy. Stents with distal protection devices have now been approved for the treatment of cervical carotid artery stenosis. Distal protection devices (e.g., balloon or basket devices) have been shown to reduce the thromboembolic complication rate and are now required for treatment in most cases. Vascular lesions located more distally and intracranial lesions are treated either with angioplasty alone or are stented following angioplasty.

Vasospasm often accompanies subarachnoid hemorrhage and results in ischemic complications, which are a common cause of morbidity and mortality following aneurysmal rupture. The endovascular therapist is often asked to treat this problem with either drugs or balloons. Direct administration of intra-arterial vasodilators, such as verapamil, nimodipine and nicardipine, has been used particularly for treatment of more distal spasm. More proximal spasm involving the arteries of the circle of Willis is often treated using high-compliance angioplasty balloons.

SUMMARY OF PROCEDURES

	Embolization	Aneurysm Therapy	Cerebral Revascularization
Position	Supine	⇐	⇐
Incision	Femoral artery, catheterization (may utilize brachial or radial artery)	⇐	⇐
Unique considerations	BP control; AVM; anticoagulation; EP monitoring	BP control; ± EP monitoring; anticoagulation	⇐
Antibiotics	Usually none; occasionally used with closure device	⇐	⇐
Procedure time	2–5 h	2–4 h	⇐
Closing considerations	Femoral artery compression or closure device	⇐	⇐
EBL	Minimal	⇐	⇐
Postop care	Ward or ICU × 24–48 h	ICU	Ward or ICU
Mortality	1–2% (vascular lesions)	⇐	⇐
Morbidity	Overall: ~5% Thromboembolic stroke Hemorrhage (AVM, AVF)	⇐ ⇐ SAH	⇐ ⇐ Vessel rupture/dissection
Pain score	1–2	1–2	1–2

PATIENT POPULATION CHARACTERISTICS

Age range	Neonatal-elderly
Male:Female	1:1
Etiology	Congenital; acquired (traumatic, infectious, degenerative, etc.)
Associated conditions	SAH ± vasospasm; ↑ ICP; HTN/CAD/PVD; blood dyscrasia

ANESTHETIC CONSIDERATIONS

PREOPERATIVE

Patients presenting for diagnostic neuroradiologic procedures frequently may require only local anesthesia and sedation. The newer nontoxic and low osmolality contrast agents have improved patient comfort and tolerance of these procedures while minimizing adverse reactions. Patients presenting for interventional neuroradiological procedures (e.g., embolization or stenting) are likely to experience more discomfort and, therefore, may require GA in order to tolerate the often lengthy procedures. The advantages of GA, however, must be balanced against the potential need for intraop neurological monitoring (e.g., speech, vision, and mental status) that requires the patient to be awake and cooperative. In this set of circumstances, close consultation between the neuroradiologist and anesthesiologist is required in formulating the anesthesia plan.

Respiratory	Access to the airway may be limited; therefore, examination should focus on the need for elective ET intubation. Patients with chronic cough may require GA to ensure immobility. **Tests:** As indicated from H&P.
Cardiovascular	Patients with recent intracranial hemorrhage may demonstrate ECG abnormalities (PVCs in 30–80%; ST-T wave changes in >50%), which need to be differentiated from new ischemic heart disease (ECHO, cardiac enzymes). **Tests:** ECG; other tests as indicated from H&P.
Neurological	Symptoms vary with the location, size, and type of lesion. Aneurysms seldom produce neurological symptoms unless they leak or rupture, whereas tumors are commonly associated with symptoms of ↑ ICP (HA, N/V, altered mental status, papilledema). Patients with recent cerebral hemorrhages are likely to be medicated with calcium-channel blockers (e.g., nimodipine, nicardipine) to ↓ arterial vasospasm. Patients with ↑ ICP or cranial trauma usually will need GA with intubation and mechanical ventilation.
Premedication	Preop sedation may mask the Sx of ↑ ICP or intracranial hemorrhage. Patients at high risk for contrast-media reactions (e.g., patients with previous contrast reaction, allergy to iodine or seafood) should receive prophylactic treatment consisting of prednisone, 50 mg po q 6 h × 3, starting 18 h before the study, and diphenhydramine, 50 mg po/im, 1 h before the procedure.

INTRAOPERATIVE

Anesthetic technique: MAC (see p. B-3) may be adequate for patients undergoing diagnostic procedures and necessary for patients requiring neurological assessment during more invasive procedures; otherwise, use GETA.

Induction	Standard induction (see p. B-2). Patients with ↑ ICP should be hyperventilated to an $ETCO_2$ of ~30 mmHg. In patients with vascular lesions that may leak or rupture, BP responses to laryngoscopy and intubation should be blunted (e.g., remifentanil: 3–5 mcg/kg iv 1–2 min in advance).	
Maintenance	Standard maintenance (see p. B-2). Muscle relaxation is usually mandatory to control ventilation and minimize the chance of movement. Hyperventilation may be necessary to ↓ ICP and may also enhance the quality of the angiogram.	
Emergence	Prompt awakening is important to permit neurologic evaluation. Ondansetron (4 mg iv) is useful to ↓ postop N/V. Extubate when airway reflexes have returned. Continuous control of BP may be necessary during emergence phase. Patients typically are transported to ICU immediately following the procedure.	
Blood and fluid requirements	IV: 18 ga × 1–2 NS @ 3–5 mL/kg/h	
Monitoring	Standard monitors (see p. B-1). Arterial line Urinary catheter	BP can be monitored from femoral line placed by radiologist. However, another arterial line often will be necessary for postop monitoring in the ICU. Place urinary catheter if procedure is lengthy (> 3 h).

Monitoring (cont'd)	± EPs	Keep isoflurane or sevoflurane < 0.5 MAC and N_2O <50% to minimize interference with EP monitoring. Supplement with remifentanil infusion, if necessary. TIVA may be requested in the erroneous belief that EP's cannot be obtained while using inhalational agents.
Control of BP	SNP (0.2–2 mcg/kg/min) Maintain normovolemia. Esmolol (50–200 mcg/kg/min)	BP control may be necessary during intracranial catheter manipulation, embolization, and postembolization. Close communication with the radiologist is important. SNP/esmolol may be infused through a second peripheral iv.
Positioning	✓ and pad pressure points. ✓ eyes.	X-ray table may not be well padded → nerve damage.
Complications, contrast-related	Common reactions: N/V Itching Urticaria Sensation of warmth Pain Anxiety Rash	These reactions occur in > 5% of patients, and may require no treatment apart from reassurance or a mild anxiolytic. Mild allergic reactions may be treated with diphenhy dramine 25–50 mg iv. Monitor patients for progression of Sx → need for more aggressive therapy.
	Neurotoxic Sx: Hemiplegia Blindness Aphasia ↓ consciousness	These reactions may be related to the hyperosmolarity of the agent. If persistent, procedure should be terminated. Rx may require steroids and vasopressors to improve perfusion. In the anesthetized patient, these Sx will be masked.
	Major allergic reactions: Bronchospasm ↓ BP Cardiac arrest Pulmonary edema Laryngeal edema Dysrhythmias	Epinephrine (0.25–0.5 mg iv) should be given immediately. **Rx of anaphylaxis** includes: eliminate antigens (e.g., contrast agent, latex, etc.); secure airway; administer 100% O_2, iv fluids, epinephrine, and diphenhydramine + ranitidine. Supplemental Rx may include steroids (e.g., hydrocortisone 5 mg/kg), atropine, $NaHCO_3$, arginine vasopressin, and epinephrine infusion.
Complications, other	Hemorrhage	Aneurysmal rupture or AVM bleeding may require immediate transport to OR for surgical repair.
	Vasospasm	Rx: vasodilators (e.g., NTG) or papaverine delivered by catheter, or balloon angioplasty.
	Occlusion of vessel	2° catheter injury of vessel wall. Rx: angioplasty. (Recanalization and stenting may be used for thrombotic occlusions.)

POSTOPERATIVE

Complications	Neurologic deficits	CT scan for evaluation, as prompt neurosurgical intervention may be required.
	Vasospasm	May require Ca^{++} channel blocker (e.g., nimodipine). Consult with neurosurgeon.

Suggested Readings

1. Arnonda R, Vo A, Dunford J, et al: Anesthesia for endovascular neurosurgery. *Neurosurgery* 2006;59:53–66.
2. Bader MK: The complexity of caring for patients with ruptured cerebral aneurysm: case studies. *AACN Clin Issues* 1997;8(2):182–95.

3. Brilstra EH, Rinkel GJE, van der Graaf Y, et al: Treatment of intracranial aneurysms by embolization with coils. *Stroke* 1999;30:470–6.
4. Cardella JF, Waybill PN: Interventional radiology: diagnostic and interventional vascular applications. In *Alternate-Site Anesthesia: Clinical Practice Outside the Operating Room*. Russell GB, ed. Butterworth-Heinemann, Boston: 1997, 115–32.
5. Fiorella D, Albuquerque PC, Deshmukh VR, et al: Usefulness of the Neuroform stent for the treatment of cerebral aneurysms: results as initial (3–6 mo) follow-up. *Neurosurgery* 2005;56:1191–201.
6. Gobin YP, Laurent A, Merienne L, et al: Treatment of brain arteriovenous malformations by embolization and radiosurgery. *J Neurosurg* 1996;85:19–28.
7. Gupta R, Vora NA, Horowitz MB, et al: Multimodal reperfusion therapy for acute ischemic stroke: factors predicting vessel recanalization. *Stroke* 2006;37:986–90.
8. Hartmann A, Mast H, Mohr JP, et al: Determinants of staged endovascular and surgical treatment outcome of brain arteriovenous malformations. *Stroke* 2005;36:2431–5.
9. Hashimoto T, Gupta DK, Young WL: Interventional neuroradiology-anesthetic considerations. *Anesth Clinics North Am* 2002;20:347–59.
10. Jayaraman MV, Marcellus ML, Hamilton S, et al: Neurologic complications of arteriovenous malformation embolization using liquid embolic agents. *AJNR Am J Neuroradiol* 2007.
11. Lai YC, Manninen PH: Anesthesia for cerebral aneurysms: a comparison between interventional neuroradiology and surgery. *Can J Anaesth* 2001;48:391–5.
12. Lakhani S, ha A, Nahser HC: Anaesthesia for endovascular management of cerebral aneurysms. *Eur J Anaesthesiol* 2006;23:902–13.
13. Marks MP, Wojack JC, Al-Ali F, et al: Angioplasty for symptomatic intracranial stenosis. *Stroke* 2006;37:1016–20.
14. Molyneux AJ, Kerr RSC, Ya LM, et al: International subarachoid aneurysm trial (ISAT) of neurosurgical clipping versus endovascular coiling in 2143 patients with ruptured intracranial aneurysms: a randomized comparison of effects on survival, dependency, seizures, rebleeding, subgroups and aneurysm occlusion. *Lancet* 2005;366:809–17.
15. Qureshi AI, Suri MF, Khan J, et al: Endovascular treatment of intracranial aneurysms by using Guglielmi detachable coils in awake patients: safety and feasibility. *J Neurosurg* 2001;94(6):880–5.
16. Reimers B, Schulter M, Castriota F, et al: Routine use of cerebral protection during carotid artery stenting: results of a multi-center registry of 753 patients. *Am J Med* 2004;116:217–22.
17. Smith WS: Safety of mechanical thrombectomy and intravenous tissue plasminogen activator in acute ischemic stroke: results of the multi Mechanical Embolus Removal in Cerebral Ischemia (MERCI) trial, part 1. *AJNR Am J Neuroradiol* 2006;27:1177–82.
18. Smith WS, Sung G, Starkman S, et al: Safety and efficacy of mechanical embolectomy in acute ischemic stroke. Results of the MERCI Trial. *Stroke* 2005;36:1432–40.
19. The n-BCA Trial Investigators: N-butyl cyanoacrylate embolization of cerebral arteriovenous malformations. Results of a prospective, randomized, multi-center trial. *AJNR* 2002;23:748–55.
20. Varma MK, Price K, Jayakrishman J, et al: Anaesthetic considerations for interventional neuroradiology. *Br J Anaesth* 2007;99:75–85.
21. Yadav JS, Wholey MH, Kuntz RE, et al: Stenting and angioplasty with protection in patients at high risk for endarterectomy investigators. Protected carotid-artery stenting versus endarterectomy in high risk patients. N *Engl J Med* 2004;351:1493–1501.

DIRECT CURRENT (DC) CARDIOVERSION

PROCEDURAL CONSIDERATIONS

Description: **Direct current (DC) cardioversion** is a treatment for cardiac arrhythmias that uses a brief, dosed discharge of electricity across the heart. This biphasic waveform energy is more efficient, requiring 20–170 J, than monophasic waveform, which requires 50–360 J. Effective depolarization of a critical mass of the heart terminates the arrhythmia, allowing NSR to resume. The electrical shock is delivered across the chest wall, using two external paddles placed in one of the standard positions (i.e., the anterior-posterior (A-P), basilar-apical, or apical-posterior). The pulse is delivered synchronous to the QRS, thus avoiding the vulnerable period for inducing malignant tachyarrhythmias. Shock to treat ventricular fibrillation is applied emergently and asynchronously (thus, the term 'defibrillation'). To avoid discomfort, cardioversion should always be performed with the patient under deep sedation or brief GA. It is unacceptable to deliver this therapy to an awake patient.

Usual preop diagnosis: Atrial fibrillation (AF); atrial flutter; other supraventricular tachyarrhythmias; ventricular tachyarrhythmias

SUMMARY OF PROCEDURE	
Position	Supine with defibrillator pads positioned A-P, basilar-apical, or apical-posterior
Unique considerations	Adequate anticoagulation (INR = 2–3) in patients with AF
Antibiotics	None
Procedure time	≤ 30 min
Postop care	Monitoring of cardiac rhythm in treatment room
Mortality	0.1%
Morbidity	Skin burns: < 15% (1st degree); 2% (2nd degree); lesser incidence with biphasic waveform Embolic event: 2% (↑ risk with mitral valve disease) Acute pulmonary edema: 1% More serious arrhythmia: 1% Myocardial damage: Incidence unknown, but estimated to be very low—proportional to delivered energy.
Pain score	2–3

PATIENT POPULATION CHARACTERISTICS	
Age range	All ages
Male:Female	3:1
Incidence	100,000/yr in the United States
Etiology	Reentry substrates (e.g., atrial flutter and fibrillation, ventricular tachycardia) from hypertensive heart disease, remote MI, cardiomyopathy; idiopathic
Associated conditions	LV dysfunction; CAD; cardiomyopathy; HTN; valvular disease; COPD; obesity; CVA; acute MI; pulmonary edema

ANESTHETIC CONSIDERATIONS

PREOPERATIVE

In general, patients presenting for cardioversion fall into one of two categories: elective or emergent. The presence or absence of hemodynamic instability will define the category. In the emergency patient, full-stomach precautions may be necessary (see p. B-5). Elective cardioversions usually are carried out on patients who have failed drug therapy.

Respiratory	Preop evaluation of the airway should focus on the need for elective ET intubation (patients with GERD, difficult mask fit, or airway compromise).
Cardiovascular	Relative contraindications to elective cardioversion include digitalis toxicity (toxic = > 3 ng/mL), ↓ K^+, inadequate anticoagulation, presence of β-blockade, AV block. The presence of significant CHF, CAD, or valvular disease may predispose this patient population to ↓↓ BP in response to anesthetic agents. Consider use of etomidate (0.1–0.2 mg/kg). Patients at ↑ risk for embolization include those with Hx of embolization within 2 yr, mitral stenosis, intraarterial thrombus, CHF, or hyperthyroidism. In these patients, ensure adequate anticoagulation (PT 1.5–2 × baseline, INR 2.0–3.0). It has been suggested that NTG patches near the electrodes be removed prior to cardioversion to avoid risk of explosion. **Tests:** ECG; TEE (✓ for thrombus and size of atrium); digitalis level (toxic = > 3 ng/mL → refractory VF following cardioversion); electrolytes; INR.
Endocrine	Hyperthyroidism → AF

Out-of-Operating Room Procedures

Gastrointestinal	Full-stomach precautions (see p. B-4) may be necessary in the emergency patient.
Neurological	✓ Hx for TIAs or CVAs →↑ risk of embolic event. Pre- and postprocedure neurologic exams should be done.
Hematologic	✓ need for anticoagulation (see above).
Laboratory	Other tests as indicated from H&P.
Premedication	Usually not needed. For the emergency patient, take full-stomach precautions (see p. B-4).

INTRAOPERATIVE

Anesthetic technique: Brief GA with mask oxygenation and ventilation

Induction	Preoxygenate patient. For hemodynamically fragile patients, etomidate (0.1–0.2 mL/kg iv) is perhaps the agent of choice (**NB:** etomidate-induced clonus → ECG artifact). For the hemodynamically stable patient, use propofol (1.0-1.5 mg/kg iv slowly) until loss of lid reflex. Additional analgesia may be provided by remifentanil (1–2 mcg/kg iv), thereby reducing anesthetic requirements.	
Maintenance	Occasionally necessary to repeat cardioversion. Additional small doses of propofol, etomidate, or remifentanil may be required.	
Emergence	Patients should awaken rapidly with full recovery of airway reflexes. Outpatients are usually discharged to home within 1–2 h.	
Blood and fluid requirements	No blood loss IV: 20 ga × 1 NS/LR @ TKO	
Monitoring	Standard monitors (see p. B-1).	Avoid placement of ECG electrodes in precordial area.
Positioning	Hospital bed, supine	Procedure takes place at patient's bedside.
Complications	Loss of airway	Use airway manipulation ± artificial airways; be prepared to intubate.
	VF	Use ACLS protocols.
	↑↑ BP/myocardial ischemia	Cardioversion → catecholamine surge → acute MI in susceptible patient population.
	Severe bradycardia	Rx: Atropine (e.g., 0.4 mg iv)
	Thermal injury	Ensure good electrode/skin contact.
	↓ CO	2° anesthetic drugs or myocardial stunning from cardioversion. Rx: inotropic support (e.g., ephedrine)

POSTOPERATIVE

Complications	Recall	Especially in hemodynamically fragile patients. Discuss possibility with patient in advance.
	Systemic embolization	Neurological exam should be repeated post-cardioversion.
	↓ BP/↓ CO/CHF New dysrhythmia	Atrial contraction may not be effective following cardioversion →↓ CO/↓ BP.
Pain management	Minimal	Myalgias not uncommon; consider ketorolac.
Tests	ECG	Verify NSR.

Suggested Readings

1. Dell'Orfano JT, Naccarelli GV: Update on external cardioversion and defibrillation. *Curr Opin Cardiol* 2001;16(1):54–7.
2. Hullander RM, Leivers D, Wingler K: A comparison of propofol and etomidate for cardioversion. *Anesth Analg* 1993;77(4): 690–4.
3. Santini L, Forleo GB, Topa A, et al. Electrical cardioversion of atrial fibrillation: different methods for a safe and effective technique. *Expert Rev Cardiovasc Ther* 2005;3(4):601–10.
4. Stoneham, MD: Anesthesia for cardioversion. *Anaesthesia* 1996;57:565–70.
5. Trohman RG, Parrillo JE: Direct current cardioversion: indications, techniques, and recent advances. *Crit Care Med* 2000;28(10Suppl):N170–3.

IMPLANTATION OF CARDIOVERTER-DEFIBRILLATOR (ICD)

PROCEDURAL CONSIDERATIONS

Description: The implantable cardioverter-defibrillator (ICD) is an effective device for the prevention of premature death from ventricular tachycardia (VT) or ventricular fibrillation (VF). The results of randomized trials involving survivors of cardiac arrest and those considered at risk for sudden death showed the superiority of ICD therapy over conventional medical therapy in lowering the incidence of sudden death and overall mortality. The most recent trial—MADIT II—showed the device therapy to be advantageous over standard medical therapy in patients with low LVEF (< 30%). Over the past decade, significant advances have occurred in ICD technology. The devices have decreased dramatically in size (now at 30–40 mL), along with substantial increases in functionality. Newer devices can incorporate the full capabilities of a permanent pacemaker for bradycardia support and resynchronization therapy, as well as hemodynamic monitoring. Therapies for atrial tachyarrhythmias (atrial tachycardia and fibrillation) are also available in select devices (e.g., Medtronic GEM AT). The more efficient biphasic waveform, which results in a much lower defibrillation threshold (DFT) and, hence, lowers required energy delivery and storage, is now standard for all ICDs, allowing for further miniaturization. Implantation of these small ICDs results in mortality and morbidity rates very similar to those associated with standard pacemaker implantation.

The device system consists of a small pulse generator and transvenous leads that are designed to record ventricular depolarizations and deliver a shock via coils or patches. ICD terminates VT/VF by sensing these rhythms and responding with an appropriate countershock. The most common ICD implantation uses endocardial leads inserted percutaneously (transvenous approach) via pectoral (or, rarely, abdominal) subcutaneous/submuscular pulse generator placement. In the unusual circumstances of difficult endocardial access or high DFT (> 25 J), additional leads can be placed either in the coronary sinus or subcutaneously. Very rarely would the leads (in the form of patches) be applied epicardially via a thoracotomy approach.

In the **transvenous approach,** the insertion of leads and pulse generator requires minimal anesthesia; however, during testing of defibrillation efficacy, VF is induced once or twice, and sometimes more frequently. Thus, in addition to continuous monitoring of VS and cardiac rhythm, the anesthesiologist should pay special attention to the patient's hemodynamic stability prior to VF induction and after the defibrillation. In the event of failed defibrillation by the programmed first shock, a somewhat prolonged VF may occur. In the case of repeated DFT testing, it is customary to give at least 5-min intervals between VF inductions to allow for sufficient hemodynamic recovery. In patients with significant LV dysfunction, ↓ BP is not uncommon, but caution should be taken with fluid administration. If recovery from ↓ BP is slow, complications such as pneumo/hemothorax or pericardial effusion/tamponade should be considered. In the absence of a PA catheter (which would interfere with ICD lead positioning), accurate assessment of hemodynamic status is limited. Thus, meticulous attention should be directed at arterial pressure, HR, and oxygenation status. Finally, it is not uncommon to encounter acute atrial fibrillation (AF) from induction and conversion of VF. Fortunately, a cardioversion can be applied easily, using the ICD itself or relying on the external rescue system (external cardioversion).

Usual preop diagnosis: Documented, induced, or high-risk ventricular fibrillation

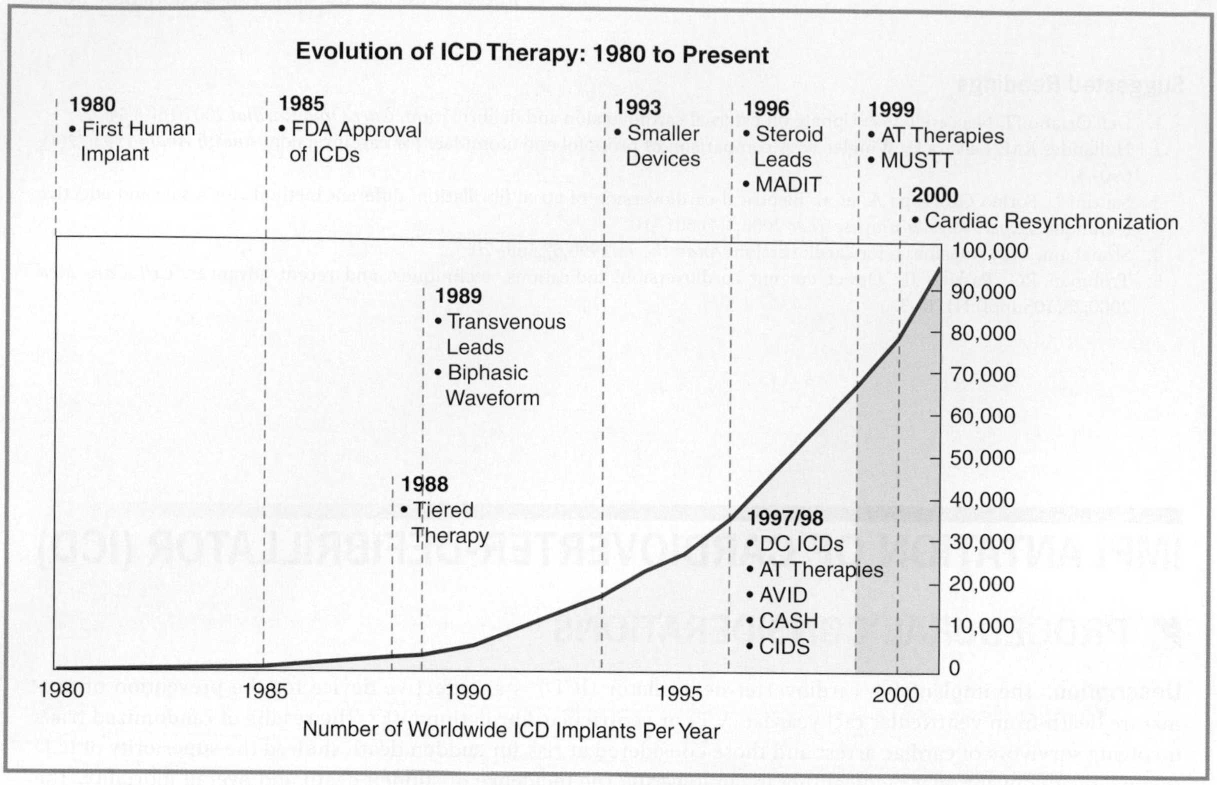

Figure 13.1-1. The annual implantation rate of ICDs is rising as the units become easier to implant and the indications for their use broadens. (Reproduced with permission from Medtronic, Inc. Minneapolis MN.)

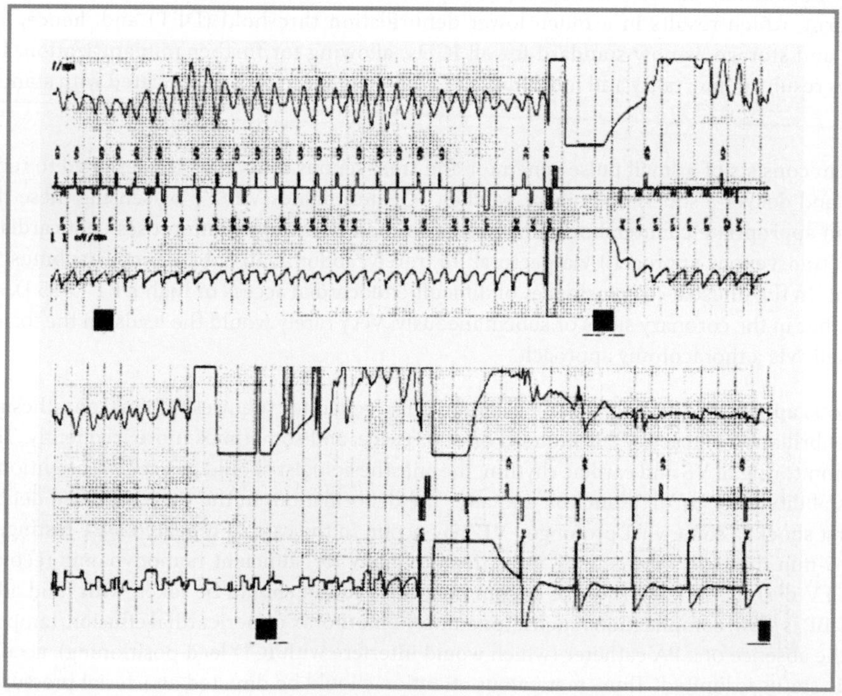

Figure 13.1-2. Induced VF (with underlying AF) is shown on top panel, whereby the first (24-J) shock failed to terminate VF but terminated AF (as indicated by the ICD annotation). The second shock (34-J) terminated VF, resulting in V-paced rhythm with underlying sinus and AV block. Total down-time during VF was 16 sec. Down-time is dependent on the detection time and charge time, which, in turn, depend on the energy programmed.

SUMMARY OF PROCEDURE	
Position	Supine with defibrillator pads positioned A-P or basilar-apical
Incision	Left pectoral or abdominal
Special instrumentation	ICD pulse generator, lead(s), and testing system (manufacturer-specific)
Unique considerations	Multiple inductions of VT/VF with associated ↓ CO, ↓ BP
Antibiotics	Standard iv antimicrobial for staphylococcus/streptococcus organism
Surgical time	1–2 h (more for ICD with cardiac resynchronization [CRT])
Closing considerations	Routine subcutaneous/submuscular pocket closure
EBL	5–20 mL
Postop care	Monitoring of arrhythmia, pocket bleeding/hematoma, pneumothorax
Mortality	0.1% (transvenous); ≤ 5% (thoracotomy)
Morbidity	New-onset arrhythmias: ≤ 5% Pneumothorax: ≤ 5% (transvenous) Pericardial effusion/tamponade: ≤ 1% (transvenous)
Pain score	3 (6–9, thoracotomy)

PATIENT POPULATION CHARACTERISTICS	
Age range	5–90 yr
Male:Female	4:1
Incidence	50,000/yr in the United States
Etiology	Reentry substrates from remote MI and cardiomyopathy; congenital anomalies (e.g., Long-QT and Brugada syndromes)
Associated conditions	LV dysfunction; CAD; cardiomyopathy; HTN; valvular disease; COPD; obesity; AF; CVA; anoxic encephalopathy

ANESTHETIC CONSIDERATIONS FOR ICD AND PACEMAKER PLACEMENT

PREOPERATIVE

Patients presenting for **ICD placement** may be divided into three populations, based on symptomatology, associated pathology, and probable outcome: (a) **Supraventricular dysrhythmias** (e.g., Wolff-Parkinson-White [WPW] syndrome): usually young and otherwise healthy patients. May be associated with Ebstein's anomaly (tricuspid valve defect → RV failure), mitral valve disease, or CAD. Low periop mortality (1%); (b) **Ventricular dysrhythmias:** usually older patients with significant ventricular dysfunction (EF = 10–35%) and other pathologies, such as CAD or cardiac failure. These patients have either survived an episode of VT/VF or are otherwise at risk for sudden death; and (c) **Congestive heart failure (CHF)** without significant dysrhythmias, usually 2° dilated cardiomyopathy. These patients have very low EFs (10–25%), left bundle branch block, and Hx of failed conventional means of CHF treatment. The ICD device is implanted in these patients to provide paced 'resynchronization' of the contractions of the LV and RV. This requires a third-pacer lead placed into the coronary sinus to pace the LV independently of the RV. In this case, the device is not placed primarily for its defibrillator function, but for its ability to pace both ventricles synchronously (biventricular pacing). Patients presenting for **permanent pacemaker insertion** may have a variety of dysrhythmias, including sick sinus syndrome (SSS), heart blocks (2nd- and 3rd-degree), and tachycardias refractory to medication.

Respiratory	May have associated pulmonary disease 2° smoking. **Tests:** CXR; consider PFT, as indicated from H&P.
Cardiovascular	**ICD:** ICD patients are left on full medication, since it usually is impossible to wean them from antidysrhythmic medications before surgery. In most studies, patients have a mean LV EF of 35% and a New York Heart Association functional class of II or III. **Supraventricular dysrhythmias:** Look for precipitating factors in the dysrhythmia, and any methods that have been used to terminate the dysrhythmia. Usually, drug therapy is terminated before surgery to make a dysrhythmia inducible. Note type of drugs used to terminate a dysrhythmia. **Ventricular dysrhythmias:** Ask about any methods that have been used to terminate dysrhythmia. Look for associated conditions, including CAD, CHF, cardiomyopathy, LV aneurysm, HTN, mitral insufficiency, diabetes. Generally, these patients have poor LV function with ↑ sensitivity to myocardial depressants. It is important to note that they may be on combinations of antidysrhythmics. Many of these drugs have significant negative inotropic effects. Of special note is amiodarone, which has been associated with intractable bradydysrhythmias, refractory vasodilation, and difficulty in weaning from CPB. **Pacemaker:** The anesthesiologist should be aware that there is an NASPE code (North American Society of Pacing and Electrophysiology) that describes pacemaker function with a three- to five-letter code. The first letter refers to the heart chamber that is paced and the second to the chamber that is sensed. These first two letters can be A (atrial), V (ventricular), or D (dual). The third letter indicates whether there is a triggering (T) or inhibiting (I) function, or both (D). For example, a VVI notation indicates that the ventricle is paced and sensed and there is inhibition by native beats. A fourth and fifth letter may be used to describe programmability and dysrhythmia control, respectively. **Tests:** ECG: ✓ dysrhythmia, ischemia, electrophysiologic report. ECHO: ✓ ventricular function, wall motion abnormalities, valvular problems. Cardiac angiography: ✓ ventricular function, CAD, valvular disease, LV aneurysm.
Renal	Patients with poor ventricular function may have associated renal compromise. Electrolyte abnormalities (K^+, Mg^{++}) may be associated with ↑ cardiac irritability and should be corrected preop. **Tests:** BUN; Cr; electrolytes
Hematologic	Hb/Hct; coag tests (PT, PTT, Plt)
Laboratory	Other tests as indicated from H&P.
Premedication	For adults: midazolam 0.5–2.0 mg iv, with careful observation and supplemental O_2.

INTRAOPERATIVE

Anesthetic technique: Local anesthesia with sedation, GA with LMA, or GETA, as indicated. Placement of most ICDs and pacemakers is done in the cardiac catheterization suite. ICDs are very small and are implanted in the same position as a pacemaker. If patients are orthopneic due to their CHF, or if the procedure is projected to be long, GA is often preferable. Also, elderly patients may become disoriented with sedation and, thus, may require GA.

Induction	Exact type of induction depends on the patient's medical condition. Sedation can be provided with small doses of midazolam (1–2 mg) ± fentanyl (25–50 mcg) titrated to effect. An alternative technique is to use a propofol infusion (e.g., 25–75 mcg/kg/min). Since local anesthesia is provided by the surgeon, the procedure usually is not painful and does not require postop pain control. It is important to avoid oversedating these patients, since they will tend to become disoriented and uncooperative. Even if local anesthesia with sedation is provided for the placement of leads and the device, a brief period of GA is always required for device testing. This can be provided easily with mask ventilation and induction with propofol (e.g., 1 mg/kg iv) or etomidate (e.g., 0.1 mg/kg iv), similar to anesthesia for cardioversion procedures. For those patients requiring GA for the entire procedure,

Induction (cont'd)	induction with STP (2–4 mg/kg), propofol (1–2 mg/kg), or etomidate (0.1–0.3 mg/kg) is often used. Muscle relaxants are not required unless intubation is planned. Narcotics usually are not required since local anesthesia is used.	
Maintenance	As previously discussed, verification of correct lead placement involves the induction of ventricular fibrillation or tachycardia and the testing of the device's capability to restore NSR. External defibrillation should be available at all times, as should antidysrhythmics (e.g., lidocaine and amiodarone). While the device is tested, the patient should be breathing 100% O_2. Multiple testing cycles can result in depressed LV function, and inotropes may be needed.	
Emergence	These patients are extubated (if GETA or LMA used). Recovery is in the PACU. If, however, multiple test shocks are needed or the heart displays evidence of injury (need for inotropes, ST segment abnormalities), then extubation may need to be deferred to ICU.	
Blood and fluid requirements	IV: 16–18 ga × 1 NS/LR @ 6–8 mL/kg/min	Care should be taken to minimize iv fluids in CHF patients.
Monitoring	Standard monitors (see p. B-1)	
	± Arterial line	
	± CVP/PA	A CVP or PA catheter may be placed according to LV function. ICD patients generally require only an arterial line.
	External defibrillation	Because antidysrhythmics may affect the testing procedure, they should be avoided when possible. Defibrillation or cardioversion are treatments of choice.
	Temperature	Normothermia should be maintained.
Positioning	Supine ✓ and pad pressure points. ✓ eyes.	
Complications	Pneumohemothorax Pericardial effusion/tamponade HTN/CHF	
	Coronary sinus rupture	Rarely, cardiac rupture may occur during lead extraction. Coronary sinus rupture has been reported during biventricular lead placement.

POSTOPERATIVE

Complications	Recurrent dysrhythmias Hemorrhage Ischemia	
Pain management	Usually managed with oral analgesics.	
Tests	CXR	✓ line/lead placement, r/o pneumohemothorax.
	ECG	✓ for ischemia, dysrhythmias.
	Electrophysiologic testing Electrolytes	

Suggested Readings

1. Abraham WT, Fisher WG, Smith AL, et al: Cardiac resynchronization in chronic heart failure. *N Engl J Med* 2002;346(24):1845–53.
2. Cox JL: Anatomic electrophysiologic basis for the surgical treatment of refractory ischemic ventricular tachycardia. *Ann Surg* 1983;198(2):119–29.

Out-of-Operating Room Procedures

3. Craney JM, Gorman LN: Conscious sedation and implantable devices. Safe and effective sedation during pacemaker and implantable cardioverter defibrillator placement. *Crit Care Nurs Clin North Am* 1997;9(3):325–34.
4. Kupersmith J: The past, present, and future of the implantable cardioverter defibrillator. *Am J Med* 2002;113(1):82–4.
5. Kusumoto FM, Goldschlager N: Device therapy for cardiac arrhythmias. *JAMA* 2002;287(14):1848–52.
6. Matthews EL, Atlee JL, Luck JC, et al: Anesthesia for patients with electrophysiologic disorders. In *A Practical Approach to Cardiac Anesthesia*, 2nd edition. Hensley FA Jr, Martin DE, eds. Little & Brown, Boston: 1995, 392–415.
7. Rozner MA. The patient with cardiac pacemaker or implanted defibrillator and management during anesthesia. *Curr Opin Anaesthesiol* 2007;20(3):261–8.
8. Swygman C, Wang PJ, et al: Advances in implantable cardioverter defibrillators. Curr Opin Cardiol 2002;17(1): 24–8.

TRANSJUGULAR INTRAHEPATIC PORTOSYSTEMIC SHUNT (TIPS)

PROCEDURAL CONSIDERATIONS

Description: Hepatic cirrhosis is a progressive disease which eventually results in portal HTN and the development of varices at a variety of sites. Bleeding from esophageal varices is a serious complication of portal HTN, occurring in 25% of patients within 1 year of diagnosis (~50% mortality). Prior to 1989, surgically placed shunts were used to direct high-pressure portal blood into the systemic venous circulation in patients with recurrent bleeding after endoscopic sclerotherapy or banding. The **transjugular intrahepatic portosystemic shunt (TIPS)** procedure has almost completely replaced surgical shunts.

TIPS is, as the name suggests, a percutaneous shunt between the portal and systemic circulations. The shunt is created between the hepatic vein and portal vein within the liver parenchyma, maintained by placement of a stent graft. This creates a low-resistance conduit to decompress the portal circulation, thereby decreasing variceal blood flow and ascites formation. Although it can be performed with conscious sedation, balloon dilation of the tract is extremely painful, typically requiring GA.

TIPS was developed initially by Rosch in dog studies in 1969. The first percutaneous portosystemic shunts were performed in humans using an angioplasty balloon in 1982, but the tract closed due to elastic recoil of the cirrhotic liver tissue. Palmaz and Richter performed the first successful TIPS in humans in 1989, using metallic stents to maintain the patency of the tract. Since then, TIPS has become the procedure of choice for patients who fail sclerotherapy and banding. In addition, it addresses another common problem associated with cirrhosis: refractory ascites.

Through the right IJ, a 10 Fr sheath is placed in the upper IVC. A catheter/guidewire combination is used to select the right hepatic vein. A wedged hepatic venogram using CO_2 is performed. Injection of iodinated contrast can result in rupture of the liver capsule and exsanguination. The wedged venogram refluxes contrast through the sinusoids and into the portal vein, thereby providing a map. The catheter is exchanged over a stiff wire for a metallic introducer/needle. A variety of needle kits are available including the Colapinto (Cook Inc., Bloomington, IN), Rosch-Uchida (Cook Inc, Bloomington, IN), and Hawkins set designed for CO_2 injections (Angiodynamics, Queensbury, NY). All include a long introducer sheath and coaxially inserted curved-tip needle or metal cannula, with directional indicator, to help steer the needle toward the right portal vein.

Portal venous pressures are measured and the pressure gradient between the portal vein and right atrium determined. Following a portal venogram, the catheter is exchanged for an angioplasty balloon, and the tract dilated (Fig. 13.1-3C). The use of covered stents for TIPS creation have led to significantly improved patency rates and for this reason, the Viatorr (Gore, Flagstaff, AZ) self-expanding covered stent has largely replaced the bare metal stents. The Viatorr is positioned across the tract and the uncovered portion is first deployed within the portal venous system (Fig. 13.1-3D). The covered portion is then pulled into the tract and deployed in a separate step. The stent may be dilated to a diameter of 8–10 mm using an angioplasty balloon, depending on the stent diameter and desired porto-systemic gradient. If necessary, a second stent is deployed to cover any remaining unstented portions of the hepatic tract. Following TIPS creating, portal venogram and pressure gradients are remeasured. Ideally, the pressure gradient following shunting should be between 6–12 mmHg. If the gradient is too high, there is a risk of

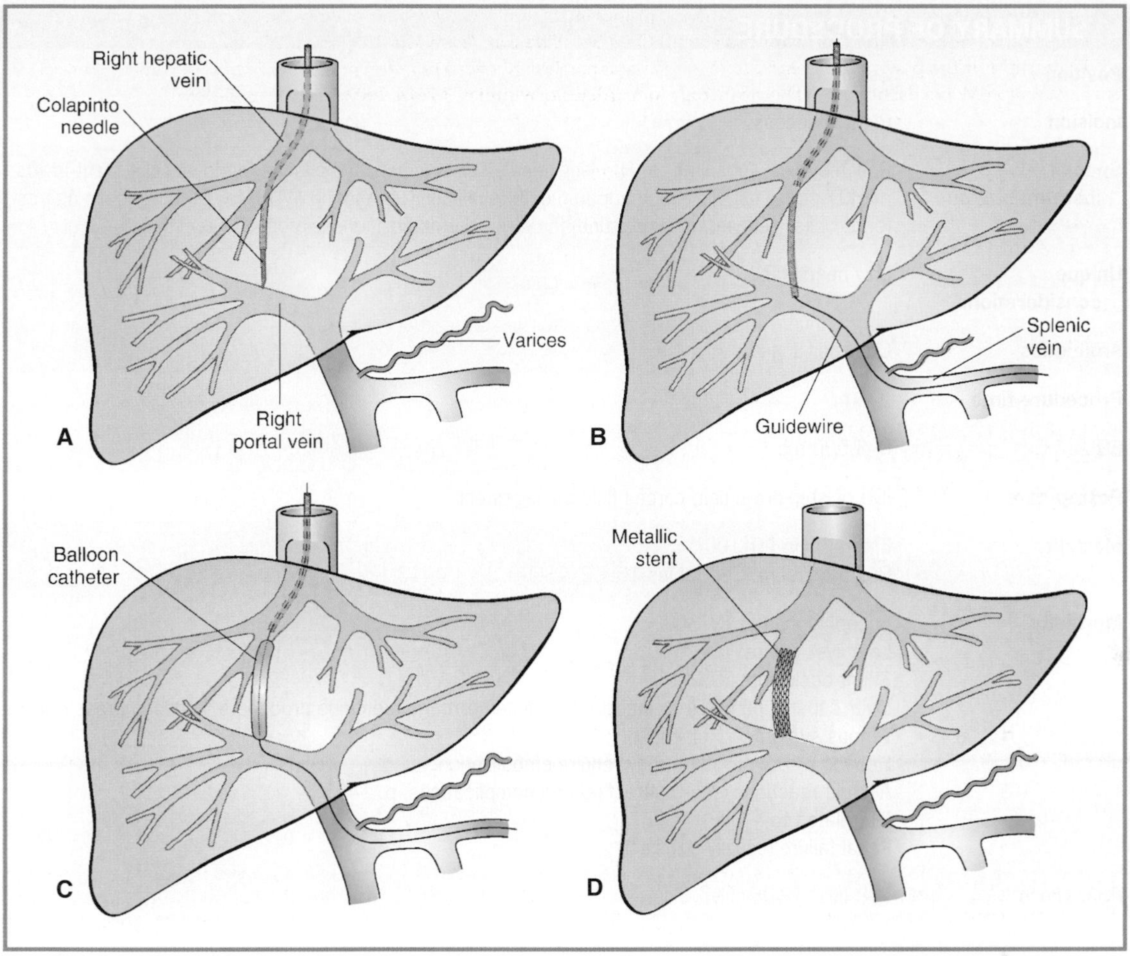

Figure 13.1-3. TIPS placement: **(A)** Sheathed Colapinto needle is advanced out of hepatic vein into portal vein branch. Varices are present. **(B)** Guide wire is advanced through the needle sheath into splenic vein. **(C)** Parenchymal liver tract is dilated using a balloon angioplasty catheter. **(D)** The metallic stent is deployed within the shunt tract. (Redrawn with permission from Haskal ZJ, Ring F: *Current Techniques in Interventional Radiology.* Current Science, Philadelphia: 1994.)

rebleeding; if too low, there is overshunting of blood, thus bypassing the entire portal venous system and increasing the risk of encephalopathy and liver failure. After successful creation of the shunt, all devices, including the right jugular sheath, are removed, and hemostasis is achieved. Patients are closely monitored in an ICU or step-down unit for 24–48 h.

DIPS (Direct IVC-to-portal shunt) is a newer alternative to TIPS. Simultaneous venous access is required from both the internal jugular vein and common femoral vein. For DIPS, an intravascular ultrasound probe is used to guide needle puncture from the IVC, through the caudate lobe, and into the main portal vein. Since the tract traverses extrahepatic regions, placement of a covered stent is mandatory. A theoretically fewer number of passes is needed to access the portal vein because the puncture is ultrasound guided; however, there is likely a greater risk of intraperitoneal hemorrhage with each puncture attempt.

If TIPS/DIPS is performed for the treatment of bleeding varices, it may be necessary to embolize and sclerose the varices if they persistently fill following shunt creation. This may be accomplished using sclerosing agents (e.g., ethanolamine) with an occlusion balloon and embolic agents (e.g., metallic coils, Gelfoam), depending on operator preference.

Usual preop diagnosis: Bleeding esophageal varices (as a result of portal HTN); ascites; Budd-Chiari and hepatorenal syndromes

SUMMARY OF PROCEDURE

Position	Supine
Incision	Right IJ access
Special instrumentation	Rosch-Uchida, Colapinto, or Hawkins needle set; angioplasty balloons; endovascular stent grafts, marker pigtail, CO_2 injection apparatus, intravascular ultrasound (IVUS) for DIPS, embolic agents (e.g., coils, gelfoam, ethanolamine) for variceal embolization/sclerosis if necessary.
Unique considerations	May need FFP.
Antibiotics	Cefazolin 1 g iv
Procedure time	2–6 h
EBL	0–3,000 mL
Postop care	ICU or step-down unit; careful fluid management
Mortality	Emergency: 50–100% Postprocedure: See Tables 13.1-2, 13.1-3, 13.1-4, 13.1-5
Morbidity	Encephalopathy: 18–30% Late liver failure: 10–25% Shunt occlusion: 10%/yr Liver capsule puncture → intraperitoneal hemorrhage (continue procedure to decompress portal venous system →↓ bleeding). Hepatic artery puncture: may require embolization. Allergic reactions (see Contrast-related complications, p. 1453). MI (related to ↑ CVP) Renal failure (usually transient)
Pain score	7–8 (first few h only)

Table 13.1-2. MELD Score Calculation

The MELD (Model for End-stage Liver Disease) score is calculated using three objective indicators—serum bilirubin, serum creatinine level (Cr), and international normalized ratio (INR)—according to the United Network for Organ Sharing modification of the original formula:

$$\text{MELD} = 9.6 \times \log e\,(\text{Cr}) + 3.8 \times \log e\,(\text{Bilirubin}) + 11.2 \times \log e\,(\text{INR}) + 6.4$$

The MELD Score can easily be calculated by accessing the following website:
http://www.mayoclinic.org/meld/mayomodel7.html

Table 13.1-3. Overall Mortality Based on MELD Score

MELD Score	No. of Patients	Mortality Rate (%) 30 days	3 months	6 months
≤ 10%	28	0 (0, 0)	0 (0, 0)	0 (0, 0)
11–17	83	7.3 (1.7, 12.9)	16.0 (8.0, 24.0)	24.9 (15.1, 34.7)
18–24	40	17.9 (5.9, 29.9)	34.8 (19.4, 50.2)	38.6 (22.4, 54.9)
≥ 25	15	42.6 (16.7, 68.4)	65.5 (39.9, 91.2)	74.2 (50.0, 98.3)

Patients undergoing elective TIPS creation with a MELD score of 18 or more had a significantly lower 3-month survival rate than those with a MELD score of 17 or less. Numbers in parentheses are 95% confidence intervals. Mortality tables reprinted with permission from Ferral H, Gamboa P, Postoak DW, et al: Survival after elective transjugular intrahepatic portosystemic shunt creation: prediction with Model for End-Stage Liver Disease Score. *Radiology* 2004;231(1):231–6.

Table 13.1-4. Mortality Based on MELD Score and Cause of Cirrhosis

			Mortality Rate (%)		
MELD Score	**Group***	**No. of Patients**	**30 days**	**3 months**	**6 months**
≤ 17	A	39	5.1 (0, 12.1)	7.7 (0, 16.1)	13.9 (2.5, 25.2
	B	72	5.6 (0.3, 11.0)	14.4 (6.1, 22.7)	21.4 (11.3, 31.4)
≥ 18	A	14	42.9 (16.9, 68.8)	57.1 (31.2, 83.1)	57.1 (31.2, 83.1)
	B	41	17.9 (5.9, 29.9)	37.9 (22.0, 53.7)	45.9 (28.1, 63.2)

A = Alcohol-induced disease, B = Non-alcohol-induced disease
Patients undergoing elective TIPS creation with a MELD score of 18 or more had a significantly lower 3-month survival rate than those with a MELD score of 17 or less. Numbers in parentheses are 95% confidence intervals. Mortality tables reprinted with permission from Ferral H, Gamboa P, Postoak DW, et al: Survival after elective transjugular intrahepatic portosystemic shunt creation: prediction with Model for End-Stage Liver Disease Score. Radiology 2004; 231(1): 231–6.

Table 13.1-5. Mortality Based on MELD Score and Ascites

			Mortality (%)		
MELD Score	**Ascites**	**No. of Patients**	**30 days**	**3 Months**	**6 Months**
≤ 17	No	48	4.2 (0, 9.8)	4.2 (0, 9.8)	4.2 (0, 9.8)
	Yes	63	6.4 (0.3, 12.5)	18.4 (8.6, 28.3)	31.3 (18.6, 43.9)
≥ 18	No	18	22.2 (3.0, 41.4)	39.8 (16.8, 62.8)	46.5 (22.6, 70.4)
	Yes	37	25.4 (11.0, 39.8)	44.4 (27.4, 61.4)	48.7 (31.1, 66.3)

Patients undergoing elective TIPS creation with a MELD score of 18 or more had a significantly lower 3-month survival rate than those with a MELD score of 17 or less. Numbers in parentheses are 95% confidence intervals. Mortality tables reprinted with permission from Ferral H, Gamboa P, Postoak DW, et al: Survival after elective transjugular intrahepatic portosystemic shunt creation: prediction with Model for End-Stage Liver Disease Score. *Radiology* 2004; 231(1):231–6.

ANESTHETIC CONSIDERATIONS

PREOPERATIVE

Patients presenting for TIPS procedures have portal HTN usually 2° end-stage liver disease (ESLD), which will affect the function of a variety of organ systems, as described below.

Respiratory	Abdominal distension → atelectasis →↑ pulmonary shunting → hypoxemia (hepatopulmonary syndrome in ESLD). Encephalopathy → hyperventilation →↓ $PaCO_2$ (respiratory alkalosis with chronic acidosis as compensation). Pulmonary effusion may be present in 5–10% of patients. **Tests:** ✓ CXR (for Sx of atelectasis); ABG and PFT, if indicated.
Cardiovascular	Cardiomyopathy (ETOH) and CAD (tobacco) occur at higher incidence in this patient population. Diuretic therapy → hypovolemia + ↓ K^+ (furosemide) or ↑ K^+ (spironolactone). Hyperdynamic circulation 2° to ↓ peripheral resistance + ↓ cardiac reserve are common findings, and correlate with poor postop outcome. **Tests:** ECG; electrolytes; cardiac ECHO, if indicated from H&P.
Neurological	Symptoms of hepatic encephalopathy range from mild confusion to coma. These patients may be very sensitive to narcotics and sedatives. A characteristic finding in liver failure is asterixis (liver flap). Hyponatremia and hypoglycemia may mimic hepatic encephalopathy. **Tests:** As indicated from H&P.
Hepatic	Drug metabolism may be markedly reduced; anticipate prolonged effect with sedative and narcotic drugs. Drugs with particularly prolonged action include midazolam, meperidine, ranitidine and lidocaine. Apparent resistance to pancuronium and all muscle relaxants is most likely due to an increased volume of distribution. Succinylcholine effects may be prolonged in patients with severe ESLD (2° ↓ plasma cholinesterase). **Tests:** Bilirubin; PT; albumin; LFTs

Gastrointestinal	Ascites →↑ intraabdominal pressure →↑ risk of aspiration. Full-stomach precautions and rapid-sequence induction are recommended (see p. B-4). Portal HTN → variceal bleeding. If possible, avoid esophageal instrumentation (e.g., TEE, esophageal stethoscope, etc.). Gastritis and peptic ulceration may be present.
Renal	Oliguric renal failure may complicate ESLD (hepatorenal syndrome). This may be reversible if liver failure improves. Differential Dx includes prerenal azotemia and acute tubular necrosis. ***NB:** Bilirubin metabolites interfere with creatinine measurement and may mask ↑ creatinine levels. **Tests:** BUN; Cr; electrolytes
Endocrine	Hypoglycemia may be present in cases of severe cirrhosis. ESLD patients may have ↓ response to catecholamines. **Tests:** Glucose
Hematologic	Patients may be anemic 2° GI bleeding. The majority of patients will exhibit coagulopathy 2° ↓ hepatic synthetic function (all factors except VIII and fibrinogen) and ↓ Plt. Patients may require vitamin K (if coagulopathy is present and time permits), FFP (if PT > 2 sec above baseline), or Plt transfusion (if Plt < 100 K) before procedure; these products should be readily available. **Tests:** CBC; Plt; PT; others as indicated from H&P.
Premedication	Patients with significant ascites will require full-stomach precautions (see p. B-4). ***NB:** Benzodiazepines should be used with caution in liver failure patients.

INTRAOPERATIVE

Anesthetic technique: In some patients (and at some centers), sedation with local anesthesia may be satisfactory; however, balloon dilation of the intrahepatic tract can be exceedingly painful. Remember, these patients may be very sensitive to narcotics → respiratory arrest. GETA is often necessary to provide adequate analgesia and airway protection.

General anesthesia:

Induction	Rapid-sequence induction (see p. B-4) is necessary in patients with encephalopathy, abdominal distention and recent variceal bleeds (blood in the stomach).	
Maintenance	Standard maintenance (see p. B-2). If muscle relaxation is to be maintained, low-dose vecuronium (1–1.5 mcg/kg/min), cisatracurium (3 mcg/kg/min infusion) or rocuronium (5–15 mcg/kg/min) may be used to maintain muscle relaxation.	
Emergence	Extubate when the patient is awake and protective laryngeal reflexes are present. Patient should be transferred to PACU accompanied by anesthesiologist.	
Blood and fluid requirements	Potential for large blood loss IV: 14–16 ga × 1–2 FFP available Plt available 2–4 U PRBC available NS/LR (as appropriate)	Glucose-containing solutions may be required for patients with hepatic failure ± CHF. ✓ blood glucose levels frequently. Vasopressor response may be impaired.
Monitoring	Standard monitors (see p. B-1)	Ventricular arrhythmias can be provoked by hepatic vein catheterization.
Positioning	✓ and pad pressure points. ✓ eyes.	Radiology tables usually are not well-padded → nerve damage.
Complications	Portal vein rupture Liver capsule perforation Complete heart block CHF	Intraabdominal hemorrhage may be massive and require emergency surgery. Patients with pre-existing LBBB may require a pacemaker pre-TIPS (2° risk of RBBB during procedure). Shunt →↑↑ venous return → CHF

POSTOPERATIVE

Complications	Portal vein thrombus	May mimic symptoms of PE or MI.
	↑ encephalopathy	2° ↓ hepatic portal blood flow
	Sepsis	May require hemodynamic support (e.g., dopamine)
	Bleeding	
	Fluid/electrolyte disturbance	Stent insertion →↑ venous return →↑ diuresis → electrolyte/fluid imbalance.
Pain Management	IV opiates	

Suggested Readings

1. Cejna M, Peck-Radosavljevic M, Thurnher S, et al: Creation of transjugular intrahepatic portosystemic shunts with stent-grafts: initial experiences with a polytetrafluoroethylene-covered nitinol endoprosthesis. *Radiology* 2001;221: 437–46.
2. Cello JP, Ring EJ, Olcott EW, et al: Endoscopic sclerotherapy compared with percutaneous transjugular intrahepatic portosystemic shunt after initial sclerotherapy in patients with acute variceal hemorrhage. A randomized, controlled trial. *Ann Intern Med* 1997;126(11):858–65.
3. Charon JM, Alaeddin FH, Pimpalwar SA, et al: Results of a retrospective multicenter trial of the Viatorr expanded polyetrafluoroethylene-covered stent-graft for transjugular intrahepatic portosystemic shunt creation. *J Vasc Interv Radiol* 2004;15:1219–30.
4. Freedman AM, Sanyal AJ, Tisnado J, et al: Complications of transjugular intrahepatic portosystemic shunt: a comprehensive review. *Radiographics* 1993;13(6):1185–210.
5. Hausegger KA, Karnel F, GEorgieva B, et al: Transjugular intrahepatic portosystemic shunt creation with the Viatorr expanded polyetrafluoroethylene-covered stent graft. *J Vasc INterv Radiol* 2004;15:239–248.
6. Huonker M, Schumacher YO, Ochs A, et al: Cardiac function and haemodynamics in alcoholic cirrhosis and effects of the transjugular intrahepatic portosystemic stent shunt. *Gut* 1999;44(5):743–8.
7. Kerlan RK Jr, LaBerge JM, Gordon RL, et al: Inadvertent catheterization of the hepatic artery during placement of transjugular intrahepatic portosystemic shunts. *Radiology* 1994;193(1):273–6.
8. LaBerge JM, Ring EJ, Gordon RL, et al: Creation of transjugular intrahepatic portosystemic shunts with the Wallstent endoprosthesis: Results in 100 patients. Radiology 1993;157(2):413–20.
9. LaBerge JM, Somberg KA, Lake JR, et al: Two-year outcome following transjugular intrahepatic portosystemic shunt for variceal bleeding: results in 90 patients. *Gastroenterology* 1995;108(4):1143–51.
10. Nicoll A, Fitt G, Angus P, et al: Budd-Chiari syndrome: intractable ascites managed by a trans-hepatic portacaval shunt. *Australas Radiol* 1997;41(2):169–72.
11. Petersen B: Intravascular ultrasound-guided direct intrahepatic portacaval shunt: description of technique and technical refinements. *J Vasc Interv Radiol* 2003;14:21–32.
12. Richter GM, Palmaz JC, Noldge G, et al: The transjugular intrahepatic portosystemic stent-shunt. A new nonsurgical percutaneous method. *Radiologe* 1989;29(8):406–11.
13. Rosch J, Keller F: Transjugular intrahepatic portosystemic shunt: present status, comparison with endoscopic therapy and shunt surgery, and future prospectives. *World J Surg* 2001;25:337–46.
14. Russell GB: Anesthesia and interventional radiology. In *Alternate-Site Anesthesia: Clinical Practice Outside the Operating Room.* Russell GB, ed. Butterworth-Heinemann, Boston: 1997, 157–71.
15. Semba CP, Saperstein L, Nyman U, et al: Hepatic laceration from wedged venography performed before transjugular intrahepatic portosystemic shunt placement. *J Vasc Interv Radiol* 1996;7(l):143–6.

IMAGING AND IMAGE-GUIDED PROCEDURES

PROCEDURAL CONSIDERATIONS

Description: Projectional imaging includes x-ray fluoroscopy, and cross-sectional imaging includes computed tomography (CT), ultrasound (US), and magnetic resonance imaging (MRI). These techniques have become indispensable in modern diagnosis. In addition, a growing number of invasive procedures are being performed using cross-sectional imaging for guidance, not only for diagnostic purposes but also for therapeutic purposes. Indications include Dx of primary or metastatic tumors; tumor staging; Dx of benign processes, such as infections; drainage of fluid collections; local regional treatment of tumors and vascular malformations, endovascular treatment of hemorrhage, aneurysms, and dissections; percutaneous treatment of urinary and biliary obstructions; and placement of venous access devices. Selection of imaging modality depends on ease of identification of the target lesion and resolution of surrounding and intervening structures. Patient compliance is crucial to success, because image resolution and spatial accuracy require the patient to be immobile during image acquisition and the procedure itself. In compliant adults, most of these procedures may be done using conscious sedation. For procedures in the pediatric population, as well as for more invasive procedures in adults, GA is frequently necessary.

Diagnostic imaging: **Pediatric:** CT scans are performed in a large, ring-shaped gantry, through which the patient is passed on an automated table. US is performed with a hand-held transducer attached to a console. Diagnostic MRI scans are performed primarily in a large, circumferential magnet with a cylindrical center bore, also incorporating an automated table. In general, conscious sedation is sufficient to ensure pediatric patient compliance for diagnostic CT, US, or MRI, but occasionally GA is necessary. **Adults:** Almost all CT, US, and MRI studies are performed without anesthesia. Approximately 5% of adult patients are too claustrophobic to complete an MRI study. Some of these may benefit from sedation, but use of GA is rare.

Image-guided procedures: **Pediatric:** Procedures performed on the pediatric patient routinely require GA. X-ray fluoroscopy-guided procedures—including angiography, angioplasty, stent placement, arterial embolization, vascular malformation sclerosis, thrombolysis, venography, renal and adrenal vein sampling, transvenous biopsy, gastrostomy and gastrojejunal tube placement, renal drainage, ureteral stent placement, biliary drainage, bronchial dilation, and placement of venous access devices (Broviacs, ports, and PICCs)—are performed in a cath-angio lab, which frequently is OR-certified. Procedures usually entail real-time x-ray imaging, requiring all personnel in the room to wear protective lead garments. For CT- and US-guided biopsies and fluid drainage, initial lesion localization images are obtained after initiation of anesthesia and immobilization of the patient. A skin entry site is then selected and marked, based on coordinates determined from the initial images. Biopsies may require multiple needle passes, either coaxially through a large-bore guiding needle, or separately without such a guide. With CT, confirmation of needle position requires interruption of the procedure to acquire images, while with US, real-time images are obtained. Ideally, adequacy of biopsy sample is determined by an on-site cytopathologist. Manipulation of a hormonally-active tumor can cause acute release of hormones. Fluid drainage may be simple aspiration or, more frequently, will result in placement of an indwelling drainage catheter. Instrumentation of infected beds (abscess, obstructed urinary or biliary system) can cause acute bacteremia and sepsis. **Adults:** X-ray fluoroscopy, CT- and US-guided procedures, such as biopsies, fluid drainage, and tissue ablation, are routinely performed under conscious sedation. More invasive and painful procedures, such as stent-graft repair of aneurysms and dissections and radiofrequency (RF) ablation of unresectable tumors (see p. 1477), frequently require GA, spinal, or epidural anesthesia. The required site of access and the positioning of the operators should be considered before the procedure. Position of the ETT and central lines can be immediately confirmed using fluoroscopy. Occasionally, iv injection of iodinated contrast medium is necessary, and adverse reactions—such as urticaria, airway edema, hormone release (e.g., from pheochromocytoma, etc.), or anaphylaxis—may occur.

The developing field of MRI-guided procedures—sometimes referred to as interventional MRI (iMRI) or magnetic resonance-guided therapy (MRT)—reflects the emergence of new magnet geometries, allowing physician access to the patient during imaging. These geometries may be C-arm configurations, parallel discs above and below the patient, or dual rings where the patient is placed either through the apertures of the rings or perpendicularly between the rings. Faster image-acquisition pulse sequences are allowing near-real-time feedback. In addition to guiding biopsies and drainage, this technology enables more aggressive procedures, such as craniotomies or percutaneous tumor ablations, to be performed with immediate feedback showing the progress of excision or ablation. Clearly, many of these procedures require GA and, accordingly, require MRI-compatible monitoring and anesthetic equipment. For safety, the anesthesiologist also is subject to the same restrictions that apply to patients, so having a pacemaker, ICD, ferromagnetic aneurysm clips, or a metallic foreign body in the orbit precludes that person's suitability to perform these cases. Hybrid systems also are being marketed, combining MRI and x-ray fluoroscopy, CT and x-ray fluoroscopy, or CT and positron emission tomography (PET). These may involve overlapping precautions and risks.

Usual preop diagnosis: Tumor, primary or metastatic; lymphadenopathy; abscess, effusion, empyema, pseudocyst, or other fluid collection; arterial occlusive disease; aneurysm or pseudoaneurysm; trauma; DVT; cirrhosis

SUMMARY OF PROCEDURES

	CT/X-ray Fluoroscopy	US	MRI/MRT
Position	Supine, prone or lateral decubitus	⇐	⇐ + sitting
Unique considerations	Metallic objects should be kept out of the CT imaging field. Exit the procedure room during scanning to avoid radiation exposure, or use protective lead garment. Contrast reaction possible.	No ionizing radiation. Room lights are frequently dimmed for better viewing of the screen.	All equipment, including monitors, valves, anesthesia machine, O_2 tanks, laryngoscopes, etc., must be nonferromagnetic. Other metals should be removed from the imaging field to avoid artifact.
Antibiotics	Indicated for open procedures or when draining infected fluid collections, including abscesses, empyemas, and obstructed biliary or urinary systems.	⇐	⇐
Procedure time	≥ 1 h	⇐	⇐
EBL	Procedure-dependent; may be internal hemorrhage, may be pre-existing hemorrhage	⇐	⇐
Postop care	PACU → room	⇐	⇐
Mortality	Rare	⇐	⇐
Morbidity	Hemorrhage Infection/sepsis Organ injury/perforation Pneumothorax Pulmonary embolus Arrhythmia Hemodynamic Collapse	⇐	⇐
Pain score	1	1	Procedure-dependent

PATIENT POPULATION CHARACTERISTICS

Age range	All
Male:Female	1:1
Incidence	Common
Associated conditions	**Fluid collections:** Patients may present with fever, sepsis, pain, or ileus. Mass effect, such as with empyema or pericardial effusion, may also affect respiratory or cardiovascular function. Instrumentation or relief of mass effect may induce a vasovagal response or acute bacteremia and sepsis. Some infections (echinococcus, entamoeba, methicillin-resistant staphylococcus aureus [MRSA], vancomycin-resistant enterococci [VRE]) may require special precautions, such as respiratory isolation, gown/glove standards, and pre- and post-procedure equipment sterilization. **Solid tumors:** Mass effect may result in obstruction of airways, blood vessels, GI/biliary tract, or urinary tract, or neural impingement. HTN may be seen with significant renal compression and, occasionally, with neuroendocrine tumors. Hematopoietic, hepatic, or renal compromise may result in coagulopathy or Plt dysfunction. **Vascular pathologies:** Aggressive anticoagulation and/or antiplatelet therapy may be used intraop. Restoration of arterial flow to kidneys may → rapid ↓ of renin production and BP. Thrombolysis of venous occlusions can → PE. Placement of central vascular access catheters can cause air embolism or cardiac arrhythmias from right atrial irritation. Sclerosis of vascular malformations may result in chemical pulmonary embolism, acute pulmonary vasospasm and hypertension.

ANESTHETIC CONSIDERATIONS

PREOPERATIVE

The adult patient population requiring anesthesia services for cross-sectioned imaging is medically quite diverse; however, many have in common the inability or unwillingness to lie still during the scanning procedure. Some of these patients are very ill, requiring the services of an anesthesiologist to maintain cardiorespiratory stability. Adult patients should be npo for 6 h preprocedure (elective). In general, US and CT scans present fewer problems for the anesthesiologist than MRI. Regardless of the method of anesthesia chosen, these patients must lie perfectly still, the airway must be protected, and IPPV may be required. Thus, children, the mentally retarded, and claustrophobic, uncooperative, or critically ill patients may all require GA.

Respiratory	As a result of limited access to the patient's airway, the preop examination should focus on the need for elective ET intubation to protect the airway. ET intubation and mechanical ventilation also may be required in trauma patients, the critically ill, or patients with GERD or sleep apnea. An LMA may be suitable for patients not at risk of aspiration.
Cardiovascular	Presence of a cardiac pacemaker or ICD is a contraindication to MRI, as are PA catheter thermistors or pacing wires.
Neurological	Patients with ↑ ICP or cranial trauma usually need GA with mechanical ventilation and intubation. The presence of aneurysm clips and/or coils may be a contraindication to MRI (✓ with surgeon or radiologist). Some of the newer aneurysm clips are nonferromagnetic and are, therefore, MRI-compatible.
Musculoskeletal	The presence of spinal instrumentation, metal plates, pins, screws, joint replacements, or other prostheses is usually not a contraindication to MRI.
Premedication	Midazolam 1–5 mg iv (titrated to effect) may be appropriate in the very anxious adult patient; alternatively, lorazepam 1–2 mg po/sl 1 h before procedure.

CONSIDERATIONS FOR MRI/MRT

The MRI/MRT suite poses many challenges to the anesthesiologist. Because of the high magnetic fields involved in MRI, any equipment containing ferromagnetic components—such as ECG monitors, anesthesia machines, etc.—cannot go near the magnet. Thus, MRI-compatible equipment is mandatory in the area of the MRI scanner. The magnetic field will destroy information on credit card/access card magnetic strips, and may damage pagers as well as mechanical devices, including wrist watches and infusion pump motors. (A microdrip infusion set is a suitable replacement for an infusion pump.)

Noise	May be very distressing for some patients and may average 95 dB in a 1.5–T scanner. Exposure to noise levels of this magnitude should not exceed 2 h/d. Ear plugs or earphones with music can be helpful.
Thermal injury	Thermal injury is caused by induced currents in metal implants or in looped conductors in contact with the skin.
Projectile effect	The magnet has a strong attraction for ferromagnetic objects that can become lethal missiles; therefore, all objects, such as pens, scissors, iv poles, O_2 cylinders, keys, stethoscopes, etc., must be removed prior to entering the scanning room.
Implanted/ foreign material	There are several reports describing problems that may occur with cardiac pacemakers (failure to pace), aneurysm clips (hemorrhage) and intravascular wires (induced currents). Metal workers may be at special risk for ocular damage 2° imbedded particles.
Contrast agent	Currently, gadolinum chelates are the only agents in use and have a higher safety margin than iodinated contrast agents. Adverse reactions, however, occur in ~2% of patients, and include HA, nausea, dizziness, hemodynamic instability, and dysrhythmias.

INTRAOPERATIVE

Anesthetic technique: Typically, iv/po sedation, often without the services of an anesthesiologist. Patients unwilling or unable to cooperate will require GA.

IV sedation	In patients with a normal airway and no Hx of GERD, sedation can be carried out most easily using a propofol infusion (25–100 mcg/kg/min), ± midazolam (0.025–0.10 mg/kg) titrated to effect. ***NB:** Infusion pumps may be damaged by the magnet. (A microdrip infusion is a useful alternative.)

General anesthesia:

Induction	Standard induction (see p. B-2) on an MRI gantry (typically in the magnet anteroom). The anesthetized patient is then transported into the magnet.	
Maintenance	Standard maintenance (see p. B-2). Most commonly, a propofol infusion provides satisfactory sedation for the procedure (see pump considerations, above). Since continuous muscle relaxation is usually not required, spontaneous ventilation may be safest.	
Emergence	Emergence and extubation are often accomplished after the patient has been moved to the adjacent anteroom, where additional airway and other support equipment are readily available. The patient should be recovered in the PACU, which may be some distance from the MRI suite. Appropriate monitoring and personnel should accompany the patient.	
Blood and fluid requirements	No blood loss IV: 20 ga × 1 NS/LR @ TKO	
Monitoring	Standard monitors (see p. B-1)	Monitoring in the MRI/MRT suite presents special problems, discussed below.
Monitoring, MRI	ECG	ECG may be distorted by magnetic fields. Use MRI-compatible electrodes. Twist leads together to avoid creating loops (↓ artifacts, ↓ burns). V5 and V6 are least likely to develop artifacts.
	Pulse oximetry	MRI-compatible oximeters are available. Locate probe outside bore of the magnet (e.g., toe). Avoid burn injury 2° induced current in looped leads.
	BP (NIBP)	Replace all ferrous connections on cuff and tubing with nylon connectors. Use tubing extensions to keep apparatus away from the field.
	± Arterial Line	If an arterial line is medically indicated, keep the transducer close to the patient to avoid recording artifacts. Use MRI-compatible transducers and connectors. Recording equipment should have radiofrequency filters.
	Precordial/esophageal stethoscope	Often unsatisfactory because of magnet noise. An MRI-compatible, infrared, wireless stethoscope is available.
	Temperature	MRI-compatible T monitors are available, although usually not necessary for adults (short procedure).
	Capnography	MRI-compatible capnographs are available. Long sample lines will distort waveforms, and $ETCO_2$ concentration may not be accurate; however, this is still useful for measuring RR and relative changes in $ETCO_2$.
	PA catheter	PA catheters with thermistors or pacing wires are an absolute contraindication to MRI.

Monitoring, MRI (cont'd)	Urinary catheter	Catheters with T probes must be removed to avoid electrical or burn hazards.
	Verbal/visual	The patient and the monitors may be viewed directly (in procedure room) or through a screened window. Contact should be maintained throughout the procedure.
Positioning	✓ and pad pressure points. ✓ eyes.	CT and MRI gantries may be poorly padded → potential nerve injury.
Complications	Contrast-related	Gadolinium → local and systemic reactions (see Contrast-related complications, p. 1453).
	Loss of airway	Patient must be promptly extracted from the magnet bore and moved beyond the range of the magnet to permit use of emergency intubation and resuscitation equipment.
	Psychological	Panic attacks and claustrophobia occur in 5–10% of patients. Use of a blindfold may be helpful in selected patients. Heavy sedation or even GA may be necessary.
	Hearing loss	Temporary hearing loss and tinnitus may be expected in 43% of patients. Prevent by using ear plugs. GA ↑ risk of hearing damage 2° stapedius muscle relaxation.
	Thermal injury	Results from induced current, heating of oximeter probe, and looping cables.

POSTOPERATIVE

Complications	Hearing loss Thermal injury	See discussion above. See discussion above.

Suggested Readings

1. Barth KH, Matsumoto AH: Patient care in interventional radiology: a perspective. *Radiology* 1991;178:11–17.
2. Bock M, Wacker FK: MR-guided intravascular interventions: techniques and applications. *J Magn Reson Imaging* 2008;27:326–38.
3. Brown TR, Goldstein B, Little J: Severe burns resulting from magnetic resonance imaging with cardiopulmonary monitoring. Risks and relevant safety precautions. *Am J Phys Med Rehab* 1993;72:166–7.
4. Douglas BR, Charboneau JW, Reading CC: Ultrasound-guided intervention: expanding horizons. *Radiol Clin North Am* 2001;39:415–28.
5. Gupta S: New techniques in image-guided percutaneous biopsy. *Cardiovasc Intervent Radiol* 2004;27:91–104.
6. Hagspiel KD, Kandarpa K, Jolesz FA: Interventional MR imaging. *J Vasc Interv Radiol* 1997;8:745–58.
7. Holshouser BA, Hinshaw DB, Shellock FG: Sedation, anesthesia, and physiological monitoring during magnetic resonance imaging: evaluation of procedures and equipment. *J Magn Reson Imaging* 1993;3:553–8.
8. Johnson JC, Blackburn TW, Russell GB: Anesthesia for computed tomography. In *Alternate-Site Anesthesia: Clinical Practice Outside the Operating Room*. Russell GB, ed. Butterworth-Heinemann, Boston: 1997, 83–100.
9. Jolesz FA, Kahn T: Interventional MRI: state of the art. *Appl Radiol* 1997;26:8–13.
10. Jorgensen NH, Messick JM, Gray J, et al: ASA monitoring standards and magnetic resonance imaging. *Anesth Analg* 1994;79:1141–7.
11. Kettenbach J, Kacher DF, Koskinen SK, et al: Interventional and intraoperative magnetic resonance imaging. *Ann Rev Biomed Eng* 2000;2:661–90.
12. Malviya S, Voepel-Lewis T, Eldevik OP, et al: Sedation and general anaesthesia in children undergoing MRI & CT: adverse events and outcomes. *Br J Anaesthesia* 2000;84(6):743–8.
13. McBrien ME, Winder J, Smyth L: Anaesthesia for magnetic resonance imaging: a survey of current practice in the UK and Ireland. *Anaesthesia* 2000;55(8):737–43.
14. Meilstrup JW, Van Slyke MA, Russell GB: Ultrasound-guided interventional diagnosis and therapy. In *Alternate-Site Anesthesia: Clinical Practice Outside the Operating Room*. Russell GB, ed. Butterworth-Heinemann, Boston: 1997, 225–42.
15. Morcos SK, Thomsen HS: Adverse reactions to iodinated contrast media. *Eur Radiol* 2001;11:1267–75.
16. Mueller PR, vanSonnenberg E: Interventional radiology in the chest and abdomen. *N Engl J Med* 1990;322:1364–74.

17. Murphy KJ, Brunberg JA: Adult claustrophobia, anxiety, and sedation in magnetic resonance imaging. *Magn Reson Imaging* 1997;15:51–4.
18. Russell GB, Taekmann JM, Cronin AJC: Anesthesia and magnetic resonance imaging. In *Alternate-Site Anesthesia: Clinical Practice Outside the Operating Room*. Russell GB, ed. Butterworth-Heinemann, Boston: 1997, 69–82.
19. Sandner-Kiesling A, Schwarz G, Vicenzi M, et al: Side-effects after inhalational anaesthesia for paediatric cerebral magnetic resonance imaging. *Paediatr Anaesth* 2002;12(5):429–37.
20. Van Slyke MA, Wise SW, Spain JW: Computerized patient imaging. In *Alternate-Site Anesthesia: Clinical Practice Outside the Operating Room*. Russell GB, ed. Butterworth-Heinemann, Boston: 1997, 35–68.
21. Zorab JS: A general anaesthesia service for magnetic resonance imaging. *Eur J Anaesth* 1995;12:387–95.

TRACHEOBRONCHIAL STENTING

SURGICAL CONSIDERATIONS

Description: **Tracheobronchial stenting** may be performed for benign or malignant strictures of upper and lower airways that are either unsuitable for surgical reconstruction or as a temporizing measure. Patients may not be considered surgical candidates due to poor medical condition (e.g., comorbidity, recent thoracic surgery, or limited life span) or certain characteristics of the stricture (e.g., active disease, airway inflammation, extensive length, or multifocality). The most common cause of tracheobronchial obstruction is bronchogenic carcinoma, with the leading benign cause being stricture secondary to prolonged intubation. Less common causes include radiation stenosis, polychondritis, tracheomalacia, and, in children, extrinsic strictures 2° vascular malformations.

Since the first lung transplant in 1963, postsurgical bronchial stenosis has joined the list of indications for tracheobronchial stenting. Bronchial stenosis is a relatively common complication of lung transplantation, occurring in single-lung, double-lung, and heart/lung transplant recipients. It is believed that this complication is 2° the lack of bronchial arterial supply, with resulting airway ischemia. These ischemic stenoses occur at the bronchial suture line and in the more distal airway, and have been reported to occur in ~10% of patients undergoing transplantation.

Stent types: There are two primary types of airway stents: silicone-based and metallic, with both bare and covered metallic prostheses available.

Silicone stents: Silicone-based stents (Silastic) are available both as straight, short tubes and as bifurcated Y-shaped devices. Straight stents are flanged on both ends to prevent dislodgement, and can remain in place in patients for extended periods. The selection of the correct size and length is critical. The stent must be long enough to enable its flanges to anchor the stent within the stricture; short enough to avoid compromise of a lobar bronchus distally or the trachea proximally; and of satisfactory diameter to maintain the caliber of the airway. The main advantage of silicone stents is that they are easily removed, either when the patient's ventilatory status has recovered sufficiently, or when reconstructive surgery is possible. In addition, the stent can be easily repositioned to obtain optimal placement. Bifurcated silicone stents are also available to accommodate the Y-shaped configuration of the carina with extension into the distal trachea and both mainstream bronchi.

Silicone-based stents do have disadvantages. Stenotic airways need to be predilated before stent insertion, whereas metallic stents can be placed within a narrow airway lumen and subsequently dilated. Silicone stents frequently become occluded with mucus plugs and granulation tissue or tumor overgrowth; therefore, regular bronchoscopic examination and treatment are necessary to keep the airway clear. Silicone stents and covered metallic stents are more likely to migrate than bare stents due to lack of incorporation into the bronchial wall. In general, silicone stents must be placed under GA because of the need for rigid bronchoscopy.

Metallic stents: The main advantages of metallic stents (e.g., Gianturco Z, Wallstent, Palmaz) are the ease of insertion, an extremely thin wall that rapidly becomes embedded in the airway, and the large gaps in the wall that allow normal ciliary function and reduced mucus impaction. The procedure can be performed using flexible bronchoscopy in the interventional room, under deep sedation. The main disadvantage of metallic stents is the inability to remove or reposition these devices once deployed. Stents become firmly embedded in the wall of the airway and incorporated into the epithelium in < 6 weeks. Removal can be accomplished by using pincers to grip the wall of the stent and applying a twisting motion to pull the stent away from the wall. Potential complications from this maneuver are catastrophic and, in our experience, once these devices are placed, they should be considered permanent. Another problem associated with metallic stents is the development of granulation tissue either at the ends of the stents or through the interstices. This requires careful follow-up by repeat bronchoscopy and may require subsequent procedures, such as bronchoplasty, restenting, and laser tissue ablation.

Because of the flexibility and low profile of the deployment systems used for metal stents, it is feasible to place them under conscious sedation; however, our practice is to utilize GA for tracheal stent placement to reduce patient movement due to the coughing that occurs with tracheal irritation. Most bronchial interventions can be performed without full GA.

Insertion Techniques: **Silicone stents** have low inherent radial force, and strictures need to be dilated before stenting. Rigid bronchoscopy is necessary to allow dilation and subsequent stent placement. Dilation can be performed with the Holinger bronchoscope, which is abutted to the stricture and advanced with a corkscrew motion. Gum-tipped Jackson dilators and various angioplasty balloons also can be used. In patients with tracheal stomas, a T-tube stent can be inserted either via the stoma or the mouth. This extends up to the vocal cords and down as far as the carina. In patients without tracheal stomas, either Y-tubes or straight stents are inserted in a similar fashion. The stent is mounted on the rigid scope, which is advanced across the stricture and then withdrawn, leaving the stent in place. A biopsy forcep is used to advance a limb of the Y-tube into the other bronchus. Placement of stents above the carina in this fashion is relatively straightforward, and the stents can be removed and repositioned until a satisfactory result is achieved. With more distal bronchial stents, the operator's vision is somewhat obscured and deployment is more difficult.

For insertion of **metallic stents,** cross-sectional and fluoroscopic imaging is used to determine the optimal length and diameter of the stent. During the procedure, selective tracheobronchography may be performed by injecting water-soluble nonionic contrast through a catheter at the level of stricture. Flexible bronchoscopy helps guide the stent placement with a soft-tipped guidewire being advanced through either the scope or the ETT into the distal airway. In the rare case where the stricture is too narrow and tight to allow passage of a small, flexible bronchoscope, the guidewire is passed, and the lesion is stented based on fluoroscopy, reconstructed CT images or bronchography. Using fluoroscopy, the stent is positioned across the stricture and visually confirmed with bronchoscopy after deployment. For tracheal stenosis, care must be taken during intubation, as the stricture often is close to the vocal cord.

Usual preop diagnosis: Bronchial compression 2° carcinoma; post-transplantation; relapsing polychondritis; sarcoidosis

SUMMARY OF PROCEDURE	
Position	Supine
Incision	None
Special instrumentation	Bronchoscope (flexible or rigid); self-expanding metallic stent (covered and uncovered); balloon-expandable, short metallic stent
Unique considerations	May have to pull the end of the tracheal tube back to the level of the vocal cords to adequately treat the entire trachea. Alternatively can stent through LMA.
Antibiotics	Not usually administered.
Procedure time	1–2 h
EBL	0
Postop care	ICU or step-down unit
Mortality	1–5%
Morbidity	Tracheobronchial irritation (usually temporary) Stent malposition → bronchial occlusion or vocal-cord paralysis
Pain score	2–4 (first few h only)

ANESTHETIC CONSIDERATIONS

PREOPERATIVE

Respiratory compromise due to airway obstruction may pose a significant management challenge. It is therefore somewhat controversial, and highly institution-dependent, whether these procedures should be performed outside of the OR. A thorough preoperative workup is necessary before anesthesia. The majority of patients present for palliation of an obstructing pulmonary malignancy or treatment of granulation tissue obstruction of lung transplant anastomosis. Some may present emergently with impending airway obstruction that precludes a complete preoperative workup. The choice of anesthesia is primarily a function of the type of stent, surgeon preference, and the comorbid conditions of the patient. In general, silicone stent placement, which requires airway dilation with rigid bronchoscopy, will necessitate GA. Metallic stents can be placed without the need for preceding airway dilatation; therefore, either topical anesthesia, with or without conscious sedation, or GA can be used. Immediate improvements in FEV_1, FVC, and PEF can be expected after stenting of an obstructed tracheobronchial segment.

Respiratory	Patients with upper or lower airway stricture may present with cough, stridor, dyspnea, and fatigue. Airway obstruction can be classified as dynamic or fixed, depending on whether the obstruction varies with the respiratory cycle. Stridor that worsens during inspiration suggests an extrathoracic dynamic obstruction, while expiratory stridor is associated with intrathoracic dynamic obstruction. Other physical findings may include bronchospasm (in COPD patients), clubbing, or cyanosis. Preop fiber optic bronchoscopic examination and/or high-resolution, thin-section CT scans will help to define the location, size, and extent of the obstruction. In patients suspected of having tracheomalacia, scans are performed at maximal inspiration and maximal expiration to unmask subtle areas of narrowing exacerbated by ↑ intrathoracic pressure on inspiration. Using this information, the appropriate size for an ETT can be estimated and potential problems with tracheal intubation can be anticipated. **Tests:** CXR; PFTs with flow/volume loops (see Fig. 5-14, Anesthetic Considerations for Mediastinoscopy, p. 322); CT scans preferably with three-dimensional reconstructions.
Cardiovascular	Directed at any underlying disease process. Restoration of intravascular volume before induction of GA is important in patients with hypovolemia 2° chronic malnutrition from malignancy. **Tests:** As indicated from H&P.
Musculoskeletal	Patients with lung cancer may have myasthenic syndrome (Eaton-Lambert) with ↑ resistance to depolarizing muscle relaxants and ↑ sensitivity to NDMRs. Post-lung transplant patients on certain immunosuppressive therapies (e.g., cyclosporine) may have prolonged muscle blockade from NDMRs.
Hematologic	Blood cross-match not necessary unless high risk of hemorrhage from injury (e.g., rigid bronchoscopy used in patients with friable tumors). Maintaining adequate O_2-carrying capacity is important in patients with poor pulmonary reserve. **Tests:** CBC; others as indicated from H&P.
Laboratory	Other tests as indicated from H&P.
Premedication	Patients in respiratory distress are extremely anxious; however, anxiolysis has to be balanced against the risk of impending respiratory arrest in some patients. Careful titration of anxiolytic medications is necessary to avoid oversedation. An antisialagogue (e.g., glycopyrrolate 0.2 mg iv) will help minimize secretions and improve visualization through the bronchoscope. Post-lung transplant patients may be steroid-dependent and stress-dose steroid supplement may be required.

INTRAOPERATIVE

Anesthetic technique: Be prepared for an airway emergency. Preparations should be made for emergency rigid bronchoscopy and/or tracheostomy below the lesion. A variety of laryngoscope blades and ETTs of all sizes, including small, uncuffed (5–6 mm) tubes, should be readily available. Endoscopic evaluation of the airway must be performed in a spontaneously breathing patient, if the airway lesion has not been defined. Muscle relaxation must be avoided until a detailed examination is completed and the operator is certain an airway can be maintained subsequently. Vocal-cord paralysis, which can mimic tracheal stenosis, can be obscured by muscle relaxation.

Topical anesthesia	Anesthetize palate, pharynx, larynx, vocal cords, and trachea with lidocaine (2–4%), using nebulizer or having the patient gargle viscous lidocaine (4%). Avoid local anesthetic overdose.

Conscious sedation	Midazolam will increase the seizure threshold in the setting of relative local anesthetic overdose. Other options include propofol (10–100 mcg/kg/min), with or without a short acting-opioid (e.g., fentanyl 25–50 mcg; remifentanil 0.05–0.1 mcg/kg/min). Caution should be exercised when mixing opioids and sedatives to avoid respiratory depression.	
Induction	Patients should be well preoxygenated. Patients may be unable to lie flat 2° respiratory distress. Low-density helium-oxygen mixtures (Heliox) reduce airflow resistance past the obstruction, which may be beneficial in optimizing the patient. Ideally spontaneous ventilation should be maintained until the airway is secured. Inhaled sevoflurane, intravenous ketamine, judicious propofol (without opioid), or awake FOB with topical anesthesia is appropriate. Optimally, the ETT is positioned ~1 cm above the lesion. Flexible bronchoscopy of the distal airways is then performed through the stricture, and the distal extent of the stricture relative to the carina is identified. In patients with a stricture near the vocal cords, the use of an LMA is a viable option, as it avoids passing an airway through the lesion and offers the ability to bronchoscopically examine the entire lesion. Avoid muscle relaxation if possible; if necessary, consider small dose of succinylcholine (in the future: rocuronium-sugammadex). Distal or mild airway stenoses may be appropriately managed with a RSI.	
Maintenance	Inhalational anesthesia is unreliable in most cases due to the limited ventilation with a bronchoscope in situ (resistance and leak). TIVA is preferable: use propofol (50–100 mcg/kg/min) and remifentanil (0.05–0.2 mcg/kg/min) infusions. Once the airway is secured, muscle relaxation can be given to avoid movement or coughing during the procedure. Succinylcholine drip (0.25–1 g/250 mL NS, titrated to twitch suppression; avoid phase II block by keeping dose < 5–6 mg/kg), or intermediate-acting (cisatracurium 0.1 mg iv, vecuronium 0.1 mg/kg iv, Rocuronium 0.15–0.3 mg/kg IV) muscle relaxant may be used. Manual IPPV through side-arm of rigid bronchoscope or via the swivel connector if fiber optic bronchoscope is used. High-flow (up to 20 L/min) O_2 or O_2 flush (barotrauma risk) may be required to compensate for leak if rigid bronchoscope is used. Hyperventilate patient in preparation for periods of apnea. Low-frequency jet ventilation (50 psi at 10/min with I:E 1:2–4) via a Sander's injector is an alternative. Barotrauma and dynamic lung hyperinflation are potential problems with this approach.	
Emergence	Patient must be fully awake before extubation with no residual neuromuscular blockade. Emergence can be 'stormy.' Patient may cough violently to clear secretions and blood. Wake-up from remifentanil infusion tends to be smoother; consider airway suctioning and lidocaine (1 mg/kg iv) to decrease airway reactivity. Postop O_2 supplementation (preferably humidified).	
Blood and fluid requirements	IV: 18 ga × 1 NS/LR @ 1–2 mL/kg/h	Transfusion unnecessary except to optimize O_2-carrying capacity or to treat hemorrhage.
Monitoring	Standard monitors (see p. B-1) ± Arterial line	$ETCO_2$ not accurate during rigid bronchoscopy Depending on patient's comorbidities.
Positioning	Supine ✓ and pad pressure points. ✓ eyes.	
Complications	Hypoxemia	Suction secretions/blood; airway instrumentation may have to be interrupted and bronchoscope removed to improve oxygenation and ventilation.
	Hypercarbia	Commonly 2° inadequate ventilation. May cause increased sympathetic drive with 2° hypertension/ tachycardia/ dysrhythmias. Simply↑ TV and RR.
	Hypertension	Ensure adequate ventilation and sedative/ anesthesia.
	Bronchospasm	Rx: bronchodilator (e.g., albuterol puff)
	Stent dislodgement	From coughing or movement. Ensure adequate anesthesia and muscle relaxation.
	Bleeding	More likely with rigid bronchoscope.

Complications (cont'd)	Tracheobronchial injury Aspiration of debris	Requires frequent suctioning. Major hemorrhage may require thoracotomy using DLT or BB to isolate and/or tamponade bleeding site. Transfusion. Patient may need to be kept intubated after the procedure.

POSTOPERATIVE

Complications	Airway edema	Rx with corticosteroids (dexamethasone 10 mg IV) and/or racemic epinephrine nebulizer. Impending airway obstruction will require reintubation.
	Airway obstruction	May be catastrophic. Secretion retention or stent dislodgement. Rigorous suction. Reintubation or restenting.
	Stent fracture/migration	May be catastrophic. May require emergent reintubation or restenting.
	Pneumothorax	Obtain CXR. May require chest tube placement if > 20%.
	Secretion retention	humidified O_2
Pain management	None	

Suggested Readings

1. Brodsky JB: Anesthesia for pulmonary stent insertion. *Curr Opin Anaesthesiol* 2003;16:65–7.
2. Conacher ID: Anaesthesia and tracheobronchial stenting for central airway obstruction in adults. *Br J Anaesth* 2003;90(3): 367–74.
3. Hautmann H, Gamarra F, Henke M, et al: High frequency jet ventilation in interventional fiberoptic bronchoscopy. *Anesth Analg* 2000;90(6):1436–40.
4. Lemaire A, Burfeind WR, Toloza E, et al: Outcomes of tracheobronchial stents in patients with malignant airway disease. *Ann Thorac Surg* 2005;80(2):434–7.
5. Lund MD, Garland R, Ernst A: Airway stenting: applications and practice management considerations. *Chest* 2007;131(2): 579–87.
6. Ochroch EA: Pro: laser endobronchial treatment does not need to occur in the operating room. *J Cardiothorac Vasc Anesth* 2005;19(1):118–20.
7. Profili S, Manca A, Feo CF, et al: Palliative airway stenting performed under radiological guidance and local anesthesia. *Cardiovasc Intervent Radiol* 2007;30(1):74–8.
8. Vaitkeviciute I, Ehrenwerth J: Con: bronchial stenting and laser airway surgery should not take place outside the operating room. *J Cardiothorac Vasc Anesth* 2005;19(1):121–2.

RADIOFREQUENCY ABLATION

SURGICAL CONSIDERATIONS

Description: **Radiofrequency ablation (RFA)** was pioneered in 1920 by Harvey Cushing for the creation of small lesions within the CNS. Since then, the technique has been refined so that precise control of lesion size can be achieved by measuring the temperature and electrical resistance within the tissues being treated. Ablating neural tissue with RF is successful in treating pain from trigeminal neuralgia, facet osteoarthritis, and failed-back syndrome. RFA has expanded treatment options for certain solid organ tumors such as hepatocellular carcinomas, colorectal metastasis to the liver, primary and secondary lung cancers, renal cell carcinoma, and painful bone lesions. Since RFA is most often done percutaneously, it is well suited for the treatment of primary and secondary malignancies in the liver, as well as other sites in patients who are not suitable for open surgery.

Mechanism of tissue destruction: In RFA, an alternating current operating in the frequency of radio waves (460–480 kHz) is emitted from the tip of an electrode or needle placed directly into tissues. This alternating current causes the local ions to vibrate, producing heat and inducing cell death by coagulative necrosis. The cytotoxic T threshold is 50°C; however, with RFA, temperatures can exceed this, and actually reach the boiling point of water (100°C). A limitation of RFA is the small lesion size it creates. Recent technical advances in RF systems have improved such that lesions > 5 cm in diameter can be created.

Techniques of radiofrequency ablation: Grounding pads are placed on the patient's thighs; if a single RF treatment probe is used, at least two and, preferably, four pads (96-cm^2 surface area each) or the equivalent (minimum total surface area = ~200 cm^2) must be used. If a three-probe cluster is used, at least four RF grounding pads or their equivalent (~400 cm^2 surface area) must be used. Presently available commercial generators usually require four grounding pads. The grounding pads and the treatment probes are connected to the RF generator. When the generator is activated, current flows between the conductive electrode tip and the grounding pads (or 'dispersive electrode'). The increase in the tissue T is proportional to the current density. Since the density is highest near the conductive electrode tip, coagulation is induced in the tissue surrounding the treatment probe. The linear extent (depth) of the resulting coagulation is determined by the length of the uninsulated probe tip, while the diameter of coagulation necrosis produced around the probe tip depends on the duration of treatment. Based on our experience using perfusion probes and pulsed current technique, areas of the tissue up to 4.5 cm diameter may be induced with a single probe and up to 7.3 cm diameter with clustered probes.

The lesion to be treated is identified and characterized by ultrasound or CT, which is used to guide the RF probe to the distal margin of the lesion. The generator is activated and output is gradually increased to a predetermined maximum, based on tip exposure and probe configuration (single vs clustered probes). Maximum power (90–120 Watts) is applied to the treatment probe cluster until tissue impedance rises. At this point, the power is turned off for 60 sec, then increased to maximum until once again impedance is seen to rise. Ultrasound monitoring of the RF site may be carried out throughout the ablation; however, it usually is limited due to the production of tissue water vapor that interferes with the transmission of the sound waves. CT can be used occasionally to check the stable position of the needle. Final tissue temperatures usually range from 60°–90°C.

Lesion size varies according to the size of the electrode, the current, duration of the treatment, and local blood flow. Tumor cells adjacent to large blood vessels may not be treated thoroughly due to the heat-sink effect of flowing blood, which carries away the RF energy as fast as it is deposited. Alternatively, cirrhotic livers with extensive fibrosis and ↓ blood flow may need fewer treatments because of increased conduction through the tumor compared to surrounding tissue, a phenomenon termed as the "oven effect" that helps achieve larger coagulation diameters.

Liver RF: The most well-known and best-studied application of RF is in the treatment of primary and metastatic liver tumors. RF has been used widely to treat HCC as well as metastases. Prospective and retrospective studies have demonstrated that complete necrosis can be achieved in 90% of tumors measuring < 3 cm in fewer than two sessions. However, the success rate drops markedly in tumors measuring > 3.5cm with complete necrosis achieved in < 50% at two sessions.

Lung RF: Recently, RF energy has been used to attempt ablation of certain primary and secondary lung tumors. The work that has been done to date has been performed in patients whose disease extent offers few therapeutic options. The results, therefore, have been understandably mixed; however, there has been a satisfying lack of major complications reported. Pneumothorax is seen in ~30% of cases (similar to rates reported during lung biopsy); and, while transcranial Doppler has demonstrated microbubbles in the brain during ablation, there have been no reported sequelae. The same basic technique is used, although lower energies are applied, since there is less solid tissue in the lung, and high levels of impedance are reached sooner.

Bone RF: RF has been applied to both benign and malignant bone tumors. The first use was for the thermocoagulation of small, painful, osteoid osteomas. The pain in an osteoid osteoma is related to prostaglandin production within the cells of the small, central, vascularized tumor nidus. Pain relief is obtained only after complete removal of the nidus, surgically or percutaneously. Surgical removal requires cortical osteotomy and a hospital stay. Recently, RF has emerged as the method of choice for treating osteoid osteoma. The ablation is done percutaneously, usually under CT guidance as an outpatient procedure. The nidus is located and a single tip RF electrode is placed in the nidus. Because the area of treatment is almost always < 1 cm, larger, multi-tined electrodes are not required. Energy required to destroy the nidus is minimal. Patients typically have 1–2 days of postprocedure pain that differs from the pain of osteoid osteoma. Relief of the osteoid osteoma pain almost always occurs within the first 24–48 hours. Cure with one session can be as high as 90% and re-treatment can be performed if the first treatment is not immediately successful or if the patient's pain returns in the future.

Preliminary studies in **malignant bone tumor treatment** with RF show promise. Previously irradiated foci of tumor, whether primary or metastatic, that are still biologically active can be treated locally with internally cooled RF electrodes. Local pain control in painful bone metastases and control of hemorrhage in both the axial and appendicular skeletons have responded well to RF ablation. In areas where tumor abuts vital structures, such as the spinal cord, RF may not be effective, since local thermal injury may not be desirable. However, spinal RF can be performed in the vertebral body when the cortex between the electrode and the spinal canal is intact.

Usual preop diagnosis: Primary or metastatic hepatic malignancy; primary or metastatic pulmonary malignancy; osteoid osteoma.

SUMMARY OF PROCEDURE

Position	Supine or prone
Incision	Over the site to be accessed
Special instrumentation	RFA probes and generator
Unique considerations	Mild ↑ T during procedure; ↑ pain as ablation continues.
Antibiotics	None usually; occasionally, ciprofloxacin 500 mg iv
Procedure time	2–4 h
EBL	None
Postop care	Step-down unit
Mortality	< 5%
Morbidity	Postprocedure pain at site Hepatic hemorrhage: Rare, due to cauterizing nature of procedure Pneumothorax (during hepatic dome lesion ablation, pulmonary ablation) Hepatic abscess (↑ incidence in patients with previous biliary manipulation)
Pain Score	5–8 (first few h only)

PATIENT POPULATION CHARACTERISTICS

Age range	Adults
Male:Female	M > F
Incidence	Uncommon
Etiology	Pain (trigeminal neuralgia; facet osteoarthritis; metastatic cancer); primary malignancies
Associated conditions	Lung cancer; cancers of the neck; polychondritis; prolonged ICU stay; lung transplantation

ANESTHETIC CONSIDERATIONS

Patients presenting for RF ablation range from those with end-stage lung cancer to otherwise healthy chronic-pain patients. In addition, analgesic/anesthetic requirements are highly variable, depending on the size and location of the target lesions. Close communication between the various care providers is essential to achieving a positive outcome.

Respiratory	Access to the airway may be limited in the typical interventional radiology suite; thus, a patient with a potentially difficult airway may require elective intubation. Appropriate airway adjuncts (LMAs, light wand, fiber optic cart, etc.) should be readily available. Intraop risks include the possibility of pneumothorax, so needle decompression supplies also should be available. Lung cancer patients presenting for tumor ablation may have compromised pulmonary function and require objective assessment of pathophysiology with PFTs and/or ABG analysis. **Tests:** PFTs, ABG, as indicated from H&P.

Cardiovascular	HTN and CHF are seen frequently in elderly patients presenting for RF procedures. These patients often have a severe disease process, which may be complicated by other significant comorbidities. The potential for cardiac ischemia should be evaluated carefully. Preop beta blockade and antihypertensive therapy may be required. **Tests:** ECG, ECHO, noninvasive stress testing as indicated from H&P.
Neurological	A thorough neurological exam is important to document neurological deficits that are present before the procedure.
Hepatic	Patients may have coagulation defects and mental status changes 2° systemic liver disease. The potential for severe hemorrhage from vascular injury, the risk of aspiration, and the lack of cooperation (encephalopathy) should all be taken into account when planning the anesthesia. Patients with severe liver disease also may exhibit hepatopulmonary or hepatorenal syndrome manifested as hypoxemia or renal failure. Consider the need for preop correction of coagulation and fluid status. **Tests:** LFTs; ammonia; INR
Endocrine	The possibility of endocrine and metabolic derangements should be assessed. Lung cancer patients may have electrolyte problems 2° SIADH, while patients with liver disease are prone to developing hypoglycemia. **Tests:** As indicated from H&P.
Hematologic	Consider the possibility of chronic anemia or hypercoagulability 2° neoplastic disease. Chemotherapy or systemic disease may have depressed bone marrow function and altered the activity of WBCs and Plts. **Tests:** Hct, Plt count, or CBC, as indicated by H&P.
Premedication	Sedation must be adjusted according to patient requirements. Small doses of midazolam, titrated to minimal sedation, are most reasonable (0.5–1 mg increments). Patients with end-stage disease often require very little premedication.

INTRAOPERATIVE

Anesthetic technique: Sedation or GA, depending on the size and location of lesions. Most ablations are well tolerated with MAC; however, large lesions may require GA. The out-of-OR site often involves working in cramped quarters with poor access to anesthesia equipment. Nevertheless, the ASA standards of monitoring should be followed.

MAC: MAC cases are performed with fentanyl (25–150 mcg) and midazolam (0.5–2 mg) boluses, combined with a propofol infusion (25–100 mcg/kg/min). The substitution of remifentanil (0.02–0.1 mcg/kg/min) for fentanyl allows rapid titration of analgesia for the brief periods of intense stimulation.

Induction	Standard induction (see p. B-2), preceding placement of an ETT or LMA.	
Maintenance	Standard maintenance (see p. B-2). Since procedures are of an unpredictable duration, short-acting muscle relaxants (e.g., mivacurium 0.2 mg/kg, rocuronium 0.6 mg/kg) are advised. Propofol (25–100 mcg/kg/min) and remifentanil (0.02–0.1 mcg/kg/min) are an appropriate combination that easily can be titrated to effect. Persistent intraop HTN may be treated with labetalol (5–25 mg) or hydralazine (5–20 mg).	
Emergence	Standard emergence (see p. B-3). Short-acting analgesics (e.g., fentanyl 25–150 mcg) should be used in outpatients. Prophylactic treatment with antiemetics (metoclopramide 10 mg and granisetron 100 mcg iv) may be beneficial, since there is a high incidence of PONV.	
Blood and fluid requirements	IV: 20–14 ga × 1–2 NS/LR: 3–5 mL/kg/h	Larger access needed for hepatic lesions.
Monitoring	Standard monitors (see p. B-1) ± Arterial line ± Urinary catheter	Foley for longer procedures (> 2 h)

Positioning	✓ & pad pressure points ✓ eyes.	Radiology tables often poorly padded.
Complications	Hemorrhage	Blood or colloid should be readily available, if the need is anticipated. Large retroperitoneal hemorrhage can develop, yet not be appreciated until blood loss is extensive.
	Pneumothorax Hemothorax	Needle decompression and/or thoracostomy tube placement may be necessary during thoracic or high hepatic procedures.
	Electrical shock Thermal injury	Electrocautery devices can produce serious injury if not properly grounded.
	Hyperthermia	Patients may develop rapid T increases 2° direct heating of large lesions.

POSTOPERATIVE

Complications	PONV	Common.
	Hemorrhage	Occult blood loss may continue for several h after the procedure is terminated.
Pain management	Standard pain management (see p. C-2)	Postprocedure pain is usually well-tolerated.
Tests	Postprocedure HCT, as indicated.	

Suggested Readings

1. Amin Z, Donald JJ, Masters A, et al: Hepatic metastases: interstitial laser photocoagulation with real-time US monitoring and dynamic CT evaluation of treatment. *Radiology* 1993;187(2):339–47.
2. De Giovanni JV: Treatment of arrhythmias by radiofrequency ablation. *Arch Dis Childhood* 1995;73(5):385–7.
3. Eagle KA, Berger PB, Calkins H, et al: ACC/AHA Guideline Update for Perioperative Cardiovascular evaluation for Noncardiac Surgery: A Report of the American College of Cardiology/American Heart Association Task Force on Practice Guidelines (Committee to Update the 1996 Guidelines on Perioperative Cardiovascular Evaluation for Noncardiac Surgery), 2002.
4. Erb TO, Hall JM, Ing RJ, et al: Postoperative nausea and vomiting in children and adolescents undergoing radiofrequency catheter ablation: a randomized comparison of propofol- and isoflurane-based anesthetics. *Anesth Analg* 2002;95(6):1577–81.
5. Goldberg SN, Solbiati L, Hahn PF, et al: Large-volume tissue ablation with radiofrequency by using a clustered, internally cooled electrode technique: laboratory and clinical experience in liver metastases. *Radiology* 1998;209:371–9.
6. Le Groupe de Rythmologie de la Societe Francaise de Cardiologie: Complications of radiofrequency ablation: a French experience. *Arch Mal Coeur Vaiss* 1996;89(12):1599–605.
7. Livraghi T, Goldberg SN, Lzzaroni S, et al: Hepatocellular carcinoma: radio-frequency ablation of medium and large lesions. *Radiology* 2000;214(3):761–8.
8. Murakami R, Yoshimatsu S, Yamashita Y, et al: Treatment of hepatocellular carcinoma: Value of percutaneous microwave coagulation. *AJR* 1995;164:1159–64.
9. Rhim H, Yoon KH, Lee JM, et al: Major complications after radio-frequency thermal ablation of hepatic tumors: spectrum of imaging findings. *Radiographics* 2003;23(l):123–34.
10. Rosenthal DI, Hornicek FJ, Wolfe MW, et al: Changes in the management of osteoid osteoma. *J Bone Joint Surg* 1998;80:815–21.
11. Rossi S, Buscarini E, Garbagnati F, et al: Percutaneous treatment of small hepatic tumors by an expandable RF needle electrode. *AJR* 1998;170:1015–22.
12. Sabo B, Dodd G, Halff G, et al: Anesthetic considerations in patients undergoing percutaneous radiofrequency interstitial tissue ablation. *AANA Journal* 1999;67(5):467–8.
13. Seki T, Wakabayashi M, Nakagawa T, et al: Ultrasonically guided percutaneous microwave coagulation therapy for small hepatocellular carcinoma. *Cancer* 1994;74:817–25.
14. Solbiati L, Ierace T, Goldberg SN, et al: Percutaneous US-guided RF tissue ablation liver metastases: long-term follow up. *Radiology* 1997;202:195–203.
15. Vogl TJ, Muller PK, Hammerstingl R, et al: Malignant liver tumors treated with MR imaging-guided laser-induced thermotherapy: technique and prospective results. *Radiology* 1995;196:257–65.

CHAPTER

13.2 Out-of-Operating Room Procedures—Pediatric

SURGEONS, CARDIOLOGISTS, RADIOLOGISTS

Sarah S. Donaldson, MD, FACR, FASTRO (*Radiation Oncology*)
Anne M. Dubin, MD (*Pediatric cardiac catheterization*)
Jeffrey A. Feinstein, MD, MPH (*Pediatric cardiac catheterization*)
Gary E. Hartman, MD (*ECMO*)
Trang H. La, MD (*Radiation Oncology*)
Stanton B. Perry, MD (*Pediatric cardiac catheterization*)
Kalyani R. Trivedi, MD (*Pediatric cardiac catheterization*)

ANESTHESIOLOGISTS

M. Gail Boltz, MD (*Pediatric cardiac catheterization*)
Rebecca E. Claure, MD (*Radiation therapy, oncology, endoscopy, imaging*)
Brenda Golianu, MD (*Radiation therapy, oncology, endoscopy, imaging*)
Chandra Ramamoorthy, MD (*Pediatric cardiac catheterization, ECMO*)
R.J. Ramamurthi, MD, FRCA (*ECMO*)
Neyssa Marina, MD (*Oncology*)

PEDIATRIC RADIATION THERAPY

PROCEDURAL CONSIDERATIONS

Trang La and Sarah S. Donaldson

Description: Modern pediatric radiation therapy (XRT) requires that the patient be in a stable and reproducible position for daily treatment. Sharply defined beams with secondary collimation are used to irradiate the tumor volume and to spare normal tissue. Patient movement may undermine techniques for sparing normal tissue and, while movement cannot be completely prevented, it must be minimized. In very young children, it is often impossible to prevent movement and achieve adequate cooperation for radiation treatment. In such cases, daily anesthesia is required. Close cooperation of the radiation oncology and anesthesia teams allows for safe and reproducible daily treatment. In general, children older than 3 or 4 years can be persuaded to lie still for radiation therapy. Children from 2.5–4 yr may cooperate during the treatment (which is usually < 15 min), but not for the treatment planning and simulation, in which an immobilization-stabilization device is made (often requiring 1–1.5 h). In most infants and young children (< 2.5 yr), anesthesia is essential.

The optimal position for XRT also must be optimal for the anesthesiologist. Ideally, the area to be treated is determined using 3-dimensional conformal techniques to optimize treatment and to minimize normal tissue exposure. This requires an imaging study (e.g., CT scan), with the patient in the same position as will be used during the radiation treatment. A series of radiographs are taken at the treatment-planning appointment, which typically lasts 1–1.5 h and requires GA. It is essential that there be no patient movement between exposures; if the patient moves, the entire procedure must be repeated. After examining the radiographs, the area to be scanned is determined; then the patient is transported (anesthetized) to the CT suite for a 3-dimensional treatment-planning CT scan. Thereafter, the specific area can be determined and individual beam-shaping devices made.

Seven to 10 days following the initial planning session, the patient has a verification procedure, which usually is of shorter duration—often requiring only 30 min. of anesthesia time. The verification procedure consists of a series of radiographs using the beam-shaping devices, which simulate the treatment to be given. When this procedure is successfully completed, the anesthetized patient is moved to the treatment room. The child is put in the identical position achieved during the planning/verification procedures and treatment is administered.

The first day or two, and weekly thereafter, a verification x-ray (called a "port film") is taken to confirm the accuracy of the treatment field. The treatment itself is only a few minutes in duration for each field; ideally, the entire procedure is completed within 15–30 min. A newer form of radiotherapy treatment planning and delivery known as intensity-modulated radiotherapy (IMRT) requires slightly longer treatment times due to the larger number and increased complexity of fields treated. A course of treatment may be only a few days, or may last for 5–6 wk, generally with treatment given 5 × per week. Occasionally, multiple (2–3) treatments per day are given at 4–8-h (usually 6 h) intervals. At the initial appointment, the patient's optimal position is determined, an immobilization device is constructed, and measurements are taken. The immobilization device is usually a body cradle or cast, and often a head/face mask is made for head and neck or brain treatment. Initially, temporary marks or Band-Aids are used; however, when the final positioning has been determined, a more permanent mark, such as a tattoo, is applied. Often, a head holder with a mask is applied to ensure the position for XRT.

In managing certain brain tumors (e.g., medulloblastoma, high-grade intratentorial ependymoma, germ cell tumors, and CNS leukemia), **cranial spinal irradiation** (CSI) is used. Conventionally, this procedure requires that the patient be placed in the prone position with the head flexed as much as possible to minimize a cervical lordosis. This positioning, however, creates special difficulties for the anesthesiologist. If the child is intubated for the setup, the radiation stabilization device must allow space for the ETT. If the child is not intubated, there must be adequate access to the airway. Newer techniques allow patients to be treated with CSI in the supine position, facilitating easier airway access for the anesthesiologist, more secure patient immobilization, and faster treatment times.

Fractionation: Pediatric protocols have been testing the efficacy of giving multiple fractions (treatments) of radiation 2–3 × per day, usually at 6-hour intervals, to allow higher total radiation doses to be administered with possible less normal-tissue morbidity. These schemes have been or are being evaluated for children with central nervous system tumors and total body irradiation (TBI) in preparation for bone marrow transplantation. Until proven to be of increased efficacy, such schemes should remain part of large protocol studies. The timing of radiotherapy may be at 4-, 6-, or 8-hour intervals 2–3 × per day, depending on the protocol. These studies provide several challenges for anesthesiologists, radiotherapists, and parents. Radiotherapy under anesthesia, however, has been successfully administered to infants undergoing multiple fractions per day. Attention must be given to potential malnutrition and/or dehydration from prolonged periods of npo status.

Total body irradiation (TBI): Although most TBI techniques are administered with the patient standing, infants and small children must lie prone and supine for the treatment. This positioning requires sedation and/or anesthesia. Retching and vomiting, sometimes provoked by the radiation, present an additional challenge for proper radiotherapy technique, as well as for anesthetic management.

Radiosurgery: The technique of using stereotactically localized radiosurgery with a highly collimated radiotherapy photon beam, as generated from a linear accelerator, is currently being employed for select patients with small CNS tumors or base-of-skull tumors. There is increasing enthusiasm for this technique for infants and children with recurrent posterior fossa and cerebral tumors, craniopharyngiomas, optic nerve and chiasmal gliomas, and small AVMs. Radiosurgery can be performed with a frame-based or frameless technique. Frame-based radiosurgery requires 6–10 h of continuous anesthesia while a patient undergoes application of a metal frame, CT localization, and multiport radiotherapy treatment. Newer technology, using image guidance, now allows frameless radiosurgery. This technique requires a 1–1.5-h treatment planning and simulation session followed by a single fraction or limited number of treatment sessions each lasting 1.5–2 h. These approaches require close coordination between the anesthesiologist, neurosurgeon, and radiotherapist.

Usual preop diagnosis: Leukemia; retinoblastoma; most of the solid tumors of childhood

SUMMARY OF PROCEDURES

	Standard XRT/ IMRT	TBI	Frameless Radiosurgery
Position	Supine or prone	Supine and prone	Supine or prone
Unique considerations	If prone: head flexed for maximal straightening of the C-spine.	May be repeated 2–3 9D at 4–6-h intervals.	Head extended for stabilization of airway.
Anesthesia time	Planning: 30–120 min Treatment: < 15 min (IMRT: 15–30 min)	45–60 min < 20 min	30–90 min 90–120 min
Postop care	PACU → home	PACU → room	PACU → home

PATIENT POPULATION CHARACTERISTICS

Age range	Usually ≤ 4 yr
Male:Female	1:1
Incidence	NA
Associated conditions:	**Brain tumors:** ↑ ICP is of concern in these patients. Postradiation edema following the first few treatments may further ↑ ICP, with potential for brain stem herniation. Some children with brain stem tumors are particularly difficult to anesthetize, perhaps because of disruption of nerve pathways in those areas of the brain stem that are affected by anesthetics. **Diabetes insipidus (DI):** It is often impossible to withhold fluids for 4-6 h prior to radiotherapy in an infant with symptomatic polydipsia from DI. **Neuroblastoma:** Neuroblastomas are capable of secreting catecholamines and related substances; hence, there is a potential for paroxysmal HTN during anesthesia induction. In these children, the principles of anesthetic management are similar to those for pheochromocytoma. **Retinoblastoma:** It is imperative that the patient be properly immobilized with no movement, as even a mm of change, as occurs with a sigh, may cause unnecessary radiation to the radiosensitive lens and anterior chamber. Optimal anesthesia prevents nystagmus and motion of the head. Even minimal lateral or rotary nystagmus may increase the risk of cataract induction.

ANESTHETIC CONSIDERATIONS

Rebecca E. Claure and Brenda Golianu

PREPROCEDURE

Orientation to the XRT suite, reassurance, positive reinforcement, and play therapy, can reduce the number of children requiring anesthesia for XRT; however, the majority of children ≤ 4 yrs will require anesthesia. A detailed preanesthesia visit is essential and is also an opportunity to gain the confidence of both child and parents. The majority of these patients will have received chemotherapy and should be evaluated for toxic side effects. The importance of NPO status needs to be stressed repeatedly, discussing the potential danger of emesis during treatment. Written instructions regarding preop protocols are extremely helpful in this context. For children with cancer, prolonged preop fasting for XRT once or twice daily could severely compromise an already marginal nutritional intake. Infants, children, and adolescents should be encouraged to drink clear liquids until 2 hours before treatment. Milk and solid foods should be held for an appropriate time interval (6 h). Reassessment before each anesthetic is recommended because the patient's medical status may change during the course of radiation therapy. Some children will have Sx of ↑ ICP which must be taken into account when designing an anesthetic plan to avoid ↑ $PaCO_2$ and other factors that may further ↑ ICP.

The most common diagnoses are: primary CNS tumor (28–33%), retinoblastoma (9–26%), acute leukemia (9–26%), neuroblastoma (2–18%), lymphoma (8%), rhabdomyosarcoma (5–7%), Wilms' tumor (5%), and Ewings (5%). The total number of treatments can range from 1–65 (median 20–24). Many patients require a mold of the head and neck. The prone position was required during 19–21% of treatments. Children can range in age from infants to adolescents, with a median age of 2.4–3.8 yr.

Respiratory	Careful evaluation for respiratory compromise due to chemotherapy. Patients with Sx of URI (rhinorrhea, cough, fever) are commonly seen during XRT treatment. If Sxs are significant, XRT should be delayed and the patient should be evaluated by primary service. Fortunately, most children can be managed without the use of an ETT, which itself can increase the risk of oxygen desaturation, laryngospasm, and bronchospasm. As always, the benefit of XRT vs. delaying treatment must be balanced against the risks of anesthesia. **Tests:** As indicated from H&P.
Cardiac	Careful evaluation for cardiac compromise due to chemotherapy. **Tests:** As indicated from H&P
Neurologic	Patients with intracranial tumors may have ↑ ICP. Postradiation edema following the first few treatments may further ↑ ICP. Sx include irritability, HA, N/V, and papilledema. Suspicion of ↑ ICP mandates ET intubation and controlled ventilation to induce hypocarbia.
Laboratory	Tests as indicated from H&P.
Premedication	Usually unnecessary in this patient group. Parents usually present for induction and majority of patients have some form of central venous access or heplock in situ. If inhalational induction necessary, midazolam 0.5–0.75 mg/kg po may be helpful. Inappropriate sedation may cause respiratory or cardiovascular depression and prolong recovery.

INTRAPROCEDURE

Anesthetic technique: Provision of anesthesia to children at sites remote from the OR is challenging. During XRT, patients must remain immobile so that the tumor can be reliably irradiated while minimizing damage to uninvolved tissue. Anesthetic goals should include: patient immobility, rapid onset, brief duration of action, and prompt recovery. The anesthetic should allow maintenance of a patent airway and spontaneous ventilation in a variety of body positions. Ketamine is a potent sialogogue and can cause nystagmus, which prevents precision radiation of retinoblastomas. It may cause prolonged or unpleasant emergence and should be avoided in patients with ↑ ICP. Choice of anesthetic technique may be limited by equipment or logistical issues. Anesthesia machines may not be available in all XRT suites.

Induction	**IV:** Propofol (2–4 mg/kg), titrated slowly to effect. Intubation is usually unnecessary, except for patients with ↑ ICP or those with potential for airway obstruction. **Inhalation:** Mask induction with sevoflurane is appropriate in children without iv access, and may be preferred by some children. Again, intubation is usually unnecessary. The airway can almost always be maintained by careful positioning and extension of the neck. It is essential that this same degree of extension/flexion be maintained for each treatment. A molded immobilization device may be placed over the patient's head and neck.

Maintenance	**IV:** Propofol (100–250 mcg/kg/min) by continuous infusion. Supplemental O_2 should be administered via nasal prongs. **Inhalation:** Sevoflurane in O_2.	
Emergence	Patients awaken rapidly following cessation of propofol infusion or sevoflurane. Extubate patient fully awake, unless there is the possibility of ↑ ICP, in which case a deep extubation may be appropriate. XRT can cause nausea/vomiting so antiemetics should be given (ondansetron 0.1–0.15 mg/kg). Avoid dexamethasone (may conflict with chemotherapy protocols and in rare cases may cause tumor lysis syndrome).	
Blood and fluid requirements	IV: NS/LR:	Majority of children receiving radiotherapy have some form of central venous access. Maintenance.
Monitoring	Standard monitors (see p. D-1).	A critical problem is the lack of access to the patient and monitors during XRT. A video camera with a zoom lens can focus on the monitors and a second camera is trained on the patient. In XRT suites with a viewing window, a small marker may be placed on the chest so that the rise and fall of chest motion is seen easily. Respiration also may be assessed by direct visualization.
Positioning	✓ and pad pressure points ✓ eyes.	Careful positioning 2° possible chemotherapy induced peripheral neuropathy.
Complications	Airway obstruction Patient movement	Respiratory obstruction may occur; it usually responds to nasal or oral airways and careful repositioning. In rare instances, intubation may be required for persistent airway obstruction. Deepen anesthesia.

POSTPROCEDURE

Complications	PONV Central line sepsis Cerebral edema	Many patients have chemotherapy induced nausea, which may be exacerbated by anesthesia, XRT, and stress. Patients may be immunocompromised following chemotherapy. Attention to sterility during access of the central venous line is critical, because repeated use by multiple health care providers ↑ risk of catheter contamination. Aseptic preparation of anesthetic iv medications, especially propofol, is important. In patients with ↑ ICP, XRT can provoke an acute ↑ ICP, with consequent ↑ HA, ↑ N/V, ↓ consciousness, and cardiac arrest. These patients should be monitored × 24-h post-XRT.
Pain management	Standard approaches	Radiation treatments are not associated with pain, but narcotics may be useful in relieving pain associated with neoplastic disease.

Suggested Readings

1. Bauman GS, Brett CM, Ciricillo SF, et al: Anesthesia for pediatric stereotactic radiosurgery. *Anesthesiology* 1998; 89(1):255–7.
2. Buehrer S, Immoos S. Frei M, et al. Evaluation of propofol for repeated prolonged deep sedation in children undergoing proton radiation therapy. *Br J Anaesth* 2007 Oct; 99(4):556–60.
3. Donaldson SS, Egbert PR: Retinoblastoma. In *Principles and Practice of Pediatric Oncology*. Pizzo PA, Poplack DG, eds, JB Lippincott, Philadelphia: 1989, 555–68.
4. Donaldson SS, Shostak CA, Samuels SI: Technical and practical considerations in the radiotherapy of children. *Front Radiat Ther Oncol* 1987; 21(1):256–69.

5. Fortney JT, Halperin EC, Hertz CM, et al: Anesthesia for pediatric external beam radiation therapy. *Int J Rad Oncol Biol Phys* 1999; 44(3):587–91.
6. Harnett AN, Hungerford JL, Lambert GD, et al: Improved external beam radiotherapy for the treatment of retinoblastoma. *Br J Radiol* 1987; 60(716):753–60.
7. Keidan I, Perel A, Shabtai E, et al: Children undergoing repeated exposures for radiation therapy do not develop tolerance to propofol. *Anesthesiology* 2004 Feb; 100(2):251–4.
8. Lo JN, Buckley JJ, Kim TH, et al: Anesthesia for high-dose total body irradiation in children. *Anesthesiology* 1984; 61(1):101–3.
9. Menache L, Eifel PJ, Kennamer DL, et al: Twice-daily anesthesia in infants receiving hyper-fractionated irradiation. *Int J Radiat Oncol Biol Phys* 1990; 18(3):625–9.
10. Motoyama EK, Davis PJ, eds: *Smith's Anesthesia for Infants and Children*, 7th edition. Mosby Elsevier, Philadelphia:2006. 849–850.
11. Murray WJ: Anesthesia for external beam radiotherapy. In *Pediatric Radiation Oncology*, Halperin EC, Kun LE, Constine LS, et al., eds. Raven Press, New York: 1989, 399–407.
12. Parker WA, Freeman CR: A simple technique for craniospinal irradiation in the supine position. *Radiotherapy Oncol* 2006; 78(2):217–22.
13. Roy WL: Anaesthetizing children in remote locations: necessary expeditions or anaesthetic misadventures? *Can J Anaesth* 1996; 43(8):764–8.
14. Seiler G, De Vol E, Khafaga Y, et al: Evaluation of the safety and efficacy of repeated sedations for the radiotherapy of young children with cancer: a prospective study of 1033 consecutive sedations. *Int J Radiat Oncol Biol Phys* 2001; 49(3):771–83.
15. Singapuri K, Russell GB: Anesthesia and radiation therapy. In *Alternate-Site Anesthesia: Clinical Practice Outside the Operating Room.* Russell GB, ed. Butterworth-Heinemann, Boston: 1997, 365–80.

PEDIATRIC CARDIAC CATHETERIZATION AND ELECTROPHYSIOLOGY

PROCEDURAL CONSIDERATIONS

Kalyani R. Trivedi, Anne M. Dubin, Stanton B. Perry, and Jeffrey A. Feinstein

Cardiac catheterization and electrophysiology testing have evolved over the recent decades from purely diagnostic tools to combined diagnostic and therapeutic procedures. Although the use of anesthesiologists and GA varies from institution to institution, higher levels of sedation are required at a minimum for critically ill patients, those requiring complex interventional strategies, small children who must remain totally still, and when TEE is used for image-guided therapy. A thorough review of diagnostic and interventional cardiac catheterization and electrophysiology is not possible in this chapter, and the interested reader is referred to the multiple textbooks available on the subject.

The placement of anesthesia equipment for these procedures must allow for: (a) proper positioning of the patient, (b) easy access to the head and neck and/or groin for the physician performing the procedure, and (c) rotation and angulation of the imaging equipment. The goal of sedation in all of these procedures is to provide a nontraumatic, safe environment for the patient. Many patients can be cared for adequately and safely using conscious sedation; however, there is a subset of pediatric patients who may require GA. This group may include patients with complex congenital heart disease, ventricular dysfunction, or airway abnormalities. It is important to understand that certain anesthetic agents may alter cardiac conduction, making arrhythmia inducibility more difficult. Catecholamine-dependent arrhythmias, such as an automatic atrial tachycardia, may be impossible to induce with the patient under GA. Furthermore, the arrhythmia itself may complicate anesthetic care, by causing sudden decreases in BP due to excessively rapid rates. In patients undergoing radiofrequency ablation (RFA) in areas close to other critical structures of the heart, GA may be necessary to keep the patient motionless during application of energy.

VASCULAR ACCESS

The modified **Seldinger technique** of cannulating blood vessels percutaneously is used to establish vascular access for cardiac catheterization. (The femoral, IJ, and subclavian veins are most commonly used for venous access.) Transhepatic access to the IVC has been used safely and successfully in patients without femoral venous access. The femoral artery is most commonly used, although the carotid and axillary arteries may be used for specific procedures or when there is bilateral femoral artery occlusion. In newborns, the umbilical artery and vein may be used. Access may be especially difficult in patients who have undergone multiple previous procedures. In the most severe cases,

reconstructive transcatheter techniques, including **balloon angioplasty** and **stent implantation** to rehabilitate the vessels, have been used to allow future catheter-based diagnostic and therapeutic interventions.

Infiltration of the skin and the subcutaneous tissues with a local anesthetic agent to reduce pain is used when the procedure is being performed under conscious sedation. With GA, infiltration of a local anesthetic agent may be deferred to the end of the procedure to alleviate pain and discomfort at vascular access sites during recovery.

HEMODYNAMIC DATA

O_2 sat measurements are made routinely in the various cardiac chambers, vena cavae, and great vessels. These measurements are used to calculate the systemic flow (CO, Q_s), pulmonary flow (Q_p), the ratio of the pulmonary-to-systemic flow (Q_p:Q_s), and PVR and SVR.

It is ideal to obtain the data with the patient awake and breathing spontaneously in room air. This is rarely possible in pediatric patients. The use of light anesthesia and sedation during the diagnostic part of the study facilitates acquisition of data in as near normal state as is possible. It is important to recognize and limit effects on intracardiac and intrapulmonary pressures and systemic and pulmonary resistances when the procedure is done under GA with IPPV. At a minimum, and when tolerated, baseline hemodynamic measurements should be performed with an FiO_2 as close to 0.21 as possible. In some cases, additional diagnostic information may be collected to study the effects of O_2, NO, vasodilators or inotropes, exercise and balloon occlusion of intracardiac or extracardiac shunts on the CO, pulmonary flow, and PVR and SVR.

From O_2 sat, dissolved O_2 (PO_2), and Hb measurements, the O_2 content (mL/dL) of the mixed venous blood and systemic arterial blood is used to calculate systemic AV O_2 content difference. Pulmonary AV O_2 content difference is similarly estimated by calculating the O_2 content of pulmonary venous and arterial blood. Systemic (Q_s) and pulmonary flow (Q_p) can then be derived using the **Fick principle:**

$$\text{Flow (Q)(L/min)} = \frac{O_2 \text{ consumption (mL/min)}}{\text{AV } O_2 \text{ difference (mL of } O_2\text{/L of blood)}}$$

When the partial pressure of dissolved O_2 is < 100, the PO_2 portion of the equation can be negated and the flow can be calculated using the O_2 consumption and sat measurements alone.

$$\text{Pulmonary Flow } (Q_p) = \frac{O_2 \text{ Consumption}}{\text{Pulmonary vein sat} - \text{Pulmonary artery sat}}$$

$$\text{Systemic Flow } (Q_s) = \frac{O_2 \text{ Consumption}}{\text{Systemic artery } SaO_2 - \text{Mixed venous } SaO_2}$$

Based on Ohm's law, which states V = IR, where V = voltage (or pressure drop) across a circuit, I = the current (or flow) through the circuit and R = the resistance in the circuit. SVR and PVR can be calculated as follows:

$$PVR = (PA_p - LA_p)/Q_p$$
$$SVR = (Ao_p - RA_p)/Q_s$$

Where PA_p = pulmonary artery pressure; LA_p = left atrial pressure; Ao_p = aortic pressure; and RA_p = right atrial pressure; pulmonary vascular resistance = PVR; systemic vascular resistance = SVR.

ANGIOGRAPHY

Biplane cineangiography is performed to delineate intracardiac or vascular anatomy and to evaluate ventricular function. Images are obtained by injection of radiographic contrast agents through angiographic catheters positioned in appropriate locations. The angiograms may be performed in postero-anterior and lateral projections or by angling the cameras to obtain cranial, caudal, left anterior, or right anterior oblique projections. Based on the site of injection and the information required, the injection may be performed with a power injector, delivering large amounts of contrast quickly, or by hand.

INTERVENTIONAL PROCEDURES

Valvuloplasty

Aortic valvuloplasty: A retrograde approach from the femoral artery generally is used, although an antegrade and transseptal approach from the femoral vein is preferred by some. In either approach, following hemodynamic evaluation and angiographic estimate of the aortic valve annulus, a wire is positioned across the valve and a balloon catheter is advanced over the wire and positioned across the aortic valve. The balloon is then inflated and deflated quickly. The inflation of the balloon leads to a transient loss of CO, ↓ SBP, and occasionally may be accompanied by ↓ HR. These hemodynamic changes recover quickly on balloon deflation. While complications of aortic valvuloplasty are rare, the anesthesiologist must be 'prepared for the worst,' which includes annular rupture and the creation of significant aortic regurgitation.

Pulmonic valvuloplasty: After femoral venous or IJ access is obtained, the technique for balloon dilation of the pulmonary valve is nearly identical to that outlined above for the aortic valve. Loss of CO and ↓ HR are seen during the time of balloon inflation with this intervention as well. While annular rupture also is a potential complication of this procedure, the creation of pulmonary insufficiency is of less concern and better tolerated than aortic insufficiency.

Angioplasty

A number of transcatheter treatment options are available for management of **pulmonary artery stenoses,** including **balloon angioplasty** and **endovascular stent implantation.** Angioplasty has been shown to be highly effective in anatomically appropriate cases with a low complication rate. Hemodynamic and angiographic assessment of the lesion is obtained, followed by selection of an optimal balloon catheter, based on both the size of the stenosis and surrounding 'normal' tissue. Using the same "over-the-wire technique," a balloon is advanced and centered over the stenosis. Hemodynamic and angiographic data are assessed following each intervention. A high index of suspicion for complications—including dissection or pulmonary artery tear, obstructive intimal flaps, thrombi, and reperfusion pulmonary edema—is justified, as management may require ventilatory manipulations and/or emergent cardiovascular resuscitation.

Balloon angioplasty of coarctation of the aorta may be performed for treatment of native or recurrent coarctation. Angiography of the aorta is performed to delineate the coarctation and estimate the dimension of the coarctated segment and the adjacent aorta. As with other angioplasty techniques, the balloon size is based on the dimensions of the stenotic area and surrounding vessel. Transient loss of lower body perfusion and ↓ HR are to be expected, as with balloon valvuloplasty, on inflation of the balloon. Pressure and angiographic data are obtained to determine adequacy of results and absence of complications. There is a 4–5% incidence of intimal tear and dissection that, in most cases, are nonprogressive. Rarely, aortic disruption may require emergent surgical repair.

Endovascular Stent Placement

Stent implantation in the pulmonary arteries or for aortic coarctation is used to maintain vessel diameter and decreased gradients in patients unresponsive to balloon dilation. Stents are mounted on balloon catheters and the balloon/stent combination is advanced over a previously placed wire. A long sheath (originating in the groin or neck) is placed across the area of narrowing to prevent the stent from slipping off the balloon catheter as it makes its way through the heart or vessels. After the stent has been properly positioned, the long sheath is withdrawn to expose the balloon/stent combination. The balloon is inflated to expand the stent and appose it to the vessel wall. Placement of long sheaths, particularly through the right ventricular outflow tract (RVOT), can be difficult and may result in transient bradyarrhythmias and loss of CO.

Closure of Congenital Defects

Atrial septal defects (ASDs): As many as 80–85% of secundum ASDs may be amenable to device closure in the cath lab. Most devices currently used include a left atrial disc with an occlusive membrane, a central spool or connecting pin, and a right atrial disc with an occlusive membrane. The membrane occludes flow through the defect and, within months, the device becomes incorporated into the septum due to endothelialization. A sizing balloon inflated across the defect permits estimation of the stretched diameter. A long sheath is then placed across the defect over a wire. The device attached to the delivery cable is loaded in the long sheath and advanced to the left atrium. The left atrial disc is opened, the device is withdrawn until the left atrial disk is in contact with the atrial septum; then the right atrial disc is opened, effectively "sandwiching" the atrial septum between the two disks. TEE is used to guide placement of the device. Intracardiac ECHO has been introduced recently and offers ECHO guidance without the requirement of GA.

Ventricular septal defect (VSD): Closure with a device can be performed in the cath lab for isolated or multiple muscular VSDs, as well as perimembranous defects. The technique requires establishment of a continuous AV guide wire loop across the defect. Most often, the wire course is from the femoral vein, through the right atrium, into the RV, across the VSD, out the aortic valve, around the aorta, and out the femoral artery. The device is then deployed via a long sheath placed across the VSD through the RV aspect. Hemodynamic compromise may be seen with tension on the wire if aortic or tricuspid insufficiency is induced. Transient arrhythmias are routine while crossing the VSD and deploying the device. Great care must be taken to avoid entrapment in the mitral, aortic, and tricuspid valves during device deployment. In addition to fluoroscopy, TEE is used to guide placement of the device. Improvements in the devices developed more recently have significantly reduced the cath lab morbidity of this procedure.

Coil occlusion: Aortopulmonary collaterals, AVMs, Blalock-Taussig (B-T) shunts, venous collaterals, coronary artery fistulae, and patent ductus arteriosi (PDA) have all been successfully occluded using the technique of coil embolization. The embolization coils consist of a metal wire, either stainless steel or platinum, ± Dacron strands, and are available in multiple sizes, lengths, and shapes. While PDA or coronary artery fistula embolization may obviate the need for surgery, most embolizations serve to either reduce the cardiac workload by decreasing the amount of shunting or simplify a planned surgical procedure.

The technique for coil closure of collaterals or other communications is straightforward. A catheter is placed in the vessel to be occluded and a selective angiogram is done to delineate the anatomy and diameter of the vessel to be closed. Coils that are slightly larger than the diameter of the vessel are used, since the vessel will distend when the coil is deployed. Using a long 'pusher' wire, the coil is advanced through the catheter and deployed in the vessel. Repeat angiography is performed to confirm complete closure. If residual flow remains, additional coils are placed. Coil dislodgement and embolization to a distal blood vessel is the most common complication. In general, the errant coil can be retrieved in the cath lab without much difficulty and a new coil of a larger size placed to occlude the vessel.

OTHER PROCEDURES

Endomyocardial biopsy is commonly performed for rejection surveillance in patients following cardiac transplantation. It also may be performed in patients presenting with acute onset of cardiomyopathy for histopathological Dx of myocarditis. The preferred site for obtaining cardiac biopsy is the RV aspect of the intraventricular septum. The specimen is obtained with a biopsy forceps advanced to the RV through a long sheath. It is usual to obtain four to five specimens to improve the diagnostic gain, as the histopathological changes can be patchy. Complications of endomyocardial biopsy include cardiac perforation and tricuspid valve damage. GA is required in patients with compromised airway and/or cardiopulmonary status from lymphoproliferative disease or obesity 2° to steroid therapy.

A variety of other transcatheter therapeutic procedures may be performed in the cardiac cath suite. **Rashkind balloon atrial septostomy, static balloon septoplasty, Brockenbrough transseptal needle puncture,** and **radiofrequency-assisted perforation** of the pulmonary valve or the atrial septum are all less commonly used than the procedures described above, but routinely are undertaken in high-volume cath labs.

ELECTROPHYSIOLOGY STUDY (EPS)

Patients with atrial or ventricular arrhythmias may require either diagnostic or therapeutic interventions in the cath lab. EP studies are catheterization procedures in which intracardiac electrical signals are recorded via specialized catheters that can both record electrical activity and stimulate the heart. These studies often are used to make a Dx of the mechanism of arrhythmia, assess the hemodynamic impact of the arrhythmia, assess efficacy of pharmacologic therapy, and map the location of abnormal conduction pathways or automatic foci. Although routine studies usually take 2–3 h, some may be quite lengthy.

Radiofrequency ablation (RFA) is a procedure in which abnormal electrical conducting pathways or automatic electrical foci (identified by EPS) are destroyed, using the application of RF energy delivered through a deflectable electrode catheter. This procedure was first described in pediatric surgery in 1991, but has rapidly become a preferred therapeutic option for supraventricular tachycardia in this population. On some occasions, RF lesions must be placed close to other critical structures in the heart (e.g., AV node).

With advances in technology and an increased understanding of high-risk pediatric patient populations, **transvenous pacemaker** and **implantable cardioverter defibrillator (ICD)** placements are becoming more common in the pediatric population. Pacemaker placement has become more common as data have accumulated regarding the risk of sudden death in patients with congenital complete heart block, as well as increased survival with postop heart block. New indications for ICD placement in patients with long QT syndrome, congenital heart disease, and hypertrophic cardiomyopathy have increased the number of ICD implantations in the last 5 yr. These procedures are commonly performed in the cath lab under GA.

ANESTHETIC CONSIDERATIONS

M. Gail Boltz and Chandra Ramamoorthy

PREPROCEDURE

Cardiac catheterization and interventional procedures in children range from those requiring simple diagnostic procedures to those requiring complex interventional procedures such as balloon angioplasties or stent placement. These patients can present a challenge, given their abnormal cardiac anatomy and physiology. Many of them have undergone repeated catheterizations and will have had multiple anesthetics. All patients require a thorough preanesthetic H&P, emphasizing cardiorespiratory function and associated comorbidities. Most children will follow the same npo protocol as they would for surgery (see NPO Guidelines, see D-1). Be cautious in single ventricle patients who are prone to clotting of shunt or are dependent on their venous return for hemodynamic stability and oxygenation. In such patients either an IV can be started for hydration or clear liquids can be given up to two hours before surgery

Previous Anesthesia	✓ Surgical and cardiological interventions; h/o difficult access; endotracheal tube size and anesthetic techniques; problems with previous anesthetics.
Family History	✓ Family history for anesthetic related problems; h/o malignant hyperthermia.
Prematurity	Will affect the decision to intubate, apnea monitoring if <55 wks, need for pre-op admission; associated clinical problems.
Neurological	✓ Head US in neonates; note preop neurological status as there is risk of embolism; for h/o seizures; h/o developmental delay. Patients are heparinized during procedure.
Craniofacial and Airway	✓ H/o difficult airway; any surgery to the airway; h/o tracheal stenosis due to multiple intubations in the past; stridor due to laryngo- or bronchomalacia; h/o loose teeth.
Respiratory	✓ H/o cyanosis, chronic cough and other chronic respiratory problems; ensure that they are under optimum control. ✓ H/o steroid use for RAD. ✓ H/o recent URI →↑ risk of adverse periop events. Patients with pulmonary HTN may have OSA. Cardiac transplant patients can develop lymphoproliferative disease, which results in redundant lymphoid tissue in the pharynx and epiglottis-possible airway obstruction. ✓ Requirement for CPAP, BiPAP, NO. Meds for pulmonary HTN should be continued. **Tests:** Assess perfusion scan for distribution of PBF. CXR to r/o infiltrates, CHF and cardiomegaly. Compare with baseline.
Cardiovascular	Review current problem, hx of all surgeries; pacemaker, ICD etc. If the patient has a pacemaker, note the settings and the reason for placing the pacemaker and when last interrogated. Identify existing shunts - will affect anesthetic plan and FiO_2. Assess cardiopulmonary reserve, (e.g., exercise tolerance, diaphoresis, and feeding difficulties). ✓ hx of syncope, hypoxic spells; note current SaO_2. Transplant patients may develop CAD. ✓ arrhythmias, palpitations, murmurs. **Tests:** ECG; ✓ recent ECHO and cardiac catheterization reports.
Gastrointestinal	Risk of reflux due to chronic use of steroids. May have G-tube/Nissen. Some single ventricle patients may have hepatic dysfunction.
Renal	Transplant recipients may develop renal dysfunction due to antirejection medication or HTN. Patients with CHF are on diuretics and could be hypovolemic. Patients may have had renal insult during previous surgery. **Tests:** ✓ BUN and Cr as these patients are also at risk for renal injury due to contrast, and also to guide hydration therapy.
Endocrine/ Steroid	✓ Transplant patients are on steroids. ✓ for other endocrine concerns.
Hematology/ Immunology	✓ History of previous transfusions and reactions. Immunological deficiency that may affect the type of blood transfusion e.g., neonates require CMV negative blood and products.
Syndromes	✓ for coexisting syndromes and associated anomalies.
Ob/Gyn	✓ Last menstrual period.
Vascular	✓ H/o vascular occlusion.
Current Medications	Stop warfarin at least three doses before cardiac cath. Heparin can be continued. Hold diuretics and ACE inhibitor starting the night before; continue all cardiac meds.

Laboratory	✓ HCT: baseline to make decision regarding transfusion; ↑HCT suggests chronic hypoxia; Severe anemia should be corrected prior to cath if possible. Type and crossmatch blood if the patient needs transfusion for anemia or any interventional procedure; blood should be available in the cath lab. ✓ Electrolytes, especially if the patient is on diuretics and or digitalis. ✓ WBC: if the child has a h/o fever and recent URI. ✓ Drug levels - e.g., digitalis, antiseizure meds to make sure they are not outside the therapeutic range. Pregnancy test: must be done the morning of surgery if patient has attained menarche.
Premedication	Midazolam 0.5–0.75 mg/kg oral. Be cautious in patients with OSA. Cyanotic kids should have O_2 sat monitored before and continuously after premedication. Antibiotics are given to patients as required for SBE prophylaxis or for those undergoing interventional procedures.
NPO	Most patients should follow the ASA guidelines for NPO. Avoid prolonged NPO in single ventricle and other shunt-dependent lesions, as the shunt flow might decrease with dehydration → ↑ viscosity.
Equipment	Transport patients to and from the cath lab with a pulse oximeter and other monitors as appropriate. Equipment to manage difficult airways and hemodynamically unstable patients should be readily available, e.g., difficult airway cart, I-stat, arterial line, blood pump, pumps to infuse vasopressors, pacemaker, defibrillator, NIRS monitor.

INTRAPROCEDURE

Anesthetic technique: The object of anesthesia and sedation in the cath lab is to maintain the patient's physiological state at rest with minimal anesthetic-related disturbance. Not all procedures require ETT placement, but all require an immobile patient. This can be achieved by varying degrees of sedation, from conscious to general anesthesia. Some interventional procedures (e.g., stenting, coiling) require a motionless field for prolonged periods of time, and are, therefore, unsuitable for sedation. Patients who require venous access via the IJ vein may not tolerate lying still for long periods of time. Critically ill neonates require intubation and controlled ventilation. Patients with moderate to severe pulmonary HTN can be managed with sedation since the physiological changes associated with intubation, and more likely extubation, might result in a pulmonary hypertensive crisis. Some older children with procedures of shorter duration where groin access is being used may tolerate incremental iv sedation with local anesthesia.

Anesthesia and sedation can be managed with propofol/ketamine (100 mg propofol + 1 mg of ketamine mixed together and infused at 150–200 mcg/kg/min) or a propofol/remifentanil infusion, as long as the patient remains normocarbic and normoxic. Hypercarbia will affect hemodynamic catheterization values.

IPPV decreases systemic venous return, particularly in the setting of depleted intravascular volume. This is particularly noteworthy in those patients with single ventricle physiology, where pulmonary blood flow is mostly passive and depends on adequate preload. When possible, patients with Fontan physiology should be allowed to breathe spontaneously. This improves pulmonary blood flow and hence systemic blood flow and cardiac output.

Induction	Standard inhalation or iv induction (see p. D-1). The choice of anesthetic drugs must include careful consideration of their effects on myocardial contractility, preload and afterload, pulmonary and systemic vascular resistance and respiration.
Maintenance	GETA with volatile agents (e.g., sevoflurane) or iv infusion (e.g., propofol with remifentanil or ketamine). Most catheterizations require the patient to be maintained on room air for accurate O_2 sat and pressure measurements. Keep $FiO_2 < 0.3$, otherwise dissolved plasma oxygen may cause an overestimate of the pulmonary blood flow, and Q_p:Q_s ratio will be correspondingly exaggerated. More importantly any FiO_2 changes should be communicated with the interventionalist so that Q_p:Q_s calculations can be corrected. Patients with pulmonary HTN presenting for cardiac catheterization are at high risk for adverse events. Avoid the routine use of anti-sialogogues so that the heart rate remains at baseline. Our institutional practice for these patients is to maintain spontaneous ventilation (uninstrumented airway) under propofol-ketamine anesthesia.

Maintenance (cont'd)	Patients requiring ASD device closure require TEE placement to guide the correct placement of the device; endotracheal intubation is necessary. TEE is not needed for PDA device closure, unless patient condition dictates it. EP studies are best managed with iv propofol 50–150 mcg/kg/min, because this agent has the least ability to induce dysrhythmias. Recent studies demonstrate that sevoflurane or isoflurane (1 MAC or lower) may be acceptable. In patients with a history of prolonged QT interval, TIVA is recommended. Overall, a slow heart rate obtained by the use of remifentanil works well with prolonged QT. Dexmedetomidine should be avoided as it prolongs the QT interval. Reversal agents can also prolong the QT interval. Heparin 50–100 U/kg is given for patients with arterial sheaths. The activated clotting time (ACT) should be in the range of >300 sec during the procedure and <175 sec when the catheters are removed. When the sheath is removed, a considerable amount of time is necessary waiting for hemostasis. NO may be required for the Rx of pulmonary HTN.	
Emergence	Do not allow child to emerge before hemostasis has been achieved at the access site. If the patient's clinical status allows deep extubation, it can be done to prevent coughing. Use of remifentanil infusion may provide analgesia during the procedure, yet allow for a rapid emergence. Consider remifentanil for patients with pulmonary HTN and controlled ventilation, where a smooth emergence is essential to prevent a hypertensive crisis. Interventional procedures and EP/ablation require overnight ICU admission for observation. Most other patients can recover in PACU.	
Blood and fluid requirements	IV: 20–22 ga × 1 NS/LR PRBCs Fluid warmer	A second volume iv may be desirable for interventional cases. The cardiologist also will have a venous access line that can be used if necessary. Interventional procedures may cause tearing of vessels and/or myocardium and can cause abrupt hemorrhage; therefore blood must be available in the room. Neonates can lose significant blood during the access and sampling and also may require transfusion. Follow serial Hcts.
Monitoring	Standard monitors, including Bair-Hugger ± Arterial line ± Foley catheter	If A-line access is required, discuss with the cardiologist. Frequently, the femoral artery is cannulated for the catheterization and may be available for use; however, access may be limited at crucial times (e.g., stenting or coiling), and therefore a peripheral arterial line may be desirable. For cases of long duration, consider Foley catheter placement. Monitor temperature. NIRS monitor (e.g. Somanetics Invos) is recommended in single ventricle and in other cyanotic lesions since pulse oximetry is a poor predictor of changes in cerebral saturation.
Positioning	✓ and pad pressure points. ✓ eyes.	Supine, arms flexed above head to allow fluoroscopy of chest. Adolescent patients are at risk of brachial plexus injury. Keep extension within 90°. All ECG leads and monitoring wires must be cleared from axilla and chest to allow fluoroscopy.
Complications	Airway obstruction Aspiration Arrhythmias	Rx: Airway support, oral/nasal airway, LMA. Intubate if necessary. Rx: Suction, secure airway if needed. Bronchodilators, H1, H2 blockers if needed. CXR. O_2 monitoring. Admit if post-op oxygen requirement persists. Determine etiology, whether hemodynamically stable or not. Cardiovert if necessary. Check electrolytes, ABG, Consult EP.

Complications (cont'd)	Hemorrhage	Rx: Fluid resuscitation with crystalloid, 5% albumin and/or blood; vasopressors as needed.
	Hypoxemia	Try to determine the cause. Check HCT in single ventricle patients. Rx: Airway support; increase FiO_2. Intubate and ventilate as needed.
	Pulmonary hypertensive crisis	Avoid hypoxia, hypercarbia, and acidosis, maintain the depth of anesthetic, and give additional anesthetic if tolerated. Consider NO, systemic vasopressors.
	Contrast reaction/anaphylaxis	Rx: Support airway, 100% FiO_2, intubate if needed: phenylephrine, volume resuscitation, steroid, antihistamine, H_2 blocker.
	Hypothermia	Especially neonates. Rx: Forced-air warming device, heat lamp. Increase environmental temperature.
	Air embolism	Rx: 100% FiO_2; identify and occlude source; Trendelenburg; fluid resuscitation; vasopressor support. Aspirate air from central access if possible.

POSTPROCEDURE

Complications	Hematoma at access site Ischemic limb Emergence delirium
Pain management	Infiltrate access sites with local anesthetic. Postop analgesia usually not required.
Tests	CXR, if indicated.

Suggested Readings

1. Alexander ME, Walsh EP, Saul JP, et al: Value of programmed stimulation in patients with congenital heart disease. *J Cardiovasc Electrophysiol* 1999; 10(8): 1033–44.
2. Baim DS, Grossman W: *Grossman's Cardiac Catheterization, Angiography, and Intervention,* 6th edition. Lippincott Williams & Wilkins, Philadelphia: 2001.
3. Baker CM, McGowan FX Jr, Keane JF, et al: Pulmonary artery trauma due to balloon dilation: recognition, avoidance and management. *J Am Coll Cardiol* 2000; 36(5):1684–90.
4. Benson LN, Nykanen D, Collison A: Radiofrequency perforation in the treatment of congenital heart disease. *Catheter Cardiovasc Interv* 2002; 56(1):72–82.
5. Chessa M, Carminati M, Cao QL, et al: Transcatheter closure of congenital and acquired muscular ventricular septal defects using the Amplatzer device. *J Invasive Cardiol* 2002; 14(6):322–7.
6. Freedom RM, Mawson JB, Yoo SJ, et al: *Congenital Heart Disease Textbook of Angiography.* Futura Publishing, Armonk, NY: 1997.
7. Friedman RA, Walsh EP, Silka MJ, et al: NASPE expert consensus conference: radiofrequency catheter ablation in children with and without congenital heart disease. Report of the writing committee. *PACE* 2002; 25:1000–17.
8. Hamid RKA: Anesthesia for nonsurgical procedures in children: cardiac catheterization and electrophysiology studies. In *Pediatric Cardiac Anesthesia,* 3rd edition. Appleton-Lange, Norwalk, CT: 1997, 165–80.
9. Hammer GB, Drover DR, Cao H et al: The effects of dexmedetomidine on cardiac electrophysiology in children. *Anesth Analg* 2008;106(1):79–83.
10. Hijazi Z, Wang Z, Cao Q, et al: Transcatheter closure of atrial septal defects and patent foramen ovale under intracardiac echocardiographic guidance: feasibility and comparison with transesophageal echocardiography. *Catheter Cardiovasc Interv* 2001; 52(2):194–9.
11. Kugler JD, Danford DA, Houston K, et al.: Radiofrequency catheter ablation for paroxysmal supraventricular tachycardia in children and adolescent without structural heart disease. The Pediatric EP Society Radiofrequency Catheter Ablation Registry. *Am J Cardiol* 1997; 80(11):1438–43.
12. Lai LP, Lin JL Wu MH, et al: Usefulness of intravenous propofol anesthesia for radiofrequency catheter ablation in patients with tachyarrhythmias: infeasibility for pediatric patients with ectopic atrial tachycardia. *PACE* 1999; 22(9):1358–64.
13. Lavoie J, Walsh EP, Burrows FA, et al: Effects of propofol or isoflurane anesthesia on cardiac conduction in children undergoing radiofrequency catheter ablation for tachydysrhythmias. *Anesthesiology* 1995; 82:884–7.

14. Lock JE, Keane JF, Perry SB: *Diagnostic and Interventional Catheterization in Congenital Heart Disease,* 2nd edition. Kluwer Academic Publishers, Nowell, MA: 2000.
15. Malviya S, Voepel-Lewis T, Siewert M, et al: Risk factors for adverse postoperative outcomes in children presenting for cardiac surgery with upper respiratory tract infections. *Anesthesiology* 2003; 98(3):628–32.
16. Maron BJ, Shen WK, Link MS, et al.: Efficacy of implantable cardioverter-defibrillators for the prevention of sudden death in patients with hypertrophic cardiomyopathy. *N Eng J Med* 2000; 342(6):365–73.
17. McCrindle BW: Independent predictors of long-term results after balloon pulmonary valvuloplasty. Valvuloplasty and Angioplasty of Congenital Anomalies (VACA) Registry Investigators. *Circulation* 1994; 89(4):1751–9.
18. McCrindle BW, Blackstone EH, Williams WG, et al: Are outcomes of surgical versus transcatheter balloon valvotomy equivalent in neonatal critical aortic stenosis? *Circulation* 2001; 104(12 Suppl 1):1152–8.
19. McCrindle BW, Jones TK, Morrow WR, et al: Acute results of balloon angioplasty of native coarctation versus recurrent aortic obstruction are equivalent. Valvuloplasty and Angioplasty of Congenital Anomalies (VACA) Registry Investigators. *J Am Coll Cardiol* 1996; 28(7):1810–7.
20. McCrindle BW, Kan JS: Long-term results after balloon pulmonary valvuloplasty. *Circulation* 1991; 83(6):1915–22.
21. Perry SB, Keane JF, Lock JE: Interventional catheterization in pediatric congenital and acquired heart disease. *Am J Cardiol* 1988; 61(14):109G–17G.
22. Perry SB, Rome J, Keane JF, Baim DS, Lock JE: Transcatheter closure of coronary artery fistulas. *J Am Coll Cardiol* 1992; 20(1):205–9.
23. Satou GM, Perry SB, Lock JE, et al: Repeat balloon dilation of congenital valvar aortic stenosis: immediate results and midterm outcome. *Catheter Cardiovasc Interv* 1999; 47(1):47–51.
24. Shaffer KM, Mullins CE, Grifka RG, et al: Intravascular stents in congenital heart disease: short- and long-term results from a large single-center experience. *J Am Coll Cardiol* 1998; 31(3):661–7.
25. Van Hare GF, Lesh MD, Scheinman M, et al.: Percutaneous radiofrequency catheter ablation for supraventricular arrhythmias in children. *J Am Coll Cardiol* 1991; 17(7):1613–20.
26. Vogel M, Berger F, Dahnert I, et al: Treatment of atrial septal defects in symptomatic children aged less than 2 years of age using the Amplatzer septal occluder. *Cardiol Young* 2000; 10(5):534–7.
27. Williams GD, Phillips BM, Boltz MG, et al: Ketamine does not increase pulmonary vascular resistance in children with pulmonary hypertension. *Anesth Analg* 2007;105(6):1578–84.
28. Yaster MY, Krane EJ, Kaplan RF: Diagnostic evaluation of congenital heart disease. In *Pediatric Pain Management and Sedation Handbook.* Mosby Yearbook, St. Louis: 1997.
29. Zimmerman AA, Ibrahim AE, et al: The effects of halothane and sevoflurane on cardiac electrophysiology in children undergoing radiofrequency catheter ablation. *Anesthesiology* 1997; 87:A1066.

PEDIATRIC ONCOLOGIC PROCEDURES

Neyssa Marina, Rebecca E. Claure, and Brenda Golianu

Most patients undergoing evaluation to rule out malignancy undergo staging procedures to determine the extent of disease at diagnosis. The staging procedures include computed tomography of the chest to evaluate the possibility of lung metastases; as well as bone scintigraphy or positron emission tomography (PET scan) to determine whether there is metastatic spread to bone. Pediatric patients with neuroblastoma also undergo staging with ^{131}I-metaiodobenzylguanine since this study appears to complement bone scintigraphy and can be useful as a therapeutic tool. Besides these studies, patients must also undergo bone marrow aspirates and biopsies to evaluate for bone marrow involvement. Patients < 5 years of age undergoing oncologic evaluation typically need sedation or GA for imaging procedures. Most bone marrow aspirates and biopsies for these patients are also performed using GA although these can also be performed using conscious sedation. In addition to these staging studies, patients with leukemia or lymphoma undergo serial spinal taps with concurrent administration of intrathecal therapy. These procedures are for both diagnostic purposes and for central nervous system (CNS) prophylaxis since about 50% of leukemia patients develop CNS disease in the absence of such prophylaxis. With current treatment protocols the incidence of CNS relapse has been drastically reduced with the use of CNS prophylaxis. Cranial irradiation is required for patients with CNS disease at diagnosis and for certain high-risk subsets. As part of the workup patients also undergo diagnostic biopsies to establish a diagnosis. If a complete resection cannot be performed the diagnostic biopsy should be performed at the most accessible site to minimize complications. However, it is essential to obtain enough tissue for diagnostic and most recently for biologic studies, because the latter can help target therapy. After a diagnosis of cancer is established, patients are given the option of inserting a central venous catheter since most pediatric cancers are systemic diseases requiring multimodality therapy to maximize outcome. Patients also require serial bone marrow aspirates and lumbar punctures. Because these procedures are painful, they are usually performed under general anesthesia unless circumstances such as the presence of upper respiratory infections (URI) complicate the clinical course. In that case, the procedure might need to be performed under conscious sedation, especially if it is a critical part of treatment (i.e., patients with relapsed disease). The diagnostic biopsies and central line placements are generally performed in the operating room under general anesthesia. The only exception occurs in patients with mediastinal masses where the patient's respiratory status is tenuous. In this circumstance, the diagnosis should be established using the least invasive procedure to minimize the complications resulting from anesthesia. This is especially true in patients with a differential diagnosis of leukemia and lymphoma where the use of steroids could jeopardize establishing a diagnosis. Line removals on the other hand, can be performed in a procedure room with sedation or GA. Pediatric oncology patients are followed very closely during their treatment, undergoing at least monthly physical exams to evaluate for side effects of therapy and determine whether proceeding with the prescribed therapy is indicated. When these patients require invasive procedures, it is essential to work with the primary oncology team to evaluate whether the requested procedure is elective or required.

PREPROCEDURE

Patients are first evaluated to determine whether the prescribed chemotherapy has produced any side effects requiring alteration of treatment or precluding continuing with the scheduled procedure. In addition, all patients undergo laboratory evaluation within 24–48 h of their scheduled procedure to make certain their blood counts are adequate for treatment administration.

A thorough preanesthetic H&P should be performed in all cases and the usual npo protocol applied (see p. D-1).

Respiratory	Major surgical procedures for patients with Sx of URI (e.g., cough, fever) are postponed unless there are circumstances (CNS disease, bone marrow relapse), which require the treatment to proceed. In those circumstances, the spinal taps and bone marrows can be performed with either light sedation or with the use of local anesthesia. Although the latter circumstance is rare there are definite situations where proceeding with therapy is definitely in the best interest of the patient. A number of chemotherapeutic agents have been associated with pulmonary toxicity: bleomycin (2–5%), BNCU (20–50%), busulfan (2.5–11.5%), cyclophosphamide (rare), methotrexate (rare). The use of these agents might require closer evaluation to make certain the patient is able to proceed with his/her procedure. **Tests:** All pediatric oncology patients undergo weekly complete blood counts to evaluate the toxicity from therapy. In addition, patients who have received any of the agents associated with pulmonary toxicity undergo pulmonary function tests at regular intervals. Although some chemotherapy agents are associated with pulmonary toxicity the cumulative doses of those agents are such that most patients are asymptomatic.
Cardiovascular	Anti-cancer treatment can produce a wider range of cardiac toxicity. Anthracycline-induced cardiomyopathy is one of the most feared conditions for pediatric oncology patients. This complication is associated with the use of cumulative doses > 300 mg/m and fortunately is rare. It is insidious in origin and most commonly presents many years following treatment with doxorubicin, daunorubicin, or amsacrine. The use of high-doses of radiotherapy is also associated with cardiac complications including: constrictive pericarditis, atherosclerosis and early myocardiac infarction. Signs of CV toxicity may include SOB, ECG changes, rhythm disturbances, pericarditis or CHF. **Tests:** Patients receiving any agents associated with cardiac toxicity are monitored at yearly interval with echocardiograms and electrocardiograms. Therefore, these tests do not need to be performed prior to a procedure requiring general anesthesia unless the preprocedure history and physical exam suggest a change in the patient's clinical condition.
Hematologic	Bone marrow suppression with all cytotoxic drugs. **Tests:** Complete blood counts are performed once to twice a week in all pediatric oncology patients. These tests help determine whether continuing with the prescribed therapy is indicated.

Neurologic	Peripheral neuropathies due to vincristine, vinblastine, cisplatin, and procarbazine may be present. Patient should be carefully positioned and padded.	
Laboratory	Most patients will have their labs checked as part of their anticancer therapy and do not generally require any additional labs.	
Premedication	Usually not required because a parent can accompany child into procedure room; however, most children will have venous access and can be given small doses of midazolam if necessary. Consider midazolam syrup 0.5–0.75 mg/kg orally for the particularly anxious child without iv access in place. For children without venous access, a peripheral iv may be placed. Prior to this, application of EMLA or ELA Max cream (1 h or 20 min, respectively) provides topical anesthesia of the skin at the lumbar puncture or bone-marrow aspiration site, as well as the peripheral iv site. Midazolam (0.5–0.75 mg/kg po) can be administered to the anxious child without iv access.	

INTRAPROCEDURE

Anesthetic technique: GA (mask or LMA) or MAC in the appropriate patient. Procedures are usually short, 10–20 min. The oncologist should infiltrate the area with lidocaine after induction.

Induction	Most children have a central venous access line in place for their oncology treatment protocol; thus, induction can proceed with iv propofol 2–3 mg/kg. Infrequently, mask induction is performed.	
Maintenance	The provider performing the procedures infiltrates the area with lidocaine. For Broviac catheter removals, heparin must be removed from the catheter and discarded before use for induction. A sufficient bolus of propofol (e.g., 0.5–1 mg/kg) must be given just prior to pulling the catheter. Additional iv usually is not warranted, because the procedure is normally ≤ 10 min. Occasionally, the catheter may break during attempted removal, and the surgeon will have to make a skin incision to allow for removal of the internal fragment. In such cases, a peripheral iv may be inserted quickly to facilitate administration of additional propofol, or mask anesthesia may be given. If the SpO_2 decreases, blow-by O_2 with gentle head and neck positioning are generally sufficient.	
Emergence	Allow child to awaken in procedure room. Ondansetron 0.15 mg/kg for patients receiving intrathecal chemotherapy during their lumbar puncture. Avoid dexamethasone, as steroids may be part of the patient's chemotherapy protocol, or may precipitate tumor lysis syndrome.	
Blood and fluid requirements	No blood loss.	Patients may require blood or factor supplementation prior to or during procedure based on preoperative laboratory values.
Monitoring	Standard monitors.	
Positioning	Lateral decubitus (lumbar puncture) Supine, seated or prone (Bone marrow aspiration, biopsy) Supine (Broviac)	
Complications	Airway obstruction Retained central venous catheter	Head and neck, reposition, jaw thrust. ℞ may require open surgical procedure.
Post-procedure Pain Management	Acetaminophen (po)	Lumbar punctures are not generally painful, whereas bone marrow aspirations and biopsies can be. Acetaminophen po is usually sufficient for analgesia. Rectal route should be avoided unless adequate Plt and WBC counts are confirmed.

Suggested Readings

1. Arndt CAS, Crist WM: Common Musculoskeletal Tumors of Childhood and Adolescence. *N Eng J Med* 1999; 341:342–52.
2. Aronin PA, Mahaley MS Jr, Rudnick SA, et al: Prediction of BCNU pulmonary toxicity in patients with malignant gliomas: an assessment of risk factors. *N Engl J Med* 1980; 303:183–8.
3. Bell MR, Meredith DJ, Gill PG: Role of carbon monoxide diffusing capacity in the early detection of major bleomycin-induced pulmonary toxicity. *Aust N Z J Med* 1985; 15:235–40.
4. Blum RH, Carter SK, Agre K: A clinical review of bleomycin--a new antineoplastic agent. *Cancer* 31:903–14, 1973.
5. Cooper JA, Jr., White DA, Matthay RA: Drug-induced pulmonary disease. Part 1: cytotoxic drugs. *Am Rev Respir Dis* 1986; 133:321–40.
6. Finklestein JZ, Ekert H, Isaacs H Jr, et al: Bone marrow metastases in children with solid tumors. *Am J Dis* Child 1970;119: 49–52.
7. Hancock SL, Donaldson SS, Hoppe RT: Cardiac disease following treatment of Hodgkin's disease in children and adolescents. *J Clin Onc* 1993; 11:1208–15.
8. Kushner BH, Yeh SD, Kramer K, et al: Impact of metaiodobenzylguanidine scintigraphy on assessing response of high-risk neuroblastoma to dose-intensive induction chemotherapy. *J Clin Oncol* 2003; 21:1082–6.
9. Lipshultz SE, Colan SD, Gelber RD, et al: Late cardiac effects of doxorubicin therapy for acute lymphoblastic leukemia in childhood. *N Eng J Med* 1991; 324:808–15.
10. Lipshultz SE, Lipsitz SR, Mone SM, et al: Female sex and higher drug dose as risk factors for late cardiotoxic effects of doxorubicin therapy for childhood cancer. *N Eng J Med* 1995; 332:1738–43.
11. Martin TM, Nicolson SC, Bargas MS: Propofol anesthesia reduces emesis and airway obstruction in pediatric outpatients. *Anesth Analg* 1993; 76(1):144–8.
12. Matthay KK, DeSantes K, Hasegawa B, et al: Phase I dose escalation of ^{131}I-Metaiodobenzylguanidine with autologous bone marrow support in refractory neuroblastoma. 1998; *J Clin Onc* 16:229–36.
13. McDowall RH, Scher CS, Barst SM: Total intravenous anesthesia for children undergoing brief diagnostic or therapeutic procedures. *J Clin Anesth* 1995; 7(4):273–80.
14. Nysom K, Holm K, Lipsitz SR, et al: Relationship between cumulative anthracycline dose and late cardiotoxicity in childhood acute lymphoblastic leukemia. *J Clin Oncol* 1998; 16:545–50.
15. Schrappe M, Camitta B, Pui CH, et al: Long-term results of large prospective trials in childhood acute lymphoblastic leukemia. *Leukemia* 2000; 14:2193–4.
16. Schrappe M, Reiter A, Ludwig WD, et al: Improved outcome in childhood acute lymphoblastic leukemia despite reduced use of anthracyclines and cranial radiotherapy: results of trial ALL-BFM 90 [In Process Citation]. *Blood* 2000; 95:3310–22.
17. Shimokawa S, Watanabe S, Sakasegawa K: Fatal complication due to a mediastinal tumor. *Ann Thoracic Surg* 2000; 70:340–1.
18. Simone J: RJAAHOHDP: "total therapy" studies of acute lymphocytic leukemia in children. Current results and prospects for cure. *Cancer* 1972; 30:1488–94.

UPPER/LOWER GI ENDOSCOPY

Rebecca E. Claure and Brenda Golianu

Diagnostic indications for gastrointestinal endoscopy include: dysphagia, odynophagia, persistent vomiting, abdominal pain with weight loss/anorexia, abdominal pain despite therapy for GERD, gastrointestinal bleeding, evaluation of inflammatory bowel disease, and significant diarrhea of unexplained origin. Therapeutic indications for gastrointestinal endoscopy include: esophageal dilation, foreign body removal, sclerotherapy or banding of esophageal varices, and polypectomy. Children presenting for endoscopy may have congenital and acquired abnormalities of the GI tract. Examples include repaired tracheoesophageal fistula (TEF) with esophageal dysmotility or strictures, ingestion of a caustic material, and presence of a foreign body.

Many endoscopy procedures are done with sedation only. Requests for anesthesia are dependent on the gastroenterologist's preference, as well as the severity of the patient's underlying illnesses. All patients must receive a complete preanesthesia H&P and follow the same NPO protocol used for surgery (see p. D-l).

ANESTHETIC CONSIDERATIONS

Gastrointestinal	Carefully evaluate for esophageal dysfunction and Sx of GERD. The stomach and bowel will be insufflated with air during the procedure, possibly increasing the likelihood of reflux.
Laboratory	As indicated from H&P. Usually none.

Premedication	If inhalation induction planned, midazolam 0.5–0.75 mg/kg po for anxious children. Parental presence may reduce the need for premedication. If iv induction is planned, EMLA cream (1 hr) or ELAMAX (20 min) should be applied for topical anesthesia. Consider midazolam for younger children requiring an iv induction.

INTRAPROCEDURE

Anesthetic technique: Upper GI endoscopy for esophageal dilation, foreign body removal, severe GERD, gastrointestinal bleeding, and banding/sclerotherapy of esophageal varices requires GETA. For children ≥ 2, with no contraindications, supplemental O_2 via nasal cannula, spontaneous respiration, and propofol infusion can be considered. Children ≤ 2 have a higher incidence of complications when not intubated due to the relatively large endoscope. Complications include partial airway obstruction, tracheal compression, laryngospasm, bronchospasm, and desaturation. Placement of the endoscope in the mouth precludes the ability to use a mask or LMA. For lower GI endoscopy (e.g., colonoscopy), supplemental O_2 via nasal cannula or mask, spontaneous respiration, and propofol infusion may be preferable.

Induction	If rapid sequence indication present, iv catheter placed prior to induction. Proceed with preoxygenation, cricoid pressure, propofol (2–3 mg/kg) or STP (3–5 mg/kg), and succinylcholine (1–2 mg/kg) or rocuronium (1 mg/kg). ETT should be well secured to the side of the mouth. If risk of aspiration relatively low, a standard pediatric iv or mask induction is appropriate (see p. D-2).	
Maintenance	GETA with inhalational agents or iv infusion of propofol (100–250 mcg/kg/min), ± remifentanil (0.05–0.10 mcg/kg/min). Alternatively, GA/sedation may be continued with supplemental O_2 via nasal cannula, spontaneous respiration, and infusion of propofol (100–250 mcg/kg/min), ± remifentanil (0.05–0.10 mcg/kg/min). Careful observation and/or holding the ETT prevents inadvertent extubation during removal of the endoscope.	
Emergence	If intubated, extubate awake. Emergence in procedure room. Patients usually transported to and recovered in PACU.	
Blood and fluid requirements	No blood loss. IV: 22 or 24 ga × 1 NS/LR @ maintenance	
Monitoring	Standard monitors (see p. D-1).	
Positioning	✓ and pad pressure points. ✓ eyes.	Lateral decubitus for upper and lower endoscopy.
Complications	Airway obstruction Hypoxemia 2° gastric insufflation Inadvertant extubation Pulmonary aspiration GI perforation	 2° endoscopist working in the mouth and pharynx

POSTPROCEDURE

Pain management	Acetaminophen (35–40 mg/kg pr or 10–15mg/kg po), hydromorphone (0.01–0.015 mg/kg) or morphine (0.05–0.1 mg/kg)

Suggested Readings

1. Disma N, Astuto M, Rizzo G, et al. Propofol sedation with fentanyl or midazolam during oesophago-gastroduodenoscopy in children. *Eur J Anaesthesiol* 2005 Nov; 22(11):848–52.
2. Gregory GA ed. Pediatric Anesthesia, 4th edition. Churchill Livingstone, New York:2002. 580–1.

3. Haight M, Thomas DW: Pediatric gastrointestinal endoscopy. *Gastroenterologist* 1995; 3(3):181–6.
4. Koh JL, Black DD, Leatherman, IK, et al. Experience with an anesthesiologist interventional model for endoscopy in a pediatric hospital. *J Pediatr Gastroenterol Nutr* 2001Sept;33(3):314–8.
5. Motoyama EK, Davis PJ, eds: *Smith's Anesthesia for Infants and Children*, 7th edition. Mosby Elsevier, Philadelphia: 2006, 850.
6. Schwartz DA, Connelly NR, Theroux CA, et al. Gastric contents in children presenting for upper endoscopy. *Anesth Analg* 1998 Oct;87(4):757–60.
7. Squires RH, Colletti RB. Indications for pediatric gastrointestinal endoscopy: A medical position statement of the North American Society for Pediatric Gastroenterology and Nutrition. *J Pediatr Gastroenterol Nutr* 1996 Aug; 23(2):107–10.
8. Squires RH, Morriss F, Schluterman S, et al: Efficacy, safety, and cost of intravenous sedation versus general anesthesia in children undergoing endoscopic procedures. *Gastrointest Endosc* 1995;41(2):99–104.
9. Sury M, Smith JH. Deep sedation and minimal anesthesia. *Paediatr Anaesth* 2008 Jan; 18(l):18–24.

CROSS-SECTIONAL IMAGING (CT, MRI)

Rebecca E. Claure and Brenda Golianu

PREPROCEDURE

A complete preanesthetic H&P should be performed in all cases and the usual NPO protocol followed (see p. D-l). For MRI, thorough questioning regarding potentially ferromagnetic implants (neurostimulators, cochlear implants, pacemakers, surgical clips, infusion pumps, etc.) is critical. Any questions regarding scanning limitations if certain implants are present should be directed to the radiologist.

Respiratory	Procedures for patients with Sx of URI (nasal congestion, cough, fever) are usually postponed for 3–4 wks unless the study is urgent. If Sx are minor, the study may proceed.
Cardiovascular	Pacemakers usually contraindicated. Prosthetic heart valves may be contraindicated (identify the type of valve present and consult with radiologist). Fresh surgical clips (e.g., recent PDA ligation) may also represent a contraindication for MRI.
Neurologic	Head CT or MRI may be performed in patients with seizure disorders or brain tumors. Review seizure meds and ✓ serum levels if appropriate. Recent drug levels may not be necessary in children with well controlled or stable seizure disorders. If ↑ ICP or ↓ intracranial compliance are present (e.g., 2° tumors or hydrocephalus), the anesthesia plan should include tracheal intubation with controlled ventilation. Metal surgical clips or coils are usually contraindications for MRI. Children with head trauma may have concurrent C-spine injuries.
Laboratory	As indicated from H&P. Usually none required.
Premedication	If inhalation induction planned, midazolam 0.5–0.75 mg/kg po for anxious children. Parental presence may reduce the need for premedication. If iv induction is planned, EMLA cream (1 hr) or ELAMAX (20 min) should be applied for topical anesthesia.

INTRAPROCEDURE

Unique considerations for MRI: See Adult Out-of-OR Procedures, p. 1470.

Anesthetic technique: **CT scans**—With current scanners, many studies can be completed in less than 15 minutes. Each set of data takes 2–3 minutes to collect, allowing many children to complete scans without any sedation. In some institutions, children undergo noninvasive CT scans with sedation by radiology personnel. For more complex cases, sedation/GA is provided by an anesthesiologist. Most commonly, noninvasive CT scans are performed with inhalation anesthesia via mask or under iv sedation with a continuous infusion of propofol (100–250 mcg/kg/min). For patients undergoing invasive CT-guided procedures (needle biopsy, placement of drainage tubes, such as thoracostomy tube, etc.), GETA is usually performed. Techniques include inhalational anesthesia and/or continuous infusion of propofol ± remifentanil.

MRI—MRI requires GA more often than noninvasive CT, since prolonged immobility is required for up to 1–2 hrs. Options include inhalational anesthesia with an MRI compatible anesthesia machine or continuous propofol infusion with an MRI compatible infusion pump. Hypothermia frequently occurs in small children. The cooling fan for the magnet can sometimes be turned off to decrease heat loss (discuss with MRI technician). One blanket over patient is usually permissible. The iv, airway circuit and monitors require extensions. Ferromagnetic objects in the MRI environment are a hazard. Objects can be propelled toward the magnet with sufficient speed and force to result in serious or fatal injury to the patient and/or health care provider.

Induction	Standard pediatric mask or iv induction (see p. D-1) can be accomplished in the CT scanner room in a special induction area outside the MRI scanner. After induction and stabilization of the airway, the patient and all personnel entering the MRI scanner should undergo a second check for removal of metal objects and equipment. Once check completed, transport patient into scanner and resume monitoring.	
Maintenance	Sedation/GA continued with supplemental O_2 via nasal cannula, spontaneous respiration, and infusion of propofol (100–250 mcg/kg/min). In children with an LMA or ETT, maintenance with inhalational agent or propofol infusion. Typically, these patients do not require muscle relaxants, and spontaneous breathing is appropriate unless controlled ventilation is required to treat ↑ ICP. Most infusion pumps need to remain a specific distance from the MRI scanner. The appropriate distance is dependent on the degree of shielding of each particular magnet. If breath holding for prolonged periods of time (e.g. several minutes for abdominal scans), intubation and/or paralysis may be required. Adequate ear protection should be routinely used during MRI.	
Emergence	Transport MRI patient back to induction area for emergence so that airway equipment is readily available. Patients usually transported to and recovered in PACU.	
Blood and fluid requirements	No blood loss. IV, if required: 22 or 24 ga × 1 NS/LR @ maintenance	
Monitoring	Standard MRI-compatible monitors (see p. D-1 for discussion of monitoring considerations).	For infants, use a child-size NIBP cuff on the leg. The length of tubing required significantly alters the values on infant-size cuffs.
Positioning	Ear protection necessary ✓ and pad pressure points. ✓ eyes.	
Complications	Airway obstruction	Repositioning, nasal or oral airway.
	Hypothermia	See adult MRI Unique Considerations and Complications, p. 1470.
	Burn injury	From inappropriate placement of pulse oximeter probe or EKG. Avoid coiling of wires and use only MRI compatible monitors.
	IV contrast reaction	
	Hearing loss (MRI)	

POSTPROCEDURE

Pain management	Noninvasive procedures are painless. Acetaminophen (35–40 mg/kg pr or 10–15 mg/kg po), hydromorphone (0.01–0.015 mg/kg) or morphine (0.05–0.1 mg/kg) as appropriate for invasive procedures

Suggested Readings

1. De Sanctis Briggs V. Magnetic resonance imaging under sedation in newborns and infants: a study of 640 cases using sevoflurane. *Paediatr Anaesth* 2005 Jan; 15(1):9–15.
2. Gregory GA ed. Pediatric Anesthesia, 4th edition. Churchill Livingstone, New York:2002. 809–18.

3. Jorgensen NH, Messick JM, Gray J, Nugent M, Berquist TH: ASA monitoring standards and magnetic resonance imaging. *Anesth Analg* 1994; 79:1141–7.
4. Levati A, Colombo N, Arosio EM, Savoia G, et al: Propofol anesthesia in spontaneously breathing pediatric patients during magnetic resonance imaging. *Acta Anaesth Scand* 1996;40:561–5.
5. Motoyama EK, Davis PJ, eds: Smith's Anesthesia for Infants and Children, 7th edition. Mosby Elsevier, Philadelphia:2006, 844-8, 851–3.
6. Usher AG, Kearney RA, Tsui B. Propofol total intravenous anesthesia for MRI in children. *Paediatr Anaesth* 2005Jan; 15(1): 23–8.
7. Young AE, Brown PN, Zorab JS: Anesthesia for children and infants undergoing magnetic resonance imaging: a prospective study. *Eur J Anaesthesiol* 1996; 13:400–3.

SURGICAL CONSIDERATIONS FOR ECMO

PROCEDURAL CONSIDERATIONS

Gary Hartman

Extracoporeal membrane oxygenation (ECMO) for prolonged periods (3–21 d) allows cardiopulmonary support for newborns and children with reversible respiratory failure. The most common indications are meconium aspiration and pulmonary HTN associated with congenital diaphragmatic hernia. The procedure is performed in the NICU with OR techniques. Patients are given anticoagulants prior to cannulation. Subsequently, repair of the diaphragmatic hernia also may be performed in the NICU on ECMO support before decannulation (Fig. 13.2-1 shows ECMO schematic).

The potential detrimental effects of the diaphragmatic repair on respiratory function can be managed with increased circuit flow. ECMO also has been helpful in some newborns with cardiopulmonary failure following correction of congenital cardiac defects. Vascular access is accomplished with one (venovenous) or two (venoarterial) cannulas. The IJ vein is cannulated in both methods with the tip of the cannula in the right atrium. In venoarterial ECMO, the common carotid artery is used with the tip of the cannula at the aortic arch. The wound is closed around the cannulas, which are secured to the infant's scalp.

Usual preop diagnosis: Meconium aspiration; diaphragmatic hernia; Bochdalek's hernia

SUMMARY OF PROCEDURE	
Position	Supine
Incision	Subcostal, right neck incision
Special instrumentation	ECMO circuit (Fig. 13.2-1)
Unique considerations	Anticoagulation
Antibiotics	Preop: ampicillin 25 mg/kg iv + gentamicin 2.5 mg/kg iv Intraop: cefazolin irrigation (1 g/500 mL NS)
Surgical time	1–2 h
Closing considerations	Assess for changes in ventilation (e.g., PIP, pre- and postductal ABG).
EBL	> 5–10 mL/kg
Postop care	Paralysis maintained; fentanyl infusion @ 2–4 mcg/kg/h
Mortality	25–30%
Morbidity	Respiratory failure sepsis
Pain score	6–7

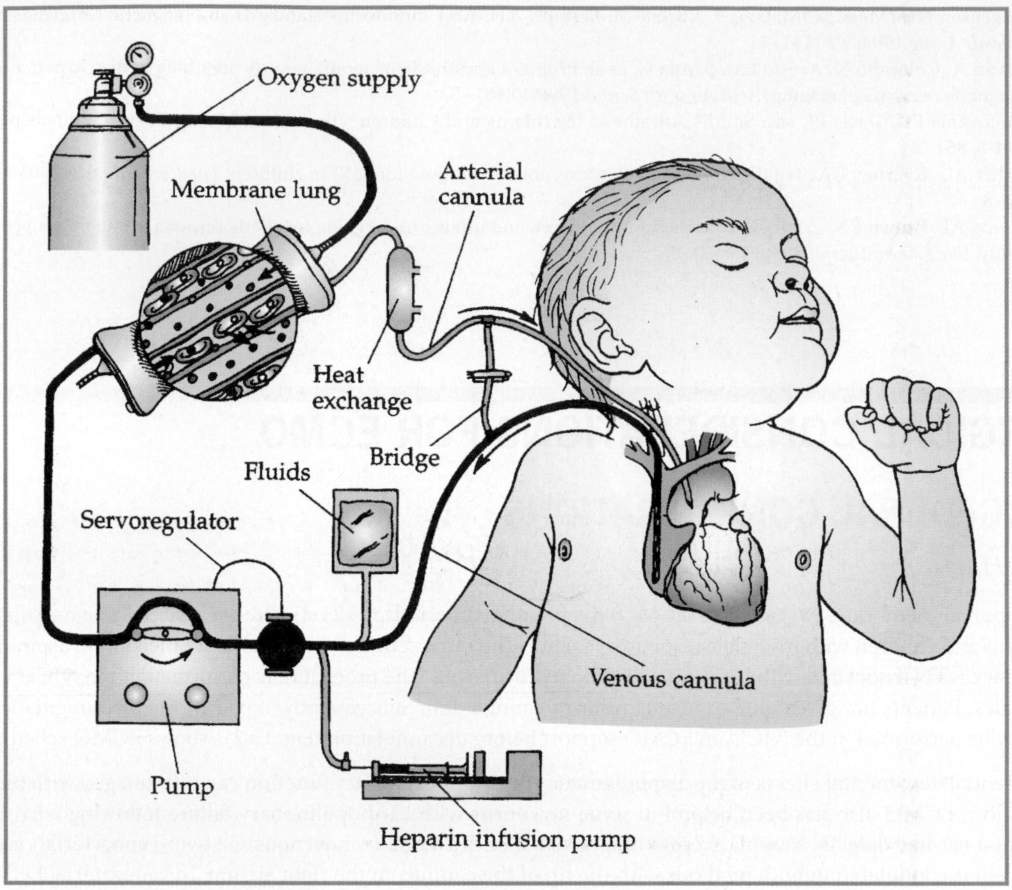

Figure 13.2-1. ECMO circuit. Venous blood is withdrawn by gravity through a servoregulator to prevent pump from actively siphoning venous return. A pump delivers blood back to the arterial cannula after it passes through the membrane oxygenator and heat exchanger. Venous return is from the right atrium, while arterial infusion is into the aortic arch in double cannula (venoarterial) or right atrium (venovenous) techniques. (Reproduced with permission from Baker RJ, Fischer JE: *Mastery of Surgery*, Vol I, 4th edition. Lippincott Williams & Wilkins, Philadelphia: 2001.)

PATIENT POPULATION CHARACTERISTICS	
Age range	Newborn–weeks or months
Male:Female	1–2:1
Incidence	1:4000 live births
Etiology	Unknown
Associated conditions	For diaphragmatic hernia: malrotation (40–100%); congenital heart disease (15%); renal anomalies; esophageal atresia; CNS abnormalities

ANESTHETIC MANAGEMENT FOR SURGICAL PROCEDURES UNDER ECMO

RJ Ramamurthi and Chandra Ramamoorthy

ECMO therapy protects the pulmonary alveoli from ventilator associated barotrauma and oxygen toxicity, while maintaining tissue oxygenation. For surgical procedures that are done on ECMO, the anesthetic management can be either TIVA or a combination of intravenous and inhalation techniques. The plastic components of the bypass circuit can sequester varying amounts of the intravenous agents, especially fentanyl, altering the plasma levels and resulting in unpredictable hemodynamic changes. Volatile anesthetics are not routinely available on ECMO circuits due to difficulties with scavenging. If ECMO is performed for systemic hypoxemia, then the decreased pulmonary flow will not favor the uptake of inhalational anesthetics.

ECLS Registry Report
International Summary
January, 2008

Extracorporeal Life Support Organization
1327 Jones Drive, Suite 101
Ann Arbor, MI 48105

Overall Outcomes

	Total Patients	Survived ECLS		Survived to DC or Transfer	
Neonatal					
Respiratory	21,916	18,638	85%	16,611	76%
Cardiac	3,266	1,899	58%	1,229	38%
ECPR	354	223	63%	134	38%
Pediatric					
Respiratory	3,693	2,368	64%	2,057	56%
Cardiac	4,036	2,465	61%	1,823	45%
ECPR	691	354	51%	269	39%
Adult					
Respiratory	1,416	833	59%	721	51%
Cardiac	825	382	46%	274	33%
ECPR	269	97	36%	70	26%
Total	36,466	27,259	75%	23,188	64%

Centers

Centers by Year

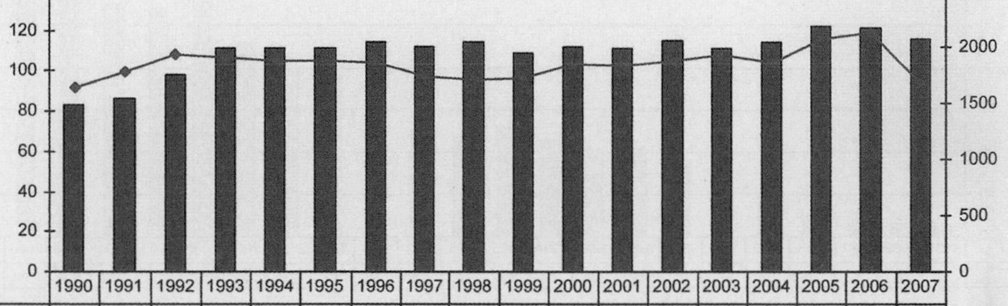

	1990	1991	1992	1993	1994	1995	1996	1997	1998	1999	2000	2001	2002	2003	2004	2005	2006	2007
Count	83	86	98	111	.111	111	114	112	114	109	112	111	115	111	114	122	121	116
Cases	1644	1775	1933	1906	1873	1870	1865	1740	1713	1718	1851	1833	1875	1929	1864	2076	2122	1675

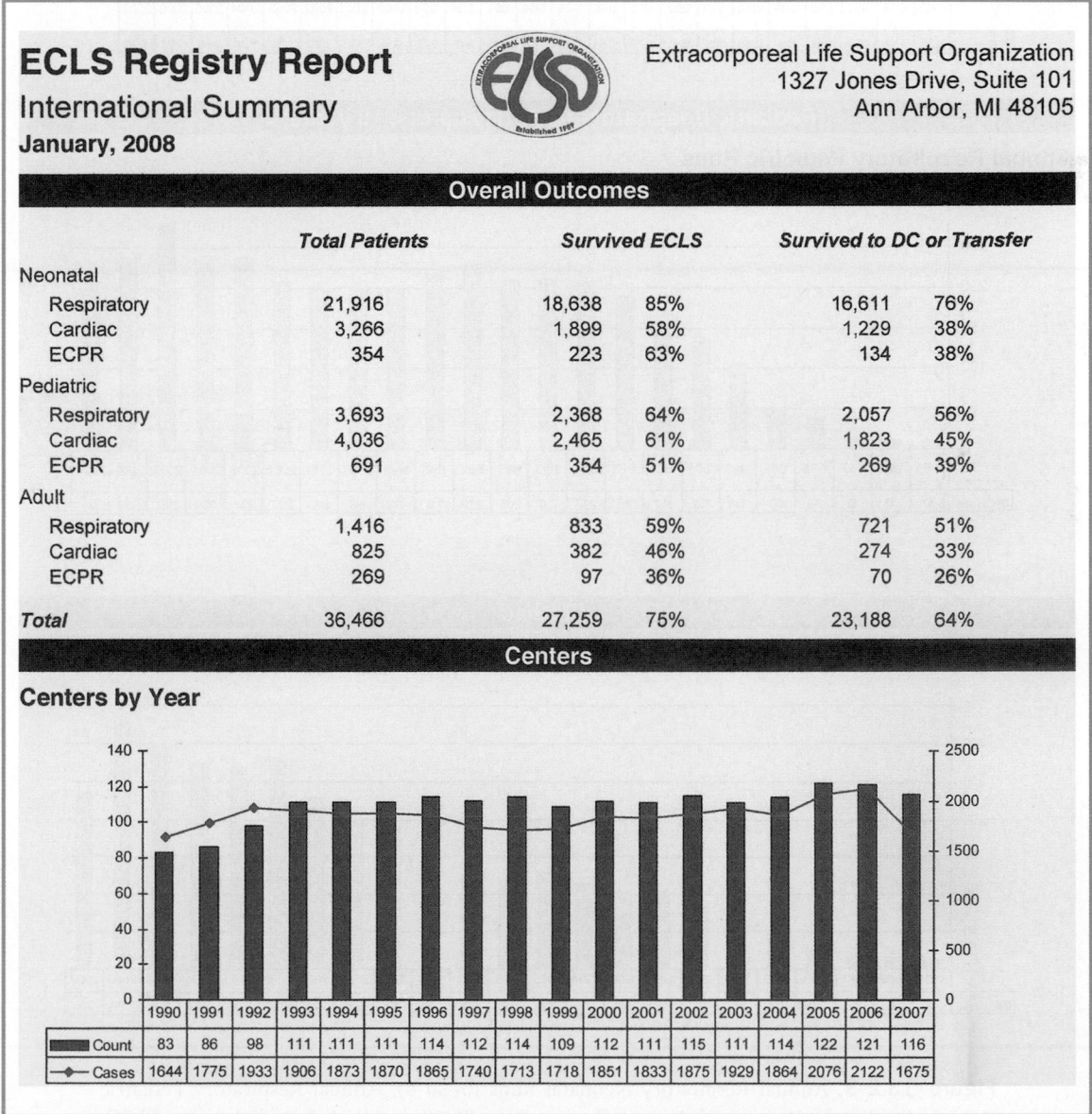

Figure 13.2-2. ECLS Registry Report January 2008. Acknowledgment: ELSO, Extracoporeal Life Support Organization, Ann Arbor, Michigan, 2008.

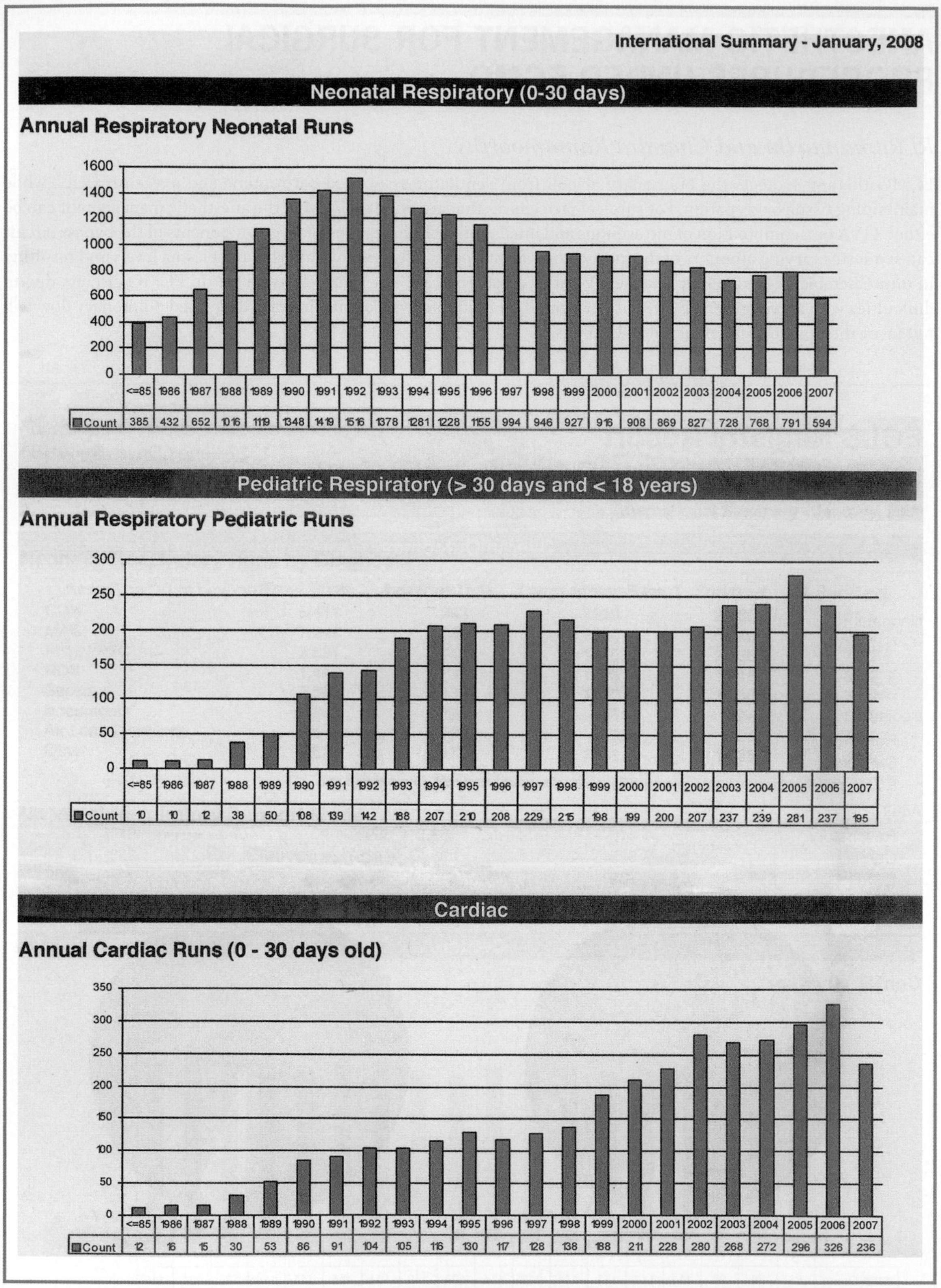

	<=85	1986	1987	1988	1989	1990	1991	1992	1993	1994	1995	1996	1997	1998	1999	2000	2001	2002	2003	2004	2005	2006	2007
Count	385	432	652	1016	1119	1348	1419	1516	1378	1281	1228	1155	994	946	927	916	908	869	827	728	768	791	594

	<=85	1986	1987	1988	1989	1990	1991	1992	1993	1994	1995	1996	1997	1998	1999	2000	2001	2002	2003	2004	2005	2006	2007
Count	10	10	12	38	50	108	139	142	188	207	210	208	229	215	198	199	200	207	237	239	281	237	195

	<=85	1986	1987	1988	1989	1990	1991	1992	1993	1994	1995	1996	1997	1998	1999	2000	2001	2002	2003	2004	2005	2006	2007
Count	12	16	15	30	53	86	91	104	105	116	130	117	128	138	188	211	228	280	268	272	296	326	236

Figure 13.2-3. Annual Respiratory Neonatal Runs (0–30 d), Annual Respiratory Pediatric Runs (> 30 d and <18 yr), and Annual Cardiac Runs (0–30 d old). Acknowledgment: ELSO, Extracoporeal Life Support Organization, Ann Arbor, Michigan, 2008.

It is important to keep in mind that altering the surgical table height will have an impact on the venous return to the ECMO circuit (passive gravity assisted drainage), hence the perfusionist must be informed before undertaking this maneuver. Anesthetic agents also cause preload and afterload changes; additional volume should be readily available to maintain adequate venous volume. Blood and products, vasoactive agents must be available to overcome transient changes in filling and blood pressure.

Diaphragmatic hernia repair is the commonest procedure done on ECMO. On the morning of surgery a trial period off bypass is used to assess the adequacy of conventional ventilation independent of ECMO. If the surgery occurs on full ECMO support, ACT is maintained at 160–200 sec by addition of heparin to the ECMO circuit.

Monitoring includes: heart rate, arterial blood pressure, temperature, pump flow rate with frequent ABGs and VBGs.

The potential detrimental effects of diaphragmatic repair on respiratory function can be managed with increased circuit flow. ECMO also has been helpful in some newborns with cardiopulmonary failure following correction of congenital cardiac defects. Vascular access is accomplished with one (venovenous) or two (venoarterial) cannulas. The IJ vein is cannulated in both methods with the tip of the cannula in the right atrium. In venoarterial ECMO, the common carotid artery is used with the tip of the cannula at the aortic arch. The wound is closed around the cannulas, which are secured to the infant's scalp. The indications for the use of ECMO have shifted over the past decade. ECMO centers and total ECMO runs peaked in 2005 and 2006 and have since declined significantly. Neonatal respiratory runs peaked in the early 1990s and have declined since, presumably due to the use of other respiratory salvage strategies. Pediatric and cardiac indications have continued to increase, especially in the last 3–4 yr. These patients are frequently on support for longer durations and cannulation may be more complex. The majority of all ECMO runs still employ VA cannulation although some centers do a significant percentage of their runs on VV ECMO.

Suggested Readings

1. American Academy of Pediatrics Section on Surgery; American Academy of Pediatrics Committee on Fetus and Newborn, Lally KP, Engle W. Postdischarge follow-up of infants with congenital diaphragmatic hernia. *Pediatrics* 2008; 121(3):627–32.
2. Falconer AR, Brown RA, Helms P, et al: Pulmonary sequelae in survivors of congenital diaphragmatic hernia. *Thorax* 1990; 45(2):126–9.
3. Stolar CJH: Congenital diaphragmatic hernia. In *Surgery of Infants and Children*. Oldham KT, Colombani PM, Foglia RP, eds. Lippincott-Raven Publishers, Philadelphia: 1997, 883–96.
4. Wilson JM, Lund DP, Lillehei CW, et al: Congenital diaphragmatic hernia: predictors of severity in the ECMO era. *J Pediatr Surg* 1991; 26(9):1028–33.

SECTION 14.0

OFFICE-BASED ANESTHESIA

SURGEONS

David A. Berman, MD (*Facial Rejuvenation*)
Vernon J. Adams, Jr, DMD (*Dental rehabilitation*)
Azeem K. Lakha, DMD (*Dental implants*)

ANESTHESIOLOGIST

Terri D. Homer, MD

INTRODUCTION—ANESTHESIOLOGIST'S PERSPECTIVE

Terri D. Homer

DEFINITION OF OFFICE-BASED ANESTHESIA

The assumption in this chapter is that office-based anesthesia (OBA) is distinct from outpatient anesthesia in a freestanding surgery facility. OBA is used in many medical specialties, including most dental subspecialties, dermatology, plastic surgery, ophthalmology, otolaryngology, and gynecology. The procedures described in this chapter are but a small sampling of the ways in which anesthesia is used in medical/dental offices. Anesthesiologists who carry out anesthetic procedures in the office setting may be sole practitioners or part of a group of anesthesiologists who have a "division" or rotation devoted to OBA. Although anesthesia practiced in an office carries the same risks, burdens of responsibility, and skill requirements as in a fully equipped surgical center, in the office setting, the anesthesiologist may be expected to arrange for the oxygen supply, suction, monitoring, and emergency equipment. They may even bring a portable anesthesia machine with them from site to site. This unique challenge for the anesthesia provider includes: working with personnel unfamiliar with anesthesia concerns, converting the office into a facility appropriate for anesthesia, selecting appropriate patients, providing safe and effective anesthesia/analgesia, and properly preparing and recovering the patients.

STATE REGULATIONS REGARDING OFFICE-BASED ANESTHESIA

Many states have laws listing strict requirements for medical facilities where anesthesia is provided for surgical procedures. Some states have regulations based on the type of surgical procedure performed. Others regulate and credential the facility based on the type of anesthesia used (i.e., GA, iv, local). Still others base regulations on the type of facility itself. In California, for example, dental offices are regulated differently than medical offices. For many years, the California Dental Board has regulated anesthesia in the dental or oral surgery office by credentialing the anesthesia provider and/or the office facility itself. An oral surgeon, dentist, or physician issued a GA permit by the Dental Board goes through a credentialing process by one or two examiners that includes direct observation of an anesthesia case, demonstration of emergency drills, and examination of required monitoring and resuscitation equipment on site. The permit allows the holder to provide GA in any dental office. The Dental Board also issues 'Conscious Sedation' permits to those dental practitioners who qualify and want to use this technique. Physicians in California wishing to have I.V. sedation or general anesthesia available in their office must first be accredited as a surgery center by one of several State agencies providing this service such as AAAHC.

EQUIPMENT NEEDED FOR OFFICE-BASED ANESTHESIA

In the office setting, the anesthesia provider may or may not have the use of an anesthesia machine or other sophisticated equipment that is readily available in a surgical center. In some respects, however, this setting is analogous to other out-of-OR locations. The ASA Guidelines for Nonoperating Room Anesthetizing Locations[1] covers all types of out-of-OR facilities, and these recommendations should be followed. Appropriate monitoring—including pulse oximetry, ECG, and BP—is required. Many portable monitors have $ETCO_2$ monitoring capability, which may be useful for the spontaneously ventilating, sedated patient. A precordial stethoscope is quite useful for monitoring respirations, especially in the dental patient, in whom airway obstruction is a frequent occurrence during the procedure. Also in accordance with the ASA guidelines, full resuscitation equipment, an adequate source of O_2 (and backup O_2), a functioning suction, adequate lighting and electrical outlets (with backup battery source), and a telephone with immediate access to a hospital ER also must be available. In the credentialed medical (nondental) facility, these items are required to be on site. In the dental facility, they may or may not be present. It is the responsibility of the anesthesia provider to make sure these items are available in the medical or dental facility before administering an anesthetic.

ANESTHETIC GOALS IN THE OFFICE SETTING

Typically, the primary anesthetic goal in the office setting is to provide moderate-to-deep sedation; however, the definition of 'sedation' in this setting varies considerably. For example, in the young or disabled pediatric patient having dental restoration work, "conscious sedation" often is not adequate and they will typically require deep sedation or general anesthesia. In the patient having dental implants, minimal or moderate sedation may be all that is required as the oral surgeon may need the patient's cooperation at times during the procedure. A patient undergoing full-face laser resurfacing most likely will require deep sedation or general anesthesia, since this procedure can be quite painful. Because sedation is a continuum and individual patient responses vary, the anesthesia provider must be prepared to resuscitate any patient receiving sedation in the office.

PATIENT SELECTION

As in all medical facilities, the patient's safety is of paramount importance. In the office setting, the ability to achieve a successful outcome is dependent first of all on appropriate patient selection. The patients presenting for OBA will fall into several categories, depending on the procedure and the patient's age and medical condition. An "appropriate patient" can be an ASA 1 or 2 patient. They may even be an ASA 3, if: (a) their medical problems are stable and well controlled with medication, and (b) the office procedure itself will not pose an undue risk to them.

PREOPERATIVE PREPARATION

An important role of the anesthesiologist is to educate the patient (or patient's parents, as appropriate) about the office anesthesia experience. A preop phone call discussing the patient's medical history, past anesthesia experience (in a hospital, surgery center, or dental office), the npo requirements, the anesthesia technique(s) to be used, postanesthesia expectations, and the anesthesia fees is essential. A written packet describing some of this information can be given to the patient in advance.

Safe and accepted npo requirements on the day of the procedure are as follows:

- A light breakfast (e.g. toast and a clear liquid), up to 6 hours before the appointment.
- Clear liquids (including Gatorade, Jell-O, fruit popsicles) up to 3 hours before the appointment.
- The patient's usual medications should be continued on the day of the procedure.

RECOVERY AND DISCHARGE

In a medical or dental office, often there is no separate recovery area designated as such. It is common practice for the patient to be recovered by the anesthesiologist in the treatment room until they can open their eyes and maintain an adequate airway without assistance. At that point, any iv or monitors that may have been used can be removed. If it is a pediatric patient, the parents may be brought into the room, although recovery remains under the supervision of the anesthesiologist. Office anesthesia patients can be discharged when they are well oriented, their pain and nausea are controlled, and they have a responsible adult to accompany them. They may still feel drowsy, but this should not prevent them from being able to walk with assistance.

Discharge instructions regarding appropriate post-op activities should be given to the responsible adult with the patient. Generally, patients are asked to adhere to the following instructions upon discharge:

- NPO except clear liquids in the first 2 hours after arriving at home. (Unless the ride is > 1 hour, we ask the patient not to drink anything in the car on the way home from the procedure facility.)
- A light meal after the first 2 hours, if the patient wishes.
- Adults should take it easy the rest of the day and have a responsible adult companion for at least 4 hours after the procedure.
- No driving for 24 hours.
- Children should stay home for the rest of the day postprocedure, under the direct supervision of a responsible adult.

The anesthesiologist also should give the responsible party (parent, friend, other relative) his/her pager or cell phone number in the event they need to contact the anesthesiologist after patient discharge.

Suggested Readings

1. American Society of Anesthesiologists: *ASA Guidelines for Nonoperating Room Anesthetizing Locations.* American Society of Anesthesiologists, 1994.
2. American Society of Anesthesiologists: *ASA Guidelines for Office-Based Anesthesia.* Available at: www.asahq.org/publicationsAndServices/office.pdf. 2004.
3. American Society of Anesthesiologists: *Continuum of Depth of Sedation, Definition of General Anesthesia and Levels of Sedation and Analgesia.* American Society of Anesthesiologists, 1994.

FACIAL REJUVENATION: LASERS AND RF TISSUE TIGHTENING

SURGICAL CONSIDERATIONS

David A. Berman

Description: In the last 13 years, a number of medical devices have been approved by the FDA to improve facial imperfections, such as wrinkles, precancerous skin lesions (actinic keratoses), acne scars, and hyperpigmentation. Today, laser skin resurfacing as well as radiofrequency tissue tightening have remained at the top of the list of popular facial rejuvenation techniques. "Super-pulsed" carbon dioxide (CO_2) lasers, erbium: YAG lasers, fractional lasers that treat the skin in a pixilated pattern, as well as deep and superficial radiofrequency (RF) devices all use heat in a controlled fashion to improve the appearance and physiology of the facial skin. Because many of these devices deliver a tremendous amount of heat to the skin surface, previous attempts at using nerve blocks and local infiltration with lidocaine were often considered inadequate, thus requiring either iv sedation or GA. Facial nerve blocks usually are performed to supplement iv sedation (added analgesia). After a Betadine prep, anesthetic eye drops are used, followed by the insertion of protective corneal shields. The treatment then begins with one or more passes performed at various energy levels. Many newer devices do not actually remove the outermost epidermal layers of the skin, but exert their beneficial effects below the surface in the dermis; however, more aggressive lasers do indeed ablate off both the epidermis and a portion of the underlying dermis, requiring postoperative care: some surgeons prefer to use only a Vaseline jelly dressing, whereas others use a more sophisticated, soothing facial dressing to prevent postoperative discomfort.

Usual preop diagnosis: Wrinkles, precancerous skin lesions (actinic keratoses), acne scars, and traumatic scars.

SUMMARY OF PROCEDURE	
Position	Supine, with shoulder roll. Surgeon at head of table.
Antibiotics	None during procedure. Antivirals and antibiotics started 1 d before procedure, and continued for 1–2 wk following.
Surgical time	45 min for full-face rejuvenation; less for regional areas
Postop care	Supine position, maintenance of facial dressing, occasional ice packs, antiviral medications, antibiotics
Mortality	None reported.
Morbidity	Bacterial infection Herpes simplex virus reactivation Delayed re-epithelialization Hypertrophic or keloid scar formation Corneal abrasion Delayed healing with redness Hyperpigmentation and hypopigmentation
Pain Score	2–5 depending on the type of medical device used.

PATIENT POPULATION CHARACTERISTICS	
Age range	18–85 yr
Male:Female	1:4
Incidence	Number of cases performed by members of the American Academy of Cosmetic Surgery/yr in the United States: 45,288 (American Academy of Cosmetic Surgery, 1085 members polled, 206 surveys returned, 19% response rate, margin of error +/– 6.15%)
Etiology	Solar radiation, acne, or trauma resulting in scars

ANESTHETIC CONSIDERATIONS

PREOPERATIVE

Many facial rejuvenation procedures are quite painful and can be very stressful to the patient; thus, local anesthesia is often inadequate. For these procedures, it is important to make sure that the patient with chronic HTN and/or other cardiovascular or respiratory disease is being adequately treated for these problems before undergoing either laser resurfacing or RF tissue tightening. A preop ECG (taken within the last yr) is recommended for those patients > 60 yr old or those being treated for HTN.

Premedication	In the adult patient, an oral premed can be given, if necessary, before the patient arrives in the office for the procedure. Diazepam 10–20 mg, or lorazepam 0.5–1.0 mg po 1 h before the appointment will help relax the severely anxious patient.

INTRAOPERATIVE

Anesthetic technique: MAC and/or GA

MAC/GA	During full-face laser resurfacing procedures, the patient will need to be under deep iv sedation, unless the surgeon is willing to use a large amount of local anesthetic (often RF tissue tightening will require less sedation, depending on the device used). Usually, a combination of intermittent doses of midazolam (1–2 mg iv), meperidine (25 mg iv), ketamine (25–30 mg iv q 1 h prn), and propofol (25–50 mcg/kg/min iv) will provide an adequate anesthetic state. If a nasal airway is inserted, nasal O_2 can be used—if the cannula is placed deep in the airway—at low flows. Otherwise, O_2 should be administered between facial passes if a laser is used. Again, the patient is not electively intubated, but an LMA may be needed if it is difficult to maintain a patent airway. Usually, patients having this procedure will require at least 75–150 mg meperidine (or its equivalent drug) to relieve the painful burning caused by multiple passes of these devices. Patients will shiver and sustain HTN and tachycardia unless an adequate level of analgesia is achieved. Because of the narcotic requirement, they should have prophylactic antiemetics during the procedure. Dexamethasone (8 mg iv) and metoclopramide (15 mg iv) are a good combination. In addition, im promethazine (25 mg) is very effective.	
Blood and fluid requirements	IV: 20 ga × 1 NS/LR @ 4–6 mL/kg/h	
Monitoring	Standard monitors (see p. B-1).	
Positioning	✓ and pad pressure points. ✓ eyes (eye shields in place).	
Complications	Laser fire	Use intermittent, low-flow O_2. Consider wrapping foil around cannula.

POSTOPERATIVE

Complications	PONV
Pain management	Oral analgesics (see p. C-2).
Recovery and discharge	The patient recovering from a full-face procedure usually has received a lot of potent anesthetic medication in a short period of time. They require at least 45–60 min to recover in the office. Vital signs should be stable (↓ BP and tachycardia must be treated). Pain and nausea also should be under control. These patients must be accompanied by a responsible adult who can stay with them at home for a few h after the procedure. A follow-up phone call to the patient by the anesthesiologist that evening is very helpful and appreciated.

OFFICE DENTAL REHABILITATION UNDER DEEP IV SEDATION

SURGICAL CONSIDERATIONS

Vernon Adams

Description: Dental rehabilitation includes the restoration of good dental health by removal of caries and decayed teeth, replacement of crowns or bridges, root canals, and periodontal treatment. Prior to treatment, the patient is placed in a supine position with a shoulder roll and the head immobilized. A throat pack is placed and a mouth prop inserted. The throat pack should be placed more anteriorly than normal since, in general, the patient will not be intubated. Dental rehabilitation is usually done in phases, starting with the operative phase. A rubber dam is placed to surgically isolate the teeth that will be treated. All dental caries are removed, the restorations are placed, and all debris is irrigated and suctioned away from the rubber dam, which is then removed. This sequence is repeated in quadrants as needed. After the operative phase of treatment is completed, the next phases (e.g., taking impressions for various appliances or dental prosthetics, dental extractions, or a dental prophylaxis) are undertaken, as necessary. Great care must be taken in maintaining the airway when taking impressions, as the bulk of impression material can compromise airway management.

Usual preop diagnosis: In-office dental rehabilitation usually focuses on treatment of the patient who is unable to be treated in a conventional setting for primarily behavioral/emotional reasons. These include dentophobia; pediatric patients who are excessively apprehensive and/or combative or who have a significant amount of dental caries; "special needs" pediatric patients—autistic, mentally retarded, developmentally delayed—and patients with mild-to-moderate forms of cerebral palsy.

SUMMARY OF PROCEDURE	
Position	Supine, with shoulder roll, head extended; surgeon at head of table (turned 90°)
Incision	Gingival or intraoral mucosa
Special instrumentation	Dental setup
Unique considerations	Nasal airway recommended; throat pack placed; forward displacement of tongue is important for airway management.
Antibiotics	None used routinely.
Surgical time	60–120 min
EBL	Minimal
Postop care	Recover in lateral position.
Mortality	Rare
Morbidity	Biting of lips or tongue 2° local anesthesia: 1% Bleeding: 1% Infection: < 1% Delayed Bleeding: Rare
Pain Score	1–2; higher for certain procedures (e.g., extraction of impacted tooth)

PATIENT POPULATION CHARACTERISTICS	
Age range	13 mo +
Male: Female	1:1
Incidence	20,000/yr in the United States
Etiology	Poor oral hygiene and/or dietary habits; lack of continuing periodic dental care

ANESTHETIC CONSIDERATIONS

PREOPERATIVE

In the pediatric dental office, the patients presenting for iv sedation are those who cannot cooperate due to age (too young) or to a preexisting mental or physical disease. Examples include a 20-month-old child with multiple "bottle caries," an 8-year-old autistic child, or a 14-year-old with cerebral palsy. Obviously, the anesthetic treatment plan must be tailored to the patient's individual needs. These patients must be screened in advance for clinical conditions that would put them at undue risk for problems 2° the anesthetic. Specifically, a patient with any cardiac, respiratory, endocrine, or neurologic problem must be evaluated. If the clinical problem is mild, stable, and under good control, the patient may be considered for anesthesia in the office. Examples of such conditions include mild nonsteroid-dependent asthma, corrected congenital heart disease, or a stable Sz disorder. The child with Down's syndrome may pose a very difficult problem in this setting, because airway obstruction can occur easily under deep iv sedation. Also, these patients frequently have concurrent congenital heart disease. Any child with a Hx of obesity, snoring, and/or sleep apnea can present a problem under iv sedation, due to airway obstruction. The child with a current or recent URI always poses a dilemma. Although there is controversy on this issue, these children generally should have their procedures postponed, because their chances of sustaining periop respiratory problems are higher than normal.

Premedication	Because there is no possibility of an inhalation induction in the office setting, as described here, the pediatric patient should receive adequate sedation as an "induction" that will allow placement of an iv with little or no emotional trauma. There are several options available for preprocedure sedation. In the older child (> 8 yr) who is psychologically mature, an iv can be placed without premedication. In a dental office that is equipped with N_2O, the patient can breathe a high flow N_2O/O_2 mix through a nasal mask for 10 min before iv placement. If the patient accepts the mask, this technique can help lessen the patient's fear of the iv. The use of a 30-ga needle for infiltration of buffered local anesthetic and, sometimes, the use of EMLA cream (placed 30 min in advance) also can be very helpful. Oral premedication is used commonly in children 4–8 yr old. Midazolam (0.5–0.7 mg/kg; maximum = 20 mg) mixed in an appropriate dose of liquid acetaminophen, given in the office 20 min before the procedure, can provide adequate sedation. In some, the addition of oral ketamine 2–3 mg/kg to the midazolam solution may result in a better sedating effect, especially in older pediatric patients. For those children who cannot cooperate with an oral premed (too young or emotionally or physically unable to do so), an im premedication is very effective. This can be administered 5 min before the procedure, in the treatment room, with the parents present. Ketamine 3 mg/kg, midazolam 0.2 mg/kg, atropine 0.02 mg/kg (or glycopyrrolate 0.01 mg/kg) can be mixed in the same syringe and given in the anterior thigh with a 23-ga needle. This has the benefits of rapid uptake and reliable achievement of an adequate level of amnesia and sedation. Because of the rapid onset, the anesthesiologist must be prepared to begin monitoring the patient immediately after injection. Additionally, the parents usually require some reassurance as they watch their child become sedated so rapidly.

INTRAOPERATIVE

Anesthetic technique: MAC. These patients are not intubated electively. A flexible LMA can be used for airway management, if needed. Following sedation, the patient is placed in the dental chair, with the head positioned to maintain an open airway. A shoulder roll may be needed to help with head extension. Monitoring—including pulse oximeter, ECG, BP cuff, and precordial stethoscope—is attached. O_2 is supplied, and $ETCO_2$ can be measured through a nasal cannula. An iv is started if not previously placed. A nasal airway is positioned with care (to avoid epistaxis) after the dental x-rays are taken. To prevent aspiration, a throat pack with a piece of dental floss attached—which remains outside the mouth—is placed, and minimal irrigation with constant suctioning is used. A rubber dam acts as a barrier between the teeth and the back of the throat. The anesthesiologist must be constantly vigilant in maintaining an open airway in these patients in the face of an oral procedure. Placing a flexible LMA may make airway management easier without interfering with the dental procedure. A propofol infusion can be started at a rate of 100–150 mcg/kg/min. Administration of a small amount of meperidine (e.g., 5–15 mg iv) may be useful in alleviating emergence delirium, especially if there is not adequate local anesthesia. Routine use of prophylactic antiemetics is recommended. In children, the use of metoclopramide (0.2 mg/kg) with dexamethasone (0.1 mg/kg) is very effective as a prophylactic antiemetic combination.

Emergence	No special considerations, except that throat packs must be removed.	
Blood and fluid requirements	IV: 20–22 ga × 1 NS/LR @ 4–6 mL/kg/h	
Monitoring	Standard monitors (see p. B-1)	
Positioning	✓ and pad pressure points. ✓ eyes.	

POSTOPERATIVE

Complications	PONV	These patients may swallow blood, with consequent PONV.
Pain management	Oral analgesics (see p. C-2).	
Recovery and discharge	In the dental office, there may not be a separate, designated recovery area. Usually, the pediatric patient is recovered by the anesthesiologist in the treatment room for at least 30 min, or until the patient is opening his/her eyes and maintaining a normal airway without assistance. At this point, the iv and monitors can be removed and the patient can continue recovering in the parents' arms, under the supervision of the anesthesiologist. The patient may need to stay another 30 min or until he/she opens his eyes without prompting, recognizes his parents, and has no nausea. Postop instructions given to the parents include: no outside or unsupervised activities for the rest of the day, no drinking or eating in the car on the way home, clear liquids for the first 1–2 h, followed by light food. The anesthesiologist should give the parents his/her pager or cell phone number so they can call with any questions that arise after they are at home. Regardless, a follow-up phone call from the anesthesiologist is always a good policy.	

DENTAL IMPLANTS AND BONE GRAFTING

SURGICAL CONSIDERATIONS

Azeem K. Lakha

Description: A dental implant consists of a tooth-root-shaped titanium post that is used to support a crown, bridge, or denture. Dental implants are inserted surgically into the mandibular or maxillary alveolar bone where teeth are missing. Single implants may be done with local anesthesia, but multiple or complex procedures are best accomplished with iv sedation. After the local anesthetic is administered, a mucoperiosteal flap is raised over the edentulous alveolus and the bone is exposed. Precise drill holes are made in the bone and the implants are screwed or tapped into place. Bone grafting may be necessary around the implants to fill in defects and is carried out using autologous, allogenic, xenogenic, or synthetic materials. In most cases, the gum tissue is closed over or around the implant. The bone is allowed to heal around the implant and 2–6 mo later the implant can be used to attach crowns, bridges, or dentures. In cases where there is insufficient bone, a bone graft is necessary **before** implants can be placed. Typically, bone grafts are allowed to heal for 6 months before implant insertion. Most minor grafting procedures are accomplished in the dental office under iv sedation and local anesthesia. Major grafts requiring extraoral donor sites may have to be done under GA via nasal ETT intubation.

Usual preop diagnosis: Acquired or congenital absence of dentition

SUMMARY OF PROCEDURE	
Position	Supine, with head tilted back, using an articulating headrest in the dental chair
Incision	Intraoral mucoperiosteal flaps
Special instrumentation	Precordial stethoscope
Unique considerations	Throat packs are used to prevent aspiration of teeth, crowns, blood, and irrigation fluids. Ensure that they are removed at the end of the case.
Antibiotics	Prophylactic antibiotics, given orally before surgery
Surgical time	1–3 h
EBL	25–100 mL
Mortality	Rare
Morbidity	Infection: 1% Bleeding: Rare Delayed Bleeding: Rare Aspiration: Rare
Pain Score	1–4, depending on procedure

PATIENT POPULATION CHARACTERISTICS	
Age range	17+ yr
Male: Female	1:1
Incidence	Becoming more common as technology improves
Etiology	Tooth loss

ANESTHETIC CONSIDERATIONS

PREOPERATIVE

Many patients having dental implant procedures are elderly and/or have multiple medical problems. The anesthesiologist should be consulted in advance about these patients so that questions about their medical conditions can be answered and a current list of medications can be obtained. Sometimes the patient's primary care physician needs to be contacted to discuss details of medical Hx. If chronic medical conditions are stable, patients often can receive "conscious sedation" and monitoring by the anesthesiologist for this procedure in the office.

Premedication Usually not necessary

INTRAOPERATIVE

Anesthetic technique: MAC. These patients are not intubated electively. In the adult patient having dental implants, the maintenance of a lightly sedated state is achieved using a combination of iv midazolam, fentanyl (or meperidine), and small amounts of ketamine (20–30 mg/dose). A pulse oximeter, ECG, BP cuff, precordial stethoscope or $ETCO_2$ monitor, and nasal O_2 should be in place. Glycopyrrolate (0.1–0.2 mg) should be given to decrease secretions. Dexamethasone 8 mg and metoclopramide 15 mg are useful as an antiemetic combination. Usually, the oral surgeon needs the patient's cooperation at some point during the procedure; therefore, propofol is not an ideal drug to use. It can be given, however, in small doses to the patient who requires more than the other drugs for sedation. Occasionally, the adult patient in this setting will require a nasal airway.

Emergence	No special considerations, except that throat packs must be removed at end of procedure.	
Blood and fluid requirements	IV: 20–22 ga × 1 NS/LR @ 4–6 mL/kg/h	
Monitoring	Standard monitors (see p. B-1)	
Positioning	✓ and pad pressure points. ✓ eyes.	

POSTOPERATIVE

Complications	PONV	These patients may swallow blood, with consequent PONV.
Pain management	Oral analgesics (see p. C-2).	
Recovery and discharge	See Recovery and Discharge for Office Dental Rehabilitation (p. 1516)	

SECTION

15.0

EMERGENCY PROCEDURES FOR THE ANESTHESIOLOGIST

ANESTHESIOLOGISTS

Frederick G. Mihm, MD

Myer H. Rosenthal, MD, FACCP

EMERGENCY CRICOTHYROTOMY

Clinical situation: Typically, this is a hypoxic patient with obstructed airway (not involving direct tracheal trauma), who cannot be mask ventilated or intubated.

Emergency "Stab" Cricothyrotomy[5]

Equipment	• Scalpel with #11 blade • Tracheal hook • Tracheostomy tubes: #6, #7 • ETTs: #6, #7 • Umbilical or twill tape for securing tube • 10-mL syringe for inflating cuff • Prep solution • 2% lidocaine • Suction device (Yankauer or Tonsil Tip) • Lubricant (lidocaine jelly or KY jelly)
Procedure	1. Prep skin. 2. Palpate cricothyroid membrane. 3. Make transverse incision through skin and cricothyroid membrane with single stab[5] (Fig. 15-1). 4. Reverse scalpel, place handle into wound, and turn 90° to expand incision. 5. Pass tracheostomy tube (or standard ETT) into trachea. 6. Inflate cuff on tracheostomy/ETT. 7. Ventilate patient. 8. Secure tube.

Emergency "Guidewire" Cricothyrotomy

Equipment	• Melker Emergency Cricothyrotomy Set (Cook Critical Care), or equivalent • Scalpel with #15 blade • 6-mL syringe half-filled with NS • 18-ga introducer needle • 18-ga iv catheter/needle • Amplatz extra-stiff guidewire 0.038" • Curved dilator • Airway catheter • Umbilical or twill tape
Procedure	1. Identify cricothyroid membrane between cricoid and thyroid cartilages (Fig. 15-2). 2. Stabilize cricothyroid membrane and make a vertical midline incision with #15 blade (Fig. 15-3). 3. Attach syringe to iv catheter and needle, and advance at a 45° caudad angle through incision until air bubbles can be aspirated (tracheal lumen). (See Fig. 15-4). 4. Remove syringe and needle, leaving catheter in place. 5. Advance soft end of guidewire into catheter several cm past end of catheter. 6. Remove catheter. 7. Assemble emergency airway device (Fig. 15-5) by inserting the dilator through the airway catheter until the handle stops against the connector of the airway catheter. 8. Advance the dilator/airway catheter assembly over the guidewire into the trachea, keeping proximal end of guidewire visible at all times (Fig. 15-6). 9. Remove guidewire and dilator, leaving airway catheter in place. 10. Ventilate patient. 11. Secure airway with umbilical or twill tape around the neck.

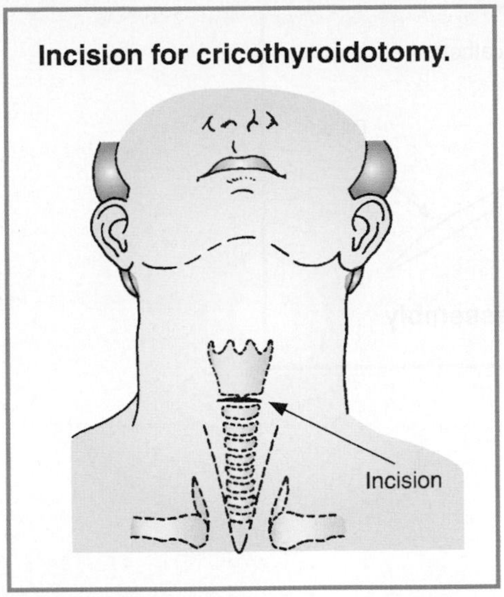

Figure 15-1. Reproduced with permission from Shackford S: Tracheostomy and cricothyrotomy. In *Clinical Procedures in Anesthesia and Intensive Care.* Benumof JL, ed. JB Lippincott, Philadelphia: 1992, 391–403.

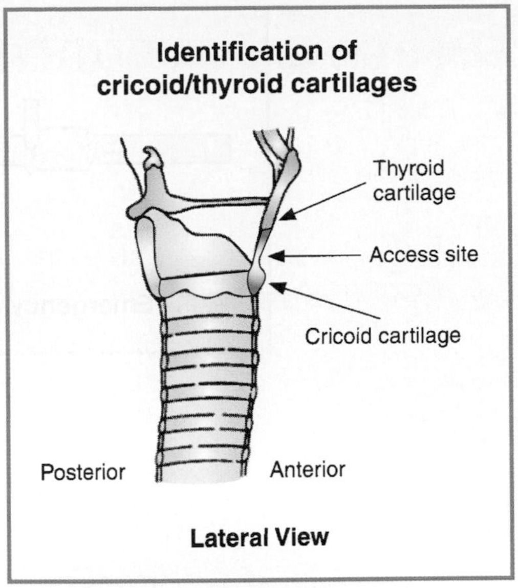

Figure 15-2.

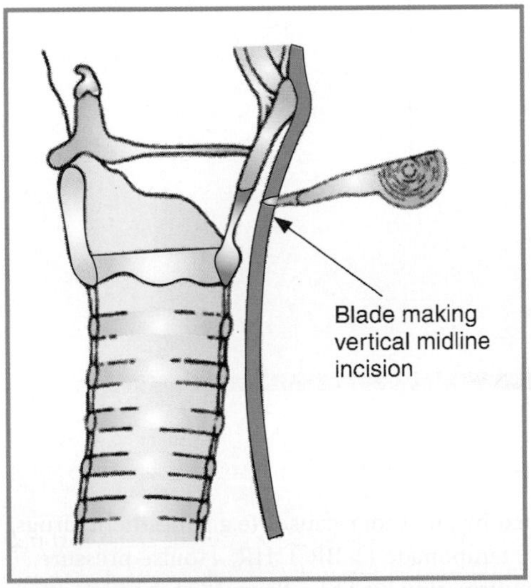

Figure 15-3.

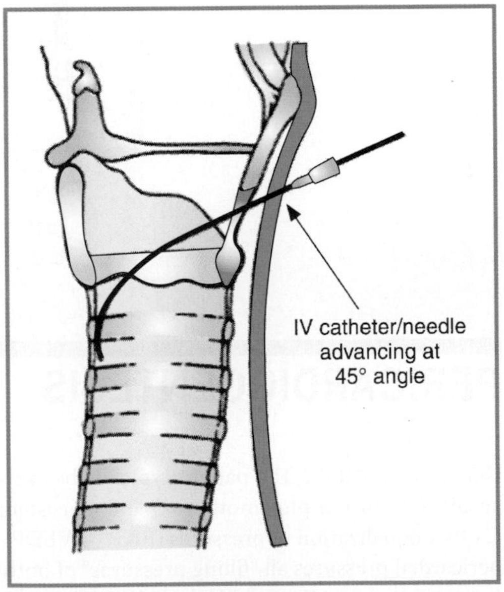

Figure 15-4.

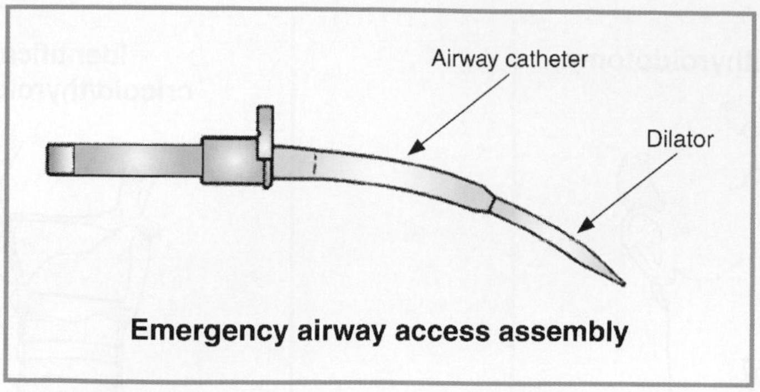

Figure 15-5.

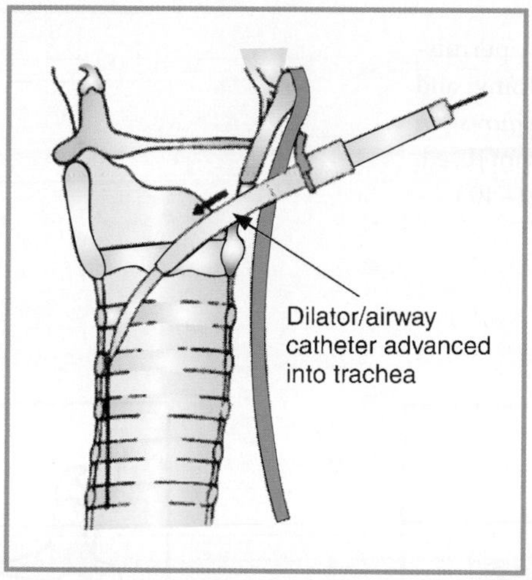

Figure 15-6.

PERICARDIOCENTESIS

Clinical situation: The patient typically has severe ↓ BP unexplained by any other causes (e.g., anesthetic drugs, autoPEEP, tension pneumothorax) and consistent with acute cardiac tamponade (↓ BP, ↑ HR, ↓ pulse pressure, ↑ CVP) ± equalization of pressures (RAP ~RVEDP ~PAD ~PAOP) ± confirmation by TEE. Because of the high intrapericardial pressures all "filling pressures" of both right and left heart appear high when preload is actually very low. In severe cases, patients will experience cardiac arrest with pulseless electrical activity (PEA).

Equipment	• 10-mL syringe • 18-ga spinal needle
Procedure[2]	1. Identify xiphoid process and point 1" below and 1" left of midline (Fig. 15-7). 2. Prep skin below xiphoid. 3. Attach needle to syringe and direct needle under rib toward left shoulder (Fig. 15-8). 4. If pericardial fluid is withdrawn, BP will ↑ immediately.

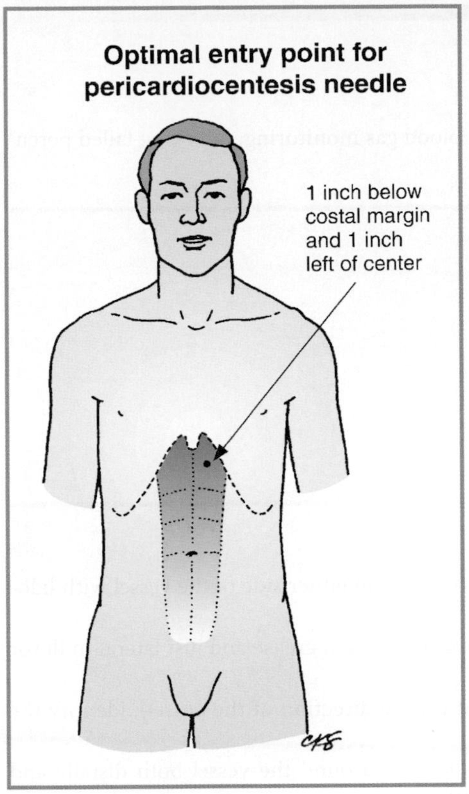

Figure 15-7. Reproduced with permission from Danforth J: Pericardiocentesis. In *Clinical Procedures in Anesthesia and Intensive Care.* Benumof JL, ed. JB Lippincott, Philadelphia: 1992.

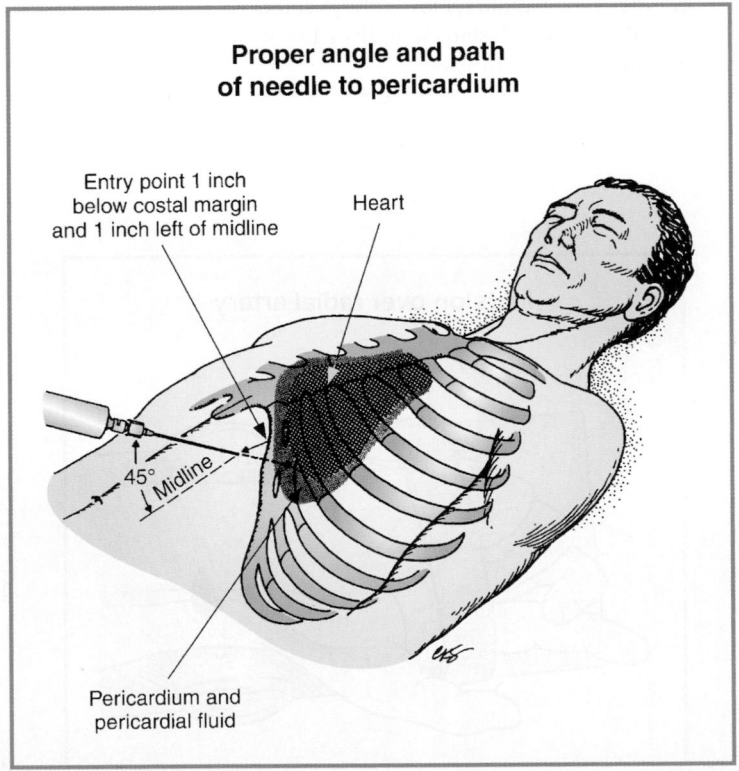

Figure 15-8. Reproduced with permission from Danforth J: Pericardiocentesis. In *Clinical Procedures in Anesthesia and Intensive Care.* Benumof JL, ed. JB Lippincott, Philadelphia: 1992.

ARTERIAL CUTDOWN

Clinical situation: A patient requires arterial catheterization for BP/blood gas monitoring, following failed percutaneous attempts, or with coagulopathy.

Equipment	• Prep solution • Wrist board • 2% lidocaine • Curved hemostat • Curved pickups • Scalpel with #10 and #11 blades • Gauze • 2–0 suture • Needle driver
Radial artery cutdown procedure[3,4]	1. Position wrist in extension on arm board. 2. Prep and drape wrist. 3. Infiltrate skin and deep tissues down to the bone on either side of the vessel with lidocaine (1–2%, 2–3 mL). 4. Make 1 cm transverse incision ~2 cm proximal to wrist crease and just lateral to flexor carpi radialis tendon (Fig. 15-9). 5. Using blunt dissection with the hemostat (in the direction of the vessel), identify the artery. 6. Blunt dissect just under artery and pass sutures around the vessel both distally and proximally (do not ligate vessel) (Fig. 15-10). 7. Use traction on the distal suture to stabilize artery for cannulation.[1] 8. After cannulation, remove sutures and close incision. (For cleaner wound closure, pass catheter through skin rather than directly into wound.) 9. Suture catheter to skin.

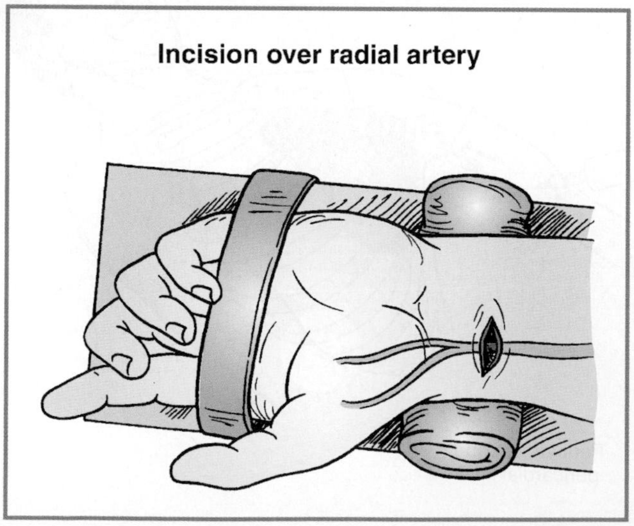

Figure 15-9. Reproduced with permission from Hirschl RB, Heiss K: Cardiopulmonary critical care and shock. In *Surgery of Infants and Children.* Oldham KT, Colombani PM, Foglia RP, eds. Lippincott-Raven, Philadelphia: 1997.

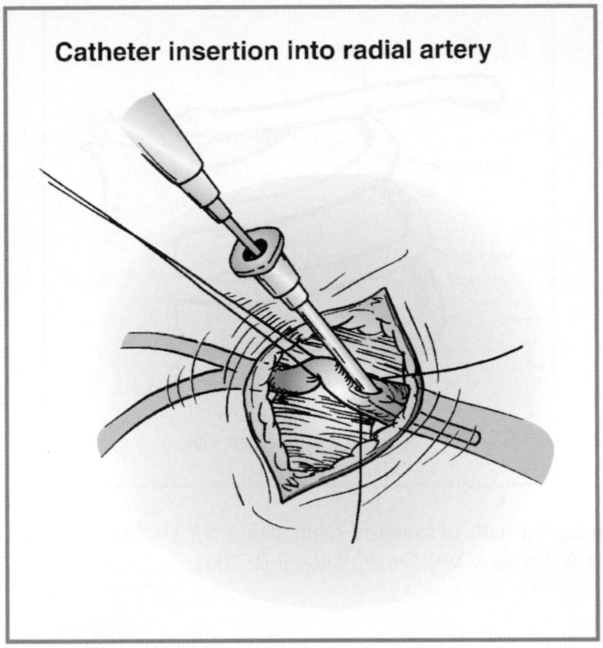

Figure 15-10. Reproduced with permission from Hirschl RB, Heiss K: Cardiopulmonary critical care and shock. In *Surgery of Infants and Children.* Oldham KT, Colombani PM, Foglia RP, eds. Lippincott-Raven, Philadelphia: 1997.

EMERGENT NEEDLE/CATHETER THORACOSTOMY

Clinical situation: A patient is experiencing severe hypotension and hypoxemia unexplained by any other cause (e.g., autoPEEP, cardiac tamponade) and consistent with acute tension pneumothorax (↑ P_{aw} ↓ movement of involved chest, ↓ breath sounds, ↑ resonance to percussion, compared to uninvolved side), and cardiovascular Sx related to ↑ thoracic pressures → ↓ preload (↓ BP, ↑ HR, ↓ pulse pressure, ↑ CVP). The CVP is artifactually elevated, reflecting the high intrathoracic pressures. Actual (transmural) CVP is very low. In severe cases, patients may experience cardiac arrest with pulseless electrical activity (PEA) because high intrathoracic pressures effectively stop venous return to the heart.

★**NB:** AutoPEEP **MUST** be ruled out first, particularly when the diagnosis is **bilateral tension PTX**. AutoPEEP is effectively ruled out (except with a ball valve airway lesion) by disconnecting the ETT from ventilator/ambu bag and allowing patient to exhale. If the patient's condition immediately improves, you have made the diagnosis of autoPEEP.

★**NB:** Release of the pressure that has built up in the chest is a life-saving maneuver. A large-bore chest tube does not need to be placed emergently. The much simpler needle/catheter thoracostomy is effective and less demanding for the nonsurgeon.

Equipment	One of the following: • 16-ga needle • 16-ga iv catheter/needle • 16-ga single-lumen CVP kit
Procedure	1. Identify the 2nd intercostal space by first identifying the Angle of Louis (union of manubrium and sternum); then move laterally to find the insertion of the 2nd rib. The interspace directly below this rib is the 2nd intercostal space. (See Fig. 15-11.) 2. Wipe skin with alcohol.

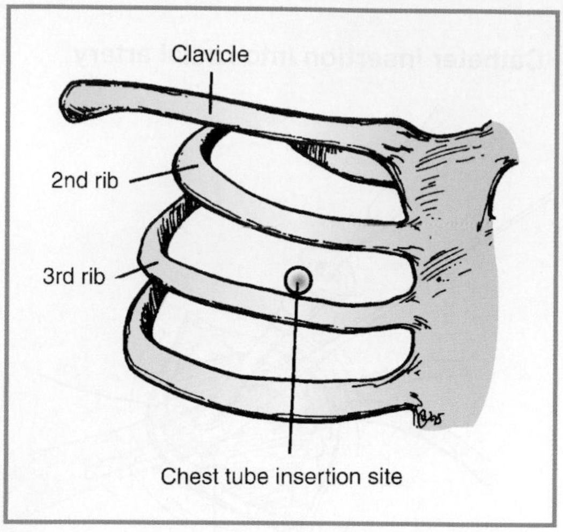

Figure 15-11. Adapted with permission from Baker RJ, Fischer JE: *Mastery of Surgery*, 4th edition. Lippincott Williams & Wilkins, Philadelphia: 2001.

Procedure (cont'd)	3. Use needle to enter the interspace anteriorly in line with a line drawn down from the clavicle at the junction of the middle and medial one-third sections. (This should be ~3 cm from the sternal margin.) 4. With entry into the pleural space, there should be an audible rush of air and immediate hemodynamic improvement in the patient.

(Note: A more permanent chest tube will still need to be placed [i.e., the patient no longer has a tension pneumothorax, but still has a pneumothorax.] This can be done in a more controlled situation by someone skilled in that procedure.)

Suggested Readings

1. Barftlett R, Munster A: An improved technique for prolonged arterial cannulation. *N Engl J Med* 1968; 279:92–3.
2. Danforth J: Pericardiocentesis. In *Clinical Procedures in Anesthesia and Intensive Care.* Benumof JL, ed. JB Lippincott, Philadelphia: 1992, 561–75.
3. Durbin CG Jr: Techniques for performing tracheostomy. *Respir Care* 2005; 50(4):488–96.
4. Grassmick B: Venous and arterial access. In *Manual of Critical Care Procedures.* Victor L, ed. Aspen Publishers, Rockville MD: 1989, 47.
5. Mackersie R: Venous and arterial cutdown. In *Clinical Procedures in Anesthesia and Intensive Care.* Benumof JL, ed. JB Lippincott, Philadelphia: 1992, 391–403.
6. Shackford S: Tracheostomy and cricothyrotomy. In *Clinical Procedures in Anesthesia and Intensive Care.* Benumof JL, ed. JB Lippincott, Philadelphia: 1992, 215–26.

APPENDICES

APPENDIX A: PREOPERATIVE CONSIDERATIONS

PREOPERATIVE LABORATORY TESTING AND DIAGNOSTIC STUDIES

Stephen P. Fischer

The value and utility of preop diagnostic studies have become central issues in evaluating cost-effective health care in the surgical patient. It is estimated that up to $3 billion is spent in the United States annually on preop laboratory and diagnostic studies. Unnecessary testing is inefficient and expensive, and it requires additional technical resources. Inappropriate studies may lead to evaluation of 'borderline' or false-positive laboratory abnormalities. This may result in unnecessary OR delays, cancellations, and potential patient risk through additional testing and follow-up.

Surgical patients require preop lab and diagnostic studies that are consistent with their medical histories, the proposed operative procedures, and the potential for blood loss. Preop lab and diagnostic testing should be ordered for specific clinical indications rather than simply because the patient is about to undergo a certain surgical procedure.

The following preop diagnostic guidelines provide basic recommendations. They are **not** intended as absolute or standard requirements. Practice guidelines should be modified based on clinical needs and individual practice, to ensure the highest quality of anesthesia and surgical patient care.

SUMMARY OF PREOP STUDIES

Chest x-ray (CXR)	**Overview:** A preop CXR should be used to assess the presence of acute, progressive, or chronic changes in cardiac/pulmonary disease. The decision to obtain a preop CXR should be individualized and based on clinical indications (see Table A-1). CXRs should not be part of a routine preop screening protocol. **Clinical indications:** Pneumonia; pulmonary edema; atelectasis; aortic aneurysm; mediastinal or pulmonary masses; tracheal deviation; pulmonary HTN; cardiomegaly; advanced COPD and blebs; dextrocardia; pulmonary embolism.
Electrocardiogram (ECG)	**Overview:** ECGs evaluate cardiac rhythm/conduction disturbances, ischemia, myocardial infarction, hypertrophy, and metabolic and electrolyte disorders. **Clinical indications:** Patients with suspected or known Hx of CAD; patient age > 50; HTN; hx of dysrhythmias, chest pain; CHF; diabetes; OSA, cerebral vascular disease and PVD; syncope or presyncope; dizziness; SOB; DOE; PND; palpitations; leg/ankle edema; abnormal valvular murmurs.
Liver function test (LFT)	**Overview:** LFTs establish the absence or presence of hepatic injury and the degree of hepatic reserve in disease states. LFTs consist of: AST(SGOT), ALT(SGPT), GGTP, alkaline phosphatase, serum albumin, and bilirubin. **Clinical indications:** Patients with suspected or known Hx of hepatitis (viral, alcohol, drugs); infiltration (tumor, immunologic); cirrhosis; portal HTN; gallbladder or biliary tract disease; jaundice; intravascular hemolysis.
Renal function testing	**Overview:** Renal function testing measures glomerular filtration and the magnitude of renal tubular dysfunction. These tests include: serum creatinine and BUN. **Clinical indications:** Renal function testing is indicated for patients with HTN; increased fluid overload (CHF/peripheral edema/ascites) associated with cardiac, hepatic, or renal impairment; dehydration; diabetes; nausea, emesis, or anorexia; polyuria; nocturia; oliguria; anuria; high-risk surgery in patients with low CO syndrome; hematuria; costovertebral angle pain: renal transplant Hx; renal disease; dialysis.
Hemoglobin (Hb), Hematocrit (Hct), CBC	**Overview:** The decision to obtain a preop Hgb, Hct, or CBC should be individualized and based on clinical indications, medical Hx, and the proposed surgical procedure. Hgb/Hct or CBC should not be part of a routine preop screening protocol. **Clinical indications:** Hematological disorder; bleeding/coagulopathy Hx; malignancy; chemotherapy; radiation therapy (CBC); renal disease; anticoagulant and steroid therapy; surgical procedures with high blood loss (> 1500 mL); highly invasive or trauma surgery; malabsorption/poor nutrition status; CNS disease.

Table A-1. Diagnosis-Based Preop Testing

Preop Diagnosis	ECG	CXR	Hct/Hb	CBC	Lytes	Renal	Glucose	Coag	LFTs	Drug levels	Ca+
Cardiac disease:											
Chronic atrial fib	X									X[2]	
CHF	X	±				±					
HTN	X	±			X[1]	X					
MI history	X				±						
PVD	X										
Stable angina	X				±						
Valvular heart disease	X	±									
CNS disorders:											
Seizures	X			X	X		X			X	
Stroke	X			X	X		X			X	
Tumor	X			X							
Vascular/aneurysms	X		X								
Coagulopathies				X				X			
Endocrine disease:											
Addison's disease				X	X		X				
Cushing's disease				X	X		X				
Diabetes	X				±	X	X				
Hyperparathyroidism	X		X		X						X
Hyperthyroidism	X		X		X						X
Hypoparathyroidism	X				X						X
Hypothyroidism	X		X		X						
Hematological disorders				X							
Hepatic disease:											
Alcohol/drug-induced								X	X		
Infectious hepatitis								X	X		
Tumor infiltration								X	X		
Malabsorption/poor nutrition	X			X	X	X	X	±			
Malignancy				X							
Morbid obesity	X	±					X				
Pulmonary disease:											
Asthma	(PFT only if symptomatic; otherwise no tests required)										
Chronic bronchitis	X	±		X							
Emphysema	X	±								X[3]	
Renal disease			X		X	X					
Select drug therapies:											
Anticoagulants			X					X			
Aspirin/NSAID	no tests										
Chemotherapy				X							
Digoxin (digitalis)	X				±					X	
Dilantin										X	
Diuretics					X	X					
Phenobarbital										X	
Steroids				X			X				
Theophylline										X	

X = OBTAIN ± = CONSIDER
1 Patients on diuretics
2 Patients on digoxin
3 Patients on theophylline

SUMMARY OF PREOP STUDIES (cont'd)	
Pregnancy testing	**Overview:** The decision to obtain a preop pregnancy test should be based on clinical Hx and examination. Several assays are available (serum hCG, urine hCG); β-hCG detectable in maternal urine and blood 8–9 d postconception. **Clinical indications:** Sexually active; time of last menstrual period; presence or absence of birth control method; patient intuition
Coagulation testing	**Overview:** Coagulation testing, or clotting function studies, should be obtained in patients with known or suspected coagulopathies as indicated from H&P and drug therapies. Tests include: prothrombin time (PT), partial prothrombin time (PTT). INR, platelet (Plt) count. **Clinical indications:** Bleeding disorder Hx; anticoagulants or other drugs affecting coagulation; critical-risk surgeries with significant blood loss expected; hepatic disease: malabsorption/poor nutrition
Urine analysis	**Overview:** Assessment of renal function, infection, intravascular volume status, metabolic disorders **Clinical indications:** There are no routine anesthesia preop requirements for a urine analysis.

Suggested Readings

1. Roizen MF, Cohn S: Preoperative evaluation for elective surgery—what laboratory tests are needed? In *Advances in Anesthesia*, Vol 10. Stoelting RK, ed. Mosby-Year Book, St. Louis: 1993, 25–47.
2. Schiff RL, Emanuele MA: The surgical patient with diabetes mellitus: guidelines for management. *J Gen Intern Med* 1995; 10(3):154–61.
3. Bapoje SR, Whitaker JF, Schulz T, et al: Preoperative evaluation of the patient with pulmonary disease. *Chest* 2007; 132(5):1637–45.
4. Cohn SL, Auerbach AD: Preoperative cardiac risk stratification 2007: evolving evidence, evolving strategies. *J Hosp Med* 2007; 2(3):174–80.

PERIOPERATIVE BETA-BLOCKER THERAPY

Cliff Schmiesing

There are new developments in the area of Perioperative Beta-Blocker (PBB) therapy, tempering the initial enthusiasm for the practice. Several recent clinical trials, retrospective reviews, and meta-analyses have not demonstrated the clinical benefit of the initial studies published nearly a decade ago, and have even demonstrated harm. The PBB issue has also taken on increased prominence and importance as it is frequently used as a measure of health care quality and benchmarking by various national organizations. Many research questions and practical considerations still remain unanswered. Identifying an individual patient likely to benefit for PBB can be difficult, especially when the risks appear intermediate or low. Choosing which β blocker, and the time frame to initiate treatment and how long to continue it remain unclear; as is the mechanism(s) underlying the therapeutic benefit of PBB. Lastly, development and evaluation of optimal care-delivery mechanisms for implementing PBB therapy are lacking.

Despite these limitations, the clinical evidence continues to favor the benefit of PBB in selected patient groups. The American Heart Association/American College of Cardiology (AHA/ACC) recently released updated recommendations for PBB in their 2007 Guidelines on Perioperative Cardiovascular Evaluation and Care for Noncardiac Surgery. The guidelines continue to recommend PBB across a wide spectrum of patients. Recommendations are divided into Class I, and Class IIa and IIb according to the strength of the supporting evidence, derived from randomized and nonrandomized clinical trials, case studies, expert opinion and the standard-of-care. A Class I recommendation is given for conditions where there is evidence and/or general agreement that PBB is beneficial, useful, and effective. Class IIa conditions are those where there is conflicting evidence and/or divergence of opinion about efficacy of PBB, but the weight of evidence favors it. A Class IIb recommendation is given when efficacy is less well established. Recommendations are stratified according to surgery type: vascular, high or intermediate risk (nonvascular), and low risk surgery, and also by the likelihood and severity of coronary heart disease (CHD). CHD is classified as low, intermediate, and high risk as determined by test results, and the presence of clinical risk factors including: known CHD, compensated or prior heart failure, diabetes mellitus, renal insufficiency, and cerebrovascular disease.

The AHA/ACC report gives a Class I recommendation for two conditions: (1) PBB should be continued in patients undergoing surgery who are already receiving β blockers to treat cardiovascular disease; and (2) β blockers should be given to patients undergoing vascular surgery who also have evidence of ischemia on preoperative testing. Class IIa (PBB ***probably*** recommended) indications include: (1) vascular surgery patients where preop assessment identifies

Table A-2. Recommendations for Perioperative Beta-Blocker Therapy (Adapted from the AHA/ACC Recommendations for Perioperative Beta-Blocker Therapy Based on Published Randomized Clinical Trials (1))

Surgery Type	No Risk Factors	≥1 Risk Factor	CHD or High Cardiac Risk (≥3 Risk Factors)	Taking β-blocker
Vascular	Consider β-blocker	Probably give β-blocker	+ Cardiac ischemia on preop testing→give β-blocker No ischemia or no prior test→probably give β-blocker	Continue β-blocker
Intermediate Risk	Inadequate data	Consider β-blocker	Probably give β-blocker	Continue β-blocker
Low Risk	Inadequate data	Inadequate data	Inadequate data	Continue β-blocker

CAD; (2) vascular surgery patients with multiple risk factors for CAD; and (3) patients undergoing intermediate- and high-risk surgical procedures who also have CAD or who have multiple risk factors for it. The Class IIb (***consider*** PBB) recommendation is given for two groups: (1) patients undergoing intermediate or high-risk surgery, including vascular surgery, who also have a single risk factor; and (2) patients undergoing vascular surgery at low cardiac risk. The AHA/ACC recommendations are summarized in Table A-2. These recommendations have not been updated since the publication of the POISE trial in 2008, which cast doubt on the benefit of PBB and showed an increased risk of death and stroke related to hypotension that effectively cancelled out the cardiovascular benefits of PBB, but of note, it excluded patients already taking β blocker medications. It is possible future recommendations will change, especially for lower risk patients in light of the POISE trial results. PBB therapy, when utilized, should be probably be started at least several days before surgery and titrated to heart rate decreasing effect—'*Start low and go slow*'. This is not always possible or practical.

In summary, PBB therapy is not beneficial for all patients, even for most patients. β blockers should be continued perioperatively for those patients taking one (unless new contraindications develop) and should be considered in the select group of vascular surgery patients with cardiac ischemia on stress testing, unless contraindicated. The need to consider a patient's risk profile and in some cases to start and manage PBB therapy underscores the importance of a timely and thorough preoperative assessment by the anesthesiologist or other physician with an understanding of this important perioperative intervention.

Suggested Readings

1. Fleisher Lee A., et al: ACC/AHA 2007 Guidelines on Perioperative Cardiovascular Evaluation and Care for Noncardiac Surgery: Executive Summary: A Report of the American College of Cardiology/American Heart Association Task Force on Practice Guidelines (Writing Committee to Revise the 2002 Guidelines on Perioperative Cardiovascular Evaluation for Noncardiac Surgery) *Circulation*; 116(17):1971–1996.
2. POISE Study Group. Effects of extended-release metoprolol succinate in patients undergoing non-cardiac surgery (POISE trial): a randomized controlled trial. *Lancet* 2008; 371:1839–47.
3. Fleisher, Lee A., et al: ACC/AHA 2006 Guideline Update on Perioperative Cardiovascular Evaluation for Noncardiac Surgery: Focused Update on Perioperative Beta-Blocker Therapy – A Report of the American College of Cardiology/American Heart Association Task Force on Practice Guidelines (Writing Committee to Update the 2002 Guidelines on Perioperative Cardiovascular Evaluation for Noncardiac Surgery). *Anesth Analg* 2007; 104:15–26.
4. Lindenauer PK, Pekow P, Wang K, et al. Perioperative ß-blocker therapy and mortality after major noncardiac surgery. *N Engl J Med* 2005; 353:349-61.
5. Fleisher, Lee A., Perioperative ß-Blockade: How Best to Translate Evidence into Practice. *Anesth Analg* 2007; 104:1–3.

APPENDIX B: STANDARD ADULT ANESTHETIC PROTOCOLS

Richard A. Jaffe, C. Philip Larson, Jr., Cliff Schmiesing, Steve Shafer

STANDARD MONITORS (NONINVASIVE)	
Blood pressure (BP)	Usually noninvasive (oscillometric) technique. Match cuff width to arm size to avoid inaccurate BP.
Capnometry/ capnography	Measurement of $ETCO_2$/display of wave form
Gas analyzer (e.g., IR, mass spectometry)	Measurement of respired gases and anesthetics
Electrocardiogram (ECG)	5-lead preferred. Usual display: lead II and $V_{4\ or\ 5}$
Esophageal or precordial stethoscope	Breath and heart sounds monitored; dysrhythmias and ΔBP may be detected. Seldom used today, because sound competes with more useful pulse oximetry sound
Nerve stimulator	Monitor status of neuromuscular blockade
Oxygen analyzer	Measurement of FiO_2
Pulse oximetry	Measurement of O_2 saturation of hemoglobin; also gives a pulse sound that indicates heart rate, rhythm, and change in saturation
Temperature	Nasal, esophageal, bladder, rectal, tympanic, or skin
Visual observation of patient	Skin color, pupils, temperature, edema, sweating, movement
Ventilator function monitors	PIP, TV, disconnect alarm, pressure-volume/flow-volume loops, etc.

STANDARD ANESTHETIC MANAGEMENT (ADULT ASA 1 & 2)

★**NB:** The following sections are guidelines only (for an otherwise healthy 70 kg adult). Specific drugs and drug dosages should be individualized, based on the physiological and pharmacological status of the patient, including factors such as age, weight, concurrent medication, and comorbidities.

PREMEDICATION

Light	Midazolam 1–2 mg iv Lorazepam 1–2 mg Hydroxyzine 25–100 mg	po 1 h preop po 1 h preop
Moderate	Midazolam 2–3 mg iv ± Fentanyl 25–100 mcg iv	Prior to induction (in patient holding area or OR) Monitor for respiratory depression or apnea.
Heavy	Diazepam 10 mg + Morphine 0.1 mg/kg with Scopolamine 0.2–0.4 mg	po 1–2 h preop im 30–60 min preop

INDUCTION TECHNIQUES

Preinduction

1. ✓ anesthesia machine, suction, airway equipment, drugs.
2. Attach monitors and verify function.
3. Administer 100% O_2 by mask × 1–3 min.
4. Administer supplemental sedation/analgesia (as appropriate).

e.g.: fentanyl	1–3 mcg/kg iv
± midazolam	0.03–0.1 mg/kg iv

Induction agents

Propofol	1.5–2.5 mg/kg iv (in increments) **NB:** Pain on injection may be lessened by prior administration of lidocaine 1% 5–10 mL.
Thiopental	3–5 mg/kg iv
Etomidate	0.2–0.4 mg/kg iv **NB:** Pain on injection; myoclonus

Muscle relaxants for intubation

Drugs	Doses	Onset	Duration
Vecuronium	0.1 mg/kg	2–3 min	24–30 min
	0.2 mg/kg (rapid onset)	< 2 min	45–90 min
Rocuronium	0.6–1.2 mg/kg	45–90 sec	30–120 min
Pancuronium	0.1 mg/kg	3–4 min	40–65 min
Mivacurium	0.1–0.2 mg/kg	1–2 min	6–10 min
Cisatracurium	0.2 mg/kg	2 min	40–80 min
Succinylcholine:	1.0 mg/kg	30–60 sec	4–8 min
If given after defasciculating dose of NMR	1.5 mg/kg	30–60 sec	4–8 min
Infusion	1 g/250–500 NS (titrated to effect)	+60 sec	While infusing (phase II block possible)

MAINTENANCE TECHNIQUES

Inhalational anesthesia

30–100% O_2
+ 0–70% N_2O
+ Isoflurane (MAC in 100% O2 = 1.17%) or Sevoflurane (MAC = 1.8%) titrated to effect
Alternatively for short procedures, consider desflurane (MAC = 6.6%)

Balanced anesthesia

30–100% O_2
+ 0–70% N_2O
+ Meperidine 0.5–1.5 mg/kg/3–4 h (intermittent bolus)
or morphine 0.05–0.15 mg/kg/3–4 h (intermittent bolus)
or fentanyl 1–10 mcg/kg prn response to surgical stimulation
or remifentanil 0.05–2 mcg/kg/min prn response to surgical stimulation (no residual analgesia)
+ Isoflurane or sevoflurane titrated to effect
or propofol 50–200 mcg/kg/min (titrated to effect)
Alternatively, for short procedures consider desflurane (MAC = 6.6%).

Total intravenous anesthesia (TIVA)[1]

Oxygen 30% in N_2O (continue 70% N_2O until end of procedure)

+ Remifentanil infusion*	Induction infusion	@ 0.5–1 mcg/kg/min × 1–2 min
(infusion off 2–5 min before end of surgery)	Maintenance infusion	@ 0.05–0.2 mcg/kg/min
+ Propofol bolus + infusion	Induction bolus	1–1.5 mg/kg
(infusion off 2–5 min before end of surgery)	Maintenance infusion	@ 40–80 mcg/kg/min

TIVA (cont'd)	*Oxygen 100%;* Can add air 50%, but it seldom offers any advantage		
	+ Remifentanil infusion*	Induction infusion	@ 0.5–1 mcg/kg/min × 1–2 min
	(infusion off 5 min before end of surgery)	Maintenance	@ 0.1–0.35 mcg/kg/min
		10 min before end surgery	@ 0.05–0.1 mcg/kg/min
	+ Propofol bolus + infusion	Induction bolus	1–1.5 mg/kg
	(infusion off 2–3 min before end of surgery)	Maintenance	@ 60–90 mcg/kg/min
		10 min before end surgery	@ 20–40 mcg/kg/min
	*No residual analgesia: postop pain management depends on type of surgery, and analgesic requirements may be substantial. Recommend having fentanyl or meperidine for quick pain relief followed by morphine or dihydromorphone for prolonged pain relief. [1]Steven Shafer, MD Source:		

If **continued muscle relaxation** is required during the above maintenance techniques, several options are available. Always use a nerve stimulator to assess block before re-dosing.

Short-acting	Mivacurium	0.1 mg/kg/10–20 min or 1–15 mcg/kg/min
Intermediate	Vecuronium	0.025 mg/kg/30 min
	Rocuronium	0.6 mg/kg/30 min
	Cisatracurium	0.2 mg/kg/40 min
Long-acting	Pancuronium	0.02 mg/kg/60–90 min

EMERGENCE

1. Reversal of muscle relaxant	As surgical conditions permit, reverse residual muscle relaxant (when at least 1 twitch is present in train-of-four) with one of the following: Neostigmine 0.05–0.07 (maximum dose) mg/kg iv + glycopyrrolate 0.01 mg/kg iv, or Edrophonium 0.5–1.0 (maximum dose) mg/kg iv + atropine 0.015 mg/kg iv.
2. Analgesia	If remifentanil was used during surgery, supplemental analgesics will be necessary and should be given promptly after emergence.
3. Nausea prophylaxis	Ondansetron (4 mg iv) (or dolasetron (12.5 mg iv), or granisetron (100 mcg iv). Also, consider adding dexamethasone 4–8 mg and/or metoclopramide (10–20 mg iv). The use of droperidol (0.625 mg iv) is unfortunately controversial because of effects on cardiac conduction at higher doses. Consider OG tube placement and suction to empty stomach. *See Prevention of PONV (below).*
4. O_2	D/C N_2O/volatile agents and administer 100% O_2.
5. Suction	Suction oropharynx thoroughly.
6. Extubation	Extubate after protective airway reflexes have returned, the patient is breathing spontaneously, and is able to follow commands.

MONITORED ANESTHESIA CARE (MAC)

1. Standard monitoring with regular verbal contact.
2. Nasal O_2 (qualitative measurement of respiratory rate, volume of ventilation, and $ETCO_2$ can be obtained by attaching a sampling catheter to the nasal cannula.)

3. Light-to-moderate levels of sedation (± analgesia) can be maintained using a propofol infusion (25–100 mcg/kg/min), or with intermittent bolus injections of midazolam (0.25–1 mg) ± fentanyl (10–25 mcg) or with a remifentanil infusion (0.025–0.07 mcg/kg/min), titrated to effect. Monitor closely for respiratory depression.
4. Alternatively, dexmedetomidine (an α–2 agonist) can produce excellent sedation and analgesia without respiratory depression. The loading dose is typically 1 mcg/kg iv over ~ 15 min (↓ BP may occur) followed by an infusion of 0.2–0.7 mcg/kg/h.
5. If the initial local anesthetic injection will be painful (e.g., retrobulbar block), then a brief period of analgesia, sedation, and amnesia can be induced with:

	Advantages:	Disadvantages:
A. Midazolam (0.5–2 mg) ± Ketamine (10–20 mg) ± alfentanil 3–7 mcg/kg or remifentanil 0.5 mcg/kg all injected 2–3 min before pain:	Profound amnesia and analgesia. Usually no apnea and airway reflexes maintained. Patient usually able to cooperate.	Patient not "asleep." Timing is important. Possible ↑BP and HR
or		
B. STP (1–2 mg/kg) or propofol (0.5–1 mg/kg) ± fentanyl (25–50 mcg/kg)	Patient "asleep"	Possible apnea with loss of airway ↓ BP Patient unresponsive.

RAPID-SEQUENCE INDUCTION OF ANESTHESIA (FULL-STOMACH PRECAUTIONS)[1]

1. ↓gastric volume/acidity	Ranitidine 50 mg iv at least 30–60 min before induction Metoclopramide 10 mg iv 30–60 min before induction 0.3 M sodium citrate 30 mL po immediately before induction
2. Induction	Preoxygenation = 3 min. Suction must be readily available. Stylet ETT. ± Defasciculate: e.g., vecuronium 1 mg iv 3–5 min before using succinylcholine. Cricoid pressure (Sellick maneuver) by assistant (8–10 lb pressure; beware of force transfer to C6 vertebra). Effective cricoid pressure makes laryngoscopy, mask ventilation, and LMA insertion difficult. Consider Trendelenburg position with graded release of cricoid pressure during laryngoscopy. Choice of induction agent depends on patient condition including hemodynamic stability. Options include: Etomidate 0.1–0.4 mg/kg Or Ketamine 1 mg/kg or for patients better able to tolerate ↓ BP: STP 2–5 mg/kg Or Propofol 1–2.5 mg/kg + Succinylcholine 1.5 mg/kg or rocuronium 1.2 mg/kg (slightly slower onset) for intubation Lungs may be ventilated while waiting for NMB—avoid airway pressure > 20 cm H_2O
3. Intubation	Intubate only when the patient is fully relaxed. Watch chest movement and auscultate for equal BBS. ✓expired CO_2 on monitor. Listen over stomach. Secure ETT and release cricoid pressure. Pass NG/OG tube and suction stomach contents.
4. Failed intubation protocol	[See Anesthetic Considerations for Cesarean Section, Obstetric Surgery, 823.]

RAPID-SEQUENCE INDUCTION (cont'd)

5. Maintenance	As indicated by patient's condition and type of surgery.
6. Extubation	Repeat NG/OG suction is often useful before emergence and extubation. Extubate when patient is awake and has active laryngeal protective reflexes. Remember, some may require postop ICU care until safe extubation can be assured.

SPECIAL PEDIATRIC CONSIDERATIONS

1. The same principles apply in children requiring surgery, and in those who may have full stomachs. Consider emptying the stomach with an OG tube prior to induction in patients with pyloric stenosis or with high-grade intestinal obstruction following po barium. If iv is placed, continue as indicated previously. If iv access is difficult, O_2/sevoflurane induction with cricoid pressure, succinylcholine (2–4 mg/kg im) will permit intubation and minimize risks of gastric aspiration.
2. Awake intubation in neonates and sick infants may be the safest method.

FIBEROPTIC INTUBATION PROTOCOL; AWAKE AND ASLEEP[2–4]

C. Philip Larson, Jr.

Premedication	If not contraindicated, patients should receive mild-to-moderate sedation with meperidine 0.5 mg/kg or fentanyl 0.3–0.5 mcg/kg and midazolam 2–4 mg iv.
Topical anesthesia	When premedication has been established, for awake FOI the oropharynx is sprayed vigorously ~ 6 times over a span of 10 min with lidocaine 4% solution using a disposable EZ spray unit powered with oxygen. Initially, the spray is directed at the front of the tongue; gradually, it is directed further back in the throat, until the entire oropharynx is numb. Having the patient inhale deeply while spraying enhances the topical effect. In reality, the lateral recesses of the oropharynx need not be anesthetized topically because both fiberoptic laryngoscope (FOL) and ETT are confined to the midline of the mouth.
Tracheal anesthesia	With patient breathing oxygen from anesthesia circuit or transport mask, transtracheal injection of cocaine or lidocaine 4% (4 mL) is made through the cricothyroid membrane, using a 5-mL syringe and a 23-ga, 3/4-inch needle. So that this injection can be made as rapidly as possible, it is important to use a small syringe, making certain that the connection between syringe and needle is tight. It is important that the operator's hand be fixed firmly against the patient's upper chest to assure that needle movement is minimized should the patient start to cough, and that the full injection is made into the trachea. When the injection is complete, the patient is urged to cough vigorously.
Laryngoscopy	After the mouth and trachea are anesthetized with local anesthetic, an oral airway with a central orifice (e.g., Tudor-Williams, Patel, Ovassapian airway) is placed in the midline of the mouth. A 7-mm orotracheal tube, without connector attached, is placed over a FOL. With the operator at the patient's side near the waist, the FOL is introduced through the hole in the airway and advanced to end of airway. At this point, the epiglottis should be visible. The tip of the fiber optic scope is flexed toward the operator about 15–20°, which should bring arytenoid cartilages and laryngeal opening into view. The scope is advanced into the larynx so that tracheal rings can be visualized. Often, the carina also can be visualized. The laryngoscopist also can place the scope in the airway by darkening the room and using the scope as a light wand, directing the light externally to the sternal notch and advancing it down the trachea. If a wire-reinforced tube is desired, use a Patel or Ovassapian airway instead of the Tudor-Williams airway for guidance, because these airways can be removed with the tube connector in place.
Intubation	The scope is placed on the patient's chest and, holding it so that it not advanced further, the orotracheal tube is advanced gently into the trachea. To facilitate passage of the orotracheal tube past the arytenoid cartilages and into the larynx, it is necessary to rotate the tube counterclockwise 90°—or even as much as 180°—several times as it is being advanced.

FIBEROPTIC INTUBATION (cont'd)

Intubation (cont'd)	Using this rotational movement, the operator should never need to push hard on the tube to position it in the larynx. After the tube is in place, the FOL and oral airway are removed, and the 15-mm connector is reattached to the tube. $ETCO_2$ confirms proper placement. The orotracheal tube is then firmly taped in place at one side of the mouth. If manual ventilation of the lungs is possible, it is often beneficial for both patient and anesthesiologist to perform FOI with the patient anesthetized. This is particularly true for patients with cervical spine injuries where manipulation of the head during direct laryngoscopy or coughing during topicalization of the airway or insertion of the tube during awake FOI may aggravate the spinal cord injury. Asleep FOI involves inducing GA, inserting an LMA, and placing the patient on controlled ventilation. Then proceed with Plan C (see ref 4). In brief, a 6.0 uncuffed tube is mounted on the FOI, the FOI is inserted into the trachea using the LMA as a guide, and the 6.0 tube is lubricated and inserted into the laryngeal opening. The FOI is removed and the lungs ventilated via the 6.0 tube. A medium sized airway exchange catheter (AEC) is lubricated on one end and inserted into the trachea via the 6.0 tube. The AEC usually meets resistance at the distal end of the 6.0 tube. If this occurs, rotate the 6.0 tube while pushing on the AEC. Once the AEC is a few cm beyond the tip of the 6.0 tube, the tube and LMA are removed en-block leaving the AEC in the airway. With the AEC in the far right corner of the mouth, thread the final endotracheal tube on the AEC and gently advance it through the mouth into the larynx, rotating it counterclockwise to avoid obstruction from the right arytenoid cartilage. Then remove the AEC and connect the ETT to the anesthetic circuit.

Suggested Readings

1. Larson CP, Steadman RH: Management of the full stomach: a reevaluation. *Curr Rev Clin Anesth* 2005; 25:253–64.
2. Larson CP: Fiberoptic intubation of the trachea, Part I. *Curr Rev Clin Anesth* 2000; 21:117–28.
3. Larson CP: Fiberoptic intubation of the trachea, Part II. *Curr Rev Clin Anesth* 2001; 21:129–36.
4. Larson CP: A safe, effective, reliable modification of the ASA difficult airway algorithm for adult patients. *Curr Rev Clin Anesth* 2002; 23:1–12.
5. Weiss M, Gerber AC: Rapid sequence induction in children—it's not a matter of time! *Pediatric* Anesth 2008; 18(2):97–9.

PREVENTION OF PONV (Adapted from Gan, et al, 2007.)

Clifford Schmiesing

PONV risk factors	Patient-related	Female gender Nonsmoking status H/o PONV/motion sickness	Simple Risk Score for PONV in Adults: assign 1 point for each of the following risk factors: female gender, nonsmoker, hx of PONV, postop opioids. Risk of PONV: point sum 0 = 10%; 1 = 20%; 2 = 40%; 3 =6 0%, and 4 = 80%.
	Anesthetic-related	Volatile anesthetics Nitrous oxide Intra/postop opioids High dose neostigmine	
	Surgical-related	Duration of surgery Type of surgery	Each 30 min ↑ in duration ↑ PONV risk by 60% Laparoscopy, laparotomy, breast, strabismus, plastic, maxillofacial, gynecologic, abdominal, neurologic, ophthalmologic, urologic
Antiemetics	**Pharmacologic Agents**	**Timing of administration**	
	Serotonin blockers	End of surgery	Ondansetron 4 mg iv, Granisetron 0.35–1.5 mg iv, Dolasetron 12.5 mg iv
	Dexamethasone 4–8 mg iv	At induction	Adverse effects not seen with single bolus dose.
	Droperidol 0.625–1.25 mg iv	30 min before end of surgery	Consider risk of Q-T prolongation and cardiac dysrhythmias especially at higher doses. Risk low at dose range of 0.625–1.25 mg iv.
	Promethazine 6.25–25 mg iv	30 min before end of surgery	Sedating and may cause local tissue damage if iv catheter infiltration occurs.

PONV (cont'd)			
Antiemetics (cont'd)	Metoclopramide 10–20 mg iv	30 min before end of surgery	Can cause anxiety, confusion, or visual changes.
	Prochlorperazine 5–10 mg iv	30 min before end of surgery	
	Scopolamine transdermal patch	2–4 h before surgery	May cause sedation, dry mouth, visual changes, and confusion, especially in the elderly
	Ephedrine 0.5 mg/kg IM	End of surgery or as rescue rx in PACU	
Nonpharmacologic	Acupuncture, acupressure	Before or after surgery	
PONV prevention strategies	↓ anesthesia-related RF's	Consider regional anesthesia where appropriate Propofol for induction/maintenance where appropriate Avoid/minimize N_2O and volatile agents Avoid/minimize postop opioids Avoid high-dose neostigmine Adequate hydration	
PONV risk stratification and management	Low risk	No prophylaxis→treat PONV when it occurs.	
	Intermediate risk	Choose 1–2 interventions	
	High risk	Choose 2 interventions	

Suggested Reading

1. Gan TJ, Meyer TA, Apfel CC, et al: Society for ambulatory anesthesia guidelines for management of postoperative nausea and vomiting. *Anesth Analg* 2007; 104:1082–89.

VENOUS THROMBOEMBOLISM (VTE) PROPHYLAXIS

(Adapted from Geerts et al, 2004)

Clifford Schmiesing

VTE Risk Factors and Prevention Strategies

Weak	Moderate	Strong
Varicose veins	Cancer or myeloproliferative disorders	Surgery (e.g., hip/leg fx)
Immobility	Central venous catheterization	Major trauma
↑Age	Hypercoagulable state	Spinal cord injury
Acute medical illness	Pregnancy postpartum	
Smoking	Estrogen therapy	
Inflammatory bowel disease	Heart or respiratory failure	
Obesity	Oral contraceptives	
Pregnancy	Previous VTE	
	Malignancy	

VTE (cont'd)

Level of risk	Successful prevention strategies	Risk profiles/examples
Low risk	No specific prophylaxis, early and "aggressive" mobilization	Minor surgery in patients < 40 yr with no additional risk factors.
Moderate risk	LDUH (q 12 h), LMWH (= 3400 U daily), GCS, or IPC	Minor surgery in patients with additional RFs or surgery in patients 40–60 yr with no additional RFs.
High risk	LDUH (q 8 h), LMWH (> 3400 U daily), or IPC	Surgery in patients > 60 yr or age 40–60 with additional RFs (prior VTE, cancer, hypercoagulable, etc.)
Highest risk	LMWH (> 3400 U daily), fondaparinux, oral VKAs (INR, 2–3), or IPC/GCS + LDUH/LMWH	Surgery in patients with multiple RFs (age > 40 yr, cancer, prior VTE), or hip or knee arthroplasty, HFS major trauma; SCI

Abbreviations: DVT: deep-vein thrombosis; GCS: graduated compression stockings; HFS: hip fracture surgery; INR: international normalized ratio; IPC: intermittent pneumatic compression; LMWH: low-molecular-weight heparin; LDUH: low-dose unfractionated heparin (aka "minidose heparin"); SCI: spinal cord injury; VKA: vitamin K antagonist.

Suggested Reading

1. Geerts, WH, Pineo, GF, Heit, JA. et al: Prevention of venous thromboembolism: the seventh ACCP conference on antithrombotic and thrombolytic therapy. *Chest* 2004; 126:S338–S400.

APPENDIX C: STANDARD PERIOPERATIVE PAIN MANAGEMENT

Sean Mackey, Ian Carroll, and Raymond R. Gaeta

INTRODUCTION

Pain during the periop period has recently become an area of significant focus. Of the > 25 million surgical procedures performed in this country each year, > 75% of patients experience pain, and > 80% of those experience moderate-to-extreme pain.[5] These observations have led, in part, to the adoption of the new Joint Commission Pain Standards recognizing the rights of patients to appropriate assessment and management of their own medical needs.

The primary goals of periop pain management include the reduction of pain and suffering with consequent improvement in function. Poor pain control leads to problems, such as a decreased ability to ambulate, which increases the risk of thromboembolic phenomenon and fatal PE. Inadequate pain control after abdominal and thoracic surgeries leads to splinting, atelectasis, and risk of pneumonia. Furthermore, activation of the neuroendocrine stress response to surgical pain stimulates the anterior pituitary gland, releasing a cavalcade of stress hormones and catecholamines, which have been shown to have deleterious effects on postop outcomes. These effects include weight loss, fatigue, immunosuppression, thromboembolism and hypercoagulability, dysrhythmias, urinary retention, and impaired pulmonary function.[2] As an additional consequence, the continuous afferent barrage of nociceptive signals induces changes in the spinal cord and brain, leading to a phenomenon of central hypersensitization or "wind-up," which is thought to play a role in the perpetuation of pain after surgery and even the transformation of acute pain states into chronic ones.[6] As we understand more of the effects of pain on organ function and the CNS during the periop period, we realize that, through optimal pain control, not only can we impact pain and suffering, but also improve the overall morbidity and mortality of our surgical patients.

MULTIMODALITY ANALGESIA

Acute pain specialists have not been particularly successful in eliminating a patient's postop pain using a single analgesic agent or technique. Instead, we have found that we can enhance patient satisfaction by using small amounts of multiple agents, each working to reduce nociception at different points along the pain processing pathways—a concept called **"multimodality analgesia."** By utilizing small amounts of opiates, COX-2Is, and neural blockade together, side effects have been reduced and pain control and patient satisfaction improved. This concept is most effective when integrated with a periop rehab approach to surgery, which involves teams of surgeons, anesthesiologists, rehabilitation specialists, nurses, pharmacists, and other health care providers, all working together. It requires that the patient be given appropriate preop education, excellent periop nociceptive blockade and attenuation of the neuroendocrine stress response, postop exercise, and early enteral nutrition.[1]

PREEMPTIVE ANALGESIA

An important component of multimodality analgesia is the notion of preemptive analgesia. This concept has been well known to the basic science researchers, but has caused much confusion, and often disappointment, in clinical practice. Part of the problem lies in how the term has been used in the past—often applied only to the administration of an analgesic agent preop or preincision. In fact, while the term does imply an intervention before surgery, it has much more stringent requirements. Specifically, it implies providing antinociceptive measures preop and postop to prevent the establishment of central sensitization caused by incisional and inflammatory injuries. Preincisional, long-acting neural blockade and administration of NSAIDs or COX-2Is have been shown to significantly reduce postop pain and opiate requirements, as compared with initiating therapy after surgery. Clinical researchers also have demonstrated improvements in postop rehab of patients by using preemptive analgesia, particularly in lower-extremity orthopedic surgery. Preemptive analgesia also may reduce the development of chronic pain syndromes following surgery, due to reduction in central hypersensitization.[4]

THE NEW ANALGESIC PARADIGM

This concept utilizes preemptive and multimodal administration of COX-2Is, neural blockade, and sustained-release opiates to replace the current overreliance on potent, short-duration opiates for postop pain management. The combination of COX-2Is, which reduce nociceptive sensitization both peripherally and centrally with a high degree of safety, and neural conduction blockade can significantly reduce pain scores, parenteral opiate dose requirements, and dose-dependent adverse events. When used in conjunction with a structured postop rehab program, these techniques can lead to decreased patient morbidity and mortality, increased patient satisfaction, decreased recovery time, and shorter hospitalization.[1,3]

Suggested Readings

1. Kehlet H: Acute pain control and accelerated postoperative surgical recovery. *Surg Clin North Am* 1999; 79(2): 431–43.
2. Kehlet H: Manipulation of the metabolic response in clinical practice. *World J Surg* 2000; 24:690–5.
3. Kirsh E. Worwag E. Sinner M. Chodak G: Using outcome data and patient satisfaction surveys to develop policies regarding minimum length of hospitalization alter radical prostatectomy. *Urology* 2000; 56(1):101–7.
4. Kissin I: Preemptive analgesia. *Anesthesiology* 2000; 93(4):1138–43.
5. Warfield CA. Kahn CH: Acute pain management. Programs in U.S. hospitals and experiences and attitudes among U.S. adults. *Anesthesiology* 1995; 83(5):1090–4.
6. Woolf CJ, Salter MW: Neuronal plasticity: increasing the gain in pain. *Science* 2000; 288(5472):1765–9.
7. Leykin Y, Pellis T, Ambrosio C: Highlights in postoperative pain management. Expert Rev Neurother 2007; 7(5):533–45.

STANDARD ADULT POSTOP ANALGESICS

Analgesics	Morphine	2 mg/10 min, up to 10 mg iv
	Meperidine	10 mg/10 min, up to 150 mg iv; not to exceed (NTE) 600 mg/d
	Hydromorphone	0.5–1 mg/10–20 min, up to 6 mg
	Fentanyl	12.5–35 μg/5 min, up to 200 mcg iv
	Ketorolac (see note 2 below)	30 mg iv slowly; then 15 mg q 6 h × 3 d max

EPIDURAL ANALGESIA

	Lumbar Epidural		Thoracic Epidural	
Loading dose	**Morphine**	**Hydromorphone**	**Morphine**	**Hydromorphone**
Lower extremities	2–3 mg	0.4–0.6 mg	—	—
Pelvis	3–4 mg	0.5–0.8 mg	1–3 mg	0.15–0.4 mg
Abdomen	5–7 mg	0.5–1 mg	2–3.5 mg	0.2–0.6 mg
Thorax	7–8 mg	0.5–1 mg	2–3.5 mg	0.4–0.8 mg
Infusion	**Morphine**	**Hydromorphone**	**Morphine**	**Hydromorphone**
Lower extremities	0.3–0.5 mg/h	0.1–0.2 mg/h	—	—
Pelvis	0.3–0.5 mg/h	0.1–0.2 mg/h	0.1–0.3 mg/h	0.1–0.15 mg/h
Abdomen	0.4–0.7 mg/h	0.2–0.3 mg/h	0.2–0.5 mg/h	0.1–0.2 mg/h
Thorax	0.5–1.0 mg/h	0.2–0.3 mg/h	0.2–0.6 mg/h	0.15–0.2 mg/h

Special considerations

1. Concentrations of opioids used for epidural infusions (in preservative-free solution):
   - Morphine, 0.15 mg/mL
   - Hydromorphone, 0.05 mg/mL
2. Ketorolac may impair hemostasis. Consult with the surgical team.

EPIDURAL ANESTHESIA/POSTOP ANALGESIA

Surgical Site	Epidural Catheter Location	Initial Bolus of 0.5% Bupivacaine	Infusion Rate of 0.125% Bupivacaine
Thoracic or upper abdomen	T6-T8	4–6 mL	5–10 mL/h
Lower abdomen	T10	10 mL	15 mL/h
Hip or knee	L2-3	8 mL	10 mL/h

Special considerations

1. Give initial bolus dose before incision. Then, if patient hemodynamically stable, give 1/2 bolus dose 30 min before end of surgery.
2. In recovery room, ✓sensory level. If no sensory block. ✓whether catheter is functioning with 8 mL 2% lidocaine bolus. (✓ vital signs.) If thoracic epidural starts with 2 mL, redose with 2 mL q 5–10 min, up to 8 mL.
3. Start infusions: If catheter is functional, as evidenced by loss of sensation, start: local anesthetic + opioid infusions (see table, above).
4. Best results: Local anesthetics and opioids are mixed in line using two separate infusion pumps. Thus, if either causes side effects, one can be stopped without the other.

PATIENT-CONTROLLED ANALGESIA (PCA) FOR INTRAVENOUS ADMINISTRATION

Loading dose	Morphine Hydromorphone Fentanyl	Titrate to comfort Titrate to comfort Titrate to comfort
Basal rate	Morphine Hydromorphone Fentanyl	0.5–1 mg/h 0.1–0.2 mg/h 5–10 mcg/h
PCA lock-out dose and time	Morphine Hydromorphone Fentanyl	1–2 mg q 10–15 min 0.1–0.2 mg q 10–15 min 5–10 mcg q 10–15 min

Typical orders

1. Call anesthesiologist with any questions about PCA.
2. Check respiratory rate q 1 h while PCA in use.
3. Call anesthesiologist if respiratory rate < 10/min. If rate < 6/min, treat with naloxone 0.1–0.2 mg iv (may repeat, to 0.6 mg), push and assist ventilation while waiting for anesthesiologist.
4. Encourage patient to ambulate 4–6 h after surgery (unless contraindicated).
5. After PCA D/C'd, start po pain medications (per surgeon).
6. If patient required a large loading dose, the PCA lockout dose may need to be increased. Expect patient to need about 1/3 loading dose q h. Change PCA dose or lockout time to permit this dosing.

PATIENT-CONTROLLED EPIDURAL ANALGESIA (PCEA)

Loading dose	Morphine Hydromorphone Fentanyl	2–3 mg 0.5–1.0 mg 50–75 mcg
Basal rate	Morphine Hydromorphone Fentanyl	0.2–0.5 mg/h 0.08–0.12 mg/h 5–10 mcg/h
PCA lock-out dose and time	Morphine Hydromorphone Fentanyl	0.1–0.2 mg q 10–15 min 0.02–0.06 mg q 10–15 min 5–10 mcg q 10–15 min

Special considerations:

1. For thoracic epidural, decrease all doses by one-third; if high thoracic, decrease by one-half.
2. Concentrations of opioids for epidural infusion (in preservative-free solution).
   - Morphine 0.15 mg/mL
   - Hydromorphone 0.05 mg/mL
   - Fentanyl 10 μg/mL
3. Bupivacaine (0.125% @ 5–8 mL/h) may be added to the previously mentioned regimen for supplemental analgesia. Typically, the bupivacaine infusion is stopped on POD 1 to facilitate early ambulation. Thoracic epidural local anesthetic may be continued if it does not interfere with ambulation.

TYPICAL ORDERS FOR POSTOP EPIDURAL/SPINAL ANALGESIA

I. EPIDURAL MEDICATIONS

_______ **1. Epidural Infusion – Opiate**
- ❑ Hydromorphone (Dilaudid) 0.05 mg/mL concentration @_______mg/h =_______mL/h
- ❑ Morphine sulfate 0.15 mg/mL concentration @_______mg/h =_______mL/h
- ❑ Fentanyl (Sublimaze) 10 mcg/mL concentration @_______mcg/h =_______mL/h
- ❑ Range: May vary infusion between_______/h to_______/h prn pain.

_______ **2. Epidural Infusion – Anesthetic**
- ❑ Bupivacaine 0.125% concentration @_______mL/h
- ❑ Bupivacaine 0.25% concentration @_______mL/h
- ❑ Turn off bupivacaine on POD # 1 @ 5 am.

_______ **3 Epidural Bolus – Opiate**
- ❑ Hydromorphone (Dilaudid)_______mg q_______h in 10 mL preservative-free NS (PFNS)
- ❑ Morphine sulfate_______mg q_______h in 10 mL PFNS

_______ **4. Breakthrough Pain**
- ❑ Fentanyl [50–100] mcg via epidural q [1] h prn pain in 10 mL PFNS
- ❑ Call MD if > 2 doses in [2] h.
- ❑ Ketorolac (Toradol) [15] mg iv q 6 h × [3] d (for a maximum of 12 doses)

II. NURSING CARE

_______ **1. Vital Signs**

❑ For opiates: T, P, BP q 4 h; RR q 2 h; then q 8 h, if stable.
Continuous O_2 sats × 24 h; then D/C if O_2 sats > 90% on room air.

❑ For anesthetics: BP & P q 2 h; then q 4 h, if stable.
Orthostatic BP before ambulation × 24 h.

_______ **2.** Label tubing, pump, infusion as "epidural." Place sign over bed; cover "Y" ports on tubing.

_______ **3.** Place naloxone (Narcan) and syringe at bedside.

_______ **4.** Administration of any additional opiates, sedatives, or antiemetics must be approved by anesthesiologist.

_______ **5.** Assess patient's pain (0–10 scale: 0 = no pain; 10 = worst pain imaginable) and level of sedation (awake, drowsy, asleep, unresponsive), along with VS.

_______ **6.** D/C Epidural Protocol when epidural D/C'd.

III. SIDE EFFECTS MANAGEMENT

_______ **1. Respiratory depression:** For RR < 6 or O_2 sat < 86% (on 2 separate occasions < 5 min apart):
Administer naloxone (Narcan) 0.1 mg–0.2 mg iv STAT; may repeat, to total of 0.6 mg.
Administer O_2 10 L/min via nonrebreathing mask. TURN OFF INFUSION. CALL ON-CALL MD STAT.

_______ **2. Excessive somnolence/sedation:**
Administer naloxone (Narcan) 0.1 mg–0.2 mg iv STAT; may repeat, to total of 0.6 mg.
Administer O_2 10 L/min via nonrebreathing mask. TURN OFF INFUSION. CALL ON-CALL MD STAT.

_______ **3. Nausea/Vomiting:**
- ❑ Metoclopramide (Reglan) [10 mg] iv q 4–6 h prn
- ❑ Ondansetron [4 mg] q 6 h prn
- ❑ Nalbuphine (Nubain) [2.5–5.0 mg] iv q 4 h prn

_______ **4. Pruritus:**
- ❑ Nalbuphine (Nubain) [2.5–5.0 mg] iv q 2–4 h prn
- ❑ Diphenhydramine (Benadryl) [10–25 mg] iv q 4 h prn

Suggested dosage shown in brackets [-]

APPENDIX D: STANDARD PEDIATRIC ANESTHETIC MANAGEMENT

STANDARD PEDIATRIC MONITORS (NONINVASIVE)	
Blood pressure (BP)	
Capnometry/capnography	Measurement of $ETCO_2$ display of wave form
Gas analyzer (e.g., Raman, IR, or mass spectroscopy)	Measurement of respired gases and anesthetics
Electrocardiogram (ECG)	5-lead preferred
Esophageal or precordial stethoscope	Breath and heart sounds monitored; dysrhythmias and ↓BP detected
Nerve stimulator	Monitor status of neuromuscular blockade
Oxygen analyzer	Measurement of FiO_2
Pulse oximetry	Measurement of O_2 saturation; 2 pulse oximeters in neonates—1 preductal; 1 postductal
Temperature	Nasal, esophageal, rectal, or skin
Visual observation of patient	Skin color, pupils, temperature, edema, sweating, movement
Ventilator function monitors	PIP, TV, disconnect alarm, etc.

STANDARD PREOP FASTING (NPO) GUIDELINES

- All solid foods and nonclear liquids (e.g., milk, infant formula, orange juice) should be withheld after midnight before scheduled surgery.
- All clear liquids (and breast milk) should be given up to 3 h before scheduled surgery. Because breast milk has a relatively short transit time through the stomach, and to simplify—therefore, to increase compliance with—these guidelines, breast milk is considered a clear liquid.
- In practice, nonemergency cases may proceed 6 h after solids and nonclear liquids and 2 h after clear liquids and breast milk have been ingested.

★**NB:** The following sections are guidelines only. Specific drugs and drug dosages should be individualized, based on the physiological and pharmacological status of the patient, including factors such as age, weight, medication, and concurrent diseases.

PREMEDICATION

- In general, patients < 9 mo of age do not need sedative premedication. Infants < 1 mo and premature infants may require atropine 0.01–0.02 mg/kg iv or 0.02 mg/kg im before intubation. Minimum iv atropine dose = 100 mcg.
- Older children (9 mo–10 yr) can be premedicated successfully by using po midazolam (0.5–0.75 mg) in syrup, grape Kool-Aid, or cherry-flavored acetaminophen elixir (10–15 mg/kg po) 20–30 min before surgery.
- For patients > 35–40 kg, po lorazepam (0.03–0.05 mg/kg) or diazepam (0.1–0.15 mg/kg) may be given 60 min before surgery with a sip of water if needed.

INDUCTION TECHNIQUES

Preinduction	1. ✓ anesthesia machine, suction, airway equipment, drugs. 2. Attach monitors and verify function. 3. Premedication: < 6–9 mo—consider atropine 0.01–0.02 mg/kg iv before laryngoscopy to prevent vagally mediated bradycardia.

INDUCTION TECHNIQUES (CONT'D)

Induction	**Routes of administration:** 1. im: ketamine hydrochloride 3–5 mg/kg (with atropine 0.02 mg/kg) 2. iv: Propofol 2–3 mg/kg STP 4–7 mg/kg 3. Inhalational: sevoflurane (MAC = 3.3% for neonates and younger infants, 2.5% for older infants and children) and halothane (MAC = 0.87% for neonates, 1–2% for infants), in N_2O (up to 70%)/O_2. Increase inspired concentration of sevoflurane incrementally every 3 breaths (up to 8%) and halothane (up to 4%). Monitor BP and HR closely, especially if using halothane.
Muscle relaxation	1. Rocuronium: 0.6–1 mg/kg iv; 1 mg/kg recommended for rapid sequence induction. If airway concerns exist, consider awake intubation, use of succinylcholine. 2. Succinylcholine: 1–2 mg/kg iv or 2–4 mg/kg im (controversial*). May be useful for rapid-sequence intubations, especially if airway concerns exist. 3. Vecuronium or pancuronium: 0.1 mg/kg iv 4. Cisatracurium 0.1 mg/kg iv 5. Deep sevoflurane or halothane anesthesia
Laryngoscope	**Blade** — **Age** Miller 0 — Neonate Miller 1 — 6–9 mo Wis-Hipple 1.5 — 9 mo–3 yr Macintosh 2 — 1–4 yr Macintosh 3 or Miller 2 — > 4 yr *Succinylcholine may trigger MH in susceptible patients or cause cardiac arrest in myopathic patients; therefore, many pediatric anesthesiologists avoid the use of succinylcholine.

TYPICAL ETT SIZE AT DIFFERENT AGES

Age	Wt	Uncuffed ETT size	Cuffed ETT size
Premature Newborn	1–3 kg 3–4 kg	2.5 or 3.0 3.5	n/a 3.0
≤ 6–8 mo	6–8 kg	3.5 or 4.0	3.0 or 3.5
≤ 8–16 mo	10–12 kg	4.0 or 4.5	3.5 or 4.0
2–3 yr	13–15 kg	4.5	4.0 or 4.5
6 yr	20	Formula (uncuffed tubes): 4+ (age/4) = ETT size (to allow for a slight leak when positive pressure is applied). For cuffed tubes, use 0.5 size smaller and inflate as necessary to attain leak of 20–30 cm H_2O.	
9 yr	30 kg		
12 yr	40 kg		

★**NB:** These ETT sizes are guidance only; prepare an ETT one size larger and one size smaller than the ETT size selected. ✓ ET placement of tube by auscultation of breath sounds bilaterally. ✓ depth of carina by auscultation over left axilla as ETT is slowly advanced. Withdraw and secure ETT 2 cm from position where diminution of breath sounds was first noted. Positive pressure leak between 20 and 30 cm H_2O is desirable. Leaks < 20 cm may result in volume loss and difficulty in providing appropriate ventilation during critical phases intraop or postop. Conversely, leaks > 30 cmH_2O may carry a higher risk of subglottic edema and/or stenosis. Cuffed ETTs may be used, provided that leak is maintained 20–30 cmH_2O. Some flexibility is required here. Consider length of case, difficulty of placing ETT, and adequacy of ventilation. A throat pack may assist in decreasing the leak if tube exchange is not desired.

MAINTENANCE TECHNIQUES

Inhalational anesthesia only	30–100% O_2 + 0–70% N_2O. In preemies and for cases where N_2O is contraindicated, air may be used to lower FiO_2. + Isoflurane, sevoflurane or halothane, titrated to effect. Consider warming and humidifying all gases for long cases. Warm room to 75–80°F for infants; 70–75°F for children.
Balanced anesthesia	30–100% O_2 + 0–70% N_2O + ~0.5% isoflurane or propofol (50–200 mcg/kg/min) **TIVA** - propofol 100–200 mcg/kg/min, + remifentanil 0.1–0.2 mcg/kg/min +/- N_2O if procedure allows. Consider including amnestic agents: midazolam, low-dose inhalational agents (e.g., sevoflurane, isoflurane). + morphine (0.05 mg/kg/h) or fentanyl (1–3 mcg/kg/h) + Dilaudid 2 mcg/kg/h + consider acetaminophen pr 30–40 mg/kg for pain control. Temperature monitoring; forced air warming; fluid warming if volume/blood/resuscitation expected. Fluid requirements LR/NS at maintenance: 0–10 kg = 4 mL/kg/h +11–20 kg = 2 mL/kg/h +>20 kg = 1 mL/kg/h (e.g., 25 kg = 65 mL/h) If continued muscle relaxation is required during the above maintenance techniques, several options are available. Always use a nerve stimulator to assess block before redosing.

Short-acting	Mivacurium	0.1 mg/kg → 6–10 min
Intermediate	Vecuronium Rocuronium Cisatracurium	0.1 mg/kg → 25–30 min 0.6 mg/kg → 30 min 0.1 mg/kg → 30 min
Long-acting	Pancuronium	0.1 mg/kg → 40–65 min

EMERGENCE

1. Reverse muscle relaxant	As surgical conditions permit, reverse residual muscle relaxant (when at least 1 twitch is present in train-of-four) with one of the following: • Neostigmine 0.05–0.07 (maximum dose) mg/kg iv + glycopyrrolate 0.01 mg/kg iv, or • Edrophonium 0.5–1.0 (maximum dose) mg/kg iv + atropine 0.01 mg/kg iv. Enlon Plus - 0.05–0.1 mL/kg is equal to edrophonium 0.5–1 mg/kg (max: 10 mg), atropine 0.007–0.014 mg/kg (max: 4 mg).
2. Nausea prophylaxis	Ondansetron 0.1 mg/kg iv or Metoclopramide 0.1 mg/kg iv (~1 h before emergence). Dexamethasone 0.1 mg/kg can be considered (avoid in oncology patients due to special protocols).
3. O_2	D/C N_2O/volatile agents and administer 100% O_2.
4. Suction	Suction oropharynx thoroughly.
5. Extubation	Laryngeal spasm is common in children; therefore, it is usual to extubate them when they are awake, moving all limbs, and breathing adequately. Infants and children with full stomachs or difficult airways must be extubated when they are fully awake. The pharynx and stomach should be suctioned thoroughly prior to extubation. If laryngeal spasm occurs, Rx with 100% O_2 and CPAP or PPV. If spasm fails to resolve and hypoxemia occurs, give succinylcholine 0.1–0.5 mg/kg and administer PPV. Consider reintubation if hypoxemia fails to resolve quickly. Consider atropine 0.01–0.02 mg/kg iv before succinylcholine, to preempt bradycardia.

PEDIATRIC EPIDURAL ANESTHESIA

Epidural anesthesia may be combined with GA for infants and children undergoing surgery involving the lower extremities, abdomen, chest, or spine. Single-dose ("single-shot") techniques may be used, or epidural catheters may be placed for longer procedures and to facilitate postop epidural analgesia (see below). Bupivacaine 0.25% ± epinephrine 1:200K is most commonly used intraop. For patients admitted following surgery, opioids (e.g., hydromorphone [Dilaudid]) are generally added, together with bupivacaine 0.1% (see p. E-6). Use saline-filled syringe for loss-of-resistance to minimize chances of VAE.

TECHNIQUES AND DOSAGES

1. Caudal

- Single-shot: 22-ga iv catheter (< 5 yr), 20-ga iv catheter (> 5 yr), or 21–23-ga iv catheter may be inserted via sacrococcygeal membrane.
- A test dose with 0.1 mL/kg (max 3 mL) lidocaine or bupivacaine + epinephrine 1:100K or 1:200K is given.
- If epidural catheter is used, add 0.8 mL to test dose volume due to dead space volume of catheter.
- Initial dose: 0.5 mL/kg for lower extremity/perineal/genital procedures; 1.0 mL/kg for abdominal procedures (max 10 mL)
- Catheter technique: in patients < 10 kg, first dilate the epidural space with 5–10 U NS; then, a 20-ga epidural catheter may be inserted through 18-ga Critikon iv catheter and advanced so that tip is located near level of incision (e.g., ~17 cm from skin to T4 in infant). If resistance is met, it may be necessary to pull the catheter back slightly, together with the needle (to avoid shearing catheter), or repeat procedure.
- Initial dose: 0.5 mL/kg, max 10 mL.

2. Lumbar

- 17- or 18-ga epidural needle inserted via L3-4 or L4-5 interspace for single-shot injection or placement of 20-ga epidural catheter.
- Use loss-of-resistance technique with fluid-filled syringe (air may cause VAE).
- Good estimate of depth to epidural space is 1 mm/kg, up to ~30 kg.
- Catheter should be threaded ~4 cm (maximum) beyond tip of needle.
- A test dose with 0.1–0.2 mL/kg lidocaine or bupivacaine + epinephrine 1:100K or 1:200K is given.
- Initial dose: 0.5 mL/kg for lower abdominal procedures; 1.0 mL/kg for upper abdominal and thoracic procedures

3. Thoracic

- The technique described for lumbar epidural catheter placement may be used between T6 and T12 in children.
- A test dose with 0.1–0.2 mL/kg lidocaine or bupivacaine + epinephrine 1:100K or 1:200K is given.
- Initial dose: 0.5 mL/kg, max 5–7 mL.
- Local anesthetic-dosing guidelines same as above (note that volume will be ~$^1/_3$ less than with caudal approach.

For indwelling catheter techniques, hourly maintenance doses of half the initial dose may be given. For continuous infusion, maximum rate for bupivacaine is 0.5 mg/kg/h (0.3 mg/kg/h for neonates).

PEDIATRIC SPINAL ANESTHESIA AND ANALGESIA

Spinal anesthesia is used primarily for procedures such as inguinal herniorrhaphy in former preterm infants at risk for postop apnea following GA. By avoiding GA, the incidence of postop apnea is reduced, but not eliminated. In most patients arriving in the OR without iv access, an iv may be inserted in a lower extremity immediately following placement of the spinal anesthetic, as little change in BP or HR occurs in infants < 6 mo of age.

After standard monitors are applied, the infant is placed in a supine or lateral decubitus position. Care is taken to avoid neck flexion, which may cause airway obstruction. The skin is infiltrated with 1% lidocaine using a 27- or 30-ga needle. Lumbar puncture is performed with a 22-ga 1.5" spinal needle to an average depth of 1.5 cm from skin. The most commonly used local anesthetic for spinal anesthesia in infants is tetracaine 1.0%, mixed with an equal volume of 10% dextrose in a dose of 0.8–1.0 mg/kg. Epinephrine 1:1000 0.01 mL/kg is added. This dose usually provides adequate anesthesia for 90–120 min for inguinal herniorrhaphy.

Complications include high spinal anesthesia requiring tracheal intubation. PDPH is very uncommon in children < 12 yr of age, and probably rare in infants.

Suggested Readings

1. Alifimoff JK, Cote CJ: Regional anesthesia. In *A Practice of Anesthesia for Infants and Children.* Cote CJ, Ryan JF, Todres ID, et al., eds. WB Saunders, Philadelphia: 1993, 429–49.
2. Sethna NF, Berde CB: Pediatric regional anesthesia. In *Pediatric Anesthesia*, 4th edition. Gregory GA, ed. Churchill Livingstone, New York: 2002, 267–316.
3. Yaster M, Krane E, Kaplan R, et al: *The Pediatric Pain and Sedation Handbook.* Mosby-Year Book, St. Louis: 1997.
4. Motoyama EK, Davis PJ: *Smith's Anesthesia for Infants and Children*, 7th edition. Elsevier, Philadelphia: 2006, 255–396.

APPENDIX E: STANDARD PEDIATRIC POSTOPERATIVE PAIN MANAGEMENT

Katie Larkin, Julie Good, and Brenda Golianu

Traditionally, children have been undermedicated for their pain because of difficulty with assessment, concerns for safety, and lack of understanding of the physiologic consequences of untreated pain. There is now strong evidence that it is not only safe, but also beneficial to treat children's procedural pain. For example, infants have adverse behavioral cardiorespiratory and neuroendocrine responses to pain, which improve when appropriate analgesia is administered.

Pain assessment	Unlike most adults, infants and children < 7 yr have difficulty understanding and using a Visual Analog Scale (VAS). A frequently used tool for assessing pain in children 3–7 yr old is the Wong-Baker Faces Scale (Fig. E-1). For infants and nonverbal children, observational scales that rely on behavioral and/or physiologic parameters are often used (e.g., the FLACC Pain Scale, Fig. E-2, PIPP, NIPS, CHEOPS, CRIES as well as appropriate translations). The "gold-standard" of pain measurement is to solicit a direct subjective report from the child whenever possible.
Oral medications	For simple outpatient procedures, such as tonsillectomy, hernia repair, circumcision, or closed reduction of a fracture, a weak oral opiate, in combination with acetaminophen, is appropriate (see chart for dosing examples, p. E-4).
Intravenous medications	**Patient Controlled Analgesia (PCA)** can be considered in patients > 5 yr who are expected to remain hospitalized overnight, especially in those who are unlikely to tolerate oral intake in the initial hours after surgery (see initial dosing chart, p. E-4). For younger children, a **Nurse Controlled Analgesia (NCA)** can be employed. When the patient begins oral medications, D/C the basal rate but continue to provide the lockout dose for several more hours to be sure that the child is tolerating the oral medication. For opioid-related side effects such as nausea and vomiting, ondansetron can be added (0.1 mg/kg q 6 h to maximum of 4 mg q 6 h), and for pruritus, diphenhydramine (0.5 mg/kg q 6 h max 50 mg), or nalbuphine (0.05 mg/kg q 6 h max 20 mg), especially effective for epidural opioid-related pruritus. For respiratory depression, naloxone can be carefully titrated beginning at 0.001 mg/kg q 1–2 min as needed to restore adequate respiratory effort and wakefulness. Care must be taken, as the naloxone will have a short half-life (10–15 minutes), and respiratory depression may recur. Reversal of analgesia may also occur if naloxone is administered for treatment of pruritus or respiratory depression.
Adjuvant medications	In addition to opiates, several adjuvant medications are useful in the periop period. **Lorazepam** (Ativan) 0.025 mg/kg iv q 6 h is useful in preventing spasms and lessening fear in an unfamiliar environment. It is important to remember that lorazepam has a half-life of up to 16 h and doses can be additive. Another useful adjuvant is ketorolac (Toradol) 0.5 mg/kg, up to a maximum of 30 mg loading dose, followed by 15 mg iv q 6 h, up to 72 h. Ketorolac is not recommended in patients with poor renal function or following surgeries where there is a large bleeding surface or complex bone repair. Ketorolac has been shown to cause delay in bony fusion in animal models, but conflicting information has been presented in humans. It also has been reported to cause acute renal failure with prolonged use, and is not recommended for use in bariatric patients due to its potential adverse impact on renal function. Given these concerns, it is helpful to observe hydration status, Plt count, and Cr, and discuss the use of this medication with the surgical team. Other adjuvants to consider include **acetaminophen** po (10–15 mg/kg/dose q 6 h) or pr (20 mg/kg/dose q 6). An initial loading dose of 30–40 mg/kg pr administration for post-op pain may be helpful. **Ibuprofen** 10 mg/kg po dose also may be used. Medications to manage side effects, such as pruritus, N/V, constipation, and respiratory depression are presented in detail on the PCA order form, p. E-5.

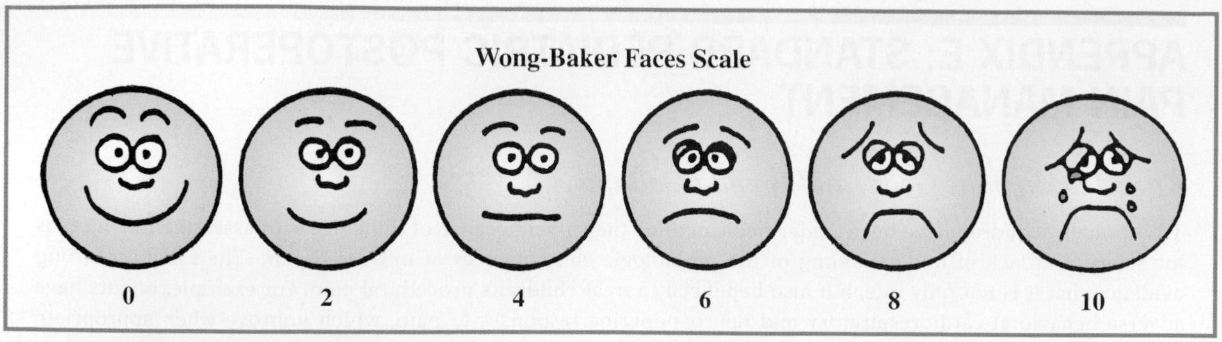

Figure E-1. Wong-Baker Faces Scale used in pain assessment in children (and other patients developmentally from 3–7 years-old). The higher the score, the greater the child's pain. (After Wong DL, Bakr CM: Pain in children: comparison of assessment scales. *Pediatr Nurs* 1988; 14:9.)

Epidural pain management	In children, it is generally considered safer to place epidurals after induction of GA to avoid movement during placement. For children 0–12 mo, a **caudal technique** can be used. The patient is placed in the lateral decubitus position, the caudal anatomy is identified, and an 18-ga iv catheter is used to enter the caudal space. The catheter is advanced and aspirated. The space is then dilated with 5–8 ml of preservative-free NS. A 20-ga epidural catheter is then advanced to the desired location, or until obstruction is felt (~10–15 cm). The catheter tip may be visualized using ultrasound or nerve stimulation, if available. The catheter is taped secured with a moisture-resistant dressing, as it can easily become dislodged with regular activity. A test dose is given (lidocaine 1.5% with 1:200,000 epinephrine 0.1 ml/kg + 0.8 ml for the dead space of the catheter). **Lumbar** and **thoracic epidurals** can be placed in children > 10–12 mo. or earlier in experienced hands. **Contraindications** for epidural catheters include infection at the local site, coagulopathy, low Plt, sepsis, progressive neurologic deficit, and refusal of patient or parent. Epidural placement should be checked by syringe aspiration before starting the infusion. Return of any bloody fluid or > 0.5 ml clear aspirant necessitates further evaluation before use of the catheter for pain control. Patients with indwelling epidural catheters may receive postop analgesia with either continuous infusion alone of continuous infusion with intermittent bolus dosing (patient-controlled epidural analgesia [PCEA]). Similar to PCA, PCEA can be used in ages ≥ 5–7 yr. Typical starting infusions are discussed in the table below. Medication dosage will depend on patient's age, location of surgical pain, catheter insertion level, and catheter tip location. A bolus dose equivalent to the hourly volume of infusion may be given when a patient is uncomfortable. Increase the infusion by 10% to maintain the new level of analgesia. Infusion should not exceed 0.3 ml/kg/h in children ≤ 6 mo or 0.5 ml/kg/h in older patients. If inadequate analgesia persists after two dosing increases, it may be appropriate to abandon this form of treatment in favor of systemic analgesia. Do not leave a patient in pain for an extended period of time trying to "fix" an epidural catheter. If in doubt, check catheter placement then bolus catheter with 2% lidocaine w/ 1:200,000 epi 0.1 ml/kg to determine if a level is able to be obtained.
Peripheral Nerve Catheters	Increasingly, peripheral nerve catheters are being employed for peri-operative pain control. Local anesthetic infusions (bupivacaine 0.1% or ropivacaine 0.2%) are continued for 3–5 days postop.

FLACC Pain Scale (For Non-Verbal Patients)			
	Scoring		
Categories	0	1	2
Face	No particular expression or smile	Occasional grimace or frown, withdrawn, disinterested	Frequent-to-constant quivering chin, clenched jaw
Legs	Normal position or relaxed	Uneasy, restless, tense	Kicking, or legs drawn up
Activity	Lying quietly, normal position, moves easily	Squirming, shifting back and forth, tense	Arched, rigid or jerking
Cry	No cry (awake or asleep)	Moans and whimpers; occasional complaint	Crying steadily, screams or sobs, frequent complaints
Consolability	Content, relaxed	Reassured by occasional touching, hugging, or being talked to; distractible	Difficult to console or comfort
Each of the five categories (F) Face, (L) Legs, (A) Activity, (C) Cry, and Consolability is scored from 0-2, which results in a total score between 0 and 10.			

Figure E-2. FLACC Pain Scale for pain assessment in non-verbal patients. By Merkel S, Voepel-Lewis T, Shayevitz JR, Malviya S. et al. *Am J Nursing* 2002; 102:55–8.

Suggested Readings

1. Anand KJ, Carr DB: The neuroanatomy, neurophysiology, and neurochemistry of pain, stress, and analgesia in newborns and children. *Ped Clin North Am* 1989; 36(4):795–822.
2. Williams DG, Patel A, Howard RF: Pharmacogenetics of codeine metabolism in an urban population of children and its implications for analgesic reliability. *Br J Anaesth* 2002; 89(6):839–45.
3. Mello SS, Saraira RA, Marques RS, et al: Posterior lumbar plexus block in children: a new anatomical landmark. *Reg Anesth Pain Med* 2007; 32(6):522–7.
4. Ecoffey C: Pediatric Regional Anesthesia–update. *Curr Opin Anaesthesiol* 2007; 20(3):232–5.
5. Giaufre E, Dalens B, Gombert A: Epidemiology and morbidity of regional anesthesia in children: a one-year prospective survey of the French-Language Society of Pediatric Anesthesiologists. *Anesth Analg* 1996; 83(5):904–12.
6. Ilfeld BM, Morey TE, Wang RD, et al: Continuous popliteal sciatic nerve block for post-operative pain control at home: a randomized, double-blinded, placebo controlled study. *Anesthesiology* 2002; 97(4):959–65.

STANDARD PEDIATRIC POSTOP ANALGESICS AND ANTIEMETICS

Analgesics	Tylenol	10–15 mg/kg po q 6 h 20–30 mg/kg po pr q 6 h	Max: 30–45 mg/kg/24 h (neo); 60 mg/kg/24 h (infants); 80 mg/kg/24 h (children)
	Lortab Elixir	7.5 mg Hydro + 500 mg APAP/15 ml	0.15 mg Hydro/kg q 6 h (e.g., 1.5 mg ≅3 ml for 10 kg child)
	Vicodin Lorcet Norco	5 mg Hydro + 500 mg APAP/TAB 10 mg Hydro + 650 mg APAP/TAB 10 mg Hydro + 325 mg APAP/TAB	Dose based on maximum acetaminophen allowed for weight (up to 15 mg/kg/dose) q 4–6 h, but not to exceed 75 mg/kg/d
	Tylenol #3	30 mg Cod + 300 mg APAP/TAB	
	Tylenol with codeine elixir	12 mg Cod + 120 mg APAP/5 ml	0.5–1 mg/kg Cod q 6 h (e.g., 5–10 mg ≅ 2–4 ml for 10 kg child)
	Oxycodone	0.1 mg/kg q 6 h	
	Percocet	5 mg oxycodone + 325 mg APAP/TAB	
Antiemetics	Metoclopramide*	0.1 mg/kg, may repeat × 1 iv	
	Ondansetron	0.1 mg/kg iv	
	***NB:** Increased incidence of extrapyramidal reactions.		

Hydro = Hydrocodone; APAP = Acetaminophen; Cod = Codeine.
Notes:
Codeine preparations are not recommended as a first-line analgesic because a substantial portion (16%) of the population cannot convert codeine to morphine, an action that is necessary to derive analgesic effect from the drug.
To prevent irreversible liver damage, it is important to D/C or supervise all other use of acetaminophen when prescribing the above medications, so as not to exceed the maximum dose of 100 mg/kg/d (60 mg/kg/d in neonates) of acetaminophen.

PATIENT-CONTROLLED IV ANALGESIA (PCA)

In a setting with trained nursing supervision, PCA can be used safely by children ≥ 5 yr old (about the age they are able to play video games). The lockout time usually is set at 10 min, but can be as short as 5 min for fentanyl. Common PCA medications and recommended starting doses in opiate-naive patients are listed below, followed by typical order for iv PCA.

Common PCA Medications

Medication	Loading dose	Basal Rate	Patient-controlled bolus
Morphine (1 or 5 mg/ml)	0.03 mg/kg	0.01 mg/kg/h	0.02–0.03 mg/kg
Hydromorphone (100 mcg/ml)	5 mcg/kg	1 mcg/kg/h	2 mcg/kg
Fentanyl (50 mcg/ml)	0.3 mcg/kg	0.1 mcg/kg/h	0.2–0.3 mcg/kg

Continuous iv infusion: When PCA is not practical (e.g., in children unable to understand PCA), continuous iv infusion of opiates may be used. Morphine infusion of 10–30 mcg/kg/h results in serum concentrations of 10–22 ng/ml and provides adequate analgesia. A common technique is to initiate iv morphine infusion with 1 mg/kg of morphine in 100 ml of D5W at 1 ml/h (the effective infusion rate is 10 mcg/kg/h). The infusion rate is slowly increased to provide adequate pain relief.

TYPICAL ORDERS FOR PATIENT-CONTROLLED IV ANALGESIA (PCA)

Patient's Name:________________________ Medical Record No.:________________________

Weight (kg):________________________ Allergies:________________________

Drug	Recommended Concentration	Loading Dose	Mode (*select one*) PCA Only	Continuous	PCA + Continuous	PCA Dose	Lockout Interval	Basal Rate
Morphine	1 mg/ml	0.03 mg/kg*				0.02–0.03 mg/kg*	6–10 min	0.01 mg/kg/h*
Hydromorphine	100 mcg/ml	5 mcg/kg*				2 mcg/kg*	6–10 min	1 mcg/kg/h*
Fentanyl	50 mcg/ml	0.3 mcg/kg*				0.2–0.3 mcg/kg*	6–10 min	0.1 mcg/kg/h*

Physician: Check all orders that apply: **Recommended starting dose for opiate-naive patients.*

Nursing Care:

❑ 1. For renewed or changed PCA orders only, continue PCA nursing are as previously ordered.

❑ 2. Do not administer any other opioids, benzodiazepines, sedatives, or antiemetics unless approved by:
Service Pager No.:

☒ 3. Continuous O_2 sat monitor. For $SaO_2 < 94\%$, administer O_2 per nasal cannula to maintain $SaO_2 \geq 94\%$.

☒ 4. Assess and record at least q 2 h: RR, O_2 sat, and level of pain, using appropriate tool. (*0–10 Scale, Wong-Baker Faces Scale, FLACC Scale, or PIPP Scale*)

☒ 5. Assess and record at least q 4 h: HR, BP, and T.

☒ 6. Bag and mask at bedside.

❑ 7. Assess for bladder retention. If no void for________________ h (since surgery or last void), may straight cath prn × 2.

Medications:

❑ 1. For renewed or changed PCA orders only, continue prn medications for PCA as previously ordered.

❑ 2. Metoclopramide (Reglan)________________mg iv q 6 h prn N/V (0.1 mg/kg/dose; max 15 mg).

❑ 3. Ondansetron (Zofran)________________mg iv q 8 h prn N/V (0.1 mg/kg/dose; max 4 mg).

❑ 4. Diphenhydramine (Benadryl)________________mg iv q 6 h prn pruritus (0.5 mg/kg/dose; max 50 mg).

❑ 5. Nalbuphine (Nubain)________________mg iv q 4 prn pruritus (0.05 mg/kg/dose; max 20 mg).

❑ 6. If no stool by________________(POD 3), administer:

- ❑ 1 pediatric glycerin suppository pr 1 or 2 × daily prn (ages 2–6 yr).
- ❑ Bisacodyl 5 mg (½ suppository) pr daily prn (ages 6–11 yr).
- ❑ Bisacodyl 10 mg (1 suppository) pr daily prn (ages > 11 yr).
- ❑ If no stool within 24 h of beginning treatment, notify physician listed above.

❑ 7. If unable to arouse or $SaO_2 < 85\%$, turn off PCA pump, administer O_2 and/or ambu-bag, stimulate patient, administer naloxone__________mg (0.001 mg/kg) q 1–2 min (obtain naloxone from floor stock) as needed to restore consciousness, and STAT page physician.

❑ 8. Other medications:____

Date: Time:	Physician's Signature: Pager:	Noted by: Date/Time:
Orders signed		RN: Date/Time:

POSTOPERATIVE EPIDURAL ANALGESIA

Patients with indwelling epidural catheters may receive postop analgesia with either continuous infusion alone or continuous infusion with intermittent bolus-dosing (patient-controlled epidural analgesia [PCEA]). The infusate may be either local anesthetic with an opioid, local anesthetic alone, or opioid alone. At Stanford, the most commonly used epidural infusate for continuous infusion is bupivacaine 0.1% with hydromorphone 3 mcg/ml. In patients receiving PCEA, bupivacaine 0.1% with hydromorphone 25 mcg/ml is often used (see Typical Orders for Continuous Epidural Analgesia and Epidural PCA, pp. E-7, E-8).

At Stanford, patients receiving epidural analgesia are managed by the Pediatric Pain Service.

Hydromorphone (Dilaudid): May bolus dose 5–10 mcg/kg or just add to continuous infusion. Reduced dose for thoracic catheters.

When opioid epidural analgesia is indicated, hydromorphone is most commonly used because:

(a) It causes less itching and nausea, compared with morphine.
(b) It is more water soluble than fentanyl (decreased systemic absorption, spread over more dermatomes).
(c) It is less water soluble than morphine (thereby minimizing late respiratory depression).

STARTING DOSES FOR EPIDURAL INFUSION

Age	Starting dose
0–6 mo	hydromorphone 3 mcg/ml + 0.1% bupivacaine @ 0.1–0.15 ml/kg/h (max bupiv 0.3 mg/kg/h); for neonates, consider 0.1% bupivacaine infusion only
6 mo–3 yr	hydromorphone 3 mcg/ml + 0.1% bupivacaine @ 0.1–0.15 ml/kg/h (max bupiv 0.5 mg/kg/h)
3–7 yr	hydromorphone 3–5 mcg/ml + 0.1% bupivacaine @ 0.1–0.15 ml/kg/h (max bupiv 0.5 mg/kg/h)
≥ 7 yr	hydromorphone 5–10 mcg/ml + 0.1% bupivacaine @ 0.1–0.15 ml/kg/h + 0.05 ml/kg/h PCEA dose q 30 min lockout (max bupiv 0.5 mg/kg/h)

Notes:
In general, use a lower concentration of opiate infusion for neonates. When spread is desired (for surgeries with incisions that cross multiple dermatomes or when catheter placement is below the level of anticipated pain), a lower concentration and higher volume infusion may be desired.

Suggested Readings

1. Alifimoff JK, Cote CJ: Pediatric regional anesthesia. In *A Practice of Anesthesia for Infants and Children.* Cote CJ, Ryan JF, Todres ID, et al., eds. WB Saunders, Philadelphia: 1993, 429–49.
2. Yaster M, Krane E, Kaplan R, et al: *The Pediatric Pain and Sedation Handbook.* Mosby-Year Book, St. Louis: 1997.
3. Ivani G, Mosetti V: Regional anesthesia for post-operative pain control in children: focus on continuous central and perineural infusions. *Paediatr Drugs* 2008; 10(2):107–14.

TYPICAL ORDERS FOR CONTINUOUS EPIDURAL ANALGESIA
(may also be utilized for Peripheral Nerve Blockade)

Patient's Name:______________________ Medical Record No.:____________

Weight(kg):__________Allergies:______________________

Drug and Concentration *(Check one)*	**Basal Rate** (0.15 ml/kg/h) (maximum 0.3 ml/kg/h for 0–6 mo)
❑ Hydromorphone 3 mcg/ml with bupivacaine 0.1% →	Epidural infusion rate__________ ml/hr
❑ Hydromorphone 3 mcg/ml with bupivacaine 0.1% → **and** Clonidine 0.5 mcg/ml	Epidural infusion rate__________ml/h
❑ Hydromorphone 3 mcg/ml with levobapivacaine 0.1% →	Epidural infusion rate__________ ml/h

Physician: Check all orders that apply:

Nursing Care:

☒ 1. Do not administer any other opioids, benzodiazepines, sedatives, or antiemetics unless first approved by Pain Management Service.

☒ 2. Maintain iv access until epidural catheter D/C'd.

☒ 3. Check epidural site q d and notify Pain Management Service if site is soiled, red, or tender.

☒ 4. Check lower extremities q 8 h while awake, and notify Pain Management if numbness or weakness exist.

☒ 5. Continuous O_2 sat monitor. For $SaO_2 < 94\%$, administer O_2 per nasal cannula to maintain $SaO_2 \geq 94\%$.

☒ 6. Assess and record at least q 4 h: RR, O_2 sat, and level of pain, using appropriate tool. (0–10/ *Numeric Scale, Wong-Baker Faces Scale, FLACC Scale, or PIPP Scale*)

☒ 7. Assess and record at least q 4 h: HR, BP. Check orthostatic BP before ambulating.

☒ 8. Assess for bladder retention. If no void for 8h (since surgery or last void) may straight cath prn × 2.

☒ 9. Bag and mask at bedside.

Medications:

❑ 1. Metoclopramide (Reglan)__________mg iv q 6 h prn N/V (0.1 mg/kg/dose; max 15 mg).

❑ 2. Ondansetron (Zofran)__________mg iv q 6 h prn N/V (0.1 mg/kg/dose; max 4 mg).

❑ 3. Diphenhydramine (Benadryl)__________mg iv q 6 h prn pruritus (0.5 mg/kg/dose; max 50 mg).

❑ 4. Nalbuphine (Nubain)__________mg iv q 4 prn pruritus (0.05 mg/kg/dose; max 20 mg).

❑ 5. If no stool by__________(POD 3), administer:

- ❑ 1 pediatric glycerin suppository pr 1–2 × daily prn (2–6 yr).
- ❑ Bisacodyl 5 mg (½ suppository) pr daily prn (6–11 yr).
- ❑ Bisacodyl 10 mg (1 suppository) pr daily prn (> 11 yr).
- ❑ If no stool within 24 h of beginning treatment, notify physician listed above.

❑ 6. If unable to arouse or SaO_2 is < 85%, turn off PCA pump, administer O_2 and/or ambu-bag, stimulate patient, administer naloxone (Narcan)__________ mg (0.001 mg/kg) q 1–2 min (obtain naloxone from floor stock) as needed to restore LOC, and STAT page pain Management Service.

❑ 7. Other medications:______________________

Date: Time:	Physician's Signature: Pager:	RN Signature: Date/Time:
Orders signed		

TYPICAL ORDERS FOR PATIENT-CONTROLLED EPIDURAL ANALGESIA (PCEA)

Patient's Name:________________________________ Medical Record No.:______________

Weight(kg):____________________Allergies:________________________________

Drug & Concentration	Mode	Basal Rate*	Epidural PCA Dose*
		(0.1–0.15 ml/kg/h)	(0.05 ml/kg/h)
Hydromorphone 5 mcg/ml with bupivacaine 0.1%	PCA + Continuous		
Hydromorphone 10 mcg/ml with bupivacaine 0.1%	PCA + Continuous		
Hydromorphone 5 mcg/ml with bupivacaine 0.1% **and** Clonidine 0.5 mcg/ml	PCA + Continuous		
	PCA + Continuous		

* When using Bupivacaine 0.1%, Basal Rate and Epidural PCA Dose combined may **not** exceed 0.5 ml/kg/h (0.3 ml/kg/h in ≤ 6 mo).

Physician: Check all orders that apply:

Nursing Care:

☐ 1. **For renewed or changed Epidural PCA orders only, continue Epidural PCA Nursing Care as previously ordered.**

☒ 2. Do not administer any other opioids, benzodiazepines, sedatives, or antiemetics unless first approved by: Pain Management Service:

☒ 3. Maintain iv access until epidural catheter is D/C'd.

☒ 4. Check epidural site q 8 h while awake, and notify Pain Management Service if site is soiled, red, or tender.

☒ 5. Check lower extremities q 8 h while awake, and notify Pain Management if numbness or weakness exist.

☒ 6. Assess and record at least q 4 h: HR and BP. Check orthostatic BP before ambulating.

☒ 7. Assess and record at least q 2 h: RR, SaO_2, and level of pain, using appropriate tool. (0–10 *Scale, Wong-Baker Faces Scale, FLACC Scale, or PIPP Scale*)

☒ 8. Bag and mask at bedside.

☒ 9. Continuous O_2 sat monitor. For $SaO_2 < 94\%$, administer O_2 per nasal cannula to maintain $SaO_2 \geq 94\%$.

☐ 10. Assess for bladder distention. If no void for h (since surgery or last void), may straight cath prn × 2.

☒ 11. For any pain management issues, notify Pain Management Service.

Medications:

☐ 1. **For renewed or changed Epidural PCA orders only, continue prn medications for Epidural PCA as previously ordered.**

☐ 2. If unable to arouse or $SaO_2<85\%$, D/C infusion, administer O_2 and/or ambu-bag, stimulate patient, administer naloxone__________mg iv (0.001 mg/kg) q 1–2 min (obtain naloxone from floor stock), as needed, to restore LOC, and **STAT page** Pain Management.

☐ 3. Metoclopramide (Reglan)________________mg iv q 6 h prn N/V (0.1 mg/kg/dose; max 15 mg).

☐ 4. Ondansetron (Zofran)__________________mg iv q 8 h prn N/V (0.1 mg/kg/dose; max 4 mg).

☐ 5. Diphenhydramine (Benadryl)________________mg iv q 6 h prn pruritus (0.5 mg/kg/dose; max 50 mg).

☐ 6. Nalbuphine (Nubain)________________________mg iv q 4 h prn pruritus (0.05 mg/kg/dose) - generally more effective for treatment of epidural opioid induced pruritus than diphenhydramine

☐ 7. If no stool by__________(POD 3), administer:

- ☐ 1 pediatric glycerin suppository pr once or twice daily prn (ages 2–6 yr)
- ☐ Bisacodyl 5 mg (½ suppository) pr daily prn (ages 6–11 yr)
- ☐ Bisacodyl 10 mg (1 suppository) pr daily prn (ages > 11 yr)
- ☐ If no stool within 24 h of beginning treatment, notify Pain Management Service.

☐ 8. When Epidural PCA is D/C'd, D/C all prn medications for Epidural PCA.

☐ 9. Other Medications:____________________

Date	Time:	Physician's Signature:	Pager:	Noted by:	Date/Time:
Orders signed				RN Signature:	Date/Time:

APPENDIX F: TABLE OF DRUG INTERACTIONS

Sandra Leigh Bardas

This table is intended only as an advisory overview of potential interactions between various drug classes that patients may be taking preop and the drugs used in anesthetic practice. It is not intended to be a comprehensive list. Drug interactions are dynamic and manifest via a variety of circumstances including dosage, duration of administration as well as the patient's genetics and current physiologic state. An excellent source for the predictive values of drug interactions due to altered metabolism can also be found in references for inhibitors, inducers, and substrates of the Cytochrome P450 Enzymes. In view of the constant flow of new drug information, the reader is strongly urged to check the primary literature of each drug or online resources, such as DRUG-REAX, Lexi-Interact and Facts and Comparisons for drug interactions and then tailor drug usage to the patient specific clinical situation.

Preop Drug or Drug Class	Anesthetic Drug or Drug Class	Interaction	Clinical Management
Adrenergic agonists (Sympathomimetics)	Inhalation anesthetics	↑ risk of dysrhythmia	Monitor rhythm.
Alteplase	Nitroglycerin	Impaired thrombolytic effect	Avoid combination.
Alfentanil	Propofol	Opisthotonus, seizure	Avoid combination.
Aminoglycosides	Fluorinated inhalation agents	↑ potential for nephrotoxicity 2° to fluoride	Monitor renal function postop.
	NMR (nondepolarizing muscle relaxants)	↑ blockade, possible prolonged respiratory depression	Support respiration.
	Succinylcholine	↑ depolarizing blockade	Delay administration of aminoglycoside for as long as possible after recovery. Support respiration.
Amiodarone	Inhalation anesthetics	Enhanced myocardial depression and conduction defects	Monitor HR and rhythm.
	Phenylpiperidone derivative opiate agonists (alfentanil, fentanyl, sufentanil)	↓ HR, ↓ BP, sinus arrest	Monitor hemodynamic function. Administer inotropic, chronotropic, and pressor agents as indicated. Large doses of vasopressors may be required. Bradycardia usually not responsive to atropine.
Amphetamines	Opiate agonists	↑ analgesia	Titrate dose of opiate.
Antacids	Oral medications	Delayed drug absorption 2° to delayed gastric emptying	Avoid administration within 2 h of each other.
Anthracyclines including doxorubicin, daunorubicin, idarubicin, epirubicin	Isoflurane	Prolonged QT interval	Monitor HR & rhythm.
Antibiotics, polypeptide (bacitracin, capreomycin, colistimethate, polymyxin B)	NMR, Succinylcholine	↑ blockade, possible prolonged respiratory depression Colistimethate and polymyxin B may have independent NMB activity.	Support respiration. Consider calcium gluconate to reverse blockade prolonged by colistimethate.

Preop Drug or Drug Class	Anesthetic Drug or Drug Class	Interaction	Clinical Management
Anticholinergics, including drugs with an anticholinergic adverse effect profile	Opiate agonists	Potential for central or peripheral anticholinergic syndrome	Monitor for effects.
Anticholinesterase inhibitors, including donepezil, galantamine, rivastigmine, tacrine + opthalmics	Succinylcholine Mivacurium	Blockade may be prolonged or antagonized.	Titrate to therapeutic effect. Monitor and support respiration.
	NMR	↓ blockade	Titrate to therapeutic effect
Antifungal agents, azole systemic (fluconazole, itraconazole, ketoconazole, voriconazole)	Alfentanil	Inhibition of alfentanil metabolism	Monitor for respiratory depression. Consider lower dosage.
	Midazolam	Prolonged CNS depression	Titrate midazolam to effect. Consider lower dosage
Aprotinin	NMR	Prolonged or recurring apnea	Monitor respiratory status.
Aprepitant	Phenylpiperidone derivative opiate agonists	↑ opiate effect	A lower dose may provide appropriate analgesia.
Aprepitant	Midazolam	↑ midazolam effect	A lower dosage may provide appropriate sedation.
Arsenic Trioxide	**Inhalation Anesthetics**	**Prelong QT Interval**	**Monitor HR & Rhythm**
Atorvastatin	Midazolam	↑ midazolam effect	A lower dosage may provide appropriate sedation.
Barbiturates	Inhalation anesthetics	↑ respiratory depression	Monitor and support respiration.
	Ketamine	↑ respiratory depression	Monitor and support respiration.
	Meperidine	Possible increase in normeperidine formation	↓ analgesic duration ↑ potential for seizure
	Midazolam	Synergy	Monitor for CNS depression.
	Opiate agonists	↑ respiratory depression	Monitor and support respiration.
Benzodiazepines	Barbiturates	Synergy	Titrate doses.
	Bupivacaine	Sz threshold raised masking signs of toxicity	Monitor for symptoms of bupivacaine toxicity.
	NMR	May prolong or antagonize blockade	Monitor and support respiration.
	Opiate agonists	May decrease respiration and BP	Monitor and support respiration and BP.
Beta Blockers	NMR	May potentiate, delay or antagonize blockade	Titrate to effect. Monitor and support respiration.
Bosentan	Propofol	Propofol is a CYP3A4 strong inhibitor	Monitor ↓ BP

Preop Drug or Drug Class	Anesthetic Drug or Drug Class	Interaction	Clinical Management
Botulinum toxins	NMR	↑ blockade	Titrate NMR to therapeutic effect.
Bupivacaine	Chloroprocaine	Enhanced bupivacaine toxicity	**Avoid combination!**
Calcium channel blockers	NMR	↑ blockade	Titrate NMR to therapeutic effect.
	Propofol	↓ BP	Monitor BP
Calcium channel blockers-nondihydropyridine (diltiazem, verapamil)	Phenylpiperidone derivative opiate agonists	Enhanced bradycardia and ↓ BP	Monitor HR & BP
	Midazolam	Enhanced midazolam effect	Consider dose reduction of midazolam
Carbamazepine	Diltiazem, Verapamil	Potential for CNS toxicity	Monitor for symptoms of CNS toxicity.
	Midazolam	↓ effect of midazolam due to enzyme induction	Titrate midazolam to effect.
	NMR	↓ blockade	Titrate NMR to therapeutic effect.
Cimetidine	Opiate	↑ CNS depression due to possible CYP 3A4 interaction	Titrate opiate to effect. If needed use naloxone.
Clindamycin	NMR	↑ blockade	Avoid combination if possible. Monitor and support respiration. Anticholinesterases or Ca^{++} may be beneficial.
Clonidine	Esmolol	Attenuation or reversal of antihypertensive effect	Monitor BP.
Clonidine, epidural	Local anesthetics	Prolonged sensory and motor blockade	Titrate dose of local anesthetics.
Conivaptan	Midazolam	Enhanced midazolam effect due to conivaptan strong CYP3A4 inhibition	Titrate to effect
	Phenylpiperidone derivative opiate agonists	Enhanced opiate effect due to conivaptan strong CYP3A4 inhibition	Titrate to effect
	Propofol	Enhanced propofol effect due to conivaptan strong CYP3A4 inhibition	Titrate to effect
Corticosteroids	Anticholinesterases	Possible antagonism of reversal agents	Monitor and support respiration.
	NMR	Altered effectiveness of blockade	Titrate NMR to therapeutic effect.
Cyclophosphamide	Succinylcholine, Mivacurium	↑ blockade, even if patient received cyclophosphamide in past few weeks	Titrate to therapeutic effect. Monitor and support respiration.

Preop Drug or Drug Class	Anesthetic Drug or Drug Class	Interaction	Clinical Management
Cyclosporine	NMR	↑ blockade	Titrate to therapeutic effect. Monitor and support respiration.
Dantrolene	Propofol	↑ muscle weakness due to inhibition of dantrolene metabolism	Monitor for hypotension.
Delavirdine	Phenylpiperidone derivative opiate agonists	↑ opiate effect	Consider dose reduction. Titrate to therapeutic effect.
Digoxin	Esmolol	↑ digoxin toxicity	Monitor for symptoms of toxicity.
	NMR	Precipitate new dysrhythmias or potentiate existing dysrhythmias	Monitor rhythm.
	Succinylcholine	Precipitate new dysrhythmias or potentiate existing dysrhythmias	Monitor rhythm.
Disulfiram	Inhalation anesthetics	Reduction in gas metabolism	Monitor for increased effect of inhalation agent.
Dobutamine	Inhalation anesthetics	Ventricular arrhythmias	Monitor HR and rhythm.
Dofetilide	Sevoflurane	Prolonged QT intervals	Monitor HR & rhythm
Echothiophate iodide (ophthalmic)	Succinylcholine	Prolonged blockade	Consider dose reduction or alternative NMB
Erythromycin (also see macrolide)	Midazolam	↑ CNS depression	Titrate dose of midazolam.
Esmolol	Alpha/Beta adrenergic agonists	↑ pressor effects	Infiltrating larger volumes of local anesthetics may have clinical relevance.
Estrogens	Succinylcholine	↑ blockade	Titrate NMR to therapeutic effect.
Ethanol	Barbiturates	Acute ingestion →CNS depression; chronic ingestion → tolerance	Avoid combination as tolerance is unpredictable.
	Benzodiazepines	Acute ingestion →CNS depression; chronic ingestion →tolerance	Titrate dose of benzodiazepines.
	Phenylpiperidone derivative opiate agonists	Chronic alcohol consumption→ pharmacodynamic tolerance	Titrate dose of opiate.
Fluvoxamine	Ropivacaine	Inhibition of CYP1A2 metabolism	Monitor for ropivacaine toxicity.
Furazolidone	Adrenergic agonists	↑ pressor sensitivity due to MAOI activity of furazolidone	**Avoid combination!** In hypertensive crisis, consider phentolamine.
	Meperidine	Risk of MAOI/meperidine interaction	**Avoid combination!**

Preop Drug or Drug Class	Anesthetic Drug or Drug Class	Interaction	Clinical Management
Gabapentin	General anesthetic agents	Case report of myotonia & dystonia	Monitor for potential adverse reactions.
Imatinib (tyrosine kinase inhibitor)	Midazolam	↑ midazolam effect	Consider dose reduction. Titrate to effect.
	Propofol	↑ effect of propofol	Consider dose reduction. Titrate to effect.
Inhalation anesthetics, halogenated	Epinephrine	Increased cardiac irritability	Limit or reduce dosage of epinephrine with local anesthetics.
	NMR	↑ blockade	Titrate dose of both agents.
Isoniazid (INH)	Enflurane	Fast acetylators of INH facilitate defluorination of enflurane → high output renal failure	Monitor renal function postop.
	Halothane	↑ hepatotoxicity	Avoid giving rifampin-INH after halothane anesthesia.
	Phenylpiperidone derivative opiate agonists	↑ opiate effect	Monitor for respiratory depression.
Ketamine	Halothane	↓ BP, ↓ CO	Monitor BP.
	NMR	↑ blockade	Monitor and support respiration.
Labetalol	Beta-2 agonists	↓ bronchodilatation	Monitor for bronchospasm.
	Inhalation anesthetics, halogenated	↓ BP	Monitor BP. Titrate anesthetic to effect.
Lidocaine	Cocaine	Possible ↓ in metabolic clearance of lidocaine	Monitor for lidocaine toxicity.
	Meperidine	Risk of MAOI/ meperidine interaction	**Avoid combination!**
Linezolid	Adrenergic agonists	↑ pressor sensitivity due to MAOI activity of linezolid	**Avoid combination!** In hypertensive crisis, consider phentolamine.
Lithium	NMR	↑ blockade	Titrate NMR to therapeutic effect. Monitor and support respiration.
Local anesthetics (large doses)	NMR	↑ blockade	Titrate NMR to effect. Monitor and support respiration.
Loop diuretics (including bumetanide, ethacrynic acid, furosemide, torsemide)	NMR	Blockade may be prolonged or antagonized; possibly dose-dependent, ↓ K^+ → ↑ blockade	Titrate NMR to therapeutic effect. Monitor and support respiration.
Macrolide antibiotics including azithromycin, clarithromycin, erythromycin	Alfentanil	↑ effect of alfentanil	Titrate dose of alfentanil. Monitor and support respiration.

Preop Drug or Drug Class	Anesthetic Drug or Drug Class	Interaction	Clinical Management
Macrolide antibiotics, including erythromycin, clarithromycin. But NOT azithromycin	Midazolam	↑ effect of midazolam	Titrate dose of midazolam. Monitor and support respiration.
	NMR	Case reports of potentiation of blockade	Titrate NMR to therapeutic effect. Monitor and support respiration.
Magnesium, parenteral	NMR	↑ blockade	Titrate NMR to therapeutic effect. Monitor and support respiration.
Mercaptopurine	NMR	May ↓ or reverse blockade	Titrate NMR to therapeutic effect.
Methotrexate	Nitrous oxide	Potentiation of cytotoxic effects	Avoid before or during methotrexate treatment
Methyldopa	Ephedrine	↓ ephedrine effect	Consider alternative pressor agent.
	Naloxone	Naloxone may precipitate a mild ↑ BP	Monitor BP.
Metoclopramide	Succinylcholine, NMR	↑ blockade	Titrate succinylcholine to therapeutic effect. Monitor and support respiration.
Monoamine oxidase inhibitor (MAOI); selective MAO Type B may have a lower risk. Antidepressants MAOI: Isocarboxazid, phenelzine, tranylcypromine. Anti-Parkinson agents MAO Type B: rasagiline, selegiline	Meperidine	Agitation, Sz, diaphoresis, hyperpyrexia, coma, apnea	**Avoid combination!** Although other opiate agonists may not have these associated problems, monitoring is prudent.
	Succinylcholine, mivacurium	↑ blockade	Titrate succinylcholine to therapeutic effect. Monitor and support respiration.
	Sympathomimetics (including local anesthetic/epinephrine combinations, and cocaine)	Indirect- or mixed-acting sympathomimetic may cause severe HA, hyperpyrexia, or hypertensive crisis. (Direct-acting sympathomimetics appear to interact minimally.)	Avoid combination! Treat ↑ BP with phentolamine.
Muscle relaxants, skeletal	Anticholinesterase inhibitors	Possible severe muscle weakness	Monitor neuromuscular blockade. Titrate dose of anticholinesterase.
Nefazodone	Midazolam	↑ effect of midazolam due to strong inhibition of CYP3A4	Monitor and titrate to effect.
	Phenylpiperidone derivative opiate agonists	↑ effect of opiate due to strong inhibition of CYP3A4	Monitor and titrate to effect.
	Propofol	↑ effect of propofol due to strong inhibition of CYP3A4	Monitor and titrate to effect.

Preop Drug or Drug Class	Anesthetic Drug or Drug Class	Interaction	Clinical Management
Nicardipine	Midazolam	↑ effect of midazolam due to strong inhibition of CYP3A4	Monitor and titrate to effect.
	Phenylpiperidone derivative opiate agonists	↑ effect of opiate due to strong inhibition of CYP3A4	Monitor and titrate to effect.
	Propofol	↑ effect of propofol due to strong inhibition of CYP3A4	Monitor and titrate to effect.
Nitrates, including NTG	Pancuronium	↑ blockade	Titrate NMR to therapeutic effect. Monitor and support respiration.
Omeprazole	Midazolam	Possible enhanced ataxia or sedation due to ↓ clearance of midazolam	Monitor for prolonged effect of midazolam.
Opiate agonists	NMBs	↑ potential for opiate toxicity	Titrate dose of opiate.
	Propofol	↓ BP	Titrate dose of each agent.
	Succinylcholine	↓ HR	Monitor HR, heart block
Oxytocic drugs (including oxytocin, ergotamine, methylergonovine)	Adrenergic agonists	↑ BP 2° to synergistic vasoconstrictive effects	Titrate dosage. Monitor BP.
Pegvisomant	Opioids	Influences therapeutic efficacy of pegvisomant	May need dosage adjustment of pegvisomant.
Phenothiazines	Alpha/Beta adrenergic agonists	↓ alpha-adrenergic effects	Potential for dysrhythmias.
	Barbiturate anesthetics	↑ neuromuscular excitation ↓ BP	Monitor BP.
	Opiate agonists	↓ analgesic effect	Titrate opiate to effect.
Phenoxybenzamine	Local anesthetics	↑ absorption of local anesthetic	Titrate dose; possibly add epinephrine to local anesthetic.
Phenytoin (including fosphenytoin)	Midazolam	Enzyme induction	Titrate midazolam to effect. May need to ↑ dosage.
	NMR	Reduced duration of blockade	Consider cisatracurium. Titrate NMR to therapeutic effect.
Phosphodiesterase 5 inhibitors (sildenafil, tadalafil, vardenafil)	Nitroglycerin	Enhanced vasodilation	Separate dose by at least 24 h (timing depends on specific agent) Half life may be prolonged by drug interactions, renal, hepatic impairment.
Piperacillin (including piperacillin/ tazobactam sodium)	NMR	↑ blockade	Titrate NMR to therapeutic effect. Monitor and support respiration.

Preop Drug or Drug Class	Anesthetic Drug or Drug Class	Interaction	Clinical Management
Probenecid	Thiopental	↑ CNS depression	Titrate dose of thiopental.
Procaine, procainamide	NMR	↑ blockade	Titrate NMR to therapeutic effect. Monitor and support respiration.
	Succinylcholine	↑ blockade 2° to competition for pseudocholinesterases	Titrate NMR to therapeutic effect. Monitor and support respiration.
Propofol	Alfentanil	Alfentanil may enhance the adverse effects of propofol	Monitor for opisthotonos and/or Sz.
	Atracurium	Bronchospasm	Anaphylactoid-type reaction
	Succinylcholine	↓ HR	Monitor HR. Consider atropine premed when propofol precedes succinylcholine.
	Vecuronium	↑ blockade	Titrate NMR to therapeutic effect. Monitor and support respiration.
Protease inhibitors except tipranavir	Phenylpiperidine derivative opiate agonists	↑ fentanyl levels due to CYP3A4 enzyme inhibition	Monitor respiration.
	Midazolam	↑ midazolam levels	Titrate midazolam to effect. Contraindicated with amprenavir and ritonavir.
QTc Prolonging Agents Public website for listing: http://www.qtdrugs.org, International Registry Drug-Induced Arrhythmias; University of Arizona Health Sciences Center, Tucson, AR	Inhalation anesthetics	Effects can be additive with enhanced/advertise/toxic profile	Conduct a risk assessment Monitor rate and rhythm
Quinine, quinidine	NMR	↑ blockade	Titrate NMR to therapeutic effect. Monitor and support respiration.
	Succinylcholine	↑ blockade	Use this combination with caution.
Ranitidine	NMR	Possible resistance to NMR	Titrate dosage. Consider another NMR.
Rasagiline	Meperidine	Risk of MAOI/meperidine interaction	**Avoid combination!**
Reserpine	Sympathomimetics	↑ direct-acting agents; ↓ indirect-acting agents	Monitor BP.
Rifamycin derivatives including rifampin, rifabutin, rifapentine	Alfentanil	↑ clearance of alfentanil	Titrate alfentanil to effect. Increased dosage may be needed.
	Halothane	↑ risk of hepatotoxicity	Avoid administration of rifampin-INH after halothane anesthesia.
	Midazolam	Enzyme induction	Titrate midazolam to effect. May need to ↑ dosage.

Preop Drug or Drug Class	Anesthetic Drug or Drug Class	Interaction	Clinical Management
Selective serotonin reuptake inhibitors (SSRIs)	Opiate agonists	Unknown mechanism	Monitor for serotonin syndrome.
	Adrenergic agonist agents	Potential for serotonin syndrome	Monitor for serotonin syndrome.
Selegiline	Meperidine	Risk of MAOI/meperidine interaction	**Avoid combination!**
Sevoflurane	Drugs that prolong the QT interval	Synergy	Monitor heart rate and rhythm.
Sibutramine	Phenylpiperidine derivative opiate agonists	Package insert caution	Monitor for serotonin syndrome.
Sotalol	Sevoflurane	Prolonged QT intervals	Monitor rhythm.
Succinylcholine	Anticholinesterase inhibitors	↑ blockade	Use combination with caution. Titrate NMR to therapeutic effect. Monitor and support respiration.
Succinylcholine	Opioids	↓ HR	Monitor for bradycardia/ heart block.
Tetracycline	NMR	↑ blockade	Titrate NMR to therapeutic effect. Monitor and support respiration.
Theophylline	Halothane	↑ catecholamine-induced dysrhythmias	Use alternative inhalation agent.
	Ketamine	Sz	Use combination with caution.
	NMR	Resistance to blockade	Titrate NMR to effect.
	Midazolam	↓ midazolam effectiveness	Titrate midazolam to effect.
	Propofol	Possibly antagonized sedation	Titrate propofol to effect.
Thiazide diuretics	NMR	↑ blockade may be 2° to hypokalemia	Correct hypokalemia. Titrate NMR to effect.
Thiopental	Succinylcholine	Possible disseminated intravascular coagulation	Use large veins. Flush tubing with saline. Wait 2–3 min between administration.
Thiotepa	NMR	↑ blockade	Titrate NMR to therapeutic effect. Monitor and support respiration.
Tricyclic antidepressants	Adrenergic agonist agents	↑ direct-acting agents;↓ indirect-acting agents	Monitor BP and rhythm. Effect unlikely in dose administered as infiltration with local anesthetics.
	Fentanyl	Potentiation of fentanyl	Titrate opiate agonist to effect.

Preop Drug or Drug Class	Anesthetic Drug or Drug Class	Interaction	Clinical Management
Trimethaphan	NMR	↑ blockade	Titrate NMR to therapeutic effect. Monitor and support respiration.
	Succinylcholine	↑ blockade	**Avoid combination!** Use nitroprusside instead.
Vancomycin	NMR	↑ blockade	Titrate NMR to therapeutic effect. Monitor and support respiration.
	Succinylcholine	↑ blockade	Avoid administering vancomycin in the postanesthesia period.
Verapamil	Etomidate	↑ respiratory depression, apnea	Monitor and support respiration.
	Midazolam	Deep and prolonged sedation	Monitor CNS and respiratory status.
	NMR	↑ blockade	Titrate NMR to therapeutic effect. Monitor and support respiration.

HERBAL AGENTS

It may be difficult to accurately predict the potential for drug interactions, because the majority of people neglect to inform health care providers of their consumption of herbal agents, natural remedies, alternative or complimentary medicines, nutritional supplements, and illicit substances. The significance of the potential interaction is also difficult to assess due to variations of botanical species, the different parts of plants that are used, assay of active ingredient(s), and product formulation. Herbs that alter hemostasis should be D/C'd 14 d before surgical, dental, or invasive procedures.

Plant	Precautions for Anesthesia and Surgery
Aloe vera	May impair hemostasis.
Bilberry (*Vaccinium myrtillus*)	May impair hemostasis.
Black cohosh (*Cimicifuga racemosa*)	Potential for hypotension.
Bladderwrack (*Fucus vesiculosus*)	May impair hemostasis.
Cat's Claw (*Uncaria tomentosa*)	May impair hemostasis.
Cayenne (*Capsicum annum*)	Has biological effect of ↑ catecholamine secretion.
Chamomile. German (*Matricaria chamomilla*)	May enhance CNS depression.
Coleus (*Coleus forskohlii*)	May impair hemostasis. Has potential for hypotension.

Plant	Precautions for Anesthesia and Surgery
Devil's claw (*Harpagophytum procumbens*)	May have chronotropic and inotropic effects. May impair hemostasis.
Dong quai (*Angelica sinensis*)	May impair hemostasis. May cause vasodilation.
Echinacea	May increase the sedative effect of midazolam.
Ephedra ma huang (*Ephedra sinica*)	Potent sympathomimetic may cause cardiac arrhythmias.
Evening primrose (*Oenothera biennis*)	May impair hemostasis.
Fenugreek (Trigonella foenum-graecum)	May impair hemostasis. Contains coumarin.
Feverfew (*Tanacetum parthenium*)	May impair hemostasis.
Fish oils	May impair hemostasis.
Garlic (*Allium sativum*)	May inhibit Plt aggregation; potential for enhanced ↓ BP.
Ginger (*Zingiber officinale*)	May → prolonged bleeding time; possible ↑ catecholamine secretion; cardioactive in large and prolonged doses.
Ginkgo (*Ginkgo biloba*)	Selective antagonist of Plt aggregation; may cause vasodilation.
Ginseng, American (*Panax quinquefolius*)	May impair hemostasis.
Ginseng, Panax (*Panax ginseng*) root	Dose-dependent effects on BP. May cause tachycardia. May impair hemostasis.
Ginseng, Siberian (*Eleutherococcus senticosus*)	May impair hemostasis. Use barbiturates with caution. May affect BP.
Golden Seal (*Hydrastis Canadensis*)	May impair hemostasis. Potential for hypotension and bradycardia. May alter liver enzymes.
Grapefruit	Cytochrome P450 (CYP3A4) inhibition. Onset of midazolam may be delayed and action increased.
Grape seed (*Vitis vinifera*)	May impair hemostasis.
Green tea (camellia sinensis)	May impair hemostasis.
Guggul (Commiphora mukul)	May impair hemostasis.
Hawthorn (*Crataegus oxyacantha*)	High doses may cause hypotension + CNS depression.
Horse chestnut (Aesculus hippocastanum)	May impair hemostasis. Has cholinergic properties.
Kava kava (*Piper methysticum*)	Synergy with midazolam.

Plant	Precautions for Anesthesia and Surgery
Licorice (*Glycyrrhiza glabra*)	May impair hemostasis. Mineralocorticoid effect
Melatonin	May enhance CNS depressants.
Passion flower (*Passiflora spp*)	Synergy with CNS depressants.
Red clover (*Trifolium pratense*)	May impair hemostasis. Contains coumarins.
Reishi (*Ganoderma lucidum*)	May impair hemostasis.
Schisandra (*Schizandra chinensis*)	Inducer of Cytochrome P450 enzyme system.
St. John's wort (*Hypericum perforatum*)	May have some MAOI activity. May reduce midazolam levels due to enzyme induction. Delayed emergence from anesthesia with propofol.
Tumeric (*Curcuma longa*)	May impair hemostasis.
Valerian (*Valeriana officinalis*)	Potentially synergistic with opiates & CNS depressants, including thiopental.
White willow (Salix alba)	Salicylate, may impair hemostasis.
Yohimbe (*Corynanthe yohimbe*) (*Pausinystalia yohimbe*)	May cause CNS stimulation. May have cardiovascular effects.

APPENDIX G: SPECIAL CONSIDERATIONS FOR LATEX ALLERGY

Naiyi Sun, Brenda Golianu, Cathy Lammers, and Alvin Hackel

Latex is the second most common cause of anaphylactic reactions under anesthesia (16.6% of cases).[9] Latex gloves are the major source of latex proteins and are implicated in most cases of latex-mediated reactions.[1] Latex exposure may occur through skin contact, mucous membrane exposure, inhalation, ingestion, or parenteral injection. Latex sensitization can lead to immune-mediated reactions, the most serious being type I IgE-mediated hypersensitivity reaction leading to life-threatening anaphylaxis.

Populations at Risk:

- Patients with history of multiple surgical procedures including those with myelomeningocele, spina bifida, and congenital genitourinary tract anomalies.
- Patients with a history of myelomeningocele and spina bifida should be treated with a "Latex precautions" regimen from birth, regardless of prior history of exposure or latex reactivity.
- Health care personnel with occupational exposure.
- Other individuals with occupational exposure such as rubber industry workers and hairdressers.
- Patients with history of atopy, hay fever, asthma, or eczema.
- Patients with history of food allergy to tropical fruits (such as avocado, kiwi, banana, mango) and chestnuts which contain cross-reacting proteins with latex.

It is currently estimated that as many as 17% of health care workers have been sensitized to latex.[11] Occupational exposure can be minimized by avoiding powdered latex gloves and limiting the use of latex-containing gloves. Applying lotion to hands before using latex gloves facilitates the transfer of latex proteins to hands and should be avoided.

In high-risk patients, latex-avoidance protocols are recommended as this may decrease the incidence of subsequent intraoperative allergic reactions. Hospitals and ORs have decreased the use of products that contain latex to the extent that some are essentially latex-free. Anesthesia carts can be assembled with latex-free products, reducing the risk of latex-sensitization for all patients and negating the need for a special "latex-free cart." The latex content of commonly used materials can be identified from external labeling, package inserts, or directly from the manufacturers. Even minimal latex exposure (e.g., an injection through a latex port of iv tubing or opening a package of powdered latex gloves) has resulted in anaphylaxis.

Diagnosis of latex allergy is based on a focused history and physical examination with positive in vivo or in vitro test. In vitro serum tests for latex-specific IgE such as RAST are highly specific but have a high false-negative rate, up to 30%.[1] Skin testing identifies patients with a high titer of IgE to latex, but must be performed with appropriate safeguards because it may induce systemic anaphylaxis.

Pharmacological prophylaxis in the acute setting is controversial for patients with documented latex allergy. Prophylaxis medications, such as diphenhydramine, ranitidine, and hydrocortisone, are not universally successful in preventing latex anaphylaxis.[12] Some authors have argued that pretreatment may mask the early immune responses leaving anaphylaxis as the first evidence of an allergic reaction.[8]

To prepare a latex-safe environment:

- Notify OR nurses, anesthesia technicians, and surgical staff of the need for a latex-free room.
- Place a sign on the door stating: "LATEX-FREE ROOM."
- Schedule the latex-allergic patient as the first case of the day to minimize the presence of airborne latex particles.
- Set up the room with latex-free materials (e.g., bag, bellows, ECG electrodes, pulse oximeter clip, iv tubing without latex ports, vinyl gloves, vinyl BP cuffs, clear micropore tape).
- Avoid bouffant surgical hair caps and shoe covers that contain latex bands.
- Wrap latex tubing on stethoscope. BP cuff, or tourniquet with Webril or cotton gauze if they contain latex derivatives.
- Removal of rubber stoppers from drug vials (instead of withdrawing through the stopper) is controversial.

Diagnosis of anaphylaxis or latex allergy:

- Skin: urticaria at site of contact with latex product or generalized urticaria, and flushing.
- Respiratory: bronchospasm, wheezing, ↑ PIP, ↓ O_2 sat, upsloping of $ETCO_2$ tracing.
- Cardiac: ↓ BP, ↑ HR, cardiac arrest.

Treatment of anaphylaxis:

- 100% O_2 and manually ventilate if needed.
- Discontinue all anesthetic agents.
- Epinephrine 0.1–1 mcg/kg iv initially, with rapid escalation as needed to support BP, may require an epinephrine infusion (0.05 – 0.1 mcg/kg/min).
- Administer iv fluid to ↑ preload and support BP.
- Stop administration of any suspected medications and remove latex products. (Instruct surgical staff to change to nonlatex gloves and remove any latex products from surgical field).
- Administer steroids (hydrocortisone 100 mg or methylprednisolone 0.5 mg/kg), antihistamine (diphenhydramine 50 mg or 0.5 mg/kg iv), H-2 blockers (ranitidine 150 mg iv).
- Administer bronchodilators (albuterol) via nebulizer for bronchospasm.
- Continue steroids and diphenhydramine for 24–48 h or until symptoms resolve.
- Consider drawing blood within 2 h of reaction to send for tryptase level (peaks at 30 min, t 1/2 is 2h) which is a mediator released from mast cells during degranulation.
- Refer patient to allergist to follow up. Skin prick test or RAST can be performed (4–6 weeks after the acute reaction resolves) to specifically test for latex allergy.
- Patients with a history of latex anaphylaxis should be advised to wear a Medic Alert bracelet.

Suggested Readings

1. ASA Committee for Occupational Health of Operating Room Personnel: *Natural Rubber Latex Allergy: Considerations for Anesthesiologists.* 2005. Available at: http://www.asahg.org/PublicationsAndServices/latexallergy.html.
2. Blum RH, Rockoff MA, Holzman RS, et al: Overreaction to latex allergy? *Anesth Analg* 1997; 84:467–8.
3. Hirshman CA: Latex anaphylaxis. *Anesthesiology* 1992; 77:223–4.
4. Holtzman RS: Clinical management of latex-allergic children. *Anesth Analg* 1997; 85(3):529–33.
5. Michael T, Niggemann B, Moers A, et al: Risk factors for latex allergy in patients with spina bifida. *Clin Exp Allergy* 1996; 26(8):934–9.
6. Rao AM, Davies MW: Syringes and latex allergy. *Anaesthesia* 1997; 52(5):506.
7. Vassallo SA, et al: Allergic reaction to latex from stopper of a medication vial. *Anesth Analg* 1995; 80(5):1057–8.
8. Hepner DL, Castells MC: Latex allergy: an update. *Anesth Analg* 2003; 96:1219–29.
9. Laxenaire MD, Mertes PM, et al: Anaphylaxis during anaesthesia. Results of a two-year survey in France. *Br J Anaesth* 2001; 87(4):549–58.
10. Zucker-Pinchoff B, Stadtmauer GJ: Latex allergy. *M Sinai J Med* 2002; 69:88–95.
11. Yassin MS, Lierl MB, Fischer TJ, et al: Latex allergy in hospital employees. *Ann Allergy* 1994; 72:245–9.
12. Setlock MA, Cotter TP, Rosner D: Latex allergy: failure of prophylaxis to prevent severe reaction. *Anesth Analg* 1993; 76:650–2.

APPENDIX H: PERIOPERATIVE ACUPUNCTURE

Jeannie Seybold, Emily Ratner, and Brenda Golianu

INTRODUCTION

Acupuncture is a treatment modality that has been practiced in China for over 3 millennia. Initially transmitted as an oral tradition, it was first described in written form in the Huang Di Nei Jing or the Yellow Emperor's Inner Cannon, the seminal text of ancient Chinese medicine dating back to the 3rd century BC.[4] Acupuncture involves placing very thin needles in the skin to stimulate the flow of qi in a complex network of meridians in the body. There are 12 principal and 8 curious acupuncture meridians that correspond to physiologic and anatomical organ functions.[4] Qi is a dynamic form of physical and spiritual energy that flows within the universe and in all organisms. One of the basic tenets of Chinese medicine is that illness and pain are caused by the stagnation or blockage of qi flow and/or the invasion of pathological influences- traditionally known as wind, heat, cold, dampness, dryness, or fire that result in imbalances of yin and yang. When a point is needled, a heavy sensation known as "deqi," or a mild paresthesia may be experienced by the patient. The practitioner may sense a gentle contraction of the connective tissue surrounding the needle, or may observe a flare developing around the needle. Needling, electrical and laser stimulation, acupressure or even herbal therapies (moxibustion or capsicum plaster) over specific points have all been documented to alleviate pain and pathological states.[11] In addition to body acupuncture, which developed in China, Japan, and Korea, many different traditions have been developed that focus on needling specific body parts, that is, the ear, scalp, or hand, as microsystems representing the entire body. Acupuncture has been used to provide analgesia during surgery since the 1950s in China. However, it was little more than a curiosity in the United States before 1971, when reporter James Reston went to China to report on the diplomatic efforts of Henry Kissinger and President Richard Nixon. While in Beijing, Reston required an emergency appendectomy and received acupuncture for postoperative ileus and pain control. The popularity of acupuncture in the United States exploded after he published his experiences in the *New York Times.* In 1997, the NIH released a consensus statement supporting the use of acupuncture for adult postoperative and chemotherapy-induced nausea and vomiting and postoperative dental pain. It also stated that acupuncture may be a useful adjunctive treatment in addiction, stroke rehabilitation, headache, menstrual cramps, tennis elbow, fibromyalgia, myofascial pain, osteoarthritis, low back pain, carpal tunnel syndrome, and asthma. During the last 10 years, acupuncture has been increasingly studied and used to treat acute postoperative pain as well as in chronic pain clinics throughout the United States.[28,29]

MECHANISMS

Several mechanisms for acupuncture analgesia have been proposed. The gate control theory by Melzack and Wall in 1965 postulated that stimulation of a-beta fibers inhibits a-delta and c fiber transmission of pain signals.[15] This may be a local mechanism of action. Other studies have shown that electroacupuncture at low (2–4 Hz) and high frequencies (100 Hz and greater) selectively induces endorphin and enkephalin release, respectively.[8] Conflicting evidence exists regarding the ability of naloxone to antagonize the analgesic effects of acupuncture. Some studies show that naloxone reverses acupuncture-induced analgesia, while others dispute this.[3,18] This suggests the analgesic mechanisms of acupuncture are more complex than the release of endorphins. Additional evidence suggests that the frequency and intensity of stimulation determine the degree of naloxone-reversibility.[9] A review of functional MRI and positron-emission tomography studies has shown that electroacupuncture exerts effects over the hypothalamus, somatosensory motor cortex, and rostral anterior cingulate cortex, with nonspecific modulation of the limbic system and hypothalamus.[16] A recent study by Tsuchiya showed that acupuncture enhanced the local generation of plasma nitric oxide, increasing regional blood flow.[24] Acupuncture may also have anti-inflammatory properties.[33]

PERIOPERATIVE USE

Acupuncture is effective for reducing PONV.[4,29] P6 (Neiguan), the most thoroughly studied acupoint, is located three fingerbreadths proximal to the wrist crease, between the flexor carpi ulnaris and palmaris longus tendons and directly over the median nerve. A Cochrane review of 26 randomized trials noted significant reduction in nausea and the need for rescue antiemetics with the use of P6 acupoint stimulation.[14] Direct electrical stimulation of this point was shown to be as efficacious as a standard dose of ondansetron for PONV in adults and resulted in a 37% reduction in nausea in children after tonsillectomy.[21] There is evidence that transcutaneous electrical acupoint stimulation

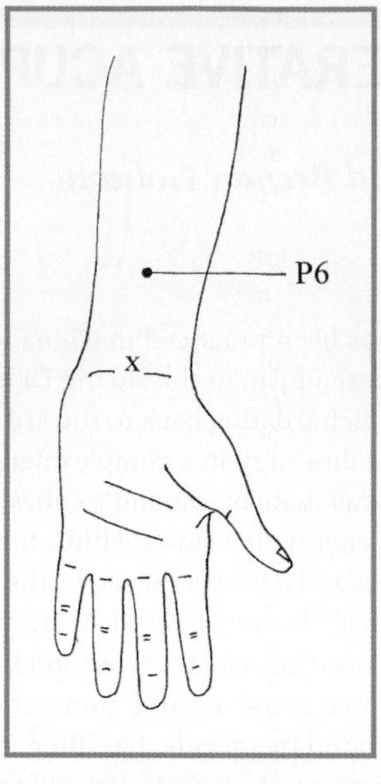

Figure H-1. P6 Acupoint. P6 is located three fingerbreadths proximal to the wrist crease directly over the median nerve and between the tendons of palmaris longus and flexor carpi radialis. For PONV prophylaxis, the two nerve stimulator electrodes can be placed over the median nerve at (1) a point proximal to the wrist crease (marked with an x) 2 cm proximal to P6, and (2) on P6 or 1 cm distal to the P6 point. Stimulus parameters: 1Hz, 0.2ms, 50 mA during anesthesia.

is also effective in reducing PONV.[10] Stimulation of P6 by twitch monitoring using a standard nerve stimulator (at 1 Hz, 0.2 ms, 50 mA) during general anesthesia for laparoscopic surgery significantly reduced PONV for 24 hours with an efficacy similar to that of commonly used antiemetic drugs.[1,22] A trained medical acupuncture practitioner would likely integrate P6 with a combination of body and ear acupuncture points to minimize PONV. Acupuncture has not been shown to eliminate the need for anesthetic medications during surgery, but it may be a useful adjuvant for perioperative analgesia and anxiolysis. In a randomized controlled trial of perioperative acupuncture for abdominal surgery, Kotani, et al. showed 50% reduction in postoperative morphine use, 20–30% reduction in postop nausea, and 30–50% reduction in plasma cortisol and epinephrine levels.[12] A reduction in postoperative pain and analgesic requirements was also seen in studies of acupuncture in patients having gynecologic, abdominal, thoracic, and orthopedic surgeries.[6,23,25,27] Acupuncture is known to produce deep relaxation and sedation, and may be useful for preoperative anxiolysis or for postoperative weaning of narcotic medications in opioid tolerant patients.[7,30] The risks of acupuncture are rare. The most common are minor bruising, limited capillary bleeding, pain or local infection at the needling site. Anesthesiologists can be trained to provide acupuncture treatment for PONV and anxiolysis. More comprehensive perioperative treatment should be performed by or under the supervision of a trained medical acupuncturist.

Suggested Readings

1. Arnberger M, Stadelmann K, Alischer P, et al: Monitoring of neuromuscular blockade at the P6 acupuncture point reduces the incidence of postoperative nausea and vomiting. *Anesthesiology* 2007; 107(6):903–8.
2. Berman BM, Lao L, Langenberg P: Effectiveness of acupuncture as adjunctive therapy in osteoarthritis of the knee: a randomized, controlled trial. *Ann Intern Med* 2004; 141(12):901–10.
3. Chapman CR, Benedetti C, Colpitts YH, et al: Naloxone fails to reverse pain thresholds elevated by acupuncture: acupuncture analgesia reconsidered. *Pain* 1983; 16:13–31.
4. Chernyak GV, Sessler DI: Perioperative acupuncture and related techniques. *Anesth Analg* 2005; 102(5):1031–78.
5. Gan TJ, Jiao KR, Zenn M, et al: A randomized controlled comparison of electro-point stimulation or ondansetron versus placebo for the prevention of postoperative nausea and vomiting. *Anesth Analg* 2004; 99(4):1070–5.
6. Gilbertson B, Werner K, Russell LC, et al: Acupuncture and arthroscopic acromioplasty. *J Orthop Res* 2003; 21(4):752–8.
7. Golianu B, Krane E, Seybold J, et al: Non-pharmacological techniques for pain management in neonates. *Sem Perinatology* 2007; 31(5):318–22.

8. Han JS: Acupuncture and endorphins. *Neurosci Lett* 2004; 361:258–61.
9. Huang C, Wang Y, Han JS, et al: Characteristics of electroacupuncture-induced analgesia in mice: variation with strain, frequency, intensity and opioid involvement. *Brain Res* 2002; 945:20–5.
10. Kabalak AA, Akcay M, Akcay F, et al: Transcutaneous electrical acupoint stimulation versus ondansetron in the prevention of postoperative vomiting following pediatric tonsillectomy. *J Alt Comp Med* 2005; 11(3):407–13.
11. Kim KS, Nam YM: The analgesic effects of capsicum plaster at the Zusamli point after abdominal hysterectomy. *Anesth Analg* 2006; 103(3):709–13.
12. Kotani NK, Hashimoto H, Sato Y, et al: Preoperative intradermal acupuncture reduces postoperative pain, nausea and vomiting, analgesic requirement, and sympathoadrenal responses. *Anesthesiology* 2001; 95(2):349–56.
13. Kundu A, Berman BM: Acupuncture for pediatric pain and symptom management. *Pediatr Clin North Am* 2007; 54:885–9.
14. Lee A, Done ML: Stimulation of the wrist acupuncture point P6 for presenting postoperative nausea and vomiting. *Cochrane Database Syst Rev* 2004; 3:CD003281. DOI:10.1002/14651858.CD003281.pub2.
15. Lewith G, Kenyon JN. Physiological and psychological explanations for the mechanism of acupuncture as a treatment for chronic pain. *Soc Sci Med* 1984; 19:1367–78.
16. Lewith GT, White PJ, Pariente J: Investigating acupuncture using brain imaging techniques: the current state of play. *eCAM* 2005; 2(3):315–9.
17. Lin YC: Perioperative usage of acupuncture. *Pediatr Anesthesia* 2006; 16:231–5.
18. Mayer DJ, Price DD, Rafii A, et al: Antagonism of acupuncture analgesia in man by the narcotic antagonist naloxone. *Brain Res* 1977; 121:368–72.
19. NIH Consensus Statement Online: *Acupuncture.* 1997 Nov 3–5; 15(5):1–34.
20. Reston J: Now let me tell you about my appendectomy in Peking. *New York Times* July 26,1971.
21. Rusy LM, Hoffman GM, Weisman SJ: Electro-acupuncture prophylaxis of postoperative nausea and vomiting following pediatric tonsillectomy with or without adenoidectomy. *Anesthesiology* 2002; 96:300–5.
22. Scuderi PE: P6 Stimulation, a new approach to an ancient technique. *Anesthesiology* 2007; 107(6):870–2.
23. Sim CK, Xu PC, Pua HL, et al: Effects of electro-acupuncture on intra-operative and post-operative analgesic requirement. *Acupunct Med* 2002; 20(2–3):56–65.
24. Tsuchiya M, Sato EF, Inoue M, et al: Acupuncture enhances generation of nitric oxide and increases local circulation. *Anesth Analg* 2007; 104:301–7.
25. Vickers AJ, Rusch VW, Malhotra VT, et al: Acupuncture is a feasible treatment for post-thoracotomy pain: results of a prospective pilot trial. *BMC Anesthesiology* 2006; 6:5.
26. Ulett GA, Han SP, Hang JS: Electroacupuncture: mechanisms and clinical application. *Biol Psychiatry* 1998; 44:129–38.
27. Usichenko TI, Dinse M, Hermsen M, et al: Auricular acupuncture for pain relief after total hip arthroplasty: a randomized controlled study. *Pain* 2005; 114:320–7.
28. Wang SM, Kain ZN, White P: Acupuncture analgesia I: the scientific basis. *Anesth Analg* 2008; 106:602–10.
29. Wang SM, Kain ZN, White PF: Acupuncture analgesia II: clinical considerations. *Anesth Analg* 2008; 106:602–10.
30. Wang SM, Peloquin C, Kain Z: The use of auricular acupuncture to reduce preoperative anxiety. *Anesth Analg* 2001; 93:1178–80.
31. White P: Use of alternative medical therapies in the perioperative period: is it time to get on board. *Anesth Analg* 2007; 104:251–4.
32. Zhang RX, Li A, Liu B, et al: Electro-acupuncture attenuates bone cancer pain and inhibits spinal interleukin-1 beta expression in a rat model. *Anesth Analg* 2007; 105:1482–8.
33. Zhang RX, Lao LX, Wang XY, et al: Electroacupuncture attenuates inflammation in a rat model. *J Alt Comp Med* 2005; 11(1):135–42.

INDEX

Page numbers followed by *f* indicate figures; page numbers followed by *t* indicate tabular material.

C

D

I

J

K

L

M

S

T

U